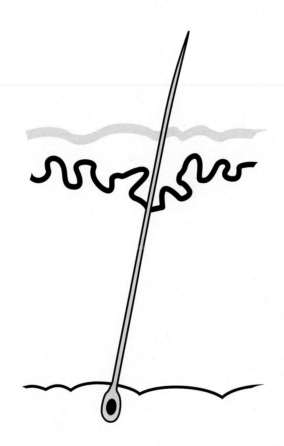

CUTANEOUS SURGERY

RONALD G. WHEELAND, M.D.

Professor and Chairman
Department of Dermatology
Chief, Mohs and Laser Surgery
University of California, Davis
School of Medicine
Davis, California

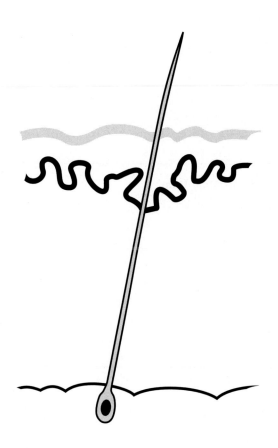

CUTANEOUS SURGERY

W.B. SAUNDERS COMPANY

A Division of Harcourt Brace & Company

Philadelphia London Toronto Montreal Sydney Tokyo

W.B. SAUNDERS COMPANY
A Division of
Harcourt Brace & Company

The Curtis Center
Independence Square West
Philadelphia, Pennsylvania 19106

Library of Congress Cataloging-in-Publication Data

Cutaneous surgery / [edited by] Ronald G. Wheeland. — 1st ed.

    p.   cm.

ISBN 0–7216–3523–7

1. Skin—Surgery.   I. Wheeland, Ronald G.
   [DNLM: 1. Skin—surgery.   2. Surgery, Plastic—methods.   3. Skin Diseases—
   surgery.   WR 650 C9884 1994]

RD520.C88 1994

617.4′77—dc20

DNLM/DLC   93-23020

Cutaneous Surgery   ISBN 0–7216–3523–7

Printed in the United States of America

Last digit is the print number: 9   8   7   6   5   4   3   2   1

A book of this magnitude cannot be written or edited in a typical workday.
Rather, it requires spending many long hours early in the mornings and late in the evenings,
as well as on weekends and holidays, to get the job done.
I would like to dedicate this book
to my loving wife,
Martha Mansur Wheeland,
and three of the best sons a father could ever hope to have,
Chris, Matt, and Jeff,
for all of the support,
understanding,
and encouragement
they provided during my many long hours of absence.
This book would simply not have been possible without them!

Contributors

DAVID M. AMRON, M.D.
Division of Dermatology, Department of Medicine, University of California San Diego Medical Center, San Diego, California
Management of Malignant Melanomas

MICHAEL J. AULETTA, M.D.
Assistant Clinical Professor, Director of Dermatologic Surgery, Division of Dermatology, Robert Wood Johnson Medical School; Dermatology Consultant, Robert Wood Johnson University Hospital, New Brunswick, New Jersey
Intraoperative Patient Monitoring, Sedation, and Analgesia

GERALD BERNSTEIN, M.D.
Clinical Professor of Medicine, University of Washington, Seattle, Washington
Surgical Anatomy

CRAIG S. BIRKBY, M.D.
Clinical Assistant Professor of Medicine, University of Washington, Seattle, Washington
Surgical Anatomy

ROBERT F. BLOOM, M.D.
Clinical Professor, Department of Dermatology, Texas Tech University School of Medicine, Lubbock, Texas
Preoperative Patient Evaluation and Preparation for Cutaneous Surgery

MARC D. BROWN, M.D.
Assistant Professor of Dermatology, University of Rochester, Rochester, New York
Conventional and Intraoperative Tissue Expansion

J. MICHAEL CARNEY, M.D.
Assistant Professor, Cosmetic Surgery Unit, Department of Dermatology, University of Pittsburgh Medical School, Pittsburgh, Pennsylvania; Assistant Clinical Professor, Department of Dermatology, University of Arkansas for Medical Sciences, Little Rock, Arkansas; Departments of Surgery and Medicine, Southwest Hospital, Little Rock, Arkansas
Chin Implants

BRUCE B. CHRISMAN, M.D.
Associate Professor of Medicine, John A. Burns School of Medicine; Kapiolani Medical Center for Women and Children, Honolulu, Hawaii
Blepharoplasty and Brow Lift

THOMAS P. CHU, M.D.
Assistant Clinical Professor, University of Arkansas for Medical Sciences, Little Rock, Arkansas; Naval Hospital, Millington, Tennessee
Hair-bearing Flaps

DAVID P. CLARK, M.D.
Associate Professor of Medicine and Surgery, University of Missouri School of Medicine; Chief, Cutaneous Micrographic Surgery, University of Missouri Hospital and Clinics, Columbia, Missouri
Management of Uncommon Malignant Tumors

ROBERT E. CLARK, M.D., PH.D.
Assistant Professor, Division of Dermatology, and Director, Dermatologic Surgery and Cutaneous Oncology, Duke University Medical Center, Durham, North Carolina
Nail Surgery

WILLIAM P. COLEMAN III, M.D.
Clinical Associate Professor of Dermatology, Tulane
University School of Medicine, New Orleans,
Louisiana; Doctors Hospital, East Jefferson Hospital,
Lakeside Hospital, Metairie, Louisiana
Liposuction

PAUL S. COLLINS, M.D.
Department of Dermatology, Lecturer, Stanford
University School of Medicine, Palo Alto, California;
Assistant Clinical Professor, Department of
Dermatology, Tulane University School of Medicine,
New Orleans, Louisiana; Dermatologic Plastic Surgery
Clinics of California, San Luis Obispo, California
Cervicofacial Rhytidectomy

THOMAS R. COWPER, D.D.S.
Head, Section of Maxillofacial Prosthetics,
Department of Dentistry, Cleveland Clinic
Foundation, Cleveland, Ohio
Facial Prosthetics in Cutaneous Surgery

JAMES Q. DEL ROSSO, D.O.
Staff Dermatologist and Director of Mohs
Micrographic Surgery, Medical Center Clinic, P.A.,
West Florida Regional Medical Center, Pensacola,
Florida
Management of Basal Cell Carcinomas

SCOTT M. DINEHART, M.D.
Associate Professor, Department of Dermatology,
University of Arkansas for Medical Sciences, Little
Rock, Arkansas
Topical, Local, and Regional Anesthesia

ZOE K. DRAELOS, M.D.
Clinical Assistant Professor, Department of
Dermatology, Bowman Gray School of Medicine,
Wake Forest University, Winston-Salem, North
Carolina; Medical Staff, High Point Regional Hospital,
High Point, North Carolina
Use of Cosmetics in Cutaneous Surgery

RAYMOND G. DUFRESNE, JR., M.D.
Assistant Professor, Brown University School of
Medicine; Director, Dermatologic Surgery and Mohs
Surgery, Roger Williams Medical Center, Providence,
Rhode Island
Mohs Surgery: Fresh Tissue Technique

DARREL L. ELLIS, M.D.
Assistant Professor, Department of Medicine, Division
of Dermatology, Vanderbilt University; Staff
Physician, Vanderbilt University Medical Center,
Nashville Department of Veterans Affairs Medical
Center, Nashville, Tennessee
Management of Dysplastic and Congenital Nevi

SALVATORE J. ESPOSITO, D.M.D.
Chairman, Department of Dentistry, Cleveland Clinic
Foundation, Cleveland, Ohio
Facial Prosthetics in Cutaneous Surgery

RAFAEL FALABELLA, M.D.
Professor and Chairman, Dermatology Section,
Universidad del Valle, and Fundacion Valle del Lili;
Chairman, Dermatology Section, Hospital
Universitario del Valle, Cali, Colombia
Surgical Repigmentation of Leukoderma

LAWRENCE M. FIELD, M.D.
Associate Clinical Professor, Dermatologic Surgery,
Department of Dermatology, University of California,
San Francisco, San Francisco, California
The Art of Cutaneous Scalpel Surgery

ALGIN B. GARRETT, M.D.
Assistant Professor and Interim Chairman,
Department of Dermatology, Medical College of
Virginia; Medical College of Virginia Hospitals,
Richmond, Virginia
Wound Closure Materials

JOHN W. GERWELS, M.D.
Associate Professor, Division of Dermatology,
University of Utah Health Sciences Center; University
of Utah Hospital, Salt Lake City, Utah
*Administrative Considerations in Office-Based
Cutaneous Surgery*

DAVID J. GOLDBERG, M.D.
Clinical Associate Professor, Chief of Dermatologic
Surgery, New Jersey Medical School, Newark, New
Jersey
Cosmetic Tattooing

MATTHEW M. GOODMAN, M.D.
Assistant Professor in Residence, Department of
Dermatology, University of California, Irvine, Irvine,
California; University of California Irvine Medical
Center, Orange, California; Long Beach Veterans
Administration Hospital, Long Beach, California
Principles of Electrosurgery

J. BLAKE GOSLEN, M.D.
Chief, Division of Dermatology, Presbyterian
Hospital, Charlotte, North Carolina
Management of Keratoacanthomas

WILLIAM J. GRABSKI, M.D.
Director, Dermatologic Surgery, Brooke Army
Medical Center, Ft. Sam Houston, Texas
Hemostatic Techniques and Materials

GLORIA F. GRAHAM, M.D.
Clinical Professor, Department of Dermatology, School of Medicine, University of North Carolina at Chapel Hill, Chapel Hill, North Carolina; Consulting Staff, Carteret General Hospital, Morehead City, North Carolina; Clinical Attending Staff, Department of Dermatology, Duke University Medical School, Durham, North Carolina, and Bowman Gray School of Medicine, Winston-Salem, North Carolina
Cryosurgery for Benign, Premalignant, and Malignant Lesions

DONALD J. GRANDE, M.D.
Associate Professor of Dermatology, Tufts University School of Medicine; Associate Dermatologist-in-Chief, New England Medical Center, Boston, Massachusetts
Lip Wedges

ALLAN C. HARRINGTON, M.D.
Mohs Surgeon, Walter Reed Army Medical Center, Washington, DC
Lip Wedges

THOMAS G. HILL, M.D.
Clinical Assistant Professor, Department of Dermatology, Emory University School of Medicine, Atlanta, Georgia; Active Staff, DeKalb Medical Center, Decatur, Georgia; Visiting Staff, Grady Memorial Hospital, Atlanta, Georgia
Skin Grafts

EDMUND R. HOBBS, M.D.
Clinical Associate Professor of Medicine, The University of Texas Health Science Center at San Antonio, San Antonio, Texas; Clinical Assistant Professor of Dermatology, Uniformed Services University of the Health Sciences, F. Edward Hebert School of Medicine, Bethesda, Maryland; Staff Dermatologist, Wilford Hall USAF Medical Center, Medical Center Hospital, Southwest Texas Methodist Hospital, Santa Rosa Northwest Hospital; Consulting Dermatologist, Humana Hospital San Antonio, San Antonio, Texas
Surgical Microbiology, Antibiotic Prophylaxis, and Antiseptic Technique

CHRISTOPHER J. HUERTER, M.D.
Assistant Professor, Head of Division of Dermatology, Creighton University School of Medicine, Omaha, Nebraska
Simple Biopsy Techniques

MANUEL IRIONDO, M.D.
Assistant Professor, Department of Dermatology, University of Miami; Jackson Memorial Hospital, Cedars Medical Center, Miami, Florida
Healing by Second Intention

R. RIVKAH ISSEROFF, M.D.
Associate Professor, Department of Dermatology, University of California, Davis, Davis, California
Autologous Skin Grafting

TIMOTHY M. JOHNSON, M.D.
Assistant Professor, University of Michigan Medical School; Dermatology, Otolaryngology, Surgery, University of Michigan Medical Center, Ann Arbor, Michigan
Conventional and Intraoperative Tissue Expansion

A. PAUL KELLY, M.D.
Professor of Medicine/Dermatology, Drew University of Medicine and Science; Associate Professor of Medicine, UCLA School of Medicine; Chief, Division of Dermatology, Drew–King Medical Center, Los Angeles, California
Considerations for Performing Cutaneous Surgery in Black Patients

GLENDA K. KILLEN, R.N.
Cleveland Clinic Foundation, Department of Dermatology-Surgery, Ambulatory Nursing, Cleveland, Ohio
Nursing Considerations in Cutaneous Surgery

JOHN Y. M. KOO, M.D.
Assistant Professor and Vice Chairman, Department of Dermatology, University of California, San Francisco, School of Medicine; Director, UCSF Psoriasis Treatment Center; UCSF Moffit Hospital, San Francisco, California
Psychiatric Aspects of Cutaneous Surgery

BRENDA L. KUNKEL, R.N., B.A.
Cleveland Clinic Foundation, Department of Dermatology, Ambulatory Nursing, Cleveland, Ohio
Nursing Considerations in Cutaneous Surgery

LARRY LANDSMAN, M.D.
Clinical Professor, Department of Dermatology, University of Miami, Miami, Florida
Scalp Reduction

PEARON G. LANG, JR., M.D.
Professor of Dermatology and Otolaryngology and Communicative Sciences, Medical University of South Carolina; Medical University Hospital (Attending), Charleston Memorial Hospital (Consultant), Charleston Veterans Administration Hospital (Consultant), Charleston, South Carolina
Management of Squamous Cell Carcinomas and Lymph Node Evaluation

PAUL O. LARSON, M.D.
Associate Professor, University of Wisconsin Medical School; University of Wisconsin Hospital and Clinics, Milwaukee, Wisconsin
Mohs Surgery: Fixed Tissue Technique

GARY P. LASK, M.D.
Clinical Associate Professor of Medicine/Dermatology, UCLA School of Medicine; Director of Dermatologic Surgery, Harbor–UCLA Medical Center, Los Angeles, California
Ear Wedges

KEAN LAWLOR, M.D.
Resident, Department of Dermatology, Cleveland Clinic Foundation, Cleveland, Ohio
Contact Allergy in Cutaneous Surgery

DAVID J. LEFFELL, M.D.
Assistant Professor of Dermatology, Yale School of Medicine; Attending Physician and Chief of Mohs Surgery, Yale–New Haven Medical Center, New Haven, Connecticut
Microanatomy, Structure, and Function of the Skin

BARRY LESHIN, M.D.
Associate Professor of Dermatology and Otolaryngology, Bowman Gray School of Medicine, Wake Forest University, Winston-Salem, North Carolina
Proper Planning and Execution of Surgical Excisions

PHYLIS A. LUDWIG, R.N.
Ambulatory Nursing Coordinator, Department of Dermatology, Cleveland Clinic Foundation, Cleveland, Ohio
Nursing Considerations in Cutaneous Surgery

WILLIAM S. LYNCH, M.D.
Assistant Professor of Dermatology, Case Western Reserve University School of Medicine; Director of Dermatologic Surgery, University Hospitals of Cleveland, Cleveland, Ohio
Surgical Equipment and Instrumentation

MARY E. MALONEY, M.D.
Associate Professor, Penn State College of Medicine; Milton Hershey Medical Center, Hershey, Pennsylvania
Management of Surgical Complications and Suboptimal Results

STEPHEN H. MANDY, M.D.
Clinical Professor, Department of Dermatology, University of Miami, Miami, Florida
Scalp Reduction

SETH L. MATARASSO, M.D.
Assistant Clinical Professor of Dermatology, Department of Dermatology, University of California School of Medicine, San Francisco; Attending Staff, University of California San Francisco Medical Center, San Francisco, California
Phenol Chemical Peels

THEODORA M. MAURO, M.D.
Assistant Clinical Professor, University of California, San Francisco; Assistant Service Chief, San Francisco Veterans Administration Medical Center, San Francisco, California
Management of Leg Ulcers

S. TERI McGILLIS, M.D.
Staff, Department of Dermatology, Cleveland Clinic Foundation, Cleveland, Ohio
Indications for and Techniques of Hair Transplantation

ANNE E. MISSAVAGE, M.D.
Assistant Professor of Clinical Surgery, University of California, Davis; Burn Director, UC Davis Medical Center, Davis, California
Autologous Skin Grafting

GARY D. MONHEIT, M.D.
Assistant Professor, Department of Dermatology, University of Alabama at Birmingham; Vice President and Chairman of Dermatology and Dermatologic Surgery, Eye Foundation Hospital; Chairman, Department of Dermatology, Health South Medical Center; Staff, Baptist Medical Center, Brookwood Medical Center; Consulting Medical Staff, St. Vincents, Veterans Administration Hospital, University of Alabama Medical Center, Birmingham, Alabama
Soft Tissue Augmentation

LAWRENCE S. MOY, M.D.
Clinical Instructor of Medicine, Division of Dermatology, UCLA School of Medicine, Los Angeles, California; Centinela Hospital, Inglewood, California; UCLA Medical Center, Los Angeles, California
Superficial Chemical Peels

RONALD L. MOY, M.D.
Assistant Professor of Medicine, Division of Dermatology, UCLA School of Medicine; UCLA Medical Center, Los Angeles, California
Superficial Chemical Peels; Management of Malignant Melanomas

HOWARD MURAD, M.D.
Assistant Clinical Professor of Dermatology, UCLA School of Medicine, Los Angeles, California
Superficial Chemical Peels

CRAIG S. MURAKAMI, M.D.
Assistant Professor, Department of Otolaryngology/ Head and Neck Surgery; Chief, Division of Facial Cosmetic and Reconstructive Surgery, University of Washington Medical Center and Hospital, Seattle, Washington
Simple Suturing Techniques and Knot Tying

CONSTANCE NAGI, M.D.
Associate Clinical Professor of Medicine; Head, Dermatologic Surgery, Mohs Micrographic Surgery, University of California San Diego Medical Center, San Diego, California
Recognition and Management of Office Medical and Surgical Emergencies

LILLIAN B. NANNEY, Ph.D.
Associate Professor of Plastic Surgery and Cell Biology, Vanderbilt School of Medicine, Nashville, Tennessee
Biochemical and Physiologic Aspects of Wound Healing

PETER B. ODLAND, M.D.
Assistant Professor, Department of Medicine, Division of Dermatology, University of Washington School of Medicine; Director, Dermatologic Surgery Service, University of Washington Medical Center, Seattle, Washington
Simple Suturing Techniques and Knot Tying

RICHARD B. ODOM, M.D.
Clinical Professor of Dermatology, Associate Chairman, Department of Dermatology, University of California, San Francisco, San Francisco, California
Topical Tretinoin for the Treatment of Photodamaged Skin

R. STEVEN PADILLA, M.D.
Professor of Dermatology, Associate Professor of Pathology, University of New Mexico School of Medicine; University of New Mexico Cancer Center, University of New Mexico Hospital, Albuquerque, New Mexico
Dermabrasion

LAWRENCE C. PARISH, M.D.
Clinical Professor of Dermatology and Director, Jefferson Center for International Dermatology, Jefferson Medical College of Thomas Jefferson University, Philadelphia, Pennsylvania; Visiting Professor of Dermatology, Yonsei University College of Medicine, Seoul, South Korea; Visiting Professor of Dermatology and Venereology, Zagazig University Faculty of Medicine, Zagazig, Egypt
Historical Aspects of Cutaneous Surgery

HARRY L. PARLETTE III, M.D.
Associate Professor of Dermatology, Plastic Surgery, Otolaryngology–Head and Neck Surgery, University of Virginia School of Medicine; University of Virginia Health Sciences Center, Charlottesville, Virginia
Management of Cutaneous Cysts

EDWARD L. PARRY, M.D.
Assistant Professor of Dermatology, Louisiana State University Medical Center; Staff, Hotel Dieu Hospital, New Orleans, Louisiana
Management of Epidermal Tumors

DANIEL PIACQUADIO, M.D.
Assistant Clinical Professor, Director of Clinical Research, Division of Dermatology, University of California, San Diego; Attending Staff Physician, University of California San Diego Medical Center; Attending Physician, Veterans Administration Medical Center, San Diego, California
Synthetic Surgical Dressings

SHELDON V. POLLACK, M.D.
Associate Professor of Medicine, and Director, Dermatologic Surgery, Faculty of Medicine, University of Toronto, Toronto, Ontario; Courtesy Staff, Women's College Hospital, Toronto, Ontario; Consultant, Meaford General Hospital, Meaford, Ontario; Consultant, Toronto-Bayview Regional Cancer Centre, Toronto, Ontario; Visiting Staff, Sunnybrook Health Sciences Centre, Toronto, Ontario, Canada
Management of Keloids

MACK RACHAL, M.D., Ph.D.
Department of Dermatology, Yale University School of Medicine, New Haven, Connecticut
Microanatomy, Structure, and Function of the Skin

BARRY I. RESNIK, M.D.
Department of Dermatology, Jackson Memorial Hospital, University of Miami School of Medicine, Miami, Florida
Management of Actinic Keratoses

SORREL S. RESNIK, M.D.
Clinical Professor of Dermatology, Department of Dermatology and Cutaneous Surgery, University of Miami School of Medicine; Active Staff, Jackson Memorial Hospital; Senior Attending and Chief of Dermatology, Miami Children's Hospital; Associate Staff, Baptist Hospital of Miami, Miami, Florida
Management of Actinic Keratoses

DIRK B. ROBERTSON, M.D.
Associate Clinical Professor of Dermatology, Emory University School of Medicine; Active Staff, and

Chief, Dermatology Service, West Paces Ferry
Hospital, Atlanta, Georgia
Dogear Repairs

JUNE K. ROBINSON, M.D.
Professor of Dermatology and Surgery, Northwestern
University Medical School; Attending Staff,
Northwestern Memorial Hospital, Veterans
Administration Lakeside Medical Center, Chicago,
Illinois
*Low-Energy Lasers for Wound Healing and Tissue
Welding*

TIMOTHY J. ROSIO, M.D.
Associate Clinical Professor, Department of
Dermatology and Cutaneous Surgery, University of
Wisconsin, Madison, Wisconsin; Director, Epstein
Photomedicine Institute, Department of Dermatology
and Cutaneous Surgery, Marshfield Clinic, Marshfield,
Wisconsin; St. Joseph Hospital, Marshfield, Wisconsin
*Revision of Acne, Traumatic, and Surgical Scars;
Techniques for Tattoo Removal*

STUART J. SALASCHE, M.D.
Associate Professor, Section of Dermatology,
University of Arizona Health Sciences Center, Tucson,
Arizona
Hemostatic Techniques and Materials

ROBERT H. SCHOSSER, M.D.
Associate Professor of Dermatology, University of
Arkansas for Medical Sciences; University Hospital,
Arkansas Children's Hospital; Chief, Dermatology,
Veterans Administration Medical Center, Little Rock,
Arkansas
Photography in Cutaneous Surgery

DANIEL M. SIEGEL, M.D.
Assistant Professor of Clinical Dermatology and
Surgery, and Head, Division of Dermatologic Surgery,
State University of New York at Stony Brook School
of Medicine, Stony Brook, New York; Attending
Staff, Stony Brook University Hospital, Stony Brook,
New York, and Northport Veterans Administration
Medical Center, Northport, New York
Use of Computers in a Cutaneous Surgical Practice

RONALD J. SIEGLE, M.D.
Associate Professor of Clinical Otolaryngology, and
Director, Mohs Micrographic Surgery and
Dermatologic Surgery, Ohio State University,
Columbus, Ohio
Management of Basal Cell Carcinomas

JON C. STARR, M.D.
Instructor, Harvard Medical School; Dermatologist,

Massachusetts General Hospital, Boston,
Massachusetts
*Use of Retinoids and Vitamin A in Cutaneous
Oncology*

THOMAS STASKO, M.D.
Assistant Professor, Division of Dermatology,
Vanderbilt University, Nashville, Tennessee
Advanced Suturing Techniques and Layered Closures

JOHN C. STEPHENS, D.P.M.
Staff, Mt. Carmel Hospital and Grant Medical Center,
Columbus, Ohio
Podiatric Soft Tissue Surgical Procedures

D. BLUFORD STOUGH III, M.D.
University of Arkansas Medical School, Little Rock,
Arkansas; St. Joseph Regional Medical Center, Baylor
Hospital, Houston, Texas
Hair-bearing Flaps

DOWLING B. STOUGH IV, M.D.
University of Arkansas Medical School, Little Rock,
Arkansas; St. Joseph Regional Medical Center, AMI
National Park Hospital, Baylor Hospital, Texas,
Wilhelmina Medical Hospital, Houston, Texas
Hair-bearing Flaps

JAMES S. TAYLOR, M.D.
Head, Section of Industrial Dermatology, Department
of Dermatology, Cleveland Clinic Foundation,
Cleveland, Ohio
Contact Allergy in Cutaneous Surgery

RUFUS M. THOMAS, M.D.
Haywood County Hospital, Clyde, North Carolina
*Recognition and Management of Office Medical and
Surgical Emergencies*

RODNEY L. TOMCZAK, D.P.M., Ed.D.
Chairman, Department of Surgery, Iowa Allied
Medical Osteopathic and Podiatry School, Des
Moines, Iowa
Podiatric Soft Tissue Surgical Procedures

WHITNEY D. TOPE, M.D.
Division of Dermatology, Duke University Medical
Center, Durham, North Carolina
Nail Surgery

ALLISON T. VIDIMOS, R.Ph., M.D.
Staff Physician, Department of Dermatology, Section
of Dermatologic Surgery and Cutaneous Oncology,
Cleveland Clinic Foundation, Cleveland, Ohio
Management of Lipomas; Ear Piercing

RICHARD F. WAGNER, JR., M.D.
Associate Professor, Department of Dermatology, University of Texas Medical Branch, University of Texas Medical Branch Hospitals, Galveston, Texas
Informed Consent and Risk Management Issues in Cutaneous Surgery

MARGARET A. WEISS, M.D.
Instructor of Dermatology, Johns Hopkins University School of Medicine, Baltimore, Maryland; Admitting and Consulting Privileges at Johns Hopkins Hospital, Baltimore, Maryland; Consultant at Mercy Hospital, Baltimore, Maryland, Fallston General Hospital, Fallston, Maryland, and Children's Hospital, Baltimore, Maryland
Sclerotherapy

ROBERT A. WEISS, M.D.
Assistant Professor of Dermatology, Johns Hopkins University School of Medicine, Baltimore, Maryland; Consultant at St. Joseph Hospital, Towson, Maryland, and Greater Baltimore Medical Center, Baltimore, Maryland; Johns Hopkins Hospital, Baltimore, Maryland
Sclerotherapy

JOHN R. WEST, M.D.
Clinical Instructor of Medicine, Division of Dermatology, University of Southern California School of Medicine, Los Angeles, California
Management of Hyperhidrosis and Bromhidrosis

RONALD G. WHEELAND, M.D.
Professor and Chairman, Department of Dermatology, and Chief, Mohs and Laser Surgery, University of California, Davis, Davis, California
Use of Retinoids and Vitamin A in Cutaneous Oncology; Basic Laser Physics and Visible Light Laser Surgery; Infrared, Ultraviolet, and Experimental Laser Surgery

DUANE C. WHITAKER, M.D.
Director of Dermatologic Surgery, Department of Dermatology, University of Iowa College of Medicine; University of Iowa Hospitals and Clinics, Iowa City, Iowa
Random-Pattern Flaps

B. DALE WILSON, M.D.
Clinical Assistant Professor of Dermatology, State University of New York at Buffalo School of Medicine; Clinician, Roswell Park Cancer Institute, Attending Physician, Buffalo General Hospital, and Millard Fillmore Hospital, Buffalo, New York
Photodynamic Therapy for Cutaneous Malignancies

Foreword

It is truly an honor for me to write this Foreword to *Cutaneous Surgery*, a book that has been edited by one of the most uniquely talented physicians in medicine, Ronald G. Wheeland. This book is solidly built on the foundation of knowledge that all dermatologists possess and that all cutaneous surgeons, even those without formal dermatology training, should attempt to learn: in-depth knowledge of all aspects of cutaneous medicine, including clinical diagnosis, normal gross and microscopic anatomy of the skin, dermatopathology, basic science, surgery, and oncology. Without an understanding of these important areas, the cutaneous surgeon's education will be incomplete, and quality patient care cannot be delivered.

In recent years, the specialty of dermatology has attracted many of the best young physicians to its residency training programs. In view of this, Dr. Wheeland has taken special care in *Cutaneous Surgery* to invite contributions from many young cutaneous surgeons who will lead the specialty into the 21st century. These carefully selected young contributors provide much new information, as well as many fresh ideas and new insights on many established topics.

Cutaneous Surgery is divided into five distinct sections. The first section, "Basic Surgical Concepts and Procedures," is the heart and soul of all that follows. It provides basic information on patient evaluation, informed consent, surgical microbiology, wound healing, and suturing techniques, among others. The second section contains chapters on essential surgical skills such as dogear repairs, layered closures, random-pattern flaps, skin grafts, and more advanced surgical procedures. The third section, "Cosmetic Surgical Procedures," consists of 15 chapters that cover many of the latest advances that have been made in cosmetic surgery in recent years, including superficial chemical peels, liposuction, and chin implants. The fourth section, "Special Surgical Procedures," includes the management of a multitude of common clinical problems such as cysts, nevocellular nevi, benign tumors, and keloids. This section also highlights many current concepts of the management of skin cancer by including multiple chapters dealing with premalignant lesions and various types of cutaneous malignancies. This is especially appropriate in view of the current "epidemic" of skin cancer, which necessitates that all cutaneous surgeons become expert in this important area. The final section, "Future Advances in Cutaneous Surgery," includes chapters on cultured epidermal allografts, low-energy lasers and wound healing, photodynamic therapy for skin cancer, and autologous skin grafts for the treatment of leukoderma.

The 1970s and 1980s were marked by the publication of four editions of the comprehensive book, *Skin Surgery,* by Ervin Epstein and Ervin Epstein, Jr., followed by the publication of a second comprehensive book by Randall K. Roenigk and Henry H. Roenigk, Jr., in 1989. The explosive growth in cutaneous surgery during these two decades was largely due to the efforts of Drs. Theodore A. Tromovitch and Samuel J. Stegman. Although many other dermatologists have certainly made significant contributions to the specialty of cutaneous surgery, Tromovitch and Stegman have been the undisputed leaders. Their lecture presentations are always well organized and superbly delivered, leaving their colleagues feeling energized and confident about the specialty. Stegman's particular gift as a public speaker had earlier resulted in his receipt of the Alexander Hamilton Award, given annually to the top high school debater in the United States.

Dr. Wheeland shares many similarities with Tromovitch and Stegman. He is a superbly organized speaker and writer who is intensely interesting and informative. He utilizes the medical literature expertly to substantiate his theses and always gives proper credit to his colleagues. He possesses superior organizational skills and a work ethic that defies comprehension. A dermatologist who is also formally trained in dermatopathology and Mohs micrographic surgery and cutaneous oncology, he is an elected member of the Board of Directors of multiple national medical specialty organizations and currently is President of the American Society for Laser Medicine and Surgery. He is a Senior Editor of the *Journal of Dermatologic Surgery and Oncology* and *Lasers in Surgery and Medicine* and has written more on laser medicine and surgery than anyone I know. The University of California, Davis recognized Dr. Wheeland's enormous potential and appointed him Chairman of the Department of Dermatology in 1991. No one in our specialty works longer hours, plans more carefully, or treats his colleagues and patients with more respect than Dr. Wheeland. He and his contributors have much to teach us, so let's get on with it!

C. WILLIAM HANKE, M.D.
Professor of Dermatology
Professor of Pathology
Professor of Otolaryngology
Indiana University School of Medicine
Indianapolis, Indiana

Preface

Remarkably rapid growth has occurred during the past several decades in the scope and sophistication of the multitude of cutaneous surgical procedures that are routinely performed. This growth has largely been the result of several interdependent factors. One of the primary factors has been the role research scientists have played in improving our basic understanding of many aspects of skin function, biochemistry, physiology, and, particularly, wound healing. For example, it is now generally accepted that wounds heal beneath occlusive dressings at a much faster rate than wounds that are left exposed to the air. This relatively simple finding not only reduced mordibity and returned patients to productivity faster than had previously been possible, but it also improved the cosmetic results in a host of surgical procedures. This research also led to the development of many new and unique synthetic surgical dressings that offered additional benefits to both cutaneous surgeons and their patients. Similar evolutionary changes can be anticipated in the relatively near future as additional basic research helps us to understand how the recently identified growth factors can be used to stimulate various aspects of wound healing. The obvious relevance of current basic research to the practice of cutaneous surgery has been stressed in this book by presenting many of the most recent advances in the physiologic, metabolic, microanatomic, and biochemical aspects of the skin in the first section. This section also serves as the foundation for a presentation of the more complex and specialized surgical procedures that follow.

A second factor responsible for stimulating a number of the rapid changes seen in cutaneous surgery is the cooperative and collaborative relationships that have been forged among dermatologic surgeons, otolaryngologists, Mohs surgeons, ophthalmologists, surgical oncologists, and oculoplastic and plastic surgeons. Each of these different groups of surgical specialists has applied the knowledge gained from basic research activities to solve many difficult clinical problems and ultimately improve the overall quality of patient care. Implementing individual techniques and sharing that information with other individuals who perform cutaneous surgery has been of integral importance to the successful evolution of cutaneous surgery. The combined knowledge, skills, and expertise of physicians from each of these specialties have allowed much more rapid incorporation and implementation of many new and creative ideas to the clinical setting than would otherwise have been possible. The net result of this collegial cooperation has been beneficial not only for the surgeon, but also for the patient who requires a specific surgical procedure. In this way, the full potential of cutaneous surgery as a subspecialty of medicine is well on its way to being realized. This book has been designed to help facilitate the acquisition of knowledge by both the beginning cutaneous surgeon and the more experienced practitioner. By starting with a presentation of some simple concepts and basic surgical procedures (e.g., antisepsis, anesthesia, biopsies, and suturing techniques), the reader will be better prepared for the presentation of the more advanced and specialized procedures that follow. The book then progresses to a discussion of the many new and improved surgical techniques that have been developed for managing a variety of different cosmetic problems.

The acquisition of new instrumentation and technology is a third factor that has been responsible for some of the recent changes that have occurred in cutaneous surgery. The multitude of technologic advances that have occurred in suture materials, anesthetic agents, electrosurgical devices, lasers, tissue expanders, materials for soft tissue augmentation, and cell culture techniques have provided many new and useful therapeutic modalities that were not even imaginable a few decades ago. These technologic advances, along with the surgical procedures that have resulted from their development, are detailed throughout this book.

The many benefits offered by these technologic advances have not only improved the results of many cutaneous surgical procedures while minimizing the risk of complications, but have also, in some cases, actually reduced the cost of the procedure by allowing it to be more safely performed in an ambulatory setting. These advances have also increased the complexity of the cutaneous surgical procedures that are now routinely being performed. The limits of what can be accomplished have certainly not yet been fully reached, and as our knowledge continues to expand, so will the clinical applications. However, with this development comes a greater need for attention to details, including meticulous preoperative patient evaluation, proper use of anesthesia and sedation to provide maximal patient comfort, and appropriate intraoperative patient monitoring. In addition, anticipation of the possible medical and surgical emergencies that may occur during a surgical procedure requires knowledge of the information presented in the early chapters of this book. In this way, the necessary precautions can be taken so the cutaneous surgeon will be prepared to effectively manage any crisis that arises in the ambulatory setting.

Many recent regulatory and fiscal changes have had a major impact on the practice of medicine and the way health care is delivered. These complex and sophisticated changes require the acquisition of much new knowledge, as well as a better understanding of the laws and regulations involved, to properly manage the outpatient cutaneous surgical practice. Consequently, detailed information on office administration and utilization of computer technology as it pertains to a cutaneous surgical practice is also provided.

This book has been designed to provide the latest and most comprehensive referenced information available related to cutaneous surgery, including some techniques that have only recently moved from the research laboratory to the clinic. By utilizing a unique mixture of innovative basic research scientists, internationally recognized senior cutaneous surgeons, and active younger authors who are keenly aware of the latest technical advances, this book is designed to be comprehensive in scope by providing much useful information for both the beginning cutaneous surgeon and the more experienced practitioner. It is hoped that this compendium will stimulate many additional evolutionary changes in cutaneous surgery so that even more effective treatments can be developed to further reduce the risk of complications while also dramatically improving the quality of patient care.

RONALD G. WHEELAND, M.D.

Acknowledgments

Much of my early interest in surgery was stimulated by the founding Dean of the College of Medicine at the University of Arizona, Dr. Merlin K. DuVal. As a surgeon, he challenged me to not merely accept the prevailing surgical dogma, but rather to question it and seek alternative explanations for the many unanswered problems that I encountered. His caring demeanor and humanism also provided me with a superb role model that has greatly influenced me throughout my career.

Along the way I have been extremely fortunate to have had the opportunity to work with some of the finest physicians and surgeons in the world. My chairman at the University of Oklahoma, Dr. Mark Allen Everett, provided me with the initial opportunity to acquire the necessary training and skills to become a cutaneous surgeon. Also at the University of Oklahoma, my colleague and good friend Dr. Walter H. C. Burgdorf demonstrated extraordinary patience in teaching me much of what I know today about scientific writing and medical editing. My first partner, Dr. Patrick E. Watson of Missoula, Montana, taught me many valuable surgical and nonsurgical skills through his meticulous technique and attention to detail. A special mention of gratitude must also be extended to Dr. C. William Hanke of Indiana University, who has personally helped advance my career by providing me with numerous speaking opportunities, committee assignments, and editorial positions at the *Journal of Dermatologic Surgery and Oncology*. Each of these individuals provided me with tremendous personal encouragement and support over the years, and I wish to acknowledge my deep appreciation for their friendship.

At W.B. Saunders Company, I would like to acknowledge the efforts of Judith Fletcher and Peter Faber, who helped keep me on schedule and also handled much of the detail work for which they generally fail to receive adequate recognition.

I would also like to thank the excellent nursing and technical staffs at both the Cleveland Clinic Foundation and the University of California, Davis for giving me the opportunity to perform cutaneous surgery in an atmosphere of warmth and concern. The efforts of these individuals have not only made my job a great deal easier and a whole lot more pleasant, but also made me realize how very lucky I am to be able to work in a profession that gives me so many personal pleasures and emotional rewards. In addition, I would like to acknowledge the positive role played by the enthusiastic, curious, and dedicated residents at the

University of Oklahoma, the Cleveland Clinic Foundation, and the University of California, Davis who continue to challenge and stimulate me to learn. They really are the best teachers one can possibly have! Finally, I would like to thank the many contributors to this book who willingly offered their expertise so that others could also learn.

Contents

PART ONE

Basic Surgical Concepts and Procedures

CHAPTER 1

Historical Aspects of Cutaneous Surgery

LAWRENCE C. PARISH

Surgical intervention has often appealed to healers of the skin. Even in ancient times, physicians found that applying a salve to a tumor could be less satisfactory than cutting away the unwanted growth. As medicine became more innovative, the practitioners of ancient Egypt used sutures to close wounds (1800 BC), while their later counterparts from the Indian subcontinent in 700 BC developed flaps to replace noses previously slashed off as punishment. Aulus Cornelius Celsus (25 BC–50 AD), a Roman gentleman and not a trained physician, suggested several cosmetic surgical procedures to repair mutilated ears and noses. He also perfected posthioplasty (replacement of the prepuce) for those who wanted to be more Roman. Accounts of ancient surgery detail the fact that man has frequently found a surgical method to correct a defect or remove a cancer.[1-3]

Early Healers of the Skin

With the emergence of modern medicine in the post-Renaissance period, surgical approaches became an integral part of cutaneous therapeutics. For example, in the first book written in English for the treatment of skin disease, Daniel Turner (1667–1740), a medical man in London, advised:

In the cutting with a Knife or Sciffars, some Authors tell us we must take heed none
of the Blood fall upon the Parts adjoining, and raise more Excrescences of the same
nature . . . and produce a new and more plentiful Crop of Warts and Corns.[4]

Thomas Bateman (1778–1821), who practiced in London

a century later, recommended intervention when nevi were observed to be enlarging:

Either their growth must be repressed by sedative applications or the whole morbid congeries of vessels must be extirpated by the knife.[5]

He was undoubtedly also reflecting the concepts of his teacher, Robert Willan (1751–1812), when he added:

The mode of extirpation is within the province of the surgeon; and the proper choice of the mode, under the different circumstances, is directed in surgical books.[5]

Until dermatology emerged as a distinct specialty a half-century later, little additional attention seems to have been paid to cutaneous surgical approaches. The dermatologists of the era appear to have been most interested in classifying, describing, and naming skin diseases. Many therapeutic suggestions concerned applications of inunctions and occasional internal medicaments. Surgery was seldom used, although lancing of boils and removal of tumors were recommended. The lack of appropriate anesthesia and a failure to understand aseptic techniques undoubtedly hampered the development of elective minor surgery.

Nineteenth Century Innovations

CUTISECTOR

Beginning in the 1870s, a flurry of new approaches to treatment and diagnosis appeared. The microscope, although infrequently used, was recognized for its meaningful input. The physician trained to use this tool could identify fungal spores and distinguish malignant from

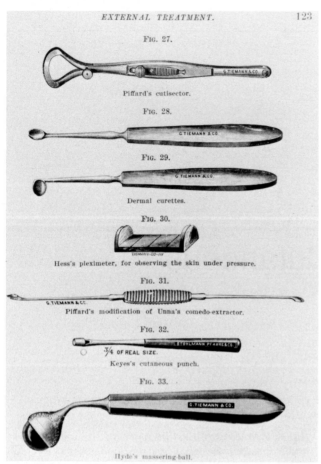

Figure 1–1. Dermatologic instruments devised and recommended by Henry Piffard. (From Piffard HG: A Treatise on the Materia Medica and Therapeutics of the Skin. Wm Wood, New York, 1881, p 123.)

benign tumors. Unfortunately, histopathologic specimens were still cut by a knife, which made them too thick and too uneven for careful study. The inventive Henry Piffard (1842–1910) of New York devised a "cutisector" to correct this problem (Fig. 1–1):

The instrument has two parallel blades which may be approximated by means of screws. The knife being held as a pen, a perpendicular incision may be made through the whole thickness of the skin, and the knife withdrawn, leaving attached a thin slice of tissue which can be easily removed with a pair of fine forceps, and placed under the microscope.[6]

Histopathology made more rapid progress with the introduction of aniline dyes for delineating cells. Physicians began to realize that they could take living tissue for study and did not need to wait until the time of the autopsy to obtain tissue specimens. Ernest Besnier (1831–1909) of l'Hôpital St. Louis, Paris, appropriately coined the term *biopsy* in 1879.[7]

KEYES CUTANEOUS PUNCH

The cutaneous punch is the prototype of cutaneous surgical inventiveness. About 1877 B.A. Watson in New

York created a discotome to remove traumatic tattoos from a patient, but his work went unnoticed. A few years later, without apparent knowledge of Watson's instrument, Edward L. Keyes (1843–1924), also of New York, invented the punch to remove gunpowder pigmentation from the face of a youth who had been careless with firecrackers:

Finding at last, when the little wounds had all healed, that my patient was marked in unseemly manner, I determined to eradicate the numerous points of disfigurement, by entirely taking away the portion of the integument involved in the colored scar. To do this I devised a number of small trephines, or punches, as they may be called with a sharp cutting edge; the diameter of the cutting edge varying from one millimetre upwards, each larger trephine having a diameter one-half a millimetre greater than the one next below it.[8]

And so this simple surgical tool became known as the Keyes punch, although this famous New York dermatologist apologized to Dr. Watson.[9] There have been many variations on its design and use. In 1924 Erich Urbach (1893–1946), then in Vienna and later in Philadelphia, used a rotary drill to make the punching procedure quicker and less painful. More recently, a disposable punch has been added to the surgical cabinet. In the 1950s L.J.A. Lowenthal (1903–1983) in South Africa chose the punch for autograft experiments.[10] He used the punch to remove lesions, covering the site with a graft removed with a punch from elsewhere on the body. This led to its use in hair transplants by Norman Orentreich (1922–   ) of New York and Samuel Ayres III (1919–   ) of Los Angeles.[11] Beginning in the 1970s, Orentreich and Waine Johnson (1928–   ) of Philadelphia each reasoned that the punch could be used to reduce or obliterate acne scars.

SKIN CURETTE

A second instrument that is a mainstay of many cutaneous surgical practices, the curette, had its origins about 1870, when Richard Volkmann (1830–1889), a surgeon in Halle, Germany, adapted a scraping spoon, or curette, for skin use. The curette, at one time called the Volkmann instrument or scharfer Löffel (sharp spoon), had been used in gynecologic procedures for many years, being created by J.C.A. Récamier, a French surgeon.[12] Louis A. Duhring (1845–1913), the distinguished Philadelphia dermatologist, later noted:

[It] may be regarded as a most valuable remedial measure. The instrument used is a small, round or oval metallic spoon or scoop [with] sharp edges. Various shapes and sizes will be found useful according to the case and the tissue to be attacked.[13]

Many cutaneous surgeons devised their own modifications of the curette. Most notable were the changes by Henry Piffard and George Henry Fox (1846–1937), of New York. Heinrich Auspitz (1835–1886) and Hans von Hebra (1847–1902) were both strong proponents of the instrument in Vienna, giving cutaneous surgeons their own instrument to practice surgical removal or *erasion*, as it was sometimes called.

Special adaptations were made in the curette for acne surgery. Piffard devised an acne instrument that had a roller to compress the papule or pustule. Jay Frank Schamberg (1870–1913) of Philadelphia and Paul Gerson Unna (1850–1929) of Hamburg, Germany, effectively improved the comedo extractor, modifications that are still popular today (Fig. 1–2). All these changes represented improvements over the contemporary recommendations of the founder of New York Skin and Cancer Hospital, L. Duncan Bulkley (1845–1928), who wrote:

> *The comedones, or clogged subaceous (sic) glands, are best emptied by pressure upon them with the end of a small tube, with an aperture of about 1/16 of an inch or a new watch key; the orifice is placed over the little black speck, and firm pressure is made perpendicular to the surface, when, in most cases, the worm like mass will rise perpendicular to the surface . . .*[14]

Volkmann's spoon was also used in scarification, whereby the skin was pierced or scraped to stimulate new tissue formation. It was thought that lupus vulgaris and sycosis barbae, among other inflammatory diseases, could then be *tamed*. Many other instruments, no longer in fashion, sprang from the scarification fad, one of the most popular being the Paquelin cautery (Claude Paquelin [1836–1905]) or thermocautery, a hot knife fueled by benzene (Fig. 1–3).[15]

Physical Modalities

The use of light and electricity has always fascinated cutaneous surgeons (Fig. 1–4). As early as 1873, William Hardaway (1850–1923) of St. Louis advocated the use of electrolysis in conditions such as sycosis barbae and lupus vulgaris. The method employed galvanic current, which was passed through needles inserted into the tissue being treated.[16] Hardaway, however, was observant enough to recognize the limitations of galvanic current, unlike some of his contemporaries.

ELECTROSURGERY

In 1893 Paul Oudin (1851–1923) invented a special resonator that made a spark gap apparatus suitable for destroying tissue. This was perfected in 1900 by another Frenchman, Joseph Rivière, who was then able to treat malignancies and cutaneous tuberculosis with his *effeuve*. In a monograph published in 1908, Walter de Keating-Hart (1870–1932) of Paris coined the term *fulguration*, as the long sparks resembled lightning (fulgur).[17] Shortly thereafter, E. Doyen placed an active electrode directly on the tissue being treated, which heated without use of sparks; thus, coagulation, or more specifically *electrocoagulation*, a word chosen by Franz Nagelschmidt,[17] was born. William Clark (1877–1936), a Philadelphia radiologist, pioneered *electrodesiccation* for treating cutaneous lesions.[18, 19] With Lee deForest's

(1873–1961) invention of the vacuum tube generator in 1907, medical instrumentation made further strides forward. Harvey Cushing (1869–1939), the famous Boston neurosurgeon, suggested to an innovative physicist at Harvard, William Bovie (1882–1958), that he create an electrosurgical unit that could coagulate and cut. With the help of two engineers, Edward Flarsheim and George H. Liebel, the modern electrosurgical unit (Bovie) was produced.[20] Soon, the Bovie was joined by the Portatherm, Multotherm, and Cauterodyne by Cameron-Miller.[19]

LASERS

Light amplification by stimulated emission of radiation (laser) began in 1896, at least in thought, when H.G. Wells suggested light energy in his novel *War of the Worlds*. Albert Einstein developed the theory of lasers in 1916, and by 1960 Theodore Maiman of the Hughes Aircraft Company had developed the ruby laser as the first operational laser. Two years later the argon laser, and 4 years later the carbon dioxide laser, were sufficiently perfected for clinical trials to begin.[21, 22]

When Leon Goldman (1909–   ) of Cincinnati learned about the ruby laser, he and Donald Birmingham (1911–   ) submitted a grant proposal to the National Institutes of Health to study its safety. As an outgrowth of this work, Goldman pioneered laser surgery. At the Laser Laboratory established in 1961, he investigated their role in melanomas and tattoos because of the presumed color specificity factor. Work continued in other areas as the technology advanced.

Goldman believes:

> *The trained cutaneous surgeon will soon use an old phrase of laser dermatology, laser non-surgical dermatology, laser diagnostics. Our current studies are in laser induced subsurface imagery. For cutaneous surgery, this imagery is in the endothelium of the superficial blood vessels and the diagnostics of intrinsic cancer in the skin and soft tissue. So, from the early days of laser development, dermatology continues to provide much for laser medicine and laser surgery today and for the future.*[23]

CRYOTHERAPY

The use of cold to ablate skin lesions had its origins in New York in 1899, when A. Campbell White (1869–1908) used liquid air. Carl Gerhardt (1833–1902) of Jena, Germany, had earlier used cold to treat cutaneous tuberculosis.[24] By 1893 Charles Tripler devised a method for liquefying air and urged its use in medicine.[25] Within a few years, George Henry Fox and Thurston Lusk (1869–1931) were treating many patients with liquid air. At first, cotton swabs were used to apply the freezing agent, as suggested by White. Later, he developed a glass cryoprobe spray, and Henry Whitehouse (1864–1938) recommended a similar spray for skin cancer destruction.[26]

In 1905 William Allen Pusey (1865–1940) of Chicago introduced carbon dioxide in stick form. This was later

Part V.

———

67 CHATHAM STREET, NEW-YORK.   **11**

Branch Store,   107 East 28th St., N Y

DERMATOLOGICAL.

Fig. 81.   Piffard's Comedone Extractor.

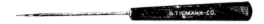

Fig. 82.   Piffard's Irido-Platinum Needle.

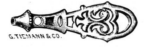

Fig. 89.   **Piffard's Sharp Spoon.**

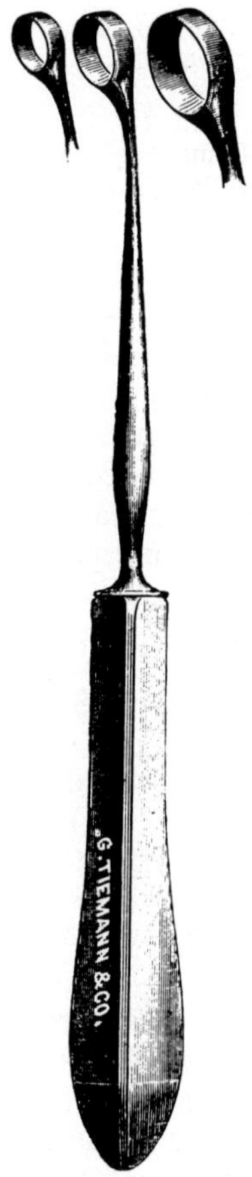

Fig. 83.   Piffard's Milium Needle.

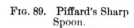

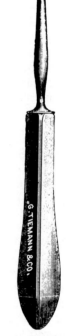

Fig. 84.   Piffard's Scarifying Spud.

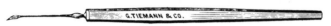

Fig. 85.   Piffard's Epilating Forceps.

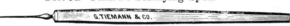

Fig. 86.   Piffard's Grappling Forceps.

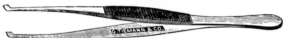

Fig. 87.   Skin Grafting Scissors.

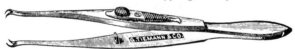

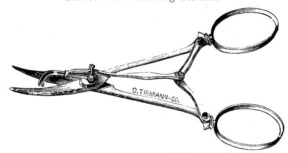

Fig. 88.   Piffard's Cutisector

Fig. 90.   Hess' Glass Pleximeter.
For observing the skin under pressure.

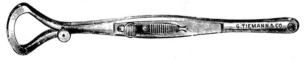

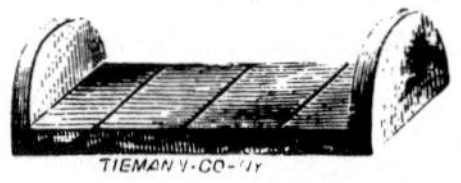

Henry's Depilating Forceps, page 46, Part III.

Piffard's Cutisector,	fig. 296, Part II.	Microscopic Instruments,	page 90, Part I.
Platina Caustic Cup,	fig. 309, Part III.	Counter Irritants,	page 63, Part I.
Fine Scissors,	figs. 110, 111, Part II.	Vaccinating Instruments,	page 66, Part I.
Scalpels,	pages 6, 46, Part I.	Hypodermic Syringes,	page 79, Part I.

Figure 1–2. Dermatologic instruments fashioned in the nineteenth century. (From the American Armamentarium Chirurgicum. Vol 11. George Tiemann & Co, New York, 1879.)

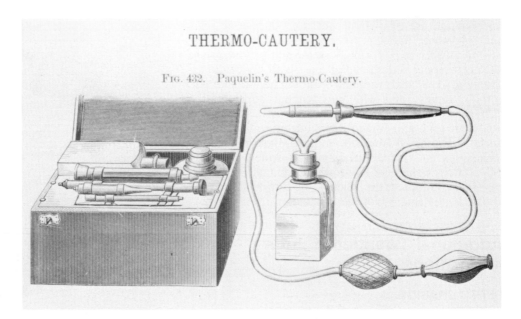

Figure 1–3. Thermocautery sold for $20 in 1879. (From the American Armamentarium Chirurgicum. Vol 1. George Tiemann & Co, New York, 1879, p 134.)

modified in 1925, by Giraudeau, who mixed it with acetone and sulfur to create a slush, advocated for the treatment of hemangiomas and acne (Fig. 1–5).

In 1950 Herman V. Allington (1906–   ) of Oakland, California, introduced liquid nitrogen. He used cotton swabs to treat a variety of skin tumors. This created a new interest in cryosurgery, a word first used by Giraudeau to replace cryocautery in 1930. Subsequently, significant advances in instrumentation were made by Setrag Zacarian (1921–   ) of Springfield, Massachusetts, who used copper discs with the liquid nitrogen, and Douglas Torre (1919–   ) of New York, who devised a closed-system cryoprobe and spray in 1967.[27]

Topical Therapy With Caustics

The pioneer cutaneous surgeons of the nineteenth century were fond of employing a wide variety of chemicals. Peeling agents, or caustics as they were often called, appear to have been introduced in the 1880s. Piffard often recommended nitric acid, acetic acid, and sulfuric acid, not only for reducing hypertrophic lesions but also for the treatment of psoriasis and eczema. Carl Heitzmann (1836–1896) of New York felt that salicylic acid was a near panacea: "No other agent softens and destroys these tissues (callosities, corns, warts) as well."[28] Additional acids became part of the armamentarium. By 1913, Charles McMurtry (1872–1914) of New York could say of salicylic acid that "there is none which possesses a wider range of usefulness."[29] Shortly thereafter, Charles N. Davis (1861–1939) of Philadelphia codified the role of trichloroacetic acid, having borrowed the idea for its use from a laryngologist about 1902.[30, 31] Around 1934, Samuel Monash of New York evaluated various concentrations of salicylic acid, reporting the most useful range to be 15 to 50%.[32] These chemicals allowed cutaneous surgeons the privilege of treating skin

conditions from three different vantage points: chemical destruction, topical chemotherapy, and chemical peeling.

CHEMICAL DESTRUCTION

The technique of chemical destruction was pioneered by Samuel Sherwell (1841–1927) of Brooklyn, New York, as early as 1873.[33] For treating skin cancer, he advocated thorough curettage followed by application of an escharotic, such as a 60% solution of acid nitrite of mercury. This concept would be developed later as a microsurgical technique in the 1930s by Frederick Mohs (1910–   ), a surgeon in Madison, Wisconsin, who pioneered modern chemosurgery. His method of cancer treatment employed zinc chloride fixative, which was applied to the base of the tumor. The tissue became an eschar and was then excised bloodlessly. The tissue could be examined under the microscope to ensure that the area was tumor free. Still later in the 1960s, Theodore Tromovitch (1932–1990) of San Francisco found that microsurgery could be performed equally successfully without the destructive pastes used as fixatives.[34, 35]

TOPICAL CHEMOTHERAPY

In 1953 Calvin Dillaha (1924–1969) and G. Thomas Jansen (1926–   ) noted that cancer patients receiving systemic 5-fluorouracil developed red blotches on the face, which faded along with the actinic keratoses. They reasoned that topical application of this agent would also destroy cutaneous neoplasms, even precancers. Thus, topical chemotherapy was developed for treating actinically damaged skin.

CHEMICAL PEELING

The concept of facial peeling dates as far back as 1903 when George Miller MacKee (1878–1955) of New York initiated the use of phenol peels to reduce acne scars and rejuvenate the skin.[36] Over the next few decades, several physicians performed "skin peeling," but its use did not become widespread at least until midcentury.[37] Trichloroacetic acid, with and without phenol, with and without taping, and with and without augmentation agents such as Jessner's solution (salicylic acid, resorcinol, lactic acid, and ethanol), was introduced or reintroduced.[38] Thomas Baker (1925–) of Miami refined the techniques and made facial peels a widely accepted procedure.[39] Baker and Howard Gordon (1927–), also of Miami, adopted the phenol mixture that became known as the Baker-Gordon formula.

Additional Twentieth Century Innovations

DERMABRASION

The concept of abrading the skin to remove scars or unwanted tissue originated with Ernst Kromayer (1862–1933), who invented the zylindermesser, which consisted of cylindric knives that punched out scars. Although some Europeans attached this instrument to a dental drill, few Americans were aware of the procedure.

After World War II, Preston Iverson (1909–1962) of Philadelphia used sterilized sandpaper to remove tattoos. The next year, 1948, William G. McEvitt (1909–1983) of Detroit adapted this method for decreasing acne scars, which resulted in the cutaneous surgical procedure known as facial sanding.

In 1952 Abner Kurtin (1912–1955) realized that ethyl chloride sprayed on the operative field reduced the pain and made the tissue stiff enough to be abraded with rotary brushes, thus allowing the procedure to become widely used. Saul Blau (1913–1987), also of New York, then coined the term dermabrasion.[40]

GRAFTS AND FLAPS

For more than a century, grafts have been used successfully. The pioneers in this area were Jacques Reverdin (1842–1929) (pinch grafts), Louis Ollier (1830–1900) (split-thickness grafts), and Kark Thiersch (1822–1895) (split-thickness grafts). Others had experimented with grafting at an earlier time, but their work was often forgotten: for example, about 1804, Guiseppe Baronio in Italy performed autografts on sheep, and in 1817 the London surgeon Sir Astley Cooper (1768–1841) grafted a patient's own skin to cover the site of an amputated thumb.[41] However, others recognized the significance of these advances, as indicated by Duhring's account of the subject:

. . . the spurs of a young cock could be "made to grow on his comb" and that a tooth could be successfully transplanted. Reverdin, however, in 1869 was the first to call special attention to the subject of grafting of epidermis, or epidermic grafting in which operation small bits of epidermis, including mucous layer, are transplanted from a healthy locality to an

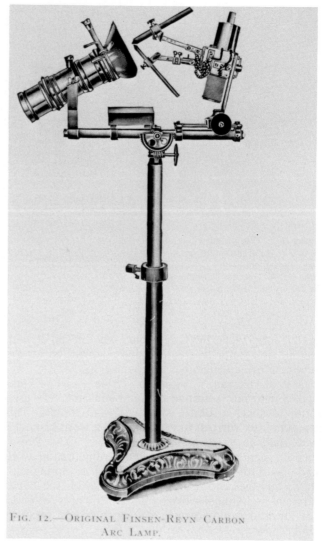

FIG. 12.—ORIGINAL FINSEN-REYN CARBON ARC LAMP.

Figure 1–4. The carbon arc lamp pioneered by Niels Finsen (1860–1904). Phototherapy followed by radiotherapy illustrates how the dermatologist rapidly adapts new technology for the treatment of skin disease. (From Hall P: Ultra-Violet Rays in the Treatment and Cure of Disease. CV Mosby, St. Louis, 1928, p 67.)

open granulating surface and there made to grow. Under favorable conditions this takes place readily with the result that a layer of epithelium spreads out from the grafts, beginning at the margins, and unites with that from other neighboring grafts.[42]

Grafting seemed such a panacea to so many ills that the public often seized upon it inappropriately. In 1891 a patient in Chicago underwent cancer surgery on his thigh; the resultant defect was so large that healing was impaired. His fraternal lodge came to the rescue when 175 of the brethren donated pieces of skin to cover the site. The amount of take is not recorded, but some volunteers were turned down for lack of cleanliness or for having other diseases.[43] During World War I three surgeons, working independently, developed the pedicle flap: V.P. Filatov performed his first flap in 1916 at the Novorossiisk Eye Clinic in Odessa, Ukraine; Sir Harold Gillies of London used a pedicle flap to repair the face

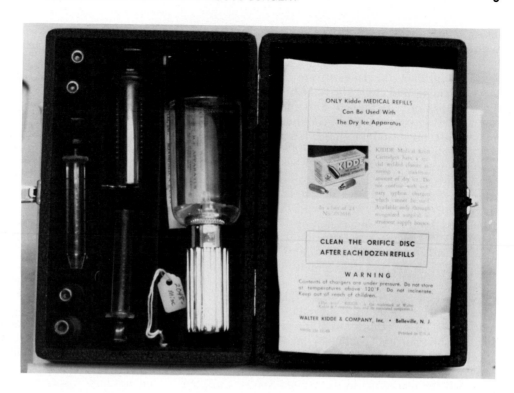

Figure 1–5. Dry ice apparatus made by Walter Kidde & Company, Inc. (Courtesy of the Mütter Museum, College of Physicians of Philadelphia, Philadelphia, PA.)

of a sailor severely burned in the Battle of Jutland; and Hugo Ganzer, a Berlin laryngologist, described the procedure to correct the damage of gunshots to the face.[44]

Z-PLASTY

The basis for the various blepharoplasties and numerous forms of incisions can be traced to the work of Charles Pierre Denonvilliers (1808–1872), a Parisian surgeon who performed a Z-plasty as early as 1854 to repair an ectropion of the lower eyelid.[45] The development of face lifts and other aspects of aesthetic surgery is another story.[46]

LIPOSUCTION

The concept of surgically eliminating fat deposits has been around for several decades; dermolipectomies consisted of excising blocks of fat. In 1964 a German surgeon, Josef Schrudde, announced that he had curetted fat through an incision. A decade later, Giorgio Fischer, an expatriate American surgeon living in Rome, and his father Arpad, also a cosmetic surgeon, developed the planotome and cellusactiotome for fat removal. The former made an intra-adipose plane, while the latter employed suction to chip off fat and then vacuum the pieces away. Yves-Gerard Illouz of Paris devised a cannula to enter the fat tissue, where it was bathed in hypotonic saline before suctioning.[47] This so-called wet method was modified to the dry method by Pierre F. Fournier (1924–), also of Paris, who eliminated the saline.[48] The procedure has been variously called lipectomy (1982), lipolysis, lipoplasty, and finally liposuction.[47]

SCLEROTHERAPY

The destruction of veins began in the middle nineteenth century with the injection of alcohol (1840) by Leory D'Etiolles or ferric chloride (1851) by Charles-Gabriel Pravaz. However, because of infection and embolism, sclerotherapy fell into disuse.[49] A serendipitous finding in the 1920s may have been responsible for stimulating a renewed interest in sclerotherapy. Patients receiving arsphenamine often developed severe sclerosis of the veins. In the 1930s Hyman Biegeleisen (1904–1991) of New York began to inject veins with chemicals.

The injection should be started in healthy tissue. The fine needle point is carried toward the offending capillary, being kept near the skin surface so that it will engage the vessel directly under the dermis. With experience, one should be able, by a gentle but firm push, to catch the needle point in the capillary wall and enter its lumen.[50]

When he created small needles (32- to 33-gauge) in 1934, Biegeleisen was able to microinject small venules, and so treatment of telangiectasia began again. He used sodium morrhuate, but other substances were subsequently introduced, including sodium tetradecyl sulfate (1946), hydroxypolyethoxydodecane (1966), and hypertonic saline and dextrose mixture (1969).[51]

SOFT TISSUE AUGMENTATION

Camouflaging scars and defects has long been a problem for cutaneous surgeons. Cosmetics have been used for centuries; sometimes a patch could conceal an embarrassing scar; other times wax might be used to fill a smallpox scar.[52] In 1899 Gersuny first injected paraffin into a youth's scrotum to replace the absent testicles. Within a few years, paraffin was being injected into the face. Despite the popularity of paraffin, which lasted in Europe until 1914, the dangers were publicized by 1906. Meyer Heidingsfeld (1871–1918) of Cincinnati wrote on the tragedies of paraffinoma. Unscrupulous practitioners, particularly in the Orient, continued to perform the miracle injections well into the 1960s.[53]

Although the use of silicones for a variety of medical purposes was studied as early as 1899, the first study relating to the skin did not appear until 1947. Initial attention was given to using silicones to prevent maceration. Over the next two decades the silicones were developed for breast augmentation. About this time, liquid silicone became available and was injected into the skin to correct defects.[53] Orentreich (1922–   ) became a pioneer in advancing its use in cutaneous surgery.[54]

In 1976 Terry Knapp (1943–   ), Edward Luck, and John Daniels of Stanford, California, found that bovine collagen could be sufficiently purified to markedly reduce its antigenicity. This finding made possible the use of collagen (Zyderm) for augmenting soft tissue deficits, both scars and aging lines.[55] By 1981, collagen was approved for marketing in the United States. Collagen has been further altered chemically to make it last longer (Zyplast), but the significant discovery, a procedure for injecting it into the appropriate skin plane, was made by Arnold Klein of Beverly Hills, California, in 1980.[56]

The development of a gelatin matrix implant began with the fractionation of plasma in 1944. A by-product was fibrin foam, which Arthur Spangler (1916–1975) of Boston began to inject into scars about 1954.[57] Subsequently, Sheldon Gottlieb (1940–   ), now of Washington, DC, conceived of using gelatin matrix to inject into scars and wrinkles. He initially referred to the lyophilized mixture of gelatin powder and aminocaproic acid as the GAP repair technique. The material is now called Fibrel and received FDA approval in 1988.[58]

SUMMARY

The role of cutaneous surgery in dermatology has become increasingly important since 1956 when the first text on the subject appeared. In the preface to *Skin Surgery*, which went through six editions, Ervin Epstein Sr. (1909–   ) wrote:

> *Some twenty years ago, I reported to a hospital to commence a residency in dermatology. My first assignment was to perform skin surgery. That first afternoon, a seemingly never ending train of patients filed by with moles, cancers, warts, etc., and I removed them with instruments that I never saw before.*[59]

Today, there are journals and societies devoted to cutaneous surgery. The American periodical *The Journal of Dermatologic Surgery and Oncology* was begun in 1975 by Perry Robbins and George Popkin (1921–   ) of New York, and the Italian journal *Giornale Italiano di Chirurgia Dermatologica e Oncologia* was founded by Antonello Tulli of Rome in 1986.

The first society devoted exclusively to dermatologic surgery, The American Society for Dermatologic Surgery, was founded in 1972, having been organized on December 5, 1970, by Leonard Lewis and Sorrel Resnick (1935–   ) of Miami. The International Society for Dermatologic Surgery was created in 1977 through the stimulus of Perry Robbins.[60] Today, there are many state societies as well as national organizations elsewhere in the world devoted to cutaneous surgery.

The University of Miami School of Medicine pioneered the concept of incorporating surgery within the name of the dermatology unit. Harvey Blank (1918–   ), Chairman of Dermatology (1956–1985) at the University of Miami School of Medicine, first conceived of the idea on November 17, 1974. He brought the concept to fruition in 1980, when the Department of Dermatology and Cutaneous Surgery became the approved name. Many schools currently have divisions or sections of dermatologic surgery, so it was only appropriate for the Association of Academic Dermatologic Surgeons to be organized in 1988.[61]

Surgery, always a part of dermatology, has become an equal partner with cutaneous medicine. Cutaneous surgery, which incorporates the therapeutic, cosmetic, and aesthetic aspects of dermatology, has a glorious future.

REFERENCES

1. Bennett RG (ed): Cutaneous surgery: history and development. In: Fundamentals of Cutaneous Surgery. CV Mosby, St. Louis, 1988, pp 1–16.
2. Majno G: The Healing Hand: Man and Wound in the Ancient World. Harvard University Press, Cambridge, 1975.
3. Marmelzat WL: History of dermatologic surgery from the beginnings to late antiquity. Clin Dermatol 5:1–10, 1987.
4. Turner D: A Treatise of Diseases Incident to Skin. J Walthoe, London, 1631, pp 284–289.
5. Bateman T: A Practical Synopsis of Cutaneous Diseases. James Crissy, Philadelphia, 1824, pp 311–312.
6. Piffard HG: Histological contribution. Am J Syphilol Dermatol 1:217–219, 1870.
7. Besnier E: Études nouvelles de dermatologie. Gaz Hebdom Méd Chir 26:645–650, 1879.
8. Keyes EL: The cutaneous punch. J Cutan Genitourin Dis 5:98–101, 1887.
9. Goodman H: Cutaneous punch. Arch Dermatol Syphilol 56:268–269, 1947.
10. Lowenthal LJA: Punch biopsy with autograft. AMA Arch Dermatol Syphilol 67:629, 1953.
11. Orentreich N: Autografts in alopecias and other selected dermatological conditions. Ann NY Acad Sci 83:463–479, 1959.
12. Wigglesworth E: The curette in dermal therapeutics. Boston Med Surg J 94:143–146, 1876.
13. Duhring LA: A Practical Treatise on Diseases of the Skin. JB Lippincott, Philadelphia, 1883, p 484.
14. Bulkley LD: Note on the local treatment of certain diseases of the skin. Arch Dermatol 2:307–310, 1876.
15. Piffard HG: A Treatise on the Materia Medica and Therapeutics of the Skin. Wm Wood, New York, 1881, pp 121–125.
16. Hardaway WA: Some further observations on electrolysis in diseases of the skin. J Cutan Genitourin Dis 15:399–403, 1897.
17. de Keating-Hart WV: Die Behandlung des Krebaes Mittelst Fulguration. Akademische Verlagsgesellschaft, Leipzig, 1980, pp 1–37.
18. Clark WL: High-frequency desiccation, fulguration and thermoradiotherapy: their uses in therapeutics. JAMA 59:916–918, 1912.

19. Pearce JA: Electrosurgery. John Wiley, New York, 1986, pp 1–15.
20. Goldwyn M: The man and the machine. Ann Plast Surg 2:135–153, 1979.
21. Wheeland RG (ed): Fundamental laser physics for the surgeon and laser-tissue interaction. In: Lasers in Skin Disease. Thieme Medical, New York, 1988, pp 1–6.
22. Wheeland RG, Walker NPJ: Lasers—25 years later. Int J Dermatol 25:209–216, 1986.
23. Goldman L: The history of development of the medical laser. In: Abela GS (ed): Lasers in Cardiovascular Medicine and Surgery: Fundamentals and Techniques. Kluwer Academic, Boston, 1990, pp 3–7.
24. Bracco D: The historic development of cryosurgery. Clin Dermatol 8:1–4, 1990.
25. Kuflik EG, Gage AA: Cryosurgical Treatment for Skin Cancer. Igaku-Shoin, New York, 1990, pp 1–13.
26. Whitehouse HH: Liquid air in dermatology: its indications and limitations. JAMA 49:371–377, 1907.
27. Torre D: New York, Cradle of cryosurgery. NY State J Med 67:465–467, 1967.
28. Heitzmann C: The value of salicylic acid in dermatology. J Cutan Genitourin Dis 6:426–428, 1888.
29. McMurtry CW: Dermatologic therapeutics: salicylic acid. J Cutan Dis 31:166–171, 1913.
30. Davis CN: Trichloracetic acid and its uses in dermatology. J Cutan Dis 33:691–695, 1915.
31. Roberts HL: The chloracetic acids: a biochemical study. Br J Dermatol Syphilol 38:323–334, 1926.
32. Monash S: The uses of diluted trichloracetic acid in dermatology. Urol Cutan Rev 49:119–120, 1945.
33. Sherwell S: The technique of an efficient operative procedure for the removal and cure of superficial malignancies. NY State J Med 8:304–308, 1908.
34. Mohs FE: Mohs micrographic surgery: a historical perspective. Dermatol Clin 7:609–612, 1989.
35. Tromovitch TA, Stegman SJ: Microscopically controlled excision of skin tumors. Arch Dermatol 110:231–232, 1974.
36. MacKee GM, Karp FL: The treatment of post-acne scars with phenol. Br J Dermatol 64:456–459, 1952.
37. Eller JJ, Wolff S: Skin peeling and scarification. JAMA 116:934–938, 1941.
38. Ayres S III: Dermal changes following application of chemical cauterants to aging skin. Arch Dermatol 82:578–585, 1960.
39. Baker TJ: The ablation of rhitides by chemical means. J Florida Med Ass 48:451–454, 1961.
40. Blau S, Rein CR: Dermabrasion of the acne pit. AMA Arch Dermatol Syphilol 70:754–766, 1954.
41. Balch CM, Marzoni FA: Skin transplantation during the pre-Reverdin era, 1904–1969. Surg Gynecol Obstet 144:766–773, 1977.
42. Duhring LA: Cutaneous Medicine. JB Lippincott, Philadelphia, 1895.
43. Buffam GBB: Mass skin grafting in the nineties. Can Med Assoc J 80:1001–1002, 1959.
44. Webster JP: The early history of the tubed pedicle flap. Surg Clin North Am 39:261–275, 1959.
45. Ivy RH: Who originated the Z-plasty? Plast Reconstr Surg 47:66–72, 1971.
46. Rogers BO: Historical development of free skin grafting. Surg Clin North Am 39:289–311, 1959.
47. Illouz Y-G: The origins of lipolysis. In: Hetter GP (ed): Lipoplasty: The Theory and Practice of Blunt Suction Lipectomy. Little, Brown, Boston, 1984, pp 25–32.
48. Otteni FM, Fournier PF: In: Hetter GP (ed): Lipoplasty: the theory and practice of blunt suction lipectomy. Little, Brown, Boston, 1984, pp 19–23.
49. Schneider W: Contribution a l'historique de traitement sclerosant des varices et a son étude anatomo-pathologique. Bull Soc Fr Phlebologie 18:177–130, 1965.
50. Biegeleisen H: Telangiectasia associated with varicose veins. JAMA 102:2092–2094, 1934.
51. Goldman MP, Bennett RG: Treatment of telangiectasia: a review. J Am Acad Dermatol 17:167–182, 1987.
52. Parish LC, Crissey JT: Cosmetics: a historical review. Clin Dermatol 6:1–4, 1988.
53. Matton G, Anseeuw A, De Keyser F: The history of injectable biomaterials and the biology of collagen. Aesthetic Plast Surg 9:133–140, 1985.
54. Selmanowitz VJ, Orentreich N: Medical grade fluid silicone: a monographic review. J Dermatol Surg Oncol 3:597–611, 1977.
55. Knapp TR, Luck E, Daniels JR: Behavior of solubilized collagen as a bioimplant. J Surg Res 23:96–105, 1977.
56. Klein AW: Implantation techniques for injectable collagen. J Am Acad Dermatol 9:224–228, 1983.
57. Spangler AS: New treatment of pitted scars: preliminary report. AMA Arch Dermatol 76:708–711, 1957.
58. Gottlieb SK: Soft tissue augmentation: the search for implantation matrials and techniques. Clin Dermatol 5:128–134, 1987.
59. Epstein E: Skin Surgery. Lea & Febiger, Philadelphia, 1956, p 5.
60. Lewis LA: The history of the American Society for Dermatologic Surgery and its impact on the specialty of dermatology. J Dermatol Surg Oncol 16:1054–1056, 1990.
61. Resnik SS: History of dermatologic surgery. In: Roenigk RK, Roenigk HH Jr (eds): Dermatologic Surgery: Principles and Practice. Marcel Dekker, New York, 1989, pp 1–4.

CHAPTER 2

Preoperative Patient Evaluation and Preparation for Cutaneous Surgery

ROBERT F. BLOOM

Although outpatient cutaneous surgery may often deal with small and relatively insignificant lesions, much larger and more complicated procedures that require tremendous surgical skill and knowledge are also now being routinely performed by cutaneous surgeons. The wide variety and tremendous complexity of some procedures[1] requires that each patient be thoroughly evaluated preoperatively in order to obtain the best possible results in all cases.[2, 3] This important process serves the primary purpose of assessing the nature of each patient's individual problem, evaluating the overall health status, and determining potential risk factors associated with performing surgery. It also provides the surgeon with an opportunity to establish rapport with patients and educate them as to the nature of their problem, the treatment options available, the associated risks and benefits, and potential complications. In addition, patients' mental and emotional status, anxiety level, and ability to perform the necessary postoperative care can also be assessed in this initial evaluation.[2] Finally, the surgeon can help prepare patients for the procedure by outlining what to expect both on the day of surgery and afterward.

Characteristics of the Patient, Staff, and Physician

THE PATIENT

Since patients may either be established in the surgeon's practice or new, they may already have a great deal of knowledge about the nature and treatment of their problem or may be totally ignorant of this important information. New patients especially require a thorough evaluation, but even established patients deserve a full and careful re-evaluation of their personal health, since many important changes may have occurred since their last visit. However, sometimes only a brief rediscussion of the problem, treatment options, and risks is necessary to refresh the memory of established patients. New patients also obviously require more time and effort to educate them about their problem and the treatment possibilities to manage it effectively.

THE STAFF

The staff should arrive at the office on time, rested, cheerful, and appropriately dressed so they can present a helpful, friendly, and cheerful attitude to patients in person or over the telephone. The primary goal of helping patients should be of ultimate importance to the office staff. The staff must be able to understand the concerns many people have regarding surgery and be willing to spend extra time to provide any assistance possible.

THE PHYSICIAN

The doctor should also be on time, rested, cheerful, and appropriately dressed. A firm handshake and directly looking into patients' eyes while speaking in a calm and reassuring tone is always a good approach in meeting them for the first time. The most important thing the physician can do during the initial patient evaluation is instill a sense of confidence. This is accomplished by thoroughly evaluating patients, providing detailed factual knowledge about the problem and the proposed procedure, and demonstrating a willingness to answer any questions they may have. This helps to dispel any fear or apprehension patients may have and eliminates any misinformation they may have received from books or magazines or discussions with well-meaning family members or friends. The cutaneous surgeon should always remember that it is an honor to have been selected to provide the necessary services required to help patients with their medical problem.

Use of Preprinted Forms for Preoperative Evaluation

Preprinted informational forms greatly aid the physician and make the initial patient evaluation more instructive, focused, and valuable. Many of these forms can be mailed to patients after their initial telephone inquiry, to be completed at their leisure at home where they have access to personal medical records, prescriptions, insurance company policy numbers and addresses, and personal calendars to confirm dates of previous medical procedures, hospitalizations, or surgeries and physicians' addresses and phone numbers. The completed forms can be thoroughly reviewed by the cutaneous surgeon at the time of the initial consultation, and items of special concern discussed in further detail. This not only provides more accurate information, but also lessens the time patients otherwise have to spend in completing forms in the waiting room on the day of consultation. While the numbers and kinds of forms needed are largely determined by the individual nature of the cutaneous surgeon's practice, the primary ones typically request general information about the patient; provide information about the location, hours, and policies of the medical practice; and seek specifics related to the patient's current medical problem and general health status. For the general questionnaire information form, usual items requested include full name and address, date of birth, sex, telephone number, insurance company, responsible party, referral source, and employment information. Some physicians, in an attempt to make the office seem appropriately friendly and cordial, also ask patients to give the name by which they prefer to be addressed (Fig. 2–1).

The health status and patient medical problem questionnaire (Fig. 2–2) should determine general information about the patients' health.[3] A clearer determination of patients' current cutaneous problem, its exact location and duration, and any previous treatment can be accomplished with the use of problem-specific questionnaires. Any allergic reactions to medications[4] should be listed as well as the use of immunosuppressive drugs,[5] beta blockers,[6, 7] neuroleptic agents, or agents such as aspirin, nonsteroidal anti-inflammatory agents,[8–10] and vitamin E that may interfere with normal coagulation. Patients should also be asked whether there have been any difficulties with bleeding[11] or excessive bruising, fainting episodes, seizures, or problems during previous surgeries, including oral surgery. Specific items should also be addressed concerning common general medical conditions that may adversely affect wound healing,[5, 12] in-

Date: _____

Patient's name: _____

Address: _____

City: _____ State: _____ Zip code: _____

Phone number: (_____) _____

Date of Birth: _____ Age: _____ Sex: _____

Employer: _____

    Address: _____

    City: _____ State: _____ Zip code: _____

    Phone number: (_____) _____

Insurance company: _____

    Address: _____

    City: _____ State: _____ Zip code: _____

    Phone number: (_____) _____

    Policy number: _____

How did you learn about our medical practice? _____

_____

Whom can we thank for referring you to our medical practice? _____

_____

I would like the doctor to address me as: _____
Thank you for completing this important information form.

Figure 2–1. General patient information form.

Date:_____

Patient's name: _____

Do you have a history of any of the following conditions?

_____ High blood pressure	_____ Gastrointestinal
_____ Heart disease	_____ Ulcers
_____ Rheumatic fever	_____ Hepatitis
_____ Pacemaker	_____ Liver problems
_____ Artificial valves	_____ Atopic disorders
_____ Diabetes	_____ Asthma
_____ Lung disease	_____ Eczema
_____ Kidney disease	_____ Hay fever
_____ Artificial joints	_____ Other disorders

Do you use any medications? _____ Yes _____ No. If yes, complete the following:

Name of medication _____ Dosage _____

Purpose _____

Name of medication _____ Dosage _____

Purpose _____

Do you have any medication allergies? _____ Yes _____ No. If yes, describe the medication and the kind of reaction _____

_____

Do you use alcohol? _____ Yes _____ No. If yes, how much? _____

Do you use tobacco? _____ Yes _____ No. If yes, how much? _____

Have you had any previous surgery? _____ Yes _____ No. If yes, complete the following:

Type of surgery _____ Date _____

Location _____ Surgeon _____

Type of surgery _____ Date _____

Location _____ Surgeon _____

Have you ever been hospitalized? _____ Yes _____ No. If yes, complete the following:

Medical problem _____ Date _____

Location _____ Physician _____

Figure 2–2. General medical history form.

crease the risk of infection, result in adverse medication interactions, or require the use of prophylactic preoperative antibiotics.[13-15] This form should also include information about medical history in regard to diabetes mellitus, the use of a pacemaker,[16] hypertension, cardiac or vascular disease, smoking history,[17] nutritional deficiency,[18, 19] or tendency toward abnormal scarring.[20-22] Specialized preoperative evaluation forms can be designed for specific conditions such as sclerotherapy, laser therapy for port-wine stains and telangiectasia, or collagen implantation (Figs. 2–3 to 2–7). Of course, whenever forms are used for these purposes, they must always be reviewed by the physician and made part of the patient's permanent medical record.

The Cutaneous Surgeon's Office

WAITING ROOM

The patient waiting room may vary in decor from very spartan to spectacular. Probably the best approach for the typical cutaneous surgeon's waiting room is to be modest in nature. Furniture and furnishings should be clean and kept in good repair. In addition to recent issues of various magazines, it is appropriate to consider providing informational material on a bulletin board in the waiting area through which patients can browse. This material may contain information about the types of services provided by the surgeon or recent advances in the specialty, such as laser surgery or the use of sunscreens to reduce the risk of premature aging or the development of skin cancer, that might be of general interest to patients or their families. A display of the physician's awards and licenses is also an appropriate decoration for the waiting room. Having a chance to look at these awards may give patients a better appreciation of the surgeon's training, skills, and expertise. Some physicians also keep a current copy of their curriculum vitae available on the bulletin board to give patients an opportunity to learn more about them. Regardless of the style or layout, which are both determined by individual preferences, the waiting room should give patients a sense of warmth and comfort. There should always be a separate area in the waiting room in which patients can be asked questions about their particular medical problem or insurance coverage, or where they can discuss billing matters or personal finances.

Text continued on page 20

Date:_____

Patient's name: _____

Do you have a history of any of the following conditions?

_____ High blood pressure   _____ Gastrointestinal
_____ Heart disease   _____ Ulcers
_____ Rheumatic fever   _____ Hepatitis
_____ Pacemaker   _____ Liver problems
_____ Artificial valves   _____ Atopic disorders
_____ Diabetes   _____ Asthma
_____ Lung disease   _____ Eczema
_____ Kidney disease   _____ Hay fever
_____ Artificial joints   _____ Other disorders

Do you use any medications? _____ Yes _____ No. If yes, complete the following:

Name of medication _____ Dosage _____

Purpose _____

Name of medication _____ Dosage _____
Purpose _____

Do you have any medication allergies? _____ Yes _____ No. If yes, describe the medication and the kind of reaction _____
_____

Have you ever been hospitalized? _____ Yes _____ No. If yes, give details _____

Please provide the following information about your port-wine stain:

Was the onset at birth? _____ Yes _____ No. If no, when did it appear? _____

Have you noticed any of the following?
_____ Color change   _____ Texture change
_____ Bleeding   _____ Infection
_____ Blebs   _____ Enlargement
_____ Impaired function   _____ Other

Have you ever had any of the following conditions or problems?
_____ Seizures   _____ Glaucoma
_____ Abnormal scars   _____ Retardation

Have you had any previous treatment? _____ Yes _____ No. If yes, describe the treatment and the results_____
_____

Does anyone in your family have a similar problem? _____ Yes _____ No

    If yes, give relationship _____

Figure 2–3. Port-wine stain history form.

Date: _____

Patient's name: _____

Do you have a history of any of the following conditions?

_____ High blood pressure   _____ Gastrointestinal
_____ Heart disease   _____ Ulcers
_____ Rheumatic fever   _____ Hepatitis
_____ Pacemaker   _____ Liver problems
_____ Artificial valves   _____ Atopic disorders
_____ Diabetes   _____ Asthma
_____ Lung disease   _____ Eczema
_____ Kidney disease   _____ Hay fever
_____ Artificial joints   _____ Other disorders

Do you use any medications? _____ Yes _____ No. If yes, complete the following:
   Name of medication _____ Dosage _____
   Purpose _____

Do you have any medication allergies? _____ Yes _____ No. If yes, describe the medication and the kind of reaction _____
_____

Have you ever been hospitalized? _____ Yes _____ No. If yes, give details _____

Do you have problems with any of the following conditions?
   _____ Easy bruising   _____ Prolonged bleeding
   _____ Clotting problems   _____ Abnormal scars
   _____ Recurrent infection _____ Low pain threshold

Have you had an excess amount of sunlight exposure in your life?
_____ Yes _____ No. Occupationally? _____ Recreationally? _____

Have you had any previous skin cancers? _____ Yes _____ No. If yes, complete the following:
   Type: _____ Location: _____
   Treatment: _____ Result: _____

Where is your current problem located? _____

How long has it been present? _____

Has this problem been previously treated? _____ Yes _____ No. If yes, describe the treatment _____

Has this area been biopsied? _____ Yes _____ No. If yes, give when, where, and your physician _____

Has anyone in your family had skin cancer? _____ Yes _____ No. If yes, provide details _____

Figure 2–4. Skin cancer history form.

Date: _____

Patient's name: _____

Do you have a history of any of the following conditions?

_____ High blood pressure   _____ Gastrointestinal
_____ Heart disease   _____ Ulcers
_____ Rheumatic fever   _____ Hepatitis
_____ Pacemaker   _____ Liver problems
_____ Artificial valves   _____ Atopic disorders
_____ Diabetes   _____ Asthma
_____ Lung disease   _____ Eczema
_____ Kidney disease   _____ Hay fever
_____ Artificial joints   _____ Photosensitivity
_____ Collagen vascular disease _____ Excess sun exposure

Does anyone in your family have a history of any collagen vascular diseases like rheumatoid arthritis, lupus, or scleroderma?
_____ Yes _____ No. If yes, give details _____
_____

Do you use any medications? _____ Yes _____ No. If yes, complete the following:
   Name of medication _____ Dosage _____
   Purpose _____

Do you have any medication allergies? _____ Yes _____ No. If yes, describe the medication and the kind of reaction _____
_____

Have you ever reacted to local anesthetics? _____ Yes _____ No. If yes, provide details _____

Have you ever been hospitalized? _____ Yes _____ No. If yes, give details _____
_____

What areas do you want treated with collagen injections? _____
_____

What is the cause of your problem?
_____ Acne? _____ Trauma? _____ Infection? _____ Aging? _____ Other?

Have you had previous treatment for this problem? _____ Yes _____ No. If yes, describe treatment _____
_____

Figure 2–5. Collagen injection history form.

Date: _____

Patient's name: _____

Do you have a history of any of the following conditions?

_____ High blood pressure	_____ Gastrointestinal
_____ Heart disease	_____ Ulcers
_____ Rheumatic fever	_____ Hepatitis
_____ Pacemaker	_____ Liver problems
_____ Artificial valves	_____ Atopic disorders
_____ Diabetes	_____ Asthma
_____ Lung disease	_____ Eczema
_____ Kidney disease	_____ Hay fever
_____ Artificial joints	_____ Stroke
_____ Easy bruising	_____ Prolonged bleeding
_____ Clotting problems	_____ Abnormal scars
_____ Recurrent infection	_____ Low pain threshold
_____ Blood clots	_____ Pulmonary emboli
_____ Phlebitis	_____ Other disorders

Do you use any medications? _____ Yes _____ No. If yes, complete the following:

  Name of medication _____ Dosage_____

  Purpose _____

Do you have any medication allergies? _____ Yes _____ No. If yes, describe the medication and the kind of reaction _____

_____

Have you ever been hospitalized? _____ Yes _____ No. If yes, give details _____

What areas do you want treated? _____

_____

What is the duration of your problem? _____ months _____ years

Does anyone in your family have a similar problem? _____ Yes _____ No. If yes, who? _____

Do you have any of the following symptoms in your legs:

_____ Aching? _____ Swelling? _____ Pain? _____ Heaviness?

Are new blood vessels continuing to appear? _____ Yes _____ No

Have you had any previous treatment? _____ Yes _____ No. If yes, describe _____

Are you currently pregnant or considering pregnancy? _____ Yes _____ No

Figure 2–6. Sclerotherapy history form.

Date: _____

Patient's name: _____

Do you have a history of any of the following conditions?

_____ High blood pressure   _____ Gastrointestinal
_____ Heart disease   _____ Ulcers
_____ Rheumatic fever   _____ Hepatitis
_____ Pacemaker   _____ Liver problems
_____ Artificial valves   _____ Atopic disorders
_____ Diabetes   _____ Asthma
_____ Lung disease   _____ Eczema
_____ Kidney disease   _____ Hay fever
_____ Artificial joints   _____ Photosensitivity
_____ Collagen vascular disease   _____ Excess sun exposure
_____ Abnormal scars   _____ Acne rosacea

Does anyone in your family have a history of any collagen vascular diseases like rheumatoid arthritis, lupus, or scleroderma?
_____ Yes _____ No. If yes, give details _____

_____

Do you use any medications? _____ Yes _____ No. If yes, complete the following:
  Name of medication _____ Dosage _____
  Purpose _____

Do you have any medication allergies? _____ Yes _____ No. If yes, describe the medication and the kind of reaction _____

_____

What areas do you want treated? _____

_____

What is the duration of your problem? _____ months _____ years

Does anyone in your family have a similar problem? _____ Yes _____ No. If yes, who? _____

Have you had any of the following:
  _____ Bleeding?   _____ Flushing with food?
  _____ Hot flashes?   _____ Flushing with alcohol?
  _____ Increasing size?   _____ Increasing number?

Have you had any previous treatment? _____ Yes _____ No. If yes, describe _____

Figure 2–7. Facial telangiectasia history form.

CONSULTATION AREA

Since the goal of the initial evaluation or consultation is a successful patient encounter in which a meaningful relationship is established, the location for performing this service must be one of the first concerns addressed. Some physicians like to have the initial consultation in their private offices; others prefer a "dedicated" consultation room. However, since many patients, especially children, adolescents, and some apprehensive adults, are extremely frightened by the prospects of surgery, it is probably unwise to carry out the initial consultation in a treatment room or operatory. However, once the consultation has been completed and satisfactory rapport established, it may be anxiety reducing to show some patients the actual operatory that will be used for their procedure. In these cases, the room should be uncluttered, with clean counters and no bloody linens or surgical instruments in plain view from surgical procedures performed earlier in the day. All possible equipment should be stored behind closed doors in cabinets or drawers.

For patients to develop a feeling of trust, the surgeon must give them complete attention without interruptions by staff, telephone calls, or pagers. After a complete history has been taken and a thorough review made of the preprinted patient historical information questionnaire, the physical examination is performed, which should include vital signs. This is of obvious importance, since it may uncover some unrecognized underlying medical disorder or condition that will require further evaluation by the patient's family physician or internist. The anatomic location may also suggest the need for obtaining preoperative laboratory studies, radiologic examination, or perhaps a consultation by another surgical specialist before the procedure is performed. In particular, the cutaneous surgeon must pay close attention to patients' overall physical and mental health, the nutritional status, the quality of healing from previous injuries or surgeries, and the anatomic location of the condition that is being evaluated for treatment.[23] This affords the physician an opportunity to consider the different treatment options available so that these may be thoroughly discussed with the patient.[24–27]

After completion of the history and physical examination, the physician must thoroughly explain the diagnosis, nature of the problem, prognosis, and treatment options available, including doing nothing in some cases. If any appropriate laboratory tests such as complete blood or platelet count, peripheral smear, prothrombin time, partial thromboplastic time or bleeding time, chest film, computed tomography (CT) scans, or magnetic resonance imaging (MRI) examinations are deemed appropriate, arrangements should be made for these to be obtained before patients' departure.[9, 11] Photographs, required by many insurance companies and always a good way to accurately document patients' preoperative appearance, can also be taken at this time so that they can be processed before the surgical procedure. If further evaluation by another surgical colleague or anesthesiologist is required, these arrangements can also be made at this time. Finally, for many surgical procedures,

a request must be submitted to the patient's insurance company to obtain preauthorization. The details of that approval process, along with the typical associated delays, should also be discussed with patients at the time of the initial evaluation.

At the completion of the consultation, patients must fully understand the prognosis of their condition along with all the ramifications of the proposed procedure, including potential complications, pain, and risks; the anticipated cosmetic result; and possible scarring. Establishing effective lines of communication between doctor and patient is necessary so that patients are fully involved in the decision-making process. Patients should always be encouraged to participate in every aspect of the interview, preparation, surgery, and recovery. Special consideration must be given to patients seeking cosmetic surgery, because these types of elective procedures are always performed at the discretion of the patient.

Unfortunately, there will be occasional situations in which conflicts develop between physician and patient, making it impossible for either party to make the necessary commitments required to proceed with treatment. In these relatively rare circumstances, it is always best to be honest and forthright. The doctor should tell the patient in clear and succinct terms what is apparently wrong with the relationship and what needs to be done. If no consensus can be reached, help should be offered to the patient in finding another doctor by providing a list of other health care professionals who could provide the requested type of service. The patient may then seek help elsewhere or may return at a later date for further discussion of the problem and reconsideration of the possible forms of treatment available. Dramatic conflicts between the patient and physician generally serve little useful purpose and should be avoided if possible.

PREOPERATIVE CONSENT FORMS

After the decision has been reached to proceed with treatment, the physician must obtain informed consent. Much of the evaluation process has been designed to inform patients of the nature of their condition, treatment options, risks, benefits, complications, and scarring, but verbal consent is insufficient to proceed with treatment and written consent should always be obtained. The written consent form should be simple and clear. At a minimum, it should contain patient's name, date, diagnosis, location, the procedure to be performed, and its associated risks, benefits, complications, and scarring. This form may be general in nature (Fig. 2–8) or specific for only one type of problem or treatment. It may also be important to include a special paragraph regarding the treatment of certain skin cancers, in which the patient consents to be responsible for seeking appropriate follow-up care. If photographs are to be taken, either preoperatively or during the procedure, a special photographic consent form should be signed. This (Fig. 2–9) should detail the purpose of taking the photographs and authorize the physician to use them in medical publications, if so desired, or in

I have had a medical consultation with _____ M.D. concerning treatment for the following medical condition:_____

_____

_____

I understand that the treatment of this condition will include the following procedure(s): _____

_____

_____

The nature, purpose, and possible complications of the procedure(s), the risks and benefits reasonably to be expected, and the alternative methods of treatment that are available have been clearly explained to me. I understand the explanation that I have received, including my right to refuse such treatment. I have had an opportunity to ask any questions I may have and have been encouraged to ask any further questions that may arise during the course of treatment.

I acknowledge that the practice of medicine and surgery is not an exact science and that reputable practitioners therefore cannot properly guarantee results. I further acknowledge that no guarantees or assurances have been given to me regarding the success or benefits that may result from the above procedure(s).

After carefully reviewing the above paragraphs, I hereby consent to be treated.

_____   _____
Patient's signature (or Patient's representative)   Date

_____   _____
Witness   Date

Figure 2–8. Treatment consent form.

Dr. _____ believes that it is essential to take photographs of the treated areas before, during, and after treatment for medical records, insurance purposes, and other limited uses as outlined below. Please read the following paragraphs and indicate your acceptance by signing and dating this form.

I hereby give my permission to be photographed before, during, and after treatment. I understand that these photographs will become part of my permanent medical records.

In addition to serving as an important part of my records, I understand that these photographs may be used for the following limited academic purposes: dissemination to other health care professionals and/or medical journals for documentation, research, teaching, publication, or presentation. I hereby give my consent to such limited additional uses. Any photographs used will contain no reference to my name.

_____   _____
Patient's signature (or Patient's representative)   Date

_____   _____
Witness   Date

Insurance Release

In the event that my insurance company requests copies of these photographs or other medical information from my record, I authorize _____ to release such information to my insurance company.

_____   _____
Patient's signature (or Patient's representative)   Date

Figure 2–9. Photograph consent form.

making professional presentations. It should also give the physician permission to send the photographs to the patient's insurance company, if requested, for obtaining preauthorization to perform the procedure.

OTHER USEFUL FORMS

Once patients have been completely evaluated and have consented to proceed with scheduling the particular surgical procedure, a number of other preprinted forms can also be beneficial. These may serve to reinforce the information provided to patients at the time of their consultation in regard to the nature of their specific problem, the prognosis, and the treatment planned. The forms can also help better prepare patients for the planned procedure (Fig. 2–10) or emphasize any specific points regarding the need to avoid preoperative use of nonprescription anticoagulants, possible need for postoperative (and in some cases, preoperative) avoidance of ultraviolet light, and the desired level of postoperative activities. Patients who require prophylactic antibiotics, because of implanted prosthetic joints, mitral valve prolapse, or other cardiac conditions, should be given the necessary prescriptions so that they can get them filled before the surgical procedure is performed and be appropriately initiated preoperatively. Although almost all cutaneous surgical procedures can be performed safely and effectively under local anesthesia without sedation, some patients should not be allowed to drive themselves home immediately postoperatively because of the nature of their dressings or because of the use of oral or intravenous sedatives during the procedure. As a consequence, these patients should be advised of the need to have someone available to drive them home after the procedure has been completed.

Written postoperative wound care instructions (Fig. 2–11) given to patients *before* surgery enable them to purchase any necessary medications or wound dressing materials or supplies that may be required postoperatively, or make arrangements to obtain appropriate family assistance (if necessary) and complete sick leave forms for their employer. These postoperative instruction forms should also indicate what patients should do if an emergency situation, such as bleeding, arises postoperatively, and should give them a phone number to call if they have any other nonemergent questions or problems. Since complications may be anticipated in any surgical procedure, albeit often of minor significance and with simple solutions, all patients must be made aware of the ones most likely to occur. These forms can be developed for many specific types of procedures (Figs. 2–12 to 2–15), if so desired.

Patients should be completely comfortable with the idea that they can always communicate any untoward occurrence with the physician as soon as possible after it has been recognized. They must be made to understand that their perception is extremely important and that they should call the physician whenever they are concerned that something may be wrong. It is important to indicate to patients that their physician *is* available, if necessary. However, since there may be times when the physician is not available, they should know which doctor to call or which facility they should attend in the event of an emergency.

Same-Day Surgery

Whenever possible, same-day surgical procedures should be performed according to patients' individual needs, since it is a great benefit to most of them. However, special procedures such as Mohs or cosmetic surgery, and those that require insurance company preauthorization or further laboratory or radiologic evaluation, obviously require scheduling well after the consultation procedure has been performed. Nonetheless, patients always appreciate maximal efficiency and effective use of their time and should be given the option of completing their procedure as soon as possible. One hidden benefit of briefly delaying performance of a cosmetic surgical procedure is that it gives patients an opportunity to evaluate their treatment options more thoroughly and not make a hasty or impulsive decision that they may later regret.

Billing

A successful patient encounter should not be marred by inaccurate or distasteful billing procedures. The goal should be to complete all paper work before patients leave the office so that they know all the details related to their procedure. Monthly billing with computerized statements is now considered standard. This task can often be completed while patients are still present, greatly reducing anxiety for the patient and work for the office staff and physician.

---

1. Avoid taking aspirin or any aspirin preparations for at least 2 weeks before surgery and for 1 week after surgery. Acetaminophen is the only pain medication that is safe to take. If you have any questions about your medications, please call at least 1 week before your surgery to obtain clarification.
2. Please notify your physician if you take warfarin (Coumadin), heparin, or dipyridamole (Persantine).
3. Please remember to notify your physician if you have an allergy to any medication, including antibiotics, anesthetics, or pain medications.
4. Also, please notify your physician if you have an artificial joint or heart valve or a past problem with rheumatic fever, of if your previous physicians have ever recommended that you take an antibiotic before any procedure, including dental work.
5. You should eat a light breakfast or lunch on the day of surgery; fasting is not required.

Figure 2–10. Preoperative surgical instructions.

1. Remove the bandage in 24 hours.
2. After bandage removal, cleanse the wound, using 3% hydrogen peroxide with cotton-tipped applicators, morning and night. The bubbling action helps remove debris from the wound.
3. Dry the wound with a clean cotton-tipped applicator.
4. First apply a thin film of an antibiotic ointment.
5. Then apply a new clean dressing over the wound.
6. Continue this care until new skin completely covers the treatment site.
7. It is important that the wound be kept dry for the first 24 hours. After that, you may take a short shower, but be sure to change the dressing immediately afterward. No swimming is permissible unless your doctor specifies otherwise.
8. Acetaminophen is the only medicine that is safe to take for pain after surgery.
9. If you have any problems or questions during the working day, call our office at (_____)_____ . After hours, weekends, or holidays, call (_____)_____ .
10. Please return as requested for wound recheck on the following date: _____ at _____ .

Figure 2–11. Postoperative care of the surgical site.

1. The area will be slightly numb for about 30 minutes after the injection of the local anesthetic.
2. The site should be kept dry for the next 24 hours.
3. The stitches must remain in place for 5 to 7 days at which time you should return for stitch removal.
4. Twice a day, remove the Band-Aid and cleanse the stitches with hydrogen peroxide and cotton-tipped applicators. Do not rub the area, but rather roll the peroxide-soaked applicators over the stitches to gently remove any crust or debris.
5. Apply a small amount of antibiotic ointment to the area and reapply a new Band-Aid.
6. Prolonged soaking of the stitches in water should be avoided, but a brief cleansing is permissible after the first 24 hours.
7. If redness, swelling, or pain develops at the biopsy area, please call and report this as soon as you notice a change.

Figure 2–12. Treatment care after skin biopsy.

General Instructions:

Immediately after treatment, for the first 24 hours:

- Avoid prolonged standing or sitting
- Elevate legs while seated as much as possible

For 24 to 48 hours:

- Avoid strenuous activity: heavy lifting, running, vigorous aerobics, jumping rope
- Avoid hot baths or hot tubs or spas
- Avoid wearing tight or constricting clothing
- The ideal types of activities include walking, bike riding, and low-impact aerobics.

Specific Treatment Site Care:

- Remove the dressings after 24 hours.
- You can expect maximal fading after 2 to 3 weeks, but some blood vessels may require up to 3 months to improve.
- You may notice some dark lines or streaks at the treatment site over the blood vessels. This is only temporary and should fade over several months.
- If you notice one of the following: scabs, blisters, ulcers, swelling, or excessive tenderness at any injection site, please call and inform us.
- In some cases you may be required to purchase and wear specially fitted support stockings. These must be worn for the first 48 hours and as much as possible for the next 3 weeks to ensure the best results; however, opaque hose can be worn over these to camouflage them.

Our telephone number is (_____)_____ .

Figure 2–13. Treatment care after sclerotherapy.

1. Keep the treatment site dry for 24 hours after treatment.
2. After 24 hours, soak the dressing in hydrogen peroxide before removal to loosen it from the wound.
3. Clean the wound with hydrogen peroxide at least once a day. Peroxide is best applied with a saturated cotton-tipped swab rubbed gently over the area to remove any residual antibiotic ointment or debris.
4. After cleaning the wound, apply antibiotic ointment and cover the wound with a clean dressing.
5. If you have any discomfort, acetaminophen is best for controlling the pain. Do not take aspirin or aspirin-containing medications for at least 1 week.
6. Do not use any cosmetics or cream on the treatment site until the scab has fallen off and the skin has healed completely.
7. Avoid sunlight exposure or use a sunscreen with an SPF of at least 15 for 6 to 8 weeks after the treatment site has healed.

If you have any questions or problems, please call our office during working hours Monday to Friday at (_____)_____ .

Figure 2–14. Carbon dioxide laser: postoperative instructions.

1. Expect a sunburn-like reaction with possible blister formation at the treatment site within the first 24 to 48 hours. Pain is usually minimal and can be relieved by applying cool tap water compresses or using acetaminophen tablets.
2. A crust or scab may form after the initial reaction and may last 7 to 14 days. It is essential that you *do not pick off the scab or crust.*
3. Keep the area clean and dry until the crust or scab comes off. This can be accomplished by gently washing with soap and water and applying a thin layer of an antibiotic ointment.
4. Once the scab or crust has come off, the area may appear pale and may look slightly depressed or indented. The area may also turn red after several weeks. This redness will gradually fade over the next several months.
5. Avoid direct sunlight or sun exposure to the treated site for 3 to 6 months. This can be accomplished by using sunscreens of SPF 15 or greater and wearing protective clothing to cover the area. Sunlight exposure can result in spotty repigmentation at the treated areas, which may be permanent or take months to fade.
6. It is important to be patient; it may take up to 3 months to evaluate the response to the laser treatment.
7. If you have any problems or further questions, call (_____)_____ . The doctor will return your call as soon as possible.

Figure 2–15. Visible light laser: postoperative instructions.

Follow-Up

Routine repeat examination of all patients after cutaneous surgery is imperative but is especially important when dealing with certain types of malignancies. As part of the consent process, many physicians make their patients sign a form confirming that they have been informed of the importance of seeking follow-up care at specified intervals. Normally, these examinations are performed at 1, 3, and 6 months postoperatively and yearly thereafter. Patients with some types of malignant melanoma may require routine CT scans, chest radiography, and laboratory evaluation as well as physical examination every 6 months for the rest of their lives, along with timely biopsy of any new or suspicious lesions at each visit.

Use of Computers in Initial Patient Evaluation

Computers can greatly assist a successful patient encounter (see Chap. 22). With appropriate software and networking of personal computers, all cutaneous surgeons have the ability to customize their system to meet their individual practice needs. This system should allow entry of all the patient information and make it possible to sort or recall groups of patients according to their diagnosis or procedure. By having a computer terminal in several different locations in the outpatient cutaneous surgical facility, patients' diagnoses, procedure, and operative notes can be entered into the central medical record so that it can be completed before they leave the office. This ensures that all the information is correct and helps eliminate the accumulation of medical records and charts awaiting dictation, typing, sorting, or mailing. With appropriate computer technology, all the day's work can usually be efficiently processed the same day. One additional benefit of computerization is that all the patient's personal and medical information can be taken from the computer at a subsequent visit in the event of a misplaced chart. A computer that can also be used to help identify patients according to diagnosis allows the cutaneous surgeon to retroactively review previous forms of treatment or to plan potentially more effective new treatment protocols. The computer system can also help confirm missed appointments and provide consultative and follow-up letters to referring physicians.

SUMMARY

Once the cutaneous surgeon has established an effective and efficient management system to assist patients in obtaining appropriate evaluation and consultation for their medical problems, it is important to constantly re-evaluate the existing plan. Any cumbersome aspects that detract from a successful patient encounter should be dropped or significantly modified. Additions and other improvements will almost certainly be required as standards of medical practice change over time because of the development of new techniques, procedures, or equipment or because of changes in policy by insurance companies or Federal agencies. The goal should always be to provide a better setting in which to practice cutaneous surgery for the benefit of the patient. Patient information sheets should be modified or clarified whenever the situation arises so as to obtain every possible advantage in clearly communicating information to the patient. A static approach to this important aspect of a surgical practice will certainly have many negative consequences. The measuring stick that should be used in determining the success of one's efforts is the ability to provide all patients with all the information required to make an appropriate and informed decision regarding their care. Efficiency is defined as the completion of a task in an orderly manner with a minimum of wasted effort or confusion. It has little relationship to the speed or number of procedures performed on a given day. Improving the efficiency of the outpatient cutaneous surgical practice will greatly enhance the likelihood of a successful patient encounter. Factors that detract from efficiently providing the best possible patient care should be eliminated and replaced by mechanisms or procedures that allow patients to benefit maximally from the interaction.

REFERENCES

1. Leshin B, Whitaker DC, Swanson NA: An approach to patient assessment and preparation in cutaneous oncology. J Am Acad Dermatol 19:1081–1088, 1988.
2. Leshin B, McCalmont TH: Preoperative evaluation of the surgical patient. Dermatol Clin 8:787–794, 1990.
3. Gross D: On history-taking before surgery. J Dermatol Surg Oncol 7:71–72, 1981.
4. Leubke NH, Walker JA: Discussion of sensitivity to preservatives in anesthetics. J Am Dent Assoc 97:656–657, 1978.
5. Pollack SV: Systemic medications and wound healing. Int J Dermatol 21:489–496, 1982.

6. Foster CA, Aston SI: Propranolol-epinephrine interaction: a potential disaster. Plast Reconstr Surg 72:74–78, 1983.
7. Dzubow LM: The interaction between propranolol and epinephrine as observed in patients undergoing Mohs surgery. J Am Acad Dermatol 15:71–75, 1986.
8. Fisher HW: Surgery on patients receiving anticoagulants. J Dermatol Surg Oncol 3:210–212, 1977.
9. Stuart MJ, Miller ML, Davey FR, Wolk JA: The post-aspirin bleeding time: a screening test for evaluating haemostatic disorders. Br J Haematol 43:649–659, 1979.
10. Amrein PC, Ellman L, Harris WH: Aspirin-induced prolongation of bleeding time and perioperative blood loss. JAMA 245:1825–1828, 1981.
11. Sharkey I, Brughera-Jones A: Evaluation of potential bleeding problems in dermatologic surgery. J Dermatol Surg 1:41–44, 1975.
12. Salasche SJ: Acute surgical complications: cause, prevention and treatment. J Am Acad Dermatol 15:1163–1185, 1986.
13. Downs JR: Joint replacement and prophylaxis. J Am Dent Assoc 94:429, 1977.
14. Hickey AJ, MacMahon SW, Wilcken DEL: Mitral valve prolapse and bacterial endocarditis: when is antibiotic prophylaxis necessary? Am Heart J 109:431–435, 1985.
15. Wagner RF, Grande DJ, Feingold DS: Antibiotic prophylaxis against bacterial endocarditis in patients undergoing dermatologic surgery. Arch Dermatol 122:799–801, 1986.
16. Sebben JE: Electrosurgery and cardiac pacemakers. J Am Acad Dermatol 9:457–463, 1983.
17. Rees TD, Liverette DM, Guy CL: The effect of cigarette smoking on skin flap survival in the face-lift patient. Plast Reconstr Surg 73:911–915, 1984.
18. Levenson SM, Seifter E: Dysnutrition, wound healing, and resistance to infection. Clin Plast Surg 4:384–388, 1977.
19. Haley JV: Zinc sulfate and wound healing. J Surg Res 27:168–174, 1979.
20. Murray JC, Pollack SV, Pinnell SR: Keloids: a review. J Am Acad Dermatol 4:461–470, 1981.
21. Reed BR, Clark RAF: Cutaneous tissue repair: practical implications of current knowledge. J Am Acad Dermatol 13:919–941, 1985.
22. Rubenstein R, Roenigk HH Jr, Stegman SJ, Hanke CW: Atypical keloids after dermabrasion of patients taking isotretinoin. J Am Acad Dermatol 15:280–285, 1986.
23. Bernstein G: Surface landmarks for the identification of key anatomic structures of the face and neck. J Dermatol Surg Oncol 12:722–726, 1986.
24. Borges AF, Alexander JE: Relaxed skin tension lines: Z-plasties on scars and fusiform excision of lesions. Br J Plast Surg 15:242–254, 1962.
25. Courtiss EH: The placement of elective skin incisions. Plast Reconstr Surg 31:31–44, 1963.
26. Bernstein L: Incisions and excisions in elective facial surgery. Arch Otolaryngol 97:238–243, 1973.
27. Spicer TE: Techniques of facial lesion excision and closure. J Dermatol Surg Oncol 8:551–556, 1982.

CHAPTER 3

Informed Consent and Risk Management Issues in Cutaneous Surgery*

RICHARD F. WAGNER, JR.

It should come as no surprise to cutaneous surgeons that an ever-increasing number of patients have high expectations about the care they receive from their physicians. Unfortunately, many patient expectations are not initially realistic, and some are based in fantasy. Whenever these expectations are not met and patients perceive that they have been harmed, some turn to the legal system for compensation. The informed consent process is an important educational opportunity for cutaneous surgeons to help patients understand their medical problems. Better patient understanding is likely to result in more realistic patient expectations. This chapter presents information about informed consent and other principles of clinical risk management as they relate to cutaneous surgery.

Tort Law

To appreciate the doctrine of informed consent, it is necessary to understand the tort of negligence. Torts are civil wrongs that arise from a duty one person owes to another.[1] Negligence is the tort most likely to be alleged by a patient if there is an adverse medical or surgical treatment outcome. The tortfeasor is the party who is alleged to be negligent. Not all negligence results in patient injury, and not all adverse outcomes are the result of negligence.

Patients must prove four demanding legal criteria in court if they are to prevail in a medical malpractice case. One publication offers a rare and valuable insight into the difficulty faced by the plaintiff's attorney in bringing this type of case to trial.[2] This article provides worthwhile background information for all cutaneous surgeons who care for patients with malignant skin tumors.

The four defined elements of negligence are:

1. A duty and/or standard of conduct on the part of the alleged tortfeasor toward the injured party.
2. Failure to conform to that duty or standard of conduct.
3. A link showing that the failure was a "proximate cause" of the injury to the complaining party.
4. Actual loss or injury that can be measured for compensation in money damages.[1]

Expert witnesses can be employed by both parties to offer testimony about what is the standard of care. Unless this standard has been set by a previous court case or is mandated by statute, the judge or jury determines the standard of care after hearing evidence. Once this standard has been established, the court determines whether the alleged negligent act falls within or outside the standard. If the act was within the standard, by definition it was not negligent; if it was outside the standard, it is determined to be negligent. The negligent act may be one of omission or commission.

Generally, the courts take a pro-patient viewpoint when adjudicating cases in which patient care was denied for economic considerations.[3] Present-day courts seem

---

*The material herein is intended as a general presentation of medicolegal issues of interest to cutaneous surgeons in the United States. Specific legal advice should be sought from a licensed attorney in the reader's jurisdiction.

more interested in preserving a high standard of care for individual patients, in contrast to a perceived governmental desire to limit health care expenditure.[3]

The next question of fact for the fact finder is the "proximate cause." Proximate cause is a difficult legal concept to define; it revolves around the question of whether the negligent act was a cause of the patient's harm. If the negligent act is so established, the patient must prove his or her damages. Some damages are easy to demonstrate, such as the cost of subsequent related medical treatments or lost wages. Other damages such as past, present, and future pain and suffering are much more subjective. In addition, punitive damages may be awarded for public policy reasons, such as trying to discourage physicians from engaging in a particular type of practice that the court thinks is contrary to the public interest. Punitive damages are usually high because their intent is to punish the physician and set an example for others. Malpractice insurance policies generally do not include coverage against an award for punitive damages, and the physician will be held personally liable for these costs.

Informed Consent

Informed consent in the nonemergency setting is the process by which the physician explains the following to the patient, the legal guardian, or both:

1. The problem to be treated or symptoms to be diagnosed.
2. The proposed test or treatment.
3. The risks, consequences, complications, and side effects.
4. The indications for the proposed test or treatment choice.
5. The expected results or goal to be achieved by the test or treatment.
6. Reasonable available alternative methods and costs of diagnosis or treatment.
7. The consequences of doing nothing.[4]

It has been observed that many physicians fail their legal duty to patients with respect to obtaining informed consent.[4]

Recent research investigated the disclosure practices of dermatologists for simulated patients with diagnoses of dysplastic nevus syndrome, malignant melanoma, neonatal port-wine stain, and recurrent basal cell carcinoma, and found these practices quite variable.[5] One surprising finding was that although 97.9% of the respondents surveyed indicated they would discuss the treatment option of Mohs micrographic surgery for recurrent alar basal cell carcinoma, only 16.7% would tell the patient about the radiation therapy option. It is true that Mohs micrographic surgery has the highest published cure rates for recurrent basal cell carcinoma,[6] but when given the spectrum of reasonable treatment options, some patients do not elect to have surgery performed. A patient who is uninformed of the radiation therapy option and who experienced a cosmetic defor-

mity after Mohs micrographic surgery could sue the treating physician on the legal theory that informed consent had not been attempted and the patient suffered damages as a result of agreeing to the only treatment option offered.

After disclosing the reasonable treatment options to the patient, cutaneous surgeons should consider other relevant factors such as absolute or relative contraindications to the various treatment interventions. They should use their special knowledge and experience to make a treatment recommendation that is specific for each patient. Once informed consent is obtained, documentation in the medical record is absolutely essential.

Medical Record Documentation

Accurate, detailed medical record keeping is essential to any medical malpractice defense and may even persuade the plaintiff's counsel that there is little merit in the claim. This knowledge is offset by physician concern about the amount of time such a medical record takes to generate.

The use of questionnaires for new patients to complete before being interviewed and examined by the physician has the benefit of providing both the patient's written complaints and a complete patient medical history. In this way, questionnaires can provide vital information and save time for the physician. For these reasons, their use has been advocated in clinical practice.[7] A questionnaire can be mailed to all new patients who make an appointment, since it is often more convenient for the patient to complete it at home before the actual visit. Returning patients can also be asked to answer the questionnaire and bring it in at their next visit. Cutaneous surgeons are able to design additional questions for the particular types of clinical problems seen in their practices in addition to using a basic questionnaire to secure information about the patient's general health. It is important that the information provided on these forms be read by the physician before initiating treatment of the patient. A few moments spent reading the completed questionnaire will provide much important information. Critical information can be highlighted so as not to escape later notice. In a similar manner, check-off lists can also be used to document that essential information has been given to the patient.

Informed consent is usually documented in writing. Either the physician writes a clinical note in the medical record about obtaining informed consent, or a standard prepared document is properly completed and becomes a part of the medical record.

Physician Liability for Nurses and Other Ancillary Personnel

Many cutaneous surgical practices use nurses and other trained personnel to render treatment that has been ordered by the physician. In the past it was common to have nurses remove sutures, change dressings, or perform acne surgery. In some modern settings, nurses and other ancillary health care providers perform electrolysis, sclerotherapy, collagen injections, laser surgery, and other time-consuming treatments. Cutaneous surgeons report that properly trained ancillary providers can obtain clinical results comparable with those of physicians in some situations. The potential benefits of this type of practice for the cutaneous surgeon and patient are easy to recognize. By the use of nurses or other physician extenders in this manner, more patients may be treated and the costs of treatment may be reduced. From a business viewpoint, this practice can also serve as a powerful economic incentive for physicians. However, there are some risks associated with this approach that should be carefully analyzed before adopting it as a practice pattern.

When a nurse or physician extender performs direct patient care under the supervision of a physician, the law usually recognizes the employee as the agent of the physician. A physician becomes legally responsible for the negligent acts of his or her agent under the doctrine of respondeat superior. When a nonphysician performs a procedure that is ordinarily performed by a physician and there is a poor outcome such as scarring, infection, hypopigmentation, or hyperpigmentation, it is not infrequent for the patient, family members, and other health care professionals to scrutinize the events and look for possible negligent behavior on the part of the treating employee and physician. Such scrutiny is often gratuitously provided by local competitors in the same or different surgical specialties who take a dim view of nonphysician patient therapy. If negligence is proved, the physician can be economically responsible for all monetary awards. A physician who decides to have nonphysician employees treat patients must make sure that the employees are well trained for the procedure and have adequate supervision.

The informed consent process should disclose to the patient who will be the person rendering treatment. A court case from New York has instructed physicians that an appropriate physical examination is necessary before they may delegate treatment to a nonphysician employee.[8] In this case a patient brought a medical malpractice action against physicians and a nurse.[8] In brief summary, the patient began receiving treatment for androgenic alopecia in January 1980. A secondary diagnosis of acne was made at that time. The patient alleged that in January 1981 a nurse, following a doctor's order, ". . . negligently performed an incision and drainage of three acne cysts and removal of blackheads on plaintiff's face causing the formation of three disfiguring, permanent depressed scars."[8] The appeals court found

There was consistent, authoritative testimony by medical experts that it was a breach of defendant's professional duty for [the nurse] . . . to be directed to perform the incision and drainage procedure when the condition being treated had not been carefully examined or diagnosed by a physician. Prescribing

treatment, particularly invasive treatment, for a condition which the physician had only noted in passing one year earlier but never previously examined or treated (and which the physician did not even view on the day of treatment) would appear to be a fundamental and serious breach of the physician's duty to exercise ordinary, reasonable care in treating his patients.[8]

The importance of this case rests with the legal analysis of a physician's affirmative duty to examine a patient before ordering invasive procedures that will not be performed by the physician. The tendency of physicians to delegate invasive procedures to nonphysicians may be tempting under some circumstances, but when this practice is used it should always be within these standards of care.

Genetic Disorders and the Cutaneous Surgeon

Cutaneous surgeons frequently treat patients with neurofibromatosis, basal cell nevus syndrome, and other genetic diseases associated with cutaneous tumors or pigmentary changes. These patients may have no knowledge about the genetic basis of their disease. Since the cutaneous surgeon may be the first to establish the genetic nature of the disease, physicians must not overlook their responsibility to disclose the hereditary nature of the condition to the patient. Because such information can have a profound effect on a patient's life, it is not surprising that the failure of a physician to reveal such information may result in a negligence lawsuit if the patient should procreate similarly afflicted children.

Wrongful birth lawsuits are often brought by the child's parents when a physician fails to provide adequate genetic counseling. This includes failing to tell a pregnant patient that a prenatal test for a suspected genetic disease is available. In a wrongful birth cause of action, the parents argue that had they been properly informed about the risk of passing a genetic disease to their child, they would have used effective birth control methods or abortion to prevent birth. If the parents are legally successful, they may be awarded the future costs of the child's medical care and compensation for pain and suffering. Damages have the potential to be astronomical.

When the parents bring a lawsuit on behalf of an afflicted child, this type of action is termed wrongful life. The idea behind this type of lawsuit is that the child's nonexistence would have been preferable to being born with the genetic disease. If the lawsuit is successful, damages are awarded to the child.

Little is known about the clinical practice of cutaneous surgeons regarding genetic counseling. A previous study found that only 39.6% of respondents would advise genetic counseling in a case presentation of the dysplastic nevus syndrome.[5] However, this same group of dermatologists overwhelmingly recommended follow-up of blood relatives (91.7%). Perhaps many dermatologists have not yet considered the issues of wrongful birth or wrongful life. The author is unaware of any wrongful birth or wrongful life cases stemming from the dysplastic nevus syndrome. It is a common experience to find that most patients who are offered genetic counseling for this condition refuse it on the basis that if their child is found to have this condition, it is relatively easy to manage. Nonetheless, the availability of genetic counseling is routinely communicated to patients with dysplastic nevus syndrome who seek consultation at the University of Texas Medical Branch pigmented lesion clinic.

Types of Medical Malpractice Insurance

The two basic kinds of medical malpractice insurance policies available to physicians are the claims-made and occurrence types. Both types of insurance coverage are usually available on an annual basis. Claims-made policies cover only claims made during the term the insurance plan is in effect, regardless as to when the incident actually occurred.[9] This type of insurance is generally less expensive. However, should the physician ever decide to cancel future insurance coverage and yet wish to remain insured against events that arose years previously, purchase of additional insurance, known as tail coverage or an extended reporting endorsement, is necessary. In contrast to a claims-made policy, an occurrence coverage policy " . . . insures against all incidents which occurred during the term of the (annual) policy, no matter how many years later they are first reported."[9]

Unapproved Drugs

Many dermatologic surgeons use or desire to use medicines for individual patient care that are not approved by the U.S. Food and Drug Administration (FDA). Special precautions are prudent when this is attempted. The following comments have been made to physicians who engage in this type of practice:[10]

1. Do not try to conceal the true nature of the drug when importing it into the United States.
2. Use the product only for the treatment of individual patients and not with the intent of doing research.
3. Obey any directives received from the U.S. FDA or U.S. Customs Service and settle any dispute with these agencies in the courts.
4. Obtain informed consent, referring to the therapy as "innovative" to distinguish it from "experimental" or "research" types of treatment.
5. Make a good faith effort to be aware of all the material facts.
6. Use the drug only if you are convinced that the benefits outweigh the risks.
7. Continue to carefully review the literature while

using the therapy and be ever vigilant to any factor that may change the risk:benefit ratio.

Approved Drugs for Unapproved Purposes

When approved medicines are used for a novel purpose, care must be taken that the patient is informed about the innovative nature of the treatment and of the known potential foreseeable risks.[10] Since the drug is being used for unapproved purposes, the patient must also be advised of the theoretical risk of unknown complications. It is important to remember that the risk:benefit analysis of a drug may change according to its potential use.[10]

Patient and Staff Risk of Iatrogenic Infection During Treatment

Some common cutaneous surgical procedures have come under scrutiny because of the risk of infection to patients and staff. The infection risks to patients of improper cryotherapy,[11] electrosurgery,[12] Med-E-Jet use[13] (Med-E-Jet Corp., Cleveland, OH), and injection technique[14] are now recognized. All known risks to patients and staff need to be reduced whenever possible. Potential risks to patient and staff from laser plumes,[15] electrocoagulation,[16] and dermabrasion aerosols[17] have also been the focus of attention in the literature. Further research is needed to determine if these potential hazards pose more than a theoretical risk.

Disclosure of Risks to Obtain Informed Consent

Some risks of cutaneous surgery are common to diverse procedures performed by cutaneous surgeons. Examples include pain; bleeding; infection; abnormal scarring such as in hypertrophic scars and keloids; poor wound healing; nerve damage resulting in permanent or temporary paralysis, loss of sensation, or both; postinflammatory hyperpigmentation and hypopigmentation; risks of local anesthesia, including anaphylaxis and death; a worsened or unsatisfactory appearance; a false-positive or false-negative biopsy leading to inappropriate treatment or nontreatment; complete or partial loss of a skin graft or skin flap; and recurrence of the original condition.

If the patient is at risk for any of these complications, they should be listed and disclosed. If there is no risk of a specific complication, it need not be disclosed. For example, the risk of local anesthesia need not be discussed when the patient will not receive it for cryosurgery of actinic keratoses. However, several caveats are in order for this analysis. First, disclosure of an uncommon risk is necessary if a patient's underlying medical condition may increase the risk of specific complications that are routinely disclosed (e.g., a patient with diabetes mellitus who has an increased risk of a postoperative wound infection). For this reason, a careful preoperative evaluation and a sound clinical knowledge base are required to gain the clinical information necessary to advise specific patients of their increased risks of complications. In addition, an underlying medical condition may predispose a patient to an unusual specific complication. An example of this is malignant otitis externa after ear surgery for a patient with underlying diabetes mellitus. In such cases it is prudent to individualize the patient's informed consent so that the increased risks due to the underlying medical conditions are understood and accepted by the patient, the legal guardian, or both before the procedure is undertaken.

The Unhappy Postsurgical Patient

A careful preoperative evaluation and consultation often remains the best insurance available for preventing a patient from having a negative experience while under a physician's care. In 1976 it was proposed that in order to practice the best possible medicine and prevent malpractice suits, the physician should be "competent, careful, candid, and concerned."[18] The importance of these four factors cannot be overemphasized and has been expanded on in greater detail.[19]

It has been observed that if a disclosed potential complication arises subsequent to a procedure, the patient is likely to cooperate with the treating physician and take corrective steps. However, if the complication is a surprise to the patient, the physician's explanation may sound like an excuse.[19]

Most of the time it comes as no surprise to the involved physician that a medical malpractice action has been initiated by an unhappy postsurgical patient. Often the first step in such a medical malpractice action is investigation by the opposing attorney. Either the patient or the patient's attorney will request a copy of the complete medical record. The opposing attorney will often hire an outside physician to review the medical record and look for evidence of negligence. By means of a thoroughly documented medical record, the defending physician has the opportunity to persuade the outside physician that the patient received quality care and that there was no negligence. When the expert witness reports this finding, the opposing attorney may realize that the suit is unlikely to be won because the patient's legal case is weak. Attorneys do not ordinarily accept medical malpractice suits on a contingency basis if there is little chance of winning or settling the claim. In addition, if the attorney estimates that the monetary damages will probably be low, he or she may not accept the case owing to the high cost of litigation.

If a poor result occurs despite delivery of high-quality patient care, a well-documented medical record may stop a medical malpractice claim. However, a poorly documented or incomplete medical record will almost invite a legal action because it may lead the plaintiff's attorney and the reviewing outside physician to suspect that negligence has occurred.

If the attorney decides to accept the medical malpractice case, the physician will receive written notification of the suit. Most medical malpractice insurance companies require notification of the lawsuit by the insured physician so that the claim can be thoroughly investigated and appropriately defended or settled. The involved physician should not discuss the matter with the opposing attorney or others. The physician's legal counsel will be able to provide further information and advice once legal action has been initiated.

Future Developments in Cutaneous Surgery Risk Management

In the past, little attention was paid to the concept of risk management in cutaneous surgery. However, current evidence points to a trend for increased litigation against cutaneous surgeons.[20] Continual attention to current medical and legal trends is necessary so that the cutaneous surgeon may develop effective risk management approaches for specific practice settings.

REFERENCES

1. Hoffman AC, Zimmerly JG, Seifert JB: Torts. *In* Legal Medicine: Legal Dynamics of Medical Encounters. American College of Legal Medicine. CV Mosby Company, St. Louis, 1988, pp 34–46.
2. Romano JF: The classic case of medical mismanagement: litigation of the failure to diagnose malignant disease cases. Am J Trial Advocacy 7:217–297, 1984.
3. Hirshfeld EB: Economic considerations in treatment decisions and the standard of care in medical malpractice litigation. JAMA 264:2004–2012, 1990.
4. Toth RS: Medical malpractice: physician as defendant. *In* Legal Medicine: Legal Dynamics of Medical Encounters. American College of Legal Medicine. CV Mosby, St. Louis, 1988, pp 482–492.
5. Shriner DL, Wagner RF Jr, Weedn VW, et al: Informed consent and risk management in dermatology: to what extent do dermatologists disclose alternate diagnostic and treatment options to their patients? J Contemp Health Law Policy 8:137–162, 1992.
6. Rowe DE, Carroll RJ, Day CL: Mohs surgery is the treatment of choice for recurrent (previously treated) basal cell carcinoma. J Dermatol Surg Oncol 15:424–431, 1989.
7. Richards RN: Specific questionnaires in medical practice: review of a 12 year experience. J Am Acad Dermatol 10:531–538, 1984.
8. 543 N.Y.S. 2d 242.
9. Gibbs RF, Moore RW: Insurance. *In* Legal Medicine: Legal Dynamics of Medical Encounters. American College of Legal Medicine. CV Mosby, St. Louis, 1988, pp 128–160.
10. Legalities important in the use, importation of unapproved drugs. Interview between Abel Torres, M.D. and Ronald Wheeland, M.D. Dermatology Times 11:40–44, 1990.
11. Jones SK, Darvile JM: Transmission of virus particles by cryotherapy and multi-use caustic pencils: a problem to dermatologists. Br J Dermatol 121:481–486, 1989.
12. Sherertz EF, Davis GL, Rice RW, et al: Transfer of hepatitis B virus by contaminated reusable needle electrodes after electrodes-

iccation in simulated use. J Am Acad Dermatol 125:212–215, 1986.

13. Hepatitis B associated with jet gun injection. MMWR 35:373–376, 1986.

14. Plott RT, Wagner RF Jr, Tyring SK: Iatrogenic contamination of multidose vials in simulated use: a reassessment of current patient injection techique. Arch Dermatol 126:1441–1444, 1990.

15. Garden JM, O'Banion MK, Shelnitz LS, et al: Papillomavirus in the vapor of carbon dioxide laser–treated verrucae. JAMA 259:1199–1202, 1988.

16. Sawchuk WS, Weber PJ, Lowy DR, et al: Infectious papillomavirus in the vapor of warts treated with carbon dioxide laser or electrocoagulation: detection and protection. J Am Acad Dermatol 21:41–49, 1989.

17. Wentzell JM, Robinson JK, Wentzell JM Jr: Physical properties of aerosols produced by dermabrasion. Arch Dermatol 125:1637–1643, 1989.

18. Dick L: Perspectives in malpractice. J Dermatol Surg 2:45–48, 1976.

19. Coleman WP, Guice WL III: Office surgery and the law. Adv Dermatol 2:202–229, 1987.

20. Hollabaugh ES, Wagner RF Jr, Weedn VW, et al: Patient personal injury litigation against dermatology residency programs in the United States, 1964–1988: implications for future risk management programs in dermatology and dermatologic surgery. Arch Dermatol 126:618–622, 1990.

Microanatomy, Structure, and Function of the Skin

DAVID J. LEFFELL and MACK RACHAL

The skin is the largest organ system of the body. It is also the most exposed to the external environment and at the greatest risk for trauma. As a consequence, its reparative powers are of paramount importance. The remarkable healing potential of the skin is largely determined by its gross and microscopic anatomy and its unique physiology. In the average 75-kg man, the skin weighs 2 kg and covers 1.8 m^2.[1] The combination of the epithelial lining (epidermis), connective tissue matrix (dermis), and appendages (hair, nails, and sebaceous and various sweat glands) allows rapid and thorough healing of the skin when external assaults violate its integrity. Through its multilayer organization the skin maintains water equilibrium and protects against ultraviolet radiation damage and invasion by foreign agents. Additional functions of the integument include immunologic surveillance, thermal regulation, excretion, sensation (heat, cold, pressure, and pain), and endocrine activities.[2-5] This review of the anatomic and physiologic bases of these functions focuses on the epidermis, dermis, and dermal-epidermal junction, with special reference to those aspects of structure and function that relate directly to wound healing.

The Epidermis

The outermost layer of the skin, the epidermis, is a continuous, self-regenerating layer of stratified squamous epithelium varying in thickness from 0.04 mm on the eyelids and genitalia to 1.5 mm on the palms and soles. The individual keratinocytes are organized into several layers within the epidermis based on distinct structural features or unique functional activities of the component keratinocytes. These layers, from deep to superficial, include the stratum germinativum, stratum spinosum, stratum granulosum, and stratum corneum. Each epidermal layer represents a distinct stage of keratinization. In this complex process, new structural proteins and organelles are synthesized while existing ones are modified, resulting in a more specialized keratinocyte. This process is manifested by a flattening of cell architecture and an increase in cell size. The end stage of this process is a dead, terminally differentiated keratinocyte composed of a plasma membrane, filamentous and matrix proteins, and lipids.

The Dermis

The dermis, or corium, is crucial in wound healing. It is an intricate connective tissue network composed of collagen and elastin fibers embedded in a ground substance matrix that accommodates collections of nerve bundles, sensory receptors, lymphatic channels, and vascular elements. The connective tissue component of the dermis provides for much of the structural integrity of the skin, including the epidermis, and protects against mechanical trauma. The nerves, receptors, and vascular elements assist in sensation, water homeostasis, and temperature regulation. Cells indigenous to the dermis include fibroblasts, macrophages, and mast cells. Other cells, like lymphocytes, plasma cells, and leukocytes, migrate into the dermis in response to various stimuli and comprise part of the dynamic physiology of this continually changing environment. The dermis and epidermis are related in a very complex structural fashion at the basement membrane zone. An understanding of the structure and regenerative capacity of the epidermis, and of the detailed components of the dermis, is essential to a grasp of the complex processes of wound healing.

COMPOSITION OF THE EPIDERMIS

The stratum germinativum, or basal cell layer, is composed of a single row of columnar epithelial cells arranged with their long axes perpendicular to the dermal-epidermal junction (Fig. 4–1). These are the mitotically active, self-regenerating progenitor cells for the more superficial layers of the epidermis. Basal cells are recognized on hematoxylin and eosin (H&E) staining by their deeply basophilic cytoplasm and dark-staining elongated nucleus. They are connected to the underlying basement membrane by the specialized cell junctions, which are composed of an electron-dense plaque and associated keratin filaments, known as hemidesmosomes; and to adjacent keratinocytes by ellipsoidal junctional discs with connecting tonofilaments, known as desmosomes.[6–9]

The cytoplasm of basal cells is dense and contains many types of keratinized fibers scattered singly as tonofilaments or arranged in bundles as tonofibrils (Fig. 4–2). To date, over 20 types of keratin fibers have been identified. Most of these fibers belong to the 100-Å class of intermediate filaments and serve a structural role.[10] Other cytoskeletal elements include the microfilaments actin, alpha-actinin, and myosin as well as the microtubules.[11] Microfilaments assist in the upward movement of differentiating keratinocytes and maintain epidermal architecture.[12] Also present within the cytoplasm are ribosomes, mitochondria, lysosomes, rough endoplasmic recticulum, Golgi apparatus, and variable numbers of melanosomes that contain membrane-bound melanin.[13]

The basal keratinocytes are active stem cells that proliferate heterogeneously. The stratum germinativum maintains homeostasis by balancing proliferating (S phase) and noncycling (G0, G1, and G2 phase) basal keratinocytes.[7, 14] Additional noncycling stem cells can be recruited by various stimuli to increase the total number of proliferating cells. Such factors can be elicited

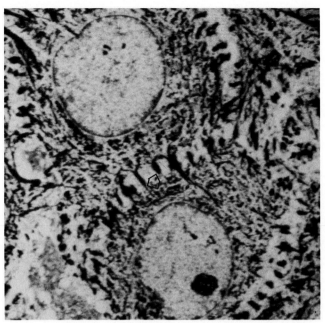

Figure 4–2. Spinous layer. Present between adjacent spinous cells are tonofilaments, visualized as electron-dense bands *(arrow)*.

by mitogens, hormones, wounding, carcinogens, or disease processes that alter normal regulatory mechanisms (Table 4–1).

Only 30 to 40% of the germinal cells are mitotically active.[15–17] Cellular synthesis of DNA takes approximately 16 hours and the average germinal cell replicates once every 19 days. Cell cycling time varies between 200 and 400 hours.[16] These actively cycling cells generate committed keratinocytes that differentiate into the stratum spinosum and stratum granulosum. Eventually, postmitotic cells emerge and give rise to the stratum corneum. The normal transit time between the stratum germinatum and stratum corneum is 40 to 56 days. Since an additional 14 days is required for corneocyte desquamation,[17] the total epidermal renewal time varies from 58 to 74 days.

The transit time from basal cell to corneocyte varies greatly among individual cells. Keratinocyte migration is a function of cell surface structures, extracellular microfilaments, and packing of epidermal keratinocytes. For example, intercellular connections temporarily dissolve and reform, allowing cells to alter both their size and shape. Movement occurs as individual cells alter their shape and slide along intercalated surfaces, assisted by contracting microfilaments.[2, 18, 19] In this manner,

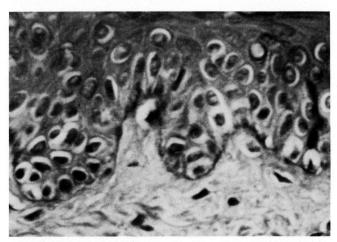

Figure 4–1. Normal epidermis (palm). Three layers of the epidermis are evident as (1) stratum basale, (2) stratum spinosum, and (3) stratum granulosum.

TABLE 4–1. **FACTORS INFLUENCING EPIDERMAL PROLIFERATION**

Extrinsic Factors	Intrinsic Factors
Epidermal growth factor (EGF)	Prostaglandins
Estrogen	Epidermal chalones
Progesterone	Cyclic nucleotides
Epinephrine	
Vitamin A	

differentiating keratinocytes can migrate toward the epidermal surface. Similarly, nonkeratinocytes in the epidermis can insert between two adjacent squamous cells.

STRUCTURE OF THE EPIDERMIS

Stratum Spinosum

The cells of the stratum spinosum have spinelike projections that protrude from the cytoplasm (see Fig. 4–1). These spinous processes result from shrinkage artifact[3] and appear where the plasma membrane attaches to desmosomes (see Fig. 4–2). Interestingly, morphologic differences exist between the layers of keratinocytes composing the spinous layer and correlate with progressive stages of keratinization. The cells of the lower spinous layer are more polyhedral and possess round nuclei, whereas the cells of the upper spinous layer are larger[20] and have elongated nuclei (see Fig. 4–1).

In addition to retaining the normal complement of housekeeping organelles, spinous keratinocytes feature a potent lysosomal system. This system probably allows the epidermis to eliminate foreign materials as they are degraded in lysosomal vesicles by acid hydrolyses and other enzymes. In contrast, nondigestible materials are enclosed in vacuoles that are transported to the stratum corneum and desquamated.[21–23] These epidermal elimination processes are probably important in the complex process of wound healing.

Stratum Granulosum

The stratum granulosum consists of the one to two layers of flattened cells immediately beneath the stratum corneum (Fig. 4–3). The component keratinocytes in this layer are noted for some characteristic basophilic granules in the cytoplasm. These granules are composed of keratohyalin, a high-molecular-weight, histidine-rich protein precursor of filaggrin.[24] Filaggrin acts as glue that cements the intercellular filaments of adjacent keratinocytes.[2, 3] Conversion of keratohyalin into filaggrin occurs during keratinocyte differentiation and plays a major role in stabilizing the epidermal structure by promoting aggregation of keratin filaments.[25] Processes that affect granule formation can have profound effects on epidermal structure. For example, in ichthyosis vulgaris, a defect exists in the production of keratohyalin granules, which alters the amount of filaggrin synthesized. An absent granular layer results in hyperkeratosis and psoriasiform changes in the skin.[26]

Two other proteins are also found in the granular keratinocytes. These include keratin filaments of 60,000 to 70,000 MW, and involucrum, a cysteine-rich protein that forms the corneocyte envelope. In addition, the lamellar granules are found at the interface of the stratum granulosum and stratum corneum, and first aggregate and then fuse with the outer cell membrane.[27, 28] Ultimately, these granules exocytose their components into the intercellular space where acid phosphatases and other enzymes partially degrade the granular cells.[29] Also, the protein and lipid contents of the granules help to create the unique barrier properties of the stratum corneum. In this way, the transition from granular cell to corneocyte requires both synthesis and modification of proteins and macromolecules that participate in autodestruction.

Stratum Corneum

The keratinocytes of the stratum corneum are characterized by their flattened, polyhedral shape and the absence of nuclei (see Fig. 4–1). High-molecular-weight keratins account for 70 to 80% of the corneocyte. The remaining balance consists of filaggrin and an uncharacterized electron-dense matrix material.[30, 31] On many light microscopic sections the lowest layer of the stratum corneum appears as a thin, homogeneous eosinophilic rim (see Fig. 4–3). This zone is referred to as the stratum conjunctivum; it is more pronounced in areas where the epidermis is thickest, such as the palms and soles.[20] The stratum lucidum differs from the rest of the stratum corneum in that its cells have Odland bodies that contain large amounts of protein-bound lipids.[32]

The cells of the stratum corneum are arranged in orderly, stacked columns. This stacking probably represents a specific type of intrinsic organization related to epidermal thickness, epidermal proliferation rates, and systematic cell movement during differentiation. Cell stacking may create a pattern for ordered desquamation at 14 days and may help prevent transepidermal water loss.[33, 34]

SPECIALIZED EPIDERMAL DENDRITIC CELLS

Melanocytes

There are three types of dendritic cells within the epidermis: melanocytes, Langerhans cells, and indeterminate cells. All are involved in wound healing at one stage or another. Melanocytes and Langerhans cells can be visualized on routine microscopic sections, but indeterminate cells are identifiable only on electron microscopy. With routine staining (Fig. 4–4), melanocytes appear to have clear cytoplasm and dark-staining nuclei, which are the result of shrinkage artifact. These pigment-producing cells are derived from the neural crest and are typically found in the basal layer between

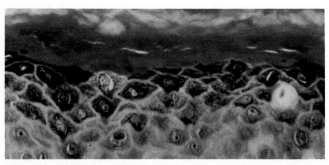

Figure 4–3. Normal epidermis (palms). The stratum granulosum and stratum corneum are highlighted by basophilic granules in cytoplasm.

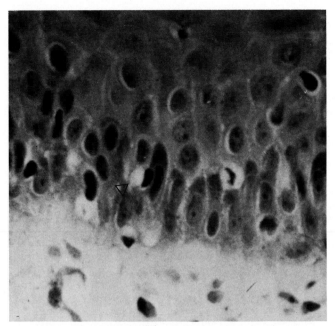

Figure 4–4. Melanocytes. Present between the basal keratinocytes are cells with clear cytoplasm and small, dark nuclei *(arrowhead)*. These are the pigment-producing melanocytes.

TABLE 4–2. STAGES OF MELANOSOME FORMATION

Stage 1
   a. 0.3-μ round vesicles containing enzymatic machinery necessary for pigment formation
   b. No detectable melanin
Stage 2
   a. 0.5-μ ellipsoid vesicles containing cross-linked longitudinal filaments
   b. Positive tyrosinase activity detected
   c. Melanin deposition on cross-linked filaments
Stage 3
   a. 0.5-μ ellipsoid vesicles
   b. Decreased tyrosinase activity
   c. Continued melanin deposition
Stage 4
   a. 0.50-μ ellipsoid vesicles
   b. No detectable tyrosinase activity
   c. Melanin completely fills vesicle and obscures internal structure

adjacent keratinocytes. Although the ratio of melanocytes to basal keratinocytes is 1:10 in vertical sections, the actual numbers of melanocytes vary with body region and ultraviolet light (UVL) exposure.[35, 36] The density of melanocytes is greatest on the face and male genitalia at approximately 2000/mm^2 and lowest on the trunk at approximately 800/mm^2. While melanocyte density is similar for white and black skin,[37] the pigmentary variation between races is due to quantitative and qualitative differences in the pigment-containing granules or melanosomes present rather than the absolute number of melanocytes.

In response to a single UVL exposure stimulus, melanocytes increase their size and functional activity.[38] Repeated UVL exposure, however, results in an increased number of melanocytes.[39] Melanogenesis itself is a complex biochemical process. An amino acid, L-tyrosine, is first converted to dihydroxyphenylalanine (dopa) and then oxidized to dopaquinone by the enzyme L-tyrosinase. In turn, dopaquinone is converted to eumelanin, mixed-type melanins, or pheomelanins, depending on the pathway used.[40, 41] Pheomelanin has a high content of sulfur compared with eumelanin, which is best characterized as a polymer of several types of pigment monomers. Melanin formation occurs within organelles called melanosomes (Table 4–2). These are membrane-bound vesicles containing structural proteins and enzymes necessary for pigment production. Melanosomes evolve[42, 43] from the spherical membrane-bound stage I vesicles containing no melanin to the melanin-filled stage IV vesicles devoid of internal structure (Fig. 4–5).

The transfer of melanosomes to keratinocytes and hair cortex cells is an active process requiring phagocytosis. On electron microscopy it appears that cytoplasmic projections of the receptor cells engulf and then pinch off the dendritic tips of melanocytes that contain numerous melanosomes. As the engulfed membrane is broken down, the melanosomes disperse into the cytoplasm.[44, 45]

Langerhans Cells

Langerhans cells appear on routine histologic staining as clear cells. They occur in the suprabasal, granular, and spinous layers of the epidermis and account for 2 to 4% of the total epidermal cell population. Their density varies between 400 and 1000 cells/mm^2.[46, 47] One organelle unique to the Langerhans cell is the Birbeck granule, also known as the Langerhans granule.[48] These granules participate in receptor-mediated endocytosis and have the characteristic appearance of a tennis racket (Fig. 4–6), which is derived from an invagination of the plasma membrane. Langerhans cells are derived from the bone marrow and express a variety of surface immunologic molecules and receptors, including HLA-Dr and Ia antigens and Fc and C3 receptors.[49–51] Langerhans cells play a critical role in the processing and

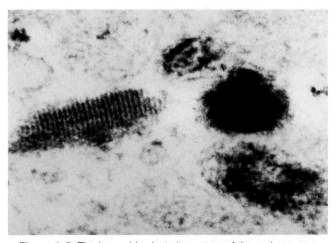

Figure 4–5. The internal laminated structure of the melanosome.

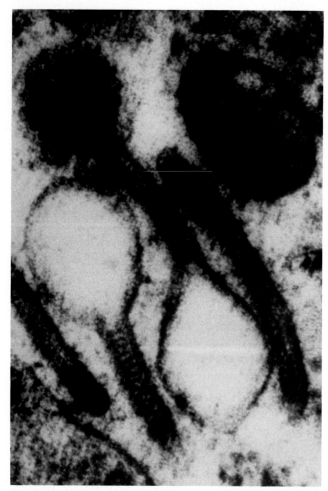

Figure 4–6. Langerhans granules. The characteristic "tennis racket" appearance of the Langerhans granules.

presentation of specific antigens to cutaneous T lymphocytes residing in the skin. They may also participate in a variety of disease processes such as allergic and contact dermatitis, cutaneous T-cell lymphoma, and graft-versus-host disease.[47]

Indeterminate Cells

A third type of epidermal dendritic cell is the indeterminate cell. Although morphologically similar to Langerhans cells, these are recognized only by electron microscopy because of the absence of Langerhans granules, and by staining with the monoclonal antibody OKT6.[52]

EPIDERMAL APPENDAGES

Hair

The hair follicle unit probably initially developed as a sensory organ. In warm-blooded animals thermal insulation remains the major function of hair. Additional functions include protection against environmental elements, pheromone dissemination, and sex delineation. Although no critical function can be ascribed to hair in

humans, scalp and body hair plays major social and sexual roles.[1-4] Hair follicles develop through interactions between the epidermis and dermis. The hair follicle (Fig. 4–7) consists of three major components: the hair bulb, the isthmus, and the infundibulum.[1-4] The hair bulb is the region that extends from the base of the follicle to the insertion site of the arrector pili muscle. The isthmus encompasses the region between the arrector pili insertion and the entrance of the sebaceous duct. The infundibulum includes the region from the sebaceous duct entrance to the hair follicle orifice.

The follicle itself is a complicated structure (Fig. 4–7). Key elements include the dermal papillae, the hair matrix, and the hair shaft. The cellular linings, from the interior to the exterior, include the cuticle, the inner root sheath, Huxley's layer, the outer root sheath, and the vitreous layer.[1-4] The histologic appearance of the

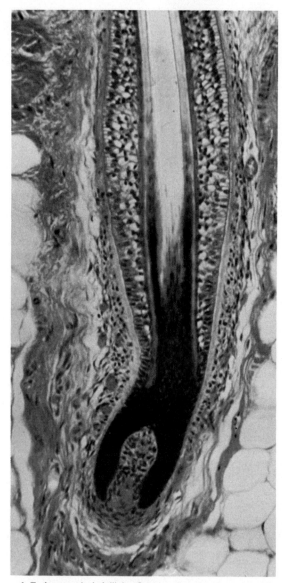

Figure 4–7. Anagen hair follicle. Surrounding the dermal papillae are the various linings of the hair bulb. From interior to exterior are the hair cuticle, the inner root sheath cuticle, the layer of Huxley, the layer of Henle, the outer root sheath, and the vitreous layer.

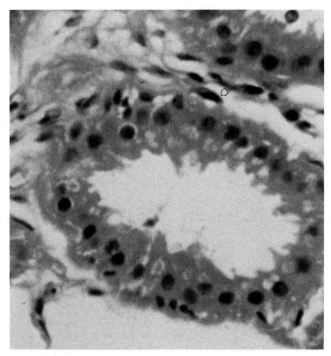

Figure 4–8. Apocrine gland, demonstrating the inner layer of secretory cells surrounded by myoepithelial cells *(arrow).*

hair follicle varies with the stage of the hair growth cycle. The anagen, or growth, phase yields to the catagen, or regression phase. The telogen, or end, phase follows just before the resumption of anagen. The anagen phase is variable and can last up to 3 years. The relatively constant catagen phase generally lasts 3 weeks; telogen, usually about 3 months. At any given time, most of the hair follicles (80 to 85%) are in anagen and the remaining follicles are in either catagen (2%) or telogen (10 to 15%).[53] The average scalp hair grows at a rate of approximately 37 mm per month.[54]

Apocrine Glands

Apocrine glands, which aid in evaporative heat loss and pheromone secretions, are found in the axillae, the anogenital area, the areolae of female breasts, and occasionally on the abdomen, face, and scalp. They consist of a secretory portion and a ductal portion with both intradermal and intraepidermal components.[55] The secretory unit is constructed of an inner single layer of secretory cells surrounded by an outer layer of myoepithelial cells (Fig. 4–8). The ductal portion is surrounded by two layers of basophilic-staining cells, with straight intradermal ducts and spiral intraepidermal ducts. The cytoplasmic secretory granules are stored on the apical surface of the secretory cells in a polar arrangement that facilitates secretion through direct partial decapitation of cytoplasm.[56]

Electron microscopy has revealed light and dark secretory granules. The dark granules are membrane bound, electron-dense vesicles that contain protein, lipid, and ferritin. Lysosomal activity is suggested by strong acid phosphatase and beta-glucuronidase reac-

tions. The light granules contain cristae and double membrane layers and are believed to originate from mitochondria.[57]

Eccrine Glands

Eccrine glands are ubiquitous on the skin except on the glans penis, inner aspect of the prepuce, nailbeds, and vermilion border of the lips. These sweat organs are most abundant in the axillae and on the palms and soles, where there are approximately $600/mm^2$. They are least numerous on the back, where there are only approximately $60/mm^2$. The average human body contains 2 to 4 million eccrine sweat glands having an excretory capacity of 10 L/day.[58] Eccrine glands permit merocrine release of a plasma ultrafiltrate in response to sympathetic stimuli. They control temperature regulation through the production of sweat, with preferential reabsorption of sodium over water. Eccrine glands allow excretion of heavy metals, organic molecules, and macromolecules.[59]

Sweat glands are structurally similar to apocrine glands. The secretory portion consists of a single layer of cells, which are either secretory or myoepithelial (Fig. 4–9). The secretory cells may be clear or dark cells. The clear cells are larger and broader at the base and contain faintly staining granules possessing large amounts of glycogen. In contrast, the dark cells are broader at the lumen and feature numerous basophilic-staining granules containing sialomucin, which is composed of neutral and nonsulfated acid mucopolysaccharides.[58] Through contraction of long fibrils, myoepithelial cells aid in the delivery of eccrine secretions.

The intradermal duct is constructed of two layers of deeply basophilic-staining cuboidal cells. The ATP-

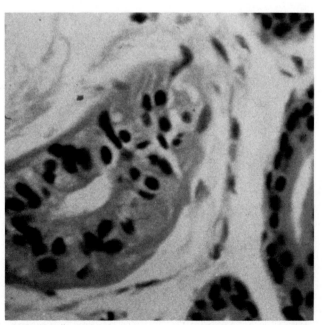

Figure 4–9. Eccrine gland, illustrating the two types of secretory cells. Dark cells are broader at the lumen and contain more granules, whereas clear cells are larger at the base.

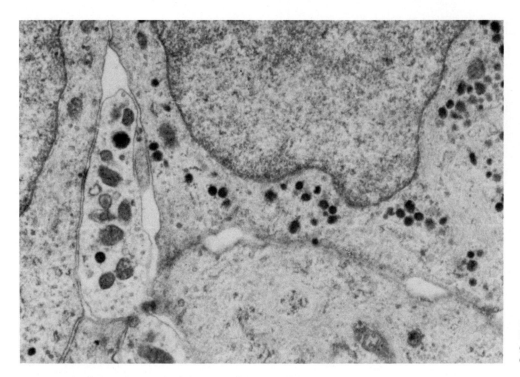

Figure 4–10. Merkel's cell. The intracytoplasmic Merkel's cell granules are evident as small, dense vesicles.

dependent preferential reabsorption of sodium and chloride over water occurs in the intradermal portion of the duct.[60] The intraepidermal duct spirals from the rete ridges to the epidermal surface, and is lined by inner layers of luminal cells surrounded by two to three layers of peripheral cells.[58] Keratinization begins at the level of the stratum granulosum.

Eccrine sweat is a mixture of water, electrolytes, macromolecules, enzymes, and inorganic substances. Nonelectrolytes include lactate, urea, ammonia, and the amino acids serine, ornithine, citrulline, and aspartic acid. In addition to water, sodium, chlorine, calcium, iodine, zinc, phosphates, sulfates, cobalt, mercury, molybdenum, and tin constitute the electrolytes and heavy metals that have been detected in human sweat.[1–4, 58, 59,] [61–64] Other macromolecules and organic substances identified in this ultrafiltrate include albumin, gamma globulin, histamine, kallikrein, and prostaglandins. The production and secretion of sweat depends on gland density, hydration status, and core body temperature.

Sebaceous Glands

Sebaceous glands occur everywhere on the skin except on the palms and soles. They are generally associated with hair follicles but may be encountered as free structures in modified skin areas such as the nipple and areola, the labia minora, and the inner aspect of the prepuce. On the lips and oral mucosa, enlarged sebaceous glands are known as Fordyce's spots. Sebaceous glands are most numerous on the face and scalp, with 400 to 900 occurring per square millimeter. Because of maternal hormones, sebaceous glands are well developed at birth. Atrophy ensues after the first few months of life until the androgens of puberty stimulate regrowth.[65, 66]

Sebaceous glands consist of one or several lobules joined by a common excretory duct lined by stratified squamous epithelium (Fig. 4–10). Each lobule bears a peripheral layer of deeply basophilic cuboidal cells, devoid of lipid droplets, which surrounds a central layer of cells containing lipid droplets composed of esterified cholesterol, squalene, phospholipids, and triglycerides.[67] Holocrine secretion occurs in which decomposing cell debris and lipid droplets are released as sebum, a skin lubricant.[68, 69]

Nerves of the Epidermis

Free nerve endings are absent in the epidermis, but intraepidermal nerve endings exist as Merkel cell–neurite complexes. These specialized epithelial cells reside just above the epidermal basement membrane and contain 100- to 200-nm thick, electron-dense, membrane-bound granules and keratin filaments that are adherent to adjacent keratinocytes (Fig. 4–11). The Merkel cells appear to sit on mitochondrium-rich, nonmyelinated axon terminals or "Merkel cell rests."[70] A neurosecretory function is suggested by neuron-specific enolase activity and synaptophysin-like immunoreactivity.[71, 72] Merkel cells may act as receptor cells that transmit stimulatory signals to the neurites through release of neuropeptides. Alternatively, they may simply provide trophic support for the neurite.

THE DERMAL-EPIDERMAL JUNCTION

Composition of the Basement Membrane Zone

The epidermis is secured to the underlying dermis by an ultrastructural array that resembles a tongue and

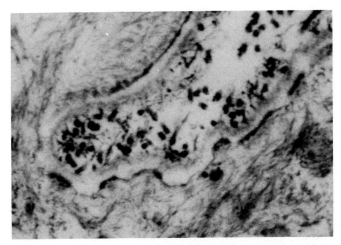

Figure 4–11. Basement membrane zone (BMZ) revealing multilayered electron-dense and lucent zones.

groove pattern. By light microscopy the basement membrane zone (BMZ) sits in the interface and appears as a thin homogeneous band (see Fig. 4–1). On electron microscopy a complex multilayer structure is obvious (Fig. 4–12). The BMZ is subdivided (Fig. 4–13) into four layers: the overlying basal cell membrane, the lamina lucida, the lamina densa, and a sublamina densa area.[73, 74] Specific BMZ macromolecules include collagen types IV, V, and VII; laminin; heparan sulfate–rich proteoglycans (BM-1); fibronectin; bullous pemphigoid antigen; cicatricial pemphigoid antigen; amidogen; and AF-1 and AF-2 antigens.[73–82]

Plasma Membrane Component of the BMZ

The plasma membrane of the basal keratinocytes, melanocytes, and Merkel cells situated along the epi-

dermal-dermal junction forms the first layer of the BMZ. Hemidesmosomes, permitting intracytoplasmic attachment, punctuate the dermal surface of these cells. Intermediate filaments (keratin) and tonofilaments extend from the hemidesmosomes, radiate toward the interior, and anchor cells to the cytoskeleton.[73, 77]

Lamina Lucida

The lamina lucida, the second layer of the BMZ, is a 20- to 40-nm thick, electron-lucent, amorphous zone. It is very complex and contains laminin, fibronectin, amidogen, and bullous pemphigoid antigen.[73, 74, 77] Laminin is a 900-kD glycoprotein that bridges basal epidermal cells and type IV collagen. It is synthesized by epithelial cells, endothelial cells, and dermal fibroblasts.[79] Nidogen is a 100- to 150-kD noncollagenous BMZ component that self-aggregates into larger units and appears strongly bound to laminin.[73, 74, 77] Bullous pemphigoid antigen (BP Ag), a 220-kD protein product of epidermal keratinocytes, is intimately associated with hemidesmosomes. BP Ag was originally defined immunologically from antibodies in the serum of patients with bullous pemphigoid.[73, 74, 77, 80] Anchoring filaments, 5 to 7 nm thick, extend vertically between the plasma membrane and the lamina densa. Other types of filaments bypass the sub-basal cell dense plaques and traverse the lamina lucida in an irregular criss-cross array.[73, 74, 77]

The Lamina Densa

The lamina densa is a 30- to 60-nm thick, electron-dense region that constitutes the third layer of the BMZ. Major structural components include type IV collagen, KF1 antigen, and heparin sulfate proteoglycans (see Fig. 4–13). Type IV collagen is a 400-kD molecule whose monomers structurally resemble hockey sticks. These

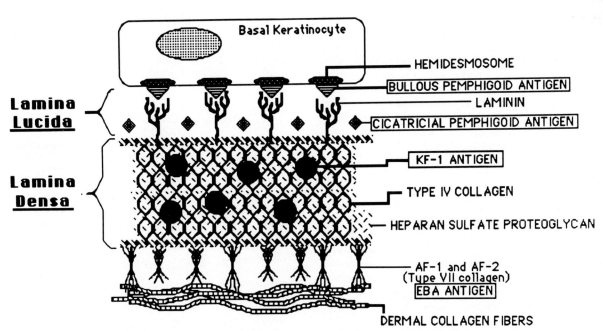

Figure 4–12. Schematic figure demonstrating the complex interconnection of BMZ components.

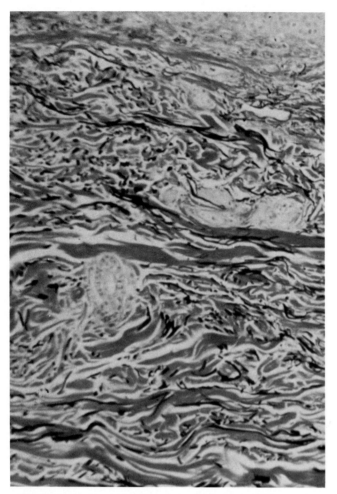

Figure 4–13. In the papillary (upper) dermis the collagen is loosely arranged, whereas in the reticular (lower) dermis the collagen is organized as large, interwoven fiber bundles.

individual monomer units align like-end to like-end to form a lattice network. Matrices of type IV collagen lack the fibrillar appearance of other collagen networks and are not degraded by skin collagenases.[73, 77, 82] The role of type IV collagen is well defined in wound healing. Extramatrix components include 120- to 750-kD species of heparin sulfate proteoglycans and KF1 antigen. Anchoring fibrils are specialized components that secure the lamina densa to the papillary dermis. These fibrils are short, curved fibrous strands that fan out biterminally and are centrally cross-banded.[72, 73, 77]

The Sublamina Densa

The deepest layer of the BMZ, or sublamina densa, contains anchoring fibrils, type VII collagen fibers, and microfibril-like elements. Here two types of fibrous structures secure the lamina densa to the underlying dermis. Anchoring fibrils composed of 20- to 60-nm thick type VII collagen fibers are the major structural connections between the dermis and epidermis.[73, 78, 82] Two immunologically indistinct molecules[73, 74, 77] within the anchoring fibrils, AF-l and AF-2 (see Fig. 4–12), have unknown structures and functions. Elastic tissues

containing oxytalan, elaunin, and mature elastin fibrils provide further support to the dermal-epidermal junction. Oxytalan fibers form a superficial lattice perpendicular to this interface and originate from a plexus of elaunin fibers in the dermis. The elaunin fibrils are connected to elastic fibers in the middle and deep dermis.[81]

In addition to its structural role, the BMZ may play a part in the differentiation and development of the epidermis. Experiments have demonstrated that in the absence of a BMZ, basal epidermal cells fail to form hemidesmosomes, and unstable binding between epidermal and dermal components results. However, reconstituted epidermis develops a high degree of differentiation independent of the presence or absence of a BMZ.[83]

COMPOSITION OF THE DERMIS

Collagen

Beneath the BMZ, collagen constitutes 75% of the dermis (Table 4–3). It is composed of three alpha-helical chains coiled into a triple helix and cross-linked. These collagen molecules are then aligned in a staggered, parallel manner to form microfibrils. Each individual alpha helix is a repeat of the monomer unit X-Y-Gly, where X and Y most commonly are represented by proline and hydroxyproline. These collagen microfibrils are assembled into bundles to form fibrils. In turn, bundles of collagen fibrils are organized into collagen fibers. In the papillary dermis (see Fig. 4–13), collagen fibers are loosely arranged and form a fine meshwork, whereas in the reticular dermis, collagen fibers are assembled into thick interwoven bundles.[82, 84, 85]

Owing to post-translational modifications and multiple genes encoding for distinct alpha chains, 20 different types of collagen representing 15 distinct gene products have been identified. Most dermal collagen (80 to 85%) is type I with a molecular weight of 290 kD. Type I collagen fibrils have a 100-nm diameter and are assembled into large, coarse fiber bundles that provide substantial tensile strength. Type III collagen fibrils make up 10 to 20% of dermal collagen and are aggregated

TABLE 4–3. **COMPARISON OF COLLAGEN AND ELASTIN**

Feature	Collagen	Elastin
Amino acid composition	1/3 are glycine	1/3 are glycine
Amino acid distribution	Every third is glycine	Random
Hydroxyproline content	10%	1%
Hydroxylysine presence	Yes	No
Glycosylated residues	Yes	No
Disulfide bonds	Yes	No
Cross-linkages	Yes	Yes
Procollagen precursor	Yes	No

into fine fiber bundles. The high content of hydroxyproline and glycine residues in type III collagen provides structural support and tissue compliance.[82, 84–86] Type IV collagen is confined primarily to the lamina densa. Its alternating collagenous and noncollagenous domains produce interruptions in the normal triple-helical structure, thereby providing flexibility.[78, 82, 84] Collagen types V, VI, and VII (anchoring fibrils) and reticulum fibers are also present in the dermis and surrounding structures. Reticulum fibers are a specialized type of thin collagen fibers (0.2 to 1.0 micron) found in sparse numbers around dermal blood vessels in association with type III collagen. Identifiable only by silver staining, they are abundant in healing tissues and in a number of pathologic states, including dermatofibromas, fibrosarcomas, and tuberculoid and sarcoid granulomas.[82, 84, 86]

Elastic Tissue

The elastic tissues in the dermis are also organized as a continuous network in a manner similar to collagen. Collagen, however, forms the dominant structural pattern, while elastic fibers surround and border the collagen bundles. Elastic fibers make up 1 to 2% of the dry weight of the skin and are distributed throughout the dermis, in the walls of cutaneous blood vessels, in the sheaths of hair follicles, and in the eccrine and apocrine glands. These fibers impart elasticity and allow tissues to return to a normal configuration after a deforming stimulus. Three types of elastic fibers are found in the dermis: mature elastic, oxytalan, and elaunin fibers. Mature elastic fibers consist of elastin and a microfibrillar protein. Elastin accounts for 85% of the mature elastic fibers. Its basic unit is tropoelastin, a soluble, electron-lucent, 72-kD protein. Tropoelastin contains 95% nonpolar amino acids rich in alanine and valine, and features various alpha-helical, large-loop, and hydrophobic domains. Desmosine and isodesmosine form covalent cross-links at 1.5 residues every 1000 amino acids that render elastin insoluble.[81, 87–90] Microfibrillar protein is a banded, electron-dense material that comprises up to 15% of the mature elastic fibers. This protein has a high content of polar amino acids and occurs as aggregations both at the periphery and within elastin fibers.[89, 90] Elastin and collagen fibers have some common properties in their composition (Table 4–3).

Oxytalan fibers are microfibrillar proteins arranged perpendicular to the dermal-epidermal interface. The microfibrillar protein and amorphous material of elaunin is arranged in a horizontal plexus that parallels the basement membrane.[87–90] Elastic fibers undergo degenerative changes as the skin ages. Specific age-induced alterations include the initial decrease and ultimate disappearance of oxytalan fibers and fragmentation of elastic fibers. Chronic UVL exposure results in hyperplasia of elastic fibers, which are histologically thicker and more tangled than the fibers seen in younger individuals. In addition, the elastic fibers assume an amorphous rather than a fibrous appearance.[81, 90]

Ground Substance

The dermal matrix consists of glycosaminoglycans and glycoproteins. This ground substance binds and stores water molecules and interacts with the filamentous proteins of the dermis. In human skin the major glycosaminoglycans are hyaluronic acid and dermatan sulfate. Various species of chondroitin sulfates are present as minor constituents.[91–93] Fibronectin is the major filamentous glycoprotein component of the dermal matrix and is produced by fibroblasts. Possessing a molecular weight of 450,000 D, fibronectin is V-shaped and features specific domains with affinities for collagen, fibrinogen, actin, heparin, heparin sulfate, DNA, and hyaluronic acid. It functions in matrix adhesion by ensheathing collagen and elastin bundles and also plays a role in the attachment of keratinocytes to the basal lamina.[93, 94] The role of fibronectin in wound healing is substantial (see Chap. 10).

STRUCTURE OF THE DERMIS

The dermis is organized into the papillary and reticular dermis. The papillary dermis (see Fig. 4–13) is the region between the BMZ and a horizontal plexus of arterioles and postcapillary venules known as the subpapillary plexus. It is composed largely of type III collagen arranged in a loose network. Type I collagen is present along the BMZ. Fibroblasts are more numerous in the papillary dermis and have an increased proliferative and synthetic capacity compared with fibroblasts of the reticular dermis. Elastic fibers in this zone are oxytalan and elaunin. The elastic tissue is primarily arranged perpendicular to the BMZ, and mature elastic fibers are generally absent. The papillary dermis and overlying epidermis are nourished by an abundance of capillary vessels.[81, 90, 95]

The reticular dermis (see Fig. 4–13) makes up the bulk of the dermis and extends from the subpapillary plexus to the hypodermis or subcutis. It is composed primarily of type I collagen fibers arranged in large interwoven fiber bundles. Mature elastic fibers surround the large collagen bundles and appear as a vast branching network. The reticular dermis is arbitrarily subdivided into three zones: the upper, intermediate, and lower reticular dermis. Collagen and elastin fibers progressively increase in size as they occur deeper in the dermis. Consequently, the upper zone of the reticular dermis, owing to the presence of intermediate-sized collagen bundles and a horizontal plexus of elastic fibers, is weakest structurally and most prone to trauma and cleavage.[81, 95]

CELLULAR COMPOSITION OF THE DERMIS

Cells indigenous to the dermis include fibroblasts, macrophages, and mast cells. While they occur in greatest number in the papillary dermis and surrounding cutaneous vasculature, they are also found in the reticular dermis. Fibroblasts are mesenchyme-derived cells that synthesize the connective tissue proteins collagen and elastin, as well as the ground substance matrix components glycosaminoglycans, glycoproteins, and fibronectin. Collagenase and gelatinase are fibroblast secretory enzymes that help degrade and remodel collagen.[1–4] Macrophages are blood-borne monocytes derived from the bone marrow that terminally differentiate after migrating into the skin. Like Langerhans cells, they express C3 and Fc receptors and HLA-Dr antigens. Macrophages phagocytose antigens, which then undergo processing by proteolytic breakdown. The resultant processed antigen fragments are presented to the helper T cells in the context of Ia surface antigens.[50, 51] Macrophages also act as effector cells. Depending on their functional capabilities, they may produce acid phosphatase, elastase, complement, interleukin-1, lysozyme, or superoxide.[96] Macrophages and fibroblasts play a central role in wound healing.

Mast cells are specialized secretory cells located most commonly around the subpapillary plexus and in the subcutaneous fat. They can be identified on routine histologic staining by their characteristic dark granules, which are both secretory and lysosomal in nature. Secretory granules contain molecular substances that induce vasodilation by slow-reacting substance of anaphylaxis (SRS-A), cause skeletal muscle contractility by histamine, and attract blood leukocytes by the release of chemotactic factors.[97] Lysosomal granules are nonsecretory in nature and contain acid hydrolases and other enzymes capable of degrading the ground substance matrix.[98, 99] Mast cells degranulate in response to light, cold, heat, trauma, vibration, pressure, and certain medications and are responsible for the immediate-type hypersensitivity skin reaction.

CELL ADHESION MOLECULES

Wound healing represents a precisely interrelated series of events that involve fibroblasts, epidermal cells, and inflammatory cells and result in the development of a mature scar. The exchange of information between these cells demands both cell-to-cell and cell-to-matrix interactions. These interactions were classically thought to be mediated by cytokines or hormones functioning in a paracrine or endocrine manner. Recent study, however, has implicated a class of molecules, designated "cell adhesion molecules" (CAMs), as the principal factors regulating cell communication. These molecules are surface proteins that can be divided into four distinct groups (integrins, immunoglobulin gene family, cadhedrins, and lectins) that interact with other cellular and matrix component molecules. These molecules play a major role in inflammatory dermatoses, the localization of neoplastic cells, and immunoregulation.[94]

Of special interest is the integrin group, which consists of heterodimers composed of an alpha and a beta subunit. The alpha subunits consist of either a single 170-kD polypeptide or a disulfide-like 20-kD light chain and a 120- to 140-kD heavy chain. Like all CAMs, integrins feature an extracellular binding domain, a transmembrane linker, and a vast intracellular domain. The intracellular domain is associated with cytoskeletal elements, and functions in signal transduction. Integrins are divided into three separate families: beta 1, 2, and 3. The beta 1 subfamily of integrins, or very late activator (VLA) integrins, currently consists of six members (VLA-1–VLA-2) and are found on keratinocytes as well as other cell types. These molecules function primarily in cell-matrix interactions. The beta 2 subfamily, or leukocyte integrins, are restricted to lymphocytes, macrophages, and monocytes. Representative family members include leukocyte function antigen (LFA-1), macrophage activation antigen (Mac-1), and p150.[95] These molecules help to regulate white cell migration, margination, opsinization, and phagocytosis, which are important in the first stages of wound repair. The beta 3 subfamily includes platelet glycoprotein IIb/IIIa, which aids in cell-to-matrix interactions.[94]

NEURAL TISSUE OF THE DERMIS

The dermis is endowed with both sensory and autonomic neural structures. The latter enervates blood vessels, arrector pili units, and apocrine and eccrine sweat glands. Sensory nerves, in addition to supplying hair follicles with fine, nonmyelinated terminal arborization, also terminate in specialized nerve-end organs known as mucocutaneous end organs, Meissner corpuscles, and Vater-Pacini corpuscles. These end organs are located at mucocutaneous junctions in the papillary dermis of the clitoris, glans penis, labia minora, perianal area, prepuce, and vermilion border of the lips.[100] These sensory units are composed of lobules that contain an array of axon terminals ensheathed by concentric lamellar processes derived from modified Schwann cells, also known as lamellar cells.

Meissner corpuscles, which mediate touch sensation, are found only in the papillary dermal tips of the palms and soles. These structures are most numerous on the hands, with their density increasing distally. On the fingertips a Meissner corpuscle is present in every fourth papilla.[101] They are composed of several layers of flattened cells arranged transversely to the long axis of the corpuscle. The corpuscles range in size from 30 to 80 microns and occupy the majority of each dermal papillae where they are located.[100, 101]

Vater-Pacini corpuscles are large, specialized nerve-end organs that mediate pressure sensation on the palms and soles, nipples, and anogenital region. They are most abundant in the tips of the fingers and toes. Vater-Pacini corpuscles[100, 102] vary in shape and are composed of a soma or body surrounded by a thick capsule with more than 30 concentric lamellar processes.

Cutaneous Circulation

The circulatory system of the skin is a complex array of subcutaneous and dermal vascular channels that supply nutrients and oxygen to both the epidermis and dermis. It also serves as an important temporary reservoir for blood and helps to regulate the core body temperature. The circulatory pathways can adapt to an ever-changing environment. Under conditions of normal hydration and internal temperature, blood flow to the skin exceeds nutritional requirements by tenfold.[2]

The circulatory system of the skin arises in the subcutaneous tissue as plexuses of small arteries and veins. Ramifying from the small arteries are bundles of arterioles that ascend into the dermis. Together with arterial and venous capillaries and postcapillary venules, these arterioles form plexuses around eccrine glands and hair follicles[103] and also in the subpapillary dermis. In addition, capillary loops derived from the horizontal subpapillary plexus supply each dermal papilla. These capillary loops are divided into intrapapillary and extrapapillary, or ascending and descending, portions. The intrapapillary and ascending extrapapillary limbs resemble arterioles because of their homogeneous basement membrane. In contrast, the extrapapillary descending limb possesses a multilayered basement membrane resembling that of veins.[104]

Ultrastructurally, the subcutaneous arteries and dermal arterioles contain a tunica intima, a tunica media, and an adventitial layer. The intima consists of endothelial cells and an internal elastic lamina. The endothelial cells express both class I and class II surface antigens, while the basement membrane contains laminin and type IV collagen. The small arteries of the subcutaneous tissue possess media composed of two or more layers of muscle cells. However, the media in arteries of the upper and lower dermis feature single and discontinuous layers of muscle cells, respectively. The adventitial layer is supported by elastic tissue and vimentin or mesenchyme-derived cytokeratin intermediate filaments.[20]

Within the reticular dermis of the palms, the soles, the fat pads and nailbeds of the fingers and toes, the ears, and the central face are specialized vascular formations known as glomus structures. The glomus is an encapsulated arteriovenous shunt that functions in temperature regulation. The arteriovenous connection is made through luminal structures 20 to 40 microns in diameter and known as Sucquet-Hoyer canals.[105] The walls of these canals are lined by a single layer of endothelial cells and possess media composed of four to six layers of large cells with clear cytoplasm, termed glomus cells. These cells are thought to represent vascular smooth muscle cells.[2, 3, 105]

Lymphatics

The dermis of human skin features lymphatic capillaries, postcapillary lymph vessels, and deep lymph vessels. On vertical histologic sections of normal skin, lymphatic capillaries are not identifiable. However, in areas of chronic lymphedema within the deep dermis, they appear as small lumina lined by endothelial cells, but lacking pericytes and a basement membrane. Both postcapillary and deep lymph vessels are located within the subcutaneous septa, between the dermis and subcutis, and in the deep dermal tissues. Postcapillary lymph vessels have wide lumina lined by occasional smooth muscle cells. A unique feature that may aid in their identification is the presence of valves lined by endothelial cells. Deep lymph vessels are similar in structure to veins and possess an internal elastic lamina, intima, and media.[2, 3, 106] Postcapillary and deep dermal vessels are identifiable only by lymphangiography. Chronic cutaneous infection and other pathologic states may adversely affect cutaneous lymphatic flow and complicate wound healing.

SUMMARY

Many of the pathologic processes that are correctable by various cutaneous surgical procedures require a complete understanding of the microanatomy of the skin to ensure a successful outcome. Knowledge of the complex mechanisms involved in wound healing, and of the important interrelationships of the structural elements of the epidermis and dermis, is also of vital importance if the cutaneous surgeon wishes to maximize the wound healing opportunities in each clinical situation.

REFERENCES

1. Farmer ER, Hood AF: Pathology of the Skin. Appleton & Lange, East Norwalk, CT, 1990, pp 3–29.
2. Fitzpatrick TB, Eisen AZ, Wolff K, et al: Dermatology in General Medicine. McGraw-Hill, New York, 1987, pp 93–455.
3. Lever WF, Schaumberg-Lever G: Histopathology of the Skin. JB Lippincott, Philadelphia, 1990, pp 1–92.
4. Arnold HL Jr, Odom RB, James WD: Andrews' Diseases of the Skin. 8th ed. WB Saunders, Philadelphia, 1990, pp 1–13.
5. Shimada S, Katz SI: The skin as an immunologic organ. Arch Pathol Lab Med 112:231–234, 1988.
6. Klein-Szarito AJP: Clear and dark cell basal cell keratinocytes in human epidermis. J Cutan Pathol 4:275–280, 1977.
7. Lavker RM, Sun TT: Epidermal stem cells. J Invest Dermatol 81:121s–127s, 1983.
8. Lavker RM, Sun TT: Heterogeneity in basal keratinocytes: morphological and functional correlations. Science 15:1239–1291, 1982.
9. Matoltsy AG: Desmosomes, filaments, and keratohyaline granules: their role in stabilization and keratinization of the epidermis. J Invest Dermatol 65:127–142, 1976.
10. Anderton B: A comprehensive catalogue of cytokeratins. Nature 301:221, 1983.
11. Bhatnager BM, Satana H: Immunofluorescent staining of myosin, actin, and alpha-actinin in normal epidermis, and cultured human epidermal cells. J Invest Dermatol 74:258, 1980.
12. Matoltsy AG: Keratinization. J Invest Dermatol 67:20–25, 1976.
13. Wolff K, Schreiner E: Trends in electron microscopy of the skin. J Invest Dermatol 67:39–57, 1976.
14. Gelfant S: Psoriasis versus cancer: adaptive versus iatrogenic human cell proliferative diseases. Int Rev Cytol 81:145–162, 1983.
15. Briggaman RA, Kelly T: Continuous thymidine labelling studies of normal human skin growth on nude mice: measurement of cycline basal cells. J Invest Dermatol 78:359, 1982.
16. Frost P, Weinstein WL, Van Scott EJ: The ichthyosiform dermatoses II. Autoradiographic studies of epidermal proliferation. J Invest Dermatol 47:561–567, 1966.
17. Halprin KM: Epidermal "turnover time": a re-examination. Br J Dermatol 86:14–19, 1972.
18. Fritsch P, Wolff K, Honigsmann H: Glycocalyx of epidermal cells in vitro. J Invest Dermatol 16:30–37, 1975.
19. Wolff K, Wolff-Schreiner EC: Ultrastructural cytochemistry of the epidermis. Int J Dermatol 16:77–102, 1977.
20. Krause WJ, Cutts JH: Concise Text of Histology. Williams & Wilkins, Baltimore, 1981, pp 213–217.
21. Wolff K, Schreiner E: Epidermal lysosomes. Electron microscopic and electron microscopic–cytochemical studies. Arch Dermatol 101:276–286, 1970.
22. Lazarus GS, Hatcher VB, Levine N: Lysosomes and the skin. J Invest Dermatol 65:259–271, 1975.
23. Wolff K, Konrad K: Phagocytosis of latex beads by epidermal keratinocytes in vivo. J Ultrastruct Res 39:262–280, 1972.
24. Lonsdale-Eccles JD, Hauger JA, Dale BA: A phosphorylated keratohyaline derived precursor of epidermal stratum corneum basic protein. J Biol Chem 255:2235–2238, 1980.
25. Christophers E: Cellular architecture of the stratum corneum. J Invest Dermatol 56:165–169, 1971.

26. Sybert VP, Dale BA, Molbrook KA: Ichthyosis vulgaris: identification of a defect in synthesis of filaggrin correlated with an absence of keratohyaline granules. J Invest Dermatol 84:191–194, 1985.

27. Green H: The keratinocyte as a differentiated cell type. Harvey Lect 74:101, 1979.

28. Elias PM: Epidermal lipids, barrier function, and desquamation. J Invest Dermatol 80:44s–49s, 1983.

29. Freinkel RK, Traczyk TN: Acid hydrolases of the epidermis: subcellular localization and relationship to cornification. J Invest Dermatol 80:441–446, 1983.

30. Dale BA: Filaggrin, the matrix protein of keratin. Am J Dermatopathol 7:65–68, 1985.

31. Tseng SCG: Correlation of specific keratins with different types of epithelial differentiation: monoclonal antibody studies. Cell 30:361–372, 1982.

32. Elias PM, Georke J, Friend DS: Mammalian epidermal barrier layer lipids: composition and influence on structure. J Invest Dermatol 69:553–546, 1977.

33. Menton DN, Eisen AZ: Structure and organization of mammalian stratum corneum. J Ultrastruct Res 35:247–264, 1971.

34. Mackenzie IC, Zimmerman K, Peterson L: The pattern of cellular organization in human epidermis. J Invest Dermatol 76:459–461, 1981.

35. Jimbow K, Quevedo WC Jr, Fitzpatrick TB, Szabo G: Some aspects of melanin biology: 1950–1975. J Invest Dermatol 67:72–89, 1976.

36. Quevedo WC, Fleischmann RD: Developmental biology of mammalian melanocytes. J Invest Dermatol 75:116–126, 1980.

37. Staricco RN, Pinkus H: Quantitative and qualitative data on the pigment cells of adult human epidermis. J Invest Dermatol 28:33–45, 1957.

38. Pathak MA, Sinesi SJ, Szabo G: The effect of a single dose of ultraviolet radiation on epidermal melanocytes. J Invest Dermatol 45:520–528, 1965.

39. Quevedo WC, Szabo G, Virks J, Sinesi SJ: Melanocytic populations in UV-radiated skin. J Invest Dermatol 45:295–298, 1965.

40. Lerner AB, Fitzpatrick TB: Biochemistry of melanin formation. Physiol Rev 30:91–126, 1950.

41. Lerner AB: On the etiology of vitiligo and gray hair. Am J Med 51:141–147, 1971.

42. Seiji M, Fitzpatrick TB, Birbeck MSC: The melanosome: a distinctive subcellular particle of mammalian melanocytes and the site of melanogenesis. J Invest Dermatol 36:243–252, 1961.

43. Szabo G, Gerald AB, Pathak MA, Fitzpatrick TB: The ultrastructure of racial color differences in man. J Invest Dermatol 54:98, 1970.

44. Cruickshank CND, Harcourt SA: Pigment donation in vitro. J Invest Dermatol 42:183–184, 1964.

45. Mottaz JH, Zelickson AS: Melanin transfer: a possible phagocytic process. J Invest Dermatol 49:605–610, 1967.

46. Wolk Basil S, Kazer AG: The Langerhans cell. Curr Probl Dermatol 4:79–145, 1972.

47. Stingl G, Tanaki K, Katz SI: Origin and function of epidermal Langerhans cells. Immunol Rev 53:149–174, 1980.

48. Hashimoto K: Langerhans cell granule: an endocytic organelle. Arch Dermatol 104:148–160, 1971.

49. Katz SI: Epidermal Langerhans cells are derived from cells originating in bone marrow. Nature 282:324–326, 1979.

50. Rowden G, Lewis MG, Sullivan AK: Epidermal Langerhans cells bear Fc and C3 receptors. Nature 268:245–248, 1971.

51. Claresky L, Tsenlund UM, Forsum M, Peterson PA: Epidermal Langerhans express Ia antigens. Nature 268:248–250, 1977.

52. Chu A, Eisinger M, Lee JS: Immunoelectron microscopic identification of Langerhans cells using a new antigenic marker. J Invest Dermatol 78:177–180, 1982.

53. Kligman AM: The human hair cycle. J Invest Dermatol 33:307–316, 1959.

54. Saitoh M, Uzuka M, Sakamato M, Koborl T: Rate of hair growth. In Montagna W, Dobson RL, eds. Advances in Biology of the Skin. Vol IX. Hair Growth. Pergamon Press, Oxford, 1969, pp 183–201.

55. Montagna W, Yun JS: The glands of Montgomery. Br J Dermatol 86:126–133, 1972.

56. Robertshaw D: Apocrine sweat glands. In Goldsmith LA, ed. Biochemistry and Physiology of the Skin. Vol I. Oxford University Press, Oxford, 1983, pp 642–653.

57. Hashimoto K, Gross BG, Lever WF: Electron microscopic study of apocrine secretion. J Invest Dermatol 46:378–390, 1966.

58. Montagna W, Chase HB, Lobitz WC Jr: Histology and cytochemistry of human skin IV. The eccrine sweat glands. J Invest Dermatol 20:415–423, 1963.

59. Sato K, Dobson RL: Regional and individual variations in the function of human eccrine sweat glands. J Invest Dermatol 54:433–439, 1970.

60. Dobson RL, Sato K: The secretion of salt and water by the eccrine sweat gland. Arch Dermatol 105:366–370, 1972.

61. Brusilow SW, Gordes EH: Ammonia secretion in sweat. Am J Physiol 214:513–517, 1967.

62. Gitlitz PH, Sunderman FW Jr, Hohnadel DC: Ion exchange chromatography of amino acids in sweat collected from healthy subjects during sauna bathing. Clin Chem 20:1305–1312, 1974.

63. Page CO, Remington JS: Immunologic studies in normal human sweat. J Lab Clin Med 69:634–650, 1961.

64. Sato K: The physiology and pharmacology of the eccrine sweat gland. In Goldsmith LA, ed. Biochemistry and Physiology of the Skin. Vol I. Pergamon Press, New York, 1983, pp 596–641.

65. Ellis RA, Henrickson RC: The ultrastructure of sebaceous glands in man. In Montagna WB, Dobson RL, eds. Advances in Biology of Skin. Vol 4. The Sebaceous Glands. Pergamon Press, New York, 1963, pp 94–109.

66. Serri F, Huber WM: The development of sebaceous glands in man. In Montagna WB, Dobson RL, eds. Advances in Biology of Skin. Vol 4. The Sebaceous Glands. Pergamon Press, New York, 1963, pp 1–18.

67. Downing DT, Strauss JS: Synthesis and composition of surface lipids in human skin. J Invest Dermatol 62:228–244, 1974.

68. Downing DT, Strauss JS: On the mechanism of sebaceous secretion. Arch Dermatol Res 272:343–349, 1982.

69. Hashimoto K: Fine structure of Merkel cell in human oral mucosa. J Invest Dermatol 58:381–387, 1972.

70. Smith KR Jr: The ultrastructure of the human Haarscheibe and Merkel cells. J Invest Dermatol 54:150–159, 1970.

71. Masuda T, Ikida S, Tajima K: Neuron specific enolase (NSE): a specific marker for Merkel cells in human epidermis. J Dermatol 13:67–69, 1986.

72. Ortonne JP, Perchot-Baaque JD, Verrando P, et al: Normal Merkel cells express a synaptophysin-like immunoreactivity. Dermatologica 177:1–10, 1988.

73. Eady RAJ: The basement membrane. Arch Dermatol 124:709–712, 1988.

74. Briggaman RA, Wheeler CE Jr: The epidermal-dermal junction. J Invest Dermatol 65:71–84, 1975.

75. Stanley JR, Hawley Nelson P, Yuspa SH, et al: Characterization of bullous pemphigoid antigen—a unique basement membrane protein of stratified squamous epithelium. Cell 24:897–903, 1981.

76. Woodley DT, Briggaman RA, O'Keefe EJ, et al: Identification of the skin basement-membrane autoantigen in epidermolysis bullosa acquisita. N Engl J Med 310:1007–1013, 1984.

77. Katz SI: The epidermal basement membrane zone—structure, ontogeny, and role in disease. J Am Acad Dermatol 11:1025–1037, 1984.

78. Leigh IM, Eady RAJ, Heagerty AHM, et al: Type VII collagen is a normal component of epidermal basement membrane. J Invest Dermatol 90:639–642, 1988.

79. Rusenko KW, Gammon WR, Fine JD, Briggaman RA: The carboxyl-terminal domain of type VII collagen is present at the basement membrane in recessive dystrophic epidermolysis bullosa. J Invest Dermatol 92:623–627, 1989.

80. Jordan RE: Basement zone antibodies in bullous pemphigoid. JAMA 200:751–756, 1967.

81. Frances C, Robert L: Elastin and elastic fibers in normal and pathologic skin. Int J Dermatol 23:166–179, 1984.

82. Bornstein P, Sage H: Structurally distinct collagen types. Annu Rev Biochem 49:957–1003, 1980.

83. Briggaman RA: Epidermal-dermal interactions in adult skin. J Invest Dermatol 83:166–170, 1984.

84. Eyre DR: Collagen: molecular diversity in the body's protein scaffold. Science 207:1315–1322, 1980.

85. Grant ME, Prockoy DJ: The biosynthesis of collagen. N Engl J Med 286:194–199, 1972.

86. Epstein EH Jr: [Alpha$_1$ (III)]3 human skin collagenase, release by pepsin digestion and preponderance in fetal life. J Biol Chem 249:3225–3231, 1974.

87. Kefalides NA, Alper R, Clark CC: Biochemistry and metabolism of basement membrane. Int Rev Cytol 61:167–228, 1979.
88. Breathnach SM, Melrose SM, Bhogal B, et al: Immunohistochemical studies of amyloid P component distribution in normal human skin. J Invest Dermatol 80:86–89, 1983.
89. Sandberg LB, Soskel NT, Leslie JG: Elastin structure, biosynthesis, and its relationships to disease states. N Engl J Med 304:566–579, 1981.
90. Varadi DP: Studies on the chemistry and fine structure of elastic fibers from normal adult skin. J Invest Dermatol 59:238–246, 1972.
91. Johnson WC, Helwig EB: Histochemistry of acid mucopolysaccharides of the skin in normal and certain pathologic conditions. Am J Clin Pathol 40:123–131, 1963.
92. Fleischmajer R, Perlish JS, Bushey RI: Human dermal glycosaminoglycans and aging. Biochem Biophys Acta 279:265–275, 1972.
93. Roden L, Horowitz MI: Structure and biosynthesis of connective tissue proteoglycans. *In* Horowitz MI, Pigmen W (eds). The Glycoconjugates. Academic Press, New York, 1978, pp 13–71.
94. Katz AM, Rosenthal D, Sauder DN: Cell adhesion molecules: structure, function, and implication in a variety of cutaneous and other pathologic conditions. Int J Dermatol 30:153–160, 1991.
95. Meigel WN: Dermal architecture and collagen type distribution. Arch Dermatol Res 251:1–10, 1977.
96. Van Furth R, Cohn ZA, Hirsch JG, et al: The mononuclear phagocyte system: a new classification of macrophages, monocytes, and their precursor cells. Bull WHO 46:845–852, 1972.
97. Soter NA: Mast cells in cutaneous inflammatory disorders. J Invest Dermatol 74:349–353, 1980.
98. Uvnas B: Chemistry and storage of mast cell granules. J Invest Dermatol 71:76–80, 1978.
99. Schwartz LB, Austin KF: Enzymes of the mast cell granule. J Invest Dermatol 60:20, 1973.
100. Orfanos CE, Mahrle D: Ultrastructure and cytochemistry of human cutaneous nerves. J Invest Dermatol 61:108–120, 1973.
101. Hashimoto K: Fine structure of the Meissner corpuscle of human palmar skin. J Invest Dermatol 60:20–27, 1973.
102. Winkelman RK, Osment LS: The Vater-Pacini corpuscle in the skin of the human fingertip. Arch Dermatol 73:116–122, 1956.
103. Yen A, Braverman IM: Ultrastructure of the human dermal microcirculation: the horizontal plexus of the papillary dermis. J Invest Dermatol 66:131–142, 1976.
104. Braverman IM, Yen A: Ultrastructure of the human dermal microcirculation II. The capillary loop of the dermal papillae. J Invest Dermatol 68:42–52, 1977.
105. Mescon H, Hurly HJ, Moretti G: The anatomy and histochemistry of the arteriovenous anastomoses in human digital skin. J Invest Dermatol 27:133–145, 1956.
106. Ryan TS, Mortimer PS, Jones RL: Lymphatics of the skin. Int J Dermatol 25:411–419, 1986.

CHAPTER 5

Surgical Anatomy

CRAIG S. BIRKBY and GERALD BERNSTEIN

It is axiomatic that surgeons must have detailed knowledge of the anatomy of the sites on which they are operating. For cutaneous surgeons, knowledge of head and neck anatomy is of prime importance since that is the area where they will be performing most of their procedures. It is also the area in which errors stemming from a lack of knowledge of the anatomy will result in serious complications. It is important that cutaneous surgeons take every opportunity to review and enhance their knowledge of surgical anatomy by dissecting cadavers as well as reviewing books[1] and monographs on the subject.

Bony Structures and Landmarks

It is uncommon for the cutaneous surgeon to encounter bone during most cutaneous operations, but the bony structures do provide important landmarks for the identification of other, more superficial anatomic structures (Fig. 5–1). The bony structures that are of great importance as surface landmarks are the zygomatic arch, the orbital rims, the mastoid process, and the mentum.[2]

The importance of the zygomatic arch is a reflection of the many soft tissue structures attached or adjacent to this structure. The zygomatic arch is a composite of the temporal, maxillary, and zygomatic bones. It is well developed and easily identified in virtually all individuals as the most prominent bone of the lateral cheek. Once the zygomatic arch has been identified, the location of the parotid gland, the parotid duct, the superficial temporal artery, and some branches of the facial nerve can generally be determined.

The orbital rim is formed by the frontal bone superiorly, the zygomatic bone laterally and inferiorly, and the maxillary bone medially and inferiorly. The lacrimal bone also contributes to the medial orbital rim near the medial canthus. The location of many sensory nerves, the lacrimal duct, and the contents of the orbit are determined by their relationship to these bones.[3]

The mastoid process is the most inferior portion of the temporal bone and is easily palpated as a rounded projection at the inferior aspect of the posterior auricular sulcus. It is important to remember that the mastoid process is not fully developed until puberty.[4] It is an important landmark for identification of the emergence of the facial nerve trunk. The inferior portion of the body of the mandible and the mandibular angle, ramus, and mentum are also landmarks that can help identify underlying structures, particularly the submandibular gland, the marginal mandibular branch of the facial nerve, and the facial artery and vein.

The three important foramina in the facial bones can be identified from the surface in most individuals. These are the supraorbital foramen, the infraorbital foramen, and the mental foramen. These three foramina are virtually always found along a vertical line extending from the supraorbital foramen (Fig. 5–2) and passing through the center of the pupil.[5] The supraorbital foramen or notch is approximately 2.5 cm, or one thumbbreadth, from the midline of the nasal root. It can be palpated in most people immediately above the orbit as a notch on the underside of the superior orbital rim. Through this opening the supraorbital artery, vein, and nerve emerge from the skull.[6]

The infraorbital foramen is found in the maxillary bone below the infraorbital rim. Through this passes the infraorbital vessels and nerve. It can usually be palpated, in all but the most obese individuals, as a small opening 1 cm below the infraorbital rim. It is on the backward slope of the maxilla as it extends into the canine fossa.

While the mental foramen is usually not palpable, it is typically present at the midportion of the mandible along the same vertical line from the supraorbital foramen. It is important to note that with age there is often a reduction in the vertical height of the mandible. As a

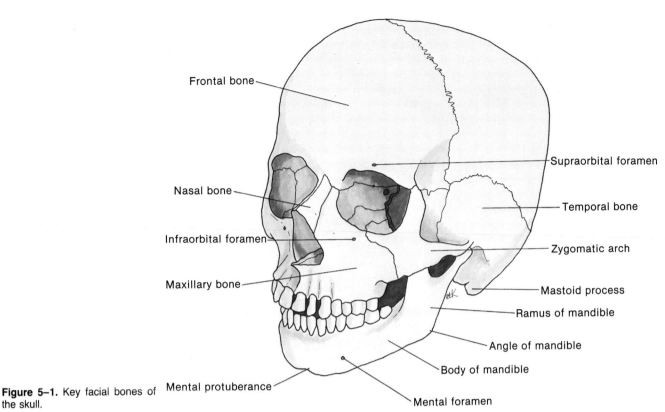

Figure 5–1. Key facial bones of the skull.

Frontal bone

Nasal bone

Infraorbital foramen

Maxillary bone

Mental protuberance

Supraorbital foramen

Temporal bone

Zygomatic arch

Mastoid process

Ramus of mandible

Angle of mandible

Body of mandible

Mental foramen

result, the mental foramen may assume a more superior location.

Surface Landmarks

With a knowledge of the bony features, many important structures of the superficial anatomy of the face can be identified before surgery (Fig. 5–3). Before beginning any cutaneous surgical procedure, the surgeon should always examine the surface landmarks and identify those structures of importance in the operative field. The masseter muscle is one of the most important soft tissue landmark structures on the face and is a reference point for locating many vital structures. This muscle originates on the zygomatic arch and inserts on the ramus, angle, and body of the mandible; it can be easily palpated in most individuals when the teeth are clenched.

The parotid gland is positioned on the posterior half of the masseter muscle and extends from the auricular meatus to just above the angle of the mandible. It has a roughly triangular configuration but may show considerable variability in size and shape. The parotid duct (Stensen's duct) emerges at the upper anterior border of the parotid. Its course is roughly from the middle third of a line connecting the earlobe to a point between the oral commissure and the nasal ala. This structure can be palpated as it runs across the masseter muscle when the teeth are clenched. At the anterior margin of the masseter muscle the duct makes a sharp right angle and passes, deeply piercing one buccinator muscle, to enter the mouth at the position of the second upper molar. Cutting into the parotid gland results in the

creation of a draining sinus that usually heals spontaneously in a few days. However, cutting the parotid duct often produces a chronic draining sinus that requires operative intervention to close.

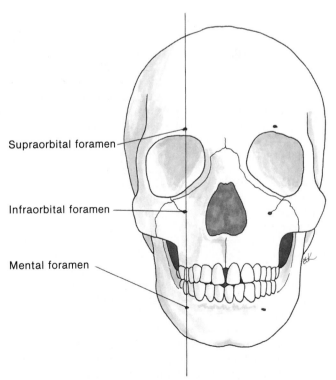

Supraorbital foramen

Infraorbital foramen

Mental foramen

Figure 5–2. A vertical line approximates the location of the foramen.

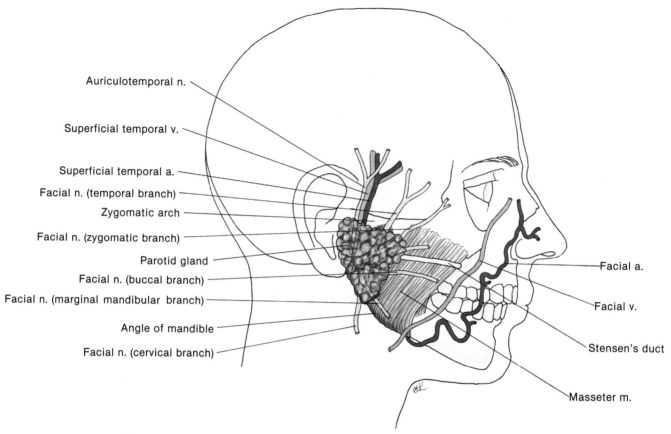

Auriculotemporal n.

Superficial temporal v.

Superficial temporal a.

Facial n. (temporal branch)

Zygomatic arch

Facial n. (zygomatic branch)

Parotid gland

Facial n. (buccal branch)

Facial n. (marginal mandibular branch)

Angle of mandible

Facial n. (cervical branch)

Facial a.

Facial v.

Stensen's duct

Masseter m.

Figure 5–3. Deeper facial structures identifiable by their relationship to surface landmarks.

Another structure associated with the parotid gland is the facial nerve. While the parotid gland protects the fibers of the facial nerve posteriorly, the branches become relatively close to the surface of the gland at its anterior margin. The branches of the facial nerve exit the anterior, superior, and inferior poles of the parotid gland deep to the superficial fascia and generally lie on the deep fascia of the masseter muscle. Although relatively deep in this area, the nerve branches are exposed to inadvertent trauma and injury.

The superficial temporal artery is the terminal branch of the external carotid artery. This artery, along with the superficial temporal vein, traverses the substance of the parotid gland and enters the subcutaneous fat at the superior pole of the parotid gland at the zygomatic arch near the level of the external auditory meatus. It can be palpated as it crosses the zygomatic arch.

The primary artery of the face is the facial artery, a branch of the external carotid artery. The facial artery can be palpated as it crosses the inferior mandibular rim immediately anterior to the insertion of the masseter muscle. This is also an important landmark for identification of the likely course of the mandibular branch of the facial nerve. The anterior facial artery and vein then follow an anterosuperior course in the direction of the oral commissure. In this region the inferior labial artery, and later the superior labial artery, branch off medially to the lower and upper lips. The facial artery then courses along the medial cheek margin near the nose as

the angular artery and enters the eye immediately above the medial canthal tendon.

The area of the temple between the zygomatic arch and the lateral tip of the eyebrow is an important landmark for identification of the course of the temporal branch of the facial nerve. The lateral margin of the frontalis muscle coincides with the lateral tip of the eyebrow. Medial to this point, the nerve branches are protected by their location beneath the muscle.

In the neck the sternocleidomastoid muscle (SCM) is the most important soft tissue structure. It originates on the clavicle and sternum and extends in a posterior diagonal direction to insert onto the mastoid process and the lateral portion of the occipital ridge. Individually, each SCM draws the head laterally and upward. Working together they flex the neck. As a prominent surface landmark the SCM divides the neck into anterior and posterior triangles. The SCM and the mastoid process are important landmarks for identifying the location of the spinal accessory nerve at its most exposed location.

Cosmetic Units, Skin Tension, and Contour Lines

The contour lines are formed by boundaries or junctions of anatomic units on the face, including the vermilion line, the eyebrows, the eyelid margins, and the contours of the nose. Other examples are the interface of the cheek and the nose, the nasolabial fold, and the junction of the ear with the cheek. These lines divide the face into cosmetic units. During surgery on the face, it is important that these contour lines be maintained to the greatest degree possible in order to minimize distortion. Moreover, contour lines can also be effectively used to camouflage scars.[7] The cosmetic units can be further divided into subunits (Fig. 5–4). Thus, the nose can be divided into the two sides, the dorsum, the alae, and the columella. Similarly, the chin is divided into the chin proper and the infralabial area. In general, when using random pattern flaps for repairing defects on the face, it is best to try to use skin from the same cosmetic unit or the same cosmetic subunit if possible.[8]

The skin tension lines (STLs), however, are more difficult to identify. Also known as Langer's lines and relaxed skin tension lines (RSTLs), they are generally thought to eventuate as wrinkle lines. It has been found that incisions placed in or parallel to the STLs produce a finer, more cosmetically acceptable scar than those placed across them (see Chapter 35). It has also been determined that the skin is three times more distensible perpendicular to the STLs than parallel to these lines. Thus, wounds are closed more easily and with less tension if they are placed in the direction of the STLs. It is generally agreed that the STLs are a result of the continuous pull of the underlying musculature on the skin, and that these skin lines form perpendicularly to the line of action of the underlying musculature.[9]

Identification of these lines is generally easy in elderly people, but it can be difficult in young people with smooth skin. Several techniques can help identify these lines. The simplest is to gently pinch the skin between the thumb and forefingers and watch for the development of the fine parallel wrinkles. Another technique is simply to have the patient smile or grimace to accentuate these lines. A more accurate maneuver to allow proper placement of incision lines is to remove the lesion as a circle. After undermining, the skin frequently becomes oval in shape with the long axis aligned with the correct STLs. The wound can then be closed accordingly.[10] STLs vary from individual to individual (Fig. 5–5), and for this reason it is not possible to effectively select the correct STLs in each case by merely referring to some preprinted, stylized contour map or diagram.

Soft Tissue Anatomy

THE INTEGUMENT

Several significant anatomic variations in the skin of the head and neck are of importance to cutaneous surgeons.[11] Dramatic changes can occur in the relationship of the skin and subcutaneous tissue in the span of just a few centimeters on the face (Fig. 5–6).

Scalp

The scalp has been classically divided into five layers that are identified by the well-known mnemonic SCALP:[12] S, skin; C, subcutaneous tissue; A, aponeurosis (galea); L, the loose connective tissue space beneath the galea; P, periosteum.

The cutaneous nerves and vessels of the scalp are in the subcutaneous fat with virtually no vessels in the subgaleal space. However, some emissary vessels that are transmitted through the skull are occasionally encountered during scalp surgery. All the nerves and vessels of the scalp originate below the level of the forehead. No motor nerves are found on the scalp.

Important structures in the integument of the scalp are fibrous bands that connect the dermis to the aponeurosis. Although also found throughout the face and body, these bands are accentuated in the scalp. Thus, during surgery in the subcutaneous fat in this area, there is significant resistance to lateral movement, and substantial undermining has to be performed to close even small wounds.[13] Also, because of the rich vascular supply of this layer, undermining is frequently associated with heavy bleeding. Fortunately, this is usually easily controlled with electrocoagulation or similar techniques. To avoid this problem, most cutaneous surgeons carry their incision through the galea. The wound edges slide easily over the periosteum and permit wound closure with little bleeding. The scalp is considered to originate on

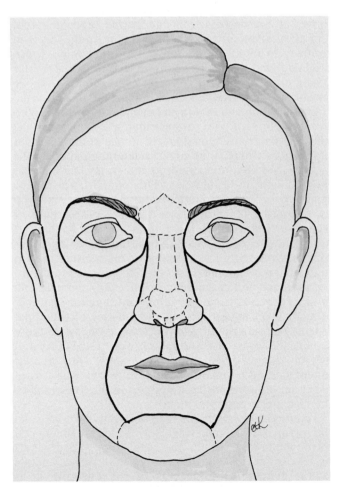

Figure 5–4. Cosmetic units (*bold lines*) and subunits (*dotted lines*).

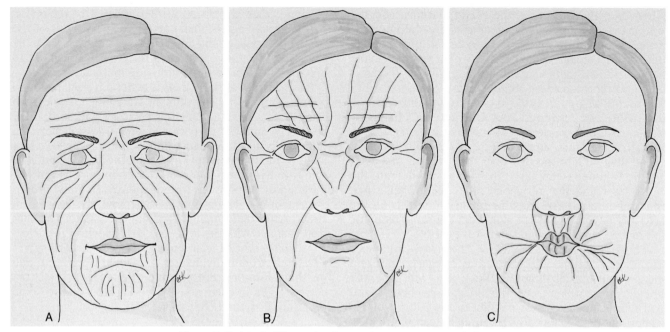

Figure 5–5. *A* to *C,* Skin tension lines and some common variations.

the eyebrows and insert into the superior occipital line. As will be seen, the galea is an aponeurosis connecting the frontalis muscle of the forehead with the occipitalis muscle of the posterior scalp.

Eyelids

The skin of the eyelids is the thinnest of the entire body and is characterized by its rich vascular supply and absence of subcutaneous fat. Thus, the skin lies directly on the muscles.[14] Caution is required during eyelid surgery because of the extreme thinness of the skin and the underlying muscles. A deep incision could conceivably carry through to the orbital septum and into the retro-orbital fat.

Lips and Chin

The skin around the lips and chin is unique in that voluntary muscles insert directly into the skin itself. The muscles are thick and large, especially on the chin, and undermining is often difficult and associated with increased bleeding. Indeed, blunt dissection on the chin is often hampered by the presence of these diagonally and vertically inserting muscular fibers. For this reason, sharp undermining is often more appropriate in these locations. By contrast, the skin of the lateral cheeks has no direct muscle insertions, and blunt undermining is quite effective. Anterior to the mastoid area the fatty layer is often rather thin. In this area lies the most posterior aspect of the parotid gland. Although the parotid gland has a grayish-tan color and is somewhat denser in consistency than adipose tissue, these two tissues can appear similar to one another, especially in a bloody operative field. For this reason, knowledge of the anatomy of this area is of paramount importance.

MUSCLES

The muscles of facial expression are unique in several ways. They are all innervated by branches of the facial nerve, all are derived from the second branchial arch, and all originate or insert into the skin itself. This is in contrast to most of the muscles of the body, which originate and insert on bony structures. The major function of the muscles of facial expression is to move the facial structures, which is important in nonverbal communication and mouth and eyelid movement.[15] With the exception of the periauricular area, most of the muscles of facial expression are in the central portion of the face.[16] Finally, the superficial musculoaponeurotic system (SMAS) interconnects, integrates, and unifies the action of these muscles. Their importance can be readily seen in the striking appearance of patients who have lost the function of the facial nerve because of trauma or a stroke.

The muscles of the face are best thought of as groups of muscles acting on particular structures rather than as individual muscles. These groups include the muscles of the forehead and periauricular skin, eyes, and nose and muscles around the mouth. Important functional considerations are apparent in that the muscles of the upper face work primarily in a vertical direction, while those around the lower face and mouth work in both vertical and horizontal directions. Consequently, the greatest functional and cosmetic deficit results from the loss of facial nerve function to the muscles in the lower half of the face and around the mouth.

The forehead muscles include the frontalis muscle and the corrugator supercilii (Fig. 5–7), which are innervated by the temporal branch of the facial nerve. The frontalis muscle originates on the supraorbital ridge, and its lateral margin is at the tips of the eyebrow. It is surrounded by a fascial SMAS envelope that comes

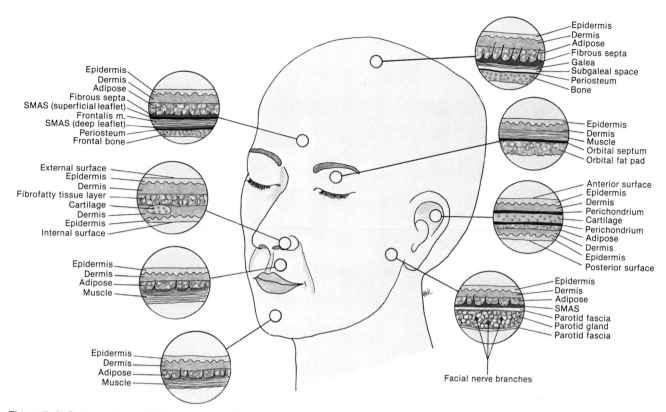

Figure 5–6. Cross sections of different areas of the face showing the variations of the integument and its relationship with the deeper layers.

together at the level of the scalp as the galea aponeurotica. The galea again splits to surround the occipitalis muscle and then comes together to insert onto the superior occipital ridge. The frontalis muscles normally function as one unit responsible for raising the eyebrows. The occipital muscles have no significant function in humans.

The major muscle around the eyes is the orbicularis oculi, which has an orbital and a palpebral component. The palpebral muscle is further divided into preseptal and pretarsal components. This muscle has a bony insertion only at the medial canthus. Contracting the orbicularis muscles closes the lids tightly and draws them medially.[17] The orbicularis muscles have no role in opening the eyes; this function is performed by the levator palpebrae superioris, a muscle that originates deeply within the orbit and is innervated by branches of the third cranial (oculomotor) nerve. Loss of function of the orbicularis muscles results in an inability to close the eye tightly. The orbicularis muscle is innervated primarily by the zygomatic branch of the facial nerve, but the upper portion of this muscle is also partially innervated by the temporal branch. This muscle lies directly beneath the skin of the eyelids. The corrugator muscle originates on the upper medial orbital crest and inserts onto the medial aspect of the eyelids. It draws the eyebrows medially and contributes to the formation of the deep vertical furrow or frown line of the glabella.

The muscles of the nose (the nasalis and procerus) have little functional importance, although they contrib-

ute to the formation of the RSTLs of the nose and medial cheeks. They are innervated by zygomatic branches of the facial nerve.[18]

The muscles of the ears are of no functional importance in the humans, but they may contribute somewhat to the formation of skin lines in these areas. They are innervated by posterior branches of the facial nerve.[19] The superior and inferior auricular muscles insert into the temporal fascia and may be important as a part of the SMAS.

The muscles of the lower face and surrounding the mouth are by far the most important. These can be divided into muscles that elevate, muscles that depress, and muscles that encircle the lips. The elevators include the levator labii superioris nasi, zygomaticus major and minor, and the levator anguli oris muscles. These muscles originate on the upper maxilla and infraorbital area, insert into the melolabial fold and upper lips, and act in a generally diagonal direction. The levator anguli oris muscles are the deepest of the elevator muscles; they originate in the canine fossa of the maxilla and insert into the angles of the mouth. They are innervated by the zygomatic and buccal branches of the facial nerve.

The depressors of the mouth include the depressor anguli oris (triangularis), depressor labii inferioris (quadratus), and mentalis muscles. These three muscles act on the lower lip and angle of the mouth. They are innervated by the marginal mandibular branch of the facial nerve. Loss of function of these muscles due to injury of this relatively vulnerable nerve produces an

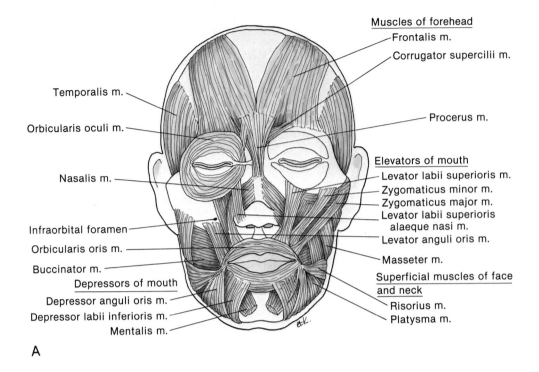

Muscles of forehead
Frontalis m.
Corrugator supercilii m.
Temporalis m.
Procerus m.
Orbicularis oculi m.
Elevators of mouth
Nasalis m.
Levator labii superioris m.
Zygomaticus minor m.
Zygomaticus major m.
Levator labii superioris alaeque nasi m.
Infraorbital foramen
Levator anguli oris m.
Orbicularis oris m.
Masseter m.
Buccinator m.
Superficial muscles of face and neck
Depressors of mouth
Depressor anguli oris m.
Risorius m.
Depressor labii inferioris m.
Platysma m.
Mentalis m.

A

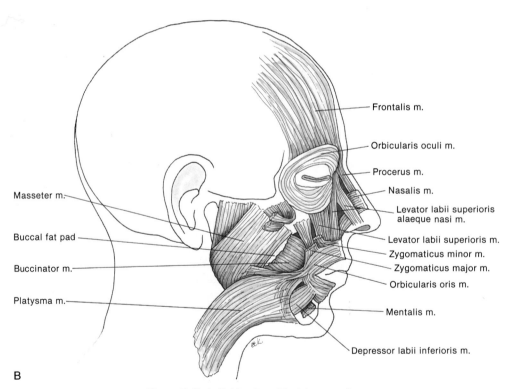

Frontalis m.
Orbicularis oculi m.
Procerus m.
Nasalis m.
Masseter m.
Levator labii superioris alaeque nasi m.
Buccal fat pad
Levator labii superioris m.
Zygomaticus minor m.
Buccinator m.
Zygomaticus major m.
Orbicularis oris m.
Platysma m.
Mentalis m.
Depressor labii inferioris m.

B

Figure 5–7. *A, B,* Muscles of facial expression.

unopposed upward and diagonal pull on the lips, causing a striking and noticeable cosmetic deficit. There is also some loss of lip function, with consequent drooling.

The orbicularis oris is the sphincter muscle of the mouth, responsible for pursing the lips. It is a circular muscle that consists of original fibers as well as fibers blending in from the elevators and depressors of the lips and the platysma and risorius muscles. Crossing fibers contribute to the formation of the philtrum, which is responsible for the exquisite control of the lips as well as for maintaining the seal of the lips to keep food and liquids within the mouth. It is innervated by the buccal branch of the facial nerve. The deep buccinator muscle, which is also innervated by the buccal branches of the facial nerve, is the fleshy part of the cheek. This muscle is also of great functional importance in that it keeps food from accumulating between the teeth and gums and forces it back into the path of the teeth.

Lateral movement of the mouth is a function of the superficial platysma and risorius. The risorius is a paper-thin muscle that originates in the fat and fascia of the lateral cheeks and inserts into the the skin and mucous membrane of the lateral lips. It draws the corners of the mouth laterally into a smile.

The platysma muscle is important from an anatomic point of view but has little functional role. It is innervated by the cervical branches of the facial nerve. Paralysis of the platysma is usually of little functional consequence. This muscle originates in the cervical fascia and inserts into the skin of the lips and chin as well as into the orbicularis muscle. Although it has a somewhat variable location, the platysma muscle crosses the jaw in most people and extends toward the lips. Only rarely does it extend as high as the zygomatic arch. It commonly presents as a broad but extremely thin muscular sheet; however, in some people it is very narrow and wispy.[20] It is responsible for tensing the skin of the neck. Its importance to the cutaneous surgeon is that it covers and protects the marginal mandibular branch of the facial nerve as well as the facial artery and vein. Therefore, for operations above the platysma muscle, it can generally be assumed that these vital structures are not at risk.

The muscles of facial expression can also be understood in terms of their depth relationships. Four layers can be appreciated: the platysma, risorius, and frontalis muscles are the most superficial; the orbicularis oris and orbicularis oculi are somewhat deeper; the elevators and depressors of the mouth are in the middle level; and the elevator anguli oris, mentalis, and buccinator are the deepest.

Despite the prominence of the temporalis and masseter, these are not muscles of facial expression but rather of mastication. They are innervated by motor fibers of the trigeminal nerve.

THE SUPERFICIAL MUSCULOAPONEUROTIC SYSTEM (SMAS)

The SMAS has been described only in the past two decades,[21] being identified as a discrete fascial and muscular system comprising the superficial fascia of the face. This system includes the fascia of the forehead and galea of the scalp, which is contiguous with the superficial fascia of the neck. While the exact anatomic details of the SMAS are still unsettled, many relationships are clear. The SMAS lies within the subcutaneous fat of the face and divides it into two distinct layers. The superficial fatty layer is pierced by fibrous bands connecting the SMAS to the lower surface of the dermis, while the deep fatty layer has no septa.[22]

The SMAS is thicker and more easily identified posteriorly, and becomes thinner and less discrete anteriorly. It terminates on the nasolabial folds and is separate from the deeper parotid, masseteric, and temporal fascia. The SMAS splits to envelop the muscles of facial expression. As a result of this, along with the discrete fibrous attachments to the overlying dermis, the SMAS serves to integrate, unify, and amplify the facial muscular actions and accounts for the wide range of facial expressions that are possible. There is, however, a functional separation of the muscles of the forehead from those of the lower face resulting from the attachment of the SMAS to the zygomatic arch.[23]

The axial arteries are found either in the superficial aspect of the SMAS or at the SMAS–subcutaneous fat border. Thus, the sub-SMAS layer is relatively bloodless. However, the branches of the facial nerve lie on the deep surface of the SMAS, so blunt dissection beneath the SMAS on the cheek is safe only to the anterior border of the parotid where the nerves are found within the body of the gland. Dissection in this plane, anterior to the gland, becomes more hazardous. In the temporal area, dissecting above the SMAS ensures the integrity of the temporal branch of the facial nerve. The unique anatomic features of the SMAS have resulted in significant innovations in cosmetic surgery, especially in face and neck lift surgery.[24, 25] Similarly, innovations in facial reconstruction and flap dynamics have resulted from an improved understanding of the anatomic relationships of the SMAS.[13]

THE VASCULATURE

Arteries

The arterial supply to the face is almost entirely derived from branches of the external carotid artery, which originates from the common carotid artery at the level of the upper border of thyroid cartilage, and passes through the neck deep to the SCM.[26] It enters directly into the parotid gland in a deep location and divides into the maxillary and superficial temporal branches (Fig. 5–8). While passing through the parotid gland, the temporal branch becomes more superficial and enters the subcutaneous space at the level of the auricular meatus. Here it can be palpated as it crosses the zygomatic arch. The superficial temporal artery then branches widely and anastomoses broadly with the other vessels of the scalp to supply blood to the lateral scalp and face.[27, 28]

The anterior facial artery exits the external carotid in the neck at the level of the mandible. It first follows an upward course deep to the stylohyoid muscle and posterior belly of the digastric muscle, and then takes an anterosuperior or diagonal course, passing beneath the submandibular gland and crossing the mandible immediately anterior to the insertion of the masseter muscle at the mandibular rim, where it can be readily palpated. It continues superiorly and anteriorly toward the angle of the mouth. Its first branch is the inferior labial artery, followed by the superior labial artery. The labial arteries of the right and left anastomose to form a continuous loop of blood around the mouth. The location of the labial arteries can be accurately predicted by measuring back ½ inch inside the mouth from the vermilion onto the mucosa. They lie in the deep subcutaneous plane directly upon the muscle. With age, however, these

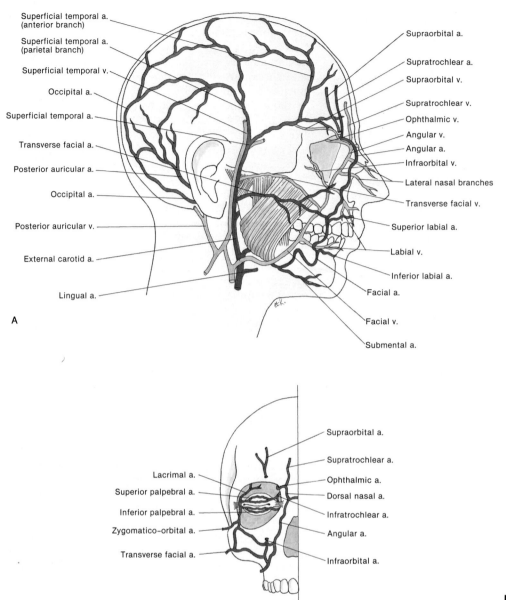

Superficial temporal a. (anterior branch)

Superficial temporal a. (parietal branch)

Superficial temporal v.

Occipital a.

Superficial temporal a.

Transverse facial a.

Posterior auricular a.

Occipital a.

Posterior auricular v.

External carotid a.

Lingual a.

Supraorbital a.

Supratrochlear a.

Supraorbital v.

Supratrochlear v.

Ophthalmic v.

Angular v.

Angular a.

Infraorbital v.

Lateral nasal branches

Transverse facial v.

Superior labial a.

Labial v.

Inferior labial a.

Facial a.

Facial v.

Submental a.

A

Lacrimal a.

Superior palpebral a.

Inferior palpebral a.

Zygomatico-orbital a.

Transverse facial a.

Supraorbital a.

Supratrochlear a.

Ophthalmic a.

Dorsal nasal a.

Infratrochlear a.

Angular a.

Infraorbital a.

B

Figure 5–8. The arteries and veins of the head.

arteries become more tortuous and often assume a more superficial location. Occasionally, they are subepidermal and can appear as nonpigmented nodules that on careful palpation often disclose a fine pulsation. In the lower face and neck the anterior facial arteries and veins are found beneath the platysma.

At the angle of the mouth the facial artery assumes a more vertical direction, passing parallel and adjacent to the nose. In this area the anterior facial artery and vein are covered by the elevator muscles of the mouth, which affords some protection from accidental trauma. The lateral nasal artery is a small branch adjacent to the lower nose at the level of the ala nasi. In this area the anterior facial artery becomes the angular artery. It continues to travel up along the nose and enters the orbit immediately above the medial canthal tendon.[29] At this point the angular artery anastomoses with branches of the ophthalmic artery, which is a branch of the internal carotid artery. It is important to note that the artery is covered only by skin in this location, since no subcutaneous fat is present. The vessels are approximately 1 cm from the nasal root.

The facial artery is always anterior to the vein. While the vein is smooth and flat, the artery tends to be thick and tortuous. It frequently bends upon itself, which makes it more difficult to identify the exact location of the transected segment of the vessel, as its direction cannot always be predicted with accuracy.

The supraorbital artery exits through the supraorbital foramen and is the terminal branch of the internal carotid artery. The supratrochlear artery exits from the medial orbit above the medial canthal tendon, where it supplies blood to the medial forehead and anterior scalp. The infraorbital artery exits from the skull at the infraorbital foramen. It is a terminal branch of the internal maxillary artery, which is derived from the external carotid. The dorsal nasal artery is another branch of the internal carotid artery and is derived from the anterior ethmoidal artery. It enters the subcutaneous layer of the skin at the middle of the nose at the junction of the bony and cartilaginous portions.

Veins

The veins of the face parallel the arteries (Fig. 5–8). They tend to be straight, thin-walled, and located posterior to the arteries.[30] It is well known that the veins of the head contain no valves, and blood can flow in either direction. Cavernous sinus thrombosis resulting from retrograde spread of midfacial infection is related to this pattern of venous flow.

The superficial temporal vein is the collecting system of the venous system of the scalp. It enters the superior pole of the parotid gland at the level of the auricular meatus and passes through the substance of the parotid, where it becomes the retromandibular vein (posterior facial). It anastomoses with the internal maxillary vein within the parotid gland. The retromandibular vein communicates with the anterior facial vein but typically flows into the external jugular vein.

The angular vein enters the face from the medial canthus and travels down the medial cheek adjacent to the nose. It anastomoses with ophthalmic veins, the veins of the eyelids and forehead, and the infraorbital vein. It also communicates with the deep facial vein, the venous companion to the buccal branch of the internal maxillary vein. It connects to the pterygoid plexus medially to the upper ramus of the mandible. The anterior facial vein is covered by the elevator muscles of the lip and inferiorly by the platysma. It is joined by veins from the nose and becomes the facial vein. At and below the level of the oral commissure, it joins with both the superior and inferior labial veins. It crosses the lower mandibular margin adjacent and posterior to the anterior facial artery. In contrast to the artery, the vein goes over the mandibular gland and enters the internal jugular vein after communicating with the retromandular veins.

Lymphatics

The vessels of the lymphatic system tend to parallel those of the venous system, but they are more variable and more numerous. They have the same general pattern of small lymphatic capillaries channeling into larger collecting vessels. The lymphatic vessels have valves every 2 to 3 mm. In general, the drainage goes from superficial to deep and from medial to lateral and caudad in a diagonal direction (Fig. 5–9). Lymph vessels of the head and neck tend to heal rapidly when transected. It has been estimated that between 20 and 50% of healthy individuals have palpable benign lymph nodes in the neck.[31] Although there is extreme variability in the location of the lymphatic vascular system, the lymph nodes tend to be arranged in a regular and predictable location. The original classification[32] is still accepted with few modifications.

The major facial lymph node groups of the head and neck are in the parotid, submandibular, and submental areas. The scalp drains to the postauricular and the occipital nodes, which then drain to the deeper cervical lymph nodes of the spinal accessory, transverse cervical, and internal jugular nodes.[33] Although the parotid nodes are identified as being both preauricular and infra-auricular in location, they are both within the gland and in the surrounding glandular fascia, and behave as a single unit. The submandibular glands also behave as a single unit but are divided into five subdivisions based on their relationship to the submandibular gland. The submental glands are in the midline with the potential to drain either to the right or left, and thus must be considered bilateral.

The major lymphatic drainage from the face consists of channels that run posteriorly in a diagonal and downward direction. The lateral and upper parts of the face, the forehead, and the lateral eyelids drain to the parotid nodes. The medial and lower face, as well as the medial eyelid and the lateral aspects of the lip, drain to the submandibular glands. Drainage to the submental nodes is from the middle two thirds of the lower lip and the chin. These nodes then drain primarily into the lateral cervical nodes (Fig. 5–9).

While examination of the parotid nodes is straightforward, the submandibular nodes are best palpated with the chin drawn medially and down to relax the muscles of the upper neck. Similarly, the submental nodes can be most effectively palpated with the chin drawn down. This procedure may be further enhanced by a bimanual examination with one finger in the patient's mouth and the fingers of the other hand pressing upward on the submental triangles. Drainage to the postauricular node is from the upper posterior aspect of the ear, and the posterior parietal, mastoid, and temporal areas of the scalp. This drains into the nodes beneath the cephalad portion of the SCM and the superior junction of the internal jugular and spinal accessory node chains. The occipital nodes drain the muscular layers of the neck and posterior aspect of the scalp.

Lateral Cervical Lymph Nodes

The lateral cervical nodes are divided into superficial and deep groups. The superficial nodes tend to be more cephalad in distribution and are found immediately below and sometimes overlapping the parotid node groups. They lie over the SCM. The deep lateral cervical nodes are divided into three main chains: spinal accessory, transverse cervical, and internal jugular. The spinal accessory chain lies in the posterior triangle of the neck and parallels the course of the spinal accessory nerve. When operating on these nodes, extreme care must be taken to avoid trauma to the spinal accessory nerve, which is in intimate contact with some of these nodes.

The transverse cervical chain is in the lower portion of the neck at the supraclavicular area. These lymph nodes are easily palpated with the fingers extended flat over the nodal chain. The internal jugular chain is divided anteriorly and laterally and is the major lymph collecting system of the head and neck.[34] The lateral internal jugular chain is the final main collecting lym-

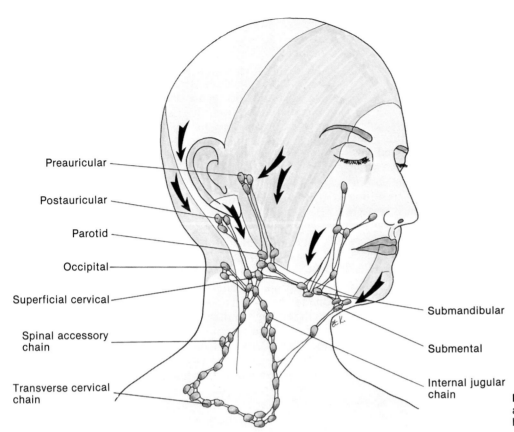

Preauricular

Postauricular

Parotid

Occipital

Superficial cervical

Spinal accessory chain

Transverse cervical chain

Submandibular

Submental

Internal jugular chain

Figure 5–9. The lymphatic drainage and major lymph nodes of the head and neck.

phatic system of the head and neck. It receives drainage from both the superficial lymphatics of the head and neck and from the deeper structures, pharynx, larynx, vocal cords, and other internal structures of the head, neck, and salivary glands. Since it lies deep to the SCM, it is most easily palpated by grasping the muscle between the thumb and fingers and turning the chin to the ipsilateral side. By flexing the neck laterally, the SCM is relaxed, which allows for greater precision in palpating this nodal chain. These nodes may be effectively examined from either the front or back of the patient, but the examination should always extend along the entire length of the neck. Careful examination of the head and neck is an essential part of all oncologic examinations. Because of individual variations in lymphatic drainage and flow, it is important that all lymph nodes be examined bilaterally.

Nerve Supply of the Head and Neck

TRIGEMINAL NERVE

The sensory innervation of the face is derived almost entirely from sensory branches of the trigeminal nerve.[35] The ophthalmic (superior), maxillary (middle), and mandibular (lower) branches exit the skull through the supraorbital foramen, infraorbital foramen, and mental foramen, respectively. All of these foramina are found along a vertical line extending from the supraorbital

foramen. Effective anesthesia using regional nerve blocks can be achieved easily in most patients after identifying the respective foramina (Fig. 5–10).

Ophthalmic Branch

The ophthalmic branch of the trigeminal nerve exits the skull through the supraorbital foramen. It extends vertically to provide sensory innervation to the forehead and anterior scalp. The lacrimal nerve exits the orbit laterally and supplies the lateral skin of the upper lids. The supratrochlear nerves exit at the medial orbit and provide sensory innervation to the area around the medial canthus, glabella, and nasal root. The infratrochlear nerve supplies sensory innervation to the nasal root and medial canthus. The dorsal nasal nerve is also a branch of the upper ophthalmic division of the trigeminal nerve. This is derived from the nasociliary branch of the anterior ethmoidal nerve and exits from the nasal cavity onto the dorsal nasal skin at the junction of the bony and cartilaginous portions of the nose. It appears midway between the cheek and the nasal dorsum.

Maxillary Branch

The second or maxillary division of the facial nerve originates from the infraorbital foramen and innervates the cheek, lower eyelid, upper lip area, and side of the nose, but not the dorsum or tip. This foramen is 1 cm below the inferior orbital rim on the "downslope" of the maxilla. The malar area is innervated by the zygo-

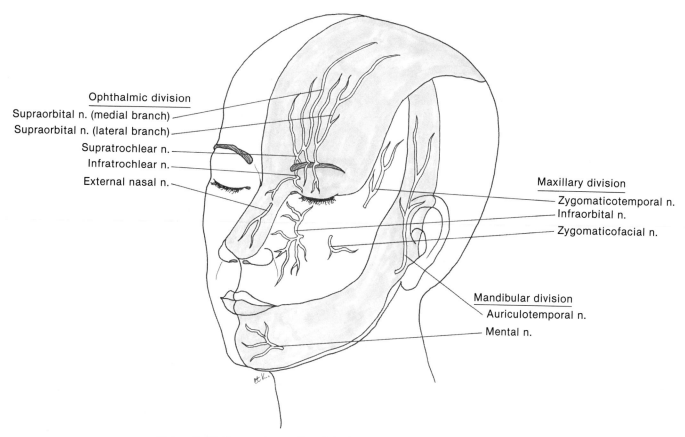

Figure 5–10. Sensory innervation of the face derived from the trigeminal nerve.

maticofacial nerve, while the zygomaticotemporal nerve supplies the temple and a small area of the adjacent temporal scalp. Both are branches of the maxillary division of the trigeminal nerve. These nerves exit onto the face through small foramina on the lower zygomatic bone and frontal process of the zygomatic bones on the lateral margin of the orbit.

Mandibular Branch

The mandibular nerve is the most inferior branch of the trigeminal nerve on the face. In addition to sensory fibers, it carries motor fibers to the muscles of mastication. This nerve has three major cutaneous branches: auriculotemporal, buccal, and mental. The auriculotemporal nerve is adjacent and deep to the superficial temporal artery and vein. It innervates the temple, the temporoparietal scalp, and part of the anterior ear.[36] It also provides sensation to the auditory canal and tympanic membrane as well as the temporomandibular joint. The buccal branch of the mandibular nerve lies deep to the parotid gland. It innervates the lower cheek over the buccinator muscle, buccal mucosa, and gingivae. These branches account for mucosal anesthesia after deeply placed injections of a local anesthetic for cutaneous surgery. The mental or most inferior branch of the mandibular division is the cutaneous terminal branch of the alveolar nerve. Emerging from the man-

dible through the mental foramen, it supplies the skin of the chin and lower lip and the mucosa of the lower lip and adjacent lower gingivae. The mental foramen is on the midvertical position on the mandible, but with age and subsequent dissolution of the upper portion of the mandible, the foramen and nerve may occupy a more cephalad position, especially in edentulous patients. The sensory innervation of the scalp, ear, and occipital skin is derived from the ventral rami of C2, C3, and C4.

FACIAL NERVE

The facial nerve innervates all the muscles of facial expression. It is a unique nerve of vital importance to cutaneous surgeons, since in many instances the branches of this nerve are superficially located and vulnerable to inadvertent trauma during surgery on the face and neck.[37] It is critical that surgeons operating in this area learn to identify those areas where the branches of the facial nerve are in greatest jeopardy (Fig. 5–11). Moreover, when surgery in these areas is planned, it is important that patients be advised preoperatively of the possibility of trauma to the nerve, rather than leave them to discover paralysis after surgery.

The facial nerve exits the skull through the stylomastoid foramen, where it is protected by the mastoid process. Since the mastoid process may not be fully

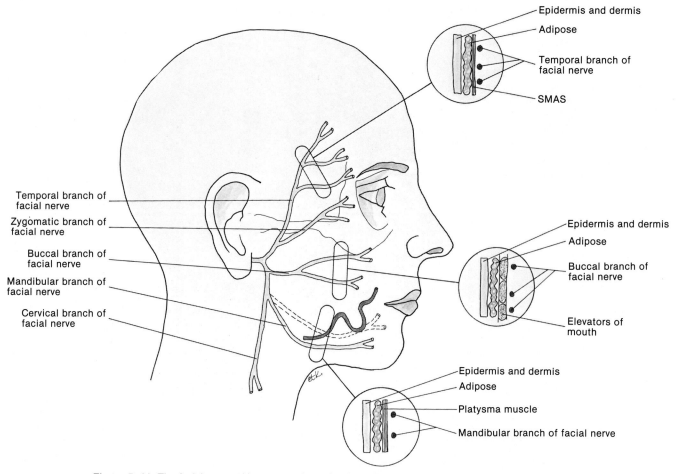

Figure 5–11. The facial nerve with cross sections showing selected relationships to the deeper structures.

developed until puberty, and the facial nerve trunk is in a subcutaneous location, it is vulnerable to inadvertent trauma from surgery performed in this area. After exiting the stylomastoid foramen, the facial nerve trunk enters the parotid gland after having first given off the postauricular branch; this is an unimportant branch supplying the postauricular muscles. After entering the posterior lobe of the parotid gland, the facial nerve assumes a more superficial location.[38] In the superficial lobe of the parotid gland, it divides into an upper temporofacial and a lower cervicofacial branch. The facial nerve exits the superior, anterior, and inferior borders of the parotid gland under the cover of the SMAS fascia.[39]

The facial nerve has five major branches: temporal, zygomatic, buccal, marginal mandibular, and cervical. These are sometimes referred to as the pes anserinus, or "goose's foot." However, five major variations in the pattern of the facial nerve have been identified,[40] and many minor variations have been recognized.[41, 42] In general, the branches of the facial nerve enter the muscles that they innervate at their posterior and deep surfaces; they are normally always covered by the SMAS fascia. If the branches of the nerve are cut anterior to a vertical line drawn from the lateral canthus, the nerve can be expected to regenerate with partial or complete recovery of function. However, nerves cut posterior to

this line are likely to show little or no recovery of function, leading to permanent paralysis.

Temporal Branch

The temporal branch is considered one of the most vulnerable branches of the facial nerve.[43] It extends from the anterosuperior portion of the parotid gland, crosses the zygomatic arch, and innervates the frontalis muscle, upper portion of the orbicularis oculi muscle, and corrugator supercilii. The major effect of cutting this nerve is flattening of the forehead and drooping of the eyebrow because of loss of the dominant frontalis muscle in the area.

After leaving the upper pole of the parotid gland, this branch is covered only by skin, subcutaneous fat, and the SMAS,[44] which leaves it vulnerable to injury, especially in thin or elderly people. The area of greatest vulnerability can be identified by drawing one line from the earlobe to the lateral tip of the highest forehead crease and a second line from the earlobe to the lateral tip of the eyebrow. The region of greatest vulnerability lies within this area, as the nerve crosses the zygomatic arch and the temple.[45] Although this nerve is commonly identified as having only one branch, making it more vulnerable to permanent paralysis from accidental section, up to four major branches of the temporal nerve are sometimes found.

Zygomatic Branches

The zygomatic branch enters the upper anterior portion of the parotid gland and travels in an almost horizontal direction to the orbicularis oculi muscle, the elevators of the lips, and the nasal muscles. It has multiple branches and also anastomoses with fibers of the buccal branch of the facial nerve. Fibers of the zygomatic nerve are also present on or over the parotid duct. This nerve tends to be less vulnerable to injury. Also, cutting branches of the zygomatic branch is usually followed by recovery, both from other fibers of the zygomatic nerve and from anastomotic fibers of the buccal branch.

Buccal Branch

The buccal branch of the facial nerve also innervates the elevators of the mouth, the orbicularis oris muscle, and the buccinator muscle, as well as the risorius muscle. This branch also has multiple fibers and tends to regenerate and recover function after sectioning. It travels deeply beneath the fat of the cheek and is not commonly traumatized during cutaneous surgery.[46]

Marginal Mandibular Branch

The marginal mandibular branch exits the inferoanterior pole of the parotid gland and crosses the angle of the mandible covered only by skin, subcutaneous fat, and the SMAS, so it is quite vulnerable to injury. It then extends along the mandible to innervate the depressors of the mouth. Trauma to this nerve can produce significant functional and cosmetic deficits, allowing lateral and upward pull on the opposite side of the mouth.[47] The ipsilateral side tends to be frozen in a persistent grimace because of the lack of apposing downward muscular contraction. Posterior to the facial artery, the marginal mandibular branch has been found 1 cm or more below the inferior rim of the mandible in 20% of cases, and at or above the lower level of the mandibular body in 80% of cases.[48] Anterior to the anterior facial artery, the nerve is always above the inferior mandibular rim. When the head is hyperextended in the opposite direction for submandibular surgery, the nerve may be as much as 2 cm or more beneath the inferior margin of the mandible. The platysma muscle is superficial to the marginal mandibular branch and thus can sometimes protect it from trauma. However, since the platysma is highly variable in size, it is an adequate landmark only when clearly identifiable. Although the marginal mandibular nerve has been generally recognized as having only a single fiber, two or more major nerve divisions of it have been identified.[48] Also, anastomoses between the buccal and marginal mandibular branches of the facial nerve can occur. In these instances, trauma to the marginal mandibular branch may be followed by recovery of function over time.

Cervical Branch

The cervical branch of the facial nerve innervates the platysma muscle.[49] It is functionally of little importance and the consequences of trauma to this nerve are rarely reported.

Surgical Anatomy of the Neck

The boundaries of the neck are the inferior margin of the mandible superiorly and the clavicle and sternum inferiorly. The skin of the neck is loose and has prominent transverse wrinkles. It is important that elective incisions be placed within these lines whenever possible to obtain an optimal cosmetic result. Because of the concave shape of the neck, especially anteriorly, vertical incisions tend to form a web, which may have functional as well as cosmetic implications.

FASCIA OF THE NECK

Beneath the skin of the neck is the superficial cervical fascia, which is continuous with the SMAS of the face and splits to envelop the platysma muscle. The platysma originates on the fascia of the upper pectoral and clavicular area and inserts into the skin and muscles of the mouth and lower face. It is innervated by the cervical branch of the facial nerve. The platysma muscle is a highly variable muscle, being thick and prominent in some individuals and thin and wispy in others. When present, it covers and protects the neurovascular structures of the neck, including the facial artery and vein and the mandibular branch of the facial nerve.[20]

The deep cervial fascia is divided into three layers. The superficial layer of the deep cervical fascia originates on the spinous process and encircles the neck; it covers the contents of the posterior triangle. The middle layer of the deep cervical fascia is only present anteriorly; it splits off from the deep cervical fascia and covers the thyroid and laryngotracheal structures. The deep layer of the deep cervical fascia also originates on the spinous process of the vertebra and encircles the neck; it covers the large deep muscles of the neck and serves as the floor of the posterior triangle.

SUPERFICIAL ANATOMIC LANDMARKS OF THE NECK

The key superficial landmarks of the neck are the hyoid bone anteriorly and the SCM laterally. The SCM divides the neck into anterior and posterior triangles.

Anterior Triangle

Four smaller triangles are found within the anterior triangle: the submental, submandibular, carotid, and muscular triangles. These are defined by the relationships of the muscles and bones of the neck and jaw (Fig. 5–12).

The carotid triangle is formed by the posterior belly of the digastric muscle superiorly, the anterior border

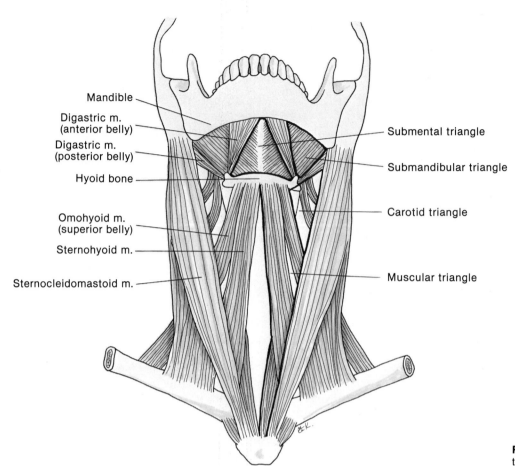

Figure 5–12. Muscles and anatomic triangles of the neck.

Labels on figure:
Mandible
Digastric m. (anterior belly)
Digastric m. (posterior belly)
Hyoid bone
Omohyoid m. (superior belly)
Sternohyoid m.
Sternocleidomastoid m.
Submental triangle
Submandibular triangle
Carotid triangle
Muscular triangle

of the SCM posteriorly, and the posterior border of the superior belly of the omohyoid muscle anteriorly. Within this triangle the common carotid artery bifurcates into the internal and external carotid arteries, slightly below the level of the hyoid bone. The carotid arteries are found within the carotid sheath along with the internal jugular vein and the vagus nerve. At this point the vessels are most vulnerable to trauma since they are covered only by the platysma muscle and the cervical fascia. This is also where the carotid pulsation can be felt most strongly. In the remainder of the neck these vital neurovascular structures are protected by the thick bellies of the SCM.

The submandibular triangle is made up of the anterior border of the digastric muscle, the posterior belly of the digastric muscle, and the mandible. It contains the submandibular gland, lymph nodes, and facial artery. The facial vein and retromandibular vein may also meet in this triangle. Of additional importance in this triangle is the possible presence of the marginal mandibular ramus of the facial nerve. The variability of the course of this nerve requires caution during surgery in the submandibular triangle. The SCM originates from the upper portion of the sternum and the middle third of the clavicle by two heads. It inserts into the mastoid process of the temporal bone and the lateral aspect of the superior nuchal line. Together the SCMs flex the neck, while individually they rotate the head caudad and turn the face upward and in the opposite direction.

Posterior Triangle

The posterior triangle of the neck is formed by the posterior margin of the SCM, the anterior surface of the trapezius muscle, and the scalene muscles. This triangle is covered by skin and the superficial fascia of the neck as well as the superficial portion of the deep cervical fascia. Covering the scalene muscles is the deep portion of the deep cervical fascia. The posterior triangle contains nerves of the superficial cervical plexus as well as the spinal accessory nerve.

The spinal accessory nerve is the most important structure in the posterior triangle since it innervates the trapezius muscle. This nerve, which is covered only by skin and fascia, is especially vulnerable to trauma and accidental sectioning during surgery.[50] Trauma to the spinal accessory nerve results in loss of function of the trapezius muscle with winging of the scapula, inability to shrug the shoulder, difficulty in initiating abduction of the arm, and chronic shoulder pain. Unfortunately, when this nerve is accidentally cut, it usually shows little tendency to recover. The spinal accessory nerve exits from behind the SCM and travels diagonally in a downward direction across the posterior triangle to enter into the space beneath the trapezius muscle. The exit from the SCM is known as Erb's point (Fig. 5–13). Coincidentally, this is the same area where the superficial cervical plexus exits from behind the SCM.

Erb's point can be identified by bisecting a horizontal line connecting the angle of the jaw to the mastoid

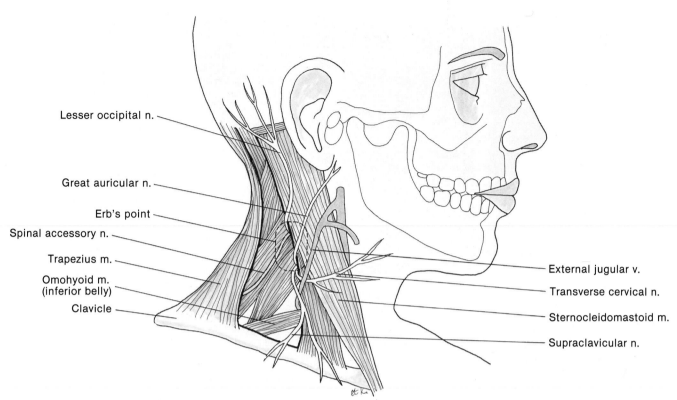

Figure 5–13. The posterior triangle of the neck and the location of Erb's point.

process with a vertical line drawn from the midpoint. The intersection of this line at the posterior border of the SCM is Erb's point. Within a short distance above and below this point, the spinal accessory, transverse cervical, lesser occipital, and greater auricular nerves all emerge from behind the SCM.[5] Another way of identifying the point of appearance of the spinal accessory nerve is to draw a horizontal line from the thyroid notch across the neck through the posterior triangle. At a point 2 cm above and 2 cm below where this line intersects the posterior margin of the SCM is the approximate area of the spinal accessory nerve as it crosses the posterior triangle of the neck.

The cervical plexus exits the posterior triangle, pierces the superficial cervical fascia, and passes across the posterior border of the SCM. This plexus is formed by sensory nerve fibers from the anterior rami of the second, third, and fourth cervical nerves.

There are four major sensory nerves of the superficial cervical plexus: lesser occipital, greater auricular, transverse cervical, and supraclavicular. The lesser occipital nerve (second and third cervical nerves) innervates the skin behind the ears and the parietal scalp; the greater auricular nerve (second and third cervical nerves) innervates the skin of the earlobe, the posterior ear, the parotid area, and the mastoid area; the transverse cervical nerve (second and third cervical nerves) passes horizontally across the SCM and fans out to provide sensory innervation to most of the anterior neck; and the supraclavicular nerves (third and fourth cervical nerves) have three branches that innervate the clavicular and sternal areas, the upper chest, and the lower neck,

and also provide sensory innervation to the clavicular deltoid area as well as to the trapezius and upper shoulder areas.

BLOOD VESSELS OF THE NECK

The major arteries of the neck are generally too deep to be of consequence to the cutaneous surgeon. They are mostly covered by the SCM but are somewhat more vulnerable in the carotid triangle. The more superficial branches of the external carotid artery are the superior thyroid, occipital, posterior auricular, and facial arteries. The last-named is of special interest since it arises at about the level of the lingual artery passing beneath the posterior belly of the digastric deep to the submandibular gland. It then crosses the lower rim of the mandible immediately anterior to the insertion of the masseter muscle.

The internal jugular vein travels with the common carotid artery and is not usually vulnerable to trauma, except possibly in the area of the carotid triangle. The superficial veins of the face are the external jugular, anterior jugular, and facial veins. The thin, straight facial vein crosses over the submandibular gland and lies posterior to the artery.

The nuchal area, or posterior neck, is bordered by the occipital scalp superiorly, the upper portion of the back inferiorly, and the anterior border of the trapezius muscles. The skin of the posterior neck is among the thickest of the body. The soft tissue structures are muscular and fascial. There are few vital structures in the posterior neck of consequence to the cutaneous surgeon.

The occipital artery enters the neck beneath the deeper muscles of the posterior neck. It soon enters the superficial layers of the deep cervical fascia and extends onto the posterior scalp to the superficial fascia of the scalp. This vessel is vulnerable to trauma during scalp reduction surgery. The greater occipital nerve is a branch of the dorsal division of the second cervical nerve. It becomes superficial in the area of the occipital scalp and supplies sensory innervation to the scalp over the vertex up to the top of the head. It communicates with the lesser occipital nerve. The third occipital nerve is another cutaneous branch of the dorsal division of the third cervical nerve that provides sensory innervation to the skin of the occipital scalp. It is located somewhat medial and caudal to the greater occipital nerve.

SUMMARY

The sheer number and variety of surgical procedures routinely performed by cutaneous surgeons, ranging from simple excisions to laser surgery to extensive Mohs surgical extirpations to complex cosmetic surgery, requires a thorough knowledge and understanding of anatomy in order to achieve the best possible results with the least amount of risk to the patient. This knowledge not only enables the surgeon to operate more safely, but may also facilitate easier wound closure, provide better cosmetic results, improve the selection of the appropriate random pattern flaps for reconstructive surgery, provide more effective pain relief from nerve block anesthesia, and allow earlier detection of lymph node involvement associated with certain neoplastic diseases. For all these reasons, all cutaneous surgeons must continually strive to review and enhance their knowledge of surgical anatomy in order to provide the best possible surgical care.

The authors wish to thank Ms. Elizabeth Kessler for the illustrations that accompany this chapter.

REFERENCES

1. Anderson JE: Grant's Atlas of Anatomy. Williams & Wilkins, Baltimore, 1983.
2. Bernstein G: Surface landmarks for the identification of key anatomic structures of the face and neck. J Dermatol Surg Oncol 12:722–726, 1986.
3. Beard C, Quickert M: Anatomy of the Orbit. Aesculapius, Birmingham, 1977, pp 2–17.
4. Hollinshead WH: Anatomy for Surgeons: The Head and Neck. Harper & Row, New York, 1968, pp 331–367, 501–504, 564–566.
5. Salache SJ, Bernstein G, Senkarik M: Surgical Anatomy of the Skin. Appleton & Lange, Norwalk, CT, 1988, pp 4–12.
6. Webster RC, Gaunt JM, Hamdan US, et al: Supraorbital and supratrochlear notches and foramina: anatomical variations and surgical relevance. Laryngoscope 96:311–315, 1986.
7. Stegman SJ: Planning closure of a surgical wound. J Dermatol Surg Oncol 4:390–393, 1978.
8. Burget GC, Menick FJ: The subunit principle in nasal reconstruction. Plast Reconstr Surg 76:239–247, 1985.
9. Borges AF: Relaxed skin tension lines (RSTL) versus other skin lines. Plast Reconstr Surg 73:144–150, 1984.
10. Bernstein G: Forces in skin tension lines of the face. In: Callen JP (ed): Current Issues in Dermatology. CK Hall, Boston, 1984, pp 213–235.
11. Dzubow LM: A histologic pattern approach to the anatomy of the face. J Dermatol Surg Oncol 12:712–718, 1986.
12. Chayen D, Nathan H: Anatomical observations on the subgaleotic fascia of the scalp. Acta Anat 87:427, 1974.
13. Dzubow LM: Facial Flap—Biomechanic and Regional Applications. Appleton & Lange, Norwalk, CT, 1989.
14. Donaxas MT, Anderson RL: Blepharoplasty: key anatomical concepts. Facial Plast Surg 1:259, 1984.
15. Rubin LR: The anatomy of a smile: its importance in the treatment of facial paralysis. Plast Reconstr Surg 53:384–387, 1974.
16. Rees TD: Aesthetic Plastic Surgery. WB Saunders, Philadelphia, 1980, pp 634–638.
17. Zide BM: Anatomy of the eyelids. Clin Plast Surg 8:623–634, 1981.
18. Zide BM: Nasal anatomy: the muscles and tip sensation. Aesthetic Plast Surg 9:193–196, 1985.
19. Weerda II: Embryology and structural anatomy of the external ear. Facial Plast Surg 2:85, 1985.
20. Cardoso de Castro C: The anatomy of the platysma muscle. Plast Reconstr Surg 66:680–683, 1980.
21. Mitz V, Peyronie M: The superficial musculoaponeurotic system (SMAS) in the parotid and cheek area. Plast Reconstr Surg 58:80–88, 1976.
22. Ruess W, Owsley J: The anatomy of the skin and facial layers of the face in aesthetic surgery. Clin Plast Surg 14:677, 1987.
23. Thaller SR, Kim S, Patterson H, et al: The submuscular aponeurotic system (SMAS): a histologic and comparative anatomy evaluation. Plast Reconstr Surg 86:690–696, 1990.
24. Cardoso de Castro C: The role of the superficial musculoaponeurotic system in face lift. Ann Plast Surg 16:279–286, 1986.
25. Owsley JQ Jr: SMAS-platysma face lift. Plast Reconstr Surg 71:573–576, 1983.
26. Hill EG Jr, McKinney WM: Vascular anatomy and pathology of the head and neck: method of corrosion casting. Adv Neurol 30:191–197, 1981.
27. Stock AL, Collins HP, Davidson TM: Anatomy of the superficial temporal artery. Head Neck Surg 2:466–469, 1980.
28. Abul-Hassan HS, Ascher GVD, Acland RD: Surgical anatomy and blood supply of the fascial layers of the temporal region. Plast Reconstr Surg 77:17–24, 1986.
29. Smith TE Jr: Surgical anatomy of the face. Otolaryngol Clin North Am 15:3–18, 1982.
30. Corso PF: Variations of the arterial, venous, and capillary circulation of the soft tissue of the head. Plast Reconstr Surg 27:160, 1961.
31. Sage H: Palpable cervical lymph nodes. JAMA 168:496–498, 1958.
32. Rouviere H: Anatomy of the Human Lymphatic System. Edwards Brothers, Ann Arbor, 1938, p 14.
33. Asarch RG: A review of the lymphatic drainage of the head and neck: Use in evaluation of potential metastases. J Dermatol Surg Oncol 8:869–872, 1982.
34. Hagensen CD: The Lymphatics in Cancer. WB Saunders, Philadelphia, 1972.
35. Panje WR: Local anesthesia of the face. J Dermatol Surg Oncol 5:311–315, 1979.
36. Bumstead RM, Ceilley RI: Local anesthesia of the auricle. J Dermatol Surg Oncol 5:448–449, 1979.
37. Baker DC, Conley J: Avoiding facial nerve injuries in rhytidectomy: anatomic variations and pitfalls. Plast Reconstr Surg 64:781–795, 1979.
38. Malone B, Maisel R: Anatomy of the facial nerve. Am J Otolaryngol 9:494, 1988.
39. Peterson R, Johnston D: Facile identification of the facial nerve branches. Facial Aesth Surg 14:785, 1987.
40. Bernstein L, Nelson RH: Surgical anatomy of the extraparotid distribution of the facial nerve. Arch Otolaryngol 110:177–183, 1984.
41. Katz AD, Catalano P: The clinical significance of the various anastomotic branches of the facial nerve: report of 100 patients. Arch Otolaryngol Head Neck Surg 113:959–962, 1987.
42. Greisen O: Aberrant course of the facial nerve. Arch Otolaryngol 101:327, 1975.

43. Grabski WJ, Salasche SJ: Management of temporal nerve injuries. J Dermatol Surg Oncol 11:145–151, 1985.
44. Ishikawa Y: An anatomical study on the distribution of the temporal branch of the facial nerve. J Craniomaxillofac Surg 18:287, 1990.
45. Ozersky D, Baek S-M, Biller HF: Percutaneous identification of the temporal branch of the facial nerve. Ann Plast Surg 4:276–280, 1980.
46. Rudolph R: Depth of the facial nerve in face lift dissections. Plast Reconstr Surg 85:537–544, 1990.
47. Moffat DA, Ramsden RT: The deformity produced by a palsy of the marginal mandibular branch of the facial nerve. J Laryngol Otol 91:401, 1977.
48. Dingman RO, Grabb WC: Surgical anatomy of the mandibular ramus of the facial nerve based on the dissection of 100 facial halves. Plast Reconstr Surg 29:266–272, 1962.
49. Ziarah HA: The surgical anatomy of the cervical distribution of the facial nerve. Br J Oral Surg 19:171, 1981.
50. King IJ, Motta G: Iatrogenic spinal accessory nerve palsy. Ann R Coll Surg Engl 65:35, 1983.

CHAPTER 6

Surgical Microbiology, Antibiotic Prophylaxis, and Antiseptic Technique

EDMUND R. HOBBS

Experience has shown wound infections to be uncommon with most cutaneous surgical procedures. Most cutaneous surgeons have wound infection rates well below the 1% standard for "clean" surgical procedures, which form the bulk of their practices. This situation probably results from the nature of the population served, the disease entities treated, and the setting in which patient care is delivered. Most procedures are relatively short and patients are generally healthy. They are not usually hospitalized and therefore not contaminated with the flora known to inhabit the hospital ward environment. The flora present are usually not the highly selected resistant organisms that typically result from antibiotic pressures within the hospital. High surgical wound infection rates may reflect poor technique, but for office cutaneous surgery the converse is not necessarily true: cutaneous surgeons cannot conclude that because their wound infection rate is low, their technique must be good.

Cutaneous surgeons are becoming increasingly involved in more sophisticated and complex outpatient procedures. As the scope of the surgical procedures broadens, cutaneous surgeons also find themselves undertaking longer and more difficult cases involving older, sicker, and more debilitated patients. They also find themselves on occasion in the hospital operating room working alongside other surgical specialists. In such scenarios, wound infection risks increase, and all reasonable, prudent, and scientifically sound steps that can be taken to reduce the incidence of wound infection should be pursued. No less can be asked in the office surgical environment, even when infection risks are fewer. When performing surgery, cutaneous surgeons are rightly held to the same standard of care that has been established for other surgeons.[1] The standards are no less applicable in the office surgery than in the ambulatory surgical facility or hospital operating room.

Determination of Relative Risk

A number of factors are important in the prevention of surgical wound infections. The literature is limited in the area of "clean" surgery. A scientific study of the importance or benefits of the many variables that exist in the surgical setting (for example, the role of the surgical cap in preventing clinical wound infection) requires an enormous study population when the prevailing infection rates are low. Such studies are unlikely to be performed, and even if they are, unlikely to be verified. This problem permeates much of this subject: antibiotic prophylaxis, hand washing, surgical attire, frequency and nature of disinfection of operatory surfaces, and surgical preparation. While there may or may not be scientific evidence of incremental benefit, standards of care nevertheless exist, and radical departure from them requires a reliable scientific basis or acceptance by the surgical community at large.

SPECIAL RISK FACTORS

The risk of developing a surgical wound infection is largely determined by three factors: host susceptibility, the condition of the wound at the end of the operation, and the amount and type of microbial contamination in the wound.[2] This chapter focuses on the third factor, which, in the "clean" surgical cases, forms the bulk of a cutaneous surgeon's practice but may not be the major factor involved in producing wound infection. A wound in healthy tissue is surprisingly resistant to infection even when contaminated with many microorganisms, but a wound containing foreign or necrotic material is highly susceptible to infection even if only a few microorganisms are present.[2] In most office surgery, improper technique is the major determinant of wound infection. Tissue must be handled gently, hemostasis achieved adequately without excessive electrocoagulation, and dead space closed with minimal use of sutures. Closure under tension, which reduces local perfusion and results in hypoxic conditions that allow bacterial proliferation, should be avoided. Probably as few as 15 microorganisms can produce septic lesions under the right conditions, whereas 100,000 bacteria per gram of tissue can be tolerated without inducing sepsis in other wounds.[3] Studies have shown that up to 92% of deep surgical wounds contain *Staphylococcus aureus* at the time of closure, with resultant clinical infection in less than 9% of the culture-positive wounds.[4]

Five factors have proved highly significant in determining the development of wound sepsis: potentially dirty types of procedures, the presence of bacteria at the end of the procedure, open multibed wards, patient age, and duration of surgery.[5] Infections in surgical patients result from exogenous or endogenous bacterial contamination.[6] Across the spectrum of surgical practice, more than 98% of surgical wound infections are considered to have originated from endogenous sources.[7] The likelihood of endogenous contamination depends on the number and virulence of the bacteria in the tissue being incised.[6] Adequate surgical preparation for cutaneous surgery eliminates transient flora and reduces resident flora to a minimum. The resident cutaneous flora that remain are not highly virulent in most situations encountered in office cutaneous surgical practices. These factors tend to reduce the threat of endogenously caused wound infections in the typical office procedure and elevate the importance of exogenous sources of infection.

Microbial Ecology

RESIDENT FLORA

Resident flora, also termed colonizing flora, are those organisms that can be persistently isolated from the skin of most persons. They are considered to be permanent residents of the skin and are not easily removed by friction.[8] As a rule, commensal bacteria are not highly virulent and help to protect the host from infection[7] by more pathogenic organisms. They do this by competing for substrates essential for the growth and survival of opportunistic bacteria, and by competing for the limited number of available tissue receptors. They also elaborate antibacterial substances and create a physiologic environment that inhibits the multiplication of transient pathogens. They may also induce an immune response that is cross reactive with other microorganisms.

The resident flora of normal human skin are the gram-positive Micrococcaceae (coagulase-negative staphylococci, *Peptococcus, Micrococcus* species), the gram-positive coryneform rods or diphtheroids (*Corynebacterium, Brevibacterium*), *Pityrosporum, Acinetobacter,* and *Propionibacterium.* Coagulase-negative staphylococci are the most prevalent resident flora, with counts as high as 10,000/sq cm on the face.[9] Of these, *Staphylococcus epidermidis* makes up more than half and preferentially colonizes the upper body.[10] *Corynebacterium* organisms also make up a significant portion of normal flora, especially in moist intertriginous areas, while *Brevibacterium* is frequently isolated from toe webs. Gram-positive *Propionibacterium* species are the most prevalent anaerobes of normal skin, with *P. acnes* the most predominant, reaching a density of 1 million/sq cm on the faces and shoulders of adults.[10] *Acinetobacter* are aerobic gram-negative rods that prefer the antecubital fossa.[9] *Pityrosporum* species are mycoflora.

Coagulase-positive *Staphylococcus aureus* can be found in intertriginous locations, especially the perineum, in up to 20% of normal persons, and may be carried in the noses of 20 to 40% of adults. From these sites, *S. aureus* may temporarily colonize other skin areas and be a source of infection, since it can survive in the environment for weeks or months.[7]

TRANSIENT FLORA

Transient flora, also termed noncolonizing or contaminating flora, are organisms that can be isolated from skin but not shown to be consistently present in most persons.[8] Organisms that are normal inhabitants of noncutaneous areas of the body may be present on the skin temporarily. Gram-negative rods that populate the GI tract, for example, may become transient flora in intertriginous areas as well as other sites.

Of greatest relevance to the cutaneous surgeon is which organisms are most likely to be pathogenic, and in what circumstances they are most likely to cause infection. Coagulase-negative staphylococci are notorious for infecting indwelling foreign devices such as prosthetic heart valves, shunts, catheters, and breast and joint implants. They are able to adhere rapidly to plastic surfaces and proliferate to form a colony. They produce an extracellular glycocalix slime that hinders antibiotic penetration, so that effective treatment may require removal of the indwelling device.[7] Coagulase-negative staphylococci may also cause osteomyelitis, urinary tract infections, and endocarditis in native valves. They may be the sole organism cultured from clinically infected surgical skin wounds. Most commonly, coagulase-positive *S. aureus* is the cause. Nasal carriage of group A streptococci occurs in less than 1% of the population, and skin carriage is most unusual.[7] When present, however, the organism may cause serious infection. Group B streptococci may colonize mucous membranes and cause recurrent erysipelas after gynecologic surgery.[10] *Pseudomonas aeruginosa,* which may be found in the ear canals and on other moist surfaces, may be implicated in severe wound infections of the external ear. *Propionibacterium acnes* can be the cause of endocarditis.[11]

The skin maintains a flora that differs remarkably little regardless of whether the host is normal or immunologically abnormal.[9] Some circumstances may alter skin flora and increase the risk of infection. Hemodialysis patients, intravenous drug abusers, diabetics, and hospital personnel are more prone to skin colonization by *S. aureus*.[10] Patients with psoriasis or atopic dermatitis also may have very high counts of *S. aureus*. Hospitalized patients typically have an increased number of gram-negative organisms. *S. aureus* colonization of the anterior nares is increased in patients taking isotretinoin. Renal transplant patients taking prednisone are at increased risk of bacterial infection. Immunosuppressed leukemia patients are more frequently and densely colonized with gram-negative bacilli.[9]

Topical Antimicrobial Agents

Topical antimicrobial agents[8] are used in two basic settings in cutaneous surgery: preoperative hand washing and surgical scrubbing of the operative site. Alcohol, chlorhexidine, and iodophors are the three agents currently used for these purposes. All have excellent killing capability for gram-positive bacteria but have variable capabilities for gram-negative bacteria, tubercle bacilli, and fungi. They also differ in rapidity of action, residual activity, degradation by organic material, and safety or toxicity.

Alcohols

Ethyl and isopropyl alcohol must be diluted with water in order to denature protein, which is their mechanism of action. Concentrations between 70 and 92% are most effective. Alcohol is the most rapidly acting agent of all for skin disinfection but has no residual activity. Nevertheless, bacterial counts continue to drop after application, probably because of the slow death of damaged organisms. Alcohol is superior to other agents in killing gram-negative bacteria, and while not sporicidal, it also kills many fungi and viruses, including cytomegalovirus and human immunodeficiency virus. The major disadvantage of alcohol is that it is both volatile and flammable, which means that it must be continually reapplied during skin preparation and must be allowed to dry thoroughly before laser or electrosurgical equipment is used, to prevent possible ignition. It dries and defats skin, but some recently marketed preparations with emollients have proved acceptable to users.[12] Although historically not popular in the United States, alcohol is the "gold standard" against which all other topical skin cleansing preparations are measured.

CHLORHEXIDINE

Chlorhexidine is inferior to other agents in killing *Mycobacterium tuberculosis* and fungi but is active against many viruses and gram-negative organisms. Its onset of action is intermediate and it acts by disrupting microbial cell membranes. Its most outstanding feature is its ability to bind to skin, remaining chemically active for at least 6 hours, which is the best persistence of any topical agent. This effect is not reduced by an alcohol wipe, an important feature if the skin is to be marked.[13] Chlorhexidine is not degraded by blood or other organic materials but is sensitive to pH effects, nonionic surfactants, and inorganic ions; it is therefore formula dependent. Chlorhexidine is not absorbed through the skin and consequently is remarkably safe and nonirritating. However, ototoxicity can result if it enters the middle ear, and it can cause keratitis if instilled into the eye. Chlorhexidine is available as a 4% detergent formulation and as an alcohol-based 0.5% hand rinse, which combines the rapid effects of alcohol with the persistence of chlorhexidine.

IODOPHORS

Iodophors kill by releasing free iodine, which penetrates cell walls, oxidizes, and substitutes for microbial contents. Approximately 2 minutes of contact time is required for free iodine release, and release is essentially stopped by drying. Moreover, its killing effectiveness is rapidly neutralized in the presence of organic material such as blood. These features tend to reduce an iodophor's effectiveness when used as a "paint" after surgical scrubbing and skin marking. Iodophors have minimal residual activity. They are as good as chlorhexidine against gram-negative organisms, but are somewhat irritating to skin and may cause allergic reactions in sensitive individuals. Toxicity by percutaneous absorption can occur. Iodophors are toxic to human cells and should not be allowed to enter the wound itself.[14, 15]

Surgical Hand Scrub

After surgical gloves, the surgical hand scrub is the second line of defense in preventing wound contamination from the surgeon's hands. Perforations may occur in gloves, as a result of either manufacturing defects or use, with such frequency that attention must be paid to the hands before gloving. Moreover, bacteria proliferate under gloves, and as procedures lengthen, the risk increases if perforation occurs. Consequently, surgical gloves are not a substitute for preoperative hand washing.[12]

Gloves are most subject to perforation at the fingertips. The periungual area harbors the most organisms, 90% of all flora found on the hands,[16] and therefore merits special attention. Nail polish should not be worn by the cutaneous surgeon because it is subject to chipping, peeling, and cracking, which create surface conditions likely to harbor microorganisms. Artificial nails should not be worn, as they discourage proper cleaning[12] and can foster the growth of gram-negative bacteria and fungi.[17, 18] Nails should be trimmed short to allow access for cleaning and to reduce risks of glove perforation. A nail stick and brush promote rapid and effective cleaning of periungual areas.

The objective of the preoperative scrub is to remove all debris and transient flora, to reduce all resident flora to minimal levels, and to inhibit the rapid rebound growth of microorganisms.[17] Hands and forearms should be free of open lesions, scratches, and breaks, which foster colonization. Rings, watches, and bracelets should be removed.

The traditional 5-minute surgical scrub of the hands and forearms with chlorhexidine or iodophor is still considered acceptable and efficacious. Chlorhexidine has proved less irritating, has much greater residual effect, and may be preferable, especially for procedures longer than 1 hour.[8, 19–21] Chlorhexidine can have greater persistence if left on the hands during surgery.[20]

It has been noted that the dermal abrasion resulting from extended surgical scrubs may promote colonization with pathogenic microorganisms. A 2-minute surgical scrub with a chlorhexidine sponge brush achieved significant bacterial count reductions, more so than povidone-iodine, and counts were further reduced with repeated use.[19] On the basis of the available evidence and cutaneous bacteriology of the hands, a preoperative scrub of at least 2 minutes using a brush on the nails and fingertip areas provides adequate disinfection.[22] A 2-minute wash with chlorhexidine detergent, followed by application of alcoholic chlorhexidine, ensures near-sterility of the hands with several hours of residual antiseptic activity.[6]

In appropriate concentrations, alcohols provide the most rapid and greatest reduction in microbial counts on skin.[8] A 1-minute immersion or scrub with alcohol has proved as effective as scrubbing for 4 to 7 minutes with other antiseptics.[21] Washing with alcohol for 3 minutes is as effective as 20 minutes of scrubbing.[8, 21] A 5-minute scrub[23] using a solution of 0.5% chlorhexidine in 70% ethyl alcohol is superior to 4% chlorhexidine and povidone-iodine in reducing bacterial counts, both immediately after scrubbing, after prolonged glove wear, and with repeated use. Commercially available agents have emollients and inert ingredients to retard alcohol evaporation.[24] They are applied without use of water and always after the fingernails, hands, and forearms have been cleaned.[8, 21] The solution is rubbed in until dry, and additional solution added for a total scrub time of 5 minutes; 10 to 30 ml of solution is required to wash the hands in this fashion.[8, 21]

It is also important for surgeons to wash their hands postoperatively to remove any blood, bacteria, or viruses that may have entered through glove perforation. In most cases 15 seconds should suffice, and particular attention is again devoted to the nails. The postoperative scrub should become a routine part of every surgical procedure.[22]

Preparing the Patient's Skin for Surgery

It is not possible to sterilize the skin, as approximately 20% of cutaneous bacteria reside beneath the surface[2, 25] in adnexal structures. Transient bacteria are easily re-

moved, and once removed do not re-establish themselves during surgery.[26] Scrubbing to remove resident bacteria carries some hazards, because skin is abraded and bacteria are exposed, contaminating the previously prepared area.[2, 25] A vigorous scrub could also theoretically cause dissemination of malignant cells from some types of skin cancers.[2]

The surgical scrub is a time-honored ritual, but evidence for its efficacy is hard to find.[25] The rationale for its use parallels the considerations for the preoperative scrub of the surgeon's hands. The selection of antimicrobial agents is also the same. Alcohols, iodophors, and chlorhexidine can be used after the patient's skin has been physically cleaned. A rapid and significant reduction in microbial counts is the major desired effect.[21] Initial bacterial kill is greater with a 1-minute alcohol cleansing than with a 5-minute iodophor scrub.[27] Chlorhexidine should not be used in periorbital areas or instilled into the ear. Working from the operative site outward, a wide skin area is thoroughly but gently scrubbed, then allowed to air dry. Most agents are as effective as they are going to be after 2 minutes of application.[22]

The only reasons to remove hair from the operative site are if it mechanically interferes with accurate anatomic approximation of the wound[22] or if it compromises effective dressing applications. Shaving also increases wound infection rates.[22, 25, 28] When it is necessary to remove hair, it should be clipped with scissors in the operatory immediately before the procedure.[25, 28]

Preoperative Showers

Repeated preoperative showering and scrubbing with chlorhexidine is more effective than use of other agents in lowering bacterial colony counts at incision sites and reducing the frequency of intraoperative wound contamination.[29–31] The efficacy of this procedure in preventing postoperative wound infection, however, continues to be debated.[2, 28, 29, 32] Perhaps its use the evening before and morning of a surgical procedure in high-risk patients such as diabetics, atopic individuals, or the immunosuppressed should be considered as an alternative to prophylactic antibiotics.[2, 22, 25]

Surgical Gloves

Sterile surgical gloves are the most important factor responsible for reducing wound infection risks in a surgical procedure.[33] However, the gloves may leak owing to manufacturing defects, are subject to puncture and tear during use, and promote bacterial growth on the hands of the surgeon. Sterile latex surgical glove standards set by the American Society for Testing and Materials allow a failure rate of 1.5% when tested by the watertight method.[34] One study showed that up to 3% of such gloves fail integrity tests for inspection, air inflation, water immersion, and water filling.[35] All failed gloves admitted a solution of safranin in alcohol applied to the surface after donning. Failure rates for nonsterile vinyl and latex procedure gloves are significantly higher. Moreover, failure rates progressively increase as the gloves are worn for longer periods. A series of manipulations designed to simulate 15 minutes of clinical activity in an intensive care unit resulted in failure rates as high as 66%.[34]

The surgeon cannot take for granted the integrity of the gloves, even when no puncture occurs. About 30% of surgical gloves become punctured during use without the surgeon's knowledge,[21, 36] increasing the risks of transmission of bacteria from the surgeon's hands to the wound. When gloves are punctured, most of the punctures occur in the fingertip portion of the glove.[22] Gloves are designed to be thin at the fingertips to allow for maximal sensitivity.[17, 37] Moreover, it is well recognized that the greatest number of microorganisms found on the hands occur around and under the fingernails, with mean numbers of bacteria per interspace exceeding 100 million colony forming units.[38] For these reasons, the surgeon's fingernails must be kept trimmed and special attention paid them during the preoperative handwash.

Bacterial counts on the hands gradually rise after gloving, as the warm moist environment created by the glove encourages bacterial proliferation.[8, 22] The longer the procedure, the greater is the bacterial load. The organism most frequently isolated is the common skin pathogen, coagulase-negative *Staphylococcus epidermidis*, in hands subjected to preoperative washing.[20] If the hands are not scrubbed adequately before gloving, the environment is well suited to gram-negative proliferation.[22]

For these reasons, surgical gloves cannot be used in lieu of a good preoperative surgical hand wash.[12] Gloves are only the frontline of defense, a line that fails often enough to render important the state of hygiene of the surgeon's hands.

Surgical Attire

It is well established that people are the major source of bacterial contamination in the operatory,[33] and the normal desquamation process plays a major role in the dispersal of airborne bacteria. The clothing worn by surgical staff should be designed to minimize bacterial shedding.[18] One-piece coverall suits or two-piece scrub attire, with tops tucked into trousers, are recommended in the hospital environment but are probably not necessary during office surgery if a cover gown is worn. It is known that use of trousers, as opposed to dresses, decreases bacterial dispersal rates, and consequently is preferable. Similarly, long-sleeved attire is advocated to contain body scurf. Clothing should be changed whenever it becomes visibly soiled or wet.

Surgical gowns have been shown to reduce bacterial dispersion rates by 30%,[39] with nonwoven fabrics about ten times more effective than cotton. Nonwoven materials are also effective in reducing the number of bacteria on the surface of the gown.[40] These fabrics are made from fibers and appear under the microscope as a random mat. They are generally very comfortable, allow easy passage of air, and work by trapping bacteria-laden particles. These gowns are disposable and should be discarded upon conclusion of a surgical procedure.

Although surgical masks, caps, and hoods have not been shown to reduce overall bacterial contamination in the operating room environment, their use by the surgical team can reduce the number of bacteria-laden particles falling onto or projected into the wound intraoperatively. Masks decrease the spread of contaminated droplets by filtration and alter the direction of dispersal from the upper respiratory tract during talking, coughing, or sneezing. They become wet and laden with microorganisms during use and should be removed and discarded upon conclusion of a procedure. Their use is also recommended as a means of reducing the surgical team's exposure to potentially infective aerosolized material from the patient.[41] For the same reason, the eyes should be protected whenever there is a risk of splashing the face. Caps or hoods help to contain hair and dander, which are major sources of particulate-carrying bacteria.[40] Shoe covers have no proved significance in reducing the incidence of postoperative wound infection and their use is not necessary.[18]

The main source of bacteria in the operatory is the people in the room, their bacteria being dispersed into the air and deposited by gravity onto surfaces.[39] Humans shed one outermost layer of skin cells per day, amounting to 1 billion squames per person per day.[39] This material may carry both transient and resident flora, both of which may cause wound infection. This is extremely important, since one in four persons carries *Staphylococcus aureus*. More important than the presence of bacteria is the tendency for them to be shed or dispersed. It is known that some people shed at higher rates than others, men more than women. A shedder can disperse up to 100,000 organisms per minute.

Regardless of staphylococcal carrier status, it is obviously important that the surgical staff maintain a high level of personal hygiene. Since scurf shedding is reduced after showering,[42] a morning shower, with sufficient mechanical abrasion to dislodge bacteria-laden squames, is advisable. Particular attention should be paid to the face, neck, and ears. It has been shown that bacterial growth on agar plates placed on the operating table during surgery consisted of the same flora isolated from facial areas of the surgical staff.[43]

DRAPES

Body drapes are necessary to keep patients warm, protect their clothing, and prevent bacteria on their skin and clothing from being transferred to the operative site. One hospital study showed a substantial reduction in sepsis after disposable drapes and gowns were used in preference to cotton, although it was not possible to determine whether the benefit derived from the drapes or the gowns.[39] A clean sheet may be satisfactory for this purpose in the office surgical setting. In the vicinity of the wound, drapes must be sterile. Their permeability and the type of fabric have little direct effect on the deposition of bacteria from the air or by direct contact. However, the use of fabrics that are more impermeable than cotton reduces the number of bacteria passing through the drape from the patient's skin.[39]

Wound Classification

Surgical wounds are classified[44] by the degree of contamination that occurs or is expected to occur. Class I, "clean" surgery, with proper aseptic technique, produces a clean wound defined as a nontraumatic, uninfected operative wound in which neither the respiratory, alimentary, or genitourinary tracts nor the oropharyngeal cavities are entered. Clean wounds are elective, primarily closed, and undrained. Most cutaneous surgery cases fall into this category. Class II is "clean-contaminated" surgery, which would be considered clean but for controlled transection of the mucous membranes that cannot be "sterilized" during the surgical preparation without unusual contamination during the course of the procedure. Wounds that are mechanically drained are also considered to be clean-contaminated; transoral surgery is one good example. Class III surgery produces "contaminated wounds" that include open, fresh traumatic wounds, the products of (1) operations in which there is gross spillage from the gastrointestinal tract, (2) surgical procedures with a major break in sterile technique such as open cardiac massage, or (3) incisions encountering acute, nonpurulent inflammation. Class IV surgery produces "dirty and infected wounds," including old traumatic wounds and those involving clinical infection or perforated viscera.

Antibiotic Prophylaxis for Wound Infections

To date, antibiotic prophylaxis, defined as the administration of antibiotics in the absence of established infection for the purpose of preventing infection, has not been proved to be of value in class I "clean" surgery except in unusual situations such as peripheral vascular reconstruction[45] or prosthetic joint insertion.[46] Controlled trials are scarce,[47] but the thrust of the literature is that the wound infection rate in most class I surgery is unmodified by antibiotic administration, to the extent that surgeons' infection rate in such procedures can be used as a measure of their surgical skill.[45, 48] The role of prophylactic antibiotics in the surgical treatment of axillary hyperhidrosis has been studied, and no difference was found in clinical wound infection rates between those receiving prophylactic antibiotics and those receiving placebo.[49] Previously, it had been shown that antibiotics were of no value in preventing wound infection in groin hernia repairs.[47] Postoperative wound infection rates in patients undergoing major class I head and neck surgical procedures such as parotidectomy, thyroidectomy, and submandibular gland excision have also been studied, and it was found that antibiotic prophy-

laxis did not reduce the risk of postoperative wound infection.[50]

In contrast, antibiotics have proved of value in some "clean-contaminated" class II surgery. A number of drugs or drug combinations have similar efficacy in preventing postoperative wound infections in major head and neck surgery patients contaminated by exposure to oropharyngeal secretions, and the use of perioperative antibiotics is now considered to be required in such cases.[51] Likewise, short-term perioperative antibiotics have proved effective in preventing postoperative wound infection in transoral orthognathic, craniofacial, and tumor surgery.[48] On the other hand, antibiotic prophylaxis is of no value in intranasal surgery such as rhinoplasty and submucous resection of the septum, even when nasal packing is left in place, in spite of the obvious contamination present in this area.[52] Similarly, prophylactic antibiotics have not been shown to be of value in routine ear and mastoid surgery.[53]

In addition, antibiotics have not proved effective in preventing infection in simple hand lacerations.[54] Lacerations of the face, scalp, feet, and trunk have also been studied[55] without showing the effectiveness of antibiotics in wound management, even in the presence of gross contamination. Good surgical wound management with debridement and irrigation is apparently all that is needed.[55]

In spite of the lack of scientific evidence supporting antibiotic prophylaxis for wound infection, its use in situations in which wound infection rates are low is common. The practice is understandable in circumstances in which the results of wound infection can be catastrophic, such as the complete hearing loss that inevitably results from postoperative infection after stapedectomy.[53] Such dire consequences are rarely associated with cutaneous surgery, in which the adverse effects of wound infection are usually limited to inconvenience, prolonged healing, and increased scarring or cosmetic deficit. In the United States, about one third of plastic surgeons customarily prescribe prophylactic antibiotics to patients undergoing cutaneous flap or graft surgery.[56] Although many plastic surgeons cite medicolegal considerations as a major motivating factor, most believe that there is a scientific basis for their decision, and the use of prophylactic antibiotics has become increasingly common.

Current practices of antibiotic prophylaxis in surgery too often result from custom, dependence on poorly designed clinical trials, or unsupported dogmatic beliefs.[47] Factors at work in the decision to administer prophylactic antibiotics include considerations of greater infection risk owing to the specific operative site (e.g., the perinasal areas), patient age, the size and vascularity of the wound, and the amount of dissection required. Prolonged procedures with local hypoxia due to poor perfusion, epinephrine use, and dehydration all increase the risk of infection,[54] as does tissue damage from poor surgical technique, excessive electrocoagulation, implantation of foreign suture material, and dead space. Surgeons may also be influenced by the standard of cleanliness maintained in the operative theatre and their estimation of the adequacy of the preoperative preparation. In the face of so many factors that appear to elevate infection risk, surgeons may be tempted to employ prophylactic antibiotics in an effort to effect some counterbalance. Proponents of this practice point to the benignity and relatively low cost of short-term antibiotic administration and argue that while controlled studies do not prove efficacy, antibiotics may successfully prevent wound infection and are therefore worth employing.

On the negative side,[52] the indiscriminate use of preventive chemotherapy may encourage laxity of good surgical technique, result in more allergic and toxic reactions, promote the selection of antibiotic-resistant organisms, be responsible for superinfection, deprive the patient of an adequate stimulus for antibody formation when administered prematurely, and increase the cost of medical care unnecessarily.

If prophylactic antibiotics are to be employed, certain principles must be applied. It is clear that to be maximally effective, the antibiotic must be present in the tissue at the time of wounding. The efficacy of antibiotics is reduced with time after wounding to the extent that if they are administered more than 3 hours after bacterial contamination, they will have no effect.[45, 48, 49, 51, 56] Because of variable gastrointestinal absorption, many recommend that antibiotics be administered parenterally just before the start of the procedure. If administered orally, antibiotics must be given in sufficient dosage and with enough lead time to generate adequate tissue levels by the time the procedure begins; however, they must not be given so early that normal microbial floral populations are altered, resulting in depression of host defense mechanisms and selection of resistant pathogens. The antibiotic level must be maintained in the tissue throughout the procedure. In practice, this means that the antibiotic should be administered an hour or two before surgery in twice the usual therapeutic dose, and repeated at half the usual therapeutic interval during the procedure.[48] For many cutaneous surgical procedures, a single preoperative dose suffices. Longer procedures may require one or two additional doses. Continuation of prophylactic antibiotics for more than 24 hours after surgery is not justified.[43, 46, 57, 58]

Antibiotic selection must take into consideration the organisms that are likely to be present and their potential for causing wound infection. In procedures contaminated with oropharyngeal secretions, wound infections are commonly polymicrobial. Anaerobic organisms that are potential pathogens include *Fusobacterium, Bacteroides,* and *Peptococcus* species,[51] and antibiotics should be used that cover these organisms. Protection against gram-negative aerobic organisms, however, is not necessary.[59] The aerobic gram-negative rods *Klebsiella, Enterobacter, Serratia,* and *Pseudomonas,* frequently isolated from postoperative wounds in oncologic head and neck surgery, more likely represent colonization than pathogenicity.[59] Thus, the addition of gentamicin to clindamycin for prophylaxis in such cases yielded no added benefit.[59] Aerobic gram-positive species cultured in such cases included streptococci, especially *S. viridans,* and coagulase-positive and -negative staphylococci. First-generation cephalosporins effectively cover

these organisms but do not address the anaerobes that may be pathogenic in such cases. Clindamycin and the third-generation cephalosporins provide adequate coverage for the entire spectrum.[51, 60]

Because of their antimicrobial spectrum and relative lack of toxicity, cephalosporins are the agents of choice for surgical procedures in which skin flora and the normal flora of the gastrointestinal and genitourinary tracts are the most likely pathogens.[54] First-generation cephalosporins are adequate and advantageous in such settings.[51, 54] However, their use is contraindicated when there is a history of immediate or accelerated reaction to penicillin. When first-generation cephalosporins are only briefly used in the perioperative period, many of the objections to prophylactic antibiotics are minimized. Allergic reactions and side effects are unlikely, cost is manageable, and there is insufficient time for superinfection or the emergence of resistant organisms.[54]

The issue of the efficacy of antibiotics in "clean" class I procedures remains, however, and the concept of a protective umbrella afforded by antibiotic prophylaxis is probably a myth.[52] In such cases the potential degree of contamination is small, its appearance episodic, the variety of potential organisms large, and the actual incidence of wound infection low.[56] It therefore seems prudent, if antibiotics are to be used at all, to reserve their use in class I cutaneous surgical procedures for patients in whom the risk of infection might be increased: e.g., patients with compromised host defenses, including poorly controlled diabetics, alcoholics, the malnourished, the obese, or the aged. Patients with end-stage renal disease or myeloproliferative disorders and those undergoing radiation or immunosuppressive therapy (e.g., with cyclosporine, steroids, or chemotherapeutic agents)[48] also fall into this category. "Clean" procedures with prolonged operative times or flap reconstruction might also be considered.[60] Antibiotics may also be warranted when artificial prosthetic materials are being implanted,[46, 58] since the number of bacteria required to cause infection is less when artificial devices are implanted.[39]

Prophylaxis of Bacterial Endocarditis

In 1990 the American Heart Association (AHA) promulgated revised guidelines for prevention of bacterial endocarditis.[61] The committee involved noted that the recommendations were based only on indirect information, since there was an absence of clinical trials. There is no evidence that antibiotic prophylaxis prevents infective endocarditis, although this appears reasonable on the basis of animal experiments.[58, 62] The guidelines have been criticized as being complicated, at times illogical, and difficult to follow.[64] Only a minority of all cases of infective endocarditis are associated with invasive surgical or dental procedures, and recommended prophylactic regimens do not cover all the known infecting organisms.[63] As a consequence, even if a perfect

TABLE 6–1. **MEDICATIONS USED TO PREVENT BACTERIAL ENDOCARDITIS FOR ORAL, DENTAL, OR UPPER RESPIRATORY TRACT PROCEDURES IN PATIENTS AT RISK**

Drug	Oral Dosage for Adults	Oral Dosage for Children
Amoxicillin	3 gm 1 hr before procedure, then 1.5 gm 6 hr later	50 mg/kg 1 hr before procedure, then 25 mg/kg 6 hr later
For Penicillin-Allergic Patients		
Erythromycin stearate	1 gm 2 hr before procedure, then 500 mg 6 hr later	20 mg/kg 2 hr before procedure, then 10 mg/kg 6 hr later
Erythromycin ethylsuccinate	800 mg 2 hr before procedure, then 400 mg 6 hr later	20 mg/kg 2 hr before procedure, then 10 mg/kg 6 hr later
Clindamycin	300 mg 1 hr before procedure, then 150 mg 6 hr later	10 mg/kg 1 hr before procedure, then 5 mg/kg 6 hr later

Note: Total pediatric dose should not exceed total adult dose.

prophylactic agent existed, the impact on the overall incidence of infective endocarditis would be small. Cost effectiveness is difficult to argue, since it costs more than $2 million to prevent one case of infective endocarditis in mitral valve prolapse.[63] It has been calculated that if the guidelines were implemented as recommended, far more people would die from penicillin anaphylaxis than from infective endocarditis.[64] Nevertheless, the existence of such guidelines creates significant pressures to conform. In California a patient with a heart defect successfully sued a dentist for not administering prophylactic antibiotics, even though infective endocarditis did not develop.[64]

The AHA guidelines contain little information applicable to cutaneous surgery. The most direct recommendation relates to surgical procedures on infected or contaminated tissues and advises the use of antibiotics "directed against the most likely bacterial pathogen."[61] This is the most probable setting in which the cutaneous surgeon is likely to be called on to use antibiotic prophylaxis for infective endocarditis. Incision and drainage of an abscess, for example, warrants use of prophylactic antibiotics in cardiac patients. Cardiac patients who have active atopic dermatitis, whose skin is likely to be heavily colonized, also appear to qualify, as do patients with eroded skin lesions. In one study, intraoperative blood cultures were performed in 35 patients with eroded tumors, and bacteremia was detected in only one, in spite of suboptimal preparation of the operative site.[65] The organisms most frequently colonizing eroded tumors were *S. aureus*, coagulase-negative staphylococci, diphtheroids, and streptococci, which are the organisms commonly found in cases of prosthetic valve endocarditis. On the basis of these findings, it was recommended that prophylaxis be used in cardiac patients with eroded tumors, but only those at high risk because of having a prosthetic valve.

The AHA guidelines recommend prophylactic antibiotics in oral and respiratory tract procedures as well as for gastrointestinal and genitourinary tract procedures on patients with certain cardiac conditions. Viridans streptococci are the most common infecting organisms in oral and upper airway cases, and enterococci (*E. faecalis*, *E. faecians*) in the gastrointestinal and genitourinary setting.[63] On occasion, the cutaneous surgeon may operate on the oral, nasal, rectal, or genitourinary mucosa, and these guidelines should be consulted (Tables 6–1 and 6–2).[61] Such guidelines have also been applied to patients with prosthetic joints.[64] The surgeon should be aware that parenteral antibiotic prophylaxis is necessary in gastrointestinal and genitourinary tract procedures in high-risk patients such as those with prosthetic valves or surgically constructed systemic-pulmonary shunts, or those who have had endocarditis previously. For those at lower risk, the standard oral regimen suffices. Patients who take continuous oral penicillin for rheumatic fever prophylaxis require an alternative regimen.[62] Intramuscular administration is to be avoided in anticoagulated patients.[61]

The overwhelming majority of cutaneous surgery

TABLE 6–2. **MEDICATIONS USED TO PREVENT BACTERIAL ENDOCARDITIS FOR GASTROINTESTINAL AND GENITOURINARY PROCEDURES IN PATIENTS AT RISK**

Drug	Dosage for Adults	Dosage for Children
Ampicillin, gentamicin, and amoxicillin	2 gm IV or IM, plus 1.5 mg/kg 30 min before procedure, then 1.5 gm orally 6 hr later	50 mg/kg 2 mg/kg 50 mg/kg; follow-up doses should be half initial dose
For Penicillin-Allergic Patients		
Vancomycin and gentamicin	1 gm IV over 1 hr, plus 1.5 mg/kg IV or IM 1 hr before procedure, then repeated in 8 hr	20 mg/kg 2 mg/kg; follow-up doses should be half initial dose
For Low-Risk Patients		
Amoxicillin	3 gm PO 1 hr before procedure, then 1.5 gm 6 hr later	50 mg/kg

Note: Total pediatric dose should not exceed total adult dose.

TABLE 6–3. CARDIAC CONDITIONS THAT REQUIRE PROPHYLACTIC ANTIBIOTICS

Prosthetic cardiac valves (including bioprosthetic and homograft valves)
Most congenital cardiac malformations
Rheumatic and other acquired valvular dysfunction, even after surgery
History of bacterial endocarditis, even in absence of heart disease
Mitral valve prolapse with valvular regurgitation
Hypertrophic cardiomyopathy

This table lists selected conditions and is not meant to be all-inclusive.

cases do not involve mucous membranes or infected or contaminated tissues, however. Antibiotics are not required, according to AHA guidelines, in cesarean section, in diagnostic cardiac catheterization and angiography, or in coronary artery bypass surgery when adequate aseptic techniques are used, because of the very low incidence of infective endocarditis. Most cutaneous surgery is analogously low risk. In four reviews that included hundreds of endocarditis cases, none was solely due to skin manipulation.[66] Blood cultures taken during surgery in 15 patients with noneroded skin tumors showed no instances of bacteremia in this small control group.[65] No current guidelines call for the use of prophylactic antibiotics in cardiac patients undergoing surgery on intact, uninfected skin. The suggestion[67] that high-risk patients receive antibiotics whenever the skin is incised is unsupported.[65, 66] It is good practice, however, to consult the patient's internist or cardiologist for recommendations before proceeding with any cutaneous surgical procedure if the patient has a cardiac condition at risk for endocarditis.

There are many cardiac conditions for which antibiotic prophylaxis is recommended (Table 6–3).[61] Note that coronary artery bypass patients do not require prophylaxis in the absence of other conditions (Table 6–4).[61] Mitral valve prolapse does not require prophylaxis unless accompanied by the systolic murmur of mitral regurgitation.[61–63, 68]

Alternative infective endocarditis prophylaxis protocols exist. A local AHA chapter is a convenient source for the most current recommendations. The Endocarditis Working Party of the British Society of Antimicrobial Chemotherapy has guidelines,[68] as does *The Medical Letter*.[62]

No specific drugs or dosing schedule recommendations are made in the AHA guidelines for the situation in which a cutaneous surgeon is most likely to be called on to administer prophylaxis for infective endocarditis: surgery in the presence of infected or contaminated tissue. Reasonable recommendations in this setting appear to be dicloxacillin, 2 gm orally 1 hour before surgery, followed by 1 gm 6 hours later; or erythromycin, 1 gm 1 hour before surgery, and 0.5 gm 6 hours later for the penicillin-allergic patient.[67] Likewise, 1 to 2 gm orally of dicloxacillin or a first-generation cephalosporin, followed by 0.5 gm orally every 6 hours for one or two doses, would also be adequate. For patients with prosthetic valves implanted within the previous 60 days, in which diphtheroids are more probably pathogenic, parenteral vancomycin was advised.

Operatory Discipline and Design

Because the fundamental source of bacteria in the operative setting is the people in the room, traffic flow into the operatory should be restricted. The room should have a door that is kept closed during the procedure, and individuals not involved in the procedure should not be permitted to enter. All surfaces, including walls and floors, should be washable. Enamel or epoxy wall paints and vinyl composition tile floors are practical and yet not expensive.

The source of airborne bacteria in the operatory is the skin of the people in the room.[69] Current operating room air standards[42] call for 20 to 25 air changes per hour, with inlets high above the floor and as remote from the exhaust outlets as possible. Air filtration requires 90% efficiency in removing particles greater than 0.5 micron, and approximately 0.005 inch of water positive pressure. Temperature and humidity ranges are 65° to 75°F and 50 to 55%, respectively. However, very little evidence supports such standards. Even though viable particle counts in the operating room are reduced significantly with such air management schemes as laminar flow, it is difficult to show a clear correlation with lower wound infection rates.[42] Joint replacement surgery, with the insertion of prosthetic materials, has become the prototype of refined clean wound surgery. Ultraclean laminar airflow systems are often employed, but even the most recent studies do not support or refute the absolute need for such systems. Laminar clean airflow rooms have not produced an abrupt, defined reduction in wound infections when put into effect, and their use is not currently thought to be necessary even for procedures that demand the highest standards of cleanliness.[42]

Cutaneous surgery does not carry the infection risks or consequences of joint replacement surgery, and the issue is not laminar flow, but the necessity for adherence to currently established operating room air standards. There are no data showing differences in wound infection rates between cutaneous surgical procedures done in such rooms and others. Wound infection rates for cutaneous surgical procedures done in outpatient clinics are not higher than the accepted rates for surgical procedures done in modern hospital operating rooms.[70] It can be convincingly argued that low wound infection

TABLE 6–4. CARDIAC CONDITIONS THAT DO *NOT* REQUIRE PROPHYLACTIC ANTIBIOTICS

Isolated secundum atrial septal defect
Previous coronary artery bypass graft surgery (CABG)
Mitral valve prolapse without valvular regurgitation*
Surgical repair without residua beyond 6 mo of secundum atrial septal defect, ventricular septal defect, or patent ductus arteriosus
History of rheumatic fever without valvular dysfunction
Cardiac pacemakers and implanted defibrillators
Physiologic, functional, or innocent heart murmurs
History of Kawasaki's disease without valvular dysfunction

*Individuals with mitral valve prolapse associated with thickening or redundancy of the valve leaflets, particularly men over 45 years of age, may be at increased risk for bacterial endocarditis.

rates in current office surgical rooms, most of which do not meet such standards, indicate that air quality is not a major issue. In wound washout studies, skin contamination has been found to contribute more to high bacterial counts than does air contamination.[42] The incremental benefit to be achieved by manipulating ventilation in the office surgical setting, while adhering to the basic tenets of perioperative discipline and good surgical technique, is probably marginal, if it exists at all. Ventilation systems should be designed for patient and operating staff comfort. Poorly designed or poorly maintained systems, however, can be responsible for outbreaks of wound infection.[42]

Disinfection of Devices and Surfaces[71]

Critical items are defined as those such as scalpels, needles, and surgical instruments that enter sterile tissue. These items require sterilization, the complete destruction of all forms of microbial life. Sterilization requires steam under pressure, dry heat, or ethylene oxide gas, most useful for the heat-labile items. Semicritical items such as anoscopes have contact with mucous membranes or with nonintact skin. These items require "high-level disinfection" destroying all microorganisms except high numbers of bacterial spores. This class of disinfectants includes demand-released chlorine dioxide, 6% stabilized hydrogen peroxide, and glutaraldehyde. High-level disinfectants must be used for more than 20 minutes to be effective. Glutaraldehyde can also sterilize when properly used; it is sporicidal when activated to a pH of 7.5 to 8.5, but then has a shelf life of only 14 days. Its efficiency is also affected by organic stress and dilution and it is irritating to the eyes and nasal passages. This agent must be rinsed from a sterilized instrument, which is a sterilization method incompatible with the use of surgical packs. It also takes 6 to 10 hours of exposure to sterilize items with this agent. For these reasons, glutaraldehyde is best restricted to use as a high-level disinfectant.[71]

Items that only come into contact with intact skin are termed noncritical and require less than 10 minutes of intermediate- or low-level disinfection, depending on the necessity for tuberculocidal activity. Intermediate-level disinfection inactivates *Mycobacterium tuberculosis*, vegetative bacteria, most viruses, and fungi but does not necessarily kill bacterial spores. Low-level disinfection cannot be relied on to kill tubercle bacilli and does not sufficiently address spores. Isopropyl alcohol 70%, phenolic germicidal detergent solutions, and iodophor germicidal detergent solutions qualify as intermediate-level disinfectants, with sodium hypochlorite and quaternary ammonium compounds added for low-level disinfection. "Quats" are not tuberculocidal or virucidal against hydrophilic viruses such as echovirus and coxsackievirus. The disadvantage of alcohol is that it tends to damage the shellac mounting of lensed instruments, swells and hardens rubber and plastic tubing, and bleaches rubber and plastic. Alcohol is also flammable and evaporates rapidly, making extended contact times difficult to achieve. Hypochlorites are relatively unstable and corrosive and are inactivated by organic matter. The phenolics are the most useful agents for decontaminating the operatory; although not sporicidal, they are bactericidal, virucidal, fungicidal, and tuberculocidal at recommended dilutions.

Regardless of the level of disinfection required, instruments used on patients should first be cleaned to remove all foreign material before disinfection or sterilization. This may be accomplished with water, mechanical action, and detergents. Any Environmental Protection Agency–registered disinfectant or detergent should be adequate for cleaning surfaces contaminated with blood. Critical items are then heat sterilized and semicritical items disinfected for at least 20 minutes with an agent such as glutaraldehyde. Operatory surfaces, including trays, tables, and counters, are best cleaned with phenolics. Amphyl, Lysol, LPH, Matar, Staphene, Backdown, and Disofect II are product brand names in this category, but should not be used on surfaces that come into contact with newborns. Patient care equipment surfaces should be disinfected between individual patient use, and linen changed. Other operatory surfaces not in direct contact with patients or specimens may be cleaned on a daily basis.

Instruments

All surgical instruments should be decontaminated immediately after a surgical procedure, ideally with a washer-sterilizer.[72] When done manually, decontamination should take place under water in a detergent or disinfectant solution. Instruments are then processed in an ultrasonic cleaner to remove any remaining bioburden from cracks and crevices. Ultrasonic cleaning of dissimilar metals may cause etching or pitting, and chrome-plated instruments may be damaged by this process. Instruments with moving parts are then lubricated with an antimicrobial, water-soluble lubricant and drained. Proper lubrication lessens the growth of bacteria and allows the penetration of steam. All instruments are then inspected before storage or sterilization.

Moist heat in the form of saturated steam under pressure is the most dependable agent for the destruction of microbial life.[44] It is also the most applicable technique used in office surgery. The process is economical, without toxic residue, easily monitored, and rapid. The microbicidal power results from two esssential actions: wetting and heating. Saturated steam at 121°C for 15 minutes kills all bacteria and spores. Chemical monitors, indicators on the autoclave pack or tape that change color when autoclaved, are useful for identifying which packs have been sterilized. Quality control is ensured by microbiologic testing, done by placing a paper strip dosed with 100,000 heat-resistant dry spores, packaged to permit aseptic retrieval and culturing, in a test location such as the least accessible part of the largest surgical pack. An alternative biologic indicator system offers on-site monitoring capability with self-contained ampules of *Bacillus stearothermophilus* spores suspended in a culture medium containing a pH indicator. Acid production during growth changes the color, facilitating detection. Biologic indicators should be used at least once a week and in every load that contains an implantable device.

Sterile packs must be kept dry and stored in closed cabinets, protected from vermin, rather than on open shelves. Safe storage time in closed cabinets is typically two to three times as long as that on open shelves.[44] Two layers of single-wrapped muslin are safe for 1 week in a closed cabinet, and two layers of double-wrapped muslin last 7 weeks. Single-wrapped two-way crepe paper, single layer, is good for at least 8 weeks in a closed cabinet. Heat-sealed paper or transparent plastic pouches are sterile for at least 1 year, even on open shelves.

Sterilization by ethylene oxide is more complex and less reliable than steam.[44] Consequently, this technique is not suited to office surgery. The process is most reliable when applied to clean, dry surfaces that do not absorb the chemical. Ethylene oxide is toxic and mutagenic; a minimum of 24 hours' aeration is necessary to ensure removal of the gas from sterilized articles. When the office surgeon requires ethylene oxide sterilization for heat-labile items, it is often best to contract with a nearby hospital or ambulatory surgical facility for the service.

Powered surgical instruments are decontaminated in accordance with the manufacturer's instructions: cleaned with a mild detergent or wiped with a disinfectant, inspected, and steam sterilized when possible. Ethylene oxide does not readily diffuse through greases and lubricants.

SUMMARY

Despite the relatively low risk of wound infection for most common elective cutaneous surgical procedures, routine observation of strict aseptic technique must be carefully followed to obtain the best results. Knowledge of the pre-existing medical conditions that require prophylactic antibiotics before a cutaneous surgical procedure is also exceedingly important. Recognition of these facts will allow the cutaneous surgeon to provide the best possible care to patients with the least risk of producing a complication as a result of surgical wound infection.

REFERENCES

1. Sebben JE: Sterile technique in dermatologic surgery: what is enough? J Dermatol Surg Oncol 14:487–489, 1988.
2. Warner C: Skin preparation in the surgical patient. J Natl Med Assoc 80:899–904, 1988.
3. Raahave A, Friis-Moller A, Bjerre-Jepsen K, et al: The infective dose of aerobic and anaerobic bacteria in postoperative wound sepsis. Arch Surg 121:924–929, 1986.
4. Davidson AIG, Smith G, Smylie HG: A bacteriological study of the immediate environment of a surgical wound. Br J Surg 58:327–332, 1971.
5. Davidson AIG, Clark C, Smith G: Postoperative wound infection: a computer analysis. Br J Surg 58:333–337, 1971.
6. Pollock AV: Surgical prophylaxis—the emerging picture. Lancet 1:225–230, 1988.
7. Emmerson AM: The role of the skin in nosocomial infection: a review. J Chemother 1:12–18, 1989.
8. Larson E: Guideline for use of topical antimicrobial agents. Am J Infect Control 16:253–266, 1988.
9. Noble WC: Skin flora of the normal and immune compromised host. Curr Probl Dermatol 18:37–41, 1989.
10. Roth RR, James WD: Microbiology of the skin: resident flora, ecology, infection. J Am Acad Dermatol 20:367–390, 1989.
11. O'Neill TM, Hone R, Blake S: Prosthetic valve endocarditis caused by *Propionibacterium acnes*. Br Med J 296:1444, 1988.
12. Larson E: Handwashing: it's essential—even when you use gloves. Am J Nurs 89:934–939, 1989.
13. Sebben JE: Sterile technique and the prevention of wound infection in office surgery. Part II. J Dermatol Surg Oncol 15:38–48, 1989.
14. Oberg MS, Lindsey D: Do not put hydrogen peroxide or povidone iodine into wounds! Am J Dis Child 141:27–28, 1987.
15. Lineaweaver W, Howard R, Soucy D, et al: Topical antimicrobial toxicity. Arch Surg 120:267–270, 1985.
16. Maley MP: Extend handwashing to the forearms? Am J Nurs 89:1437, 1989.
17. Proposed recommended practices: surgical scrubs. AORN J 51:226–228, 230–234, 1990.
18. Recommended practices: surgical attire. AORN J 51:828, 830, 832, 835, 837, 1990.
19. Aly R, Maibach HI: Comparative antibacterial efficacy of a 2-minute surgical scrub with chlorhexidine gluconate, povidone-iodine, and chloroxylenol sponge-brushes. Am J Infect Control 16:173–177, 1988.
20. Dahl J, Wheeler B, Mukherjee D: Effect of chlorhexidine scrub on postoperative bacterial counts. Am J Surg 159:486–489, 1990.
21. Laufman H: Current use of skin and wound cleansers and antiseptics. Am J Surg 157:359–365, 1989.
22. Masterson BJ: Skin preparation. Clin Obstet Gynecol 31:736–743, 1988.
23. Larson E, Butz AM, Gullette DL, Laughon BA: Alcohol for surgical scrubbing? Infect Control Hosp Epidemiol 11:139–143, 1990.
24. Morrison AJ, Gratz J, Cabezudo I, Wenzel RP: The efficacy of several new handwashing agents for removing non-transient bacterial flora from hands. Infect Control 7:268–272, 1986.
25. Mackenzie I: Preoperative skin preparation and surgical outcome. J Hosp Infect 11:27–32, 1988.
26. Johnston DH, Fairclough JA, Brown EM, Morris R: Rate of bacterial recolonization of the skin after preparation: four methods compared. Br J Surg 74:64, 1987.
27. Geelhoed GW, Sharpe K, Simon GL: A comparative study of surgical skin preparation methods. Surg Gynecol Obstet 157:265–268, 1983.
28. Craig CP: Preparation of the skin for surgery. Infect Control 7:257–258, 1986.
29. Garibaldi RA, Skolnick D, Lerer T, et al: The impact of preoperative skin disinfection on preventing intraoperative wound contamination. Infect Control Hosp Epidemiol 9:109–113, 1988.
30. Kaiser AB, Kernodle DS, Barg NL, Petracek MR: Influence of preoperative showers on staphylococcal skin colonization: a comparative trial of antiseptic skin cleansers. Ann Thorac Surg 45:35–38, 1988.
31. Leclair JM, Winston KR, Sullivan BF, et al: Effect of preoperative shampoos with chlorhexidine or iodophor on emergence of resident scalp flora in neurosurgery. Infect Control 9:8–12, 1988.
32. Newsom SWB, Rowland C: Studies on perioperative skin flora. J Hosp Infect 11:21–26, 1988.
33. Ritter MA, Marmion P: The exogenous sources and controls of microorganisms in the operating room. Orthop Nurs 7:23–28, 1988.
34. Korniewicz DM, Laughon BE, Butz A, Larson E: Integrity of vinyl and latex procedure gloves. Nurs Res 38:144–146, 1989.
35. Yangco BG, Yangco NF: What is leaky can be risky: a study of the integrity of hospital gloves. Infect Control Hosp Epidemiol 10:553–556, 1989.
36. Lowbury EJL, Lilly HA: Disinfection of the hands of surgeons and nurses. Br Med J 5184:1445–1450, 1960.

37. Parker ME, Williams H: Cross-infection and cross-contamination: the relationship between subungual bacteria and fingernail length. Dent Hyg 61:68–72, 1987.
38. Leyden JJ, McGinley KJ, Kates SG, Myung KB: Subungual bacteria of the hand: contribution to the glove juice test; efficacy of antimicrobial detergents. Infect Control Hosp Epidemiol 10:451–454, 1989.
39. Whyte W: The role of clothing and drapes in the operating room. J Hosp Infect 11:2–17, 1988.
40. Silo HMS: Perioperative nursing research. Part V: Intraoperative recommended practices. AORN J 49:1627–1636, 1989.
41. Update: universal precautions for prevention of transmission of human immunodeficiency virus, hepatitis B virus, and other blood-borne pathogens in health-care settings. MMWR 37:377–382, 387–388, 1988.
42. McQuarrie DG, Glover JL, Olson MM: Laminar airflow systems: issues surrounding their effectiveness. AORN J 51:1035–1047, 1990.
43. Hodge WR, Trepal M, Woolf WH, Piccora R: Effect of desquamation of facial skin during surgery. J Am Podiatr Med Assoc 80:83–85, 1990.
44. Altemeier WA (ed), American College of Surgeons. Manual on Control of Infections in Surgical Patients. JB Lippincott, Philadelphia, 1982.
45. Fry DE: Antibiotics in surgery. Am J Surg 155:11–15, 1988.
46. Young EJ, Sugarman B: Infections in prosthetic devices. Surg Clin North Am 68:167–180, 1988.
47. Chodak GW, Plaut ME: Use of systemic antibiotics for prophylaxis in surgery. Arch Surg 112:326–334, 1977.
48. Peterson LJ: Antibiotic prophylaxis against wound infections in oral and maxillofacial surgery. J Oral Maxillofac Surg 48:617–620, 1990.
49. Ma S, Chiang SS, Fang RH: Prophylactic antibiotics in surgical treatment of axillary hyperhidrosis. Ann Plast Surg 22:436–439, 1989.
50. Johnson JT, Wagner RL: Infection following uncontaminated head and neck surgery. Arch Otolaryngol Head Neck Surg 113:368–369, 1987.
51. Johnson JT, Yu V: Antibiotic use during major head and neck surgery. Ann Surg 207:108–111, 1988.
52. Weimert TA, Yoder MG: Antibiotics and nasal surgery. Laryngoscope 90:667–672, 1980.
53. Johnson JT: Prophylaxis in surgical procedures. Am J Otolaryngol 4:433–434, 1983.
54. Kaiser AB: Antimicrobial prophylaxis in surgery. N Engl J Med 315:1129–1138, 1986.
55. Sacks T: Prophylactic antibiotics in traumatic wounds. J Hosp Infect 11:251–258, 1988.
56. Krizek TJ, Gottlieb LJ, Koss N, Robson MC: The use of prophylactic antibacterials in plastic surgery: a 1980's update. Plast Reconstr Surg 76:953–963, 1985.
57. Bergamini TM, Polk HC Jr: Pharmacodynamics of antibiotic penetration of tissue and surgical prophylaxis. Surg Gynecol Obstet 168:283–289, 1989.
58. McCue JD: Medical and surgical use of prophylactic antibiotics. Hosp Pract 21:167–170, 1986.
59. Johnson JT, Yu VL, Myers EN, Wagner RL: An assessment of the need for gram-negative bacterial coverage in antibiotic prophylaxis for oncological head and neck surgery. J Infect Dis 155:331–333, 1987.
60. Rubin J, Johnson JT, Wagner RL, Yu VL: Bacteriologic analysis of wound infection following major head and neck surgery. Arch Otolaryngol Head Neck Surg 114:969–972, 1988.
61. Dajani AS, Bisno AL, Chung KJ, et al: Prevention of bacterial endocarditis: recommendations by the American Heart Association. JAMA 264:2919–2922, 1990.
62. Antimicrobial prophylaxis in surgery. Med Lett Drugs Ther 31:105–108, 1989.
63. Bisno AL: Antimicrobial prophylaxis for infective endocarditis. Hosp Pract 24:209–214, 219–221, 224–246, 1989.
64. Pogrel MA: Prophylactic antibiotics. Br Dent J 188:446–447, 1990.
65. Sabetta JB, Zitelli JA: The incidence of bacteremia during skin surgery. Arch Dermatol 123:213–215, 1987.
66. Lycka A: Antibiotic prophylaxis and dermatologic surgery. Arch Dermatol 123:424–425, 1987.
67. Wagner RG Jr, Grande DJ, Feingold DS: Antibiotic prophylaxis against bacterial endocarditis in patients undergoing dermatologic surgery. Arch Dermatol 122:799–801, 1986.
68. Antibiotic prophylaxis of infective endocarditis. Recommendations from the Endocarditis Working Party of the British Society for Antimicrobial Chemotherapy. Lancet 335:88–89, 1990.
69. Hambraeus A: Aerobiology in the operating room—a review. J Hosp Infect 11:68–76, 1988.
70. Whitaker DC, Grande DJ, Johnson SS: Wound infection rates in dermatologic surgery. J Dermatol Surg Oncol 14:525–528, 1988.
71. Rutala, WA: APIC guideline for selection and use of disinfectants. Am J Infect Control 18:99–117, 1990.
72. Recommended practices: care of instruments, scopes, and powered surgical instruments. AORN J 47:556–558, 560–563, 566–569, 1988.

CHAPTER 7

Contact Allergy in Cutaneous Surgery

KEAN LAWLOR and JAMES S. TAYLOR

Contact dermatitis, a relatively common problem that can contribute significantly to perioperative morbidity, may arise in cutaneous surgery as a consequence of the surgery itself or of the perioperative care. Surgical patients are at particular risk from exposure to a number of cutaneous irritants and allergens, especially topical antibiotics, local anesthetics, latex and adhesives, metallic instruments, preoperative scrubs and antiseptics, and dressing materials. Also of importance is the contact dermatitis that occurs in surgeons, nurses, and other medical personnel. The potential sequelae of dermatitis in health care workers include inconvenience, lost work time, and in some severe cases career change or modification of work habits.

Patch Testing

Although patch testing performed and interpreted by experienced individuals offers a reasonably scientific and accurate method of diagnosing allergic contact dermatitis, it is almost certainly underutilized[1] and probably inaccurately diagnosed in most cases.[2] Patch testing offers a uniform and reproducible method of diagnosis and is far superior to the "trial and error" method, which frequently fails to determine the actual cause of dermatitis.[1] This procedure is cost effective and provides both patient and physician with valuable information regarding etiology.[3] Results of testing may also have medicolegal importance.

Categories of Contact Dermatitis

Contact dermatitis encompasses three general categories: irritant, allergic, and immediate or type I reactions. Of these, the most common is irritation.[4-7] By definition, irritant contact dermatitis is elicited on first exposure to the offending agent in most of the exposed population. In reality, however, irritant thresholds vary greatly among patients tested with known irritants.[5] The two major subtypes are acute and cumulative irritation, each of which may be indistinguishable from allergic contact dermatitis. Delayed, pustular, and other forms of irritation have also recently been described.

In contrast, allergic contact dermatitis[8-9] occurs in individuals as a type IV Gell and Coombs allergic response. The development of allergic contact dermatitis involves both an induction and an elicitation phase. Induction usually occurs after a refractory period of at least several days and involves antigen penetration and conjugation with epidermal protein, migration to lymph nodes, and production of circulating effector and memory cells. The duration of the induction phase varies from 5 days to several weeks but is usually 14 to 21 days. After this initial sensitization, subsequent exposure elicits recall and recognition at the skin site by effector cells and a T-cell mediated inflammatory response ensues. This results in an eczematous dermatitis usually occurring between 12 and 96 hours after exposure, occasionally as long as 1 week, with sensitization usually persisting for years.

The third group of contact eruptions is the immediate type or type I Gell and Coombs reaction. This occurs when an antigen cross-links mast cell membrane-bound IgE antibodies. This cross-linking results in degranulation, which releases tissue active mediators, including histamine, kinins, and slow-reacting substance of anaphylaxis.[9] Clinically, this may be manifested by contact urticaria or the more serious symptoms of anaphylaxis with airway obstruction, hypotension, or shock.

Very little published information exists on contact

dermatitis in the surgical setting. In a prospective study of 100 consecutive hospitalized adult surgical patients,[6] contact dermatitis was found to occur commonly. Twelve patients developed postoperative irritant dermatitis from rubber-based adhesive tape, and two patients had allergic contact dermatitis, one from benzoin and the other from rubber-based adhesive tape. Another prospective study of cutaneous surgical patients[10] found a 4.2% incidence of sensitization to topical antibiotics among 215 patients. This chapter discusses the most frequent causes of contact dermatitis in cutaneous surgeons and their patients, as well as the uncommon reactions that occur as a result of commonly used materials.

Principal Causes of Contact Dermatitis

The principal causes of contact dermatitis in cutaneous surgery are topical antibiotics, local anesthetics, gloves, adhesives, nickel and chrome, and antiseptics. Each of these will be discussed separately.

ANTIBIOTICS

Neomycin

Among the topical antibiotics,[11–40] neomycin is the best known and most frequent cause of sensitization.[11–27] It was the fourth most common sensitizer among the standard allergens tested by the North American Contact Dermatitis Group, after nickel, paraphenylenediamine, and quaternium 15.[12] As cutaneous surgeons have become more aware of the sensitizing potential of neomycin, its use has become somewhat supplanted in postoperative wound care by antibiotic preparations free of this agent. However, it is still widely available in both nonprescription and prescription preparations (Table 7–1).[13]

Sensitization to neomycin usually follows prolonged application to a nonhealing ulcer or some other erosion. Other predisposing conditions include application to chronic eczematous dermatoses, otitis externa, and eyelid eczema with conjunctivitis. Sensitivity often presents clinically with a worsening of the pre-existing eczema, or the sudden eruption of eczema around the site of a nonhealing ulcer.[14, 15] Corticosteroids, present in some neomycin preparations, may help to partially suppress the dermatitis.[14] In several large studies the prevalence of neomycin sensitivity has varied. In one study of 158 patients in a general U.S. population,[19] a sensitization rate of 1% was found. In patch test clinics the prevalence has varied from a low of 1.7% in Poland[16] to a high of 19% reported from Finland.[17] It was found that the prevalence of neomycin sensitivity remained relatively constant during a 5-year period in about 4% of patients studied.[14] This is similar to the rate of approximately 6% reported by the North American Contact Dermatitis Group.[12] In patients with stasis dermatitis and leg ulcers, the rate of sensitization may be much higher. It was found that 34% of leg ulcer patients were allergic to neomycin.[18] Similarly, it was noted that any patient with

a history of applying a neomycin-containing product to inflammatory dermatitis for longer than 1 week was at substantially increased risk of developing sensitization.[19] However, patients with little exposure to neomycin or those who used neomycin prophylactically were unlikely to develop an allergic dermatitis. On the basis of these data, it is possible to divide patients into high- and low-risk groups for developing neomycin sensitivity. After a recent prospective study of topical antibiotic allergy in cutaneous surgery patients, the avoidance of neomycin was recommended in postoperative wound care instructions.[9]

Unfortunately, allergy to neomycin often precludes the use of other aminoglycoside preparations, as cross-reactions are frequent.[14, 20, 21] Two separate studies of patients with positive neomycin patch tests found that 60% also reacted to tobramycin[20] and 55% to gentamicin.[20, 21] As these drugs currently have an important role in the treatment of many systemic infections, allergy to neomycin may carry important therapeutic implications for patients if treatment of life-threatening infection is required. Systemic administration of neomycin or cross-reacting aminoglycoside to neomycin-sensitive patients may cause systemic contact dermatitis manifested as a severe eczematous dermatitis, a drug eruption, or a flare of positive neomycin patch test sites.[13]

It is also of clinical relevance that approximately half the neomycin-allergic patients were found to be allergic to another preservative, base, or medication.[14] In particular, simultaneous sensitization with bacitracin has often been reported.[15, 22–24] Most bacitracin-sensitive pa-

TABLE 7–1. PARTIAL LIST OF NEOMYCIN-CONTAINING PRODUCTS

Ak-Spore	Neomycin (generic)
Ak-Trol Suspension	Neomycin corticosteroid
Bactine	Neo-Polycin
Coly-Mycin	Neo-Rx
Dexacidin Suspension	Neo-Thrycex
Dexasporin Suspension	Neotricin
Infectrol Suspension	Nisopyn
Kaomycin	Nivromycin
Lanabiotic	Pediotic Suspension
LazerSporin-C Solution	Septa
Maximum Strength Neosporin	Spectrocin
Maxitrol	Trimycin
Medi-Quik	Triple antibiotic (generic)
Mycifradin	Triple antibiotic with hydrocortisone
Myciguent	
Mycimist	**Combination Products**
Myclinicin	Cordran-N
N.B.P.	Cortisporin
Neocidin	HC-Neomycin (generic)
Neo-IM	Myco-Biotic II
Neomal	Neo-Cortef
Neomin	NeoDecadron
Neomix	Neo-Medrol
Neomixin	Neo-Synalar
Neomycane	

Compiled from Handbook of Nonprescription Drugs. 9th ed. American National Pharmaceutical Association, Washington, D.C., 1990; Drug Facts and Comparisons. Updated monthly. Facts and Comparisons, Inc., St. Louis, 1993; and Index Nominum, International Drug Directory. Medpharm, Stuttgart, 1990–1991.

tients have been found to be neomycin sensitive as a result of "cosensitization."[15, 22, 24, 25] It has been argued effectively that since neomycin and bacitracin are not structurally related, positive coincident reactions in patients represent cosensitization rather than cross-reaction between these antibiotics.[22] Most patients in two studies who were allergic to bacitracin were also allergic to neomycin.[9, 24] For this reason, bacitracin-polymyxin B–containing preparations may not be a safe alternative in neomycin-sensitive patients.[25] In contrast, another study found no clear correlation between bacitracin and neomycin allergy.[18]

Bacitracin

The incidence of bacitracin allergy without neomycin cosensitization appears to be increasingly common. Several years ago it was thought that bacitracin was a rare sensitizer.[13, 14] However, in Finland, where antibiotics have been available without a prescription for many years, the incidence of bacitracin allergy appears to be high. One study found bacitracin allergy in 7.8% of 17,600 patients tested during an 11-year period.[27] This increase in frequency of bacitracin allergy correlated with the increased consumption of bacitracin- and neomycin-containing products by the public. A total of 13% of patients with stasis dermatitis and leg ulcers were found to be allergic to bacitracin. In 1987 it was reported that bacitracin sensitivity was becoming common in the postsurgical setting, with nine cases reported in a single year.[28] In seven of these patients, dermatitis followed a surgical procedure such as electrodesiccation and curettage or excision. No cases resulted from the application of bacitracin to stasis or chronic ulcers. Only one person coreacted with neomycin. Interestingly, only three patients had a positive patch test at 48 hours; the rest demonstrated a positive reaction at 96 hours. Therefore, a single 48-hour patch test reading could indeed overlook bacitracin sensitivity; 96-hour readings are essential if bacitracin allergy is suspected. Delayed readings for neomycin should also be performed, since they also may take up to 1 week to react.[14] A significant number of allergic reactions to Polysporin has led some cutaneous surgeons[39, 40] to stop using this agent because of frequent contact allergy after its use (Table 7–2).

Immediate hypersensitivity has also been reported in patients using topical bacitracin. One patient was reported to develop anaphylactic symptoms after application of bacitracin to a stasis ulcer.[29] After a negative prick test, the patient underwent intradermal testing during which she experienced anaphylactic shock. Similarly, anaphylaxis was described in a 14-year-old girl who had applied bacitracin ointment to infected atopic eczema.[30] Her Prausnitz-Küstner reactions were positive, and circulating antibodies to bacitracin were demonstrated in the serum, but not in controls. Another young female developed anaphylaxis resulting from the application of bacitracin to a chronic foot dermatitis.[31] A review of six cases of anaphylaxis to topical medications[32] described four patients who applied bacitracin to the skin with "chronically impaired" barrier function, which was felt to be responsible. In the same

TABLE 7–2. PARTIAL LIST OF BACITRACIN-CONTAINING PRODUCTS

Ak-Spore	N.B.P.
Ak-Spore H.C.	Neomixin
Ak-Tracin	Neo-Polycin
Baciguent	Neosporin
Baci-IM	Neo-Thrycex
Baci-Rx	Ocu-Tracin
Bactine	Ortega-Otic
Cortisporin	Otocort
Cortitrigen	Otomycin
Drotic	Polysporin
Lanabiotic	Septa
Maximum Strength Neosporin	Topitracin
My Cort Otic	Trimycin
Mycitracin	Triple antibiotic

Compiled from Handbook of Nonprescription Drugs. 9th ed. American National Pharmaceutical Association, Washington, D.C., 1990; Drug Facts and Comparisons. Updated monthly. Facts and Comparisons, Inc., St. Louis, 1993; and Index Nominum, International Drug Directory. Medpharm, Stuttgart, 1990–1991.

report the authors described a patient with coexistent type I (anaphylaxis) and type IV (contact dermatitis) hypersensitivity to bacitracin. They suggested that anaphylaxis occurs only when a topically applied drug can enter the systemic circulation in large quantities through impaired skin. Although type I reactions are rare with bacitracin, cutaneous surgeons should be aware of this phenomenon and manage patients at risk accordingly.

Mafenide and Nitrofurazone

Although allergic contact dermatitis has occurred with most topically applied antibiotics,[13] several in particular deserve special mention. Topical sulfonamide, or mafenide, allergy may result in cross-reactivity to para-aminobenzoic acid (PABA) sunscreens, benzocaine, hair dyes, and systemically administered sulfa drugs. The use of nitrofurazone and mafenide for the treatment of burns has declined in the United States. Although nitrofurazone is a potent sensitizer, some cases of contact allergy from nitrofurazone-containing products have resulted from polyethylene glycol present in the vehicle of the topical preparation.[38]

Erythromycin

Delayed hypersensitivity to erythromycin sulfate[34] and types I and IV reactions with erythromycin stearate have been reported . It has been advocated that erythromycin base ointment is a good nonsensitizing alternative to neomycin- and bacitracin-containing preparations.[26, 36, 37] There are descriptions of how to obtain or compound erythromycin ointment.[28] To date, no cases of allergic contact dermatitis to erythromycin base have been reported.

Mupirocin

Mupirocin (Bactroban, pseudomonic acid), a new, widely used topical antibiotic, is principally active against gram-positive organisms. A few cases of allergic contact dermatitis to this medication have been cited.

LOCAL ANESTHETICS

Contact sensitivity to local anesthetics[41–63] is one of the most frequent causes of dermatitis due to medicaments.[2, 41] Local anesthetics may be classified into three chemically unrelated families: esters, amides, and a miscellaneous group.[42, 43] This classification is based on the chemical moiety linking the nonpolar and the polar portions of the anesthetic molecule.[42]

Esters

Contact dermatitis from the ester group of local anesthetics is most often due to benzocaine.[43] This is because of the wide variety and general availability of over-the-counter compounds containing benzocaine. This ingredient is found in over 700 products, including sunscreens,[44] astringents, wart medications, toothache and teething remedies, vaginal creams, ear drops, lozenges, and antibacterial and antifungal agents.[45] Application of benzocaine to chronic eczema, burns, or nonhealing ulcers also predisposes to sensitization.[42]

Benzocaine and chemically related compounds are also commonly employed in injectable forms as local anesthetics. Cross-reaction between benzocaine and other ester-type antibiotics is common. In a series of benzocaine-sensitive patients, all were also found to be procaine sensitive.[46] In addition to ester anesthetics, cross-reactions may occur with other drugs derived from benzoic acid such as sulfonamides, thiazides, sulfonylureas, and PABA-containing sunscreens.[44] Application or ingestion of these agents has resulted in severe widespread contact dermatitis in individuals previously sensitized with topical benzocaine.[42] Application of paraphenylenediamine, the active ingredient of most permanent hair dyes, may also result in severe dermatitis in the benzocaine-allergic patient. Use of the orally administered sulfonylureas can produce generalized dermatitis in sulfonamide-sensitive patients but not in those sensitized to benzocaine or paraphenylenediamine.[47] Injection of ester-type anesthetics in benzocaine-allergic individuals may lead to localized swelling at the site of injection[48] or (rarely) generalized urticaria or anaphylactoid reactions. Coexistent nonimmunologic contact urticaria and type IV contact sensitivity to benzocaine was reported in one patient.[50]

Amides

Contact sensitivity to the amide group of local anesthetics is much less common, despite widespread use of lidocaine both as a topical and injectable anesthetic and as a antidysrhythmic agent. In one review, 17 patients were described with patch test–proved delayed-type hypersensitivity to lidocaine.[52] One other case has been reported,[53] but none have been described in the United States. Contact sensitization may manifest as delayed local swelling[52] or as a rash[53] at the site of injection or at the site of application. As with the ester-type anes-

thetics, cross-sensitization within the amide group of anesthetics (prilocaine, mepivacaine, and bupivacaine) is common.[52, 54]

Miscellaneous Anesthetics

EMLA. This topical emulsion of lidocaine and prilocaine is also known as an *e*utectic *m*ixture of *l*ocal *a*nesthetics. It has proved a safe and effective topical anesthetic for minor surgical and laser procedures[58] or venous cannulation.[59] Anticipated to become available in the United States, its rate of sensitization will probably be similar to that of amide-type anesthetics.

Pramoxine. This topical anesthetic is structurally unrelated to the amide or ester anesthetics.[45] It is effective and carries a low risk of topical sensitization and no risk of cross-sensitization.[48]

Injectable Anesthetics

Most systemic reactions from injectable local anesthetics are due to nonimmunologic phenomena such as vasovagal collapse, inadvertent intravenous injection, alpha or beta effects of epinephrine, and nonimmunologic histamine release.[49] Immediate IgE-mediated reactions to local anesthetics may also occur but account for only 1% of the injectable local anesthetic reactions. Clinical manifestations of IgE allergy range from urticaria and angioedema to bronchospasm and anaphylaxis.[55–57] At least 38 reported cases of IgE-mediated local anesthetic reactions have been reported; more than one third were from lidocaine or related agents.[63] The approach to the local anesthetic–sensitive patient includes taking a detailed history and performing invasive skin testing with incremental challenge.[49, 63]

In addition to the active ingredient in the injectable anesthetics, allergic reactions to the additives sulphites, benzoates, and parabens have been reported. Sensitization to methylparaben, found as a preservative in multidose vials of injectable anesthetics, must be considered when evaluating a patient with suspected anesthetic allergy.[60] Parabens may primarily sensitize but may also manifest as a cross-reaction to benzocaine, as the two compounds are structurally similar.[61] Benzocaine- and other ester-allergic patients with contact dermatitis can tolerate injections of paraben-free amide anesthetics without being skin tested, since the ester and amide groups do not cross-react.

In one report, delayed hypersensitivity from injectable amide anesthetics, including lidocaine presented clinically as local swelling of delayed onset and was diagnosed by positive patch tests to the anesthetics; intradermal testing was not performed.[52] In another case,[53] after a reaction to a lidocaine-containing injectable preparation, patch tests with lidocaine were positive; intradermal tests were negative. As anesthetics are often employed systemically and topical sensitization may preclude use of an entire class of medication, it is important that physicians try to limit the use of topical anesthetics to those not used systemically.[46]

TABLE 7–3. CLASSIFICATION OF GLOVE REACTIONS

Irritation from occlusion, friction, and maceration; worse with dermographism
Allergy to glove material
    Contact dermatitis
    Contact urticaria, angioedema, and anaphylaxis to latex
Aggravation of pre-existing dermatoses by gloves
Penetration of chemicals through gloves, especially epoxy and acrylic resins
Other reactions
    Endotoxin reaction
    Ethylene oxide reaction
    Chemical leukoderma

GLOVE REACTIONS

Allergic Contact Dermatitis. Glove reactions among health care workers are often overlooked, but the incidence is rising with mandatory glove usage.[64–71, 73–75] Although irritation from occlusion, friction, maceration, and frequent hand washing is more common than allergy, anyone with hand eczema who wears latex gloves should be considered to have allergic contact dermatitis until it is proved otherwise.[65, 66] The diagnosis is often difficult because of the delayed onset and chronicity of the dermatitis. Many patients have a nonspecific patchy or diffuse eczema on the dorsa of the hands or fingers, without a sharp cut-off above the wrist. Most patients can be accurately diagnosed by patch testing with the major rubber allergens on a standard patch test screening tray. Patch testing with both sides of postage stamp–size glove pieces sometimes produces false-negative reactions, and occlusion for 72 to 96 hours may be required to increase the yield.[66]

If patch testing with a piece of glove is positive in the absence of a positive reaction from a standard tray rubber chemical, the allergen may be other rubber chemicals. These include accelerators, antioxidants, and additives. Specific examples are 4,4′-thiobis(6-*tert*-butyl-m-cresol)(Lowinox 44S36), 2-*tert*-butyl-4-methoxyphenol (BHA), and certain thioureas.[66, 69]

"On Call" Dermatitis. Eyelid dermatitis in the absence of hand eczema has been reported in physicians and nurses allergic to latex gloves who are required to change gloves frequently. Prolonged eyelid contact with the rubber accelerator thiuram, which leaches into the glove powder, occurs despite the fact that the accelerator is removed from the hands because of frequent washing.[66]

Other Glove Reactions. There are numerous causes of glove reactions (Table 7–3). Vinyl glove allergy has been reported and the allergen is usually a dye or a plasticizer.[66, 70]

Latex Allergy. Patients with putative rubber glove allergy should also be evaluated for contact urticaria to latex, which is being reported with increasing frequency. Latex allergy is a potentially serious occupational problem for health care professionals and may be accompanied by angioedema, asthma, and even anaphylaxis, several cases of which have been fatal.[72, 73] In 1991 the Food and Drug Administration issued a medical alert on the problem to the medical profession[73] and also notified all latex manufacturers.[74] Although latex surgical gloves have been worn since 1890, it was not until 1979 that the first case of contact urticaria to latex gloves was described. Since then, numerous other cases have been reported, and recent epidemiologic studies, which included skin testing, showed the incidence among operating room physicians to be 7.4% and among nurses 5.6 to 10%.[67, 68, 76] Less frequent reactions occur in other health care personnel, homemakers, and industrial workers. Contact with numerous other medical and consumer latex devices places these patients at risk. Cutaneous surgeons should ask these high-risk patients about latex allergy.[73]

Contact urticaria to latex is an IgE-mediated, type I allergic reaction in which the allergen is usually a protein in the natural latex.[67, 68, 75] In contrast, the allergen in type IV allergic contact dermatitis is an accelerator or antioxidant that is added during latex curing (Table 7–4).[64–71, 75, 76] Type I reactions may have clinical findings that vary from pruritus alone to erythema, or wheal and flare reactions at the site of latex contact, usually occurring within 5 to 20 minutes. The reaction usually resolves without treatment within 30 minutes to 2 hours. The diagnosis is often difficult with concomitant hand eczema masking the urticaria. The patient typically suspects glove powder or soap as the culprit.[68] Predisposing factors include atopy, pre-existing hand eczema, frequent latex glove use, and spina bifida, probably as a result of latex exposure during multiple medical and surgical procedures in these patients.[68, 73]

Severe accelerated type I allergic reactions with angioedema, generalized urticaria, asthma, and anaphylaxis have been reported in a number of patients simply after use of latex or surgical gloves, inflating a balloon, undergoing a barium enema or surgery, or even exposure to condoms. These patients are at further risk from contact with other latex medical devices such as gloves

TABLE 7–4. ALLERGENS* IN MEDICAL/SURGICAL GLOVES

Rubber
    Latex proteins of 6-34-kD
    Accelerators
        Thiurams
        Mercaptobenzothiazoles
        Carbamates
        Thioureas
        Others
    Antioxidants
        Paraphenylenediamines
        4,4′-thiobis(6-*tert*-butyl-m-cresol) (Lowinox 44S36)
        2-*tert*-butyl-4-methoxyphenol (BHA)
        Others
    Flavors/fragrances
        Mint
        Cinnamon
Vinyl
    Plasticizers
    Color

*Latex proteins produce only type I (contact urticaria) allergy; the others mainly produce type IV (contact dermatitis) allergy, but occasionally type I allergy.
BHA, Butylhydroxyanisole

worn by dentists, physicians, and other health care professionals; catheters; intubation; intravenous and other tubes; sphygmomanometer tubing; anesthesia masks; and dental polishers and dams. These patients may also react to other latex products such as rubber bands and soft rubber balls. Mucosal exposure to latex is more likely to be associated with anaphylaxis. Latex can also be an aeroallergen, since it leaches into glove powder and can become airborne during glove changes, resulting in mucosal or other systemic symptoms.[64, 67, 68, 71–76]

The diagnosis of contact urticaria to latex can be confirmed with the following evaluation and work-up.[68, 76] First, it is important to differentiate between symptoms and signs of immediate and delayed reactions. Separating contact urticaria from coexisting irritant or allergic contact dermatitis may be difficult. Delayed-onset contact urticaria of 2 to 8 hours has been reported. During the initial evaluation of the patient's history, questions about itching, swelling, or wheezing after wearing latex gloves or inflating a balloon are especially useful. A properly performed positive prick or scratch test to latex remains the diagnostic gold standard. Latex items producing the strongest skin test reactions are usually the patient's own disposable latex gloves and dried raw latex. The latter confirms the allergen as natural latex since most patients do not react to cornstarch. Although rare, severe allergic reactions may occur during skin testing, and epinephrine and resuscitation equipment should be available. At present, no commercially prepared latex allergen is available for skin testing. Wear or use tests are performed to confirm doubtful reactions or when the patient refuses skin tests. Since anaphylaxis has occurred from wearing an entire glove, the patient should wear only one glove finger on the moistened hand. The appearance of one or more urticarial wheals at 20 minutes is considered a positive test. If the one-finger test is negative, one whole glove should be worn on one hand and a vinyl glove worn as a control. A repeat or extended wear test should be carried out in doubtful cases. The wear test is nearly as sensitive as the skin test. Evaluation with a radioallergosorbent test (RAST) using Phadizym latex allergen discs can be performed on a small blood sample by a radioimmunoassay laboratory. However, the latex RAST is less sensitive and is positive in only about 60% of cases of latex allergy.

High-pressure liquid chromatography (HPLC) has revealed allergenic protein fractions with peaks at molecular weight between 2000 and 30,000 daltons in natural rubber as well as latex surgical and examination gloves. Skin prick tests with the HPLC fractions have been positive.[68] Quantitative, rather than qualitative, differences exist between the allergenicity of various latex gloves and condoms. Recent immunoelectrophoresis and radioimmunoblotting studies have identified similar 6 to 34 kDa molecular weight latex allergens of either IgE or IgG4 antibody class.[75]

Since hyposensitization to latex is not yet feasible, latex avoidance or substitution becomes mandatory. Preprocedure allergy prophylaxis, which is sometimes used for radiocontrast allergy, should not be used in place of latex avoidance. Some gloves can be worn by latex-sensitive individuals (Table 7–5). Latex avoidance is especially important in outpatient clinics, operating rooms, radiology units, and other health care facilities (Table 7–6). It should be recognized that vinyl gloves may not provide adequate primary barrier function against infectious diseases,[77] since problems such as leak rate and viral passage were noted in one study. Alternative use of both nonlatex and latex gloves has been outlined in a FDA alert (Table 7–7).

ADHESIVES, GUMS, AND RESINS

Adhesives

Most medical adhesives are pressure-sensitive adhesives (PSAs), natural resins, or gums.[78] The classification and chemistry of medical adhesives has been detailed.[78] Most PSA tape is used in a dry state to hold a dressing in place by application of light pressure. Medical PSAs are commonly used to pull or hold tissues together. Most skin reactions to adhesive tape are irritant in nature, with allergic reactions infrequently reported and probably largely overlooked. Of these, skin stripping injury by repeated application and removal of tape, chemical injury from trapped chemicals such as benzoin between skin and adhesive, and tension blisters from tape pulled too tight are among the most common reactions (Table 7–8).

Allergic contact dermatitis from surgical adhesives is most commonly caused by rubber-based adhesives and less often by the newer single-component, acrylic-based PSAs. In contact allergy the entire area under the adhesive is eczematous and edematous with intense pruritus, unlike the patchy, less pruritic irritant contact dermatitis. The most common allergens in the rubber-based adhesives are tackifiers derived from rosin (colophony). Other sensitizers are terpene tackifiers, plasticizers, lanolin, antioxidants, and accelerators. Rubber-based adhesives are still used in surgical tapes and other dressings, including ostomy products.[78–81]

Four cases of allergic contact dermatitis to rubber-based Band-Aid Sheer Strips have been identified, one patient being allergic to 2,5-di(tertiary-amyl)-hydroquinone (DTAHQ), the antioxidant in the adhesive, and another to tricresyl phosphate, the plasticizer in the backing. The other two cases were unexplained. DTAHQ is also present in other brands of adhesives.[89]

Since the polymers used in acrylic PSAs are not very sticky, small amounts of rosin are often added to improve the "tack." In a 1984 report, allergy to Foral 85, a wood rosin derivative, in the acrylic-based adhesive of some skin closure tapes was identified.[94] As a result, 3M removed Foral 85 from Steri-Strips. Acrylic PSAs are less allergenic than rubber-based tapes because the amounts of uncured monomers present are negligible. Nevertheless, contact allergy to acrylics occurs and has been reported from Curad adhesives (2-ethylhexyl acrylate [2-EHA], N-dodecyl maleamic acid, and derivatives) and Scanpore tape (2-EHA) among others.[78]

Patch testing for PSA tape allergy should be done by applying a postage stamp–size piece of both the adhesive

TABLE 7–5. **SELECTED GLOVES THAT LATEX GLOVE–SENSITIVE PATIENTS MAY WEAR***

		Rubber Accelerators		
Glove	*Manufacturer*	MBT	Thiuram	Carbamates
Type I Allergy (Contact Urticaria)				
Vinyl				
1. BD Tru-Touch Vinyl (Examination and sterile)	Becton Dickinson & Co.	–	–	–
2. Triflex vinyl (Examination and sterile)	Baxter Pharmaseal	–	–	–
Synthetic nonlatex				
Tactyl 1 (examination and sterile)	Allerderm	–	–	–
Synthetic latex				
1. Neolon	Becton Dickinson	–	–	+
2. Dermaprene	Ansell	–	–	–
Type IV Allergy (Allergic Contact Dermatitis)				
Vinyl				
As above	As above		As above	
Synthetic nonlatex				
As above	As above		As above	
Synthetic latex				
As above	As above		As above	
Latex "hypoallergenic"				
1. Eudermic	Becton Dickinson	–	–	+
2. See article by Rich et al[69] for a more complete list.				

*Vinyl gloves may not provide adequate primary barrier protection.[77]

MBT, (2-mercaptobenzothiazole); –, not present; +, present.

Adapted from Rich P, Belozer ML, Norris P, Storrs FJ: Allergic contact dermatitis to two antioxidants in latex gloves: 4,4′-thiobis(6-*tert*-butyl-meta-cresol) (Lowinox 44S36) and butylhydroxyanisole. Allergen alternatives for glove-allergic patients. J Am Acad Dermatol 24:37–43, 1991.

side and backing to look for contact urticaria and dermatitis. Simultaneously, one should also test with the standard screening tray to identify allergens such as rubber, rosin, epoxy resin, or *p-tert*-butylphenol-formaldehyde resin (Table 7–9). Finally, one should also test with PSA tape components from a plastics and glue tray or from the manufacturer to identify other allergens, including specific rosin derivatives, acrylics, antioxidants, and backing components.

Elastoplast and Transpore adhesive allergy from rosin may be avoided by substituting tape with acrylic adhesives such as Micropore and Dermalite. Routine 24-hour preoperative patch tests with five brands of adhesive tape by a British orthopedic unit identified several

cases of allergy every month. Other PSA allergies in hospital and office practice have also been reported. These include electrode gels and pastes that cause a contact allergy of the chest and hands corresponding to sites of contact with *p*-chlorometaxylenol–containing electrode gel and hospital liquid soap;[91] transdermal drug delivery systems in which, in addition to the

TABLE 7–6. **LATEX AVOIDANCE IN OUTPATIENT CLINICS, ANESTHESIA, SURGERY, RADIOLOGY, AND OTHER HEALTH CARE UNITS FOR PATIENTS WITH TYPE I LATEX ALLERGY**

Gloves: use vinyl or synthetic latex gloves

Drugs: use ampules in place of bottles with latex diaphragms, use glass syringes

IV fluids and tubing: plastic bottle; nonrubber injection ports, connectors, and three-way stopcocks

Endotracheal tube: plastic

Anesthesia: disposable Bain circuit with plastic tubing and vinyl mask, use ventilator with silicone bellows

Anesthesia: rubber reservoir bag lined with a thin plastic bag

Avoid all latex medical and nonmedical devices (occult latex exposure may still occur); look for silicone substitutes for catheter products

TABLE 7–7. **ALLERGIC REACTIONS TO LATEX-CONTAINING MEDICAL DEVICES: RECOMMENDATIONS TO HEALTH PROFESSIONALS**

1. Question all patients about latex allergy, especially surgical, radiology, and spina bifida patients and health care workers
   a. History of itching, rash (swelling), or wheezing after wearing latex gloves or inflating balloons is useful
   b. Flag charts of allergic patients
2. For suspected latex allergy, consider devices made of alternative materials, e.g., plastic
   a. If patient is allergic, health professional could wear nonlatex glove over latex glove
   b. If both patient and health professional are allergic, latex *middle* glove could be used; latex gloves labeled "hypoallergenic" may not prevent reactions
3. Be alert to allergic reactions from all latex-containing medical devices, especially those with mucous membrane contact
4. If a suspected latex reaction occurs, advise patient and consider an allergy evaluation
5. Advise patients to inform health professionals and emergency personnel about latex sensitivity before undergoing procedures, and to consider wearing a medical identification bracelet

From U.S. Food and Drug Administration Medical Alert of March 29, 1991.[73]

TABLE 7–8. **ADHESIVE TAPE REACTIONS**

Irritation
  Skin stripping injury
  Chemical injury
  Tension blisters
  Folliculitis
  Miliaria
  Maceration
  Adhesive residue reaction
  Nontension mechanical injury
  Contact urticaria
  Dermographism
Allergy
  Contact urticaria
  Contact dermatitis

Adapted from Bryant RA: Saving the skin from tape injuries. Am J Nurs 88:189–191, 1988.

adhesive, contact dermatitis may occur from the active drug or backing; ostomy devices in which, in addition to the cementing materials, contact allergy may occur from topical medications and the ostomy devices themselves; and wart plasters that contain rosin or other derivatives, which are the allergens in 40% salicylic acid plasters and one wart gel.[85–87]

Resins

Contact allergy to the natural resins rosin (colophony) and benzoin, and to natural gums, is particularly relevant to cutaneous surgery. A variety of materials are considered in this category, including rosin, benzoin, podophyllum, cantharidin, and karaya gum. Each of these materials will be discussed separately.

Rosin, a complex mixture of many chemicals,[2, 78, 80–90] is used ubiquitously as an adhesive and is also a common component of many PSAs. Occlusion increases the risk

TABLE 7–9. **SELECTED ALLERGENS IN MEDICAL ADHESIVES, GUMS, AND RESINS**

Adhesives
  Antioxidants: DTAHQ
  Accelerators: thiurams, MBT,
    carbamates
Rubber
  Tackifiers: rosin (colophony)
  Acrylates: 2-EHA, N-DMA
  Plasticizers: tricesyl phosphate
  Other resins and synthetic rubbers
    Urethane
    Chloroprene
    p-tert-Butylphenol-formaldehyde resin
  Others
Gums
  Karaya
  Gum tragacanth
Resins
  Rosin (colophony)
  Benzoin
Other
  p-Chlorometaxylenol*

*Present in an electrode gel.[66, 78, 91]
DTAHQ, 2,5-di(tertiary-amyl)-hydroquinone; 2-EHA, 2-ethyl-hexyl acrylate; N-DMA, N-dodecyl maleamic acid.

of sensitization. Patients sensitized to adhesive rosin may also react from many other sources of exposure, since large quantities are used in paper, solder flux, cutting oils, printing inks, and rubber paperboard sizing. Rosin is modified before being used in technical products, and this may act to influence its allergenicity compared with that of unmodified rosin. Accordingly, it is important to also test with the patient's own rosin, since patch test tray rosins are often unmodified and may not always react positively.

Benzoin[78] is present in tincture of benzoin, which contains 10% alcohol. Compound tincture of benzoin contains 10% benzoin, 2% aloe, 8% storax (styrax), and 4% tolu balsam in ethyl alcohol. Benzoin is still widely used in cutaneous surgery either as an adhesive alone or as a tincture to reinforce PSA tape. It is also used as an adhesive for other medicaments such as podophyllum. Benzoin cross-reacts with balsam of Peru, tolu balsam, storax, myrrh, and related resins. Because of its sensitizing capacity, use of benzoin as a surgical adhesive is not recommended. Sensitivity often occurs in medical personnel and patients who have frequent exposure. Reactions may be locally severe or associated with generalized flares. An open patch test with a benzoin concentration of 10% in alcohol is first made to document contact allergy. If this is negative, it is followed by closed patch testing.

Podophyllum and cantharidin[78] are strong vesicant resins used primarily to treat warts. Both may cause serious systemic toxicity if used over large areas.

Other resins and gums[78, 84] can also cause contact allergy. Reports of allergies to resins and gums often used in surgical adhesives, such as Manila, karaya, dammar, and copal, are relatively common.[93] The principal natural gums used in medicine have been reviewed.[78] Although karaya, acacia, and tragacanth gums are the most common sensitizers, reports of contact allergy are infrequent.

METALS

Nickel

Nickel is the most frequently identified cause of contact dermatitis among individuals patch tested in North America.[12] Since nickel is present in many older surgical instruments, vascular clips, needles, and other objects in the cutaneous surgical setting, it is a significant cause of dermatitis among health professionals and their patients. A high incidence of nickel dermatitis (26%), which was equal to the female population was found in German health care workers.[95] In these workers, 70% of cases were not occupationally acquired but thought to be secondary to jewelry, pierced earrings, or clothing buckles. It was concluded that important risk factors for the development of hand dermatitis in previously nickel-allergic patients included an atopic diathesis; occupational contact with nickel, especially when it involved "wet work"; and contact with various disinfectants.

Although nickel-allergic individuals may safely work with most surgical stainless steel objects,[96] there is a risk of nickel leaching from other steel alloys, which often contain substantial quantities of nickel.[97] An acidic pH, sweat, and blood may liberate nickel ions from stainless steel alloys.[98] In general, the dimethylglyoxime (DMG) spot test is useful in detecting those items that freely liberate nickel. When added to a metallic object, a strawberry red precipitate is indicative of the presence of nickel ions, which may be freely liberated.[101] Instruments, tools, or other items that elicit a positive spot test should be avoided by nickel-sensitive patients.

Although fixed orthopedic implants such as pins and rods[99, 100] account for most of the reported reactions to implanted nickel, there are also anecdotal accounts of reactions from other sources.[105] A case of severe neck dermatitis after thyroidectomy with the use of stainless steel skin clips has been reported.[97] The patient was strongly patch test positive to both nickel sulfate and the surgical clip. Dermatitis has also followed exposure to nickel-plated cannulas and retractors, shrapnel, acupuncture needles, pacemakers, and heart valves. A local reaction occurred at the site of a Dermajet injection, presumably as a result of release of nickel from the device into the injection solution.[105]

Overall, the development of nickel allergic dermatitis from implanted metal is rare, given its high incidence in the general population and the relatively common nature of nickel in the modern surgical setting. It does seem prudent, however, to use surgical stainless steel tools and surgical instruments that have a negative DMG spot test for performing cutaneous surgical procedures in nickel-allergic patients.

Chrome

Although much less common, allergy to chrome may also occur. Chromic gut suture materials have been reported to cause eczematous dermatitis at the operative site in a patient who underwent knee surgery.[103] Previous surgical procedures that also used chromic catgut suture had evoked similar allergic episodes of eczematous dermatitis. The patient was found to be patch test positive to potassium dichromate as well as a piece of chromic gut suture. Among chrome-sensitive physicians, two gynecologists and two surgeons were reported to consider chromic catgut as the cause of their dermatitis.[104] All the physicians had handled the chromic suture without gloves at some time before the onset of their eruption. It has been suggested that preoperative testing be performed in suspected chrome-sensitive patients using the presumed causative chromic suture material and a control suture of another material, such as nylon or polypropylene. The two sutures are left in place for 7 days to identify any reactivity. This same testing technique could also be used to determine possible reactions to metal surgical clips. Finally, there have been anecdotal reports of allergic reactions to chromic catgut, silk, and polyglycolic acid suture materials.[39]

CHLORHEXIDINE

Chlorhexidine is a broad-spectrum disinfectant agent used widely in the cutaneous surgical setting. It is also a primary constituent[107] of many creams and solutions (see Table 7–1) in its digluconate form. It is also widely used in Europe as an impregnated gauze in its diacetate form (Bactigras).[108] In cutaneous surgery it is commonly used as a preoperative scrub or a skin preparation for patients. Several reports[108, 111-114] suggest that contact dermatitis to chlorhexidine may be more common than previously thought.[109, 110] A total of 1063 patients were patch tested with chlorhexidine;[108] of these, approximately 5% were initially positive, but positivity was confirmed in 72% on retesting. Most of these positive test reactions were thought to be relevant, since most patients could recall previous exposure to chlorhexidine either through application to a leg ulcer or as a preoperative surgical scrub. Of 551 patients patch tested to chlorhexidine gluconate, 14 showed a clinically relevant reaction.[111] This study, along with another reported series,[114] indicates that patients with leg ulcers or stasis dermatitis are at increased risk of developing contact sensitivity. Immediate reactions to chlorhexidine may take the form of contact urticaria[107, 113, 115] or true anaphylaxis.[113] Six patients were described who developed urticaria and anaphylactic shock after topical application of chlorhexidine in concentrations of 0.05 to 1%.[113] Scratch or intradermal testing was positive in all patients and closed patch testing produced wheals in two patients. While most patients reported having chlorhexidine applied directly to mucous membranes or open wounds, four could not recall any previous contact. Irritant dermatitis may also result from topical application of chlorhexidine solution,[104] and photosensitivity has also been proved by photopatch testing.[116] A potential delay in wound healing caused by chlorhexidine has also been reported.[117] A 1% aqueous solution of chlorhexidine should be used for epicutaneous testing, since chlorhexidine in petrolatum has been shown to produce false-negative patch tests.[118]

GLUTARALDEHYDE

Glutaraldehyde (pentanedial) is a naturally acidic dialdehyde agent.[119] However, in an alkaline buffered solution, it is commonly found in solutions used for cold sterilization of surgical and medical instruments. It is also found in tissue fixatives, cosmetic preparations, wart remedies, and antifungal agents.[120] Contact sensitivity to glutaraldehyde is reported with increasing frequency, especially among health care workers.[119, 121, 122] This may be partially attributable to the increasing use of glutaraldehyde as a sterilizing agent or to its potency as an allergen.[119] Two cases have been reported of contact dermatitis of the hands in cleaning personnel within 6 months of first using a glutaraldehyde-containing cleaning solution.[121]

Cross-reactions between glutaraldehyde and formaldehyde probably do not occur.[123, 124] However, concomitant sensitization with formaldehyde was reported in three of 13 glutaraldehyde-sensitive patients.[125] In the same series, five of 15 patients were also rubber, thiuram, or carbamate sensitive, which suggests that concurrent sensitization with formaldehyde, latex gloves, or other allergens is common and may be an important factor. Persistence of hand dermatitis secondary to glutaraldehyde is common. In one report, all patients with glutaraldehyde allergy had persistent dermatitis and half had to leave their job as a result.[125]

Glutaraldehyde penetrates common latex or vinyl gloves. Only the "4-H glove" may be protective against glutaraldehyde.[122] Topical sensitization to glutaraldehyde may be site dependent. Application of a 2.5% solution to the antecubital area in glutaraldehyde-sensitive patients caused severe dermatitis, but when a 25% solution was applied to the soles of the same patients twice a day for a week, no dermatitis was produced.[126] Glutaraldehyde concentrations above 0.13% may irritate the skin; 2% glutaraldehyde solutions commonly cause yellowing.[122]

POVIDONE-IODINE

Contact dermatitis to povidone-iodine (polyvinylpyrrolidone), is an uncommon occurrence, given its frequent use in the surgical setting.[127] Povidone-iodine is a germicidal solution that acts as an iodophor. It consists of 10% bound and 1% free iodine and is available in many forms, including solution, ointment, gel, shampoo, douche, vaginal gel and dressing. It is also the most frequently employed surgical scrub.[128] True cutaneous allergy seems to occur often when povidone-iodine is applied to compromised skin,[129, 130] such as postoperative sites,[127] or leg ulcers.[129] Sensitivity among physicians and nurses may be promoted by abrading the skin with surgical brushes and then occluding the hands with latex gloves.[127] The offending allergen is usually povidone-iodine itself,[127] less often the surface-active agents, nonoxynols, or plain iodine.[129] Contact allergy has been proved by patch testing with 10% povidone-iodine in petrolatum. Scrub solutions may produce false-positive irritant reactions.

Irritant reactions to povidone-iodine products may also occur.[132, 133] In one report, erythema and tissue necrosis were attributed to the addition of stabilizing reagents, later omitted, to the povidone-iodine preparation.[132] Extensive erythema of the back and buttocks was reported after contact of these areas with a 10% povidone-iodine solution during an 8-hour cardiac operation.[133]

In addition to causing dermatitis, absorption of povidone-iodine solutions may occasionally result in systemic toxicity.[130, 134, 135] Severe metabolic acidosis was reported in two patients with extensive burns as a result of povidone-iodine absorption.[134] Substantially increased serum iodine levels have also been reported after use of a povidone-iodine vaginal douche.[135]

ALCOHOLS

Alcohols are frequently used in cutaneous surgery as solvents for various dyes and as antiseptic skin preparations. True contact sensitivity is a rare occurrence, although it has been reported.[136, 137] Similar patients have been described who are allergic to isopropyl alcohol found in prepackaged swabs.[143, 144] Cross-sensitivity between lower aliphatic alcohols is also common.[138–140]

Ingestion of ethanol may cause flares of hand dermatitis in individuals with alcohol contact allergy.[139, 141]

If contact dermatitis to alcohols is suspected, patch testing should be performed to all alcohols in their purified and unpurified forms. Two types of patch test reactions to alcohols may occur:[142] an immediate-type urticarial reaction consisting of bright red erythema with or without urticaria, and a delayed eczematous reaction. Alcohols should also be tested in their unpurified form, as the denaturing agents found in alcohol infrequently cause sensitization. As organic solvents, alcohols are more often responsible for an irritant-type dermatitis than true allergic sensitization.[142]

HYDROGEN PEROXIDE

Although reported to be nonsensitizing, hydrogen peroxide[145] can cause contact allergy in postoperative wounds. A 3% hydrogen peroxide solution is the proper patch test concentration.[146]

THIMEROSAL

Contact dermatitis from thimerosal is common among the general population[147] but rare in the cutaneous surgical setting. Thimerosal and other related organic mercurial compounds were formerly used as skin antiseptics, but this practice has declined with the development of other antiseptics such as chlorhexidine and povidone-iodine. However, thimerosal is still used as a preservative in many parenteral preparations, including vaccinations, antitoxins, medications,[148] ophthalmic preparations,[149] and diluting fluids for antigens used in skin testing.[148]

Thimerosal has been implicated in a variety of allergic reactions, including allergic contact dermatitis[148] and conjunctivitis,[149] immediate-type reactions such as acute urticaria[150] or angioedema of the airway,[151] and systemic contact dermatitis.[152] The type I and systemic dermatitis reactions have been due largely to thimerosal-containing parenterally administered vaccines or skin tests.[147] Many thimerosal-allergic patients also react to the thiosalicylic acid portion of the chemical. It has been reported that contact allergy to thiosalicylic acid is a marker for patients at high risk for developing piroxicam (Feldene) photosensitivity.[153] Surgical personnel allergic to thimerosal or other organic mercurials should be aware of preparations containing these products so that proper avoidance measures may be taken.

POST-TRAUMATIC ECZEMA

The entity of dermatitis in loco minoris resistentiae or dermatitis in the path of diminished resistance was coined in 1982[154] to describe the phenomenon of eczematous dermatitis occurring in surgical or burn scars. The issue of eczema arising in sites of previous injury or trauma has been characterized in great detail.[155] Post-traumatic eczema is defined as eczematous dermatitis caused by a physical agent within 1 month at the site of previous trauma. Eczematous dermatitis from infection, foreign body reaction, or topical contact allergy must be ruled out to verify the diagnosis.

Two general subclassifications of post-traumatic eczema are the isomorphic or Koebner type, in which eczema develops at the site of trauma identical in morphology to pre-existing or subsequently developing cutaneous lesions in nontraumatized skin; and the idiopathic type, in which eczema develops at a traumatized site without a history of eczema elsewhere on the body. This eruption usually occurs on the extremity several weeks after a traumatic insult such as thermal burn, laceration, or abrasion. This type of eczema may respond to local measures such as topical steroids, but is often recurrent or persistent.[155]

Irritant dermatitis can be the result of repeated low-grade frictional trauma in which the eczematous dermatitis may be a reaction pattern to injury of the skin.[156] Irritant dermatitis of the face has been described after use of a rotating brush for the treatment of acne; the patient was patch test negative to her acne remedy and soaps.[157]

MINOXIDIL

Until recently, topical minoxidil (Rogaine) was infrequently reported to cause contact dermatitis. However, contact dermatitis has been described in ten of 1050 patients presenting with an acutely pruritic vesicular dermatitis or local erythema and edema of the scalp.[158] Six of ten patients were patch test positive to minoxidil in various concentrations. One patient was also positive to propylene glycol, present as a solubilizing agent in commercial preparations. Of the patch test negative patients, all were able to reinstate therapy successfully after a period of abstinence. Only one case of allergic and one case of irritant contact dermatitis were reported among 777 patients enrolled in an open study using minoxidil for treatment of androgenic alopecia.[159] A patient with photocontact dermatitis to minoxidil proved by photopatch testing has also been described.[160]

There have been other reports of allergic reactions as well as irritant dermatitis to both minoxidil and propylene glycol.[159, 162, 163] The package insert for Rogaine 2% topical solution lists a 5% incidence of allergic and irritant dermatitis, but no distinction is made regarding the incidence of each, or which reaction is more common.[161]

In another report,[164] 7.5% of 161 patients had irritant dermatitis that necessitated discontinuing treatment, and 3.7% had allergic contact dermatitis. It was found that propylene glycol and methylethyl ketone were the best vehicles for the patch testing of minoxidil. Petrolatum and alcohol were thought to be unsuitable bases for testing, which may have accounted for false-negative test reactions in previous studies.

5-FLUOROURACIL

Topical fluorouracil has become widely used as a treatment for actinic keratoses but has also been used for other premalignant skin lesions, warts, and early squamous and basal cell carcinoma.[165] Fluorouracil is a pyrimidine nucleotide analog that acts through inhibiting DNA thymidylate synthetase.[166] It is relatively specific for abnormal tissue and rarely produces an adverse reaction in normal tissue.[165] Reports of true allergic sensitization are uncommon, although an irritant dermatitis invariably occurs during the course of treatment.[167] Allergic contact dermatitis was demonstrated in six patients using fluorouracil for actinic keratoses.[168] All sensitized patients had undergone at least two courses of treatment, and sensitization was manifested as an allergic type of dermatitis, differing in morphology from the usual irritant dermatitis. Allergy was confirmed by positive patch or intradermal test. Widespread "systemic-type" eczema developed in three patients. The following criteria can be used to help differentiate between irritant and allergic contact dermatitis from 5-fluorouracil: development of a severely pruritic, eczematous eruption either localized to the site of application or remote sites, positive patch or intradermal test to preservative-free 5-fluorouracil, correlation between intracutaneous and epicutaneous test results, and compatible histologic findings on biopsy of the eczematous rash. The overall incidence of contact dermatitis secondary to 5-fluorouracil in this study was 8.6%.[168]

Use of 5% 5-fluorouracil in petrolatum is recommended for patch testing.[172] However, in view of 25% false-negative results, 1% 5-fluorouracil should be used for intradermal testing of these patients.

Pustular contact dermatitis with persistent rosacea as a sequela occurred in one patient.[169] This eruption was morphologically similar to pustular patch test reactions seen from heavy metals or halogen salts. Patch testing with 1% fluorouracil in water produced a pustular reaction. The mechanism of this eruption was not clear.

Irritant dermatitis was reported in normal scrotal skin where 5-fluorouracil had inadvertently been applied by four patients undergoing treatment for warts or other premalignant skin conditions.[170] The reaction was not allergic, and enhanced absorption of fluorouracil through the scrotal skin was postulated as the cause of the dermatitis. As with many other topical medicaments, it is important to rule out sensitivity to parabens, propylene glycol, or other preservatives found in fluorouracil preparatons as a cause of the dermatitis.[171]

BIOSYNTHETIC SURGICAL DRESSINGS

The emergence of biosynthetic occlusive or semiocclusive dressings has provided the cutaneous surgeon with many superior alternatives in the treatment of various types of ulcers, abrasions, burns, or wounds.[173–181] The occlusive dressings can be divided into those made from films of polyurethane and polyethylene; hydrogels of cross-linked polyethylene oxide or povidone-iodine; composite polymers; and hydrocolloids of gelatin, pectin, and carboxymethyl cellulose. In controlled situations, these dressings have been proved to speed reepithelialization, decrease pain, and absorb water, serum, or blood through expansion of the dressing matrix.[173, 177] Adhesives are not used in all these dressing formulations, but when present may consist of acrylics, latex, rosin, or other components. Reports of contact dermatitis resulting from the use of these dressings have been rare.[176, 178, 179, 181] Two cases of allergic contact dermatitis to Synthaderm have been reported.[178] Individual components were not available for patch testing, but the allergen was proved to be an isocyanate component. Contact dermatitis from Allevyn, a hydrophilic polyurethane dressing, was briefly mentioned,[181] although patch testing was not performed. Because these dressings are often used on leg ulcers and few patch test studies have been performed, contact allergy to biosynthetic dressings, including their adhesives, may be a largely overlooked phenomenon.

MARKING DYES

Dermatitis due to marking materials used in cutaneous surgery is rare. A single case of dermatitis due to brilliant green has been documented.[182] Cutaneous allergy to a marking pen containing gentian violet used on a patient undergoing patch testing has also been demonstrated;[183] the patient could recall no previous exposure to gentian violet. Most cases of allergic contact dermatitis from gentian violet have occurred after application of this dye to chronic eczematous conditions or to nonhealing ulcers.[184] Immediate hypersensitivity reactions consisting of asthma and rhinitis after exposure to various reactive dyes has also been seen.[185, 186] Triketohydrindene hydrate (Ninhydrin), a constituent of the blue gentian-violet surgical marking pens, has also been reported to cause dermatitis in skin areas marked during patch testing.[187] In general, these dyes are weak sensitizers,[188] and allergy is more likely to result from their application to eczematized or ulcerated skin.[184, 188]

SUMMARY

The cutaneous surgeon must always be alert to the possibility of contact allergy in the surgical setting. If a patient should develop an intervening reaction to one of the multitude of surgical preparation solutions, topical anesthetics, surgical adhesives, dressing materials, or topical antibiotics, the desired results could be compromised. Early recognition and treatment of these types of reactions is therefore of tremendous importance. In addition, the apparent rapid increase in the incidence of allergic reactions to surgical gloves also requires that the cutaneous surgeon be aware of this potential problem and how best to manage it should it arise.

REFERENCES

1. North American Contact Dermatitis Group: Patch testing in allergic contact dermatitis. Am Acad Dermatol 1984, pp 1–3.
2. Ancona A, Arevalla A, Macotela E: Contact dermatitis in hospital patients. Dermatol Clin 8:95–105, 1990.
3. Rietschel R: Is patch testing cost effective? J Am Acad Dermatol 21:885–887, 1989.
4. Wilhelm K, Maibach H: Factors predisposing to cutaneous irritation. Dermatol Clin 8:17–22, 1990.
5. Bergstresser P: Immune mechanisms in contact allergic dermatitis. Dermatol Clin 8:3–11, 1990.
6. Marks J, Rainey M: Cutaneous reactions to surgical preparations and dressings. Contact Dermatitis 10:1–5, 1984.
7. Lammintausta K, Maibach HI: Contact dermatitis due to irritation—general principles, etiology, and histology. In: Adams RM (ed): Occupational Skin Disease. WB Saunders, Philadelphia, 1990, pp 1–15.
8. Wood GS, Abel EA: Immunologic aspects of allergic contact dermatitis. In: Adams RM (ed): Occupational Skin Disease. WB Saunders, Philadelphia, 1990, pp 31–35.
9. Katchen BR, Maibach HI: Immediate type contact urticaria reaction: immunologic contact urticaria. In: Menne T, Maibach HI (eds): Exogenous Dermatoses. CRC Press, Boca Raton, FL, 1991, p 53.
10. Gette MT, Marks JG, Maloney ME: The frequency of postoperative allergic contact dermatitis to topical antibiotics. Arch Dermatol 128:365–367, 1992.
11. Fisher A, Adams R: Alternative for sensitizing neomycin topical medicaments. Cutis 28:491–498, 502–503, 1981.
12. Storrs FJ, Rosenthal LE, Adamas RM, et al: Prevalence and relevance of allergic reactions in patients patch tested in North America—1984–1985. J Am Acad Dermatol 20:1038–1045, 1989.
13. Fisher A: Reactions to topical antibiotics. In: Contact Dermatitis. Lea & Febiger, Philadelphia, 1986, pp 195–211.
14. Cronin E: Medicaments. In: Contact Dermatitis. Churchill Livingstone, New York, 1980, pp 203–204, 210–214.
15. Pirila V, Rouhunkosky S: On sensitivity to neomycin and bacitracin. Acta Derm Venereol (Stockh) 39:470, 1959.
16. Rudzki E, Kleniewska D: The epidemiology of contact dermatitis in Poland. Br J Dermatol 83:543, 1970.
17. Forstrom L, Pirila V: Cross sensitivity within the neomycin group of antibiotics. Contact Dermatitis 4:312, 1978.
18. Fraki J, Peltonen L, Hopsu-Havu K: Allergy to various components of topical preparations in stasis dermatitis and leg ulcer. Contact Dermatitis 5:97–100, 1979.
19. Prystowsky S, Nonomura J, Smith R, et al: Allergic hypersensitivity to neomycin. Arch Dermatol 115:713–715, 1979.
20. Schorr W, Ridgway H: Tobramycin-neomycin cross sensitivity. Contact Dermatitis 3:133–137, 1977.
21. Schorr W, Hegedus S: Cross sensitivity in aminoglycoside antibiotics. Arch Dermatol 107:533–539, 1973.
22. Binnick A, Clendenning W: Bacitracin contact dermatitis. Contact Dermatitis 4:180, 1978.
23. Epstein S, Wenzel F: Cross sensitivity to various mycins. Arch Dermatol 86:183–191, 1962.
24. Bjorkner B, Moller H: Bacitracin: a cutaneous allergen and histamine liberator. Acta Derm Venereol (Stockh) 53:487, 1973.
25. Held JL, Kalb RE, Ruszkowski AM, DeLeo V: Allergic contact dermatitis from bacitracin. J Am Acad Dermatol 17:592–594, 1987.
26. Fisher A, Adams R: Benzocaine and bacitracin as sensitizers. J Am Acad Dermatol 16:1055–1057, 1987.
27. Pirila V, Forstrom L, Rouhunkoski S: Twelve years of sensitization to neomycin in Finland. Arch Dermatol Venereol (Stockh) 47:419–425, 1967.
28. Katz B, Fisher A: Bacitracin: a unique topical antibiotic sensitizer. J Am Acad Dermatol 17:1016–1024, 1987.
29. Comaish J, Cunliffe W: Absorption of drugs from venous ulcers: a cause of anaphylaxis. Br J Clin Pract 21:97, 1967.
30. Roupe G, Strennegard O: Anaphylactic shock elicited by topical administration of bacitracin. Arch Dermatol 100:450–452, 1969.
31. Elsner P, Pevny I, Burg G: Anaphylaxis induced by topically applied bacitracin. Am J Contact Derm 1:162–164, 1990.
32. Schecter J, Wilkinson R, Carpio J: Anaphylaxis following the use of bacitracin ointment. Arch Dermatol 120:909–911, 1984.
33. Fisher A: Adverse reactions to bacitracin, polymyxin and gentamicin sulfate. Cutis 32:510–512, 520, 1983.
34. Lombardi P, Campolmo P, Spallanzani P, Sertoly A: Delayed hypersensitivity to erythromycin. Contact Dermatitis 8:416, 1982.
35. van Ketel W: Immediate and delayed type of allergy to erythromycin. Contact Dermatitis 2:363, 1976.
36. Fisher A: Is topical erythromycin base nonallergenic? Contact Dermatitis 9:243, 1983.
37. Fisher A: The safety of topical erythromycin. Contact Dermatitis 2:43–44, 1976.
38. Lo JS, Taylor JS, Oriba H: Occupational allergic contact dermatitis to airborne nitrofurazone. Dermatol Clin 8:165–168, 1990.
39. Bennett RG: Fundamentals of Cutaneous Surgery. CV Mosby, St. Louis, 1988, pp 166, 304.

40. Taylor WB: Personal communication. Ann Arbor, MI, December 1990.
41. Fisher A: Topical medicaments which are common sensitizers. Ann Allergy 49:97–100, 1982.
42. Dripps RD, Eckenhoff JE, Vandam LD (eds): Local anesthetics. In: Introduction to Anesthesia: The Principles of Safe Practice. 7th ed. WB Saunders, Philadelphia, 1988, pp 214–220.
43. Fisher A: Local anesthetics. In: Contact Dermatitis. Lea & Febiger, Philadelphia, 1986, pp 220–227.
44. Fisher A: The presence of benzocaine in sunscreens containing glycerol PABA (Escalol 1:6). Arch Dermatol 113:1299, 1977.
45. Physicians' Desk Reference. 45th ed. Medical Economics Co., Oradell, NJ, 1991, p 1159.
46. Adriani J, Dalili H: Penetration of local anesthetics through epithelial barriers. Anesth Analg 50:1, 1971.
47. Angelini G, Meneghini C: Oral tests in contact allergy to para-amino compounds. Contact Dermatitis 7:311–314, 1981.
48. Fisher A: Allergic reactions to topical (surface) anesthetics with reference to the safety of Tronothane (pramoxine hydrochloride). Cutis 25:584, 586, 589–591, 625, 1980.
49. Galletly D, Gibbs J: Anaphylactoid reacion during anesthesia. In: Nunn JF, Utting JE, Brown BR Jr (eds): General Anesthesia. Butterworths, London, 1989, pp 639–648.
50. Ryan M, Davis B, Marks J: Contact urticaria and allergic contact dermatitis to benzocaine gel. J Am Acad Dermatol 2:221–223, 1980.
51. Schwartz G, Covino B: Local anesthetics. In: Miller RD (ed): Anesthesia. Churchill Livingstone, New York, 1990, pp 454–466.
52. Curley R, Macfarlane A, King C: Contact sensitivity to the amide anesthetics lidocaine, prilocaine, and mepivacaine. Arch Dermatol 122:924–926, 1986.
53. Fernándes de Corres L, Leanizbarrutia I: Dermatitis from lignocaine. Contact Dermatitis 12:114–115, 1985.
54. Fregert S, Tegner E, Thelin I: Contact allergy to lidocaine. Contact Dermatitis 5:185–188, 1979.
55. Lynas R: A suspected allergic reaction to lidocaine. Anesthesiology 31:382–383, 1969.
56. Chin T, Fellner M: Allergic reaction to lidocaine hydrochloride. Int J Dermatol 19:147–148, 1980.
57. De Shazo R, Nelson H: An approach to the patient with a history of local anesthetic hypersensitivity: experience with 90 patients. J Allergy Clin Immunol 63:387–394, 1979.
58. Ashinoff R, Geronemus R: Effect of the topical anesthetic EMLA on the efficacy of pulse dye laser treatment of port-wine stains. J Dermatol Surg Oncol 16:1008–1011, 1990.
59. Philip B: Local anesthesia and sedation techniques. In: White PF (ed): Outpatient Anesthesia. Churchill Livingstone, New York, 1990, pp 263–271.
60. Aldrete J, Johnson D: Allergy to local anesthetics. JAMA 207:356–357, 1969.
61. Schorr W: Paraben allergy. JAMA 204:107–110, 1968.
62. Fisher A: Propylene glycol dermatitis. Cutis 21:166–167, 174–177, 1978.
63. Glinert RJ, Zachary CB: Local anesthetic allergy. J Dermatol Surg Oncol 17:491–496, 1991.
64. Taylor JS, Cassettari J, Wagner W, Helm T: Contact urticaria and anaphylaxis to latex. J Am Acad Dermatol 21:874–877, 1989.
65. Estlander T, Jolanki R: How to protect the hands. Dermatol Clin 6:105–114, 1988.
66. Taylor JS: Rubber. In: Fisher AA (ed): Contact Dermatitis. Lea & Febiger, Philadelphia, 1986, pp 603–643.
67. Turjanmaa K, Reunala T, Alenius H, et al: Allergens in latex surgical gloves and glove powder. Lancet 336:1588, 1990.
68. Turjanmaa K: Latex glove contact urticaria (thesis). University of Tampere, Finland, 1988.
69. Rich P, Belozer ML, Norris P, Storrs FJ: Allergic contact dermatitis to two antioxidants in latex gloves: 4,4'-thiobis (6-tert-butyl-meta-cresol) (Lowinox 44S36) and butylhydroxyanisole. Allergen alternatives for glove-allergic patients. J Am Acad Dermatol 24:37–43, 1991.
70. Estlander T, Jolanki R, Kanerva L: Dermatitis and urticaria from rubber and plastic gloves. Contact Dermatitis 14:20–25, 1986.
71. Percquet C, Leynadier F, Dry J: Contact urticaria and anaphylaxis to natural latex. J Am Acad Dermatol 22:631–633, 1990.
72. Ownby DR, Tomlanovich T, Sammons N, McCullough J: Fatal anaphylaxis during a barium enema associated with latex allergy. J Allergy Clin Immunol 87:268, 1991.
73. Gaffey C: Allergic reactions to latex-containing medical devices. FDA Medical Alert March 29, 1991. US FDA, Center for Devices and Radiological Health, HFZ–70, Rockville, MD.
74. Stigi J: To all manufacturers of latex devices. Letter of May 1, 1991. US FDA, Division of Small Manufacturers Assistance, HFZ 220, Rockville, MD.
75. Makinen-Kiljunen S, Turjanmaa K, Alenius H, et al: Characterization of latex allergens with immunoelectrophoresis and immunoblotting. J Allergy Clin Immunol 87:270, 1991.
76. Turjanmaa K. Personal communication. June 1991.
77. Korniewicz D: Leakage of virus through used vinyl and latex examination gloves. J Clin Microbiol 28:787–788, 1990.
78. Taylor JS: Adhesives, gums and resins. In: Fisher AA (ed): Contact Dermatitis. Lea & Febiger, Philadelphia, 1986, pp 644–674.
79. Bryant RA: Saving the skin from tape injuries. Am J Nurs 88:189–191, 1988.
80. Soderberg TA, Elmros T, Gref R, Hallmans G: Inhibiting effect of zinc oxide on contact allergy due to colophony. Contact Dermatitis 23:346–351, 1990.
81. Hausen BM, Krohn K, Budianto E: Contact allergy due to colophony (VII). Contact Dermatitis 23:352–358, 1990.
82. Ehrin E, Karlberg A-T: Detection of rosin (colophony) components in technical products using an HPLC technique. Contact Dermatitis 23:359–366, 1990.
83. Hausen BM, Mohnert J: Contact allergy due to colophony (V). Contact Dermatitis 20:295–301, 1989.
84. Karlberg AT, Boman A, Hacksell U, et al: Contact allergy to dehydroabietic acid derivatives isolated from Portuguese colophony. Contact Dermatitis 19:166–174, 1988.
85. Veraldi S, Schianchi-Veraldi R: Allergic contact dermatitis from colophony in a wart gel. Contact Dermatitis 22:184, 1990.
86. Lachapelle JM, Leroy B: Allergic contact dermatitis to colophony included in the formulation of flexible collodion BP, the vehicle of salicylic and lactic acid wart paint. Dermatol Clin 8:143–146, 1990.
87. Karlberg AT: Colophony-free wart removers in Sweden. Contact Dermatitis 18:254, 1988.
88. Karlberg AT: Air oxidation increases the allergenic potential of tall oil rosin. Colophony contact allergens also identified in tall oil rosin. Am J Contact Derm 2:43–49, 1991.
89 Norris P, Storrs FJ: Allergic contact dermatitis to adhesive bandages. Dermatol Clin 8:147–152, 1990.
90. Satyawani Oranje AP, van-Joost T: Perioral dermatitis in a child due to rosin in chewing gum. Contact Dermatitis 22:182–183, 1990.
91. Ranchoff RE, Steck WD, Taylor JS: Electrocardiograph electrode and hand dermatitis from parachlorometaxylenol. J Am Acad Dermatol 15:348–350, 1986.
92. Hindson C, Sinclair S: Contact allergy to self-adhesive dressings. Lancet 1:1224, 1988.
93. Kitchen N: Adhesive dressing allergy. Lancet 2:111, 1988.
94. James WD: Allergic contact dermatitis to a colophony derivative. Contact Dermatitis 10:6–10, 1984.
95. Schubert H: Nickel dermatitis in medical workers. Dermatol Clin 8:45–47, 1990.
96. Fisher A: Safety of stainless steel and nickel sensitivity. JAMA 221:1279, 1972.
97. Samitz M, Katz S: Nickel dermatitis hazards from prostheses. Br J Dermatol 92:287–290, 1975.
98. Nurse D: Nickel sensitivity induced by skin clips. Contact Dermatitis 5:497, 1980.
99. Kubba R, Taylor JS, Marks KE: Cutaneous complications of orthopedic implants. Arch Dermatol 117:554, 1981.
100. Roed-Petersen B, Roed-Petersen J, Dreyer Jorgensen K: Nickel allergy and osteomyelitis in a patient with metal osteosynthesis of a jaw fracture. Contact Dermatitis 5:108–112, 1979.
101. Waterman A, Schrik J: Allergy in hip arthroplasty. Contact Dermatitis 13:294–301, 1985.
102. Wilkinson J, Hamboy E: Nickel spot testing at home. Contact Dermatitis 4:114–115, 1978.
103. Gola M, Francalanci P, Campoli P: Catgut dermatitis. Contact Dermatitis 15:104, 1986.

104. Rudzki E, Rebandel P, Grzywa Z: Patch test with occupational contactants in nurses, doctors, and dentists. Contact Dermatitis 20:247–250, 1989.

105. Wilkinson JD: Cutaneous reactions from other sources of implanted metal. In: Maibach HI, Mennet T (eds): Nickel and the Skin: Immunology and Toxicology. CRC Press, Ocala, FL, 1989, pp 151–153.

106. Fisher AA: The nylon suture material test for an allergic reaction. Am J Contact Derm 1:69, 1990.

107. Fisher A: Contact urticaria from chlorhexidine. Cutis 43:17–18, 1989.

108. Lasthein Andersen B, Brandrup F: Contact dermatitis from chlorhexidine. Contact Dermatitis 13:307–309, 1985.

109. Fisher A: Chlorhexidine. In: Contact Dermatitis. Lea & Febiger, Philadelphia, 1986, pp 186–187.

110. Cronin E: Chlorhexidine (Hexamethylene bis-chlorphenyl biguainde; Hibitane; Nolvasan; Rotersept; Sterilon). In: Contact Dermatitis. Churchill Livingstone, New York, 1980, pp 696–697.

111. Osmundsen P: Contact dermatitis to chlorhexidine. Contact Dermatitis 8:81–83, 1982.

112. Shoji A: Contact dermatitis from chlorhexidine. Contact Dermatitis 9:156, 1983.

113. Reynolds N, Harman R: Allergic contact dermatitis from chlorhexidine acetate in skin swab. Contact Dermatitis 22:52, 1990.

114. Bechgaard E, Ploug E, Hjorth N: Contact sensitivity to chorhexidine? Contact Dermatitis 13:53–55, 1985.

115. Okano M, Nomura M, Hata S, et al: Anaphylactic symptoms due to chlorhexidine gluconate. Arch Dermatol 125:50–52, 1989.

116. Wahlberg J, Wennersten G: Hypersensitivity and photosensitivity to chlorhexidine. Dermatologica 143:376–379, 1971.

117. Mobacken H, Wengstrom C: Interference with healing of rat skin incisions treated with chlorhexidine. Acta Derm Venereol (Stockh) 54:29, 1974.

118. Ljunggren B, Moller H: Eczematous contact allergy to chlorhexidine. Acta Derm Venereol (Stockh) 52:308, 1972.

119. Goncalo S, Menezes Brandao F, Pecegueiro M, et al: Occupational contact dermatitis to glutaraldehyde. Contact Dermatitis 10:183–184, 1984.

120. Fisher A: Glutaraldehyde (Pentanedial). In: Contact Dermatitis. Lea & Febiger, Philadelphia, 1986, pp 155–157.

121. Hansen K: Glutaraldehyde occupational dermatitis. Contact Dermatitis 9:81–82, 1983.

122. Fisher A: Allergic contact dermatitis of the hands from Sporicidin (glutaraldehyde-phenate) used to disinfect endoscopes. Cutis 45:227–228, 1990.

123. Cronin E: Glutaraldehyde (Pentanedial). In: Contact Dermatitis. Churchill Livingstone, New York, 1980, pp 795–797.

124. Maibach H: Glutaraldehyde and cross reaction to formaldehyde. Contact Dermatitis 1:326, 1975.

125. Nethercott J, Holness D, Page E: Occupational contact dermatitis due to glutaraldehyde in health-care workers. Contact Dermatitis 18:193–196, 1988.

126. Maibach H, Prystowsky S: Glutaraldehyde (Pentanedial) allergic contact dermatitis. Arch Dermatol 113:170–171, 1977.

127. van Ketel WG, van den Berg WHHW: Sensitization to povidone-iodine. Dermatol Clin 8:107–109, 1990.

128. Ancona A, Suarez de la Torre R, Macotela E: Allergic contact dermatitis from povidone-iodine. Contact Dermatitis 13:66–68, 1985.

129. Dooms-Goossens A, Gidi de Alam A, Degreef H: Contact sensitivity to nonoxyls: a cause of intolerance to antiseptic preparations. In: Current Topics in Contact Dermatitis. Springer-Verlag, Berlin, 1989, pp 104–107.

130. Marks J: Allergic contact dermatitis to povidone-iodine. J Am Acad Dermatol 6:473–475, 1982.

131. Lachapelle J: Occupational allergic contact dermatitis to povidone-iodine. Contact Dermatitis 11:189–190, 1984.

132. Shroff AP, Jones JK: Reactions to povidone-iodine preparation. JAMA 243:230–231, 1980.

133. Okano M: Irritant contact dermatitis caused by povidone-iodine. J Am Acad Dermatol 20:860, 1989.

134. Pietsch J, Meakins J: Complications of povidone-iodine absorption in topically treated burn patients. Lancet 1:280–282, 1976.

135. Vorherr H, Vorherr UF, Pushpa M, et al: Vaginal absorption of povidone-iodine. JAMA 244:26–29, 1980.

136. Wasilewski C: Allergic contact dermatitis from isopropyl alcohol. Arch Dermatol 98:502–504, 1968.

137. Ludwig E, Hausen B: Sensitivity to isopropyl alcohol. Contact Dermatitis 3:240–244, 1977.

138. van Ketel WG, Tan-Lim KN: Contact dermatitis from ethanol. Contact Dermatitis 1:7–10, 1975.

139. Drevets C, Seebohm P: Dermatitis from alcohol. J Allergy 32:277–282, 1961.

140. Haxthausen H: Allergic eczema caused by ethyl alcohol—elicited both by epicutaneous and by internal application. Acta Derm Venereol 25:527–528, 1944.

141. Cronin E: Alcohols and glycols. In: Contact Dermatitis. Churchill Livingstone, New York, 1980, pp 805–809.

142. Fisher A: Alcohol. In: Contact Dermatitis. Lea & Febiger, Philadelphia, 1986, pp 525–526, 538–539.

143. Richardson D: Allergic contact dermatitis to "alcohol" swabs. Cutis 5:1115, 1969.

144. Kurwa A: Contact dermatitis from isopropyl alcohol. Contact Dermatitis News 8:168, 1970.

145. Cronin E: Hydrogen peroxide. In: Contact Dermatitis. Churchill Livingstone, New York, 1980, p 126.

146. Fisher A: Hydrogen peroxide. In: Contact Dermatitis. Lea & Febiger, Philadelphia, 1986, p 880.

147. Fisher A: Antiseptics and disinfectants. In: Contact Dermatitis. Lea & Febiger, Philadelphia, 1986, pp 178–181.

148. Fisher A: Allergic reactions to merthiolate. Cutis 27:580–587, 1981.

149. Tosti A, Tosti G: Thimerosal: a hidden allergen in ophthalmology. Contact Dermatitis 18:268–273, 1988.

150. Tosti A, Nelino M, Bardazzi F: Systemic reactions due to thimerosal. Contact Dermatitis 15:187–188, 1986.

151. Maibach H: Acute laryngeal obstruction presumed secondary to thimerosal (merthiolate) delayed hypersensitivity. Contact Dermatitis 1:221, 1975.

152. Novak N, Kvicalova E, Friedlanderova B: Reactions to merthiolate in infants. Contact Dermatitis 15:309–310, 1986.

153. Serrano G, Bonillo J, Aliaga A, et al: Piroxicam-induced photosensitivity and contact sensitivity to thiosalicylic acid. J Am Acad Dermatol 23:479–483, 1990.

154. Zuehlke R, Rapini R, Puhl S, Ray T: Dermatitis in loco minoris resistentiae. J Am Acad Dermatol 6:1010–1013, 1982.

155. Mathias GT: Post-traumatic eczema. Dermatol Clin 6:35–42, 1988.

156. Freeman S, Rosen R: Friction as a cause of irritant contact dermatitis. Am J Contact Derm 1:165–170, 1990.

157. Ayres S, Mihan R: Facial dermatitis following friction treatment of acne. Cutis 24:610–611, 1979.

158. Camarasa J, Serra-Baldrich E, Garcia-Bravo B, et al: Contact dermatitis to minoxidil. In: Current Topics in Contact Dermatitis. Springer-Verlag, Berlin, 1989, pp 261–263.

159. Roenigk H, Pepper E, Kuruvila S: Topical minoxidil therapy for hereditary male-pattern alopecia. Cutis 39:337–342, 1987.

160. Tosti A, Birdazzi F, De Padova M, et al: Contact dermatitis to minoxidil. Contact Dermatitis 13:275–276, 1985.

161. Package insert. Rogaine topical solution (minoxidil 2%). Upjohn, Kalamazoo, MI, 1990.

162. Degreef H, Hendricks I, Dooms-Goossens A: Allergic contact dermatitis to minoxidil. Contact Dermatitis 13:194–195, 1985.

163. van der Willigen A, Dutree-Meulenberg R, Stolz E, et al: Topical minoxoidil sensitization in androgenic alopecia. Contact Dermatitis 17:44–45, 1987.

164. Wilson C, Walkden V, Powell S, et al: Contact dermatitis in reaction to 2% topical minoxidil solution. J Am Acad Dermatol 24:661–662, 1991.

165. Jansen G, Dililaha C, Honeycutt W: Bowenoid conditions of the skin: treatment with topical 5-fluorouracil. South Med J 69:185–188, 1967.

166. Eaglestein W, Weinstein G, Frost P: Fluorouracil: mechanism of action in the human skin and actinic keratosis. Arch Dermatol 101:132–139, 1970.

167. Sams W: Untoward response with topical fluorouracil. Arch Dermatol 97:14–22, 1968.

168. Goette D, Odom R: Allergic contact dermatitis to topical fluorouracil. Arch Dermatol 113:1058–1061, 1977.

169. Sevadjin C: Pustular contact hypersensitivity to fluorouracil with rosacea-like sequela. Arch Dermatol 121:240–242, 1985.

170. Shelley W, Shelley E: Scrotal dermatitis caused by 5-fluorouracil (Efudex). J Am Acad Dermatol 19:929–931, 1988.

171. Fisher A: 5-Fluorouracil. In: Contact Dermatitis. Lea & Febiger, Philadelphia, 1986, pp 153–154.

172. Epstein E: Contact dermatitis to 5-fluorouracil with false negative patch tests. Contact Dermatitis 6:220–221, 1980.

173. Eaglstein W: Experiences with biosynthetic dressings. J Am Acad Dermatol 12:434–440, 1985.

174. Falanga V, Eaglstein W: Therapeutic approach to venous ulcers. J Am Acad Dermatol 14:777–784, 1986.

175. Curreri W, Desai M, Bartlett R, et al: Safety and efficacy of a new synthetic burn dressing. Arch Surg 115:925–927, 1980.

176. Spence W, Bates I: Synthetic dressings for the injured skin. Presentation at the Texas Medical Association, 1981 Annual Session, Forum of Original Research, May 28, 1981.

177. Barnett A, Berkowitz R, Mills R, Bistnes L: Comparison of synthetic adhesive moisture vapor permeable and fine-mesh gauze dressings for split-thickness skin graft donor sites. Am J Surg 145:379–381, 1983.

178. Helland S, Nyfors A, Utne L: Contact dermatitis to Synthaderm. Contact Dermatitis 9:504–506, 1983.

179. Eaglstein WH: Personal communication. November 12, 1990.

180. Mertz PM: Intervention: dressing effects on wound healing. In: Eaglstein WH (ed): New Directions in Wound Healing. Bristol-Myers Squibb, Princeton, NJ, 1990, pp 83–96.

181. Young JR, Terwoord BA: Stasis ulcer treatment with compression dressing. Cleve Clin J Med 57:529–531, 1990.

182. Shehade S, Foulds I: Allergic contact dermatitis to brilliant green. Contact Dermatitis 14:186–187, 1986.

183. Cox N, Moss C, Hannon M: Compound allergy to a skin marker for patch testing: a chromatographic analysis. Contact Dermatitis 21:12–15, 1989.

184. Lawrence C, Smith A: Ampliative medicament allergy: concomitant sensitivity to multiple medications including yellow soft paraffin, white soft paraffin, gentian violet, and Span 20. Contact Dermatitis 8:240–245, 1982.

185. Alanko K, Keskinen H, Bjorksten F, Ojanen S: Immediate hypersensitivity reactive dyes. Clin Allergy 8:25–31, 1978.

186. Thoren K, Meding B, Nordlinder R, Belin L: Contact dermatitis and asthma from reactive dyes. Contact Dermatitis 15:186, 1986.

187. Roesler J, Kleinhans D: Contact allergy towards Ninhydrin in a marking pen for patch testing. In: Current Topics in Contact Dermatitis. Springer-Verlag, Berlin, 1989, pp 342–344.

188. Fisher A: Antiseptics and disinfectants. In: Contact Dermatitis. Lea & Febiger, Philadelphia, 1986, pp 191–192.

CHAPTER 8

Surgical Equipment and Instrumentation

WILLIAM S. LYNCH

O ver the past several decades, the trend in health care delivery has been to perform more surgical procedures in outpatient settings. Ambulatory surgery by definition does not require a hospital stay and may be performed in an outpatient surgical center within a hospital, in a freestanding surgical center, or in a surgical suite within the physician's office.[1,2] For years cutaneous surgeons have performed surgical procedures in an ambulatory setting.[3] This has proved more personalized and efficient, less expensive, and more convenient for both patient and physician.[4,5] With careful adherence to appropriate standards, quality of care and patient safety are not compromised.[6,7]

The Surgical Suite

The design and layout of an operating suite are extremely important. It must provide an atmosphere for efficient, comfortable, state-of-the-art care. The setting should be pleasant and reassuring for both patient and the surgical staff.[8] The surgical suite should contain a surgical sink and also be large enough to accommodate strategically placed furniture and equipment such as operating tables, lights, instrument stands, electrosurgical and suction equipment, and waste containers. Adequate storage within the room should also be provided to facilitate easy access to commonly used instruments and supplies. For more complex surgical procedures, special additional accommodations and equipment are required for general anesthesia, laser surgery, liposuction, and other cosmetic procedures.[9]

Surgical Equipment

OPERATING TABLE

High-quality surgical tables are strongly recommended for a busy surgical practice, to provide comfort for the patient and easy access for the surgeon. In addition to comfort, adjustability and overall dimensions are the most important considerations to keep in mind when purchasing an operating table. Power tables with foot-operated or fingertip controls are the most desirable. Tables are manufactured with multiple joints to allow great flexibility (Fig. 8–1). Most tables are fully electric, while others have hydraulic components. The degree of adjustability, as well as smoothness and speed, varies greatly among models. Table elevation limits are fairly uniform, but the lowest position is also important for ease of patient access. Adjustments in back and foot elevation are essential for individual patient comfort. Attention should be given to specific medical conditions such as cardiopulmonary disease and neck or back problems. It is often desirable to have pillows available to further refine positioning and maximize patient comfort. The tilt positioning of the table is important, enabling the angle of the table to be adjusted. This not only enhances patient comfort, but is also essential if a patient must be placed in the Trendelenburg position during the procedure.

Surgical tables are manufactured in various dimensions. A wider table more easily accommodates heavier patients, while a narrow table occupies less space and provides better access for the surgeon. Head-rest size may vary and is an important consideration for comfort

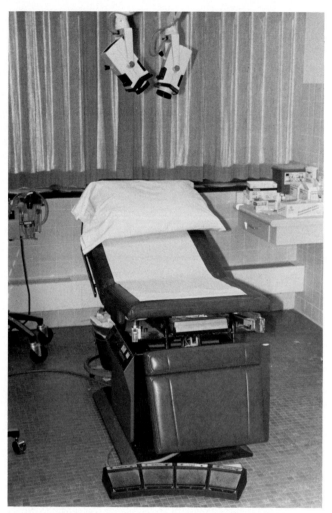

Figure 8–1. Power surgical table (Midmark Corp.).

OPERATING ROOM LIGHTS

Optimal illumination of the surgical field is essential, especially during precise surgical procedures. A wide range of surgical lights are available and should be closely matched to the needs of the procedures to be performed. Specific considerations include the intensity of the light, the field size illuminated, heat production, shadows produced, and maneuverability. The intensity of the light relates to the type of bulbs and filters: it is expressed in foot-candles, with the range between 3000 foot-candles for smaller lights and 8000 foot-candles for the larger models. A common model consists of a single lamp centrally placed in a concave reflective shell (Fig. 8–2); these are available in single or dual mountings. More expensive, larger designs are available that provide multiple lights set in a concave reflective shell, each aligned at a slightly different angle to widen the illuminated area and minimize shadows. The diameter, shape, and composition of the concave reflective surface determine the focused depth of field as well as the shadow and glare produced. More expensive models are equipped with a focusing adjustment to help sharpen the intensity of the illumination.[11]

Heat production can be an important consideration, especially in lengthy surgical procedures. The heat is related to the type of bulb as well as to filtering and ventilation. Reflective light is cooler than direct light. Some manufacturers use enhanced ventilation- and heat-absorbing materials in the reflective surface. One popular type of light with intensity and field size adjustments contains a halogen lamp with a cooling fan.

In addition to field size and illumination, maneuverability is a vital consideration. The greatest range of

and access. Arm rests are another option that may be important, especially for older or anxious patients. Finally, many tables may be purchased with detachable arm boards, restraint straps, Mayo tables, and stirrups. These items are purely a matter of personal preference and must be individualized for a specific surgical practice.

These functions may be obtained in the two basic types of table designs. In addition to the standard configuration surgical table (see Fig. 8–1), a chair design may be chosen to provide improved access to the upper torso and head and neck. However, it will often be too narrow to accommodate the heavier patient comfortably. The chair design chosen should provide all the functions listed above, with special attention to the ability to lie completely flat and convert into the Trendelenburg position. It is strongly recommended that surgeons actually lie on the table themselves for 5 to 15 minutes, to best evaluate the many options available. This will provide a practical assessment of design comfort, padding, and contour. Cost is always a consideration, but it is usually advisable to buy the best, most versatile table, with functions and options tailored to the specific type of surgical practice.[10]

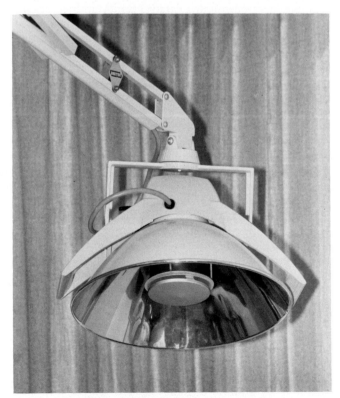

Figure 8–2. Surgical operating light (Burton Corp.).

motion is provided by ceiling-mounted track lighting, which can allow for 360 degrees of flexibility as well as full illumination of the head and feet. Ceiling-mounted fixed units are perhaps the most commonly employed. They should be situated over the table to illuminate the largest field possible. All operating lights should be equipped with handles to allow positioning during the procedure. These handles should be capable of being sterilized. Sterile, disposable handle covers are available from most manufacturers. Wall-mounted units are less desirable as they generally have more limited access. Movable floor units are cumbersome, occupy crucial floor space, and should be used only as ancillary lighting. Finally, a fiberoptic headlight may be preferred for procedures performed in confined spaces such as the ear canal or deep cavities. These may be unwieldy at first but can provide excellent lighting in certain circumstances.

ELECTROSURGICAL EQUIPMENT

This discussion is devoted only to electrocautery; a more detailed review of electrosurgery is presented in Chapter 19. Thermal cautery pertains to conduction of heat from a heated instrument to tissue resulting in desiccation, coagulation, and necrosis. Various pieces of equipment are available, some with electrocautery capabilities only and some with additional high-frequency electrosurgical and electrolysis capabilities.[12, 13]

The older units, such as the Geiger or National, provide only heat cautery. The heat is generated in a hot metal tip that is applied to tissue. The unit will cauterize despite the presence of small amounts of tissue fluid and blood and is safe to use even in patients with pacemakers.[14] A battery-powered portable unit is currently available and is very convenient for use during inpatient consultations or in nursing home settings. Another commonly used unit is the Birtcher hyfrecator (Fig. 8–3). This device does not provide a cutting current and is used only as a coagulating instrument. For effective use, a dry field is necessary. The units are relatively small and can be mounted on the wall or placed on a movable stand. New models provide for fingertip control of the on-off setting as well as power setting. The Bovie electrosurgical unit is a reliable, multifunctional unit providing both coagulation and cutting features. Newer models are smaller and less cumbersome and are useful in an outpatient setting.

A new electrosurgical unit manufactured by the Ellman International Manufacturing Co., the Surgitron F.F.P.F.,[15] uses radiowave frequency and provides four currents for specific indications. The fully filtered current allows microsmooth cutting, the fully rectified current provides blended cutting and coagulation, the partially rectified current allows enhanced coagulation, and the fulgurating current may be used for spark-gap desiccation. The unit offers a number of options, including a finger-switch control, autoclavable handpieces, and a variety of different electrodes.

It is essential that an electrosurgical handle and electrode tip be used in a sterile environment. For some

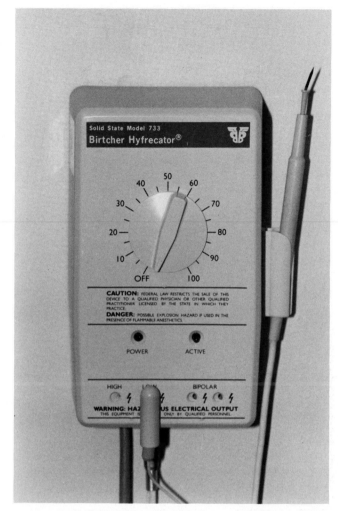

Figure 8–3. Birtcher hyfrecator with fingertip controls (Birtcher Corp.).

devices the entire handle may be sterilized, necessitating that a number of handles be available, or a sterile sleeve, such as a Penrose drain, may be used to cover the handle for each procedure.[16] The tips can be purchased as reusable, autoclavable electrodes or as disposable cautery tips such as the Electrolase (Birtcher Corp.).

A specialized electrosurgical instrument used by many is the Shaw scalpel,[17] which has a heated, sharp scalpel blade that provides true electrocautery as it cuts. The blade has special sensors so that the temperature can be adjusted with a control on the handle within the range of 120° to 270°C. The handle can be sterilized, but the disposable, sterile blades are prepackaged. This instrument is particularly valuable for performing procedures in vascular areas such as the nose or scalp.

SUCTION EQUIPMENT

Suction equipment is essential for safety in extensive surgical procedures such as Mohs fresh tissue micrographic surgery or complex flaps. Institution-based ambulatory surgery suites may have wall suction available.

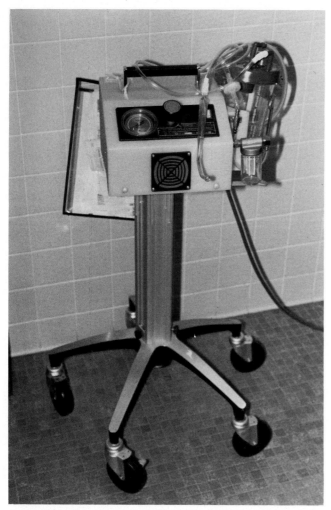

Figure 8–4. Aeros aspirator (Aeros Instrument Manufacturers).

However, portable units such as the Gomco or Aeros aspirator (Fig. 8–4) are also commonplace. The suction tubing can be purchased presterilized. Suction tips are available in a variety of sizes and shapes and can be purchased in reusable autoclavable styles or disposable plastic models.

MAYO STAND

The Mayo stand is universally required. It allows for easy, convenient access of equipment and supplies and is adjustable in height. A table unit with four or six wheels is most maneuverable and can be moved during the procedure.

WASTE DISPOSAL

Well-equipped surgical suites should include kick-bucket waste containers. These are stainless steel wastebaskets on wheels with a protective hard rubber and steel rim that can be used to move the bucket with the feet during a procedure. They can be lined with heavy plastic that can be sealed for disposal after each procedure. In view of the risk of infectivity, all supplies and disposable surgical equipment should be handled according to stringent guidelines established for the safe disposal of bodily fluids and tissue.

ANCILLARY EQUIPMENT

An ambulatory cutaneous surgical unit requires additional, specific high-performance equipment. Electrosurgical, cryosurgical, and resuscitation equipment are standard; the availability of lasers and ancillary equipment such as hand engines and liposuction, hair transplantation, and dermabrasion equipment depends on the size and nature of the surgical practice. A common piece of equipment in a cutaneous surgical practice is the hand engine used for performing hair transplantations and dermabrasions.[18] Popular models include the Bell hand engine (Fig. 8–5) and the Osada handpiece; these operate in the range of 5000 to 20,000 rpm. They accept various sizes of punches for hair transplantation procedures and diamond fraises for dermabrasion.

Every practice in which surgical procedures are performed should have the full spectrum of emergency equipment available, including oxygen, intravenous equipment, emergency medications, airway and blood pressure monitoring equipment, and a defibrillator. The essential supplies and equipment can be obtained in a prepackaged kit such as the STAT KIT by Banyan Instrument Corp. (see Appendix I). It is important that all surgical personnel be trained in emergency procedures and that physicians and nurses maintain current Life Support certification. All equipment should be regularly checked and medications updated in a timely fashion. It is also advisable to practice resuscitation procedures on a regular basis through simulated emergencies.

ARRANGEMENT OF EQUIPMENT

The equipment in the surgical suite must be arranged in a manner that allows optimal convenience, accessibility, and freedom of movement for the surgical staff. The operating table should be centrally located with

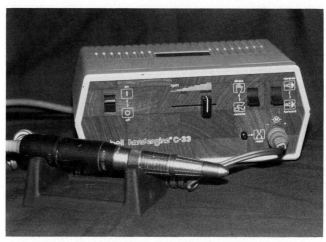

Figure 8–5. Bell hand engine.

free access from all sides. Surgical lights should be positioned to provide maximal illumination. Movable equipment such as Mayo stands, electrosurgical equipment, and waste containers should be placed to enhance flexibility during the procedure.

Surgical Instrumentation

Modern surgical instrumentation dates back to the early 1900s with the advent of stainless steel equipment. As sterilization procedures became more advanced, durable, reusable equipment evolved. In recent years, however, there has been a trend toward disposable instruments. While these may offer certain advantages and conveniences, the surgeon should always select instruments that provide greatest comfort for precision and control. Surgical stainless steel contains carbon alloy (up to 1.7%), which contributes to hardness. To prevent corrosion, chromium (12 to 18%) and nickel (8%) are also incorporated. With function in mind, the exact concentration of these alloys is adjusted to achieve the desired sharpness, hardness, and corrosion resistance for a particular piece of equipment. Newer materials, such as tungsten carbide, are being incorporated into instruments to enhance function and durability.[11] With the wide variation in cost and quality, the purchase of surgical instruments is an important task that is best performed by the surgeon. A reputable manufacturer and distributor wishes to have satisfied customers and will be very responsive to a surgeon's specific needs. A close working relationship between physician and dealer proves mutually beneficial and promotes optimal patient care.

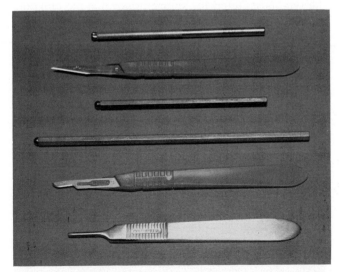

Figure 8–6. Scalpel handles. *Top to bottom*: round Beaver handle, disposable handle with No. 11 blade, hexagonal Beaver handle (short), hexagonal Beaver handle (long), disposable handle with No. 15 blade, Bard-Parker No. 3 handle.

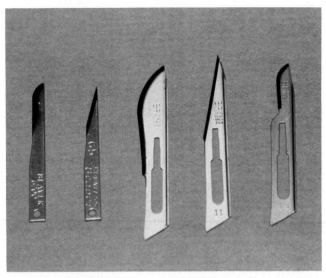

Figure 8–7. Scalpel blades. *Left to right*: Beaver No. 6700 blade, Beaver No. 65 blade, Bard-Parker No. 10 blade, Bard-Parker No. 11 blade, Bard-Parker No. 15 blade.

SCALPELS AND BLADES

The selection of a scalpel, composed of a handle and blade, is a matter of personal preference. The commonly used scalpel handle in routine cutaneous surgical procedures (Fig. 8–6) is a No. 3 with a No. 15 blade. A useful feature is a centimeter scale on the scalpel handle, which allows easy measurement of lesions and surgical defects and aids in flap planning. Handles vary both in shape (flat, round, or octagonal) and weight distribution. Most handles accept all standard sizes of blades. For delicate work, some surgeons prefer a Beaver handle, which may be hexagonal or round and comes in different lengths and diameters. Some cutaneous surgeons find the ability to roll the Beaver handle with the fingertips provides greater flexibility and control. Disposable scalpel handles with attached blades are also available, but they are lighter and weighted differently so may be less suitable for fine work.

The scalpel blade is composed of stainless steel or the sharper carbon steel. The sharpest portion of a curved blade is the belly, not the tip, so that most cutting is performed with that part of the blade. The most commonly used blade is the No. 15, the No. 10 blade being used for larger excisions (Fig. 8–7). For stab incisions or nicking tissue, a No. 11 blade is commonly used. Beaver blades are smaller and fit only Beaver handles. The most commonly used blades are Nos. 65 and 67, which are designed for performing precise and delicate surgery. Commonly, the blades on disposable handles are made of stainless steel and may be less sharp than carbon steel blades. Safe attachment and removal of scalpel blades is vitally important. A hemostat or blade extractor may be used to minimize injury to all personnel handling scalpel blades.

An economical sharp cutting edge for performing

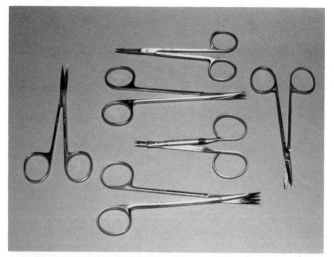

Figure 8–8. Scissors. *Left to right, top to bottom*: curved iris scissors (4¼ inch), straight iris scissors (4¼ inch), curved Stevens tenotomy scissors (5 inch), straight Gradle tissue scissors with overlapping shank (4 inch), Kilner undermining scissors (5½ inch), Spencer suture removal scissors (4½ inch).

simple procedures such as shave biopsies can be provided by a safety razor blade such as a Gillette Super Blue Blade. To use these blades, a blade breaker and holder is usually necessary. The Castroviejo model provides a sliding lock for holding a piece of the blade, enhancing both safety and control.[19]

SCISSORS

In cutaneous surgery, scissors are used for the four basic functions of cutting tissue, undermining, suture removal, and bandage removal. Tissue scissors have many different optional features and come with straight or curved blades, long or short shanks, sharp or blunt tips, and serrated cutting edges or diamond cutting edges.[19] Popular models for working with delicate tissue include the Stevens tenotomy scissors, the Gradle and Gibbs-Gradle scissors, and the iris scissors (Fig. 8–8).[20] An invaluable instrument for finer tissue work is the spring-tipped Castroviejo scissors with sharp tips (Fig. 8–9). In most cases, undermining scissors have longer

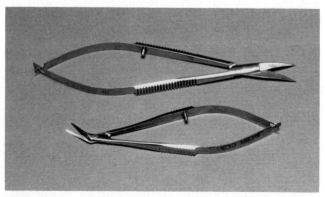

Figure 8–9. Delicate tissue scissors. *Top to bottom*: curved Castroviejo scissors (4½ inch), Castroviejo corneal scissors (3¾ inch).

shanks and blunt tips. Stevens tenotomy scissors provide excellent control for undermining in delicate areas such as the face. Other useful undermining tools include the Metzenbaum, Ragnell, Shea, and Kilner scissors. Specially designed scissors are also available for removing especially fine suture material. Many of these have a small hooked tip that helps catch the suture and reduces the risk of nicking the skin. They are also available in straight or curved models of varying lengths. The Short-bent and Spencer scissors are some of the most versatile and popular in cutaneous surgery. Bandage scissors are a mainstay in any surgical office; the classic scissors for this purpose is the Lister, usually the 5½-inch model. It is made with angled blades and a large blunt tip to slide under the dressing without damaging the skin. The heavy-duty Universal scissors is another popular model with serrated edges and larger ring sizes for greater power.

FORCEPS

The handling of tissue in cutaneous surgery is greatly facilitated by forceps or pick-ups (Fig. 8–10). A variety of tips are available for different tissues and functions. Small, toothed forceps having one to three teeth can be used for gentle tissue manipulation. The most popular models include iris, Bishop-Harman, Foerster, Semken, and Adson forceps. Forceps with fine serrated jaws are commonly called dressing forceps. Adson or Brown-Adson forceps can be used for handling tissue, but excessive pressure will result in significant tissue damage. In general, smooth-jawed forceps do not provide enough tissue traction to be useful for most cutaneous surgery. Another useful type in cutaneous surgery is the splinter forceps, which comes with fine, extra-fine, or superfine tips. It may be used for spot coagulation with the bipolar electrosurgical equipment and for placement of minigrafts during hair transplantation procedures. The type best suited for suture removal is the epilating

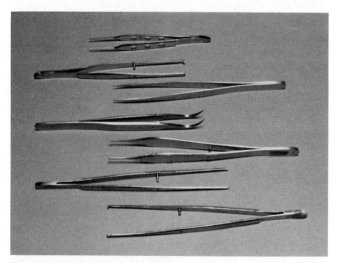

Figure 8–10. Forceps. *Top to bottom*: Bishop-Harman forceps 1 × 2 teeth; straight iris forceps 1 × 2 teeth; plain splinter forceps; curved jeweler's forceps with fine tip; Adson forceps 1 × 2 teeth; Semken forceps, delicate with serrated tips; Semken forceps 1 × 2 teeth.

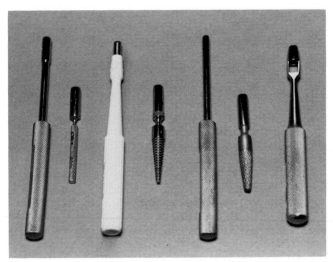

Figure 8–11. Punches. *Left to right*: Australian punch 4.0 mm, Orentreich manual hair transplant punch 4.5 mm, Acu-derm disposable punch, Stough hair transplant punch 4.0 mm, Australian punch 2 mm, manual hair transplant punch 3.5 mm, Keyes punch 4.0 mm.

forceps, which provides firm pressure with little effort. The Bergh forceps has an angled tip; the Barraquer forceps, a rounded tip.

PUNCHES

Cutaneous surgeons have popularized the use of the skin punch for cutaneous surgery (Fig. 8–11).[21] The original Keyes punch has a heavy handle, with slanted sides and a beveled cutting edge. The piece of tissue removed thus possesses less dermis than epidermis. With the advent of punch graft hair transplantation procedures and hand engines, a number of useful punches have been designed. Hair transplantation punches are very sharp and do not have slanted sides. The Orentreich punch has a straight inner wall and a beveled outside wall; the Australian punch has a beveled inner surface and a straight outside wall. These are available in both hand-held and power versions. Punches can be obtained in a wide variety of sizes, ranging from 1 to 6 mm in diameter, with selection determined by the specific procedure being performed. Keyes punches are available in larger sizes from 10 to 20 mm in diameter in 1.0-mm increments. All the above punches must be sterilized and become dull and slightly irregular with use.

Disposable punches are also now available and provide the advantage of always being sharp. They are not reusable, but many cutaneous surgeons find them suitable for a single biopsy procedure. They are especially applicable when suspected infected tissue is being removed. The disposable punches, manufactured by Acuderm and Baker-Cummings, are available in the standard diameter sizes of 2.0, 3.0, 3.5, 4.0, 4.5, and 6 mm.

CURETTES

Another useful instrument for superficial lesions is the skin curette, available in an assortment of sizes and shapes of the cutting head, as well as lengths, shapes, and weights of the handle (Fig. 8–12). A common example is the Fox curette, which has a round cutting head and a straight or angled handle. The Piffard curette is broader and much heavier with an oval cutting head. The Cannon and Rein curettes are other popular models with oval heads. In most cutaneous surgical practices the commonly used sizes have cutting heads of 3 to 4 mm in diameter, although smaller and larger sizes should also be available. Smaller curettes are available for identifying small pockets of tumor or for working in small cavities such as cysts; the Skeele, Heath, and Meyhoeffer models are particularly suited for this purpose.[22]

NEEDLE HOLDERS

Comfortable and functional needle holders are essential to the precision required in cutaneous surgery. A wide variety of models are available, with both smooth and finely serrated jaws (Fig. 8–13). Alloy inserts such as tungsten carbide may be added to increase the hardness and strength of the jaws and prolong the life of the instruments. The Webster or Halsey holders with smooth jaws are ideal for smaller needles and fine suture material. For larger needles the Halsey or Baumgartner holders provide excellent control for proper suture

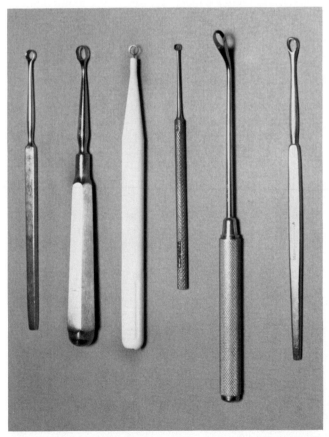

Figure 8–12. Curettes. *Left to right*: Fox curette 4 mm, Piffard curette 4 mm, Acu-derm disposable curette 3 mm, Heath curette 2 mm, Coakley curette 60-degree angle, Cannon curette size 3.

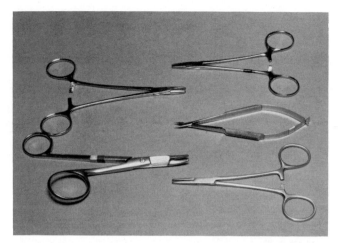

Figure 8–13. Needle holders. *Top to bottom, left to right*: Baumgartner needle holder with horizontal serrations, Gillies-Sheehan curved needle holder and scissors combination, Brown needle holder with rounded jaws, Castroviejo needle holder with smooth jaws, Halsey needle holder with smooth jaws.

placement. The Olsen-Hegar needle holder has the advantage of having scissors behind the jaws. Although initially they may be difficult to use, these instruments can save valuable time if an assistant is not constantly present during a surgical procedure. Finally, for extremely delicate work with very small needles, the Castroviejo holder is ideal. The small tips do not damage fine needles, and function with spring action as the instrument is held between the fingers.

HEMOSTATS

Hemostats are essential in cutaneous surgery for clamping blood vessels (Fig. 8–14). The Halsted and Hartmann instruments provide precision and accuracy. They can be obtained with straight or curved tips, depending on personal preference. The Halsted model

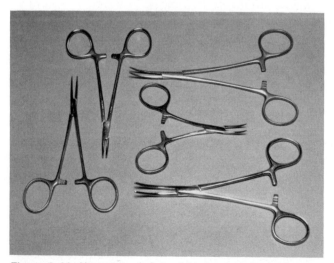

Figure 8–14. Hemostats. *Left to right, top to bottom*: Hartmann straight hemostat 4½ inch, Hartmann curved hemostat 4½ inch, Skillman curved clamp 5½ inch, Halsted curved mosquito hemostat 3½ inch, curved Kelly clamp 5½ inch.

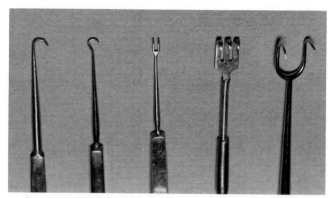

Figure 8–15. Skin hooks. *Left to right*: Frazier single skin hook, Frazier single shepherd skin hook, sharp double-pronged Guthrie skin hook, triple-pronged flexible rake retractor, double-pronged heavy sharp retractor.

is commonly called a mosquito forceps. The tips of both these forceps are finely serrated throughout their entire length. The standard Kelly hemostat is heavy and cumbersome and has little application in most cutaneous surgical procedures, except when a strong, secure hold is required.

SKIN HOOKS

Skin hooks provide invaluable assistance in handling tissue with a minimum of trauma, especially during undermining and moving skin flaps.[23] They may have single, double, or triple prongs and the tips may be sharp or blunt within varying radii (Fig. 8–15). Sharp-pointed hooks are preferable and single-pronged hooks are the ones used most frequently. The double-pronged hooks give a better hold on tissue, providing better eversion and visualization. Commonly used skin hooks include the Frazier, Tyrrell, and Guthrie double-pronged hooks. The Joseph skin hook has two prongs that may be ordered with different amounts of separation from 2 to 12 mm.

COMEDO EXTRACTORS

Many cutaneous surgeons express comedones as part of the routine treatment of acne. The Schamberg extractor is commonly used for this purpose (Fig. 8–16).

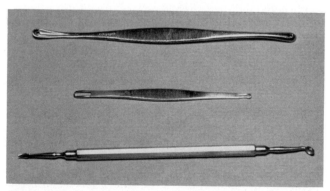

Figure 8–16. Comedo extractors. *Top to bottom*: Unna expressor, Schamberg expressor, Zimmerman-Walton expressor.

Each end is angled and the opening allows for adequate extrusion of the expressed tissue. The central portion is ribbed to promote a more secure grasp. Some comedo extractors have a lancet on one end to remove the top of the lesion; these need to be sterilized before each use. An alternative is the Zimmerman-Walton extractor, which accepts a sterile needle on one end for each procedure.

MISCELLANEOUS INSTRUMENTS

A number of specialized pieces of equipment have found valuable application in cutaneous surgery.[24] Chalazion clamps (Fig. 8–17) are of great help in immobilizing tissue and providing hemostasis on the lips and eyelids. The Desmarres model has an oval opening and can be obtained in three sizes.[25] The nail splitter and nail elevator are essential instruments for nail surgery. The nail splitter has a spring action, allowing easy cutting of even very thick nails. For precise cutaneous surgical procedures, a caliper can be useful. The Jameson model with tips that can be placed in a wound provides more accuracy than flat rulers.

Instrument Care

To ensure extended usefulness and maximal function for expensive surgical instruments, special attention must be devoted to their handling and care. Regular sharpening and lubrication are required to maintain precision. Appropriate cleaning, sterilization, and packaging are necessary to maintain both safety and function.

SHARPENING

Despite the popularity of some disposable instruments such as scalpels and punches, some surgical instruments require sharp surfaces in order to function properly. Scissors, curettes, and punches must be either sharpened in the office or sent back at regular intervals to the manufacturer. Most surgeons do not like to spend time

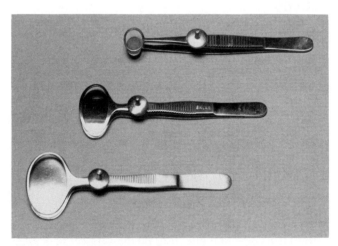

Figure 8–17. Chalazion clamps. *Top to bottom*: Desmarres clamp—small, medium, large.

sharpening their own equipment, but there are specialized machines available for this purpose (Honing Machine Corp.). Instruments should be marked for identification purposes and their maintenance catalogued.

LUBRICATION

All instruments with moving parts need lubrication. Lubricating oil may act as a protective barrier to organisms if steam sterilization is used. Therefore, instruments are best lubricated with silicone oil compounds or oil-in-water emulsions such as instrument milk. Some of these solutions may prevent corrosion, prolonging the life of the instrument.

CLEANING

Instruments should be cleaned as soon as possible after use. Ideally, they should be rinsed in cold water, brushed vigorously with a bristled brush and detergent in warm water, and allowed to dry before sterilization. Alternatively, they may be rinsed and placed in an ultrasonic cleanser. These cleansers act by a process called cavitation, in which sonic waves create minute bubbles that implode because of hydrostatic pressure, dislodging debris that may be in small or tight spaces. These ultrasonic chambers can be purchased with rinsing and drying chambers. They are expensive and space-occupying, but when used properly can be beneficial. The main disadvantage is that an aerosol is inevitably produced, which may be a source of contamination. In addition, the detergent solution used should be changed daily.

DISINFECTION

Disinfection describes the process of destroying infectious agents, but not necessarily bacterial spores, tubercle bacilli, or non–lipid-containing viruses. Sterilization describes the process of totally destroying all forms of microbial life: bacteria, fungi, and viruses.[26] A number of chemical agents are available for disinfection, including quaternary ammonium compounds, chlorine compounds, iodine solution, formaldehyde, glutaraldehyde, alcohols, and phenols (see Chapter 6). Glutaraldehyde is commonly used in sterile covered stainless steel pans as a holding solution for instruments. Sterile precautions must be strictly observed and the solution changed every 2 weeks.[27]

STERILIZATION

Various means are available to destroy all forms of microbial life:[28] dry heat, steam, chemical vapor, and gas sterilization (see Chapter 6). Dry heat is a useful but relatively inefficient method of sterilization. The instruments are placed in a type of oven and heated at a specific temperature for a defined period. A small unit is available for ambulatory surgical suites: the Cox Rapid Heat Sterilizer (Cox Sterile Products, Inc.), which rapidly heats individual instruments in as little as 6 minutes without damaging the sharp instruments. Steam-pressure sterilization is most commonly used in ambulatory surgical practices. Steam under pressure kills microorganisms by coagulation of proteins. Steam autoclaves are best operated with distilled water, which is a minimal added expense. Routine cleaning is necessary to prevent a build-up of deposits in the sterilization chamber. The main disadvantage of the steam sterilization process is the gradual dulling of cutting surfaces. Higher-quality instruments resist this insult much better than more inexpensive instruments. Popular office units are available, such as the Harvey steam autoclave (MDT Corp.) and the Ritter steam autoclave (Fig. 8–18).

Chemical vapor sterilization uses a chemical instead of distilled water in the steam autoclave process. With this chemical process, there is less tendency to dull the sharp-edged instruments. The inclusion of formaldehyde, which is an alkylating agent and carcinogenic, is a matter of concern. Environmental guidelines to prevent potential atmospheric contamination must be closely followed.[29] The commonly used models of chemical vapor sterilizers, which include the Harvey Chemiclave (MDT Corp.), available in three different sizes and are very functional. Gas sterilization is a modality most often found in hospital settings. This process uses ethylene oxide to destroy microorganisms in a relatively complicated, expensive process that requires extensive safety measures. Before it was realized that ethylene oxide is a carcinogen, mutagen, and neurotoxin, portable sterilization units were developed for office use.[30] This process is now highly regulated and is limited to large institutional settings.[31]

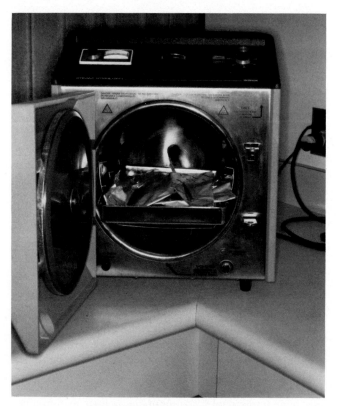

Figure 8–18. Ritter steam sterilizer.

PACKAGING

Before sterilization, instruments are normally packaged in an appropriate wrapping material of paper or cloth. It is often most efficient to design instrument packs for the most commonly performed procedures, such as punch biopsy, excision, or suture removal. The packs are sealed with special autoclave tape and dated. This may require the purchase of more individual instruments, but the cost is often worth the savings in time and convenience.

Miscellaneous Surgical Supplies

NEEDLES AND SYRINGES

The infiltration of local anesthetic agents is a necessary but uncomfortable experience. Pain can be minimized to some extent by selection of the proper equipment and by technique. Syringes may be disposable or reusable glass. They exist in various sizes, commonly 1, 3, 5, and 10 ml. Assuming a constant needle size, the smaller the plunger diameter, the easier is the injection. A Luer-Lok hub is essential for safety and convenience. Specialized glass syringes with rings for two fingers and thumb are advantageous for sclerotherapy and injection into sclerotic areas.

Needles are also available in various sizes and are disposable or reusable. Most needles are disposable, but fine 32- to 33-gauge needles for delicate areas or sclerotherapy can be sterilized. The smaller the caliber of the needle, the smaller is the puncture wound, and consequently the less trauma inflicted. Large-bore needles of 18 to 20 gauge are used to draw up medication, and needles of 27 to 30 gauge are commonly used for injection. The ½-, ⅝-, and ¾-inch needles are most popular for injection. Long needles of 1, 1½, and 2 inches are more flexible and may be desirable if a greater distance under the skin can be reached through a single injection site.

GLOVES

Gloves should be worn by all personnel, not only for the surgical procedure but also for dressing change, handling tissue specimens, and cleaning after the procedure.[32] Nonsterile gloves are usually supplied in small, medium, and large sizes; sterile gloves come in specific sizes from 5 to 8½. Sterile gloves are commonly made of latex, but vinyl and hypoallergenic gloves are also available. Gloves may be ordered with powder, but powder-free gloves are becoming more popular. The hypoallergenic gloves are comfortable but expensive.

MASKS, GLASSES, AND GOGGLES

The main purpose of a surgical mask is to protect the patient from possible infection by the surgical personnel and to protect the surgical team from inhalation of discharge from the surgical site. Masks should be worn over both the mouth and nose, since the nasopharynx is a common site for harboring microorganisms. Masks are available in different qualities, and special masks have been developed for laser surgical procedures. This has become necessary as a way to provide protection against possible inhalation of living viral particles in the laser plume.[33] Eye protection is also important during surgical procedures. Adequate protection for the surgical team can be achieved if glasses with side protectors or wraparound goggles are worn.

DRAPES AND GOWNS

Drapes are commonly used for large cutaneous surgical procedures. They protect the surgical field from contamination and provide a sterile backdrop for instruments, sutures, and other surgical materials. Reusable drapes are made from a woven material such as muslin or cotton. These are not effective when they become wet because of a wicking effect for microorganisms. Disposable drapes are nonwoven and usually made of plastic or some other synthetic material. These are also commonly treated with fire-retardant chemicals that provide an extra margin of safety during electrosurgery or carbon dioxide laser surgery. Surgical gowns are also commonly worn in the ambulatory surgical setting. They help to protect the surgical staff and contribute to the professional atmosphere of the surgical suite. Reusable cotton gowns and scrub suits are available as well as disposable, waterproof surgical clothing.

GAUZE AND SWABS

Absorbent gauze and cotton-tipped applicators are often used during a surgical procedure to clear the surgical field and provide better visualization. Gauze is manufactured in varied sizes from 2×2 to 4×4 inches and can be obtained in presterilized packs or in larger quantities of nonsterile packages that can be used as part of a wrapped tray or set of instruments to be sterilized later. Cotton-tipped wooden applicators can also be sterilized as part of a surgical tray and provide excellent assistance during surgery.

SUMMARY

High-quality equipment and instruments for cutaneous surgery allow the surgeon to practice with maximal skill. A thorough knowledge of equipment and instrument manufacture, design, function, and maintenance is essential. From experience, a cutaneous surgeon will learn to select the most appropriate instrument for a particular procedure to provide the best clinical results. Finally, the progressive surgeon should always be alert for newly developed instruments, equipment, and other technologic innovations that may further improve or refine a specific procedure, allowing it to be performed with greater ease, safety, and skill.

REFERENCES

1. Burns LA: Ambulatory Surgery: Developing and Managing Successful Programs. Aspen Systems Corp, Rockville, MD, 1984.
2. Hill GJ: Outpatient Surgery. 3rd ed. WB Saunders, Philadelphia, 1988.
3. Kopf A, Baer R: Yearbook of Dermatology: Dermatologic Office Surgery. Year Book, Chicago, 1964.
4. Simms RL: The office surgical suite: pros and cons. Otolaryngol Clin North Am 13:391–397, 1980.
5. Terino EO: A cost analysis of office plastic surgery. Plast Reconstr Surg 63:355–358, 1978.
6. Davis JE: The need to redefine levels of surgical care. JAMA 251:2527–2528, 1984.
7. Webster RC: Credentialing in dermatologic surgery. J Dermatol Surg Oncol 14:155–157, 1988.
8. Tobin HA: Office surgery: the surgical suite. J Dermatol Surg Oncol 14:247–255, 1988.
9. Chrisman BB: Planning and staffing an appropriate outpatient facility. J Dermatol Surg Oncol 14:708–711, 1988.
10. Maloney ME: The Dermatologic Suite: Design and Materials. Churchill Livingstone, New York, 1991.
11. Bennett RG: Fundamentals of Cutaneous Surgery. CV Mosby, St. Louis, 1988.
12. Elliott JA Jr: Electrosurgery: its use in dermatology with a review of its development and technologic aspects. Arch Dermatol 94:340–350, 1966.
13. Sebben JE: Electrosurgery principles: cutting current and cutaneous surgery—Part I. J Dermatol Surg Oncol 14:29–31, 1988.
14. Krull EA, Pickard SD, Hall JC: Effects of electrosurgery on cardiac pacemakers. J Dermatol Surg Oncol 1:43–45, 1975.
15. Ellman Int. Mfg., Inc.: What's New in Office Electrosurgery? Radiosurgery 1989.
16. Stoner JG, Swanson NA, Vargo N: Penrose sleeve. J Dermatol Surg Oncol 9:523–524, 1983.
17. Fee WE, Jr: Use of the Shaw scalpel in head and neck surgery. Ontolaryngol Head Neck Surg 89:515–519, 1981.
18. Stegman SJ, Tromovitch TA: Cosmetic Dermatologic Surgery. Year Book, Chicago, 1984.
19. Arista Surgical Instruments: Arista Surgical Supply Co., Inc., New York, 1990.
20. Gibbs RC: A love affair with the Gradle scissors. J Dermatol Surg Oncol 7:771, 1981.
21. Stegman SJ: Commentary: the cutaneous punch. Arch Dermatol 118:943–944, 1982.
22. Krull EA. Surgical gems: the little curet. J Dermatol Surg Oncol 4:656–657, 1978.
23. Popkin GL: Surgical gems: another look at the skin hook. J Dermatol Surg Oncol 4:366–368, 1978.
24. Stegman SJ, Tromovitch TA, Glogau RG: Basics of Dermatologic Surgery. Year Book, Chicago, 1982.
25. Bartlett RE: Use of the Desmarres clamp in major eyelid surgery. Ann Ophthalmol 9:360–362, 1977.
26. Sebben JE: Avoiding infection in office surgery. J Dermatol Surg Oncol 8:455–458, 1982.
27. Block SS: Disinfection, Sterilization and Preservation. Lea & Febiger, Philadelphia, 1977.
28. Simmonds WL: Sterilization. Cutis 25:78–80, 1980.
29. Sebben JE: Sterilization and care of surgical instruments and supplies. J Am Acad Dermatol 11:381–392, 1984.
30. Hazard Alert No. 3: Ethylene oxide. California Department of Health Services, Hazard Education System and Information Service, Sacramento, July 1982.
31. Znamirowski R, McDonald S, Roy JE: The efficiency of an ethylene oxide sterilizer in hospital practice. Can Med Assoc J 83:1004–1006, 1960.
32. Gross DJ, Jamison Y, Martin K, et al: Surgical glove perforation in dermatologic surgery. J Dermatol Surg Oncol 15:1226–1228, 1989.
33. Garden JM, O'Banion MK, Shelnitz LS, et al: Papillomavirus in the vapor of carbon dioxide laser–treated verrucae. JAMA 259:1199–2021, 1988.

CHAPTER 9

Topical, Local, and Regional Anesthesia

SCOTT M. DINEHART

Most cutaneous surgical procedures are performed with the aid of some form of local anesthesia. Local anesthesia is more popular for cutaneous surgery than general anesthesia, since studies have shown that patients at high risk for complications from general anesthetics tolerate local anesthesia with less morbidity.[1] The use of local anesthesia for cutaneous procedures also conforms to recent trends toward cost containment and a greater emphasis on outpatient surgery. In addition to safety and cost effectiveness, local anesthesia provides a convenient and reliable means of reducing pain during these procedures.

Safe and effective use of local anesthetics depends on a thorough understanding of physiology, side effects, dosage, and proper technique. This chapter is designed to provide an understanding of these fundamentals.

History

The use of cold and pressure for anesthesia has been known since ancient times,[2] but it is only during the last 100 years that anesthetic pharmacologic agents commonly used today have been developed. Cocaine was isolated from the leaves of the South American bush *Erythroxylon coca* in 1860 by Niemann, who noted that this extract produced numbness of the tongue.[3] In 1880 the anesthetic qualities of cocaine after subcutaneous infiltration were reported.[4] In 1884 Koller and Freud were the first to use cocaine in clinical practice when they showed that ocular instillation of this substance produced topical ophthalmic anesthesia.[4] Finally, Halsted performed the first peripheral nerve block using cocaine in 1885.[4]

No satisfactory alternative to cocaine was available until procaine was produced in 1904.[3] An ester of para-aminobenzoic acid (PABA), procaine (Table 9–1) gained immediate popularity despite its tendency to produce allergic reactions in some patients. In 1930 tetracaine was introduced as a more potent PABA ester, but it also had a propensity to produce allergic reactions.[3] A major breakthrough came when an amide derivative of diethylaminoacetic acid, lidocaine, was synthesized in 1943.[3] Lidocaine has been shown to be relatively free of the sensitizing properties of the ester anesthetics and has become the standard against which all new local anesthetics are measured. In addition to lidocaine, a number of amide anesthetics have been developed (Table 9–2).

TABLE 9–1. **COMMONLY USED ESTER LOCAL ANESTHETICS**

Generic Name	Trade Name
Cocaine	None
Procaine	Novocain
	Neocaine
Chloroprocaine	Nesacaine
Tetracaine	Pontocaine
	Pantocaine

TABLE 9–2. **COMMONLY USED AMIDE LOCAL ANESTHETICS**

Generic Name	Trade Name
Lidocaine	Xylocaine
	Seracaine
Bupivacaine	Marcaine
	Sensorcaine
Mepivacaine	Carbocaine
Prilocaine	Citanest
Etidocaine	Duranest

TABLE 9–3. **PHYSIOLOGY OF ESTER LOCAL ANESTHETICS**

Generic Name	Metabolism	Onset	Duration (min)		Maximal Recommended Dose (70-kg person)	
			w/out epi	w/epi	w/out epi (mg)	w/epi (mg)
Cocaine	Plasma	Fast	45	N/A	200	N/A
Procaine	Plasma	Fast	15–30	30–90	500	600
Chloroprocaine	Plasma	Fast	30–60	N/A	800	1000
Tetracaine	Plasma	Slow	120–240	240–480	100	N/A

N/A, Not available.

Mechanism of Action

All currently existing pharmacologic agents act by blocking peripheral nerve function. Stimulation of a nerve produces an impulse or action potential that results from movement of both sodium and potassium ions across the nerve membrane. Local anesthetics act by preventing sodium channels in the axon membrane from opening, so that depolarization does not occur and action potentials are not propagated.[5] However, the resting charge across the nerve membrane remains unaffected. Several mechanisms have been postulated for preventing the influx of sodium ions. The most likely mechanism for the action of amide anesthetics involves binding of the cationic form of the anesthetic to a receptor in the sodium channel.[6] The vasoconstrictive properties of cocaine are due to its ability to prevent the reuptake of norepinephrine.[7]

Structure and Physiology

All pharmacologic agents that have activity as local anesthetics have similar chemical structures made of three components: an aromatic portion, an intermediate chain, and an amine portion. Changes in any one of these three parts of a local anesthetic modify its potency, time of onset, and duration of action (Tables 9–3, 9–4). The aromatic portion is responsible for lipid solubility, an important property that helps anesthetics diffuse through the highly lipophilic nerve membrane.[5] The amine portion of the anesthetic is hydrophilic and largely responsible for the desired property of water solubility.[5] The intermediate chain contains the ester (Fig. 9–1) or amide (Fig. 9–2) linkage by which anesthetics are classified.

Most local anesthetics are weak bases that are prepared as solutions of a salt to enhance their water solubility. The relative proportions of base and its cation depend on the dissociation constant (pKa) of each anesthetic and the hydrogen ion concentration (pH).[8] If the pH of an anesthetic solution is lowered, such as when antioxidants are added to prevent degradation of epinephrine, less base and more ionized forms become present, which increases the difficulty for diffusion across nerve membranes. In addition to the pH of the solution, the pH of the tissue being injected can also affect the anesthetic function. Local anesthetics do not work well in inflamed or infected acidic tissue environments.[9] Injection of an acidic anesthetic solution into normal tissues may, after the initial anesthetic effect wears off, produce tolerance to subsequent injections because of lowered pH at the operative site.[10]

Classification of Anesthetics

As mentioned, local anesthetics can be classified into two groups depending on the linkage in the intermediate chain. Ester anesthetics have an ester linkage in the intermediate chain, while amide anesthetics have an amide linkage. Besides differences in the linkage of the intermediate chain, the two types of anesthetics also differ in their metabolism and potential for sensitization.

Ester anesthetics include procaine (Novocain) and are hydrolyzed by an enzyme in plasma, pseudocholinesterase (see Table 9–3).[11] Some individuals with atypical forms of this enzyme may be subject to overdosage if a large quantity of an ester anesthetic is given.[11] Lidocaine

TABLE 9–4. **PHYSIOLOGY OF AMIDE LOCAL ANESTHETICS**

Generic Name	Metabolism	Onset	Duration (min)		Maximal Recommended Dose (70-kg person)	
			w/out epi	w/epi	w/out epi (mg)	w/epi (mg)
Lidocaine	Liver	Fast	30–120	60–400	300 (30 ml of 1%)	500 (50 ml of 1%)
Bupivacaine	Liver	Slow	120–240	240–480	175	225
Mepivacaine	Liver	Slow	30–120	60–400	300	500
Prilocaine	Liver	Slow	30–120	60–400	400	600
Etidocaine	Liver	Slow	200	240–360	300	400

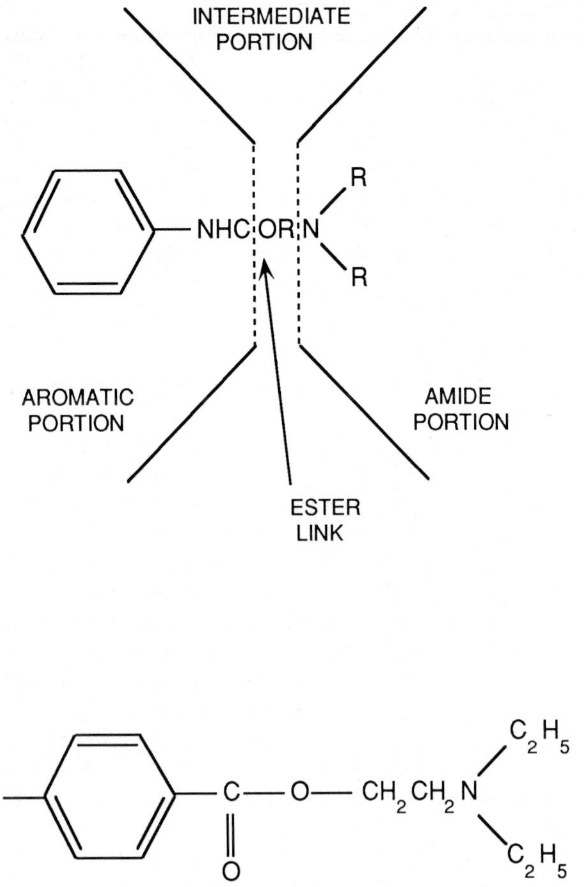

AROMATIC
PORTION

INTERMEDIATE
PORTION

AMIDE
PORTION

ESTER
LINK

$NHC \cdot OR \cdot N$
R
R

Use of Anesthetics During Pregnancy and in Childhood

Occasionally, there is a need to perform minor surgical procedures during pregnancy. These may include treatment of malignancies or surgical management of infected, inflamed, or bleeding lesions.[14] It is always best to keep the number of pharmacologic agents used during pregnancy to a minimum and to consult with the patient's obstetrician or general physician before any cutaneous surgical procedure. Sterile water or normal saline can be effectively used for anesthesia in very small procedures; however, the local anesthetic of choice during pregnancy is generally lidocaine. Although over 50% of lidocaine is eliminated by the first pass through the liver, lidocaine permeability of the placental membranes ensures that the fetus will receive some exposure

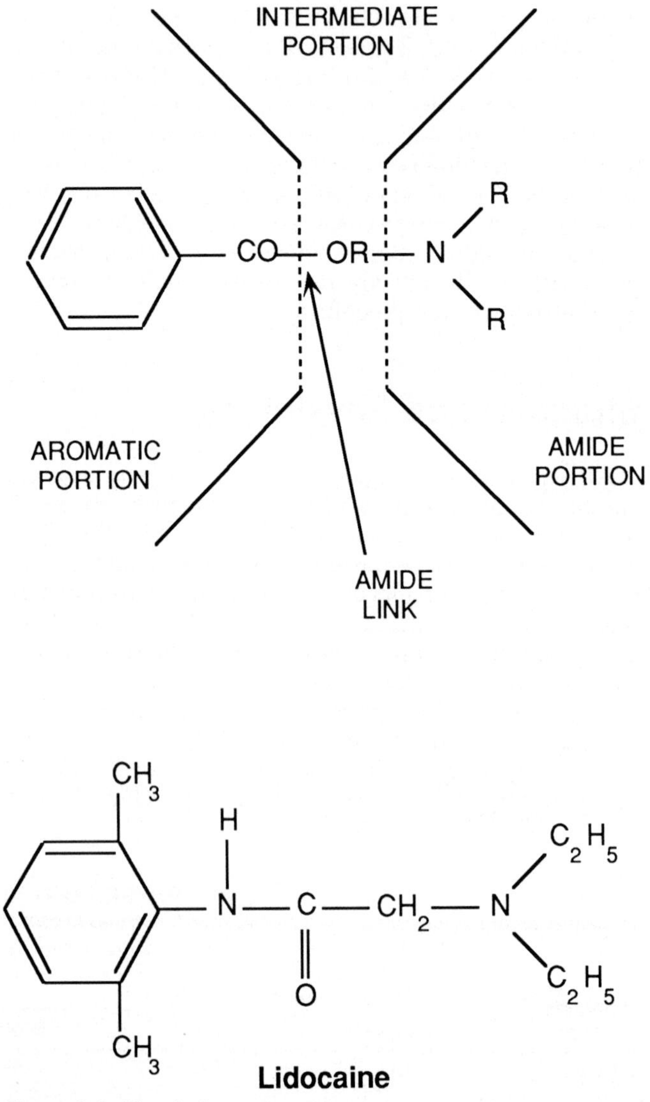

Procaine

Figure 9–1. Chemical structure of the ester group of local anesthetic agents.

(Xylocaine) is among the amide anesthetics. Amide anesthetics are metabolized in the liver and excreted by the kidneys (see Table 9–4). For this reason, individuals with poor liver function have a reduced tolerance to amide anesthetics and consequently are more susceptible to overdosage.[12] There are many commonly used amide and ester anesthetics (see Tables 9–1, 9–2).

Dosage, Onset, and Duration

In general, the long-acting anesthetics are more toxic and have lower maximal safe dosages as a result. Onset of action is usually slower for long-acting anesthetic agents. The maximal safe dosages for local anesthetics are well established (see Tables 9–3, 9–4). It should be remembered that peak plasma levels are highly dependent on the concentration of the injected anesthetic, a slow or long duration time of infiltration, the vascularity of the injected site, and the ability of the body to metabolize the anesthetic.[13]

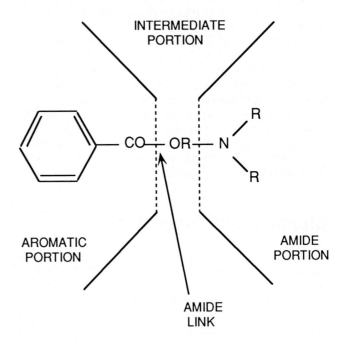

AROMATIC
PORTION

INTERMEDIATE
PORTION

AMIDE
PORTION

AMIDE
LINK

$CO \cdot OR \cdot N$
R
R

Lidocaine

Figure 9–2. Chemical structure of the amide group of local anesthetic agents.

to this agent.[14] It is suggested that local anesthetics not be used in the first 3 to 4 months of pregnancy during the period of greatest organogenesis. Although it is best to avoid all pharmacologic agents during this time, studies have shown no association between mothers exposed to local anesthetics during the first 4 months of pregnancy and the existence of anatomic deformities in newborns.[15] In general, lidocaine can be regarded as a nonteratogen and safe for use in pregnancy if nontoxic doses are given.[14] Although there is some concern over the use of epinephrine in high doses during pregnancy, this agent can be safely added to anesthetics in dosages commonly used in cutaneous surgery.[14] The addition of epinephrine generally reduces plasma levels of anesthetic and expedites the procedure.

As in pregnancy, the use of lidocaine for local anesthesia is considered safe in children. Suggested maximal dosages of lidocaine for children over 3 years of age are 1.5 to 2.0 mg/kg for lidocaine without epinephrine[16] and 3.0 to 4.5 mg/kg when epinephrine is added. Lidocaine is metabolized by the immature liver of newborns,[17] but precautions should be taken in jaundiced neonates. Parabens, the preservatives found in most commercially prepared anesthetic solutions, competitively bind albumin and theoretically can displace bilirubin.[18] For this reason, it is suggested that paraben-free solutions of anesthetics be used in newborns. General anesthesia or delay in a procedure should be considered when complex or long procedures are necessary in newborns or children. Topical anesthetics, such as the eutectic mixture of prilocaine/lidocaine (EMLA), are also useful in a variety of cutaneous surgical procedures in children.[19, 20]

Additions to Local Anesthetics

Several substances are frequently added to local anesthetics to modify the effect (Table 9–5). These substances may be added by the pharmaceutical manufacturer before commercial sale or by the physician just before use. It is important to understand the appropriate usage and be aware of the risks of adding various substances. Knowledge of these added substances may also be useful when evaluating adverse reactions.

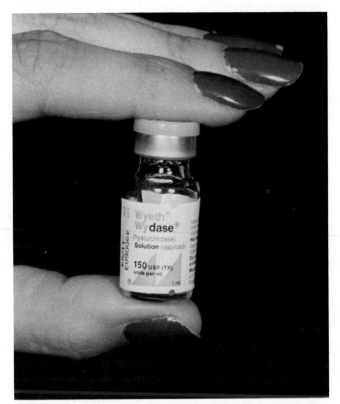

Figure 9–3. A bottle of hyaluronidase solution at a concentration of 150 units per milliliter.

HYALURONIDASE

Hyaluronidase (Wydase), an enzyme that depolymerizes hyaluronic acid, is sometimes added to injectable local anesthetic solutions (Fig. 9–3) to facilitate diffusion of the anesthetic through tissue and to keep anatomic distortion to a minimum.[21] Hyaluronidase is most useful for procedures around the orbit where distortion of tissues is otherwise frequent. The addition of hyaluronidase may also be useful when performing nerve blocks in which spreading of anesthetic is desirable, or when harvesting large split-thickness skin grafts using local anesthesia. Dosage is one ampule (150 units) in 30 ml of anesthetic. Hyaluronidase contains a small amount of the preservative thimerosal, a reported contact sensitizer. It should be remembered that hyaluronidase can accelerate absorption of lidocaine and thus increase peak plasma lidocaine levels. The duration of anesthesia is also likely to be shorter when hyaluronidase is added. However, the addition of epinephrine can increase the duration of action of lidocaine with hyaluronidase to that of a lidocaine-epinephrine mixture without hyaluronidase.[21] Although rare, allergy to hyaluronidase is possible. Consequently, a small amount is injected intradermally, as in a tuberculosis skin test, 10 to 15 minutes preoperatively. If an urticarial wheal with pseudopods forms, use of hyaluronidase is contraindicated.

VASOCONSTRICTORS

Vasoconstrictors are added to anesthetic solutions for several reasons. First, most anesthetics, with the excep-

TABLE 9–5. **ADDITIVES TO LOCAL ANESTHETICS**

Additive	Dosage	Purpose
Epinephrine	1:100,000 or less	To decrease bleeding, prolong anesthesia, reduce anesthetic toxicity
Hyaluronidase	150 units added to every 30 ml of anesthetic	To promote spreading, decrease tissue distortion
Sodium bicarbonate	1 ml (1 mEq/ml) for every 10 ml of 1% lidocaine with or without epinephrine	To decrease pain with infiltration of acidic solution

tion of cocaine, cause vasodilation by direct relaxation of vascular smooth muscle. Since vasodilation enhances bleeding at the operative site, vasoconstrictors are added to decrease bleeding. Also, vasoconstrictors decrease the absorption of anesthetic agents, enabling the use of smaller amounts of drug while prolonging the duration of action. Vasoconstrictors are less effective in prolonging the more lipid-soluble, long-acting anesthetics such as etidocaine and bupivacaine because these agents are so tightly bound to tissues.

Epinephrine is the most common vasoconstrictor added to local anesthetics, although phenylephrine[22] or a 2% solution of ornithine-8-vasopressin[23] has been used to avoid the cardiac effects of epinephrine. Epinephrine is premixed commercially with anesthetics at a concentration of 1:100,000. Studies have shown that epinephrine retains some vasoconstrictive effects at concentrations as low as 1:500,000[24] and that concentrations greater than 1:200,000 are probably not necessary.[25] Epinephrine concentrations greater than 1:100,000 are also associated with an increased risk of side effects.[26] It should be remembered that it takes 7 to 15 minutes for epinephrine to produce full vasoconstriction,[8] and the blanching of the skin caused by epinephrine usually, but not always, delineates the anesthetized area.

Acidic preservatives, including sodium metabisulfite and citric acid, are added to commercial anesthetic solutions containing epinephrine. Because an alkaline pH can degrade epinephrine over time, lidocaine with epinephrine solutions are adjusted to a lower pH (3.3 to 5.5) than lidocaine without epinephrine (5.0 to 7.0). This is important because acidic solutions produce more pain on injection than neutral or alkaline solutions.[27] Freshly prepared solutions of lidocaine with epinephrine are less painful upon injection because of a higher pH.[8] Epinephrine can be mixed freshly each day with local anesthetic by using ampules of epinephrine produced at a concentration of 1:1000. A total of 0.1 ml 1:1000 epinephrine added to 20 ml lidocaine results in a solution having a 1:200,000 concentration of epinephrine and a higher pH than commercial preparations.

SODIUM BICARBONATE

The pain of infiltrating commercially prepared lidocaine with epinephrine into the skin can be reduced by adding sodium bicarbonate.[27, 28] Lidocaine is a very stable compound, but epinephrine can be quite labile in alkaline and neutral pH solutions. To prevent degradation of epinephrine, commercial agents are prepared at an acid pH that causes more pain than those having a neutral pH.[27, 28] The pH of lidocaine with epinephrine solutions can be neutralized by adding 1 ml of 8.4% sodium bicarbonate for every 10 ml of anesthetic solution. Because epinephrine in the neutralized solutions declines at the rate of 25% per week,[28] it is suggested that such prepared solutions be discarded after 1 week. Although lidocaine concentration is not reduced, it may appear to be less effective over time because of the decline in epinephrine concentration.

OTHER ANESTHETICS

Sometimes, several different local anesthetics are mixed together to try and take advantage of various useful properties of each agent. Generally a long-acting anesthetic that has a prolonged time of onset, such as bupivacaine, is mixed with a shorter-acting, quick-onset anesthetic, such as lidocaine. In a study evaluating such a combination, it was concluded that mixtures of anesthetics generally take on the exclusive properties of only one of the pharmacologic agents.[29] It appears, therefore, that there is little advantage in mixing anesthetics. Although mixing anesthetics before injection may not be beneficial, a common strategy is to inject a longer-acting anesthetic into an operative site that has previously been anesthetized with a short-acting anesthetic when a prolonged procedure is anticipated.

Topical Anesthetic Agents

The stratum corneum presents a formidable barrier to the absorption of drugs through the skin. Innovative delivery systems or vehicles are often needed to enhance penetration of anesthetics through intact skin. Tape stripping of the outer layer of the skin before application of the anesthetic increases penetration and efficacy but is often impractical.[30] In addition to cryoanesthesia, a physical means of producing topical anesthesia, the most common agents for topical use include the three ester anesthetics cocaine, tetracaine, and benzocaine and the two amide anesthetics lidocaine and prilocaine.

Topical freezing agents such as ethyl chloride or dichlorotetrafluoroethane sprays can also be used to anesthetize superficial lesions, such as molluscum, before curettage. Dichlorotetrafluoroethane spray is commonly used during dermabrasions. Anesthesia for scalpel incision and drainage of infected cysts or furuncles can be provided by refrigerant sprays or liquid nitrogen. When the skin is infected, cryoanesthesia is generally more useful than injected anesthetics because of the negative effect the acidic environment of infected tissues has on anesthesia. Ice cubes may also occasionally be helpful for minor procedures in children.

One useful pharmacologic agent for topical anesthesia is cocaine. In contrast to other local anesthetics, cocaine is a potent vasoconstrictor that decreases bleeding during surgery. This property makes it a highly effective agent for upper airway procedures, including the resection of some cancers. Cocaine is usually prepared as a 2 to 4% solution that is applied with cotton balls or Gelfoam strips. The peak anesthetic effect occurs after 3 to 5 minutes and lasts about 30 minutes. The maximal dosage for a 70 kg person is 200 mg (5 ml of a 4% solution), although severe toxic reactions may occur with as little as 20 mg. Central nervous system stimulation, bradycardia in small doses, and tachycardia and hypertension in high doses are commonly reported systemic side effects.[31] Myocardial infarction has been reported after anesthesia for nasal surgery.[31] The potential for recreational abuse and systemic side effects makes cocaine a less than ideal topical anesthetic.

Benzocaine, another ester anesthetic, is poorly soluble in water and therefore is not used as an injectable anesthetic. However, it is commonly used as a topical anesthetic, particularly when anesthesia of mucous membranes is desired. It is available as a 20% aerosol or gel and in solutions of up to 20%. The 20% solution or aerosol takes only 15 to 30 seconds to become effective and has a relatively short duration of action (12 to 15 minutes). Contact sensitivity to benzocaine is seen commonly enough to dissuade some physicians from using this formulation.

Tetracaine was introduced as a long-acting ester anesthetic and has been used mostly as a topical anesthetic for ophthalmic procedures. It can also be combined with other agents to produce an effective topical preparation for obtaining anesthesia before repair of pediatric lacerations.[32] This formulation, termed TAC, includes *te*tracaine, epinephrine (*A*drenalin), and *c*ocaine. Tetracaine alone, encapsulated into phospholipid membranes (liposomes), has shown promise as a topical anesthetic for intact skin but is not yet available commercially.[33] Other vehicles that have tetracaine as an active agent have produced unacceptable side effects.[34]

The use of commercially available 2 to 4% lidocaine mixtures in conventional vehicles for mucous membrane anesthesia is common. However, these mixtures are not useful for anesthesia of intact skin. EMLA (2.5% lidocaine combined in a eutectic mixture with prilo-

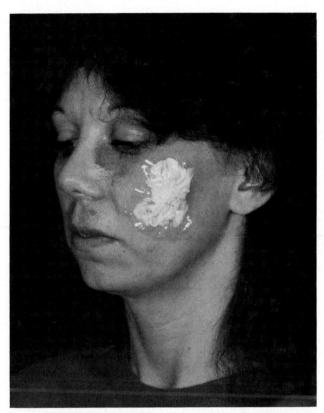

Figure 9–5. Clinical appearance of the patient in Figure 9–4 with 30% lidocaine topical anesthetic cream under an occlusive dressing before laser photocoagulation.

caine 2.5%) has found use in superficial cutaneous surgery.[19, 20] Topical application for 45 minutes under occlusion provides sufficient anesthesia[19, 20] to perform a variety of superficial procedures (Figs. 9–4, 9–5) but not excisional surgery. FDA approval of this product should provide easier access and more widespread use.

A formulation of 30% lidocaine in acid mantle cream was first described and tested in 1964 but has only recently enjoyed increasing popularity as a topical anesthetic.[35] Although the mixture is not available commercially, it can be prepared easily and economically by any pharmacist. Anesthesia on facial skin is achieved after occlusion for 20 to 30 minutes, but significant anesthesia in other areas requires a minimum of 45 minutes under occlusion. Rare contact sensitivity to lidocaine in lower concentrations is well documented; however, use of this compound in over 7000 patients without a significant adverse reaction has been reported.[35] Mild erythema of the skin, which does not interfere with treatment of vascular lesions, has been the only adverse reaction described. Anesthesia is adequate for superficial procedures such as shave biopsy or pulsed dye laser treatment, but other procedures such as punch or excisional biopsy require additional anesthesia. This compound, as well as the lidocaine-prilocaine cream, can be applied to the skin of anxious patients before injecting other anesthetics.

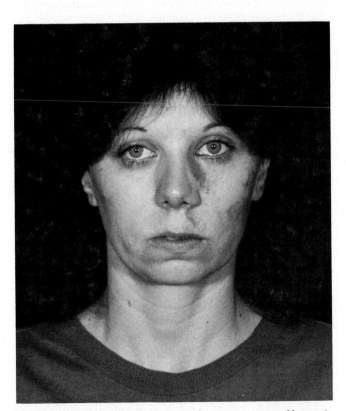

Figure 9–4. Preoperative appearance of a young woman with a port-wine stain.

Iontophoretic induction of anesthetics, particularly lidocaine, has received increasing notice in recent years.[36] Solutions of 1 to 4% lidocaine and 1:10,000 to 1:50,000 epinephrine are used to produce superficial topical anesthesia. Useful anesthesia is produced in 3 to 5 minutes with 1 milliamp of current. The primary disadvantage of this technique is the additional equipment needed.

Infiltrative Anesthesia

Infiltrative anesthesia involves direct inhibition of nerve ending excitation by an anesthetic and is the most frequently used local anesthetic technique. It is most commonly accomplished using lidocaine in a 1% concentration. For larger procedures requiring great volumes of anesthetic or in children, 0.5% lidocaine is suggested. When longer procedures are anticipated, 0.25% bupivacaine or etidocaine formulations are often infiltrated into areas previously anesthetized with lidocaine. Epinephrine- and non–epinephrine-containing solutions of lidocaine should always be available. Procaine and chloroprocaine are rapid-acting ester anesthetics but are seldom used because of the possibility of allergic reactions.

Infiltrative anesthesia involves placement of anesthetic directly into the surgical site, injected intradermally or subcutaneously. Intradermal injection is similar to the procedure in a tuberculosis skin test (Fig. 9–6) and results in a rapid onset of anesthesia that lasts longer than deeper injections.[37] The disadvantages of this technique include increased pain and distortion of tissues. Subcutaneous placement of anesthetic is slower in onset and has a shorter duration but is less painful.[37] Subcutaneous placement is advisable for larger procedures or for very anxious patients. Regardless of the type of infiltrative technique used, all injections are probably best begun by placing a small amount of anesthetic

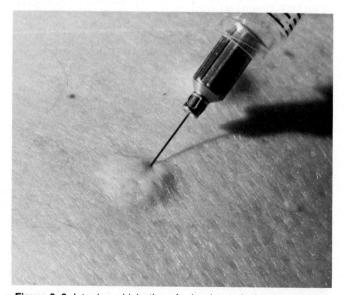

Figure 9–6. Intradermal injection of a local anesthetic agent creates a wheal similar to that produced by a tuberculosis skin test.

intradermally to produce a wheal or bleb. If subcutaneous placement is then desired, injection through the wheal or bleb will decrease patient discomfort.

Some pain is always felt when local anesthetics are injected. Good technique and careful planning can diminish this pain and keep patient discomfort to a minimum.[37] Patients generally feel a "stick," which represents the needle piercing the skin, and a "sting" or "burn," indicating actual infiltration of the anesthetic. Placing the needle into the skin in a quick definitive manner hurts less than a slow, hesitant advancement. If 30-gauge needles are used for injection, the "stick" felt by the patient can be reduced even further. Although claims have been made of reduced pain when the needle is inserted through pores or follicular openings in the skin, this technique is not particularly useful. In extremely anxious patients or children, topical anesthetics before initial injection may be helpful.

As mentioned previously, the "sting" of local anesthesia occurs as the anesthetic is infiltrated. The "sting" may be lessened by subcutaneous rather than intradermal injection of anesthetic.[37] Much of the pain is produced by rapid distention of tissues.[37] It is for this reason that slow injection is desirable. The use of as small a volume of anesthetic as possible will help keep distention of tissues to a minimum. However, there is controversy over the effect that warming anesthetic solutions to body temperature has on the amount of pain felt.[37, 38] One study demonstrated markedly reduced pain on injection when the local anesthetic solution was first warmed to body temperature.[39] Finally, the use of freshly prepared anesthetic solutions containing epinephrine or the use of bicarbonate to buffer commercial solutions can greatly reduce the pain associated with infiltration.[27, 28]

FIELD BLOCK

A special type of infiltrative anesthesia is the field or ring block. This type of anesthesia involves placement of a ring of anesthetic around the operative site (Fig. 9–7). The center of the ring is anesthetized even though no solution has been injected into the area. Field blocks are particularly useful for procedures such as cyst removal where injection of the anesthetic immediately adjacent to the cyst can sometimes cause rupture of the cyst contents. For extensive procedures, a field block can help diminish the total amount of anesthetic needed.

TUMESCENT TECHNIQUE

The tumescent technique of local anesthesia for liposuction surgery deserves special mention as a type of infiltrative anesthesia. In this technique, large volumes of very dilute solutions of lidocaine (0.05%) and epinephrine (1:1,000,000) in saline are infiltrated into the subcutaneous fat before liposuction.[13] A safe upper limit for lidocaine dosage with this technique is estimated to be 35 mg/kg.[13] It appears that delayed absorption of anesthetic produces lower peak plasma lidocaine levels than would be expected from using equivalent doses with other infiltrative techniques. The tumescent tech-

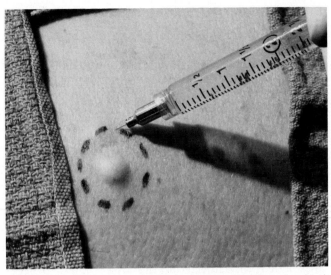

Figure 9–7. Field block anesthesia involves injection of a local anesthetic in a ring distribution around the operative site.

nique has the additional advantages of providing prolonged anesthesia, which obviates the need for postoperative analgesia,[13] and replenishing fluids lost during the procedure.

Peripheral Nerve Block Anesthesia

Injection of a small amount of local anesthetic around a nerve whose anatomic distribution is known produces anesthesia of the skin that the nerve supplies (Fig. 9–8). This type of injection is known as nerve block anesthesia. It is particularly useful when anesthesia is needed for large anatomic areas, since a smaller amount of anesthetic is required; this in turn reduces the risk of anesthetic toxicity. Another advantage of nerve block anesthesia includes absence of distortion at the operative site, since it is not being directly infiltrated. Nerve block anesthesia also usually results in less discomfort to the patient than infiltrating the entire distribution of the nerve.

There are some disadvantages to nerve block anesthesia, however. First, the technique requires greater skill and a complete knowledge of anatomy. Second, nerve block anesthesia does not produce vasoconstriction of the operative site, since this area is usually distant from the injection site. Third, because anesthetic is placed in close proximity to the nerve, there is an increased risk of inadvertent laceration of the nerve by the injection needle.[40] This can result in long-lasting dysesthesia, but in most cases the nerve regenerates and sensation returns to normal in time. Because nerves and blood vessels are sometimes located along similar anatomic areas in neurovascular bundles, there is a risk of vessel laceration with resultant hematoma or ecchymosis.[40]

Anesthetics of the amide type, similar to those used in infiltration anesthesia, are most commonly used for nerve blocks. Vasoconstrictors are seldom added for

cutaneous surgery procedures because of the increased risk of vascular compromise. Furthermore, vasoconstrictors are not useful in decreasing bleeding during a nerve block because anesthesia is not placed directly into the operative site. Higher concentrations of anesthetics, such as 2% lidocaine, are useful because they provide a greater concentration gradient of anesthetic and promote diffusion. This is particularly important when the anesthetic is placed close to, but not directly around, a nerve. Although it must be remembered that a toxic dose will be reached more quickly with a higher concentration of anesthetic, smaller amounts of anesthesia are needed when performing nerve blocks.

The technique of nerve block anesthesia is similar to that of the subcutaneous type of infiltrative anesthesia, since most major nerves are located subdermally. A 1-inch, 30-gauge needle is sometimes desirable, depending on the anticipated depth of the nerve. The use of 25-gauge needles is sometimes recommended so that intravascular injection can be more easily detected. Regardless of the needle size used, larger vessels may be encountered more often when placing nerve blocks, so intravascular injection is determined by pulling back on the plunger of the syringe before injection. The needle is generally advanced either close to the nerve or within the same fascial plane, and anesthetic is allowed to diffuse around the nerve itself. Hyaluronidase can be

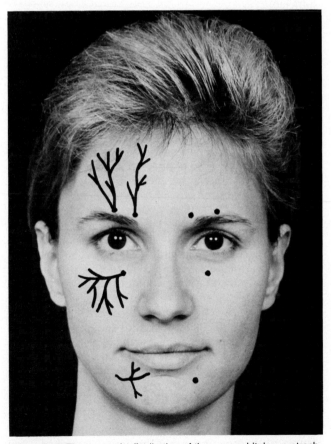

Figure 9–8. The anatomic distribution of the supraorbital, supratrochlear, infraorbital, and mental nerves is shown (left) along with the injection sites for performing nerve blocks for each of these nerves (right).

added to anesthetics to promote diffusion. Injection into the nerve itself is not desirable, and elicitation of paresthesia before injection is not recommended for most nerve blocks used in cutaneous surgery. Nerve block anesthesia takes longer to develop, so 15 to 20 minutes should be allowed before testing the quality of anesthesia.[8]

DIGITAL NERVE BLOCK OF FINGERS OR TOES

The easiest and perhaps most frequently used peripheral nerve block is the digital block. Each digit is supplied by two superior and two inferior digital nerves. Placement of anesthetic medially and laterally around these nerves at the base of the digit provides complete anesthesia of the digit. The use of epinephrine is not recommended, since an avascular field for digital surgery can be provided by using a tourniquet.

To anesthetize a digit, the needle is inserted into the side of the digit and a small amount of anesthetic is injected. The skin is entered first from the dorsolateral aspect of the digit; this is less painful than entering from the palmar or plantar aspect. Using one insertion point, anesthetic can be placed along both superior and inferior digital nerves. The needle is then withdrawn and the procedure repeated on the opposite side. A total of 1 to 3 ml of anesthetic, commonly 2% lidocaine, is usually sufficient.

Although complications are unusual with digital blocks, it should be noted that large volumes (more than 8 ml) of anesthetic injected into this closed space can result in regional circulatory difficulties, particularly when vasospastic disease or a swollen digit is present before injection.[8]

SUPRAORBITAL-SUPRATROCHLEAR NERVE BLOCK OF FOREHEAD

The medial portion of the forehead above the eyebrows to the scalp can be anesthetized by blocking the supraorbital and supratrochlear nerves. The supratrochlear nerve exits the skull along the upper medial corner of the orbit. The supraorbital nerve exits the skull through the supraorbital foramen, which lies along the supraorbital ridge in the midpupillary line.

The supratrochlear nerve is blocked by injecting 1 to 2 ml of anesthetic at the junction of the root of the nose and the upper rim of the orbit. The supraorbital nerve is blocked by injecting 1 to 2 ml of anesthetic at the supraorbital notch. If anesthesia of the entire forehead is required, injection of the subcutaneous tissue underlying the eyebrow will result in blockage of the lacrimal and occasionally the zygomaticotemporal nerves, as well as the supratrochlear and supraorbital nerves.

Swelling and ecchymosis of the upper and lower eyelid can follow this type of nerve block. These difficulties usually resolve rapidly, but the use of pressure immediately after injection can help limit hemorrhage and subsequent ecchymosis.

INFRAORBITAL NERVE BLOCK OF CHEEK

The lower eyelid, the upper lip, and part of the medial cheek and nose can be anesthetized by blocking the infraorbital nerve. The infraorbital nerve exits the infraorbital foramen in the midpupillary line about 1 cm inferior to the infraorbital ridge. For proper injection of anesthetic, the infraorbital foramen can usually be easily palpated. The needle is advanced to this area, and approximately 2 ml of anesthetic is injected around but not into the canal. The addition of hyaluronidase can be very useful in successfully executing this nerve block. An alternative technique, which may be preferable for some patients, is to inject the foramen through the oral cavity after the mucous membranes have been topically anesthetized. While the foramen is palpated, the needle is advanced through the superior labial sulcus until it is in close proximity to the canal. A total of 2 ml of anesthetic is then injected in this area.

Common complications include swelling of the lower eyelid and ecchymosis. A less common complication is transient vision loss from ophthalmic nerve block if the needle is advanced too far up in the canal.

MENTAL NERVE BLOCK OF CHIN

Anesthesia of the chin, lower lip, and mucous membranes can be produced by blocking the mental nerve. The mental nerve exits the mental foramen approximately 2.5 cm from the midline of the face in the midpupillary line. This nerve can be blocked by advancing the needle to the area of the mental foramen and injecting 2 ml of anesthetic. An alternative oral approach to the mental foramen involves advancement of the needle through the inferior labial sulcus at the apex of the first bicuspid. Again, hemorrhage and ecchymosis can be prevented by applying pressure immediately after injection.

Adverse Reactions

Adverse reactions to anesthetic solutions can be produced by the anesthetic itself or, more often, by additives such as epinephrine. Local reactions to epinephrine are uncommon, but tissue necrosis due to vasoconstriction has been reported.[41–43] Most cases of tissue necrosis involve the digits, particularly in patients with peripheral vascular disease or diabetes. Because of this, it is recommended that solutions containing epinephrine not be used on the fingers or toes. Other distal anatomic areas, such as the tip of the nose or earlobes, are quite vascular and can be directly infiltrated with epinephrine without causing complications.

Short-term systemic reactions to epinephrine are common and include tremor, tachycardia, diaphoresis, restlessness, palpitations, headache, increased blood pressure, and chest pain.[8, 44] These reactions are attributed to beta-adrenergic stimulation by epinephrine. Hyperthyroid patients are particularly sensitive to even small doses of epinephrine. An uncommon, but potentially dangerous interaction between epinephrine and propranolol has been reported.[45] Injection of epinephrine into a patient receiving propranolol can result in vasoconstriction, probably mediated by alpha$_1$ receptors. Clinically, this may result in hypertension, bradycardia, and even possible cardiac arrest. This reaction has been reported in patients receiving small quantities of each drug,[45] but most individuals taking propranolol do not experience this reaction.[46]

Systemic reactions to local anesthetics can appear when toxic levels are reached. Toxic blood levels result from the injection of larger than recommended quantities, inadvertent direct vascular injection, or abnormalities in metabolism. Toxicity to the amide anesthetics is typically characterized by central nervous system (CNS) inhibition at low blood levels followed by CNS excitation at high blood levels.[47–49] At the lower toxic doses of lidocaine (3 to 6 µg/ml) digital and circumoral paresthesias, lightheadedness, drowsiness, slurred speech, and restlessness occur. As blood levels increase (5 to 9 µg/ml), muscle twitching, irritability, blurred vision, and nystagmus appear. Further increases can cause seizures, respiratory arrest, or death (Table 9–6).

Toxicity reactions caused by inadequate metabolism can be prevented by inquiring about liver disease or pseudocholinesterase deficiency. Direct vascular injection should be avoided, and the minimal amount of anesthetic that is adequate for the procedure should always be used. The use of vasoconstrictors such as epinephrine can reduce the total amount of anesthetic needed for a given procedure. If a toxic reaction occurs, oxygen and intravenous diazepam can help reverse the reaction.[50]

Allergic reactions to anesthetics are uncommon and occur more frequently with ester preparations.[51, 52] Procaine is rarely used today because it is highly sensitizing. Reactions to procaine can be of either type I, immediate or anaphylactic, or type IV, delayed hypersensitivity or contact dermatitis. Procaine can cross-react with other ester anesthetics, procaine penicillin preparations, and paraben preservatives. No cross-reactivity exists between ester and amide anesthetics.

Reports of allergy to amide anesthetics are rare and most are unsubstantiated.[51, 53–60] Many of the allergic reactions to amide anesthetic solutions are caused by additives, typically the paraben preservatives.[61] Single-dose vials of preservative-free lidocaine are available and may be useful if such a sensitivity is suspected. Although infrequent, topical sensitization to lidocaine has also been reported.[62]

The approach to patients with a history of anesthetic allergy is difficult. True type I allergic reactions presenting with pruritus, rhinorrhea, urticaria, angioedema, or anaphylaxis should be differentiated from psychogenic reactions presenting as hyperventilation, apprehension, syncope, nausea, or other vasovagally induced symptoms. If a clear history of procaine sensitivity is elicited, use of amide anesthetics is recommended. Often the history is unhelpful and other diagnostic tests become necessary. Unfortunately, patch testing has not been helpful in identifying patients with type 1 hypersensitivity,[63] and there is considerable disagreement over the value of intradermal testing.[64]

Often the most practical solution to local anesthetic allergy is to use alternative anesthetics or other means of anesthesia. Both water[65] and sterile saline[66] have been advocated for small cutaneous surgical procedures, but diphenhydramine is probably the most often used alternative anesthetic when amide anesthetic allergy is possible.[67] A 1% solution of diphenhydramine is recommended and can be used for shave or punch biopsies or to treat small malignancies. Diphenhydramine causes some sedation, so patients should always have a friend or relative escort them home after the procedure. Epinephrine can be added to diphenhydramine solutions during operations in vascular areas. Sedation can also be a useful adjunct to anesthesia produced by diphenhydramine; when larger procedures are anticipated, general anesthesia should be considered.

SUMMARY

For most procedures in cutaneous surgery, local anesthesia is ideal and preferable. The pharmacologic agents used to produce this anesthesia are generally easy to administer, effective and inexpensive. Awareness and respect for local anesthetic allergies and side effects is necessary for quality clinical care of patients undergoing cutaneous surgery. It is hoped that the expanded use of local anesthetic agents for many cutaneous procedures will promote the development of new agents, delivery systems, and formulations that will have an even greater safety profile.

TABLE 9–6. LIDOCAINE LEVELS AND SYMPTOMS OF TOXICITY

3–6 µg/ml	Subjective toxicity: lightheadedness, euphoria, digital and circumoral paresthesias, restlessness, drowsiness
5–9 µg/ml	Objective toxicity: nausea, vomiting, tremors, blurred vision, tinnitus, confusion, excitement, psychosis, muscular fasciculations
8–12 µg/ml	Seizures, cardiopulmonary depression
12–20 µg/ml	Coma, respiratory arrest, cardiac standstill

REFERENCES

1. Backer CL, Tinker JH, Robertson DM, Vliestra RE: Myocardial infarction following local anesthesia for ophthalmic surgery. Anesth Analg 59:257–262, 1980.
2. Münch RT, Absolon KB: Carl Ludwig Schleich and the development of local anesthesia. Rev Surg 33:371–380, 1976.
3. Wildsmith JAW, Strichartz GR: Local anaesthetic drugs—an historical perspective. Br J Anaesth 56:937–939, 1984.
4. Fink BR: Leaves and needles: the introduction of surgical local anesthesia. Anesthesiology 63:77–83, 1985.
5. Covino BG: Local anesthesia. N Engl J Med 286:975–983, 1972.

6. Hille B: Local anesthetics: hydrophilic and hydrophobic pathways for the drug-receptor reaction. J Gen Physiol 69:497–515, 1977.
7. Baker JD, Blackmon BB: Local anesthesia. Clin Plast Surg 12:25–31, 1985.
8. Grekin RC, Auletta MJ: Local anesthesia in dermatologic surgery. J Am Acad Dermatol 19:599–614, 1988.
9. Bieter RN: Applied pharmacology of local anesthetics. Am J Surg 34:500–510, 1936.
10. Cohen EN, Levine DA, Colliss JE, Gunther RE: The role of pH in the development of tachyphylaxis to local anesthetic agents. Anesthesiology 29:994–1001, 1968.
11. Covino BG: Local anesthesia. N Engl J Med 286:1035–1042, 1972.
12. Selden R, Sasahara AA: Central nervous system toxicity induced by lidocaine: report of a case in a patient with liver disease. JAMA 202:908–909, 1967.
13. Klein JA: Tumescent technique for regional anesthesia permits lidocaine doses of 35 mg/kg for liposuction. J Dermatol Surg Oncol 16:248–263, 1990.
14. Gormley DE: Cutaneous surgery and the pregnant patient. J Am Acad Dermatol 23:269–279, 1990.
15. Heinonen OP, Slone D, Shapiro S: Birth Defects and Drugs in Pregnancy. Publishing Sciences Group, Littleton, MA, 1977, pp 357–365.
16. Physicians' Desk Reference. 45th ed. Medical Economics Co., Montvale, NJ, 1991, p 624.
17. Kuhnert BR, Knapp DR, Kuhnert PM, Prochaska AL: Maternal, fetal and neonatal metabolism of lidocaine. Clin Pharmacol Ther 26:213–220, 1979.
18. Rasmussen LF, Ahlfors CE, Wennberg RP: The effect of paraben preservatives on albumin binding of bilirubin. J Pediatr 89:475–478, 1976.
19. Hallen B, Uppfeldt A: Does lidocaine-prilocaine cream permit painfree insertion of IV catheters in children? Anesthesiology 57:340–342, 1982.
20. Rosdahl I, Edmar B, Gisslen H, et al: Curettage of molluscum contagiosum in children: analgesia by topical application of a lidocaine/prilocaine cream (EMLA). Acta Derm Venereol (Stockh) 68:149–153, 1988.
21. Lewis-Smith PA: Adjunctive use of hyaluronidase in local anaesthesia. Br J Plast Surg 39:554–558, 1986.
22. Aellig WH, O'Neil R, Laurence DR, et al: Cardiac effects of adrenaline and felypressin as vasoconstrictors in local anaesthesia for oral surgery under diazepam sedation. Br J Anaesth 42:174–176, 1970.
23. Davis J: Vasoconstrictor for facelifting. Aesthetic Plast Surg 12:33–34, 1988.
24. Grabb WC: A concentration of 1:500,000 epinephrine in a local anesthetic solution is sufficient to provide excellent hemostasis. Plast Reconstr Surg 63:834, 1979.
25. Winton GB: Anesthesia for dermatologic surgery. J Dermatol Surg Oncol 14:41–54, 1988.
26. Moore DC, Bridenbaugh DL, Thompson GE, et al: Factors determining dosage of amide-type local anesthetic drugs. Anesthesiology 47:263–268, 1977.
27. McKay W, Morris R, Mushlin P: Sodium bicarbonate attenuates pain on skin infiltration with lidocaine, with or without epinephrine. Anesth Analg 66:572–574, 1987.
28. Stewart JH, Cole GW, Klein JA: Neutralized lidocaine with epinephrine for local anesthesia. J Dermatol Surg Oncol 15:1081–1083, 1989.
29. Galindo A, Witcher T: Mixtures of local anesthetics: bupivacaine-chloroprocaine. Anesth Analg 59:683–685, 1980.
30. Monash S: Location of the superficial epithelial barrier to skin penetration. J Invest Dermatol 29:367–376, 1957.
31. Chiu CY, Brecht K, DasGupta DS, Mhoon E: Myocardial infarction with topical cocaine anesthesia for nasal surgery. Arch Otolaryngol Head Neck Surg 112:988–990, 1986.
32. Bonadio WA, Wagner V: Efficacy of TAC topical anesthetic for repair of pediatric lacerations. Am J Dis Child 142:203–205, 1988.
33. Gesztes A, Mezei M: Topical anesthesia of the skin by liposome-encapsulated tetracaine. Anesth Analg 67:1079–1081, 1988.
34. Brechner VL, Cohen DD, Pretsky I: Dermal anesthesia by the topical application of tetracaine base dissolved in dimethyl sulfoxide. Ann NY Acad Sci 141:524, 1967.
35. Lubens HM, Ausdenmoore RW, Shafer AD, Reece RM: Anesthetic patch for painful procedures such as minor operations. Am J Dis Child 128:192–194, 1974.
36. Sloan JB, Soltani K: Iontophoresis in dermatology: a review. J Am Acad Dermatol 15: 671–684, 1986.
37. Arndt KA, Burton C, Noe JM: Minimizing the pain of local anesthesia. Plast Reconstr Surg 72:676–679, 1983.
38. Peterson DS, Kein DR: Pain sensation related to local anesthesia injected at varying temperatures. Anesth Prog 25:164–165, 1978.
39. Bainbridge LC: Comparison of room temperature and body temperature local anaesthetic solutions. Br J Plast Surg 44:147–148, 1991.
40. Laskin DM: Diagnosis and treatment of complications associated with local anesthesia. Int Dent J 34:232–237, 1984.
41. Garlock JH: Gangrene of the finger following digital nerve block anesthesia. Ann Surg 94:1103–1107, 1931.
42. Ruben JA: Sloughing in local anesthetics—its causes and prevention. Penn Med 23:713, 1920.
43. Serafin FJ: A precaution in the uses of procaine-epinephrine for regional anesthesia. JAMA 91:43–44, 1928.
44. Miller HC, Dick PG, Stuart CW: Clinical and electrocardiographic findings following the use of various local anesthetic solutions. Anesth Analg 17:207–210, 1938.
45. Foster CA, Aston SJ: Propranolol-epinephrine interaction: a potential disaster. Plast Reconstr Surg 72:74–78, 1983.
46. Dzubow LM: The interaction between propranolol and epinephrine as observed in patients undergoing Mohs surgery. J Am Acad Dermatol 15:71–75, 1986.
47. Binnion PF, Murtagh G, Pollock AM, Fletcher E: Relationship between plasma lidocaine levels and induced haemodynamic changes. Br Med J 3:390–393, 1969.
48. Benowitz NL, Meister W: Clinical pharmacokinetics of lidocaine. Clin Pharmacokinet 3:177–201, 1978.
49. Mather LE, Cousins MJ: Local anaesthetics and their current clinical use. Drugs 18:185–205, 1979.
50. deJong RH: Toxic effects of local anesthetics. JAMA 239:1166–1168, 1978.
51. Brown DT, Beamish D, Wildsmith JAW: Allergic reaction to an amide local anaesthetic. Br J Anaesth 53:435–437, 1981.
52. Verrill PJ: Adverse reaction to local anesthetics and vasoconstrictor drugs. Practitioner 214:380–387, 1975.
53. Morrisset LM: Fatal anaphylactic reaction to lidocaine. US Armed Forces Med J 8:740–744, 1957.
54. Mulvey, PM: Allergy to local anaesthetics. Med J Aust 1:386, 1980.
55. Noble DS, Pierce GFM: Allergy to lidocaine: a case history. Lancet 2:1436, 1961.
56. Aldrete JA, Johnson DA: Evaluation of intracutaneous testing for investigation of allergy to local anesthetic agents. Anesth Analg 49:173–183, 1970.
57. Barer MR, McAllen MK: Hypersensitivity to local anaesthetics: a direct challenge test with lignocaine for definitive diagnosis. Br Med J 284:1229–1230, 1982.
58. Holti G, Hood FJC: An anaphylactoid reaction to lignocaine. Dent Pract 15:294–296, 1965.
59. Lynas RFA: A suspected allergic reaction to lidocaine. Anesthesiology 31:380–382, 1969.
60. Eyre J, Nally FF: Nasal test for hypersensitivity, including a positive reaction to lignocaine. Lancet 1:264–265, 1971.
61. Nagel JE, Fuscaldo JT, Fireman P: Paraben allergy. JAMA 237:1594–1595, 1977.
62. Fregert S, Tengner E, Thelin I: Contact allergy to lidocaine. Contact Dermatitis 5:185–188, 1979.
63. Aldrete JA, O'Higgins JW: Evaluation of patients with history of allergy to local anesthetic drugs. South Med J 64:1118–1121, 1971.
64. Incaudo G, Schatz M, Patterson R, et al: Administration of local anesthetics to patients with a history of prior adverse reaction. J Allergy Clin Immunol 61:339–345, 1978.
65. Wiener SG: Injectable sodium chloride as a local anesthetic for skin surgery. Cutis 23:342–343, 1979.
66. Sperling LC, Weber CB, Rodman OG: Toward less painful anesthesia: water, saline, and lidocaine. J Dermatol Surg Oncol 7:730–731, 1981.
67. Roberts EW, Loveless H: The utilization of diphenhydramine for production of local anesthesia: report of a case. Texas Dent J 97:13–15, 1979.

CHAPTER 10

Biochemical and Physiologic Aspects of Wound Healing

LILLIAN B. NANNEY

Many recent advances have had a major impact on the field of wound repair. The areas of growth regulation and molecular biology have heralded a new focus on the whole subject of wound healing. Accordingly, this chapter reviews cutaneous wound healing and the various peptide growth factors that function as modulators of this process (Table 10–1).

Wound healing consists of a complex, integrated sequence of events that are initiated at the time of injury and proceed through repair and remodeling. Although various peptide growth factors have been shown to stimulate or accelerate wound repair in crude experiments, definitive pathways and molecular mechanisms for these cytokines have not been clearly elucidated in vivo. This review brings together the selected pieces of the wound healing puzzle.

Animal Models for Studying Wound Repair

The field of cutaneous wound healing is diverse because there are many different types of wounds and modes of injury (Table 10–2). Wounds may range from the shallowest of injuries such as blisters, superficial abrasions, and first-degree burns to moderate injuries such as second-degree burns and partial-thickness excisions and incisions, and ultimately to severe injuries or wounds such as third-degree burns, full-thickness excisions, and chronic cutaneous ulcers. The variety of wound healing models popularized by investigators reflects this diversity (Table 10–2). Each individual model of wound repair has its own unique advantages and disadvantages.

The existing in vivo wound healing data must be interpreted in light of possible differential responses to various stimuli in differing circumstances. For example, a wound under an occlusive dressing (see Chapter 11) that is bathed in wound fluid containing growth factors or proteases may differ substantially in its cellular composition, receptors, or rate of collagen synthesis from a wound dressed with a nonocclusive bandage. Another significant hindrance to solving the mysteries of wound repair is the fact that the common chronic cutaneous ulcers found in humans have no real counterpart in animal wound healing experiments. While the avascular rabbit ear excision or the ischemic rabbit ear may be close animal model approximations, no animal model truly mimics the poor rates of wound repair that are unique to certain humans. Another problem confounding wound repair research is the fact that normal young animals, frequently used in laboratory research on wound healing, have a rapid intrinsic rate of healing. Only the most potent cytokine formulations could produce significant differences above baseline healing rates when they are being evaluated in young animals in their prime of life. In addition, laboratory animals do not typically exhibit significant hypertrophic scarring or keloid formation, which has greatly retarded progress in the development of procedures and techniques directed toward the elimination of scars.

Phases of Wound Repair

INFLAMMATORY PHASE

Although the inflammatory period has classically been described as the first phase of wound repair, it is

TABLE 10–1. **IN VIVO ACTIONS OF SELECTED GROWTH FACTORS**

Action	EGF	TGFα	TGFβ	PDGF	FGF	IL-2	TNF	IGF
Epithelialization	S	S	S	U	S	U	U	U
Cellular influx (cellularity or DNA)	S	U	S	S	S	U	O	O
Angiogenesis	S	S	S	U	S	U	S	U
Breaking strength	S	U	S	U	S	S	S	U
Collagen content	O	U	S	S	U	S	O	U
Granulation tissue thickness	S	U	S	S	S	U	U	O
Endogenous growth factor production of wound fluid	S	S	S	S	U	O	S	S
Reversal of impaired healing	S	U	S	S	U	O	S	U

EGF, Epidermal growth factor; TGF, transforming growth factor; PDGF, platelet-derived growth factor; FGF, fibroblast growth factor; IL, interleukin; TNF, tumor necrosis factor; IGF, insulin-like growth factor; S, stimulatory; O, no effect; I, inhibitory; U, unknown.

apparent that the clotting cascade is the first event to occur after wounding. After an initial injury that penetrates into the dermis, blood vessel integrity is breached and hemorrhage occurs. Extravasation of serum, deposition of a provisional matrix of fibrin, release of protein factors from platelet granules, and resultant hypoxia are all characteristics of this early wound environment. Minimal tissue injury, as occurs in an abrasion or blistering injury, results only in local leakage of plasma and its components. While wound repair may be somewhat different under these circumstances, the aesthetic results are certainly more favorable.

In surgical or traumatic wounds a complex clotting cascade is initiated by the action of platelets and their subsequent degranulation. Platelets are of proved importance owing to their contribution of soluble clotting factors, but they undoubtedly also exert a profound influence on the next stage of wound repair. Upon their arrival in the wound, platelets release a whole host of growth factors, including transforming growth factor alpha (TGFα), TGFβ, epidermal growth factor (EGF), fibroblast growth factor (FGF), and platelet-derived growth factor (PDGF) into the wound. Studies have not yet answered the mechanistic questions of how PDGFs, either individually or collectively, regulate wound healing events. However, clinical trials with autologously derived platelets suggest that endogenous growth factors are capable of regulating wound repair.[1]

The inflammatory phase of wound healing is characterized by the presence of blood-derived cells, which readily infiltrate the fibrin-fibronectin provisional matrix to enter the wound environment. A host of factors have been implicated in both the early and late influx of inflammatory cells such as neutrophils and macrophages into the wound site. This inflammatory phase, which may be long or short depending on the type of wound and its bacterial population, is usually followed by the development of a granulation tissue containing fibroblasts, endothelial cells, macrophages, and a few T lymphocytes.

TABLE 10–2. **MODELS OF CUTANEOUS REPAIR**

Type of Injury	Animal Model
I. Normal wound healing	
A. Epidermal component	
1. Blistering (suction, vesicants)	Humans, guinea pigs
2. Tape stripping	Humans
3. Light energy (laser ultraviolet wavelength)	Humans, mice
B. Mesenchymal component	
1. Polyvinyl alcohol sponge	Rats
2. PFTE tubes	Humans, rats
3. Stainless steel wire mesh chamber	Rats
C. Epidermal and dermal components	Pigs, rats, guinea pigs, rabbits
1. Burns (scalds, metal templates, lasers)	Pigs, rats, mice
2. Linear incisions	Humans, pigs, rats, guinea pigs
3. Excisions	
a. Partial thickness	Humans, pigs, rats, guinea pigs
b. Full thickness	Pigs, rats, mice, rabbit ears, fetal rabbits
II. Impaired healing	
A. Radiation therapy	Rats, dogs
B. Drug therapy	
1. Corticosteroid	Pigs, rats
2. Doxorubicin	Rats
3. Alloxan/streptozotocin	Db/Db mice, rats
C. Ischemia	Rabbit ears, rat flaps
D. Malnutrition	Rats, mice, guinea pigs
E. Aged	Rats, mice

The respective roles of growth factors as inflammatory mediators are under extensive scrutiny. Although many peptide candidates have been identified through in vitro experiments, their respective roles within the in vivo wound environment have not been fully elucidated.

The early hours after wounding are characterized by the rapid entrance of neutrophils into the wound. Their well-defined activation and killer functions are vital to host defense. Evidence suggests that neutrophils are attracted into the wound by a variety of chemoattractants. One current hypothesis is that the original degranulation of proteins from platelets at the time of injury may serve as the natural source of these chemoattractants. Neutrophils have been shown to contain TGFβ,[2] which suggests yet another source of TGFβ and other cytokines that would continue to deliver endogenous peptides during the first 48 hours after injury. In vivo studies to date have not directly shown the secretion of neutrophil-derived TGFβ into the cutaneous wound, but the recruitment of TGFβ-containing neutrophils has been demonstrated in the inflammatory condition rheumatoid arthritis.[3] Thus, it now seems plausible that growth factors are present at the early stages of wound healing and may serve as potent initiators of the repair process.

GRANULATION TISSUE PHASE

During the continuum of wound repair, the inflammatory phase gives way to the formation of granulation tissue. This tissue was named because of its gross appearance, which is caused by an exuberant production of new blood vessels. The formation of granulation tissue is characterized histologically by an increasing accumulation of macrophages, the formation of new blood vessels (angiogenesis), and a period of active synthesis of matrix proteins.

The requirement to create a highly cellular, well-vascularized connective tissue is normally met fairly rapidly. This phase of wound repair has been extensively studied because it lends itself well to biochemical analysis. Certain wound healing models (Table 10–2), such as polyvinyl alcohol (PVA) sponges or Hunt-Schilling chambers, are designed to isolate a standardized quantity of granulation tissue for subsequent analysis. For this reason, a great deal of knowledge has been developed about collagen synthesis after introduction of growth factors or mediators into these controlled wound repair models (see Table 10–1).

The focus of research is now expanding to probe other factors that influence the granulation tissue phase of wound repair. The renewed interest in structural protein interactions with cells will undoubtedly lead to an understanding of how the provisional matrix of fibrin and fibronectin facilitates cellular migration and influx. It is also becoming increasingly evident that the inflammatory cells and their growth factor products may be the driving forces that convert a nascent, loosely organized, highly cellular granulation tissue into a relatively acellular, dense, irregular connective tissue.

Macrophages

As mentioned, platelets and neutrophils are the first cells to enter the wound environment during the inflammatory stages after the initial injury. In the normal wound repair process, these two cell types are quickly followed by monocyte infiltration, which suggests that this cell population also plays a pivotal role in cutaneous repair. The first piece of evidence implicating macrophages in the stimulation of granulation tissue formation came from studies in which the depletion of macrophages produced a marked delay in the onset and extent of granulation tissue formation.[4] In vitro studies have since shown that activated macrophages express and secrete TGFβ[5] as well as a number of other growth factors.[6, 7]

In humans, alveolar macrophages release PDGF, so this peptide may be a causal factor in the excessive mesenchymal accumulations that accompany idiopathic pulmonary fibrosis.[8] Additional in vitro observations suggest that the macrophages act as the producing cell type in a paracrine mode of interaction. This same mechanism may also prove to be operative in cutaneous wound repair.

There is increasingly strong evidence that the macrophage plays a major role during the formation and development of granulation tissue during healing. Wound repair has actually been shown to be promoted in aged mice by the local injection of macrophages.[9] In a porcine excisional model, exogenous application of TGFβ induced a macrophage population to express even more endogenous TGFβ in a dose-responsive manner.[10] Under TGF stimulation, this same cell population showed increased expression for a host of extracellular matrix proteins including collagens I and III, elastin, and fibronectin but not stromelysin. Indirect studies using an incisional wound model have shown that administration of glycan, an activator of macrophages, can produce an increase in collagen cross-linking.[11] More and more studies are evaluating the role of macrophages as major factories for the production of growth factors. Perhaps the most critical test of the importance of macrophage-derived factors will come when specific antagonists are used to block their effects.

Reepithelialization

When a defect is created in the epidermis, the basal keratinocytes at the wound margin, as well as the keratinocytes in damaged hair follicles and sweat glands, begin to flatten and migrate into the wound. Increased mitotic figures are detected at the edges of the wound.[12] If the wound is kept moist and protected from the external environment so that desiccation and crust formation do not impede this migrating sheet of epithelium, resurfacing will occur at a more rapid rate than normal.[13] During the past decade, various occlusive dressings have been successfully introduced into routine clinical practice. The positive effects of occlusion on the rate of epidermal resurfacing in noninfected superficial wounds have been proved multiple times with various types of synthetic surgical dressings.

During reepithelialization, the keratinocytes must directly contend with the dermal extracellular matrix. It is possible that keratinocytes may actually regulate the maturation of granulation tissue by the production and release of growth factors. Keratinocytes are known to produce growth factors that may function in a paracrine or autocrine fashion. TGFα is produced by rapidly growing keratinocytes in certain proliferative conditions such as those found in tissue culture or in newborn foreskin.[14] PDGF is also expressed by keratinocytes that are actively involved in the resurfacing of a wound.[15] Another growth factor, bFGF, is mitogenic for keratinocytes[16, 17] and is produced by these same cells in culture.[18]

A new family of cell surface adhesion receptors, collectively termed integrins, has been defined.[19, 20] It is now apparent that many different types of cells can attach to their surrounding matrix via their integrin receptors. Integrin-mediated adhesion to extracellular matrix proteins involves their recognition of a specific amino acid sequence such as arginine-glycine-aspartic acid.[19, 20] A wide variety of cell types involved in wound repair, such as keratinocytes, endothelial cells, platelets, and lymphocytes, have specific integrin receptors on their surfaces. Although the details are still lacking, there is much to learn about the interaction of integrin receptors and matrix proteins during all phases of wound repair. Such receptors can mediate the entrance of cells into the wound during the early inflammatory phase of healing. These cellular receptors also affect epithelialization and angiogenesis during the formation of granulation tissue. The last phase of wound healing, contraction and remodeling, when matrix molecules link with myofibroblasts, may someday be eliminated by the use of blocking antibodies against specific integrin receptors.

Some studies have suggested that growth factors can play an active role in wound repair. Experiments with keratinocyte colonies have shown that these cells grow by a combination of cell multiplication and cell migration in the presence of either TGFα or EGF.[21] A number of soluble growth-modulating peptide factors also influence keratinocyte motility in vitro. These enhancers include TGFβ, EGF, and somatomedin-C.[22] Studies using porcine skin explant cultures showed that TGFβ did not increase mitosis but rather facilitated keratinocyte migration.[23] Furthermore, the combination of EGF and TGFβ produced additive effects on migration and mitosis[23] that may be related to cellular adhesion.[24] These studies merely suggest a few of the potential directions or targets for growth factors.

To date, some growth factors have demonstrated an ability to accelerate epithelialization in a variety of in vivo wound studies (see Table 10–1). Clinically, EGF stimulated resurfacing of human donor site wounds,[25] while studies in a pig model have also shown an acceleration of epidermal healing.[26, 27] Other studies of EGF using differing drug delivery formulations and timing have sometimes failed to show significant improvement

in the rates of resurfacing.[28] Acceleration of the rate of epithelialization was reported with a single application of bFGF.[29] Another growth factor, named "epidermal cell–derived factor," also significantly stimulated extensive migration and proliferation of the epidermis after surgical wounding.[30] Recent data also indicate that during epithelialization of pig wounds, PDGF and its receptor are expressed in the healing epidermis.[15] While it is abundantly clear that growth factors are present and can exert a significant impact on the epithelialization stages of wound repair, the complex interplay of both the known and the as yet uncharacterized growth factors is not understood.

Whenever growth factors are added into a dynamic system, the possibility that uncontrolled growth will be stimulated must be considered. Fortunately, the proliferative response of the epidermis appears to be self-limiting in nearly all wounds. Once the surface of the wound is covered, the keratinocytes undergo a normal pattern of differentiation, and certain signals to turn off the evoked wound healing response must undoubtedly be generated. One such signal may be the downmodulation of either EGF/TGFα receptors after exposure to TGFβ.[31] Although this signaling pathway is operational in cultured keratinocytes, this mechanism has not yet been demonstrated with in vivo repair models.

Fibroplasia

It is clear from cell culture studies that the fibroblast functions best when associated with extracellular matrix proteins. Certain peptides have been identified as probable participants in the recruitment of new fibroblasts into granulation tissue, but the mechanisms involved are much more complex than previously thought. With a PVA sponge model, it was noted that sustained slow release of EGF resulted in enhanced collagen accumulation owing to an increased number of fibroblasts.[32] This increase did not reflect a specific stimulation of the rate of collagen synthesis, but instead was caused by an increase in the fibroblast population in the sponge. In the same sponge model a single dose of bFGF produced a remarkable increase in collagen, protein, and DNA content.[33] The injection of bFGF into incisional wounds also showed an increase in collagen maturation or cross-linking.[34]

In wound chambers, PDGF, bFGF, and TGFβ all produced fibroplasia, but EGF did not.[35] The fact that these responses were observed at day ten of healing suggests that secondary mechanisms were at work. In the porcine excisional model, two different groups of data suggest that the dermis responds to bFGF treatments with an increased thickness or an increase in collagen deposition in the granulation tissue.[27, 29]

Wound healing experiments with yet another "epidermal cell–derived factor" showed a stimulation of epithelialization but a significant inhibition of contractility of fibroblasts both in vitro and in vivo.[30] Such studies underscore the interdependence of epidermal and dermal repair, which most typically occur simultaneously. Most research performed to date indicates that the granulation tissue stage in wound repair can be significantly modulated by growth factors.

Neovascularization

The process of angiogenesis is critical to wound repair, for the ingrowing vascular supply must provide the continued nourishment for the granulation tissue. In optimal wound healing situations, endothelial buds are noted by the second day after injury. The quality and quantity of angiogenesis can be modulated by a number of different mediators (Table 10–3).

Endothelial cells are known to produce their own angiogenic growth factors and can operate from an autocrine mode. One such growth factor, bFGF, is conveniently deposited and stored in the subendothelial extracellular matrix.[36] While bFGF is believed to initiate endothelial cell migration during the neovascularization phase of wound healing, this autocrine action by bFGF has been demonstrated only in denuded culture plates of endothelial cells.[37] Angiogenesis can also be modulated by other mediators, including PDGF, bFGF and TGFβ.[35] An acceleration of angiogenesis after a single dose of bFGF in a porcine excisional model has been reported.[29] Furthermore, the role of the matrix proteins may be germane to this process. Support for this can be seen by the onset of angiogenesis, which is significantly accelerated if a sponge implant is coated with either laminin or fibrinogen.[38] Not addressed as yet is the resorption of capillaries during the regression of granulation tissue, since a salient feature of scars is a paucity of blood vessels with relative cellularity amid a dense collagenous matrix.

MATRIX FORMATION OR REMODELING PHASE

Granulation tissue proceeds to acquire more and more collagen. The early accumulation of type III collagen gives way to a predominance of type I collagen. In addition, a number of extracellular matrix molecules are deposited in granulation tissue by a variety of cell types. A few, such as fibronectin, collagen, and proteases, seem at this time to be regulated by growth factors. The life span of the granulation tissue period is variable. For incisional injuries, it is limited in both volume and time. For full-thickness injuries, the other end of the spectrum, both the volume and time period of existence for granulation tissue are greatly extended. However, all granulation tissue that goes on to complete the healing process gradually loses its cellularity and vascularity. It is clear that the three-dimensional meshwork present in granulation tissue plays an essential role in guiding or impeding cellular influx and the subsequent deposition of matrix molecules.

Collagen

Certain peptide growth factors are proved mediators in the formation of new collagen and other matrix proteins (see Table 10–1). TGFβ was the first to be identified when subcutaneous injections induced a transient yet extreme fibrosis in normal skin.[39] Historically, wound healing studies have focused on either the collagen content or the tensile strength in tissues during this period of wound repair. It has been shown that growth factors can accelerate collagen synthesis so that peak values are reached several days earlier than untreated wounds. PDGF has also shown promise in this regard, for in wound chambers an increase in collagen deposition was noted after treatment with it.[40] In rat incisions, PDGF or TGFβ had a major impact on tensile strength. Others have noted that in incisional wounds, EGF or TGFβ[41, 42] in appropriate vehicles could stimulate an early transient increase in tensile strength.[43]

In an excisional model, TGFβ increased matrix expression of collagens I and II, elastin, and fibronectin[10] in a dose-response way. TGFβ treatment enhanced the expression of TGFβ in the same macrophages, which showed a dose-responsive increase in the expression of all matrix proteins. Another experiment, one of the first to address the intrinsic functions of growth factors in wound repair, used neutralizing antibody to bFGF to suggest that endogenous bFGF is intrinsically involved during wound repair.[44] In the absence of active bFGF, significant reductions in collagen, DNA, and protein content were noted in comparison with controls.

The collagens are not the only important matrix proteins to play an integral role in wound repair. Historically, much more is known about collagen biochemistry than about any of the other matrix proteins. The availability of newer probes and antibodies is rapidly expanding the field of wound repair beyond this narrow focus, and much has been learned about fibronectin, laminin, and other components of basement membranes as well as proteoglycans.

Although the pieces of the puzzle do not fit into a clear picture at this time, fibronectin research offers another avenue for understanding wound healing mechanisms. In vitro studies show that keratinocyte migration is stimulated by fibronectin and thrombospondin, but inhibited by laminin.[22, 45] All the current data indicate that the many interactions of keratinocytes with matrix proteins are tightly regulated by a family of integrin receptors.[19, 20] This rapidly expanding field will offer new insights into the areas of wound repair, early stages of development, and other proliferative conditions such as neoplasia.

For now, the in vivo evidence of keratinocyte–matrix protein interaction is still vague yet remains very intriguing. At least two growth factors (bFGF and TGFβ) are

TABLE 10–3. **PROVED IN VIVO MODULATORS OF ANGIOGENESIS**

Mediator	Model	References
TGFα	Sponge, hamster cheek	38, 81
TNF	Sponge, mouse injection	38, 39
EGF	Hamster cheek	81
IL-1α	Sponge	38
FGF	Sponge, pig, diabetic rat	29, 33, 44, 57
TGFβ	Mouse, pig	10, 39, 76

selectively retained within basement membranes where they could serve as a reservoir for growth factor delivery.[46, 47] In a porcine model, TGFβ treatment has been shown to increase the expression of fibronectin in the upper region of the granulation tissue.[10] This evidence suggests that complex feedback mechanisms regulate the delivery of mediators.

Degradation Enzymes

It is clear that the rate of degradation and generation of matrix proteins must be optimally regulated during wound repair. Major restructuring of the extracellular matrix must be accomplished in the conversion of granulation tissue during scar formation and remodeling. In normal skin the extracellular connective tissue is largely degraded through the action of the matrix metalloproteinases.[48] This enzyme family consists of collagenases, gelatinases, and stromelysins.[49] The degradation of the normal and altered matrix is tightly regulated by a balance in the action of TIMP I (tissue inhibitor of metalloproteinases) and these proteases.[50]

A number of proteases secreted from transitory and resident cells have been implicated in wound repair. Collections of fluid from a variety of different types of chronic wounds will soon lead to a greater understanding of wound healing and the factors responsible for slow-healing or nonhealing wounds. To date, efforts to ascertain the role of metalloproteinases have been primarily directed toward either in vitro assays or tumorigenesis.[51] Several lines of evidence have implicated growth factors in the regulation of the expression of collagenase and TIMP. For example, bFGF is a strong stimulator of collagenase production in cultured cells derived from granulation tissue.[52] In this way, collagenase could potentially degrade the extracellular matrix components, thereby allowing cells to migrate through the matrix. PDGF appears to stimulate the production of collagenase by normal fibroblasts.[53] Exogenous applications of TGFβ were inhibitory to the expression of stromelysin in excisional wounds.[10] Certainly, protease-catalyzed restructuring of collagen and other extracellular matrix proteins is critical to both the movement of cells and the remodeling of granulation tissue. With the availability of appropriate probes, the degradative aspects of wound repair will be amenable to extensive evaluation in the near future.

ABNORMAL REPAIR

Scarring

The pathogenesis of hypertrophic scarring and keloids remains enigmatic. In addition, the pathology of scarring and chronic wounding extends well beyond the boundaries of cutaneous repair (Table 10–4). Many of the mechanisms at work in hepatic cirrhosis or rheumatoid arthritis are parallel to the events occurring in cutaneous repair. Human wounds typically heal by contraction and formation of scar tissue rather than by regeneration, as found in amphibians. Although an excessive accumulation of collagen is the apparent cause of hypertrophic

TABLE 10–4. EXAMPLES OF ABERRANT HUMAN WOUND REPAIR

Hypertrophic scars	Arteriosclerosis
Keloids	Rheumatoid arthritis
Dupuytren's contractures	Pulmonary fibrosis
Contractures surrounding breast implants	Scleroderma
Peritoneal adhesions	Neuromas
Hepatic cirrhosis	Ankylosis of joints

scars and keloids, the mechanisms driving these pathologic conditions remain unknown. In vitro studies with collagen gels seeded with fibroblasts have suggested that growth factors are implicated in contraction. Certainly, bFGF was capable of inhibiting gel contraction in vitro.[54] Other experiments with keloid-derived fibroblasts have shown a reduced requirement for growth factors.[55] This suggests that keloids are regulated by unknown mechanisms. In the clinical arena, the carbon dioxide laser has been effectively used for the revision of hypertrophic full-thickness skin grafts on a limited basis.[56] Eventually, such studies may have therapeutic implication in the prevention of scar contractures. However promising these studies may be, there have been no major breakthroughs in discovering the mechanisms that might modify or eliminate scar formation.

Chronic Wounds

A number of studies have been designed to address the problematic wound repair characteristic of diabetic patients. Impaired wound healing is frequently studied in genetically engineered or drug-induced diabetic mice and rats (see Table 10–2). Growth factors have proved effective in restoring many wound healing parameters in these animals to normal levels (see Table 10–1). The introduction of PDGF into wound chambers stimulated the formation of granulation tissue in diabetic rats.[40] The ability of PDGF to restore the decreased rate of repair in diabetic wounds suggests that it may be a limiting endogenous factor at chronic wound sites. This is the major rationale behind the exogenous application of pharmacologic doses of peptide growth factors in situations in which wound healing is compromised. Similar stimulatory effects after TGFβ treatments were also observed in a diabetic rat model.[57] Exogenous growth factors may be able to compensate for some tissue deficiency and prime the system that induces the release of endogenous factors that in turn subsequently stimulate wound healing. Certainly, some chronic slow-healing wounds such as irradiated wounds and decubitus and venous stasis ulcers may benefit from this growth factor research in the near future.

SKIN SUBSTITUTES, CULTURED AUTOGRAFTS, AND ALLOGRAFTS

Promising developments that have therapeutic potential for burn victims with extensive cutaneous losses are no longer elusive.[58] A partially artificial product has proved satisfactory in clinical trials,[59, 60] as have cultured epithelial autografts.[61, 62] Histologic evaluation of these new procedures has produced many insights regarding critical events that influence scarring, as well as the long-term suitability of these new forms of treatment. A short-term study of only eight patients noted adequate permanent coverage yet no anchoring fibrils at the dermal-epidermal junction.[61] Long-term studies with cultured autografts after burns showed that long-term graft fragility is not a major pitfall. On the contrary, a new and functionally satisfactory dermis actually regenerated during a 6-month to 5-year period.[62] The previously cultured epidermis developed rete ridges, and the new dermis contained elastin as well as the normal architecture of blood vessels and collagen. This process would also explain the reports of successful use of composite allogenic dermis with autologous keratinocytes.[63] However, this evidence must be balanced against the reported difficulties in achieving a "take" with cultured autografts.[64]

An artificial matrix polymer containing type I collagen–chondroitin-6-sulfate seeded with autologous keratinocytes (Integra) has been evaluated in a multicenter trial and proved to be an effective treatment for severely burned victims.[59] The physical characteristics of this collagen-glycosaminoglycan copolymer successfully modulated cellular events so that wound contraction was inhibited, yet stable dermal restoration was achieved.[65] Continued experimentation with perturbations of artificial matrix polymers have the added potential to foster a clearer understanding of mesenchymal regeneration. Although the frontier of artificial skin has always been alluring, only the first steps have been taken in this direction.

RELATIONSHIP OF WOUND REPAIR AND TUMORIGENESIS

Wound repair is characterized as controlled cellular proliferation, which is in stark contrast to the uncontrolled cellular proliferation associated with neoplasia. However, considerable similarities have been uncovered to link these two processes. This is why many of the advances in the field of wound healing are due in part to discoveries in cancer research. The fields of wound repair and tumor development were first linked together well over 200 years ago[66] and only resurfaced in 1986 when it was proposed that tumors are wounds that do not heal.[67] There are many similarities between stroma generation by tumors and wound healing phenomena such as granulation tissue and wound maturation.

For years, scientists have examined malignant cells in culture to elucidate the mechanistic actions of the various peptide growth factors. Many of the growth factors involved in the initiation of cell replication in the malignant state are identical to those involved in wound healing. An old association between wound repair and malignant transformation can be seen in the condition known as Marjolin's ulcer. These invasive carcinomas occur with increased frequency in chronic wounds that have failed to achieve complete healing or are injured after many years.[68] It has been suggested that Marjolin's

ulcers are immunologically privileged owing to the destruction of lymphatic channels and obstruction due to scarring,[69] but the mechanisms controlling the conversion of an old scar to an aggressive invasive tumor are still unknown.

In recent years, enhanced tumor growth in animals with healing wounds has been reported by at least three groups.[70–72] These data show that fewer tumorigenic cells are necessary to produce a tumor in a wounded area than in a nonwounded area. The best explanation for these results is that stimulation of tumor cell proliferation is produced by growth factors in the microenvironment of the wound. This phenomenon has been demonstrated in a variety of tumorigenic cell types. For this reason, an understanding of the endogenous interactions of growth factors in wounds could have major clinical impact on therapies aimed at the prevention of local tumor recurrence.

FUTURE DIRECTIONS: SYNERGISM OF GROWTH FACTORS

Therapeutic uses of combinations of growth factors in various wound repair situations must await better characterization of the individual roles and interactions of each factor. Several in vivo animal studies have already embarked on this course. In a porcine partial-thickness injury, PDGF in combination with insulin-like growth factor 1 (IGF–1) resulted in significantly thicker granulation tissue associated with stimulatory effects on the epidermis.[73] Later work by this same group showed that PDGF and TGFα could cause a similar increase in connective tissue volume, collagen content, and maturity.[74] As suspected, some combinations of growth factors showed no synergy in their effects; others, like tumor necrosis factor alpha (TNFα) and TGFβ,[75, 76] have proved inhibitory. As evidence accumulates regarding the mechanisms of action of the growth factors, it may be possible to initiate healing with one factor and modify the later phases of repair with another factor.

A combination of growth factors in the form of platelet releasate,[1] an autologous mix from platelets composed of at least nine different growth-mediating agents, has shown promise in chronic ulcers. However, work is continuing to isolate the specific growth factors actually responsible for wound repair. Several clinical trials using solitary growth factors are now nearing completion. When these results are analyzed, patients may finally begin to benefit from years of laboratory studies in wound repair.

SUMMARY

Recent developments in growth factors and cutaneous wound repair are currently undergoing exponential growth. This information explosion is accruing from fields such as developmental biology, cancer research, and immunology.

Many problematic conditions in wound repair, such as chronic ulcers, irradiated wounds, and aesthetically unsatisfactory scarring, still represent formidable challenges. However, there is every indication that peptide growth factors will serve as the basis for numerous therapeutic applications to help restore the normal healing process after trauma, after surgery, or in compromised patients.

_____

This work was supported in part by the Veterans Affairs Health Services and Public Health Service Grants GM 40437.

REFERENCES

1. Knighton DR, Ciresi KF, Fiegel VD, et al: Classification and treatment of chronic non-healing wounds. Successful treatment with autologous platelet-derived wound healing factors (PDWHF). Ann Surg 204:322–330, 1986.
2. Grotendorst GR, Smale G, Pencev D: Production of transforming growth factor beta by human peripheral blood monocytes and neutrophils. J Cell Physiol 140:396–402, 1989.
3. Fava R, Broadley K, Davidson JM, et al: Intra-articular injection of rTGF/β1 in rat knee joints mimics events associated with early stages of arthritis. In: Dinarello CA, Kluger MJ, Powanda MC, Oppenheim JJ (eds): The Physiological and Pathological Effects of Cytokines. Wiley-Liss, New York, 1990, pp 99–104.
4. Leibovich SJ, Ross R: The role of the macrophage in wound repair. A study of hydrocortisone and antimacrophage serum. Am J Pathol 78:71–91, 1975.
5. Assoian RK, Fleurdelys BE, Stevenson HC, et al: Expression and secretion of type β transforming growth factor by activated human macrophages. Proc Natl Acad Sci USA 84:6020–6024, 1987.
6. Rappolee DA, Mark D, Banda MJ, Werb Z: Wound macrophages express TGFβ and other growth factors in vivo: analysis by mRNA phenotyping. Science 241:708–712, 1988.
7. Madtes DK, Raines EW, Sakariassen KS, et al: Induction of transforming growth factor-α in activated human alveolar macrophages. Cell 53:285–293, 1988.
8. Martinet Y, Rom WN, Grotendorst GR, et al: Exaggerated spontaneous release of platelet-derived growth factor by alveolar macrophages from patients with idiopathic pulmonary fibrosis. N Engl J Med 317:202–209, 1987.
9. Danon D, Kowatch MA, Roth GS: Promotion of wound repair in old mice by injection of macrophages. Proc Natl Acad Sci USA 86:2018–2020, 1989.
10. Quaglino D, Nanney LB, Kennedy R, Davidson JM: Transforming growth factor-β stimulates wound healing and modulates extracellular matrix gene expression in pig skin. Lab Invest 63:307–319, 1990.
11. Browder W, Williams D, Lucore P, Pretus H: Effect of enhanced macrophage function on early wound healing. Surgery 104:224–230, 1988.
12. Winter GD: Effects of air drying and dressings on the surface of a wound. Nature 197:91–92, 1963.
13. Eaglstein WH, Davis SC, Mehle AL, Mertz PM: Optimal use of an occlusive dressing to enhance healing: effect of delayed application and early removal on wound healing. Arch Dermatol 124:392–395, 1988.
14. Coffey RJ Jr, Derynck R, Wilcox JN, et al: Production and auto-induction of transforming growth factor in human keratinocytes. Nature 328:817–820, 1987.
15. Antoniades HN, Galanopoulos T, Neville-Golden J, et al: Injury induces in vivo expression of platelet-derived growth factor (PDGF) and PDGF receptor mRNAs in skin epithelial cells and PDGF mRNA in connective tissue fibroblasts. Proc Natl Acad Sci USA 88:565–569, 1991.
16. O'Keefe EJ, Chiu ML, Payne RE: Stimulation of growth of keratinocytes by basic fibroblast growth factor. J Invest Dermatol 90:767–769, 1988.
17. Shipley GD, Keegle WW, Hendrickson JE, et al: Growth of normal human keratinocytes and fibroblasts in serum-free medium is stimulated by acidic and basic fibroblast growth factor. J Cell Physiol 138:511–518, 1989.
18. Halaban R, Langdos R, Birchell N, et al: Basic fibroblast growth factor from human keratinocytes as a natural mitogen for melanocytes. J Cell Biol 107:1611–1619, 1988.
19. Hynes RO: Integrins: a family of cell surface receptors. Cell 48:549–554, 1987.
20. Ruoslahti E, Pierschbacher MD: New perspectives on cell adhesion: RGD and integrins. Science 238:491–497, 1987.
21. Barrandon Y, Green H: Cell migration is essential for sustained growth of keratinocyte colonies: the roles of transforming growth factor-α and epidermal growth factor. Cell 50:1131–1137, 1987.
22. Nickoloff BJ, Mitra RS, Riser BL, et al: Modulation of keratinocyte motility. Am J Pathol 132:543–551, 1988.
23. Hebda PA: Stimulatory effects of transforming growth factor-β and epidermal growth factor on epidermal cell outgrowth from porcine skin explant cultures. J Invest Dermatol 91:440–445, 1988.
24. Ignotz RA, Massague J: Cell adhesion protein receptors as targets for transforming growth factor-beta action. Cell 51:189–197, 1987.
25. Brown GL, Nanney LB, Griffen J, et al: Enhancement of wound healing by topical treatment with epidermal growth factor. N Engl J Med 321:76–79, 1989.
26. Brown GL, Curtsinger L, Brightwell JR, et al: Enhancement of epidermal regeneration by biosynthetic epidermal growth factor. J Exp Med 163:1319–1324, 1986.
27. Nanney LB: Epidermal and dermal effects of epidermal growth factor during wound repair. J Invest Dermatol 94:624–629, 1990.
28. Chvapil M, Gaines JA, Gilman T: Lanolin and epidermal growth factor in healing of partial-thickness pig wounds. J Burn Care Rehabil 9:279–284, 1988.
29. Hebda PA, Klingbeil CK, Abraham JA, Fiddes JC: Basic fibroblast growth factor stimulation of epidermal wound healing in pigs. J Invest Dermatol 95:626–631, 1990.
30. Eisinger M, Sadan S, Silver IA, Flick RB: Growth regulation of skin cells by epidermal cell–derived factors: implications for wound healing. Proc Natl Acad Sci USA 85:1937–1941, 1988.
31. Massague J: Transforming growth factor-β modulates the high-affinity receptors for epidermal growth factor and transforming growth factor-α. J Cell Biol 100:1508–1514, 1985.
32. Buckley A, Davidson JM, Kamerath CD, et al: Sustained release of epidermal growth factor accelerates wound repair. Proc Natl Acad Sci USA 82:7340–7344, 1985.
33. Davidson JM, Klagsburn M, Hill KE, et al: Accelerated wound repair, cell proliferation and collagen accumulation are produced by a cartilage-derived growth factor. J Cell Biol 100:1219–1227, 1985.
34. McGee GS, Davidson JM, Buckley A, et al: Recombinant basic fibroblast growth factor accelerates wound healing. J Surg Res 45:145–153, 1988.
35. Sprugel KH, McPherson JM, Clowes AW, Ross R: Effects of growth factors in vivo. I. Cell ingrowth into porous subcutaneous chambers. Am J Pathol 129:601, 1987.
36. Vlodavsky I, Fridman R, Sullivan R, et al: Aortic endothelial cells synthesize basic fibroblast growth factor which remains cell associated and platelet-derived growth factor-like protein which is secreted. J Cell Physiol 131:402–408, 1987.
37. Sato Y, Rifkin DB: Autocrine activities of basic fibroblast growth factor: regulation of endothelial cell movement, plasminogen activator synthesis, and DNA synthesis. J Cell Biol 107:1199–1205, 1988.
38. Mahadevan V, Hart IR, Lewis GP: Factors influencing blood supply in wound granuloma quantitated by a new in vivo technique. Cancer Res 49:415–419, 1989.
39. Roberts AB, Sporn MB, Assoian RK, et al: Transforming growth factor type β: rapid induction of fibrosis and angiogenesis in vivo and stimulation of collagen in vitro. Proc Natl Acad Sci USA 83:4167–4171, 1986.
40. Grotendorst GR, Martin GR, Pencev D, et al: Stimulation of granulation tissue formation by platelet-derived growth factor in normal and diabetic rats. J Clin Invest 76:2323–2329, 1985.
41. Pierce GF, Mustoe TA, Lingelbach J, et al: Platelet-derived growth factor and transforming growth factor-β enhance tissue repair activities by unique mechanisms. J Cell Biol 109:429–440, 1989.
42. Pierce GF, Mustoe TA, Lingelbach J, et al: Transforming growth factor β reverses the glucocorticoid-induced wound healing deficit

in rats and is regulated by platelet-derived growth factor in macrophages. Proc Natl Acad Sci USA 86:2229–2233, 1989.

43. Brown GL, Curtsinger L, White M, et al: Acceleration of tensile strength of incisions treated with EGF and TGF-β. Ann Surg 208:788–794, 1988.

44. Broadley KN, Aquino AM, Woodward SC, et al: Monospecific antibodies indicate that basic fibroblast growth factor is intrinsically involved in wound repair. Lab Invest 61:571–575, 1989.

45. O'Keefe EJ, Payne RE, Russell N, Woodley DT: Spreading and enhanced motility of human keratinocytes on fibronectin. J Invest Dermatol 85:125–130, 1985.

46. Folkman J, Klagsbrun M, Sasse J, et al: A heparin-binding angiogenic protein-basic fibroblast growth factor is stored within basement membrane. Am J Pathol 130:393–400, 1988.

47. Fava RA, McClure DB: Fibronectin associated transforming growth factor. J Cell Physiol 131:184–189, 1987.

48. Harris ED, Welgus HG, Krane SM: Regulation of mammalian collagenases. Collagen Rel Res 4:493–512, 1984.

49. Chin JR, Murphy G, Werb Z: Stromelysin, a connective tissue–degrading metalloendopeptidase secreted by stimulated rabbit synovial fibroblasts in parallel with collagenase. J Biol Chem 260:12367–12376, 1985.

50. Stricklin GP, Welgus HG: Human skin fibroblast collagenase inhibitor: purification and chemical characterization. J Biol Chem 258:12252–12258, 1983.

51. Childers JW, Hernandez AD, Kim JH, Stricklin GP: Immunolocalization of collagenase inhibitor in normal skin and basal cell carcinoma. J Am Acad Dermatol 17:1025–1032, 1987.

52. Buckley-Sturrock A, Woodward SC, Senior RM, et al: Differential stimulation of collagenase and chemotactic activity in fibroblasts derived from rat wound repair tissue and human skin by growth factors. J Cell Physiol 138:70–78, 1989.

53. Bauer EA, Cooper TW, Huang JS, et al: Stimulation of in vitro human skin collagenase expression by platelet-derived growth factor. Proc Natl Acad Sci USA 82:4132–4136, 1985.

54. Finesmith TH, Broadley KN, Davidson JM: Fibroblasts from wounds of different stages of repair vary in their ability to contract a collagen gel in response to growth factors. J Cell Physiol 144:99–107, 1990.

55. Russell SB, Trupin KM, Rodriguez-Eaton S, et al: Reduced growth-factor requirement of keloid-derived fibroblasts may account for tumor growth. Proc Natl Acad Sci USA 85:587–591, 1988.

56. Wheeland RG: Revision of full-thickness skin grafts using the carbon dioxide laser. J Dermatol Surg Oncol 14:130–134, 1988.

57. Broadley KN, Aquino AM, Hicks B, et al: The diabetic rat as an impaired wound healing model: stimulatory effects of transforming growth factor beta and basic fibroblast growth factor. Biotech Ther 1:55–68, 1989.

58. Gallico GG, O'Connor NE, Compton CC, et al: Permanent coverage of large burn wounds with autologous cultured human epithelium. N Engl J Med 311:448–451, 1984.

59. Stern R, McPherson M, Longaker MT: Histologic study of artificial skin used in the treatment of full-thickness thermal injury. J Burn Care Rehabil 11:7–13, 1990.

60. Heimbach D, Luterman A, Burke J, et al: Artificial dermis for major burns. A multi-center randomized trial. Ann Surg 208:313–320, 1988.

61. Herzog SA, Meyer A, Woodley D, Peterson ND: Wound coverage with cultured autologous keratinocytes: use after burn wound excision, including biopsy follow-up. J Trauma 28:195–198, 1988.

62. Compton CC, Gill JM, Bradford DA, et al: Skin regenerated from cultured epithelial autografts on full-thickness burn wounds from 6 days to 5 years after grafting: a light, electron microscopic and immunohistochemical study. Lab Invest 60:600–612, 1989.

63. Cuono CB, Langdon R, Birchall N, et al: Composite autologous-allogeneic skin replacement: development and clinical application. Plast Reconstr Surg 80:626–635, 1987.

64. Eldad A, Burt A, Clark JA: Cultured epithelium as a skin substitute. Burns 13:173–180, 1987.

65. Murphy GF, Orgill DP, Yannas IV: Partial dermal regeneration is induced by biodegradable collagen-glycosaminoglycan grafts. Lab Invest 63:305–313, 1990.

66. Sporn MB, Roberts AB: Peptide growth factors and inflammation, tissue repair, and cancer. J Clin Invest 78:329–332, 1986.

67. Dvorak HF: Tumors: wounds that do not heal: similarities between tumor stroma generation and wound healing. N Engl J Med 315:1651–1659, 1986.

68. Fleming MD, Hunt JL, Purdue GF, Sandstad J: Marjolin's ulcer: a review and reevaluation of a difficult problem. J Burn Care Rehabil 11:460–469, 1990.

69. Bostwick J 3rd, Pendergrast WJ Jr, Vasconez LO: Marjolin's ulcer: an immunologically privileged tumor? Plast Reconstr Surg 57:66–69, 1975.

70. Weese JL, Ottery FD, Emeto SE: Do operations facilitate tumor growth? An experimental model in rats. Surgery 100:273–275, 1986.

71. Eggermont AMM, Steelar EP, Sugarbaker PH: Laparotomy enhances intraperitoneal tumor growth and abrogates the antitumor effects of interleukin–2 and lymphokine-activated killer cells. Surgery 102:71–78, 1987.

72. Baker DG, Masterson TM, Pace R, et al: The influence of the surgical wound on local tumor recurrence. Surgery 106:525–532, 1989.

73. Lynch SE, Nixon JC, Colvin RB, Antoniades HN: Role of platelet-derived growth factor in wound healing: synergistic effects with other growth factors. Proc Natl Acad Sci USA 84:7696–7700, 1987.

74. Lynch SE, Colvin RB, Antoniades HN: Growth factors in wound healing. Single and synergistic effects on partial thickness porcine skin wounds. J Clin Invest 84:640–646, 1989.

75. Steenfos HH, Hunt TK, Scheuenstuhl CS, Goodson WH: Selective effects of tumor necrosis factor-α on wound healing in rats. Surgery 106:171–176, 1989.

76. Lawrence WT, Sporn MB, Gorschboth C, et al: The reversal of an Adriamycin induced healing impairment with chemoattractants and growth factors. Ann Surg 203:142–147, 1986.

77. Franklin JD, Lynch JB: Effects of topical applications of epidermal growth factor on wound healing: experimental study on rabbit ears. Plast Reconstr Surg 64:766–770, 1979.

78. Niall M, Ryan GB, O'Brian BJ: The effects of epidermal growth factor on wound healing in mice. J Surg Res 33:164–169, 1982.

79. Schultz GS, White M, Mitchell R, et al: Epithelial wound healing enhanced by transforming growth factor alpha and vaccinia growth factor. Science 235:350–352, 1987.

80. Buckley A, Davidson JM, Kamerath CD, Woodward SC: Epidermal growth factor increases granulation tissue dose dependently. J Surg Res 43:322–328, 1987.

81. Schreiber AB, Winkler ME, Derynck R: Transforming growth factor-α. A more potent angiogenic mediator than epidermal growth factor. Science 232:1250–1253, 1986.

82. McGee GS, Broadley KN, Buckley A, et al: Recombinant transforming growth factor β accelerates incisional wound healing. Curr Surg 46:103–106, 1989.

83. Barbul A, Kund-Hanson J, Wasserkrug HL, et al: Interleukin-2 enhances wound healing in rats. J Surg Res 40:315–319, 1986.

84. Mooney DP, O'Reilly M, Gamelli RL: Tumor necrosis factor and wound healing. Ann Surg 211:124–129, 1990.

85. Grotendorst GR, Grotendorst CA, Gilman T: Production of growth factors (PDGF and TGFβ) at the site of tissue repair. Prog Clin Biol Res 266:47–54, 1988.

86. Ford HR, Hoffman RA, Wing EJ, et al: Characterization of wound cytokines in the sponge matrix model. Arch Surg 124:1422–1428, 1989.

87. Spencer E, Skover G, Hunt TK: Somatomedins: do they play a pivotal role in wound healing? Prog Clin Biol Res 266:103–116, 1988.

CHAPTER 11

Synthetic Surgical Dressings

DANIEL PIACQUADIO

Historical Aspects

The search for an ideal wound dressing is probably as old as man. The instinctive desire to "cover" a wound was founded in a need to protect it from further injury. With time, the role of such coverings or dressings has changed to emphasize healing. Chinese and Egyptian archeologic records from 3000 to 2500 BC document some of the earliest work in wound healing. The Chinese Red Emperor Shen Nung is credited with compiling the first medical herbal, the Pen-tsao (2800 BC).[1] Herbs were perceived as vital in correcting the imbalance within the body produced by wound infections. The Egyptians used splints of palm fiber and reed bundles to immobilize injured limbs.[1] The early Egyptians are also well known for their use of "dressings" in the mummification process and for wound care adjuvants of potential aseptic or antibacterial value such as green copper and mercury.[2] Unfortunately, other salves or ointments included animal waste products and botanical concoctions that probably did more harm than good.

The Papyrus Ebera, an ancient Egyptian medical document, contains detailed information on tending for the sick and bandaging wounds.[3] Included in this document are details of the use of gum-impregnated linen strips to close gaping wounds, much as modern tape is used today, 4000 years later. Another wound dressing favored by Galen (129–200 AD), the prominent Greek physician and author of over 300 texts, was cobwebs. It was thought that the webs formed a matrix that aided clot formation and healing; their use persisted well into the fourteenth century.[2]

In 400 BC Hippocrates laid down the principles of asepsis. He recommended that wounds be washed out with tepid water, with or without vinegar, and then left to dry. Wine or vinegar, with its high alcohol content, probably served as the first antiseptic.[4] Unfortunately,

the true value of such therapy was not fully appreciated for the next 2000 years. Rather, Galen's theory of "laudable pus" dominated wound care.[1, 2] This theory advocated pus as an integral and important component of healing. Only in the nineteenth century did Joseph Lister discover the association between pus and bacterial infection in a wound. In 1867 he published his findings advocating the use of antiseptic carbolic acid spray during surgical procedures.[1] Although not initially accepted, Lister's work eventually established the need for keeping wounds free of contamination.

To this end, dressings were thought to make a significant contribution. Until the mid-1800s linen fabrics dominated as dressing materials. At that time, dressings made of woven and nonwoven materials, such as cotton gauze, gradually became available. Over the next 100 years many variations using these materials appeared, including tulle gras, a nonadherent dressing made by impregnating gauze with soft paraffin or oil.[2] Eventually, advancing technology and an improved understanding of wound healing gave rise to a host of new synthetic and semisynthetic surgical dressing materials.

Practical and Theoretical Considerations

Numerous factors are important in the proper selection of an ideal surgical dressing for any clinical situation. Unfortunately, in many cases the decision is based on habit and standard practice rather than on a true understanding of the processes involved in wound healing. While the ideal dressing material is not yet to hand, many new methods are now available that improve the rate and quality of healing. Several important basic considerations must be kept in mind in order to choose the best dressing for each clinical situation.

ADHERENCE

Adherence is one of the most important characteristics of a dressing material. Adherence to the skin surrounding a wound is desirable in that it keeps the dressing in place, aids in bacterial barrier function, and may minimize loss of wound exudate.[5, 6] However, in clinical settings in which the surrounding tissues are inflamed, edematous, or compromised,[7] nonadherent wound dressing materials are often preferable.

The choice of an adherent dressing sometimes depends on the type of wound. One of the new surgical dressings, made of a hydrocolloid material, does not stick to moist surfaces. In addition, incorporation of wound exudate into the dressing results in a viscous gel that also does not adhere to the wound.[8] Conversely, many film dressings have a uniform adhesive backing that does adhere to newly epithelializing surfaces.[9] However, if the wound is wet or heavily exudative, this is not a problem. Adherence can also result from interaction between the wound and the dressing material. In this way, the dressing may adhere to the wound bed by fibrin or protein exudates and become mechanically incorporated into the healing wound.[10, 11] In these situations, dressing changes may strip away newly healed epithelium and disrupt the healing process.[9, 12, 13] To minimize this problem, dressing materials with an ointment or nonadherent absorbent inner layer should be used.

OCCLUSION

In addition to preventing wound desiccation,[7] occlusive dressings appear to have a much broader effect on wound healing. Occlusion is one of the features common to most new biosynthetic surgical dressings. In the late 1950s it was observed that a blister healed faster if it was left unbroken. These observations were supported in studies of epithelialization rates in burns, in which healing rates were noted to be 40% faster when blisters were left intact rather than being broken.[14] In a 1962

landmark study, the first step in applying this knowledge to improve wound care was taken. In this study, a polyethylene film (Polythene) dressing was shown to more than double the wound epithelialization rate in an animal model.[15] Since these initial studies, the clinical value of a moist healing environment has been fully established.[7, 16, 17] However, the mechanisms by which moist wound healing is beneficial remain complicated and controversial. In original studies, the deleterious effects of eschar formation and wound desiccation were emphasized.[15, 18–21] The eschar acts as a mechanical obstruction to migrating epithelial cells, while desiccation leads to greater tissue loss (Fig. 11–1). Improved healing rates in occluded wounds[19, 20] were due to accelerated epidermal migration rather than increased mitotic rates. In one study, occlusive dressings were actually found to reduce the magnitude and duration of the mitotic response compared with the situation in open wounds.[19] These findings were confirmed by human stratum corneum stripping studies.[22] All these studies dealt with superficial injuries in which the use of occlusive dressings minimizes tissue loss by preventing desiccation. Some investigators have hypothesized that this preservation of tissue is reflected by the decreased mitotic activity seen in occluded wounds.[17]

As further evidence for their tissue sparing effects, an occlusive dressing (Op-Site) was shown to preserve underlying structures better after a burn injury.[23] All test sites received uniform burn injury and then were covered with either Op-Site or a gauze dressing. Sites treated with occlusive dressings healed with less scarring and the appendageal structures were preserved. Since these preliminary studies, numerous other human and animal studies have been performed using various types of commercially available biosynthetic dressings. Uniformly, all these dressing materials have shown superior rates of reepithelialization and decreased healing times by 25 to 40%.[17, 24–27] Even full-thickness wounds show a similar benefit with occlusion.[28–30]

In full-thickness wounds the rate of reepithelialization is also partially a reflection of the ability of the wound

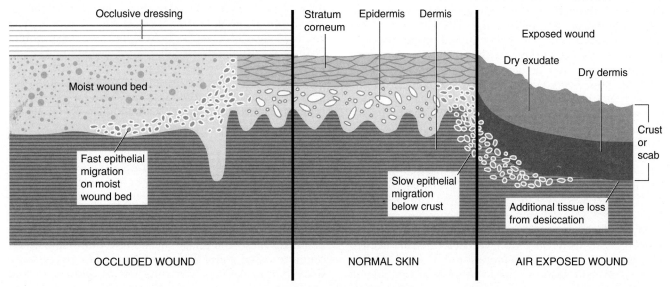

Figure 11–1. Occluded compared with air-exposed wound healing. (Redrawn from Winter GD: Formation of scab and the rate of epithelization of superficial wounds in the skin of the young domestic pig. Nature 193:293–294, 1962.)

to contract. Early studies suggested that a loss of moisture from the wound would enhance contraction.[31, 32] However, more recent evidence favors the use of occlusive dressings in full-thickness defects to promote wound contraction. An increased rate of contraction has been observed in several animal models.[21, 31, 33] A study of 58 Mohs surgery patients with full-thickness defects reported that healing was facilitated by a polyurethane film (Bioclusive), which was superior to traditional antibiotic gauze dressings. A 50% reduction in defect size was seen at the 6-month follow-up evaluation in 17 of 26 patients treated with occlusion, compared with eight of 25 patient given traditional dressings.[30] The mechanism for this increased rate of contraction is not well understood. However, more organized fibroblast infiltrates, suggestive of contractile myofibroblasts, have been noted in occluded wound sites.[33]

Occlusive dressings also appear to alter collagen production as well as the character of the inflammatory infiltrate in wounds. Initial studies showed increased collagen production in superficial wounds treated with occlusive dressings,[12] but subsequent studies showed decreased production.[34-36] The significance of this possible decrease in collagen production is unclear. Wound strength, which is related to collagen deposition and degree of cross-linking, is delayed with occlusion.[34] However, this appears to be of no clinical importance. When large abdominal wounds were closed using a sutureless skin closure technique,[37, 38] there were fewer complications, less inflammation, and a cosmetically superior result compared with clip or sutured closures. Several other investigators noted similar cosmetic improvement when occlusive dressings were used in other applications.[30, 34, 37]

This change in collagen production is probably related to the alteration in the inflammatory cell infiltrate that occurs in wounds treated with occlusive dressings. The lymphokines and growth factors elaborated by these cells undoubtedly play a key regulatory role. In general, inflammation appears to be reduced when occlusive dressings are used.[34, 36] This correlates with a decrease in erythema, pain, and tenderness seen clinically.[7, 17 37] One study showed an elevation in neutrophils, monocytes, fibroblasts, and endothelial cells with moist healing.[33] This difference may be attributed to the model or possible technical variations. Interestingly, this same study demonstrated an acceleration in the phases of healing, both histologically and by the content of the cellular infiltrate,[33] when occlusion was used.

The mechanism by which occlusive dressings influence the cellular infiltrate in a wound site is complex. The availability of oxygen was initially thought to be of primary importance to the rate of wound healing.[39, 40] This influenced the development of an oxygen-permeable membrane as one of the first available occlusive dressings (Op-Site).[41] Evidence from more recent studies[12, 42-46] showed that the oxygen requirement for optimal fibroblast proliferation is quite low, only 5–10 mm Hg.[43] Similarly, only low levels of oxygen are needed to accelerate vascular proliferation.[44, 45] Macrophage-derived growth factors appear to play a key role in

modulating these events. Release of these factors is regulated by the oxygen tension of the wound.[45, 47] Clinically, investigators have documented very low levels of oxygen tension in the fluid beneath occlusive dressing. Surprisingly, the oxygen-permeable synthetic surgical dressings also maintain only very low levels of oxygen underneath the dressing.[42] In these situations, other factors, including bacterial and inflammatory cell infiltrates, probably play an important role. The proved efficacy of these dressings is probably associated with their ability to establish an environment conducive to wound healing. However, it should always be recognized that adequate oxygen provided by wound perfusion is vital to the normal wound repair process.[47, 48]

MICROBIOLOGY AND OCCLUSIVE DRESSINGS

One of the most important issues concerning occlusive dressings is the effect they have on the microbial population of the wound. Historically, the formation of an eschar was advocated because of the antimicrobial effects produced by desiccation, even though it was a bacterial reservoir.[49] All occlusive dressings have been found to promote bacterial growth. The rate of growth and type of bacterial growth vary with the type of dressing.[6, 42, 50-52] One example of this is the shift to gram-negative organisms that is seen with film and hydrogel dressings.[51, 53] Other factors, including hydration, pH, PO_2, skin surface lipids, neutrophils, and other bacterial antagonists, also contribute to differences in bacterial growth. Even in the presence of bacterial overgrowth, increased rates of reepithelialization and healing are consistently seen with the biocclusive dressings,[54] despite the inverse relationship between bacterial counts and healing reported by several investigators.[55, 56] Since the type of bacteria detected may prove important[57] as our understanding of this complex relationship grows, it is possible that wound healing could be successfully modified by manipulating the bacteria present in a wound. Despite concern about the possibility of promoting infection, the occlusive dressing has been shown, after well over three decades of clinical use, to be a safe and effective way to promote healing and not cause infection. A 1990 review of clinical wound healing reported an overall clinical infection rate of 2.6% for wounds treated with occlusive dressings and 7.15% for those given conventional dressings (Fig. 11–2).[54] Several occlusive dressings may also be effective in reducing clinical infection by acting as barriers to outside pathogens.[53]

Traditional Wound Dressing Materials

Traditional wound dressing materials are natural, synthetic, or semisynthetic materials used in wound care. Some of these materials, including cotton and other cellulose-based gauze materials, have been in existence since before 1960. Over time, many variations and

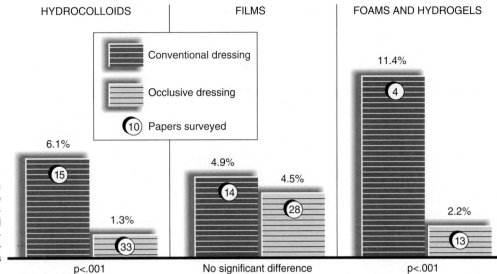

Figure 11–2. Infection rates with conventional versus occlusive dressings. (Redrawn from Hutchinson JJ: Prevalence of wound infection under occlusive dressings: a collective survey of reported research. Wounds 1(2):125, 1989.)

combinations of these materials have been designed to optimize their clinical value.

TULLE GRAS

Lumière, a French surgeon during the Great War, developed tulle gras. This paraffin-impregnated cotton or silk gauze dressing was one of the first nonadherent materials used for dressing wounds.[2] Today, several other impregnated gauze dressing materials are available (Table 11–1). These nonadherent dressings are used at the interface layer of the wound to minimize trauma to reepithelializing wounds.

TABLE 11–1. TYPES OF OCCLUSIVE DRESSINGS

Polyurethane films	Op-Site, Bioclusive, Tegaderm, Ensure-It, Blisterfilm, Acu-derm, Polyskin, Uniflex, Co-Film, Visulin, Omiderm
Hydrocolloids	DuoDerm, J&J Ulcer Dressing, Comfeel Ulcus, Actiderm, Restore, Intact, Ultec, Tegasorb, DuoDerm-CGF, HydraPad, Intrasite
Alginates	Algosteril, Algiderm, Kaltostat, Sorbsan
Foams	Synthaderm, LYOfoam, Allevin, Epilock, Cutinova Plus, Epigard
Hydrogels	Vigilon, Geliperm, Elastogel, Cutinova Gelfolie, Nu-gel
Composites	Viasorb, Tegaderm Pouch
Impregnates	Adaptic, Vaseline Gauze, Biobrane Gauze, Xeroflo, Jelonet, Scarlet Red Gauze, Aquaphor Gauze
Pastes/Gels	Carrington Gel, Spand-Gel, Geliperm Granulat, Debrisan Wound Cleaning Paste, Envisan Paste, Hydron, Curasol Wound Gel
Absorption powders	Bard Absorption Dressing, Hydrogran, Hollister Exudate Absorber, Debrisan Beads, Comfeel Powder, DuoDerm Granules
Unique types	N-terface, Biobrane

Adapted from Alvarez O: Moist environment of healing: matching the dressing to the wound. Ostomy/Wound Management 21:65–83, 1988.

COMPOSITE DRESSING MATERIAL

Another product designed as a nonadherent dressing material is Telfa, a composite dressing made of two discrete components that have different purposes. This dressing is composed of a thin, perforated, polyester film placed on both surfaces of a central, absorbent cellulose core. Studies concerning the benefits of Telfa are controversial, and no consensus exists on the value of this dressing.[58–60] When used on wounds having heavy exudates, the dressing can easily become adherent. Nonetheless, Telfa remains a popular dressing material and is most commonly used as a wound interface or contact dressing material that is covered by an absorbent layer of gauze.

MONOFILAMENT DRESSING MATERIAL

Another nonadherent interface dressing material is N-terface, a thin, woven dressing material made from a high-density monofilament plastic. The dressing is intended as an interpositional material[61] that is applied directly to the wound bed. This material acts as a permeable nonadherent junction between the wound and an outer absorbent dressing. Although the product does not enhance wound healing directly, it reduces pain associated with dressing changes and prevents mechanical disruption of the reepithelializing surface of the healing wound.

GAUZE DRESSINGS

Conventional 4-inch × 4-inch gauze dressing has also gone through a great deal of change. These simple dressing materials were initially made from cotton but today are frequently made of semisynthetic materials, such as cellulose acetate, that are more absorbent. Composite gauze dressings, such as Topper, are also now available. These dressings provide bulk for compression and also have a highly absorbent cellulose filler core. Although gauze dressing materials are well tolerated during normal clinical use, they are not metabolized by the body. Foreign body reactions to retained dressing fragments or lint are well documented but fortunately do not pose a serious problem.[62]

Traditional Dressing Techniques

LAYERED DRESSINGS

Conventional dressings are often conceptualized as having distinct layers or zones, each with a specific purpose or function (Fig. 11–3). The interface or contact layer is applied directly to the wound. Ideally, this layer should be nonadherent, permeable to wound fluids, and capable of conforming to the wound contours. The body of the dressing should provide bulk for absorption and hemostasis by external pressure.

TAPE

External to both of these layers is an outer layer that is required for dressing retention. Tape is most often used for this layer. However, alternatives (Kerlix or burn net gauze dressings) may also be used, especially for the extremities. While there is a wide variety of tape available, paper tape is generally preferred because it is less irritating and is associated with lower levels of bacterial growth.[63] Regardless of the type of surgical or wound dressing applied, it should be placed securely and neatly over the wound. Often, patients may not appreciate the difficulty or expertise required to treat their condition surgically, but all patients and those who have contact with them will view the dressing as a reflection of the quality of care delivered.

TAPE ADHESIVES

Tape adherence to the skin can be improved simply by first cleaning the site with an alcohol wipe. Alterna-tively, agents that improve tape adherence to the skin, such as Mastisol (a gum mastic-based product that contains storax), or tincture of benzoin (which contains benzoin, storax, balsam of tolu, and aloe) may be used. Allergic contact dermatitis does occur with these products, as may cross-reactivity.[64, 65] In general, because Mastisol is colorless, it may be preferred by patients.

INTERFACE DRESSINGS

With traditional gauze dressings, one of several types of products such as Telfa can be used as a nonadherent interface with the wound (Fig. 11–3). However, these dressings may become adherent with exudative wounds. Use of impregnated gauze or antibiotic ointments with Telfa can help minimize this problem. Impregnated gauze or antibiotic ointments are often a popular and effective choice as an interface material and many products of this type are currently being sold for this purpose. Unfortunately, little is known about the true value of these materials (Table 11–2). In general, toxicity associated with antibacterial ointments has not been a problem,[66] but with the exception of a few controlled studies, their effects on wound healing have not been established.[67, 68] The mechanism by which these medications work is also unclear.

TOPICAL ANTIBIOTICS

Topical antibiotic ointments are frequently used, but there is considerable doubt over whether the antibacterial effect of these products is responsible for their activity. Work comparing the effects of Neosporin ointment, Silvadene cream, Pharmadine, and Furacin in a swine model[67] suggests that the effect of these agents is not related to their antimicrobial action. This study further demonstrates that many of the vehicles for these products may also affect wound healing. In the past, the

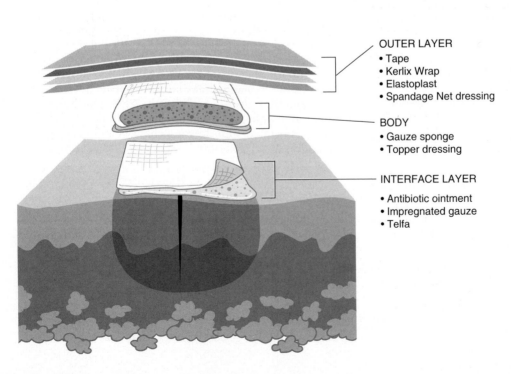

OUTER LAYER
• Tape
• Kerlix Wrap
• Elastoplast
• Spandage Net dressing

BODY
• Gauze sponge
• Topper dressing

INTERFACE LAYER
• Antibiotic ointment
• Impregnated gauze
• Telfa

Figure 11–3. Anatomy of a dressing. (Redrawn from Bennett RG: Fundamentals of Cutaneous Surgery. CV Mosby, St. Louis, 1988, p 402.)

TABLE 11–2. AGENTS AFFECTING EPIDERMAL RESURFACING

Dressing	Relative Rates of Healing (%)
Silvadene	+ 25
Silvadene base	+ 21
Neosporin	+ 25
Neosporin base	+ 5
Bacitracin zinc	+ 30
Petrolatum USP	+ 17
Dakin's solution (1%)	− 6
Povidone-iodine solution	− 10
Hydrogen peroxide (3%)	− 8
Hibiclens	− 7
Triamcinolone acetonide (0.1%)	− 34

Adapted from refs. 16, 67, and 69.

vehicles were thought to be inactive or inert.[68] For this reason, products that appear to be similar may not perform in an identical fashion (Table 11–2). Petrolatum, the primary constituent of all ointment-based products, can differ widely in its properties and biologic activities in a wound. For example, USP petrolatum when compared with the petrolatum vehicle of Neosporin ointment resulted in a 17% reduction versus 5% increase in relative healing rates.[69] For some bases, the relative difference in the rate of healing can be as high as 28%. However, newer occlusive dressings produce superior cosmetic results and healing rates (Table 11–3) compared with traditional surgical dressings.[30, 70–72]

Sensitization to topical antibiotic ointments is also of concern. This may be related to the antibiotic or another component of the ointment. Of all the topical antibiotics, neomycin is the most sensitizing.[73] Although bacitracin and neomycin are not related chemically, cross reactivity to these agents is frequently seen. The reason for this is unclear, but may be related to concurrent sensitization.[74] Sensitization to these products is usually characterized by a local contact dermatitis. However, well-documented cases of associated systemic complaints and even anaphlylaxis have also been reported.[75, 76]

TABLE 11–3. COMPARISON OF POLYURETHANE DRESSING AND ANTIBIOTIC GAUZE DRESSING IN FULL-THICKNESS MOHS MICROGRAPHIC SURGERY DEFECTS

	Antibiotic Gauze (N = 25)	Polyurethane (Bioclusive) (N = 26)
Healed completely by day 24	9	19
Wound contracture, 50% or more	8	17
Anatomic deformity at 6 mo	14	5
Cosmetic results, excellent at 6 mo	20%	62%
Pigmentary changes	Same	Same
Scar surface	Same	Same
Patient subjective evaluation	N/A	Better

Compiled from Hien NT, Prawer SE, Katz HI: Facilitated wound healing using transparent film dressing following Mohs micrographic surgery. Arch Dermatol 124:903–906, 1988.

TOPICAL ANTISEPTICS

Topical antiseptics also play a significant role in wound care and wound dressings (see Table 11–2). The initial use of this class of agents was advocated by Lister.[1] In the mid-1800s, the introduction of the antiseptic carbolic acid made a significant impact on surgical infection rates. During World War I, Dakin's solution (sodium hypochlorite) was introduced as a chemical means to debride and disinfect wounds.[76] Since that time, other antimicrobial solutions have been introduced, including Betadine (1% povidone-iodine), 3% hydrogen peroxide, and Hibiclens (4% chlorhexidine gluconate). Unfortunately, a great deal of controversy surrounds the potential value of these products. Initially, they were enthusiastically embraced by physicians with little scientific evaluation, but in time reports of toxicity and delayed wound healing began to surface. Decreases in wound strength and rates of epithelialization, along with fibroblast toxicity, were reported with varying concentrations of Dakin's solution.[66] Lower concentrations (0.5%) were found to preserve fibroblast function yet maintain bactericidal activity. Later, cell culture studies suggested that all concentrations of Dakin's solution cause tissue toxicity.[77] Clinically, however, Dakin's continues to be used successfully without significant local adverse events or systemic difficulties. This solution has broad antimicrobial activity and is also effective against fungi and viruses, including the human immunodeficiency virus (HIV).[78] Dakin's wet-to-dry dressings can be effectively used to clean and debride a wound. Conversely, some surgeons advocate replacement of Dakin's with saline, given the toxicity of this soulution.[77] However, once the necrotic tissue has been debrided from the wound, Dakin's solution should be discontinued and replaced with a dressing that promotes healing. The key function of wet-to-dry dressings is to clean and debride a wound, even though they may stimulate granulation tissue formation.[79] Long-term use of such dressings delays healing, even when compared with open-air controls.[12] A prospective study demonstrated superior healing in pressure sore patients treated with hydrocolloid dressings compared with those given 0.5% Dakin's wet-to-dry dressings.[80]

The effect of povidone-iodine on wound healing is also controversial. Fibroblast toxicity and delayed wound reepithelialization has been seen at clinically relevant concentrations.[68] Similarly, studies in bacterially challenged wounds in guinea pigs showed that povidine-iodine solutions offered no therapeutic benefit compared with control wounds treated with saline.[81] In contrast, other investigators have noted no delay in healing when povidone-iodine solutions are used.[82, 83] Overall, however, the Food and Drug Administration has not found sufficient evidence to approve povidone-iodine solutions or scrubs for use in wounds.[84] Scrub solutions such as Betadine scrub appear to be more problematic for wounds. The detergent base is cytotoxic and has proved deleterious to wound healing.[81] In general, these detergent-containing solutions should be reserved for surgical skin preparations. Hibiclens, another common surgical prep solution, is also not trouble free; ocular toxicity

TABLE 11–4. **PROPERTIES OF BIOSYNTHETIC DRESSINGS**

	Polyurethane Films	Hydrocolloids	Hydrogels	Alginates
Transmits oxygen	+	−	+ (?)	+ (?)
Transmits moisture vapor	+	−	− (?)	+
Excludes bacteria	+/−	+	−	−
Absorbs fluids	−	+	+/−	+
Transparent	+	−	+/−	−
Adhesive	+	+	−	−
Wound pain reduction	+	+	+	+

+, Yes; −, No; +/−, somewhat.
Adapted from Eaglstein WH: Experiences with biosynthetic dressings. J Am Acad Dermatol 12:434–440, 1985.

manifested by keratitis, pain, and scarring has been reported, usually from presurgical preparation.[85] Inadvertent or accidental exposure should be treated immediately with copious irrigation, and an ophthalmologic consultation obtained.

A solution of 3% hydrogen peroxide exhibits some mild toxicity but does not appear to affect epithelialization rates.[66] Tissue catalases cause rapid decomposition and effervescence on contact. The overall germicidal activity is brief and weak.[86] Other than providing a cleansing action, hydrogen peroxide probably offers little benefit over normal saline.

Biosynthetic Dressings and Moist Wound Healing

Several different types of biosynthetic dressings are commercially available today (see Table 11–1), each with different properties (Table 11–4). Each type of dressing has its own unique features, indications, and qualities, but several unifying characteristics are common to all these materials.

OCCLUSION

The first of these common characteristics is the occlusive quality of these biosynthetic dressings, which creates a moist healing environment. Even though the film dressings are only semipermeable, they allow for oxygen and water vapor exchange but not the loss of all wound exudate. Both intradermal and full-thickness wounds have been shown to heal faster in this environment.[17, 24–27, 30] The reasons for this accelerated healing are numerous but not fully understood. Moist wound healing limits additional tissue loss from desiccation, alters the influx of inflammatory and mesenchymal cells, affects collagen production, and possibly affects wound strength. Clinically, the wounds appear less inflamed, edematous, and crusted and pain is also significantly reduced. In general, pain reduction is a consistent finding with all occlusive dressings; it can occur almost immediately with application of the dressing or may improve gradually over time. As a rule, pain reduction is one feature patients uniformly appreciate about these dressings.

WOUND DEBRIDEMENT

The occlusive environment is also ideal for wound debridement. Crusts and debris are easily loosened by the moisture under the dressing. Also, lytic enzymes contributed by polymorphonucleocytes and other cellular debris create an autolytic type of cleansing action. This process can be so effective that wounds may at first appear to be enlarging, but in fact it indicates that the sites have just been cleared of residual necrotic debris.

EFFECTS ON WOUND BACTERIA

One of the greatest concerns regarding the use of occlusive dressings is the increase in bacteria and purulent material that occurs under the dressing (Table 11–5). However, numerous studies have shown enhanced reepithelialization rates without an increase in wound infection.[17, 54] Bacterial counts frequently exceed what is classically defined as an infection (more than 10^5 colonies per gram of tissue).[87] The clinical appearance and associated signs and symptoms are therefore the best guides to assessing the wound for the possibility of an infection. These features include edema, tenderness, increasing erythema, fever, lymphadenopathy, and elevated white blood cell count. To ensure compliance, patient education is particularly important given the purulent, foul-smelling exudates that are commonly seen with use of

TABLE 11–5. **ADVANTAGES AND POTENTIAL DISADVANTAGES OF OCCLUSION**

Advantages	
Reduced pain	Waterproof
Rapid healing	Fewer dressing changes
Rapid debridement	Cost effective
Easy to use	Bacterial barriers
Better cosmetic results	

Potential Disadvantages	
Accumulation of pus	Silent infection
Hematoma or seroma	Folliculitis
Adherence to new tissue	Reinjury upon removal
Increased bacterial counts	Retarded wound strength
Bacteria shift to gram-negative organisms	

Adapted from Alvarez O: Moist environment of healing: matching the dressing to the wound. Ostomy/Wound Management 21:65–83, 1988; and Eaglstein WH: Experiences with biosynthetic dressings. J Am Acad Dermatol 12:434–440, 1985.

occlusive dressings. These dressings should be used carefully in immunocompromised patients and are contraindicated for clinically infected wounds.

COST EFFECTIVENESS

Another concern is the cost effectiveness of occlusive dressings for wound care. Dressing changes with the new occlusive surgical dressings are far more expensive, up to 50% more, than with traditional dressings. However, the true cost of therapy must also address the frequency of dressing changes and the assistance required to perform them. In this regard, numerous studies have shown that occlusive dressings are much more cost effective than traditional dressings. In a study evaluating ulcer patients, hydrocolloid dressings were found to be significantly less expensive.[80] The cost of wet-to-dry Dakin's dressings compared with hydrocolloid on a weekly basis was $52.50 ($2.50 per dressing, changed three times a day) and $6.20 ($3.10 per dressing, changed twice a week), respectively. It was also estimated that 7 hours per week of nursing time was required for the wet-to-dry dressings compared with 10 minutes for the hydrocolloids.

Obviously, there is a great deal of variability in determining such comparisons because of differences in the frequency of dressing changes, dressing types, cost of labor and dressing, and the extent of home self-care. However, even taking into account all these factors, a survey of the literature reveals that occlusive dressings have proved at least 50% less costly than traditional dressings.[27, 70, 80] There is also the additional benefit of more rapid healing seen with these materials. Such cost and time savings are obviously of great value in today's health care environment.

TYPES OF BIOSYNTHETIC SURGICAL DRESSINGS

Unna Boots

Many consider Unna boots a traditional dressing since they have been in existence for well over 100 years. However, in many ways they were the first biocclusive dressing. In the early 1880s, Paul Gerson Unna (1850–1929) began to experiment with a zinc oxide, gelatin, and glycerin paste that could be impregnated into a cotton dressing. The zinc oxide was found to be particularly beneficial in neutralizing the acid plaster in such dressings, making them less irritating.[88] Unna experimented with the clinical use of these dressings and found them beneficial in the treatment of various types of dermatitis and venous stasis ulcers.

Since that time, Unna's original formula has been slightly modified, but the basic dressing remains unchanged. Over the past century the Unna boot has been considered by many to be the dressing of choice for venous stasis ulcers.[89] The dressing offers the benefits of a semiocclusive dressing material and venous compression. An alternative use in skin graft recipient sites has also been exploited.[90] More recently, Unna boot dressings, used in combination with newer occlusive dressing materials such as alginates and hydrocolloids, have demonstrated even greater benefits.

Film Dressings

The first of the most recently developed biosynthetic dressings was a film made from polyurethane or copolyester. These adhesive dressings are semipermeable and allow for the exchange of oxygen, carbon dioxide, and water vapor across the dressing membrane.

Ideally, films provide a moist healing environment and prevent skin maceration. When these dressings were first introduced, oxygen permeability of the dressing was thought to be important.[39, 40] However, more recent evidence favors low PO_2 levels under the dressing to promote healing.[12, 43–46] Ironically, low PO_2 levels were found under film dressings despite their permeability.[42] Dressing pore size is limited to prevent bacterial penetration or loss of wound exudate. In heavily exudative wounds, excess fluids may accumulate beneath the film and cause difficulties with maceration, leakage, and skin irritation.[5] Excess accumulation of fluids under the dressing may be managed by aspiration of the fluid, using a 27- or 30-gauge needle, or more frequent dressing changes. Consideration should also be given to switching to a dressing designed to absorb wound exudate. In general, films are better suited for minimally exudative wounds.

Numerous animal and human studies have established the value of film dressings.[5, 12, 17, 24, 30, 90] These studies show an increase in healing rates of 25 to 40% compared with untreated controls. However, some problems have been noted with the adhesive found on the film dressing.[5, 17] Initially, when the wound bed is moist, adherence is not a problem, but as the wound epithelializes, the newly formed epithelium may be stripped away by subsequent dressing changes. To avoid this, some film dressings, such as Blisterfilm, are made with a central, adhesive-free zone.[16] A composite dressing using Vigilon or impregnated gauze overlying the wound covered by a film dressing can also be used. Another dressing, Omiderm, a copolymer polyurethane film, has no adhesive at all and clings to the wound by the surface tension of the fluid layer between the wound and dressing material. This material has been shown to be nontoxic to tissue and, like other films, it promotes would healing.[91, 92] Proper placement of a film dressing can be difficult. Firm uniform tension on the dressing is needed during placement to avoid wrinkling and self-adhesion. Wrinkling provides avenues for bacterial penetration and leakage of irritating wound exudate.[53] A 2- to 3-cm zone of adhesion in all directions beyond the wound is recommended.[5] As for all occlusive dressings, numerous studies have documented increased bacterial growth underneath,[42, 51, 52, 63] and with time a shift toward gram-negative organisms has been noted.[51, 53] An increased rate of infection has not been reported, but the transparent nature of these dressings offers a distinct advantage, allowing monitoring of the wound site without removal of the film.

Hydrocolloids

The value of hydrocolloids as dressing materials evolved from their initial use in ostomy products. Patients with erosions and nonhealing areas around their ostomy site were noted to heal when covered by their ostomy barriers. A wide variety of different hydrocolloid dressings are commercially available (see Table 11–1). Although these dressings are not identical, they have similar formulations. A hydrophilic colloid base composed of pectin, carboxymethyl cellulose, karaya, or quar is mixed with an adhesive component containing polyisobutylene or elastomeric substances such as styrene isoprene or ethylene vinyl acetate. The outer layer of the dressing is composed of a thin layer of impermeable material such as polyurethane. The adhesive quality of this dressing is enhanced when exposed to a moist surface. The hydrophilic nature of the dressing leads to particle swelling, and eventually an adherent matrix forms. Hydrocolloids are easy to use because of their ability to adhere and conform to a wound site. They are also advantageous because of their protective and cushioning effects. Their application as a pressure-relieving dressing, especially over bony prominences, is becoming popular.[93] Dressing changes are based on the time required for the dressing to leak, up to a 7-day maximum. During the early exudative phase, dressings may require changing two or three times a day, but dressings may later remain in place for several days at a time. Taping at the dressing borders is recommended to minimize leakage and increase the life of the dressing.[94]

When the dressing is removed, a yellow-brown viscous gel with a foul smell is evident. This can easily be confused with a purulent exudate if one is unfamiliar with the material (Fig. 11–4). Patients must be warned of these changes or they may become uncomfortable with the use of these dressings. As with other occlusive dressings, bacterial counts do increase over time, but no increased risk of wound infection has ever been documented.[52, 54] In addition, several investigators have reported a decrease in *Pseudomonas* growth. This has been attributed to low pH or low Po_2 levels under the

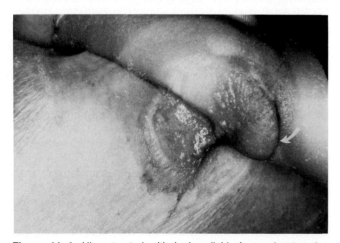

Figure 11–4. Ulcer treated with hydrocolloid. Arrow denotes the hydrated portion of the dressing, which yields a yellow-brown viscous gel.

dressing, or the organism's sensitivity to desiccation.[52] However, the clinician must maintain an awareness regarding infection and check for other signs and symptoms such as erythema, tenderness, induration, and fever. Although this gelatinous material does improve the dressing seal, it does not cause disruption of newly epithelializing tissues as the dressing is removed, although some residual gel may remain on the wound. Saline soaks with light gauze swabbing usually remove this material.

A number of studies have established the value of hydrocolloid dressings.[11, 17, 80, 95] Rates of healing appear to be increased by about 40% compared with open-air controls. Studies comparing hydrocolloids with conventional saline or Dakin's wet-to-dry dressings in over 150 patients with pressure sores significantly favored the hydrocolloids.[80, 96] Similarly, a blinded bilateral comparative study of cardiac surgery chest wounds was used to compare hydrocolloids and petrolatum gauze dressings.[70] At the tenth postoperative day, 13 of 21 versus six of 21 sites were healed using the hydrocolloid and gauze dressings, respectively. In addition, the patients preferred the occlusive dressing because of greater comfort.

Alginates

Although alginates were discovered over a century ago, they are the least well known of the biocclusive dressings. Their use as a wound dressing material became popular in the 1950s, but their use declined because of product limitations and manufacturing difficulties.[97] Fortunately, recent innovations in the formulation and manufacturing of alginate dressings have renewed interest in alginates as wound dressing materials. Alginate dressings are derived from salts of alginic acid. Various types of kelps or algae serve as the source for this complex polysaccharide, including the giant kelp *(Macrocystis pyrifera)* and the horsetail kelp *(Laminaria digitata).* When the material is extracted from the plant, it is in a soluble sodium salt form. During manufacturing, sodium ion exchange occurs with elements such as calcium magnesium and zinc, which leads to the formation of alginate fibers. These fibers are then used in the manufacture of the dressing material.

Currently, several alginate-based dressing materials are available (see Table 11–1). Clinical and scientific evaluation has shown that these dressings promote wound healing.[27, 97, 98] However, exudate from the wound is required to transform this gauzelike material into a therapeutic gel matrix. The exudate contains the necessary sodium ions to exchange with the insoluble salt form. Sodium from the blood and wound exudate provides the basis for the ionic exchange that leads to the formation of the soluble sodium alginate gel. With a calcium alginate dressing material, free calcium ions are released during this exchange, providing one of the essential elements of the clotting cascade.[99] It has been hypothesized that this mechanism may play a role in the hemostatic properties of this material. From a clinical standpoint, several investigations have established the hemostatic properties of this material,[100, 101] which is of particular value in dressing full-thickness surgical sites and split-thickness graft donor sites, where bleeding may be of concern. A new alginate dressing, Algiderm, contains alginic salts of zinc and magnesium, in addition to calcium. Clinically, the hemostatic properties of this dressing appear equivalent to one made of just calcium alginate. The value of the other ionic components remains to be seen. However, studies have cited zinc as being beneficial to wound healing.[102, 103] Finally, evaluation of a new alginate-based surgical gauze has shown superior absorbency, a decrease in surgical blood loss, and a reduction in operating time.[101]

Alginate-based dressings have proved effective in a wide variety of clinical settings, including ulcers, pressure sores, split-thickness graft donor sites, and full-thickness surgical defects.[27, 95, 104] The one unifying characteristic of all these wounds is that they are exudative. Hydration of the dressing with saline may be effected at the time of placement for less exudative wounds, but this decreases the overall absorbency of the dressing. If the wound loses its exudative quality and a moist environment cannot be maintained, an alternative dressing material should be used. Alginate dressings, if not properly hydrated, can be very irritating and will adhere to the wound bed.[98] They are easy to use, since they readily conform to the shape and contour of the wound bed, but must be held in place by an overlying secondary gauze dressing. Dressings are changed when wound exudate seeps through the secondary dressing. When the dressing is changed, the material will appear as a yellow-brown gel (Fig. 11–5). However, because it is soluble, it can be readily removed by saline irrigation. This technique can provide for pain-free dressing changes. Any trace material left behind is of no concern since it will be broken down and metabolized by the body.[98, 105] Although there has been some question regarding the potential toxicity of alginates, the material has been used extensively over the past 40 years without complications.[104]

Hydrogels

In contrast to film dressings, hydrogels can absorb exudate from the wound yet maintain a moist healing environment. Although they are not adhesive, they remain in place if not disturbed. An overlying secondary gauze dressing is often used to maintain their location and to absorb excess exudate. Several hydrogel dressings are commercially available (see Table 11–1). Hydrogels, as their name implies, are composed primarily of water, often 90% or more (see Table 11–4). The gel is formed by a cross-linked polymer network such as polyethylene-oxide (Vigilon), polyacrylamide (Geliperm), or polyvinyl alcohol (Cutinova Gelfolie). Some dressings have a supportive inner gel mesh or are covered with a thin film. Vigilon, for example, is a 4% polyethylene oxide gel sandwiched between two thin layers of polyethylene film. When the dressing is applied, the film on the contact side is always removed. With the outer film in place, the dressing is oxygen permeable only and the gel can absorb its own weight in exudate. If the outer film is removed, excess exudate will pass through the gel into the outer gauze dressing.

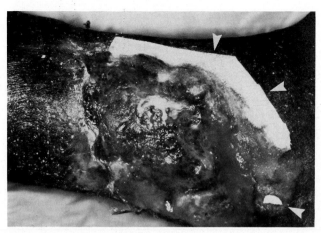

Figure 11–5. Leg ulcer treated with an alginate dressing showing the wound base covered with yellow-brown gel. The wound margin shows focal areas of original dressing material *(arrowheads).*

Facilitated wound healing has been demonstrated with hydrogels. In one study of split-thickness wounds in pigs, 100% of wounds treated with a hydrogel were healed by the fourth postoperative day compared with only 32% of air-exposed controls.[106] Another study showed superior results when a hydrogel was used as a dressing material for hair transplantation in 26 patients and for dermabrasion in 10 patients.[26] Hair transplant donor and recipient sites appear to heal faster than with the standard Telfa dressings, and dermabrasion sites fully epithelialized in 4 to 5 days with Vigilon dressings compared with 6 to 7 days with Adaptic and Telfa dressings. Hydrogels are also very effective in reducing pain. They possess a high specific heat and are therefore cool and soothing.[16] Refrigeration before application can further enhance this quality.

Bacterial growth under hydrogels is well documented and, with time, gram-negative organisms are favored.[53] As with other occlusive dressings, no increase in infection has been documented.[26, 54] Barrier function to outside bacterial contamination is not ideal and probably reflects the nonadherent nature of this material.[53] Dressing change schedules vary with the clinical application and manner in which the gel is used. In general, dressing changes are more frequent than with other occlusive dressings.

Foam Dressings

Of all the types of occlusive dressings available, foams are the least well studied in animals or humans, but clinical case series have established their potential value.[7, 107] Foam dressings are silicon- or polyurethane-based, nonadhesive materials. In general, the inner surface adjacent to the wound is both absorbent and gas permeable, and functions to absorb wound exudate and maintain a moist environment. The outer layer is a nonabsorbent foam that limits bacterial penetration and desiccation of the underlying layer. The dressing material is conformable but not to the same extent as other dressings. An overlying secondary gauze dressing is needed to ensure proper placement and create a good edge seal. If the seal is poor the dressing will leak, possibly dry out, and create problems with adherence. The ability of these dressings to absorb wound exudate is limited, so dressings should be changed frequently, every 1 or 2 days.

Dressing Selection and Application

One of the most confusing issues regarding surgical and wound dressings is the choice of which dressing to use.[7] Unfortunately, there are no absolute rules to guide the cutaneous surgeon in selecting an ideal dressing for any given situation. In fact, there may often be several reasonable options available. Another issue is how to best use the currently available dressings to obtain optimal results. Little work has been done in this area because dressings have only recently been appreciated for their potential therapeutic value. Initial studies implied some temporal relationship between dressing application and its clinical impact.[34] Studies have shown that fibroplasia, as indicated by wound-breaking strength, was only significantly affected if the film dressing was in place during the first 2 or 3 days of healing. A subsequent study evaluated intradermal wounds treated with polyurethane film dressings.[108] It was found that to promote optimal healing the dressings must be applied within 2 hours after wounding. The dressings also needed to remain in place for at least 24 hours. Obviously, the results of these studies closely relate to the mechanisms of action of occlusive dressing materials, which currently are poorly understood. For now, cutaneous surgeons must rely on the information available in the literature and their own clinical experience as the basis for selecting the best dressing for each clinical situation.

Alternative Use of Surgical Dressings

As our understanding of biocclusive dressings has increased, so have their potential applications. One study examined the potential benefit of these dressings as a means to dress sutured wounds.[34] In 19 patients with elective abdominal incisions, one half of each incision was covered with a film composite dressing, Surlyn, with rayon gauze at the periphery for absorbency; the other half of the incision was covered with rayon or cotton gauze alone. The film composite dressing yielded faster reepithelialization, decreased eschar formation, less inflammation, and better wound edge apposition in 70% of the cases, and were cosmetically superior even after 6 months. Subsequent studies evaluated Vigilon as a primary dressing material in 45 patients with sutured wounds. These findings concurred with the earlier study, showing similar benefit with the hydrogel dressing. Hydrocolloids or foams may also be used with similar results. Care must be taken, however, if the wound is exudative, since film dressings could produce maceration and increase the risk of infection. In these situations, an absorbent dressing such as a hydrogel or hydrocolloid should be used. Films and hydrocolloids offer the additional advantage of being waterproof so that the patient may shower and bathe more freely.

Film dressings have also been used as a primary skin closure. In a series of 110 patients undergoing elective or emergency abdominal surgery, patients were randomized to one of three methods of closure: sutureless using only Op-Site, sutures, or staples.[37] In all cases the fascia was closed and simple interrupted sutures were placed to close the dead space if the subcutaneous fat was greater than 1 cm, but no dermal sutures were placed. Overall, the film closures (Table 11–6) displayed less inflammation and no increase in infection, and were judged to be cosmetically superior by the patients and an independent investigator. An equivalent degree of skin overlap was noted with each method of closure, a likely reflection of the surgical technique. In addition, both nurses and patients preferred the film dressing. Patients could shower after 24 hours, and the wound could be easily monitored through the transparent film. No dressing changes were required until removal at the seventh postoperative day. A retrospective study of 350 patients with abdominal wounds closed with tape as the sole method of skin closure yielded similar results.[38] The

TABLE 11–6. **COMPARISON OF SUTURELESS SKIN CLOSURE WITH CONVENTIONAL CLOSURE TECHNIQUES**

	Polyurethane Film (N = 55)*	Nylon Suture (N = 40)*	Clips (N = 15)*
Postoperative wound infection	1	4	1
Soundly healed, no inflammation	48	24	2
Soundly healed, with inflammation	1	15	2
Skin dehiscence	0	1	1
Skin overlap	3	2	2
Cosmetic results (rated excellent)			
Independent investigator	36	6	1
Patient	45	13	4

Compiled from Eaton AC: A controlled trial to evaluate and compare a sutureless skin closure technique (Op-Site skin closure) with conventional skin suturing and clipping in abdominal surgery. Br J Surg 67:857–860, 1980.
*Numbers shown indicate patient(s)

lower rate of wound infection may be attributed to the absence of suture and suture tracks, which provide additional foci and paths for infection.

Many other uses for the occlusive dressings have been developed (Table 11–7). Clinically, these techniques have proved beneficial in cutaneous surgery. Once the technique of application is mastered, this method of closure can yield impressive and gratifying results (Fig. 11–6).

The Future

Before 1960 the wound dressing materials available were only variations of traditional gauze dressings. In 1962 the value of moist wound healing was unequivocally established. Since that time, many animal and human studies have validated this principle. Despite this work, the mechanisms of how the new bioocclusive dressings

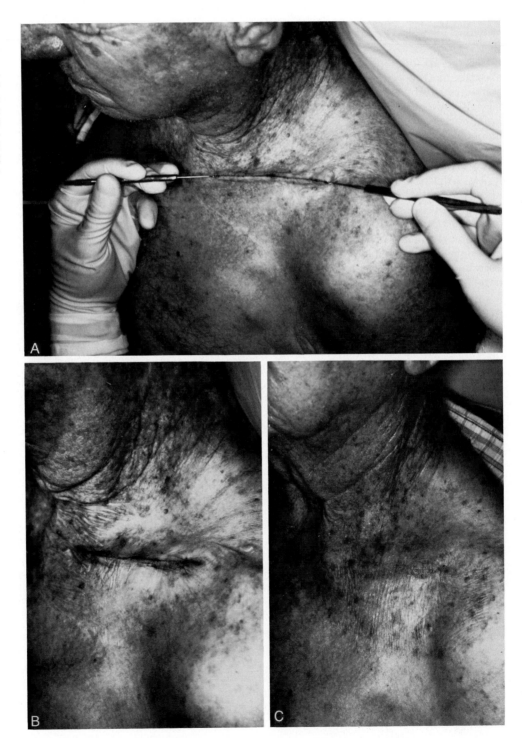

Figure 11–6. Sutureless wound closure. *A,* Supraclavicular skin graft donor site with the wound edges aligned with skin hooks. Transcutaneous needles just beyond the ends of the incision may also be used in place of skin hooks. *B,* The site covered with film dressing; the skin edges must be aligned without gaps or wrinkles in the dressing. *C,* Wound appearance at 14 days without inflammation and showing a well-epithelialized incision.

TABLE 11–7. ALTERNATIVE USES FOR OCCLUSIVE DRESSINGS

Prevention of contact dermatitis
Prevention of factitial disease
Hair growth in trichotillomania
Prophylactic use of pressure areas
Earlier re-harvesting of skin graft donor sites
Intravenous catheter care

From Eaglstein WH: Experiences with biosynthetic dressings. J Am Acad Dermatol 12:434—440, 1985.

work remain largely unclear. Most recently, investigators have begun to explore the potential use of the growth-regulating peptides, epidermal and platelet-derived growth factors, and fibroblast-derived growth factor, as therapeutic tools in wound healing.[109] The wound exudate under occlusive dressings is now known to contain many of these factors,[110] and in tissue culture models these exudates have been shown to increase keratinocyte proliferation. The retention of these elements within the healing wound matrix made possible by occlusive dressings is probably responsible for at least some of the beneficial effects observed with these materials. Clinical trials incorporating these regulatory factors in biosynthetic dressings are already under way and have produced some promising early results. These and other innovations yet to come have set the stage for the development of another generation of wound dressing materials that will allow the cutaneous surgeon to be even more effective in manipulating wounds in order to optimize healing.

SUMMARY

A number of useful generalizations can be made about the care of cutaneous wounds. First, the use of wet-to-dry and wet-to-wet dressings is valuable in wound debridement. However, after the wound is clean, consideration should be given to switching to a different dressing. Second, there is special merit in using the occlusive dressings for pain relief, since essentially all occlusive dressings reduce pain. An occlusive dressing should not be applied to an infected wound. When perilesional tissues are compromised by edema or inflammation, a nonadherent dressing material should be used. If biomechanical factors, such as pressure over a bony prominence, are of concern, the cushioning effect of a hydrocolloid surgical dressing may be of value. The patient should always be carefully evaluated for signs of infection. Purulent, foul-smelling drainage may be seen with the occlusive dressings, but associated fever, redness, edema, induration, or tenderness is indicative of infection. Patient education is an absolute requirement in these types of clinical situations. In many cases, patients are participating in their own care, and they need to know what to expect and how to evaluate their wound.

It should be remembered that all ointments and creams used for conventional dressings are not equivalent and allergic reactions can occur. Wound healing is a dynamic process and the type of dressing required for each of its phases changes frequently. To do this most effectively, the wound should be constantly re-evaluated during healing, in the realization that there is no one ideal dressing available, and the use of each material should be based on the needs of the wound at that point in time.

REFERENCES

1. Lyons AS, Petrucelli RJ: Medicine, An Illustrated History. Harry Abrams, New York, 1978.
2. Bibbings J: The history of wound dressing. Nursing (Lond) 3(5):169–174, 1986.
3. Elliott IMZ, Elliott JR: A short history of surgical dressings. Pharmaceutical Press, London, 1964.
4. Lawrence JC, Payne MJ: Historical landmarks. In: Wound Healing User's Guide. Update Group, London, 1984, pp 8–19.
5. Alper JC, Welch EA, Maguire P: Use of the vapor permeable membrane for cutaneous ulcers: details of application and side effects. J Am Acad Dermatol 11:858–866, 1984.
6. Katz S, McGinley K, Leyden JJ: Semipermeable occlusive dressings. Arch Dermatol 122:58–62, 1986.
7. Falanga V: Occlusive wound dressings. Arch Dermatol 124:872–877, 1988.
8. Data on file. ER Squibb & Son, Princeton, NJ.
9. Zitelli JA: Delayed wound healing with adhesive wound dressings. J Dermatol Surg Oncol 10:709–710, 1984.
10. Noe JM, Kalish S: The problem of adherence in dressed wounds. Surg Gynecol Obstet 147:185–188, 1978.
11. Scales JT: Wound healing and the dressing. Br J Ind Med 70:82–94, 1963.
12. Alvarez OM, Mertz PM, Eaglstein WH: The effect of occlusive dressings on collagen synthesis and re-epithelialization in superficial wounds. J Surg Res 35:142–148, 1983.
13. Odland G: The fine structure of interrelationship of cells in the human epidermis. J Biophys Biochem Cytol 4:529–535, 1958.
14. Gimbel NS: A study of epithelization in blistered burns. AMA Arch Surg 74:800–802, 1957.
15. Winter GD: Formation of scab and the rate of epithelization of superficial wounds in the skin of the young domestic pig. Nature 193:293–294, 1962.
16. Alvarez O: Moist environment of healing: matching the dressing to the wound. Ostomy/Wound Management 21:65–83, 1988.
17. Eaglstein WH: Experiences with biosynthetic dressings. J Am Acad Dermatol 12:434–440, 1985.
18. Hinman CD, Maibach HI: Effects of air exposure and occlusion on experimental human skin wounds. Nature 200:377–378, 1963.
19. Rovee DT, Kurowsky C, Labun J: Effect of local wound environment on epidermal healing. In: Maibach HI, Roovee DT (eds): Epidermal Wound Healing. Year Book, Chicago, 1972, pp 152–181.
20. Rovee DT, Kurowsky CA, Labun J: Effect of local wound environment and epidermal healing. Mitotic response. Arch Dermatol 106:330–334, 1972.
21. Rovee DT, Linsky CB, Boothwell JW: Experimental models for evaluation of wound repair. In: Maibach HI (ed): Animal Models in Dermatology. Churchill Livingston, New York, 1975.
22. Fisher LB, Maibach HI: Physical occlusion controlling epidermal mitosis. J Invest Dermatol 59:106–108, 1972.
23. Lawrence JC: The perinecrotic zone in burns and its influence on healing. Burns 1:197–199, 1975.
24. Barnett A, Berkowitz RL, Mills R, Vistnes LM: Comparison of synthetic adhesive moisture vapor permeable and fine mesh gauze dressings for split-thickness skin graft donor sites. Am J Surg 145:379–381, 1983.
25. Friedman S, Su DWP: Hydrocolloid occlusive dressing management of leg ulcers. Arch Dermatol 120:1329–1336, 1984.
26. Mandy SH: A new primary wound dressing made of polyethylene oxide gel. J Dermatol Surg Oncol 9:153–155, 1983.

27. Attwood AI: Calcium alginate dressing accelerates split skin graft donor site healing. Br J Plast Surg 42:373–379, 1989.
28. Rakallio J, Mottonen M, Nieminen L: Evaluation of three synthetic films as wound covers. Acta Chir Scand 139:1–14, 1973.
29. Smith KW, Oden PW, Blaylock WK. A comparison of goldleaf and other occlusive therapy. Arch Dermatol 96:703–705, 1963.
30. Hien NT, Prawer SE, Katz HI: Facilitated wound healing using transparent film dressing following Mohs micrographic surgery. Arch Dermatol 124:903–906, 1988.
31. Linsky CB, Rovee DT: Influence of the local environment of the course of wound healing in the guinea pig. In: Gibson T (ed): Wound Healing. Foundation for International Cooperation in Medical Science, Montreux, l975, p 211.
32. Zahir M: Contraction of wounds. Br J Surg 51:456, 1964.
33. Dyson M, Young S, Pendle CL, et al: Comparison of the effects of moist and dry conditions on dermal repair. J Invest Dermatol 91:434–439, 1988.
34. Linsky C, Rovee D, Dow T: Effects of dressings on wound inflammation and scar tissue. In: Hildick-Smith NP (ed): The Surgical Wound. Lea & Febiger, Philadelphia, 1981, pp 191–204.
35. Banes AJ, Compton DW, Bomhoeft J, et al: Biologic, biosynthetic, and synthetic dressings as temporary wound covers: a biochemical comparison. J Burn Care Rehabil 7:96–104, 1986.
36. Ksander GA, Pratt BM, Desilets-Avis P, et al: Inhibition of connective tissue formation in dermal wounds covered with synthetic, moisture vapor–permeable dressings and its reversal by transforming growth factor-beta. J Invest Dermatol 95:195–201, 1990.
37. Eaton AC: A controlled trial to evaluate and compare a sutureless skin closure technique (Op-Site skin closure) with conventional skin suturing and clipping in abdominal surgery. Br J Surg 67:857–860, 1980.
38. Pepicello J, Yavorek H: Five year experience with tape closure of abdominal wounds. Surg Gynecol Obstet 169:310–314, 1989.
39. Hunt TK, Pai MP: The effect of varying ambient oxygen tensions on wound metabolism and collagen synthesis. Gynecol Obstet 135:561–567, 1972.
40. Rovee DT (ed): Epidermal wound healing. Year Book, Chicago, l972, pp 291–305.
41. Grim PS, Gottlieb IJ, Boddie A, Batson E: Hyperbaric oxygen therapy. JAMA 263:216–220, 1990.
42. Varghese MC, Balin AK, Carter MD, Caldwell D: Local environment of chronic wounds under synthetic dressings. Arch Dermatol 122:5257, 1986.
43. Balin AK, Fisher AJ, Carter DM: Oxygen modulates the growth of human cells at physiologic partial pressures. J Exp Med 160:152–160, 1984.
44. Knighton DR, Hunt TK, Scheuenstuhl H, et al: Oxygen tension regulates the expression of angiogenesis factor by macrophages. Science 221:1283–1285, 1983.
45. Knighton DR, Silver IA, Hunt TK: Regulation of wound healing angiogenesis: effect of oxygen gradients and inspired oxygen concentration. Surgery 90:262–270, 1981.
46. Horikoshi T, Balin AK, Elsinger M, et al: Modulation of proliferation in human epidermal keratinocyte and melanocyte cultures by dissolved oxygen. J Invest Dermatol 80:411, 1984.
47. Knighton DR, Fiegel VD: Macrophage-derived growth factors in wound healing. Regulation of growth factor production by the oxygen microenvironment. Am Rev Respir Dis 140:1108–1111, 1989.
48. Orgill D, Demling RH: Current concepts and approaches to wound healing. Crit Care Med 16:899–908, 1988.
49. Rabell G, Pillsbury DM, Phalle G, et al: Factors affecting the rapid disappearance of bacteria placed on the normal skin. J Invest Dermatol 14:247–263, 1950.
50. Aly R, Maibach HI: Aerobic microbial flora of intertriginous skin. Appl Environ Microbiol 33:97–100, 1977.
51. Mertz PM, Eaglstein WH: The effect of a semiocclusive dressing on the microbial population in superficial wounds. Arch Surg 119:386–389, 1984.
52. Gilchrist B, Reed C: The bacteriology of chronic venous ulcers treated with occlusive hydrocolloid dressings. Br J Dermatol 121:337–344, 1989.
53. Mertz PM, Marshall DA, Eaglstein WH: Occlusive wound dressings to prevent invasion and wound infection. J Am Acad Dermatol 12:662–668, 1985.
54. Hutchinson JJ, McGuckin M: Occlusive dressings: a microbiologic and clinical review. Am J Infect Control 18:257–268, 1990.
55. Lookingbill DP, Miller SH, Knowles RC: Bacteriology of chronic leg ulcers. Arch Dermatol 114:1765–1768, 1978.
56. Alinovi A, Bassissi P, Pini M: Systemic administration of antibiotics in the management of venous ulcers. J Am Acad Dermatol 15:186–191, 1986.
57. Marshall DA, Mertz PM, Eaglstein WH: Occlusive dressings. Arch Surg 125:1136–1139, 1990.
58. Gillman T, Hathom M: Profound modification by dressings of wound healing and site behavior of donor and recipient sites. Transplantation 4:64, 1957.
59. Knudsen EA, Snirker G: Wound healing under plastic-coated pads. Acta Derm Venereol 49:348, 1969.
60. Winter GD: A note on wound healing under dressings with special reference to perforated film dressings. J Invest Dermatol 45:299, 1965.
61. Salasche SJ, Winton GB: Clinical evaluation of a nonadhering wound dressing. J Dermatol Surg Oncol 12:1220–1222, 1986.
62. Sturdy JH, Baird RM, Cerein AN: Surgical sponges: a cause of granuloma and adhesion formation. Ann Surg 165:128, 1967.
63. Marples RR, Kligman AM: Growth of bacteria under adhesive tapes. Arch Dermatol 99:107, 1969.
64. Marks JR Jr: Cutaneous reactions to surgical preparations and dressings. Contact Dermatitis 10:1, 1984.
65. James WD, White SW, Yanklowitz B: Allergic contact dermatitis to compound tincture of benzoin. J Am Acad Dermatol 11:847, 1984.
66. Lineaweaver W, Howard R, Soucy D, et al: Topical antimicrobial toxicity. Arch Surg 120:267–270, 1985.
67. Geronemus RG, Mertz PM, Eaglstein WH: Wound healing. Arch Dermatol 115:1311–1314, 1979.
68. Alvarez OM, Goslen JB, Eaglstein WH, et al: Wound healing. In: Fitzpatrick T, Eisen A, Wolff K, et al (eds): Dermatology in General Medicine. McGraw-Hill, New York, 1987, pp 321–336.
69. Eaglstein WH, Mertz PM: "Inert" vehicles do affect wound healing. J Invest Dermatol 74:90–91, 1980.
70. Alsbjörn BF, Ovesen H, Walther-Larsen S: Occlusive dressing versus petroleum gauze on drainage wounds. Acta Chir Scand 156:211–213, 1990.
71. Barnett A, Berkowitz RL, Mills R, Vistnes LM: Comparison of synthetic adhesive moisture vapor permeable and fine mesh gauze dressings for split-thickness skin graft donor sites. Am J Surg 145:379–381, 1983.
72. Gilmore WA, Wheeland RG: Treatment of ulcers on legs by pinch grafts and a supportive dressing of polyurethane. J Dermatol Surg Oncol 8:177–183, 1982.
73. Fisher AA, Adams RM: Alternative for sensitizing neomycin topical medicaments. Cutis 28:491, 1981.
74. Fisher AA (ed): Reactions to topical antibiotics. In: Contact Dermatitis. 3rd ed. Lea & Febiger, Philadelphia, 1986, pp 195–210.
75. Comaish JS, Cunliffe WJ: Absorption of drugs from varicose ulcers: a cause of anaphylaxis. Br J Clin Pract 21:96, 1967.
76. Roupe G, Strannegard O: Anaphylactic shock elicited by topical administration of bacitracin. Arch Dermatol 100:450, 1969.
77. Kozol RA, Gillies C, Elgebaly SA: Effects of sodium hypochlorite (Dakin's solution) on cells of the wound module. Arch Surg 123:420–423, 1988.
78. Olin BR (ed): Drugs: Facts and Comparisons—1991. JB Lippincott, Philadelphia, 1991.
79. Cuzzell JZ: Wound care forum: artful solutions to chronic problems. Am J Nurs 85:162–166, 1985.
80. Gorse GJ, Messner RL: Improved pressure sore healing with hydrocolloid dressings. Arch Dermatol 123:765–771, 1987.
81. Rodeheaver G, Bellamy W, Kody M, et al: Bactericidal activity and toxicity of iodine-containing solutions in wounds. Arch Surg 117:181–186, 1982.
82. Dennis D: Does PVP-iodine interfere with wound healing? Infect Surg 2:371, 1983.
83. Faddis D. Daniel D, Boyer J: Tissue toxicity of antiseptic solutions: a study of rabbit articular and periarticular tissues. J Trauma 17:895–897, 1977.

84. O-T-C topical antimicrobial products: Over the counter drugs generally recognised as safe, effective and not misbranded. Federal Register 43:1220–1249, 1978.

85. Phinney RB, Mondino BJ, Hofbauer JD, et al: Corneal edema related to accidental Hibiclens exposure. Am J Ophthalmol 106:210–215, 1988.

86. McEvoy GK: AHFS Drug Information. American Society of Hospital Pharmacists, 1989, pp 1535–1536.

87. Robson MS, Heggars JP: Quantitative bacteriology and inflammatory mediators in soft tissues. In: Hunt TK, Heppenstall RB, Pines E, Rovee D (eds): Soft and Hard Tissue Repair: Biological and Clinical Aspects. Praeger, New York, 1984, pp 483–507.

88. Kaplan D: Unna's boot. The names and faces of medicine. N C Med J 50:103, 1989.

89. Kikta MJ, Sculer JJ, Meyer JP, et al: A prospective randomized trial of Unna's boots versus hydroactive dressing in the treatment of venous stasis ulcers. J Vasc Surg 7:478–486, 1988.

90. Harnar T, Engrav LH, Marvin J, et al: Dr. Paul Unna's boot and early ambulation after skin grafting the leg: a survey of burn centers and a report of 20 cases. Plast Reconstr Surg 69:359–360, 1982.

91. Rosily M, Clauss LC: Cytotoxicity testing of wound dressing using normal human keratinocytes in culture. J Biomed Materials Res 24:363–377, 1990.

92. Limova M, Roth H, Shannon N, Rovee D: Clinical experience with a new non-adhesive film dressing. Wounds 2:Nov/Dec, 1990.

93. Stoker FM: Evaluation of Comfeel pressure relieving dressing. Prof Nursing 5:644–653, 1990.

94. Duoderm Clinical Application Guide, Convatec Squibb, 1988.

95. Van Rijswik L, Brown D, Friedman S, et al: Multicenter clinical evaluation of a hydrocolloid dressing for leg ulcers. Cutis 35:173–176, 1985.

96. Hornmark A, Fall PA, Linder L, et al: Care of pressure sores: a controlled study of the use of hydrocolloid dressing compared with wet saline gauze compresses. Am Derm Venereol (Stockh) Suppl 149:3–10, 1989.

97. Thomas S: Use of a calcium alginate dressing. Pharmaceut J 235:188–190, 1985.

98. Barnett SE, Varley SJ: The effects of calcium alginate on wound healing. Ann R Coll Surg Engl 69:153–155, 1987.

99. Jarvis PM, Galvin DAJ, Blair SD, McCollum CN: How does calcium alginate achieve hemostasis in surgery? XIth International Congress of Thrombosis and Hemostasis, Brussels, July, 1987.

100. Groves AR, Lawrence JC: Alginate dressing as a donor site haemostat. Ann R Coll Surg Engl 68:27–28, 1986.

101. Blair SD, Jarvis P, Salmon M, McCollum C: Clinical trial of calcium alginate haemostatic swabs. Br J Surg 77:568–570, 1990.

102. Soderberg T, Agren M, Tengrup I, et al: The effects of an occlusive zinc medicated dressing on the bacterial flora in excised wounds in the rat. Infection 17:27–31, 1989.

103. Agren MS: Percutaneous absorption of zinc from zinc oxide applied topically to intact skin in man. Dermatologica 180:36–39, 1990.

104. Barnett AH, Odugbesan 0: Seaweed-based dressings in the management of leg ulcers and other wounds. Intens Therapy Clin Monitor May/June 1988.

105. Burrows T, Welch MJ: The development and use of alginate fibres in nonwovens for medical end-users. In: Cusick GE (Ed): Nonwoven Conference Papers. UMIST, 1983.

106. Geronemus RG, Robins P: The effect of two new dressings on epidermal wound healing. J Dermatol Surg Oncol 8:850–852, 1982.

107. Lyofoam Clinical Experiences. Acme United Corporation, Fairfield, CT, 1990.

108. Eaglstein WE, Davis SC, Mehle AL, Mertz PM: Optimal use of an occlusive dressing to enhance healing. Arch Dermatol 124:392–395, 1988.

109. Atri SC, Misra J, Bisht D, Misra K: Use of homologous platelet factors in achieving total healing of recalcitrant skin ulcers. Surgery 108:508–512, 1990.

110. Madden MR, Nolan E, Finkelstein JL, et al: Comparison of an occlusive and semi-occlusive dressing and the effect of the wound exudate upon keratinocyte proliferation. J Trauma 29:924–931, 1988.

CHAPTER 12

Nursing Considerations in Cutaneous Surgery

GLENDA K. KILLEN, BRENDA L. KUNKEL,
and PHYLIS A. LUDWIG

The best approach to the patient undergoing a cutaneous surgical procedure often involves a team effort to provide the most comprehensive care possible. This requires effective use of the combined knowledge and skills of the cutaneous surgeon as well as the administrative and nursing staff. Despite the rapidity with which technologic changes have occurred in medicine over the past several decades, the traditional role of the nurse as a liaison between patient and physician has not decreased in importance. However, largely because of these advances, the nurse has had to acquire many new skills to deal effectively with complex new monitoring devices, emergency procedures, laser systems, medications, and sophisticated new surgical instrumentation for recently developed procedures. With the acquisition of these new skills, the role of the nurse in cutaneous surgical procedures has undergone dramatic changes. For the greatest benefit from this new knowledge and skill, it is important that cutaneous surgeons understand the importance of nursing considerations in caring for patients undergoing cutaneous surgery.

Communication Skills

The art of communication enhances all good nursing care as well as other types of interpersonal relations. For this reason, it is important for the nurse to remember, when speaking to patients about their medical problem or postoperative care, to use understandable terms and always maintain good eye contact. The nurse is often the first member of the surgical team to create an effective bond with the patient or the patient's family. One of the most important roles of the operative nurse is serving as a liaison between physician and patient, patient and family, and patient and health care facility. This sometimes complicated role requires the nurse to convey a unique blend of empathy, support, compassion, and concern. The patient often relies heavily on the nurse to provide comfort throughout the procedure as well as during the recovery phase.

It is vital to realize that when patients seem angry, difficult, or abusive, they often may be merely trying to convey the apprehension, pressure, or outright fear they are feeling about the planned surgical procedure. By establishing good lines of communication and demonstrating an appropriate sense of care and concern, the surgical nurse may be able to provide invaluable assistance to the patient in this time of need. Sometimes, just sitting and talking with patients or holding their hand is all that is necessary to establish a bond of trust.

During some of the longer cutaneous surgical procedures such as Mohs surgery or hair transplantation, the nurse must also be aware of the need to serve as a communication link with the patient's family or friends by providing updates on the progress being made throughout the course of the surgery. Patient education by the nurse is also an important part of the communication process and should be provided whenever the opportunity arises. In this way, it is possible to assess whether patients understand the information being presented by having them repeat the instructions or otherwise verbalize their comprehension of the facts presented.

General Preoperative Nursing Care

Preoperative care begins on the day of consultation. Patients may have little or no knowledge about the nature of their problem or the procedure needed to manage it most effectively. Unwittingly, many patients receive much misinformation from well-meaning family members or friends about their problem or its treatment, which may be the source of significant apprehension or stress. The surgical nurse is often the first individual patients ask about their problem and what they can expect from the treatment. A reassuring attitude and a brief explanation of the proposed procedure often helps to put anxious patients at ease.

Many older patients require some nursing evaluation on the day of consultation. A quick determination of vital signs (pulse, respirations, and blood pressure) may uncover an undiagnosed or poorly controlled cardiac disorder or hypertension[1] requiring further evaluation or treatment by the primary care physician before the surgical procedure. This initial determination also serves as a useful baseline for subsequent comparison on the day of surgery. This is especially true when patients are very anxious and present for surgery with a rapid pulse and elevated blood pressure that might otherwise be difficult to evaluate without the previous normal recording in the medical record.

It may be advisable to inform patients at the time of consultation that for some cutaneous surgical procedures in which intravenous sedation is used or in which postoperative dressings may interfere with vision, it will be necessary for them to have someone drive them home. For the Mohs surgical procedure, in particular, in which there may be relatively long delays while tissue is being processed in the laboratory, it is often beneficial to have a family member or friend present to provide emotional support and comfort. Significant benefit will also result from having someone accompany an elderly patient with poor hearing acuity or diminished mental capacity to the office on the day of surgery, so that complete comprehension of the postoperative instructions can be assured.

Obviously, for patients who are deaf or have some other language barrier, interpreting services must be provided to ensure that they understand the nature of their problem, the treatment options available, and what to expect both on the day of surgery and postoperatively. If these types of interpreting services are not readily available, necessary arrangements should be made.

MEDICATION REVIEW

Despite the fact that the cutaneous surgeon will have already elicited a complete medical history at the time of the initial consultation, it is always proper for the surgical nurse to review these medications before the patient's departure, to reduce the risk of medication interaction.[2] It is important to emphasize to patients the necessity of continuing to take their regular medications up to and including the day of surgery. In addition, it is important to provide patients with a written list of the often overlooked nonprescription medications that should be avoided before surgery (Table 12–1), including aspirin and nonsteroidal anti-inflammatory agents, because of their effect on clotting.[3, 4] Also, while this substance is not traditionally thought of as a medication, patients should be advised to abstain from drinking alcohol for 48 to 72 hours before surgery, since it causes vasodilatation, which can increase bleeding.[5] Lastly, it is always important to document in the medical record any medication allergies patients may have.

NEED FOR PROPHYLACTIC ANTIBIOTICS OR OTHER SPECIAL CARE

One commonly overlooked medical problem requiring special precautions before surgery is the presence of joint prosthetics.[6] Even though the risk of infection from most cutaneous surgical procedures is extremely low, it is considered good medical practice to place patients with prosthetic joints on prophylactic antibiotics. Since prosthetic joints are becoming increasingly common and may provide such good functional results that affected patients may have no outward sign of their previous surgery, they may fail to report this information to the physician. Thus, it is always appropriate for the nurse to reconfirm the possible existence of prosthetics.

Another condition that may occasionally go unreported, especially if the physical examination performed by the physician is limited to the exposed parts of the skin, is the presence of a cardiac pacemaker.[7] Again, even though the risk is small, it may be appropriate to avoid using bipolar electrocautery during a surgical procedure to control bleeding in patients with pacemakers. In these cases, it may be appropriate, if possible, to perform the operation using the carbon dioxide laser to obtain hemostasis, since this does not adversely affect the function of the pacemaker.[8] For all these reasons, careful preoperative evaluation of cutaneous surgery patients is of vital importance.[9–11]

Surgical Preparations

PREOPERATIVE PREPARATIONS

It remains the responsibility of the nurse to prepare the operative environment on the day of surgery. The anticipated surgical tools, devices, and equipment must all be in good working order, sterilized (if appropriate for the planned procedure), and immediately available. The nurse must also anticipate the possible need for emergency equipment if some unforeseen circumstance should arise. This includes having a well-established plan and all personnel familiar with their specific role in case an emergency should occur. This requires that all basic resuscitative supplies and equipment be current

TABLE 12–1. MEDICATIONS TO AVOID BEFORE SURGERY

Prescription and Nonprescription Drugs

Advil	Dinol Tablets	Motrin
Alka-Seltzer Effervescent Tablets	Disalcid Capsules	Nalfon
Alka-Seltzer Plus Cold Medicine	Doan's Pills	Naprosyn
Anacin Maximum Strength	Duoprin-S Syrup	Naproxen
Anaprox	Duoprin Capsules	Neocylate Tablets
Anodynos Tablets	Duradyne Tablets	Norgesic
Argesic Tablets	Durasal Tablets	Norgesic Forte
Arthralgen Tablets	Dynosal Tablets	Nuprin
Arthritis Pain Formula	Easprin	Orudis
Arthritis Strength Bufferin	Ecotrin Tablets	Os-Cal Gesic Tablets
Arthropan Liquid	Efficin Tablets	Pabalate
A.S.A. Tablets	Emagrin Tablets	Pabalate-SF Tablets
A.S.A. Enseals	Empirin Tablets	Pepto-Bismol
Ascriptin with Codeine	Empirin with Codeine	Percodan
Ascriptin Tablets	Equagesic Tablets	Percodan-Demi
Ascriptin A/D Tablets	Excedrin	Persistin Ascriptin
Ascriptin Extra-Strength	Feldene	A/D Tablets
Asperbuf Tablets	Fenoprofen	Ponstel
Aspergum	Fiorinal Tablets	Propoxyphene Compound 65
Axotal Tablets	Fiorinal with Codeine	Proxican
Bayer Aspirin Tablets	Four-Way Cold Tablets	Robaxisal Tablets
Bayer Children's Aspirin	Gaysal-S Tablets	Rufen
Bayer Children's Cold Tablets	Gemnisin Tablets	S-A-C Tablets
Bayer Timed-Release Aspirin	Goody's Headache Powder	St. Joseph Aspirin for
BC Tablets and Powder	Ibuprofen	Children
Buff-A Comp	Indocin	St. Joseph Cold
Buff-A Comp #3 with Codeine	Indo-Lemmon Capsules	Tablets for Children
Buffaprin Tablets	Indomethacin	Saleto Tablets
Bufferin Tablets	Ketoprofen	Salocol Tablets
Bufferin Arthritis Strength	Lanorinal Tablets	Sine-Off Sinus Tablets
Bufferin Extra-Strength	Magan Tablets	SK–65 Compound Capsules
Bufferin with Codeine #3	Magsal Tablets	Stanback Tablets
Buffets II Tablets	Marnal Capsules	Stanback Powder
Buffinol Tablets	Maximum Bayer Aspirin	Supac
Buf-Tabs	Measurin Tablets	Synalgos Capsules
Cama Arthritis Pain Reliever	Meclofenamate	Synalgos-DC Capsules
Congespirin Chewable Tablets	Meclomen	Talwin Compound Tablets
Cope Tablets	Medipren	Tolectin
Cosprin Tablets	Mefenamic	Tolmetin
CP–2 Tablets	Methocarbamol with Aspirin	Trendar
Darvon with Aspirin Pulvules	Micrainin Tablets	Triaminicin Tablets
Darvon Compound Pulvules	Midol Caplets	Trigesic
Darvon Compound–65	Mobidin Tablets	Trilisate Tablets
Darvon N with Aspirin	Mobigesic Tablets	Trilisate Liquid
Dasin Capsules	Momentum Muscular	Uracel
	Backache Formula	Vanquish Caplets
	Tablets	Verin
		Zorpin Tablets

Anticoagulants (Blood Thinners)
Coumadin
Persantine (dipyridamole)
Heparin

and available, including defibrillator, oxygen, emergency medications, intravenous fluids, and respiratory bag-valve devices, and that the staff be knowledgeable in their use.

Patients should be greeted cordially and promptly in a confident and professional manner to demonstrate that the nurse is a knowledgeable caregiver. The operatory should always be uncluttered, neat, and clean for patients' arrival. It helps reduce apprehension if patients know that every attempt will be made to explain each step of the planned procedure before it is actually performed and that they should feel free to ask questions at any time. If the procedure is expected to be lengthy, it is appropriate to ask patients if they need to use the bathroom before getting started.

The patient should remove all clothing necessary to permit easy visualization of and access to the treatment site. The use of a hospital gown is often appropriate even for the treatment of lesions found on the head or neck, since surgical preparation solutions may inadvertently spill on patients' clothes and permanently stain them. Also, there is always the possibility that excessive bleeding or some other emergency condition may occur that could be impeded by regular clothing. However, many patients feel more secure if they are allowed to wear as much of their personal clothing during the procedure as possible.

Whenever patients have partially or fully disrobed, it is beneficial to preserve as much of their modesty as possible by covering any exposed portions of their body with blankets or towels while keeping the operatory doors closed and restricting traffic in the area. Furthermore, since the temperature of many operatories is quite cool, many patients need blankets to maintain their warmth and comfort. All extraneous noises should be kept to a minimum. If patients are being treated at a teaching institution, it is often best for the nurse to let them know in advance whether medical students, residents-in-training, or visiting physicians will be observing the procedure. If the patient registers strong objection to this, the faculty member primarily involved in the care of the individual should be informed as soon as possible.

The nurse can often set the tone for the entire procedure during the initial moments of interaction with the patient. As the vital signs are taken and recorded, the nurse should re-establish lines of communication. The pulse and blood pressure should be compared with earlier readings. If either is elevated, this should be noted in the medical record and reported to the attending physician. If the previous blood pressure reading was normal and patients admit to being anxious, it is often best to have them recline in a comfortable position with the lights turned down for 10 to 15 minutes while they try to relax. After that interval, the blood pressure should be rechecked. If it remains elevated but has improved somewhat and the patient remains apprehensive, it may be necessary for the surgeon to prescribe 5 to 10 mg of sublingual diazepam before proceeding.[10]

After the initial vital signs have been recorded, the nurse should fully review the procedure with patients to provide further reassurance as to what they can expect. In some surgical practices, after patients have been properly positioned, the nurse obtains initial measurements of the affected area and takes appropriate preoperative photographs of the anticipated treatment site. At this point, if local anesthesia is to be used, patients often become very anxious. As the anesthetic is injected, it is helpful for the nurse to provide support by gently holding patients' hands, talking in a reassuring tone, and encouraging them to take slow, deep breaths to relieve the discomfort.

Once the injection has been completed and the treatment site prepared with chlorhexidine or povidone iodine, 10 to 15 minutes are usually given to allow time for the maximal vasoconstriction by the epinephrine found in many local anesthetic agents. During this time, the nurse should make sure that the operating room table is at the proper height, the side rails are up and locked into proper position, and the electrosurgical grounding plate (if it is likely to be needed) is in place. Patients should be visually monitored closely and the vital signs rechecked several times during this "rest" interval to ascertain whether there has been any adverse reaction to the local anesthetic.

INTRAOPERATIVE ASSISTANCE

In some cases the nurse may serve either as the surgeon's assistant or as a circulator. As the assistant, the nurse provides primary help in controlling any bleeding with pressure or blotting with cotton-tipped applicators for small, delicate procedures, or 4-inch × 4-inch cotton gauzes for larger procedures. The nurse also hands surgical instruments to the surgeon, uses the suction equipment, and applies traction to the operative site to provide better exposure or make smoother incisions. When nurses function primarily as a circulating nurse, their primary roles are to monitor the vital signs, record the use of all intraoperative medications, adjust the surgical lights as needed, provide continual reassurance to the patient, and obtain any additional instruments or supplies required to complete the procedure. If the procedure is lengthy, the circulating nurse should keep the waiting family or friends informed of the patient's status and constantly try to make the patient as comfortable as possible.

Postoperative Nursing Care

Once the procedure has been completed, most patients experience a significant amount of relief. By conveying a positive attitude, the surgical nurse can offer patients reassurance that the procedure was successful and that their cooperation was at least partially responsible for this favorable outcome. The most important part of the postoperative nursing responsibilities is to instruct patients in proper wound care.

WOUND CARE INSTRUCTIONS

It is best for wound care instructions to be presented to patients in a clear, concise, and well-organized fashion. It is often beneficial to demonstrate each step of the wound care process. However, it may be unwise to show patients their wounds as part of this demonstration process. Written instructions should be given them to follow as the demonstration is performed, so that they can ask any questions that may arise. A small packet of the required wound care materials should be provided for the convenience of patients to initiate the care at home until additional supplies can be purchased. It is essential that patients and their families feel free to call the nurse or any other member of the operative team at any time if questions arise postoperatively. The written wound care instructions should provide emergency telephone numbers to use if necessary.

If the treatment site is large, if the amount of wound care required is expected to be great, or if the patient is elderly or lives alone, it may be worthwhile for the nurse to suggest several return visits early in the postoperative period at which time the quality of care and healing can be evaluated and appropriate changes instituted. If travel presents a hardship to patient or family, phone calls should be encouraged and the suggestion made to use a local visiting nurse who can assist patients on a daily basis until they are able to manage their care alone. If an elderly patient resides in a nursing home or some other type of boarding facility, the surgical nurse should send written wound care instructions to the medical personnel at that facility and follow up with a telephone call later in the day to make sure the instructions have been received and fully understood.

Finally, the importance of patients performing proper wound care in order to obtain the best functional and cosmetic results possible should be stressed. If patients understand what to do in caring for their wounds and why it is important, they will become more effective members of the "team" and perhaps feel more secure in calling the surgical nurse to clarify the wound care instructions or seek reassurance about some other aspect of their particular problem. The value of this two-way communication cannot be stressed too highly. Before patients leave the facility on the day of surgery, they should be given a specific time and date to return for re-examination, suture removal, or routine follow-up.

PAIN MANAGEMENT

One of the most frightening aspects of cutaneous surgery for many patients is the postoperative pain they are likely to experience. Some simple maneuvers are worth mentioning to help patients reduce the pain and also speed healing. If the treatment site is on a dependent part of the body such as the hand or leg, it is important to keep the affected part elevated above the level of the heart as much as possible during the first 24 to 48 hours in order to reduce swelling. This in turn reduces discomfort and minimizes the risk of infection or interference with wound healing. If the treatment site is on the head or neck, keeping the head elevated with an extra pillow or two at night for 4 to 5 days will lessen the tendency for the patient to develop significant periorbital edema or a "black eye." Other simple measures to help reduce pain and swelling are use of an ice bag (with a cloth wrapping so the ice is not immediately adjacent to the skin) on the affected site for 10 to 15 minutes each hour for the first few hours after treatment.

Physical activities should be reduced in accordance with the type of surgical procedure being performed. At a minimum, patients should be encouraged to rest at home and remain quiet for the first 24 hours after the procedure. They can eat or drink anything they like, with the exception of alcoholic beverages. If facial nerve blocks were used to provide anesthesia for the procedure, or if the surgical procedure was performed on the lips, on the tongue, or inside the mouth, patients should be cautioned to avoid hot foods or beverages until normal sensation returns. Soft foods that can be chewed easily or foods that can be broken into small bites should be recommended for the first 1 to 2 days or until patients can open their mouths fully and chew food without difficulty.

The need for postoperative pain medications usually cannot be accurately predicted. Seemingly minor procedures that typically are unassociated with significant postoperative pain may be interpreted by some patients as being "unbearable." Conversely, some intrinsically painful procedures may be tolerated without complaint by other patients. In most cases, it is prudent to recommend that patients first try acetaminophen tablets. If these do not relieve the pain, acetaminophen plus codeine is usually successful. All patients should be encouraged to take their pain medications at the onset of their discomfort and not wait for it to become intolera-

ble. In addition, taking the appropriate dosage of pain medication at bedtime often provides a restful night's sleep.

Nursing Considerations for Mohs Micrographic Surgery

GENERAL DESCRIPTION OF THE SURGICAL TECHNIQUE

Mohs micrographic surgery, more simply referred to as Mohs surgery, is a surgical technique that uses histologically prepared frozen sections, which are interpreted by the cutaneous surgeon to evaluate the surgical margins of excisions performed for the removal of skin cancers.[12–14] By means of microscopic control and horizontal excisions of cutaneous neoplasms, this procedure is able to maximally conserve the greatest amount of normal tissue and at the same time provide the highest cure rate possible. This is true even for anatomic locations at high risk of recurrence such as the central face, nose, eyelids, and ears; for recurrent tumors that have failed to respond to previous treatment; and for sclerosing or morpheaform types of basal cell carcinomas.[15]

SPECIAL PREOPERATIVE CONSIDERATIONS

All the communicative skills discussed above must frequently be brought into play in dealing with patients about to undergo Mohs surgery. This is largely a result of the general apprehension most people have in dealing with cancer of any kind, especially when they may have an underlying fear of disfigurement or death. The surgical nurse can eliminate much of this apprehension by rediscussing the surgical options available as well as the important benefits that the Mohs surgical technique offers. Since the typical Mohs surgery patient is an older individual and the procedure is commonly rather lengthy, it helps to explain to patients at the time of the initial evaluation the value of having someone accompany them to the facility on the day of the surgery. The family may provide important emotional support during the long and tiring procedure, and it may be necessary to have someone drive the patient home, since the postoperative dressing may interfere with normal vision.

A review of medications, especially nonprescription arthritis drugs, is also worthwhile, since many patients in this age group require them.[3, 4] Direct inquiries should be made about prosthetic joints,[6] pacemakers,[7] or previous drug allergies.[11] Finally, patients should be encouraged to eat a light breakfast on the day of surgery to reduce the risk of hypoglycemia, and to take all their routine prescription drugs as they normally do.

PREOPERATIVE CONSIDERATIONS

The standard considerations, as previously mentioned, should be routinely followed in the Mohs surgery patient. Vital signs are taken and recorded, and the cancer to be treated should be measured and photographed. A surgical diagram or anatomic "map" is created to help the Mohs surgeon accurately determine the location of residual tumor found after viewing the histologic specimens, so that subsequent stages of Mohs surgery will harvest tissue only from the areas of residual disease.

OPERATIVE CONSIDERATIONS

During the procedure the vital signs should be intermittently monitored by the circulating nurse. In some high-risk patients a pulse oximeter may be required to monitor the pulse and oxygenation constantly throughout the procedure. After the tissue has been harvested, the nurse is responsible for preparing anatomically correct blotters that allow transportation of the specimen for subsequent subdivision and color coding by the surgeon without the loss of proper orientation.

After completion of the first stage of Mohs surgery the nurse remeasures the wound, records its size, photographs the defect, and places a temporary dressing on the treatment site while the tissue is being processed in the laboratory. At this time it is important for the nurse to keep patients and their families informed of the status of the procedure and to provide as much comfort and reassurance as possible. If the procedure is lengthy and multiple stages of Mohs surgery are required, patients may become exhausted, both emotionally and physically, from the repeated long periods of waiting, the painful reinjections, and the frustration of not knowing what to expect. If the nurse recognizes these possible feelings and offers appropriate support and comfort, much of the patients' apprehension and tension can be reduced. During the long waiting periods, the nurse can also provide patient education about postoperative wound care, the need to avoid additional sunlight exposure with use of sunscreens and clothing, the warning signs and symptoms of skin cancers, and the importance of frequent follow-up visits.

POSTOPERATIVE CONSIDERATIONS

Once the Mohs surgical procedure has been completed, considerable relief may initially be expressed by patients and their family. However, patients now must face the reality of the wound or defect for the first time. By presenting a positive attitude, the surgical nurse can often relieve their insecurity.

Most skin cancers treated with the Mohs surgical technique are on the head and neck. For this reason, it is important that the nurse discuss with patients the benefits of keeping the head elevated as much as possible to reduce postoperative edema and pain. Intermittent ice bag applications to the treatment site may also help reduce swelling during the first 12 to 24 hours after surgery.

Wound Care Instructions for Surgically Repaired Mohs Wounds

Whether the Mohs defect is repaired by primary closure, random pattern flaps, or skin grafts, patients normally begin wound care after about 24 hours. They are generally told to apply a layer of antibacterial ointment to the reconstructed defect two or three times a day after first gently cleansing the wound with 3% hydrogen peroxide and cotton-tipped applicators. Products that contain neosporin should be avoided, since sensitization to this agent is common.[16, 17] The dressing consists of a nonstick material and several layers of absorbent cotton gauzes, held in place by paper tape. Patients should be instructed to keep the wound dry for the first 24 hours. Thereafter, they can generally shower carefully or even bathe as long as the treatment site does not get soaking wet. Immediately after bathing, the dressing should be changed, the wound cleansed, and a new dressing applied. This care is followed until patients return for suture removal. They should be told to immediately call the cutaneous surgeon if there is a continuing problem with pain, if dramatic swelling develops under the reconstructed wound, or if a purulent discharge occurs from its surface.

Wound Care Instructions for Second-Intention Healing

There are many advantages associated with allowing some Mohs surgery wounds to heal gradually over time by second intention.[18, 19] The most important one is that, in certain select circumstances, the final functional and cosmetic results obtained will be comparable or better than wounds that have been surgically reconstructed. Furthermore, if the skin cancer being treated was particularly aggressive or had recurred after previous treatment,[15] wound healing by second intention will facilitate earlier detection of any recurrent growth. This is because there has been no distortion of the tissue planes from undermining, and visualization or palpation of the site is not impeded by a thick flap or skin graft. For many patients, especially those with arthritis or other internal medical conditions, the long process of performing Mohs surgery is so exhausting that they may prefer not to have any more surgery performed and may choose to let the wound heal "naturally." In these cases, this is a very cost-effective method to manage acute wounds as long as patients accept first the time required for second-intention healing, which may be 3 to 5 weeks in some cases, and second the appearance of the round, flat, hypopigmented scar that is normally likely to result. The biggest disadvantage of this technique is that patients must be willing to participate actively in their care by performing the vital cleansing and dressing changes over prolonged periods.

Immediately after completion of Mohs surgery the wound is typically packed with gelatin foam to provide hemostasis. However, once patients return home, if there is bleeding that cannot be controlled by firm external pressure for 10 minutes, they should notify the surgeon immediately. The care required for second-intention healing is similar to that for a closed wound, but patients should be cautioned about several important features. First, they must understand the vital necessity of keeping the wound completely covered at all times with a layer of antibiotic ointment to prevent desiccation.[20, 21] They should be informed that a dried crust or scab is undesirable for wound healing and may actually slow down the rate of healing, increase the risk of infection, and worsen the final appearance of the scar.[22-24]

Patients should understand that for the first few days it may appear that no changes have occurred in the wound, and that it is very easy to get discouraged or frustrated with their progress. However, the first sign of healing is often a slight increase in the vascularity of the wound edges, manifested as a light pink color, which is due to an increase in the number of blood vessels that are integral to the subsequent phases of healing. The base of the wound will initially appear white or slightly yellow in color, especially after cleansing with hydrogen peroxide. Patients should be told that this is not a sign of infection but a normal progression in the healing process. However, if patients notice "heat," pain, redness, increased drainage, or swelling around the wound, the surgical nurse or surgeon should be called immediately. Patients should be told that the wound will gradually contract in size and heal from the edges. Patience is a distinct virtue when wounds are allowed to heal in this manner. Consequently, patients should be encouraged to call if any questions arise over the status of their healing, or if their frustration is becoming significant.

FOLLOW-UP VISIT

If patients return after their wound has healed but are unhappy with the result, it is important for the surgical nurse to offer comfort as well as provide additional information. It is common for wounds that have been allowed to heal by second intention to be slightly red, swollen, and raised at first, but with time and light daily external finger massage by the patient, most scars show dramatic improvement. The same is true for wounds that were reconstructed immediately after surgery. However, if despite the passage of time and use of massage the patient still feels that the final appearance of the treatment site is suboptimal, scar revision can be performed at a later date to provide further improvement.

At the first postoperative visit, it is important for the nurse to stress the need for patients to prevent further damage caused by additional sun exposure through the use of sunscreens or clothing. Patients should be made aware that even though the previous ultraviolet light damage cannot be reversed, there still remains value in limiting additional exposure. The warning signs and symptoms of skin cancer should be rediscussed and the patient encouraged to keep future follow-up appointments on a regular basis because of the importance of (1) treating premalignant lesions before they become malignant, (2) identifying any recurrences as soon as possible, and (3) monitoring the possible development of new cancers.

Nursing Considerations for Hair Replacement Surgery

GENERAL DESCRIPTION OF THE SURGICAL TECHNIQUES

Surgical techniques used for the permanent correction of male-pattern baldness and traumatic alopecia include scalp reductions,[25] flaps, and hair transplantation.[26-30] Of these, hair transplantation is the most common form of hair replacement surgery and is typically performed under local anesthesia with sedation in an outpatient setting. The benefits of permanent hair replacement surgical procedures have now been well established. To obtain the best possible results, expertise is required of the cutaneous surgeon as well as the surgical nurse. The surgical nurse plays a vital role in the preoperative evaluation of patients seeking hair replacement surgery as well as in successfully performing the procedure in a smooth, efficient, and well-orchestrated manner in which the needs of patient and surgeon are anticipated in advance. The nurse acts as a resource person and source of information for the patient in addition to often serving as an operative assistant during the procedure.

SPECIAL PREOPERATIVE CONSIDERATIONS

As with most cosmetic surgical procedures, in order to obtain the best possible cosmetic results, patients must be full and willing participants in all aspects of their care. This cooperation begins at the time of the initial evaluation, since all patients must demonstrate that they have realistic expectations and that they believe that these goals can be met by the proposed procedure. Some patients are so desirous of seeking improvement in their appearance that they fail to recognize the potential problems, complications, or limitations that are intrinsic to many of the procedures available. This is certainly true for hair replacement surgical procedures. The surgical nurse can often help provide additional clarification of the treatment options presented by the cutaneous surgeon. Furthermore, the nurse may often help evaluate the patients' rationale for having hair replacement surgery performed. Often, patients may seek this type of surgery at the request of a girlfriend, wife, or parent despite being neither eager nor interested in it themselves. Obviously, if this is true, full cooperation during the subsequent phases of the procedure is unlikely to be obtained.

PREOPERATIVE NURSING CONSIDERATIONS

After initial evaluation and consultation by the cutaneous surgeon, a plan is outlined for the patient's subsequent care. In most cases this consists of a series of interdependent procedures that are most appropriately staged in sequential fashion over a protracted period in order to obtain the best results by minimizing vascular impairment, surgical trauma, and blood loss. Since patients do not always comprehend the process, even after the consultative appointment, it is important for the nurse to rediscuss the various stages of the procedure and what patients can expect after each phase.

As for virtually all other cutaneous surgical procedures, the nurse should elicit from patients a list of their current prescription and nonprescription medications, drug allergies, and other significant medical problems. There are many specific preoperative patient recommendations relevant to hair replacement surgery (Table 12–

TABLE 12–2. PREOPERATIVE INSTRUCTIONS FOR HAIR REPLACEMENT SURGERY

1. Allow the donor site hair to grow longer than normal
2. Do not get the hair cut before the procedure
3. Shampoo the scalp and hair on the day of surgery
4. Avoid conditioners, hair spray, dyes, or oils on the hair after shampooing, since they may cause irritation
5. Avoid topical use of minoxidil on the scalp for 6 weeks preoperatively, since it will increase bleeding
6. Do not consume alcoholic beverages for 48 hours before the surgery, since it can increase bleeding
7. Do not take aspirin, aspirin-containing preparations, or nonsteroidal anti-inflammatory agents for at least 1 week preoperatively
8. Make arrangements to have someone drive the patient home or to stay overnight in a nearby hotel; operation of a motor vehicle is prohibited for 1 day postoperatively
9. Eat a moderate meal before surgery (there is no reason to fast); this should include several large glasses of water, juice, or soda
10. Wear clothing with buttons or zippers that do not have to be pulled over the head for removal
11. Wear no necklaces, chains, or other jewelry on the day of surgery

2) that will allow the procedure to be performed more effectively and with less interference with normal activities postoperatively. Particular attention should be given to avoiding salicylates and nonsteroidal agents that can interfere with clotting and increase the risk of bleeding. In most cases, before the first stage of hair replacement surgery, patients are asked to undergo several important blood tests of their blood counts and ability to clot normally. They should be told why these tests are being performed and that it is unnecessary to be fasting for these procedures.

Finally, patients should be prepared for their postoperative appearance. They should understand that they are likely to leave the operatory with a full-head, turban-style dressing. Many patients feel less conspicuous if they bring a colored wool knit or ski-type cap to pull on over the dressings for the trip home or to a nearby hotel for the first postoperative night.

OPERATIVE NURSING CONSIDERATIONS

The two most important aspects of the hair transplantation procedure relate to the size and number of plugs being harvested. After the surgeon has marked the recipient site with a surgical marking device, the number of plugs required should be recorded in the patient's medical record. Once the number of plugs to be harvested has been determined by the surgeon, the appropriate donor site should be prepared. This is done by trimming the hair at the donor site very short, but not shaving the area, so as to allow proper orientation of the plugs into the recipient sites. All hair fragments that result from this procedure can easily be removed by lightly touching the area with tape, which is then discarded. The area should then be prepared with chlorhexidine or povidone-iodine solution.

Next, the nurse should ascertain the size of punch the cutaneous surgeon wishes to use for harvesting the grafts. It is vital that the nurse check to be sure the correct size of punch is attached to the electrically driven punch, so that the proper-sized plugs are cut for subsequent implantation. The size of the punch is usually stamped on the side of the punch in millimeters. For the recipient site, if a hand-held punch is to be used, it is typically 0.5 mm smaller than the size of the punch used to harvest the grafts. The size is usually stamped on the side of the punch or on the handle.

Another of the important nursing responsibilities during the harvesting procedures is to ensure an accurate count of the plugs as they are cut. Often, during the course of the harvesting, several small arteries are cut, which necessitates a brief interruption of the procedure while the surgeon obtains hemostasis. At these times the surgeon may lose track of the number of plugs that have been cut up to that point. The number of plugs harvested should be rechecked as they are removed from the donor site and placed in a chilled saline bath for holding until ready for implantation. The thickness of the donor plugs is often greater than the recipient site can easily accommodate. For this reason, the excess subcutaneous fatty tissue, debris, and hair fragments that result from the harvesting procedure must be removed before implantation. This portion of the procedure is often performed by the surgical nurse. Obviously, care must be taken not to transect any hair bulbs as this is done. In addition, the nurse can "grade" the quality of the plugs as each one is carefully inspected so that the best plugs can be implanted most advantageously to provide the greatest degree of coverage.

POSTOPERATIVE NURSING CONSIDERATIONS

After the full-head dressing is applied, patients typically receive an intramuscular injection of short-acting steroids to reduce postoperative swelling. The reason for this should be fully explained. The nurse should emphasize the success of the procedure and thank patients for their cooperation during the procedure. The patients' level of responsiveness should be assessed and the nurse should check that they have someone to drive them home. Postoperative instructions are again provided in both written and verbal form, emphasizing the need to keep the head elevated, limit physical activity, and apply ice to the recipient area intermittently the first night. A follow-up appointment is made for the next day.

The day after surgery, patients return for wound check and dressing change. Before proceeding, the nurse should ask about postoperative pain, bleeding, or other problems. Next, the nurse should always check the dressings before removal for any sign of excess bleeding. The outer bulky dressing material can usually be removed without difficulty. However, to remove the inner layers most easily and atraumatically, it is best to first soak the dressings with sterile saline or 3% hydrogen peroxide solution. Once all the dressings have been removed, any dried blood or other debris should be carefully cleaned before having the surgeon check the plugs for proper alignment and the donor site for a hematoma. Usually at this time a smaller dressing is applied but is removed once the patients return home. Patients are given additional wound care instructions to soak the donor and recipient sites with hydrogen peroxide on the third postoperative day and lightly shampoo on the fourth day. Excess physical activity should be strongly discouraged for at least 2 weeks to reduce the risk of bleeding or displacement of plugs. A follow-up appointment is made for the removal of sutures from the donor site (if they were used) and to recheck the recipient site. Patients should again be encouraged to call immediately if excess pain, bleeding, redness, heat, swelling, or discharge arise.

FOLLOW-UP NURSING

Often by the next visit the transplanted hairs have entered the telogen effluvium phase and have been lost. Since this is of obvious concern to patients, it is important to emphasize that this is a normal occurrence, neither unexpected nor indicative of a poor prognosis. Reassurance by another member of the operative team is often comforting and valuable. A limited further discussion about the features of the next stage of the proposed hair replacement surgery should be given to patients at this time and arrangements made for the subsequent procedure. Emphasis should again be placed on the necessary preoperation precautions and the continuing availability of the surgeon and surgical nurse to answer any questions that may arise.

Nursing Considerations for Dermabrasions and Chemical Peels

GENERAL DESCRIPTIONS OF THE TECHNIQUES

Dermabrasions[31–33] and chemical peels[34] are typically performed to improve the cosmetic appearance of certain types of facial defects such as surface irregularities or scars resulting from trauma, acne, or viral infection; and fine wrinkling and irregular pigmentation resulting from aging, excess ultraviolet light exposure, pregnancy, or use of birth control pills or other hormones. The objective of both procedures is to provide a more acceptable appearance and improve patients' self-image. Skilled nursing personnel can greatly assist the cutaneous surgeon in both of these procedures by carefully assessing patients' needs,[35] providing comprehensive care, serving as an important resource of information for patients, and reinforcing the wound care requirements. In this way, the surgical nurse can play a vital role in helping to achieve optimal results.

SPECIAL PREOPERATIVE NURSING CONSIDERATIONS

As with other procedures performed for cosmetic purposes, a thorough evaluation of patients' psychological makeup, mental stability, and motivation must be made. In this regard, the surgical nurse can offer much important assistance to the surgeon in selecting the patients best suited to these types of procedures.

PREOPERATIVE NURSING CONSIDERATIONS

Patients must be carefully counseled and informed about all aspects of the proposed procedure. Particular emphasis must be placed on the sequence of events they will experience on the day of surgery as well as their appearance, the postoperative wound care, and the level of assistance that may be required from family members or friends after completion of the procedure. A complete list of medications, allergies, and health problems should be determined and duly recorded in patients' medical record, and the vital signs taken and recorded. Full-face, oblique, and lateral photographs should be taken, after obtaining written consent by the patient, so that these will be available before the day of surgery.

Patients should be advised to eat a light breakfast on the day of the procedure and to try to get a good night's sleep. They should avoid use of alcoholic beverages for at least 48 hours preoperatively, but should drink plenty of juices, water, or other liquids for several days before the procedure. They should avoid aspirin or aspirin-like medications for at least 7 days before the procedure.

On the day of surgery, patients should thoroughly wash the face and apply no makeup before coming to the health care facility. Contact lenses and jewelry should not be worn on the day of surgery, and all clothing should button or zipper and not require removal over the head. Because the full-face postoperative dressing may interfere with vision and sedation is also frequently used during the procedure, a family member or friend should accompany patients to the facility on the day of surgery to assist them home.

OPERATIVE NURSING CONSIDERATIONS

The procedure begins by covering patients' hair with a surgical cap and thoroughly cleansing their face with an antibacterial soap. This is followed by removing any residual facial oil with alcohol or acetone. The area to be treated by dermabrasion is appropriately marked with a surgical marking device or gentian violet. Next, an intravenous sedative such as diazepam is administered. The eyes and hairline are covered by application of a thick sterile ointment, and eyepads and goggles are placed over the eyes for protection. Ice packs are applied to pre-chill the areas to be treated. For dermabrasions, the nurse should ascertain that the correct fraise or wire brush is attached to the electrically powered motor. If a chemical peel is to be performed, the proper solution and concentration should also be double-checked before beginning. For dermabrasions, all surgical personnel

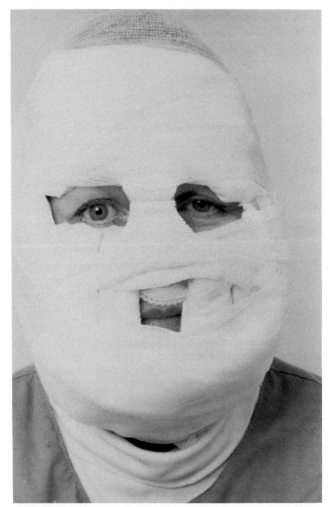

Figure 12–1. Clinical appearance of the full-face dressing applied immediately after dermabrasion.

must wear protective surgical gowns, caps, and plastic face shields to protect against any airborne debris.

POSTOPERATIVE NURSING CONSIDERATIONS

After the procedure has been completed, the surgical dressing is applied. An antibacterial ointment or synthetic surgical dressing made of a hydrogel is most frequently used.[36] A full face absorbent (Fig. 12–1) dressing is then applied and left in place until the patient returns the following day for re-examination. Patients are reminded to refrain from all vigorous activity, stay at home, and rest as much as possible. They should keep their head elevated above the level of their heart when lying down by using several extra pillows. Ice packs can be applied to the face on top of the bulky dressing to reduce swelling, which may be severe. Patients should be warned that, despite these maneuvers, the eyes may become swollen shut or their face may appear greatly enlarged; they may be reassured that this is fully anticipated and not a cause for alarm. If there is excessive drainage, the dressing should not be removed

but merely reinforced as necessary with a clean towel or cloth so that it remains in place until the next day. If there is significant discomfort, patients should be encouraged to take the prescribed pain medication as directed every 4 to 6 hours as needed, but should also be reminded that this may impair the ability to function. In the event of any problems or questions, patients should be told to immediately call the emergency telephone numbers where the surgeon or surgical nurse can be reached at any time.

FOLLOW-UP NURSING

When patients return the day after surgery, they should be prepared for the anticipated unpleasant appearance of their face. The face will be markedly swollen in most cases and the skin will appear eroded, light pink, or whitish-gray, depending on the procedure performed. Because of this appearance and not because of physical discomfort, most patients should be prepared for about 10 days of total or relative incapacitation, which will preclude most social, physical, or business activities. Postoperative wound care instructions should be provided both verbally and in writing. These instructions should specifically detail the need to clean the skin gently with dilute antibacterial soap and water at least 3 or 4 times a day, to be followed by application of a thin film of antibiotic ointment, which helps to reduce discomfort, speed healing, and maintain function by allowing the skin to retain flexibility. The wounds should *not* be allowed to form dry crusts or scabs. This wound care should continue until all the treated sites have healed, leaving a slightly pink appearance to the skin. At this time, patients may cautiously restart the use of makeup. They should be cautioned to meticulously avoid exposure to ultraviolet light for at least 3 to 6 months in most cases, to reduce the risk of irregular pigmentation forming.[37] This can be accomplished by applying a quality sunscreen having a sun protection factor of at least 15. Patients should be advised that the pink color will typically fade and be replaced by normal skin color and texture over 6 to 12 weeks.

Nursing Considerations for Laser Surgery

GENERAL DESCRIPTION OF THE SURGICAL TECHNIQUES

Use of various laser systems has provided an entirely new dimension in the effective management of many cutaneous conditions for which there was once only ineffective treatment or none at all.[38] For purposes of this discussion, the various lasers will be described according to whether they emit invisible or visible light.

Over the years, the most common laser system used to treat cutaneous disorders was the carbon dioxide laser, which emits invisible infrared energy having a wavelength of 10,600 nm. Its common use was largely related to the fact that it was relatively inexpensive to purchase, required only limited maintenance, and could

TABLE 12–3. VISIBLE LIGHT LASERS IN CUTANEOUS SURGERY

Laser System	Wavelengths (nm)	Application
Argon	488–514	Vascular lesions, benign pigmentation
Argon-pumped tunable dye	488–638	Vascular lesions, benign pigmentation, photodynamic therapy
Flashlamp-pumped pulsed dye	585	Vascular lesions
Copper vapor	511, 578	Vascular lesions, benign pigmentation

be used in two entirely different modes of operation: focused to precisely and bloodlessly make incisions,[39, 40] even in anticoagulated patients; and defocused to superficially ablate a host of appendageal tumors,[41] warts,[42] and even tattoos.[43] It remains an extremely useful laser in cutaneous surgery, even today, for a variety of other conditions as well.[44]

The visible light lasers (Table 12–3) have long been used to treat vascular conditions of the skin and internal organs. One of the first to be used for treating port-wine stains and telangiectasia was the argon laser, which emitted blue-green light.[45] Since the initial development of the argon laser, numerous other laser systems have been developed that emit yellow light,[46–50] which increases precision, reduces the risk of scarring, and also permits the effective treatment of children.

SPECIAL PREOPERATIVE CONSIDERATIONS

Carbon Dioxide Laser Surgery

As in virtually all other cutaneous surgical procedures, the procedure should be explained in detail to patients. Many do not know much about lasers except what they see in movies or on television, and as a result experience much apprehension, misunderstanding, and fear. It is important to dispel the notion many patients have that lasers are like "x-rays" and can cause cancer. In view of more than 30 years' clinical experience with laser use in medicine without a problem developing after exposure, plus the fact that the currently available medical laser systems are incapable of causing ionization, patients should be told that this is an inappropriate concern.

Visible Light Laser Surgery

Since many of the visible light laser surgical procedures are performed without either local or general anesthesia, the biggest worry most patients have relates to the discomfort of the procedure. To help best prepare them for the procedure, they should be reassured that the pain is usually quite tolerable and generally short-lived. One commonly used description of the discomfort associated with treatment is that of a rubber band being snapped on the skin. Given reassurance that they can control the rate at which the cutaneous surgeon delivers the laser light, most patients find comfort in the fact that the procedure will at least be tolerable.

Patients should be told to limit their preoperative sunlight exposure, since the melanized epidermis may interfere with penetration of some of the visible wavelengths of light and cause damage to the skin surface. They should be asked to not wear makeup on the day of the procedure, or if they feel particularly self-conscious about their appearance, to wear makeup but be prepared to remove it before the procedure.

PREOPERATIVE NURSING CONSIDERATIONS

Carbon Dioxide Laser Surgery

The details of the operative procedure should be discussed with patients to reduce any anxiety they may have about undergoing laser surgery. The need for eye protection with goggles, glasses, or eye shields should be explained.[51] The use of the laser smoke evacuator and laser surgical mask by patients should also be explained.[52, 53] They should be warned about the strange and unusual mechanical noises from the equipment used in this surgery.

Visible Light Laser Surgery

Many visible light laser surgical procedures are performed for both cosmetic and functional improvement. It is therefore imperative to obtain high-quality preoperative photographs to document both treatment pattern and response. It is also beneficial for the nurse to re-emphasize preoperatively that many visible light laser treatment protocols use small representative test sites to confirm that patients can tolerate the procedure, will perform the necessary postoperative care, and will obtain the desired level of improvement before treatment of larger areas of involvement is begun.

OPERATIVE NURSING CONSIDERATIONS

Carbon Dioxide Laser Surgery

Before having the patient enter the laser operatory, the nurse has several primary concerns that relate to safety. First, it is important to confirm that appropriate warning signs are placed on the outside door stating that the carbon dioxide laser is in use. Also, a pair of safety glasses or goggles should be available outside the operatory. Normally, prescription glasses provide adequate eye protection as long as side guards are attached to the arms of the glasses. Contact lenses do not offer sufficient protection. Next, it is important to ascertain that the laser smoke evacuator is operational, with a new filter, clean tubing, and a sterile nozzle for use. The laser should be activated to determine that the helium-neon laser aiming is coaxial with the carbon dioxide laser light by impacting a moistened tongue blade with one or two short pulses. The proper lens system should be inserted into the laser handpiece for the particular procedure to be performed, and the laser placed in the "stand-by" mode for subsequent use.

After being brought into the operating room, patients should be told what to expect from the particular procedure. Photographs of the treatment site should be taken, and the patient should be given a special laser surgical mask and protective eyewear to wear. Frequently, for procedures to be performed on the superior cheeks or around the orbit, wet gauzes held in place with tape or plastic eye protectors are required for safety. Less commonly, stainless steel laser scleral eye shields may be required if the procedure is to be performed directly on the eyelids or inner canthal areas.[51] Proper eye protection and laser surgical masks for all members of the operative team are also required.[52, 53] Moistened surgical towels must be placed around the treatment site before the procedure to protect the adjacent tissue from inadvertent exposure to stray laser light. This may require use of sterile saline or sterile water, depending on the type of procedure.

Visible Light Laser Surgery

Again, patients should be told what to expect from the particular treatment to be performed. Photographs of the treatment site should be taken to document the effectiveness of the therapy. However, to prevent inadvertent eye injury, safety must be the chief concern during visible light laser surgical procedures. Appropriate signs must be posted on the door of the operatory, and proper eyewear donned by the patient and the entire surgical team. This is of particular concern today with the newer laser systems, such as the argon-dye and copper vapor lasers, which can deliver more than one wavelength of light. The fact that the visible light lasers do not generate a laser plume means that a smoke evacuator and laser surgical masks are not required.

POSTOPERATIVE NURSING CONSIDERATIONS

For both carbon dioxide and visible light lasers, detailed written and verbal wound care instructions must be provided.

Carbon Dioxide Laser Surgery

The wound care for carbon dioxide laser incisions is identical to that for traditional surgical procedures. For the vaporizational procedures, in which the superficial wounds will be allowed to heal by second intention, patients should always be shown their wound immediately after surgery. Generally, wound care begins the day after surgery with cleansing, using 3% hydrogen peroxide to remove any surface debris. The wound is then covered with a thin film of antibiotic ointment, and a nonstick gauze and absorbent dressing applied. This procedure is usually repeated two or three times a day until reepithelialization is complete. This may require 2 to 6 weeks, depending on the nature of the original problem and the depth of the treatment. Pain is not a factor in most cases because the nerve endings are sealed as the laser removes tissue. However, especially for large lesions such as tattoos or for those on dependent areas of the body such as plantar warts, narcotic analgesics may sometimes be required.

Visible Light Laser Surgery

Patients should be told that a sunburn-like sensation will usually last for a few hours. Immediate postoperative application of aloe vera gel and ice will reduce much of this discomfort. In addition, for treatment sites on the head and neck, patients should be told to keep their head elevated for several nights to reduce edema. If vesicles or bullae form, they are generally best left intact. However, if they rupture, normal wound care consists of application of an antibiotic ointment until reepithelialization has occurred. If peeling or scaling occurs, which is much more common, topical application of an emollient cream or moisturizing lotion is usually all that is required. Patients should be told not to use cosmetics on the treatment site until healing is complete and to avoid sunlight exposure as much as possible.

FOLLOW-UP NURSING

Carbon Dioxide Laser Surgery

For laser-incised wounds, the development of normal tensile strength may be somewhat delayed.[54] It is therefore imperative that surgical tapes be used to provide support after suture removal. Usually, by the first postoperative visit, laser vaporization treatment sites will have healed, but they may remain somewhat erythematous. Patients should be told that this is a normal consequence of healing and that progressive lightening may be anticipated with time. If the site is on an exposed area, caution should be used with sunlight exposure for several months. For the treatment of verrucae, in particular, of which recurrences may be anticipated in some patients, it may be beneficial to discuss a suitable time for repeat treatment.

Visible Light Laser Surgery

After initial visible light laser testing of port-wine stains, patients return for the sites to be evaluated in regard to the quality of healing and the response to the various test doses. This enables the laser surgeon to more accurately choose the proper parameters for subsequent treatment. After treatment, the sites remain somewhat pink, but patients may be reassured that either spontaneous improvement will occur with time or repeat treatment can be performed if so indicated. The need to prevent additional sunlight exposure remains of paramount importance.

SUMMARY

Nursing personnel play an important role in the performance of many cutaneous surgical procedures. Not only do nurses contribute substantially to the skill and efficiency with which the procedure can be performed, but they also play a vital part in educating patients about the various preoperative, operative, and postoperative aspects of the surgery. The expertise provided by the cutaneous surgical nurse greatly contributes to the overall successs of many procedures in providing optimal results for each patient. As surgical equipment and techniques continue to evolve with time, the role of the nurse is almost certain to increase in importance.

REFERENCES

1. Dzubow LM: Blood pressure as a parameter in dermatologic surgery. Arch Dermatol 122:1406–1407, 1986.
2. Dzubow LM: The interaction between propranolol and epinephrine as observed in patients undergoing Mohs surgery. J Am Acad Dermatol 15:71–75, 1986.
3. Amrein PC, Ellman L, Harris WH: Aspirin-induced prolongation of bleeding time and perioperative blood loss. JAMA 245:1825–1828, 1981.
4. Ferraris VA, Swanson E: Aspirin usage and perioperative blood loss in patients undergoing unexpected operations. Surg Gynecol Obstet 156:439–442, 1983.
5. Salasche SJ: Acute surgical complications: cause, prevention, and treatment. J Am Acad Dermatol 15:1163–1185, 1986.
6. Jacobson JJ, Matthews LS: Bacteria isolated from late prosthetic joint infections: dental treatment and chemoprophylaxis. Oral Surg 63:122–126, 1987.
7. Krull EA, Pickard SD, Hall JC: Effects of electrosurgery on cardiac pacemakers. J Dermatol Surg 1:43–45, 1975.
8. Koranda FC, Grande DJ, Whitaker DC, Lee RD: Laser surgery in the medically compromised patient. J Dermatol Surg Oncol 8:471–474, 1982.
9. Gross D: On history-taking before surgery. J Dermatol Surg Oncol 7:71–72, 1981.
10. Leshin B, Whitaker DC, Swanson NA: An approach to patient assessment and preparation in cutaneous oncology. J Am Acad Dermatol 19:1081–1088, 1988.
11. Leshin B, McCalmont TH: Preoperative evaluation of the surgical patient. Dermatol Clin 8:787–794, 1990.
12. Robins P: Chemosurgery: my 15 years' experience. J Dermatol Surg Oncol 7:779–789, 1981.
13. Cottell WI, Proper S: Mohs surgery, fresh-tissue technique: our technique with a review. J Dermatol Surg Oncol 8:576–587, 1982.
14. Swanson NA: Mohs surgery. Arch Dermatol 119:761–773, 1983.
15. Lang PG, Maize JC: Histologic evolution of recurrent basal cell carcinoma and treatment implications. J Am Acad Dermatol 14:186–196, 1986.
16. Pirilä V, Förström L, Rouhunkoski S; Twelve years of sensitization to neomycin in Finland. Acta Derm Venereol (Stockh) 47:419–425, 1967.
17. Fisher AA, Adams RM: Alternative for sensitizing neomycin topical medicaments. Cutis 28:491, 1981.
18. Zitelli JA; Wound healing by secondary intention. J Am Acad Dermatol 9:407–415, 1983.
19. Ellner KM, Goldberg LH, Sperber MA: Comparison of cosmesis following healing by surgical closure and second intention. J Dermatol Surg Oncol 13:1016–1020, 1987.
20. Winter GD: Formation of scab and the rate of epithelialization of superficial wounds in the skin of the young domestic pig. Nature 193:293–294, 1962.
21. Hinman CD, Maibach HI: Effects of air exposure and occlusion on experimental human skin wounds. Nature 200:377–378, 1963.
22. Alvarez OM, Martz PM, Eaglstein WH: The effect of occlusive dressings on collagen synthesis and reepithelialization in superficial wounds. J Surg Res 35:142–148, 1983.
23. Katz S, McGinley K, Leyden JJ: Semipermeable occlusive dressings. Arch Dermatol 122:58–62, 1986.
24. Falanga V: Occlusive wound dressings. Arch Dermatol 124:872–877, 1988.
25. Alt TH: Scalp reduction as an adjunct to hair transplantation, review of relevant literature, presentation of an improved technique. J Dermatol Surg Oncol 6:1011–1018, 1980.
26. Orlentreich N: Autografts in alopecias and other selected dermatologic conditions. Ann NY Acad Sci 83:463–479, 1959.
27. Farber GA; The punch scalp graft. Clin Plast Surg 9:207–220, 1982.
28. Unger WP: Construction of the hairline in punch transplanting. Facial Plast Surg 2:221–230, 1985.
29. Knowles RW: Hair transplantation: a review. Dermatol Clin 5:515–530, 1987.
30. Norwood OT, Taylor BJ: Hair transplant surgery: innovative designs. J Dermatol Surg Oncol 16:50–54, 1990.
31. Kurtin A: Corrective surgical planing of skin. Arch Dermatol Syphilol 68:389–397, 1953.
32. Fulton JE: Modern dermabrasion techniques: a personal appraisal. J Dermatol Surg Oncol 13:780–789, 1987.
33. Yarborough JM, Jr: Dermabrasion surgery. State of the art. Clin Dermatol 5:75–80, 1987.
34. Duffy DM: Informed consent for chemical peels and dermabrasion. Dermatol Clin 7:183–185, 1989.
35. Yarborough JM: Preoperative evaluation of the patient for dermabrasion. J Dermatol Surg Oncol 13:652–653, 1987.
36. Pinski JB: Dressings for dermabrasion: new aspects. J Dermatol Surg Oncol 13:673–677, 1987.
37. Ship AG, Weiss PR: Pigmentation after dermabrasion: an avoidable complication. Plast Reconstr Surg 75:528–532, 1985.
38. Wheeland RG, Walker NPJ: Lasers—twenty-five years later. Int J Dermatol 25:209–216, 1986.
39. Slutzki S, Shafir R, Bornstein LA: Use of the carbon dioxide laser for large excisions with minimal blood loss. Plast Reconstr Surg 60:250–255, 1977.
40. Sacchini V, Lovo GF, Arioli N, et al: Carbon dioxide laser in scalp tumor surgery. Lasers Surg Med 4:261–269, 1984.
41. Wheeland RG, Bailin PL, Kronberg E: Carbon dioxide (CO_2) laser vaporization for the treatment of trichoepitheliomata. J Dermatol Surg Oncol 10:470–475, 1984.
42. McBurney EL, Rosen DA: Carbon dioxide laser treatment of verrucae vulgares. J Dermatol Surg Oncol 10:45–48, 1984.
43. Reid R, Muller S: Tattoo removal by CO_2 laser dermabrasion. Plast Reconstr Surg 65:717–728, 1980.
44. Whitaker DC: Microscopically proven cure of actinic cheilitis by CO_2 laser. Lasers Surg Med 7:520–523, 1987.
45. Achauer BM, vander Kam VM: Argon laser treatment of telangiectasia of the face and neck: 5 years' experience. Lasers Surg Med 7:495–498, 1987.
46. Scheibner A, Wheeland RG: Argon-pumped tunable dye laser therapy for facial port wine stain hemangiomas in adults—a new technique using small spot size and minimal power. J Dermatol Surg Oncol 15:277–282, 1989.
47. Walker EP, Butler PH, Pickering JW, et al: Histology of port wine stains after copper vapour laser treatment. Br J Dermatol 121:217–223, 1989.
48. Garden JM, Polla LL, Tan OT: The treatment of port-wine stains by the pulsed dye laser. Arch Dermatol 124:889–896, 1988.
49. Tan OT, Sherwood K, Gilchrest BA: Treatment of children with port-wine stains using the flashlamp-pulsed tunable dye laser. N Engl J Med 320:416–421, 1989.
50. Goldman L, Taylor A, Putnam T: New developments with the heavy metal vapor lasers for the dermatologist. J Dermatol Surg Oncol 13:163–165, 1987.
51. Wheeland RG, Bailin PL, Ratz JL, et al: Use of scleral eye shields for periorbital laser surgery. J Dermatol Surg Oncol 13:156–158, 1987.
52. Walker NPJ, Matthews J, Newsom SWB: Possible hazards from irradiation with the carbon dioxide laser. Lasers Surg Med 6:84–86, 1986.
53. Garden JM, O'Banion MK, Schelnitz LS, et al: Papillomavirus in the vapor of carbon dioxide laser–treated verrucae. JAMA 259:1199–1202, 1988.

Recognition and Management of Office Medical and Surgical Emergencies

CONSTANCE NAGI and RUFUS M. THOMAS

I n 1992 Guidelines of Care for Office Surgical Facilities were published that included facility, equipment, and staff requirements for classes I, II, and III facilities.[1] Class I facilities are those performing cutaneous procedures under local, regional, or topical anesthesia. Class II facilities may also use sedative or analgesic drugs, including intravenous administration thereof. Class III facilities perform procedures under general anesthesia with the external support of vital body functions. Specific recommendations regarding emergencies for all facilities include availability of a source of airway maintenance and oxygen, training of the physician and assistants in current basic cardiopulmonary resuscitation (CPR) techniques, and an established plan of notification and patient transport in the event of an emergency.

In classes II and III facilities the physician and staff should be prepared to provide cardiac life support, at least one operating room should be equipped with oxygen, and resuscitation equipment with the appropriate medications for CPR should be within reasonable proximity.

These guidelines make it clear that the cutaneous surgeon must become thoroughly familiar with the recognition and proper treatment of office emergencies. Although emergencies are rare in the office setting, the risk becomes more likely with the increasingly older patient population and the greater complexity of the procedures being performed. Proper training of staff, planning, and ready availability of basic emergency equipment and medications are essential to the successful management of these situations.

Training and Planning

Training in Basic Life Support (BLS) and Advanced Cardiac Life Support (ACLS) is required for physicians to obtain privileges at many hospitals. Excellent BLS and ACLS courses are offered through the Red Cross, the American Heart Association, and local hospitals in most communities. All physicians and nursing personnel should minimally receive training in BLS with an annual refresher course.[2] The BLS course can be given to the entire office staff in familiar surroundings using the resuscitation mannequin. Training in ACLS is also recommended for the cutaneous surgeon.

Planning for an emergency situation begins with the development of a written plan that details each staff member's role. These roles should include activating the emergency medical system; accurately recording the time of events, vital signs, and medications; performing basic CPR; and starting intravenous infusions. Office drills simulating emergency situations can sharpen the skills, confidence, and response time of the office staff.[3]

The main goal in managing an emergency is to stabilize and transport the patient to an emergency care facility as quickly as possible. The phone number for the local emergency medical system (EMS) should be posted by all office telephones. Sometimes, arrangements can be made in advance with a nearby internist or critical care specialist to assist in the care of emergency patients.

TABLE 13–1. EMERGENCY MEDICATIONS AND EQUIPMENT

Essential Pharmaceuticals

Injectables
Epinephrine 1:1000
                  1:10,000
Lidocaine   1% or 2%
Atropine
Diazepam (Valium)
Diphenhydramine (Benadryl)
Methylprednisolone (Solu-Medrol)
Dextrose 50%

Optional Injectables
Sodium bicarbonate
Calcium chloride
Bretylium
Dopamine
Aminophylline

Injectables should be available in single-dose syringes for ease of use during emergencies; expiration dates of all drugs should be reviewed on a regular basis; appropriate adult and pediatric dosages should be listed in table form and kept in the emergency cart.

Noninjectables
Nitroglycerin tablets
Metaproterenol inhaler (Alupent)

Basic Equipment
Oxygen tank with adapter and tubing
Bag-valve mask or pocket mask
Suction apparatus and tubing
Intravenous catheters, tubing, and fluids
Backboard
Monitor-defibrillator unit

Optional Equipment
Laryngoscope
Endotracheal tubes

Equipment and Medications

Basic emergency equipment and medications must be readily available (Table 13–1). Oxygen that can be given by mask is an essential part of the basic emergency equipment. A small portable oxygen tank with regulator, tubing, and some type of mask or nasal cannula is sufficient.[4] Surgical tables that can be manually or automatically placed into a Trendelenburg position are also highly recommended. If the surgical table is firm, a cardiac board may not be needed. Cardiac monitor and defibrillation units, laryngoscopes, and endotracheal tubes are important additional pieces of equipment that should be restricted to medical personnel trained in their use.

Essential pharmaceuticals along with other equipment can be conveniently kept in an emergency tray or rolling cart (Fig. 13–1). Intravenous fluids, tubing, and catheters are necessary for the delivery of medications. A listing of appropriate adult and pediatric dosages for the various medications should be attached to the emergency cart. The contents, expiration dates, and patency of all drugs should be reviewed regularly, as should equipment checks such as testing the power supply to the monitor-defibrillator, and checking the pressure and volume of the oxygen tank and oxygen delivery system.

A log book should be kept to document that medications are current and all emergency equipment is in working order and functioning well.

Treatment of Specific Noncardiac Emergencies

SYNCOPE

The most common emergency encountered in cutaneous surgery is vasovagal syncope. This may occur during or after even minor surgical procedures such as a shave biopsy. Often, patients exhibit extreme apprehension or arise too quickly from the recumbent position. Patients frequently report previous syncopal episodes associated with vaccinations, venipuncture, or even seeing blood. A family history of similar episodes is not uncommon. Physiologically, syncope is caused by excessive vagal stimulation, which results in loss of peripheral vasomotor tone with secondary visceral blood pooling and inadequate return to the heart. Without an adequate increase in cardiac output, cerebral hypoperfusion and unconsciousness occur.

Certain measures can effectively prevent syncopal episodes. The most important step is to always provide a detailed explanation to patients of what to expect in regard to the procedure, especially any discomfort that may be experienced. Speaking in a calm, reassuring tone is always helpful. Procedures should be carried out with patients recumbent, and they should not be allowed to view the procedure or the pathology specimen.[5] Any family members or friends who accompany patients should also be prevented from viewing the procedure, as they too may experience syncope. After the procedure, patients should be slowly assisted into a sitting position and observed for signs and symptoms of syncope before standing is allowed.

Signs of syncope include pallor, diaphoresis, initial tachycardia followed by bradycardia, hypotension, and loss of consciousness. The loss of consciousness is usually very brief if appropriate measures are taken. Treatment includes protecting patients from falling, immediately placing them in the Trendelenburg position, applying cool compresses to the face, loosening restrictive clothing, and administering oxygen at 4 to 6 L/min, if readily available. Spirits of ammonia may be used to stimulate patients. Vital signs should be taken and recorded. Atropine, 0.5 mg given intravenously, should be considered if the syncopal episode is severe or prolonged.[6] If patients do not promptly return to full mental and cardiopulmonary status, more serious conditions such as stroke, seizure, myocardial infarction, and cardiac arrhythmia must be considered.[7]

CONVULSIONS

Convulsions may occur as a result of a variety of disorders, including drug reactions, insulin shock, cerebrovascular accidents, anesthetic toxicity, and primary convulsive disorders. Signs and symptoms include auras, excessive salivation, convulsive movements of the ex-

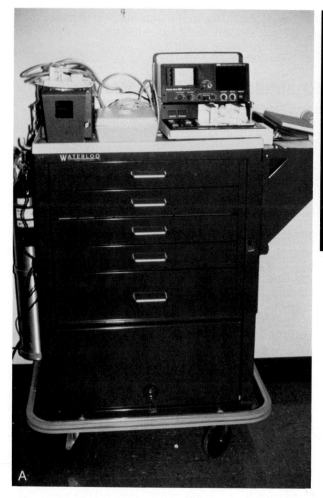

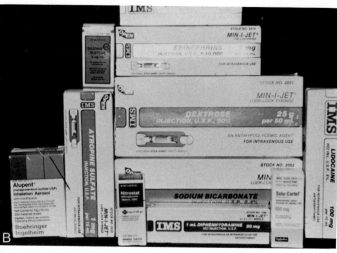

Figure 13–1. *A*, Emergency cart with portable suction unit, oxygen tank, and cardiac monitor-defibrillator unit. *B*, Emergency medications available in the cart.

tremities, and loss of consciousness. Therapy is primarily aimed at protecting patients from personal injury. They should be placed in a position in which they cannot hurt themselves during their convulsive movements. If possible, they should be kept lying on their side so that mucus and saliva will flow freely and not block the airway. A plastic airway can also be inserted between the teeth to prevent trauma to the tongue and cheeks.[8] Most convulsions are self-limited, and intervention may be unnecessary. However, status epilepticus, a condition in which patients do not completely regain consciousness during a series of continuous major motor seizures, constitutes a potentially life-threatening medical emergency.

In 50% of patients with status epilepticus, no previous seizure is reported.[9] It is therefore essential to search for and correct metabolic disturbances such as hypoglycemia, hyponatremia, hypomagnesemia, and hypocalcemia. Blood samples should be drawn for glucose, various blood chemistries, and anticonvulsive drug levels. A dose of 50 ml of 50% dextrose in water should be given intravenously to treat possible hypoglycemia before administering anticonvulsive therapy. Diazepam is the drug of choice for effective control of status epilepticus. It should be given intravenously: 5 to 10 mg at a rate of no more than 1 to 2 mg/min for adults.[10] If

the seizures have not stopped within 10 minutes, another 5 to 10 mg should be administered. Blood pressure and respirations must be closely monitored. If the seizures are not terminated, administration of phenobarbital or phenytoin should be considered.

HEMORRHAGE

Significant hemorrhage occurring intra- or postoperatively is usually caused either by a pre-existing bleeding disorder or by inadequate intraoperative hemostasis. A pre-existing bleeding disorder can most often be determined before surgery by taking an adequate history and performing a careful physical examination. Inquiry should be made as to a family history of bleeding problems or a personal history of prolonged bleeding after trauma, unprovoked nose bleeds, or bleeding from the gums. A complete list of medications, including all over-the-counter products that may contain aspirin, should be reviewed. Petechiae and ecchymoses found on physical examination may indicate a significant bleeding diathesis.

Screening laboratory tests should be used to evaluate hereditary or acquired coagulopathy.[11] These tests include complete blood count, platelet count, peripheral smear for platelet morphology, prothrombin time, partial thromboplastin time, and bleeding time. If the patient's history or physical examination raises doubts, a simple bleeding time test performed in the office effectively screens for most major potential bleeding complications.

Aspirin, nonsteroidal anti-inflammatory drugs (NSAIDs), and anticoagulants are common causes of drug-induced coagulopathy. Patients undergoing parenteral anticoagulation with heparin are not candidates for elective cutaneous surgery. Patients requiring chronic anticoagulation with a coumarin-type drug may be able to undergo most cutaneous surgical procedures with certain precautions. Coumarin may be stopped 4 days before a surgical procedure and reinstituted after surgery, but only in consultation with the patient's primary physician. When the patient's medical condition does not warrant discontinuation of the anticoagulant, the procedure may often still be performed, but in this case meticulous attention should be given to intraoperative hemostasis and application of a postoperative pressure dressing. Use of the focused carbon dioxide laser as a cutting instrument may be an alternate surgical method, since small capillary vessels are sealed immediately, resulting in a relatively bloodless incision. Oral or parental vitamin K can also be administered to control persistent bleeding.

Aspirin and NSAIDs such as ibuprofen should be avoided for 7 to 14 days before surgery and 2 to 7 days after surgery in order to diminish problems with hemorrhage. The length of time to discontinue these medications should be determined by the complexity of the surgical procedure and the underlying medical condition. Alcohol is another drug that should be avoided during the perioperative period, as it is a potent vasodilator.[11]

Hemorrhage secondary to inadequate intraoperative hemostasis is a preventable complication.[2] Before closure, careful and thorough cautery or ligation of all bleeding points should be accomplished. Adequate closure of all dead space should be performed using subcutaneous, dermal, and skin sutures as necessary. Special attention should be given to the application of an effective pressure dressing during the first 24 hours after surgery. Postoperative hemorrhage necessitating a return visit to the physician requires a complete examination of the surgical wound and may include evacuation of a hematoma and ligation of any bleeding points. Antibiotic therapy is indicated at that time, if not already instituted.

DRUG TOXICITY

During cutaneous office surgery, toxic reactions to drugs are most commonly related to local anesthetics, and may be either local or general.

Local Reactions

Local toxicity involves the tissue at the site of injection and includes cellulitis, ulceration, abscess formation, and tissue slough. Local toxicity is uncommon and may be due to contamination of the anesthetic agent, trau-matic administration of or reaction to the anesthetic itself, the added preservatives, or vasoconstrictors.

Systemic Reactions

The systemic reactions of general toxicity may be due to excessive dosage, rapid absorption, inadequate metabolism or redistribution, or unintentional intravascular injection. Systemic toxic reactions to local anesthetics are almost always due to overdosage and are entirely preventable. The physician should be thoroughly familiar with the toxic dose of the anesthetic being used. Aspiration should be performed before injecting, especially in mucous membranes. The anesthetic should be injected slowly and the dosage should be compatible with the body weight of the patient. For example, the toxic dose of the most commonly used anesthetic, 1% lidocaine, is 300 mg or 30 ml when used without epinephrine, and 500 mg or 50 ml when used with epinephrine in a healthy adult patient having an average weight of 150 pounds (70 kg).

Systemic toxicity to local anesthetics often presents with early symptoms that should alert the physician to a possible toxic reaction. These include yawning, drowsiness, coughing, twitching, restlessness, or numbness of the tongue and perioral tissues.[12] The central nervous system is the primary target of toxic levels of anesthetics. This is manifested with biphasic excitatory and depressant stages.[13] In addition, lightheadedness, nervousness, apprehension, euphoria, confusion, dizziness, tinnitus, diplopia, vomiting, tremors, and convulsions may all characterize the initial excitatory stage, which may be brief or may not occur at all. The first manifestation of toxicity may be the depressant stage characterized by extreme drowsiness merging into unconsciousness, respiratory depression, and arrest. Respiratory arrest is the most common cause of death directly attributable to reactions to local anesthetics. The cardiovascular manifestations of anesthetic toxicity are usually the depressant effects. These include myocardial depression with peripheral vasodilatation, hypotension, bradycardia, and cardiovascular collapse leading to cardiac arrest.

Management of Anesthetic Toxicity

Management of local anesthetic emergencies begins with careful monitoring of vital signs and mental status after each local anesthetic injection. If an abnormality is detected, immediate attention should be given to maintenance of a patent airway,[4] administration of oxygen, and starting an intravenous infusion.[14] Intravenous diazepam, 2.5 to 5.0 mg, may be given very slowly for persistent seizures. However, as this medication may inhibit respirations, close attention should be given to the patient's respiratory pattern. Circulatory depression may require intravenous fluids and a vasopressor. In severe toxic reactions in which there is respiratory or cardiac arrest, standard CPR measures should be instituted immediately.

Reactions to Vasoconstrictive Agents

Toxic reactions may also occur with vasoconstrictive agents, which are frequently administered along with local anesthetics. Vasoconstrictive agents, most commonly epinephrine, prolong the duration of local anesthesia, lessen bleeding at the surgical site, and inhibit absorption to minimize the possibility of systemic toxicity. However, toxic reactions can occur with epinephrine when a high dosage is used or with accidental intravascular injection. Some of the manifestations include palpitations, throbbing headache, tremor, tachycardia, tachypnea, and cardiac arrhythmias. Fortunately, the half-life of epinephrine in serum is short, and usually supportive therapy is all that is needed.

Some patients are very sensitive to the effects of epinephrine, and in these it is probably best to avoid epinephrine entirely. Absolute contraindications to epinephrine are hyperthyroidism and pheochromocytoma. Epinephrine should also be used with caution in patients with a history of cardiac disease. In addition, a possible interaction with epinephrine-containing local anesthetics given to patients receiving propranolol has been described.[15] The proposed mechanism of the interaction is thought to be propranolol-induced blockade of the beta$_2$ vascular bed receptors, with resultant unopposed alpha-pressor effect. This pressor effect may lead to malignant hypertension, stroke, and cardiac arrest. Since the most serious reported reactions have occurred primarily with higher doses of epinephrine, the lowest effective dosage and concentration of epinephrine should always be used. Epinephrine concentrations of 1:200,000 or less should be used whenever a large volume of anesthetic is needed, since higher concentrations add little to the degree of vasoconstriction, but can be associated with more serious side effects.

ALLERGIC REACTIONS AND ANAPHYLAXIS

In the office setting, the most common cause of allergic reactions is injected medications or local anesthetics. A wide spectrum of clinical manifestations can occur, ranging from very mild ones such as pruritus and urticaria to very severe ones such as angioedema, laryngeal edema, bronchospasm, hypotension, and cardiovascular collapse. Anaphylaxis is the most severe form of allergic reaction in which death may occur within minutes.

The older anesthetic agents, which are rarely used for local anesthesia of the skin, are associated with allergic reactions at a rate of 1%.[16] These agents are from the ester linkage group and include procaine, chloroprocaine, and tetracaine. The newer amide linkage group of local anesthetics (lidocaine, bupivacaine, mepivacaine, etidocaine, and prilocaine) are used almost exclusively today, and true allergic reactions to this group appear to be rare. As the ester and amide anesthetic groups are chemically dissimilar, cross-reactivity does not occur. Of the few allergic reactions to the amide group of anesthetics that have been reported, most may in fact be attributable to the preservative methylparaben contained in multidose vials.[17] Single-dose vials do not

contain parabens, and lidocaine ampules used in cardiac resuscitation contains neither epinephrine nor preservatives. It may be used as a local anesthetic in cases of documented or suspected allergic reactions to an amide anesthetic. Normal saline or diphenhydramine may also be used effectively in smaller procedures such as shave or punch biopsy[18] in patients with a suspected anesthetic allergy.

Epinephrine is the initial drug of choice for pharmacologic treatment of allergic reactions.[19] In adults, 0.3 to 0.5 ml of a 1:1000 solution should be administered subcutaneously every 20 to 30 minutes as needed for up to three doses; the dose for children is 0.01 ml/kg of a 1:1000 solution administered subcutaneously. For life-threatening anaphylactic reactions, 5 ml of a 1:10,000 solution should be given intravenously and repeated every 5 to 10 minutes as needed. If an intravenous line cannot be immediately established, sublingual or endotracheal epinephrine may be given. In addition, if an injected medication is the source of the allergic reaction, a venous tourniquet proximal to the injection site can be used to delay absorption of the antigen. Similarly, epinephrine, 0.3 ml of a 1:1000 solution, may be injected subcutaneously into the site.

Maintenance of a patent airway along with the administration of oxygen is critical. With signs of upper airway compromise, endotracheal intubation should be performed; in cases of severe laryngeal edema, cricothyrotomy or tracheostomy may be necessary. Bronchospasm should be treated with aminophylline, 6 mg/kg infused intravenously over 20 to 30 minutes. Initially, however, inhaled bronchodilators such as metaproterenol may also be effective. Volume expansion with normal saline or Ringer's lactate solution may be needed, as large losses of fluid from the intravascular compartment are common.[20] Hypotension unresponsive to volume expansion may require infusion of dopamine hydrochloride, titrated by being given at a rate of 2 to 50 µg/kg/min. Antihistamines and corticosteroids, of little value in treating the acute episode, should both be considered for early use, as they may shorten the duration of the reaction and prevent relapse. Diphenhydramine hydrochloride, 25 to 50 mg intravenously over several minutes, can be administered, although intramuscular or oral routes may also be used. Hydrocortisone sodium succinate, 500 mg, or its equivalent is administered intravenously. All patients experiencing anaphylaxis should be admitted to the hospital for careful monitoring and observation.

Recognition and Management of Cardiac Emergencies

MYOCARDIAL INFARCTION

Myocardial infarction is an emergency requiring immediate recognition and appropriate management. Classic signs and symptoms of acute myocardial infarction include crushing substernal chest pain, diaphoresis, cyanosis or pallor, and nausea or vomiting. Pain may be mild or severe, central or diffuse, and may radiate to one or both shoulders or arms, or to the neck, mandible, or back.[21] If myocardial infarction is strongly suspected, the surgery should be immediately terminated and the emergency medical system activated. Most deaths occur during the first few hours and are due to ventricular fibrillation.

Because of the high incidence of life-threatening arrhythmias during the early hours of infarction, electrocardiographic monitoring should be initiated immediately, if available. Oxygen should be administered by mask or nasal cannula at a flow rate of 4 to 6 L/min, as administration of oxygen may minimize the extent of myocardial damage. Intravenous lines should be established promptly. Vital signs should be measured frequently and recorded by one member of the office team. If the patient is normotensive or hypertensive, a trial of 0.4 mg nitroglycerin should be given sublingually in an attempt to relieve the pain. If this is unsuccessful or if the pain is severe, morphine sulfate can be administered intravenously at titrated doses of 2 to 5 mg as often as every 5 minutes. As ventricular fibrillation may occur suddenly without preceding arrhythmias, initiation of prophylactic therapy with lidocaine as early as possible is often recommended, even in the absence of ventricular ectopy.[22] An intravenous bolus of 1 mg/kg 1% lidocaine is administered initially, followed by a continuous infusion at 2 μg/min. This dosage should be reduced by 50% in the presence of decreased cardiac output, in patients older than 75 years, and in those with hepatic dysfunction.

CARDIAC ARREST

Cardiac arrest is the most feared emergency in cutaneous office surgery. In patients who suffer cardiac arrest, pre-existing coronary artery disease is most commonly responsible for precipitating the arrest. However, cardiac arrest may also occur as the unexpected result of an administered medication or a toxic dose of local anesthetic. The chances of survival are dramatically improved when early CPR is coupled with an efficient EMS and advanced cardiac life support capability. As noted earlier, training and retraining in the BLS and ACLS courses are essential. It is also important to note that significant changes in both the BLS and ACLS courses were made by the 1985 National Conference on Standards and Guidelines for Cardiopulmonary Resuscitation and Emergency Cardiac Care.[22]

The sequence of BLS includes opening the *a*irway, rescue *b*reathing, and external chest *c*ompression, also known as the "ABCs." The assessment phase begins with determination of unresponsiveness, breathlessness, and pulselessness, in that order. The degree of unresponsiveness can be assessed by gently tapping or shaking the patient and shouting "Are you OK?" Determination of unresponsiveness is important to prevent injury from attempted resuscitation of a patient who is not truly unconscious. If the patient is unresponsive, a member of the office team should be directed to activate the EMS.

In unconscious patients the airway should be opened immediately using the head tilt–chin lift maneuver (Fig.

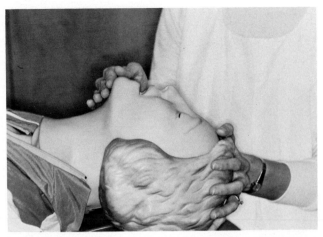

Figure 13–2. Head tilt–chin lift maneuver, used to open the airway in an unconscious patient.

13–2). The head tilt–neck lift maneuver is no longer recommended. Assessment for breathlessness should take no more than 5 seconds by looking for the rise and fall of the patient's chest, listening for air escaping during exhalation, and feeling for the flow of air from the nose or mouth. This should be done while the airway is opened and maintained. In patients with no signs of spontaneous respirations, two initial breaths of 1 to 1.5 seconds each should be given.[23] Formerly, four "quick" initial ventilations were recommended. An alternative to mouth-to-mouth treatment is mouth-to-mask ventilation. A properly fitted face mask equipped with a one-way valve that diverts the patient's exhaled air away from the rescuer is an effective, simple method of providing ventilation (Fig. 13–3).[22] A bag-valve-mask device with supplemental oxygen may also be used for ventilation, but proper training and practice in its use is required.

Pulselessness should be assessed carefully, checking the carotid pulse for 5 to 10 seconds. If a pulse is present but there is no breathing, rescue breathing should be done at a rate of 12 times per minute, once every 5 seconds, after the initial two breaths. If no pulse is palpable, the diagnosis of cardiac arrest is confirmed. The EMS should be activated and external chest compressions begun.

Proper hand positioning and chest compression technique are important for effective CPR. The heel of the hand nearest the patient's head is placed over the lower half of the sternum, and the other hand is placed on top of the hand on the sternum. Elbows are locked and the shoulders positioned directly over the hands so that each chest compression is directed down onto the sternum. The sternum must be depressed 1½ to 2 inches for normal-sized adults. External chest compressions must be released completely, allowing the chest to return to its normal position after each compression.

A compression rate of 80 to 100 per minute for both single- and two-rescuer CPR is now recommended. Proper compression to ventilation rate for one rescuer is 15:2, and for two rescuers 5:1. The mnemonic "one and two and three and four and" helps establish the

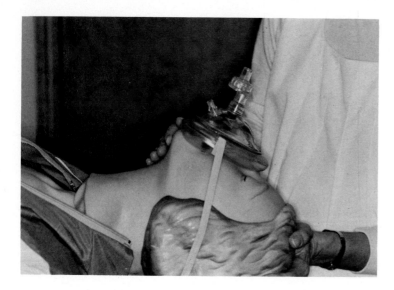

Figure 13–3. Pocket mask with one-way valve for ventilation. A separate port is provided for supplemental oxygen.

proper compression rate of 80 to 100 per minute. After compressions, the airway should be opened again and rescue breaths delivered, two for the single rescuer and one for two rescuers. Ventilation should be 1 to 1.5 seconds long. Four cycles of 15 compressions and two ventilations should be performed before checking the carotid pulse.

Placement of an oropharyngeal, nasopharyngeal, or endotracheal airway combined with an oxygen delivery system will facilitate the best delivery of oxygen to the lungs. Proper training in the use of airway equipment is essential. Ventilations should not be interrupted for more than 30 seconds when placing an airway. A suction apparatus should be available to remove oral and gastric secretions before placement of an endotracheal tube. Once an endotracheal tube is in position, ventilation need not be synchronized to chest compression, but should be performed at a rate of 12 to 15 per minute. Endotracheal intubation should be attempted only by personnel highly trained in this technique.[21]

Cardiac arrest is a life-threatening emergency that must be diagnosed and treated immediately. ACLS training provides hands-on experience in the use of specific drug and defibrillation therapies. The most common electrocardiographic patterns of cardiac arrest include ventricular fibrillation, pulseless ventricular tachycardia, asystole, and electromechanical dissociation. A monitor-defibrillator unit is necessary to determine which cardiac arrest pattern is present. To administer medications, a reliable intravenous line must be established early. If difficulty is encountered in establishing a line, epinephrine, lidocaine, and atropine can be administered via an endotracheal tube if one is in place.[24] Antecubital veins should be the first choice to establish venous access, since cannulation of either the jugular or subclavian veins not only interrupts CPR, but also is associated with a significant number of complications if improperly performed. A solution of 5% dextrose in water is generally used to keep the intravenous line open.

The three drugs of greatest value in the acute man-agement of cardiac arrest are epinephrine 1:10,000, lidocaine 1% or 2%, and atropine (Table 13–2). These should be available in premixed, ready-to-inject syringes. Two medications, calcium chloride and sodium bicarbonate, which were previously used routinely in the treatment of cardiac arrest, are now employed infrequently or only in very specific settings. Calcium chloride is indicated only in specific situations such as cardiac arrest related to hyperkalemia, profound hypocalcemia, or toxic reaction to calcium channel blocking drugs.[24] Sodium bicarbonate should be given only after defibrillation, chest compressions, ventilatory support with intubation, epinephrine, and antiarrhythmics have all been used, and then only when blood gases are available and indicate a profound acidosis with pH less than 7 despite effective ventilation.[24]

Ventricular fibrillation or pulseless ventricular tachycardia are arrhythmias diagnosed by means of a cardiac monitor. Approximately 70 to 80% of outpatient arrests are probably due to ventricular fibrillation. CPR should be performed until a defibrillator is available; immediate defibrillation is then critical (Table 13–3). Initial defibrillation should be done with 200 joules. If there is no change in cardiac defibrillation, the strength of the second shock should be increased to 200 to 300 joules. If the first two shocks are ineffective in establishing a life-sustaining rhythm, a third shock not exceeding 360 joules should be delivered immediately. Proper paddle electrode positioning is of critical importance. One electrode should be placed to the right of the upper sternum and below the clavicle; the other should be placed to the left of the nipple with the electrode in the center of the midaxillary line (Fig. 13–4). In patients with permanent pacemakers, the electrode should not be closer than 5 inches to the pacemaker generator.

A precordial thump has been shown to convert ventricular fibrillation and is recommended in patients with monitored ventricular fibrillation or in witnessed cardiac arrest when a defibrillator is unavailable. If initial defibrillation is unsuccessful, epinephrine, probably the most important drug in cardiac arrest, should be administered

TABLE 13–2. **BASIC CARDIOPULMONARY RESUSCITATION DRUGS**

Drug	Dosage	How Supplied	Remarks
Epinephrine	5–10 ml	1:10,000	IV or endotracheal administration is preferable to intracardiac; give every 5 min during resuscitation attempt
Lidocaine	1 mg/kg	10 mg/ml (1%)	Only bolus therapy should be used in cardiac arrest setting; repeat at 0.5 mg/kg every 8–10 min as needed to a total of 3 mg/kg
Atropine	0.5–1.0 mg	0.1 mg/ml	1.0 mg IV for asystole; repeat in 5 min if asystole persists

immediately after establishing an intravenous line: 5 to 10 ml of a 1:10,000 solution every 5 minutes during resuscitation. Intracardiac administration of epinephrine should be avoided unless neither intravenous nor endotracheal routes are readily available, because of a significant risk of coronary artery laceration, cardiac tamponade, or pneumothorax. Intracardiac epinephrine also causes interruption of external compressions and ventilation. Epinephrine is the first drug used in cardiac arrest because of its potent alpha-adrenergic receptor stimulating properties, which increase myocardial and central nervous system blood flow during ventilation and chest compression.

Lidocaine is the drug of choice for ventricular ectopy, including ventricular tachycardia and ventricular fibrillation. It is recommended when the arrhythmia is resistant to defibrillation, since it may improve the response to the electrical therapy. An initial dose of 1 mg/kg lidocaine is administered via intravenous push; thereafter, additional boluses of 0.5 mg/kg can be administered every 8 to 10 minutes if necessary, up to 3 mg/kg.

TABLE 13–3. **TREATMENT SEQUENCE FOR VENTRICULAR FIBRILLATION (VF) AND PULSELESS VENTRICULAR TACHYCARDIA (VT)**

Begin CPR until a defibrillator is available.

If monitor confirms VF or VT, defibrillate with 200 joules; repeat a second time with 200–300 joules and a third time with up to 360 joules if VF persists

Continue CPR if no pulse; establish IV if possible and give epinephrine, 1:10,000, 5–10 ml IV push; repeat every 5 min as needed

Intubate if possible but do not interrupt CPR for more than 30 sec

Defibrillate again with up to 360 joules

If unsuccessful, give lidocaine 1 mg/kg IV push and defibrillate again with up to 360 joules

If unsuccessful, give bretylium 5 mg/kg IV push, or repeat doses of lidocaine 0.5 mg/kg every 8 min to a total dose of 3 mg/kg; defibrillate again with up to 360 joules

Consider use of bicarbonate at this time

If unsuccessful, give bretylium 10 mg/kg IV push; defibrillate again with up to 360 joules

Boluses of lidocaine or bretylium may be repeated at recommended intervals to maximal limit; each bolus should be followed by defibrillation of up to 360 joules

CPR, Cardiopulmonary resuscitation.

In a cardiac arrest, only bolus therapy should be used. Continuous infusion of 2 to 4 µg/min should be started only after successful resuscitation. The dose should be reduced to half the normal bolus dose in the presence of decreased cardiac output, in patients over 70 years of age, and in those with hepatic dysfunction. If signs of lidocaine toxicity such as slurred speech, altered consciousness, muscle twitching, and seizures are observed, the drug dosage should be reduced immediately.

In ventricular fibrillation refractory to defibrillation and lidocaine, bretylium is administered in an intravenous bolus of 5 mg/kg, followed by a single electrical defibrillation of up to 360 joules. The bretylium dosage can be increased to 10 mg/kg and administered at 15- to 30-minute intervals until a maximum dose of 30 mg/kg has been administered. Bretylium is used only in refractory ventricular fibrillation and is very expensive, so it is probably not an essential addition to the office emergency kit.

In cardiac arrest due to ventricular asystole, epinephrine should be given in the same dosage and frequency as for ventricular fibrillation (Table 13–4). Atropine is then administered in a 1.0-mg intravenous push. As a parasympatholytic agent, atropine enhances sinus node automaticity and atrioventricular conduction through its direct vagolytic effect.[21] If asystole persists, a second intravenous dose of 1.0 mg is repeated in 5 minutes. Full vagal blockade occurs after a total dosage of 2.0 mg.

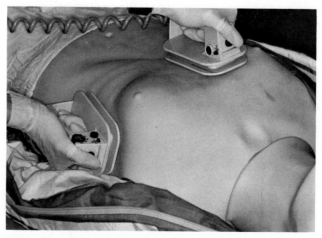

Figure 13–4. Correct paddle electrode positioning for cardiac defibrillation.

TABLE 13–4. TREATMENT SEQUENCE FOR VENTRICULAR ASYSTOLE

Begin CPR until a defibrillator is available

If rhythm is unclear and there is possible VF, defibrillate as for VF

Once diagnosis of asystole is confirmed, establish IV and give epinephrine 1:10,000, 5–10 ml IV push while continuing CPR; repeat epinephrine every 5 min as needed

Intubate if possible but do not interrupt CPR for more than 30 sec

Give atropine 1.0 mg IV push; repeat in 5 minutes if asystole persists

Consider use of bicarbonate at this time

If no response, consider a pacemaker

CPR, Cardiopulmonary resuscitation.

Epinephrine should be administered before atropine and repeated every 5 minutes if ventricular asystole persists.

Electromechanical dissociation is the cardiac arrest sequence in which the electrocardiogram shows organized electrical activity, but without effective myocardial contraction. This rhythm disturbance is frequently fatal and can have many causes, including severe acidosis, hypovolemia, hypoxemia, tension pneumothorax, and pulmonary embolism. This is a very difficult rhythm disturbance to treat. Meticulous CPR should be maintained, intravenous line established, and epinephrine administered 5 to 10 ml intravenous push every 5 minutes while attempts are made to identify a correctable cause (Table 13–5).

SUMMARY

Assessment and management of office emergencies require expertise in basic supportive care and CPR techniques, proper use and maintenance of emergency equipment and supplies, and immediate access to the local EMS. The time and effort spent in planning and training and in practicing these emergency techniques

TABLE 13–5. TREATMENT SEQUENCE FOR ELECTROMECHANICAL DISSOCIATION

Owing to multiple causes of this rhythm disturbance, make an aggressive attempt to identify a correctable cause while maintaining scrupulous CPR

Establish IV and give epinephrine 1:10,000, 5–10 ml IV push; repeat every 5 min as needed

Intubate if possible but do not interrupt CPR for more than 30 sec

Consider use of bicarbonate

Atropine 1.0 mg IV push may be helpful if bradycardia exists concurrently

CPR, Cardiopulmonary resuscitation.

will ensure the best possible patient outcome should an emergency occur.

REFERENCES

1. Guidelines of Care for Office Surgical Facilities. Part I. J Am Acad Dermatol 26:763–765, 1992.
2. Amonnette RA, Thomas RM: Emergencies in skin surgery. In: Roenigk RR, Roenigk HH Jr (eds): Dermatologic Surgery: Principles and Practice. Marcel Dekker, New York, 1989, pp 71–84.
3. Krull EA, Danbe DT: Diagnosis and treatment of surgical emergencies. In: Epstein E, Epstein E Jr (eds): Skin Surgery. Charles C Thomas, Springfield, IL, 1982, pp 114–132.
4. Nagi C, Greenway HT: Emergency airway assessment and management: guide for office practice. J Assoc Milit Dermatol 9:66–72, 1985.
5. Castrow FF: Office emergencies. Dialog Dermatol 12:4, 1983.
6. Bennett RG: Fundamentals of Cutaneous Surgery. CV Mosby, St. Louis, 1988, pp 781–783.
7. Schultz KE: Vertigo and syncope. In: Rosen P, Baker FJ, Braen GH, et al (eds): Emergency Medicine. CV Mosby, St. Louis, 1983, pp 1359–1388.
8. Tomlanovich MC, Yee AS: Seizure. In: Rosen P, Baker FJ, Braen GH, et al (eds): Emergency Medicine. CV Mosby, St. Louis, 1983, pp 1339–1358.
9. Pruitt AA: Neurologic emergencies. In: Wilkins EW Jr (ed): Emergency Medicine. Williams & Wilkins, Baltimore, 1989, pp 336–384.
10. Fox PT: Neurologic emergencies in internal medicine. In: Orland MJ, Saltman RJ (eds): Manual of Medical Therapeutics. Little, Brown, Boston, 1986, pp 394–410.
11. Salasche SJ: Acute surgical complications: cause, prevention and treatment. J Am Acad Dermatol 15:1163–1185, 1986.
12. Donohue JH, Schrock TR: Emergencies in outpatient skin surgery. In: Epstein E, Epstein E Jr (eds): Skin Surgery. 6th ed. Philadelphia, WB Saunders, 1987, pp 71–77.
13. Luikart R: The treatment of emergencies which occur in office practice. In: Epstein EH, Epstein EH Jr (eds): Techniques in Skin Surgery. Lea & Febiger, Philadelphia, 1979, pp 24–30.
14. Stegman SJ, Tromovitch TA, Glogau RG: Basics of Dermatologic Surgery. Year Book, Chicago, 1982, pp 125–127.
15. Dzubow LM: The interaction between propranolol and epinephrine as observed in patients undergoing Mohs surgery. J Am Acad Dermatol 15:71–75, 1986.
16. Giovenniti JA, Bennett CR: Assessment of allergy to local anesthetics. J Am Dent Assoc 98:701–706, 1979.
17. Leubke NH, Walker JA: Discussion of sensitivity to preservatives in anesthetics. J Am Dent Assoc 97:656–657, 1978.
18. Thomas RM: Local anesthetic agents and regional anesthesia of the face. J Assoc Milit Dermatol 8:28–33, 1982.
19. Stine RJ, Marcus RH: Medical Emergencies. In: Orland MJ, Saltman RJ (eds): Manual of Medical Therapeutics. Little, Brown, Boston, 1986, pp 411–435.
20. Ellenhorn MJ, Barceloux DG: Medical Toxicology. Elsevier Science, New York, 1988, pp 183–185.
21. Textbook of Advanced Cardiac Life Support: American Heart Association, 1987.
22. Standards and Guidelines for Cardiopulmonary Resuscitation (CPR) and Emergency Cardiac Care (ECC). JAMA 255:3905–2974, 1986.
23. Jaffee AS: Cardiac arrest and cardiopulmonary resuscitation. In: Orland MJ, Saltman RJ (eds): Manual of Medical Therapeutics. Little, Brown, Boston, 1986, pp 141–147.
24. Hayes HR: Cardiopulmonary resuscitation. In: Wilkins EW Jr (ed): Emergency Medicine. Williams & Wilkins, Baltimore, 1989, pp 10–24.

CHAPTER 14

Simple Biopsy Techniques

CHRISTOPHER J. HUERTER

The ability to perform simple skin biopsies successfully is essential for the diagnosis and treatment of many cutaneous disorders. The three types of simple skin biopsies that the cutaneous surgeon must master include the shave, punch, and scissor biopsies. Several factors must be weighed when considering which type of biopsy is most appropriate. Lesion location, morphology, and differential diagnostic possibilities are all important considerations in selecting the best type of biopsy. For the pathologist to make an accurate diagnosis, it is critical to obtain a specimen that is adequate. For example, certain inflammatory conditions of the skin or subcutis will be missed if a superficial shave biopsy is performed.[1] Clinical clues from the appearance of a lesion also may dictate which biopsy is most appropriate. Some types of skin disorders require a more complicated biopsy procedure to ensure that adequate tissue has been obtained for an accurate diagnosis. The more knowledgeable the cutaneous surgeon is about the nature of various skin disorders, the better is the chance that a representative biopsy specimen will be obtained.

Preoperative Considerations

As with all surgical procedures, the patient's general health should be briefly reviewed before any skin biopsy. Information obtained should include a list of medications and any history of allergies, possible anticoagulation, cardiac disturbances, and hypertension. In addition, diabetes, peripheral vascular disease, peripheral edema, and clinical evidence of vasculitis (palpable purpura) indicate a need for caution when considering biopsies of acral sites. Use of anticoagulants, especially aspirin, obviously increases the risk of postoperative hemorrhage. Severe hemorrhage has also been reported after a small punch biopsy in a patient with hemophilia.[2]

The use of epinephrine in local anesthetics may result in tachycardia, heart palpitations, and increased blood pressure.[3]

Simple skin biopsies are generally short, straightforward procedures, but common sense and attention to detail can help avoid unnecessary complications.

Skin Preparation

The skin at a biopsy site must be clean before the procedure. This can easily be accomplished with 70% isopropyl alcohol. Studies on facial skin have shown that a 10-second scrub with isopropyl alcohol is as effective in reducing aerobic microflora in 5 minutes as a 60-second scrub with alcohol, povidone-iodine, or chlorhexidine.[4] For this reason, the short alcohol scrub is a convenient and effective antiseptic skin preparation before simple skin biopsy procedures.

Anesthesia

There are many useful local anesthetics that differ in time of onset, duration of action, and potency (see Chap. 9). The most commonly used agent is lidocaine because it has many features that make it ideal for performing small skin biopsies: rapid onset of action, adequate duration, excellent safety profile, and low cost.[5] Lidocaine is available as a plain solution or with epinephrine added in a concentration of 1:100,000 to provide vasoconstriction,[6] prolonged duration, and decreased absorption.[7] For most simple skin biopsies, the addition of epinephrine is not critical, but at vascular anatomic sites such as the head and neck it provides better hemostasis. One potential interaction between epinephrine and propranolol that leads to uncontrollable hypertension followed by reflex bradycardia is worth noting.[8] Since this potentially disastrous consequence has been reported only with the use of large amounts of local anesthetic, the small amount of local anesthesia required for simple skin biopsies makes the probability of this interaction very unlikely.[5] To keep epinephrine stable in a lidocaine solution, a lower pH is required. Unfortunately, the lower pH also increases the pain of injection. For particularly sensitive areas, the addition of bicarbonate to raise the pH can decrease the pain of injection.[9] It should also be noted that plain lidocaine without epinephrine is less painful to inject[10] and can be used for initial anesthesia with a lidocaine and epinephrine mixture added after a few minutes, if the benefits of epinephrine are desired.

Injection Technique

Good injection technique can yield a more rapid onset of anesthesia with minimal discomfort. Knowledge of some simple details can make local anesthesia for simple skin biopsies minimally painful, allowing patients to remain more calm during the procedure and improving their confidence in the cutaneous surgeon. This can be particularly important when dealing with the pediatric population: if children become upset during the administration of anesthesia, they often remain so throughout the procedure, regardless of pain.

The use of a small 30-gauge needle can also significantly reduce the pain of injection. This needle is typically attached to a 1-ml syringe, as most cases of simple skin biopsies require 1 ml or less of local anesthetic. A locking syringe is preferable, particularly in areas where there is modest tissue resistance to infiltration, such as the nose. Raising a small wheal in the skin with a superficial dermal injection can provide rapid anesthesia and allow subsequent advancement of the needle through the wheal with less pain. A slow, steady injection technique is also considerably less painful than a rapid injection. Another helpful technique to decrease the pain of injection is to pinch the skin to be injected between the index finger and thumb (Fig. 14–1). Stimulating the sensory nerves in the area blocks transmission of other painful sensations.[11]

The use of a needle angulated at 30 to 45 degrees with the hub and the bevel directed downward causes a reduction in pain with injection.[12] The angled needle allows for smoother and easier application of pressure as the needle punctures the skin. With the bevel down, local anesthetic is also pushed deeper into the dermis, away from the superficial nerve plexus. Local anesthetic should be injected into the dermis for simple skin biopsies. Choice of the correct site for skin infiltration will result in blanching of the skin followed by onset of anesthesia within minutes.

Adverse reactions to lidocaine are uncommon.[13] Reactions to local anesthesia are often incorrectly determined to be "allergic" when they actually result from a vasovagal response with lightheadedness, sweating, pallor, and nausea.[14] If allergy is suspected, undiluted solutions of diphenhydramine and chlorpheniramine[5] or

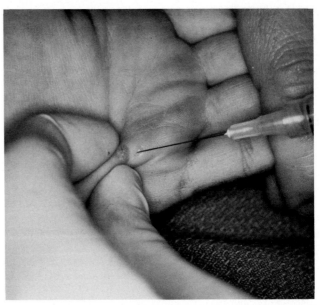

Figure 14–1. Pinching the skin before injection of local anesthetic can decrease the pain of injection.

intradermal injection of 0.9% sodium chloride solution[15] may provide sufficient anesthesia of short duration for the performance of simple biopsy procedures.

Skin Biopsy Techniques

Once the decision has been made to biopsy a cutaneous lesion, careful consideration must be given to the most appropriate technique. Lesion location and morphology are most important factors. For example, since the skin over the palms and soles has a greatly thickened stratum corneum, a superficial shave biopsy would probably be inadequate to permit an accurate histologic diagnosis. Conversely, elevated or pedunculated skin growths are often best treated with superficial shave or scissor biopsy techniques and do not require a more invasive procedure.

Some general rules may be used as a guide to determine the best form of biopsy. Inflammatory lesions are best sampled with full-thickness punch biopsies.[16] A more superficial biopsy may miss the diagnostic pathology that is often in the deep dermis. All indurated lesions, either benign or malignant, typically require a punch biopsy procedure to ensure adequate sampling depth for diagnosis. Flat or atypical pigmented lesions clinically suspected of being melanoma are also best managed by deeper types of biopsies. Superficial, clinically benign lesions are more amenable to superficial techniques such as shave or scissor biopsies.

Cosmesis is also an important factor and should always be considered before any biopsy is performed. A good cosmetic result can be achieved with any of the simple biopsy techniques, but each lesion and patient should be evaluated individually. For a patient with a superficial benign lesion, such as a small seborrheic keratosis on the face, a small shave biopsy will remove the growth completely, heal quickly, and provide a better cosmetic result than a deeper punch excision. A knowledge of the biology and histopathology of various skin lesions allows the cutaneous surgeon to make the most appropriate choice of skin biopsy technique in each clinical situation.

Shave Biopsy

Shave biopsies are an indispensable part of the armamentarium of any surgeon involved in the management of skin disease. When done correctly, shave biopsies provide tissue for pathologic diagnosis, and remove lesions with good cosmetic results. Superficial, exophytic skin lesions such as seborrheic keratoses, verrucae, certain types of nevi, actinic keratoses, and small papular angiomas are amenable to shave excision. Shave biopsies of suspected small skin cancers such as basal cell or squamous cell carcinomas offer a rapid and appropriate means of confirming the diagnosis. This form of biopsy allows for later treatment of the tumor by other techniques, including excision or electrodesiccation and curettage.[17] Shave excision leaves behind a firm, flat dermis on which to perform electrodesiccation and curettage,[18] a highly effective form of therapy for superficial skin cancers in low-risk sites. On the other hand, a punch biopsy creates a full-thickness defect in the skin that makes subsequent therapy with electrodesiccation and curettage technically more difficult to perform and may result in an unsatisfactory cosmetic result.[19]

There are different ways to perform shave biopsies. One method employs a razor blade, which has the advantages of being very flexible as well as extremely sharp.[20] The Gillette Super Blue Blade has been advocated for this procedure because of its consistently sharp edge and ready availability. The blade can be broken in half by bending along its longitudinal axis. This provides two blades, each with a single sharp edge that can be secured between the fingers and thumb. Holding the blade without use of a hemostat or blade handle gives the cutaneous surgeon great flexibility in appropriately curving the blade as needed to facilitate excision. With this blade, superficial lesions are removed by means of a horizontal sawing motion to the desired depth within the dermis. For very small and superficial epidermal lesions, this technique can even be performed without anesthesia.

The most common technique for a shave biopsy employs a No. 15 scalpel blade attached to a standard handle. This is held in the hand much like a pencil, with the index finger and thumb of the opposite hand placed around the site to be biopsied to provide traction (Fig. 14–2). This allows for an easier, sawing-type motion. If a lesion is minimally elevated, it may be helpful to pinch the perilesional skin between the fingers to bunch it up. Additional local anesthetic can be injected to slightly elevate the lesion to be removed (Fig. 14–3). Forceps may be gently used on exophytic lesions to provide upward traction, allow clear visualization of the base of the skin lesion, and provide a taut surface for cutting.

It may be difficult to begin the excision at the desired horizontal plane. To start cleanly, it may be helpful to cut the skin slightly, using the tip of the scalpel blade. Once the skin is perforated, the belly of the blade can be employed to complete the biopsy. Gently grasping the tissue being removed during the procedure helps to provide traction and improve visualization. It is not uncommon to find remnants of the lesion at the edges of a shave biopsy site. For example, small pieces of a seborrheic or actinic keratosis may be left behind after initial shave biopsy. These may be rapidly and effectively removed by curettage. In this way, benign lesions can be completely removed at the time of biopsy.

Once the biopsy has been completed, hemostasis must be obtained. For superficial shave biopsies, this is easily accomplished by several means. The simplest of these is chemical cautery using either aluminum chloride solution or Monsel's solution (20% ferric subsulfate). Aluminum chloride at a concentration of 20 to 40% in alcohol can be applied directly to the wound with cotton-tipped applicators. Hemostasis usually occurs within seconds, probably by activation of the extrinsic pathway of coagulation.[21] Aluminum chloride has the advantages of being simple, inexpensive, and effective. However, histologic studies have revealed delayed wound healing after its use.[22] Monsel's solution is also an effective agent but can produce tattooing of the skin secondary to iron deposition.[23] This deposition results in tissue artifacts that can cause histologic confusion when a previously biopsied pigmented lesion undergoes subsequent excision.[24] Monsel's solution also has a cytotoxic effect on healing wounds.[21] For these reasons, aluminum chloride is often the preferred agent for chemical cautery. Another simple method of providing hemostasis is electrosurgery,[21] which allows for more rapid hemostasis of larger biopsy sites.[25]

Punch Biopsy

The punch biopsy is a simple technique that may result in an incisional or excisional removal, depending on the lesion size and the size of the punch. It offers a quick, safe procedure with excellent cosmetic results while providing a good specimen for histopathologic diagnosis. The two types of skin lesions best suited for punch biopsy involve inflammatory and neoplastic processes. This technique also can be used to obtain tissue for bacteriologic cultures, immunofluorescence, and electron microscopy. A punch excision with primary suture repair can frequently provide better cosmetic results and ensure adequate depth of removal for certain exophytic benign lesions on the face.

Skin preparation for punch biopsy also requires a 10 second scrub with 70% isopropyl alcohol (Fig. 14–4). A wheal of 1% lidocaine with or without epinephrine is raised beneath the site to be biopsied. The use of epinephrine greatly assists in hemostasis at more vascular sites such as the head and neck. Typical punch biopsies vary in size from 2 to 10 mm in diameter, the 3- and 4-mm punch sizes being the most commonly

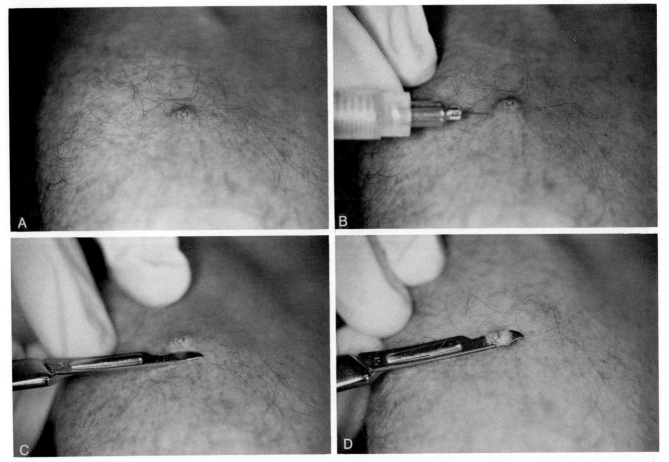

Figure 14–2. *A,* Clinical appearance of a keratotic lesion on the forearm. *B,* A local anesthetic agent is injected to raise a wheal around the biopsy site. *C,* Shave biopsy with the fingers placed around the lesion for traction while the scalpel blade is held horizontally. *D,* The lesion is removed superficially.

employed. The punches are either disposable after one use or reusable. The advantages of disposable punches are consistent sharpness and sterility. Reusable punches dull after several uses and may need to be resharpened, because a dull punch produces torsion in the specimen, which can distort the histologic appearance.

The index finger and thumb are placed about the lesion site to provide traction on the skin. These two digits should be placed opposing one another with the force of traction in opposite directions (Fig. 14–5). This results in the creation of an oval defect in the skin, which facilitates suture repair. With proper planning, the resultant scar can be properly aligned with facial lines or creases. With direct vertical pressure, the punch is rotated between the fingers to produce a biopsy of full skin thickness. As the punch moves from the deep dermis into the subcutaneous fat, a decrease in tissue resistance is typically palpable. This tells the cutaneous surgeon that sufficient depth has been reached.

It is extremely important to remove the biopsy specimen from the skin correctly. Excessive force with forceps on the edges of the biopsy specimen during removal may create a tissue artifact that distorts the histologic appearance and make diagnosis more difficult.

Tissue artifacts can be avoided by using peripheral downward pressure on the skin around the cut tissue, which elevates the biopsy specimen above the surrounding skin. Removal can then easily be accomplished by "spearing" the biopsy[26] with the same needle used to obtain anesthesia (Fig. 14–6).

Hemostasis is best achieved by the placement of one or two nonabsorbable interrupted epidermal sutures.[27] On occasion a small amount of blood may ooze from the biopsy site after suturing; slight pressure for several minutes will control this. Chemical cautery (aluminum chloride or Monsel's solution) or electrosurgery (electrocautery or electrodesiccation) without suturing, to achieve hemostasis at small punch biopsy sites, is sometimes used in cosmetically unimportant areas. Simple suturing has several advantages: no tissue destruction to impair healing, no open wounds to increase the risk of subsequent hemorrhage or infection, and better cosmesis in most cases.

With larger skin lesions, consideration must be given as to the best site for biopsy. Areas of active disease, for example at the edge of an expanding border of a lesion, are preferable biopsy sites in most situations. When biopsying ulcerated tissue, it is helpful to obtain

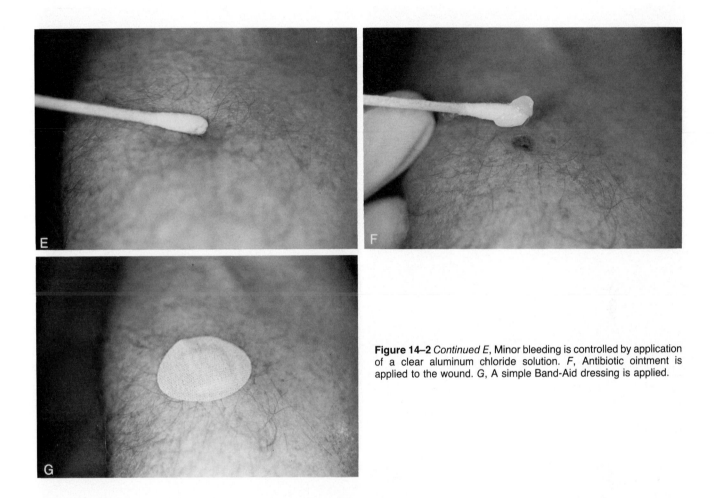

Figure 14–2 *Continued E*, Minor bleeding is controlled by application of a clear aluminum chloride solution. *F*, Antibiotic ointment is applied to the wound. *G*, A simple Band-Aid dressing is applied.

Figure 14–3. Injection of local anesthetic into the superficial dermis may elevate flat lesions for easier shave biopsy.

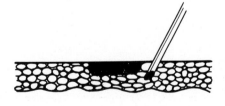
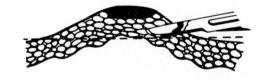

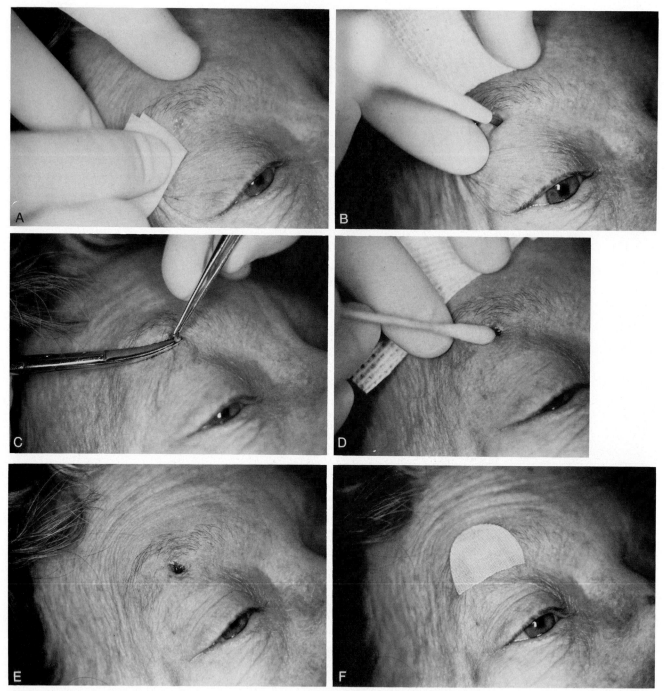

Figure 14–4. *A,* Clinical appearance of a translucent papule in the right eyebrow being prepared for biopsy by wiping with an alcohol pad. *B,* A 3-mm punch is rotated while the skin is held taut between the fingers of the opposite hand. *C,* The plug of tissue is gently lifted with forceps as the attachments at the base are divided with iris scissors. *D,* Aluminum chloride solution is applied to stop the minor bleeding. *E,* Appearance of the wound immediately after the bleeding has been controlled. *F,* Postoperative dressing consists of a simple Band-Aid.

Figure 14–5. *A*, An ill-defined plaque on the left temple is prepared for biopsy with an alcohol pad. *B*, Firm traction in opposing directions provides a taut skin surface to create an oval defect that will facilitate closure. *C*, The biopsy specimen is gently lifted with forceps for removal. *D*, Simple interrupted nylon epidermal sutures are used to close the wound in the direction of the adjacent folds or wrinkles.

Illustration continued on following page

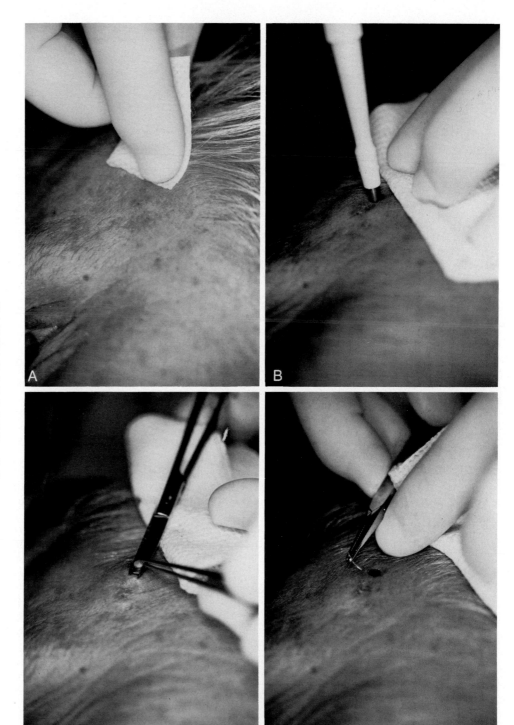

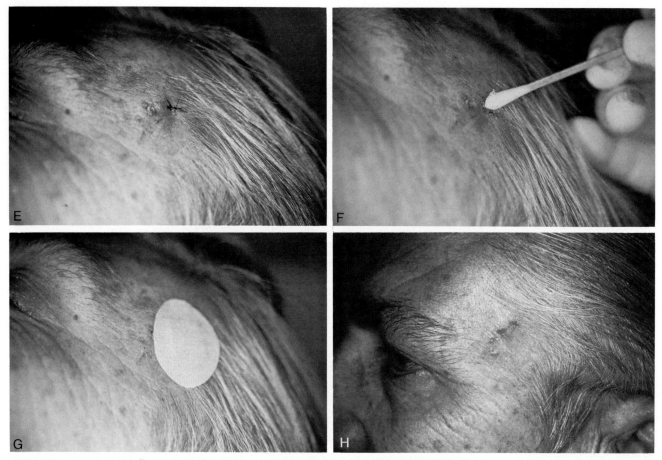

Figure 14–5 *Continued E,* Clinical appearance after sutures have been placed to repair the wound in linear fashion. *F,* Antibiotic ointment is applied to the sutured wound. *G,* A simple Band-Aid dressing is applied. *H,* The biopsy site has completely healed at the time of suture removal 1 week later.

some of the surrounding epithelium at an edge of the wound. Similarly, a punch biopsy of necrotic tissue will obviously provide little useful information.

Scalp biopsies require some additional attention to technique. It is critical to perform the biopsy in a direction parallel to hair growth to avoid transecting

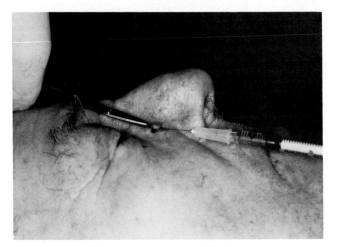

Figure 14–6. "Spearing" the punch biopsy with a 30-gauge needle minimizes tissue trauma when removing the biopsy specimen.

hair follicles and producing inadvertent alopecia.[28] It is also important to extend the biopsy well into the subcutis to ensure that the terminal bulbs of the hair follicle are included.

There are some important limitations to the punch biopsy technique. Skin lesions suspected of involving inflammation of the fat or deeper tissues such as fascia will require larger, deeper, fusiform incisional biopsies to obtain adequate tissue. In addition, irregularly pigmented lesions greater than 5 mm in size are usually best managed by complete excisional biopsy whenever possible. However, punch biopsy is a valuable tool that can be easily and quickly mastered by even the novice cutaneous surgeon. Attention to details of technique and knowledge of the best means of application are essential in order to maximize the benefits from this type of biopsy.

Scissors Biopsy

Scissors biopsy is indicated for pedunculated and very superficial skin growths such as acrochordons, papular seborrheic keratoses, and small filiform verrucae or nevi. These types of growth most commonly occur on the eyelids, neck, axilla, and groin. Depending on lesion size and morphology, anesthesia may or may not be necessary. Often, large numbers of acrochordons and seborrheic keratoses may be rapidly removed with minimal discomfort without anesthesia. For larger lesions that have a wide base, local anesthesia is indicated.

As with any skin surgery, good lighting is essential to allow for clear visualization of the base of pedunculated lesions. Small forceps with teeth and a pair of sharp curved or straight iris scissors are the only surgical instruments required. The lesion to be removed is lightly grasped with forceps (Fig. 14–7). By gently pulling upward, traction provides a firm cutting surface and allows clear visualization of the lesion base. Small, minimally elevated skin tags or seborrheic keratoses may frequently be removed without use of forceps.

Bleeding after such procedures is usually minimal and easily controlled by application of 35% aluminum chloride solution. When treating large numbers of lesions, it is helpful to have an assistant apply the topical hemostatic to those biopsy sites that require it. Brisk bleeding sometimes occurs after scissors biopsy and cannot be adequately controlled with chemical cautery. In these circumstances, it may be necessary to inject a local anesthetic and control bleeding with electrosurgery.

The need to submit scissors-biopsied tissue for histopathologic diagnosis is a matter of clinical judgment. Many lesions removed by this technique do not require this. However, if there is concern about the possibility of malignancy or underlying skin disease, any tissue removed should be submitted for routine pathologic examination. More importantly in these situations, a different type of biopsy technique should probably be considered.

Oral Biopsy

Biopsy of the oral cavity can be accomplished using the same techniques employed for skin biopsy. Histologically, the mucous membranes are very similar to skin except for an absence of stratum corneum over most of the oral mucosa. Nonetheless, performing biopsies in the oral cavity can be intimidating to those without experience in this type of surgery.

There are several obstacles to performing an adequate biopsy within the oral cavity. First, this area is quite vascular, and it may be more difficult to obtain hemostasis. Second, access is more difficult, being complicated by the enclosed cavity. Finally, achieving adequate

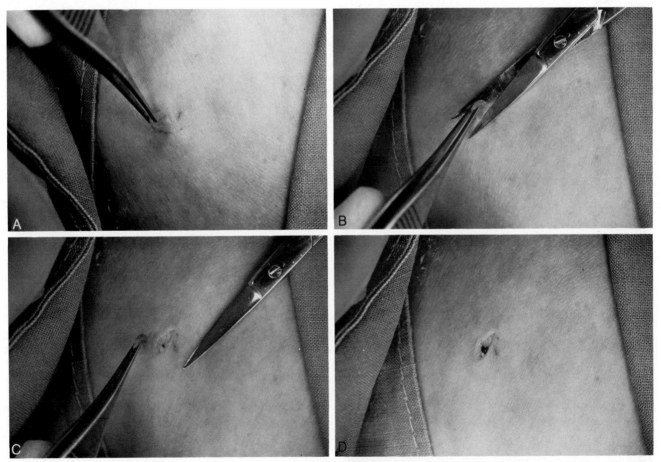

Figure 14–7. *A,* For performing a scissors biopsy, gentle upward traction with forceps allows visualization of the base of the lesion and provides a firm cutting surface. *B,* Iris scissors are positioned to remove the lesion so that its base is flush with the surrounding skin. *C,* The base is cleanly divided with minimal bleeding. *D,* Clinical appearance of the postoperative defect.

lighting presents more of a challenge than with routine skin biopsy.

Most simple oral biopsies are best performed with the punch biopsy technique. This allows for a full-thickness specimen, and suture repair greatly facilitates hemostasis. As a rule, wounds of the oral mucous membranes heal rapidly and with few complications. Larger, exophytic, or dome-shaped lesions such as oral fibromas or myxoid cysts may be better managed with shave excision or full-thickness scalpel excision, and these possibilities should be considered in advance. Preparation of the biopsy site is minimal. The extensive microflora within the oral cavity and the moist conditions produced by saliva make an antiseptic scrub pointless. Anesthesia is best accomplished with 1% lidocaine and epinephrine 1:100,000. By waiting approximately 10 minutes, the maximal vasoconstricting effects of epinephrine can be achieved. This hemostatic effect greatly facilitates performance of the biopsy.

The chalazion clamp, used by ophthalmologists in chalazion removal from the eyelids, is a helpful tool for oral biopsies on the oral lips, anterior buccal mucosa, or tongue. This clamp, with a solid metal back and ringlike opening anteriorly, is tightened in place around the lesion to be biopsied (Fig. 14–8). It performs the two important functions of providing a firm surface upon which to work and yielding nearly complete hemostasis. Sutures can be placed in the center of the ringed opening before the clamp is loosened. Conversely, hemostasis with chemical or electrocautery can be accomplished before removing the clamp.

Another simple tool that provides better access to the oral cavity is a plastic or metal cheek retractor. It is placed over the buccal mucosa and, by means of simple traction, greatly facilitates visualization of lesions on the gingiva or buccal mucosa. It also allows for much improved lighting throughout the oral cavity. Grasping oral tissues with a dry, cotton gauze can be very helpful

and improves access, lighting, and traction for certain surgical sites. Routine surgical lamps can provide adequate lighting for the oral cavity, as overhead lamps can usually be positioned to create a clear surgical field. A surgical table with tilt capability can also assist with lighting and allow more comfortable positioning of the patient. When suturing simple biopsies of the oral mucosa, it is best to use silk sutures. This type of suture is easy to work with in cramped spaces, but more important, it remains soft and nonirritating to the mucous membranes. Healing of the oral mucosa occurs rapidly, and sutures can usually be removed within 7 days.

A knowledge of the oral anatomy is important before biopsies are undertaken. The opening of the parotid duct is on the buccal mucosa, opposite the upper second molar; this area should be avoided during oral biopsies. Similarly, biopsies of the floor of the mouth in the area of the sublingual salivary gland should be approached cautiously. Lesions that are more posterior in the oral cavity are more difficult and more potentially dangerous to reach for a biopsy. It is important that the cutaneous surgeon recognize these limitations and refer these patients to oral surgeons or otolaryngologists for biopsies not easily performed with simple biopsy techniques.

Punch biopsy of gingival tissues may be necessary to differentiate between gingivitis and blistering disorders such as pemphigoid or Behçet's disease. The interdental papilla is a good location for this type of biopsy. The papilla between the incisors should be avoided, however, as they tend to heal more slowly than lateral sites. Simple oral biopsies offer quick and safe diagnosis of many oral disorders such as lichen planus, leukoplakia, squamous cell carcinoma, pemphigoid, and pigmented lesions. It is important that the cutaneous surgeon become comfortable and proficient with these type biopsies.

Biopsy of Pigmented Lesions

The appropriate biopsy method to diagnose cutaneous melanoma has been an area of controversy, despite the tremendous importance of performing a biopsy to confirm the possible presence of this malignancy. There is no place for shave biopsy of an irregularly pigmented lesion suspected of being a melanoma,[1, 16] for several reasons. If the biopsy is too superficial, a deeper melanoma may be missed and adequate measurement of the depth of invasion is impossible. Without viewing the full depth of the specimen, Spitz's nevus may be mistaken for a melanoma or vice versa. Another reason is the risk of the development of atypical histologic changes with benign pigmented lesions that recur.[29] The name "pseudomelanomas" has been coined for these lesions because of their alarming histologic appearance, similar to superficial spreading melanomas.[30] The use of Monsel's solution as a hemostatic agent after shave biopsies may further add to the dysplastic appearance of benign lesions.[29] Any regrowth of benign pigmented lesions after shave biopsy may lead to later unnecessary wide excision, with its attendant risks and morbidity.

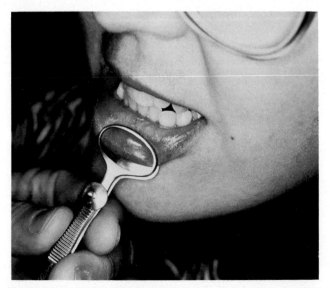

Figure 14–8. A chalazion clamp is positioned over the anticipated biopsy site on the lower lip.

Another area of controversy concerns whether an incisional biopsy is an appropriate way to diagnose melanoma. Those in favor of a primary excisional biopsy argue that the punch biopsy procedure may dislodge tumor cells and force melanoma cells deeper into the dermis or subcutaneous fat, or into the surrounding lymphatic or vascular structures, increasing the risk of metastatic spread.[31, 32] Theoretically, this might convert a Clark's level II melanoma into a level III or IV. This view has been criticized as being speculative with no evidence based on prospective controlled studies.[33] Other studies suggest that there is no difference in patient outcome regardless of the type of biopsy performed,[34] and many retrospective studies have been published that essentially agree with this view.[33] It has also been effectively argued that complete excision provides the pathologist with the best specimen for making an accurate diagnosis.[31]

To summarize, there are no clear-cut data to suggest the best type of biopsy to perform on suspicious pigmented lesions. Common sense can best assist the cutaneous surgeon with this problem. Lesions that are clinically very suspicious are probably best managed with initial total excision, if possible. Lesions that are of lower clinical suspicion or are found in areas where cosmesis is of great concern are probably best managed by a smaller, incisional punch biopsy. Regardless of the approach used, re-excision of biopsy-proved melanomas to obtain acceptable margins is always appropriate on the basis of pathologic examination.[35]

Postoperative Care

The postoperative care of wounds created by punch, shave, or scissors biopsy is essentially the same. The wound is cleaned with a 3% hydrogen peroxide solution to help remove dried blood and any debris from the wound site. This is followed by application of a thin coat of antibiotic ointment (Neosporin, Polysporin, or bacitracin) directly on the wound. This routine should be followed twice a day until the skin is completely reepithelialized. Studies have shown that Neosporin ointment increases reepithelialization of wounds by 25%.[36] Many patients have the misguided notion that the quick formation of a "scab" or eschar is good. However, a dried-out wound is more uncomfortable and heals more slowly than a wound kept moist with antibiotic ointment.[37]

Shave and punch biopsies are covered immediately after surgery with a simple Band-Aid dressing or gauze and paper tape. Small scissors biopsies may not require any dressings at all. If a dressing is used, it should be left in place for 24 to 36 hours. After this interval, dressing the wound is optional for most sites provided that the area is adequately covered with antibiotic ointment. Wounds exposed to constant friction such as beneath clothing, under eyeglasses, or on the feet or hands heal more quickly if kept covered. Patients may generally shower the day after simple skin biopsy; antibiotic ointment should be reapplied immediately after showering. If sutures have been used for wound closure, they may be removed 7 to 14 days after punch biopsy.

Surgical Complications

Unfortunately, complications may occur even with simple skin biopsies. Hemorrhage, infection, unsightly scar formation, slow-healing wounds, and pain are uncommon occurrences that the cutaneous surgeon must strive to avoid. Postoperative hemorrhage should not be a significant problem with minor skin biopsy. If a thorough medical history is taken, most patients who use anticoagulants or have an underlying coagulopathy can be readily determined. It is important to ask specifically about use of aspirin or over-the-counter nonsteroidal anti-inflammatory agents, since these drugs impair normal clotting. Small amounts of oozing may be noticed after the epinephrine has worn off or after inadvertent trauma, but firm pressure to these sites for 5 to 10 minutes should control this. It is useful to give patients preprinted instructions on how to handle postoperative bleeding and list of phone numbers to call if problems develop.

Good antiseptic technique helps to keep postbiopsy infection rates low. Factors that increase the risk of infection include shaving, distant infection elsewhere on the body, certain medications such as corticosteroids or immunosuppressive agents, and metabolic disorders such as renal or liver failure and diabetes.[38] Shave biopsies normally heal with a wound exudate that patients frequently mistake for infection. If there is any doubt about possible infection, the patient should be reexamined.

Scar formation is an inevitable part of many skin biopsies. Those areas of the skin that are exposed to greater stress from breathing or normal body movement, such as the chest and upper back, predictably heal with poor cosmetic scars. At suture removal, a typical wound will have only 3 to 5% of its original strength; this increases to 15 to 20% by 3 weeks and ultimately to 70 to 80% of original strength by 6 weeks.[38, 39] This may lead to scar spread and elevation. The absolute need for biopsy should be carefully assessed in patients with a history of keloid formation, and the least injurious technique possible should be used for performing the biopsy.

Pain from simple skin biopsies is usually minimal, but may become significant if a hematoma or wound infection develops. Patients need to know that simple biopsies do not typically require use of any type of analgesia postoperatively. However, any deviation from the normal course, including excess pain, should be reported to the cutaneous surgeon so that any possible complication related to the procedure can be determined.

SUMMARY

Simple skin biopsies are invaluable tools to the cutaneous surgeon. They may be performed quickly and safely while providing essential tissue for the diagnosis of a large variety of cutaneous disorders. The nature, location, and morphology of a cutaneous growth are all important factors in determining which type of biopsy to perform. Attention to the details of the procedure and technique helps keep complications to a minimum.

REFERENCES

1. Ackerman AB: Training residents in dermatopathology: why, when, where and how. J Am Acad Dermatol 22:1104–1106, 1990.
2. Maytin EV, Levine JD, Dover JS: Severe hemorrhage from a 4 mm punch biopsy site in a hemophilia patient with acquired immunodeficiency syndrome. J Am Acad Dermatol 21:1033–1034, 1989.
3. Miller HC, Dick PG, Stuart CW: Clinical and electrocardiographic findings following the use of various local anesthetic solutions. Anesth Analg 17:207–210, 1938.
4. Dzubow LM, Halpern AC, Leyden JJ, et al: Comparison of preoperative skin preparations for the face. J Am Acad Dermatol 19:737–741, 1988.
5. Grekin RC, Auletta MJ: Local anesthesia in dermatologic surgery. J Am Acad Dermatol 19:599–614, 1988.
6. Graham WP: Anesthesia in cosmetic surgery. Clin Plast Surg 10:285–287, 1983.
7. Robinson JK: Ask the experts. J Dermatol Surg Oncol 5:944–945, 1979.
8. Foster CA, Aston SJ: Propranolol-epinephrine interaction: a potential disaster. Plast Reconstr Surg 72:74–78, 1983.
9. Stewart JH, Cole GW, Klein JA: Neutralized lidocaine with epinephrine for local anesthesia. J Dermatol Surg Oncol 15:1081–1083, 1989.
10. Knowles WR: Minimizing pain due to local anesthesia. J Dermatol Surg Oncol 16:489, 1990.
11. Wall PD: The gate control theory of pain mechanisms: a re-examination and re-statement. Brain 10:1–18, 1978.
12. Robinson JK: Advantages and technique of inducing local anesthesia with small-bore angulated needle. J Dermatol Surg Oncol 5:465–466, 1979.
13. Ruzicka T, Gerstmeier M, Przybilla B, Ring J: Allergy to local anesthetics: comparison of patch test with prick and intradermal test results. J Am Acad Dermatol 16:1202–1208, 1987.
14. Incaudo G, Schatz M, Patterson R, et al: Administration of local anesthetics to patients with a history of prior adverse reaction. J Allergy Clin Immunol 61:339–345, 1978.
15. Wiener SG: Injectable sodium chloride as a local anesthetic for skin surgery. Cutis 23:342–343, 1979.
16. Ackerman AB: Shave biopsies: the good and right, the bad and wrong. Am J Dermatopathol 5:211–212, 1983.
17. Roenigk RK: Mohs micrographic surgery. Mayo Clin Proc 63:175–183, 1988.
18. Kopf AW, Popkin GL: Shave biopsies for cutaneous lesions. Arch Dermatol 110:637, 1974.
19. Bart RS, Kopf AW: Techniques of biopsy of cutaneous neoplasms. J Dermatol Surg Oncol 5:979–987, 1979.
20. Shelley WB: The razor blade in dermatologic practice. Cutis 16:843–845, 1975.
21. Larson PO: Topical hemostatic agents for dermatologic surgery. J Dermatol Surg Oncol 14:623–632, 1988.
22. Sawchuk WS, Friedman M, Manning T, et al: Delayed healing in full-thickness wounds treated with aluminum chloride solution. J Am Acad Dermatol 15:982–989, 1986.
23. Camisa C, Roberts W: Monsel solution tattooing. J Am Acad Dermatol 8:753–754, 1983.
24. Olmstead PM, Lund HZ, Leonard DD: Monsel's solution: a histologic nuisance. J Am Acad Dermatol 3:492–498, 1980.
25. Boughton RS, Spencer SK: Electrosurgical fundamentals. J Am Acad Dermatol 16:862–867, 1987.
26. Ackerman AB: Biopsy: why, where, when, how. J Dermatol Surg Oncol 1:21–23, 1975.
27. Lever WF, Schaumburg-Lever G (eds): Technic for Biopsy. In: Histopathology of the skin. JB Lippincott, Philadelphia, 1983, pp 1–2.
28. Headington JT: Transverse microscopic anatomy of the human scalp. Arch Dermatol 120:449–456, 1984.
29. Duray PH, Livolsi VA: Recurrent dysplastic nevus following shave excision. J Dermatol Surg Oncol 10:811–815, 1984.
30. Kornberg R, Ackerman A: Pseudomelanoma: recurrent melanocytic nevus following partial surgical removal. Arch Dermatol 111:1588–1590, 1975.
31. Rampen FHT, van der Esch EP: Biopsy and survival of malignant melanoma. J Am Acad Dermatol 12:385–388, 1985.
32. van der Esch EP, Rampen FHT: Punch biopsy of melanoma. J Am Acad Dermatol 13:899–902, 1985.
33. Chanda JJ, Callen JP: Adverse effect of melanoma incision. J Am Acad Dermatol 13:519–520, 1985.
34. Lederman JS, Sober AJ: Does biopsy type influence survival in clinical stage I cutaneous melanoma? J Am Acad Dermatol 13:983–987, 1985.
35. Zitelli J: Melanoma update. J Dermatol Surg Oncol 15:881–882, 1989.
36. Geronemus RG, Mertz PM, Eaglstein WH: Wound healing, the effects of topical antimicrobial agents. Arch Dermatol 115:1311–1314, 1979.
37. Harris DR: Healing of the surgical wound. J Am Acad Dermatol 1:197–207, 1979.
38. Salasche SJ: Acute surgical complications: cause, prevention, and treatment. J Am Acad Dermatol 15:1163–1185, 1986.
39. Clark RAF: Cutaneous tissue repair: basic biologic considerations. J Am Acad Dermatol 13:701–725, 1985.

CHAPTER 15

Proper Planning and Execution of Surgical Excisions

BARRY LESHIN

The simple fusiform (elliptical) excision is the cornerstone of cutaneous surgery. Proper planning of this procedure requires knowledge of superficial anatomy, awareness of many functional considerations of the head and neck, and, in the treatment of cutaneous malignancies, understanding of tumor biology. Although seemingly complicated, once the fundamentals have been learned, the fusiform excision is a relatively simple procedure that can be performed expeditiously while simultaneously providing an excellent cosmetic outcome. Vital to any surgical procedure is adequate preoperative evaluation.[1, 2] This evaluation must include patient assessment, consideration of risk factors for complications, and patient education.

Before excisional surgery is performed, adequate attention to superficial anatomy is imperative.[3, 4] This includes determining the favorable lines of closure, as well as evaluating the affected cosmetic subunits.

Planning the Ellipse

FAVORABLE LINES OF CLOSURE

One of the most important initial steps in planning the elliptical excision is determining proper orientation. More specifically, the ellipse should be designed so that the scar is least noticeable and not likely to affect function.[5-7] Orientation of an ellipse in the most favorable lines of excision yields not only a less conspicuous thin scar, but also one that heals faster and has a higher tensile strength. This will result in an incision line that runs parallel to imaginary lines known as maximal skin tension lines (MSTLs).[7] Typically, but not always, congruent with relaxed skin tension lines,[8-12] MSTLs conform to wrinkle lines and to folds resulting from

contraction of underlying muscles. Although numerous diagrams of these lines exist, there is considerable individual variation.

There are a variety of ways of making an assessment of the underlying MSTLs around a particular lesion. The simplest approach is to pinch the skin in all directions to determine where the tension on the skin is least. Maximal wrinkling occurs with pinching in the direction of the short axis of the planned excision. Alternatively, having the patient move the underlying muscles by grimacing or smiling may also unmask these lines. Finally, it may be best in some cases to simply excise the lesion as a circle rather than as an ellipse, undermine the wound margins, and observe the direction in which the wound assumes an oval shape. The oval configuration can then be converted to a fusiform ellipse for wound closure.[5, 13]

COSMETIC UNITS

When performing excisions on the face, it is critical that consideration be given to cosmetic units. Conceptually, the face can be subdivided into multiple topographic units. A scar confined to a single unit will ultimately be less conspicuous than one that crosses the boundary between two contiguous units.[6, 14] In many instances this principle takes priority over MSTLs or even the configuration of the lesion being removed. A longer scar contained within a single cosmetic subunit may be less conspicuous than a scar that crosses the boundary between two subunits.

NATURE OF LESION REMOVED

If the lesion being removed is benign, it is critical that the ultimate scar be less conspicuous than the lesion being removed and that the amount of normal tissue sacrificed be minimal. On the other hand, management of cutaneous malignancies adds an additional consideration to the proper planning of an ellipse.[9] First, it is imperative that an excision provide for the complete removal of the tumor. In addition, when excising a melanoma, attention should also be paid to the direction of draining lymph nodes. This is particularly important if a wider resection or subsequent regional lymphadenectomy might become necessary. An improperly oriented initial excision may ultimately mean the difference between primary closure or a wound graft after the definitive surgical procedure.[15]

The configuration of the lesion may be the key determinant of orientation of the ellipse. If the lesion being excised is oval in shape, then by placing the long axis of the ellipse parallel to the long axis of the lesion, the overall length of the scar will be shortened (Fig. 15–1). In some settings, this compromises the principle of keeping the scar within a single cosmetic unit, and the final analysis may depend on the orientation that yields the least noticeable scar.

FUNCTIONAL CONSIDERATIONS

When planning an excision, attention should also be given to important functional considerations.[6, 10, 14] Two examples of this include the need to avoid lower eyelid malposition when excising a lesion in the periorbital area and undesirable lip retraction with excisions in the perioral region. In a similar fashion, a fusiform excision that is placed in a skin crease on the forehead may inadvertently elevate the brow. Also, proper orientation of a fusiform excision on the extremities avoids contracture of an underlying joint.

DIMENSIONS

As a general rule, the length of a fusiform excision should be three times the width, but the ratio of length to width may vary from 3:1 to 4:1. The length of the short axis of the ellipse is predetermined by the size of the lesion being removed. For instance, a 4-mm malignant tumor to be excised with 3-mm margins will leave a short axis of 10 mm, and the long axis will be approximately 30 mm in length. It is important to recognize that even a proportionate and properly designed ellipse may produce a closure with small standing cones, or "dogears," at each pole that must be removed. It is also important to recognize that the inherent elasticity of the skin and the geometry of an ellipse make a 30-degree angle optimal for the tips of the ellipse.

MARGINS

No fail-safe guidelines exist for determining adequate margins. Obviously, the amount of normal tissue included in the excision of a benign lesion should be minimized. When excising a nonmelanoma malignant skin tumor, a very rough guideline of 3 to 4 mm of normal-appearing skin is typically recommended. The margins of resection for melanomas require special consideration.[9, 15, 16]

FUSIFORM EXCISION VARIATIONS

There are two very useful variations on the classic fusiform excision, the S-plasty and the crescentic excision. The S-plasty is a fusiform excision in which the two sides of the ellipse are "lazy Ss." The ultimate effect of an S-plasty is to increase the length of the scar between the two end points of the wound. This is particularly useful over convex surfaces such as the cheek or extremity in which horizontal contraction on the scar may result in a depressed scar. By lengthening the scar, the horizontal forces of contraction will pull and straighten the "S," rather than depress the scar (Fig. 15–2).[17]

The crescentic excision can be accomplished in two different ways. The simplest technique is to design the ellipse so that one side is substantially longer than the other. By then closing the defect using the "rule of halves," a slightly curved scar is produced.[18] Another means to achieve a gently curved scar that matches a curved line of facial expression is to create a "belly" in the midportion of the ellipse. This results in the wound having sides of equal length but in a configuration that yields a gentle curve to the ellipse.[19, 20]

SKIN PREPARATION AND MARKING THE ELLIPSE

Before designing and marking the proposed skin incision lines, it is desirable to clean the operative site with a detergent antiseptic surgical scrub. The incision lines may then be drawn using any of a variety of skin markers such as gentian violet, brilliant green, Bonney blue or Berwick's solution. These may be applied with a toothpick or a broken wooden applicator stick. Some surgeons favor a sterile surgical marking pen or a Sharpie permanent marker.[21] It is critical that the incision lines be drawn before injection of anesthetic, because vasoconstriction may substantially obscure the clinical clues that guide margin assessment and the anesthetic will distort the tissue.

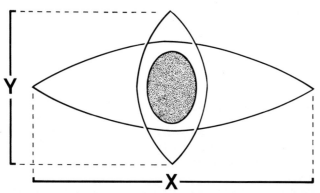

Figure 15–1. By orienting the ellipse so that the long axis of the lesion parallels the long axis of the ellipse, the length of the scar is significantly shorter (Y is much shorter than X).

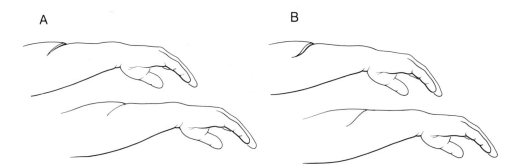

A   B

Figure 15–2. *A,* When a lesion is excised on a convex surface, scar contraction will result in a depressed scar. *B,* Scar contraction after S-plasty results in straightening of the S. (Modified from Zitelli JA: TIPS for a better ellipse. J Am Acad Dermatol 22:101–103, 1990.)

After marking the skin and infiltrating local anesthetic, the skin is then ideally repainted with an aqueous antiseptic surgical prep solution. Before incision, any residual surface wetness should be removed with a gauze sponge.

Removing the Specimen

Although seemingly simple, several aspects of specimen removal require close attention to provide the best cosmetic outcome.

AVOIDING CROSS-HATCHING

To avoid unnecessary injury, it is desirable that the tips of the ellipse meet at a fine point, without unnecessary extension of the incision beyond that point (Fig. 15–3).[7, 18] When using the standard No. 15 blade, the incision is initiated with the scalpel handle held perpendicular to the skin. After the incision is made, the scalpel handle is then gently tilted to a 45-degree angle for incising the remainder of the margin until the other tip is reached. At that point the blade is then returned to the perpendicular position. When performing very

small excisions, it is often advantageous to use a smaller blade such as a No. 15c or, alternatively, a No. 11 blade.

AVOIDING BEVELED EDGES

When incising the skin, it is preferable to make an incision perpendicularly through the dermis into the underlying subcutaneous fat[7, 18] (Fig. 15–4A). By so doing the wound margins will be more likely to evert appropriately for a cosmetically acceptable closure. If the edges are beveled inward, the base of the specimen can be compromised, bringing the resection margins unnecessarily close to the edges of the lesion being excised. In hair-bearing regions, it is preferable to angle the incision lines so that they are parallel to follicles (Fig. 15–4B)[5, 7, 18] to avoid follicle transection and permanent hair loss around the scar.

MINIMIZING PASSES THROUGH THE DERMIS

The amount of pressure or force used when incising the skin is learned only by experience. The force necessary to incise through the dermis obviously depends on the thickness of dermis. It is desirable to minimize the number of passes the scalpel makes through the dermis to avoid "staircasing" the wound margins (Fig. 15–5) and compromising the approximation of the edges.

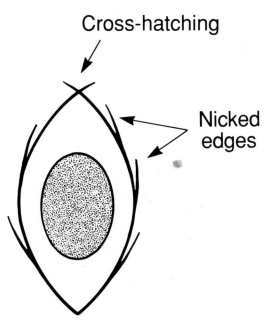

Cross-hatching

Nicked edges

Figure 15–3. Careful incision technique avoids cross-hatching the tips and nicking the wound edges.

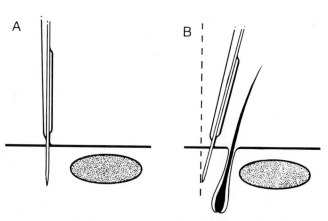

A   B

Figure 15–4. *A,* An incision is carried out perpendicular to the skin surface. *B,* In terminal hair-bearing skin, the incision is angled parallel to the hair follicles to avoid transection. (Modified from Swanson NA: Atlas of Cutaneous Surgery. Little, Brown, Boston, 1987, p 19.)

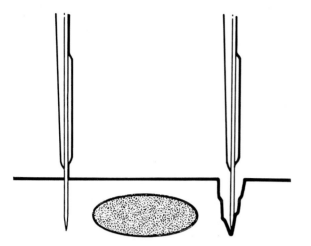

Figure 15–5. Minimizing passes through the dermis during incision avoids a staircased wound margin *(right)*.

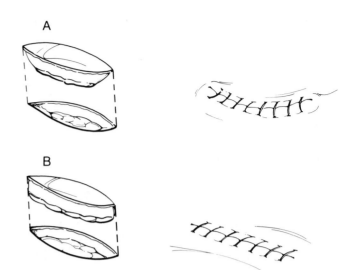

Figure 15–6. *A,* A boat-shaped specimen that leaves additional tissue at the wound tips may result in pseudo-dogears. *B,* A specimen of uniform thickness avoids this problem. (Modified from Zitelli JA: TIPS for a better ellipse. J Am Acad Dermatol 22:101–103, 1990.)

UNIFORM THICKNESS

There is a common tendency when removing an excisional specimen to reduce the amount of tissue removed at the two ends. This results in a boat-shaped specimen (Fig. 15–6). More importantly, the residual tissue left in the defect may cause protrusions at the two tips, creating "pseudo-dogears."[17] The assistant can put traction on the skin perpendicular to the direction of the incision to help provide a smooth contour to the incision, thereby decreasing the effort required to make the incision to the desired level. After careful incision, the base of the tissue can be transected at the desired depth with either a scalpel or scissors.

Undermining the Defect

BREADTH OF UNDERMINING

Undermining the defect after removal of the specimen minimizes tension on the wound margins, facilitates closure, avoids unnecessary vascular compromise, everts the wound margins, enhances the cosmetic outcome after scar contraction, and provides a horizontal scar plate to help minimize the spread of scars at sites of high wound tension.[7] Dead space can result from undermining that produces a seroma or hematoma. Some surgeons favor obliteration of this dead space,[22] although this is not imperative.[7]

The amount of tissue that needs to be undermined is that which is sufficient to allow minimal tension on the wound margins so they may be everted without compromising vascularity. It is important to undermine completely around the defect, including the two ends. By missing the two ends, these areas become unnecessarily tethered and may ultimately protrude upward with scar contraction (Fig. 15–7).[17]

DEPTH OF UNDERMINING

The recommended depth of undermining varies with the anatomic site. In general, undermining should be

carried out using blunt-tipped scissors as superficially as possible to avoid unnecessary damage to blood vessels and nerves. Undermining on the scalp is best carried out below the galea to avoid transection of hair follicles. The loose areolar tissue beneath the galea is an easily identified, bloodless plane, and the galea aponeurotica easily supports the suture tension required for closure of scalp wounds. The forehead is best undermined in the deep subcutaneous tissue, since deeper undermining threatens sensory innervation to the scalp. To avoid injury to the superficial motor nerves, undermining on the temple, cheeks, and chin should be carried out in the superficial subcutaneous tissue. On the trunk and extremities, undermining can be carried out at any level above the muscle fascia, the middle to deep subcutaneous adipose layers usually being optimal. At sites of minimal subcutaneous tissue, such as the hands and feet,

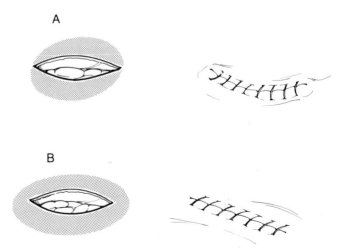

Figure 15–7. *A,* Failure to undermine the wound tips may result in tissue protrusion after closure. *B,* Undermining the tips avoids this problem. (Modified from Zitelli JA: TIPS for a better ellipse. J Am Acad Dermatol 22:101–103, 1990.)

undermining should be carried out just below the dermis.[7]

During undermining, it is also important that the wound margins be handled gently. Unnecessary crushing of the wound edges with serrated or multitoothed forceps may compromise the ultimate cosmetic outcome. The importance of handling the wound margins gently with forceps or a skin hook cannot be overstated.[23]

HEMOSTASIS

During incising and undermining of the skin, blood vessels are inevitably transected or nicked. To prevent hematoma formation, hemostasis should be achieved by clamping and ligating large vessels or by pinpoint electrocoagulation or electrodesiccation. It is also important to avoid excess electrosurgery, which results in the creation of nonvital, charred tissue that may impede wound healing or serve as a nidus for wound infection. Minor bleeding from transected dermal capillaries is effectively stopped by sutures used for wound closure.

Closure

SUTURE TECHNIQUES

Closure technique varies substantially from site to site and from patient to patient. For example, a wound in heavily sun-damaged skin on an elderly person's face might yield an excellent outcome with a running continuous 5-0 monofilament suture. However, the same wound in a younger individual might best be closed with a 6-0 polypropylene subcuticular suture. Whatever the patient setting, the closure technique—including wound closure materials, suture techniques, and timing of suture removal—should be modified to achieve a well-approximated, everted wound with minimal suture tracking. A variety of suture techniques (Fig. 15–8) may be useful in cutaneous surgery, with each having clear advantages and disadvantages.[18, 24–29]

Postoperative Care

DRESSING THE WOUND

After cleansing the skin surface immediately postoperatively to remove any dried blood or residual antiseptic, the wound dressing is applied. Typically, this consists of four layers: an occlusive antibacterial ointment, a nonadherent gauze material, an absorbent cushion to wick blood away from the wound, and tape.

Patients should be instructed to remove the postoperative pressure dressing after 24 to 48 hours, cleanse the wound surface with hydrogen peroxide, and reapply the occlusive ointment. This wound care is repeated two to three times daily until the sutures are removed. A light gauze dressing is optional depending on the site of the wound and need for a protective dressing.

SUTURE REMOVAL

The timing of epicutaneous suture removal is of critical importance. Obviously, sutures should be left in

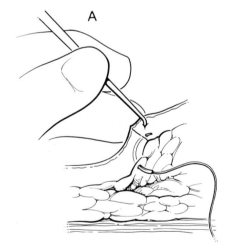
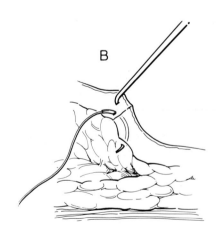
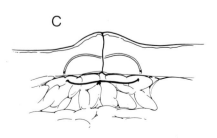

Figure 15–8. *A* to *C*, A buried vertical mattress suture produces prolonged eversion of the wound margin. (Modified by permission of the publisher from Zitelli JA, Moy RL: Buried vertical mattress suture. J Dermatol Surg Oncol 15:17–19, 1989. Copyright 1989 by Elsevier Science Publishing Co., Inc.)

long enough for epithelialization across the wound margins to be complete. However, they should be removed early enough to avoid unnecessary suture tracking. Typically, sutures are removed from the face at 7 days, although some surgeons favor earlier removal at 5 days. Suture removal on the trunk and extremities is usually performed at 10 to 14 days. Certainly there is significant individual variability in wound healing. For example, young, healthy, nonsmoking patients can have their sutures removed earlier than older, less healthy, smoking patients because of problems with delayed healing. To bolster the wound margins after suture removal, it is advisable to use wound closure tapes for 5 to 7 days.

Complications

Although complications are relatively infrequent in cutaneous surgery, they do occur.[30] It is imperative that patients be informed of the potential complications before surgery and educated as to how such complications might be manifested immediately after surgery. When problems are encountered, the surgeon must be able to recognize and manage them adeptly.

HEMATOMA

Hematomas typically occur during the first 48 to 72 hours after surgery and are manifested as swelling, erythema, and tenderness at the wound site. Hematomas should be evacuated early by partially or completely opening the wound, controlling any active bleeding, and, if treated within 48 to 72 hours of surgery, resuturing the wound. Alternatively, after evacuation of the hematoma, the open wound may be left to heal by second intention with scar revision performed at a later date, if necessary. In some instances, small hematomas may be managed conservatively with warm compresses until resolution occurs.

INFECTION

Infection is a rare event in cutaneous surgery, having a rate of occurrence of less than 1%.[31] When a wound is frankly infected, it is imperative that all sutures, including buried sutures, be removed and the patient begun on antibiotics. Consideration should be given to culturing an infected wound before initiating antibiotic therapy.

DEHISCENCE

Dehiscence is the easiest of the complications to recognize, since the wound pulls apart. If there is no underlying infection, the dehiscent wound can simply be resutured if dehiscence has occurred within 48 to 72 hours after surgery. Dehiscence is more typically a complication of an underlying wound infection or hematoma, and these underlying problems must obviously be managed first. A dehiscent wound can be allowed to heal by second intention with delayed scar revision performed later, if necessary.

NECROSIS

Wound necrosis after fusiform excisional biopsy is rare. It most typically occurs when a wound is closed under significant tension, which compromises the vascularity of the wound margins. In this setting, it is important to remove suture material, debride the necrotic tissue, and allow the wound to heal by second intention.

SUMMARY

The proper planning and execution of a surgical excision are of fundamental importance to the cutaneous surgeon. Essential ingredients of successful surgery include a mastery of a wide array of principles that involve anatomy, anesthesia, tumor biology, wound healing, and surgical technique. With attention to these details, this procedure can provide an exceptionally good cosmetic and functional result both safely and efficiently and can also yield an appropriate specimen for subsequent histologic analysis.

REFERENCES

1. Leshin B, McCalmont TH: Preoperative evaluation of the surgical patient. Dermatol Clin 8:787–794, 1990.
2. Leshin B, Whitaker DC, Swanson NA: An approach to patient assessment and preparation in cutaneous oncology. J Am Acad Dermatol 19:1081–1088, 1988.
3. Bernstein G: Surface landmarks for the identification of key anatomic structures of the face and neck. J Dermatol Surg Oncol 12:722–726, 1986.
4. Salasche SJ, Bernstein G, Senkarik M: Surgical Anatomy of the Skin. Appleton & Lange, East Norwalk, CT, 1988.
5. Spicer TE: Techniques of facial lesion excision and closure. J Dermatol Surg Oncol 8:551–556, 1982.
6. Webster RC, Smith RC: Cosmetic principles in surgery on the face. J Dermatol Surg Oncol 4:397–402, 1978.
7. Bennett RG: Fundamentals of Cutaneous Surgery. CV Mosby, St. Louis, 1988, pp 353–444.
8. Borges AF, Alexander JE: Relaxed skin tension lines. Z-plasties on scars, and fusiform excision of lesions. Br J Plast Surg 15:242–254, 1962.
9. Bart RS, Kopf AW: Techniques of biopsy of cutaneous neoplasms. J Dermatol Surg Oncol 6:979–987, 1979.
10. Bernstein L: Incisions and excisions in elective facial surgery. Arch Otolaryngol 97:238–243, 1973.
11. Courtiss EH: The placement of elective skin incisions. Plast Reconstr Surg 31:31–44, 1963.
12. Kneissel CJ: The selection of appropriate lines for elective surgical incisions. Plast Reconstr Surg 8:1–28, 1951.
13. Davis TS, Graham WP III, Miller SH: The circular excision. Ann Plast Surg 4:21–24, 1980.
14. Stegman SJ: Planning closure of a surgical wound. J Dermatol Surg Oncol 4:390–393, 1978.
15. Balch CM, Milton GW, Shaw HM, Seng-Jaw S: Cutaneous Melanoma. JB Lippincott, Philadelphia, 1985, pp 71–90.
16. Veronesi U, Cascinelli N, Adamus J, et al: Thin stage I primary cutaneous malignant melanoma: comparison of excision with margins of 1 or 3 cm. N Engl J Med 318:1159–1162, 1988.
17. Zitelli JA: TIPS for a better ellipse. J Am Acad Dermatol 22:101–103, 1990.
18. Swanson NA: Atlas of Cutaneous Surgery. Little, Brown, Boston, 1987.
19. Lapins NA: The crescentic ellipse revisited. J Dermatol Surg Oncol 14:935–936, 1988.
20. Manstein CH, Manstein ME, Manstein G: Creating a curvilinear scar. Plast Reconstr Surg 83:914–915, 1989.

21. Sebben JE: Sterile technique and the prevention of wound infection in office surgery—Part II. J Dermatol Surg Oncol 15:38–48, 1989.

22. Ocampo J, Camps A: The application of the tie-down suture to the excision of cutaneous tumors. J Dermatol Surg Oncol 14:1357–1360, 1988.

23. Popkin GL, Gibb RC: Another look at the skin hook. J Dermatol Surg Oncol 4:366–367, 1978.

24. Stegman SJ: Suturing techniques for dermatologic surgery. J Dermatol Surg Oncol 4:63–68, 1978.

25. Perry AW, McShane RH: Fine tuning of the skin edges in the closure of surgical wounds: controlling inversion and eversion with the path of the needle—the right stitch at the right time. J Dermatol Surg Oncol 7:471–476, 1981.

26. Robinson JK: Even coaptation of wound edges of unequal thicknesses or unequal heights. J Dermatol Surg Oncol 5:844, 1979.

27. Coldiron BM: Closure of wounds under tension: the horizontal mattress suture. Arch Dermatol 125:1189–1190, 1989.

28. Zitelli JA, Moy RL: Buried vertical mattress suture. J Dermatol Surg Oncol 15:17–19, 1989.

29. Bennett RG: Selection of wound closure materials. J Am Acad Dermatol 18:619–637, 1988.

30. Salasche SJ: Acute surgical complications: cause, prevention, and treatment. J Am Acad Dermatol 15:1163–1185, 1986.

31. Whitaker DC, Grande DJ, Johnson SS: Wound infection rate in dermatologic surgery. J Dermatol Surg Oncol 14:525–528, 1988.

CHAPTER 16

Simple Suturing Techniques and Knot Tying

PETER B. ODLAND and CRAIG S. MURAKAMI

The skill and art of suturing date back thousands of years to the Smith Papyrus.[1] Although techniques and materials have changed, the fundamental reasons for using sutures have not. In cutaneous surgery, sutures should be used for gentle closure of wounds until the tissues re-establish their inherent tensile strength. This should be done in a way that promotes a functional and aesthetic outcome while minimizing the risks of both acute and late complications. The old adage "approximation without strangulation" clearly states the most important point about proper suturing technique.

Suturing is defined as the "surgical uniting of two surfaces by means of stitches."[2] Suturing is an incredibly simple concept, yet correct application requires a high level of concentration, attention to detail, and discipline. An understanding of basic wound healing, the nature of suture materials, and general principles regarding excision and closure of wounds are all very important to obtaining a satisfactory outcome. Failure to recognize these important concepts will yield surgical results that are less than adequate, thereby frustrating both the surgeon and the patient and making the entire experience unsatisfying and unrewarding.

Basic Terms and Concepts

MATERIALS AND INSTRUMENTS

The suture needle[3] most commonly used in cutaneous surgery can be subdivided into several parts. The tip is a fine, delicate point used to penetrate tissue surfaces. The swage is where the needle is clamped to the suture material; this represents the broadest point of the entire suture. The remaining portion, where the needle is grasped with instruments, is the body. The basic instru-ments used in cutaneous suturing include a needle driver (holder), tissue forceps, and skin hooks.

The standard needle holder has a ratchet-type locking mechanism that stabilizes the needle securely in the jaws. When a needle is in the jaws, one should avoid locking beyond the first snap. Locking the needle be-yond this position causes flattening of the needle and "denting" the opposing surfaces of the jaws of the instrument. This frequently results in slippage of fine suture materials during subsequent use.

Tissue forceps with fine teeth allow for gentle handling and stabilization of the tissues being sutured and for grasping the emerging needle tip during suturing. How-ever, if they are not used carefully and gently, trauma to the wound edge may occur and compromise wound healing. Alternatively, a skin hook can be used to stabilize tissue and, in skilled hands, is less traumatic to soft tissue than forceps.

The needle holder should be grasped with the thumb and ring finger in the loops of the instrument (Fig. 16–1A). The tip of the first finger is extended and rests on the arms of the instrument at or near the hinge, while the middle finger flexes gently to secure the base of the loop (Fig. 16–1B, C). None of the fingers are inserted past the first knuckle to allow maximum dexterity and rotation. Some surgeons choose to "palm" the needle holder and avoid placing fingers in the loops altogether (Fig. 16–1D). Both techniques can be learned and used effectively, although it is normal to feel awkward when using either technique initially. A great deal of practice is necessary before one becomes facile in the use of these techniques. Forceps should be held somewhat like a pencil, but this may vary depending on the particular use.

A skin hook can be effectively held between the

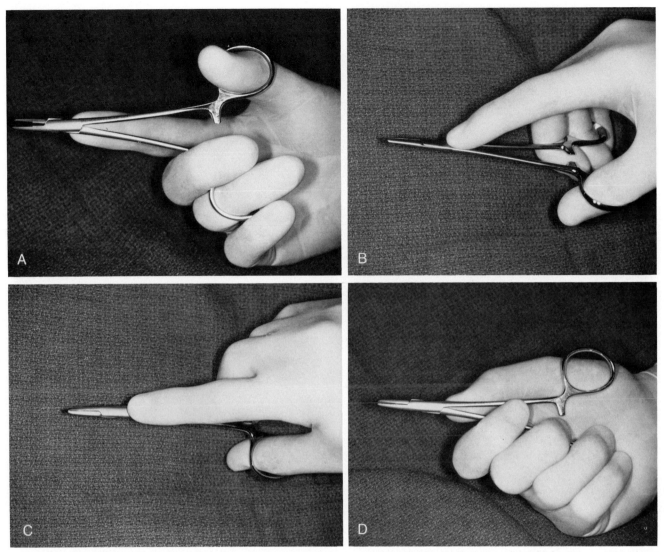

Figure 16–1. Technique for grasping the needle holder. *A,* Fingering the instrument. *B,* Supporting the instrument at the fulcrum (oblique view). *C,* Supporting the instrument at the fulcrum (vertical view). *D,* Palming the instrument.

thumb and the first finger.[4] "Choking" up on the handle nearer to the hook will allow for more accurate handling of the instrument by the surgeon.

NEEDLE AND INSTRUMENT PLACEMENT AND ORIENTATION

The needle must be placed in the needle driver at the end of the jaws with proper orientation. This will achieve optimum utilization of the instrument. Correct placement of the needle toward the end of the jaws allows for greater accuracy and precision in suturing. Furthermore, because the surface area at the end of the jaws is smaller, there is less chance of crushing the needle and flattening its curve. Orientation in the vertical axis (tilt) and along the longitudinal axis of the needle driver (twist) must be exact (Fig. 16–2). Failure to properly orient the needle will prevent effective advancement of the needle through tissue. Positioning the needle in the jaws of the needle driver ideally is done with a forceps.

At first it may be a frustrating technique, but mastering it will minimize the risk of needle sticks and with experience will actually reduce operating time. Most surgeons place the needle holder one half[1, 5] to three fourths[6] of the way from the tip to the swage on the body of the needle. Placement closer to the tip may limit advancement of the needle through the full thickness of the skin being sutured, while placement closer to the swage frequently results in bending of the needle. If a needle is unnecessarily bent several times, it becomes weakened to the point where it may break.

SUTURING STEPS

Proper wound closure requires precise suture placement to re-establish the original anatomic configuration of the various skin components (Fig. 16–3). The needle should always penetrate the surface perpendicularly to obtain ideal wound edge approximation with mild eversion (Fig. 16–4*A*). The needle tip is the sharpest point.

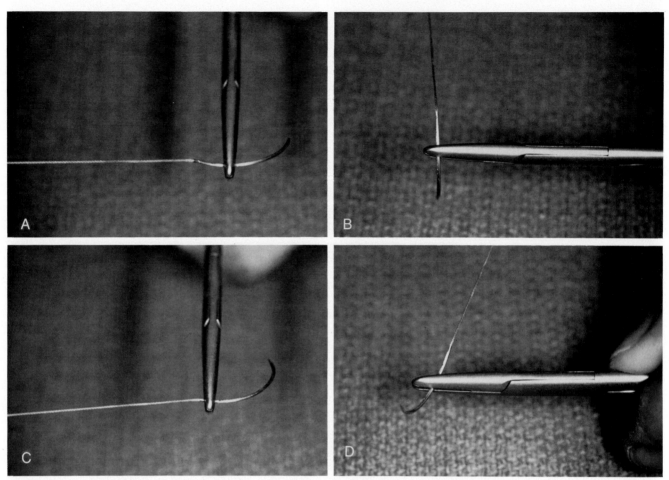

Figure 16–2. Placement of the needle in the needle holder. *A,* Correct placement at the proximal flat portion of the needle body. *B,* The needle is oriented perpendicularly to the holder. *C,* Incorrect placement at the rounded hub or swaged portion of the needle. *D,* The needle can be misplaced in the needle holder by a tilting or twisting movement.

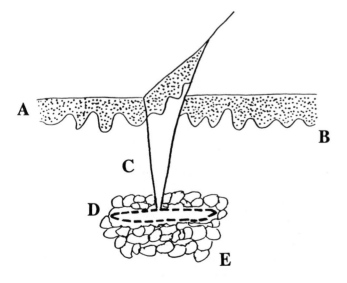

Figure 16–3. Cutaneous wound anatomy. A, Epidermal layer. B, Papillary dermal layer. C, Reticular dermal layer. D, Undermining plane. E, Subcutaneous fat layer.

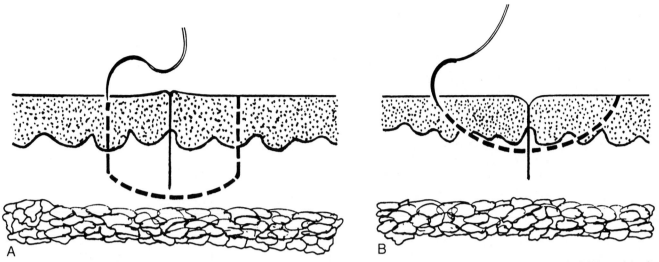

Figure 16–4. Needle penetration. *A,* Correct technique with square or flask-shaped passage through tissue. *B,* Incorrect superficial, semicircular passage through tissue.

Its effectiveness in overcoming the resistance of initial penetration is reduced if the needle is introduced tangentially. In addition, a superficial wound will be larger and more visible (Fig. 16–4*B*). The point of penetration should be mentally selected very carefully before applying pressure with the needle. Selection of this point depends on the type of suturing technique being used and the spacing between sutures. Unnecessary punctures are always undesirable and will result in excessive tissue trauma. As increasing pressure is applied, the initial resistance to penetration will result in a temporary depression of the surface of the skin. The depth of this depression depends on the anatomic area, the laxity of the skin, and the size and tip design of the needle being used. With increasing pressure, the resistance suddenly ceases, and needle penetration occurs. The suddenness of this penetration may be somewhat startling to inexperienced surgeons and may result in a reflexive withdrawal of the needle. For this reason, stabilizing the needle-driving hand on the patient or with the surgeon's opposite hand may be helpful. After initial penetration, the needle should be driven to the appropriate depth for the particular stitch being used. The next movement is a twisting one, with the needle driver being rotated around its long axis. This advances the curved needle in a horizontal plane so that the tip emerges in the defect at the desired depth. The tip of the needle is then gently but securely grasped with fine forceps or stabilized with a skin hook. The latter may be slightly more difficult. However, by placing the hook deep to the needle, the needle can be stabilized by pulling up gently at the point where it emerges from the tissue. Rotating the hook may provide even more stability by capturing the needle in the opposing end of the semicircular arc of the hook.

The needle should be released from the jaws of the needle driver without moving the needle itself. If the amount of tissue through which the needle has passed is large, then securing the needle or surrounding tissue with forceps or a skin hook is important and will prevent backward retraction of the needle into the tissue. The needle should be grasped with the needle driver, with close attention paid to the tilt and twist of the needle at the tip of the jaws. By rotating the needle driver in the same arc as the needle, the rest of the needle will emerge from the tissue and the attached suture material will follow. The needle must be repositioned in the jaws of the needle driver in preparation for penetrating the deep tissue of the opposing wound edge. For correct vertical and horizontal alignment of the wound edges, the needle must penetrate the opposing side at precisely the same depth as the side from which it emerged (Fig. 16–5*A*). A completed knot should provide a level surface with a symmetric, small amount of eversion of the edges. The sides of the wound should be well aligned so that redundant tissue does not develop at the end of the incision line and cause vertical or horizontal malalignment (Fig. 16–5*B*). To accomplish this, the opposing wound edge is gently stabilized with forceps or skin hook for penetration into the deep tissue. Resistance will generally be less than was encountered at the surface of the skin. After introduction and advancement of the needle into the tissue horizontally, rotation will direct the tip of the needle through the surface of the skin. This should be at a point that is equidistant from the wound edge when compared with the opposite side.

These very basic steps apply to almost all suturing techniques. Modifications in suture orientation and the type of material used can produce a variety of desired effects.

Simple Suturing Techniques

The most important basic principles in suturing include gentle handling of tissue at all times, using appropriate instrumentation, and always burying dermal or subcutaneous sutures when closing a wound that is under tension.[7]

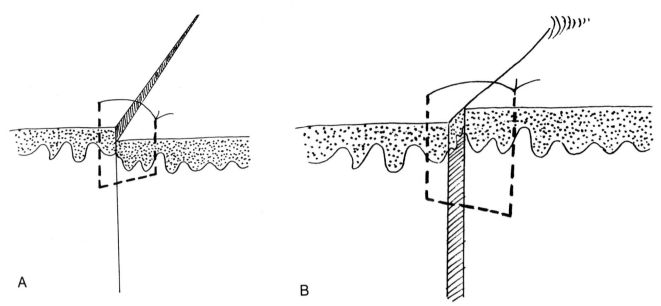

Figure 16–5. Alignment of wound edges. *A,* Vertical malalignment. *B,* Horizontal malalignment.

SIMPLE INTERRUPTED SUTURE

The simple interrupted suture is undoubtedly the most commonly used suturing technique because of its versatility and relative ease of use. The technique for employing this stitch to evert the wound edge requires that the needle enter the skin at a 90-degree angle[8] approximately 1 to 2 mm from the wound edge.[1] After penetration, the needle should be redirected to proceed in a slightly oblique fashion away from the wound edge to the desired depth and then across to the other side of the wound, where its course should follow a mirror image of the first side. This can be facilitated by grasping the deep tissue with forceps, then passing the needle through the skin.[9] Either of these techniques should create a loop that encircles a broader base of tissue at its depth than at the surface so that the outline of the suture pathway looks somewhat like a flask (Fig. 16–6A). Eversion of the wound edges is a result of a greater amount of tissue being pushed together deeply, causing the surface to be displaced (Fig. 16–6B). Eversion is desirable, because wounds contract as they heal. The vertical component of this contracture may result in a depressed scar at the suture line if the edges are not initially everted.[7, 10–12]

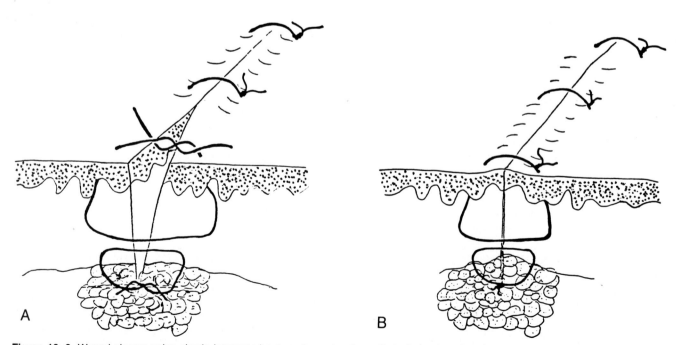

Figure 16–6. Wound closure using simple interrupted sutures in conjunction with buried suture (nearly reapproximated wound) *(A). B,* Final appearance of the approximated wound.

In some anatomic areas, inversion of the wound edges may be desirable. When this is the case, passage through the tissue is just the opposite of the eversion stitch, with the suture pathway encircling more tissue superficially than at the depth.[11] This is accomplished by penetrating the skin perpendicularly, as always, and then directing the needle obliquely toward the wound edge. Exiting the tissue through the other side of the defect is again done in a mirror-image fashion. It should also be noted that the suture loop must be placed in such a way that it is wider than it is deep.

The advantages of the simple interrupted stitch are multiple and include the following:

1. It is useful for making gross or minute adjustments to the wound edges for proper alignment and tension.[7]
2. It is easy to perform.
3. It allows expression of serum or blood from between sutures.[13]
4. It is useful for approximating both large and small amounts of tissue.
5. It is helpful as a tacking stitch for flaps or large irregular wounds.[7]
6. It has greater security than a running stitch.[14]

If the basic requirements of suturing are observed and practiced, it is unlikely that a simple interrupted stitch will cause any problems. However, if placed incorrectly or inappropriately, these sutures can cause wound inversion, which in the vast majority of cases is undesirable. The principal disadvantage of this stitch is "railroad track," or cross-hatch, scarring. This can be avoided by removing sutures before 7 days or by using a more advanced suturing technique such as a running subcuticular technique. Also, compared with the running stitch, this suture is a time-consuming way to close a wound.[7]

BURIED ABSORBABLE SUTURE

There are essentially three variations of buried absorbable sutures that are used in surgery of the skin: subcutaneous (Fig. 16–7A), dermal-subdermal, and dermal (Fig. 16–7B). Buried sutures are primarily used to close any dead space that may have been produced by the surgical excision, to reapproximate the wound edges, and to help prevent wound dehiscence. Buried sutures are especially important to use if a wound has been closed under significant tension. In this situation cutaneous surgeons try to prevent epithelialization of the suture tracks by removing the nonabsorbable epidermal stitches within 7 to 10 days. However, this removal occurs at a time when the wound has developed very little tensile strength (Fig. 16–8) and is highly susceptible to separation.[15] By using buried sutures, especially if their composition gives them a relatively long half-life, wound integrity will be maintained even if the epidermal sutures are removed. The buried sutures are usually oriented vertically but can also be oriented horizontally.[1, 7, 8, 11, 13, 16] Placement of buried sutures generally follows adequate undermining and hemostasis. The type of buried suture used depends on the thickness of the defect, the tension on the wound, and the amount of dead space.[17] A relatively broad excursion of the needle is required to pass the suture through enough fibrous septae to maintain security. Small "bites" often tear through the subcutaneous tissue as they are being tightened. It should always be kept in mind that it is particularly easy to strangulate subcutaneous tissue. There is no significant advantage to burying the knot for this stitch (see Fig. 16–7A).

The dermal-subdermal stitch[16] is passed first through the deep side of one of the undermined edges of the defect so that the suture pathway is through a small

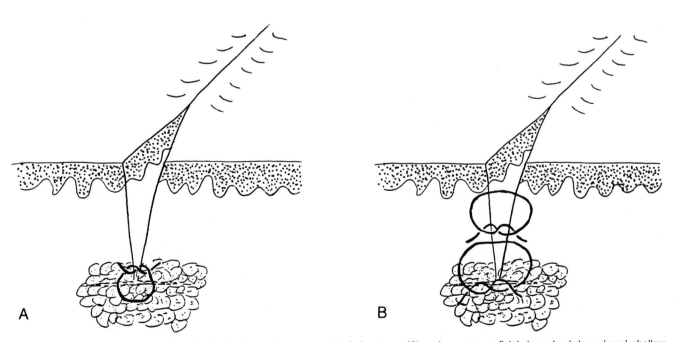

A   B

Figure 16–7. Full-thickness wound closed with deep subcutaneous buried sutures *(A)* and more superficial dermal-subdermal and shallow dermal sutures *(B)*. Note that these knots are always buried as deeply as possible in tissue.

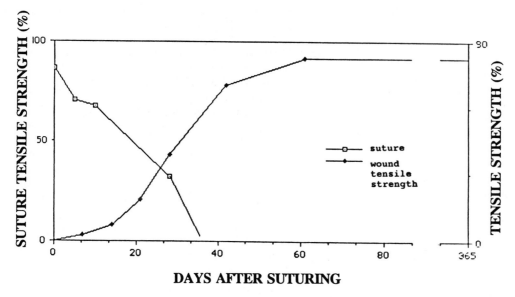

Figure 16–8. Wound tensile strength compared with suture tensile strength.

amount of both subcutaneous and dermal tissue. If the dermis is thick, it is unnecessary to bury the knot. This suture is necessarily vertically oriented. As the name implies, the dermal stitch is placed exclusively within the dermis. For relatively thin skin, the wound edge is reflected to expose the undermined surface of the dermis. The needle penetrates this surface 2 to 5 mm away from the wound edge and is directed obliquely toward the edge and the surface such that the epidermal edges will be everted. With few exceptions, the knot should be buried (Fig. 16–7*B*), which is accomplished by passing the stitch from deep to superficial and then from superficial to deep. Occasionally a fine, horizontally oriented, absorbable dermal suture can be placed. The utility of such a stitch to relieve tension at the surface must be balanced against the risk of suture abscess or tattooing.

A multilayered deep closure is required in the case of a full-thickness wound. First the deep fascial and muscular tissues are approximated with buried sutures. Then, in a layered fashion, the subcutaneous tissue and superficial layers of the dermis are closed. If a significant amount of tension is anticipated, a dermal-subdermal suture should be used, but if there is no tension, a dermal stitch should be used.

Buried sutures are very useful for relieving tension in wounds, closing dead space, and ensuring proper realignment of anatomic layers. There are very compelling reasons to use buried stitches in nearly all full-thickness cutaneous surgery; noted exceptions are wounds that are without tension and some selected procedures on thin-skinned areas of the body such as the eyelids. The tensile strength of a wound at the time of suture removal is less than 5% of what it ultimately will be. Without deep suture reinforcement, the risk of wound dehiscence after suture removal is great. In addition, ideally placed deep sutures will appose the skin edges so well that fewer skin stitches will be required, yielding a better cosmetic result.[1]

Although there are both theoretical and real disadvantages to using deep sutures, the benefits generally outweigh them. The potential pitfalls of buried sutures include possible strangulation and necrosis of tissue, promotion of infection, and prolonged inflammation as the result of the presence of foreign material.[17]

Difficulties encountered in placement of buried sutures often result from the small working area. Ideally, the first stitch is placed in the exact middle of the two sides of the wound. This is possible in most instances by having an assistant gently, physically coapt the edges of the wound as the first two throws of a knot are secured. When tension on the wound is great, an alternative technique is to begin the deep closure at one of the apices of the wound. However, there is a potential problem in this situation: by the time the opposite apex is reached, the sides may have become unequal in length, requiring a redundant tissue repair.[1, 7, 8, 11, 13, 16]

Knots

There are many knot configurations used to approximate soft tissues. In selecting suture material and knot types, it must be remembered that the ultimate goal of suturing is to provide adequate approximation of the tissues with the least amount of trauma and inflammation. Thus, the surgeon selects a suture material with an appropriate tissue half-life and knots that will be secure long enough to keep the wound approximated until adequate intrinsic tensile strength has been established. The larger the suture diameter and knot volume, the greater the risk of tissue inflammation and infection.[18] On the other hand, choosing suture or knots that are too weak for a given wound will result in wound dehiscence and surgical complications. Studies have shown that the security of a knot is related to the surface coefficient of friction[19, 20] and the stiffness of the suture material.

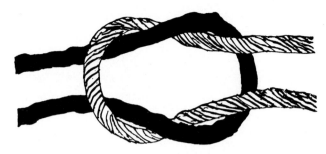

Figure 16–9. Square knot.

SQUARE KNOT

The most common knot used is the square knot. In optimal circumstances this knot will provide 80 to 90% of the tensile strength of an intact suture. When examining a square knot, it can be seen that each strand begins and ends on the same side of the knot (Fig. 16–9). Because of its symmetric design, it tends to tighten and remain secure when tension is applied equally to both strands. However, this is somewhat dependent on the type of suture material being used. Some suture materials are too slippery and will not hold with a simple square knot. Sutures are often coated with silicone or wax to allow easier passage through the soft tissues, but this decreases the holding capacity of the knot.[21] In addition, suture material becomes more slippery when covered with blood and serum. If the knot is not placed flat or if the tension on each strand is uneven, the square knot twists into a half-hitch knot, which slides and is extremely unstable.[22] For this reason, the square knot is usually reinforced with an additional throw, and with slippery materials such as monofilament nylon, two to three extra throws may be necessary.

SURGEON'S KNOT

Many surgeons prefer the surgeon's knot, which is a double throw followed by a single throw in parallel, as in the square knot (Fig. 16–10). Like the square knot, the surgeon's knot is usually reinforced with an additional throw. The initial double throw provides increased friction to hold the wound together until the second throw can be placed. This is especially helpful in closing wounds that are under mild tension. A triple throw can also be placed to provide even more tension. However,

if this becomes necessary, tension on the wound may be sufficient to warrant use of other measures to reduce the tension.

INSTRUMENT TIE

Closure of soft tissue defects in cutaneous surgery is usually accomplished using an instrument tying technique. The two-handed tie technique that is often seen in a general surgical practice is rarely used for soft tissue surgery of the skin. Instrument tying is quick, effective, easy to perform, and suture sparing (Fig. 16–11). To use the instrument technique to tie a square knot or a surgeon's knot, the needle is first passed through the tissue. This task is completed when the suture is pulled through the wound until 2 to 3 cm of tail suture remains. Leaving a longer tail results in cumbersome aggravation and unnecessary suture wastage. Starting with the needle holder between the two strands of suture, the holder is rotated clockwise around the suture, the short end of the suture is clamped, and the knot is placed flat across the wound by crossing the hands. The second throw is begun by again placing the needle holder between the two strands, but this time the holder is rotated counterclockwise around the suture and the throw placed flat by crossing the hands in the reverse direction. The needle holder always rotates around the suture; the suture does not rotate around the needle holder, as this technique is cumbersome, time consuming, and distracts attention from the tail of the suture. When the second throw is placed, it is important to be especially careful not to overtighten the knot and strangulate the wound. Some surgeons prefer to place a second double throw to stabilize the knot (Fig. 16–12). Poor technique will lead to pressure necrosis and prominent suture marks.

Figure 16–10. Surgeon's knot.

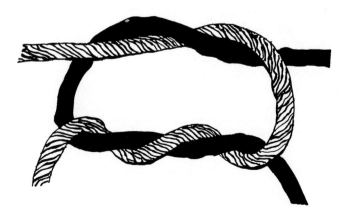

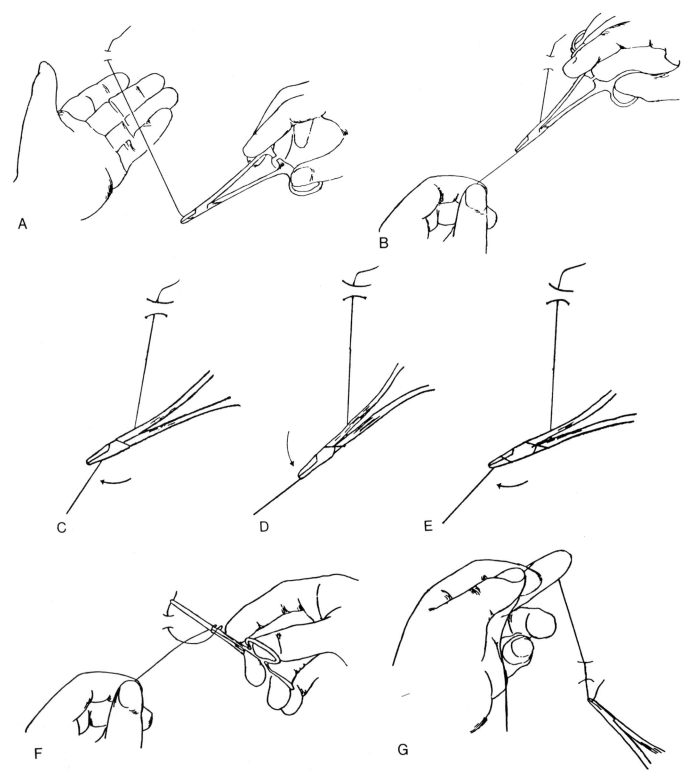

Figure 16–11. Instrument knot-tying technique. *A,* Needle is regrasped after first passing through tissue. *B,* Initiating the surgeon's knot. *C,* First wrap of suture is made around needle holder. *D,* Initiating the second wrap. *E,* Completing the second wrap. *F,* Preparing to make the first (forehand) throw. *G,* Completing the first throw. (Courtesy of Dr. T. McCulloch.)

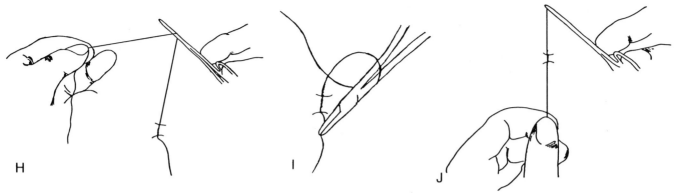

H, I, J

Figure 16–11 *Continued H,* Initiating the second (backhand) throw. *I,* Grasping the free end of the suture to complete the second throw. *J,* Completing the second throw of a surgeon's knot. (Courtesy of Dr. T. McCulloch.)

Instrument tying is easy and quick if the surgeon concentrates on conserving motion and eliminating extraneous maneuvers. As with most other surgical procedures, suturing should be a smooth flow of progressive steps that proceed in an accurate, logical, and rapid manner.

If the needle holder is not alternately rotated in a clockwise and then a counterclockwise direction, a "granny" knot is created. This type of knot slips more than the square knot and is therefore less desirable. Simple placement of additional throws will help secure this knot, but it is preferable to develop a consistent tying technique that results in predictably more reliable and secure square knots.

If the hands are not alternately crossed with each throw, a sliding knot is created (Fig. 16–13). For thick wounds under tension, such as scalp defects, this knot allows the suture to slide and tighten, much like a lasso does around a post. To secure this knot, two or three additional throws must be placed, depending on the suture being used.[23, 24] This increases the overall volume of the knot and increases the risk of inflammation and infection when this knot is used subcutaneously.[18, 23]

In cutaneous soft tissue surgery, the subcutaneous suture bears the majority of the tension. There should be minimal or zero tension on the epithelial edges if optimal results are to be obtained. If there is no tension on the epithelial margins, one may use surface-supporting tape strips or a knot technique that is tension free. The Straith loop, one such knot, is a double throw followed by a small 4 to 5-mm gap and secured with a square knot. The advantages of this knot are that it prevents postoperative edema from strangulating the wound around the suture, it prevents overtightening the second throw, and it makes suture removal easier. Simply cutting the base of the loop allows atraumatic removal of fine suture. If the wound is free of tension, the surgeon can also use an interlocking slip knot.[25]

Once the cutaneous knots are placed, they should be moved to one side or the other and not left directly over the wound. This prevents the tails of the suture from becoming imbedded in the wound and allows easier access and removal.[26] The knot should also be placed away from structures that might become irritated (e.g., the eyes and nose) and away from the edges of a flap.[27]

SUMMARY

A variety of wound healing studies[28, 29] have shown the importance of using meticulous technique in performing simple knot tying for wound closure. Despite the apparent simplicity of the technique, knowledge of

Figure 16–12. Double surgeon's knot.

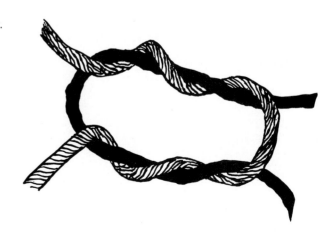

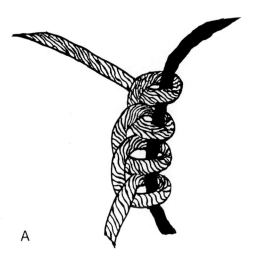

A

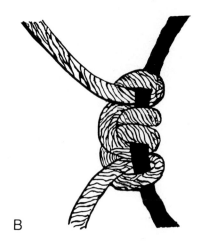

B

Figure 16–13. Two different types of sliding knots.

suture materials, needles, and different types and uses of various knots[30] is vital to a good outcome in all cases.

REFERENCES

1. Bennett RG: Fundamentals of Cutaneous Surgery. CV Mosby, St Louis, 1988, pp 382.
2. Stedman's Medical Dictionary. 23rd ed. Williams & Wilkins, Baltimore, 1976.
3. Trier WC: Considerations in the choice of surgical needles. Surg Gynecol Obstet 149:84–94, 1979.
4. Popkin GL, Gibbs RC: Another look at the skin hook. J Dermatol Surg Oncol 4:366–368, 1978.
5. White JH, Stern RU: A theoretical consideration of suturing technique. Ann Opthalmol 3:509, 1971.
6. Holt GR, Holt JE: Suture materials and technique. Ear Nose Throat J 60:12, 1981.
7. Stegman SJ: Suturing techniques for dermatologic surgery. J Dermatol Surg Oncol 4:63–68, 1978.
8. Jankauskas S, Cohen IK, Grabb W: Basic techniques of plastic surgery. In: Smith J, Aston S (eds): Plastic Surgery. Little, Brown, Boston, 1991.
9. Dushoff IM: A stitch in time. Emerg Med 1:16, 1973.
10. Lober CW: Suturing techniques. In: Roenigk RK, Roenigk HH Jr (eds): Dermatologic Surgery. Marcel Dekker, New York, 1989, pp 205–217.
11. McCarthy JG: Introduction to plastic surgery. In: McCarthy JG (ed): Plastic Surgery. WB Saunders, Philadelphia, 1990, pp 1–68.
12. Zitelli JA: TIPS for a better ellipse. J Am Acad Dermatol 22:101–103, 1990.
13. Chang W: Wound management. In: Chang W (ed): Fundamentals of Plastic and Reconstructive Surgery. Williams & Wilkins, Baltimore, 1980.
14. Stephenson KL: Suturing. Surg Clin North Am 57:863–873, 1977.
15. Odland PB, Whitaker DW: Wound dehiscence. In: Salasche SJ, Whitaker DW, Zitelli JA (eds): Complications in Cutaneous Surgery. WB Saunders, Philadelphia. In press.
16. Albom MJ: Dermo-subdermal sutures for long, deep surgical wounds. J Dermatol Surg Oncol 3:504–505, 1977.
17. Milewski PJ, Thomson H: Is a fat stitch necessary? Br J Surg 67:393–394, 1980.
18. Elek SD, Conen PE: The virulence of *Staphlyococcus pyogenes* for man: a study of the problems of wound infection. Br J Exp Pathol 38:573, 1957.
19. Gupta BS: Effect of suture material and construction on frictional properties of sutures. Surg Gynecol Obstet 161:12–16, 1985.
20. Taylor FW: Surgical knots. Ann Surg 107:458–468, 1938.
21. Becker J, Davidoff MR: The physical properties of suture materials as related to knot holding. S Afr J Surg 15:105–113, 1977.
22. Flinn RM: Knotting in medicine and surgery. Practitioner 183:322–328, 1959.
23. Trimbos JB, Brohim R, van Rijssel EJC: Factors relating to the volume of surgical knots. Int J Gynecol Obstet 30:355–359, 1989.
24. van Rijssel EJC, Brand D, Admiraal C, et al: Tissue reaction and surgical knots: the effect of suture size, knot configuration, and knot volume. Obstet Gynecol 74:64–68, 1989.
25. van Rijssel EJC, Trimbos JB, Booster MH: Mechanical performance of square knots and sliding knots in surgery: a comparative study. Am J Obstet Gyncol 162:93–97, 1990.
26. Noe JM: Where should the knot be placed? Ann Plast Surg 5:145, 1980.
27. Lucid ML: The interlocking slip knot. Plast Reconstr Surg 34:200, 1964.
28. Ordman LJ: Studies in the healing of cutaneous wounds. Arch Surg 93:883–910, 1966.
29. Vistnes LM: Basic principles of cutaneous surgery. In: Epstein E, Epstein E Jr (eds): Skin Surgery. WB Saunders, Philadelphia, 1987, pp 44–55.
30. Trimbos JB, van Rijssel EJC, Klopper PJ: Performance of sliding knots in monofilament and multifilament suture material. Obstet Gynecol 68:425–430, 1986.

CHAPTER 17

Hemostatic Techniques and Materials

WILLIAM J. GRABSKI and STUART J. SALASCHE

The precise control of bleeding is paramount to performing complication-free surgery. Many hemostatic agents and methods are available to the cutaneous surgeon, and each has its own particular set of advantages and disadvantages and applications in specific situations. While no ideal hemostatic method or material currently exists, some desirable characteristics include minimal tissue damage, convenience and ease of use, low cost, and biodegradability.[1]

During cutaneous surgery the most common and useful methods to obtain hemostasis include the use of epinephrine in the local anesthetic, application of pressure to the bleeding site, ligation of the larger vessels, application of an escharotic agent such as aluminum chloride, electrocoagulation or electrodesiccation, and compression dressings.

Some of the more expensive and cumbersome topical hemostatic agents, such as topical thrombin, oxidized cellulose, an absorbable gelatin sponge, a collagen hemostatic sponge, and fibrin glue, have limited application in cutaneous surgery but may be useful in some select situations. For example, they may be beneficial in neurosurgery in which it is necessary to control diffuse bleeding from multiple vessels on the extremely delicate surface of the brain or the dura mater.[2] In addition, these agents are often valuable in controlling bleeding from internal organs such as the liver or spleen.

There is no ideal way to group the various hemostatic agents and methods. However, for purposes of this discussion they will be divided into three basic categories: mechanical, thermal, and chemical.[2]

Mechanical Agents

The mechanical methods and agents used to control bleeding have no inherent hemostatic ability, but instead act through tamponade.

DIRECT PRESSURE

Direct pressure is one of the simplest and most atraumatic methods of achieving hemostasis. Pressure collapses blood vessels to allow platelet aggregation, plug formation, and release of platelet granules and mediators that initiate fibrin clot formation. Unfortunately, direct pressure may require considerable time. The application of direct, firm pressure is especially valuable when there is a briskly oozing surface, such as muscle, or when there is persistent oozing from the needle puncture site while placing surface stitches. Firm, direct pressure over the bleeding site with a gauze sponge for 5 minutes will usually control the bleeding. However, it is best to maintain the pressure for the entire period and avoid repeatedly removing the gauze pad to check the site.

LIGATION

Most small bleeding vessels can be controlled by electrocoagulation, but larger vessels should be tied off to prevent postoperative bleeding. Bleeding may not be readily apparent when the blood vessel is cut because of the epinephrine effect in the local anesthetic and the natural vasoconstriction that occurs in the injured vessel. Even though a dry field is evident at the time of closure, these larger blood vessels may begin to bleed several hours after the procedure. As a consequence, if a blood vessel is large enough to be readily identified at the time an incision is made, it should be clamped with a hemostat and then ligated with a suture.[3, 4]

Several methods can be used to ligate blood vessels. If a moderately long portion of the vessel can easily be separated from the surrounding tissue, it should be isolated with a hemostat and tied off without the inclusion of any surrounding nonvascular tissue (Fig. 17–1).

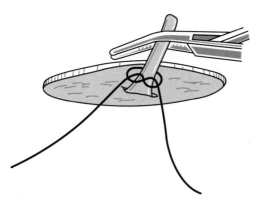

Figure 17–1. When a moderate length of a blood vessel can be isolated from the surrounding tissue, it can be ligated by tying it off just below the tip of the hemostat with a square knot. (Redrawn courtesy of Mrs. Janici Salasche.)

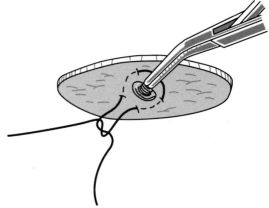

Figure 17–3. A "pursestring" stitch takes longer to place but gives extra security for the ligation of larger vessels. (Redrawn courtesy of Mrs. Janici Salasche.)

It is occasionally difficult to isolate the vessel from the surrounding tissue, especially when it is on the lateral margin of a wound. Thus, to ligate this type of vessel securely, some of the surrounding tissue should be included in the knot, which can be accomplished with a "stick-tie" (Fig. 17–2). Another method used to securely ligate larger vessels is a "pursestring" stitch, which envelops a larger amount of adjacent tissue in the knot (Fig. 17–3) than the stick-tie.

TOURNIQUETS

A tourniquet can be quite helpful when performing surgery on cylindrical anatomic parts such as the fingers or toes. The use of local anesthetic agents without epinephrine and the rich vascularity of the digits frequently result in brisk hemorrhage during surgery. Excessive bleeding can interfere with visualization of the surgical site, which is especially important when performing surgical procedures on the nail unit. For example, a dry field is absolutely necessary when performing chemical matricectomy for nail ablation. In these situations, a dry field can easily be obtained by wrapping a wide Penrose drain around the base of the digit and

clamping it dorsally with a hemostat (Fig. 17–4). Kinking of the tourniquet should be avoided to prevent uneven or excessive pressure. The tourniquet generally should not be left in place for longer than 15 minutes. Alternatively, intermittent firm lateral digital compression by the surgeon or the surgical assistant can provide relatively good hemostasis. An inflated brachial blood pressure cuff can be used as a tourniquet when a bloodless field is required while performing surgery on the hand.[5–8]

COMPRESSION DRESSINGS

Compression or pressure dressings can be used during the first 24 hours after surgery to help prevent postoperative hemorrhage. These dressings are especially helpful (1) after surgery on patients who require medications that may interfere with normal clotting, (2) to provide proper care of wounds created on vascular anatomic locations, (3) following excision of vascular lesions, or (4) in patients with internal medical problems that may make them particularly susceptible to bleeding. Pressure dressings are fashioned by adding bulky loose gauze, gauze pads, petrolatum-impregnated gauze, cotton balls, or dental rolls to the standard dressing. Additional pressure can also be produced by using elastic bandages, tubular gauze, or elasticized tape.[9]

Fashioning an appropriate dressing for the ear or nose requires skill and innovation. The nasal ala is a very vascular area and prone to postoperative hemorrhage. Unfortunately, a pressure dressing applied to this area is not effective, because the nostril has a tendency to collapse. There are, however, several ways to fashion an effective pressure dressing for the nose. A plug can be cut from a cotton dental roll and covered with a thin layer of petrolatum-impregnated gauze. This is then placed inside the nostril to apply counterpressure to the external cutaneous dressing. A more elegant, commercially available nasal tampon is made of synthetic sponge material that expands when saturated with liquid. The tampon is covered with an antibiotic ointment to allow easy insertion into the nostril. Once in place, the sponge is irrigated with saline or water, which causes expansion

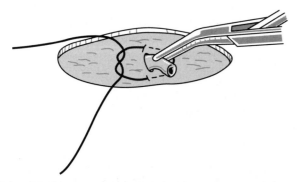

Figure 17–2. A vessel not easily isolated from the adjacent tissue is ligated using a "stick-tie." A small amount of adjacent tissue is sewn into the ligation so that the tie will not be dislodged from the end of the vessel. (Redrawn courtesy of Mrs. Janici Salasche.)

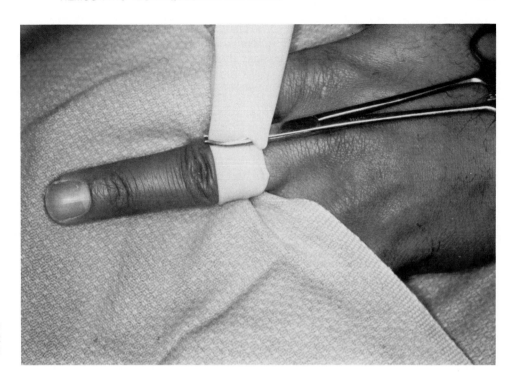

Figure 17–4. A Penrose drain clamped dorsally with a hemostat makes an ideal tourniquet for nail surgery.

of the sponge. The nasal tampon and pressure dressing can usually be discontinued after 24 hours.

After extensive scalp surgery such as a hair transplant, a turban scalp dressing can be fashioned by applying two interwoven elastic gauze rolls. The two gauze rolls are wrapped sequentially with one circling the scalp and interlocking repeatedly with the other, which is placed back and forth across the crown. These help compress the underlying dressing against the vascular surgical site. Tape placed along the forehead, temple, and posterior neck helps to anchor the dressing in place (Fig. 17–5).

Sometimes patients are unable to change their own

dressings but are also unavailable to return the day after surgery. In these situations, a combination dressing can be fashioned with an outer compression component, which is removed by the patient after 24 hours, and an inner portion that remains intact until the time of suture removal. This inner component consists of a thin layer of antibiotic ointment applied to the incision site and liquid adhesive applied to the adjacent area. Several layers of flesh-colored paper tape are then placed over the wound, and a compression dressing is applied with the tape running perpendicular to the orientation of the primary dressing. This dressing works well in select

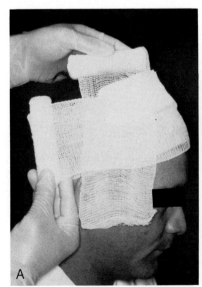
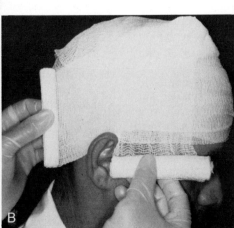
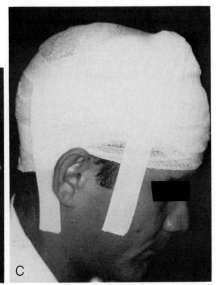

Figure 17–5. *A*, A turban compression dressing is fashioned by interweaving two elastic gauze rolls. *B*, One roll circles the scalp and repeatedly interlocks with the other, traversing back and forth across the crown. *C*, The dressing is anchored in place with tape.

situations and helps to obviate the need for unnecessary dressing changes. It should always be remembered that the use of pressure or compression dressings should be only an adjunctive step in proper wound care and not a substitute for obtaining meticulous hemostasis during the surgical procedure.

ACRYLATES

Acrylates are rapidly polymerizing plastics found in super glues that quickly adhere to tissue and can be used to provide a mechanical blockage of hemorrhage.[10] They are not routinely used as hemostatic agents because of their difficult handling characteristics and associated tissue toxicity, which can result in inflammation, fibrosis, and neurotoxicity when they are applied directly to nerve tissue.[11–13] The development of less toxic analogs in the future may make the routine use of acrylates more feasible.

Thermal Agents

The thermal methods and agents employed for hemostasis all utilize heat to seal the bleeding vessels.

ELECTROSURGERY

When an electric current passes through a material, heat is produced as a result of resistance to the flow of current. Electrosurgery uses high-frequency alternating current to generate heat through tissue resistance. The active electrode remains cold, but the concentrated electrical activity creates molecular heat within each cell it touches. By varying the electrode, the intensity, and the current, it is possible to produce different effects on tissue, including electrodesiccation, electrocoagulation, and electrosection (cutting).[14–18] The higher output electrosurgical units that use lower voltage will not operate without the use of a dispersive electrode.[19] The current passes from the active electrode through the patient and is collected through the dispersive plate back to the machine to complete the circuit.

Electrodesiccation and electrocoagulation are the primary hemostatic modes. Electrocoagulation is often used for the sealing of actively bleeding blood vessels within a surgical wound. Electrosurgical energy should always be applied to a relatively dry surface. If the electric current is conducted through blood, it will be effectively distributed over a much wider area, and little or no effect will be noted. A much higher current will then be required to achieve hemostasis, resulting in a larger amount of tissue damage.[4] Vascular areas such as the nose, ear, and lip can be compressed between the surgeon's thumb and index finger to temporarily stop all bleeding and allow electrosurgical coagulation to be performed on a dry field. Bleeding can also be controlled while electrocoagulation is being performed by directly compressing the bleeding site with a gauze pad or cotton-tipped applicator. A small suction unit can prove valuable when performing extensive surgical procedures. Small capillary bleeding can best be stopped by touching

the area directly with the active electrosurgical electrode (Fig. 17–6). Unfortunately, if the bleeding vessel is large, this tends to produce excessive char and tissue damage.

A less traumatic and preferred method for medium-sized vessels is to carefully isolate the bleeding point and grasp it with a pair of fine hemostats or delicate forceps.[4] The curved Halsted mosquito hemostat is one of the most popular and useful hemostats for cutaneous surgery because hemostasis can be achieved with minimal damage to the surrounding tissue (Fig. 17–7). It is often helpful to isolate the bleeding vessel from the surrounding tissue by slightly elevating the clamped vessel while lifting up on the instrument. This helps prevent inadvertent damage to the wound edge if the hemostat also touches this portion of the wound. If the applied current does not seem to be effective, it may be because too much tissue is being grasped in the instrument. In this situation, reclamp as small an area as possible that includes the bleeding vessel and reapply the current.

Sterility must be maintained when using electrosurgical instruments to avoid wound contamination. A sterile electrode tip should be used for each procedure. Disposable electrodes and electrodes that can be resterilized and used multiple times are both readily available. Another option is to use an adapter that plugs into the handle of the electrosurgical unit and allows the attachment of disposable metal-hubbed needles.[20] An assistant can handle the nonsterile electrosurgical equipment, which has a sterile electrode tip so that it can be touched to the hemostat without contaminating the surgical field. The current is conducted through the hemostat to the point of tissue contact. This technique is the simplest for minor bleeding because a sterile electrosurgical handle and cord are not required.

When it is necessary for the surgeon to handle the electrosurgical equipment, several techniques are avail-

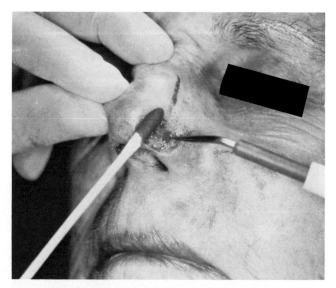

Figure 17–6. Small capillary bleeding can be controlled by applying electrosurgical current directly to the site with a sterile electrode. A cotton-tipped applicator is rolled back and forth over the site to temporarily produce a dry field.

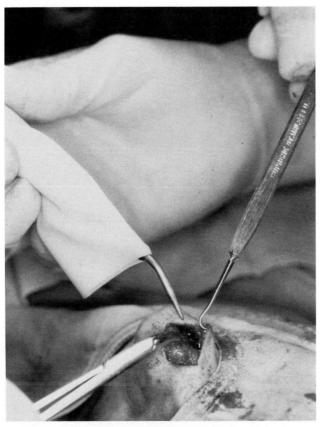

Figure 17–7. For pinpoint electrocoagulation with minimal tissue damage, the bleeding vessel is clamped with a hemostat and the active electrode is applied to the instrument.

able for maintaining a sterile surgical field. Sterile plastic sleeves are available to place over the electrosurgical handle to allow the surgeon to manipulate the equipment without contamination. A sterile Penrose drain can also be slipped over the handle and cord to maintain sterility (Fig. 17–8).[21] Alternatively, the electrosurgical handle can be placed inside a sterile glove with the active sterile tip protruding through one of the fingertips. Another option is to have an extra supply of electrosurgical handles and cords that can be resterilized for individual use.

For longer or more complicated procedures, bipolar electrosurgical forceps can be used. The forceps connect to an electrosurgical cord, and the bleeding site is grasped and coagulated directly by the two active electrodes with one wire going to each side of the forceps. In this way coagulation is localized to the area grasped between the tips of the forceps, as the current passes only from one tip to the other.[22–24] The use of pinpoint, localized electrocoagulation on bleeding sites is a good method to achieve hemostasis, because it causes minimal heat production and reduces thermal damage to the surrounding tissue. It is more time consuming than other methods but usually results in faster healing and more cosmetically acceptable scars.

ELECTROCAUTERY

Electrocautery is not the same as electrocoagulation, although the two terms are often confused. Electrocautery uses electrical current to heat only a filament tip so that no electric current is actually transferred to the patient. The heated tip turns red hot and is applied directly to the bleeding site. The intense heat coagulates the tissue and results in hemostasis.[25, 26] However, significant heat damage to the adjacent tissue, which may result in delayed wound healing and scarring, is possible.[27, 28] Small, inexpensive, disposable, battery-operated cautery units are available (Fig. 17–9).

One advantage of electrocautery is that it can be used on nonconductive tissues such as nail, cartilage, and bone. In addition, no electrical current is conducted to adjacent areas, and the method is effective even in a bloody surgical field.[26] It may also be used on patients with cardiac pacemakers that should not be exposed to electrical current.[29] Because of their portability, the disposable cautery units are especially useful for performing small procedures at the bedside.

ELECTROSECTION, LASER, HOT SCALPEL

Electrosurgical cutting current (electrosection), lasers, and hot scalpels (Shaw scalpel) can all be used in select situations to combine excisional capability with instant coagulation of small- and medium-sized blood vessels.

Figure 17–8. This electrosurgical handle has a finger switch and can be placed inside a sterile Penrose drain to allow the surgeon to maintain sterility.

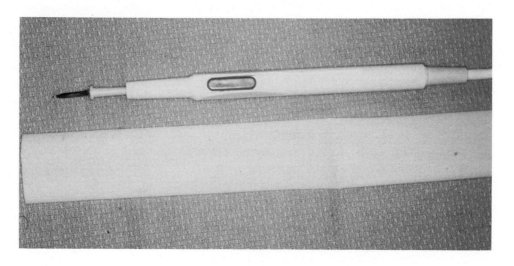

The Shaw scalpel utilizes a Teflon-coated scalpel blade that contains a heating element. The sharp blade cuts through the tissue as the heated sides seal the blood vessels. The Shaw scalpel may be useful for excisions on vascular areas such as hair-bearing scalp where cosmesis is not critical.[30–32]

True electrosection or cutting current produces very focused heating that ruptures the tissue. Unfortunately, such cutting current must be blended with some coagulation current; otherwise it has no advantage over a scalpel incision. This adds the benefit of hemostasis to the cutting current, but also results in the lateral spread of heat into the surrounding normal tissue, which may damage the wound edges, delay wound healing, and result in increased scarring.[33–35] In select situations, such as rhinophyma repair, the use of cutting current has proved valuable.[36–38]

The carbon dioxide laser with its focused, high-intensity beam can also be used for cutting tissue. This seals small- to medium-sized vessels up to 0.5 mm in diameter. The primary drawback of these methods is that they all utilize heat to achieve hemostasis, which results in more damage than that caused by cold steel excision. This heat-induced damage may result in slower wound healing and increased scarring.[39, 40] However, these methods may offer advantages in the medically compromised patient with bleeding tendencies.[41]

Chemical Agents

The chemical agents utilized to achieve hemostasis can be subdivided into caustic and physiologic types. The escharotic, or caustic, agents produce hemostasis at the expense of tissue damage, whereas the physiologic agents affect the clotting mechanism to enhance hemostasis with minimal tissue injury.

ESCHAROTIC (CAUSTIC) AGENTS

Aluminum Chloride

Aluminum chloride is one of the most popular topical hemostatic agents used to control bleeding after superficial procedures such as shave biopsies or curettage. It is commonly available as 20 to 40% concentrations in water or alcohol. It can also be purchased as a ready-mixed product in a 20% concentrated solution of ethyl alcohol known as Drysol. Drysol is marketed for the control of hyperhidrosis. The hemostatic effect is probably due to protein precipitation by the aluminum ion and the acidic nature of the solution.[10, 42, 43] With this technique, a solution-soaked cotton-tipped applicator is applied to the wound surface in a rolling back-and-forth motion until hemostasis is obtained (Fig. 17–10). It must be applied to a relatively dry field to be effective. Pressure or traction on the wound edges will temporarily help control the hemorrhage while the solution is being applied. Aluminum chloride should not be used on deep wounds because, being a caustic agent, it damages tissue and can result in delayed healing and increased scarring in full-thickness wounds.[42, 44]

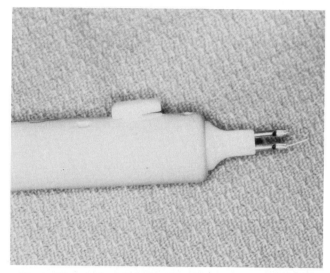

Figure 17–9. A disposable, battery-operated electrocautery unit.

Some of the less popular escharotic agents include Monsel's solution, silver nitrate sticks, phenol, and dichloroacetic or trichloroacetic acid. Although quite effective, all of these agents denature and agglutinate protein and damage surrounding tissue to a greater extent than aluminum chloride. These agents are useful when it is advantageous to destroy an extra rim of tissue surrounding a wound, such as during the treatment of a wart or in a wound containing excessive granulation tissue.[43] Monsel's solution (20% ferric subsulfate) can cause tissue tattooing and greater postoperative discomfort, which has resulted in a decline in its popularity.[10]

Hydrogen Peroxide

Hydrogen peroxide has a mild hemostatic effect when applied to bleeding sites.[10] The mechanism is not clear,

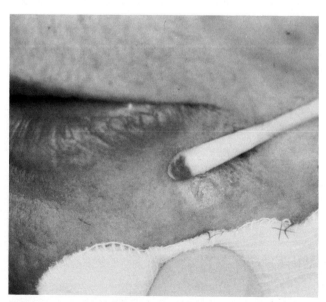

Figure 17–10. Aluminum chloride is applied to a shave biopsy site with a cotton-tipped applicator, using a rolling back-and-forth motion. Traction on the surrounding skin produces a relatively dry field.

but it is a nonallergenic, nontoxic, and inexpensive method to obtain limited hemostasis. Tissue catalase rapidly degrades hydrogen peroxide to oxygen and water.[45] Hydrogen peroxide–soaked surgical gauze can be placed on the bleeding site and removed when hemostasis is achieved, or a gelatin sponge can be saturated with the solution and left in place.

PHYSIOLOGIC AGENTS

Epinephrine

Epinephrine is often added to local anesthetics to decrease bleeding, because plain lidocaine can cause vasodilation. Epinephrine produces vasoconstriction in the skin and mucosa and acts to significantly decrease bleeding during surgery. In addition, epinephrine prolongs anesthesia and reduces the risk of systemic anesthetic toxicity.[46] To maximize vasoconstriction, it is best to wait at least 10 minutes after local infiltration before starting the surgery. Epinephrine should be avoided in procedures involving the fingers and toes because of the theoretic risk of tissue necrosis and gangrene as a result of intense vasoconstriction of the main arterial supply.[10] Toxic side effects of epinephrine overdose can be seen if it is injected too rapidly or if accidental intravascular injection occurs. These side effects include nausea, tachycardia, hypertension, tremors, anxiety, palpitations, headache, and arrhythmias.[46]

Standard commercially available lidocaine preparations typically contain either a 1:100,000 or a 1:200,000 concentration of epinephrine. Patients who are susceptible to the side effects of epinephrine can be treated with more dilute concentrations such as 1:400,000 or 1:500,000 without causing a significant loss of vasoconstriction.[46–49] This can easily be accomplished by diluting the epinephrine-containing anesthetic with plain lidocaine and then waiting the required l0 to l5 minutes after injection for the vasoconstrictive effect to be achieved.

Epinephrine solutions in concentrations of 1:1000 to 1:10,000 have been used as topical hemostatic agents on skin graft donor sites and after tangential excision of burn wounds.[50] In this technique, a syringe is used to squirt the solution on the surface of the oozing site. There are conflicting reports on the efficacy of topical epinephrine as a hemostatic agent.[51]

Absorbable Gelatin Sponges

There are several hemostatic agents whose physical meshwork acts to facilitate blood clotting. Gelatin foam (Gelfoam) is a sterile, nonantigenic, pliable surgical sponge prepared from animal skin gelatin (Fig. 17–11). This sponge can be applied to a bleeding site either dry or soaked with saline or thrombin solution. Gelatin foam is quite porous and capable of absorbing and holding many times its weight in whole blood. Its hemostatic action is nonspecific and may be a result of the concentration of clotting factors in the sponge.[2, 10, 52, 53]

When implanted, the gelatin sponge is completely absorbed in 4 to 6 weeks. The same agent is also

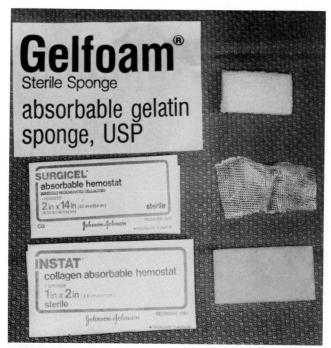

Figure 17–11. *Top,* Absorbable gelatin sponge. *Middle,* Oxidized cellulose absorbable fabric hemostat. *Bottom,* Absorbable collagen sponge hemostat.

available as a powder, the powder being much more difficult to handle than the sponge. The sponge is supplied as sheets or smaller dental packs and can be easily cut to the appropriate size. Gelatin sponge can be applied to the nailbed after surgery or can be placed in punch biopsy sites to help control diffuse bleeding. However, because it is a foreign body, gelatin sponge may increase the rate of infection in surgical wounds in which it is implanted.[54–56]

Oxidized Cellulose

Oxidized cellulose (Oxycel, Surgicel) is an absorbable material made from cellulose that has been subjected to oxidation by nitrous oxide (Fig. 17–11). This process makes the material soluble under physiologic conditions so that it is absorbed after being implanted into tissues. Like gelatin sponge, oxidized cellulose absorbs uncoagulated blood in its interstices. However, its acidic pH may also play an important role in its hemostatic properties.[10, 52, 53]

This material is generally used to control oozing from broad surfaces. On reacting with blood, its low pH produces a brownish-red gelatinous mass. Oxidized cellulose possesses mild bactericidal properties, so it may be a good choice to use in possibly contaminated surgical wounds.[2, 54–56] Oxycel is available as a gauze pad or pledget, and Surgicel is manufactured as a knitted fabric strip that has superior handling qualities

Thrombin

Thrombin is a physiologic hemostatic agent produced by the activation of bovine prothrombin. Thrombin

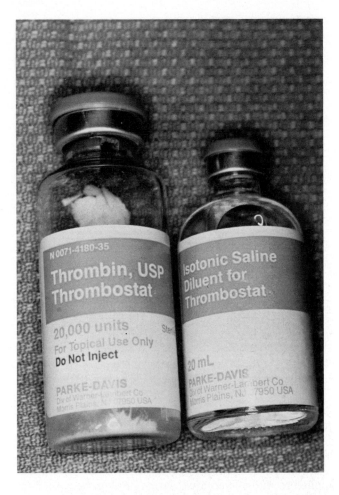

Figure 17–12. Thrombin comes in vials of freeze-dried powder, which can be combined with sterile saline and sprayed onto a site.

activates fibrinogen to form a fibrin clot that results in almost instantaneous coagulation. It is available in vials containing freeze-dried powder (Fig. 17–12) and can be dusted on or made into a solution with sterile saline and squirted onto the bleeding site with a syringe. Thrombin solution can also be added to an absorbable gelatin

sponge to produce a very effective hemostat. Care must be taken to ensure that thrombin is not allowed to enter any major blood vessels, as it can cause extensive intravascular clotting.[2, 10, 52] Because of its relatively high cost and difficult handling properties, its applications in cutaneous surgery have been greatly limited.

Figure 17–13. Microfibrillar collagen hemostat (Avitene) is supplied as a fluffy, loose, fibrous material that can be applied to bleeding sites.

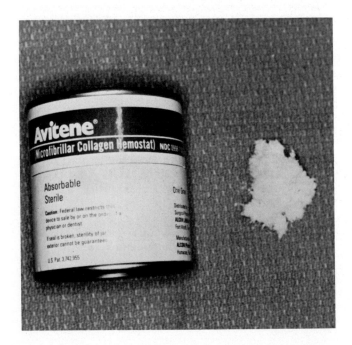

Fibrin Sealant and Glue

Fibrin glue, composed of two separate solutions of fibrinogen and thrombin, is widely used in Europe. By taking advantage of the final stages of the clotting cascade, fibrin glue components coagulate within 15 seconds. It is especially effective in heparinized patients or those with hemostatic disorders. Simultaneous application of the thrombin and fibrinogen using a double-barrel syringe (Duploject system) creates an effective, thin, sealant film.[57, 58] This product has not been approved for routine use in the United States because of the risk of disease transmission from the fresh frozen plasma that is used to isolate the fibrinogen. A safer, but more complicated, way to make tissue glue would be to use the patient's own blood to extract the fibrinogen; the thrombin component is extracted from bovine sources. Applications for fibrin sealant or glue have been limited in cutaneous surgery.

Bovine Collagen

Topical application of bovine collagen induces hemostasis by providing a surface to which platelets can adhere. It is available as a white, fluffy, compressible, loose, fibrous material (Avitene) (Fig. 17–13) and in a sponge form (Instat) (see Fig. 17–11). The application of collagen mimics the physiologic situation after vascular injury in which exposed collagen interacts with platelets, leading to the formation of a clot. Bovine collagen is a highly effective hemostatic agent that resorbs within 3 months, causes minimal tissue reaction, and is relatively nonantigenic.[2, 10, 52, 53] The biggest disadvantage is its relative expense compared with other hemostatic agents.

Collagen hemostatic sponges are available as 6-mm cylindrical plugs that can be used to control bleeding after punch biopsy in place of suture closure (Fig. 17–14). The hemostatic sponge can also be used in the base of a wound healing by second intention. The collagen

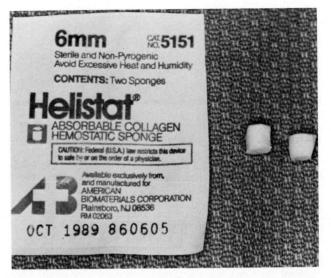

Figure 17–14. These 6-mm plugs of absorbable collagen hemostatic sponge (Helistat) are available for placement in punch biopsy sites.

sponge significantly decreases postoperative bleeding and also simplifies wound care. The sponge is kept moist with antibiotic ointment applied daily until healing is complete (Fig. 17–15). Bovine collagen is an effective physiologic chemical hemostatic agent that has found multiple useful applications in cutaneous surgery.

SUMMARY

A large number of hemostatic agents and modalities are available to the cutaneous surgeon. Each of these can provide unique advantages in select situations. Electrocoagulation remains the primary method to achieve hemostasis in routine cutaneous surgery. However, its use should be as precise as possible to avoid excessive injury to normal tissue, since charred, thermally injured tissue must be enzymatically debrided from the wound

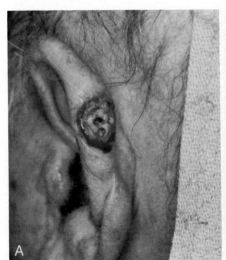
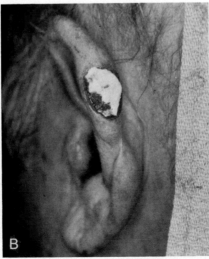
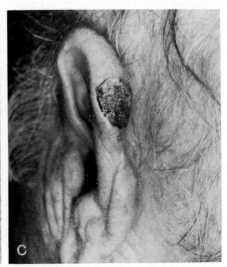

Figure 17–15. *A*, An oozing surgical wound of the ear. *B*, Collagen absorbable hemostatic sponge is trimmed and placed over the site. *C*, The next day the wound is dry, and since the collagen hemostat is absorbable it can be left in place.

as part of the wound healing process. This increased inflammation slows healing, decreases local host defenses, and increases the risk of adverse scarring. For all these reasons, a complete understanding of the techniques and methods of providing hemostasis is vital to the proper performance of cutaneous surgery.

REFERENCES

1. Chvapil M, Owen JA, DeYoung DW: A standardized animal model for evaluation of hemostatic effectiveness of various materials. J Trauma 23:1042–1047, 1983.
2. Arand AG, Sawaya R: Intraoperative chemical hemostasis in neurosurgery. Neurosurgery 18:223–233, 1986.
3. Johnson H: The Hyfrecator—a useful device for conserving time in surgery. Plast Reconstr Surg 34:630, 1964.
4. Sebben JE: Blood vessel coagulation for incisional surgery. J Dermatol Surg Oncol 15:1050–1053, 1989.
5. Reid HS, Camp RA, Jacob WH: Tourniquet hemostasis. J Clin Orthop Res 177:230–234, 1983.
6. Cramer LM, Chase RA: Hand. In: Schwartz SI (ed): Principles of Surgery. McGraw-Hill, New York, 1974.
7. Salasche SJ. Surgery. In: Scher RK, Daniel CR (eds): Nails: Therapy, Diagnosis, Surgery. WB Saunders, Philadelphia, 1990.
8. Baran R: Surgery of the nail. Dermatol Clin 2:271–284, 1984.
9. Winton GE, Salasche SJ: Wound dressings for dermatologic surgery. J Am Acad Dermatol 13:1026–1044, 1985.
10. Larson PO: Topical hemostatic agents for dermatologic surgery. J Dermatol Surg Oncol 14:623–632, 1988.
11. Lehman RAW, Hayes GH, Leonard F: Toxicity of alkyl 2-cyanoacrylates. Arch Surg 93:441–450, 1966.
12. Bessermann YL: Cyanoacrylate spray in the treatment of prolonged oral bleeding. Int J Oral Surg 6:233–240, 1977.
13. Lehman RAW, Hayes GH: The toxicity of alkyl 2-cyanoacrylate tissue adhesives: brain and blood vessels. Surgery 61:915–922, 1967.
14. Sebben JE: High frequency electrosurgery. In: Sebben JE (ed):Cutaneous Electrosurgery. Year Book Medical, Chicago, 1989.
15. Boughton RS, Spencer SK: Electrosurgical fundamentals. J Am Acad Dermatol 16:862–867, 1987.
16. Sebben JE: Electrosurgery: high-frequency modalities. J Dermatol Surg Oncol 14:367–371, 1988.
17. Elliott JA: Electrosurgery. Arch Dermatol 94:340–348, 1966.
18. Blankenship ML: Physical modalities: electrosurgery, electrocautery, and electrolysis. Int J Dermatol 18:443–452, 1979.
19. Sebben JE: Patient "grounding." J Dermatol Surg Oncol 14:926–931, 1988.
20. Stegman SJ, Tromovitch TA, Glogau RG: The Bernsco adapter. J Dermatol Surg Oncol 10:680–681, 1984.
21. Stoner JG, Swanson NA, Vargo N: Penrose sleeve. J Dermatol Surg Oncol 9:523–524, 1983.
22. Sebben JE: The status of electrosurgery in dermatologic practice. J Am Acad Dermatol 19:542–549, 1988.
23. Sebben JE: Physics and circuitry of electrosurgery. In: Sebben JE (ed):Cutaneous Electrosurgery. Year Book Medical, Chicago, 1989.
24. Cherazi B, Collins WF: A comparison of effects of bipolar and monopolar electrocoagulation in brain. J Neurosurg 54:197–203, 1981.
25. Stegman SJ, Tromovitch TA, Glogau RG: Hemostasis. In: Sebben JE (ed):Basics of Dermatologic Surgery. Year Book Medical, Chicago, l982.
26. Sebben JE: Galvanic surgery and electrocautery. In: Sebben JE (ed): Cutaneous Electrosurgery. Year Book Medical, Chicago, 1989.
27. Sebben JE: Treatment technique. In: Sebben JE (ed): Cutaneous Electrosurgery. Year Book Medical, Chicago, 1989.
28. Liu D, Stasior OG: Thermal orbital injuries from disposable cauteries. Plast Reconstr Surg 74:1–9, 1984.
29. Sebben JE: Electrosurgery and cardiac pacemakers. J Am Acad Dermatol 9:457–463, 1983.
30. Levenson SM, Gruber DK, Gruber C, et al: A hemostatic scalpel for burn debridement. Arch Surg 117:213–219, 1982.
31. Tromovitch TA, Glogau RG, Stegman SJ: The Shaw scalpel. J Dermatol Surg Oncol 9:316–319, 1983.
32. Millay DJ, Cook TA, Brummett RE, et al: Wound healing and the Shaw scalpel. Arch Otolaryngol Head Neck Surg 113:282–287, 1987.
33. Kalkwarf KL, Krejci RF, Edison AR, et al: Subjacent heat production during tissue excision with electrosurgery. J Oral Maxillofac Surg 41:653–657, 1983.
34. Kalkwarf KL, Krejci RF, Edison AR, et al: Lateral heat production secondary to electrosurgical incisions. Oral Surg 55:344–348, 1983.
35. Fry TL, Gerbe RW, Botros SB, et al: Effects of laser, scalpel, and electrosurgical excision on wound contracture and graft "take." Plast Reconstr Surg 65:729–731, 1980.
36. Albom M: Surgical gems. Electrosurgical treatment of rhinophyma. J Dermatol Surg Oncol 2:189–191, 1976.
37. Linehan J, Goode R, Fajardo L: Surgery vs. electrosurgery for rhinophyma. Arch Otolaryngol 91:444–448, 1970.
38. Greenbaum SS, Krull EA, Watnick K: Comparison of CO_2 laser and electrosurgery in the treatment of rhinophyma. J Am Acad Dermatol 18:363–368, 1988.
39. Keenan KM, Rodeheaver GT, Kenney JG: Surgical cautery revisited. Am J Surg 147:818–821, 1984.
40. Hambley R, Hebda PA, Abell E, et al: Wound healing of skin incisions produced by ultrasonically vibrating knife, scalpel electrosurgery, and carbon dioxide laser. J Dermatol Surg Oncol 14:1213–1217, 1988.
41. Koranda FC, Grande DJ, Whitaker D: Laser surgery in the medically compromised patient. J Dermatol Surg Oncol 8:471–474, 1982.
42. Epstein E: Topical hemostatic agents for dermatologic surgery. Letter. J Dermatol Surg Oncol 15:342–343, 1989.
43. Larson PO: Dr. Larson replies. Letter. J Dermatol Surg Oncol 15:343, 1989.
44. Sawchuk WS, Friedman KJ, Manning T, et al. Delayed healing in full-thickness wounds treated with aluminum chloride solution. J Am Acad Dermatol 15:982–988, 1986.
45. Hankin FM, Campbell SE, Goldstein SA, et al: Hydrogen peroxide as a topical hemostatic agent. J Clin Orthop Res 186:244–248, 1984.
46. Winton GB: Anesthesia for dermatologic surgery. J Dermatol Surg Oncol 14:41–54, 1988.
47. Grabb WC: A concentration of 1:500,000 epinephrine in a local anesthetic solution is sufficient to provide excellent hemostasis. Plast Reconstr Surg 63:834, 1979.
48. Graham WP: Anesthesia in cosmetic surgery. Clin Plast Surg 10:285–287, 1983.
49. Siegel RJ, Vistnes LM, Iverson RE: Effective hemostasis with less epinephrine. Plast Reconstr Surg 51:129–133, 1973.
50. Glasson DW: Topical adrenalin as a hemostatic agent. Plast Reconstr Surg 74:451–452, 1984.
51. Snelling CFT, Shaw K: The effect of topical epinephrine hydrochloride in saline on blood loss following tangential excision of burn wounds. Plast Reconstr Surg 72:830–834, 1983.
52. Collins PA: Hemostatic agents. JORRI 3:8–12, 1983.
53. Landry JR, Kanat IO: Considerations in topical hemostasis. J Am Podiatr Med Assoc 75:581–585, 1985.
54. Dineen P: Antibacterial activity of oxidized regenerated cellulose. Surg Gynecol Obstet 142:481–486, 1976.
55. Hinman F, Babcock KO: Local reaction to oxidized cellulose and gelatin hemostatic agents in experimentally contaminated renal wounds. Surgery 26:633–640, 1949.
56. Lindstrom PA: Complications from the use of absorbable hemostatic sponges. Arch Surg 73:133–141, 1956.
57. Thompson DF, Letassy NA, Thompson GD: Fibrin glue: a review of its preparation, efficacy, and adverse effects as a topical hemostat. Drug Intell Clin Pharm 22:946–952, 1988.
58. Malviya VK, Deppe G: Control of intraoperative hemorrhage in gynecology with the use of fibrin glue. Obstet Gynecol 73:284–286, 1989.

CHAPTER 18

Wound Closure Materials

ALGIN B. GARRETT

Newer sutures are designed with high tensile strength and low tissue reactivity. To take advantage of these properties, the surgeon should have a basic knowledge of the healing properties of the skin to be closed and an understanding of the condition of the wound that is being treated. Knowledge of the biologic response and the physical properties of sutures is important in selecting the most ideal wound closure material.[1, 2]

History

Over the centuries, many different approaches have been used to close wounds.[3] Egyptian literature as far back as 2000 BC describes the use of string and animal sinews for suturing. As early as only 25 years ago, the choice of suture was simple, because only a few were available. Several different types of sutures with varying needle sizes are currently available, and it is incumbent on the surgeon to become familiar with the various types of sutures so that a logical decision can be made concerning the most suitable suture for a particular surgery.

Characteristics of Sutures

The ideal suture should consist of inexpensive material that can be used in any operation, tensile strength being the only variable. Tissue reaction should be minimal, and the suture material should not promote bacterial growth. There should be no detrimental effects in wound healing. Handling should be favorable and knot tying easy. The suture should be nonallergenic, noncarcinogenic, and resorbed with minimal tissue reaction once the wound has healed. There is no one suture that meets all of these criteria, and unfortunately the ideal suture does not currently exist.[4–6]

The physical characteristics ascribed to sutures are defined by the United States Pharmacopeia (USP).[7] This organization is also responsible for setting the standards for manufacturing and packaging sutures.[8] Tensile strength, capillarity, and suture configuration are features of sutures that provide a basis for suture evaluation. Tensile strength is defined as the amount of tension or pull, expressed in pounds, that a suture will withstand before it breaks. Tensile strength is proportional to the diameter of the suture. Generally, as suture diameter increases, tensile strength increases. However, the type of suture material also contributes to its tensile strength. In addition, a knotted suture has only about one third the tensile strength of an unknotted suture, although this varies with the type of knot and the suture material used.[9]

Capillarity reflects the ability of fluid to travel along the axis of a suture. The physical configuration, either monofilament or multifilament, affects the capillarity of sutures. Multifilament sutures such as braided sutures have shown an ability to take up bacteria at a higher frequency than monofilament sutures.[10]

Other physical properties of sutures such as memory, which is the tendency of a suture to retain its natural position or configuration, and knot security are influenced by the elasticity, plasticity, and physical configuration of the suture material. Elasticity refers to the intrinsic property of a suture material to regain its original length after being stretched, and plasticity is the ability of a suture material to retain its new length after being stretched. These features are important in situations in which there is swelling of tissue, as those sutures with a high degree of plasticity will stretch to accommodate the swelling and not cut into it.[11]

The pliability and coefficient of friction determine the ease with which any suture can be used. For example, braided suture material is very pliable and bends easily, so it is readily capable of being tied into a knot. The coefficient of friction determines the ease with which a suture will slide through tissue. Thus, a suture with a low coefficient of friction will slide easily through tissue, making it an excellent choice for use as a running subcuticular stitch. However, this same characteristic will cause the knots tied with this material to be less secure.

SIZE OF SUTURES

The size of suture materials follows standards set by the USP. Suture size is determined by the diameter of the suture material. Generally, the number of zeros determines the size of the suture: the more zeros, the smaller the suture. Conversely, as the strand size increases, the number of zeros decreases. For example, the designation 8–0 refers to a very fine suture, while 3–0 refers to a thicker suture. As the size of the suture decreases, the tensile strength, a measure of the tendency of knotted suture to break under weight, decreases. Conversely, if the diameter of a suture is doubled, the tensile strength will quadruple.

TISSUE REACTION TO SUTURE

All foreign materials, including sutures, evoke a cellular response when implanted into tissues. The degree of this tissue reaction is determined by the nature of the material implanted and the tissue type. The intensity of the reaction is also determined by the condition of the tissue at the time of implantation. The use of monofilament versus braided or twisted suture has been shown to influence the rate of wound infections.[12, 13] It has also been shown that the presence of infection at the time of suturing may evoke a significant reaction that may result in delayed healing, decreased wound strength, and dehiscence.[12, 14]

An uncomplicated tissue reaction to suture material changes in 3 to 4 days from a cellular infiltrate that is populated primarily by neutrophils to one that contains mostly monocytes, plasma cells, and lymphocytes. Beginning about the fourth day, fibroblasts, and macrophages begin to appear. Proliferation of the fibroblasts results in the production of fibrous tissue, and by approximately the seventh day, chronic inflammation begins. The intensity of the tissue reaction is influenced by the absorptive characteristics of the suture material. Histochemical studies have shown that cellular enzyme activity is an important factor in suture tissue reactions. Several authors[2, 15] have shown that silk evokes more tissue reaction than either nylon or polypropylene. Reaction to chromic gut suture is greater than that for monofilament sutures but is not as intense as reaction to cotton or silk sutures.

Types of Suture Material

Sutures are divided into two categories: absorbable and nonabsorbable. Sutures that can be digested by enzymes or hydrolyzed by tissue fluids are classified as absorbable. Sutures that cannot be dissolved by hydrolysis or are not digested by enzymes are classified as nonabsorbable sutures. However, most nonabsorbable sutures, except for stainless steel, polypropylene, and polyester, lose a significant amount of their tensile strength over time when implanted under the skin.[16] Sutures can be further subdivided into single strand, or monofilament, types and multifilament types, which are composed of several strands that are either braided or twisted together. The configuration of the suture has been shown to affect performance in tissue. Monofilament sutures resist infection[15, 17] and organisms, whereas twisted or braided sutures have better handling and tying qualities.[12, 18]

NATURAL ABSORBABLE SUTURES

Surgical gut (plain gut or catgut) is made from the submucosal layer of sheep intestine or the serosa layer of cow intestine. This material is treated so that it becomes highly purified collagen that is then made into a monofilament strand. Plain gut is digested by neutrophils, causing it to lose its tensile strength in 7 to 10 days and to be totally digested in 60 to 70 days. Plain gut is used primarily as a ligature for superficial blood vessels and can also be used where minimal tissue support is required for a short period (e.g., in the closure of a small punch biopsy wound to provide immediate hemostasis). There is also a fast absorbing surgical gut suture that is heat treated to facilitate loss of tensile strength and to speed absorption.[19]

Chromic gut, also called surgical gut, is plain gut that has been treated with chromic salt solutions to increase its resistance to body enzymes. The concentration of chromium salts used to treat the surgical gut determines the speed at which the suture material is absorbed. The tensile strength of chromic gut typically lasts for only 10 to 14 days, but some strength is retained even at 21 days. The suture is completely absorbed at 80 days.[2, 20, 21] The suture can be used to support tissue for a longer period of time than plain gut. A mild chromic gut is also manufactured that is absorbed very rapidly (50% in 3 to 5 days) and is used primarily in ophthalmic surgery.

SYNTHETIC ABSORBABLE SUTURES

Polyglactin 910 (Vicryl) is one of the more commonly used types of absorbable sutures currently available (Table 18–1). This is a braided suture made as a copolymer of lactide and glycolide.[22] The water-repelling properties of lactide slow down the penetration of water into the suture filaments, thus delaying the loss of tensile strength. Vicryl retains 60% of its tensile strength at approximately 14 days and 30% at 21 days and is completely absorbed in 60 to 90 days.[1] Vicryl is coated with a second type of polyglactin, polyglactin 370, and calcium stearate, which allows for easy passage through tissue and easier knot placement.

Vicryl is absorbed without enzymatic action.[23] Occasionally, it is extruded without inflammation and rarely may persist as a small nodule in the suture line. This suture should be buried deeply in the subcutaneous

TABLE 18–1. **COMMONLY USED ABSORBABLE SUTURES**

Material	Configuration	Tensile Strength	Knot Tying	Knot Security	Tissue Reaction	Absorption Time	Uses
Surgical gut (plain)	Twisted	Poor at 7–10 days	Fair	Poor	Moderate	6–8 wk	Subcutaneous closure
Surgical gut (fast-absorbing)	Twisted	50% at 3–5 days	Fair	Poor	Low	2–4 wk	Closure of punch biopsies
Surgical gut (chromic)	Twisted	Poor at 21–28 days	Poor	Poor	Less than plain	8–10 wk	Subcutaneous closure
Polyglactin (Vicryl)	Braided	60% at 14 days; 30% at 21 days	Good	Fair	Low	8–12 wk	Subcutaneous closure, vessel ligature
Polyglycolic acid (Dexon)	Braided	50% at 21 days	Good	Good	Low	7–14 wk	Subcutaneous closure, vessel ligature
Glycolic acid (Maxon)	Monofilament	70% at 14 days; 55% at 21 days	Fair	Good	Low	26 wk	Subcutaneous closure, vessel ligature (high-tension areas)
Polydioxanone (PDS)	Monofilament	70% at 14 days; 50% at 30 days, 25% at 42 days	Poor	Poor	Low	24–26 wk	Subcutaneous closure (high-tension areas), contaminated tissue

tissue, as it is not rapidly absorbed when used as a percutaneous suture. A comparison of tissue reaction to Vicryl with tissue reaction to other sutures in this group has shown that Vicryl produces less reaction postoperatively. Although this suture material is available in both purple and undyed colors, only the colorless type should be used when closing wounds in thin skin so that the suture will not be visible.[24]

Polyglycolic acid (Dexon) is a braided absorbable suture composed of a polymer of glycolic acid. This suture was introduced in 1970 as the first synthetic absorbable suture.[25] It is similar to Vicryl in that its absorption occurs primarily by hydrolysis, which results in minimal tissue reaction.[26] However, because polyglycolic acid has been shown to persist longer in a wound, it generates more tissue reaction than Vicryl but less than plain gut or chromic gut. While Vicryl has proved stronger than polyglycolic acids up to day 35, the absorption rate for both is between 60 and 120 days.[26]

Although the physical configuration of the suture should allow for easy tying, polyglycolic acid often catches on itself to make knot tying and movement through tissue difficult. To help alleviate this problem, a smaller, more tightly braided suture, as well as a coated suture, is now available. The suture does not tolerate wound infections well and should not be placed in a contaminated wound.[27, 28] Like Vicryl, this suture should be placed deeply in the wound and not used as a percutaneous suture.

Glycolic acid (Maxon) is a complex suture material composed of glycolic acid and trimethylene carbonate. It is a monofilament suture with a long half-life, retaining 70% of its tensile strength for 14 days and 55% for 21 days, much longer than the linear chain polymer of glycolic acid. It is removed by hydrolysis resulting from the action of tissue enzymes that are released from macrophages and other inflammatory cells that participate in wound healing.

Polydioxanone (PDS) is a monofilament synthetic absorbable suture made from polyester poly (p-dioxanone).[29] This suture retains 70% of its tensile strength at 2 weeks, 50% at 4 weeks, and 25% at 6 weeks. It is completely absorbed by hydrolysis at 6 months with minimal tissue reaction. Like Maxon, PDS is a monofilament suture that can be safely used in a contaminated wound, since it does not appear to potentiate infection and essentially eliminates the formation of sinus tracts.[30, 31]

NONABSORBABLE SUTURES

Although there are many commonly used nonabsorbable sutures (Table 18–2) made from naturally occurring materials such as silk, cotton, and linen, many have been totally replaced by the introduction of newer synthetic products.[32] To best understand the potential uses of these products, each will be discussed individually.

Cotton suture, as the name implies, is made from cotton fibers. This is the weakest of the nonabsorbable sutures but has good knot security. It produces marked tissue reaction[33] and has significant capillarity, making it unsuitable for use in contaminated wounds. For all these reasons, cotton suture material is not commonly used in cutaneous surgery.

Linen suture is derived from the flax plant, which has very irregular fiber diameters. It also is not commonly used in cutaneous surgery.

Silk suture is a widely used suture material. Its important role in cutaneous surgery is partly attributable to its long-standing use. It is the standard by which the new synthetic sutures are measured. The braided configuration of silk allows for good knot stability and tying ease, but also results in a high coefficient of friction. Silk has been shown to generate an intense tissue reaction and does not provide tensile strength comparable with that of the newer synthetic sutures.[1] After 7 days there is a moderate zone of inflammatory response around the suture that consists of macrophages and giant cells. By as early as 7 days, the suture filaments are widely separated, and by 21 days fibroblasts, as well as giant cells, can be seen invading the filaments.

TABLE 18–2. **COMMONLY USED NONABSORBABLE SUTURES**

Suture	Type	Tensile Strength	Knot Tying	Tissue Reaction	Uses
Cotton	Twisted	Fair	Good	Marked	None
Silk	Braided/twisted	None in 365 days	Excellent	Moderate	Mucosal surfaces
Nylon					
Ethilon	Monofilament	20% per year	Good to fair	Low	Skin closure Blood vessel ligature
Dermalon	Monofilament	Good	Good to fair	Low	Skin closure Blood vessel ligature
Surgilon	Braided	Similar to monofilaments	Good	Low	Skin closure
Nurolon	Braided	Good	Good	Low	Skin closure
Polypropylene					
Prolene	Monofilament	Extended	Good to fair	Minimal	Skin closure Subcuticular
Surgilene	Monofilament	Extended	Good to fair	Minimal	Skin closure Subcuticular
Polyester					
Mersilene	Braided	Indefinitely	Very good	Minimal	Skin closure
Ethibond	Braided	Indefinitely	Very good	Minimal	Skin closure
Polybutester					
Novafil	Monofilament	Extended	Good to fair	Low	Skin closure
Stainless steel	Monofilament braided or twisted	Indefinitely	Poor	Extremely low	Sternal closure, tendon repair, subcuticular skin closure (pull-out)

Because the suture is braided, it is soft and handles extremely well. It is useful in the periocular area, on the oral lips, and on other mucosal surfaces, because it remains soft and pliable. It also does not easily cut through tissue.[34] Silk suture is also useful for intertriginous areas where the prickly nature of other suture materials can be extremely annoying. Very small suture sizes, 8–0 and 9–0, are available for use in ophthalmic surgery.

Nylon suture is made of an inert polyamide polymer. The suture is available in clear, black and green colors and either as a monofilament or as multiple monofilaments. The suture is widely used because of its low tissue reactivity[35] and high tensile strength.[1] Nylon suture is also manufactured as a braided white or black nylon suture called Nurolon. The pliable characteristic of nylon allows for easy handling, but because it is a monofilament suture, it has a tendency to return to its original shape or become untied. Monofilament nylon can be used as a ligature for large blood vessels or as a percutaneous suture to close incisions. The buried suture loses approximately 20% of its strength yearly through hydrolysis and has a low incidence of infection.

Polypropylene suture is a crystalline stereoisomer of a linear hydrocarbon.[36] The suture is extremely inert[1] and retains high tensile strength in tissue. Like most monofilament sutures, it is more difficult to tie than braided sutures but is more pliable and easier to handle than most other monofilament sutures. The suture resists infection and has been successfully used in contaminated wounds.[18]

The three polypropylene sutures are Dermalene, Prolene, and Surgilene. These sutures are very popular in skin surgery and, because of their smooth surfaces and low coefficients of friction, are often used as "pull-out" or running subcuticular sutures. Because this suture material is very plastic, it will not cut through swollen tissues. However, it may allow the wound edges to separate once the swelling has subsided, as it will remain stretched.[37]

Polyester sutures are made from tightly braided, multifilament fibers of polyester or polyethylene terephthalate. The polyester suture has been shown to last indefinitely in the body.[38] Two common types of polyester suture are the white- or green-colored Mersilene and Ethibond. Mersilene is uncoated and has significant tissue drag. Both are easy to handle, with good knot-tying ability. Ethibond is braided polyester suture that is coated with polybutilate. This suture provides a low infection rate, secure knot tying, smooth removal, low reactivity and easy passage through tissue. This is an excellent suture for skin surgery but is more expensive than other sutures with similar indications for use.

Polybutester suture is composed of polyglycol terephthate and polybutylene terephthate and is considered to be a modified polyester suture. Novafil, a monofilament suture with very low tissue reaction, has demonstrated excellent handling qualities with cosmetically superior scars in wound closure.[39] The popularity of this suture in cutaneous surgery is gradually increasing.

Stainless steel suture has as its main attractions very high tensile strength and low tissue reactivity because of its inert nature. However, this suture has a potential to corrode or break at points of bending, twisting, or knotting,[40] making it very difficult to handle. Both monofilament and twisted or braided multifilament stainless steel sutures are available. The difficulty in handling this suture and its tendency to cut through tissue makes it very unpopular for cutaneous surgery.

Surgical Needles

The surgical needle does not play a direct role in wound healing, but the selection of an undesirable needle may lengthen the operative time of a given procedure or result in local tissue necrosis.[41] Needles are designed to carry suture material through tissue with minimal trauma. The needle should be sharp enough to cause minimal injury and should be sturdy but flexible enough to endure stress without breaking. The best needles are made of stainless steel, as carbon steel needles may corrode. There are many types of needles available, and proper selection is determined by the tissue to be sutured, anatomic location, accessibility, suture size, and surgical preference. Another important consideration is the tensile strength of the tissue, since suture tensile strength should not exceed that of the tissue.

All surgical needles have three basic components: the point, the body, and the eye. The eye of the needle is usually either closed or swaged. The closed eye needle is similar to the traditional sewing needle so that the suture is placed through the needle opening. Most sutures currently used have swaged or eyeless ends. The suture is inserted into the hollow end of the needle and is then mechanically crimped to hold the suture securely in place. The body of the needle can be round, triangular, oval, or trapezoidal in cross-sectional configuration. Occasionally, ribs are made along the convex surface of the needle to assist in grasping it. The curved needle is used most commonly, as it provides for easy maneuverability in small spaces; straight needles are sometimes used in areas of easy accessibility. Needles are available in different curvatures. The portion of a circle that makes up the arc of the needle defines its curve. It can be of several different types, but the ⅜- and ½-circle needles are the most frequently used (Fig. 18–1).

There are two types of cutting needles used primarily for cutaneous surgery: conventional and reverse. The conventional needle has a triangular tip with two opposing cutting edges and a third cutting edge on the inside curved surface of the needle (Fig. 18–2). The reverse-cutting needle has two opposing cutting edges and a third cutting edge on the outer curved surface of the needle. The round needle has limited use in cutaneous surgery but is commonly used in suturing muscle, dura, fascia, and aponeurosis.

The nomenclature used to identify needles is confusing, because several different series of needles are available. The major manufacturers of needles are Davis & Geck and Ethicon. Both companies make a variety of needles to be used in various types of tissue. The Ethicon needles for skin closure include the FS, PS, P, CPS, and PC series. The FS ("for skin") and PS ("plastic skin") are very basic needles with reverse-cutting edges, but the PS needle is sharper than the FS needle. The P ("plastic") needle is sharper and smaller than the PS and FS needles. The P series needle is also available as a reverse-cutting needle. The CPS ("conventional plastic surgery") needle is a higher quality needle than the FS, PS, and P series needles. The design of these needles is such that the triangular cutting edge occupies only one third of the arc of the needle. The body is flattened to allow for good grasping with the needle holder and to limit twisting of the needle while suturing. The PC

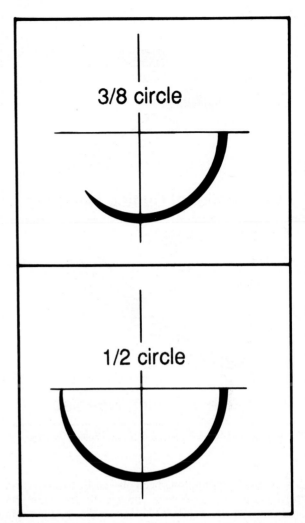

Figure 18–1. Needles with a ⅜-circle and a ½-circle are most commonly used.

("precision cosmetic") needle represents Ethicon's superior skin surgery needle. This needle has a conventional cutting edge with a square body, as opposed to the more triangular body used for the other needle types. The design of this needle causes less damage during its passage through the skin.

The Davis & Geck needles are the PRE, CE, DP, SC, and SBE series and are all available with a reverse-cutting edge. The "E" signifies a ⅜-circle needle. The number that follows in the needle name indicates the length of the needle itself. The DP ("diamond point"), CE ("cutting ⅜-circle"), and SC ("skin closure") needles are basic needles used for skin surgery. The SC needle has a conventional cutting edge. The PRE ("plastic reverse") is Davis & Geck's superior quality skin surgery needle for delicate tissue, because it is finely honed and extra sharp. The SBE ("slim blade") needles are premium, hand-honed, reverse-cutting needles with very thin bodies.

Staples

The use of skin staples has become increasingly popular since its introduction into the United States in the

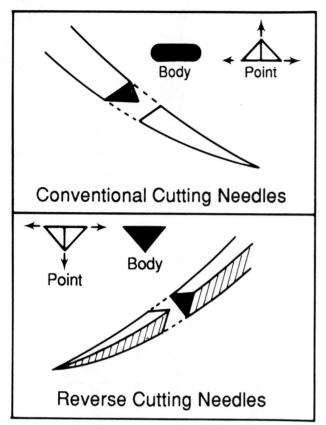

Figure 18–2. Conventional and reverse cutting needles.

early 1970s.[42] Stapling has been shown to be faster than suturing and to cause less damage to the skin than nonabsorbable sutures.[43, 44] Until recently, the packaging of staples was very limited, and staples were primarily available in packages of 25 or 35 staples. Because most cutaneous surgery produces wounds that require fewer staples for closure, wastage was unavoidable. However, over the past several years, new packaging of disposable staples has improved their availability to the cutaneous surgeon. The 3M Company has packaged skin staples in units that contain two to 35 staples. Although this certainly makes staples more convenient for surgery, the use of staples remains largely limited to the extremities, abdomen, trunk, and scalp, because they are not readily accepted by most patients. The advantages that stapling provides over traditional suturing are speed, less tissue damage, greater wound edge eversion, less tissue strangulation, and reduced expense.[45, 46] Even though the cosmetic results of stapling may be better than those of suturing, their efficacy on the face has not been proved.

Skin Closure Tapes

Excisions that are shallow and with little tension in cosmetically sensitive areas or locations where it is important to minimize tissue trauma may be closed with adhesive tapes. Such tapes are generally used for closing wounds after the skin edges have been well approximated with placement of dermal sutures or when no tension exists on the wound edges. It is important to first obtain good hemostasis and eversion of the wound edges before using the tapes for closure. This technique employs adhesive-backed strips such as Steri-Strips that are placed across the wound edges. Before application of the tape, an adhesive solution such as Benzoin or Mastisol is applied to the skin so that the tapes will remain in place for 3 to 7 days.

One advantage of tape closure is the sustained mechanical support it provides for the wound edges. Because no percutaneous sutures are used, there is also no opportunity for producing epidermal ingrowth along the sutures that could cause "railroad track" scarring. The disadvantages occur when these conditions are not met, and wound separation or inversion occurs. Occasionally, the strips become occlusive and result in skin maceration. The strips also have less mechanical strength than that provided by sutures. However, if used in appropriate circumstances, wound closure tapes can be very helpful. They are also beneficial in providing support for the healing wound after percutaneous sutures have been removed.

One relatively new wound closure tape is the E-verter strip. Each self-adhering strip has a central U-shaped area that flattens as it is applied across the wound edges under slight tension. After placement, the inherent elasticity of the strips results in eversion of the wound edges as they try to regain their original shape. To properly use these new wound closure tapes, the same conditions applicable to other wound closure tapes must also be met.

SUMMARY

There are many suture choices for the cutaneous surgeon. Several factors may affect the suture selection. The first concern should be to choose a suture that will sustain adequate tensile strength during the healing process with little risk of knot slippage and minimal tissue reaction. Obviously, an understanding of the healing process in the area where the sutures will be placed is important, as healing can differ with anatomic location. For example, the face generally heals rapidly, but in the lower leg, wound healing may be protracted. The age and health of the patient are also quite important. Increasing age does not necessarily imply delayed healing. In fact, the healthy elderly patient can tolerate cutaneous surgery very well. However, patients in poor health, regardless of age, may have delayed healing. The presence of infection or contamination at the site of surgery may adversely affect wound healing and also influences suture choice.[47] Often, small monofilament sutures are best suited for wound closure where cosmesis is the primary concern. If percutaneous sutures are not required, the value of skin closure tapes should not be underestimated. Staples for wound closure offer the advantage of speed and the possible benefit of cost containment, as the cost of suture material is not inconsequential and may also influence suture choice.

Once a surgeon becomes comfortable with the performance of the various sutures available for cutaneous surgery, the choice of sutures and needles generally becomes less difficult. Experience will allow the cutaneous surgeon to choose a few select absorbable and nonabsorbable sutures that provide reproducibly excellent results in virtually all clinical situations.

REFERENCES

1. Van Winkle W, Salthouse TN: Biological Response to Sutures and Principles of Suture Selection. Ethicon Research Foundation, Somerville, NJ, 1976.
2. Bennett RG: Selection of wound closure materials. J Am Acad Dermatol 18:619–637, 1988.
3. Majno G: The Healing Hand: Man and Wound in the Ancient World. Harvard University Press, Cambridge, 1977.
4. Ulin AW: The ideal suture material. Surg Gynecol Obstet 133:475, 1971.
5. Postlethwait RW: Wound Healing in Surgery. Ethicon, Somerville, NJ, 1971, pp 8–9.
6. Anscombe AR, Hira N, Hunt B: The use of a new absorbable suture material (polyglycolic acid) in general surgery. Br J Surg 57:917–920, 1970.
7. The United States Pharmacopeia. 20th rev. Convention, Inc, Rockville, MD, July 1, 1980.
8. Swanson NA, Tromovitch TA: Suture materials, 1980's: properties, use and abuses. Int J Dermatol 21:373–378, 1982.
9. Herrmann JB: Tensile strength and knot security of surgical suture materials. Am Surg 37:209–217, 1971.
10. Bucknall TE: Factors influencing wound complications: a clinical and experimental study. Ann R Coll Surg 65:71–77, 1983.
11. Holmlund DEW: Physical properties of surgical suture materials: stress-strain relationship, stress-relaxation and irreversible elongation. Ann Surg 184:189–193, 1976.
12. Usher FC, Allen JE, Crostwait RW, Cogan JE: Propylene monofilament: a new biologically inert suture for closing contaminated wounds. JAMA 179:780–782, 1962.
13. Stillman RM, Bella FJ, Seligman SJ: Skin wound closure. Arch Surg 115:674–675, 1980.
14. Botsford TW: The tensile strength of sutured skin wounds during healing. Surg Gynecol Obstet 72:690–697, 1941.
15. Postlethwait RW, Willigan DA, Ulin AW: Human tissue reaction to suture. Ann Surg 181:144-150, 1975.
16. Edlich RF, Ponek PH, Rodeheaver GT, et al: Surgical sutures and infections: a biomaterial evaluation. J Biomed Mater Res 8:115–126, 1974.
17. Alexander JW, Kaplan TZ, Attemeier WA: Role of suture materials in the development of wound infection. Ann Surg 165:192–199, 1967.
18. Sharp WV, Belden TA, King PH, Teague PC: Suture resistance to infection. Surgery 91:61–63, 1982.
19. Webster RC, McCullough EG, Giandello PR, Smith RC: Skin wound approximation with new absorbable suture material. Arch Otolaryngol 111:517–519, 1985.
20. Jenkins HP, Hudina LS, Owen FM Jr, Swisher FM: Absorption of surgical gut (cat gut). III. Duration in the tissue after loss of tensile strength. Arch Surg 45:74–102, 1942.
21. Birdsell DC, Gavelin GE, Kemsley GM, Hein KS: "Staying power"—absorbable vs. nonabsorbable. Plast Reconstr Surg 68:742–745, 1981.
22. Conn J Jr, Oyaso R, Welsh M, Beal JM: Vicryl (polyglactin 910) synthetic absorbable sutures. Am J Surg 128:19–23, 1974.
23. Blomstedt B, Jacobsson S: Experiences with polyglactin 910 (Vicryl) in general surgery. Acta Chir Scand 143:259–263, 1977.
24. Aston SJ, Rees TD: Vicryl sutures. Aesthetic Plast Surg 1:289–293, 1977.
25. Postlethwait RW: Polyglycolic acid surgical suture. Arch Surg 101:489–494, 1970.
26. Craig PH, Williams JA, Davis KW, et al: A biologic comparison of polyglactin 910 and polyglycolic acid synthetic absorbable sutures. Surg Gynecol Obstet 141:1–10, 1975.
27. Eilert JB, Binder P, McKinney PW, et al: Polyglycolic acid synthetic absorbable sutures. Am J Surg 121:561–565, 1971.
28. Williams DF: The effect of bacteria on absorbable sutures. J Biomed Mater Res 14:329–338, 1980.
29. Ray JA, Doddi N, Regula D, et al: Polydioxanone (PDS), a novel monofilament synthetic absorbable suture. Surg Gynecol Obstet 153:497–507, 1981.
30. Rodenheaver GT, Powell TA, Thacker JG, Edlich RF: Mechanical performance of monofilament synthetic absorbable sutures. Am J Surg 154:544–547, 1987.
31. Lerwick E: Studies on the efficacy and safety of polydioxanone monofilament absorbable suture. Surg Gynecol Obstet 156:51–55, 1983.
32. Postlethwait RW: Long term comparative study of nonabsorbable sutures. Ann Surg 171:892–898, 1970.
33. Castelli WA, Nasjleti CF, Diaz-Perez R, Caffesse RG: Cheek mucosa response to silk, cotton and nylon suture materials. Oral Surg Oral Med Oral Pathol 45:186–189, 1978.
34. Adams IW, Bell MS, Driver RM, Fry WG: A comparative trial of polygylcolic acid and silk as suture materials for accidental wounds. Lancet 2:1216–1217, 1977.
35. Nilsson T: Mechanical properties of Prolene and Ethilon sutures after three weeks in vivo. Scand J Plast Reconstr Surg 16:11–15, 1982.
36. Miller JM, Kimmel LE Jr: Clinical evaluation of monofilament polypropylene suture. Am Surg 33:666–670, 1967.
37. Nilsson T: Mechanical properties of Prolene, Ethilon and surgical steel loops. Scand J Plast Reconstr Surg 15:111–115, 1981.
38. Hermann JB: Tensile strength and knot security of surrounding suture materials: Am Surg 37:209–217, 1971.
39. Bong RL, Mustafa MD: Comparative study of skin closure with polybutester (Novafil and polypropylene). J R Coll Surg (Edinb) 34:205–207, 1989.
40. Clark DE: Surgical suture materials. Contemp Surg 17:43, 1980.
41. Bernstein G: Needle basics. J Dermatol Surg Oncol 11:1177–1178, 1985.
42. Campbell JP, Swanson N: The use of staples in dermatologic surgery. J Dermatol Surg Oncol 8:680–690, 1982.
43. Johnson A, Rodeheaver GT, Durand LS, et al: Automatic disposable stapling devices for wound closure. Ann Emerg Med 10:631–635, 1981.
44. Stegmaier OC: Use of skin stapler in dermatologic surgery. J Am Acad Dermatol 6:305–309, 1982.
45. Bucknal TE, Ellis H: Skin closure: comparison of nylon, polyglycolic acid and staples. Eur Surg Res 14:96–97, 1982.
46. Brickman KR, Lambert RW: Evaluation of skin stapling for wound closure in the emergency department. Ann Emerg Med 18:1122–1125, 1989.
47. Barham RE, Butz GW, Anwell JS: Comparison of wound strength in normal, radiated and infected tissues closed with polyglycolic acid and chromic catgut sutures. Surg Gynecol Obstet 146:901–907, 1978.

CHAPTER 19

Principles of Electrosurgery

MATTHEW M. GOODMAN

Electrosurgery is an integral and indispensable part of many cutaneous surgical procedures. A proper understanding of the principles and applications of electrosurgery and electrosurgical equipment not only contributes to better patient care, but also greatly reduces the risk of undesirable results.

Terminology

Because of occasional confusion with the definitions and usage of terms relating to electrosurgery, a brief explanation of terminology is required. *Electrosurgery* is a general term used to encompass all methods in which electricity is used during the performance of surgery, including electrocautery, electrolysis, electrofulguration, electrodesiccation, electrocoagulation, and electrosection (cutting). *Cautery* is derived from the Greek word *kauterion,* meaning "hot iron," and refers to the direct application of a hot metal element on tissue to cause necrosis or coagulation of tissue. *Electrocautery* is the process by which an electrically heated element or "hot tip" is brought directly into contact with tissue to transfer heat and burn the tissue, without passing any current through it. *High-frequency electrosurgery* refers to any technique that uses high-frequency alternating current (AC) electricity ("cold tip") to burn, coagulate, or cut tissue, as in electrofulguration, electrodesiccation, electrocoagulation, and electrosection (cutting). As alternating current passes through tissue, resistance produces heat and thermal damage.

Electrolysis is the process by which low-flow direct current (DC) electricity is passed through tissue between two electrodes, resulting in tissue damage by a chemical reaction that occurs at the tip of one of the electrodes.

It is commonly used to destroy hair follicles. *Thermolysis* uses high-frequency alternating current at low voltage and low current to thermally destroy or epilate hair follicles. *Electroepilation* is another term for thermolysis. *Electrofulguration* is a process by which a monoterminal, high-frequency electrosurgical electrode is held at a distance of 1 to 3 mm from the tissue surface, resulting in a coarse spark that crosses the gap and causes tissue damage and carbonization. *Electrodesiccation* is the process by which a monoterminal high-frequency electrosurgical electrode is held in contact with the tissue, resulting in fine sparks that are absorbed by the tissue, causing thermal injury with less carbonization than that produced by electrofulguration. *Electrocoagulation* is the process by which a biterminal high-frequency, high-current electrosurgical electrode is placed on or near tissue, resulting in significant electrical current passing through the tissue, thermally coagulating it. *Electrosection* (cutting) is a process by which a biterminal high-frequency, high-current electrosurgical electrode is physically passed through tissue, cutting as it goes. The very high local temperatures at the point of contact between the electrode and the tissue result in separation or "cutting" of the tissue. *Diathermy* is a general term meaning the passage of heat through a tissue or some other substance. When applied to surgery, it usually describes the process of heat production and tissue necrosis from monoterminal or biterminal electrosurgery. Passage of high-frequency alternating current through tissue from a small, active electrode to a large, dispersive electrode causes a concentration of the current at the tip of the small, active electrode with consequent tissue necrosis. *Radiosurgery* is occasionally used to refer to high-frequency electrosurgery in which very-high-frequency current reaches radiowave levels of 500,000 to 3,000,000 hertz.

MONOPOLAR-BIPOLAR AND MONOTERMINAL-BITERMINAL TERMINOLOGY

Some terms used in electrosurgery may be confusing. "Monopolar" and "bipolar" are often used to describe how many points of contact are made with the patient by an electrosurgical device. However, "polarity" classically is a term used only in direct or galvanic electric current systems where there are constant positive and negative "poles," as in electrolysis. Therefore, the use of "monopolar" and "bipolar" in high-frequency alternating current devices is technically incorrect, because the "poles" are reversing positions literally thousands or millions of times per second. However, since use of the terms monopolar and bipolar persists in the surgical literature and even appears on the instrumentation of some commercial high-frequency devices, they must be recognized.

Although monopolar and bipolar are often used synonymously with monoterminal and biterminal when referring to high-frequency electrosurgery, the latter terms are more correct. These terms usually refer to the number of contacts made with the tissue or patient by the electrosurgical device. The term monoterminal should be reserved for instances in which only one electrode or terminal comes into contact with the patient (Fig. 19–1A), while the term biterminal should be used when two electrodes or terminals come in contact with the patient (Fig. 19–1B, C).

There are two types of biterminal electrosurgery. The first is when a small active electrode and a large dispersing electrode plate are used (e.g., during electrocoagulation or electrosection) (Fig. 19–1B). The second is when two small, active electrodes are held together in contact with a small amount of tissue (e.g., when fine electrocoagulating forceps are used to seal blood vessels between the two active prongs of the forceps) (Fig. 19–1C). Some authors reserve the term biterminal for this latter application only.[1]

History of Electrosurgery

In ancient times, hot cautery was used by the Egyptians and Greeks to treat tumors and abscesses and to stop bleeding.[2,3] In the nineteenth century, direct battery current or galvanic current was used to heat an electrosurgical device, similar to a soldering iron; this was called electrocautery.[4] In 1891, d'Arsonval discovered that alternating current at greater than 10,000 cycles per second (cps) produced local heat in tissue without causing muscle tetany or other obvious harm to the body.[5,6] His circuit device for producing high-frequency alternating current is still used and is known as the d'Arsonval coil. In 1893, Oudin refined the use of a secondary coil that greatly increased the voltage output of the d'Arsonval coil, producing a fine spray of sparks that was found to be suitable for the monoterminal treatment of skin lesions. In 1908, deKeating-Hart discovered that holding a high-frequency-current electrode a small distance from the tissue caused a coarse spark resembling lightning. He is credited with originating the term *fulguration* (from the Latin *fulgur,* meaning "lightning").[7] In 1911, William Clark found that using low current and high voltage with a monoterminal electrode held in direct contact with tissue resulted in marked superficial tissue drying, or desiccation (from the Latin *desiccare,* meaning "to dry"), of the immediate area.[8] In 1908, Doyen apparently was the first to develop a method for delivering lower voltage, higher current electrical energy to patients by placing a large indifferent or dispersive electrode under them. This resulted in higher temperatures at the point of electrode contact, a biterminal process known as *electrocoagulation* (from the Latin *coagulare,* meaning "to clot"),[9] and the ability to seal off larger, deeper vessels than was previously possible.

In 1926, William Bovie, a physicist, collaborated with Harvey Cushing, a neurosurgeon, to develop a high-frequency electrosurgical instrument that allowed a variable amount of "damping" as well as variable voltage and current output. This instrument could coagulate vessels of many sizes with or without cutting tissue and was the direct forerunner of modern electrosurgical devices.[10] In 1932, the Birtcher corporation introduced its spark gap–based Hyfrecutter, which has become popular for office-based monoterminal and biterminal electrofulguration, electrodesiccation, and electrocoagulation.

Currently, there are numerous commercially available

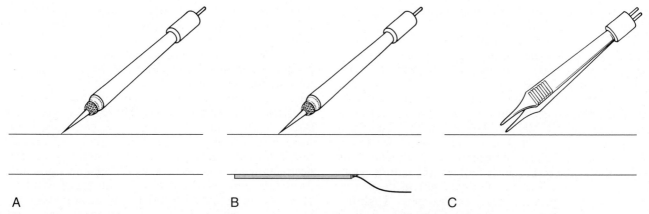

Figure 19–1. *A,* Schematic of a monoterminal electrode. *B,* Schematic of a biterminal electrode with active and dispersive electrodes. *C,* Schematic of a biterminal electrode with two active electrodes in a pair of forceps. (Redrawn courtesy of Mr. Bill Touchton.)

A   B   C

TABLE 19–1. **EXAMPLES OF ELECTROSURGICAL UNITS**

Unit	Manufacturer	Monoterminal	Biterminal	Cutting	Wattage
Solid state					
Hyfrecator 733 (discontinued)	Birtcher Corp. El Monte, CA	+	+	−	22
Hyfrecator Plus	Birtcher Corp. El Monte, CA	+	+	−	22
Surgitron FFPF	Ellman Hewlitt, NY	+	+	+	140
ESU-30	Elmed, Inc. Addison, IL	+	+	+	30
ESU-60	Elmed, Inc. Addison, IL	+	+	+	60
Cameron-Miller	Cameron-Miller Chicago, IL	−	+	+	80
Surgistat	Valley Lab Corp. Boulder, CO	−	+	+	25
SSE 2-L	Valley Lab Corp. Boulder, CO	−	+	+	375
Force 2, 4	Valley Lab Corp. Boulder, CO	−	+	+	300
Spark gap					
Cameron-Miller Electrosurgery Unit 26–230	Cameron-Miller Chicago, IL	−	+	+	60
Cameron-Miller Electrosurgery Unit 26–0345	Cameron-Miller Chicago, IL	+	+	+	95

electrosurgical devices (Table 19–1). Before purchasing any unit, the particular strengths and specific clinical applications of the unit should be thoroughly evaluated.

Principles of Electrosurgery

ELECTRICAL CURRENT–TISSUE INTERACTION

Heat is generated when an electrical current flows through any substance, including living soft tissue, that offers resistance to its passage. The active electrode or terminal remains cold during high-frequency electrosurgery, unless the tissue heat is conducted back to the electrode by holding the two in contact. Heat production in tissue results in dehydration and shriveling of cells, local necrosis, and coagulation. The intensity of the current and the power of the electrical field determine how much heat is produced. Therefore, the treatment site must be kept relatively small to achieve maximal effect with minimal current.[11]

The most common form of electrosurgery employs high-frequency alternating current. Modern electrosurgical devices increase standard outlet current to very-high-frequency and voltage levels while at the same time reducing the current. For example, standard 110-volt, 60-hertz alternating current is increased to several thousand volts and 500,000 to 3,000,000 hertz. These high frequencies have resulted in the use of the term "radiosurgery," since the electromagnetic waves produced fall within the medium-frequency radio wavelength range of 100 to 600 m[12] and thus are interfered with by the nearby operation of high-frequency electrosurgery. High-frequency, high-voltage, low-amperage current has little if any effect on the body as it passes through. However,

if the treatment terminal or electrode is small, the electrical energy generates a great amount of heat at the treatment site.

WAVE FORM

All high-frequency electrosurgical devices generate an oscillating radiowave known as a sine wave. Early high-frequency electrosurgical devices were of the mechanical spark gap type or triode vacuum type. The spark gap method generated a *damped* sine wave, while the vacuum tube method produced a *pure* sine wave (Fig. 19–2). The damped current was empirically found to be superior for electrofulguration, electrodesiccation, and electrocoagulation. The pure sine wave devices were found to be effective for electrosection but not for coagulation or hemostasis. Combinations of the two sine wave forms, damped and pure, provide varying degrees of coagulation with hemostasis and cutting and are called blended waves. The older spark gap and vacuum tube devices have now been largely replaced by solid-state, transistor circuits that have been electronically adapted to produce all these different wave forms.

The mechanical nature of the early spark gap units produced not only the fundamental frequency necessary for electrocoagulation, but also multiple unwanted frequencies. These latter were uncontrollable and resulted in increased tissue destruction. Through the use of solid-state circuits, the spark gap–type electrodesiccation wave form could be reproduced without all the additional unwanted frequencies. The result was less tissue destruction and increased control. Reliability and reproducibility were also enhanced. The latest solid-state electrodesiccation devices offer near linear power output at lower as well as higher powers, providing greater precision and control.

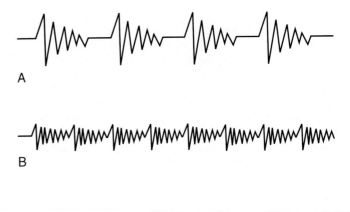

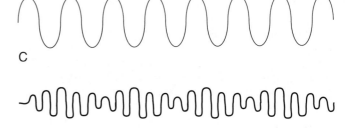

Figure 19–2. The four variations of high-frequency electrosurgical wave forms *A,* Damped wave, electrofulguration, electrodesiccation and electrocoagulation. *B,* Lightly damped wave, less electrocoagulation, less damage. *C,* Pure sine wave, pure electrosection without electrocoagulation. *D,* Blended sine wave, electrosection with electrocoagulation. (Redrawn courtesy of Mr. Bill Touchton.)

ELECTROSURGICAL DEVICES: BASIC DESIGN

Electrosurgical devices are designed to convert ordinary wall outlet electric current into surgically useful energy. This requires converting a low-voltage, low-frequency power source into high-voltage, high-frequency electrical energy. This can be done in a variety of ways, but the basic process is rather simple (Fig. 19–3). The standard power source for electrosurgery is wall outlet electricity or alternating current (110 to 120 volts, and 60 hertz, or cps). Voltage is increased to approximately 550 volts by a step-up transformer that contains two or more adjacent coils of wire. Through electromagnetic conduction, voltage in the second coil is increased in direct proportion to the number of loops in it. Frequency is increased in a more complicated way. Most modern devices are solid state and use transducers to duplicate the wave forms of electromagnetic energy produced by the older spark gap and vacuum tube devices.

HISTOLOGIC AND TISSUE EFFECTS

High-frequency electrosurgery causes shriveling of cells, producing elongated, dense nuclei. Thrombosis of smaller blood vessels occurs with little associated hemorrhage. Healing is associated with a mild exudate and the formation of a crust. Scarring generally depends on the amount of power used.[13]

Electrolysis and Thermolysis

Epilation, or permanent hair removal, is currently performed by either electrolysis or thermolysis.[14, 15] Elec-

trolysis is defined as an electrochemical process using direct or galvanic current for hair removal. It is quite effective and associated with little pain and low risk of scarring, but is relatively slow. In electrolysis, as direct current is passed through tissue between two DC electrodes, a chemical reaction occurs at the negative electrode. Electrons are released at this pole, which produces hydrogen gas and hydroxide ions from water. The

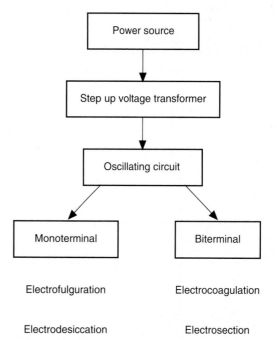

Figure 19–3. Basic design of high-frequency electrosurgical devices. (Redrawn courtesy of Mr. Bill Touchton.)

resultant hydroxides then chemically destroy the adjacent tissue or, in this case, the hair follicle.

Thermolysis is defined as high-frequency electroepilation of hair follicles using low voltage and low current to destroy hair follicles thermally. Nonphysician personnel performing epilation generally use pure galvanic electrolysis or blended galvanic and high-frequency electroepilation techniques, while medical professionals tend to prefer faster high-frequency electroepilation. Currently, 27 states require licensing for an individual to perform permanent hair removal.[16]

EQUIPMENT

Most needles used in epilation are very fine, either tapered or untapered, and have rounded or bulbous tips. An insulated needle for epilation was introduced in 1983, limiting heat generation to the base of the follicle only.[17] The insulated probe produces greater damage to the deep peribulbar tissue and less necrosis of the upper perifollicular dermis, which reduces the chance of scarring (Fig. 19–4); however, correct placement of the insulated needle remains very important (Fig. 19–5). The effectiveness and safety of the insulated epilating needle technique was confirmed in 1985.[18] Most modern epilating devices have very accurate timers so that insulated and noninsulated epilating needles are still in use.

Pure galvanic electrolysis devices are most often used by nonmedical personnel. These devices are safer, less likely to produce scarring, and less painful, but are slower than high-frequency electroepilation devices. A hand-held electrolysis unit (Perma-Tweez) is available without a prescription and may be satisfactory for home use.[19] Blended electrolysis-electroepilating devices are also being used by electrologists. Sophisticated high-frequency, automatically timed devices such as the Fischer, Hoffman, and Instantron & Kree devices are more often preferred by cutaneous surgeons. These destroy the hair follicle by the production of heat that results from tissue resistance to the passage of rapidly oscillating alternating current.

EPILATION TECHNIQUE

For hair removal to be complete and permanent, the hair follicle root or base must be destroyed.[14] The risk of scarring can be minimized or eliminated if the superficial portion of the hair follicle is not treated. All methods of epilation require good lighting and clean skin; magnification may also be helpful. The epilating needle is attached to the negative electrode for electrolysis or to the active electrode for thermolysis (high-frequency electroepilation). The blunt or bulbous tip prevents perforation of the hair follicle. The needle is inserted into the follicular infundibulum parallel to the hair shaft and advanced slowly until the base of the follicle is reached and resistance is felt, usually at a depth of 3 to 4 mm. Some operators advance the needle an additional 1 mm to increase the probability of hair root destruction. Correct insertion of the needle is relatively smooth and painless. Pain may indicate perforation of the follicle wall or inappropriate placement of the needle tip. After insertion of the needle to the desired depth, the device is activated. Premature activation of the electrode or premature withdrawal of an activated electrode is usually painful and may damage the superficial skin and cause scarring.

Galvanic electrolysis units are usually set at 0.5 to 1.0 mA and activated for 15 to 20 seconds. A small bubble of hydrogen gas usually appears at the follicular orifice, indicating that chemical hydroxides have formed at the base of the follicle to cause the desired chemical destruction. The end point and sign that the hair papilla has been destroyed is the ability to remove the hair shaft using forceps with only gentle traction. If the hair cannot be easily pulled out, the device should be briefly reactivated and gentle hair removal reattempted. Rarely is more than a total of 60 seconds of direct current per hair necessary. After the first few hairs have been treated, the optimal time and current parameters can be established for the patient. In general, coarse hair requires a longer exposure time and higher power for removal than fine hair.

Thermolysis, also known as high-frequency electro-

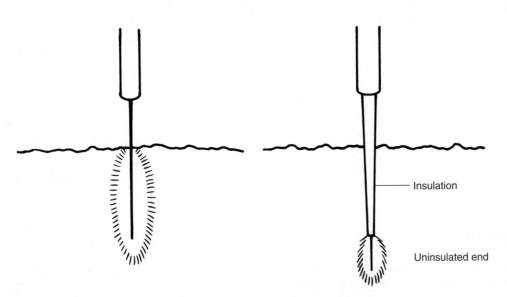

Figure 19–4. Tissue damage resulting from uninsulated *(left)* and insulated *(right)* epilating needles. (Redrawn courtesy of Mr. Bill Touchton.)

Insulation

Uninsulated end

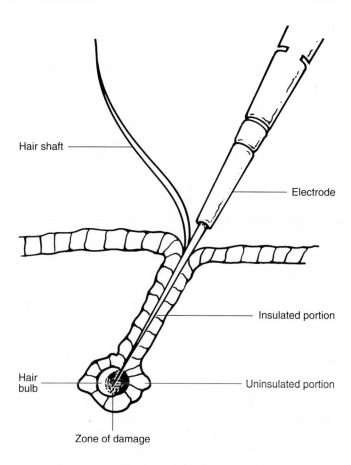

Figure 19–5. Diagram showing proper placement of insulated epilating needle for thermolysis. (Redrawn courtesy of Mr. Bill Touchton.)

epilation, has a somewhat higher risk of scarring and pain. Modern electroepilating devices have precise automatic timers that reduce the risks of scarring. However, precise power output in milliamperes is not usually indicated in these units, and the operator must first estimate a "safe" power. Again, the desired end point is easy removal of the hair with gentle traction. Some operators prefer repeated short bursts to a longer sustained one, to reduce pain and the chance of scarring. Maximal concentration of high-frequency alternating current usually occurs at the needle tip, especially if short bursts are used. However, prolonged activation of current flow will cause a cylindrical zone of tissue injury around the inserted needle, resulting in unwanted damage and possible scarring. In addition, the needle should be cleaned often, since conductive tissue debris may stick to the needle and cause damage more superficially, resulting in less effective hair follicle destruction.

It is preferable not to treat adjacent hair follicles within 3 to 4 mm of each other to reduce thermal build-up. As many as 100 hairs can be removed in 20 minutes with thermolysis. The rate of permanent follicle destruction with thermolysis is 70 to 80%, compared with 80 to 90% with the slower galvanic electrolysis techniques.[14]

APPLICATIONS OF EPILATION

Epilation is indicated in all instances when permanent hair removal is desired, including cases of hirsutism, familial hypertrichosis, and pseudofolliculitis barbae.

Electrolysis and thermolysis techniques, both with and without insulated needles, have also been employed in the removal of unwanted telangiectasia and spider angiomas.[20] Electroelimination of sweat glands in patients with bromhidrosis and hyperhidrosis, using an insulated needle with the thermolysis technique, has also been reported to be successful.[21]

Electrocautery

Electrocautery uses an electric current to heat a metal element that is then placed in direct contact with tissue to produce coagulation and hemostasis or necrosis. No electrical current passes through the tissue. Strict electrocautery is usually applied with battery-operated wire loop devices for pinpoint hemostasis. This technique is useful in periorbital skin to avoid conduction or channeling of high-frequency AC current to the optic nerve and involuntary twitching of periorbital musculature when activating high-frequency electrodes.

Until recently, electrocautery had been largely replaced by high-frequency electrosurgery among cutaneous surgeons. However, with the advent of the Shaw scalpel and sterile, disposable, battery-operated ophthalmic hot-loop cautery units, electrocautery is becoming somewhat more common. Electrocautery continues to be especially widely used in the United Kingdom.[13]

SHAW SCALPEL

The Shaw scalpel is a true electrocautery or "hot-tip" device. It has been used widely in all fields of surgery, including cutaneous surgery,[22] since its introduction in the early 1980s. A specially designed scalpel blade is heated to between 110° and 270°C, using pulsed DC electricity. This heat is thermally conducted to the tissue by direct contact through the blade, sealing small blood vessels up to 2 mm in size while simultaneously cutting through the tissue. No electrical current enters the patient.

The Shaw scalpel (Oximetrix, Inc., Mountain View, CA) uses blades of conventional size and shape (No. 15 and No. 10) but constructed of surgical steel, with an inner copper and outer Teflon coating (Fig. 19–6). The outer Teflon coating is an important adjunct, allowing coagulated tissue and blood to be wiped off easily during the procedure. Between the copper and Teflon are situated three individually regulated heating and sensing elements that precisely and rapidly control the blade temperature. Most cutaneous surgical procedures are done at 130° to 150°C. If a larger vessel is transected, the temperature may be immediately raised to 270°C and the blade tip used to seal the bleeding vessel with hot cautery.

The Shaw scalpel has been successfully used in routine cutaneous surgical procedures, cosmetic surgery (e.g., scalp reduction), and Mohs micrographic surgery.[22] In addition, it has been used in combination with the carbon dioxide laser and dermabrasion for treatment of rhinophyma.[23] It causes very little thermal damage to surrounding tissue while providing excellent hemostasis. Some Mohs surgeons prefer to incise the epidermis with a standard scalpel blade or with the cold Shaw scalpel blade first and then complete the incision through the

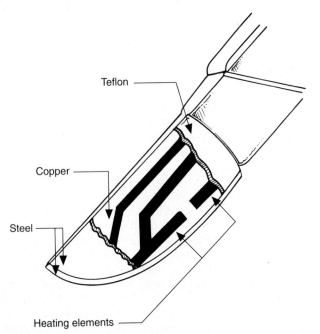

Figure 19–6. Schematic showing Shaw scalpel construction. (Redrawn courtesy of Mr. Bill Touchton.)

dermis and subcutaneous tissue with the heated blade. The heat occasionally causes the epidermis to separate from the underlying dermis.[22] Of course, if left in contact with the tissue too long, coagulation and necrosis occur, and the histologic margins of tissue are obscured.

Studies comparing cold steel surgery with Shaw scalpel surgery in an animal model have shown that healing times and relative tensile strengths are similar.[24] Similar studies of the carbon dioxide laser with regard to amount of bleeding and healing time have not yet been performed.

The obvious advantages of the Shaw scalpel include the reduced time required to obtain hemostasis, the decreased need for suction vacuum apparatus, and the incorporation of the standard scalpel design, which requires little adaptation for use by the cutaneous surgeon. In addition, because no electrical current enters the tissue, no distracting muscle stimulation or twitching occurs while coagulating tissue. The main disadvantages are the potential for thermal damage to the surrounding tissue with consequent histologic distortion of margins and possible suboptimal wound healing.

Techniques and Applications of High-Frequency Electrosurgery

High-frequency electrosurgery can be simplified by subdividing it into four basic processes: electrofulguration, electrodesiccation, electrocoagulation, and electrosectioning or electrocutting.

ELECTROFULGURATION AND ELECTRODESICCATION

Because electrofulguration and electrodesiccation are very similar in technique and application, they will be discussed together. They differ mainly in the distance the active electrode is held from the skin surface, the respective depths of destruction, and the degree of precision and localization of damage. Both electrofulguration and electrodesiccation usually employ a monoterminal active electrode without a dispersive electrode (Fig. 19–7). By far the most commonly used device is the Birtcher Hyfrecutter.[25] In electrofulguration, a coarse spark is generated that literally "arcs" or "jumps the gap" from the electrode to the tissue. The electrical energy in the spark is converted by resistance in the tissue into heat, but only very superficially. This is because the wave form is damped and much of the energy is lost as the spark travels between electrode and tissue. This fulgurating effect produces very superficial tissue damage while giving the surgeon the ability to carefully control the depth of destruction and scarring. The disadvantage of the electrofulguration technique is that the lateral direction of sparking is difficult to control, so that small or well-defined lesions are difficult to remove precisely without damaging the adjacent normal skin.

The most common applications for electrofulguration are removal of epidermal lesions such as seborrheic

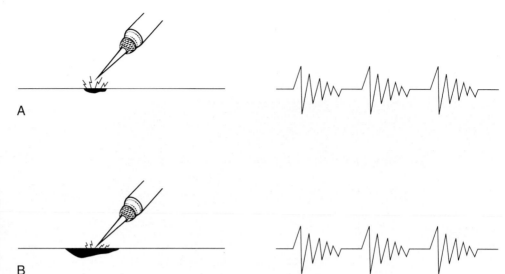

Figure 19–7. High-frequency electrosurgical monoterminal techniques and their respective electrical wave forms. *A,* Electrofulguration with damped sine wave. *B,* Electrodesiccation with damped sine wave. (Redrawn courtesy of Mr. Bill Touchton.)

keratoses, skin tags, warts, molluscum, and condylomata.[1, 26] Cure rates for condyloma have been reported to be higher with electrodesiccation than with cryotherapy or podophyllin.[26] Additional benign lesions treated with electrofulguration or electrodesiccation include actinic keratosis, pyogenic granuloma, sebaceous hyperplasia, and syringomata.[1, 27] Monoterminal electrodesiccation has also been reported to be a useful adjunct in blepharoplasty procedures to remove adipose tissue without extensive dissection.[28] Together with curettage, electrofulguration and electrodesiccation are also used to treat keratoacanthomas and small, superficial skin cancers such as primary basal cell carcinomas and actinically induced squamous cell carcinomas less than 1 to 2 cm in diameter.[29–35]

For superficial benign lesions, electrofulguration is usually done alone or in conjunction with curettage. The technique varies slightly from device to device but usually begins with initial infiltration of local anesthesia. The device is then turned to a low or medium power output, and the hand holding the handpiece is stabilized by resting it on the patient or the table. The electrofulgurating electrode is held approximately 1 to 3 mm from the lesion, and the electrode is activated. A blue-white spark is immediately seen, and light charring of the lesion can be observed. The electrode is moved in a back-and-forth fashion or in a circular motion with continuous or intermittent bursts until the entire lesion is equally charred. Wet gauze is then used to remove the char. Cosmetic results are usually excellent, with only occasional hypopigmentation or atrophy of the treated site.

It should be noted that treatment of cutaneous malignancies should always be done with the intent of completely removing the involved tissue while preserving maximal function and cosmesis. Very high cure rates for treatment of primary basal cell carcinomas and squamous cell carcinomas less than 2 cm in diameter have been reported with curettage and electrosurgery, and properly selected cases should continue to be treated with this convenient and easily learned technique.[29–35]

Electrodesiccation is used in conjunction with curettage to treat basal cell and squamous cell carcinomas. In this technique, the curetted skin surface is desiccated and carbonized by holding the electrode in direct contact with the curetted surface to destroy any remaining cancer cells (Fig. 19–8). This procedure is usually repeated two or three times.[34] Some surgeons prefer electrofulguration, holding the electrode 1 to 3 mm from the surface of the tissue while moving the electrode. Others use a combination of electrofulguration and electrodesiccation or even electrocoagulation.[36]

Other uses of electrodesiccation include hemostasis by coagulation of small (less than 1 mm) vessels, pinpoint destruction of telangiectases (Fig. 19–9), cherry angiomas (Fig. 19–10), spider angiomas, skin tags, angiofibromas, syringomas, angiokeratomas, warts and condylomata, lymphangiomas, molluscum contagiosum, sebaceous hyperplasia, and pyogenic granulomas. One study[37] showed that monoterminal electrodesiccation was also effective in the treatment of actinic cheilitis. In this bilateral comparison study, seven patients with biopsy-proven actinic cheilitis of the lower lip were treated on one side with low-power electrodesiccation and on the contralateral side with the carbon dioxide laser. The final clinical result was excellent with both modalities. Time for complete healing was approximately 2 to 3 weeks on the electrodesiccation side and approximately 4 weeks on the laser-treated side. A posthealing biopsy showed no evidence of residual actinic cheilitis, and after a follow-up period of 1 year there was no recurrence.

ELECTROCOAGULATION

Electrocoagulation is a deeper-penetrating form of biterminal high-frequency electrosurgery in which lower-voltage, higher-amperage current is used. Its principal use is in obtaining hemostasis of larger blood vessels. The active electrode is usually employed in conjunction with a large dispersive "grounding" plate, which is held in contact with the patient to help direct the current

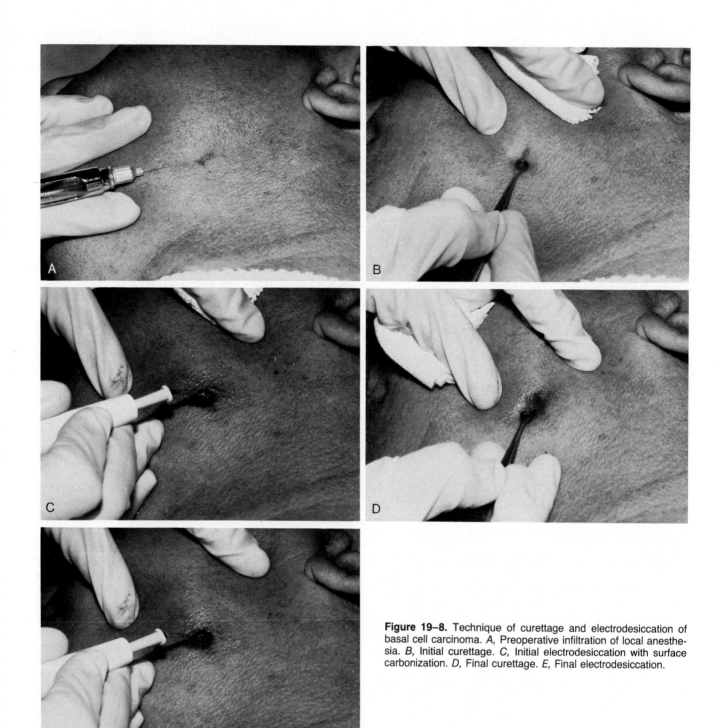

Figure 19–8. Technique of curettage and electrodesiccation of basal cell carcinoma. *A,* Preoperative infiltration of local anesthesia. *B,* Initial curettage. *C,* Initial electrodesiccation with surface carbonization. *D,* Final curettage. *E,* Final electrodesiccation.

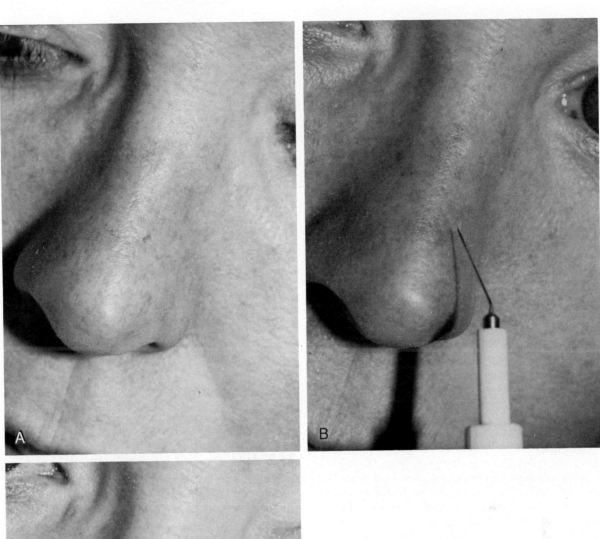

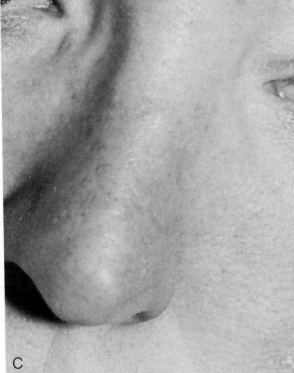

Figure 19–9. Electrodesiccation of fine facial telangiectasia. *A,* Preoperative clinical appearance. *B,* Electrodesiccation with fine needle tip held lightly in contact with the skin surface. *C,* Immediate postoperative clinical appearance.

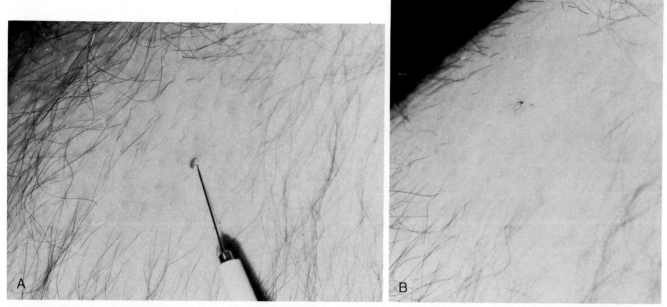

Figure 19–10. Electrodesiccation of cherry angioma. *A,* Preoperative clinical appearance. *B,* Immediate postoperative clinical appearance. (Courtesy of Mr. Bill Touchton.)

flow (Fig. 19–11). The higher amperage, or current flow, from the active electrode produces greater tissue heat that can be used to coagulate larger vessels. An alternative device for electrocoagulation is the biterminal forceps, in which both "poles" of the forceps are alternating active electrodes. The tissue between the two active electrodes receives very concentrated, high-current flow, and coagulation is thorough (Fig. 19–1C).

The application of electrocoagulation was described in 1928 by Cushing,[38] who noted that bleeding vessels were effectively coagulated as a result of tissue dehydration. Although electrocoagulation is superior to electrodesiccation for hemostasis in bloody fields, even electrocoagulation cannot produce effective heat in very wet or bloody operative fields because of the dispersive effect of the fluid on the current. Hemostasis by electrocoagulation is achieved by holding the active electrode in direct contact with the blood vessel or using a clamp or forceps to hold the blood vessel while contact is made with the active electrode. This second technique is not very useful for monoterminal devices, because the current is usually too low and too dispersed to generate sufficient heat to coagulate the vessel. Proper technique involves the delivery of just enough mechanical pressure

and electrical energy to fuse the vessel walls. However, all too often, because of its deep-penetrating, destructive ability, electrocoagulation causes inadvertent damage and necrosis of deeper adjacent tissue, which may affect wound healing and nerve function.

ELECTROSECTION OR ELECTROCUTTING

Electrosection is used to incise, divide, or separate tissue. This is made possible by generating high-frequency, high-voltage, high-amperage electrical energy with a very uniform sine wave oscillating pattern (Fig. 19–2). Pure electrosection current provides little or no coagulation and is therefore of little value in cutaneous electrosurgery (Fig. 19–12). Therefore, it is usually modified or "blended" with a coagulation current to provide both cutting and coagulation actions (Fig. 19–13).

Electrosection can be performed with a variety of electrodes, the most common of which are thin wire loops. Blade-shaped electrodes are also available but tend to produce excessive thermal injury because of the greater power required and the greater surface area of the flat electrode that is in contact with the tissue as it

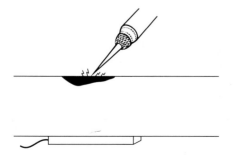

Figure 19–11. High-frequency electrosurgical technique of biterminal electrocoagulation with moderately damped electrical sine wave form. (Redrawn courtesy of Mr. Bill Touchton.)

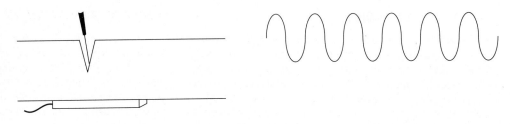

Figure 19–12. High-frequency electrosurgical technique of biterminal electrosection (pure) with pure electrical sine wave form. (Redrawn courtesy of Mr. Bill Touchton.)

cuts. A wire loop electrode also produces greater thermal injury than a straight line wire electrode because of the increased electrical power required to produce cutting power density. Electrosection is performed as a biterminal modality, with a dispersive plate keeping the patient in the circuit and directing the flow of high current. Because of the higher current flow, the dispersive plate electrode must be placed properly to avoid burning the patient.

Electrosection should be done at a steady, brisk speed. The optimum speed will cause clean separation with little or no charring. Charring produces better hemostasis but causes a larger zone of thermal damage. A cutting rate of 5 to 10 mm per second[39, 40] has been recommended. The technique of electrosection is more similar to carbon dioxide laser incision than to cold steel incision, because little or no tissue resistance to cutting is felt by the surgeon. For this reason, considerable practice is required to produce straight, even, uniform cuts. The blend of cutting and coagulating current is usually fixed by the machine and does not pose a problem to the operator. Because a small amount of charred tissue may adhere to the cutting electrode, thereby interfering with the cutting or coagulating action, the electrode should be cleaned regularly during the procedure. If char build-up seems excessive, the power may be too high or the cutting speed too slow.

Applications of cutting current include benign and malignant cutaneous tumors, scalp incisions, and rhinophyma.[1, 41] It should be noted that healing may be delayed in electrosection wounds. However, moderate to severe rhinophyma responds well to electrosection. A study of 13 patients with rhinophyma treated with electrosection indicated that the risk of scarring was low and the final cosmetic result excellent.[41] Another study showed comparable results between carbon dioxide laser and electrosurgery for rhinophyma.[42]

Risks of Electrosurgery

There are few risks to the patient from properly applied electrosurgery. However, potential hazards should be understood so they can be minimized. More emphasis is currently being placed on the potential risks to the surgeon and the operating room personnel.

BURNS

Burns represent the most obvious hazard in electrosurgery. They may result from the inadvertent contact of the electrode with the skin of the patient or the surgeon, but the most common burn injury in electrosurgery occurs when there is inadequate contact between the patient and the dispersive electrode plate.[43] Occasionally, the patient or the surgeon may inadvertently touch a grounding element such as the metal on the treatment table, resulting in a burn or shock. If the dispersive electrode plate is well placed, this "ground" burn or shock usually does not occur.

CHANNELING

There are reports that high-frequency electrosurgical current can be conducted along neurovascular bundles.[44] This must be kept in mind, especially when using high-frequency electrosurgery around larger nerves, since tissue damage distant from the local site may occur. This so-called "channeling" is rarely a problem at the lower power settings used in most office-based cutaneous surgical practices. Channeling is always avoided by use of bipolar forceps or electrocautery devices.[45, 46]

FIRE HAZARD

Fire may be a hazard if alcohol is used as a preparation solution for electrosurgery. For this reason, nonflammable antiseptic solutions such as povidone-iodine or chlorhexidine should be used. Dry gauzes, oxygen, and some anesthetic gases can also be ignited, so extreme care or avoidance of electrosurgery is recommended in these situations. Common fire hazard prevention and extinguishing techniques must be thoroughly understood.[46]

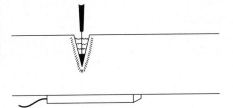

Figure 19–13. High-frequency electrosurgical technique of biterminal electrosection (blended) with modulated electrical sine wave form. (Redrawn courtesy of Mr. Bill Touchton.)

CARDIAC PACEMAKERS

Most modern pacemakers operate in a demand mode, requiring sensing and output circuits. Any of these circuits may be interfered with by high-frequency electrical current, which may have adverse effects on pacemaker function. Despite the fact that most modern pacemakers are normally well shielded and filtered to avoid interference from outside electrical current, high-frequency electrosurgery should be avoided in patients with pacemakers. However, limited electrodesiccation of small lesions probably poses no risk to the relatively healthy pacemaker patient.[47] "Hot-tip" electrocautery is an acceptable substitute, since no electrical current passes into the patient.

PLUME

The risks to the surgeon in the course of performing any type of electrosurgery are no longer trivial and deserve close inspection. The smoke from electrosurgery has been shown to have mutagenic potential, much like the smoke from cigarettes.[48] However, of potentially greater concern is the possible presence of infectious particles on the electrode or in the plume or splatter of electrosurgery cases. Infective hepatitis B virus has been demonstrated to be present on the electrode tips after electrodesiccation.[49] This strongly argues against using the same unsterilized electrode on consecutive patients.[50]

Electrodesiccation has been shown to produce a fine aerosol and splatter of blood droplets for at least several centimeters around the electrodesiccated site.[50, 51] If inhaled, this aerosol may be infectious. Herpes virus particles have also been shown to be dispersed by the Hyfrecutter.[52] Transfer of bacteria during electrodesiccation has also been demonstrated in a laboratory setting.[53]

The presence of human papillomavirus (HPV) particles in the plumes from carbon dioxide lasers and electrosurgery has also been investigated.[54] Infectious bovine papillomavirus and HPV DNA have been found in the plumes from both electrocoagulation and carbon dioxide laser vaporization. HPV is now known to be present in certain types of cutaneous carcinomas.[55] Although surgical masks have been shown in the laboratory to filter out HPV, complete filtration without leakage in a clinical setting cannot be ensured. This fact has caused many physicians to re-evaluate their preferred methods for the treatment of viral warts and condylomata and to reduce the number of electro- or laser surgeries they perform for these cases. A graver implication of these HPV studies is that other viruses such as the human immunodeficiency virus and the hepatitis viruses may also remain intact in the plume and be inhaled by the surgeon or operating room personnel. No laboratory or clinical evidence for this exists as yet, and additional studies are needed. Use of a commercial smoke evacuator device is suggested for all but the briefest electrosurgical procedures.[56]

RECOMMENDED SAFETY PROTOCOL

An outline for the safe operation of electrosurgical equipment has been compiled and published.[1] Emphasis should be placed on keeping the equipment well maintained and grounded, avoiding carbon build-up on the active electrode, using sterile electrodes with each patient, ensuring uniform skin contact with the dispersive electrode, avoiding alcohol or flammable gases during electrosurgery, keeping a fire extinguisher appropriate for electrical fires nearby, and always wearing gloves. When performed in this manner, electrosurgical procedures should pose no additional hazard to the patient or the surgeon when compared with traditional surgical procedures.

SUMMARY

For most effective use of electrosurgery in any cutaneous surgical procedure, a thorough understanding of the equipment and technique used is required. The recent introduction of many new pieces of electrosurgical apparatus has greatly facilitated the surgeon's ability to limit unwanted thermal damage and maximize precise electricity-tissue interaction in many different types of cutaneous surgical procedures.

REFERENCES

1. Sebben JE: Cutaneous Electrosurgery. Year Book Medical, Chicago, 1989.
2. Breasted JH: The Edwin Smith Surgical Papyrus. Vol 1. University of Chicago Press, Chicago, 1930.
3. Mitchell JP, Lumb GN: A Handbook of Surgical Diathermy. John Wright and Sons, Ltd, Bristol, 1978.
4. Bryant T: Clinical lectures on bloodless operating and bloodless operations as illustrated by the use of galvanic cautery. Lancet 1:469, 1874.
5. d'Arsonval A: Action physiologique des courants alternativs. Soc Biol 43:283–286, 1891.
6. d'Arsonval A: Action physiologique des courants alternatifs a grande frequence. Arch Physiol Norm Pathol 5:401–408, 1893.
7. Pozzi M: Remarques sur la fulguration. Bull Assoc Franc Cancer 2:64–69, 1909.
8. Clark WL: Oscillatory desiccation in treatment of accessible malignant growths and minor surgical conditions. New electrical effect. J Adv Ther 29:169–183, 1911.
9. Doyen D: Sur la destruction des tumeurs cancereuses acessibles par la methode de la voltaisation bipolaire et de l'electro-coagulation thermique. Arch Elec Med 17:791–795, 1909.
10. Goldwyn RM: Bovie: the man and the machine. Ann Plast Surg 2:135–153, 1979.
11. Kalkworf KL, Krejci RF, Edison AR, et al: Subjacent heat production during tissue excision with electrosurgery. J Oral Maxillofac Surg 41:653–657, 1983.
12. Bennett RG: Fundamentals of Cutaneous Surgery. CV Mosby, St Louis, 1988.
13. Rook A, Wilkinson DS, Ebling FJG: Textbook of Dermatology. 4th ed. Blackwell Scientific, London, 1986.
14. Moschella SL, Hurley HJ: Dermatology. 3rd ed. WB Saunders, Philadelphia, 1992.
15. Wagner RF, Tomich JM, Grande DJ: Electrolysis and thermolysis for permanent hair removal. J Am Acad Dermatol 12:441–449, 1985.

16. Wagner RF: Physical methods for the management of hirsutism. Cutis 45:319–321, 1990.

17. Kligman AM, Peters L: Histologic changes of human hair follicles after electrolysis: a comparison of two methods. Cutis 34:169–176, 1984.

18. Kobayashi T: Electrosurgery using insulated needles: epilation. J Dermatol Surg Oncol 11:993–1000, 1985.

19. Sternberg TH: Clinical study of Perma Tweez self use electrolysis. General Medical Company, Los Angeles, 1972.

20. Kobayashi T: Electrosurgery using insulated needles: treatment of telangiectasias. J Dermatol Surg Oncol 12:936–942, 1986.

21. Kobayashi T: Electrosurgery using insulated needles: treatment of axillary bromhidrosis and hyperhidrosis. J Dermatol Surg Oncol 14:749–752, 1988.

22. Tromovitch TA, Glogau RG, Stegman SJ: The Shaw scalpel. J Dermatol Surg Oncol 9:316–319, 1983.

23. Eisen RF, Katz AE, Bohigian RK, et al: Surgical treatment of rhinophyma with the Shaw scalpel. Arch Dermatol 122:307–309, 1986.

24. Fee WE: Use of the Shaw scalpel in head and neck surgery. Otolaryngol Head Neck Surg 89:515–519, 1981.

25. Sebben JE: The status of electrosurgery in dermatologic practice. J Am Acad Dermatol 19:542–549, 1988.

26. Stone KM, Becker TM, Hadgu A, Kraus SJ: Treatment of external genital warts: a randomised clinical trial comparing podophyllin, cryotherapy, and electrodesiccation. Genitourin Med 66:16–19, 1990.

27. Stevenson TR, Swanson NA: Syringoma: removal by electrodesiccation and curettage. Ann Plast Surg 15:151–154, 1985.

28. Bisaccia E, Scarborough DA, Swensen RD: A technique for blepharoplasty without incising or "puncturing" orbital septum. J Dermatol Surg Oncol 16:360–363, 1990.

29. Knox JM, Lyles TW, Shapiro EM et al: Curettage and electrodesiccation in the treatment of skin cancer. Arch Dermatol 82:197–204, 1960.

30. Sweet RD: The treatment of basal cell carcinoma by curettage. Br J Dermatol 75:137–139, 1963.

31. Freeman RG, Knox JM, Heaton CL: The treatment of skin cancer. A statistical study of 1,341 skin tumors comparing results obtained with irradiation, surgery, and curettage followed by electrodesiccation. Cancer 17:535–538, 1964.

32. Tromovitch TA: Skin cancer: treatment by curettage and desiccation. Calif Med 103:107–108, 1965.

33. Knox JM, Freeman RG, Duncan WC: Treatment of skin cancer. South Med J 60:241–246, 1967.

34. Spiller WF, Spiller RF: Treatment of basal cell epithelioma by curettage and electrodesiccation. J Am Acad Dermatol 11:808–814, 1984.

35. Shanoff LB, Spira M, Hardy SB: Basal cell carcinoma: a statistical approach to rational management. Plast Reconstr Surg 39:619–624, 1967.

36. Whelan CS, Deckers PJ: Electrocoagulation for skin cancer: an old oncologic tool revisited. Cancer 47:2280–2287, 1981.

37. Diwan R, Skouge JW: A comparison of electrosurgery and the CO_2 laser for the treatment of actinic cheilitis. Presented at the 17th Annual Clinical and Scientific Meeting, Am Society of Dermatologic Surgery, Maui, Hawaii, February 17, 1990.

38. Cushing H: Electro-surgery as an aid to the removal of intracranial tumors; with a preliminary note on a new surgical-current generator by W.T. Bovie. Surg Gynecol Obstet 47:751, 1928.

39. Honig WM: Mechanisms of cutting current in electrosurgery. IEEE Trans Biomed Eng 22:58–62, 1975.

40. Kalkworf KL, Krejci RF, Edison AR, et al: Lateral heat production secondary to electrosurgical incisions. Oral Surg Oral Med Oral Pathol 55:344–348, 1983.

41. Clark DP, Hanke CW: Electrosurgical treatment of rhinophyma. J Am Acad Dermatol 22:831–837, 1990.

42. Greenbaum SS, Krull EA, Watnick K: Comparison of CO_2 laser and electrosurgery in treatment of rhinophyma. J Am Acad Dermatol 18:363–368, 1988.

43. Mitchell JP, Lumb GN, Dobbie AK: A Handbook of Surgical Diathermy. 2nd ed. John Wright & Sons, Bristol, England, 1978.

44. Sebben JE: The hazards of electrosurgery. J Am Acad Dermatol 16:869–872, 1987.

45. Dujovny M, Vas R, Osgood CP: Bipolar jeweler's forceps with automatic irrigation for coagulation in microsurgery. Plast Reconstr Surg 56:585–587, 1975.

46. Sebben JE: Fire hazards and electrosurgery. J Dermatol Surg Oncol 16:421–424, 1990.

47. Sebben JE: Electrosurgery and cardiac pacemakers. J Am Acad Dermatol 9:457–463, 1983.

48. Tomita Y, Mihashi S, Nagata K, et al: Mutagenicity of smoke condensates induced by CO_2-laser irradiation and electrocauterization. Mutat Res 89:145–149, 1981.

49. Sherertz EF, Davis GL, Rice RW, et al: Transfer of hepatitis B virus by reusable needle electrodes after electrodesiccation in simulated use. J Am Acad Dermatol 15:1242–1246, 1986.

50. Berberian BJ, Burnett JW: The potential role of common dermatologic practice technics in transmitting disease. J Am Acad Dermatol 15:1057–1058, 1986.

51. Sebben JE: Contamination risks associated with electrosurgery. Arch Dermatol 126:805–808, 1990.

52. Colver GB, Peutherer JF: Herpes simplex virus dispersal by Hyfrecator electrodes. Br J Dermatol 117:672–679, 1987.

53. Bennett RG, Kraffert CA: Bacterial transference during electrodesiccation and electrocoagulation. Arch Dermatol 126:751–755, 1990.

54. Sawchuck S, Weber PJ, Lowy DR, et al: Infectious papillomavirus in the vapor of warts treated with carbon dioxide laser or electrocoagulation: detection and protection. J Am Acad Dermatol 21:41–49, 1989.

55. Moy RL, Eliezri YD, Nuovo GJ, et al: Human papillomavirus type 16 DNA in periungual squamous cell carcinoma. JAMA 261:2669–2673, 1989.

56. Karaca AR: Using the suction apparatus of the laser machine to get rid of smoke from electrocoagulation. Plast Reconstr Surg 84:372, 1989.

CHAPTER 20

Photography in Cutaneous Surgery

ROBERT H. SCHOSSER

Whether the purpose is record keeping, documentation, monitoring therapeutic response, or medical education, the ultimate goal of clinical photography is to record an image containing maximal, clinically significant detail while avoiding unnecessary or distracting elements. Cutaneous surgeons strive to translate the ideal features from a three-dimensional clinical subject into an effective two-dimensional representation.

Light and Its Qualities

While it is true that photographers are image recorders, they are also light manipulators. Without the successful manipulation of the reflected light that forms images, we would never be able to achieve the goal of recording them with maximal clinical detail. For photographic purposes, two types of light exist: available light and photographic light. Available light, in turn, is composed of natural and artificial light. Natural light is sunlight that has been modified by various natural conditions,[1] while artificial light comes from a variety of sources, including fluorescent fixtures, tungsten bulbs, and metal vapor lamps. As a rule, available light sources cannot be filtered, repositioned, or otherwise controlled.

If available artificial light is viewed as undisciplined light, photographic light is just the opposite. Photographic light is defined as artificial light of controlled diffusiveness, color temperature, and direction that is produced by equipment designed for use with image-recording systems.[1] The three qualities of photographic light that are of concern are color temperature; "hard" versus "soft" light; and flat, contour, and texture light.

COLOR TEMPERATURE

When some materials are heated beyond a certain temperature, they become *incandescent,* which means that they radiate light. We use the temperature of a radiant object to specify the color of light that it radiates. When so used, it is called *color temperature* and is stated using the absolute temperature scale—*degrees Kelvin* (K).[2] It should be remembered that all incandescent objects radiate a continuous spectrum.

Light may also be produced by methods other than heating a substance. Rather than producing an infinitely variable range of color temperatures, these other techniques tend to produce peaks of light at various wavelengths. Fluorescent lamps are one such light source, as are the different metal vapor lamps. It is difficult, even impossible at times, to balance these light sources effectively for the limited range of color films.

Video cameras can be "white balanced" for many different light sources. No matter what the light source, objects appear to be their proper color: lemons are yellow, and red apples are red. The human eye perceives the sun, various fluorescent lamps, and incandescent lamps with other light sources as producing "white light."

Film, however, is very rigid in this respect. Films are "balanced" for very few color temperatures. Daylight films expect to "see" light with a color temperature of 5500°K. Another type of film is balanced for tungsten light with a color temperature of 3200°K, and a few types of film are balanced for tungsten light of a slightly higher color temperature, 3400°K. If films record light of a color temperature other than what their emulsion is balanced for, the color of objects reflecting that light will be misrepresented.

TABLE 20–1. **COMMON REPRODUCTION RATIOS**

Reproduction Ratios (Magnification)		Area of Coverage	
		Centimeters	Inches
1:1	(life size)	2.4 × 3.6	0.96 × 1.44
1:1.25		3.0 × 4.5	1.20 × 1.76
1:1.50		3.6 × 5.4	1.44 × 2.16
1:2	(1/2)	4.8 × 7.2	1.92 × 2.88
1:3	(1/3)	7.2 × 10.8	2.88 × 4.32
1:4	(1/4)	9.6 × 14.4	3.84 × 5.76
1:5	(1/5)	12.0 × 18.0	4.80 × 7.20
1:6	(1/6)	14.4 × 21.6	5.76 × 8.64
1:7	(1/7)	16.8 × 25.2	6.72 × 10.08
1:8	(1/8)	19.2 × 28.8	7.68 × 11.52
1:9	(1/9)	21.6 × 32.4	8.64 × 12.96
1:10	(1/10)	24.0 × 36.0	9.60 × 14.40
1:15	(1/15)	36.0 × 54.0	14.40 × 21.60
1:20	(1/20)	48.0 × 72.0	19.20 × 28.80
1:30	(1/30)	72.0 × 108.0	28.80 × 43.20
1:40	(1/40)	96.0 × 144.0	38.40 × 57.60
1:50	(1/50)	120.0 × 180.0	48.00 × 72.00

HARD VERSUS SOFT LIGHT

Hard light produces sharp-edged, dense shadows. Light sources producing hard light are relatively small with respect to the size of the subject. They behave as single-point sources of light, and the rays of light they produce are essentially traveling parallel to one another. Soft light, on the other hand, is characterized by less dense shadows with diffused or less-defined borders. Soft light is produced by light sources that are relatively large compared with the size of the subject. The rays of light they produce emanate from many points on their surface and travel in different directions, striking a subject and its edges at many different angles.

FLAT, CONTOUR, AND TEXTURE LIGHT

Flat, contour, and texture light are related to the length and direction of shadows produced by photographic light sources. Flat light has an even intensity across a subject's surface; raised areas on a subject's surface produce minimal shadows. Single sources of flat light are located near the optical axis of the photographic lens. Paired sources of flat light are of equal intensity and located at angles of no more than 45 degrees on either side of the optical axis.

Contour light causes a subject's larger contours to cast enough of a shadow that a viewer may perceive the contour as being raised or sunken with respect to its surrounding surface. Because of shadows, an ulcer would appear to be depressed, and a nodule or tumor would appear to be raised above the surrounding surface. Contour light is produced by a "main light" located at an angle of 45 degrees with the optical axis. The main light may be used with a "fill light" of lower intensity located on the opposite side of the lens but close to its axis. The purpose of the fill light is to reduce the density of the shadows cast by the main light. It "fills in" or restores detail that would be lost in the shadow. A white "fill card" may be used in place of the fill light. The fill card is placed as close to the subject as possible on the side opposite the main light. The fill card reflects light onto the subject, reducing shadow density.

A main light angled about 85 degrees with the lens axis produces "texture light," also known as "skim light." As with contour light, a fill card or light is usually included in the lighting system. The term texture light comes from the fact that small surface variations have a relatively fine roughness, or texture, when the fingers are rubbed across them. Skim lighting is particularly useful in causing small surface variations such as tiny follicular papules to cast sufficient shadows that they are recognizable. However, when used with larger surface irregularities, skim lighting produces excessively long shadows that tend to be distracting.

Reproduction Ratios and the Domain of Cutaneous Photography

Reproduction ratios are nothing more than the ratio of the size of an object's image on film to its actual size, and thus represent magnification ratios. If a 1-cm image is made of an object 10 cm in size, a reproduction ratio of 1:10 exists. The image is 1/10 life size.

The dimensions of a 35-mm image are 2.4 × 3.6 cm. At 1/10 life size, those dimensions will provide an area of coverage of 24 × 36 cm, or 9.6 × 14.4 inches. An effective way of approaching cutaneous photography is to consider what anatomic parts will fit into a given area of coverage. This allows the photographer to apply the concept of reproduction ratios to infants or adults with equal effectiveness. The many commonly used reproduction ratios and their areas of coverage for the 35-mm format are given in Table 20–1.

Domain of Dermatologic Photography

Most dermatologic photography is "close-up" (Table 20–2) or "ultra close-up" photography.[3] Dermatopathologists use sophisticated photomicroscopes to take photomicrographs of histopathology specimens, but the photographs of skin lesions taken through a culposcope or equipment used for what has been referred to as "epiluminescence microscopy"[4] are known as photomacrographs.

TABLE 20–2. **PHOTOGRAPHIC DOMAINS**

Type	Reproduction Ratio
Common photography	≤1:10
Close-up photography	1:10–1:4
Ultra close-up photography	1:4–1:1 (life size)
Photomacrography	1:1 (life size)–30:1
Photomicrography	30:1 and higher; degrees of magnification usually recorded through a compound microscope

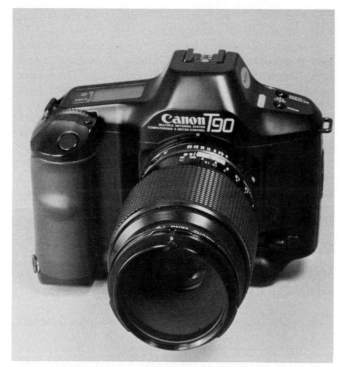

Figure 20–1. The Canon T90 is a modern 35-mm single lens reflex camera offering manual, aperture priority, shutter priority, and program modes. It features TTL metering for flash and continuous light. A 100-mm macro lens is mounted on the T90 in this photograph.

Equipment for Clinical Photography

CAMERA BODIES AND DESIRABLE FEATURES

The portability and versatility of the 35-mm single lens reflex (SLR) camera make it the instrument of choice for most cutaneous photography (Fig. 20–1). In recent years, 35-mm SLR camera bodies have evolved tremendously and now are available from all major camera manufacturers with a variety of exposure modes and automatic metering systems.

A number of features should be considered when selecting a 35-mm camera body (Table 20–3); few, if any, cameras provide them all. A photographer must decide which features are important for the types of photographs to be taken and select the equipment on the basis of those requirements.

Manual Exposure Capability

All current 35-mm SLR cameras have in-camera metering systems. In many newer cameras, computer chips interpret the meter reading in concert with the speed of the film being used and set the aperture, shutter speed, or both. Many cameras allow the user to set both the aperture and shutter speed for manual exposure capability when strobe units are used for lighting purposes. Despite the sophistication of current automatic metering systems, manual exposure techniques are still thought to yield the most consistent results in clinical photography.

Studio strobe lighting systems must be used with manual exposure techniques. Portable strobe units that are attached to the camera either directly or through a bracket also yield the most consistent results when used in conjunction with a pre-established manual exposure system.

Continuous light produced by special tungsten lamps is often used to take photographs of specimens, surgical instruments, and other equipment, because it is easy to see where shadows fall. The lamps may be moved around to get desired effects. Fewer current camera models allow manual exposure control with continuous light.

Through-The-Lens Flash Metering

While all modern 35-mm cameras meter continuous light through the lens (TTL), it was not until the mid-1980s that all major manufacturers marketed at least one camera capable of metering burst or flash lighting through the lens. TTL flash metering is generally accomplished by having a tiny sensor read a percentage of the light reflected off the film itself[5] (hence the designation, Through-The-Lens Off-The-Film [TTL-OTF] metering). TTL flash metering is necessary if one is to effectively use an automatic exposure mode in clinical photography, particularly photography of cutaneous lesions.

Aperture Priority Exposure Mode

Programmed automatic modes allow the camera to set both the aperture size and shutter speeds at the same time according to one or more programs built into a small computer system in the camera. Aperture priority exposure mode allows the user to determine the size of the opening that will allow light into the camera and to select the proper shutter speed, depending on the speed of the film used and the light available. Aperture priority exposure mode is the most effective automatic exposure mode for clinical photography, because the photographer may select an aperture small enough to give the necessary depth of field.

High Shutter Speed Flash Synchronization

Normally, the intensity of strobe lighting overpowers ambient, artificial light sources, providing correct color

---

TABLE 20–3. USEFUL SLR CAMERA FEATURES

Manual exposure control mode
TTL flash metering with aperture priority exposure mode
High shutter speed flash synchronization
User-interchangeable focusing screens
Effective ergonomics
Power winder or motor drives
Depth-of-field preview capability (stopped-down metering capability)
Miscellaneous
    Mirror lock-up
    Multiple exposure
    High eyepoint finder

balance for daylight color films. Available bright artificial lighting, such as that found in an operating room, can cause aberrant color balance and ghost images. Camera bodies providing flash synchronization speeds of $\frac{1}{125}$ second or less minimize this problem, because the fast shutter speed markedly reduces the quantity of available light striking the film.

User-Interchangeable Focusing Screens

A matte surface screen with an etched grid is very useful in aligning a subject for standardized anatomic views and for general lesion photography as well. A double–cross hair reticle screen is of great assistance when taking pictures of subjects magnified greater than life size, particularly with photographs taken through the microscope. The split-image screen is difficult to use in ultra close-up photographs. Because of magnification factors and relatively low intensity ambient lighting, half of the split image will often black out, since less than average amounts of light are available for focusing. Split-focusing screens are generally most helpful when trying to focus at distances sufficient to photograph the entire body of an adult.[3]

Ergonomics

A comfortable camera "feel" is more than just size or weight. A small pair of hands should not necessarily be matched with a small or lightweight camera, and large hands do not need a large or heavy camera. What is important is how the camera fits the user's hand, which includes whether the user is comfortable with the location of various controls on the camera body. The sensation of "camera fit" should be thoroughly tested before any system is purchased.[3]

Depth-of-Field Preview Capability

Depth-of-field preview capability is also known as "stopped-down metering." During focusing and composition, a camera lens is usually open to its maximal aperture. As the shutter release is pressed, the lens will close to the correct size for a given exposure. Depth of field is important for the near–life-size magnification ratios commonly encountered in clinical photography; therefore, the ability to actually see how much of the image is in focus can be very useful. The depth-of-field preview capability provides this function. Stopped-down metering also permits a camera to be used with nonautomatic lens systems, as in photomicroscopy.

LENSES

A "standard" lens is a lens that provides a field of view roughly equal to that in which the eyes produce a sharp image. Standard lenses are also known as "normal" lenses. Another definition of the standard lens is a lens whose focal length approximately equals the diagonal of the image formed at the film plane. The diagonal of a 35-mm film frame is 43 mm. However, 50

mm is usually considered a standard lens for the 35-mm format. Lenses whose focal length is less than twice the diagonal of the film plane are often considered "short" lenses.[6] In that sense, a standard lens is one kind of short lens. A "long" lens has a focal length greater than twice the diagonal of the film plane for a given format. Thus, any lens with a focal length greater than 86 mm can be considered a long lens for the 35-mm format.

Lenses that have some application in dermatologic photography include macro lenses, both short and long types; conventional fixed-focal-length lenses; and zoom lenses.

Macro Lenses

Macro lenses (Fig. 20–1) are commonly characterized by several features. First, the long focus travel allows the lens to achieve reproduction ratios of up to at least 1:2 (Fig. 20–2). Most macro lenses are capable of producing life-size (1:1) images, but some lenses require an adapter (extension ring) to bridge the gap from 1:2 to 1:1. The reproduction ratios are marked on the lens barrel. Second, these lenses have flat (edge-to-edge) focus at all apertures. Most macro lenses offer very small (often f/32) minimum apertures. The final characteristic of a macro lens is freedom from distortion such that straight lines are not curved in or out by the lens.

Standard macro lenses are less expensive than their longer counterparts, but they have only one half to one fourth the free working distance from the subject. Short working distances may make effective lighting difficult and occasionally put the photographer closer to some subjects than is desirable. More importantly, standard macro lenses produce an inaccurate representation of facial features at reproduction ratios commonly used for those views. The nose may appear to be disproportionately large compared with the overall size of the face.

Most long macro lenses have focal lengths between

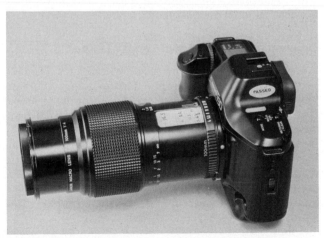

Figure 20–2. This Canon 100-mm macro lens will produce a reproduction ratio of 1:2 when fully extended as in this illustration. It is capable of reproduction ratios as big as 1:1 with an added extension ring. Note the label tape affixed to the barrel. The shutter speeds and reproduction ratios are standardized for use with the Canon ML1 lighting system (not shown).

90 and 105 mm. These lenses provide double the free working distance of a 50- or 55-mm macro lens and offer a much more accurate representation of facial features. On the negative side, the longer working distance makes it nearly impossible to obtain a full-length view of an adult in an average examination room. For most dermatologic photographers, this view is not often required, and on the rare occasion when it is, an inexpensive, short, conventional fixed-focus lens or short zoom lens may be used in its place. Even though long macro lenses have slightly less depth of field than standard lenses, this is too insignificant to be a practical handicap. Perhaps the greatest drawback of the long macro lens is its cost, which is usually twice that of a standard macro lens.

A few 200-mm macro lenses are currently being marketed. Although they provide the most normal-appearing facial features, because of their exceedingly long working distances and great expense, they are not commonly used in cutaneous photography.

In addition to macro lenses, other techniques for achieving image magnification exist. Extension rings may be connected to conventional lenses. Reverse-mounted short conventional lenses can produce extremely crisp, magnified images but can only be used in the stopped-down manual-metering mode. Because the rear lens element has been turned around to become the front of the lens, the connecting pins and rear lens surface itself are exposed to potential damage.

Macro-focusing teleconverters exist, and some can achieve life-size images when attached to conventional lenses. However, this usually occurs at a cost of an additional loss of two exposure steps, or f stops. The sharpness of the image they produce is usually less than acceptable.

Supplementary (diopter) lenses are an inexpensive way of achieving some magnification. Most of the time, this is done at a definite cost of image quality. However, because these are simple magnifying lenses, there is no light loss. High-quality coated diopter lenses, when used with high-quality conventional lenses, may have some application in cutaneous photography.[7]

Conventional Fixed-Focal-Length Lenses

Until the advent of the modern computer-designed zoom lens, conventional (nonmacrofocusing) standard lenses (50 mm) were considered to be the most useful lens for routine photography. The maximum magnifying power of a conventional fixed-focal-length lens is usually in the vicinity of 1/10 life size. Conventional fixed-focal-length lenses are not as closely corrected for distortion as macro lenses. A conventional 50-mm lens is useful for taking half- and full-body-length views in confined areas such as the average examination room. These lenses are usually exceedingly inexpensive.

Zoom Lenses

Zoom lenses are variable-focal-length lenses. Early models usually produced inferior images when compared with fixed-focal-length lenses. Now, however, even very long zoom lenses rival their fixed focus counterparts in image sharpness. Some zoom lenses are referred to as "macro zoom lenses," but this reference is inappropriate, because such lenses offer a maximum magnification of only 1/4 life size. Short zoom lenses—35- to 70-mm or 28- to 85-mm lenses, for example—may be used like the standard conventional fixed-focal-length lens for taking half- and full-body-length views in confined areas.

FILM

Films used in clinical photography include both conventional and instant process types. Conventional process films are generally of two types: print (negative) film, in both black and white (monochrome) and color; and transparency (reversal) film in black and white (monochrome), color, Kodachrome, and E-6 process films. Instant process films are also of two types: print film and transparency film.

Print Film

Monochrome print film is primarily used for images planned for publication on the printed page, with fine-grain, panchromatic films being preferred. Panchromatic films are sensitive to all visible wavelengths. The so-called orthochromatic films are not particularly sensitive to red and tend to see pinks and reds as dark gray or black. For this reason, orthochromatic films darken lesions characterized by the predominance of these colors. A cyan or green filter used with panchromatic film achieves essentially the same result. When red filters are used with panchromatic films, lesions characterized by red or pink shades tend to become much lighter.[3]

Color print film is infrequently used in clinical photography. However, because of readily available rapid processing and new, fine-grain, color-saturated film such as Kodak's Ektar, color print film may begin to enjoy expanded use in medical record keeping. A photograph of a color standard such as the Macbeth Color Checker should be included on all rolls of color negative film, since errors in color reproduction may be generated during the printing step unless some reference point is present.

Transparency Films

Monochrome transparency films are also rarely used in clinical photography but have wide application in graphic arts. Continuous tone and line films are available as both negative and reverse process films.

Color transparency films are the gold standard of clinical imaging. The Kodachrome process has been virtually unchanged since it was originally introduced in 1939. Kodachrome is a very simple film, although the processing is exceedingly complex. Unfortunately, since Kodak franchised Kodachrome processing, the reliability of the processing has become quite variable.

The E-6 process as it is known today was introduced in 1976. This process is associated with Kodak's Ektachrome line of films. The first Ektachrome films were marketed in 1946 as E-1 process sheet film. The E-2 process and roll film versions of Ektachrome were introduced in 1955. In 1966, improvements were made, and new films and the E-4 process were introduced.[8]

Many manufacturers currently offer E-6 process–compatible films (Ektachrome, Fujichrome, and Agfachrome) and even their own versions of E-6 processing systems. While we may think that the evolution of film has come to a standstill and that all true advances are being made in the area of electronic imaging, this is simply not true. A staggering number of new films of all types have been marketed over the last few years, and there appears to be no end in sight.

There is no single "right" transparency film for clinical photography. Kodachrome 25 has enjoyed a large loyal following for many years. The reduced reliability of Kodachrome processing and problems with the inherent red bias of this film, particularly when converting Kodachrome images to electronic images, have placed added emphasis on the use of E-6 process films in clinical photography. Ektachrome professional film (EPN) 100 ISO is touted currently as being the most accurate transparency film available.[3]

Instant Process Films

Polaroid markets a variety of monochrome and color instant print films. Some are used with medium- or large-format cameras for checking complex lighting configurations before a final exposure is made on conventional print or transparency film. Others are designed for use with one of the many special use instant photography systems marketed by Polaroid. Instant-prints are commonly used by cutaneous surgeons for record keeping and documentation for insurance companies.

A series of 35-mm "instant" slide films is also marketed by Polaroid. The films are exposed in conventional 35-mm SLR cameras. Each roll of film is supplied with its own chemical processing packet, and the exposed film and the processing packet are inserted into a small, portable processing unit. The processed roll of film is ready for cutting and mounting in plastic slide mounts within a few minutes. Processing time varies slightly depending on the film type. The processing unit and a small film-cutting and slide-mounting device are marketed separately by Polaroid.

The currently available films include Polagraph, a black-and-white line film that produces black letters on a white or clear background and is useful for making quick graphic slides; Polapan, a panchromatic, continuous-tone, black-and-white transparency film that is particularly useful for making copies of continuous-tone, black-and-white images such as clinical photographs from journals or books to be used in presentations; Polablue, an "instant" method of making white-on-blue text, chart, and graph slides for presentation; Polachrome, a color transparency film often used for making last-minute photomicrographs or gross specimen photographs for conferences; and Polachrome HC, a new, higher contrast version of Polachrome.

Although all these films may have particular uses, they are not intended to replace their conventional film counterparts. In addition, their archival quality is questionable, as is their ability to withstand repeated projection. The color films in particular will produce a dimmer on-screen image than conventional films. Because the instant films also reflect different amounts of light than conventional films, TTL-OTF camera metering systems do not work well with them.

Professional Films

Films intended for general use are not manufactured to meet the close tolerance of film lines designated as "professional films."[9] As all emulsions age, the manner in which they render colors will also change. The warmer the ambient temperature, the more rapidly the changes occur. Amateur films are intended for storage at room temperature, since a range of color renditions is accepted as satisfactory.

For some applications, more consistent color rendition is necessary. The color balance of professional films is engineered to very close tolerance. Professional film is kept refrigerated from manufacture until close to the time it is used. All films continue to age after exposure, so they should be processed as soon as possible.

LIGHTING EQUIPMENT

Because clinical photographers are not interested in recording motion, they have the option of using either continuous light or short bursts of light. These bursts, called flash lighting, trace their beginnings to "flashes" of light produced by the ignition of magnesium powder. Later, the first flash bulbs consisted of glass envelopes containing fine strands of magnesium. Most burst lighting today is produced by strobe lights, which were invented by Dr. Harold Edgerton in the 1930s. Regardless of their size, these repeatable flash units all work by current discharge in a xenon-charged vacuum tube. The unit is ready to fire again as soon as its capacitor is recharged. Two types of strobe lighting are used in clinical photography. One type is a small, portable unit often mounted directly on the camera or the lens. The second variety is a much less portable but more powerful, and inherently more consistent, studio flash system. Each of these types will be discussed separately.

Continuous Lighting

The major advantage of continuous light is that one is able to see exactly where shadows will fall and how intense they will be. Fluorescent lights produce a low-intensity, continuous-spectrum output and have much higher discontinuous peaks of light. No fluorescent unit is accurately balanced for use with color photographic film, but reasonably good color correction can be achieved with "daylight" fluorescent bulbs and use of magenta color-compensating filters. They are not, as a rule, used for patient photography but find some application in specimen and other small object photography.

Most sources of continuous photographic light are incandescent tungsten filament lamps. The two types of tungsten light sources currently used are flood lights and tungsten halogen lamps. Conventional photoflood lights look like slightly large household light bulbs. They are color balanced for 3200° or 3400°K and are mounted in reflector bowls, the same way one would screw a household light bulb into its socket. Most of these are rated at between 250 and 500 watts. Because of their tremendous electrical requirements, these lights should be connected directly to wall receptacles. For safety reasons, if extension cords are used, they should be rated for carrying heavy electrical loads. The "reflector flood" is a variant of the glass-enveloped bulb. The glass envelope is shaped like a funnel with a clear lid, and the sides are coated with a reflecting agent so that these may be used without a bowl reflector. Common ratings for these lamps are between 125 and 250 watts.

The second type of tungsten light is the tungsten halogen lamp, also known as a quartz halogen lamp because of the material that composes its envelope. These small, powerful lamps are evacuated and filled with an inert halogen gas. They require a special receptacle and are color balanced for 3200°K.

The effective life span of photofloods is quite short. Although they may burn for 4 to 6 hours, their color temperature may begin to noticeably shift after only 2 hours of use. The life expectancy of a quartz halogen bulb is 10 to 20 times that of a standard photoflood. It retains its constant color temperature throughout its lifetime, because the tungsten vapor generated during use is redeposited on the filament after the current is turned off. Conventional photofloods gradually deposit tungsten vapor on the glass envelope, which alters the color temperature and reduces light output. Despite a greater initial cost, tungsten halogen lamps and fixtures are often a better long-term investment. Compared with strobe lights, tungsten lamps are exceedingly inefficient, but one of the main drawbacks to all forms of tungsten illumination is the tremendous amount of heat that is generated. Indeed, these units are often generically referred to as "hot lights." In addition to the discomfort that would be poorly tolerated by sick patients and many children, significant thermal burns can occur if the photographer or patient happens to touch the hot bulb or the reflector.

Burst Lighting: Portable Strobe Lighting Systems

Portable strobes may be categorized as point sources or ring lights. Point sources can be either shoe mounted or near-axis mounted. The ring lights can be either a true ring light or a ring light variant.

Portable strobes may be used in either a manual mode or, with many modern camera systems, in one of several automatic metering modes. There are differences between older generic "automatic" strobes and current TTL metered units.[5] The earliest automatic strobe lights had their own sensors that shut down the unit when an approximation of the correct exposure was perceived. The photographer was responsible for both setting the film speed on the flash and selecting the proper aperture on the camera. With various combinations of apertures and film speeds, some degree of automated flash pho-

tography was available, particularly at reproduction ratios greater than 1/10 life size. These units were particularly useful with color negative film because of its wide exposure latitude. As a rule, these early "automatic" strobes were mounted directly on the camera, either in a hot shoe or triggered by a synchronization cord that connected to the X-sync socket on the camera body. Some had remote sensors that could be mounted on or near the camera while the strobe itself was positioned away from the camera to create special lighting effects.

"Dedicated" strobes soon evolved, along with more automated camera bodies. All dedicated strobes were able to communicate with the particular camera system, which in turn could communicate its aperture and flash speed settings to the strobe. If a camera system had TTL-OTF flash metering, it could shut the strobe off when the camera determined that sufficient light had reached the film. Camera systems without TTL-OTF flash metering also had dedicated strobes, but the sensor remained outside the camera, either on the strobe or attached to it via cable. These units were similar to the older automatic units in the sense that the strobe was responsible for shutting itself off. For the close-up and ultra close-up views that characterize dermatologic photography, TTL-OTF flash metering is by far the most effective automatic method.

One of the most problematic characteristics of portable strobe lighting is that it is usually not fixed in its distance from the subject. When mounted on the camera or lens, the strobe moves either closer to or farther away from the subject, depending on the working distance of the lens at a given magnification. Because light obeys the inverse square law, the decrease in flash intensity is dramatic as the strobe is moved farther away from the subject. This is particularly true of smaller, low-powered units. The farther a strobe is from the subject, the smaller is the relative size of the strobe with respect to its subject. Light also gets progressively "harder" the farther a strobe is from its subject. This is particularly important for small, raised lesions.

Portable point sources consist of a small flash unit with a single tube that may be mounted in the hot shoe (Fig. 20–3) or held near the lens axis by a bracket. Unless modified by a diffusion or reflecting device, small point sources tend to produce hard light.

A ring light is usually a low-powered circular strobe tube mounted in a housing attached to the front of the lens by a threaded ring.[10] The tube surrounds the optical axis of the lens, producing flat, soft light. Although true ring lights are uncommon, ring light variants with a flash tube that is not ring shaped (Fig. 20–4) attach to the lens like a true ring light. These variants have two to four point sources that are mounted around the lens. When all the flash tubes are fired simultaneously, the end result is nearly identical to the lighting configuration produced by a true ring flash. Depending on the number and size of the individual lamps, some degree of directional lighting can also be accomplished when only one of the lamps is fired. Ring lights or their variants are most useful at reproduction ratios between 1:10 and life size.

With various connecting cables and off-camera shoes,

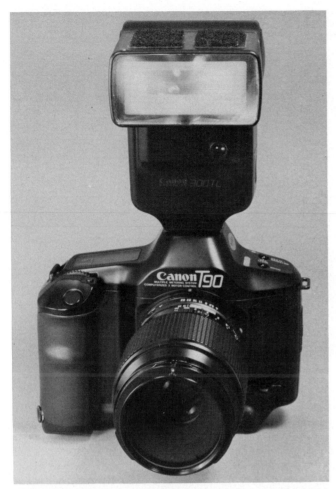

Figure 20–3. The Canon 300TL portable strobe was designed primarily for use with the Canon T90. The 300TL is a dedicated, fully automatic strobe, but it also has high- and low-power manual modes.

portable, it is also true that because of the increasing complexity of procedures performed by cutaneous surgeons and the consistency of image quality required for pre- and postoperative studies, studio lighting systems may be the most effective. The lack of portability can become an asset in terms of reproducible quality by partially dedicating an examination room to photography. Using a studio lighting system is the single most important step one can take toward maximal consistency in clinical photography. Total body surveys for the dysplastic nevus syndrome or preoperative cosmetic surgery such as liposuction are much more readily accomplished with studio strobe lighting. Photographs of medium- or smaller-sized lesions may be quite adequately performed with portable lighting systems, but when these images become the preoperative portion of a comparative study, studio lighting provides the most consistent result. Whenever a photograph of half or more of the length of an adult patient is necessary to show multiple lesions or the extent of one large lesion such as a giant hairy nevus, the overall even illumination and shadow control that can be provided by studio

point sources may be hand held, mounted on tripods, or attached to light stands away from the lens axis in an effort to obtain lighting patterns that produce desired specialized shadow patterns and density. With some automatic systems, multiple strobe lights may be connected to a single camera. Depending on cable length, a remote strobe may not have to move with the camera. Optical sensors known as "slaves" may be used to trigger small portable strobes that are not physically connected to the camera system.

Studio Strobe Lighting Systems

There are two different methods of studio strobe lighting.[11] One uses self-contained strobe units, each with its own power supply, and the other consists of several flash heads connected to a power pack by means of electrical cables. Physician photographers have traditionally avoided using studio strobe lighting, probably because the systems were thought to be prohibitively expensive, unnecessarily complex, and not portable. These reasons are neither true nor valid with respect to the needs of today's physician photographer.

While it is true that studio strobe systems are not

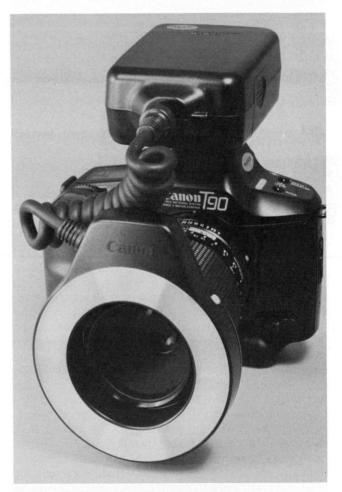

Figure 20–4. The Canon ML2 is a dedicated ring light variant designed for automatic TTL controlled function with the T90. It functions in aperture priority, shutter priority, and program modes. It may also be used as a manual strobe. The ML2's power source mounts in the hot shoe of the T90 as shown here. There is one flash tube on either side of the ring-shaped flash head.

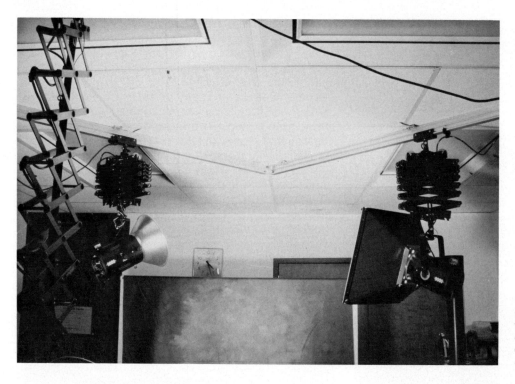

Figure 20–5. These self-contained studio strobes are mounted on ceiling tracks to keep them out of the way, yet ready for use in an instant.

systems are superior. Intraoperative photography in the office surgical suite can also be performed with self-contained studio strobes mounted on a movable ceiling track system to give a rapid and effective method for obtaining procedural photographs (Fig. 20–5).

Photographic Background Materials

An effective photographic background should remain in the background and be unnoticeable. The materials from which backgrounds are constructed depend somewhat on whether studio lighting systems or portable strobe systems are being employed. Seamless background paper may be used with studio lighting when space availability allows the subject to be far enough away from the background for proper shadow control. Cloth background materials may be particularly useful with portable equipment, but they should not exhibit an obvious woven pattern, should not have sufficient sheen to produce unwanted reflections, and must always be kept free of lint and other debris. Some background materials tend to produce interference patterns when film images are converted to National Television Systems Committee (NTSC) (Standard American Television) signals. Velvet and velveteen have been touted as excellent light traps but are generally less effective as background materials because a wrinkle in the material produces specular highlights even with very dark or black material. Polyester/cotton fleece material such as used in the manufacture of sweatshirts has also proven to be an excellent background material. The fleece side is nonreflective and exhibits no weave pattern. This material is inexpensive and may be washed several times and still be an effective background material.

With respect to white or light background colors, dense distracting shadows tend to be a problem unless extra lighting is trained on the background. Glare is also a potential problem as are marks, stains, and dirt. Medium and darker gray backgrounds can be very effective, since shadows are not striking. However, what appears to be gray to the eye may be recorded as a shade of blue on the film. For this reason, color consistency from one apparently gray background material to another is difficult to obtain.

Black is preferred by many physician photographers because it is the most consistent background color, and it gives a dramatic appearance. Black polyester/cotton fleece makes a durable, consistent background and is a very effective light trap. Lint removal is occasionally necessary. The major negative feature of black background materials is that without some degree of side or edge lighting, dark-skinned subjects tend to blend in with them.

Flat black matte board makes an excellent background for preoperative photographs of the hands. It reproduces as a dark charcoal gray and also absorbs shadows.[3] Standard mat board is 32 × 40 inches, so that four equal pieces of 16 × 20 inches can be cut from a single sheet. If the surface develops shiny areas or other minor defects, it may be repaired by spraying the surface with flat black paint. If the board becomes contaminated with body fluids, it should obviously be discarded.

If other background materials are used, saturated colors and multicolored backgrounds should be avoided. Saturated colors, including blue, tend to alter the perception of image color and, by reflecting light, may actually alter the color of adjacent skin. In addition, saturated color backgrounds transfer to electronic images rather poorly, as they tend to "bleed" into the image. Muted colors such as olive green are particularly effective backgrounds since, if subtle color shifts occur during transfer of film images to electronic images, they are less noticeable.

Clinical Photographic Technique

It has been said that standardization is the key word in all discussion of clinical photography.[12] A system of standardization enables the reasonable comparison of images taken at different times in one patient or of different patients.[13–15] Any such system requires the establishment of consistency in several areas[12]: film type, lighting technique, background control, patient and camera position, reproduction ratio, and film handling, including processing, printing, and viewing. Clinical photography must be considered in the context of standardized, reproducible technique.

The term standard view refers to an established set of patient positions for images of various areas of the body. Having a standard format for facial photography is of particular importance to the cutaneous surgeon.[14] Standard views are useful for pre- and postoperative comparisons, for serial studies, and as localizing views in lesion photography. As a general rule, the camera should be centered on the anatomic part being photographed. The optical axis should be perpendicular to the major plane of the subject.

STANDARD VIEWS FOR CUTANEOUS SURGERY

Face and Nose

The four suggested standard facial views include[12] anterior, right and left oblique, right and left lateral, and inferior.

Facial views are taken at a reproduction ratio of 1:10 (Fig. 20–6*A–D*). If the photographs are intended for record keeping purposes only, the vertical format is used. For use in education, a horizontal format may be preferred. For true anterior views, the tip of the nose should be aligned with the earlobes (i.e., a line connecting the nasal tip and the earlobes should be parallel to the floor). The distance between the outer canthi and the ear should be bilaterally equal. The optical axis of the lens should be centered on the nasal tip.

Oblique views are captured by rotating the subject 45 degrees. A line drawn between the visible earlobe and the tip of the nose should be parallel to the floor. For lateral views, the medial edge of the opposite eyebrow is visualized and then the head is rotated slightly away from the camera, stopping at the estimated midline of the glabella. The visible earlobe and tip of the nose should be in position such that a line connecting them would be parallel with the floor. The image should be centered in the view finder with the optical axis at the level of the tip of the nose. It is important to note that when using the vertical format at $\frac{1}{10}$ life size, the back of the head may not fit into the image frame.

The inferior view shows the thickness and alignment of the columella, as well as the inferior aspect of the alae. This view is obtained by having the patient lean slightly backward, tilting the head backward as well until the tip of the nose is positioned between the eyebrows. The lens axis is centered on the insertion of the columella. Special views, such as photographs of facial expressions such as smiling, frowning, or closing one or both eyes, should be taken in addition to standard views if they accentuate certain elements of pathology. For individuals who wear makeup, surgical preoperative and postoperative studies should include a series with and without makeup as a demonstration of the practical effectiveness of a procedure. All facial photographs should be taken with long macro lenses, because standard lenses tend to exaggerate the size of the nose with respect to the rest of the face.

Head and Alopecia Series

Standard views of the head include a posterior view in addition to the standard facial views (Fig. 20–7). For consistent posterior views, the patient should be set up for an anterior view and then rotated 180 degrees. In hair transplant patients or in serial studies of any disorder characterized by alopecia, a view of the vertex should also be included. Consistent vertex views may be obtained by having the patient lean slightly forward and flex the neck until the tip of the nose is the only visible facial feature when the top of the head is centered in the viewfinder (Fig. 20–8).

Oral Photography

For views of normal bite alignment, use the standard anterior facial view set-up guidelines. Plastic or metal oral retractors should be used. A 1:4 reproduction ratio and horizontal format are best for these photographs. A ring flash may be used, but to show fine shadows (e.g., between the teeth), a camera-mounted portable strobe will provide even illumination if a long macro lens is used.

Plastic or metal oral retractors are not used for oral cavity views, because they may actually limit a patient's ability to open the mouth. The preferred lighting is a ring flash or ring flash variant[3, 10] with the patient set up for an inferior facial view and the mouth open as wide as possible. Most views are taken at reproduction ratios of 1:4 or 1:2. When retraction is necessary, a gloved finger is used.

Eye

Individual preferences for special views of the external eye and lids abound. Standard views include the routine facial series plus a life-size or ½ life-size view of each eye with the lids opened normally and with the lids closed. Eye or lid positions that accentuate anterior eye or lid pathology should also be photographed in addition to any standard series.

Ear

Suggested routine views of the ear include the standard alopecia series plus selected ¼ to ½ life-size views, at the discretion of the physician.

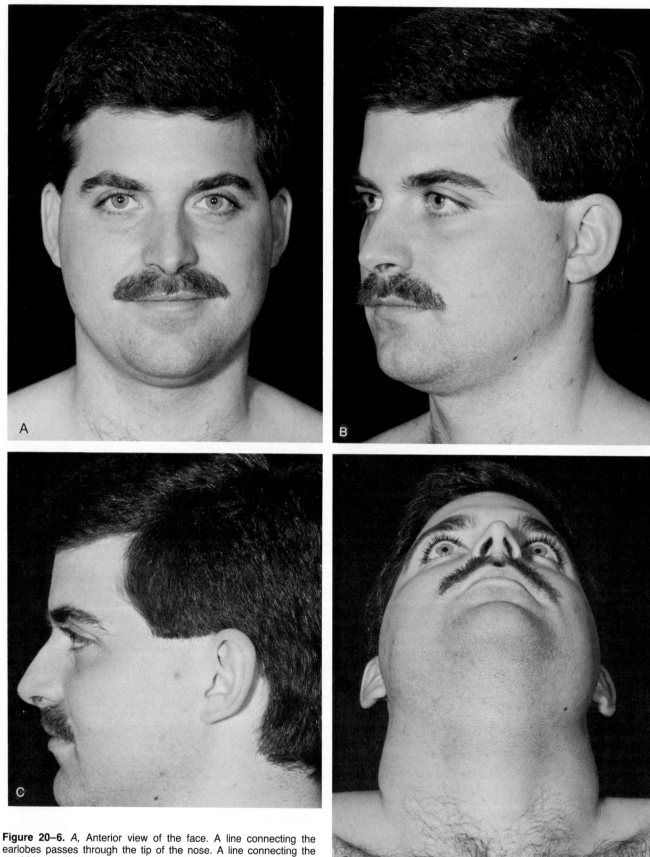

Figure 20–6. *A,* Anterior view of the face. A line connecting the earlobes passes through the tip of the nose. A line connecting the canthi is parallel to that line, and both lines are parallel to the floor. The distance between the outer canthi and the ears is equal bilaterally. *B,* An oblique view of the face is produced by turning the patient 45 degrees from the anterior. A line connecting the visible earlobe and the nasal tip is parallel to the floor. *C,* A lateral view of the face is produced by turning the patient 90 degrees from the anterior. At 1/10 life size the back of the head will not fit in a vertical format view most of the time. Note that the glabella is just visible. *D,* Inferior view of the face. Note that the tip of the nose lies between the eyebrows. The configuration of the columella and inferior aspect of the alae is readily visible.

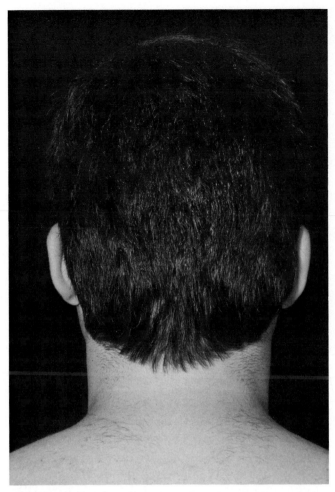

Figure 20–7. In this posterior view of the head, both ears are equally visible.

Neck

The neck is included in vertical format views of the head. If photographs of the neck only are required, anterior lateral oblique and posterior views of the neck may be obtained by posing the subject for a corresponding facial view using a 1:8 reproduction ratio and centering the camera perpendicular to the neck.

Trunk

Anterior, posterior, and occasionally lateral or oblique views of the trunk are commonly used as localizing views for larger lesions such as congenital melanocytic nevi. A reproduction ratio of 1:30 taken in the vertical format works well for most adults. Midbody views cover an area from the umbilicus to the midthigh. An anterior view may be used as a localizing view for groin lesions, while anterior and posterior views are useful for large "bathing trunk" lesions such as congenital nevi. Anterior, posterior, lateral, and oblique views combined with contour or texture lighting are useful for preoperative and postoperative liposuction surgery. For this purpose, a studio lighting system is most effective.

Extremities

Anterior and posterior views of the upper extremities held in anatomic position are included in standard views of the trunk reproduced at ⅓₀ life size. The same reproduction ratio and vertical format will work for full-length views of the lower extremity. Because the camera should be held at knee level, it is easier to have the patient stand on a footstool that has been draped with old pieces of black fleece background material saved for this purpose.

For photographs of the hands and distal forearms, a piece of black matte board is placed between the forearms and the trunk. The matte board is held in place by slight backward pressure from the patient's forearms and hands. Vertical format and a reproduction ratio of 1:15 are used, as are views in pronation and supination.

Hands

Anterior and posterior views of both hands are usually taken in horizontal format at ¹⁄₁₀ life size (Fig. 20–9). When a portable strobe mounted on the camera or lens is used for lighting, the lens axis should be tipped slightly toward the ends of the fingers to cause shadows to recede into the web spaces. These views are used as localizing views to document dorsal or palmar lesions and disorders that affect multiple joints and nails. Some

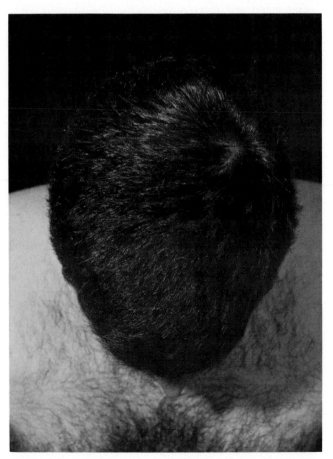

Figure 20–8. Vertex view of the scalp. The tip of the nose is the only visible facial feature.

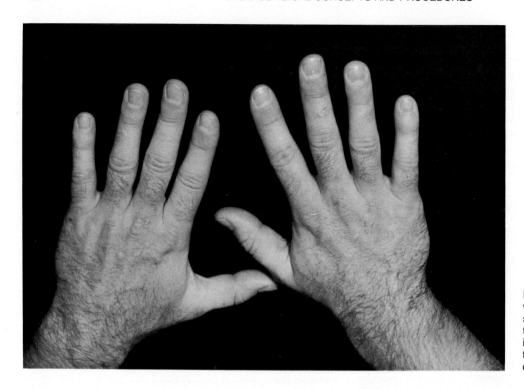

Figure 20–9. This photograph was taken using a pair of studio strobes located 30 degrees from the lens axis. Black matte board is the background material. Note that the matte board renders a dark charcoal gray.

disorders affecting the hand are best illustrated by including the patient's hand and the hand of a "normal" volunteer in the same photograph.

One hand and distal forearm may be photographed ⅛ life size in the vertical format, while nails are photographed life size.[16] A horizontal-format, ¼ life-size view is often useful for comparing three or four nails.

Feet

Photographs of the plantar surface are usually taken with the patient in the prone position and the feet extended beyond the edge of the examining table. Black fleece draped over the edge of the table is held in place by the anterior surface of the patient's legs. Another piece of fleece is draped over the ankles from above to make contact with the lower piece. An alternative is to prepare a piece of fleece with two parallel vertical slits 6 inches apart. The slits are just large enough to slide the feet through them, with the top of the slit resting on the ankle. A 1:10 reproduction ratio and horizontal format are used.

The same reproduction ratio and format are used for an anterior view that includes the tops of the feet and ankles. This view is obtained by tipping the optical axis toward the tops of the feet. The patient may be standing on a footstool draped with black fleece or seated on background cloth at the edge of an examining table with legs and cloth hanging over the edge. If the latter method is chosen, care must be taken to make sure the feet are parallel to the floor.

Views of the lateral or medial aspect of a foot and ankle may also be taken with the patient seated or standing. Vertical format and a 1:8 reproduction ratio are used. Format and reproduction ratios used for toes and toenails are the same as those used for distal fingers

and nails. The patient should be seated and posed in the same fashion as for an anterior view of the top of the feet and ankles, except that the feet are comfortably plantarflexed to get the nails parallel to the film plane.

Total Body Surface Surveys

Body surface surveys are most commonly used to follow dysplastic nevus or basal cell nevus syndrome patients. There is no generally agreed on technique.[3, 17, 18] A suggested method is to divide the anterior, posterior, and lateral body surfaces, as well as the medial aspects of the extremities, into ⅒ to ⅟₁₅ life-sized units, photographing each unit as a part of a series using a 35-mm camera. These ⅒ life-size views are essentially localizing views for discrete lesions. Suspicious lesions should be numbered with a marking pen before taking the survey views. Intermediate views and ultra close-up views of individual lesions and small groups of lesions are performed where appropriate. A size scale is usually added to the photographs of individual lesions and small groups of lesions. Studio lighting is particularly useful for body surface surveys because of its consistency and ability to cover large areas with even light. These systems recycle very rapidly, allowing these multiple views to be taken in an expeditious fashion.

Lesion Photography

Two or sometimes three views are often necessary to properly document many skin lesions.[3] The first view establishes the location of the lesion by showing its relationship to adjacent landmarks. Localizing views are usually taken at reproduction ratios between 1:10 and 1:4. Additional views consist of ultra close-up images from ¼ life size up to life size, depending on the lesion, to demonstrate fine detail. Intermediate-range views may be useful for large congenital nevi, since it may be helpful to demonstrate a specific region in a large lesion from which closer life-size images will be taken.

In most instances, one of the previously discussed standard views should be used as a localizing view. Photographs of small- to medium-sized lesions on the midthigh, leg, arm, or forearm may present a problem if the photographer attempts to center the lesion in the localizing view, because the small reproduction ratio will make the lesion difficult to find. It is usually better to use a ratio of 1:10 or 1:8 and locate an anatomic landmark near one edge of the photograph and the lesion near the opposite edge. In any event, the reproduction ratios and angles of view that reveal the greatest amount of significant detail should always be selected.

Makeup, jewelry, or street clothing should not generally be included in clinical photographs except as mentioned previously, as they serve as distractions for the viewer.

Lighting techniques in lesion photography are dictated by the nature of the disease process and the particular features the photographer wishes to illustrate. Flat lighting is effective for whole- and half-body views, as well as any localizing view. Flat lighting is also the most effective lighting technique for demonstrating ultra close-up features of macular lesions. The diameter and height of a raised lesion may help the photographer choose between texture or contour lighting. Texture lighting is particularly effective at separating multiple tiny lesions from surrounding skin. Contour lighting, on the other hand, provides the dimensional quality needed in photographs of larger, more elevated lesions. If texture light were to be used for larger, raised lesions, the length of the shadow would be distracting.

Intraoperative Photography

Planning is important if different stages of a surgical procedure are to be photographed. The process of obtaining photographs should be built into the planned sequence of steps included in the procedure itself. Intraoperative photography is actually action photography, with the primary goal to document a process rather than producing standardized images that can be effectively compared with another set of images taken at another time. For this reason, tiny bits of static detail are not as important as they might be in lesion photography.

The focal length of lenses used in intraoperative photography should be matched with the type of procedure being performed. Vertical views taken while leaning over a recumbent patient are most effective when a short lens is used. A long lens is particularly effective for head and neck procedures performed on seated or semirecumbent patients. A close-focusing zoom lens covering ranges from slightly less than 50 mm up to 100 mm may be used to crop out unwanted detail. Although autofocus systems may have limited applicability in clinical photography, because surgical defects

tend to be centered in the film frame and depth-of-field constraints are less of a problem, they may be useful for intraoperative photography. This is particularly true when used in conjunction with a close-focusing zoom lens and an automatic exposure system. The servo or continuous-focus autofocus mode is probably the best mode for intraoperative photography. A ring flash or ring flash equivalent provides even light over the operative field and is powerful enough for the relatively short working distances that are encountered in intraoperative photography. A point light source mounted near the lens axis can also be effective. Ceiling-mounted self-contained studio strobe lighting systems are used effectively for head and neck procedures performed on seated or semirecumbent patients. They must, of course, be used with manual exposure systems. Since the strobe does not move when the camera is repositioned, exposure calculation is much easier.

Minor considerations can dramatically improve the quality of photographic images taken during procedures. Clean drapes and gloves put in place immediately before the photograph is taken are highly effective. While background control is more difficult in intraoperative photography, all unnecessary instruments and bloody sponges should be removed from the operative field. Depending on the angle of view, other surrounding elements in the room may come into view. An assistant may hold a sheet or background cloth behind the surgeon to effectively eliminate cluttered backgrounds.[3]

Instant photography systems are often used to record Mohs' surgery defects. A close-up adapter that will produce ½ life-size images at a camera-to-subject distance of 10 inches is available for the Polaroid Spectra System. A ½ life-size view is a full-face image in this format. The adapter disables the sonar focusing system while correcting view finder and flash parallax. The close-up adapter costs approximately $25.00.

Under license from Polaroid, Minolta markets a Spectra system clone called the Instant Pro, and the close-up adapter is included in its purchase price of approximately $125.00. Lester Dine, Inc., also markets a close-up modification of a Polaroid camera that uses standard Polaroid 600 or 779 film. It has three defined magnifications and costs about $300.00.

All these systems produce noticeable perspective distortion, but for instant documentation they have a definite place in intraoperative photography. Several systems are also available that make instant prints on standard Polaroid film from conventional slides. For photographers who use same-day processing services for their transparencies, these systems can provide an instant print that can be included in a letter to a referring physician. The cutaneous surgeon retains the original slide so that additional prints may be made as necessary. The Vivitar Instant Slide Printer is the least expensive of these units. Its price is typically less than $100.00.

Calibrating a Manual Exposure System

Once a manual exposure system is calibrated for each intended magnification ratio, only minor subject-related adjustments will be necessary. The steps for calibrating such a system are as follows:

1. Read the flash guide number (GN) from the instruction book. Guide numbers are related to the flash intensity and are specific for a given film speed. In the United States, the guide numbers are usually listed for ISO (ASA) 100 speed film with the flash-to-subject distance listed in feet. In Europe, guide number units are usually listed as DIN° meters. The relationship is:

$$GN = f\ stop \times Flash\text{-}to\text{-}subject\ distance$$

The GN concept presumes that the quantity, not quality, of light is of concern; that ambient light is *not* an exposure factor; that the subject has average reflectance; and that the flash is used indoors and some reflection off walls will occur, an unimportant factor when the flash is very close to the subject. If the instruction book is not available, set the ISO number to 100. Multiply any f-number on the scale by the distance in feet adjacent to it. This will yield the GN in feet when ISO 100 film is being used.

2. Calculate the corrected GN for the speed of film to be used. As stated above, GNs are usually listed in feet for ISO 100 film. If film rated at a speed other than ISO 100 is being used, the following formula may be used to determine the correct GN[2]:

$$GN_2 = GN_1 \sqrt{\dfrac{New\ film\ speed}{Published\ film\ speed}}$$

where GN_1 = known GN (usually for ISO 100 film), GN_2 = new GN to be determined, published film speed = known ISO rating (usually 100), and new film speed = rating to be used for film.

For most manual strobe units, these calculations will be unnecessary. Merely set the desired ISO on the strobe, select any f stop listed on the dial, and multiply by the adjacent flash-to-subject distance in feet. The calculations will be needed when a dedicated TTL meter-controlled strobe is used in manual mode.

3. Determine the flash-to-subject distance for each reproduction ratio to be used by measuring from the center of the face of the strobe to the subject with a tape measure or yardstick. On most macro lenses, both distances and reproduction ratios are listed on the lens barrel. Any reproduction ratio not listed by the manufacturer may be approximated by matching the height of a focused viewfinder image of a tape measure with the actual distance on the tape measure. Consider the following example. For a desired ratio of 1:10,

$$\frac{1}{10} = \frac{2.4\ cm}{X}, \text{ where } X = 24\ cm.$$

The desired image size (or reproduction ratio) is $\frac{1}{10}$, 2.4 cm is the size of the vertical aspect of the viewfinder image, and X is the vertical distance on the tape measure. Another way of looking at this is that when an in-focus, 24-cm subject just fills the vertical distance in the viewfinder, the reproduction ratio approximates $\frac{1}{10}$. Mark this location on the lens barrel,

TABLE 20–4. EXPOSURE CORRECTIONS

Magnification (Reproduction Ratio)	Stop Correction
1:1	2 stops
1:2	1 stop
1:4	1/2 stop

and then read the distance adjacent the mark. Using this method, reproduction ratios may be established for any lens, including zoom lenses.

If the strobe is camera-mounted, the distance listed on the lens may be used as the flash-to-subject distance, since the strobe is very close to the film plane. If the strobe is mounted on a bracket in front of the film plane, subtract the difference.

4. Using the GN and the flash-to-subject distance, calculate the preliminary f stop (f) using the following formula:

$$f = \frac{GN}{Flash\text{-}to\text{-}subject\ distance}$$

5. Add the exposure correction for high magnification factors using a bellows or lens extension factor (Table 20–4). If the preliminary f-number works out to be 22, the desired reproduction ratio is 1:1, and two f stops will be lost. The final estimated exposure becomes f/11.

6. Expose a test roll using a normal subject. In ½-stop increments, bracket one stop over and one stop under the final exposure estimate, and keep an accurate exposure record. Use the same color background material that will be used for clinical photographs.

7. Select the most accurate exposure at each reproduction ratio and record it on the lens barrel or strobe. Self-adhering paper label tape usually works well.

8. A final exposure correction will be necessary for patients with very light or dark complexions. Very light subjects will need one stop less exposure than normal subjects. Very dark subjects will require one to two stops more exposure. It is best to bracket all exposures ½ stop over and under the final estimated exposure to get one perfect exposure. The additional exposures are often usable and virtually eliminate the need for expensive duplicates. Slightly underexposed slides usually project better than the most correct exposure, and better prints may be made from a slightly overexposed slide.

Standardized Photography With an Automatic Exposure System

Automatic exposure systems expect subjects to reflect, on the average, 18% of the light that strikes them. Clinical subjects are often lighter or darker than average, and a single subject may have very light as well as very dark areas. The ultimate uncertainty with automatic exposure systems is: What will the meter decide is the correct exposure? Despite this uncertainty, automatic exposure techniques may be employed with success, and some degree of standardization is obtainable using the following sequence:

1. Select aperture priority mode to optimize depth of field and image sharpness, using apertures as close to f/16 as possible.
2. Use set reproduction ratios for all serial studies and lesion photography.
3. Bracket all exposures at least ⅓ stop over and under the baseline exposure by varying the ISO setting. Some systems offer autobracketing features. It should be remembered that automatic exposure techniques cannot be used with studio strobe systems.

Medicolegal Considerations

It has always been important to protect the patient's right to privacy.[3, 19] As electronic media become more prominent in education and record keeping, it is more important than ever to obtain a patient's written permission to take and use photographs. Permission forms should list possible uses for the images, and patients should be asked to designate which they approve. Some of the possible uses include medical record keeping; education of medical students, physicians, and paramedical and lay audiences; and publication in medical journals, textbooks, or paramedical or lay literature.

Storage, Retrieval, and Record Keeping

The choice of storage and retrieval systems depends to a degree on whether photographs are taken primarily for record keeping or instructional purposes. Slides are presently the universal instructional photographic medium. If an individual needs frequent access to those images, many commercial systems are available. Polypropylene or polyethylene folio pages may be used, with the pages kept in archival binders or suspension file cabinets. If file cabinets are used, they should be high-quality units painted with baked-on or dry spray enamel. If only infrequent access is needed, archival boxes may be used for bulk storage.

Color or black-and-white prints may be stored in patients' charts, but negatives should be stored separately. To reduce the likelihood of loss or damage, if slides are used as medical records and as instructional tools, it is best that folio pages not be kept in patients' charts. A note may be entered in the chart as to the slides' exact location. Permission forms should always be kept in patient charts.

SUMMARY

The goal of clinical photography is to produce images that contain a maximum amount of clinically significant detail. All major camera manufacturers market manual and automatic photographic systems capable of achieving this goal. Manual systems used with studio strobe lighting provide the maximal degree of standardization. Manual or automatic exposure systems using portable strobe lights are effective tools for lesion photography. Automatic exposure systems with autofocusing capability have potential use in intraoperative photography. Instant print systems are particularly used by surgeons using Mohs technique. Obtaining a patient's written permission to take and subsequently use the photographs is a priority.

REFERENCES

1. Freeman M: Light. Amphoto, New York, 1988.
2. Shipman C: SLR Photographer's Handbook. 2nd rev ed. HP Books, Tucson, AZ, 1985.
3. Schosser RH, Kendrick JP: Dermatologic photography. Dermatol Clin 5:445–461, 1987.
4. White JW: Close-up Photography. Publication KW-22, Kodak, Rochester, NY, 1984.
5. Wildi E: Dedicated flash and OTF in functional photography. Funct Photogr 22:38–41, 1987.
6. Pehmberger P, Steiner A, Wolff K: In vivo epiluminescence microscopy of pigmented lesions. I. Pattern analysis of pigmented skin lesions. J Am Acad Dermatol 17:571–583, 1987.
7. Lefkowitz L: The Manual of Close-up Photography. Amphoto, New York, 1979.
8. Eastman Kodak Company. Progress in Reversal Color Processing Process E-6. Publication E-63, Kodak, Rochester, NY, 1977.
9. Burian PK: Are "pro" films worth it? Outdoor Photogr 6:21–24, 1990.
10. Weiss CH: A new breakthrough in ringflash design: the Minolta macro 80 PX auto-electroflash. J Biol Photogr 5:21–24, 1986.
11. Buff PC: Lighting for still photography. Paul C. Buff, Nashville, TN, 1984.
12. Williams AR: Positioning and lighting for patient photography. J Biol Photogr 53:131–143, 1985.
13. Vetter JP: Standardization for the biomedical photographic department. J Biol Photogr 47:3–18, 1979.
14. Davidson TH, Hoffman HT, Webster RC: Photographic interpretation of facial plastic and reconstructive surgery. J Biol Photogr 48:87–92, 1980.
15. Shue W Jr: Photographic cures for dermatologic disorders. Arch Dermatol 125:960–963, 1989.
16. Weiss CH: Dermatologic photography of nail pathologies. Dermatol Clin 3:543–556, 1985.
17. Shue W, Kopf AN, Rivers JK: Total-body photographs of dysplastic nevi. Arch Dermatol 124:1239–1243, 1988.
18. Schosser RH, Michaels KV, Giannavola S, et al: Total body photographs of dysplastic nevi. Arch Dermatol 125:566–567, 1990.
19. Tarcinale MA: Medical photographer's role in protecting a patient's right to privacy. J Biol Photogr 48:183–185, 1980.

CHAPTER 21

Administrative Considerations in Office-Based Cutaneous Surgery

JOHN W. GERWELS

Dealing with the many mundane administrative aspects that pertain to the day-to-day operations of the cutaneous surgical practice is an important, but often neglected, element of physician education. The suggestions that follow are the product of readings, discussions with physicians who are particularly surgically oriented, personal experiences, and opinions held by the author. There are many practitioners who could provide additional beneficial suggestions and also those who could appropriately take issue with some of the recommendations made, based on their particular experience, location, and practice mix.

Basic suggestions pertinent to administering the office-based surgical practice are made. These views should be taken in the context that while generally applicable, specific circumstances—including location, type of practice (e.g., solo, clinic, or partner corporation), personal preferences, and local statutes—necessarily affect ultimate implementation of some recommendations.

An important first concept to consider is that of "permission." It seems very few physicians take hands-on control of all aspects of their practice. Reasons for partial to total noninvolvement include lack of knowledge of business practices; a desire to practice only medicine and surgery; discomfort with certain aspects of administration (e.g., personnel issues or firing employees); and a lack of understanding of financial reports. However, on consideration, most physicians find they do have the talent to run their own practice but don't, because they may feel they do not have the "permission" of their employees to do so. This can occur because employees may "stake out their turf" and rebuff all attempts to change or influence their responsibilities, even by the physician. In some cases, the physician acquiesces to this situation, as it is easier to accept the situation than change it. In other instances,

the physician may have been "educated" in the way medical practices should be run, and no tampering with the situation is allowed.

Whether the physician functions as a solo practitioner or in concert with other physicians (as in most circumstances), there should be a realization that the practice does function as a business; that the physician is a proprietor; and that the physician does not need the "permission" of the employees to be involved in the details of the business if so desired. Once cutaneous surgeons realize that they have the ultimate responsibility for the practice and are the ultimate authorities within the practice, they can elect to assume or delegate as much responsibility for the nonmedical portion of the practice as their comfort level allows.

Physical Plant

The physical layouts of many cutaneous surgical practices often share some general characteristics. Typically, there is a separate (but sometimes shared) reception area. This is generally adjacent to the front office or business area. Within the business work area are stations at which the various employees carry out their daily tasks. This area also generally houses the office equipment necessary for day-to-day operations. Chart storage may be within this area or, at worst, adjacent to it. The back practice area includes the examination rooms, procedure rooms, separate consultation rooms (if utilized), and the laboratory preparation area, where medically related supplies, microscope, surgical instruments, and sterilization equipment are housed. In addition, if intravenous sedation, nitrous oxide sedation, or general anesthesia is used in the practice, a recovery area should be present. The physician's private office facilities are usually in or adjacent to the medical practice area. It is ideal to have a separate entry to, and exit from, the practice area. It is particularly beneficial for patients who have undergone certain procedures, particularly of a cosmetic nature, to have a separate exit that does not require transit through the reception area. This helps protect the patient's privacy and avoids the apprehension that may be generated when an assortment of bandages, some quite impressive, are paraded through the waiting area. In the event that a separate exit is available, it is wise to have a portion of the business office located on or adjacent to this exit to facilitate rescheduling and to settle accounts. If possible, there should also be a private entry for the physician. In addition, access to the treatment area should be adequate to allow for entry and use of emergency equipment, including a gurney, if needed.

Specifics regarding the layout and design of the physical plant are obviously limited by the available space and whether remodeling is feasible or desirable under the constraints of lease or rental arrangements. Each physician may have slightly different priorities as to what is necessary and useful.[1] Because of this, no specific ideal layout plans exist. It is generally accepted that 1200 to 1500 square feet of office space are needed for each physician.

Personnel

A common estimate regarding the number of employees needed for a practice is 2.5 employees per physician. Factors that influence exactly how many are necessary depend on patient flow, the practice mix, the number of procedures, and the use of ancillary workers involved with medical transcription or stenography. The responsibilities allocated to each employee and the attention demanded of the employee by a particular task also influence the number of employees needed. However, employing an excess number of personnel does not necessarily solve "people" problems. Finally, there is also a "comfort" level at which a particular office just seems to function most smoothly. This may vary within a specific office, depending on the mix of employees at any given time.

Front Office Employees

The number of employees required for successful operation of the front office varies with the size of the practice, particularly the number of patient encounters during the day. The size of the practice also influences the number of telephone calls received. The minimal number of front office employees is one. If patient traffic in the office is low because of the nature of the surgical practice, it is entirely possible that a single employee can fill the multiple roles of receptionist, clerk, cashier, typist, and insurance secretary. While this may seem to be a substantial burden, many successful offices function in just such a fashion. In some circumstances, back office employees can also assist in some of these duties, which otherwise might be the sole responsibility of the front office person. Such tasks may include answering the telephone, making appointments, refiling charts, and other tasks that do not compromise the responsibilities of the back office employee.

When patient flow is high, smooth functioning of the front office may require a second person. How the duties are shared depends entirely on the desires of the surgeon and the talents of the individuals. Both front office workers should possess good telephone skills, as should anyone else who has the responsibility of telephone contact with the public. In such a front office situation, it is wise, if a computer is employed, to have both individuals skilled in operating all the necessary functions for the office computer. Although such skills are not necessarily uniformly available, capable employees can usually be trained to perform at least some functions on the computer, including data entry for charges and collections, making appointments, recalling information from the memory regarding status of accounts, and answering queries regarding whether the insurance company has paid or checks have been received. Sometimes, to avoid employing more full-time personnel than necessary, it may be desirable to delegate some of the simpler and more menial tasks to part-time employees. Such duties as filing laboratory reports, pathology reports, and correspondence into charts, and filing charts into their proper alphabetical order can be delegated to these personnel. If they are going to answer the telephone, they must also be trained in the appropriate techniques used to characterize the practice.

There are several advantages to using part-time employees. Part-timers provide a reservoir of talent that can be used when full-time employees become ill, are out of the office for personal time off, or are on vacation. A disadvantage of using part-timers is that frequently, because of task division, responsibilities, or lack of motivation, the total effectiveness of two part-time employees may be less than a single full-time employee.

It is always prudent to use employees who are bondable so that they may be covered by the general liability insurance policy. This can provide security in the event of fiscal impropriety.

Typed notes are strongly recommended for patient charts. This eliminates the problem of legibility and generally provides more complete notes pertaining to the patient's history and physical examination, progress notes, and procedure notes. It is beneficial to use either an existing in-office staff member for typing or, if convenient, a separate, part-time person who can type in the office or at home. The responsibilities of the typist can be limited to typing notes in a specified fashion and placing them in the appropriate charts when the typing is completed. These individuals should be thoroughly screened during the application process in a fashion similar to that used for other office employees. They should also be aware of the contents of the personnel manual, their particular role, and their responsibilities pertaining to the care of the patient and, in particular, issues of patient privacy.

If the size of the practice increases to the point where

more than two full-time employees are needed, consideration should be given to acquiring an office manager.

Medical (Back Office) Staff

The selection of the medical assistance staff is as critical to the medical practice operation as the selection of the front office staff is to the financial operation of the practice. The mix of the practice may help determine the type of personnel selected for the medical and surgical portion of the practice. Medical assistants without nursing degrees may be as satisfactory as more highly trained individuals, provided that the level of their performance meets the needs of the surgeon. Untrained individuals can receive on-site training to teach them to perform the functions desired by the physician. One may also elect to use medical assistants who have been trained in a 1- or 2-year medical assistant training program provided through private training schools, vocational training programs, community colleges, or, in some instances, 4-year colleges with associated vocational training programs. These individuals are already established in the basics of medical assistance. Their skills can then be tailored to the specific needs of the practice. A disadvantage of using medical assistants, whether professionally trained or trained on site, is that they cannot provide some of the functions that nursing personnel are trained and licensed to perform. Their medical background is also likely to be limited. Ideally, if more complex surgical procedures are performed, it is prudent to have at least one trained nursing member on the staff, either a registered nurse or a baccalaureate nurse. A nurse with a surgical background would be very advantageous, but these nurses are generally in short supply, as they are coveted by surgeons performing procedures similar to those that cutaneous surgeons perform. However, it is sometimes possible to acquire a nurse with operating room experience, even one with surgical assistance skills, since on occasion they wish to alter their routine from that demanded by hospital management (e.g., shifts and time on call). Such nursing personnel usually command a prime salary compared with nurses without surgical experience, but in the long run they are well worth it.

The assistants to the physician should be capable of eliciting the essentials of a history from the patient. Their judgment will obviously be heightened with previous experience and background training. The better the qualifications of the staff, the more assistance they will be able to provide the surgeon in patient education, questions regarding medications and prescriptions, telephone inquiries about problems, and requests for medication refills. How much latitude is allowed depends on the talent of the individual employees, the degree of responsibility the physician wishes to give them, and the limitations imposed by state law.

Duties that should reasonably be assumed by these personnel include daily examination of the premises and treatment rooms to ensure general orderliness and cleanliness and a safety check for all equipment within each room to ensure it is in operating order and has not been inadvertently jostled or mispositioned by ancillary personnel such as the cleaning staff. They should also ensure that all the supplies necessary for the day's schedule are available and in their proper place; these include bandages, topical medications, injectable medications, and patient information handouts pertinent to the procedures, wound care, and limitations of activities postoperatively.

One individual should be responsible for assessing supplies and placing orders for appropriate materials, checking deliveries and comparing them with the invoices, and then ensuring that the invoices are submitted to appropriate front office personnel for payment. This person can also meet with pharmaceutical company sales representatives and, if desired, deal with them exclusively, unless the physician wishes to be involved.

Responsibilities pertinent to the direct care of patients, in addition to obtaining and recording a pertinent history, include escorting the patient to the examination or procedure rooms and ensuring that the anatomic areas requiring evaluation are readily accessible and that the patient is appropriately draped and positioned when the surgeon arrives. The time spent by the physician with the patient should ideally be limited to effective elicitation of additional important historical information, examination of the patient, discussion of the diagnosis and treatments available, acquisition of informed consent, and performance of the indicated procedure.

If a procedure has been planned, the necessary equipment and supplies for performing such a procedure should already be prepared and ready for the surgeon to use. How much direct assistance will be necessary depends, of course, on the nature of the procedure. It is almost always best to have the assistant available in the room to provide surgical assistance if required or to provide additional bandages or medications as the need arises. For procedures in which direct assistance is required and in which an assistant is to be sterilely gloved, the presence of an additional assistant to circulate and provide additional supplies, instruments, or materials is advisable. This assistant can also monitor the patient, if necessary, and provide documentation during the ongoing surgery. How much responsibility the surgeon wishes to delegate in bandaging the wounds and providing postoperative care instructions for the patient is at the discretion of the surgeon. In many instances, assistants can perform valuable functions that free the surgeon to see other patients or perform other procedures.

Staff Role and Emergencies

The size of the staff will depend on the nature of the practice. It may need to be expanded depending on the number of patients seen and the number and types of procedures performed. All medical assistance personnel should have basic cardiopulmonary resuscitation (CPR) training, and at least one individual should be well versed in basic cardiac life support. It is advisable that front office personnel also be familiar with CPR (see Chap. 13). All personnel should have ready access to emergency phone numbers and should know whom to contact in the event an emergency requiring additional assistance develops. Before any untoward event, the physician and the nursing staff should identify nearby physicians who are willing and able to assist in the event of an emergency.

The amount and type of monitoring that is done during surgery depends to a great extent on the types of procedures being performed and also on the physical condition of the patient. It is obviously imprudent to perform complex procedures in the office on a patient whose medical condition is critical or marginal, unless provision for advanced life support is available. These types of procedures are best performed in either an ambulatory surgical facility or a hospital operating room. Good practice would dictate that vital signs be recorded before starting the procedure and checked at appropriate intervals both during the procedure and afterward. A pulse oximeter is a convenient and helpful tool to accurately assess the patient's oxygen saturation (see Chap. 13). The decision to utilize cardiac monitoring devices depends on the nature of the cases being treated. Their use requires that the physician be capable of interpreting the data generated and of acting appropriately in response to it. It is also prudent to have cardioversion equipment nearby, if not on the premises.

The surgeon and staff must be able to quickly treat the patient who undergoes a syncopal episode or becomes hypotensive as a result of the procedure or medications administered. While "shock blocks" can provide necessary assistance in elevating the legs and increasing venous return, a third staff member should be designated to retrieve and place them, since the surgeon and assistant may be occupied in caring for the well-being of the patient. A better solution is to ensure that all the tables used for performing procedures can be moved quickly to a head-down or leg-elevated position. This allows the on-site personnel to better attend to the other needs of the patient.

Sterilizing Instruments

Depending on the facilities in which the physician works, the processing of instruments, particularly sterilization, determines how such a function is carried out (see Chap. 6). It is usually preferable to have on-site sterilization capacity commensurate with the instrumentation available. The responsibility for cleaning and preparing instruments should rest with one or more of the medical assistants, and all instruments should be sterilized promptly after use so that they will be available.

It is valuable to have one sterile tray always assembled and readily available at the end of the day in case a patient sustains a complication that requires treatment after office hours.

Capable and enthusiastic assistants can make cutaneous surgery a pleasure for the surgeon, rather than something to be endured, and can provide a higher level of care, safety, and satisfaction for the patient. A harmonious, efficient, and congenial team is essential to providing a satisfactory outcome for the patient and the practice.

Telephone Procedure and Etiquette

Most patients have their initial contact with the physician's office by telephone rather than in person. Therefore, it is important that proper telephone procedure and etiquette be followed by all personnel who will be answering the telephone. How this is specifically to be done should be included in the personnel manual.

Three phone lines are recommended per practitioner, using two lines for incoming calls and the third for outgoing calls and for personnel. The local telephone company can do peak load and busy-signal studies, generally at no cost, as frequently as necessary. This is done automatically, without invasion of privacy and without interrupting incoming telephone traffic. If busy signals exceed 10%, another line is needed.[2] The telephone should have a "ring-back" feature in which a call that has been placed on "hold" will, at a preset time such as 30 seconds, emit a distinctive ring to alert the receptionist that a caller is still waiting. Another hardware feature worth considering is the use of the newer, lightweight, and less expensive headset-microphone combinations. These are less fatiguing for personnel to use and also frees both hands, allowing the answerer to be more effective in caller-related or other tasks.

Employees answering the telephone should do so in a way that conveys courtesy, cordiality, and professionalism. Telephone calls should be answered within three rings, and the caller should be greeted warmly with the name of the physician, partnership, or corporation (not "doctor's office") and an offer of assistance such as "How may I help you?" If there are multiple phone lines and more than one line rings, a caller should be put on hold, preceded by the request, "Can you hold, please?" with time allowed for the caller to affirm whether they will or will not wait. Simply asking the caller to hold and then switching them off is impolite and may invite repercussion, particularly if the call happens to be urgent or the caller cannot wait for some reason. Ideally, more than one person in the office will answer the telephone, particularly if there are multiple lines.

The attitude of the person answering the telephone is readily apparent to the caller and may determine the success of the interaction. The person answering should provide an upbeat introduction to the office, as this can foster a feeling of confidence for the caller. If the call is hostile, maintaining a positive attitude and supplementing it with concern, empathy, and a willingness to assist the caller can defuse a potentially unpleasant interchange and reverse the caller's attitude.

When responding to inquiries, it is preferable to give the caller an impression of what can be done for them, rather than what cannot. Rather than say, "The doctor is with a patient," it is preferable to reply, "The doctor can return your call," stating a specific time and reaffirming the number at which the caller can be reached. If, for example, the caller is requesting the results of a biopsy report, rather than indicate that the results are not available yet, suggest that the results will be available at a certain time and that the office will call the patient back with the information desired. This approach will serve well for virtually all forms of inquiries an office might receive. However, it is important that the person answering the telephone respond only to those inquiries for which the answerer is qualified. Requests for assistance beyond those abilities should be delegated to another, more appropriate person.

A log of incoming telephone calls should be kept in duplicate, using telephone log forms readily available from a variety of office form suppliers, to provide a record of calls and messages. The telephone log duplicate copies should be kept as part of the permanent office records. The original should be delivered to the appropriate person who is not able to take the call immediately. A system must be in place ensuring that calls that require a response have been returned by the end of each working day. All responses from office personnel of any medical import should be duly logged in the patient's chart and made part of the permanent record.

Rather than looking on the telephone as a nuisance, it should be regarded as the communication lifeline for the practice and used positively as a tool that will enhance the practice's image and relationship with patients.

There are multiple sources for outlining and developing a proper telephone technique. Textbooks for medical assistants include at least one section on this topic. The American Medical Association has booklets as well as audiocassette courses with workbooks that may be valuable to have as a resource for current and new employees.

Office Manager

The need for an office manager varies among practices. There is no doubt that in offices requiring three or more front office employees, one individual should be designated as "in charge." In larger practices, such as those composed of several physicians or in clinics, there may be even more front office personnel. Coordinating the various job functions and seeing that they are carried out in an expeditious manner generally requires the presence of an individual who functions as the manager for that section.

In some multiphysician offices, the responsibilities for various aspects of managing the office may be delegated to a team of physicians who assume responsibility for a particular area, or perhaps to a senior physician who has had experience in office management. There are numerous drawbacks to the physician-team management concept, not the least of which is that ultimately the

team tends to function ineffectively. It is better to select a single physician who has the talent and the interest to act as a managing partner and to compensate that person accordingly for the time and effort required. If such an individual is not available, then a distinct, nonphysician office manager may be needed.

The purpose of an office manager should be thoroughly defined in a written job description (Fig. 21–1). In addition to administering the day-to-day functioning of the front office personnel, the office manager should also relieve physicians of problems demanding their time that may not strictly be related to the practice of surgery. It is more expeditious to use the talents of the physician for practicing medicine, rather than supervising receptionists or bookkeepers.

The amount of responsibility given the office manager also varies. This may range from simply supervising the effective implementation of day-to-day business in the office to assuming overall administrative control of all but patient care matters. The requirements for the position therefore vary considerably, but an office manager should not be hired to be used as a personal secretary.

Some physicians pride themselves on having a grasp of every detail of the function of their practice, whereas others may wish to sever themselves from all but the most important business aspects of the practice functions. Involvement in the minutiae of the day-to-day function of the office requires time, expertise, and tolerance. It can also be a source of substantial frustration, particularly if problems are extant in the office workings. In most offices in which there are multiple physicians or an extremely busy single physician, it is probably prudent to either designate or hire an office manager.

An office manager can be obtained from one of several sources depending on the demands of the position. In a small office, a responsible, long-term, loyal employee might be promoted. In other instances, recruitment outside the office may be necessary. It may be prudent, considering the complexity of the position, to enlist an outside consultant to find and possibly train a person for the position. Some very capable office managers can be acquired from situations that, although not providing experience in a medical office, gave them sufficient background and training such that, once they are conversant with the demands of the position, they function exceptionally well.

How much responsibility and latitude are given to the manager depends on the circumstances of the practice, the talent of the manager, and how much responsibility the physician is willing to delegate. This can range from merely supervising the other employees to functioning as travel and meeting coordinator, promoting the practice, suggesting and coordinating changes in the function of the office, and serving as intermediary between the physician and the various legal or accounting advisors to the practice. The office manager either should be the responsible party or should assign someone in the office to contact insurance companies in the event that preauthorization is necessary for admission to the hospital or for performance of a procedure. Ideally, the salary

1. FINANCIAL
    a. Prepare in-house monthly financial statements (not practical in a small practice).
    b. Maintain checkwriting and payroll.
    c. Undertake special financial studies and reports as necessary.
    d. Provide liaison with advisors.
    e. Provide assistance relative to proposed annual budget.
    f. Monitor practice savings and checking accounts.
2. PERSONNEL
    a. Recruit, hire, and fire staff (subject to final approval by physicians).
    b. Supervise staff, including job delegation.
    c. Maintain control and records of hours worked, vacations, and sick leave.
    d. Provide performance evaluation for salary review purposes.
    e. Determine and change personnel assignments and job descriptions as necessary.
    f. Train staff.
    g. Organize and set agendas for regular office meetings.
3. SUPPLIES
    a. Order all clerical and business supplies.
4. COLLECTIONS
    a. Supervise systems for delinquent account follow-up.
    b. Handle difficult collection matters.
5. OFFICE FACILITIES
    a. Assure proper maintenance of present office, including ordering new equipment and services.
    b. Coordinate with landlords.
    c. Investigate and act as agent for physicians in office building ownership and the development of plans for office changes.
6. AUDIT CONTROLS
    a. Review and supervise internal systems.
    b. Deal with audit control systems devised by accountants.
7. COORDINATE PHYSICIANS
    a. Attend physician meetings, record decisions, implement ideas, pursue options and report back.
    b. Coordinate physician activities on a daily basis.
8. INSURANCE
    a. Handle all office insurance coverage needs.
9. PERSONAL FOR PHYSICIANS
    a. Act as agent for physicians to save their time for clinical work.
    b. Perform physicians' civic, medical, and committee responsibilities.

Figure 21–1. Suggested job description for an office manager. (After Kalogredis JD: Effective Practice Management: Legal and Financial Issues. MacMillan, Florham Park, NJ, 1989.)

expense of a manager should be offset by better efficiency, improved collections, and fewer write-offs. In addition, intangibles such as improved office atmosphere, a more smoothly run office, fewer impositions on the physician's time, or relief from the mundane responsibilities of overseeing personnel may be sufficient rewards in themselves. Ideally, the office manager will be removed from the performance of day-to-day chores in the office and can function as an administrator with time for conceptualization, planning, and implementation; however, this depends on the nature of the practice. Also, the manager can serve as a buffer between the physicians and the staff and between the physicians, advisors, and outside interlopers, but for this to occur, the manager must be given commensurate authority for these responsibilities by the physician or physicians. After arriving at a decision to use an office manager, the physician must also make a commitment to support the manager's actions and decisions. This is done by communicating with the manager and having him or her execute decisions that have been mutually made. Intercession in the day-to-day working of the office should then be made not by the physician, but by the manager. The manager must be provided with not only the responsibility, but also the authority to implement strategies that will benefit the practice.

The manager serves as a conduit through which decisions by the physician(s), in concert with the manager, are implemented and staff problems, procedural problems, or financial concerns are brought to the physicians.

Rather than have a haphazard arrangement in which the physician periodically communicates concerns to the manager, regular weekly meetings between the manager and the physician should be scheduled using an agenda, with input from both the manager and the physician, to best use time constructively. Ideally, particularly in a practice involving multiple physicians, the manager should be present at all physician meetings. Meetings scheduled on a monthly basis should be adequate to get input from the manager on practice finances, other problems, and personnel issues. This is also an ideal venue for analysis of the monthly financial report. It is at this meeting that managers should provide minutes of previous meetings, take notes on the current meeting, and discuss pertinent business or problems. Unless the manager has been involved in these physician meetings, it is difficult to carry out these responsibilities.

The time to acquire an office manager is when it is necessary, not "when I can afford it." An effective manager should be able to generate the funds for the practice to pay the salary, benefits, and more. Ultimately, an office manager will benefit the practice by expediting efficient functioning of the office and practice and freeing the physicians to do what they do best: practice medicine and perform surgery.

Practice Advisors

Every practice, regardless of size, requires at least two advisors: an accountant and an attorney. The primary responsibilities of the accountant are to review and supervise the practice's bookkeeping and to provide tax advice. A prime consideration is whether the accountant can communicate effectively with the physician. To some extent, the selection of an accountant depends on the financial sophistication of the physician and the nature of the practice. In any event, the accountant must be able to communicate clearly in lay language, rather than "accountantese," with the physician. Too often, accountants make presumptions regarding the physician's financial and economic sophistication that, if not clarified, can ultimately result in misunderstandings and wrong decisions. When interviewing accountant candidates, the physician should identify the needs of the practice. Ideally, an accountant can serve as a tax advisor, as well as a financial advisor regarding cash flow, equipment leasing versus purchasing, and the tax consequences of any decisions made pertinent to the financial aspects of the practice. The accountant should be able to provide input regarding business decisions in which financial problems arise and ultimately should be available to answer other questions that might occur. It is prudent to determine whether the advisor tends to be conservative or aggressive in tax matters and to select one whose philosophy parallels that of the physician or the group. It is also important to check references, particularly physicians whom the accountant is working for or has previously served.

Concerns about how to decrease overhead, increase collections, and increase production are frequently misdirected to accountants. Although some may have the knowledge and the inclination to assist with these problems, few will. These matters are bettered addressed by practice consultants or advisors, who may also be able to address most, if not all, questions pertinent to the nonmedical portions of the practice.

An important note: all practice consultants are not the same! Once a consultant has been identified as possibly being capable of providing assistance, he or she should be contacted, a resumé obtained, and references contacted. The prospective advisors should be interviewed, and the same scrutiny that would be accorded a potential employee should be applied to a potential advisor.

Depending on the geographic location of the practice, a lawyer practicing general law may have the satisfactory expertise and experience for the needs of the office. Ideally the same attorney can provide advice in the physician's transactions in both practice and personal life. It is mandatory that the attorney be consulted in matters regarding personnel, particularly termination, and in matters of corporate practices, including maintaining corporate minutes, negotiating matters of partnership with physician-employees, buy-sell agreements, leases, division of income, practice sale and retirement, restrictive covenants, and dissolution of practice or partnership. Other matters in which the attorney should be consulted include real estate transactions or agreements, practice mergers, amendment of retirement plans, developing fringe benefits for employees, relations with third-party payers, hospital medical staff issues, and prudent future planning of the business practice.

Other situations in which advisors may be of assistance include matters related to insurance. Ideally, one advisor may be available to assist with all aspects of personal insurance such as automobile and homeowner's insurance, including fire, theft, liability, and "umbrella" coverage. In addition, assistance with insurance pertinent to the practice—including liability, contents, professional liability, disability, and health and life insurance—is desirable. Not all individuals or agents have access to all types of insurance, but when they do, it is convenient to consolidate these policies. Coverage should be evaluated on the contents of the proposed policies, coverage, costs, and availability of assistance in case of a claim. Before making an ultimate decision, it is prudent to examine each of the proposals before acquiring insurance. The advice of an attorney may also be beneficial.

From time to time, counsel in other matters may be necessary. A general rule is: if important decisions need to be made in an unfamiliar area, seek help from a knowledgeable source. One example is found in smaller practices, where the details of doing staff payroll with the accompanying requirements for tax withholding, paying social security, filing quarterly reports, and filling out various forms are probably best, and most economically, performed by an outside payroll service. If the medical practice enlarges, it may be worthwhile to bring the service in house.

Personnel Issues

HIRING

The hiring process begins when replacement of an existing employee or addition of another employee becomes necessary. It is essential that the responsibilities involved in the available position be fully identified. This is necessary in developing a job description that accurately outlines the responsibilities for the person being sought. As a consequence of this, inclusionary and exclusionary criteria for screening and evaluation of applicants are developed. If the position is a replacement and the previous employee was not terminated but left under good graces, it may be beneficial to have the former employee, if he or she is willing, participate in an exit interview. It should be made clear to the former employee that such an interview is voluntary, without the implication of any sanctions or retributions. This interview, if candid and forthright, can sometimes identify dissatisfactions, conflicts, or other problems within the office that may not have been apparent to the employer and as such should be considered for correction before selecting a replacement.

There are many ways to reach the available pool of talent the employer is seeking: word of mouth regarding the position; posting of notices on hospital bulletin boards; queries to local medical assistant training programs; and advertisements in a local newspaper or professional journals. The notice should outline the available position, describe the necessary qualifications and the salary or hourly wage, and state whether the salary is negotiable commensurate with qualifications and experience. It is best to have responses to the notices or advertisements directed to a post office box number. This allows the applications to be gathered and screened without numerous potential applicants coming to the office requesting interviews or asking about the job and without handling an unnecessary number of phone calls. A disadvantage is that potentially valuable employees may not apply, being fearful of applying unwittingly to their current employer.

Applying to a blind box requires the applicant to develop a cover letter and submit a resumé. Evaluation of the contents of this initial contact can be extremely helpful in screening applicants. The cover letter should be scrutinized to see whether it is organized and reflects thoughtful consideration on the part of the applicant. It should be well written and preferably typed without spelling or grammatical errors. Some suggestion as to the applicant's career goals should be contained in the letter. If present, these goals should be examined to determine whether they are consistent with the position available. For instance, an applicant for a receptionist position who indicates an ultimate desire to obtain a master's in business administration and own a business is not likely to be employed with the practice very long.

The resumé should be neat, easy to read, and concise. The content of the resumé should be analyzed to identify the potential applicant's previous education and whether it was completed in a reasonable amount of time. Previous experience should be reviewed to determine whether it is compatible with the position being offered (Fig. 21–2). These work experiences should be examined to determine whether the applicant's position has been static or there has been a demonstration of growth with promotions to positions of higher responsibility. If an applicant has, in previous employment, ascended to responsibility greater than that offered by the available position, one should ask, why are they applying? The job responsibilities outlined should be consistent with the education of the individual, the positions held, and the length of time in the work place. Finally, salary expectations, if listed, should be within the range of the position. The resumé should, however, be viewed in its proper perspective as an introduction to the applicant, and it should be remembered that it always presents the candidate in the best possible light. The resumé is a basis for determining whether an interview would be worthwhile. The interview can then be used to substantiate and amplify the facts contained in the resumé and the application.

Once the initial inquiries have been evaluated, those candidates who are considered potential employees should complete an application form. The application should be designed to elicit information considered necessary to assess the applicant's qualifications for the job. Legal restraints prevent use of race, national origin, gender, family status, age, or religion as a basis for evaluating potential employees. Handicaps alone cannot be used to disqualify an applicant, unless they would prevent the applicant from performing the duties of the position. Inquiry regarding previous legal problems must be limited to criminal convictions only. If an applicant has had a criminal conviction, obtaining relevant information may be pursued, but it would be prudent to examine local statutes before interviewing an applicant with a criminal record. The financial status of the candidate cannot be used as a criterion for evaluation, although a credit check on the applicant is allowed.

After the application has been reviewed and the candidate appears qualified, and references have been examined, an interview should be scheduled. Interviews should always be conducted in person and in the office of the employer. All initial employee candidates for a new practice should be interviewed and selected by the physician. Subsequently, with expansion or turnover, some of the screening and interviewing may be delegated. In some instances, prescreening of applicants by an office manager, personnel director, or an employee with similar responsibilities may be carried out, but the final judgment should be made by the physician. Screening of front office personnel by another office employee or office manager raises the possibility of conflicts arising when a well-qualified and talented applicant is screened out, because the initial interviewer identifies the applicant as a potential threat to the interviewer's job or "power." Avoiding this may be difficult, particularly if

	Yes	No
I. Cover Letter		
Typed, well-written, no spelling or grammatical errors.	—	—
Conveys organized thinking and career goals.	—	—
II. Appearance of Resumé		
Clean, well-organized, and easy to read.	—	—
Concise (two pages or less).	—	—
III. Content		
Applicant has necessary education, training, or experience for the position.	—	—
Education completed in a reasonable time.	—	—
Work experience shows career growth and increasing responsibility (if applicable).	—	—
Dates of work experience continuous, without unexplained gaps.	—	—
Job responsibilities listed seem consistent with positions, education, and length of experience.	—	—
Salary requirements within range.	—	—

Figure 21–2. Ten points in evaluating a resume. (Modified from Derm Marketing and Practice Management. Dermatology Services, Inc., in cooperation with the American Academy of Dermatology, Evanston IL, 1991.)

the screening interviewer feels that confidence in their ability to perform their job has been impugned. The alternatives are to have an outside party, such as a practice consultant, or the physician do the initial screening interviews.

The interview should be standardized to avoid violation of legal statutes, the penalties for which can be severe. The constraints described regarding the application also pertain to the interview process. The guidelines should be reviewed and understood in advance by the interviewer. The questions to be asked of the applicant should be determined in advance and the same questions asked of all candidates. Any deviation from this format should be in pursuit of work-related background information only. As the last part of the application, there should be an attached waiver whereby the applicant authorizes the prospective employer to contact previous employers. This waiver should include a "hold harmless" statement in which the applicant agrees to indemnify and hold harmless the former employers and the prospective employer from any and all liability as a result of references given by former employers. Another useful provision that can be attached to this waiver is a statement that any false information provided on the application is sufficient grounds for dismissal at any time the misrepresentation is identified.[3] The application should be signed by the prospective employee.

Testing applicants for skills necessary to perform the job is both allowed and well advised, provided it can be established that these talents are critical to proper job performance. The status of polygraph use in applicant evaluation is controversial and probably not a prudent tool. Other tests such as blood tests, genetic evaluation, and drug screening, all of which may have some merit, are relatively new techniques, and their use should be restricted to situations in which strong justification exists and should only be implemented with concurrence of legal counsel. It is important to say nothing during the interview that could be construed as a binding contract (e.g., indicating promotion schedules, regular bonuses, or benefits).

After identification of an applicant who appears to meet the necessary qualifications and who may mesh well with the existing office staff, employment may be offered. The individual who offers the job and hires the applicant should be the physician, since employee allegiance lies with the individual who gives them the job. In small offices, a simple verbal agreement as to starting time, hours, and wages should be sufficient to institute employment. In some instances, one may wish to formalize the employment by use of a formal employment agreement. Such an agreement spells out the responsibilities and expectations between employer and employee. In small offices, this may not be necessary, but it is encouraged for positions of significance such as an office manager. The decision of whether to use a formal employment contract should be discussed with an attorney. A copy of the personnel and procedures manual should be provided to employees at the time of hiring, and they should sign a form indicating that they have received it.

PERSONNEL MANUAL

There must be a clear understanding immediately after initiation of employment regarding the employee's job description and responsibilities and the obligations of both the employee and the employer. These are the "rules" of the office. Although this can be accomplished orally, it may become a focus of contention in the event of conflict with the employee or termination. The legal status of written personnel manuals and office policies may vary, but if the rules are in writing, the content will never be in dispute. These manuals are always subject to interpretation by the courts, particularly whether such a document can be construed to be part of an employment contract. Although there is no obligation to have such a document, the numerous advantages to both employee and employer should warrant its development.

This manual should be constructed with great care and with the overview and consultation of legal counsel. Once implemented, the policies and procedures therein must be followed. The manual can and should be updated to reflect legal changes and the changing needs or nature of the practice. When such changes are made, they should be made known to the employees, and the distribution of that information should be documented.

The manual should be written in a succinct and understandable fashion. Its purpose is to serve as an educational tool and guide, and it should not be prepared as a legal tome. It is important at the beginning of the manual to indicate that it is informational and is not to be construed as contractual. Its purpose is to provide guidelines for employees to understand conditions of their employment, their tasks and responsibilities, office organization and hierarchy, and standards for office and clinical procedures and to ensure fair and consistent treatment for each employee.

The content of the manual will vary somewhat from practice to practice, with some information deleted and other information added. A brief job description should be given for each position, with references to cross-training, allowing some employees to also carry out the functions of others, included.

The code of conduct that is to be observed within the office should be spelled out. In this area, methods of address and courtesies to patients and coworkers can be described. The manner and deportment of employees in the office should be maintained at all times, even when no patients are physically present in the area. Appearance, grooming, dress, or uniform requirements and the use of name tags, if desirable, should be outlined. Restrictions involving cosmetics, perfume, nail polish, or jewelry should also be addressed. Use of the office facility for religious, political, or charitable activities should not be permitted.

Working hours for the employees, both full-time and part-time, should be explained. Care should be taken to indicate that because of unforeseen circumstances or emergencies, it is not always possible to function on a regular clocklike basis, and time worked will be restricted to a 40-hour week. No overtime should be allowed without the specific approval of the office manager or the physician. Work is not to be taken home, nor is the employee to come in after hours to carry out activities without obtaining permission. It should be stressed that employees who elect to eat lunch in the office should not be allowed to work during that time, as this can be construed as overtime. It is particularly important that this section of the manual be clear and definitive, as overtime tends to be a focus of disagreement, particularly in the event that an employee is terminated. It should be specified that if the physician elects to take a half or full day off during the week, the office will still be open for business, and preparation of equipment, billing, collection calls, and insurance forms will be carried out.

Observed holidays should be identified. The six commonly observed holidays are New Year's Day, Memorial Day, Independence Day, Labor Day, Thanksgiving, and Christmas. Guidelines regarding additional holidays that might be recognized by federal or state governments must also be spelled out. These holidays are usually paid holidays for full-time personnel. If part-time personnel are being used, compensation for these days should be proportional to the average number of hours they work compared with full-time employees. It is a good general policy to require that the business day before and after the holiday must be worked to receive compensation for the holiday. For employees whose religious beliefs mandate other holidays, such holidays should be considered and honored on an individual basis.

Established sick leave policies should clearly state that sick leave should be used only for illnesses that prevent employees from actively and responsibly carrying out their duties. In some circumstances, although an employee may feel well enough to work, the nature of the illness and its potential effects on coworkers and patients should also be considered. It should be clearly established that verification of illness may be required. The manner in which sick leave is accumulated should also be identified. Generally speaking, 5 paid working days per year are allowed. Paid sick leave should not be made cumulative from one year to the next and it should not be utilized before it has been earned. Exceptions to this should be made only rarely and only with the approval of the physician or office manager. A decision must be made and a clear policy established regarding compensation of employees who have not used all of their sick leave at the end of an employment year. If it is elected to provide such "wellness" compensation, it must be uniformly applied to all eligible employees.

Paid personal time off (PTO) may be considered in addition to sick leave. PTO can be legitimately used for family emergencies or funerals. In general, 2 to 4 of these paid days per year may be allowed. Each circumstance in which PTO is requested should be considered on an individual basis. In the event that absence exceeds the established limits, rules should state clearly that such leave is generally unpaid but may be granted on an individual basis.

Unfortunately, the illness and PTO policy suggestions are stated in a manner that might suggest that employees cannot be trusted and therefore close scrutiny of all absences is warranted. In reality, most employees do not fit in such a category. A more considerate approach to sick leave and PTO is to lump the two together as PTO and to indicate that the time is to be used when the employees feel they cannot properly function or carry out their assigned responsibilities. It still may be possible to reward those who do not find it necessary to use all the time available to them. Those who choose to abuse this situation will also abuse other personnel policies and may become subject to dismissal.

Vacation policy applies to full-time employees only, and arrangements for part-time employees should be individualized. The manner in which vacation time accumulates varies greatly, but it should be specified that vacation time accumulates only after a specific period of employment. Generally speaking, 10 working days of vacation are usually granted after 1 full year of employment. Increased amounts of vacation time after specified periods of service can be designed to reward long-term employees. Except in special circumstances, vacation time should be used as it is accrued and not carried over to subsequent years, nor should employees be compensated for vacation time unused during their employment.

To have employee vacation time cause the least disruption of normal office routine, some policy should be developed to encourage employees to have vacation time coincide with physician absences while on vacation or attending meetings. Providing first priority to employees who select vacation time that coincides with periods of physician absence may promote this policy. Giving stronger consideration to requests for vacation during slack time than for that during busier times should also be standard. Requests for vacation time should be submitted in writing, preferably 2 to 3 months in advance. In the event that conflicts in vacation periods arise, employee seniority, the date of the request, or a rotational preference system may be used. If an employee requests vacation, usually to coincide with the spouse's vacation, before that time has been earned it may, at the physician's discretion, be granted as unpaid vacation. It may also be granted as paid vacation, with the stipulation that if the employee resigns or is terminated before the vacation time has been earned, such pay will be deducted from final compensation. Provisions for civic duties (e.g., election day or jury duty) should also be specified. In addition, maternity and possibly paternity leave should be addressed. This is an area of great current legal flux, and investigation of state and local statutes, as well as consultation with an attorney, is advisable.

It should be noted that attendance and hours worked are chronicled. In small offices, the use of time sheets is usually satisfactory (Fig. 21–3). In larger offices, the use of a time clock may be necessary. Punctuality should be emphasized, and specifics as to how chronic abuse will be treated must be made clear. It is the employee's responsibility to advise the employer as far in advance as possible if they are unable to work on a particular day. The manual must spell out how failure to communicate inability to work on a particular day will be handled. Dealing with brief absences, such as parent-teacher conferences and dental or physician visits, should be defined. Perhaps allowing the employee to

Employee _____

SSN _____

Position _____

Entitled To:
Sick Days _____

Personal Time Off _____

Vacation Days _____

Date Hired _____

	1	2	3	4	5	6	7	8	9	10	11	12	13	14	15	16	17	18	19	20	21	22	23	24	25	26	27	28	29	30	31	Monthly Totals				
																																	S	P	V	L	O
January																																				
February																																				
March																																				
April																																				
May																																				
June																																				
July																																				
August																																				
September																																				
October																																				
November																																				
December																																				

Annual Summary

*May wish to arrange calendar to correspond to fiscal year

Code: S = Sick
P = Personal
V = Vacation
L = Late
O = Absent, Other

Comments: _____
_____
_____
_____

Figure 21–3. Personal attendance record.

make up the time by working a comparable amount of time during the same week can be arranged. The employee should not be allowed the latitude of arriving early so as to leave early unless specific previous arrangements are made. Even then, this can place a substantial burden on the remaining employees, and its use should be discouraged or disallowed.

Salaries and how they are determined should be described in general terms. The dates for employee performance review and salary adjustments should be identified. The basis for raises, cost-of-living adjustments, and bonus determination should be specified. The interval for payment of wages should be indicated as weekly, semimonthly, or monthly. It should be emphasized that salary and wages are individual and confidential. Disclosure of such information between employees who have unequal remuneration, for whatever reason, can contribute to substantial friction and in-office rancor. Violation of the confidentiality of this information can be grounds for termination. Benefits beyond salary that may be available to employees, such as health insurance, life insurance, worker's compensation insurance, disability insurance, parking allowance, expenses for pertinent educational programs, and uniform allowance should be identified (Fig. 21–4). Participation in a retirement or profit sharing plan should be indicated, but this is usually addressed in specific separate documents as required by statute. Details of the various plans and the contact people for these plans may be appended to the manual.

Performance evaluations should be done on a regular basis, either once or twice annually. This should be a formal procedure whereby predetermined criteria are used in the evaluation of each employee (Fig. 21–5). It is valuable to have employees rate themselves before the employer does so. The evaluation should be discussed forthrightly and honestly with the employee, and an opportunity should be provided for "give-and-take" regarding the evaluation. A copy of the evaluation sheet signed by the evaluator and the employee should be maintained in the employee's file and a copy provided to the employee.

If an employee elects to terminate employment, it should be required that 2 weeks' notice be given. If the employee fails to comply, the customary 2 weeks' separation pay can be waived or reduced. Additionally, accumulated vacation time may be forfeited without 2 weeks' notice.

A grievance process should be available for employees in the event a problem is identified. This can be initiated informally by the employee with written or verbal notice to the office manager or to the physician. Each grievance should be handled on an individual basis.

Termination of an employee can be a wrenching and emotional experience for the employee as well as the employer. It is also fraught with numerous potential legal hazards. Some of the necessary procedures are outlined by statute, and therefore this portion of the personnel manual must be designed with legal counsel. Situations that justify termination without notice, benefits, or severance pay should be identified. Generally these include dishonesty; misuse of controlled sub-

stances; working under the influence of mind-altering substances, drugs, or alcohol; gross negligence; violation of patient confidentiality or confidential information; and unprofessional conduct.

Confidentiality, although addressed briefly earlier, should be emphasized. All information regarding a patient, including medical records, letters, and even appointment times, is included in the concept of confidentiality, and it is improper to reveal any of this information to anyone, including members of the patient's family, without the expressed written or witnessed verbal permission of the patient. The only exception is information about a child given to the child's parents, but in some instances, the privacy of juveniles must be maintained also. Any conversation regarding the condition of patients or information regarding patients within the front office setting, particularly over the telephone, is unjustified unless the conversation can be conducted remote from unauthorized listeners.

A formal master copy of the personnel manual should be maintained, copies distributed to each employee, and receipt of such a manual acknowledged by signature of the employee. This acknowledgment should be maintained in the employee's file. It is a good practice to have a final paragraph in the manual reiterating its purposes and possibly soliciting any suggestions, alterations, or questions that the employee might have.

The preparation of a personnel manual can be time consuming, particularly when the physician has had no previous experience preparing one, but it is well worth the effort to establish an effective employee-employer relationship. Various guides to the development of these manuals are available,[4] and examination of several of them may enhance the quality of the procedure manual produced.

TERMINATION

At some point during a physician's practice, it will probably be necessary to terminate one or more employees. This situation tends to be unpleasant, emotional, and distasteful but must be executed in a fashion that complies with existing legal statutes, which are designed to protect the employee and, to a certain extent, the employer. Compliance with these rules is necessary to avoid retaliation and possible legal action by the employee. To be on the soundest possible footing, the grounds for dismissal should have been set forth in the personnel manual, and periodic personnel evaluations with written documentation and acknowledgment of their performance by the staff should be used.

The simplest form of termination is probably that in which a reduction in staff is made necessary by reduced patient flow owing to a change in the nature of a practice or simply a diminished case load. In these instances, the reality of decreased need for the services of an employee can usually be documented simply and used as the basis for termination. The selection of which employee must be released under these circumstances should be based, as much as possible, on objective considerations of the services required. The least capable employee is then let go. In such a circumstance, despite its being an

FISCAL YEAR _____

EMPLOYEE _____

SN _____

	BENEFIT	ADDITIONAL EMPLOYER COST
W-2 Salary	_____	
Social Security	_____	_____
Workmen's Compensation Insurance		_____
Federal unemployment		_____
State unemployment		_____
Retirement plan _____ %	_____	
Insurances		
Health	_____	
Disability	_____	
Life	_____	
Bonuses	_____	
Uniform allowance	_____	
Sick leave and personal time off	_____	
Educational programs	_____	
Family medical care provided	_____	
TOTAL	_____	

Vacation days: Earned _____ Used _____ Remaining _____

Nonpaid days off _____

Figure 21–4. Employee benefit report.

emotional blow to the employee, it is probably the most understandable of reasons to that employee and is the least likely to produce rancor, although this is certainly not assured.

In termination for cause, as outlined in the personnel manual, there should be documentation as to the specific cause or causes. In addition, the employer must be certain that the use of a progressive disciplinary system, if stated in the personnel manual, has been followed. The specific situation must be reviewed to ensure that violation of state or federal statutes has not occurred. An employee may not be terminated on the basis of race, color, sex, religion, or national origin. Furthermore, some states prohibit discrimination based on political affiliation, personal appearance, civic activities, juvenile criminal records, marital or family status, fertility, pregnancy, sexual orientation, military service (or lack thereof), wage garnishment, voting, or jury duty. Violation of any of these rules can put the employer at risk for future legal action by the employee. Employees cannot be terminated for exercising their legal rights. For instance, employees cannot be terminated for filing a worker's compensation claim, or for reporting violations of an employer under the Occupational Safety and Health Administration (OSHA) statute. Laws also pro-

tect employees who engage in union-organizing activities.

If it seems apparent that an employee must be terminated, it is often wise to consider an alternative to dismissal, particularly if there are circumstances that might suggest that the termination could be tainted. It is possible that an additional warning, a temporary suspension, or placement on probation could solve the problem. A change of duties might relieve the individual of tasks he or she is incapable of performing. A leave of absence could also be considered if it might possibly improve the performance of the individual. If it appears that none of the foregoing alternatives will be successful in remediation, then termination should proceed expeditiously, as it is better to terminate an unsatisfactory employee sooner than later. Most terminations ultimately prove to be a result of personality conflicts or interpersonal relationship problems within the business.

The use of a checklist has been suggested[3] to aid in determining whether potential legal liabilities for the employer might exist. Personal employee information should be reviewed regarding age, sex, minority group status, term of service, and the extent of vested pension rights, if any. If the employee has filed any complaints regarding work place safety or services provided or has

EMPLOYEE_____

DATE HIRED:_____

DATE LAST REVIEW:_____

Skill/Attribute	Rating		Reviewer Comments
	Emp	Rev	
Accepts Instruction/Criticism			
Adaptability			
Appearance			
Attitude Toward Job			
Attitude Toward Others			
Cross-training Skills			
Improves Skills			
Initiative			
Job Knowledge			
Leadership			
Patient Relations			
Performance Quality			
Reliability			
Telephone Demeanor			
Works Well With Others			
			Total Previous Reviews:

Employee Comments:_____

_____

_____

_____

Recommended Action:_____

_____

_____

_____

_____

_____   _____   _____
Employee's Signature   Date   Reviewer's Signature

Ratings: 0 = Unsatisfactory
          1 = Improvement Necessary
          2 = Adequate
          3 = Above Average
          4 = Outstanding

Figure 21–5. Performance review.

initiated any job-related legal claims, such as those covered under OSHA or workmen's compensation, termination should be considered very carefully.

Specific reasons for discharge should be documented as though legal action might be taken against the employer. Improper behavior or exercise of responsibilities should be identified and noted. Failure to correct previous shortcomings, as identified in the job performance review, should be noted, as should any previous warnings or reprimands for which compliance was lacking.

There should be documentation, particularly if the employee's performance is unsatisfactory, that compliance with the disciplinary procedures outlined in the employee's personnel manual have been followed, that the employee was informed of the potential consequences of poor performance, and that discharge is justified on the basis of the employee's actions. There should be a trail of documentation of the shortcomings and evidence that an opportunity for the employee to explain or justify these items was provided. There should be a timely relationship between the triggering event or inadequacy of the employee and the decision to terminate. In the event the review of this information makes it questionable as to whether termination is advisable at this point, or if there is any doubt lingering in the mind of the employer, legal counsel should be sought. In virtually all actions of termination, pertinent advice should be sought from legal counsel.

Once the decision to terminate the employee has been reached, it will, in all likelihood, fall on the physician to perform this task personally. In a larger office this can sometimes be delegated to the office manager or the staff person with the closest relationship to the employee, but only after the foregoing admonitions have been reviewed and the physician is in concurrence with the decision.

The termination should be effected in private and in person, in a face-to-face meeting with the employee. The reasons for the dismissal should be outlined, and the employee should be given an opportunity to respond. After this, the physician should not engage in a dialogue or discussion meant to give reassurance or otherwise give an indication of uncertainty as to the dismissal. The employee should then be provided with a prepared check for severance pay, generally 2 weeks. The employee should then be escorted to the desk, where personal belongings can be gathered under supervision and keys retrieved. The employee is then escorted from the premises to avoid retribution. It is imprudent to allow the employee to continue to work or complete unfinished tasks, particularly if a computer is available for part of his or her duties. In addition, it is wise to have the locks changed or re-keyed.

When it becomes probable that an employee will have to be terminated, if time exists and the situation warrants, it may be wise to consider drafting and signing a termination agreement with the employee. This type of an agreement generally outlines the potential legal rights of an employee and then states that the employee agrees to release all potential legal claims relating to the dismissal. To make such an agreement workable, some additional consideration beyond that to which the employee is normally entitled is necessary. This can be as simple as an increase in the amount of severance pay normally provided. Such a document should always be drafted by an attorney.

Confidentiality regarding termination of employment is required in some states; this requirement should be determined and respected. Unfortunately, this may place the employer in an untenable position if the terminated employee solicits a recommendation or if a potential future employer requests information regarding previous employment. Such a situation, should it arise, must be clarified with an attorney, if such a release was not included on the job application form.

Scheduling Patients

Scheduling is an exercise in time management for both the patient and the surgeon. The practice mix will determine which type of scheduling format will ultimately be most beneficial. As staff members gain experience in the length of time required to treat various problems, they are better able to optimally schedule patients. There may be a tendency by the physician to underestimate how effectively and quickly a problem can be solved or a procedure can be done, and an experienced nurse or assistant will probably have a better estimate.

Four major scheduling systems have generally been employed. The "free-for-all" system is basic chaos: patients arrive at the physician's office and are seen sequentially until all of those who can be accommodated within a period of time have been attended. Fortunately for the patient, staff, and physician, this system is little used except in some types of indigent care clinics.

Two types of "wave scheduling" have been employed. In one system, a modified "free-for-all," a certain number of patients are scheduled in the morning and a certain number in the afternoon, and patients are seen in order of arrival as the physician can attend to them. This works only slightly better than the "free-for-all" system. A "modified wave" system involves smaller waves of patients scheduled at the beginning of each hour; these are seen as they arrive. None of the foregoing would serve satisfactorily or gracefully for a cutaneous surgical practice.

The so-called "stream scheduling" allots a specific appointment time to each patient, who is seen at the time of arrival. This requires some degree of accuracy in estimating the amount of time each patient will require and assumes that the patient's arrival will be prompt and the physician's treatment can be carried out within the allotted time. As with other scheduling systems, this system is at the mercy of events such as late patient arrival, extra time needed to see preceding patients, emergencies, telephone interruptions for the physician, and complications that may lengthen the time required to perform a procedure.

Any system that is devised must fit not only the needs of the staff and the surgeon but also those of the patient. Patients are quite aware of their time constraints and rightfully resent spending time waiting for the doctor. It behooves the physician and the reputation of the practice to see patients expeditiously. In the long run, it is better to see fewer patients on time and to have them exit happily than to overschedule in an effort to see as many patients as possible during the day.

To this end, use of a system in which new patients are scheduled on the basis of information provided to the receptionist at the time of initial contact is often helpful. Information given to the receptionist can also allow a reasonable estimate of the time required for established patients to be seen on subsequent visits. When a patient is seen and a problem requiring surgical intervention is indicated, that procedure may be scheduled in advance for the requisite amount of time.

There are several confounding factors that must be considered in all offices. One problem is patients who present with the assumption that all the issues that concern them can be discussed and solved at the time of the appointment. Sometimes this can be accomplished, particularly if the problems are minor or can be expeditiously treated (e.g., warts, skin tags, or pedunculated or irritated lesions). If this is not the case, however, the patient may require much more time than expected, and sometimes it is best to schedule an additional appointment as necessary.

Another problem, particularly in a referral or consultative practice, is a patient who may have come a great distance and cannot conveniently return for a procedure. Common sense and good judgment indicate that the procedure should be carried out at the time of the initial visit, if possible. Fortunately, receptionists can generally identify most of these patients at the time the initial inquiry is made by telephone. One point should be made, however: if the patient is traveling a substantial distance, the receptionist must inquire as to *all* the problems for which the patient is seeking help.

The following system may work for the benefit of both the surgeon and the patient. Once the nature of the problem has been discreetly identified by the receptionist, most new patients are given an "A" appointment. This is a 30-minute appointment during which the initial acquaintance with the patient, evaluation of problems, and treatment of as many of these as possible can be accomplished. "B" appointments of 15 minutes are used for follow-up patients. During these, a problem can be evaluated, additional therapy instituted, minor procedures such as cryosurgery or laser ablation of lesions performed, and reassurance and instructions provided. "C" appointments are 7.5 minutes each and are used for interim examination of previous surgical procedures, removal of sutures, and rebandaging and treatment that can be expeditiously provided (e.g., cryosurgery of actinic keratoses or seborrheic keratoses). The final appointment category does not have a letter designation, since the time required depends on the specific problem necessitating surgery. The amount of time alloted is left to the discretion of the surgeon, nurse, or assistant and varies with the magnitude of the procedure. Previous experience with the individual surgeon's operating time for various procedures, the amount of assistance available, and possible complications all help determine the amount of time needed. Excision and primary closure of a nevus, for example, will obviously require less time to perform than more complex procedures such as transposition or rotation flaps or scalp reductions. It is better to allow more time than too little in case problems are encountered during the surgical procedure, thus delaying the examination of patients scheduled later.

It is beneficial to have new patients and scheduled surgery patients arrive at the office 10 to 15 minutes early so that the necessary paperwork can be completed beforehand and the start of the procedure is not delayed. This also allows time for answering any questions the patient might have, for providing adequate information so that informed consent is obtained from the patient, and for surgical preparation before the start of the procedure. It is usually far preferable to be ahead of schedule than behind schedule.

Of all the procedures performed by cutaneous surgeons, as many as possible should be done in the office, provided facilities are adequate for their safe performance. Use of facilities in ambulatory surgical sites or hospital operating rooms may be necessary at times. In scheduling procedures at such sites, it is imperative that adequate physician travel time be allowed and that best use is made of this time by sequentially scheduling as many patients for that facility as possible. Nevertheless, the surgeon is at the mercy of previously scheduled procedures by other doctors, emergencies, late patient arrivals, slow room-turnover time, and a host of other factors.

Communication of the time necessary for scheduling patients can be done by the physician or the assistant, indicating in the appropriate area on the "superbill" or attending physician's statement (APS) the same codes: "A", "B," or "C". If a procedure requires a specific amount of time, such as 30 minutes, 60 minutes, or 3 hours, this can be indicated. It may be prudent to provide a buffer time of from 15 to 30 minutes at late midmorning and midafternoon to allow for errors in the schedule. This also will provide for emergencies and drop-in patients with urgent problems, as well as the expeditious examination or treatment of out-of-town patients who were scheduled earlier in the morning or afternoon.

Requests for consultations to deal with elective or cosmetic procedures are generally scheduled for an "A" appointment. These consultations should be done in an unhurried and comfortable manner, allowing adequate time for evaluation and discussion of alternative remedies and the advantages, disadvantages, risks, and known possible complications. If a known problem may warrant additional time, this can be determined by the receptionist or individual responsible for scheduling.

It is mandatory that patients be called as a reminder, preferably 48 hours before any scheduled appointment. This provides an opportunity to possibly answer any questions that may have developed and to reconfirm, cancel, or reschedule the appointment, thus freeing the appointment time for another patient in the event of a cancellation or rescheduling. This call before the appointment can also be used to remind patients who are having a surgical procedure to bring a companion who can be responsible for transporting them safely home, if this is deemed prudent by the surgeon. It is also wise to maintain a list of patients who are scheduled for future appointments and who desire to be seen sooner, if possible. These individuals may then be called to fill appointments that are canceled or rescheduled.

As much as possible, patients' wishes regarding preferred appointment times should be honored. Depending on demand, it may be necessary to make off-hours appointments available in the early morning, during lunch, or in the early evening 1 or 2 days per week or on weekends to accommodate school schedules, work hours, or long travel distance.

Although rules provide a solid basis for scheduling patients, it remains something of an art that is constantly evolving and should be suitably flexible to allow for modification. This system (Fig. 21–6) will work satisfactorily whether appointments are logged in a book or a computer.

Patient Information Booklets

One of the most important pieces of information that can be provided to both patients and prospective patients is the patient information booklet, which is a synopsis of information regarding the physician's practice that is of interest and importance to patients, including office hours, specialty areas of practice, fees, and policies regarding insurance. This booklet should be a part of every practice; in addition to being of interest to prospective patients, it functions as a valuable marketing tool. The booklet can be very simple or a multipage color extravaganza. It is most suitable for the brochure to be designed to fit easily in a regular mailing envelope.

From a practical standpoint, the basics of the patient information booklet can be designed by the doctor with staff input. Because an inordinate amount of office time is spent in answering the same questions, this booklet should be prepared in a fashion to answer them in a more efficient manner. It is frequently useful to examine brochures from other medical practices, including those in other specialties, as ideas may be encountered that would be beneficial for inclusion in the proposed publication. After the content has been determined, placed in order, examined, and found to be complete in fitting the needs of the practice and tailored to the profile of the practice's patients, it can be taken to a professional printer who will also advise, make suggestions, assist with layout, and ultimately print it.

Once produced, one pamphlet should be given to every new patient who visits the office, any interested parties who accompany a patient, and prospective patients who inquire of the office regarding types of procedures the physician performs, the physician's credentials, or other policies of the practice. The address of the potential patient should be obtained and the booklet mailed. For patients who may be uncertain as to whether a service they desire is available, at what cost, or at what inconvenience, the pamphlet may persuade them to make an appointment and pursue the matter further.

The patient information booklet generally must be custom designed for each practice; however, there are individuals who are willing to design these pamphlets. Some practice consultants also have had experience in these matters and may have examples of what they feel to be a good design. It is prudent in designing the booklet to make several rough drafts and discuss these with the various members of the front office and medical staff, as they are a major information source for patients and are well versed in the types of questions they encounter frequently. It is often wise to set forth categories one may wish to include in the patient information booklet and then circulate this among the staff to see which items they feel should be included and to provide the opportunity for any additional comments they might have. All of these ideas should be taken into consideration when preparing the final design of the pamphlet.

CONTENT

The first portion of the booklet should be a welcome to the patient. The practice should be identified by name and the address and phone numbers given. If the practice is in an area where access might be a problem, directions or a map should be provided.

The objectives and philosophy of the practice should be given in the welcoming statements. After this paragraph, the nature of the practice should be identified. In a cutaneous surgery practice, the particular procedures that the surgeon emphasizes should be listed in consecutive fashion in a sentence, paragraph, or tabular format, whichever best suits the nature and image the physician wishes to project in the brochure.

A description of the surgeon should be given, including a recent photograph, if possible; educational background, including residency, specialty, and subspecialty training; and any other credentials. If specific study or apprenticeship for certain procedures has been done, this should also be mentioned. The function and responsibilities of the staff should be described. It is not prudent to include photographs of the entire staff, as turnover could render the pamphlet inaccurate within a short period of time. The surgeon's staff appointments and privileges at hospitals should be noted, along with addresses and phone numbers of those hospitals.

The method for scheduling appointments should be identified, delineating the hours in which patients are seen from the hours in which the office is attended only by secretarial and receptionist help. The policy that new patients should arrive 10 or 15 minutes before their appointed time to complete necessary paperwork should be stated, along with polite emphasis that established or follow-up patients should be on time for their appointments. This should be accompanied by a statement to the effect that the physician respects the patient's time, and for the appointment system to work to everyone's benefit, promptness is necessary.

The pamphlet should specify whether 24- or 48-hour advance notification is required to cancel an appointment. If a policy of charging a fee for a missed appointment or failure to cancel in a timely fashion is in existence, it should be spelled out clearly. Some advisors feel that use of such a policy is antagonistic to the patient and might dissuade a potential patient from making an appointment. Such a policy should be implemented in a thoughtful, fair, and discretionary fashion. However, it should be noted that there is no evidence that existence of such a policy diminishes the number of missed appointments. If a 24- or 48-hour reminder

C-double (7 1/2 min.)
B-15 minute
A-30 minute

DR _____ Day _____ Date _____

DATE	NAME	PHONE	PROBLEM
7:30			
8:00			
8:00			
8:15			
8:30			
8:30			
8:45			
9:00			
9:00			
9:15			
9:30			
9:30			
9:45			
10:00			
10:00			
10:15			
10:30			
10:30			
10:45			
11:00			
1:00			
1:00			
1:15			
1:30			
1:30			
1:45			
2:00			
2:00			
2:15			
2:30			
2:30			
2:45			
3:00			
3:00			
3:15			
3:30			
3:30			
3:45			
4:00			
4:00			

Figure 21–6. Patient-scheduling format.

system for calling scheduled patients and reconfirming their appointment is in existence, this should be noted in the pamphlet as well.

In addition to indicating what appointment hours are available, there should also be a statement indicating the times the physician accepts telephone calls during office hours. The procedure for having the calls screened and answered by ancillary personnel should be explained whenever possible. Those calls that should be directed to the physician, if not emergencies, should be designated to a certain "call-back" time. The doctor's philosophy on telephone requests for prescription refills should be spelled out in this section. Special testing or procedures that can be provided for the patient by the physician, either in the office or in an ancillary facility, should be outlined in the pamphlet. The methods for having those tests accomplished should be specified.

It is helpful to describe the types of situations the doctor considers to be emergencies and the sequence for attempting to contact the doctor or obtain other help. During the day, of course, the office phone number should be used; after hours, an answering exchange can be used. The specific types of medical problems or conditions for which the cutaneous surgeon provides telephone coverage should be made available to the physician's answering exchange. If back-up coverage or the doctor is not available, the telephone numbers for paramedics, the local poison center, and the emergency department of the nearest hospital should all be identified.

A statement regarding determination of professional fees and collection policies should be given. The policy on payment at the time of service should also be made clear. If billing is necessary, the dates on which bills are sent should be indicated. It is wise to specify when accounts are considered past due, what collection services are used, and how they are implemented. It is essential to indicate that the office policies on collections conform to the Federal Truth In Lending Act. If interest will be charged on the unpaid portion of a fee, this should be spelled out. (If four or more payments are made, the requirements laid out by the Federal Truth In Lending Act must be followed, and the patient must be given an appropriate statement indicating the annual interest rate percentage. However, although this is information the patient ultimately must have, it need not be spelled out in the pamphlet.) If there is a billing charge for sending out statements, either beginning with or after the first statement, this should be stated. Any fees for preparing insurance forms beyond the first should be specified. It is wise to indicate that if patients have a question regarding a fee or bill, they are able to discuss this with the physician or an appropriate assistant.

A section on health insurance should be included. In this, the physician should indicate those insurance companies, health maintenance organizations (HMOs), preferred provider organizations (PPOs), or independent practice associations (IPAs) in which he or she is a participant. The physician's policy as to insurance being a contract between the patient and the insurance company should be stated. It should also be stipulated that the relationship between the physician and the patient is distinct from the relationship between the insurance company and the patient, and the patient is ultimately responsible for the fee. This information should not be dispensed in a heavy-handed fashion, but can be accompanied by a statement that there may always be exceptions to the rule, and the staff is willing to provide information, respond to questions, and assist patients in completion of insurance forms. If a superbill (APS) is used in the office, this is a good place to indicate that simple attachment of the completed superbill to the insurance form will generally satisfy most insurance companies. If a physician participates in Medicare or Medicaid, this should be so specified; if not, it is wise

to indicate this and perhaps also give the reasons for not participating. The local medical society can be contacted for suggestions as to how to best phrase this statement. Participation in worker's compensation insurance should also be identified in a similar fashion.

It is useful to have a section regarding medical records and the fact that all aspects of a patient's medical care within the office are considered confidential, and for this reason, information will not be released without the specific permission of the patient or responsible adult. An explanation of how to request a release form and to whom appropriate information is to be directed should be identified here as well. This is a good place to state that additional reports and summaries to various insurance companies, particularly those requesting background health information on a candidate applying for life insurance, as well as attorneys, will be issued with appropriate release by the patient, but for an appropriate fee that must be received in advance.

The last item in the booklet should indicate that the booklet has been prepared for the benefit of the patient and should be retained for future reference. In addition, suggestions from patients regarding other items that might be beneficially included in the booklet should be solicited.

Medical Records

A separate medical record should be maintained for each patient. The basic purpose of the medical record is to assemble adequate information for patient care. In addition, it is a chronicle of ongoing care and services provided to the patient. Although the physical elements of the medical chart belong to the physician, the information contained within it has been legally determined to also be the property of the patient. Because the patient is within legal boundaries in requesting to see the chart or to be furnished with the information it contains (unless, in the physician's opinion, the information could be detrimental to the patient), it is imperative that the information be accurate, complete, and objective. If such information is requested by the patient for personal use or for use by others, it is necessary to determine the time frame or period for which the records are requested. Providing information in excess of that requested may be considered a violation of privacy. It is also mandatory to obtain the patient's written request to release the records and to identify the parties to whom the records are being provided.

The medical record should contain results of the history and physical examination obtained at the first encounter. If the patient provides a supplemental history or records from another physician, it is necessary to review these documents and make note of it on the copies. Rather than store the supplied information in the patient's record, it may be more prudent to make a summary of the salient features of that record, including laboratory tests, pathology reports, or operative notes, to insert in the patient medical record and store the copies provided in a separate file. Notes for each patient encounter should be dutifully and accurately logged as soon after the encounter as possible and practical. Some surgeons prefer to dictate these notes and have them transcribed and placed in the chart; others may prefer handwritten entries. Although the latter at times may be more convenient, in an effort to make the notes concise because of time constraints, information that could later prove pertinent may be inadvertently deleted. In the event that handwritten entries are elected, these must be legible, not only to the writer, but also to others who may have a need to use the chart. Once in the record, notes of any sort should not be altered unless proper procedure is used. This consists of striking through erroneous information with a single line and initialing and dating the correction. Other integral parts of the chart include the documentation of informed consent for surgical procedures and nonstandard treatments, as well as releases for photography, videotape, and disposition of specimens and tissue and written releases to provide portions of the chart to other parties. In addition, if copies of the entire record or portions of the record are forwarded to another party, an entry to that effect should be made by the office personnel responsible for copying and sending them.

Other useful components of the chart include the laboratory studies requested and reported, pathology reports, consultations and communications with other physicians regarding the patient, copies of prescriptions provided to the patient, and reports of radiologic examinations. Anatomic diagrams are extremely helpful for charting the distribution and exact location of disorders, abnormalities, lesions, biopsy sites, operative sites, and even tissue movement, including flap design for reconstruction. In each instance where an anatomic diagram is utilized, the site of the lesions or procedures should be identified and dated. Pertinent measurements can also be placed on this diagram. Ideally, a separate diagram for each visit can be made, but in some instances multiple entries can be made on the same diagram as long as the lesion site and the date are made clear.

Some physicians prefer to use a narrative description wherein all information gathered during a visit and procedures accomplished are documented sequentially. For any major procedure, it is often preferable to generate a separate operative note. In this way, information regarding a procedure can be provided simply by copying the requested procedure note and forwarding it to the party requesting it. This allows the request to be filled more effectively and protects against the possible violation of privacy that might occur if a comprehensive note regarding other problems not pertinent to the requested information is provided.

When any telephone communication regarding a medical problem transpires, whether it is handled by an assistant or personally by the physician, an entry pertinent to the discussion should be made in the chart by the person involved, with documentation as to the date, time, and content of the discussion. This should be signed or initialed by the staff person involved. Entries regarding telephone contact with the patient after surgery should be made in a similar fashion by the person communicating with the patient.

Although medical records should be available in the office at all times to provide accurate information regarding the patient, accomplishing this is often difficult. Charts may be removed from the file for a variety of reasons and taken to various places in the office. The best way to prevent misplaced charts is to require that they be immediately refiled after their use for any purpose.

Regardless of the size of the practice, old records accumulate. From time to time, purging these records is necessary. This can be accomplished in several ways. One way is refiling them in a long-term storage area reserved for patient records that have had no activity for a specified time. This interval may vary, but the records should not be destroyed or permanently disposed of unless statutorily allowable, again with concurrence of legal counsel. State statutes vary regarding record retention requirements, and the required storage period for adults may differ from that for minors. An attorney should be consulted before disposing of any patient records.

Thinning a chart is, in effect, another form of purging. In this instance the portions of the records removed should also be saved and subject to the same constraints outlined earlier. Portions or entire charts can be placed on microfilm and stored in much less space, but a special viewer is required to later read the microfilm, and the process is expensive.

A frequent occurrence is a request, usually by telephone, from an interested or concerned relative or friend regarding the condition or test results of a patient. Again, this information should not be released, even verbally, to anyone without the consent of the patient or the responsible adult. This may lead to some concern or anger on the part of the calling party, particularly if it is a spouse, mother, daughter, or son; nevertheless, time should be taken to politely explain the patient's right to privacy. From a practical standpoint, if the caller is in a position to be allowed such information, the caller can contact the patient, who can then personally decide whether he or she wishes to provide such information. Although this may sound unduly harsh or impolite, the office staff has no way of establishing the identity of the caller, and providing any patient information without authorization is justifiably indefensible.

The requirements for detailed documentation may seem to be excessive, but solid, accurate, complete medical records benefit both the patient and the physician.

Patient Education

Patient education has always been important, but with more sophisticated consumers and a greater demand for information about medical treatments and procedures for various conditions, it is mandatory that a provision be made for meeting these needs. Providing adequate information benefits not only the patient, but also the physician and staff. This is because the better educated the patient is regarding the problem, the alternative forms of therapy available, and the various ramifications of accepting or using a particular form of treatment, the more likely it is that the needs of the patient will be satisfied. This also provides a solid basis for discussion regarding proposed and completed procedures, which may provide substantial protection for the physician in the event an untoward result develops. Patient education is the basis, but not a substitute, for obtaining informed consent in treatment.

There are three different ways to provide such education: discussion between the patient and the staff and physician, written materials pertinent to the disease process and possible forms of therapy, and other media such as photographs, slides, and video presentations. In some instances, one method may be preferable, but all forms of education should be complementary.

Written educational materials can be developed by the surgeon to satisfy personal needs and tastes. These materials may include information about a specific surgical procedure, the indications for using the procedure, how it is performed, the benefits it is likely to provide, and its limitations and possible side effects. Postoperative wound care instructions, limitations on activities, and circumstances that require immediate contact with the office personnel can also be included. In addition, published pamphlets are available for purchase from many professional societies and from the National Institutes of Health. Prepared information regarding many prescription medications is available from the American Medical Association and can be used as an adjunct to oral instructions given to the patient. These materials serve to educate the patient and can help dispel misinformation and "myths" that surround some medical problems and surgical procedures. The time at which these materials are used is at the surgeon's discretion, but generally they are provided at the time the patient is seen in the office.

Ideally, when the patient arrives at the office, the nature of the problem is already known. If not, it can be determined by a medical assistant when the patient is in the examination room. It may be appropriate at that time to provide the patient with some written information regarding the diagnosis, particularly if there will be a waiting period before seeing the surgeon. During this time, the patient can examine the information and use the material as a foundation to ask pertinent questions of the surgeon. The information can also be used to supplement the discussion after consultation and examination.

In some instances, it may be appropriate to supply written material to a patient who has requested an appointment for a specific problem, provided there is enough time to mail such material to the patient before the scheduled appointment. However, it may happen that providing such material in advance without the opportunity for direct discussion can generate unwarranted concern on the part of the patient and possibly result in cancellation or failure to keep an appointment. The manner in which written materials are used in the practice should be established as office policy.

Proper use of ancillary personnel such as medical assistants and nurses can greatly expedite essential verbal communication. It also can beneficially limit the amount of time the physician must spend responding to some of the more mundane concerns and questions posed by the patient. This makes the physician's time with the patient more effective, and although it certainly does not absolve the surgeon from the responsibility of communicating effectively with the patient, it allows more time to be spent on items the physician feels to be important. The use of discussion, as well as written information provided to the patient, should be recorded in the chart notes, as this will help supplement any contentions that might arise later regarding the adequacy of information and informed consent.

The use of visual aids can be beneficial, but if event photographs or slides are used to describe procedures or suggest possible results that could be attained, appropriate authorized releases from the patients whose photographs are used should be obtained and documented before use. In addition, it should be made clear that these pictorial representations are for educational purposes only and are not a guarantee that similar or better results may be obtained. The same policy also pertains to the use of videotape presentations involving patients. Educational video presentations can be an extremely effective, concise method of providing information about the technical aspects of a procedure without requiring the presence of the physician, nurse, or assistant. After the patient has viewed these presentations, an opportunity to discuss them is essential. While educational video cassettes on some surgical subjects are available on a commercial basis, the entire array of procedures the surgeon performs may not necessarily be available. Therefore, if certain procedures are performed frequently by the surgeon, it may be prudent to make a videotape of each procedure to be used as an educational tool in the practice setting.

The effectiveness of all of these methods of patient education depends on the participation of the physician and the assistant staff and the effort made by the patient to use the materials provided.

Fees

In the past, physicians could establish their fees by simply identifying what they felt was a reasonable charge for the procedure and using this as the basis for their remuneration. This has been made more complex by a number of uncontrollable outside influences: rental of office space; rental, lease, or purchase of equipment; personnel-related expenditures (salaries and attendant benefits); and the cost of supplies, utilities, and taxes. All of these contribute to determining what will be the ultimate fees. The easiest way for a physician to determine fees in a particular locale is to simply ask other physicians. However, this approach is not condoned by various statutes and is fraught with perils, including the imposition of legal sanctions, penalties, fines, possible loss of license, and even incarceration. Therefore, inquiry regarding such matters, if done at all, should be done judiciously and in such a fashion that it cannot be construed to resemble price fixing or establishment of a noncompetitive atmosphere.

From a practical standpoint, the intrusion of third-party payers may limit the fees that can be charged for various services, since ceilings for many procedures may have been set. Information can be obtained in an indirect fashion by making inquiry of various insurance companies, providing them with a schedule of the proposed fees for certain procedures, and asking them to indicate whether these are within the allowable limits. Insurance companies will generally indicate which fees exceed their limits but not those that are below the limit they impose. Nevertheless, some information can be derived in this fashion. Additionally, some HMOs, PPOs, and IPAs can provide information regarding their allowances for various procedures. In fact, if a surgeon is considering establishing a relationship with one of these groups, it is mandatory that such information be obtained before making a reasonable decision about participation. It is not necessary to participate in any or all of these plans to have a successful and profitable practice.

In dealing with Medicare, the physician should contact the Professional Relations Department of the carrier for the state's Medicare program, utilizing professional letterhead stationery to file a request for the customary fee profile for the area. If the physician has not been established as a Medicare provider in the area, the Freedom of Information Act requires the carrier to provide a list of the procedures and services, with attendant "customary" fees in certain percentile groups. Although these fees will, in almost all instances, be less than those accepted by other third-party payers, there tends to be a relative relationship from procedure to procedure, and a rough estimate of the fees of others in the area can be made. One very useful document, *Determination of Reasonable Charges Under Part B Medicare, BHI 029,* can be obtained from the government by requesting a copy from either the local Medicare carrier or from the Health Care Financing Administration, Department of Health and Human Services, Baltimore, Maryland, 21207. This document reiterates the steps and procedures used by Medicare in determining allowable charges. This can be used with modifications as a guide for establishing fees. An additional source of information on established fee schedules can be obtained from workman's compensation insurance in each state. *Medical Economics* also publishes an annual issue profiling fees across the country, divided by region and specialty. Although not exhaustive, it is fairly complete, and perusal of the most recent issue can be enlightening.

Another third-party arrangement known as managed care consists of groups who administer various insurance plans for employers. These act as intervenors, contractors, reviewers, and administrators for the various employers who are their clients. Like HMOs and PPOs, they attempt to enlist physician participation and offer their clients, who pay for their services, more effective use of the financial resources being expended on behalf of the employees. These groups seek to reduce the financial expenditures of the employer while getting the best medical care for the employees. Obviously, the only way the administrators of such programs make money is by saving money for their clients, and this usually comes in the form of reduced fees offered to the physician. In exploring such offers, copies of their allowances for various procedures should also be obtained.

Whether dealing with an HMO, PPO, or a managed care program, it is mandatory that, when an offer to participate is made, the entire document be examined carefully regarding the duration of the contract; the time frame for fee payment; whether fees are held pending year-end analysis of the program; the methods for appeal of denied or reduced fees; and whether the program requests the physician to sign a "hold harmless" agreement, in which medicolegal liabilities for the patient may fall on the physician and release the organization from any responsibility. These agreements are binding contracts and as such should be read carefully. Some state medical societies provide review of these documents as a service to their members. Although they do not generally advise participation or nonparticipation, they can identify pitfalls for the physician and possibly suggest alternative terms or methods for negotiating changes before signing the document. Even if such an analytical service is available, it is prudent to have each of these proposals examined by an attorney who can point out any potential problems that might ensue from participating.

The physician should be familiar with two major sources of information that can affect fees and the ability to collect them. These are the *International Classification of Diseases Clinical Modification,*[5] currently in its ninth revision. This is also known as the *ICD-9-CM.* The other book is *Physician's Current Procedural Terminology (CPT).*[6]

The *ICD-9-CM* is based on the official version of the *World Health Organization's International Classification of Diseases,* ninth revision (*ICD-9*), which is designed to classify morbidity and mortality data for statistical purposes. It is also used to index hospital records according to disease and surgical procedures for the purposes of data storage and retrieval. The clinical modification, the *ICD-9-CM,* is intended for use by physicians and hospitals. The compilation is published in three volumes. Volume 1, *Diseases,* is a tabular listing that classifies diseases and injuries according to their causes and anatomic system. Volume 2, also called *Diseases,* contains an alphabetical index of diseases and injuries, tables of chemicals and drugs, and an index to external causes of injuries and poisonings. These initial two volumes are necessary for physician use. Volume 3, *Procedures,* contains both tabular and alphabetical listings of procedures by anatomic site and is intended for hospital use. The procedure information necessary for physicians is contained within the *CPT.*

The *ICD-9-CM* has been implemented by Medicare as the official coding method to be utilized on Medicare claims. Most insurance companies prefer, if not require, the use of *ICD-9-CM* codes for diagnostic purposes. These codes expedite the manner in which claims can be processed. In some instances, failure to use the codes may result in rejection of the claim. In the case of

Medicare, if a physician fails to provide the required diagnostic codes, the claims will be denied for assigned claims. For unassigned claims, if the physician does not provide the appropriate code on the initial claim, processing will be suspended and the physician requested to provide such information. If the physician does not promptly reply with the code, the physician may then be subject to civil monetary penalties of up to $2000. In repeated instances, additional sanctions can be imposed by the Medicare carrier.

The carriers insist that the codes used for a patient's condition be used at "the highest level of specificity." This order of specificity is represented by a five-digit code or subclassification. In instances in which a five-digit code is not available, the most appropriate four-digit code is to be used. In the absence of adequate information or lack of diagnostic specificity, a three-digit code may be used. In addition to diagnostic specificity, most insurers require that the diagnostic code be linked to the procedure or appropriate visit code. In the case of multiple diagnoses, the most prominent diagnosis should be listed first, followed by the appropriate procedural code and then by other diagnoses, listed in descending order of importance, with the appropriate procedural codes correlated with them. The *ICD-9-CM* should be available as a reference in the office for appropriate coding, and at least one office staff member should be familiar with its importance and utilization.

The *CPT* is an annual publication of a work that initially appeared in 1966 and provides the most widely accepted nomenclature used to report physician services and procedures to government and private insurance programs. It is used by these groups for administrative management of insurance claims processing. Because it is used nationwide, it can provide a basis for regional comparison. The codes mainly represent procedures, but because new procedures are constantly being added while others are falling into disuse, the coding scheme is a dynamic entity and is constantly being modified to provide more specificity. In addition, as procedures are modified by practice or technology, the changes are ultimately identified. Input from various subspecialty groups is provided to the *CPT* editorial panel. These suggestions are considered and implemented on a consensus basis by incorporating them into subsequent revisions.

The importance of this publication lies in the use of these *CPT* codes by insurers and administrators to determine compensation for the procedures and services provided by the physician. An intimate understanding of this code book is essential to provide accurate claims that are processed expeditiously, without rejection or return for modification. The instructions for use of the *CPT* are contained within the manual. It is imperative that the introduction and guidelines for each pertinent section be examined and understood. Proper use of the *CPT* codes can provide not only more accurate information, but also more appropriate remuneration. The surgeon should also be aware that there may be a variety of methods for coding the same procedure. For example, a skin biopsy can be coded as 11100; however, provision is made whereby skin biopsied in specific anatomic areas

may qualify under a different code, with possibly a different and higher fee (e.g., biopsy of the eyelid, coded as 67810). Additionally, destructive therapy for warts, for example, is generally coded under the 17100 series, but treatment of the same lesions on the penis uses a 54050 series code. Some helpful clues to alternative coding suggestions are found in a small handbook, *Another 101 Hiding Places to Find Profits in your Practice*, by Inga Ellzey (Practice Profitability Associates, Inc.; distributed free by Glaxo Dermatology). All staff members involved in coding, billing, filing of insurance forms, and collections, as well as the physician, should be familiar with the foregoing series of publications, as they are essential to the financial health of the practice.

Once decisions regarding fees and participation with various insurers or groups have been made, the fee schedule should be established, but always with an eye toward periodically revising it. It is prudent to examine the fee schedule once or twice a year. When requested, fees should be discussed openly with the patient before performing procedures. If the surgeon feels there might be some concern or inability on the part of the patient to pay for a particular service, the fees should be discussed before performing the procedure so that there is no question or subsequent conflict about it. Fees are a major source of complaint by patients, and unpleasant situations can develop when the amount of obligation has not been made clear. This applies to all procedures, but particularly to cosmetic procedures, where it is unlikely that third-party reimbursement will be available. Discussion of fees allows the physician the opportunity to establish procedures for payment of the fees either through scheduled partial payments or, preferably, through advance payment before surgery.

Collections

The ideal system for collection of professional fees is to obtain payment at the time services are rendered. However, this is rarely feasible and may dissuade some who would ultimately prove to be grateful and reliable patients. Ultimately there must be a balance between payment at the time of service (tight credit), with a potentially smaller patient practice, and delayed payment (loose credit), with increased accounts receivable and a larger patient volume. A suggested reasonable distribution is to collect 25% at the counter, 25% from monthly statements, and 50% from insurance. If possible, an effort should be made to increase on-site collections and decrease the other two categories.

To accomplish this, the collection policy must be firmly established and understood both by the patients and office personnel who are dedicated to implementing that policy. This ideal, although seldom accomplished, is a worthwhile goal in several respects. The main benefit is that every account collected at the time of service is an account that does not require the additional time and expense of billing. As the time since provision of professional services grows, there is an increasing disinclination to pay for those services, so that after 90 days have elapsed, some feel these accounts are almost uncollectible.

The pamphlet on the physician's office policy should clearly state the expectations for payment. In addition, collecting the fee for service should begin with the initial office appointment and can be implemented tactfully and effectively by those staff members making appointments. When a request for an appointment is made, the reason for the visit is identified, and after the details of patient's name, phone number, and insurance coverage are logged, the person making the appointment should indicate that the office policy is for the fee to be paid at the time of the visit. Most patients will simply accept this information. Others, however, may state that they have insurance, and the insurance company is responsible for the payment. At this point, the receptionist can indicate whether the doctor does or does not participate with that particular insurance group and, if the latter, that the staff will be happy to assist in the filing of insurance claims. At this point, the potential patient may inquire as to what the fee might be. In some instances this information may be provided with some accuracy, but in most instances, particularly if the nature of the problem is unclear or a surgical procedure may be required during an office visit, only a range of fees may be provided. A statement can be made to the effect that the professional fee for the visit may vary depending on the nature of the problem, the time involved, and whether laboratory tests or procedures may be necessary. Many times patients simply want to be prepared to take care of the charges. In other instances, the prospective patient may be comparing physician fees and not seriously seeking assistance. It may also be appropriate at that time to indicate to the prospective patient, particularly one who may not have insurance coverage, that the office also accepts credit cards.

Patients who plan to come to the office for evaluation for elective cosmetic procedures (particularly evaluation for tattoo removal, dermabrasion, chemical peel, and others) should be advised that payment for the evaluation is necessary at the time of the visit. This is the physician's only protection from being burdened by the time lost and expertise expended in consulting with the patient when, after the discussion, the patient decides that the procedure is not something to be pursued. When these patients arrive at the office, the nature and purpose of their visit should be reconfirmed, and at that time, before the physician has seen them, the fee indicated and collected. If individuals elect to pursue the procedure after consultation, some surgeons deduct the fee for the initial consultation from the fee for the procedure. Such a decision is an individual matter.

When a patient has consulted with the physician and an elective cosmetic procedure is to be scheduled, it is appropriate to request that a certain percentage of the fee be paid at the time the appointment for surgery is scheduled. This financially commits the patient to the procedure and makes failure to keep the subsequent surgical appointment less likely. Because a significant amount of time may be required for such a procedure, it is imperative that all efforts be made to ensure that such an appointment is kept. In addition, make it clear to the patient that cancellation of the appointment must be done more than 72 hours in advance, and failure to do so may result in forfeiture of all or part of the advance portion of the fee. If the patient resists such an effort to collect part of the fee in advance, it should be explained that failure to keep the appointment results in a substantial loss of time committed by the surgeon and staff and is unfair to other patients who wish to be scheduled for care. In the event that patients indicate that they are not able to make such a commitment at that point, the best procedure is to suggest that when they can comply with the policy, they should call back to schedule the appointment. If an individual patient has had a previous satisfactory financial relationship with the surgeon, other arrangements for payment may be made, but these should be made in writing, which constitutes a contract by the patient to pay for specified services within a specified time. Such commitments must correspond to rules outlined by the Federal Truth in Lending Act. The balance of the surgical fee is paid at the time of the scheduled procedure, and the patient should be reminded of this during the reminder call 48 hours before surgery.

For services that are not likely to be considered cosmetic and when the patient has insurance coverage, it is prudent to contact the insurer to determine that the patient's coverage is current and will be in force at the time the procedure is to be performed. This is also an opportunity to determine the nature of the coverage and what copayment or percentage of the fee will be the patient's responsibility. When this is determined, it is appropriate to request the patient to pay the balance calculated at the time the procedure is performed. Knowing the financial obligation in advance allows the patient to plan appropriately, but it is always wise to collect the fee at the time of service. Such knowledge also counters the frequent patient request for the physician to bill the insurance company and send the patient the bill after finding out what the insurance pays.

Even for established patients, fees should be collected at the time of service. If patients indicate they wish to be billed, it is ideal to have a bill ready, hand it to them with a self-addressed envelope, and ask them to please return payment by week's end. This approach has been effective for those patients who have forgotten their checkbook or credit cards. It can be mentioned to them that if it is necessary to mail them a bill, an appropriate billing charge may be assessed for each bill tendered. It is unwise to approach this in such a fashion unless it has been previously mentioned in the physician's office pamphlet or the patient has a good track record with the practice.

There are several reasons why some practices send more monthly statements than others. First, insurance forms are not completed in a timely or accurate fashion. Second, communication to an insurance company was not answered. Third, patients who have made a commitment to pay have not complied. In those instances where statements must be sent, there is variation among experts as to when those bills should be tendered. Some contend that they should be submitted on exactly the same calendar date each month, but this can conflict with weekends and holidays. Others suggest using a business day such as the 24th or the 25th of the month to ensure that the statement will arrive before the end of the month and thus precede billings sent by other creditors that may arrive at the first of the month. This doesn't prevent the patient from giving the physician's bill a low priority, but at least it arrives early enough to merit some attention. When possible, billings should be submitted at the end of the day's business. This coincides more closely with the patient's time of visit, since they receive the bill shortly after the services are provided and there is no 1-month lag time. This also expedites cash flow in the office, with receipts occurring on a more uniform basis rather than in waves related to monthly billings. Other alternatives include weekly or bimonthly billings. The most workable system often depends on the availability of a computer to handle more frequent disbursement of statements.

When payment is not received and a second statement is required, the patient must be reminded the account is already past due, and attention to the bill is mandatory. The most effective collection tool is a telephone call to the patient, which can be used initially and as an adjunct to other collection techniques. Various methods of communicating this message to the patient have been devised, including the use of rubber stamp imprints on the bill and the use of stickers on the statement, but probably the most effective method is a written notice on the bill, which can be generated with little difficulty by a computerized system but also can be handwritten. Inquiry as to why the bill has not been paid, whether the patient is having some financial difficulty in meeting the obligation, and an offer to assist in such a situation can be made, along with a request to contact the office. If there is no response after two billings, it is prudent to advise the patient that the third statement is the final opportunity to clear the account and failure to do so will result in turning the account over to a collection agency, with possible attendant harm to the patient's credit reputation. Although these may seem like harsh measures, sometimes they are necessary to get the late payer's attention. The office should be willing and ready to turn such an account over to a collection agency after the appropriate amount of time has passed. However, before doing so, it is incumbent that the physician personally review the patient's record to identify any circumstances in which potential professional liability might exist. After being assured that the likelihood of such an untoward event is low or unjustified, the decision to send an account for outside collection can be made.

At this point, the likelihood of collecting accounts due has diminished substantially. It also can change the relationship with the patient. When a patient account is turned over to a collection agent, some physicians choose to terminate provision of professional services to the patient and family except for emergency care related to existing problems, until the claim has been satisfied. At this time, indication of other available sources of medical care should be provided to the patient in a letter sent by certified mail with a return receipt re-quested. Before pursuing the use of a collection agency or termination of the relationship with the patient, it is wise to have previously cleared the proper methodology for doing so with an attorney, as there may be state or local statutes that govern appropriate procedure.

It is very important at the initial visit to always obtain the patient's actual address, not just a post office box. It can be explained that if it is necessary to contact patients in an urgent situation, the actual address will be required. Individuals who maintain that they are protecting their privacy or that they are avoiding a previously damaged relationship are usually using this as cover to avoid payment of bills. If they maintain that privacy is an issue or they fear that this information will fall into the hands of another individual, they should be reassured that all records in a medical office are confidential and information will not be released without their expressed consent. If patients persist in their refusal to provide a geographic address, it is highly recommended that those patients be treated on a cash basis only. In perusing uncollectible accounts, it usually does not take long to identify the significant percentage of problems this requirement can prevent. It should be noted, however, that one obvious exception occurs in rural areas of the country where residents go to a central post office to collect their mail because rural delivery is not provided. It is not unreasonable to expect, taking into consideration adjustments for specific contractual arrangements with Medicare, Medicaid, and some third-party providers, that a 95% collection rate should be achieved in a cutaneous surgical practice.

Financial Records for the Office

It is an absolute necessity that a sound system be in place for detailing the financial transactions of the practice. This includes having records for receipts and disbursements of all kinds and methods for recording and tracking them. Whether this system is manual, using pegboard systems or a posting or billing machine, or computerized, certain items must be in place to provide a record of financial activities.

There must be a "day sheet" on which the record of charges and payments received for the day is kept. This must be separate from the appointment book. The day sheet should reconcile payments made at the time of service, mailed payments, and insurance payments with the daily bank deposit. The bank balance, including the day's deposit, should be known daily. A separate journal or record for disbursements from the practice—including refunds to patients; payments for supplies, medications, and personnel; and other expenses—should be maintained. This journal should have sufficient space for identifying, in categories, the various expenditures. A coding system may be used for this purpose and computerized spreadsheet programs make this task much easier. The completeness and accuracy of these entries should be checked on a daily basis by a responsible front office person, the office manager, or the physician. It is advisable at the end of the day to have two employees present when closing out the day's business. This provides a doublecheck to avoid erroneous entries and a safeguard against possible embezzlement. The amount of cash in the cash drawer must be reconciled with the day's record. Any inaccuracies or inconsistencies should be pursued until the entry error, or a satisfactory explanation for a discrepancy, can be identified. It is important to ensure accuracy in these records for accounting and income tax purposes. Consultation with an accountant is advisable when establishing these procedures. Also, should the need or desire arise to make changes in the procedures of financial record keeping, an accountant's advice should be solicited before implementing a new procedure. It is easier to prevent problems than to go back and correct them.

An integral part of the record keeping and collection system is the type of system selected to implement collections. There are several different types of systems: a pegboard system, an accounting machine, sometimes also known as a posting machine; off-site data processing; and computerized accounting systems.

Pegboard systems are in common use and are particularly valuable for single practitioners or practices with low patient volume. They require hand-written entries in a comprehensive record that, in one operation, enables posting to the patient's ledger record, the patient's statement, and the receipt and disbursement sheets. When the payment is recorded, a receipt is automatically generated for the patient, and an entry into the bank deposit slip is made. The use of this system reduces the number of documents that must be handled, which decreases the opportunities for error or loss of document. Additionally, it provides an ongoing record of accounts receivable by adding the day's charges to the balance carried forward from the previous day, after subtracting payments received from the total. This system helps to encourage payment at the time of service, as the patient's previous balance, if any, and the charges for the day's visit can be quickly tallied. Patients can be advised of the amount and asked how they would like to take care of the fee. The main drawbacks to the system are that it can take up a significant amount of counter space, and it requires transfer of information from the APS to the document; hand entry of all the data, including calculations at the time entries are made (a relatively time-consuming process); and ultimately, transferral of information to ledger cards. In addition, no useful management data are generated. There are numerous suppliers of these systems. Additional sources of information regarding the pegboard system can be obtained by querying other physicians who use them and soliciting the opinions of the staff who use these particular systems. In this way, the advantages and disadvantages of each particular product can be elicited.

The APS (Fig. 21–7) consolidates a large amount of information on a two- or three-part form. This saves a substantial amount of time and enhances accuracy by having the physician identify the diagnoses and procedures performed. It also can consolidate other information, such as laboratory studies requested and the date and duration of the next appointment. It can include an entry for the existing balance of the patient's account, space for entering the day's charges, and the balance due. Space is provided to indicate what portion of the account has been paid. Another advantage of the APS is that it can be tailored to the individual physician's type of practice, using diagnoses most commonly encountered and procedures most commonly performed while leaving spaces for entry of less commonly used procedures and diagnoses. The three-part form generates a copy for the office, a copy for the patient, which serves as a receipt and income tax record; and a copy that can be used either by the patient for insurance reimbursement or by the office filing the insurance claim by attaching it to the insurance claim form.

An accounting or posting machine will reduce hand entry work and is beneficial if large numbers of patients are seen. It posts the debit and credit transactions on a statement or ledger card and maintains a running balance of the day's activity. This machine has largely been supplanted by microcomputers or larger computer systems.

Off site data processing may be an attractive alternative to in-office bookkeeping, but it does not supplant the need for a basic amount of data entry to provide adequate information for the processor. In some instances, a copy of the day sheet can be provided; in other instances, a transmitting device in the office connects with a computer via a telephone hook-up, and data entered by the office assistant are then transmitted to the central processing site. Another method used is a form of adding machine or calculator that punches data onto a tape, which is then provided to the processor. A final and less desirable method is to send actual charge slips to the processor, which runs the risk of the slips being lost or misplaced. The advantages of an off-site system are (1) office bookkeeping is reduced; (2) summary forms generated by the processor are readily available and can be examined efficiently; and (3) investment in expensive office equipment is avoided. Its disadvantage is that the operation is not immediately available for scrutiny by the physician or office manager. Depending on the firm handling the account, larger clients may get preferential and more expeditious treatment, thus delaying prompt patient statements to smaller clients. If errors occur in posting and billing, it may be very difficult to track and correct them.

Currently, the most effective method of bookkeeping is the use of some form of computer system. There are innumerable vendors of both the hardware and software necessary for implementing such a system. Costs vary depending on what tasks are delegated to such a system and the number of work stations involved. Overall, the benefits strongly outweigh the drawbacks. Investigating and implementing such a system in the office can be complex and confusing, with peril for the uninitiated. In such instances, one may be at the mercy of the veracity of the vendor. It is prudent to investigate different systems, preferably viewing the system actually functioning on a daily basis and not in a demonstration. The systems examined should parallel as closely as possible the actual flow and volume of the practice. It may be more efficient to have a practice advisor, office manager, or other consultant who has expertise in such

ATTENDING PHYSICIAN STATEMENT

Copyright 1992 John W. Gerwels, M.D.

DERMATOLOGY

Office Services	New	Establ.
Brief	99201	99211
Limited	99202	99212
Intermediate	99203	99213
Extensive	99204	99214
Comprehensive	99205	99215
Consultation, Outpt	**New**	**Confirm**
Limited	99241	99271
Intermediate	99242	99272
Extensive	99243	99273
Comprehensive	99244	99274
Complex	99245	99275
Consultations, Inpt	**New**	**F/U**
Limited	99251	99261
Intermediate	99252	99262
Extensive	99253	99263
Comprehensive	99254	
Complex	99255	
Emergency Room		
Limited	99281	
Intermediate	99282	
Extended	99283	
Comprehensive	99284	
Complex	99285	
Telephone conslt/managmnt		
Brief	99371	
Intermediate	99372	
Extended	99373	

Surg Destruction: Cryotherapy, Chem, Elec	Benign	Premal/face	Elec
*Single Lesion	*17100	*17000	
Second Lesion	17101	17001	
Third Lesion	17102	17002	
Additional			17104

Excision	Benign	Malig
Torso/Leg/Arm		
0-5 mm	11400	11600
6-10 mm	11401	11601
11-20 mm	11402	11602
21-30 mm	11403	11603
31-40 mm	11404	11604
Scalp/Hand/Foot/Neck/Genital		
0-5 mm	11420	11620
6-10 mm	11421	11621
11-20 mm	11422	11622
21-30 mm	11423	11623
31-40 mm	11424	11624
Face/Ear/Eyelid/Nose/Lip		
0-5 mm	11440	11640
6-10 mm	11441	11641
11-20 mm	11442	11642
21-30 mm	11443	11643
31-40 mm	11444	11644
Shave Excision		
One	11060	
2 to 4	11061	
5+	11062	

INPATIENT

Injections & Infusions	
Intralesional 1-7	*11900
8+	*11901
Therapeutic	90782-26
Infusion, chemo	96410
IV infusion prlgd	96414
Special Derm. & Surg. Proced.	
Acne Surgery	*10040
Cryotherapy	17340
I&D Abscess	
Simple	*10060
Complex	10061
I&D Paronychia	*10100
Debridement	*11000
Biopsy, Skin	11100
Each additional	11101
Lip	40490
Eyelid	67810
Ear	69100
Skin Tags 1-15	*11200
Each additional	11201
Unna Boot	29580
Patch Test 1-10	95040
11-20	95041
21-30	95042
>30	95043
Phototest	95056

Miscellaneous	
Modifier*	
Unusual Service	-22
Reduced fee	-52
Photo, Spot	1657
Photo, Tot. Body	1659
Last Srgry, Vasc	
Repair Intermediate	
Scalp/Ax/Torso/Extrem	
<2.5 cm	*12031
2.6-7.5 cm	*12032
7.6-12.5 cm	12034
Neck/Hand/Feet/Genital	
<2.5 cm	*12041
2.6-7.5 cm	12042
7.6-12.5 cm	12044
Face/Ear/Ld/Nose/Lip/Muc Membr	
<2.5 cm	*12051
2.6-5 cm	12052
5.1-7.5 cm	12053
Lab/Path	
Micro. Exam	87205
Wet Mount	87210
Tzanck	87207
Froz Sectn 1st	88331
2nd	88332
Surg. Path.	88304
Surg. Path. Complx	88305
Int. Outside Slide	88317
Follow-up Surgery	

Special	FEE
Industrial	90620
Apheresis	36520
Photopheresis	36522
Phototherapy	
PUVA general	96912
PUVA hd/foot	96912-52
Destructn, Malig	
Torso/Extremity	
0-5 mm	17260
6-10 mm	17261
11-20 mm	17262
21-30 mm	17263
31-40 mm	17264
Sclp/Nk/Acr/Gen	
0-5 mm	17270
6-10 mm	17271
11-20 mm	17272
21-30 mm	17273
31-40 mm	17274
Face/Muc Mem	
0-5 mm	17280
6-10 mm	17281
11-20 mm	17282
21-30 mm	17283
31-40 mm	17284

REFERRING DOCTOR
AUTHRZN #   99025

Date: ___
Physician's Name: ___   PBO # ___
Physician's Signature ___
Ordered Tests: ___
Return: ___ Days ___ Weeks ___ Months
Next Appointment: ___ month ___ date ___ day ___ time ___ am/pm

DIAGNOSIS	ICD.9.CM		
Acne	706.1	Dermatophyt.	110.
Actinodermatosis	692.7	Dermographism	708.3
Alopecia Areata	704.01	Drug Reaction	995.2
Alopecia, Other	704.09	Dysplastic nevus	238.2
Androgenic Alopecia	704.09	Erythema Multiforme	695.1
Balanitis	607.1	Erythema Nodosum	695.2
Basal/Sq. Ca.	173.	Folliculitis	704.8
Capillariasis	127.5	For. Bod., Superficial	919.6
Carbuncle	680.	Granuloma Annulare	695.89
Cellulitis	682.	Granuloma/For. Body	709.4
Cheilitis Actinic	692.79	Granuloma Pyogenicum	686.1
Chondrodermatitis	380.00	Hemangioma Skin	228.01
Corns/Callus	700.	Herpes, Simplex	054.9
Cyst, Epithelial	706.2	Herpes, Zoster	053.9
Cyst, Mucinous	528.4	Hidradenitis Suppurativa	705.83
DERMATITIS		Hyperhidrosis	780.8
Asteatotic	706.8	Impetigo	684.
Atopic (hereditary)	691.8	Insect Bite, Nonvenom	910.4
Contact, Allergic	692.9	Keloid/Hypert. Scar	701.4
Contact, Irritant	692.4	Keratosis Pilaris	757.39
Dyshidrotic	705.81	Keratosis, Seb. or Benign	702.1
Factitial	698.4	Leukoplakia/Act. Ker.	702.
Herpetiforms	694.0	Lichen Planus	697.0
Inf. or Seborrheic	690.	Lupus Eryth. (Discoid)	695.4
Intertriginous	709.8	Lupus Eryth. (Systemic)	710.0
Nummular	692.9	Lymphomatoid Papulosis	696.2
Other	690.	Melanoma, Malgnt	172.
Perioral/Rosacea	695.3	Melasma	709.0
Plant	692.6	Miliaria	705.1
Stasis	454.1	Molluscum Contagiosum	078.0
Dermatofibroma	216.	Moniliasis	112.
		Morphea	701.0

Mycosis Fungoides	202.1	Stomatitis, Aphthous	528.2
Nail Disease	703.9	Sweat Gland Dis.	705.9
Necrolysis, tox. ep.	695.1	Tattoo	709.0
Neoplasm, Skin Unspec.	239.2	Telangiectasia	448.1
Neoplasm, Skin, Benign	216.	Tinea Versicolor	111.0
Neurodermatitis	698.3	Ulcer, Leg	707.1
Onychomycosis	110.1	Ulcer, Stasis	454.2
Panniculitis	729.30	Undiagnosed Disease	799.9
Parapsoriasis	696.2	Urticaria	708.
Parasitic Skin Infest.	134.9	Vasculitis	447.6
Paronychia	681.9	Allergic	287.0
Pemphigoid	694.5	Cryoglobulinemic	273.2
Pemph. Muc. Membr.	694.60	Nodular	695.2
Pemphigus	694.4	Verruca (all types)	078.1
Photosensitivity Derm.	692.79	Viral Exanthem	057.9
Pigment Abnorm.	709.0	Vitiligo	709.0
Pityriasis Alba	696.5	Xanthoma	272.2
Pityriasis Lichenoides	696.2	Xerosis	706.3
Pityriasis Rosea	696.3	Previous Balance	
Pityriasis Rubra Pilaris	696.4	Today's Charge	
Prurigo Nodularis	698.3	Amount Paid	
Pruritus, Other	698.9	New Balance	
Psoriasis	696.1		
Pyoderma	686.0		
Rhagades	701.8		
Scabies	133.0		
Scar	709.2		
Scleroderma	701.0		
Skin Tags	701.9		
Spider Veins	454.9		
Stomatitis	528.0		

INSURANCE COMPANIES: This form contains information necessary to process claim. If forms or other reports are needed, send $20

Figure 21–7. Example of a comprehensive attending physician statement. (Courtesy of the author, John W. Gerwels, M.D.)

matters (but no relationship whatsoever with the vendors being considered) evaluate the needs of the practice and make recommendations. It is also important that the office staff be capable and willing to implement such a system. Employees sometimes view a computer as a threat to their job and resist its introduction. In reality, some of the claims made by computer vendors for reduction in the work force are substantially overstated, and it is likely that any staff reduction will be minimal. The computer ultimately makes the office operation more efficient and less prone to errors, provides data for analysis of how the practice is operating, provides more accurate information regarding billing and accounts receivable, and ultimately frees some employees for more efficient pursuit of the other needs of the office, such as transcription, record compilation, chart filing, telephone assistance, and collections.

The array of services that can be provided by a computer are sometimes spectacular. The potential purchaser needs to identify what functions the computer should perform and avoid, as much as possible, some of the unnecessary features that may be attached at significant cost. The basic functions the computer should serve are the same as those of any other bookkeeping system, but they can be performed much more expeditiously and accurately than can be done in any other fashion. Ideally, the patient returning to the front desk with the APS can have the data from the APS immediately entered into the computer to generate an on-site statement for the patient. Depending on whether charges are paid at that time, a receipt of payment can be generated and the patient provided with an instant statement of account that can be given to them before they leave the office. The data regarding this encounter are then automatically stored in the computer and are available to generate a monthly statement of account balances due.

Programs are also available for scheduling patients. If such a program is used, the next appointment can be scheduled while the patient is present and indicated on the form provided before the patient leaves the office. A wide variety of appointment programs are available, but in a one-physician office, this may not be a necessary function for the computer to perform. If multiple front office employees are doing various tasks, separate computer work stations are necessary. It is important that the computer have multitask capability, in which the computer can be accessed by different personnel performing different tasks at the same time (e.g., a receptionist making appointments, a staff member answering questions regarding an account balance, another employee entering a current transaction, and perhaps another posting accounts or generating end-of-the-month statements).

Other benefits of the computer include the ability to generate reminder notices to important follow-up patients (e.g., recall appointments for cancer patients or other patients in whom re-examination is critical), to add reminders to monthly statements, and to generate form letters or health update advisories that can be enclosed with monthly statements. The computer can be used in conjunction with word processing for letter writing, publishing a newsletter, and sending reports requested by insurance companies.

One of the great advantages of a computerized system is that much more financial data regarding the practice can be generated on a daily, weekly, biweekly, or monthly basis, as desired. At the end of the day's office activity, a computer can provide a summary of the accounts, the day's activity, deposits, total of accounts receivable, types of patients seen, and charges for laboratory or pathology services, as desired. Monthly statements as to the status of all accounts, including those past due; a summary of all patients seen; and a summary of categories of charges can also be generated. These are invaluable in monitoring the day-to-day and month-to-month activity of the practice. With such information available, decisions regarding certain aspects of the practice that may be enhanced or diminished can be more intelligently considered.

Because purchase of a computer system may entail a substantial financial outlay, the decision should be carefully considered after consultation with an accountant and other appropriate advisors. The reliability of the equipment, back-up for hardware, availability of qualified vendor personnel for training and corrections, on-going costs for support and supplies, and future availability of service are all important considerations. Overall the benefits of computer use in the office more than outweigh the space requirements, training, and expense involved.

For accounts payable, an important safeguard is that only the physician is authorized to sign checks. Prior to signing a check, the purpose should be determined by examination of the attached invoice or bill, ledger card, or statement of account. This simple precaution can prevent unauthorized disbursement of funds.

Financial and accounting records should always be kept for 3 to 5 years, except for the general books of accountants, which should be permanent. Payroll and related records such as employees' deduction authorizations, payroll register, records of payments and reports to the government, and individual personnel files have various retention requirements that should be clarified with the accountant or attorney.

SUMMARY

An active cutaneous surgery practice can be a complicated business to properly administrate for the benefit of both the patient and the physician. With knowledge of some common business concepts, selection of quality employees, and attention to details, a successful and enjoyable environment can be created in which quality surgical services can be provided in an efficient and friendly atmosphere.

Acknowledgment

The author wishes to express appreciation to Richard E. Carter (The Carter Consulting Group) for his straightforward criticisms and suggestions that have assisted the preparation of this chapter.

REFERENCES

1. Bennett RG: Fundamentals of Cutaneous Surgery. CV Mosby, St. Louis, 1988.
2. Donohugh DL: Practice Management for Physicians. WB Saunders, Philadelphia, 1986.
3. Carlson RJ: How to Avoid Employee Lawsuits. Enterprise Publishing, Wilmington, DE, 1980.
4. Ehrlich A: Medical Office Procedures Manual. Colwell Systems, Champaign, IL, 1986.
5. ICD-9-CM—The International Classification of Diseases. 9th rev.—Clinical Modification. Publication No. (PHS) 89-1260. US Department of Health and Human Services, Washington, DC, 1989.
6. CPT 1991, Physicians' Current Procedural Terminology. American Medical Association, Chicago, IL, 1990.

GENERAL SOURCES OF INFORMATION

Certified Professional Business Consultants (CPBC)

The Society of Professional Business Consultants, 321 North LaSalle Street, Chicago, IL 60601; (312) 346–1600.
The Society of Medical and Dental Management Consultants, 4959 Olson Memorial Highway, Minneapolis, MN 55422; (612) 544–9621.

Office Supplies, Records, and Forms

Bibbero Systems, Inc., 1300 North McDowell Boulevard, Petaluma, CA 94953.
Colwell Systems, Inc., 201 Kenyon Road, Champaign, IL 61820.
Control-O-Fax; Creative Systems, Inc., 3070 West Airline Highway, P.O. Box 778, Waterloo, IA 50704.
Histacount Corporation, Walt Whitman Road, Melville NY 11747.
NEBS, Inc., 500 Main Street, Groton, MA 01471–0002.
Medical Arts Press, 3440 Wynnett Avenue North, Minneapolis, MN 55408.
Physicians Record Company, 300 South Ridgeland Avenue, Berwyn, IL 60402.
Safeguard Business Systems, 470 Maryland Drive, Fort Washington, PA 19034.

Patient Information Pamphlets

Department of Practice Management, American Medical Association, 515 North State Street, Chicago, IL 60610.
American Academy of Dermatology, P.O. Box 3116, Evanston, IL 60204–3116.
American Society for Dermatologic Surgery, P.O. Box 3116, Evanston, IL 60204–3116.
National Cancer Institute, 9000 Rockville Pike, Bethesda, MD 20892.
Photodamage and Photoprotection, Westwood Skin Care Information Center, 301 East 57th Street, New York, NY 10022.
Skin Phototrauma Foundation, P.O. Box 6312, Parsippany, NJ 07054.
Skin Wellness Program, Mary Kaye Cosmetics, Inc., 8787 Stemmons Freeway, Dallas, TX 75247–9985.
Superintendent of Documents, U.S. Government Printing Office, Washington, DC 20402. (This is the source for International Classification of Diseases (ICD); The National 5-Digit Zip Code and Post Office Directory, 1992 ($15.00); and U.S. Postal Service Domestic Mail Manual (DMM).
The Carter Consulting Group, 11590 Summerfield Circle, Sandy, UT 84092.

Bibliography

Current Procedural Terminology, 1990. American Medical Association, Book and Pamphlet Fulfillment, OPO 54191, P.O. Box 2964, Milwaukee, WI 53201.
Donohugh DL: Practice Management for Physicians. WB Saunders, Philadelphia, 1986.
Frederick PM, Ken ME: The Medical Office Assistant. WB Saunders, Company, Philadelphia, 1988.
ICD-9-CM—The International Classification of Diseases. 9th Rev—Clinical Modification. Publication No. (PHS) 89-1260. US Department of Health and Human Services, Washington, DC, 1989.
Levesque JD: Manual of Personnel Policies, Procedures and Operations. Prentice Hall, Englewood Cliffs, NJ, 1986.
Medical Office Handbook. G&C Merriam. Soykhanov AH: Webster's Medical Office Handbook. G & C Merriam, Springfield, MA, 1979.

CHAPTER 22

Use of Computers in a Cutaneous Surgical Practice

DANIEL M. SIEGEL

Computers are an integral part of American life and medicine in the 1990s. Computers serve multiple uses in the medical world and in our private lives. They can be used for documentation, storage and retrieval of data, streamlining paperwork, and integration of multiple activities. It is unlikely that there are any individuals in the United States whose life is not touched in some way by a computer, be it the receipt of computer-generated advertising, a paycheck, or other documents pertaining to their health and well-being. This chapter represents the personal opinion of the author regarding computer applications in cutaneous surgery. For that reason, before a significant amount of money is invested in any computer system, it is always wise to seek additional advice from someone who is familiar with specific individual needs.

Most cutaneous surgeons were in practice before the computer became established as a tool for the physician and consumer. Computer sales personnel and complex manuals on the shelves of bookstores can easily intimidate an individual who was not gradually exposed to the development of the personal computer during the 1980s. This is unnecessary, as personal computers (PCs), minicomputers, or home computers can be made "user friendly" and can assist cutaneous surgeons in many aspects of their practice.

Computer Development

The initial encouragement for cutaneous surgeons to use computers came in the form of a brief series of articles published in the early and mid-1980s.[1-5] The first of these articles appeared only a few months after the release of the first IBM PC, the computer that took computing from the domain of electronics technicians and hobbyists to American consumers. In the ensuing decade, major advances in hardware and software, along with a reduction in the cost of computers, have brought this technology to the forefront in both medicine and daily living. This chapter will acquaint the neophyte with computer technology and software availability, as well as give the experienced user some suggestions for computer implementation in clinical practice.

IBM VERSUS APPLE PCs

In the 1990s, the two major choices in personal and minicomputing are the IBM-compatible machines and the Apple Macintosh. A number of other possible hardware and operating systems such as UNIX and Xenix also exist, but the utilization of these is relatively small compared with the IBM and Macintosh user base. However, many of these systems are becoming increasingly popular and, as prices drop, may make inroads into the currently popular systems.

Many people believe that the IBM route offers a greater variety of available software through a wide range of applications at a more affordable price. Furthermore, there has been relatively slow development of the graphic user interface that is the hallmark of the Macintosh. In addition, it has always been possible to obtain more hardware capability for a given amount of money in the IBM-compatible format, as this technology is spread over a broad array of manufacturers and competition keeps the price low. Apple has a monopoly on the Macintosh bios, and no other manufacturer has been able to successfully clone the Macintosh without violating Apple's copyrights. Much of what will be presented here in the IBM line has parallels in the

Macintosh format, with regard to developmental evolution of processors and software. The ultimate choice of IBM or Macintosh should be based on the available software and hardware that best meet the needs of the practitioner.

Computer Basics

The explanations and analogies used to discuss basic concepts of computers are easily grasped by most individuals who are unfamiliar with their operation. For those desiring greater detail, there are two excellent recommended texts: *The Winn Rosch Hardware Bible* (Brady, New York, 1989), by Winn L. Rosch, one of the contributing editors of *PC Magazine*, and *Upgrading and Repairing PC's* (Que, Carmel, IN, 1988), by Scott Mueller. The former is an excellent technical reference written for use by both experienced users and newcomers, while the latter is a complete presentation of computer hardware from the perspective of upgrading and repairing machines and is essentially a home repair book for computers.

OPERATING SYSTEM

The operating system lays down the framework for the smooth functioning of the computer, including the way information will be written to storage devices, the priorities the computer will obey, and the way the computer will interact with software and peripheral equipment. As a sort of "parliamentarian," the operating system determines which types of computer data will address which parts of the system and in what order, and it will "lock up" and freeze the computer if these rules are disobeyed. The operating system also "mandates" ordinances that determine "property ownership" with respect to areas of memory; this is necessary to allow the operating system and software running under it to function properly. Transgressions here can also lock up the system, causing a situation known in computer slang as a "crash."

A variety of operating systems are in current use, some of which will run on a variety of machines. IBM computers primarily run on some version of DOS, or disk operating system. The name *DOS* is usually preceded by "PC" (for personal computer) or "MS" (for Microsoft, a company that produces both products [PC-DOS and MS-DOS] for almost all computer manufacturers). A few DOS "clones" have been produced over the years, the most versatile being a product called Dr DOS, a variety that emulates DOS and seems to have many of the features that the other current versions of DOS leave out. DOS is usually described with a version number following it (e.g., DOS 1.0, DOS 2.0, DOS 3.1, DOS 3.3, or DOS 4.01). Each digit change denotes a major change in DOS capabilities, and each decimal point change indicates a more useful product with less dramatic alteration than a full digit change. The improvements seen during the decade since the initial sale of DOS 1.0 have included support for multiple types of storage, support for bigger storage devices, background processing that allows printing to proceed simultaneously with foreground or on-screen activity, network support to allow personal computers to communicate with other personal computers through cables in efficient and reliable ways, and control of the size and number of lines of text.

One hallmark of operating systems from DOS 2.0 onward is that any software written for a given version of DOS will run on newer versions. This allows the user to benefit from improvements in the operating system without having to give up a favorite software package. This "upward compatibility" has been one of the major selling points of the Microsoft DOS product and has been emulated by competitors.

Operating systems are necessary for the use of a computer and frequently are part of a computer purchase. The vendor should provide choices among a few of the latest available. In 1991, the operating system of choice was DOS 5.0 with enhanced management of extended memory. Digital Research's product, Dr DOS version 6.0, is an alternative, as it is supposed to be 100% compatible with MS DOS and functions in a more user friendly manner than MS DOS. MS DOS version 5.0 offers an even better interface, or appearance on the screen, and enhanced capabilities within the operating system.

COMPUTER HARDWARE

Microprocessors (Central Processing Units)

The "brain" of the IBM PC is the microprocessor chip, which usually resides on the "motherboard," the "skeleton" of electronic components around which the PC is built. To understand the evolution of the microprocessor, one must appreciate the meaning of the term "bus." Envision the microprocessor chip as a large factory. The first chip used commercially in IBM was the Intel 8086, which had a 16-bit bus both internally and externally. The "factory" can thus be perceived as having a 16-lane highway system that allows materials and products to be received and shipped away. Inside the factory, the materials and products move about on 16-lane conveyor belts. The Intel 8088 chip, which followed the Intel 8086, had an external (also known as data) 8-bit bus and an internal 16-bit bus. It was less expensive to make, took less power to run, and made the IBM PC more affordable. Both of these chips could "address," or communicate normally through their external "highways," with 1 million bytes, or individual yes/no or on/off pieces, of "real" memory. Memory might be looked at as a warehouse and peripheral plant for the main factory. The microprocessor, or factory, is limited in the number of the remote sites it can have under its control. Memory was extremely expensive in the early systems, and access to a full megabyte of memory (1 million bytes) was usually limited by this factor.

With the introduction of the 80286 microprocessor, more than 1 megabyte of "real" memory, or virtual memory, could be tracked. Virtual memory is a data storage location that can be used as memory for certain applications. Imagine an encyclopedia having 26 volumes; one could carry only one volume to work each day and return home with it at the end of each day. This would be one's working memory. The 25 volumes that remained at home would be the data storage site. To convert this to "virtual" memory, one could get 25 fast book carriers to produce an exact volume when it is wanted, at any time; this would be like using a hard disk for virtual memory. If all 25 of the book carriers memorized their volumes and could provide access to the data very rapidly, even though one could only work with small amounts at a time, the situation would be analogous to "expanded" memory. Additionally, the 80286 chip has 16-lane external highways and 16-lane internal conveyor belts, as well as a host of other features that are beyond the scope of this chapter's discussion.

The 80386 microprocessor and those that follow, the 80486 and the soon-to-be-released 80586, are chips with external 32-lane highways and 32-lane internal conveyor belts. The 80486 chip, to continue using the factory analogy, is much like the 80386 but has an integral coprocessor, a chip that speeds up certain mathematic calculations using software that can communicate with the coprocessor. It also has a memory cache, a portion of memory used as a repository for frequently accessed information. Imagine a library with 10,000 books that must be retrieved by the librarian. Each time a borrower asks for a book, the librarian must locate the book, go to the shelf to retrieve it, and carry it to the borrower. The librarian, or microprocessor, obtains a small bookshelf that will hold 100 books. Each returned book is kept on this small shelf on the assumption that a popular book will be wanted more frequently than any other random book. The librarian can easily retrieve this nearby book faster than searching the rest of the library. As the shelf fills up, the least recently used book on the little bookshelf is returned to the main shelves. It becomes obvious that the larger the cache, the easier it is to retrieve popular books quickly. If the shelf becomes too large to locate the book with a quick visual check, a new filing system must be set up for the shelf itself, a process known as cache management. Additionally, these chips have even more enhanced memory management capabilities, including the ability to allow multitasking so that multiple programs can run simultaneously.

A compromise chip, a hybrid of the 80286 and 80386, is considered by many to be the current "entry level" microprocessor. This is the 80386SX, which has 32 "conveyor belts" inside but communicates with the outside world through 16 "highways." This chip offered an intermediate price between the 80286 and 80386 at a time when prices were higher than they are currently.

When buying a computer, one selects a microprocessor chip and a "bus" speed in units of megahertz. Available chips include 8086/8088 (range of speeds, 4.77 to 8 MHz), which are slower than 80286 (8–20 MHz), which are slower than 80386SX (16–25 MHz), which are slower than 80386 (16–33 MHz), which are slower than 80486 (25–50 MHz) chips. The higher the number, the faster the computer will work, the more it will cost, the

more power it will consume, and the more heat it will generate. Power and temperature are important considerations. One should be sure that a 33-MHz 80386 machine has a true 80386-33 chip in it, since some unscrupulous vendors may push a slower chip to this speed and deal with the excess heat by attaching a comblike aluminum heat dissipator to the chip. Chips used in this manner are more prone to early failure. Chips are plainly marked with the chip speed, and the vendor should be happy to show it if the buyer desires to see it.

The 80386SX microprocessor-based system should currently be considered the most basic computer to purchase. However, the 80386 system should also be given consideration, as the price differential is only a few hundred dollars. This allows access to the newer products that are being written specifically to take advantage of the multitasking and large memory-handling abilities of these machines. Clinicians who have less powerful machines should not despair, however, as these can still be workhorses for data entry and word processing.

Coprocessor chips, mentioned earlier, are mainly used by database, spreadsheet, and computer-aided drafting and design programs that perform frequent, complex mathematic calculations. Unless the software used specifically addresses or "talks to" these chips, they are unnecessary.

Mass Storage

The most commonly used form of mass storage in PCs is the hard disk drive, which is basically a metal platter that stores information electronically like a recording tape. The platter (or platters) in most systems runs under a series of read-write heads that allow information to be read, written, and erased. To appreciate the precision of this disk-head interaction, imagine a fighter plane traveling a few inches above a flat, well-groomed golf course, picking up and dropping golf balls in precise locations.

A variety of hard disk mechanisms, encoding schemes, and controller mechanisms exist; in order of decreasing cost, speed, and reliability, these are:

- Enhanced Small Device Interface (ESDI).
- Small Computer Systems Interface (SCSI, pronounced "scuzzy").
- Run Length Limited (RLL).
- Modified Frequency Modulation (MFM).

Although none of these is bad, the minimum size to consider for any application in an office is 40 to 65 megabytes of storage. Prices for storage in terms of dollars per megabyte decrease with increasing size into the 200- to 300-megabyte range. There are no firm guidelines for size requirements, but the need can be roughly determined by adding how much space the planned software will use plus how much space the data files will need, and then doubling this calculated number.

Another cost-determining feature is hard disk speed, which is measured in milliseconds and known as the "seek" speed. The lower the number, the faster the disk. In 1991, a seek speed of more than 45 ms was considered very slow, 17 to 28 ms was considered normal, and 9 ms was state-of-the-art speed that could easily be found in PCs. Speed is most important for disk-intensive applications that require frequent readings from and writings to the disk, such as databases and spreadsheets. It is less important for word processing and other software programs in which most activities occur in memory.

Another mass storage option is the optical disk, which is notably slower than many hard disks, having a current speed in the 45- to 65-ms range. They are quite useful for storing lots of information in a small and easily transportable form. The most widely used optical disks are in the CD-ROM format, which can be read but not written to. Software and reference works such as medical books, encyclopedias, business materials, and literature can be purchased on these disks, which are physically the same size as compact disks used in music systems. Also available are Write Once, Read Many (WORM) drives, which can record but cannot be erased. They may have some use as archiving devices if their price decreases. Erasable optical drives are still relatively expensive for the small business user, and many problems still need to be worked out. Uniformly accepted standards for optical disks do not yet exist, which may have played a role in slowing their ultimate acceptance. This obstacle should be overcome in the next few years, and prices should diminish as usage increases, a recurring phenomenon in the PC environment.

Floppy disk drives, available in 3½- and 5¼-inch sizes, are the most popular media for transport of information and programs. Both are thin films of magnetic coated media that can be easily moved from location to location. All computers should have at least one, and preferably both, formats for convenience. The 3½-inch format, which can hold more data in less space and has its own protective shell, is rapidly becoming the standard, although the 5¼-inch disk is a long way from obsolescence.

Memory

Memory utilization has been previously discussed in general terms. MS DOS allows the use of 640 kilobytes of memory. The microprocessor uses part of the next 384 kilobytes, which can be visualized as a brick wall with different colored bricks above the 640 kilobytes marker, for controlling the video system and other housekeeping chores. It should be noted that 384 + 640 = 1024, not 1000. However, despite this imprecision, 1024 kilobytes is still referred to as a megabyte.

Extra memory can be used on 80286 and higher machines as either "extended" or "expanded" memory depending on the application, the specific microprocessor, and the software "drivers" that allow configuration of the memory. The two types of memory are quite different, although both are brought into the computer system by the addition of additional memory chips. Extended memory is a true extension of the first megabyte of memory (i.e., the "brick wall" is built higher),

but special software is needed to access it. Expanded memory is not attached to the top of the 1-megabyte "wall," but instead is reached through a "hole" in the portion of the wall above the 640-kilobyte mark and below the 1-megabyte mark. Extended memory is the current state-of-the-art memory configuration for which software is written.

Expanded memory was an excellent fix when the amount of memory directly accessible was limited, making possible the swapping out or paging of data. Expanded memory has evolved under a series of compatibility standards known as either LIM (for Lotus, Intel, and Microsoft, the three companies that set the initial standard) or EEMS (for Enhanced Expanded Memory Specification, which is followed by a version number). Expanded memory will probably be of minimal significance to computing in the next decade.

In addition to application software-specific uses for this extra memory, extended or expanded memory is used to create the "cache." Random access memory (RAM) "disks" can be used to store frequently used software and data; these are different from a cache in that they can be treated like another disk drive, addressed by software, and read from and written to at a much faster rate. Changes to a RAM disk must be saved to the hard disk before turning the computer off to avoid losing the changes made during that work session. In addition, extended memory can be used for the creation of "print spoolers" that allow one to "dump" information from the "working" memory (i.e., the bottom 640 kilobytes) into a holding area that feeds it to the printer while the user goes back to work. Without this, the computer may "freeze" the keyboard until the printing job has been completed. Caches, RAM disks, and spoolers usually consist of software that can "talk to" or address memory, be it the first 640 kilobytes or expanded or extended memory. Many newer programs can read the system, determine what type of memory is available, and configure themselves for the task.

Memory is packaged in a variety of physical forms, and the one used is the one designed for the specific system. The cost of memory is determined by speed, with lower numbers representing faster speeds and greater cost. Currently, 80 ns is considered an average speed, and 100 ns is considered slow. Memory that is rated faster than the system can handle does no harm, except in terms of cost, but slow memory can slow the system down. Memory has become relatively inexpensive since 1990, and a few extra megabytes for caches, RAM disks, and spoolers are useful. Memory beyond this is only of value if the user is doing multitasking or networking or has software that will directly benefit from it.

Video

The video monitor is an important feature of every computer. A variety of video options are widely used; these are, in order of decreasing cost and resolution:

- Video Graphics Array (VGA).
- Enhanced Graphics Adapter (EGA).

- Color Graphics Adapter (CGA).
- Monochrome Display Adapter (MDA).

Other uncommon options are also available. Some of the newer, higher resolution video configurations are not supported by many software companies and may not be utilized to their full capability by most commercial software.

The most important single concept to use when choosing a monitor is resolution. The finer the resolution, the less eye strain the user will experience. A number of specific parameters are important when deciding on a monitor. Resolution is expressed in pixels; for example, "1024 × 768" is better than "640 × 480," currently the most popular VGA display. Dot pitch is a measure of the space between dots on the screen; 0.28 is better than 0.40, because the spaces are smaller and the image looks "crisper." The video capabilities of the system are also related to the video controller, a hardware device that determines the palette of available colors and the time it takes a screen to rewrite, such as when moving from one data entry screen to another, from one page in a report to another, or from one picture to another. Video controllers often have their own memory capacity to speed up these tasks.

Other factors that can influence monitor and video controller selection include compatibility, since some software requires high-resolution video such as EGA or VGA to run, and on-unit controls such as contrast and brightness. For data entry, some individuals prefer a monochrome screen consisting of a white background with black letters and shades.

Networking

Networking allows multiple workstations, such as PCs with less power and less storage, to use one central "brain," known as the "server," for storage and data manipulation. This approach costs less than multiple freestanding PCs with similar capabilities. For example, an 80386 33-MHz server with a 300-megabyte hard disk could network a number of 80286 12-MHz workstations for less than the cost of a similar number of stand-alone 80386 machines whose speed and capacity may not be needed for all tasks. For office management, the data entry person and transcriptionist will only need a machine that can accept data faster than it can be typed, while the office manager and accounting personnel will need a faster machine for analytic purposes. However, if everyone can access the central storage device, or server, there is no concern about data availability. Many software packages have network versions that enable the network to function smoothly. A large number of network connection systems are available. Networks are potentially the most complex part of setting up an office computer system, and the choice of network type should be based on the software being used.

The decision to develop a network in a medical office should also include a consideration of security issues. Networks can be set up that limit access to certain files or disks to maintain privacy over financial, patient, or other information. For specific information and implementation of security, one should consult the vendor. It should be kept in mind that even the most sophisticated systems can be violated. If high security is essential, a removable hard disk or other removable mass storage device that allows physical separation of the data one wishes to protect from the computer network itself is a good solution.

Printers

One or more printers are essential for the use of a computer in a typical medical practice. For preprinted or multicopy forms, such as insurance claims, a dot matrix (impact) printer is optimal. For rapid, quiet output on either plain or letterhead paper, a laser printer is the printer of choice. Daisy wheel printers that use preformed characters, much like the impacting letters in a regular typewriter, give high-quality print but are slow.

Both electromechanical and software switches are available to allow multiple printers to be used by one or more computers and for one printer to be used by multiple computers. The former situation is optimal in a situation where all operative reports and office notes are printed on a high-speed dot matrix or laser printer, all consultation letters are printed on a laser printer, and all claim forms and monthly statements are printed on dedicated dot matrix printers that allow continuous-feed forms to be left in place. Software is also available that will allow duplication of forms and generation of completed copies on the laser printer. Letterhead paper can be scanned electronically into a software program and printed out on a laser printer for some applications.

Communications

All communications from one computer to a computer at a remote site take place via a modem (MOdulator-DEModulator), a device that connects computers via a telephone line and sends and receives information in the form of electronic signals. Modems come in internal and external varieties. Internal modems fit into a slot on the motherboard; external modems, which cost a few dollars more, use one of the serial ports or connectors on the back of the computer. The route to take is a personal choice, but many individuals feel more secure if they can see the status lights of an external modem to confirm that the modem is connected. Modems have a variety of speeds, given in units of 300, 1200, 2400, or 9600 bits per second. Most communication is currently done at 2400 bits/sec, but 9600 bits/sec is becoming more widely used. Various error correction and compression schemes are used to minimize the chance of data disruption or distortion and to send more data over a phone line in a shorter time. The V42bis and MNP5 formats are currently the state of the art in each of these areas, respectively. Dedicated data lines, with less static and a higher usage cost, are available from most telephone companies for those who need the 9600-bits/sec transmission rate.

A modem is especially useful for software support. A vendor, using the correct software, can control a remote computer from a distant site to help solve a problem without an on-site visit and the cost and delay inherent with an on-site service call. Some manufacturers now produce fax-modem boards that allow one to fax directly from many software programs, a useful device if this is important to the medical practice (e.g., if dermatopathology reports are sent to referring physicians).

Back-up

The most important thing to remember when using any computer is to *always back up the files*. Computers are not perfect, and if they "crash" or get "zapped" by an electrical surge, important data can be lost. Therefore, frequent back-ups are a very important consideration. The most widely used mass storage back-up medium is tape. The two most popular formats currently are DC-600 and DC-2000. The first is considered to be the gold standard, while the second is favored by some because of its exceedingly small size. A variety of brands and formats of tapes are available, and the frequency and type of back-up done and rotation of tapes will be determined by individual needs. Rotation schedules allow frequent back-ups to be kept on and off site in case of fire or theft. Most back-up systems—be they software for disk back-up alone or hardware-software combinations with tape drives or other media—should include a manual discussing rotation strategies. For large medical practice applications, configurations with two hard disks continuously mirroring each other offer the greatest degree of data protection. An end-of-day tape back-up for safe, remote storage will complete the security measures. Other options for back-up include floppy disks, which are considered unwieldy because of the large numbers needed; removable storage such as optical drives; and Bernoulli boxes, which can be thought of as high-volume, floppy-hard disks that provide 44 megabytes of storage in a paperback book–sized container. An excellent strategy for determining what back-up equipment is best is available in *PC Magazine* (Miller CD: DC 2000 tape drives: backup on a personal scale. PC Magazine 8:192, 1989).

Power

Electric current from the wall outlet can vary widely depending on output from the local power company, other appliances used in the office and building, and a variety of other factors that are often difficult to control. If the computer is in the middle of a write-to-disk operation during a power loss, the user may have to restore the entire back-up, as the file being written to may be irretrievably corrupted. Surge protectors, which can be purchased rather inexpensively, protect sensitive circuitry from these surges. They can also be purchased to provide modem protection as well. This approach is the lowest level of protection and should be considered only in regions where power surges are rare and voltage dips or outages are even rarer.

The next step up are line conditioners, which take incoming voltage, often 105 to 135 volts, and transform it to 120 volts. In this way, a wide range of both surges and dips in power will be stopped from harming the computer. However, if there is more than a momentary outage, loss of data may still occur. A bank of batteries that provide an uninterruptible power supply will protect the computer in the event of power loss. This is the ultimate protection available. The size and capabilities of the protection system purchased must be individualized for each computer system.

Static discharge pads placed by keyboards are also important for the protection of the computer from very high voltage, low-amperage static sparks, especially in very dry environments. Touching these items prior to working on the computer should become a reflexive action. Special conductive flooring to help minimize this problem is also available but is much more expensive.

Miscellaneous

A number of miscellaneous hardware devices, such as mice, trackballs, and light pens that perform tasks without using the keyboard, are available; their use is software dependent. A scanner that allows conversion of a printed image into a computer file can be useful for capturing text and images from journals and other documents.

HARDWARE ACQUISITION SUMMARY

Several important generalizations can be made about the acquisition of new computer hardware. First, one should always buy as much as one can reasonably afford. The computer hardware industry is undergoing constant change, with newer and faster systems and configurations constantly being developed. A system with a given configuration may drop in price 5% to 25% over a 12-month period if current trends continue. The current entry level machine for practice management should at least contain an 80386 processor so it can serve as a single workstation or the "server" for an office network. The marginal cost of an 80386-based machine, when viewed from the expected 3- to 5-year life span, is only pennies per day. This same philosophy holds true with respect to chip speed, memory size and speed, storage devices, and video quality.

Second, the whole integrated system is only as good as its lowest quality component. For example, a database program for practice management and billing is usually disk intensive, meaning that information must frequently be obtained from the hard disk. A slow hard disk will noticeably slow down the function of the system, regardless of the speed of the central processing unit (CPU). Alternatively, the fastest hard disk will stand idly by with a slow CPU microprocessor.

Third, it should be remembered that a number of hidden factors play a role in determining cost:

1. The size of the internal power supply, usually 200 to 250 watts, which plays a role in determining how many accessories can be added to the system without overloading.

2. The number of available slots or receptacles for devices that allow communications, control extra printers, and access optical disk drives.

3. The type of slots—8-bit XT, 16-bit AT, or 32-bit 386 type—which allows a given accessory to keep pace with the microprocessor.

4. The number of available bays or places for additional internal storage devices such as extra hard drives, optical drives, and tape drives.

Much like any purchase, one can pick and choose the exact system wanted, with the desired options.

It is always exceedingly important to find an honest hardware vendor. Much controversy exists as to whether to purchase a computer locally or from a mail-order vendor. On any given day, a variety of local vendor advertisements can be found in any large city newspaper, usually in the business section. The listed or advertised prices usually are higher than those advertised in *PC Magazine, Computer Shopper*, or other computer publications. The decision to use any particular vendor must be based on a number of easily determined factors. If one is electronically inclined or has access to such vendors, an inexpensive system purchased through the mail may be sufficient. This method provides no technical support and users are often on their own after the purchase.

The next step up is the mail-order system offering on-site service or overnight replacement of parts in the event of a breakdown. On-site service is often contracted through a local firm or a national corporation that offers this type of service. Of importance is the duration of the service offered; a period of 90 days to 1 or 2 years is typical, but some plans can be extended. The response time also varies, with the norm being 24 to 72 hours depending on geographical area. Overnight service offers the opportunity to have the malfunctioning part sent via overnight mail, assuming the purchaser is comfortable working inside the computer. While the internal components of a computer are designed to "plug and play," some users are intimidated by even removing the cover of the computer. For these users, a scheme that lets them ship the entire system back to the vendor is preferable, but of course, this leaves one without a functioning machine until the replacement arrives. If the medical practice cannot afford any interruption, a local vendor who offers emergency service may be the best solution but at a significant cost. However, this cost may well be less than the expense of being without a system for 1 or more days.

SOFTWARE

Software, the "maps" along which computers run, is available from a variety of sources. Mass market products purchased from local or mail-order vendors; shareware, which can be tried out for a low price and "rented" for a reasonable fee if one decides to use it; and custom-designed software are the major forms available. It is illegal to obtain "bootleg" copies of software from friends or colleagues, as it deprives programmers of their livelihood and decreases the likelihood that a good package will survive and prosper with frequent and valuable upgrades. It is also dangerous, as this software may have acquired a "virus" along the way that can infect, distort, or destroy the user's data. Software that detects and destroys computer viruses does exist, and no incurable computer virus has yet been created; however, the best way to avoid this problem is to avoid accepting "bootlegged" software.

The actual decision as to which products should be purchased should be based on need, capabilities, and comfort with the way the product works.* Within a given group of quality products, the final decision is personal and truly cannot be criticized.

Word Processing and Desktop Publishing

Word processing software is primarily responsible for the "computer revolution," because it took an everyday task and automated it. At its simplest, it can be used for generating form letters, forms, and other documents with easy revision and customization. Illegible scrawls in patient charts that can be misconstrued in the courtroom become a thing of the past. Spelling and grammar checkers allow automated evaluation of the generated documents. Major programs in this group include Wordperfect, Microsoft Word, Wordstar, and Displaywrite.

Desktop publishing software is word processing software that allows the integration of text with graphics. This permits generation of pamphlets, newsletters, and brochures of professional quality. The leader in this field is Pagemaker, but many programs with fewer features, such as Publish-It!, can also meet the needs of a cutaneous surgical practice.

Graphics and Presentation Software

Packages exist for generating high-quality, high-resolution graphics used primarily for generating slides for projection. Harvard Graphics, a leader in the field, is one of many programs that will allow one to output images to a device such as the Polaroid Palette to make high-quality slides in the office. If the clinician is unwilling to invest in such a device, services are widely available that will take slide data files from floppy disks or via modem and make the slides in their facility.

Additionally, if high-quality video components exist in the computer system, very good slides can be made directly from the screen with a camera and a tripod. This is done by formatting the screen in the graphics program or word processor to fit the 3:2 width-to-height ratio of 35-mm slides. The farther the image is from the screen edge, the less distortion will occur from the screen edge curvature. One can format the pages in the word processor to one slide per page or set the graphics program as for a slide show; the transition from slide to slide can be quite rapid.

The edges of the video monitor should be masked with nonreflective black tape to minimize reflection from the screen. The 35-mm camera is mounted on a tripod to stabilize it. A cable release and power winder or

---

*Widely used, commercially available products are mentioned by name for informational purposes. This author has no current association with any software producer except the publishers of Medfile/R (Delasco, Inc.).

motor drive are useful accessories. The macro lens, used for clinical photos, is excellent for this purpose. An E-6 process film such as Ektachrome should be used for shooting the slides, as Kodachrome does not give good results in this application. The photographer should work in a totally dark room to eliminate screen reflections. A test roll should be shot to determine proper exposures and acceptable color palettes, as not all computer-generated colors will project or photograph well. One should keep track of the camera settings, along with the settings on the video monitor brightness and contrast controls. An intermediate contrast level and maximal brightness are generally best, but this should be individualized. The test exposures are begun at ⅟₁₅ second using manual exposure mode and the largest aperture. The aperture can be varied, but it is best not to increase the camera shutter speed, since this can result in uneven illumination of the slide and cause visualization of the photon beam tracking across the screen. After determining the test exposures, one can advance the text or graphic slide on the computer and photograph the image. A 36-exposure roll of slides can be exposed in 5 to 10 minutes in this manner. If slides are changed frequently, a laptop computer and a liquid crystal display (LCD) projection screen can be used with an overhead projector to directly project the video images.

On-Line Information Services

A variety of on-line information services are available for both medical[6] (COLLEAGUE, MEDLINE, DERM/INFONET) and nonmedical (Prodigy, CompuServe) purposes. Some allow the user to interact with others through electronic mail, obtain public domain software ("download"), or retrieve information from well-defined databases. To access these databases, the user must have a modem; subscribe via flat monthly fees, on-line time fees, or database use fees; and have communications software such as PROCOMM, GTCOM, or CROSS-TALK to connect with these services. Available services include journal article abstracts and full texts, textbook excerpts, and drug information.

Practice Management and Enhancement

A large variety of software packages exist for managing billing; preparing Health Care Financing Administration (HCFA) forms for insurance companies; performing in-house analysis of a practice by demographic features such as ZIP code, age, or referring physician; and appointment scheduling. Other features such as prescription writing and electronic storage of medical records are also present in some packages. These can be potentially controversial, since an interested third party such as an insurance agency or pharmaceutical company could obtain data regarding prescribing habits, which could be an invasion of patient privacy. The medical record application also generates concerns, because electronic information can be erased and rewritten, and accusations of alteration of the "electronic chart" might result.

Regardless of which practice management software one decides to purchase, it is important to buy good quality software. The decision should be based on the ability of the software to do what is necessary, the ease with which it can be learned by the staff, and the quality of the support offered by the vendor. Unlike word processing packages, which are often used by millions, most practice management programs have only a few dozen or a few hundred or thousand users. A vendor with a single program with a small user base is in greater danger of fiscal mayhem than a larger, more established firm with a broader business base. If a small medical software company goes out of business, the clinician may be left with a program that can no longer be supported or maintained. With current government regulations mandating changes in forms and documentation on an almost annual basis, the physician could be left with data that can only be manually transferable to another system.

Alternatively, if a large medical software company supports a large base of users who express satisfaction with the service and function; if the company has a group of programmers who work on updates; and if the computer source code is held in escrow so that if any problems arise with the company, the program does not have to become "deadware," or unsupported outdated software, one should seriously consider the product.

A system that is to be used in the office should be one that can easily be mastered by the personnel. The system should be as self-explanatory as possible to minimize "down time" and adaptation time. A system that can be operated after minimal formal training by an individual who has no computer experience is ideal. On-screen prompting for commands or data entry are important features of a good medical practice program. A menu-driven program, in which the next choice or step to be taken can be chosen from a menu that appears in the middle of the screen, is helpful, because the need to refer to manuals or other instruction material is minimized. Context-sensitive information, or helpful information relevant to the situation in question at the time of inquiry; on-screen help; or a video manual that opens to the correct page is a valuable feature. The system should be flexible enough to deal with the needs of the practice, be it university based or private, with regard to expansion, remote offices, and changing styles of both hard copy documentation and electronic transmission. The system should also guide the user through its use in plain English. This is more easily accepted than a high-technology system requiring memorization of large amounts of technical data by the user. (For example, a home video cassette recorder, a form of computer, falls into this category: the less complex the remote and timer settings, the more likely it is to be used.)

An important overall consideration when computerizing a practice is to determine how the computer will streamline many repetitive processes without forcing the user to change the way in which data are collected or the style in which documents are generated. In this respect, the computer should be a "friendly black box" that facilitates the task it was designed to do, which

DATE

FIRST NAME, LAST NAME, M.D.
ADDRESS LINE 1
ADDRESS LINE 2
CITY   STATE   ZIP

Dear **(FIRST NAME OR DR. LAST NAME)**:

Thank you for sending **(PATIENT-FIRST-NAME PATIENT-LAST-NAME)** to me for evaluation of a **(DISEASE)** of **(his/her ANATOMIC SITE)**. I have examined **(him/her)** and discussed the best therapeutic approach with **(MR(S) PATIENT-LAST-NAME)** and will proceed with surgery shortly. I will keep you informed of our progress.

Thank you for allowing me to assist you in this patient's treatment.

Sincerely,

(CUTANEOUS SURGEON), M.D.

Figure 22–1. Standard referral letter.

justifies the cost. A computer system that does not make its intended tasks faster and easier to perform will not be used optimally and may well be abandoned by those who are supposed to be using it. A simple example of this is HCFA forms. Taking these from the typewriter to the computer minimally requires a one-time entry of demographic data, with less chance of invoking errors from eye strain or a mispunched key that must then be corrected on three copies with correcting fluid. This time savings alone justifies the computer cost for many practices. If one adds to this the convenience of electronic claims made via modem, the system may actually generate revenue. If the HCFA implements a plan to penalize paper claims with a filing fee and reward electronic transmission of claims with more rapid payment, the cost-effectiveness will increase even further.

The medical office staff may initially be afraid that a computer will replace them or that they may damage something. However, if it is introduced to them in the correct fashion, they will rapidly learn that their lives will be better and work will be done more efficiently with less strain by using the computer. Initially, they must be encouraged to understand that their job will be made better, not lost. The person who buys the computer system should be able to understand what it does so that the investment and the practice can be protected, but it is not necessary to understand the intricacies of programming languages and hardware design.

Examples of Computer Use in Surgical Practice

There are numerous specific examples of how computers help to streamline paperwork. One of the more common is the use of macros, or short keystroke sequences, that allow the input of preformed blocks of text, dates, salutations, and letter closings to produce a customized document for each individual patient or referring doctor. Templates, or document "shells," are another commonly used method to reduce paperwork. In this situation, previously created blanks in a standard document are filled in with individual patient information so as to produce a customized, letter-perfect, aesthetically pleasing finished document.

DOCUMENTATION

Documentation is a critically important part of medicine. While much of what makes medicine exciting is the unique nature of every patient, some facets of the documentation process are largely boring, repetitive, and redundant. Examples include referral letters, initial evaluations, operative reports, and some follow-up visits. Despite the theory that a unique report is dictated for every encounter, most physicians find that there are fixed and variable portions of each report. Most consultations break down into simple forms (Fig. 22–1). Each form has variable portions in most circumstances, and a limited number of logical choices are left to be filled in. This letter can be relayed to the secretary in a brief dictated note or worksheet as, "CONSULT FORM 1; PATIENT-FIRST-NAME   PATIENT-LAST-NAME; DISEASE; ANATOMIC SITE." Radiologists and pathologists often use a similar system for generating their reports. Clinicians who argue that their work cannot be categorized in the same way often have not gone far enough down the "fixed and variable" tree to see otherwise. Other, more complex consultation letters can also be developed (Fig. 22–2). The pertinent specific information can be relayed to the secretary as, "CONSULT FORM 2; PATIENT-FIRST-NAME PATIENT-LAST-NAME; DETAIL (which may include, e.g., a

DATE

FIRST NAME, LAST NAME, M.D.
ADDRESS LINE 1
ADDRESS LINE 2
CITY   STATE   ZIP

Dear **(FIRST NAME OR DR. LAST NAME)**:

Thank you for sending **(PATIENT-FIRST-NAME PATIENT-LAST-NAME)** to me for evaluation of a **(DISEASE)** of **(his/her ANATOMIC SITE)**.

(EXTENSIVE DISCUSSION OF HISTORY, PHYSICAL EXAMINATION and THERAPEUTIC OPTIONS. This is a variable section but can be subdivided into further fixed and variable subsets, such as presence or absence of risk factors for skin cancer, prewritten paragraphs about the risks and benefits of soft tissue augmentation, the side effects of leg vein injection.)

I will keep you informed of our progress.

Thank you for allowing me to assist you in this patient's treatment.

Sincerely,

(CUTANEOUS SURGEON), M.D.

Figure 22–2. Complex referral letter format.

Patient name:_____

Date of procedure:_____ Surgery time:_____ minutes

Surgeon: Daniel Mark Siegel, M.D.

Pre-op Dx: (This is captured from what was circled above) of the (anatomic site entered above), _____ by _____.
Post-op Dx: (This is captured from what was circled above) of the (anatomic site entered above), _____ by _____.

Title of operation: Excision of _____
of the _____.

Anesthesia: **(1%w/EPI PLAIN 50:50 SALINE)**
(The anesthetic circled above directs the secretary to enter a macro that inputs "1% lidocaine with epinephrine 1:100,000," "1% plain lidocaine," "equal amounts of 0.5% bupivacaine and 1% lidocaine with epinephrine 1:100,000," or "nonbacteriostatic normal saline," respectively.)

Procedure: Following a discussion of the risks and benefits of the procedure, the planned excision was designed along relaxed skin lines with a _____ margin of normal tissue. Local anesthesia was administered. Thereafter the area was cleansed with chlorhexidine scrub and draped with sterile towels. The lesion was excised down to **(DEEP DERMIS SUBQ FAT PERICHONDRIUM PERIOSTEUM MUSCLE CARTILAGE BONE OTHER_____).**

_____Hemostasis was obtained with **(ELECTROCAUTERY THERMAL CAUTERY).** The specimen was placed in formalin with a suture at the superior margin for orientation.

_____The wound **(BLUNTLY   SHARPLY)** undermined subdermally in all directions for _____ mm.

_____The depth of the wound was then closed with _____ dermal sutures for strength and wound edge eversion.

The skin surface was closed with _____
(SIMPLE   RUN   RUNLOCK   RUNSUBQ) sutures.

The wound was closed in one layer with _____
(SIMPLE   RUN   RUNLOCK   VERTMAT) sutures.

There were no complications, and the procedure was well tolerated. Blood loss was negligible.

The wound was dressed with antibiotic ointment, nonstick gauze, and a pressure dressing. Routine written postoperative instructions were given to the patient and reviewed with (him/her) by the nurse. Follow-up will be in _____ **(WEEK   DAYS).**

_____
Daniel Mark Siegel, M.D.

cc: _____

Figure 22–3. Excisional surgery worksheet.

SUNSCREEN PARAGRAPH, a MOHS SURGERY PARAGRAPH, or a SCLEROTHERAPY RISK PARAGRAPH at a defined point.)"

Operative reports can also be automated to a great extent. Blanks in a standard operative note template worksheet (Fig. 22–3) can be filled in or appropriate capitalized responses can be circled on a hard copy. The secretary then transfers this information to a simple word processor template form (Fig. 22–4), which allows the generation of a clean and simple operative report.

Should any complex changes or additions be needed, they can be dictated or directly edited on screen by the surgeon.

Variable portions of documents can have only a few possibilities (closures such as "Sincerely yours" or "Best regards"), a few dozen possibilities (referring physicians, types of grafts and flaps, or antibiotics), a large number of possibilities (all patients in the practice, medical record numbers) or infinite possibilities (symptom complexes, patient self-perceptions noted in a cosmetic surgical consultation). The more effectively a variable can be defined with a specific list of responses, the easier it will be to study groups of patients for academic or other reasons. For many procedures, the *Surgical Procedure Logbook*, distributed by the American Academy of Dermatology and the American Society for Dermatologic Surgery, can serve as an ideal model of development for templates.

MOHS SURGERY TEMPLATES AND FORMS

For Mohs micrographic surgery, a custom-designed software package called PATRAK (for PAtient TRAcKing) was developed by Gateley and Associates of Jacksonville, Texas, in 1986. It allows generation of

OPERATIVE REPORT

Joan Doe
Medical record number: 12345678
Date of procedure: 8/15/92   Surgery time: 15 minutes

Surgeon: Daniel Mark Siegel, M.D.

Pre-op Dx: Nevus of the left side of the neck, 8 × 6 mm.
Post-op Dx: Nevus of the left side of the neck, 8 × 6 mm.

Title of operation: Excision of changing nevus of the left side of the neck.

Anesthesia: 1% lidocaine with epinephrine 1:100,000.

Procedure: Following a discussion of the risks and benefits of the procedure, the planned excision was designed along relaxed skin lines with a 2-mm margin of normal tissue. Local anesthesia was administered. Thereafter the area was cleansed with chlorhexidine scrub and draped with sterile towels. The lesion was excised down to subcutaneous fat. Hemostasis was obtained with electrocautery. The specimen was placed in formalin with a suture at the superior margin for orientation. The wound was bluntly undermined subdermally in all directions for 10 mm. The depth of the wound was closed with 5-0 polyglycolic acid dermal sutures for strength and wound edge eversion. The skin surface was closed with 6-0 polypropylene running locked sutures. There were no complications, and the procedure was well tolerated. Blood loss was negligible.

The wound was dressed with antibacterial ointment, nonstick gauze, and a pressure dressing. Routine written postoperative instructions were given to the patient and reviewed with her by the nurse. Follow-up will be in 1 week.

_____
Daniel Mark Siegel, M.D.

cc: **Primus Doctorus,** M.D.

Figure 22–4. Completed operative report.

operative reports, referral letters, demographic and risk factor studies, and insurance statements, as well as rapid location of specific cases by searching for a number of features, such as diagnosis, age, or anatomic location. A series of data entry screens and an array of templates can be filled out and entered into the database at the time of surgery. The dramatic feature of this system is its simple menu-driven data entry screens that allow mastery of the system in a short time by almost any user. This system is based on the case numbering system in use at Baylor College of Medicine at the time of development. In its original form, the software did not run as a fully integrated practice management package, but in 1989, Richard Rice of Delasco, Inc., redesigned the original patient tracking system and incorporated the best features into a practice management software package, Medfile/R, while maintaining the simplicity of the data entry screens. The current version has greatly expanded the facility of the original system.

At the patient's initial visit, an intake sheet is used to determine general medical history, specific skin cancer information, risk factors for skin cancer, and family history, all of which become part of the permanent record. The demographic record portion follows the intake screen of the Medfile/R Surgery Tracking System input screens. On the day of surgery, an "operative worksheet" is filled out on all patients (Fig. 22–5) after completion of surgery. The sequence number is a five-digit number that gives the year, followed by a case number. All microscope slides and photographs are filed according to this number. The information from the worksheet is entered into screens for storage of information (Fig. 22–6). After all screens containing demographics, lesion detail, histologic sections, and comments have been filled in, operative reports and referral letters can be generated. The templates for the repairs are customized for second-intention healing, primary closure, flaps, and full- and split-thickness grafts. Additional reports, including operative reports, can be created as needed and used as desired (Fig. 22–7). The variables are replaced by information obtained from the database entered from the operative worksheet. Paragraphs labeled "FIRST" are used one time in the report, while the "REPEAT" paragraphs may be used once for each Mohs excision beyond the first, except the last stage. If the case is only two stages, the "FIRST" and "LAST" paragraphs are each used once. The "REPAIR" paragraph describes an uncomplicated flap repair, but the report template could be rewritten to meet any number of clinical situations. From a practical perspective, whenever a situation is encountered in which the existing reports need extensive modification, a new template report should be generated. Referral letters can be prepared in a similar fashion (Fig. 22–8).

All data entered into the database are available for study and review at any time so that an office-based tumor registry can be created. The potential exists for creating a national tumor registry if agreement on a standard for data entry can be reached. This same approach could be used for a variety of procedures, including hair transplants, chemical peels, laser surgery, or virtually any other procedure where data accumulation can be standardized.

Simple letters, as discussed earlier, can be generated on a word processor. If the operator is comfortable with the computer, macros can be used to generate elaborate and extensive documentation in an orderly manner. Estimates are that this approach can save up to 30 minutes/day in dictation based on the performance of six surgical cases per day.[7]

UTILITIES

Utilities are programs that are designed to keep things running correctly. Major programs in this category include Norton Utilities, PC TOOLS, and Mace Utilities. All are excellent, and owning at least one is imperative. Even though it is only rarely necessary to reconstruct lost data, the benefits of having one of these loss-prevention programs will be readily obvious if this type of recovery becomes required. At other times, these programs can be used with cache software and disk clean-up utilities to optimize the functioning of the system. As the hard disk goes spinning along with more and more data, data can be spread around the disk and take longer to be retrieved than before fragmentation. This time lag may be a blink of an eye on a defragmented, optimized system or seconds or even minutes on a badly fragmented disk. Defragmentation or optimization utilities can be used to perform these housekeeping functions at times of low utilization on a regular basis to keep the system running at peak performance levels.

OTHER SOFTWARE

A host of other software is available for a variety of uses. Spreadsheets such as Lotus 1-2-3, Quatro, and Excel serve as electronic replacements for the accountant's columnar pads; databases such as dBase, R:Base, or Foxbase are electronic replacements for address books, index cards, library card catalogs, and manual mailing lists; all-in-one packages such as Framework and Microsoft Works and graphic user interfaces such as Windows and GEOS allow users to pick commands by choosing electronic pictures called "icons" instead of typing commands.

If one wants to computerize the payroll in a medical practice, a payroll (PAYROLL USA) or accounting program (Peachtree, DAC-Easy) is probably the best way to proceed. Starting from scratch with a spreadsheet is generally not cost effective for a small business. For personal finances, integrated programs such as Managing Your Money are bargains in view of their capabilities and low cost. This type of program frequently allows "exporting" data in such a way that one can examine and manipulate it within a more powerful spreadsheet or database program if desired or necessary. Also, it allows data to be shared with the accountant in a standardized form that can be used when performing tasks for the medical practice. Formats such as Lotus 1-2-3 for spreadsheets and dBase for databases have become industry standards, and most software packages will convert to or from these programs.

Unless programming is a hobby or pasttime, it is wise

PATIENT_____DATE_____ SEQ#_____

ANESTHESIA   1 with epi   2 plain   3 bupivacaine   4 50:50 mix

PRE & POST OP DX   1 BCE   2 SCCA   3 BOWENS   4 MM   5 XMAMPAGETS   6 DFSP   7 LM   8
ECCRINECA   15 DESMOTRICHOEP   98 LESION   99

POST OP LENGTH_____   POST OP WIDTH_____

INVASION   1 PARTIAL   2 FULL   3 FOCAL FULL   4 SOFT>PERICH   5 SOFT>CART   6 MUSCLE
               7 SOFT>PERIO   8 FT>MUCOSA   9 SOFT>FASCIA   10 SOFT>BONE   11 FT-LID
               12 FT-ANAT REGION   13 FAT   14 SOFT>TENDON

ANAT LOC   _____

CHEMO CHECK   NO   YES
L1____/____   L2____/____   L3____/____   L4____/____   L5____/____   L6____/____
L7____/____

REPAIR 0   1 ROTATE   2 ADVAN   3 TRANSP   4 NL-TRANSP   5 PTSG   6 FTSG   7 COMPSITE
                 8 ELLIPSE   9 COMPLEX   10 MUCOSAL ADV   11 SUBQISLAND   99_____

DRESSING   3 ABX-PRESS   4 OXYCEL-ABX   5 GELFOAM   6 SURGICEL-ABX   7 HYDROCOLLOID
                14 COLLODION   15 EUTRA

DONOR SITE_____(IGNORE IF LEFT BLANK ON THIS SHEET)

SUBCUT SUTURE   1 5POLYDIOX   2 6NUR   3 5FAST   4 6FAST   5 5CHROM   6 6CHROM
                     7 4CHROM   8 6NYLON   9 5POLYPROP   10 5POLYGLYC   11 6POLYGLYC
                     12 3POLYGLYC   13 4POLYGLYC   99 MISC

SKIN SUTURE   1 5POLYDIOX   2 6NUR   3 5FAST   4 6FAST   5 5CHROM   6 6CHROM
                   12 3POLYGLYC   13 4POLYGLYC   99 MISC

ADDIT SUTURE   1 5POLYDIOX   2 6NUR   3 5FAST   4 6FAST   5 5CHROM   6 6CHROM
                    12 3POLYGLYC   13 4POLYGLYC   99 MISC

COMMENTS (ALL CIRCLED)   1 CAUTERY   2 CHROMIC TIES   3 NEURAL-CA   4 BX   5 ACETA/COD   7
BX-TCA   8 BX-CAUTERY   99 _____

_____
Daniel Mark Siegel, M.D.

Figure 22–5. Mohs surgery operative worksheet.

to obtain a commercially available program for as many needs as possible. Purchasing a program such as Lotus 1-2-3 or dBase and planning to run a medical practice from it is sheer folly. These programs cannot do all the functions that are wanted, and it is generally not cost or time effective for the busy practitioner to do this from scratch. Purchasing the software and hiring a programmer to write the specific applications needed is by far the best tactic to take in most cases.

RANDOM-ACCESS FREE-FORM DATABASES

A useful computer tool in the cutaneous surgical practice is the random-access free-form database. Productivity may be defined as attempting to optimize results in a fixed amount of time or getting the most benefit with the least amount of time invested. This is true in most aspects of daily existence, from personal interactions to a business or medical practice. Some

CAPTURE LESION DETAIL   DANIEL M. SIEGEL, M.D.

ACCOUNT: 123456   FIRST: John   Q LAST: PATIENT

```
LESION #: 1          1—PREOP LEN:22      3—POSTOP LEN:44
                     2—PREOP WID:11      4—POSTOP WID:33      5—DEBULK:y
             6—PREV TRTMNT:N
       7—PRE-OP DX:[173.9  BCC] [BASAL CE                  ]
       8—POST-OP DX:[173.9  BCC] [BASAL CE                 ]
       9—ANESTHESIA:1          :1% lidocaine with epinephrine 1:100,000
      10—INVASION:1            :partial thickness of the dermis
      11—ANATOMY:1             :left occipital scalp
      12—REPAIR:1              :rotation
      13—REP REFER:            :
      14—DRESSING:1            :antibiotic ointment, gauze and pressure
      15—DONOR LOC:1           :left parietal scalp
      16—SKIN SUTURE:9         :5-0 polypropylene
      17—SUBCUT. SUTURE:13     :4-0 polyglycolic acid
      18—             :        :
      19—             :        :
      20—             :        :
Trx {#}N:{1} SIEGEL           Version:  3.00              Today:  11/23/90
```

Enter field # to change, ⟨RETURN⟩ To accept and continue, ⟨HOME⟩ To quit now

⟨F1⟩—Help   ⟨Home/Esc⟩—Quit now

Figure 22–6. Data storage sheet for Mohs surgery.

common examples include the use of stamp pads or self-stick name and address labels for postage. The computer can also be used as a productivity device in a number of novel tasks to minimize storage space, paper clutter, and retrieval time in a variety of forms. A class of software that allows performance of these tasks is known as Personal Information Managers, or PIMs. These productivity tools ultimately allow a piece of information to be dealt with one time and then manipulated, retrieved, or acted on without a search for paper at each step. A variety of these software programs exist, with list prices beginning at less than $100.00. Types include telephone dialers that dial a number on the video screen through a modem, "things-to-do" calendars, and formal address books. Some of the newer products work with graphic user interfaces such as Microsoft Windows and are very powerful, allowing the incorporation of text and graphics. The disadvantage of these programs is that they appear to be slow because of the need for constant "rewriting" in memory of complex graphic screens. However, they are the wave of the future, and the material entered can easily be moved into one of these programs if so desired. One product, Memory-Mate, can be used successfully and even enjoyably. Technically, it is a random-access database that can retrieve data from any record. It currently sells for $79.00 but can be purchased in many discount software outlets for $39.00 to $50.00. It is very versatile and simple. Many of the PIMs can emulate the capabilities of this software, but none are as simple and intuitive to use. This program, along with others like "Instant Recall" and "Info-Select," can be run as Terminate and Stay Resident (TSR) programs, which means that they can be accessed from within other applications or programs. TSR programs do consume memory, but usually this consumption is small or can be shifted into expanded or extended memory to avoid eating into the DOS 640-kilobyte barrier.

The user is led through the command set and logic for the program using the basic MemoryMate screen (Fig. 22–9). The command section is at the top of the screen and the "time stamps" are at the bottom. At any point during use of the program, context-sensitive help is available by pressing the F1 key, one of the 10 to 12 function keys found on all IBM-compatible keyboards. If text is imported from another application, the "help" screen will be specifically relevant to that situation. If printing, the "help" screen will walk through the choices available in that area as well. Each screen may reveal up to 19 lines of text at a time, and each record may contain up to 120 lines of 80 characters/line.

The actual commands are accessed from the command menu by simultaneously pressing the CTRL ("control") key and the first letter of the command desired or by pressing the ESC ("escape") key followed by the first letter of the command desired. These commands include the following:

FIND. This command searches for a word or phrase typed into the computer and retrieves all records containing that word or phrase from that part of the file being searched. Searches can also be done by date of creation or modification of the record. Searches are case insensitive, meaning that capital letters and small letters will not be differentiated by the software. "Wild cards," or characters that can define any number of possibilities, can be used in searches where the precise spelling is unknown. For example, a search for "flap" would find only "flap" in a case-insensitive program. A search for "flap?" using the universal wild card symbol, "*", would retrieve all occurrences of "flap" (e.g., flapping, flapper, flappers, etc.). A search for "flap?"

NAME: **&PN&**\

MEDICAL RECORD NUMBER: **&AC&**\

ENCOUNTER #: **&U1&**\

SURGEON: Daniel Mark Siegel, M.D.

DATE OF OPERATION: **&SD&**

OPERATIVE REPORT

REFERRING PHYSICIAN: **&RD&**

PREOPERATIVE DIAGNOSIS: **&PD&** of the **&AN&.**

POSTOPERATIVE DIAGNOSIS: **&OD&** of the **&AN&**, **&OL&** mm by **&OW&** mm in diameter. Ulcer of the same area secondary to tumor removal.

TITLE OF OPERATION: Excision of **&OD&** of the **&AN&** with micrographic control by the method of Mohs surgery. The defect was repaired with a **&RE&.**

FIRST

The patient's **&AN&** was anesthetized with **&ARE&** and cleansed with chlorhexidine scrub and draped with sterile towels. The tumor was excised and a representative frozen section prepared for evaluation. Thereafter, the borders of the tumor were excised as a horizontal layer 2 to 3 mm in thickness. This tissue was cut into **&HP&** pieces that were marked with dyes and mapped on the Mohs micrographic surgery map, frozen, cut, and stained with toluidine blue. On microscopic examination, **&OD&** was seen in the deep and outer borders of **&PO&** pieces of tissue.

REPEAT

The patient's **&AN&** was reanesthetized with **&ARE&**, reprepped, and redraped in a sterile fashion. The tumor was re-excised as a horizontal layer 2 to 3 mm in thickness. This tissue was cut into **&HP&** pieces that were marked with dyes and mapped on the Mohs micrographic surgery map, frozen, cut, and stained with toluidine blue. On microscopic examination, **&OD&** was seen in the deep and outer borders of **&PO&** pieces of tissue.

LAST

The patient's **&AN&** was reanesthetized with **&ARE&**, reprepped, and redraped in a sterile fashion. The tumor was re-excised as a horizontal layer, 2 to 3 mm in thickness. This tissue was cut into **&HP&** pieces that were marked with dyes and mapped on the Mohs micrographic surgery map, frozen, cut, and stained with toluidine blue. On microscopic examination, no further **&OD&** was seen in the deep or outer borders of the excised pieces of tissue, and the tumor was considered to be completely excised. The final size of the defect of the **&AN&** was **&OL&** mm by **&OW&** mm in diameter, infiltrating through the **&IN&.**

REPAIR

Following the removal of the tumor, treatment options for the resultant defect were reviewed with the patient, who had previously discussed these with me during our consultation and read about them in my routine preoperative patient information pamphlet. Following this discussion, a **&RE&** was designed. The **&RE&** was moved from the **&DS&** to the **&AN&**. The **&RE&** was sewn into place with buried **&SU&** sutures and **&SK&** cutaneous sutures. The secondary defect was closed with buried **&SU&** and **&SK&** cutaneous sutures. The donor site was dressed with **&DR&**, and the recipient site was dressed with **&DR&.**

COMMENTS

Daniel Mark Siegel, M.D.

Figure 22–7. Operative note—flap repair, multiple stages.

&DT&

&RD&

&A1&

&A2&

&RC&, &RS& &RZ&

Dear **&SL&**:

Enclosed are the operative pictures and operative report on **&PN&**, whom you referred to me.

I excised the **&OD&** of the **&AN&** with micrographic control by the method of Mohs. The defect was closed using a **&RE&** flap.

Thank you most kindly for referring the patient to me and for asking me to assist you with the treatment.

Sincerely,

Daniel Mark Siegel, M.D.

Figure 22–8. Mohs surgery referral letter.

using the character wild card symbol, "?", would retrieve all occurrences of "flap" where the word or the word with one extra character occurs (e.g., flaps, flap1, flape, flapx, etc.). The words "and" and "or" may be used to contract or expand an initial search.

NARROW. This narrows a "find" command down if an unwieldy number of records have been found. The command follows Boolean logic principles, so the "flap" search, as in the preceding example, can be narrowed to "flap and advancement" to search for records where the two words only occur together. Further narrowing using the word "and" is also possible. The word "or" may be used to expand the search as above in FIND without retyping the whole command. A search for "flap" and "[nasolabial or advancement]" would locate any records with both flap and either of the other two words in it.

JUMP. With a given list of retrieved records, one may "jump" over records to a specific record. This is useful when retrieving chronologic records to get to the vicinity of a desired record in a large number of retrieved records.

REJECT. This allows the user to eliminate retrieved records without eliminating them from the database, which is useful for printing out groups of records.

IN. This allows the user to bring data into the system from an ASCII, or "plain" English, file. This is one of the most valuable commands, as it can import text from a variety of other applications.

OUT. This allows the user to export data to an ASCII file either as records that have a distinct breakpoint or as continuous text. Much like "IN," this is useful for sharing records between formats of different software applications.

GO. This allows the user to change the database file that is currently being worked with. For example, separate databases can be used for articles, slides, general use, clinical therapeutics and pearls, personal filing, computer searches, and forms. The creation of a new database takes only a few keystrokes, and the program walks through the procedure. The size of the database is limited by the size of the hard disk. A database of about 200 typed pages will occupy approximately 1 megabyte of space.

ZAP. This allows the elimination of unwanted records from the database.

UNDO. This brings back the last ten records that were zapped in case one decides after the fact to undo a "ZAP."

CUT. This deletes material from a record permanently and allows it to be placed elsewhere using the "paste" command.

DITTO. This highlights and copies material from a record and allows it to be copied ("pasted") elsewhere in another MemoryMate database or another application with the PASTE command.

PASTE. This allows the placement of material that has been previously cut, or dittoed, either into the program or out into another application.

VIEW. This allows the user to capture a screen in another program he or she is working on while using MemoryMate in its TSR mode.

TYPE. This allows the printing of retrieved records or parts that have been dittoed.

EXIT. This allows the user to leave MemoryMate but reminds him or her to save any new records that were created.

SAVE. This allows the user to save a record and tie

```
Find    Narrow   Reject   Cut   Ditto   Paste   Jump    Go      F1 for Help
Save    View   Type In   Out   Hyper   Zap    Undo   Exit     Working Record
```

Figure 22–9. The basic MemoryMate screen.

NAME:

COMPANY:

ADDRESS:

OFFICE PHONE:

HOME PHONE:

COMMENTS:

Figure 22–10. Simple card file form.

it to a reminder date. The reminder will be brought up continuously after the date is reached until it has been changed or removed.

HYPER. This is a way of linking together records (hypertext) that may not be retrieved by simple search. It uses links between one record and another to permit jumping from one point in a record to a specified point or group of records, even in another database. The user can create hierarchies of hypertext links to allow rapid movements between records, such as jumping from a record locating an article on basal cell carcinoma in the article database to a record on grafts in the clinical pearls database and then to a group of records locating slides in the photography collection.

The " + " and " − " keys of the numeric keyboard and the F9 and F10 function keys allow the user to scroll through retrieved records. The cursor, or arrow, keys and "PgUp" and "PgDn" keys allow the user to scroll within a record. The function keys F2 through F8 can be used as "hot keys" to link single records or groups together for immediate retrieval. If the user wishes to maintain a group of records together when writing an article, these records can be retrieved through the use of FIND, NARROW, and REJECT and then linked together with a hot key. Each database can have multiple assigned hot keys, which can be reassigned at any time.

Specific Uses of MemoryMate

RANDOM MEMOS

The little scraps of paper that tend to pile up on one's desk can be input into the computer with reminder dates when necessary. Such reminders may include personal calls, airline and hotel incentive programs, meetings, and plane reservations, among others. The program can be set to give an automatic reminder about that material at a particular time so that the user is reminded every day until that date arrives.

CARD FILE

A form can be easily produced with a few keystrokes, and data can be entered into it with defined "fields," or areas with specific information such as name, address, and phone number, to allow easy access to these mate-

rials. The form (Fig. 22–10) can be "called" whenever it is needed with a few keystrokes. This eliminates the need to retain business cards that clutter the office. Each field or data entry break point in a database is ended with a colon. The user moves from field to field in the blank form and fills in the blanks. This can be elaborated on or changed at any time, as it is still randomly accessible. A more precise form (Fig. 22–11) facilitates the transfer of this information into a form used by any other database with a simple maneuver. All desired records are retrieved and "exported" as a plain text file. This file can then be imported into a word processor and "labels" such as LAST NAME, FIRST NAME can be removed and replaced with field delimiters, such as "," or ";". The file can be saved as plain text and imported into the appropriate database program.

SLIDE FILE

It can be time consuming to store patient photographs or slides so that they can be quickly retrieved for use in presentations or publications. One system used for this purpose is based numerically on Stanford Lamberg's "Retrieval System for Dermatological Photographs," which is produced as a public service by Westwood Pharmaceuticals in conjunction with the Dermatological Photographic Society and incorporates additional information when available. However, other approaches are also compatible with many current filing systems already in use (Fig. 22–12). The form could leave out any of the fields and still be useful for the record. The record can easily be searched according to diagnosis, Lamberg-coded condition, descriptive terms, or date and the retrieved slide records exported for manipulation in a word processor or direct printing. A more specific record (Fig. 22–13) can be used to describe a group of slides on, for example, a particular patient with a malignancy and can be retrieved easily for a talk or presentation on Mohs surgery, flaps, or nasal lesions. If a group of retrieved slides is used in a talk, they can be linked by a "hot key" for easy replacement in the master collection after presenting or duplicating the talk. If a particular picture is published or loaned out, this information can also be added to the record.

ARTICLE FILE

Previously, articles, reprints, and clippings were usually stored in folders and listed alphabetically by topic.

LAST NAME: FIRST NAME: MI:

ADDRESS1:

ADDRESS2:

CITY: STATE: ZIP:

OFFICE PHONE:

HOME PHONE:

Figure 22–11. Precise card file form.

SEQUENCE #: **3456**

DIAGNOSIS: **BULLOUS TINEA PEDIS**

LAMBERG #: **10-01**

DATE: **11/3/84**

PT NAME:

PROCEDURES:

COMMENTS: **SCALING PLANTAR PATCH**

Figure 22–12. General photographic file system.

However, dilemmas were often encountered as to where a specific publication should be most appropriately filed. When using the computer to maintain an article file, the best approach is to have all retrievable material accessed under many different topics, or "concepts." In this way, the material can easily be located by searching for many different terms, words, or phrases in the listing, including the year or even the journal. For articles entered using this system, a standard form can be set up (Fig. 22–14).

This approach is very useful if one is unsure of the correct spelling of an author or entity. For example, if one were looking for an article written by Dr. Perry Robins, but there was some uncertainty whether "Robins" was spelled with one "b" or two, one could initiate a search in the article database under "Rob*" which would retrieve all occurrences of "Rob" (for example, "Robins, Robbins, Robert, Robin, Robinson, Robertson, and Robot"). The few dozen records could be narrowed down and retrieved by asking for the author and topic, "Rob* and cart,*" if one were unsure of the spelling of cartilage, which might retrieve only one record. The record could even be followed by a short discussion if the title was not self-explanatory, so as to aid in subsequent retrieval.

A scanner can be used to scan the table of contents from a series of journals into a plain text file, import it into the word processor, standardize its form, add delimiters, save it as a plain text file, and import it into MemoryMate for an inexpensive electronic index. The entire text of articles can also be imported, if required. If this is done on a regular basis, the purchase of CD-ROM equipment would probably be a better approach.

SEQUENCE #: **88345**

DIAGNOSIS: **Basal cell carcinoma (BCC) of the nasal bridge**

LAMBERG #: **17-51**

DATE: **8/3/88**

PT NAME: **Ima Tumor**

PROCEDURES: **Mohs preop postop advancement flap 2 weeks 1 year**

COMMENTS:

Figure 22–13. Specific photographic file system.

OFFICE FORMS

MemoryMate can also be used for generating and storing standardized forms, such as drug information sheets and postoperative care sheets, that can be easily customized for individual patients. In this way, MemoryMate acts like a simple word processor. Rather than printing up large numbers of information sheets, forms can be printed and updated as often as needed. Please note that the computer record does not take the place of printed documentation for medicolegal purposes, so it is still best to have a copy of any instructions given to patients placed in their chart or on file so that distribution of any "standard" instruction sheet can be referenced to that particular time period.

COMPUTER LITERATURE SEARCHES

Computer literature searches on BRS COLLEAGUE, MEDLINE, or other databases are becoming commonplace. Frequently the search is designed to find a specific article. On occasion, however, the database may need to be searched for any relevant information available. A compromise is to download the search into a text file, a capability available on all communications software such as PROCOMM or GTCOMM, and import this text file into its own MemoryMate database for perusal at some later time. This lets one get "off line" as rapidly as possible and minimizes the cost of performing a search. Many medical libraries now subscribe to MEDLINE on CD-ROM and are willing to download searches to a floppy disk to conserve paper. These same searches, often available at no cost to an end user, can easily be input into the database. Most searches have a delimiter built into them that is very unlikely to be reduplicated in the body of the text (e.g., "AN 12345678" for a retrieval accession number or "AU *Smith -J-Q*"). Using the word processor, it is possible to substitute one of these sequences for a sequence that is unlikely to show up in the search, such as "~~" and save it as a plain text file. Then simply import IN to the database using the "~~" as a break point for each record. MemoryMate will only use one- or two-character record break points, so that if the original "AN 12345678" or "AU *Smith -J-Q*" was left and used "AN" or "AU" for break points, a record might be split in the middle of a word such as "hANd" or "cAUtery," an easily fixable error if this route is

SEQUENCE #: **1934**

AUTHOR: **Goldberg LH, Collins SAB, Siegel DM**

TITLE: **The Epidermal Nevus Syndrome: Case Report and Review**

JOURNAL: **Pediatric Dermatology 4:27–33**

YEAR: **1987**

COMMENTS: **30 + female with generalized epidermal nevus with sebaceous and verrucous lesions and basal cell carcinomas BCC.**

Figure 22–14. Standard publication listing form.

chosen. As records are input in order, simply CUT and PASTE the offending records back together and continue with the search.

RANDOM-ACCESS FREE-FORM DATABASE TEXTBOOKS

At the 1988 American Academy of Dermatology meeting, a scientific exhibit entitled "The High-Speed Peripheral Brain: A Computerized Random Access Dermatology Textbook" was presented. This consisted of a "textbook" of clinical and basic science "pearls of wisdom" that had been collected over 30 years by Stuart M. Brown, M.D., along with a variety of forms and brief reports by Daniel Mark Siegel, M.D., and Denis Lee Beaudoing, M.D., all of which was input into MemoryMate to demonstrate the function of a random-access, easily searched textbook. Thomas Hoffmann, M.D., supplied a database consisting of abstracts for all articles occurring in *Archives of Dermatology* and the *Journal of the American Academy of Dermatology* during the preceding 3 years. This approach demonstrates an application that could benefit all physicians immediately. After reading a journal or returning from a professional meeting, the physician summarizes and enters into an easily retrieved record the pertinent clinical points or techniques that were learned from the educational activity; the information can be easily retrieved at a later date for future reference.

SUMMARY

References for this information are unfortunately quite thin, as this is a rapidly evolving field and most of the evolution is outside the literature of refereed medical journals. However, several resources can be suggested to provide reliable information. Computer magazines, such as *PC Magazine, Byte, Info World*, and *Computer Shopper*, offer frequent reviews of software and hardware, as well as columns and editorials relating to all aspects of computer technology. Reading one of these for several months will allow one to pick up the language of the computer age and become aware of what is on the market. All new products are typically reviewed in one of the major computer magazines at least every 12 to 18 months, usually coincident with a flurry of upgraded versions. These magazines will also give a good starting point for determining a "fair" price, which changes rapidly. Unfortunately, medical practice management software is not reviewed in these publications, and other sources of information about them must be consulted.

Computer user support groups exist in many parts of the country and provide a way for information to be shared among users with similar interests in a given area. One can learn about these groups from local computer stores, from local high school or college computer science departments, and often by attending a local computer "swap meet." *Computer Shopper* has a list of electronic bulletin boards (BBS), which are an excellent source of information about local users groups. While most software comes with documentation, it is not always very useful. A large number of manuals now exist for a wide variety of software and can be very valuable for different types of applications. QUE and Brady are among the major publishers of books in this area. These manuals are generally well written and easy to follow and complement the original software documentation. A number of guidebooks to the purchase of computer hardware and software are also available. One general guide is the *Personal Computer Buying Guide: Foolproof Advice on How to Buy Computer Software and Hardware*, by O. Pearson and the Editors of Consumer Reports Books. Like all *Consumer Reports* products, the authors have no vested interest in any of the commercial products and are very objective in their assessments. These are all excellent ways to learn more about computers and how to effectively incorporate this established technology in a cutaneous surgical practice. It may initially be hard to get started computerizing a medical practice, but it will certainly be worth the effort!

REFERENCES

1. Rigel DS: Is it time for a computer in your practice? I. Introduction. J Dermatol Surg Oncol 7:964–965, 1981.
2. Rigel DS: Is it time for a computer in your practice? II. What tasks your computer can perform. J Dermatol Surg Oncol 8:168–170, 1982.
3. Rigel DS: Is it time for a computer in your practice? III. Types of computer systems for medical offices. J Dermatol Surg Oncol 8:532–534, 1982.
4. Rigel DS: Is it time for a computer in your practice? IV. Which practices benefit? J Dermatol Surg Oncol 9:961–962, 1983.
5. Rigel DS: Is it time for a computer in your practice? V. How to evaluate if a computer is appropriate for your practice. J Dermatol Surg Oncol 11:215–216, 1985.
6. Kopf AW, Rigel DS, White R, et al: DERM/INFONET: A concept becomes a reality. J Am Acad Dermatol 18:1150–1157, 1988.
7. Swinehart JM: Computer-generated operative reports. J Am Acad Dermatol 23:508–512, 1990.

PART TWO

Advanced Surgical Procedures

CHAPTER 23

Intraoperative Patient Monitoring, Sedation, and Analgesia

MICHAEL J. AULETTA

Much of cutaneous surgery has traditionally been performed using only local anesthesia. However, there are times when the use of adjunctive agents such as sedatives or analgesics may be helpful in making the surgical procedure more pleasant or tolerable for the patient.[1] These agents are typically required when an anxious patient or child[2] is undergoing a long or complex procedure. Mild sedation can also be of benefit for those with poor cardiac status, since the anxiety associated with the induction of local anesthesia and the surgical procedure itself can increase the heart rate and possibly lead to extra systoles.[3] Although effective in relieving anxiety, sedatives and analgesics should not be used by the surgeon as a substitute for taking time to explain the surgical procedure to all patients and answering any questions they may have.[1]

Preoperative Evaluation

Because these agents differ in their effects, it is best to tailor the use of sedatives or analgesics in cutaneous surgery to the individual patient. Many considerations should be kept in mind during the preoperative evaluation.

TYPE AND LENGTH OF PROCEDURE

Simple procedures such as skin biopsies rarely require the use of adjunctive agents, except in a very young or anxious patient. However, even the most stoic of patients may require sedation for procedures lasting longer than 90 minutes. Generally, procedures requiring the injection of fairly large amounts of local anesthetic or those being performed on the head or neck are more comfortably carried out by incorporating the use of these agents.

PHYSICAL STATUS OF THE PATIENT

A pertinent medical history and physical examination must be performed before considering the use of any medication,[4, 5] as many pre-existing medical conditions can affect the metabolism of some agents.[6] Because most anesthetics are metabolized in the liver and excreted by the kidneys, caution must be exercised in patients with dysfunction of these organs.[7] In the elderly or debilitated patient, the dosage should often be reduced.[7] A history of alcohol or sedative use can also affect the metabolism of these agents. In pregnant women, the use of these agents should be avoided unless absolutely necessary.

MEDICATIONS, ALLERGIES, AND ADVERSE REACTIONS

There is a potential drug-drug interaction with some of these agents, and it is important to be familiar with this possibility before prescribing any sedative or analgesic.[5, 8] It is also important to know if the patient has ever received one of these agents before, as it is not uncommon for patients to have had a bad experience with an analgesic such as codeine or a sedative in the past.

Intraoperative Patient Monitoring

GENERAL CONCEPTS

The use of preoperative sedation or analgesia, especially when administered intravenously, is associated with a definite increased risk of morbidity and mortality,[9] particularly in children.[10] Failure to properly monitor patients for signs of toxicity from sedatives is the most common error resulting in fatality.[11] Thus, it is important to be knowledgeable of the proper way to monitor patients receiving sedatives.

SIMPLE MONITORING OF VITAL SIGNS

Monitoring should be adjusted to the individual patient. The degree of monitoring depends on the medication used, the dosage, the route of administration, and the status of the patient. Assigning a nurse to observe for signs of distress is the minimum requirement for all patients. In addition, it is best not to allow any patient who has received a sedative or opioid analgesic to be left unattended, even for short periods of time. Although oral administration of these agents is usually safe, there is always the possibility that a patient may experience some adverse reaction such as emesis, especially if receiving the medication for the first time. Parenteral administration of these medications usually requires that a staff member stay with the patient until the patient departs for home.

FUNCTION OF MONITORING DEVICES

Although devices exist to assist in monitoring patients, they do not serve as a substitute for constant personal contact.[10, 12] Before receiving any medication preoperatively, all patients should have their baseline resting blood pressure, pulse, and respiration rate recorded.[12] Vital signs should be checked periodically during both the administration of the sedative and the operative procedure.[5] The frequency with which this is done depends on the patient and the agent used. One member of the surgical team should be free to converse with the patient during this process and to record changes in vital signs, in addition to noting the time, dosage, and route of administration of any medication given and documenting any adverse events. Voice contact is reassuring to the patient and also serves as an additional way to monitor the patient for signs of distress.

Some surgeons advocate monitoring patients even when only local anesthesia is used,[13] but monitoring is especially important whenever intravenous sedation is given.[14] Monitoring devices serve two main purposes. First, they supply continuous information on the patient's vital signs. Monitors can provide a constant readout and a permanent record of changes in heart and respiration rates[15] and blood pressure.[10, 16] Second, they provide an alternative method of evaluating the patient, including continuous heart monitoring and pulse oximetry.

ELECTROCARDIOGRAPHIC MONITORING

Continuous electrocardiographic (ECG) monitoring devices should provide a visual display on an oscilloscope that can indirectly help to detect early signs of hypotension or respiratory depression resulting from preoperative medications.[12] Occasionally, arrhythmias

may also develop directly from the use of preoperative medications.[5] The use of ECG monitors has been shown to significantly reduce the chance of death from agents used for sedation and analgesia.[17] However, it must be understood that the electrocardioscope only provides information on the electrical activity, standard leads I and II, of the heart.[5] It does not offer information on the strength of myocardial contraction and therefore must be used in combination with other data, such as blood pressure and mental status.[12] ECG monitors should provide a permanent record from a built-in recorder; this record can be placed in the patient's chart.[5]

PULSE OXIMETRY

The pulse oximeter represents a significant advance in the noninvasive monitoring of patients[18] (Fig. 23–1). It makes use of the observation that the color of blood is directly related to the relative oxygen saturation of hemoglobin. A noninvasive probe attached to the finger, toe, or ear emits a low-intensity laser light that spectrophotometrically determines the oxyhemoglobin concentration of pulsatile (arterial) blood in the appendage.[19] Along with the heart rate, this information is continuously updated, processed, and displayed on a monitor as the percent oxygen saturation of blood (SaO_2). A normal SaO_2 is between 95 and 100%. The SaO_2 values given by this device have been correlated with arterial blood gas measurements and are reliable at saturations between 70 and 100%.[20, 21] A pulse oximeter can determine the presence of hypoxemia sooner than other noninvasive methods of monitoring patients,[19] which allows for earlier adjustment in the delivery of sedatives or analgesics that affect respiration and helps avoid serious complications.

The accuracy of a pulse oximeter to determine SaO_2 can be adversely affected if blood flow to the appendage is decreased. For this reason, the probe should not be placed on the same arm as the blood pressure cuff, if possible.[19] Other causes of reduced peripheral blood flow, such as vascular disease or hypothermia from a

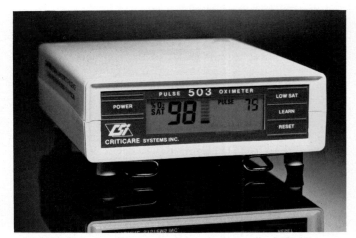

Figure 23–1. Pulse oximeter. (Courtesy of Criticare Systems Inc., Milwaukee, WI.)

cold room, will affect the accuracy of the device. Whenever there is a sudden change in the readings by the device, the probe should first be checked for proper positioning, since it can be dislodged by movement.[19] Pulse oximeters are available from several manufacturers and differ somewhat in their ability to reject extrinsic signals that can give false readings.[19] Other features to consider when choosing an oximeter include screen readability, probe design, and the presence of a low SaO_2 value alarm.

RESUSCITATION EQUIPMENT

Because an anaphylactic drug reaction or cardiopulmonary arrest occurring during the surgical procedure is always a possibility, the current standard of care requires that an emergency kit be readily available.[5] The essential equipment of an emergency cart should include an Ambu bag, airway or intubation equipment, a resuscitation board, oxygen, and emergency drugs (see Chap. 13). All office personnel should receive yearly certification in cardiopulmonary resuscitation (CPR) and be familiar with their role and proper course of action in case of an emergency.[22] In addition, physicians using intravenous sedation should have knowledge of Advanced Cardiac Life Support (ACLS) and ready access to cardioversion equipment (defibrillator).[5]

Preoperative Sedatives and Analgesics

Agents used preoperatively can be divided into two broad categories: analgesics and sedatives, such as tranquilizers and hypnotics. Which category of drugs is most appropriate is dependent on the patient and the procedure to be performed. For most relatively small procedures, only a sedative may be necessary. Larger procedures or those that require only minimal use of local anesthetics, such as dermabrasion or chemical peels, may require use of a potent analgesic. It may even be occasionally necessary to combine both a sedative and an analgesic to achieve the proper combination of sedation and pain relief.

ROUTE OF ADMINISTRATION

Most patients prefer oral to parenteral administration of preoperative medications. As a general rule, while oral administration offers a certain degree of safety, it is usually at the expense of being somewhat less effective and with a slower onset of action.[23] For this reason, oral medication usually needs to be administered at least 30 to 60 minutes before beginning the procedure. Depending on individual circumstances, it may be desirable for the patient to take the medication at home before arriving at the office. In any event, it is absolutely necessary that patients arrange for someone to drive them whenever any medication is used that is sedating in nature or capable of adversely affecting their ability to drive. In addition, it is desirable for a family member

or friend to stay with the patient the evening after surgery, especially when medication is administered parenterally. Because children often have an exaggerated fear of needles, preoperative medication should always be administered orally to pediatric patients if possible.[2]

Intramuscular injection of preoperative medication offers some advantages over oral dosing, especially when analgesics are given. It tends to result in a more rapid onset of action, with higher effective blood levels.[23] Preoperative medications should be injected deeply into a large muscle mass, such as the buttocks, using a Z-technique,[24] since certain medications can be very irritating to tissues when they are injected more superficially. A degree of safety is also obtained from this technique, as absorption from a deep muscle mass is usually slow and continuous. Care should be taken to aspirate before injection to avoid inadvertent intravenous (IV) administration.

IV infusion is usually the most effective method of administering preoperative medication. It offers the most rapid onset of action and a finer degree of control over the desired[8] level of sedation and analgesia. However, these advantages are countered by the fact that complications secondary to overdosing are much more likely to occur with IV administration and require closer patient monitoring for signs of respiratory depression. The best rule to follow is that IV administration of sedatives or analgesics should be performed only by persons familiar with the use of these agents and the management of the potential respiratory depression associated with them. A continuous IV infusion should be maintained for the entire period of time that the patient is being sedated. Sedatives and analgesics are more safely administered intravenously in an office setting by intermittent dosing rather than by continuous drip. It must also be recognized that the drug dosages given in this chapter are to be used only as a general guideline in deciding the proper dosage for any particular patient. Dosage must be individualized, always evaluating the patient's age, weight, physical status, general health, use of other drugs, and the surgical procedure being performed.

TYPES OF SEDATIVES

Any surgical procedure, especially when complex or located on the face, can be stressful for the patient. The goal of preoperative sedation is to relieve anxiety and possibly induce some degree of amnesia for the procedure.[25] This is most safely accomplished with a minimum of drowsiness, although a certain amount may be needed in some patients. Depending on the agent chosen, the dosage, and the route of administration, varying levels of anxiety relief and drowsiness can be achieved. One risk of oversedating a patient is difficulty in determining the adequacy of nerve blocks.[26]

Benzodiazepines

The benzodiazepines are generally considered the preferred preoperative sedative for adults.[1] They offer a high degree of safety and are generally very well tolerated. In addition, they are capable of inducing some amnesia, depending on the dose, for the surgical procedure.[27] Although any of the benzodiazepines may be useful as preoperative sedatives, two agents are generally preferred: diazepam and midazolam.

Diazepam. Diazepam (Valium) is the preferred agent when oral or sublingual administration is desired.[28] An additional benefit from the use of diazepam is that it may raise the seizure threshold to local anesthetics, which may be desirable when larger amounts of local anesthetics are required.[29]

Sublingual administration of benzodiazepines tends to produce a more rapid effect compared with the oral route.[30] Diazepam is available in 2-, 5-, and 10-mg tablets. The usual oral or sublingual starting dose for adults is 5 mg to 10 mg (0.1 to 0.2 mg/kg),[28] which is administered 30 to 60 minutes before surgery. Either route of administration will produce a mild to moderate calming effect adequate to make the injection of local anesthesia less stressful for the patient. The effect can last up to 3 hours. This dosage may be repeated every 3 to 4 hours as needed. Some recommend use of a higher initial dose of diazepam, 0.25 mg/kg,[31] but this is more likely to have an hypnotic effect. Patients who chronically take diazepam may need twice the usual dose to achieve a similar effect.[32] Diazepam is unpredictably absorbed from intramuscular injection,[32] and therefore that route of administration is not recommended. The recommended oral pediatric dosage for children more than 5 years old is 1 to 2.5 mg (0.2 mg/kg),[2] starting at the lowest dose.

IV administration of diazepam offers more predictable results in relieving anxiety[33] but is somewhat more likely to produce respiratory depression,[34] especially when the dosage exceeds 0.2 mg/kg.[28] While IV dosing is more likely to result in antegrade amnesia,[28, 32] it is the route of choice when more intense levels of sedation are desired. The solution for injection contains 5 mg/ml of diazepam. IV administration can cause pain, phlebitis,[35] and venous thrombosis at the injection site, which can be minimized by injecting slowly, allowing 1 minute for each 5 mg; by injecting into a rapidly flowing IV tube; and by avoiding the use of relatively small veins, such as those located on the dorsum of the hand.[32] Some surgeons advocate injecting lidocaine with diazepam to alleviate this pain.[2] The usual initial IV dose for adults is 2.5 to 5 mg injected slowly into a supine patient until signs of sedation such as slurred speech, blepharoptosis to the midpupillary level, or drowsiness are observed.[28] This initial dosage may be repeated at 15-minute intervals until a maximum of 20 mg is delivered. Most healthy patients require 5 to 10 mg to achieve the desired sedative effect. Pediatric intravenous dosing is 0.25 mg/kg injected slowly over 3 minutes. This may be repeated at 15- to 30-minute intervals until the desired level of sedation is achieved, up to a maximum dose of 0.75 mg/kg.[36]

Midazolam. The second most commonly used sedative is midazolam (Versed), a benzodiazepine designed for parenteral use. It has distinct advantages over diazepam in that it has a rapid onset of action and a much shorter recovery time.[28, 37] It is relatively rapidly cleared from the blood by the liver and is 1½ to 2 times more potent than diazepam. Another advantage is that it is much better absorbed after intramuscular (IM) injection than diazepam.[38] The IM use of midazolam is better able to induce sedation and amnesia for perioperative events than oral diazepam,[1, 37] and as stated earlier, it should be injected deeply into a large muscle. The usual pediatric or adult intramuscular dosage is 0.07 to 0.08 mg/kg.[2, 28] Sedative effects begin to appear in 15 minutes and peak in 30 to 60 minutes.[28] This dosage rarely has an effect on respiration.[36]

Antegrade amnesia for the operative event is often associated with parenteral use of this medication.[36] A potential hazard of amnesia is a failure to remember the postoperative instructions, which necessitates that written instructions be provided for these patients.[39] Patients should not be allowed to drive until the day after the procedure has been performed.[36] Intravenous administration of midazolam has an advantage over diazepam in that it has a faster onset of action with a relatively short duration. However, it can produce a slight decrease in blood pressure.[37] The more rapid onset of action makes it easier to titrate to the desired clinical end point.[9] Another advantage of midazolam is that it is less likely to produce venous complications than diazepam.[37] Midazolam is supplied in concentrations of 1 and 5 mg/ml; the lower concentration should be used for IV administration.[36]

To avoid overdosage in adults, 1 mg of midazolam should be given intravenously over 2 minutes, allowing an additional 2 minutes to determine the sedative effect.[36] This dosage may be repeated until the desired level of sedation, manifested by slurred speech or ptosis, is obtained.[40] The anxiolytic effects appear within 1 to 2 minutes and persist for 30 minutes.[37] A dose of 1 to 2.5 mg of midazolam will produce conscious sedation in most normal adults.[36] This is equivalent to an oral dose of 5 to 10 mg of diazepam. If a higher degree of sedation is desired, a total dose of 5 to 10 mg (0.1 mg/kg) is usually required.[37] This will produce adequate sedation for most procedures, with minimal risk of respiratory depression. Higher dosing (0.15 mg/kg given intravenously) may cause significant respiratory depression.[37] Because midazolam has a much narrower therapeutic range than diazepam, it should never be administered rapidly or as a single bolus.[36] Concomitant use with narcotic premedications may also increase the risk of apnea.[28] The pediatric IV dosage of midazolam is 0.08 mg/kg.[2]

Barbiturates

Barbiturates are primarily used when a hypnotic effect or drowsiness is desired. Because this group of drugs causes nonselective central nervous system depression, anxiety reduction usually occurs in association with some degree of drowsiness[41] and respiratory depression. Barbiturates with a short onset of action and short duration, such as pentobarbital and secobarbital, are preferred as preoperative sedatives.[32] The sodium salt form of the drug is rapidly absorbed orally,[41] and the rate of absorption is increased by administering it on an empty stomach. Its usual onset of action is 20 to 60 minutes.

Because barbiturates are metabolized predominantly in the liver, they may be useful in patients with reduced kidney function. Both pentobarbital (Nembutal) and secobarbital (Seconal) are available in 50- and 100-mg capsules. For preoperative sedation, the oral dosage for adults is 100 to 200 mg (1.5 mg/kg) and for children, 2 mg/kg,[25] with the effect lasting 3 to 4 hours. IM injection is painful and results in erratic absorption.[2] Phenobarbital has a longer duration than secobarbital but has the advantage of being excreted through the kidney, so it may be useful in patients with altered hepatic function.[5] The dosage for phenobarbital is the same as for secobarbital and pentobarbital. Patients who use sedatives chronically, smoke, drink heavily, or take anticoagulants may require higher dosages. Administration of barbiturates in children and the elderly may produce paradoxical excitement.[32, 41]

Chloral Hydrate

Chloral hydrate is probably the best sedative for infants and small children, because it rarely produces paradoxical excitement,[5] is well tolerated, and offers a high degree of safety. It is available as a syrup (500 mg/10 ml), which can be mixed with milk to counter its bitter taste, reducing its tendency to cause nausea when taken on an empty stomach.[41] Chloral hydrate should be used with caution in patients with renal or liver disease.[41] The pediatric oral or rectal dosage is 20 to 40 mg/kg, with onset of action in 30 to 60 minutes. For adults, the oral dosage is 500 mg to 1 gm,[32] and the sedative effect can last 5 to 6 hours.

Methoxyflurane

Methoxyflurane (Penthrane), a volatile liquid with a fruity odor, provides sedation and analgesia[42] when breathed through a hand-held inhaler. The inhaler, called the Analgizer, is a plastic cylinder with a mouthpiece and containing a felt wick that is saturated with methoxyflurane by pouring 2 to 3 ml of fluid into the cylinder. The inhaler may be refilled every 10 minutes. Self-administration by breathing through the inhaler produces a feeling of lightheadedness within 5 to 10 minutes. Constant dosing requires a conscious effort by the patient, so overdosing is unlikely. Because the material is exhaled by the patient, adequate ventilation is important.

The total dosage for administering methoxyflurane with the inhaler should not exceed 15 ml,[42] and administration should be limited to the preoperative period. Methoxyflurane may produce a dose-dependent nephrotoxicity, which generally occurs when it is used as a general anesthetic for long periods of time.[42] This side effect is unlikely with the hand-held inhaler. Concurrent use in patients taking tetracycline can produce fatal renal toxicity. Hepatic toxicity, unrelated to dose, is also possible,[36] and for this reason, methoxyflurane use is contraindicated in patients with hepatic or kidney disease.[42] Because inhalation of methoxyflurane occasionally results in temporary loss of the gag reflex, the patient should fast after the procedure and be observed until the gag reflex returns.

PREOPERATIVE OPIOID ANALGESICS

Although cutaneous surgical procedures are often performed under local anesthesia, it is sometimes desirable to use a potent analgesic before surgery, especially if a complex procedure requiring multiple nerve blocks is planned. Opioid analgesics are usually necessary to provide an adequate degree of analgesia. Parenteral administration is often necessary, either by IM or IV injection. Opioids such as morphine or meperidine can produce nausea, vomiting, hypotension, and respiratory depression that can last for several hours.[43] Constipation can also be a problem after their use. In addition, they are usually poorly tolerated by patients with chronic breathing problems such as asthma and emphysema, and dosages must be adjusted in patients with liver or kidney dysfunction.[8] Opioids differ in their potency, duration of action, and tendency to produce side effects. For example, fentanyl is 50 to 100 times more potent than morphine[8] and approximately 750 times more potent than meperidine. Depending on the dosage, pain can be partially or completely relieved.[44] Opioids should not be used parenterally unless an opioid antagonist, such as naloxone, and resuscitative equipment are available.[8]

Morphine

Morphine has both sedative and analgesic properties that can last 6 to 10 hours,[5] and it commonly produces a feeling of euphoria.[45] Nausea is also common, especially after the first dose.[46] Morphine is available in dosage strength of 10 mg/ml. The usual dosage is 10 to 15 mg, injected intramuscularly or subcutaneously, in adults and 0.1 to 0.2 mg/kg in children.[44] Peak respiratory depression occurs within 30 minutes after IM injection and 90 minutes after subcutaneous injection[44] and can last up to 5 hours.

Meperidine

Meperidine (Demerol) produces less euphoria and nausea[23] than morphine with a shorter onset of action[2] and a shorter half-life.[45] Meperidine is administered intramuscularly or subcutaneously in a dose of 50 to 100 mg in adults[5] and 1 to 2 mg/kg in children[47] every 3 to 4 hours. Analgesia begins to occur at 15 minutes and peaks at 45 to 60 minutes.[44] Respiratory depression is maximal within 1 hour of an IM injection and persists for up to 4 hours.[44] When administered intravenously with slow infusion, the full analgesic effect is observed in 15 minutes. IV administration can produce tachycardia,[44] and higher doses can depress cardiac contractility.[45] Meperidine is available in a variety of different concentrations for parenteral use.[36]

Fentanyl

Fentanyl (Sublimaze) is a very potent opioid analgesic that possesses little sedative activity at low doses (1 to 2 μg/kg).[45] An advantage over other opioids is that it is less likely to induce nausea or vomiting than either meperidine or morphine.[36] The analgesic effect is rapid in onset with a shorter duration of action.[45] Unlike other opioids, fentanyl does not cause the release of histamine[44] but can stimulate a strong cholinergic action resulting in bradycardia, which occasionally requires the coadministration of atropine.[5]

Respiratory depression from administration of fentanyl, although of shorter duration,[44] occurs much more rapidly than with other narcotics.[5] Rapid injection of fentanyl should be avoided, since generalized muscle rigidity can occur.[44] Excessive dosing of fentanyl can produce apnea, with the peak effect on ventilation being seen within 5 to 15 minutes after a single IV injection.[36] Because it is metabolized by a number of different pathways, fentanyl can even be used cautiously in patients with renal or liver disease.[8]

Although not yet available for general use, fentanyl citrate at a dose of 5 to 20 μg/kg has been shown to produce sedation and analgesia within 30 minutes after transmucosal dosing using a "lollipop."[48, 49] The analgesic effect has been shown to last 1 to 2 hours with little respiratory depression. The onset of analgesia is significantly delayed, more than 60 minutes, if the medication is administered orally.[48]

Fentanyl is usually administered parenterally in an IM dosage of 50 to 100 μg.[5] It is available in ampules containing 50 μg/ml of fentanyl base.[36] The analgesic effect begins within 7 to 8 minutes after injection and lasts 1 to 2 hours.[36] IV administration produces an almost immediate analgesic effect that peaks 3 to 5 minutes after injection.[5] The adult IV dosage is 2 μg/kg (100 to 200 μg),[45] which provides adequate analgesia for most procedures and may be repeated every 30 to 60 minutes as needed. The analgesic effect can last up to 1 hour and is usually of shorter duration than the effect on ventilation.[45] IV doses greater than 200 μg can produce respiratory depression[46] and should only be given with ventilatory support. The pediatric dosage of fentanyl is 0.5 to 2.0 μg/kg IV or IM.[45]

Adjunctive Agents

ANTIHISTAMINES

Antihistamines are somewhat less effective than other agents in producing sedation.[1, 32] Their main use as a preoperative agent is as an antiemetic, which is helpful in countering the nausea and vomiting that may be induced by the opiates.[32] Antihistamines also offer a fairly high degree of safety, which makes them sometimes useful as sedatives for children. In addition, they produce a bronchodilatory effect that may be helpful in patients with asthma or bronchitis or to help counter certain allergic reactions.[36]

Hydroxyzine

Hydroxyzine (Vistaril) is rapidly absorbed from the gastrointestinal tract and manifests clinical effects usually within 15 to 30 minutes,[5] with a peak effect in 1 to 2 hours.[32] It frequently causes a slight decrease in heart rate[50] and may potentiate the effect of opiates.[51] It is available for oral administration as a capsule (25 and 50 mg) and as an oral suspension (25 mg/5 ml). The dosage as a preoperative sedative is 50 to 100 mg in adults[5] and 0.6 mg/kg in children. Parenterally, hydroxyzine is administered by deep IM injection, usually in a dosage of 25 to 100 mg in adults and 1 mg/kg in children.[25]

Promethazine

Promethazine (Phenergan) is also well absorbed when administered orally, having an onset of action of 20 minutes. Although it usually has a significant sedative effect in adults, paradoxical hyperexcitability reactions have been reported to occur after relative overdosage in children. In addition to being available in tablet forms of 12.5, 25, and 50 mg and as a syrup of 6.25 mg/5 ml for pediatric use, it is also available as rectal suppositories of 12.5, 25, and 50 mg. The rectal suppository is especially useful postoperatively to control nausea or vomiting induced by pain or use of opiates. Dosage for sedation is 25 to 50 mg in adults and 0.5 mg/kg in children. Dosage for postoperative nausea in adults is a 25-mg rectal suppository twice a day and for children, 0.5 mg/kg twice daily. Promethazine is also available for IM administration in a dosage of 25 to 50 mg in adults and 0.5 mg/kg in children.[25]

ATROPINE

Atropine is occasionally indicated to reduce salivary and bronchial secretions and overstimulation of vagus reflexes induced by preoperative agents.[25, 46] It produces dilation of the pupil, blurred vision, dryness of the mouth, and tachycardia.[46] The usual IM or subcutaneous adult dosage is 0.3 to 0.6 mg 30 to 60 minutes before surgery, although it may also be given intravenously at the induction of anesthesia. The pediatric dosage is 0.02 mg/kg intramuscularly or intravenously.[2, 25]

NALOXONE

Naloxone (Narcan) is the preferred opioid antagonist for respiratory depression induced by opioids,[45] as it reverses the sedative and analgesic effects[44] while producing minimal side effects.[46] The usual IV dosage for adults is 0.2 to 0.4 mg, which is titrated at a rate of 0.2 mg every 2 minutes to the desired clinical response.[5, 45] Reversal of respiratory depression occurs within 1 to 2 minutes.[44] Because it has a relatively short half-life, it must be readministered every 1 to 2 hours to maintain its antagonistic effects.[8, 36] If IV administration is not possible, naloxone may be given intramuscularly or subcutaneously.[47] The usual IV pediatric dosage is 0.01 to 0.1 mg/kg, starting at the lowest dose and then increasing in a stepwise manner until the desired effect is achieved.[47]

Combined Drug Regimens

ADULTS

Many different combinations of drug regimens for adults exist, usually combining a sedative with an opioid analgesic. The choice of a particular drug regimen is often a personal one, largely based on previous experience with the different agents. Caution should be exercised with combined drug regimens, since drugs can have synergistic effects resulting in respiratory depression.

Several different regimens have been found to be useful in adults. One combines the use of diazepam (5 to 10 mg sublingually) 30 to 60 minutes before surgery and meperidine (50 to 100 mg) with hydroxyzine (25 to 50 mg) intramuscularly 20 to 30 minutes before surgery. This is a generally well-tolerated regimen that provides adequate sedation and analgesia, even for fairly complicated procedures. Another regimen uses an IM injection of midazolam (5 mg) 30 to 60 minutes before surgery and fentanyl (100 µg) intravenously 3 to 5 minutes before surgery. This combination provides a good mixture of sedation and analgesia preoperatively for more involved procedures. The substitution of oxymorphone (1 mg intravenously) instead of fentanyl has been shown to result in significant postoperative analgesia.[52] The combined use of either diazepam or midazolam with fentanyl should be used with caution in patients with cardiovascular disease.[45]

Another drug that is sometimes used in combination therapy is ketamine,[53] a phencyclidine derivative that can produce intense analgesia without significant respiratory depression.[46, 54] For this reason, it is sometimes preferred over opioid analgesics. In cutaneous surgery, this analgesic effect can significantly lessen the discomfort from injections of local anesthetics.[53] The major drawback of ketamine, however, is that it frequently produces bizarre hallucinations, confusion, violent behavior, hypertension, and tachycardia,[46] which necessitates concomitant use of a sedative such as diazepam or midazolam.[53] A combination regimen with these drugs begins with IV injection of midazolam (0.075 mg/kg). After 3 to 5 minutes, ketamine is subsequently infused in a dose of 0.5 mg/kg over 2 to 3 minutes[53] to produce anesthesia that will last for 15 to 30 minutes.[46] If additional analgesia is required, a supplemental dose of ketamine (10 mg) can be administered. This combination with a local anesthetic can provide adequate sedation and analgesia for most larger cutaneous surgery procedures with a minimal risk of cardiorespiratory depression.[53] Analgesia begins within 1 minute of IV administration and 3 to 8 minutes after IM injection.[28] IM dosing of ketamine at 0.4 mg/kg will produce analgesia for approximately 90 minutes.[28] Ketamine should not be used in patients with hypertension, coronary artery disease, or psychiatric disorders.[28, 53]

CHILDREN

Chloral hydrate, as a single agent, is often adequate for most procedures in children. If sedation and analgesia are both desired, oral premedication with atropine (0.02 mg/kg), meperidine (1.5 mg/kg), and diazepam (0.1 mg/kg) is reported to be very effective.[55]

Other Methods of Sedation

MUSIC

Music can be a useful distraction for many patients undergoing surgical procedures. This is most effectively accomplished with a portable radio or cassette player to which headphones are attached.

HYPNOSIS

Hypnosis can also be effective in relieving a patient's feeling of anxiety for the surgical procedure.[56] The hypnotic technique, which requires special training, takes only about 3 minutes to perform. However, patients need to be screened preoperatively for their ability to undergo hypnosis. Courses for physicians interested in learning hypnotic techniques are conducted by many local or regional professional dental societies.

Postoperative Analgesics

Some degree of pain is an inevitable consequence of surgery. Its severity is often predicated on the complexity and location[8] of the surgery. In large part, the personality of the patient determines the ability to tolerate pain, which varies considerably. For these reasons, the approach to postoperative pain should be tailored to meet the individual needs of the patient.

Postoperative pain from cutaneous surgery has multiple causes. Tissue injury during surgery results in the production of various substances such as eicosanoids that either sensitize nerves to painful stimuli or mediate the sensation of pain.[8] Pain is often more prominent when there is pressure from edema or bleeding, when the tissue is ischemic, or when there is intervening infection. Pain is also more likely after large or complex procedures, especially when performed on the head or neck.

Because the severity of pain can be made worse by anxiety,[8] much of the apprehension about postoperative pain can be relieved by providing the patient with a simple preoperative explanation of the degree of discomfort that can be reasonably expected from the procedure. Written instructions detailing the prescribed treatment plan for postoperative discomfort are also helpful and should include a discussion of the common side effects associated with analgesics.

Treatment of Postoperative Pain

The treatment of postoperative pain begins with good postoperative wound care. The application of a pressure dressing and the use of an ice bag during the first 24 hours will help to relieve pain, reduce swelling, and decrease the chance of bleeding complications. For relatively minor procedures, this may offer sufficient relief to obviate the need for analgesics in many patients.

Patients who can be expected to have moderate to severe pain as a result of the nature of their problem or the procedure should be offered analgesics routinely. Because it is easier to prevent than to treat pain,[8] analgesics should be offered at regular 4- to 6-hour intervals during the first 12 to 24 hours after surgery. Intermittent or "as-needed" dosing of analgesics during this period is less effective in relieving pain and anxiety than regular dosing[8] and should be avoided unless the need for analgesics seems doubtful. Because pain normally decreases over time, it is appropriate to adjust dosing accordingly after 24 to 48 hours. For most cutaneous surgical procedures, it is unusual for patients to require analgesics after 48 hours in the absence of complications such as bleeding or infection. Patients who complain of intensified pain after this time should be evaluated by the physician.

The choice of analgesics should be dictated by the severity of the pain expected after surgery and the ability of the patient to tolerate discomfort. A patient with a relatively low tolerance for pain will require analgesics for even minimal discomfort. For mild pain, a nonsteroidal anti-inflammatory drug (NSAID) such as acetaminophen should be sufficient. If moderate to severe pain is expected, an NSAID containing an opioid analgesic is usually required. Because cutaneous surgery is frequently done on an outpatient basis, oral dosing is preferable. The dosage of pain medications must be adjusted according to the age,[8] weight, and physical status of the patient. Pain relief should be achieved with minimum sedation. Infants and children often receive insufficient analgesics,[44] and regular dosing of analgesics, every 4 to 6 hours, should be routine for patients in this age group for the first 24 hours, as it is often difficult to tell when they are having pain.[47]

NSAIDs

NSAIDs are the cornerstone for the treatment of postoperative pain. They reduce pain by affecting the generation of prostaglandins both peripherally at the site of surgery and centrally in the central nervous system.

ACETAMINOPHEN

Acetaminophen is the NSAID of choice for treatment of mild to moderate postoperative pain, as it is the least likely to alter the hemostatic action of platelets and is generally well tolerated by all patients. Acetaminophen has antipyretic activity and will mask a fever if taken regularly. It is available in 325- and 500-mg tablets; a pediatric oral solution of 160 mg/5 ml is also available. The normal adult oral dosage is 325 mg to 1 gm every 4 to 6 hours, while the pediatric dosage is 10 mg/kg every 4 to 6 hours.[47] If stronger analgesia is required,

acetaminophen is often prescribed in combination with opioid analgesics.

ASPIRIN

Aspirin should be avoided because of the chance of bleeding complications.

IBUPROFEN

Ibuprofen has less tendency to affect platelet coagulation than aspirin and may be considered for use in an attempt to avoid opioid analgesics. The usual adult oral dosage is 200 to 600 mg every 4 to 6 hours.

Opioid Analgesics

Severe pain, especially when associated with anxiety, often requires the use of opioid analgesics. Opioids act peripherally at the site of surgery to induce analgesia by a direct stabilizing effect on the sensory nerve terminals.[8] They also can inhibit the release of substance P and other peptides from primary afferent nerves.[8, 44] However, sensory nerve pathways in the central nervous system are most sensitive to opioids and are generally felt to be more important sites clinically for analgesia of postoperative pain.[8]

Common side effects of opioids include euphoria, dependence liability, respiratory depression, sedation, nausea, vomiting, constipation, urinary retention, and pruritus.[8] Opioid analgesics are often prescribed in combination with acetaminophen, as the two agents have a synergistic effect in reducing pain.[8, 44] It should be noted that if opioids are used parenterally during the preoperative period, the dose of the medication should be reduced to as low as one fourth of that usually recommended during the immediate postoperative period to decrease the risk of overdosage.

CODEINE

The analgesic action of codeine is thought to occur in part by its metabolism in the liver to morphine,[8, 44] which makes it effective in treating moderate pain.[44] It has good oral efficacy as a result of lower first-pass metabolism by the liver.[44] Analgesia begins within 20 minutes of administration and is maximal at 1 to 2 hours[47]; its duration is 4 to 6 hours.[44] The usual adult oral dosage is 15 to 60 mg every 4 to 6 hours. A higher dosage does not significantly increase analgesia.[46] Codeine is available in 15-, 30-, and 60-mg tablets. It is often prescribed as Tylenol #3, which combines acetaminophen 325 mg with 30 mg of codeine in each tablet. The usual adult oral dosage is 1 to 2 tablets every 4 to 6 hours. A pediatric elixir is also available containing 12 mg of codeine and 120 mg of acetaminophen/5 ml.[36] The pediatric oral dosage of codeine is 0.5 to 1.0 mg/kg every 4 to 6 hours.[47]

OXYCODONE

Oxycodone, a derivative of morphine, is equipotent to morphine[44] and ten times more potent than codeine. It is indicated for the relief of moderate or moderately severe pain,[45] but because it is metabolized in part to codeine, it should be avoided in patients intolerant of codeine. Oxycodone is available in 5-mg tablets, and the usual adult dosage is 5 to 10 mg every 4 to 6 hours. It is commonly prescribed as Percocet, which combines acetaminophen (325 mg) with oxycodone (5 mg) in each tablet. The usual adult oral dosage is one tablet every 6 hours.[36]

HYDROCODONE

Hydrocodone is a semisynthetic opioid analgesic that is very effective when given orally. It is indicated for the relief of moderate or moderately severe pain.[36] Hydrocodone is available in 5-mg tablets and in a syrup (5 mg/5 ml). Vicodin is a commonly prescribed form that combines hydrocodone (5 mg) with acetaminophen (500 mg) in each tablet. The usual adult dosage is one to two tablets every 4 to 6 hours,[36] while the dosage for children 6 to 12 years of age is 2.5 mg every 4 to 6 hours.[36]

LEVORPHANOL

Levorphanol is a very strong oral analgesic that is equipotent to morphine but is less likely to produce nausea,[44] constipation,[36] or sedation. It is indicated for the treatment of severe pain.[36] Its fairly long duration of action, 6 to 8 hours,[36] means that it may only need to be given one to two times per day.[46] It is available in 2-mg tablets, and the usual adult oral dosage is 2 to 3 mg every 6 to 8 hours.[36] The use of more potent analgesics such as levorphanol is rarely indicated for treatment of pain secondary to cutaneous surgery. If pain is so severe as to warrant the use of this medication, other causes of pain, such as infection or bleeding, should be investigated.

Postoperative Nausea

Nausea is a fairly common problem after extensive surgery of either the face or scalp, and there are multiple possible causes. The first is pain, especially when moderate to severe. Usually, adequate treatment of postoperative pain by regular dosing with an analgesic will help reduce this tendency. Another common cause of postoperative nausea is extensive surgery of the scalp, especially when the galea is manipulated; this may reflexively produce nausea several hours after surgery, even in the absence of significant pain. Use of opioid analgesics, especially codeine, commonly produces nausea by a direct effect on the central nervous system.

Treatment of nausea is usually with either prochlorperazine or promethazine.[46] Because oral dosing often compounds the problem, prescribing a rectal suppository is prudent. Both agents are available in a 25-mg sup-

pository, and the usual adult dosage is 25 mg every 12 hours.[36] Prochlorperazine is also available in a 5-mg suppository for children 6 to 12 years of age. The usual rectal dosage is 5 mg every 12 hours.[36]

SUMMARY

An extra margin of safety is derived from performing many cutaneous surgical procedures under local, rather than general, anesthesia. However, it is important to recognize that many patients, especially children, will have significant levels of anxiety preoperatively that could have an adverse impact on the skill with which the procedure can be performed.

For this reason, a thorough understanding of the various types and uses of sedatives and analgesics is vital to the success of the operation. When these agents are used appropriately, most patients can be expected to have a more pleasant experience with minimal discomfort and the least amount of anxiety possible.

REFERENCES

1. White PF: Pharmacologic and clinical aspects of preoperative medication. Anesth Analg 65:693–694, 1986.
2. Krane EJ, Davis PJ, Smith RM: Preoperative preparation. In: Motoyama EK, Davis PJ (eds): Smith's Anesthesia for Infants and Children. CV Mosby, St. Louis, 1990.
3. Edmondson HD, Roscoe B, Vickers MD: Biochemical evidence of anxiety in dental patients. Br Med J 4:7–9, 1972.
4. Spiro SR: Physical evaluation prior to conscious-sedation (parenteral) administration. In: Spiro SR (ed): Pain and Anxiety Control in Dentistry. Jack K. Burgess, Englewood, NJ, 1981.
5. Snow JC: Manual of Anesthesia. Little, Brown, Boston, 1982.
6. Henefer EP: Physical evaluation prior to general anesthesia administration. In: Spiro SR (ed): Pain and Anxiety Control in Dentistry. Jack K. Burgess, Englewood, NJ, 1981.
7. Wood AJJ: Drug disposition and pharmacokinetics. In: Wood M, Wood AJJ (eds): Drugs and Anesthesia: Pharmacology for Anesthesiologists. Williams & Wilkins, Baltimore, 1990.
8. Alexander JI, Hill RG: Postoperative Pain Control. Blackwell Scientific, Boston, 1987.
9. White PF, Vasconez LO, Mathes SA, et al: Comparison of midazolam and diazepam for sedation during plastic surgery. Plast Reconstr Surg 81:703–710, 1988.
10. Steven JM, Cohen DE: Anesthesia equipment and monitoring. In: Motoyama EK, Davis PJ (eds): Smith's Anesthesia for Infants and Children. CV Mosby Co, St. Louis, 1990.
11. Memery HN: Anesthesia mortality in private practice. A ten-year study. JAMA 194:1185–1188, 1965.
12. Blitt CD: Monitoring during outpatient anesthesia. Int Anesthesiol Clin 20:17–25, 1982.
13. Williams JE: Plastic surgery in an office surgical unit. Plast Reconstr Surg 52:513–519, 1973.
14. Singer R, Lewis CM: Rhytidectomies in office operating rooms. Plast Reconstr Surg 63:173–175, 1979.
15. Grande DJ, Koranda FC, Guthrie D: Monitoring respirations for outpatient surgery. J Dermatol Surg Oncol 9:338–339, 1983.
16. Shimada K, Ogura H, Kawamoto A, et al: Noninvasive ambulatory blood pressure monitoring during clinic visit in elderly hypertensive patients. Clin Exp Hypertens 12:151–170, 1990.
17. Mazel MS, Bolton HE, Tapia FA, et al: Prevention of cardiac arrest during surgery. Dis Chest 45:639–645, 1964.
18. Singer R, Thomas PE: Pulse oximeter in the ambulatory aesthetic surgical facility. Plast Reconstr Surg 82:111–115, 1988.
19. Alexander CM, Teller LE, Gross JB: Principles of pulse oximetry: theoretical and practical considerations. Anesth Analg 68:368–376, 1989.

20. Yelderman M, New W Jr: Evaluation of pulse oximetry. Anesthesiology 59:349–352, 1983.
21. Brodsky J, Shulman MS, Swan M, et al: Pulse oximetry during one lung ventilation. Anesthesiology 63:212–214, 1985.
22. Standards and guidelines for cardiopulmonary resuscitation (CPR) and emergency cardiac care (ECC). JAMA 244:453–508, 1980.
23. LaSalle AD: Suggested agents, dosage and routes of administration. In: Spiro SR (ed): Pain and Anxiety Control in Dentistry. Jack K. Burgess, Englewood NJ, 1981.
24. Hays D: Do it yourself the Z-track way. Am J Nurs 74:1070–1071, 1974.
25. Wood M: Anticholinergic drugs: anesthetic premedication. In: Wood M, Wood AJJ (eds): Drugs and Anesthesia: Pharmacology for Anesthesiologists. Williams & Wilkins, Baltimore, 1990.
26. Kawar P, McGlimpsey JG, Gamble JAS, et al: Midazolam as a sedative in dentistry. Br J Anaesth 54:1137, 1982.
27. Clarke PRF, Eccersley PS, Frisby JP: The amnesic effect of diazepam (Valium). Br J Anaesth 42:690–697, 1970.
28. Wood M: Intravenous anesthetic agents. In: Wood M, Wood AJJ (eds): Drugs and Anesthesia: Pharmacology for Anesthesiologists. Williams & Wilkins, Baltimore, 1990.
29. deJong RH, Bonin JD: Benzodiazepines protect mice from local anesthetic convulsions and death. Anesth Analg 60:385–389, 1981.
30. Gale GD, Galloon S, Porter WR: Sublingual lorazepam: a better premedication? Br J Anaesth 55:761–765, 1983.
31. Jakobsen H, Hertz JB, Johansen JR, et al: Premedication before day surgery. Br J Anaesth 57:300–305, 1985.
32. Peterson LJ, Topazian RG: Ataractics and sedatives. In: Spiro SR (ed): Pain and Anxiety Control in Dentistry. Jack K. Burgess, Englewood, NJ, 1981.
33. Steen SN, Hahl D: Controlled evaluation of parenteral diazepam as preanesthetic medication: a statistical study. Anesth Analg 48:549–554, 1969.
34. Dundee JW, Haslett WH: The benzodiazepines: a review of their actions and uses relative to anesthetic practice. Br J Anaesth 42:217–234, 1970.
35. Conner JT, Bellville JW, Wender RH, et al: Evaluation of intravenous diazepam as a surgical premedicant. Anesth Analg 56:211–215, 1977.
36. Barnhart ER (ed): Physician's Desk Reference. Medical Economics, Oradell, NJ, 1991.
37. Reves JG, Fragen RJ, Vinik R, et al: Midazolam: pharmacology and uses. Anesthesiology 62:310–324, 1985.
38. Crevoisier CH, Eckert M, Helzmann P, et al: Relation between the clinical effect and the pharmacokinetics of midazolam following I.M. and I.V. administration. Arzneimittelforschung 31:2211–2215, 1985.
39. Philip WK: Hazards of amnesia after midazolam in ambulatory surgical patients. Anesth Analg 66:97–98, 1987.
40. Benvenuti D: Benzodiazepine for ambulatory surgery. Plast Reconstr Surg 79:1008–1009, 1987.
41. Rall TW: Hypnotics and sedatives, ethanol. In: Gilman AG, Rall TW, Nies AS, Taylor P (eds): The Pharmacological Basis of Therapeutics. Pergamon Press, New York, 1990.
42. Marshall BE, Longnecker DE: General anesthetics. In: Gilman AG, Rall TW, Nies AS, Taylor P (eds): The Pharmacological Basis of Therapeutics. Pergamon Press, New York, 1990.
43. Downes JJ, Kemp RA, Lambertsen CJ: The magnitude and duration of respiratory depression due to fentanyl and meperidine in man. J Pharmacol Exp Ther 158:416–420, 1967.
44. Jaffe JH, Martin WR: Opioid analgesics and antagonists. In: Gilman AG, Rall TW, Nies AS, Taylor P (eds): The Pharmacological Basis of Therapeutics. Pergamon Press, New York, 1990.
45. Wood M: Opioid agonists and antagonists. In: Wood M, Wood AJJ (eds): Drugs and Anesthesia: Pharmacology for Anesthesiologists. Williams & Wilkins, Baltimore, 1990.
46. Vickers MD, Schnieden H, Wood-Smith FG: Drugs in Anaesthetic Practice. Butterworths & Co, Boston, 1984.
47. Yaster M, Deshpande JK: Management of pediatric pain with opioid analgesics. J Pediatr 113:421–429, 1988.
48. Stanley TH, Hague B, Mock DL, et al: Oral transmucosal fentanyl citrate (lollipop) premedication in human volunteers. Anesth Analg 69:21–27, 1989.
49. Feld LH, Champeau MW, Steennis CA, et al: Preanesthetic medication in children: a comparison of oral transmucosal fentanyl citrate versus placebo. Anesthesiology 71:374–377, 1989.
50. Andersen TW, Gravenstein JS: Cardiovascular effects of sedative doses of pentobarbital and hydroxyzine. Anesthesiology 27:272–278, 1966.
51. Beaver WT: Comparison of the analgesic effects of morphine sulphate, hydroxyzine and their combination in patients with postoperative pain. In: Bonica JJ (ed): Advances in Pain Research and Therapy. Raven Press, New York, 1976.
52. Shafer A, White PF, Urquhart ML, et al: Outpatient premedication: use of midazolam and opioid analgesics. Anesthesiology 71:495–501, 1989.
53. Scarborough DA, Bisaccia E, Swensen RD: Anesthesia for outpatient dermatologic cosmetic surgery: midazolam–low dosage ketamine anesthesia. J Dermatol Surg Oncol 15:658–663, 1989.
54. Campbell RL: Dissociative drugs. In: Spiro SR (ed): Pain and Anxiety Control in Dentistry. Jack K. Burgess, Englewood, NJ, 1981.
55. Brzustowicz RM, Nelson DA, Betts EK, et al: Efficacy of oral premedication for pediatric outpatient surgery. Anesthesiology 60:475–477, 1984.
56. Goldmann L, Ogg TW, Levey AB: Hypnosis and day care anesthesia. Anaesthesia 36:10–15, 1981.

CHAPTER 24

Dogear Repairs

DIRK B. ROBERTSON

A skin protrusion present at the end of an excision is commonly referred to as a dogear. Although this term is not particularly descriptive, it has, in the period since the 1960s, become firmly rooted in the surgical literature.[1] A number of alternative terms have been suggested to describe this fold of excess skin that protrudes above the surface. These include pucker,[2] lentoid,[3] and tricone.[4] Concerns regarding possible patient misconception with the term dogear are clearly justified, and uniform acceptance of an alternative term is highly desirable. In an attempt to avoid further confusion in nomenclature, the descriptive term "tissue protrusion" will be used in place of "dogear" in this chapter.

Tissue Dynamics

Tissue protrusions are caused by the presence of redundant skin at the ends or sides of an excision. Before selecting the best modality for their removal, the cutaneous surgeon should assess the causative factors responsible for their development. The amount of tissue protrusion formed in a given wound is fundamentally determined by the amount of rotation and advancement of the surrounding skin. The intrinsic tissue elasticity of the surrounding skin and the local surface contours also contribute to the final degree of tissue protrusion.[5]

When the angle present at the apex of an excision is closed by rotation around the pivot point, a "standing cone" (Fig. 24–1) is formed.[6] The pivot point is forced out of the plane of closure and, in usual circumstances, rises above the surface of the skin. Occasionally, the pivot point may be forced below the plane of the skin surface, resulting in an "inverted cone." In most anatomic sites, the intrinsic elasticity of the skin is sufficient so that if the angle of closure is less than 15 degrees, tissue protrusion will be minimal. When the rotational angle of closure is greater than 30 degrees, a noticeable tissue protrusion will usually be produced.

Suturing wound edges of unequal length into apposition results in the linear advancement of excess surrounding tissue, which creates a tissue protrusion. In fusiform elliptical excisions, the opposing skin edges are moved toward a central line of closure. The wound edges may be conceptualized as arcs whose lengths are greater than that of the final closure line. When the sides of the wound are brought into apposition, tissue along each edge is compressed. When the limits of the

Figure 24–1. Closing a wound by rotation around a pivot point *(left)* will create a standing cone *(right)*.

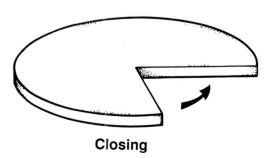

Closing

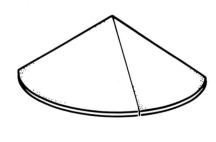

Standing Cone

local tissue compression characteristics are exceeded, tissue protrusions form.[5]

The intrinsic elasticity, or "stretchability," of skin contributes significantly to the formation of tissue protrusions. In areas where the dermis is relatively inflexible and lacks elasticity, even small degrees of tissue rotation may result in protrusion of the pivot point. In areas where the skin possesses significant elasticity, larger angles of rotation are absorbed by tissue compression without causing significant protrusion. The elasticity of a given area may be estimated by lifting and stretching the skin between the surgeon's index finger and thumb.

Intrinsic tissue elasticity is related to the patient's age, amount of actinic damage, and anatomic site. In general, younger patients possess greater tissue elasticity for a given anatomic site than older patients. Skin that demonstrates marked actinic damage will possess less elasticity than photo-protected skin. In some anatomic sites, such as the back of the hand or elbow, the skin is easily movable but quite inelastic, and even a 30-degree angle of closure may produce a noticeable tissue protrusion.[7]

Circumferential closures performed on highly convex surfaces, such as the arm, will result in tissue protrusions at the ends of the closure. This occurs because the edges of the wound at the midpoint along the long axis of closure lie at a higher elevation than the ends of the wound. As the suture line is closed over the convexity, it is drawn into a lower elevation than the original plane of the excision, and tissue protrusions are produced at the ends. Tissue protrusions present on convex surfaces may be minimized by utilizing an S-plasty design (Fig. 24–2), which allows the terminal ends to continue on a relatively horizontal plane, eliminating large height differentials.[5, 8, 9]

If excess subcutaneous fat is present at the apex of an excision, the resultant elevation of the angle of closure may mimic a tissue protrusion. Removal of the excess fat, with adequate undermining of the apex, will invariably result in resolution of this "pseudo-dogear."[7] In a similar fashion, swelling caused by infiltration of a local anesthesic may mimic a true tissue protrusion, especially in areas where there is loose or easily distensible subcutaneous tissue. This artifactual tissue protrusion will resolve spontaneously, and care should be taken to proceed with surgical correction of only those tissue protrusions that are not expected to resolve with time.

Figure 24–2. Circumferential closure of a wound on a convex surface *(A)* will create tissue protrusions at the ends *(B)*. An S-plasty design *(C)* allows the terminal ends to remain in the same horizontal plane *(D)*.

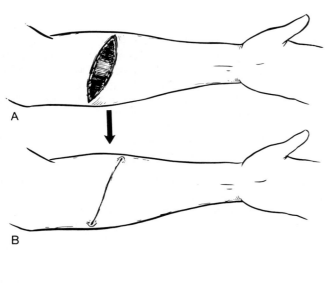

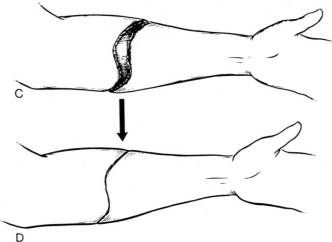

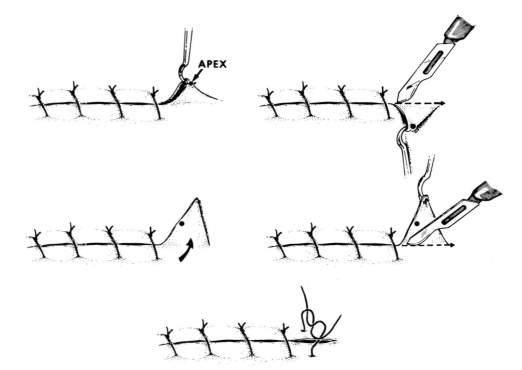

Figure 24–3. The linear repair of a tissue protrusion begins with lifting the apex with a skin hook *(top left)*, drawing the tissue to one side *(top right)*, and incising the base. The triangular wedge is then draped over the wound edge *(middle left)*, and the base is incised *(middle right)* before closing the wound in a straight line *(bottom)*.

Methods of Tissue Protrusion Correction

Several methods have proven useful in the surgical correction of tissue protrusions. Before planning the removal of a protrusion, it is often beneficial to partially close the wound edges to determine whether a tissue protrusion will form. This also helps define the degree of excess tissue that will need to be removed and allows the surgeon to design the repair to be certain that the excision lines are aligned with the relaxed skin tension lines.

LINEAR REPAIR

Linear repair is conceptually simple, easily performed, and particularly useful when it is desirable to extend the excision in a straight line. The apex of the tissue protrusion is elevated with a skin hook to define the geometry of the tissue protrusion in the shape of a standing cone (Fig. 24–3). The apex of the cone is drawn to one side so that the base of the tissue protrusion is in line with the long axis of the anticipated wound closure. The base is incised and undermined to free up a triangular wedge of tissue. The triangular section is then draped over the underlying wound edge with gentle tension, and the base is incised over the line of closure. The wound is then repaired in a straight line.

An alternative method to correct a tissue protrusion in a linear fashion is to remove it in two smaller triangular segments.[2, 10] After elevation of the apex of the tissue protrusion, a scalpel is placed in the center of the excess tissue with the cutting edge placed upward (Fig. 24–4). The tissue protrusion is then incised into two halves. Each respective triangle of tissue is elevated and its base incised in a line continuous with the long axis of the wound. The resulting incision is then closed in linear fashion.

CURVED REPAIR

The curved tissue protrusion repair is particularly useful when an oblique extension of the excision line will match an existing adjacent wrinkle, fold, or crease. The excess tissue at the apex is lifted with a skin hook to form a standing cone (Fig. 24–5). The excess tissue is gently pulled to the side so that a curved incision may be placed in the desired location (e.g., the final line of extension from the excision end). The triangular portion is then undermined and gently draped over the opposing side of the wound, and the base of this triangle is then incised, utilizing the underlying cut edge as a template. The wound is then closed in standard fashion.

HOCKEY-STICK REPAIR

In instances when an acute angle may be required to fit a tissue protrusion excision into a resting skin tension line, a hockey-stick repair often proves helpful. Again, the tissue protrusion is lifted with a skin hook (Fig. 24–6), and an incision is made tangential to the base of the standing cone and oblique to the long axis of the main incision. This incision should be precisely placed in the desired line of closure of the tissue protrusion repair. The triangular portion of tissue is then undermined and draped over the wound with gentle tension. The underlying cut edge serves as a template for making the incision along the base of the draped triangle. The defect is repaired in traditional fashion.

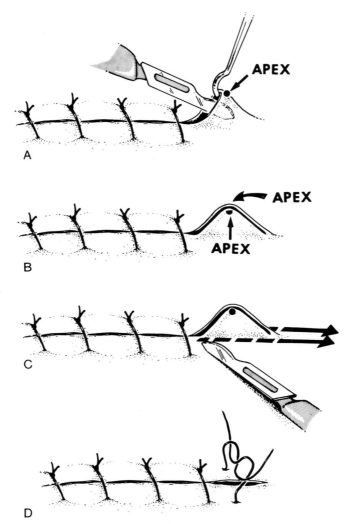

Figure 24–4. An alternative method incises the excess tissue in the middle *(A)* to create two small triangles *(B)*, which are both incised at their bases *(C)* before closing the wound in a straight line *(D)*.

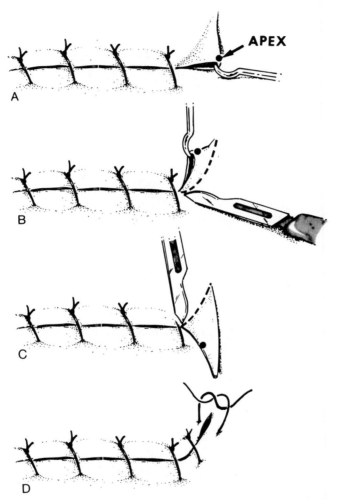

Figure 24–5. In the curved repair, the excess tissue is lifted at the apex *(A)* and pulled to one side so a curved incision can be made *(B)*. The tissue is draped over the wound *(C)*, and the triangle of tissue is removed along the cut edge of the incision *(D)* before final closure.

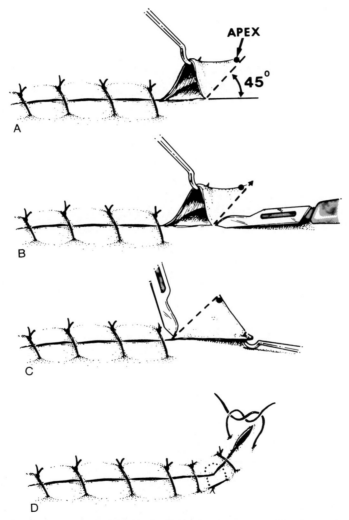

Figure 24–6. To perform a hockey-stick repair, an apex of tissue is lifted with a skin hook *(A)*, and an oblique incision is made at the base *(B)*. The excess tissue is draped over the wound *(C)*, and the triangle of tissue is removed along the cut edge of the incision *(D)* before final closure.

L-SHAPED REPAIR

When the tissue protrusion is predominantly unilateral as a result of closure of wounds of unequal length, the longer side may be reduced by using the concept of Burow's triangulation. This results in an L-shaped tissue protrusion repair. The excess tissue is picked up with a skin hook to form a lying half-cone (Fig. 24–7). The tissue protrusion is then incised from the distal cut edge of the excision to the apex of the lying half-cone. The triangle of tissue is undermined sufficiently to allow it to drape across the freshly cut edge, and a second cut is made at its base to permit standard wound closure.

T-SHAPED CORRECTION

When excess tissue is present on both sides at the end of an excision, use of bilateral Burow's triangulation repairs will result in a T-plasty. Conceptually, each side of the wound should be considered a lying half-cone (Fig. 24–8). The final closure to create a T-shaped repair is performed with a four-point tip stitch.

M-PLASTY REPAIR

Correcting tissue protrusions using an M-plasty is a variation of the Burow's triangulation T-plasty repair.[11] The tissue protrusion is elevated at the apex with a skin hook (Fig. 24–9), and incisions are made on both sides, tangential to the base, at 30- to 45-degree angles from the long axis of the excision line. The apron of tissue is then unfolded and draped over the newly incised wound edges, forming two new triangles overlying the lateral tissue. The bases of these triangles are then incised to match the cut edge of the tissue below. The resulting M-plasty is closed with a three-point suture.

SUMMARY

Closure of even the most carefully planned and executed excision may result in the development of tissue protrusions. The proficient cutaneous surgeon should have a basic understanding of the dynamics of tissue movement and skin elasticity, which will allow anticipation and subsequent correction of tissue protrusions

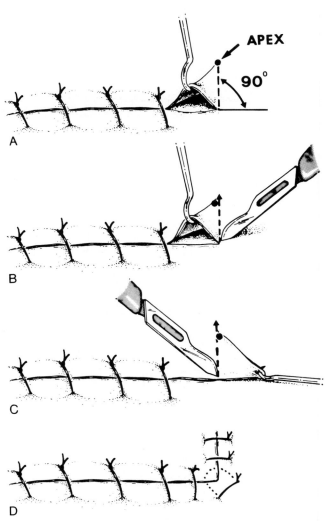

Figure 24–7. In an L-shaped repair, the tissue is lifted *(A)*, and a 90-degree-angle incision is made at its base *(B)*. The triangle is cut after draping the excess tissue over the incision line *(C)*, and the wound is closed in standard fashion *(D)*.

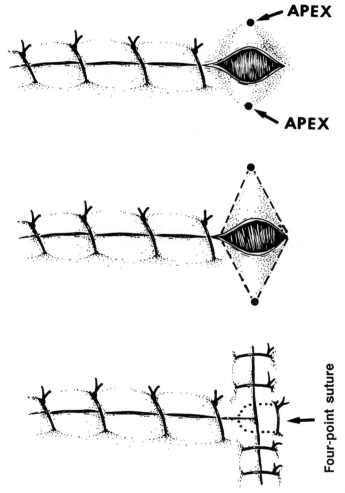

Figure 24–8. The T-shaped correction of tissue protrusions *(top)* creates two Burow's triangles *(middle)*. Closure is made with a tip stitch *(bottom)*.

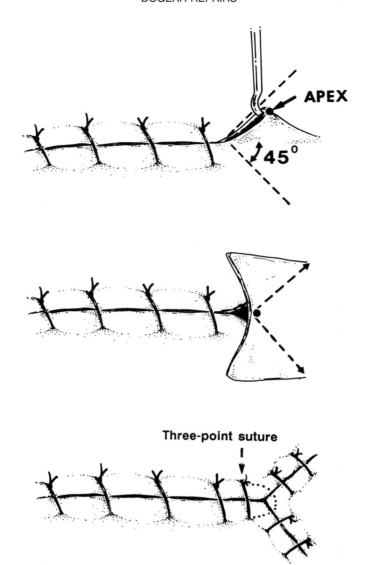

Figure 24–9. For M-plasty repair, the excess tissue is lifted at the apex *(top)* so that two tangential incisions can be made. The tissue that drapes over the lines *(middle)* is removed and the wound closed with a three-point stitch *(bottom).*

in the most expeditious fashion. An attempt should always be made to place the final incision line parallel to relaxed skin tension lines, preferably hidden in a nearby wrinkle, fold, or crease. Proper design and execution of these techniques may provide the critical difference that separates an average result from a superb cosmetic outcome.

REFERENCES

1. Limberg AA: Design of local flaps. In: Gibson T (ed): Modern Trends in Plastic Surgery. Butterworth & Co., London, 1966, p 2.
2. Bennett RG: Fundamentals of Cutaneous Surgery. CV Mosby, St. Louis, 1988.
3. Markley JM Jr: Lentoid. Plast Reconstr Surg 81:298–299, 1988.
4. Vaughan KT, Samlaska CP, Mulvaney MJ: Hello tricone; goodbye "dog-ear." Arch Dermatol 126:1366, 1990.
5. Dzubow LM: The dynamics of dog-ear formation and correction. J Dermatol Surg Oncol 7:722–728, 1985.
6. Davis WE, Renner GJ: Z-plasty and scar revision. In: Thomas JR, Holt R (eds): Facial Scars—Incision, Revision & Camouflage. CV Mosby, St. Louis, 1989.
7. Stegman SJ, Tromovitch TA, Glogau RG: Basics of Dermatologic Surgery. Year Book Medical, Chicago, 1983.
8. Zitelli JA: TIPS for a better ellipse. J Am Acad Dermatol 22:101–103, 1990.
9. Borges AF: Dog-ear repair. Plast Reconstr Surg 69:707–713, 1982.
10. Zachary CB: Basic cutaneous surgery. Churchill Livingstone, New York, 1991.
11. Salasche, SJ, Roberts LC: Dog-ear correction by M-plasty. J Dermatol Surg Oncol 10:478–482, 1984.

CHAPTER 25

Advanced Suturing Techniques and Layered Closures

THOMAS STASKO

The ultimate goal of suturing in cutaneous surgery is to reapproximate the skin surfaces in the most precise way possible that will result in the least noticeable scar. Although the simple interrupted suturing technique is the most common one utilized in skin surgery, many other advanced suturing techniques are also available. Although these techniques can successfully meet many specific objectives, each is associated with several intrinsic advantages and disadvantages that must be fully recognized to choose the best one for a given clinical situation.

Terminology

An understanding of suturing terminology is important in determining how each technique can be most beneficially used. Except for adhesive tape strip skin closures, all suture techniques involve the placement of suture material below the skin surface. If any of the suture material lies above the skin surface, the technique is referred to as partially buried. Such sutures can vary from the simple suture, in which less than 50% of the suture material is buried, to the removable running subcuticular suture, in which only the knotted suture ends remain above the skin surface. In a completely buried suture, such as an interrupted subcutaneous stitch, no part of the suture is above the skin surface. The general advantages of partially buried sutures include ease of placement and the relative lack of foreign body material in the wound. The more buried suture that is used, the fewer entrance and exit points that will

be required on the skin surface. By decreasing these puncture wounds, the risk of infection, formation of epithelial tracks, and "railroad track" scarring will be substantially reduced.[1-3]

The name of a suturing technique also often contains a description of the tissue level at which the suture is placed. A deep suture may be used to approximate muscle, fascia, cartilage, or subcutaneous fatty tissue. More superficial sutures may be subcuticular,[4] intradermal,[5-7] percutaneous, or epidermal. Suturing techniques may be referred to as simple or running. In a simple suture, each loop of suture is placed and tied individually and is separate from the next. In running sutures, each loop of suture is linked to the next in a continuous fashion. Simple sutures are generally easier to place and provide greater wound security, so that if one loop of the suture breaks, the others will maintain their position independently. Running sutures can be placed more rapidly, because fewer knots are tied. In addition, a running suture may be able to better distribute tension along the entire length of the wound.

Buried Sutures

Deeply placed buried sutures are commonly utilized to reapproximate the cut edges of deep structures such as muscle, cartilage, or fascia to restore the functional integrity and contours of the anatomic site. They may also be used to provide long-term support of a wound closed under tension (Fig. 25–1). In some deep wounds, buried sutures can be used to reduce the wound size[8] by simply plicating the fascia, which allows pleating and folding of the fascia on itself even if it has not been violated. This technique results in a substantial decrease

---

All the illustrations in this chapter, with the exception of Figures 25–4 and 25–12, have been redrawn courtesy of Mary Ann Stasko.

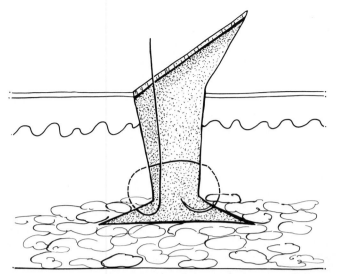

Figure 25–1. The buried suture includes the dermis and a significant amount of subdermal tissue to lend strength to the closure of the subcutaneous fat while providing initial epidermal approximation.

in the size of the wound, as well as a reduction in the surface tension on the wound edges.

Slight variations in placing buried sutures may help accomplish other specific goals as well. Increased wound eversion may be obtained by modifying the placement of the intradermal component of the suture. By arching closer to the skin surface in the superficial reticular dermis, a buried vertical mattress suture is created[7–9] (Fig. 25–2). If the wound is excessively long, a running buried suture may be placed.[10] This suture is initiated by placing the first loop of suture at the end of the wound in the usual manner. After tying the knot, only the free end of suture is cut, and additional loops of suture are placed in a running fashion. At the end of the wound, a buried slipknot is placed by tying the free end of the suture to the last loop. If space limitations make placement of a vertical buried suture difficult, the

suture may be placed in a horizontal fashion[11] (Fig. 25–3). Because the pursestring-like suture also offers the advantage of enclosing a large amount of tissue with each single stitch, care must be taken not to cause strangulation.

At times it is necessary to fix a wound margin in a specific position with regard to underlying structures or surface features. Such fixation allows proper distribution of tension across the wound to avoid distortion of adjacent structures and can also help to re-create surface and subsurface contours.[12] An example is the repair of a defect that crosses the nasofacial sulcus to involve two separate anatomic units (Fig. 25–4). A proposed closure might repair the cheek portion of the defect using tissue mobilized from the cheek. Meanwhile, the nasal portion of the defect is repaired using tissue mobilized from the nose. If the tissues from these two sites are simply sutured together, the skin with the greatest laxity will be stretched across the nasofacial sulcus, causing tenting and obliteration of the normal contours. However, by suturing the subcutaneous and deep dermal tissue to an underlying fixed structure such as the periosteum, both advancing skin edges can be stabilized in their proper positions. The skin edges of the two properly positioned tissues may then be finely approximated under minimal tension with simple skin sutures. This type of suture, known as a "pexing" suture, is placed by starting deep on the wound edge and advancing superficially into the fibrous tissue of the deep dermis. The suture may then exit the flap either through the cut edge or through a second point proximal to the cut edge. By pulling the advancing tissue with this first loop of suture, the wound margin can be advanced into the desired position to ascertain the proper position for placing the loop of suture into the deep structure. The suture is then placed securely in the deep structure and tied, taking care not to strangulate any tissue included in the loop. Such a deeply placed suture may also be used to re-create contours away from the advancing wound edge margin. This is done by placing a deep stitch that fixes the dermis to the periosteum in the lateral portion of a nasolabial

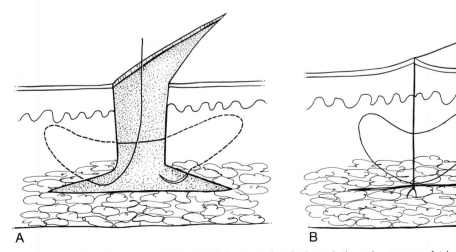

A   B

Figure 25–2. *A,* An alternative buried suture where the stitch enters deeply through the subcutaneous fat but arches toward the skin surface. *B,* When the suture is tied, this maneuver increases wound edge eversion.

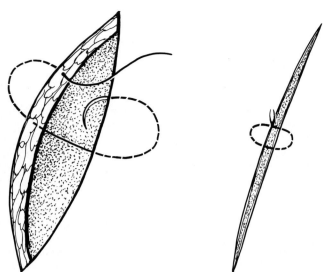

Figure 25–3. In the horizontal buried suture the suture enters and exits the dermis at the same level, encompassing as much tissue as necessary *(left)* to facilitate wound closure *(right)*.

flap so that a normal-appearing nasofacial sulcus can be re-created.[13]

Modifications of Simple Suturing Techniques

The simple interrupted percutaneous suture is the most commonly utilized of all skin closure methods, and its ease of application and adaptability to various clinical circumstances make mastery of this stitch critical to every cutaneous surgeon. However, modification of the simple interrupted suture provides the basis for many alternative sutures.

LEVELING STITCH

Perhaps the most direct modification is the use of simple sutures to level the surface of uneven wounds. If the sides are uneven, the suture should exit the dermis high on the high side and low on the low side[14] (Fig. 25–5). This technique levels the epidermal surface.

SIMPLE RUNNING STITCH

The running simple suture is a continuous linking of simple sutures. After a simple interrupted suture is placed at one end of the incision, the end of the suture that is attached to the needle is not cut. Instead, the suture remains attached to the first knot as continuous loops of simple sutures are made along the length of the wound (Fig. 25–6). When the end of the wound is reached, a knot is tied, using the free end of the suture and the last previous loop. This running simple suture allows for rapid placement of many closely spaced sutures in an area of minimal tension. Most commonly, nonabsorbable suture material such as polypropylene or nylon is used and removed at the normal time interval. On wounds already well approximated with buried su-

tures, some surgeons prefer to use an absorbable suture (e.g., mild chromic or fast-absorbing gut) and allow the suture material to be gently removed from the site by the patient as it breaks down. Similarly, a running simple suture can also be used to fix the edges of a full- or split-thickness skin graft to the defect margins.

RUNNING LOCKED STITCH

Each loop of a running suture can be locked on itself to allow the use of a running suture in areas under slightly more tension. The locking is performed by looping the suture through the suture from the previous loop (Fig. 25–7). One problem with this stitch is that fine edge approximation is difficult to obtain. In addition, the tension applied by the suture, combined with the pressure produced by the external loops of suture on the skin surface, can compromise the blood supply and possibly result in focal necrosis. As a result, this suturing technique is often used only for closure of areas of limited cosmetic sensitivity (e.g., postauricular full-thickness skin graft donor sites).

Vertical Mattress Sutures

The vertical mattress suture (Fig. 25–8) is probably the most commonly used advanced suturing technique. It is often used to evert skin edges in situations where they naturally tend to infold, to align wounds in which the edges of the tissues are of unequal thickness, to provide extra strength and security to a wound closure, and to help approximate the deeper tissue while also eliminating dead space.[11] The suture consists of two loops, one placed 4 to 8 mm from the skin edges ("far-far") and the second placed 1 to 2 mm from the wound edges ("near-near"). Classically, the "far-far" loop is placed first, similar to a widely based simple suture. The direction of the needle is then reversed, or "back-

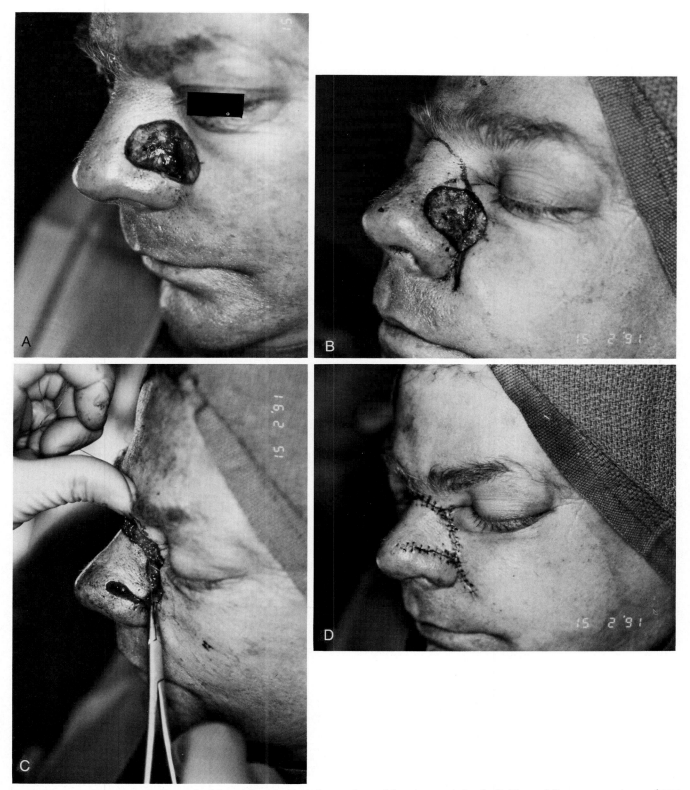

Figure 25–4. *A*, Clinical appearance of a large defect that includes portions of the nose and cheek. *B*, Planned flap movements are drawn. *C*, Deep sutures are used to fix the dermis of the advancing cheek flap to the periosteum in the nasofacial sulcus. *D*, The final repair demonstrates the distribution of the closure, which maintains the nasofacial sulcus.

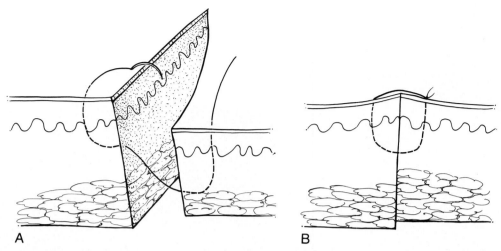

Figure 25–5. *A,* The simple percutaneous suture is used to level the skin edge by linking low on the "low side" to high on the "high side." *B,* Final appearance, showing a level skin surface.

handed," and the "near-near" loop is placed, similar to the placement of a fine epicuticular suture and encompassing only the papillary dermis, at most.

As the suture is pulled tight and the free ends tied together, the skin edges are everted. The relatively large amount of tissue contained in these loops provides for greater closure strength and better distribution of the wound tension. However, if the wound is tied too tightly, necrosis of the epidermis under the externalized loops may result. Care must be taken to tie vertical mattress sutures with only the minimal amount of tension necessary to avoid "railroad track" scarring. Everting the epidermal edges allows better dermal apposition, which appears to result in faster wound healing and more rapid development of wound strength. In many cases, only a few vertical mattress sutures, interspersed with simple interrupted sutures, may be needed along the length of an incision to obtain this effect.

A potential problem with wound dehiscence may occur with the use of this suturing technique if it is used to close a wound under tension without combining it with a buried suture to provide long-term support. This is a result of the fact that vertical mattress sutures are often removed in 7 to 10 days to avoid epithelialization of the suture tracks; at this time the wound has not had sufficient time to develop significant tensile strength. If the wound is insufficiently supported by placement of deep buried sutures or by meticulous postoperative application of adhesive tape strips on the surface by the patient, wound dehiscence may result.

ONE-HALF BURIED VERTICAL MATTRESS STITCH

When one of the external loops of the vertical mattress suture must be placed in a location in which the external loop of the suture is undesirable, (e.g., on the lip or eyelid), a half-buried vertical mattress suture may be used (Fig. 25–9). After entering the wound to place the first half of the "far-far" component, the loop through

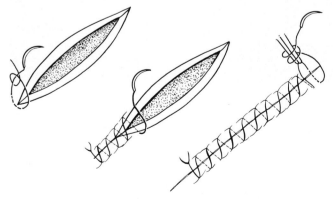

Figure 25–6. The running simple suture begins with a simple suture placed at one wound edge *(left),* followed by continuous loops of simple suture *(middle),* and completed with the final knot placed by tying the suture on itself *(right).*

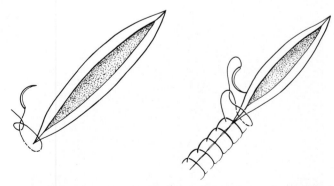

Figure 25–7. The running locked suture is begun in a similar fashion to the running simple suture *(left),* but each pass is "locked" by looping it through the loop of suture from the previous pass *(right).*

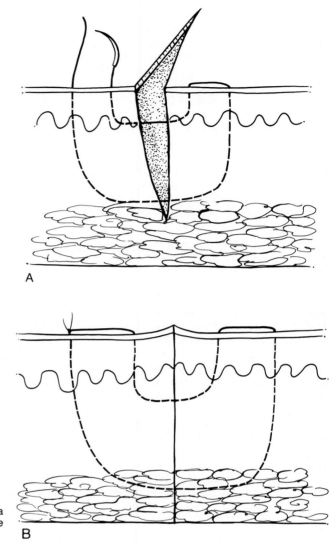

Figure 25–8. *A*, In the vertical mattress suture the loops are placed in a "far-far," "near-near" manner. *B*, Tying the suture produces wound edge eversion.

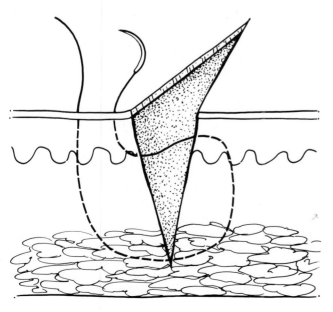

Figure 25–9. For the half-buried vertical mattress suture, one loop is buried completely within the dermis.

the opposite side of the wound does not exit through the skin surface but is placed similarly to a buried mattress suture. This loop enters the dermis deeply, as in a regular mattress suture, but exits through the wound edge at the level of the midreticular dermis. The first side is then re-entered at the same level, and the suture exits through the skin surface, where it is tied in the usual manner.

Vertical mattress sutures are often time-consuming to place. It has been proposed that reversing the sequence of loop placement to "near-near" and "far-far" might significantly decrease the placement time.[15] The loop near the skin edge is placed first. Gentle lifting of this loop then facilitates placement of the far-far loop, and the suture is then tied in the usual manner.

MODIFIED VERTICAL MATTRESS SUTURING TECHNIQUES

When the goal of using a vertical mattress suture is to add strength to the wound closure, a small modification may provide a mechanical advantage[16] (Fig. 25–10). After completing, but not tying, the knot of the vertical mattress suture, the suture is looped back through the external loop on the opposite side of the incision and pulled across before being tied normally. This maneuver allows the new loop to function as a pulley, which places less tension on each of the other strands.

Another modification that allows for a similar mechanical advantage is the "far-near," "near-far" suture[17] (Fig. 25–11). The double loops of suture are produced by placing the first loop of suture 4 to 6 mm from one wound edge, but exiting only 1 to 2 mm on the opposite side. The suture is then looped again across the incision

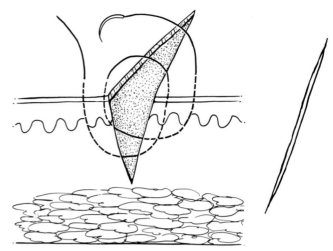

Figure 25–11. The "far-near," "near-far," or "pulley" suturing technique.

line, and a "near" suture is placed, followed by a "far" suture on the opposite side. This suturing technique also creates a pulley effect as it is tied across the wound. Both of these techniques allow greater stretch of the wound edges, but these must not be stretched to the point of vascular compromise.

The "near-far," "far-near" suture presents a distinct mechanical and tensor strength advantage such that it is very useful in creating the stretch needed for intraoperative tissue expansion. This suture can also be invaluable in initiating the closure of large wounds with significant tension (Fig. 25–12). One or two pulley stitches can be placed to begin approximation of the wound. Buried sutures can then be easily positioned without having to struggle against the wound tension with each suture. Skin edges can then be finely approximated in the usual manner. At this point, the pulley stitch can be left in place to help reduce wound edge tension or removed if tension has been sufficiently redistributed over the other sutures.

The large amount of tissue encompassed by mattress sutures obviously aids in the reduction of subcutaneous dead space. To further reduce such dead space, the deep loop of the suture may make an additional pass through the underlying deep tissue[11] (Fig. 25–13). In addition, if the deep structure is relatively fixed in position (e.g., as with periosteum or deep muscle fascia), this additional loop may aid in re-creating contours and distributing the tissue stretch equally between the two sides of the wound.

Horizontal Mattress Sutures

The horizontal mattress suturing technique is useful for repairing wounds that must be closed under significant tension. It is also useful as the first stitch in movement of a flap,[11] particularly for wounds on the hand. It can also be effectively used in conjunction with simple interrupted sutures to support the closure of a

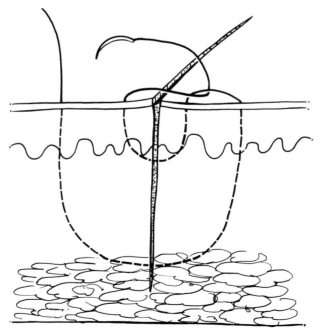

Figure 25–10. A pulley effect is created by looping the suture back through the external loop on the opposite side.

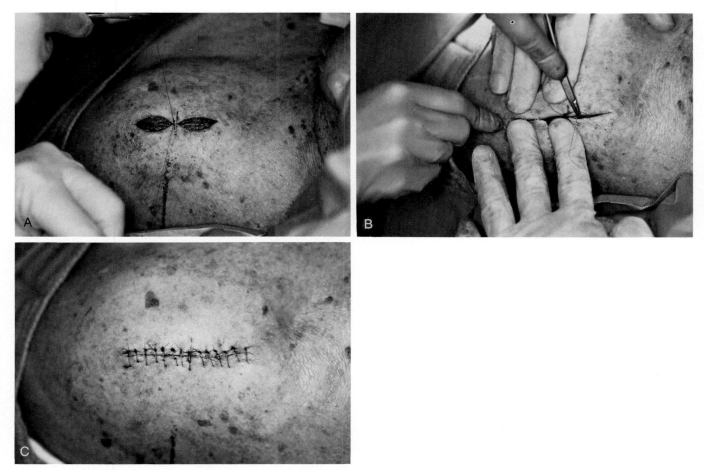

Figure 25–12. *A,* The pulley suture is used to initiate wound closure. *B,* Regular buried sutures can then be placed with ease. *C,* The final wound approximation is done with simple and vertical mattress sutures.

Figure 25–13. The vertical mattress suture has included deep tissue in the "far-far" pass to help close any dead space.

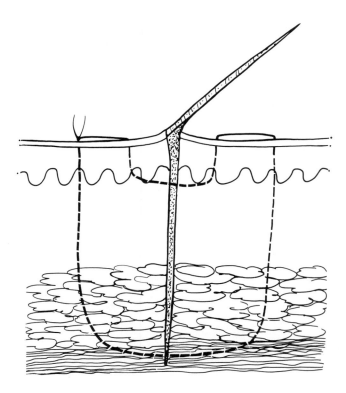

broad wound to provide hemostasis[1] after punch biopsy on a vascular anatomic location, and to close dead space.

If the double loop of suture is applied parallel to the wound instead of perpendicular to it, as in the vertical mattress suturing technique, a horizontal mattress suture is created (Fig. 25–14). This somewhat complex stitch is composed of four segments: two vertical (or deep) segments and two horizontal (or exposed) segments. The vertical segments are perpendicular to the wound axis, and the horizontal segments are parallel with it. The initial penetration of the needle occurs 5 to 10 mm away from the wound edge and follows a path deep into the dermis. It then crosses the defect, enters the opposite side of the wound at the same depth, and penetrates the epidermis at an equal distance from the wound edge. The continuation of the stitch is the exposed epidermal, or horizontal, segment. The length of the exposed segment varies, but the length is generally equal to the distance from the wound edge. The second vertical segment is performed in an identical fashion, but in reverse order. This requires placing the needle backward in the jaws of the holder and then penetrating and advancing in a reverse or "backhanded" fashion. The free end of the suture is then tied to the loose end of the original loop.

Relatively large amounts of tissue are encompassed by this suture. Because the pressure is distributed across the dermis between the loops of suture, a pursestring effect is created so that bleeding from dermal vessels can be controlled by tamponade. However, excess pressure may also significantly compromise the blood supply and lead to necrosis. In addition, the pressure placed on the epidermis by the external loops of suture may lead to epidermal necrosis and produce suture marks. For this reason, some type of padding material or bolster is used to help spread the pressure over a larger area and minimize this potential problem. Any sterile material can be used as a bolster, including cotton dental rolls, cardboard suture packaging, and the plastic tubing used to protect instrument tips. Even with the pressure

distributed across the bolster, necrosis under these externalized portions of the suture may still result. Consequently, the suture should be tied with the minimal amount of tension necessary and the stitch removed as soon as possible.

To help close large wounds under significant tension, one or more widely spaced horizontal mattress sutures may be placed 1 to 2 cm from the wound edge to help remove tension from the wound edge sutures.[18] The skin edges themselves are then reapproximated with simple sutures or other appropriate closure methods. A large-caliber suture (e.g., 2–0 or 3–0 polypropylene) is needed for strength, and a bolster is almost always necessary to help distribute the tension. Sterilized plastic clothing buttons may an ideal bolster for widely placed horizontal mattress sutures.[19]

In a similar attempt to minimize the amount of suture marking caused by the pressure of the exposed loops of suture, all but the very corners of a tension mattress suture may be buried.[20] The vertical pass is initiated into one of the wound margins. By re-entering the skin near the exit point of the vertical pass, the horizontal pass can also be buried. Using an absorbable suture, the knot is tied and buried deeply in the wound.

RUNNING HORIZONTAL MATTRESS SUTURES

The horizontal mattress suture can also be placed in a running manner. The first loop is placed as a simple suture, but only the free end is cut at the knot. The suture is then moved as a continuous loop of horizontal mattress sutures until the final loop is tied on itself as in other running sutures.

ONE-HALF BURIED HORIZONTAL MATTRESS SUTURES

A one-half buried horizontal mattress suture can also be created (Fig. 25–15). Like the half-buried vertical mattress suture, this stitch is useful in locations where

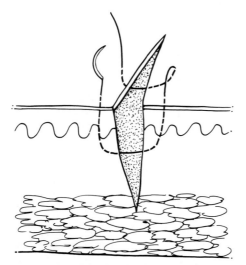

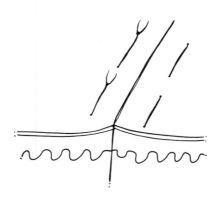

Figure 25–14. The horizontal mattress suture: entrance and exit points *(left)* and final appearance of tied knot *(right)*.

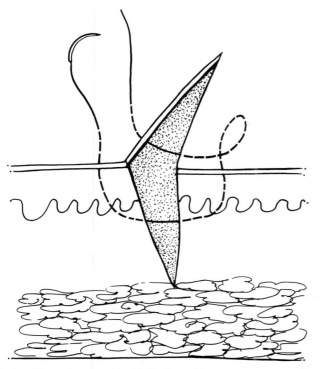

Figure 25–15. In the half-buried horizontal mattress suture, one loop is completely buried under the skin surface.

it is undesirable to place an externalized loop of the horizontal stitch. The stitch is initiated in the usual manner, but on the opposite side of the wound, the stitch is placed completely within the dermis in a horizontal fashion. The loop then crosses back to the original side and is again brought to the surface as in a usual horizontal mattress suture.

CORNER OR TIP STITCH

A particularly useful variation of the half-buried horizontal mattress suture is the corner or tip stitch (Fig.

25–16). This stitch allows gentle approximation of a V-shaped corner with less risk of tip strangulation. The suture is started on the side of the "V" that is opposite the V-shaped tip. The entrance point is slightly away from the apex of the "V" and exits through the mid-dermis. The stitch is then carried onto the V-shaped tip, taking care to enter the tip at the same level as the previous exit point to ensure a smooth surface on closure. The stitch passes through the tip, exiting on the opposite side of the apex before it is taken back to the recipient bed at the same level in the dermis where it exits. The suture is then gently tied to provide fine approximation. The importance of keeping the tip level with the surrounding tissue cannot be overemphasized. In addition, the suture must be placed far enough back from the apex that the suture on the skin surface does not cross the tip. Although this is an elegant solution to fine approximation of V-shaped tips, the corner stitch may not increase tip survival. Indeed, wounds closed with a simple stitch placed vertically across the tip show similar tip viability.[21] The half-buried mattress suture may also be used to close areas in which two, three, or four flap points[11] come together (Fig. 25–17).

Running Intradermal Suture

The running intradermal suture, also known as the running subcuticular suture, can provide fine epidermal approximation while minimizing scarring.[1, 2] The use of this stitch is somewhat limited, because it is only appropriate in special circumstances (e.g., a wound with good initial epidermal approximation and only minimal wound tension). This requires either a shallow wound with minimal loss of tissue or a wound in which buried sutures have already been placed. The wound edges should be relatively straight and of even length and even thickness. In these circumstances, this suture technique offers unique advantages with the possibility of decreased scarring.

Classically, the suture is begun by entering the skin beyond the wound edge on the long axis and exiting

Figure 25–16. The corner stitch allows accurate placement of the V-shaped tips *(left)* and also levels the skin surface *(right)* after knot is tied.

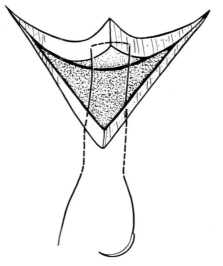

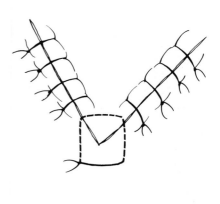

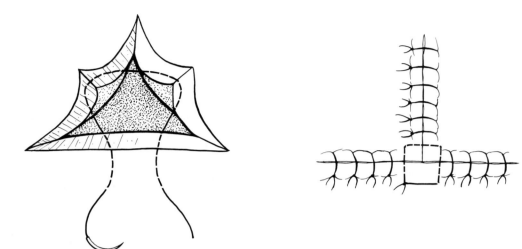

Figure 25–17. Two flap points *(left)* are approximated with a half-buried horizontal mattress suture *(right).*

through the apex in the mid to upper dermis (Fig. 25–18). Horizontal loops are then carried from side to side at the same level in the mid-dermis. Each entrance site in the dermis is backtracked slightly from the opposite exit point. When the end of the wound is reached, an exit loop is placed in the mid-dermis and brought out through the skin surface at the apex. Both ends of the suture are then pulled to tighten the closure and approximate the wound edges. Ideally, there will be little tension present, and the ends can simply be fixed in place with tape closures. If some tension does exist, each end of the suture can be tied on itself. Unfortunately, the tying of these knots can cause tissue bunching at the ends of the wounds and may result in burying them, which may make removal difficult. A stainless steel spring device (tensor), tied to the loose ends of the running intradermal suture, has been used to keep tension on the suture without creating the problems inherent with tying knots at each end.[22] Small gaps that

remain in the wound surface after placement of the intradermal suture may be closed with superficially placed simple sutures, which may be removed in a few days. Alternatively, the entire wound edge may be reinforced with tape closures.

There are many variations on how to start and end the suture. Instead of starting at the apex, the stitch may be started at one side of the wound edge.[11] This arrangement places the force produced by the final loop in the same direction as that produced by the other loops of suture and helps avoid bunching at the ends of the wound when the suture is pulled tight. The initial pass begins at the site of the apex and exits through the mid-dermis, from which the running intradermal suture begins. The suture may also be continued as an initial first simple suture to fix one end of the suture.[11] With only the loose end cut, the suture re-enters the skin and exits through the mid-dermis of the wound as the running intradermal suture is continued. A simple suture may be placed at the terminal end of the suture to fix it in place.

The running intradermal suture may be removed at the usual interval or left in place for a prolonged period if needed for wound support. The lack of puncture sites and loops of suture over the wound is possible without the usual formation of suture tracks. Unfortunately, removal of running intradermal sutures left for prolonged periods may be difficult, as the sutures may adhere to the healing tissue or the knots at the ends may become buried. For this reason, it is best to use monofilament polypropylene suture material, as this presents the least drag[23] and slips through the tissue more easily than any other suture material. If the wound is long, suture removal may be aided by the placement of escape loops. To place such loops, the suture is passed through the epidermis at intervals instead of the usual intradermal loop. The suture can then be passed over the wound, just as a simple suture would be, and the running stitch restarted on the opposite side (Fig. 25–19). Alternatively, the loop may be placed horizontally, just as the intradermal loop would have been placed. This arrangement helps avoid tracking across

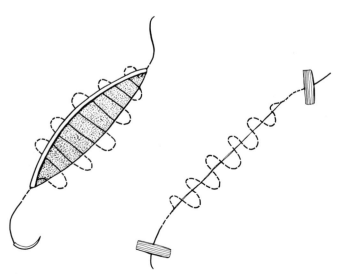

Figure 25–18. In the running intradermal suture *(left),* the loose ends can be held in place with tape strips *(right)* when little tension is present.

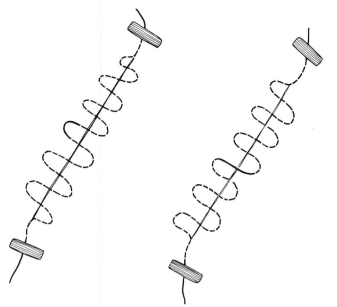

Figure 25–19. Escape loops in a long running intradermal suture may be placed vertically across the wound *(left)* or horizontally along the wound *(right)*.

the wound margin. If this alternative method is used, it may be helpful to tie a loop of free suture under the escape loop to help locate it after prolonged placement. With either method, at the time of suture removal, the loop is elevated and cut and the suture removed by applying tension to both ends. Escape loops should be placed every 2 to 3 cm. One method for removing running intradermal sutures that stubbornly resist removal[23, 24] uses a small hemostat attached to both one end of the suture and a rubber band. Firm tension is

applied to the rubber band by fixing it to a location distal to the suture. This force is gently transferred to the suture and, after a few minutes, results in gradual release of the stubborn material.

Another way to avoid problems with removal is to leave the suture buried in the wound. Most often this is accomplished by using synthetic absorbable suture. The knots may be buried by starting the suture in a way similar to that used to place a horizontal buried suture at the apex. The suture may also be started and ended through the skin in the usual manner. One to 2 weeks later these ends are cut at the skin surface and the residual suture allowed to retract into the wound. If prolonged support is desired, relatively nonreactive permanent suture material such as nylon or Prolene may be used in a similar manner.

Pursestring Sutures

Another modification of the running intradermal suture is the use of the pursestring suture to reduce the size of a wound before placement of a full- or split-thickness skin graft[25–27] (Fig. 25–20). A suture of appropriately sized polypropylene enters the wound from the skin surface and exits through the mid-dermis. Continuous horizontal loops of intradermal suture are made, with appropriate escape loops placed at intervals around the wound. Near the original entry point, the suture is again passed through the skin surface. Both suture ends are then pulled tightly to reduce the wound size as much as possible without distorting the surrounding tissue. A full- or split-thickness skin graft may then be used to cover the remaining defect, or the wound may be allowed to heal by second intention. This pursestring suture is left in place for 2 to 3 weeks.

Figure 25–20. To facilitate removal of the "pursestring" suture, escape loops are placed at appropriate intervals *(left)* so that when the suture is pulled tightly to reduce the overall size of the wound *(right)*, it can still be easily removed.

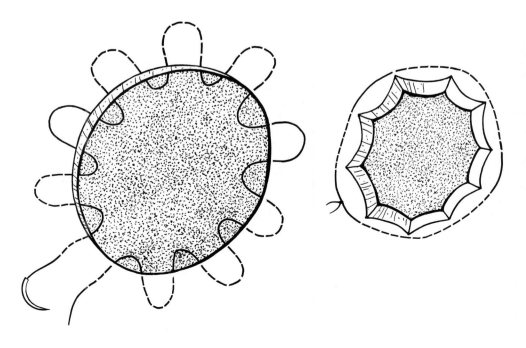

Tissue-Conserving Sutures

A combination of two different suturing techniques has been proposed as a way to reduce the need for removal of "dogears" in excisional surgery (Stuart J, personal communication, March 17, 1991). In this procedure, a variation of the horizontal buried suturing technique, a suture is passed from the central portion of the defect toward the apex to reduce the redundancy. This horizontal oblique suture (Fig. 25–21) is initiated by entering the deep dermis near the center of the wound. The suture is moved horizontally and obliquely toward the apex and exits the wound high in the dermis. The suture then crosses the wound and enters the opposite side high in the dermis, where it is again moved horizontally and obliquely to exit opposite the original entry point. As the suture is pulled tight, the apex of the wound is pulled toward the center of the wound and slightly down. This movement distributes the redundant tissue from the apex around the entire wound. If any redundancy remains, an apex suture may be used to flatten the bulge. This is performed at a 45-degree angle to the line of wound closure and even with the center of the redundancy. The suture enters the skin and is directed along the 45-degree angle toward the wound edge just proximal to the apex. The stitch is then mirrored on the opposite wound edge. Gentle tying of the suture helps to provide additional flattening of the redundancy.

Layered Closures

The layered closure of a surgical defect is simply an attempt to re-create in three dimensions an area that has been altered by a surgical procedure. This is done while simultaneously maintaining the functional and cosmetic integrity of the involved anatomic structures. The suturing techniques range from deep buried sutures to superficial skin sutures. The goal is simply to close and re-create the various skin layers. Each layer is closed progressively, using suturing techniques that are most appropriate to that layer.

To ensure optimal results, the site must first be prepared for closure by performing appropriate undermining as necessary to either mobilize sufficient tissue to close the defect or free the skin edge for suture placement. After the undermining has been completed, the surgeon must assess the feasibility of closing the wound in the manner that had been originally planned. Approximating the wound using two skin hooks will permit a rough determination as to whether there is sufficient tissue movement for closure and whether the lines of closure are cosmetically and functionally appropriate. If a problem is encountered, the planned closure must be re-evaluated and alternative closures using flaps or grafts considered.

The first step in actual closure is to assess the need for deep sutures. If deep tissues such as muscle or fascia have been violated, they should be closed. Contours can be re-created by using buried sutures or placing sutures into deep structures such as periosteum or fascia.

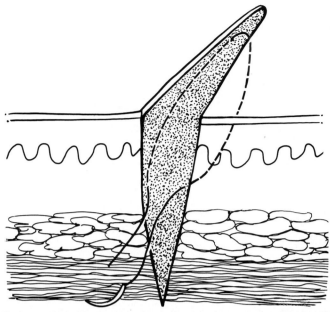

Figure 25–21. The buried horizontal oblique suture is used to pull the apices of an incision with dogears down and toward the center of the wound.

Any dead space should be appropriately closed to aid in wound healing and prevent potential complications such as hematoma or seroma formation. As the closure moves closer to the surface, approximation of the dermis will remove tension from the wound edges and provide prolonged wound support. In each of these situations, buried sutures are used in a progressive manner to reapproximate the structures appropriately. The final step in a layered closure is the selection of the suture for epidermal approximation.

SUMMARY

The nature of a wound and its anatomic location will help determine the best suturing technique for proper wound closure. Closure of the entire wound should be thought out before the first suture is placed, considering all of the simple and advanced suturing techniques available. Obviously, as the closure progresses, changes can be made as circumstances dictate, but advanced planning will help ensure that all the goals of wound closure will be fulfilled.

REFERENCES

1. Angelini GD, Butchart EG, Armistead SH, Breckenridge IM: Comparative study of leg wound skin closure in coronary artery bypass graft operations. Thorax 39:942–945, 1984.
2. Taube M, Porter RJ, Lord PH: A combination of subcuticular suture and sterile Micropore tape compared with conventional interrupted sutures for skin closure. Ann R Coll Surg Engl 65:164–167, 1983.
3. Pepicello J, Yavorek H: Five year experience with tape closure of abdominal wounds. Surg Gynecol Obstet 169:310–314, 1989.
4. Aitken RJ, Anderson EDC, Goldstraw S, Chetty U: Subcuticular skin closure following minor breast biopsy: Prolene is superior to polydioxanone (PDS). J R Coll Surg Edinb 34:128–129, 1989.

5. Hartman LA: Intradermal sutures in facial lacerations. Arch Otolaryngol 103:542–543, 1977.
6. Albom MJ: Dermo-subdermal sutures for long, deep surgical wounds. J Dermatol Surg Oncol 3:504–505, 1977.
7. Zitelli JA, Moy RL: Buried vertical mattress suture. J Dermatol Surg Oncol 15:17–19, 1989.
8. Dzubow LM: The use of fascial plication to facilitate wound closure following microscopically controlled surgery. J Dermatol Surg Oncol 15:1063–1066, 1989.
9. Davidson TM: Subcutaneous suture placement. Laryngoscope 97:501–504, 1987.
10. Ftaiha Z, Snow SN: The buried running dermal subcutaneous suture technique. J Dermatol Surg Oncol 15:264–266, 1989.
11. Stegman SJ: Suturing techniques for dermatologic surgery. J Dermatol Surg Oncol 4:63–68, 1978.
12. Salasche SJ: The suspension suture. J Dermatol Surg Oncol 13:973–978, 1987.
13. Zitelli JA: The nasal-labial flap as a single stage procedure. Arch Dermatol 126:1445–1448, 1990.
14. Perry AW, McShane RH: Fine tuning of the skin edges in the closure of surgical wounds. J Dermatol Surg Oncol 7:471–476, 1981.
15. Snow SN, Goodman MM, Lemke BN: The short hand vertical mattress stitch—a rapid skin everting suture technique. J Dermatol Surg Oncol 15:379–381, 1989.
16. Gault DT: Loop mattress suture. Br J Surg 74:820–821, 1987.
17. Bernstein G: The far-near, near-far suture. J Dermatol Surg Oncol 11:470, 1985.
18. Coldiron BM: The closure of wounds under tension: the horizontal mattress sutures. Arch Dermatol 125:1189–1190, 1989.
19. Adnot J, Salasche SJ, West RW: Button bolsters in dermatologic surgery. J Dermatol Surg Oncol 15:59–61, 1989.
20. Epstein E: The buried horizontal mattress suture. Cutis 24:104–106, 1979.
21. McQuown SA: Gillies' corner stitch revisited. Arch Otolaryngol 110:450–453, 1984.
22. Weber PJ, Dzubow LM, Wulc AE: Suture tensor. J Dermatol Surg Oncol 16:535–537, 1990.
23. Mangus DJ: Reversing the antilock braking system theory for suture removal. Plast Reconstr Surg 79:987–989, 1987.
24. Hockly G: Easy removal of the obstinate subcuticular suture. Plast Reconstr Surg 63:275–276, 1979.
25. Peled IJ, Zagher U, Wexler MR: Purse-string suture for reduction and closure of skin defects. Ann Plast Surg 14:465–469, 1985.
26. Hodgson K, Hughes L: A simple technique for improving the cosmesis of excision of a melanoma and skin grafting. Surg Gynecol Obstet 163:491–492, 1986.
27. Katz AE, Grande DJ: Delayed reconstruction of large facial defects after Mohs surgery. In: American Academy of Otolaryngology: Instructional courses. Vol 2. CV Mosby, St. Louis, 1989.

CHAPTER 26

Skin Grafts

THOMAS G. HILL

The history of skin grafting may have begun as early as 900 AD in India,[1] although this fact is poorly documented. The scientific description of the technique originated much later, with G. Baronio during the "age of enlightenment," in the late 1700s; Baronio described skin grafting in animals,[2] but Bunger, in 1823, provided the first report of skin grafting in humans.[3] The evolution of the procedure has been slow but progressive, beginning with its use as a last-choice option by earlier surgeons,[4] and continuing to its present-day status as a primary surgical option in many situations and a strong secondary alternative in many others.

Graft Survival and Bacteriology

The survival of any skin graft (Table 26–1) depends on the complex interplay of many factors, including simultaneous dependence on inosculation[5] and angioneogenesis[6] for early survival of the graft, reinnervation,[7] and immediate resistance to an extremely variable spectrum of resident skin bacteria.[8] The return of vasomotor function[9] and preservation of the original character of grafted skin and appendages[10] ensures both a relatively normal appearance and physiologic function even after the initial stages of healing. In most circumstances it is advisable to utilize postoperative antibiotics after grafting, using either a cephalothin derivative[11] or erythromycin to reduce potentially harmful resident skin flora that may have been carried with the graft, originally existed adjacent to the wound site, or been transmitted to the area by incidental contact. Heroic measures, particularly the use of hyperbaric oxygen,[12] have been demonstrated to be valuable to the survival of compromised grafts, although this particular adjunct is very expensive and unavailable to most cutaneous surgeons. Although most mild staphylococcal infections can be easily managed, streptococcal infections seem to be the most vexing bacterial problem. A very small tissue load of beta-hemolytic streptococci can often destroy an otherwise excellent graft.[13]

Classification of Grafts

Originally, skin graft thicknesses (Fig. 26–1) were roughly defined by the instruments used to harvest them. By current definition, thin split-thickness grafts are 0.006 to 0.012 inch thick; intermediate split-thickness grafts are 0.012 to 0.018 inch thick; thick split-thickness grafts are 0.018 to 0.024 inch thick; and essentially any thicker graft is classified as full thickness.[14] Several different

TABLE 26–1. **FEATURES OF THE VARIOUS TYPES OF SKIN GRAFTS**

	Nutritional Needs	Infection Risk	Cosmesis	Durability	Technical Skill	Donor Sites	Size
Full-thickness grafts	High	Moderate	Good	Good	Moderate	Limited	Medium
Split-thickness grafts	Low	Low	Fair	Fair	Low	Many	Large
Pinch grafts	Moderate	Moderate	Poor	Good	Low	Many	Medium
Composite grafts	Very High	High	Good	Good	High	Few	Small

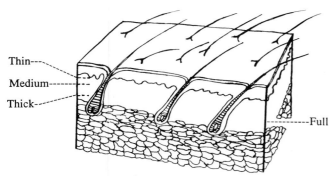

Figure 26–1. Schematic showing the two common types of skin grafts: split-thickness (*left*) and full-thickness (*right*).

types of specialty grafts also exist. The pinch graft is a full-thickness graft centrally but only a split-thickness graft peripherally. Composite grafts consist of full-thickness skin plus a thin layer of subcutaneous fat, as well as another tissue such as cartilage. Hair transplant grafts include skin and portions of the subcutis containing hair follicles. Incidental skin grafts, such as the full-thickness "dogear" graft that is made from excess tissue removed from the ends of a linear wound, can be employed to fill small residual defects in a complex reconstruction in some special circumstances.

Patient Preference: Flaps or Grafts

Most scientific discussions of surgical treatment fail to include the most basic consideration of all: patient preference. Obviously, every type of surgical reconstruction will result in some scarring, contour defects and color change in the skin. Currently, the reconstructive technique preferred by many cutaneous surgeons for most defects is some variation of the random pattern flap. Many flaps, however, either cross dominant re-

gional boundaries or produce multiple scars resulting from local tissue movement.

When all issues are addressed and discussed, many patients choose skin graft reconstruction over the distortion of natural facial landmarks or multiple secondary scars that will result from random pattern flaps. In many instances, a well-chosen skin graft (Fig. 26–2) can be a more conservative procedure than a complicated, but geometrically satisfying, random pattern flap. Making the patient an equal partner in the decision-making process may result in greatly increased use of skin grafts for reconstructive surgery (Fig. 26–3).

Full-Thickness Skin Grafts

GENERAL CONSIDERATIONS

Full-thickness skin grafts remain the workhorse of facial defect reconstruction for many cutaneous surgeons. Important technical points crucial to the success of this procedure are donor site selection, selection of appropriate defects, and use of meticulous technique to avoid the major causes of graft failure. The full-thickness skin graft may be unique among facial reconstructive procedures in that a failure in any one of the above areas can often spell disaster or disappointment for physician and patient alike. Because a full-thickness graft includes all skin layers except subcutaneous fat, it is generally limited in its use to small- or medium-sized defects that are impractical to close primarily and for which skin flap reconstruction would result in excessive scarring or transgression of natural skin surface boundaries.

If the donor tissue is harvested so that it is large enough to "drape" into the defect, wound contracture can be essentially eliminated. The cosmetic appearance, both in terms of skin color and skin surface texture, is maximized with full-thickness grafts, unlike with split-thickness grafts. Because of these features, the full-thickness skin graft remains the most useful graft in cutaneous surgery. However, because of tissue thickness

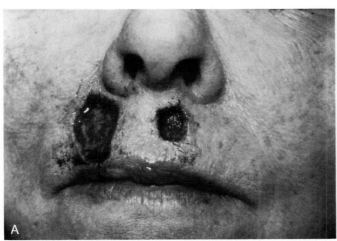
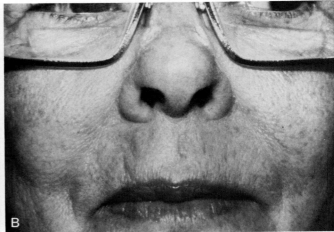

Figure 26–2. *A,* Preoperative clinical appearance showing two defects on the upper lip. *B,* Postoperative appearance following placement of full-thickness skin grafts.

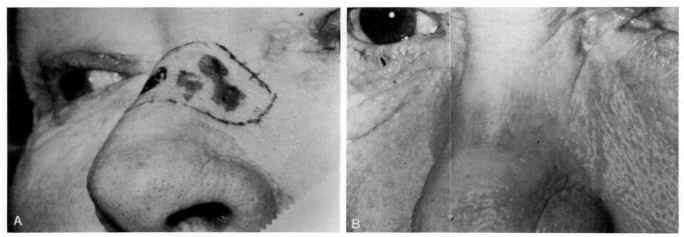

Figure 26–3. *A,* Preoperative clinical appearance of a planned excision site on the nasal bridge. *B,* Appearance after placement of a full-thickness skin graft.

and bulk,[15] full-thickness grafts have greater metabolic requirements. This may increase the failure rate unless absolute attention is given to all technical requirements of the procedure.

DONOR SITES

For many years, the postauricular donor site (Fig. 26–4) seemed to be the only site considered for facial reconstruction. More recently, however, many other alternate grafts and donor sites have been described (Figs. 26–5, 26–6), including eyebrow-to-eyebrow grafts,[16] eyelid-to-eyelid grafts,[17] preauricular grafts,[18] trapezius-to-nosetip grafts,[19] adjacent nasal donor sites,[20] and others. Other donor sites recognized in recent years are the glabellar area for the chin and upper lip, the nasolabial fold for lateral nasal defects, the thinner

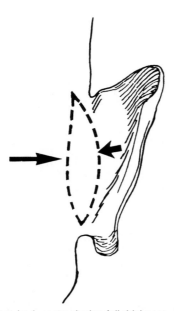

Figure 26–4. Standard postauricular full-thickness skin graft donor site.

portions of the postauricular area for the eyelid, and the lateral neck for a variety of areas. Automatic choices of donor site should never be made, because local variations in skin texture, color, and sebaceous quality are usually much better guides to use in selecting the best match for donor and recipient areas. As a general rule, the surgeon should attempt to use a donor site as near as possible to the recipient site, provided that site is practical and will not result in noticeable secondary scarring. The thickness of the donor skin is another important consideration in donor site choice because of the desirability of extra skin thickness, which can be precisely sculpted to match the exact contours in the graft bed. This capacity offers the best opportunity for creating normal skin surface geometry after healing and a more pleasing final cosmetic result.

FULL-THICKNESS SKIN GRAFT TECHNIQUE

Because the full-thickness skin graft is deprived of its original blood supply, considerable care must be taken in designing the graft, obtaining hemostasis, preparing the graft bed, and approximating the graft to its recipient bed to ensure a good result.

Choosing the Donor Site

Choosing the ideal donor site is the first step in the process. The surgeon should select donor skin that matches the recipient site as closely as possible in color, texture and tissue thickness to prevent a depressed final appearance. Incision lines should be made either in a natural fold or parallel to relaxed skin tension lines. Some surgeons use various materials as templates for accurately determining the size of the donor specimen. Sterilized x-ray film, the imprint of the graft bed on a cotton gauze, a piece of sterile glove paper, or nonstick dressing material may all be used successfully. It should be remembered that the tension produced by the natural elastic fibers in skin will both shrink the size of the donor skin and slightly enlarge the defect. Therefore, if

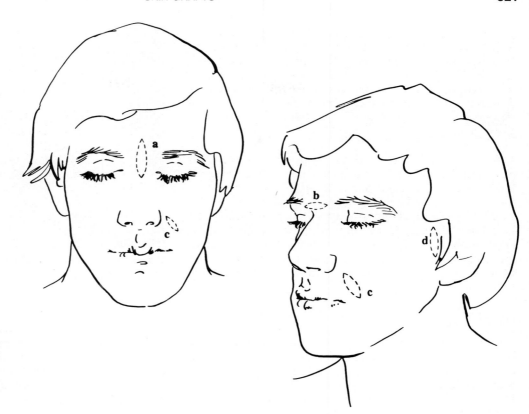

Figure 26–5. *Left*, Anterior view of some full-thickness skin graft donor sites on the face. a, Vertical glabella; c, nasolabial fold. *Right*, Oblique view. b, Horizontal glabella; c, nasolabial fold; d, preauricular.

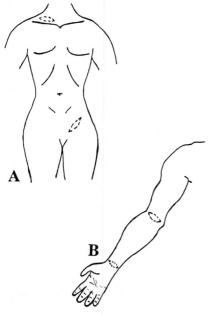

Figure 26–6. Alternate full-thickness skin graft donor sites on the trunk. *A*, Supraclavicular and inguinal. *B*, Antecubital fossa and volar wrist. *C*, Trapezius.

a template is to be used, it should be cut approximately 10% larger than the graft bed so that the graft can be loosely "draped" into the recipient site rather than stretched to fit. Stretching a graft to fit the graft bed may compromise the natural revascularization processes of inosculation and angioneogenesis.[21]

Preparing the Recipient Site

An excellent tissue bed for grafting must also be prepared for successful full-thickness grafting. Meticulous hemostasis, performed without creating excessive tissue char or devitalizing large amounts of tissue by electrosurgery or chemical cautery, and a vascularized tissue bed, such as fascia, muscle, periosteum, or perichondrium, are essential to graft survival. Postoperative bleeding, infection, and shearing or tearing of the graft from its bed are the most common causes of partial or total skin graft failure.

Harvesting the Graft

Once a good graft bed has been prepared, the proper donor site chosen, and anesthesia accomplished, the donor site is incised and dissected in the usual appropriate dissection plane at the midsubcutaneous fat layer for the face and just above the muscle fascia in most other locations. After harvesting, the donor tissue is placed on a gauze sponge in a cold, sterile saline bath to maintain viability. The donor site is then undermined and closed as carefully as would be done for a cosmetic surgical defect to maximize patient satisfaction.

Preparing the Graft

Trimming and contouring the graft is arguably the most important technical operation to ensure survival, contour match, and patient satisfaction. The donor skin specimen is retrieved from its saline bath and placed on a sterile gauze sponge held in the surgeon's nondominant hand. All subcutaneous fatty tissue and any remaining hair follicle bulbs are trimmed from the underside of the donor skin (Fig. 26–7), followed by trimming through the pinkish dermal layer to the whitish dermal layer. Care should be taken at this stage not to remove excess dermal tissue. A careful inspection of the various surface contours in the graft bed is then made, and the graft is trimmed circumferentially to precisely fit the recipient site. Multiple trimming operations are usually necessary[22] to achieve the perfect reverse contour[23] in the donor skin that will exactly match the graft bed. Care must be exercised not to "buttonhole," or perforate, the graft specimen during this operation.

Fixating the Graft

Fixating the donor skin to the recipient bed is the next step in full-thickness skin grafting. Many different methods have been described by numerous surgeons, but all successful techniques share several characteristics: the graft must be securely approximated to its recipient bed, a method to minimize hematoma or

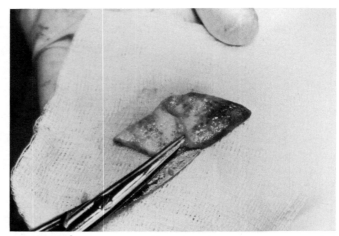

Figure 26–7. Trimming a full-thickness graft with iris scissors (left half already completed).

seroma formation must be used, careful approximation of the graft to the graft bed edges is required, and some means of maintaining external pressure is employed.

A simplified approach to all these issues has been described[24] and consists of placing interrupted sutures of Teflon-coated braided suture material at 1-cm intervals around the graft edge for the first 180 degrees, leaving one end long for the tie-over dressing. This step is followed by placement of multiple basting sutures of the same material through the grafted skin and into the graft bed to fixate it and prevent the formation of a hematoma or seroma. Basting sutures must be placed no closer than 1 cm apart for best results. The remaining 180 degrees of the graft circumference can then be roughly approximated with interrupted sutures at 1-cm intervals, leaving one end long to help secure the tie-over dressing. A running suture is then employed to exactly approximate the graft to the edges of the bed, taking care to invert tissue edges and not strangulate the tissue with excessive tension.

Applying the Dressing

Providing even compression to the completed graft is done with a variety of different dressing techniques. External stents composed of dental stent material were employed early in the history of full-thickness skin grafting. These have been replaced by more common materials such as sterile cotton balls or gauze soaked in saline and sterilized orthopedic cast foam that has been precisely carved to match each graft.[24] A stent simply provides consistent external pressure to the graft, both to fixate the graft and to facilitate revascularization in the early postoperative period. In addition to basting sutures and stents, external compression dressings are used by many surgeons to further ensure stability of grafted skin.

Postoperative Care

Postoperative antibiotics appropriately chosen to minimize streptococcal and staphylococcal infections are helpful to prevent graft loss. The use of any particular medication is the individual choice of each surgeon based largely on prior experience. A 5-day course of oral antibiotics will usually suffice, but longer therapy may occasionally be desired, especially in diabetic patients.

The most nagging controversy in postoperative graft care is when to inspect the graft. Some surgeons prefer to examine the site at 24 to 48 hours to ensure that no hematoma or seroma has formed. If strict hemostasis was obtained and all three fixation methods were employed, a first look at the new graft at 7 days is usually a safe practice. Several basting and interrupted sutures are usually left in place to ensure continued graft adherence for several additional days.

Miscellaneous Considerations

Additional miscellaneous considerations for successful full-thickness skin grafting include prohibition of aspirin for 2 weeks before the operation, elimination of alcoholic beverages for 2 days before and 1 week after grafting,[25] advising patients with facial grafts to sleep in an upright position on several pillows for several days, and avoidance of strenuous activities and lifting for several weeks. The most important considerations for ultimate patient happiness still remain the proper selection and management of the donor site.[26]

Dermabrasion Revision of Full-Thickness Grafts. After a lesion has been removed and the skin graft site has healed, most patients have a tendency to take for granted the skills and biology involved in their operation and shift their concern to the visual appearance of the graft. Although most grafts will improve in appearance over time, most full-thickness skin grafts can be further improved by skillful revision using dermabrasion.[22] Dermabrasion revision of primary scars is most effective when performed within 2 to 4 weeks after surgery or injury. Skin grafts, however, require much more time for growth and maturation of nourishing vessels and

may be partially or completely destroyed by early dermabrasion. No adequate study on the ideal time to dermabrade grafts exists. However, if at least 2 months have elapsed after skin graft surgery, results from dermabrasion are usually excellent. A second dermabrasion revision may be required 3 to 6 weeks later to obtain an optimal cosmetic result.

Split-Thickness Skin Grafts

Split-thickness skin grafts consist of epidermis and varying partial thicknesses of dermis. They are usually classified into thin (0.012 inch, 0.30 mm), intermediate (0.018 inch, 0.46 mm) and thick (0.024 inch, 0.61 mm). These sizes are somewhat arbitrary and were developed from the settings of older split-graft instruments, particularly the Padgett dermatome, which is rarely used today.

The split-thickness graft has both advantages and disadvantages compared with full-thickness grafts. The primary advantages include the ability to cover relatively large areas, especially when meshed; a very high "take" or success rate, even when placed on poor quality or infected graft beds; and a lower level of technical skill required by the surgeon. The disadvantages of split grafts are contraction, which adversely affects both function and appearance; the need for specialized equipment to harvest these grafts; the increased fragility of split grafts; and poor color and texture match compared with the surrounding normal skin.

INSTRUMENTS FOR HARVESTING SPLIT-THICKNESS GRAFTS

A Weck blade is the simplest of instruments to use but requires steady technique and a good eye to cut acceptable split grafts. It is difficult to cut a continuous sheet of skin by this method (Fig. 26–8), and these grafts are never uniform.

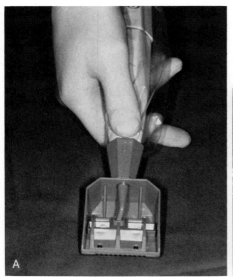
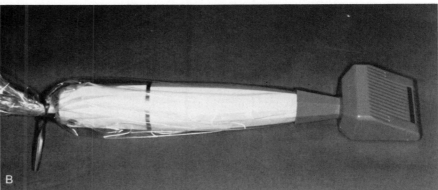

Figure 26–8. A, The Davol-Simon dermatome with sterile disposable head. B, The Davol-Simon dermatome in its sterile, transparent bag.

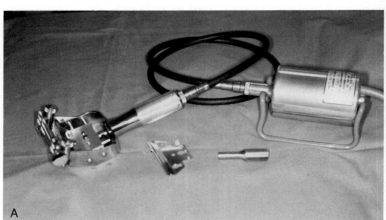
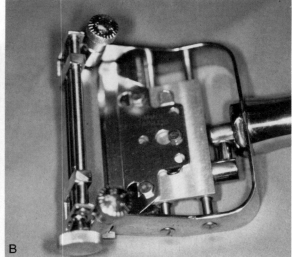

Figure 26–9. *A,* The Brown dermatome and its electric motor. *B,* Adjustable head of the Brown dermatome that can be used to vary both the width and the thickness of the grafts.

The Davol-Simon dermatome consists of a battery-powered handle, which can be placed in a sterile plastic sleeve, and a disposable sterile cutting head with fixed settings of 0.015-inch thickness and 1¹⁵⁄₁₆-inch width. This is a very inexpensive and useful instrument for small defects. The lack of adjustability and the narrow graft width, however, somewhat limit the usefulness of the Davol-Simon instrument.

For harvesting larger grafts, the electric or gas-operated Brown dermatome (Fig. 26–9) is most commonly used.[27] This instrument is adjustable for cutting very thin up to very thick split-thickness grafts and is generally employed at a setting of 0.018 inch (0.46 mm). It is somewhat difficult to calibrate and set the thickness on this instrument accurately, requiring minimum adjustments of at least 0.005 inch (0.13 mm) to prevent breakage. However, graft width can be varied with this machine.

TECHNIQUE FOR HARVESTING SPLIT-THICKNESS GRAFTS

The donor and recipient sites are first anesthetized in preparation for grafting. Usual donor areas for harvesting split-thickness skin grafts include the abdomen, back, buttocks and anterior thighs (Fig. 26–10). Sterile lubricant is generously spread on the donor site before cutting the graft. Op-Site, a synthetic polyurethane surgical membrane, can first be placed on the donor site to increase the ease of tissue handling and prevent the graft from contracting and rolling up after being cut. Use of the membrane will decrease graft thickness by 0.002 inch, which is the average membrane thickness. No other preparation of the site is necessary, unless shaving the area is appropriate.

Cutting a uniform split graft requires at least one assistant to hold the surrounding skin very taut while the graft is cut (Fig. 26–11). As cutting proceeds, it is

ideal to have another assistant pick up the first portion of the graft to prevent fouling of the blades and to ensure a more uniform specimen. The graft is then loosely placed directly into the defect. Often more than one graft is necessary to cover a wound adequately, and the graft edges should overlap onto normal surrounding skin. That portion of graft that overlies epidermis will not survive. A running suture is used to join the split graft to the graft bed edges. Multiple basting sutures or a running basting suture may be placed to secure the graft, and a sterile external compresssion dressing is placed. The dressing is not disturbed for 7 days, by which time the graft has usually taken. The area may be re-dressed daily if any doubt exists as to the success.

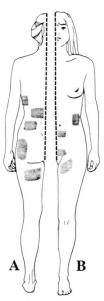

Figure 26–10. Common split-thickness skin graft donor sites on the posterior *(A)* and the anterior *(B)* aspects of the body.

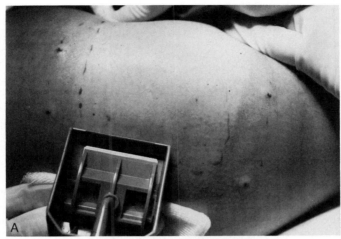

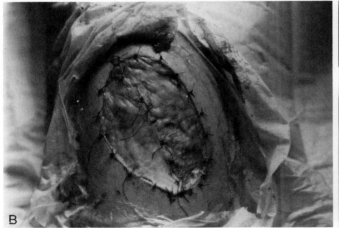

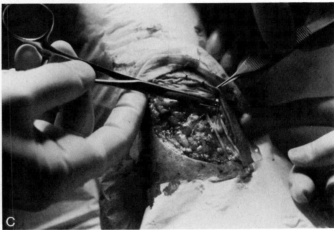

Figure 26–11. *A,* Split-thickness skin graft being cut with the Davol-Simon dermatome. *B,* Suturing the graft into the graft bed. *C,* Appearance of the completely sutured graft.

Donor site management includes pressure to control bleeding, followed by application of an Op-Site membrane, which is left in place until the skin has healed.[28] A few slits in the membrane and daily dressing changes at the donor site will control fluid exudation from the area.

A mechanical cutter is occasionally used to mesh or cut many small slits in the graft when there is a need to cover large areas or only a limited donor area exists. A meshed graft can cover many times the area of a standard split-thickness skin graft, can be used over mobile areas, and will easily fit into body folds and creases such as the axilla.

Specialized Types of Skin Grafts

A number of specialized skin grafts have been developed for use in unique cosmetic or reconstructive situations. Different principles govern choosing, harvesting, constructing, and caring for each of these grafts.

COMPOSITE GRAFTS

The composite skin graft[29–31] is essentially a technique that was developed to solve the surgical problem of alar

rim reconstruction. Because of the fibrofatty cartilaginous tissue that supports the ala, a semirigid structure must be created when reconstructing defects in this area. This type of graft is used when full-thickness loss of the alar rim is encountered.

The exclusive donor site for composite grafts is the ear (Fig. 26–12). This obviates any problem of donor site choice in most patients. Skin and cartilage are harvested en bloc, taking care to harvest a larger donor specimen than the defect requires to allow for shrinkage. Almost any segment of the ear may be used for com-

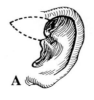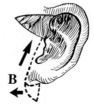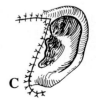

Figure 26–12. Schematic diagram showing a composite skin graft. *A,* Planned excision lines marked on the donor site. *B,* Appearance of the defect after excision of the graft and the anticipated repair using an inferiorly based advancement flap that excises the Burow's triangle below the earlobe; *C,* Appearance after closure of the defect.

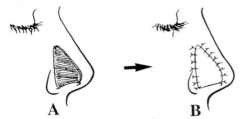

Figure 26–13. *A,* Appearance of a full-thickness defect of the ala. *B,* After reconstruction using composite graft from ascending helical rim.

posite grafting. After harvesting, the composite graft is sutured into the defect with minimal-width suture, taking care not to strangulate tissue (Fig. 26–13). The very high metabolic needs of this graft make a complete take unlikely. Unfortunately, the tissue most often lost is the cartilage needed to support and stabilize the alar rim. Because nourishment of this graft depends solely on the peripheral vasculature, a practical upper size limit is generally only 1 cm. Dressings to immobilize the grafted site are used as in other grafts. A successful composite graft often requires secondary revisional procedures, which are performed at a later date.

PINCH GRAFTS

Although pinch grafts have usually been described as split-thickness grafts,[32] in practice most cutaneous surgeons actually cut a graft that is full thickness centrally and tapers to very thin split thickness at the periphery.[33] Pinch grafts are almost always used to resurface intractable leg ulcers, and the common donor sites are the abdomen, thighs, and buttocks (Fig. 26–14).

The technique for harvesting pinch grafts is simple. Wheals are raised using intradermal injections of local anesthetic. The tops of these wheals are shaved off with a scalpel and then placed directly onto the prepared ulcer bed. Graft bed preparation can be accomplished by sharp scalpel dissection, soaking with a 1% vinegar-and-water solution (1:3 mixture), or the use of other local wound care that promotes the formation of granulation tissue. These grafts take as well on granulation tissue as on a normal bed. After grafting, an external compressive dressing coated with an antibacterial ointment is applied for 7 to 10 days. The patient should remain at rest with the extremity elevated as much as is practical during the postoperative period.

Several sessions of pinch grafting may be necessary to provide complete coverage of the ulcer, because all of

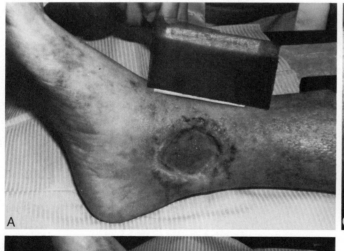

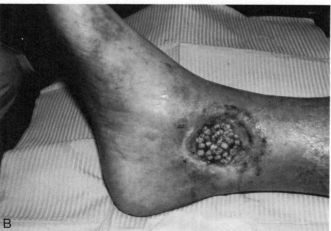

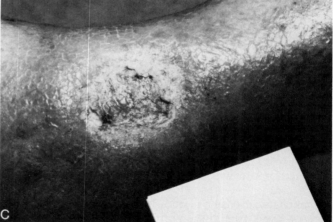

Figure 26–14. *A,* Clean leg ulcer site with granulation tissue ready for pinch grafts. *B,* Pinch grafts applied to wound bed. *C,* Clinical appearance 2 months postoperatively.

the grafts are not expected to take. This method of skin grafting is designed to close an ulcer defect only; it does not serve as a cosmetic graft. Virtually all these grafts will exhibit color variation, surface pebbling, and an uneven appearance.

DELAYED GRAFTING

An interesting variation of grafting can be successfully used with full-thickness grafts.[34] Delayed grafting simply offers the opportunity to apply a full-thickness graft to a poor-quality graft bed. In this procedure, the graft bed is left ungrafted for several days to allow granulation tissue to form. The tremendous vascularity of the granulation tissue then allows application of a full-thickness graft onto an otherwise ungraftable bed. For selected defects, this technique can be invaluable.

PUNCH GRAFTS

Punch grafts have been used for many years, and hair transplantion surgery currently relies largely on this method. From the original application of punch grafting for hair transplantation, other uses have developed over the years. Punch excision of deep "ice-pick" acne scars, followed by the insertion of punch grafts in the small defects, can significantly improve the final result in many patients after dermabrasion. A new application of this technology is punch grafting skin to repigment vitiliginous skin.[35] The technique in punch grafting is elementary, involving only punch excision of a small segment of skin with various punch instruments, followed by positioning the grafts in punch excision graft beds. The grafts can be secured by sutures or by skin-adhesive strips, and healing occurs without difficulty. These small grafts serve as a source of melanocytes, which can repopulate the vitiliginous areas and produce normal pigmentation.

TUNNEL GRAFTS

Wearing a hairpiece is a vexing problem for many patients. Adhesive tape systems tend to lose effectiveness over several hours because of the natural oiliness of the scalp. A sudden gust of wind can then remove the hairpiece, to the great embarrassment of the owner. Tunnel grafts[36] were designed to eliminate this problem for hairpiece users. To create the graft, a strip of scalp skin is incised and elevated in three sectors of the bald scalp. Full-thickness skin grafts are chosen from any area, harvested, and formed into a strip circle to exactly fit the defect formed by elevating the incised scalp skin. It is much like fitting a circular graft, raw side to raw side, into a slit defect. The innate vascularity in the scalp usually allows complete survival of this graft, and it is ready for use in about 2 months to anchor the hairpiece securely in place.

DOGEAR GRAFTS

The dogear graft is formed by using the excess normal tissue that is excised from the ends of a linear wound.

This excess tissue is defatted and used as a full-thickness graft wherever required to close a large or complicated defect. The low metabolic needs of this small graft generally ensure success, as well as a good cosmetic match. This ancillary maneuver can be useful anywhere on the body.

EPIDERMAL SUCTION GRAFTS

Epidermal grafting is another technique that has been successfully used in the repigmentation of vitiliginous skin (see Chap. 77). The depigmented area is deepithelialized with a scalpel blade or suction cup. Pigmented donor skin is then raised as a suction blister using a suction cup and negative pressure. The donor skin is then immediately placed on the recipient site. A compression dressing applied for 7 to 10 days helps to ensure a successful graft take. The centrifugal spread of pigment can be anticipated from these grafts over time. The singular problem seen with this method is lack of pigment uniformity in the final result.

Graft Failure

The main causes for graft failure are bleeding, infection, and shearing motion of the graft that disrupts the vascular supply (Table 26–2). Systemic diseases can also interfere with graft survival, particularly diabetes mellitus and immunodeficiency disorders. Incidental trauma, as when patients roll over in their sleep, can unavoidably destroy an otherwise successful operative procedure. Failure to physically elevate the grafted part can cause improper healing, as well as retard the normal regenerative processes. An incorrect assessment of the graft

TABLE 26–2. **COMMON CAUSES OF GRAFT FAILURE**

Poor wound care
   Excess physical activity
   Dependent position
   Motion causing shearing action
   Inadvertent trauma
Poor donor site
   Fat, bone, cartilage, tendon
   Necrotic debris in wound
   Excess electrocoagulation
   Inadequate granulation tissue
Infection
   Staphylococcus sp.
   Streptococcus sp.
   Pseudomonas sp.
Systemic disease
   Diabetes
   Immunosuppression
   Collagen-vascular disorders
Technical errors
   Inadequate size
   Excess thickness
   Tension
   Incomplete hemostasis causing hematoma formation
   Improper dressing
      Too tight
      Not immobilizing
   Rough handling leading to trauma

bed quality and choice of an inappropriate graft thickness can also doom the graft to fail in some instances.

SUMMARY

Skin grafting can provide an effective method for the reconstruction of many wounds. Attention to meticulous hemostasis without producing devitalized graft bed tissue, proper choice of graft donor site and thickness, stabilization of the graft on its bed, and appropriate use of postoperative antibiotics will prevent most potential problems from occurring. Other factors, such as the surgeon's experience, knowledge, and good judgment, are also of vital importance in determining the successful outcome of any skin graft procedure.

REFERENCES

1. Limova M, Grekin RC: Synthetic membranes and cultured keratinocyte grafts. J Am Acad Dermatol 23:713–719, 1990.
2. Baronio G: On Grafting in Animals. JB Sax, Boston, 1985.
3. Bunger C: Gelungener versuch einer Nasenbildung aus einem volig getrennten aus dem beine. J Chir Ausgenh 4:569, 1823.
4. Hill TG: The evolution of skin graft reconstruction. J Dermatol Surg Oncol 13:834–835, 1987.
5. Henry L, Marshall DC, Friedman EA, et al: A histologic study of the human skin autograft. Am J Pathol 39:317–323, 1961.
6. Converse JM, Smahel J, Ballentyne DL Jr, Harper AD: Inosculation of vessels of skin graft and host bed: a fortuitous encounter. Br J Plast Surg 28:282–285, 1975.
7. Waris T, Rechardt L, Kyosola K: Reinnervation of human skin grafts: a histochemical study. Plast Reconstr Surg 72:439–447, 1983.
8. Kearney JN, Harnby D, Gowland G, Holland KT: The follicular distribution and abundance of resident bacteria on human skin. J Gen Microbiol 130:797–801, 1984.
9. Freund PR, Brengelmann GL, Rowell LB, et al: Vasomotor control in healed grafted skin in humans. J Appl Physiol 51:168–171, 1981.
10. Martin DL, Chang PS, McGrouther DA: Full thickness graft of haemangiomatous skin. Br J Plast Surg 38:588, 1985.
11. Alexander JW, MacMillan BG, Law EJ, Krummel R: Prophylactic antibiotics as an adjunct for skin grafting in clean reconstructive surgery following burn injury. J Trauma 22:687–690, 1982.
12. Gonnering RS, Kindwall EP, Goldman RW: Adjunct hyperbaric oxygen therapy in periorbital reconstruction. Arch Ophthalmol 104:439–443, 1986.
13. Converse JM (ed): Reconstructive Plastic Surgery. 2nd ed. WB Saunders, Philadelphia, 1977, p 180.
14. Wheeland RG: Skin grafts. In: Roenigk RK, Roenigk HH Jr (eds): Dermatologic Surgery: Principles and Practice. Dekker, New York, 1989, pp 323–346.
15. Ostrovskjv NV: Selection of the skin graft thickness with regard to structure of the donor skin site. Acta Chir Plast 27:145–151, 1985.
16. English FP, Forster TD: The eyebrow graft. Ophthalmic Surg 10:39–41, 1979.
17. Holmstrom H, Bartholdson L, Johanson B: Surgical treatment of eyelid cancer with special reference to tarso-conjunctival flaps. Scand J Plast Reconstr Surg 9:107–115, 1975.
18. Breach NM: Pre-auricular full-thickness skin grafts. Br J Plast Surg 31:124–136, 1978.
19. Hill TG: Reconstruction of nasal defects using full-thickness skin grafts: a personal reappraisal. J Dermatol Surg Oncol 9:995–1001, 1983.
20. Vecchione TR: The use of proximal nasal tissue in nasal reconstruction. Aesthetic Plast Surg 6:177–178, 1982.
21. Wullstein HL, Wullstein SR: The altered metabolism of the full thickness skin graft. Laryngoscope 82:1990–1999, 1972.
22. Hill TG: Enhancing the survival of full-thickness grafts. J Dermatol Surg Oncol 10:639–642, 1984.
23. Hill TG: Contouring of donor skin in full-thickness skin grafting. J Dermatol Surg Oncol 13:883–888, 1987.
24. Hill TG: A simplified method for closure of full-thickness skin grafts. J Dermatol Surg Oncol 6:892–893, 1980.
25. Buckley RM, Ventura ES, MacGregor RR: Propranolol antagonizes the anti-inflammatory effects of alcohol and improves survival of infected intoxicated rabbits. J Clin Invest 59:554–559, 1978.
26. Rigg BM: Importance of donor site selection in skin grafting. Can Med Assoc J 117:1028–1029, 1977.
27. Skouge JW: Techniques for split-thickness skin grafting. J Dermatol Surg Oncol 13:841–849, 1987.
28. Barnett A, Berkowitz RL, Mills R, Vistnes LM: Comparison of synthetic adhesive moisture vapor permeable and fine mesh gauze dressings for split-thickness skin graft donor sites. Am J Surg 145:379–381, 1983.
29. Bennett JE, Thurston JB: Cancer of the nose: ablation and repair. Clin Plast Surg 3:461–469, 1976.
30. Vecchione TR: Reconstruction of the ala and nostril sill using proximate composite grafts. Ann Plast Surg 5:148–150, 1980.
31. Vecchione TR: The use of proximal nasal tissue in nasal reconstruction. Aesthetic Plast Surg 6:177–178, 1982.
32. Wheeland RG: The technique and current status of pinch grafting. J Dermatol Surg Oncol 13:873–880, 1987.
33. Stegman SJ, Tromovitch TA, Glogau RG: Basics of Dermatologic Surgery. Year Book Medical, Chicago, 1982, pp 105–106.
34. Ceilley RI, Bumsted RM, Panje WR: Delayed skin grafting. J Dermatol Surg Oncol 9:288–293, 1983.
35. Selmanowitz VJ: Pigmentary correction of piebaldism by autografts II. Pathomechanism and pigment spread in piebaldism. Cutis 24:66–71, 1979.
36. Bendl BJ: The tunnel graft procedure for attachment of a hairpiece. Cutis 18:559–562, 1976.

CHAPTER 27

Random-Pattern Flaps

DUANE C. WHITAKER

Dermatologists, plastic surgeons, head and neck surgeons, orbital surgeons, and general surgeons all commonly perform cutaneous surgery. The body of knowledge about skin surgery is a combination of contributions from these specialties, as well as from the basic sciences of anatomy, biochemistry, physiology, anatomic pathology, and others.[1] Many disciplines have contributed to our understanding of the science of wound healing, which has improved surgical technique and postoperative wound care, rehabilitation of the wound or injured site, and management of complications and revisions of adverse outcomes.

A complete preoperative evaluation is important to the full understanding of the biology and pathology of the disease being treated and is essential if the procedure is to be performed with the best possible judgment and technique. Recognition of the concepts, skills, and techniques of tissue movement is also vital to obtaining the best results when using local skin flaps to repair a surgical defect. The cutaneous surgeon must understand the nature of the disease, and if the lesion removed was malignant, the likelihood for recurrence must be evaluated. In cutaneous oncology, a margin-control method of removal should be used before performing complex or local flap closure. Margin clearance using Mohs technique, multiple frozen sections, or permanent sections with delayed closure gives the best assurance of tumor-free margins. It is unacceptable to close a cutaneous defect with a flap if there is risk of tumor-positive margins. The additional defect and scar embellishment created by the flap make re-excision much more difficult and may subject the patient to unnecessary surgery. There is also a risk of spreading residual tumor, which may make the precise location of any foci of residual tumor difficult, if not impossible. This may in turn result in a larger and more disfiguring scar than would have otherwise been required. In addition, when treating multiply recurrent tumors, the surgeon should recognize that regardless of the quality of treatment, there is still a significant risk of recurrent disease. When this is the case, it will affect not only the type of flap chosen but also whether a flap closure is even appropriate. However, if the surgeon is removing a benign lesion and recurrence of the disease presents no harm to the patient, the very best functional and cosmetic outcomes must be the guiding elements.

Wound Closure Options

Most cutaneous defects are amenable to the four following wound closure options: primary closure with variations, second-intention healing, skin grafts, and local or distant flaps. The surgeon should consider all four options when presented with a cutaneous defect and, using a mental checklist, take into account not only these broad categories, but also the options within each category. Many skin defects can be closed primarily or with some minor variation or modification[2-4] such as M-plasty, S-plasty, broken-line closure, and others. Second-intention healing allows the wound to epithelialize without formal repair. Nearly all cutaneous wounds that are not full thickness have an acceptable recipient bed that can be skin grafted. Delayed skin grafting can also be combined with second-intention healing by waiting from 48 hours to several weeks before proceeding with full- or split-thickness skin grafts to enhance graft survival. When a tumor at high risk for recurrence is treated, grafting or second-intention healing may be the management of choice. When properly chosen, these two techniques can achieve good long-term functional and cosmetic results,[3] although scar tissue or poor tissue match may make the site noticeable.

Flaps, on the other hand, provide a unique opportunity for wound closure that may not be apparent or even considered by the nonsurgeon.[5] Very simply, flaps are dependent on a relative excess amount of adjacent tissue that can be moved into the defect. One or more secondary incisions extending beyond the primary surgical defect allow this tissue to be advanced, rotated, or transposed into the defect. The well-designed flap, when applied expertly, can achieve nearly "perfect" wound closure. This can give the patient who has a surgical loss of tissue a functional and cosmetic outcome that may be imperceptible from normal. On the other hand, a poorly chosen flap can create a deformity beyond that that was required to treat the original disease. The surgeon who performs flap surgery is obliged to have sufficient expertise and experience in choosing and executing the best closure for the patient. Ill-chosen and poorly executed flaps not only create unnecessary pain and expense but also may ultimately injure the patient.

Weighing the Wound Closure Options

The surgeon must understand the disease process being treated and recognize the importance of the patient's age and medical condition and the location and size of the defect.[6] The expectations and capacity of the patient to comply with good postsurgical care must also be considered. An identical defect in two different patients will not necessarily be managed the same way. For a full-thickness defect of the ear or lip, a complex layered or flap closure is necessary. A more superficial defect gives more latitude to the surgeon. Cutaneous oncologists probably have greater experience with second-intention healing of wounds than any other surgical specialty. Open wounds that are properly cared for have a very low complication rate of both infection and hemorrhage.[7] Any closed wound has a higher risk of infection because of the presence of a foreign body in a closed area, which promotes colonization by bacteria. When tissue undermining is required to accomplish a closure, the risk of inadvertent injury to other structures, prolonged dysesthesias, and postoperative bleeding increases. For some patients, no closure may be the best option.

Bleeding under a flap usually requires evacuation of the hematoma, which sometimes results in loss of the flap as well as the area undermined. This complication does not occur in wounds that heal by second intention.

An undesirable event, bleeding under a skin graft, may result in loss of the graft. Therefore, the patient who is on anticoagulants or antiplatelet medications or has some other bleeding diathesis may be a poor candidate for flap reconstruction if the defect can be managed in another way. The heavy smoker with chronic pulmonary disease and poorly vascularized peripheral tissue may also be a poor candidate for flap reconstruction because of the tenuous vascularity inherent in all local flaps. Flaps from neck tissue are difficult to immobilize in ambulatory patients, as all patients will inadvertently move the neck, even after a painful surgical procedure. For this reason, neck flaps should be performed with care because of the additional risk of hematoma formation and the possible emergency situation produced by an enlarging mass in the neck.

Considering the Intangibles

All surgeons have their own standards of excellence that they strive to equal or exceed in all surgeries they perform. This is derived partially from training, partially from the desire to give the best care to the patient, and partially from emulation of peers or mentors. However, in addition to these standards, it is important to understand the patient's own expectations. Some patients arrive for the consultation appointment well informed and appropriately prepared for what the surgery involves. More typically, however, patients have a combination of unrealistic fear and almost magical expectation of what modern medicine can perform. When faced with cutaneous surgery, some patients say to the physician, "I really don't care about a scar" or even, "It doesn't matter what I look like, I'm too old," but few patients actually mean this. Despite the differences among patients, all patients want to retain maximal function and present an "acceptable" face or profile to the public. Regardless of the patient's words, it is the physician's responsibility to determine what the patient thinks the surgery involves and what the outcome may be.[6] The physician must realistically portray the range of outcomes and the risks involved. Patients must understand that it is not always possible to return them to their original anatomic state; this depends on the location and size of the defect and the severity of the disease treated. When malignancy is treated, patients must understand the priorities of treatment and also recognize that the more severe or neglected the disease, the fewer reconstructive options that are available. Most patients can accept a cosmetic defect if they understand in advance that this may be necessary to improve the likelihood of complete cure of the disease. Since no one likes unhappy surprises, the physician must have sufficient empathy to understand the patient's viewpoint. Too frequently, patients are seen who have had surgery competently performed but are unhappy because they did not expect the surgical outcome.

Tissue Movement

ANATOMY

Skin surgery requires both a biologic and a practical understanding of skin anatomy and the underlying subcutaneous tissue.[8] Even though surgery of the skin and the superficial adipose tissue does not usually place motor nerves at risk of injury in most instances, the cutaneous surgeon must be aware that terminal branches of the facial nerve, cranial nerve XI (spinal accessory nerve), and the digital nerves are located relatively superficially. Surgery must be done with care and with knowledge of the underlying anatomy. Two other structures located relatively superficially in the face and neck are the parotid gland and the great auricular nerve.

That portion of the parotid gland located anterior and inferior to the lobule of the ear is protected only by skin and subcutaneous tissue; there is no overlying musculature. The sensory great auricular nerve, traversing the sternocleidomastoid in the mid and lower neck, is protected only by skin and subcutaneous fat. Since sensory nerves terminate in the skin and subcutaneous tissue, any surgery will result in temporary numbness, tingling, and dysesthesias. These are usually of short duration, as long as the main nerve trunk is not transected. Sensory aberration usually will diminish 3 to 6 months after the surgery. Occasionally, patients are bothered by dysesthesias that persist longer than would be expected from the simple nature of the surgery.

CONCEPTS OF TISSUE MOVEMENT

Because fusiform or elliptical excisions and closures of the skin utilize a straightforward logic, they are generally understood by all surgeons. Flaps, however, are different and require a conceptual three-dimensional view of the skin that is not always readily apparent. Good flap closures require both knowledge of the anatomy and technical skill. Successful flap surgery also depends on the capacity of the surgeon to develop a mental image of how the donor tissue can be used to close the presenting defect. The surgeon must have significant experience to fully understand the components and symmetry of the head and neck region as well as the operative area under consideration. The surgeon determines this by very carefully assessing each patient. Most surgeons begin this process first with careful observation and then with testing using experienced hands, fingers, or skin hooks to determine the laxity of adjacent skin that might be used to reconstruct the defect. At the same time, the surgeon must also consider how much donated tissue will be necessary to close the primary defect, whether the secondary defect can be closed primarily and what will be the resultant scar, and whether significant distortion of adjacent structures will result. The surgeon combines visual and conceptual experience with knowledge gained by gentle palpation and sliding of tissues by hand or skin hook.

Although each face is composed of the same basic anatomic structures, the quality and mobility of skin vary greatly from one individual to another. Older patients have more relaxed tissue than younger patients. However, there are many significant interage variations of this general rule. No matter how many surgeries a surgeon has been performed, he or she knows that the ultimate benefit of the flap can be determined only by performing it, as flap surgery is not a totally predictable art or science. With experience, the surgeon also will have alternative plans in mind. If the first attempt at closure has different results from those predicted, modifications can be employed. Training in flap surgery should be extensive so that surgeons can develop creative ways of adapting to the problems that occur when the planned tissue movement does not provide the desired result.

Early published articles on flap surgery were very closely tied to specific geometric standards of flap surgery (e.g., the traditional rhomboid flap). Other published flap articles showed very simplistic two-dimensional diagrams of flap correction of defects in various parts of the face and neck. Although these publications helped to stimulate thought and were useful in teaching, the diagrams were rarely directly transferrable to any one patient. For this reason, flap surgery is best learned through a combination of studying the available literature and working by the side of an experienced surgeon. Soft tissue surgery has come a long way since the presentation of a predetermined number of flaps, when the goal always appeared to be stretching the patient's skin to fit a picture in the book. To facilitate this rigid geometric approach, templates were manufactured so that the surgeon could apply the outline to the patient and then draw and cut along the lines. These techniques have fallen from favor because they fail to provide the surgeon with the best closure for each patient.

The best flaps are usually developed by pressing and stretching the tissues along with some undermining, followed by further stretching of the tissue with skin hooks. Then, using removable tissue markers, the first outlines for the flap design are created. A rigid predetermined plan rarely works. More important than creating an accurate geometric template is respect for the facial units and boundaries between facial units and recognition of the course of relaxed skin tension lines.[9–12] For example, a perfectly designed bilobed flap that obliterates the melolabial fold is a failure. A flap that can confine and hide a scar within the unit of the cheek itself, within the unit of the lip, or within that fold or junction of tissue between the two units is superior.[13, 14] Flap design has evolved in a way that respects the face and its units, unlike a geometric or precisely angulated flap that exists without regard to either the anatomy or the tissues themselves.

SCAR MATURATION IN TISSUE MOVEMENT

The scar maturation process is very important in local flaps. All closures should be considered from both the long- and the short-term view of the defect and the scar that is created. Young scars are composed of immature collagen, excess ground substance, and excess fluid. With scar maturation, the most obvious clinical change is a decrease in scar volume with time.[1] Because of this, suture lines should always be slightly elevated and everted and never depressed.[15] Because the skin of older patients is generally more "forgiving," a mediocre flap of only average design can be expected to improve with maturation and time. However, the skin of younger patients is not likely to be so forgiving. Therefore, the long-term view should be taken when designing and executing a flap. Incisions and flaps should be placed away from the center of the face and hidden in facial creases, in junctions between two different qualities of skin, or even in a depressed or angulated part that will tend to shadow and obscure any scar. Good scar outcome depends on the technical skill of the surgeon, as well as the ability of the patient to camouflage the location and visibility of the scar as much as possible.

Surgical Technique

HANDLING TISSUE

Special care should always be used when handling flaps. There is no substitute for gentle and fine handling of tissues in all such manipulations and surgical interventions. Forceps should be fine in caliber, and the tissues must not be crushed. A small amount of pressure applied with the hand or the wrist, when transmitted through the mechanical advantage of the instrument, can damage the tissue. In general, because the use of skin hooks helps prevent the surgeon from inadvertently damaging tissues, many skilled surgeons choose and prefer them over tissue forceps. However, when handled with finesse and care, either instrument can provide very satisfactory results.

UNDERMINING AND HEMOSTASIS

Most local flaps and closures require undermining. This allows the skin and the vascular subcutaneous layer to slide more freely over the deeper attachments so that tissues can be stretched, pulled, or slid in the desired direction to help accomplish closure. Undermining tissues also allows them to heal and contract in a more homogeneous fashion,[16] which may prevent scar contracture from occurring along the flap edge, resulting in a pouched appearance. However, undermining to facilitate wound closure also creates potential dead space and causes additional injury to tissue. Because the undermining plane is usually in the superficial subcutaneous tissues overlying fascia, cartilage, or bone, motor nerves are not commonly injured. However, undermining increases bleeding, which results in greater potential for hematoma formation. Thus, it should not be done without due consideration, and it must be performed in the correct plane and with a specific purpose in mind.

Hemostasis is critical to the ultimate success of all closures. Any time undermining is done, the surgeon is obliged to carefully establish hemostasis. This can be done with an electrosurgical instrument of choice or a hemostat and suture ligature. Bipolar coagulation, in which the current simply passes between the two tips of a pair of forceps, causes minimal tissue damage. Monopolar electrocoagulation is also effective, although it causes slightly more tissue necrosis.

SUTURING TECHNIQUE

Suturing skills for flaps rely less on the use of specific sutures and more on the knowledge and technique necessary to achieve good subcutaneous closure and very fine dermal apposition without strangulation of tissues. Flaps are frequently closed with absorbable buried sutures and simple, interrupted, vertical mattress and half-buried mattress skin sutures. A running stitch or combination of running and interrupted sutures can also be used as long as skin apposition and eversion of the wound edges are obtained and the sutures removed in a timely manner.

Flap Classification

Local flaps are classified in several ways.[2, 5, 17] A useful way to understand flap nomenclature is to consider the three broad categories of dominant flap movements: advancement, rotation, and transposition. However, most flaps actually represent a combination of one or more of these types. Axial-pattern flaps are based on a specific artery, such as the temporal or supratrochlear arteries. Most local flaps are not classified by vascular pattern but are random in their vascular supply. The vascular supply of most local flaps is not derived from a single arterial supply but rather from the general arterial and capillary pattern of blood flow to that region of tissue. Distant flaps are frequently classified by their vascular supply, donor site (e.g., deltopectoral), whether the flap was delayed, and the use of special techniques to transfer the flaps (e.g., microvascular reanastomosis). Flap configuration can further differentiate a flap, so advancement flaps may be single or double, and rotation flaps may be bilobed or single lobed. The name of a flap may also refer to a particular classic region of use (e.g., nasolabial or melolabial flap). For purposes of this discussion, flaps will be referred to primarily by their dominant movement.

Tissue Advancement Flaps

PLANNING AND CONCEPTUALIZATION

Most flaps are planned around an existing defect. In primary closure of a fusiform defect, tissue advancement is used to close the defect, and no additional incisions are made to free tissue and achieve closure. For practical purposes, flaps require preplanning and additional incisions beyond the primary defect to achieve closure. When a closure cannot be achieved primarily, a flap may offer advantages that result in a superior closure.

Tissue advancement, which is the direct act of sliding, stretching, and pushing tissue into a defect, is used in almost all closures and is the simplest method of movement. It differs from primary closure in that the tissue moved will often glide more freely if it is undermined and incised free from the adjacent dermis. In some defects (Fig. 27–1), a strip of tissue only 1 cm wide often will actually advance farther than tissue three or four times larger. The extension and outcome of an advancement flap can be easily visualized. This also allows for little secondary movement. In general, advancement flaps are predictable and provide what the eye and the hand can help to determine by testing the tissue before actual closure. Very seldom do such flaps provide more movement than is perceived during preplanning.[6, 18]

TYPES OF ADVANCEMENT

The single advancement flap and double advancement flap (Fig. 27–2) utilize tissue movement that is equal on its inferior and superior dimensions. The tissue imme-

lateral brow. This flap has to be carefully developed deep to the hair follicles so that preservation of the hair-bearing tissue can be maintained. This advancement flap is useful when existing skin lines run parallel to the incisions of the flap. Single or double advancement flaps generally are not very useful for the scalp, cheek, or chin region. However, single-arm bilateral advancement flaps (Fig. 27–4) are useful in the forehead and temple region.

Once the technique and the concept of advancement flaps have been mastered and the effect on surrounding tissues can be visualized, it is no longer necessary to confine the flap to certain geometric shapes.[11, 20] It is more useful to think simply of the general advancement of tissue. If possible, the advancement of tissue should coincide with facial topographic features that can help to camouflage the incisions required to create the flap (Fig. 27–5). A single advancement flap can often meet the requirements of the defect and preserve the overall surrounding architecture, while a single rectangular advancement flap would create noticeable scars and provide an inferior long-term outcome. Simple advancement of tissue is designed so the scar conforms to a facial junction (Fig. 27–6), making it adaptable to many different clinical situations.

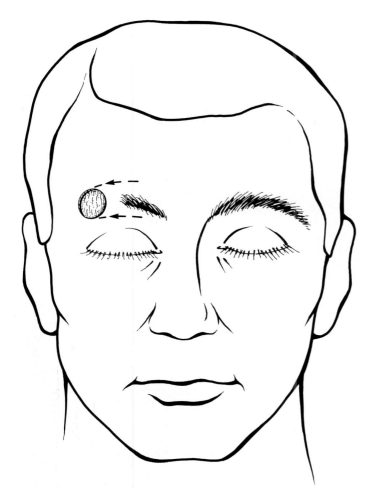

Figure 27–1. Schematic showing typical tissue advancement. (Redrawn courtesy of Frank Syndelar.)

diately adjacent to the flap moves somewhat less than the flap itself, so there is pouching or redundancy of tissue at the farthest extent of the advancement flap incisions. The most common way to deal with this redundancy is excision of a small piece of tissue, referred to as Burow's triangle. If a single advancement flap does not provide enough laxity to close the defect, then a second flap from the opposite side can be created. The resultant scar is roughly H shaped. If this flap is planned with no greater than a 3:1 length:width ratio in the head and neck skin, then flap survival is excellent. Other parts of the body may not tolerate a ratio as high.

The result of a single advancement flap is to stretch a band or strip of tissue farther than the surrounding nonflap tissue, leaving the dogears distant to the defect. The advancement flap distorts the surrounding tissue very little, because there is very little secondary movement. The key to evaluating whether this flap is appropriate lies in the capacity to see not only the defect but also how the scar will look and where the dogears will lie.[19] For a defect of the lateral eyebrow (Fig. 27–3) in which a portion of the hair-bearing tissue has been lost, a single advancement flap is used to close the defect and at the same time re-create the original length of the

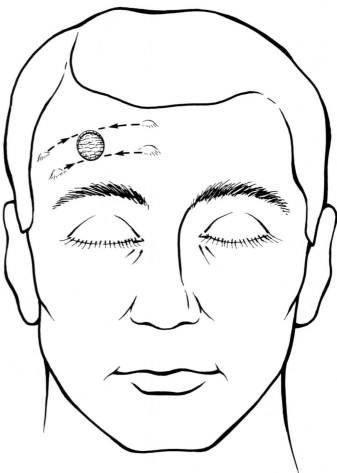

Figure 27–2. Schematic of a single and double advancement flap. (Redrawn courtesy of Frank Syndelar.)

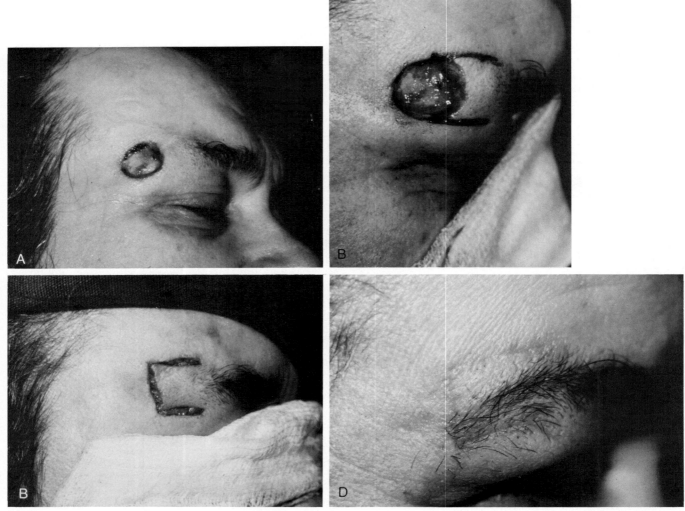

Figure 27–3. *A*, Defect of the lateral brow. *B*, A single advancement flap is outlined. *C*, Tissue is advanced into the defect with placement of subcutaneous sutures and then skin sutures. *D*, Early result after 1 month.

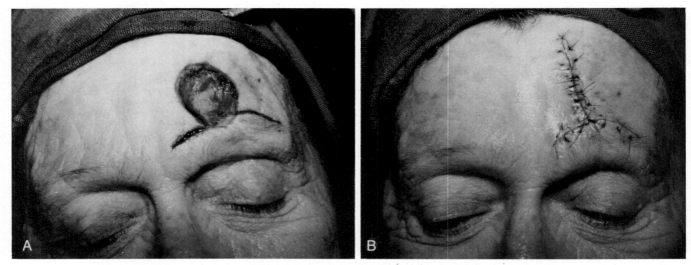

Figure 27–4. *A*, Single arm bilateral advancement flaps of the forehead. *B*, Flaps sutured into place.

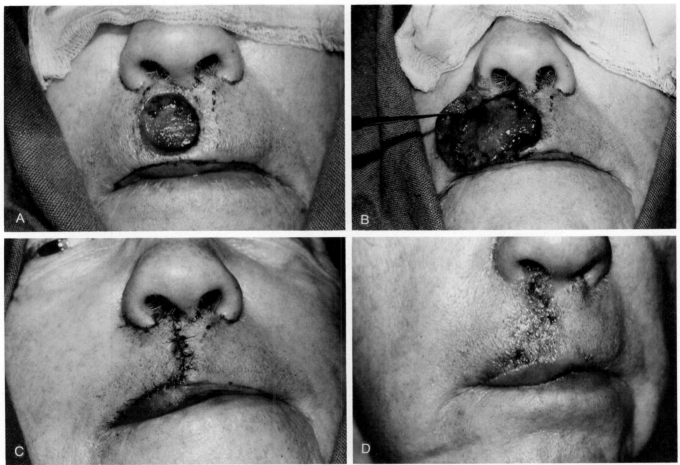

Figure 27–5. *A,* Defect of the upper lip. *B,* Advancement of the lip based on the vermilion and alar margins. *C,* Advancement flap sutured into place. *D,* Appearance after 1 week. The temporary edema of the vermilion resolves over time.

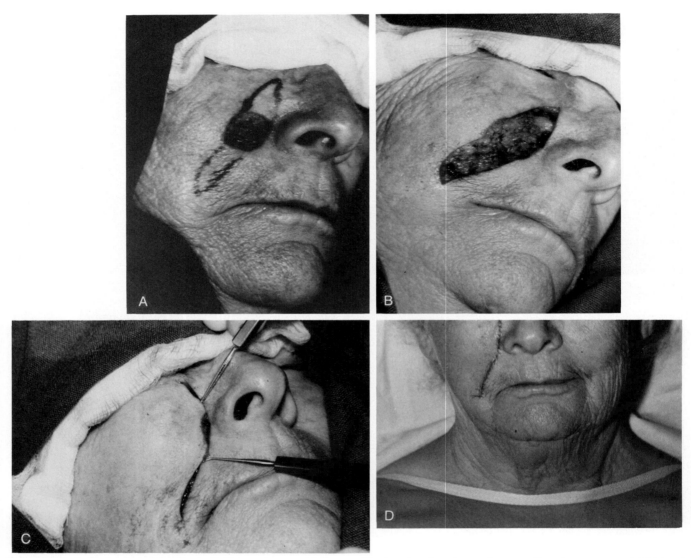

Figure 27–6. *A,* Oval defect of the cheek. *B,* Tissue above and below sacrificed so that the advanced tissue will conform to the melolabial and melonasal junction. *C,* Tissue is advanced into the wound. *D,* Tissue is sutured into place.

Island Pedicle Flaps—Advancement of Pedicle Tissue

Island pedicle flaps and grafts[21–24] utilize the concept of tissue advancement (Fig. 27–7). Once sutured into place, this flap looks like an oval, diamond-shaped, or triangular skin graft. While the adjacent tissues are undermined, the flap itself is not. Rather, the flap is advanced into the defect with V-Y type of closure to assist the sliding motion of the pedicle of this tissue. The utility and quality of this flap should be judged on the flap's outcome and whether it presents a significant cosmetic and functional advantage over other repairs (Fig. 27–8). Because this flap nearly always has a rather notable geometric shape, it is important that it be used in an area where that geometry will be hidden in a fold, crease, line, or some other facial irregularity. The island pedicle flap is useful in certain limited applications in which it can provide a good tissue match in terms of color and texture. If selected and applied carefully, island pedicle flaps do not require revision or grafting any more often than other types of surgical repair.

APPLICATIONS AND ADVANTAGES OF ADVANCEMENT FLAPS

Advancement flaps are particularly useful in the lateral brow and temple area but can also be beneficial in the forehead, lip region, and preauricular area. The main limitation of this type of flap is that it often does not give much extra tissue beyond what primary closure would provide. This is not always true, however, as there are regions of variable laxity in the skin, and an advancement flap can capitalize on such variations. In addition, double advancement flaps tend to "sink" at the ends, so the suturing technique must be directed toward eversion of the advancement point of the two flaps.

An advantage of the advancement flap is minimal secondary movement of adjacent tissues or distortion of adjacent structures. The point of greatest tension of an advancement flap closure is usually obvious and unidimensional. Therefore, an advancement flap can be used when it is especially important to pull a structure in one direction only. For example, defects in the infraorbital region can be closed by direct medial advancement below the lid. A lid that is somewhat lax will be tightened, neither pulled down nor out.

If an advancement flap is planned, the surgeon may consider whether a single or double flap is required. If a double flap is anticipated, one flap can be created and mobilized, and if it is sufficient for proper closure, then the second flap does not need to be performed. The surgeon should decide if a more conservative single flap can close the defect before proceeding with the double procedure. While a preplanned, geometric advancement flap is not used very frequently in cutaneous surgery, pure advancement of tissue to close a defect is very commonly used.

Rotation Flaps

Many flaps that are referred to as advancement flaps actually employ a combination of advancement and rotational motion. Nearly all transposition flaps rotate

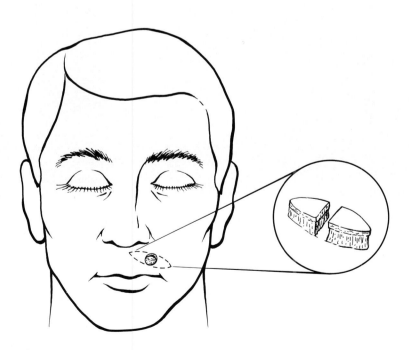

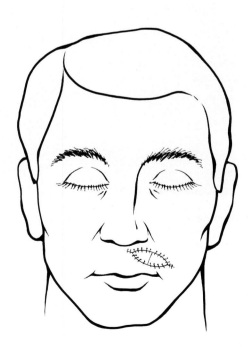

A   B

Figure 27–7. *A,* Schematic of a vascular island pedicle flap. *B,* The pedicle advanced and sutured into place. (Redrawn courtesy of Frank Syndelar.)

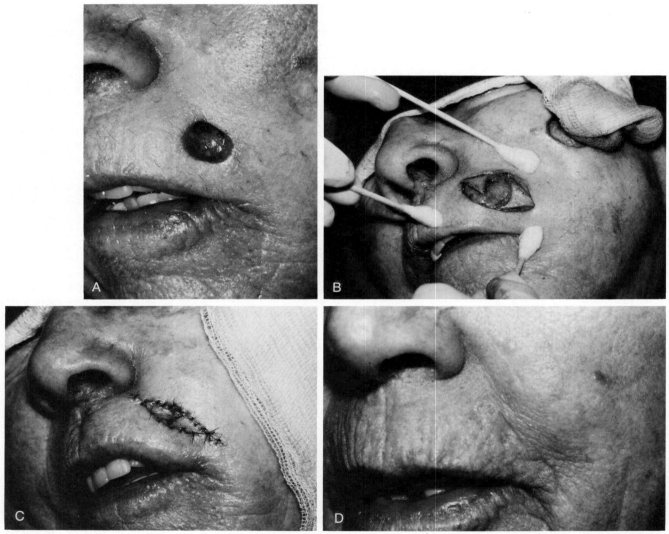

Figure 27–8. *A,* Defect of the upper lip. *B,* Two vascular pedicles are freed from surrounding tissue. *C,* The islands are sutured and advanced into place using V-Y closures. *D,* Clinical appearance after 1 month.

at their vascular base. Advancement and rotation across the underlying subcutaneous tissue are the only two basic types of movement available to skin. Pure rotation and rotation combined with advancement are very useful in closing cutaneous defects in certain anatomic locations such as the scalp.

The classic rotation flap consists of a triangle or two radians from a portion of a circle (Fig. 27–9). Rotation always takes place about a vertex or fulcrum and can be visualized as degrees of movement of radians in a circle. It is often difficult to apply the concept of this triangulated diagrammatic defect to a rotation flap in a clinical situation, since defects very rarely present with a triangulated shape. The surgeon who is trying to duplicate a diagram in a textbook may decide to triangulate or increase the size of the defect to accommodate the rotation flap. This is unnecessary and creates a larger defect without good reason.[14] Most defects in cutaneous surgery present with some variation of a circular or oval shape. For planning purposes, the surgeon should conceptualize all defects as though they were circular (Fig. 27–10). If the surgeon is contemplating a rotation flap, this diagram can easily be transposed onto the basic defect to help visualize the rotational motion and more easily determine the exact point of rotation. It also should be apparent that the curvature of the incision creating the rotation flap will determine the vertex of the arc of rotation. Even after the flap is cut, the way the flap is rotated can be altered about the point of rotation.

In an advancement flap, all tissue must come from straight-line movement of the flap. If the flap is cut and does not fill the defect, the only option is to undermine further and extend the length of the flap, which may provide extra laxity and permit closure of the defect. In the rotation flap, there is more than one option available, which is one of its strengths. Not only may the flap be designed larger, but the length of the curved incision may also be extended to free more tissue for rotation, thereby giving the flap greater versatility. If the rotation flap still does not close the defect, an additional maneuver that may be employed is a back-cut to the arc of the flap (Fig. 27–11). The biggest

disadvantage of the back-cut is that it decreases the width of the vascular pedicle, which may compromise the blood supply to the tip. However, the chief advantage is that the flap can be rotated or angulated more at the point of the back-cut. All rotation flaps create redundant tissue, which usually can be removed anywhere on the outside portion of the arc (Fig. 27–12). It is most commonly evident at the farthest extent of the rotation flap incision. The length of the advancing front of the flap can be increased to provide extra donor tissue.[25]

The single rotation flap does not have any letter designation as many common flaps do. The double rotation flap is frequently referred to as an O-to-Z flap (Figs. 27–13, 27–14). This concept is illustrated as an O with two arms, resulting in an approximately Z-shaped scar after tissue movement has been completed. The O-to-Z flap can be especially useful on the scalp. The bilateral rotation flap has the advantage of allowing the surgeon to plan for a double advancement by initially creating a single rotation flap. If more tissue is needed to close the defect, it can be accomplished in stages as the need becomes apparent during surgery. A rotation flap with a planned back-cut can provide excellent tissue movement for reconstructing many defects.[26] This flap is a combination of rotation and advancement and usually requires a long, slightly curved arc to create the original rotation flap. The secondary defect created by the flap is closed primarily.

Rotation flaps call for careful design, planning, and good technique in undermining and hemostasis in preparation for flap movement. One special feature of the rotation flap is that even after the flap has been designed, the surgeon has an option in how far the flap is rotated. The surgeon should check all dimensions of the defect and determine where the greatest tension lies (Fig. 27–15). The rotation should carry the flap to the point where the tissue is needed most. Wherever there is least distortion of adjacent tissue, the flap should be rotated or reverse rotated to that point of least tension and a tacking suture placed. Obviously, the flap can only be rotated a fixed amount without kinking the base or creating excess redundant tissue that will compromise the outcome. There is a safe range in which the flap can be rotated and secured after design. Essentially, once the rotation flap is in place, the primary defect has been divided into two fusiform defects. Such defects are then closed in a way that shares the flap. A temporary tacking suture is the first stitch placed and is placed before any of the subcutaneous stitches. This stitch is very helpful in establishing the overall plan and execution and can be left in place until the flap starts to take shape. This can be done with any suture material, but silk is a good choice as a temporary suture, because it has less cutting potential than nylon or other synthetic suture materials.

All flaps cause redundant tissue buckling, and additional modifying procedures may be necessary to correct this. Surgeons vary in their opinions about buried sutures and flap surgery. Clearly, large flaps or flaps under tension need solidly placed subcutaneous sutures or deep dermal sutures to secure them adequately without constricting the full-thickness dermis. It is probably best to

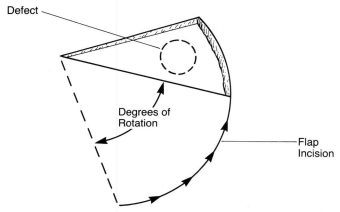

Figure 27–9. Schematic of a classic rotation flap. (Redrawn courtesy of Frank Syndelar.)

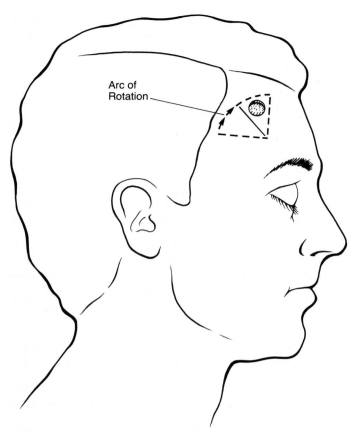

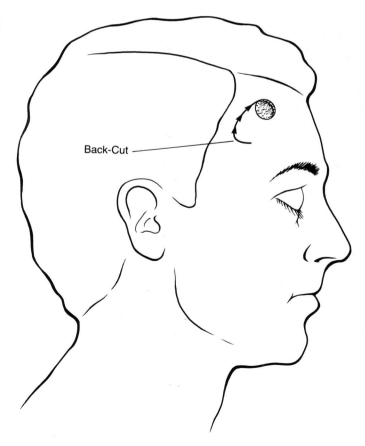

Figure 27–10. The concept of using a rotation flap to reconstruct a circular defect on the temple. (Redrawn courtesy of Frank Syndelar.)

Figure 27–11. Schematic of a back-cut to increase motion of a rotation flap. (Redrawn courtesy of Frank Syndelar.)

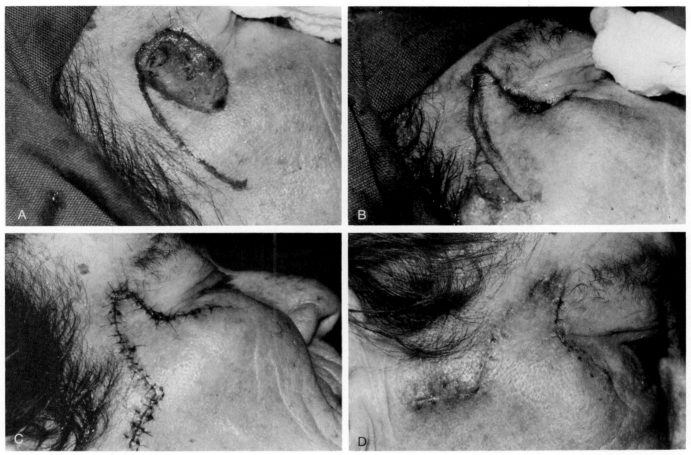

Figure 27–12. *A,* Defect on the temple with the rotation flap marked. *B,* The flap is incised and rotated into place. (Note that redundant lateral tissue will be excised.) *C,* The flap is sutured and the dogear has been repaired. *D,* Appearance 1 week after suture removal.

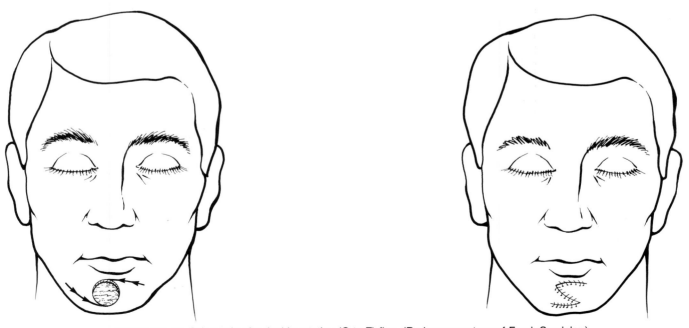

Figure 27–13. Schematic of a double rotation (O-to-Z) flap. (Redrawn courtesy of Frank Syndelar.)

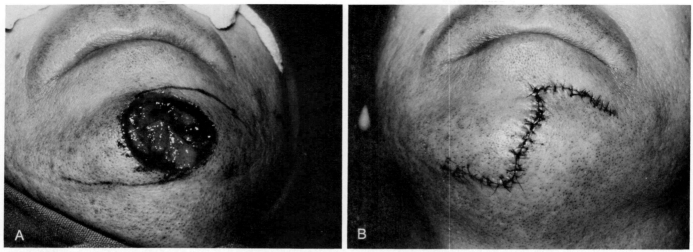

Figure 27–14. *A,* Bilateral rotation flap with the superior arm in the mental crease and the inferior arm below the mandible. *B,* The flaps are sutured into place.

determine the requirements of the flap and then work forward from there. If tension produced by the skin stitches strangulates tissue, then deep buried dermal sutures are necessary. All dead space should be eliminated, and buried sutures must be used for that purpose. Well-placed subcutaneous sutures have a very helpful hemostatic effect. Normally, synthetic absorbable suture that retains tensile strength for at least 20 days is preferred. Because skin stitches will be taken out after 5 to 9 days in facial closures, there is no logic in using buried sutures with an equivalent or shorter absorption time. Once the point of rotation has been secured and subcutaneous sutures have been placed, the technical skill of suturing combined with an overall sense of the aesthetics determines the success of the skin closure. The smallest effective suture material should be used to

Figure 27–15. Schematic showing various movements of a rotation flap. (Redrawn courtesy of Frank Syndelar.)

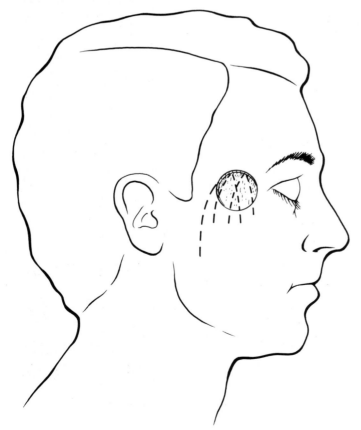

prevent strangulation of skin. The dermal and epidermal edges should be well apposed, both vertically and horizontally, without overlap. Bulges and puckers should be excised and repaired as needed. Finally, the tacking suture is removed and replaced with interrupted sutures or a half-buried mattress tip stitch, if necessary.

APPLICATION AND ADVANTAGES OF ROTATION FLAPS

Rotation flaps tend to be particularly useful in the lateral face, the preauricular cheek, inferior auricular region, and lateral temple area. The arc of rotation will be placed in the lateral face whenever possible, which has the advantage of placing the new incision lateral to the center of the face so that it will be less noticeable. Redundant tissue is usually created along the arc of rotation and will require some type of dogear repair; this must be recognized when designing the flap. Even if the first steps of a flap are very well planned, the aesthetics can be defeated by an ill-placed dogear repair.[19] The best camouflage is provided when the dogear is carried into a facial junction. Examples are the groove between the lateral cheek and the ear, and a defect that partially encircles the nasal ala (Fig. 27–16), a structure that cannot be moved without causing some deformity. This closure takes tissue from two different locations, the lip and cheek. The important structures to preserve

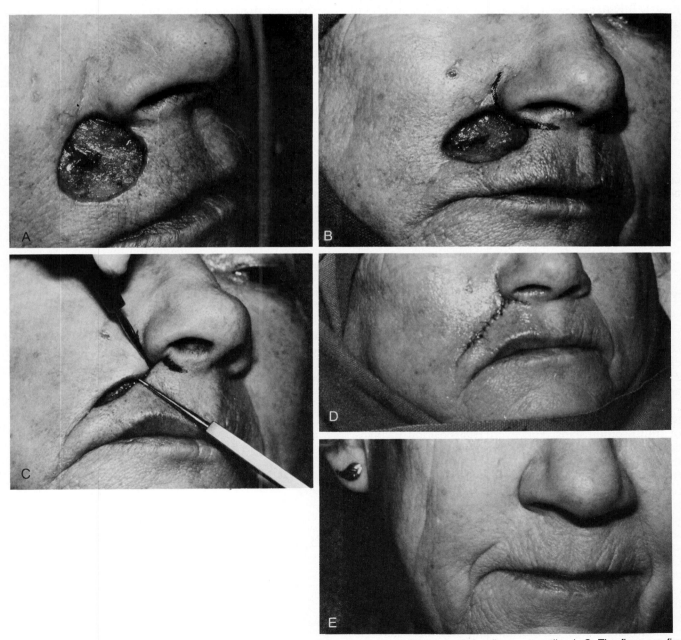

Figure 27–16. A, Defect of the lip-cheek junction at the base of the nasal ala. B, Bilateral rotation flaps are outlined. C, The flaps are first rotated. D, Sutures are placed. E, Clinical appearance after 3 months.

in position are the lip and nasal ala. Also, both the alar cheek groove and mesolabial fold must be maintained if the patient is to have normal facial symmetry. If there is obliteration or blunting of the cheek fold, the patient will have noticeable facial dysfunction of lip movement and impairment of the muscles of facial expression. The animation and movement of these muscles of facial expression, although not essential for life, are extremely important for their aesthetic and social value. To preserve these two structures, it is best to close the defect by sharing tissue from more than one donor region. In this case, the closure is accomplished on the lip portion of the defect with lip tissue and on the cheek portion of the defect with cheek tissue. The vertex of the rotation overlies the nose, but the vertex of rotation of both flaps is slightly different. This example represents useful application of a symmetric bilateral rotation flap.

Limitations of this flap include resistance of some tissues to rotation and the rather large dogear that is sometimes created. Both scalp and cheek tissue tend to rotate well. Forehead skin can be advanced from the lateral forehead slightly medially and then rotated downward. The limitation to the back-cut is potential vascular compromise, but a back-cut also adds more donor tissue. The greater the length of the cut, the greater the additional rotation that is possible. This must be balanced against vascular compromise created by any back-cut. The tip of the nose and lateral nasal tissue on the ala tend to rotate very poorly. However, lateral tissue superior to the ala sometimes rotates quite well. The ability to rotate is the basis for successful use of bilobed and glabellar flaps to repair defects of the lateral nasal tissue and the bridge of the nose, respectively.[27]

Transposition Flaps

Transposition flaps are the most difficult to visualize conceptually and require the most experience to apply effectively. Transposition flaps borrow tissue that is separated from the defect by intervening normal tissue and transposed over the normal tissue into the defect. The concepts and knowledge of tissue movement learned from rotation flaps are critical to the execution of transposition flaps. However, transposition involves another step of complexity: an understanding of how the intervening tissue functions in the performance of this flap. Transposition flaps capitalize on areas of differential tissue movement around skin defects. If there is an equal amount of tissue movement from all directions, then advancement or rotation based on any vertex should close the defect. The transposition flap requires sufficient donor tissue nearby so that it can be incised, freed up, rotated, and then transposed into the primary defect. Transposition flaps create secondary defects because of their considerable secondary movement, and the redundant tissue often requires repair. Here the secondary defect created, as well as the intervening normal tissue, is very important and must be visualized

in tandem with the entire flap plan. Transposition flaps first close defects with inapparent nearby tissue. Second, and most importantly, this intervening island of tissue is key in closing the secondary defect that is created. This is difficult for some surgeons to visualize in three dimensions. The fact that the secondary defect is closed by the intervening tissue underscores the special benefit of transposition flaps. This is not always emphasized in texts and must be appreciated before the full advantages of transposition flaps are realized. The challenge and technique of flap design is to close the secondary defect aesthetically and functionally. Nothing is achieved if the secondary defect cannot be fully closed or must be skin grafted.

Another important concept of the transposition flap is realizing that the surgeon makes a major decision in flap design and its effectiveness when choosing the angle at which the transposition flap will be created and rotated into the defect (Fig. 27–17). The angle varies from 30 to 120 degrees in most transposition flaps. The 30-degree version has been referred to as the Webster flap, while the standard transposition at 90 degrees is referred to as the rhombic flap. Neither flap is applicable in all situations, and the surgeon must determine the best variation for each application. The ability to transfer the textbook image to the clinical situation is critical. Textbooks frequently depict diamond-shaped defects and sharply angulated transposition flaps that close the diamond. This depiction can only be effectively transferred to the clinical situation (Fig. 27–18) by mentally or diagrammatically converting circular and oval defects to the diagram. Templates are not necessary to precisely measure the degrees of angulation, but some physicians may find them useful. Generally, precise measurement of an angle is not the key to creating a successful flap. The critical features are determining whether there is sufficient tissue that can be moved to close the defect and effectively closing the primary defect with the intervening tissue (Fig. 27–19). Once surgeons understand and can apply these concepts, the transposition flap will prove to be one of the most useful and best conceived closures in their cutaneous surgery armamentarium.[28]

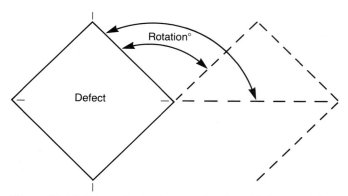

Figure 27–17. Schematic of a transposition flap. (Redrawn courtesy of Frank Syndelar.)

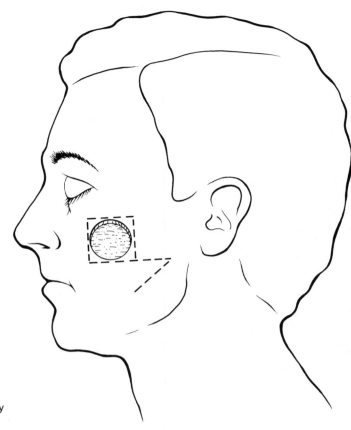

Figure 27–18. Clinical use of a transposition flap. (Redrawn courtesy of Frank Syndelar.)

SPECIAL TYPES OF TRANSPOSITION FLAPS

Nasolabial Flap

Traditionally, transposition flaps have been applied to the nasolabial or cheek-to-nose flap.[29] This has been the easiest flap for surgeons to apply, because it uses an area of considerable laxity—the cheek—to close defects on the nose, an area that has very little laxity. The nasolabial flap can be used to transfer excess cheek tissue to the nose when no other options are apparent. Without cheek flaps, many defects of the nose require use of skin grafts or must heal by second intention.

Many nasolabial flaps done in the past did not always give superior long-term results. One of the common flaws is obliteration of the nose-cheek junction resulting in an aesthetically unpleasing deformity. Another is a trapdoor or pincushion type of defect of the flap as the scar matures. Both are unsightly and may be functionally and aesthetically inferior to skin grafting.

With many refinements, the nasolabial flap has re-emerged as a useful and frequently applied type of transposition flap (Fig. 27–20). Certain refinements make it the flap of choice for closure of particular nasal defects.[30] Trapdoor defects can be greatly decreased if the entire perimeter of the original defect is undermined and the flap sutured to undermined tissue. It appears that the tissue then heals as a single unit, lessening any accentuation of the flap outline.[16, 31]

Glabellar Flap

A glabellar transposition flap is frequently used to repair nasal defects (Fig. 27–21). Nearly all individuals, regardless of age, have some donor tissue available in the glabellar region. Fortunately, this donor site has vertical furrows as well as a very good blood supply from the supratrochlear and supraorbital vessels, making it an excellent donor tissue site. In addition, the donor site can be closed primarily. Glabellar tissue can be donated as a single transposition flap or donated to a second flap, as in bilobed repairs. Even though glabellar tissue is sometimes thicker than tissue on the bridge of the nose, this is usually not a cosmetic limitation if good technique is used in fixation of the flap.

Bilobed Flap

The two keys to performing superior bilobed transposition flaps are creation of the second flap at a site where primary closure eliminates the defect and recognition that a greater degree of rotation is required at the base, sometimes as much as 180 degrees. Therefore, tissue must be well vascularized and flexible enough to undergo this degree of rotation (Fig. 27–22). Transposition flaps are usually revised (i.e., the vascular base is trimmed) much later after surgery rather than at the time of surgery.[16] Even though most local flaps are done in a single stage, the patient must understand that a later revision may be necessary to give the best outcome.

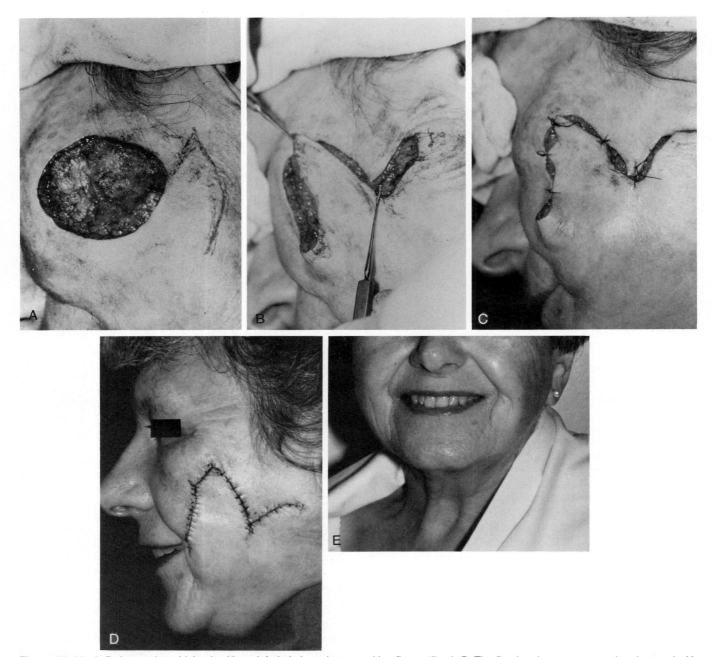

Figure 27–19. *A,* Defect at the midcheek with an inferiorly based transposition flap outlined. *B,* The flap has been transposed and rotated with the intervening tissue filling the secondary defect. *C,* Tacking sutures are placed. *D,* The flap is sutured. *E,* Clinical appearance 6 months after surgery.

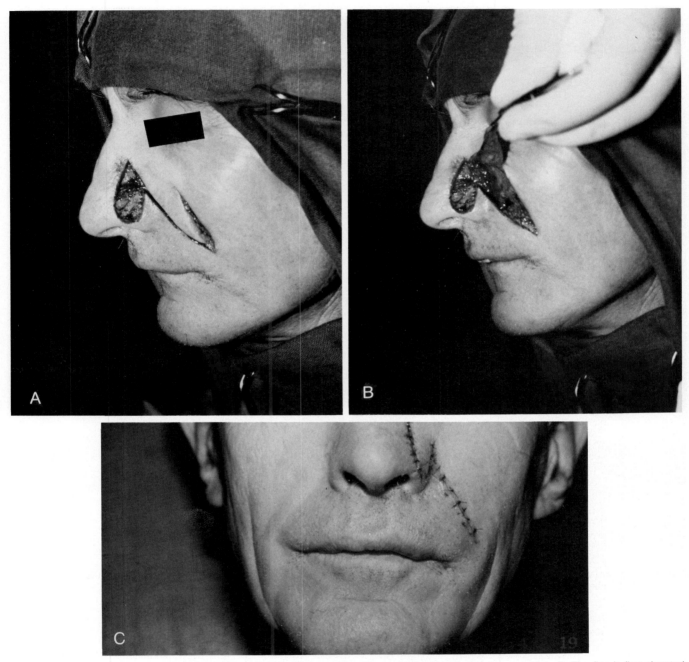

Figure 27–20. *A,* Defect of the nasal ala and lateral nose with a superior dogear excised before flap transposition. *B,* The flap is first elevated. *C,* Sutures are placed.

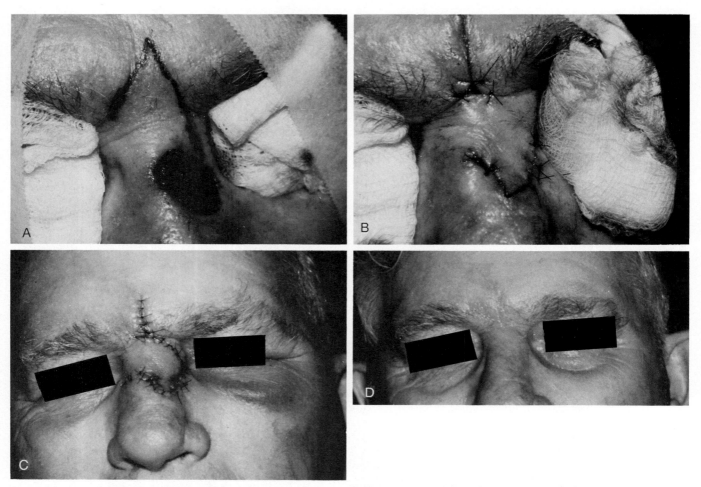

Figure 27–21. *A,* Defect of the lateral bridge of the nose with the planned rotation-transposition flap outlined. *B,* The flap is rotated into the defect. *C,* Appearance 3 days postoperatively. *D,* Appearance after 2 months.

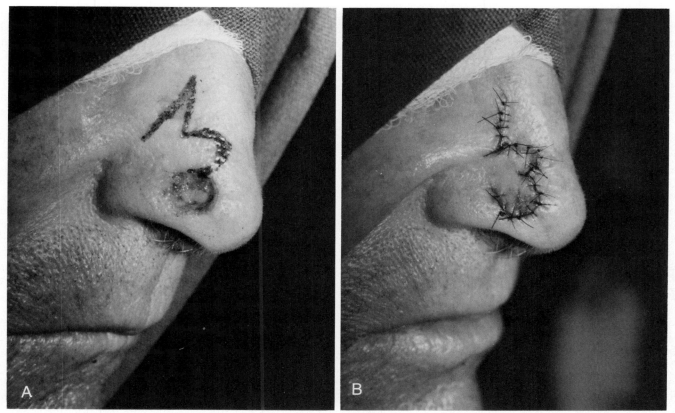

Figure 27–22. *A,* Defect of the nasal ala with a bilobed flap outlined. *B,* The flap sutured into place with the tertiary defect closed primarily.

SURGICAL TECHNIQUE

Initially, surgeons may have difficulty with both the size and placement of transposition flaps. Placement is determined by where the transposition flap will most easily rotate without compromising the base. Some surgeons design the size of the flap to equal the width of the surgical defect. In practice, though, this can be varied, and precise measurements are not necessary in most cases. Before making incisions, skin hooks or a gloved hand can be used to palpate the tissue to determine maximal rotational laxity. Also, pinching the tissue in all directions is necessary to determine how much tissue can be donated. If the surgeon is certain that a transposition flap will be used, the entire defect should be undermined and an attempt made to close the wound primarily or by advancement from the direction of the transposition flap. If, for example, the defect could be reduced 30% by primary closure, then the width of the transposition flap could also be reduced by approximately 30%. The flap should be wide enough to allow closure of both defects without producing excess tension on either the primary or secondary closure. This method is quite reliable for determining correct flap width. The most challenging parts of performing the transposition flap are closure of the secondary defect and rotation of the flap into the primary defect.

Once the tissue is undermined and the flap is designed, the next steps are similar to those used for a rotation flap. In planning the flap, it is useful to remember that most of the movement of a transposition flap is rotational. Tissue should be transposed and rotated using two temporary stay sutures. One is used to tack the flap, and the other is used to tack the intervening island of tissue into the secondary defect. Again, buried stitches should be used as needed.

Initially, skin closure should not be directed toward the tips, since they are often trimmed or revised as the flap takes shape. Suturing should start near the tips and then be directed away from them. This leaves tip suture placement as the last step. It also has the advantage of pushing any redundant tissue to the far edges of the flap. These redundancies can be repaired without readjusting the flap. The surgeon should avoid the practice of starting to suture a rotation flap and then changing the degree of rotation, removing sutures, and readjusting the flap. Determination of the best rotation and transposition flap placement should be done at the beginning of the procedure. The surgeon should be satisfied with flap tip placement before any extensive suturing and should not neglect this important part of the process.

APPLICATIONS AND ADVANTAGES OF TRANSPOSITION FLAPS

The transposition flap has very broad applications, depending on the preferences of the surgeon. Such flaps can be used in situations in which there is an excess of differential donor tissue near a defect. They can also be used when the surgeon believes the type of "broken-up" scar produced by the transposition flap will ultimately offer a superior closure. Transposition flaps require more vascularity, since there are always two tips and some rotational tension on the base. Consequently, they should be chosen carefully and used only in well-vascularized tissue.

Limitations of the flap are the additional incisions required for creation. A certain amount of experience is necessary to judge whether the additional scars created by the transposition flap will ultimately give the patient a better outcome. The transposition flap has the benefit of moving tissue into a defect that could not otherwise be closed primarily. It also can obscure and break up a single scar line, yielding a better aesthetic and functional outcome.

Postoperative Care of Random-Pattern Flaps

The requirements for postoperative wound care as well as follow-up visits should be discussed with patients before surgery. They do not need all details at that time, but they do need a general idea of wound care and follow-up requirements. They also need to know if there is a possibility of a multistaged procedure and should be well informed regarding special activity limitations after surgery, potential postoperative pain, and any dietary or other restrictions. Wound care for flaps is similar to that for other cutaneous surgical procedures and primary closures. In flap surgery, undermining is increased, and the procedure may be prolonged, increasing the risk of postoperative bleeding. Occasionally a 24- to 48-hour wound check is judicious.

Surgeons utilize a wide variety of postoperative instructions, and it is clear that there are many workable options. If the patient is healthy and a good technique has been used, perhaps the only essential requirement for good healing is relative immobilization of the part and application of a sterile dressing. If the wound is contaminated during surgery and therefore susceptible to infection, it is doubtful whether any type of topical care after wound closure will deter the infection. Many surgical specialties have traditionally practiced dry wound care after suturing. However, research during the 1980s clearly showed that in an uninfected wound, moist wound care results in earlier repair and faster healing.

The traditional preference for dry wound care became established because all infected wounds develop either serous or purulent drainage. For many surgeons, a wet state was synonymous with a breeding ground for infection. However, a moist wound in the absence of infection heals extremely well. What is less well established is the ideal medium for maintaining a moist wound. It appears that many dressings work well. An antibiotic or antiseptic medium that is part water and part lipid seems ideal. Wounds heal equally well, however, when covered with synthetic polyurethane occlusive films. Wounds also heal well if a pure lipid substance, such as petroleum jelly, is used for occlusion. Uninfected dry wounds heal well, although experimental studies show they heal with slower epithelialization and reduced collagen synthesis. Within these general principles, surgeons can choose the type of wound care they prefer.

One good technique for wound care is to dress sutured wounds with an antibiotic ointment, cover this with a sterile gauze and an occlusive dressing of padded gauze, and then secure it with tape or wrap it with an elastic net. If extra pressure is required, a sponge can replace the gauze or be added to it. With practice, pressure can be applied quite effectively with tape stretched tightly across the wound. Patients are always instructed to leave dressings on and keep them dry for 48 hours. The bandage is then removed and the area cleansed twice daily with hydrogen peroxide or a diluted antiseptic solution. Antibiotic ointment is then applied to coat the wound before re-dressing it with gauze sponges. It is often satisfactory to simply apply the antibiotic ointment without use of other occlusive dressings. Most patients, however, prefer a bandage on top of the sutures. The primary reason for cleansing before application of the antibiotic is to saturate the crust with an antimicrobial solution and to thoroughly hydrate it. Once-daily cleaning is adequate for these purposes.

In children, an occlusive polyurethane dressing can be applied to the wound and left on for 48 hours. Patients then return for dressing removal and wound check. With this technique, many wounds can be managed with a dressing change only once every 2 to 3 days, and no other wound care is needed.

Drains are used very infrequently for local facial flaps. Very uncommonly, if a patient has postoperative bleeding, a drain can be used immediately after hematoma evacuation for 24 or 48 hours and the patient placed on prophylactic antibiotics. However, prophylactic antibiotics are not needed in healthy patients for a same-day procedure. Use of prophylactic antibiotics for 3 to 5 days is probably useful when performing delayed skin grafts. When flaps are delayed, prophylactic antibiotics are not used unless there is some medical indication for the patient. The antibiotic chosen for most patients is either erythromycin or penicillinase-resistant penicillin.

The timing of suture removal must be gauged to anatomic location and the amount of tension placed on the flap. The sutures from facial flaps are nearly always removed after 6 to 9 days. Cross-hatching suture marks are very uncommon if good wound care is practiced. Maintaining a moist wound allows much better epithelialization in repair of suture perforations in the skin. Removing sutures too early can result in dehiscence, which is a serious problem. Whenever the sutures are removed, the wounds should always be taped for at least 2 weeks, because the tensile strength of wounds at 2 weeks is only 10% of their ultimate tensile strength, and wounds can be separated easily by minor trauma in the early period after surgery. Taping not only secures the edges of the wound, but also (and more importantly) serves as a constant reminder for the patient to be careful of the part and not exert pressure that might pull the wound apart. An alternative to taping is to rebandage the wound with a light layer of gauze and secure it completely with tape. The patient can then be allowed to change the dressing on a daily basis. He or she must be shown how to remove the tape properly so the wound edges are not disturbed.

Follow-up Evaluations of Random-Pattern Flaps

Most patients should be scheduled for a return visit for suture removal between 6 and 9 days after surgery. If there is concern about hemorrhage, infection, or some other complication, the wound should be checked after 48 to 72 hours. If the flap is healing properly with no evidence of complications, then follow-up examinations should be performed approximately 1 month after suture removal and then again 2 to 3 months later. Follow-up by the operating surgeon is recommended for at least 3 months, and subsequent follow-up can then be performed by the referring physician. Additional follow-up visits are usually scheduled for 6 and 12 months after the surgery. However, if the patient experiences any complication or is dissatisfied or concerned about the outcome, follow-up should be tailored to that individual's needs. All facial surgery should be followed closely, as the postoperative outcome can be expected to remodel with time. Many patients need emotional support and may require more frequent wound checks. Because all scar tissue matures and generally improves over time, the surgeon should monitor this process and reassure the patient if necessary. Wounds can continue to remodel for 2 years or even longer after surgery. The ultimate length of follow-up can be tailored to the disease treated and the degree of patient satisfaction with the outcome.

Revisionary Work

Before any surgery, patients should be informed that revisionary work may be necessary at a later date to improve the result. Surgeons vary greatly on the frequency and timing of this revisionary work. The most common revisionary technique is to refine the base of a flap or excise redundant tissue. Even in this instance, most patients should be advised to wait at least 6 months after the surgery, since maturation of the scar usually works to the patient's advantage. The exception to this, of course, is scar hypertrophy. When this develops, the earlier treatment is initiated, the better. The first line of treatment is injection of intralesional steroids. Scar massage is also helpful for indurated scars and some elevated flaps. This is usually begun at about 6 weeks postoperatively and continued for a maximum of 2 months. The scar massage technique consists of simple digital pressure applied by the patient to the scar with massage in a circular motion done to a count of 50 twice daily. Dermabrasion of flap edges is somewhat controversial.

Depending on the disease or tumor initially treated, revisionary work may need to be delayed. If a tumor with a high local recurrence rate is treated, a functional but aesthetically unpleasing repair such as skin graft or second-intention healing may be the best initial management.[32] Once the patient has been followed for 1 to 2 years without cancer recurrence, a more elegant reconstruction can be safely performed in most cases.

SUMMARY

All cutaneous defects should be viewed critically and the options of second-intention healing, skin grafts, random-pattern flaps, and other closures considered. When primary closure cannot be accomplished, random-pattern flaps give the surgeon the opportunity to close defects with adjacent skin that offers good color and texture match. Random-pattern flaps also allow for the preservation of important facial boundaries and may yield cosmetic and functional results that are superior to those provided by skin grafts. When carefully considered, planned, and executed, random-pattern flaps provide the opportunity for excellent reconstruction and rehabilitation that are impossible to achieve by any other means.

REFERENCES

1. Bennett RG: Fundamentals of Cutaneous Surgery. CV Mosby, St. Louis, 1988.
2. Tromovitch TA, Stegman SJ, Glogau RG: Flaps and Grafts in Dermatologic Surgery. Year Book Medical, Chicago, 1989.
3. Stegman SJ, Tromovitch TA, Glogau RG: Basics of Dermatologic Surgery. Year Book Medical, Chicago, 1982.
4. Swanson NA: Atlas of Cutaneous Surgery. Little, Brown, Boston, 1987.
5. Dzubow LM: Facial Flaps Biomechanics and Regional Application. Appleton & Lange, Norwalk, CT, 1990.
6. Leshin B, Whitaker DC, Swanson NA: Preoperative evaluation in dermatologic surgery. J Am Acad Dermatol 19:1081–1088, 1988.
7. Whitaker DC, Grande DJ, Johnson S: Wound infection rate in dermatologic surgery. J Dermatol Surg Oncol 14:525–528, 1988.
8. Salasche S, Bernstein G, Senkarik M: Surgical Anatomy of the Skin. Appleton & Lange, Norwalk, CT, 1988.
9. Burgett GC, Minick FJ: The subunit principle in nasal reconstruction. Plast Reconstr Surg 176:239–247, 1985.
10. Dzubow LM: Tissue movement—a macrobiomechanical approach. J Dermatol Surg Oncol 15:389–399, 1989.
11. Dzubow LM, Zak L: The principle of cosmetic junctions as applied to reconstruction of defects following Mohs surgery. J Dermatol Surg Oncol 16:353–355, 1990.
12. Burgett GC: Aesthetic restoration of the nose. Clin Plast Surg 12:463–480, 1985.
13. Whitaker DC, Goldstein GD: Lateral nose and perinasal defects: options in management following Mohs micrographic surgery for cutaneous carcinoma. J Dermatol Surg Oncol 14:1177–1183, 1988.
14. Dzubow LM: Defects subdivision as a technique to repair defects following Mohs surgery. J Dermatol Surg Oncol 6:426–430, 1990.
15. Zitelli JA, Moy RL: Buried vertical mattress suture. J Dermatol Surg Oncol 15:17–19, 1989.
16. Zitelli JA: Bilobed flap for nasal reconstruction. Arch Dermatol 125:957–959, 1989.
17. Wheeland RG: Random pattern flaps. In: Roenigk RK, Roenigk HH Jr (eds): Dermatologic Surgery Principles and Practice. Marcel Dekker, New York, 1989, pp 265–322.
18. Dzubow LM: Chemosurgical report: indications for a geometric

approach to wound closure following Mohs surgery. J Dermatol Surg Oncol 13:480–486, 1987.

19. Dzubow LM: The dynamics of dog-ear formation and correction. J Dermatol Surg and Oncol 11:722–728, 1985.

20. Whitaker DC, Birkby CS: An approach to cutaneous surgical defects of the forehead and eyebrow following Mohs micrographic surgery. J Dermatol Surg Oncol 13:1312–1317, 1987.

21. Eliezri YD: Variations in Burow's grafts. J Am Acad Dermatol 18:1143–1145, 1988.

22. Zitelli JA: Burow's grafts. J Am Acad Dermatol 17:271–279, 1987.

23. Tomich JM, Wentzell MJ, Grande DJ: Subcutaneous island pedicle flaps. Arch Dermatol 123:514–518, 1987.

24. Dzubow LM: Subcutaneous island pedicle flaps. J Dermatol Surg Oncol 12:591–596, 1986.

25. Dzubow LM: The dynamics of flap movement: effect of pivotal restraint on flap rotation and transposition. J Dermatol Surg Oncol 13:1348–1352, 1987.

26. Snow SN, Mohs FE, Olanski DC: Nasal tip reconstruction: the horizontal J rotation flap using skin from the lower lateral bridge and cheek. J Dermatol Surg Oncol 16:727–732, 1990.

27. Zimany A: The bi-lobed flap. Plast Reconstr Surg 11:424–434, 1953.

28. Dzubow LM: Design of an appropriate rhombic flap for a circular defect created by Mohs microscopically controlled surgery. J Dermatol Surg Oncol 14:124–126, 1988.

29. Spear SL, Kroll SS, Romm S: A new twist to the nasolabial flap for reconstruction of lateral alar defect. Plast Reconstr Surg 79:915–920, 1987.

30. Zitelli JA: The nasolabial flap as a single-stage procedure. Arch Dermatol 126:1445–1448, 1990.

31. Davis JS, Kitlowski EA: The immediate contraction of cutaneous grafts and its cause. J Arch Surg 23:954, 1931.

32. Zitelli JA: Wound healing by secondary intention: a cosmetic appraisal. J Am Acad Dermatol 9:407–415, 1983.

CHAPTER 28

Conventional and Intraoperative Tissue Expansion

MARC D. BROWN and TIMOTHY M. JOHNSON

Tissue expansion refers to the unique ability of the skin to stretch and grow to accommodate an enlarging mass beneath it. A typical example is the protuberant female abdominal skin seen with pregnancy, as well as the exotic African customs of lip, earlobe, and neck expansion. Another example of slow tissue expansion is how the skin overlying a large lipoma or epidermoid cyst is redundant and freely movable at the time of surgical excision. Tissue expansion relies not only on the innate elastic properties of the skin, but also, most importantly, on the creation and growth of new tissue.

This natural ability of human skin to adapt to intrinsic or extrinsic forces by increasing in surface area led Neumann in 1957 to place an expanding rubber balloon subcutaneously for the purpose of reconstructing an ear.[1] It was approximately 20 years later that Radovan and Austad began to pioneer the use of controlled tissue expansion[2-5] using a silicone expander inflated by percutaneous injection through a distant injection valve for breast reconstruction following mastectomy. Since the late 1970s, the technique of tissue expansion has been greatly refined and has gone through many advances. Tissue expanders have been placed in virtually every area of the body, attesting to the many advantages offered by this unique procedure.

In its basic form, tissue expansion involves the placement of an inflatable silicone balloon under normal skin in close proximity to a planned surgical site or an existing traumatic or surgical defect. The major advantage of tissue expansion is the creation of new skin immediately adjacent to a surgical site, which allows for an excellent match in terms of color, consistency, texture, and hair-bearing qualities. This is particularly important in reconstruction of the scalp (with hair bearing being most important) and face (with color and texture being predominant). In most cases, no significant donor defect is created, because the expanded tissue will cover both donor and recipient sites. The balloon-like implant is gradually inflated over a period of weeks to months until the desired degree of skin stretching has been achieved. The implant is then removed, and the expanded tissue is used to reconstruct the surgical defect. Although the procedure may sound simple and straightforward, it requires experience and careful planning, as well as an understanding of the proper surgical technique for controlled tissue expansion, its indications and advantages, and its potential risks and complications, to achieve the desired cosmetic result.

Advantages of Tissue Expansion

The advantages of tissue expansion are multiple (Table 28–1). Its major advantage and primary purpose is to provide expanded tissue that will cover both the donor and recipient site so as to eliminate a significant donor defect. Tissue expansion will often circumvent the need for large skin grafts, multiple-stage excisions, or complex flaps. For example, the potential functional disability that results from a large musculocutaneous flap might be avoided with the use of controlled tissue expansion.[6] Tissue expansion is indicated when there is inadequate adjacent tissue to allow primary closure of a defect or when the defect can be repaired only by a flap or graft that results in a significant donor or recipient site deformity. Tissue expansion will often allow primary closure, which would otherwise have been impossible, of a very large defect.

There may also be cost benefits with tissue expansion.[7] Although expansion does require at least two surgical

TABLE 28–1. **ADVANTAGES OF TISSUE EXPANSION**

Outpatient procedure
Generally well tolerated
Good tissue match
Minimal or no donor defect
May be used in almost any area of the body
Increased flap survival as a result of neovascularization and
    increased length-to-width ratio
Increased flap strength because of fibrous capsule formation
Adnexal structures unchanged
Sensation usually normal
Eliminates potential need for skin grafts, distant flaps, staged
    excisions
Eliminates need for multiple surgical procedures
Can be performed before the ablative or reconstructive procedure
Can be repeated

procedures and multiple office visits, it avoids multistage procedures and prolonged hospitalizations, since it can be performed as an ambulatory surgical procedure. Patient discomfort is variable, but tissue expansion is generally well tolerated. Expansion works best when it is performed preoperatively before the definitive ablative or reconstructive procedure is performed. Of course, tissue expansion is used postoperatively when a larger-than-expected defect is produced, such as following Mohs micrographic surgery. In this case, a temporary skin graft can be placed initially, to be followed at a later time by controlled tissue expansion and eventual reconstruction.

One of the great advantages of tissue expansion is that it provides the best donor skin in terms of color, texture, and adenexal structures. Because tissue expansion occurs immediately adjacent to the surgical site, the skin has basically the same characteristics and consistency of the original tissue. Adnexal structures remain intact so that, for example, scalp reconstruction will contain hair, and facial reconstruction in the male will permit growth of a normal beard.[8, 9] Likewise, normal sensation usually persists in the expanded tissue, because cutaneous nerves are preserved.

Expanded tissue has the additional advantage of being more viable, primarily because it is highly vascular.[10–13] Rapid angiogenesis occurs in expanded tissue, and this increased vascularity allows for increased flap survival. Expanded tissue also leads to an increased flap length-to-width ratio, which improves flap viability.[14, 15] Finally, the fibrous capsule that develops around the implant adds strength to the flap.[16] Expansion can also be repeated, with the same tissue being expanded a second or third time, if necessary.[6]

Tissue expanders can be placed in almost any area of the body. Various sizes and shapes have been designed to accommodate the anatomic site at which the implant will be placed. Much of the original work with tissue expansion related to breast reconstruction after mastectomy. However, tissue expansion is currently being used on the scalp, forehead, nose, eyelid, ear, cheek, neck, trunk, extremities (including hand and foot), and scrotum.[17]

Indications for Tissue Expansion

Although tissue expansion was initially developed for breast reconstruction after mastectomy,[3, 18–19] new indications for tissue expansion have been subsequently developed, including many specific applications for cutaneous surgery.[18–22] Even if a cutaneous surgeon chooses not to employ this procedure, it is important to understand the potential uses of tissue expansion to counsel and educate patients adequately.

SCALP

Tissue expansion holds great promise in scalp surgery because of the relative tightness of the skin in this area and the desire to maintain the normal hair-bearing qualities of the scalp. Tissue expansion has been adapted to treat cicatricial alopecias when scalp reduction by itself is insufficient.[6, 15, 23, 24] The goal is to remove the entire scar in one procedure after expansion instead of performing multistage procedures. The expanders are inserted in the subgaleal space, which later serves as the advancing edge of the flap. Although there may be a decrease in hair density during large scalp expansions, hair growth continues, as the hair follicles are not injured.[17] Hair loss does not occur, and the pattern of hair growth remains the same. Reduction in hair density is usually not noted until density has decreased by approximately 50%. This allows for scalp expansion of two to three times the original surface area before a change in hair density becomes evident.[6] When treating scarring alopecias that are associated with an inflammatory component such as discoid lupus erythematosus, pseudopelade, and lichen planopilaris, it is important to proceed cautiously, in that any remaining active inflammatory disease could affect wound healing and the final cosmetic result, as well as reactivate the disease.[23]

Scalp expansion is also used for male pattern baldness, usually in assisting with scalp reduction surgery.[25–28] The scalp is normally very tight, and excessive tension on the wound edges can produce a wide, unattractive scar sometimes seen with scalp reduction surgery. The goal of tissue expansion is to provide more hair-bearing scalp with less resultant wound tension and to minimize the number of scalp reduction procedures that are necessary. Expanders are usually placed in a temporal-parietal location well away from the hair line. Incisions for expander placement are made at the hairline. Multiple expanders are recommended to provide maximal tissue gain[6, 17]; typical volumes are 200 to 500 ml. There is an initial 2- to 3-week lag in which scalp expansion proceeds slowly, probably because of the resistance of the strong galea. Typically, scalp expansion takes 6 to 8 weeks. Use of galeotomies at the time of expander placement can hasten the process of expansion but can also increase the risk of extrusion of the expander. The area of alopecia is excised only after advancing or rotating the expanded scalp to be certain it is large enough to close the defect. The capsule surrounding the expander is not excised, as this provides strength and vascularity.[6] Expansion has also been used in conjunction with scalp flaps such as the Juri flap and occipital-based flaps, because it provides for larger and more highly vascularized hair-bearing flaps.[29]

FACE AND NECK

When dealing with tissue expansion on the face and neck, careful planning is required to provide expanded skin with a good match in terms of color, sebaceous gland content, thickness, texture, and hair-bearing qualities. Expanded forehead skin is employed for reconstruction of adjacent forehead defects or, more often, for nasal reconstruction with the use of a forehead flap.[8, 30, 31] Large nasal defects are fairly common following Mohs micrographic surgery and are a challenge to reconstruct, often requiring a forehead flap. Tissue expansion of the forehead is utilized to create a forehead flap for nasal reconstruction when there is insufficient tissue for a primary closure of the donor site.[32, 33] Flaps as wide as 6 to 7 cm can be developed with the use of expanded skin and still allow for primary closure with a single vertical midline scar.[8] Incisions for forehead expansion are placed 3 to 4 cm posterior to the hairline. The recipient pocket should be extended to the level of the supraorbital rim. A 250-ml rectangular expander is commonly used. Expansion for purposes of nasal reconstruction usually requires approximately 8 weeks and may be more painful than other types because of pressure on the supraorbital and supratrochlear nerves. Because the expanded flap is more vascular, it permits more aggressive thinning of the subcutaneous fat and removal of frontalis muscle at the time of transposition. This provides a thin, flexible flap. The surrounding fibrous capsule usually needs to be removed to allow contouring on the nose.[8]

Expansion of the cheek and neck is indicated for reconstruction of defects of this area when local flaps are inadequate.[30, 34, 35] Expanded tissue can provide a flap with a better length-to-width ratio and a better vascular pedicle. The expander is placed subcutaneously and deep to the platysma muscle in the neck. Because of gravitational forces, inferior migration of the expander can occur.[8, 35] This can be minimized by securing the base of the expander to the underlying tissue with the use of permanent sutures. Complications with neck expansion are more frequent, with extrusion of the expander occurring in as many as 50% of patients.[35] This is most likely because of the thinner skin and subcutaneous tissue of the area and the lack of an adequate bony foundation on which to rest the implant. When possible, the base of the expander should be over the malar eminence or mandible in the cheek and over the transverse process of the cervical spine in the neck.[8]

Tissue expansion is being creatively used for ear and eyelid reconstruction as well.[36, 37] When used in ear reconstruction, the tissue expander should be placed through a remote incision within the postauricular scalp line. The pocket for the expander should be dissected above the fascia. A crescent-shaped 60- to 100-ml expander appears to work best. Expansion should proceed slowly, increasing by only 5 to 10 ml each week. At the time of expander removal, it is advisable to excise the capsule to allow tight skin-to-cartilage approximation.[36] For eyelid surgery, a cigar-shaped 1.2-ml silicone expander has been developed that is placed in a subcutaneous pocket extending from medial to lateral canthus. The incision for expander placement extends laterally from the lateral canthus. To avoid pressure on the globe of the eye, the expander is positioned inferior to the inferior orbital rim. However, the risk of implant extrusion can be high.

EXTREMITIES

Tissue expansion on the arms and legs has been successfully performed for multiple purposes.[38-41] In cutaneous surgery, it can be used to assist in removal of large congenital nevi, cosmetic removal of large tattoos, or treatment of hypertrophic scars and scar contractures.[42, 43] Again, the goal is to avoid a multistage procedure and to provide a larger and more viable flap for closure. The complication rate of lower leg expansion is higher, possibly because of the decreased vascularity in this area.[17, 39]

DISTANT SKIN FLAPS

One of the purposes of tissue expansion is to avoid the use of distant flaps. At times, however, expansion of local tissue is not sufficient to reconstruct a defect, and regional or microsurgical flaps are necessary. The use of these flaps often requires the use of a skin graft to close the donor site. Preoperative tissue expansion of the proposed regional flap could potentially allow a simpler linear closure of the donor site while simultaneously providing for a more viable flap.[8, 44]

Technique of Tissue Expansion

Tissue expanders are available from various manufacturers in multiple shapes and sizes. The expander is composed of a balloon type implant and reservoir dome connected by tubing (Fig. 28–1). It is important to choose the correct expander, which is usually determined by the size, shape, and location of the defect. Expanders can be round, oval, elliptical, rectangular, or even custom made in other shapes. Volumes vary from 1.2 ml to 2000 ml. In general, rectangular expanders allow for a greater increase in surface area than do round expanders.[14] Expander size can be roughly estimated as follows: the base of the expander should be approximately 2½ times the size of the defect.[8] Expanders can be used singly or in combination. At times, multiple expanders are used to maximize tissue gain and decrease the apparent deformity that results from the use of a single larger expander. The use of an expander with a distant valve is preferred to decrease the risk of expander perforation. This also allows placement of the injection port away from the defect and planned reconstructive site.

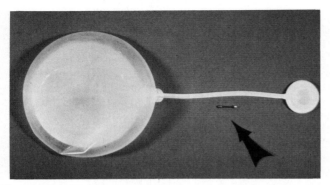

Figure 28–1. The tissue expander is composed of a balloon-type implant *(left)* and a reservoir dome *(right)* connected by tubing. The arrow points to a metal joint that can be placed at the junction of the reservoir and tubing to help prevent kinking of the silicone tube. (Courtesy of Michael Sullivan, M.D., Ohio State University, Columbus, OH.)

Careful planning is critical for an ultimate successful outcome in tissue expansion procedures. Choosing the proper site for placement of the expander and reservoir is imperative. Placement must be carefully designed so as not to interfere with any incision required for subsequent reconstruction. Placement should also not interfere with eventual rotation or transposition of a planned flap. The donor area selected should be compatible with the recipient site in consistency, texture and color. Care must be taken to avoid important underlying anatomic structures such as major nerves and arteries in the expanded region. Prophylactic antibiotics are usually recommended, with cephalosporins being most commonly used preoperatively and continued for 48 hours postoperatively. Antibiotics are usually not recommended for the entire period of expansion.

At the time the expander is implanted, a subcutaneous pocket is created, usually above the level of the fascia. Exceptions are the scalp (subgaleal) and breast (subpectoral). A submuscular location is sometimes used in the neck and chest area. The size of the pocket should be large enough to accommodate the implant easily and without significant tension; otherwise, extrusion of the implant may occur. Direct contact of the implant with the suture line will also increase the risk of extrusion. Meticulous hemostasis must be maintained to decrease the risk of hematoma formation and subsequent infection. Insertion of the expander is usually performed under local anesthesia in an ambulatory outpatient surgical setting using strict aseptic technique.

The injection port and inflation reservoir should be placed 4 to 6 cm away from the expander to avoid accidental trauma to the implant. The injection port should be placed in an area where it can be easily palpated for percutaneous access. The tunnel between the reservoir and expander through which tubing passes should be as small as possible to prevent migration of the reservoir dome. When possible, the reservoir should be placed over a firm area, such as a bony prominence, to provide stability at the time of percutaneous puncture and injection. Permanent monofilament sutures are used to close the skin and may be left in place during

expansion to minimize the risk of extrusion.[9] In the scalp, permanent sutures are also used to close the galea.[8] At the time of implantation, the expander is filled with only enough saline to obliterate the dead space, usually about 10 to 15% of the fully expanded volume. Some surgeons instill a small amount of methylene blue at the same time to help in later distinguishing postoperative seromas from leaks in the expander.[45]

There are no absolute time schedules for initiating inflation, but 2 to 3 weeks are usually allowed for healing of the surgical site before the initial inflation begins. Most inflations then proceed at approximately weekly intervals, with a range of 3 to 14 days between expansions. Full expansion is usually completed in 6 to 8 weeks, depending on the size of the expander and the location. More rapid expansion over 1 to 2 weeks has been attempted but has not become the standard of practice.[46, 47] At time of inflation, the skin over the reservoir is prepped and draped in a sterile manner. A 23- or 25-gauge needle is placed at the back wall of the reservoir and then withdrawn 1 to 2 mm. Saline is slowly injected until the skin overlying the expander becomes tense. This is usually associated with some discomfort, which subsides quickly. If blanching of the overlying skin occurs, some saline should be immediately withdrawn. The amount of saline able to be injected depends on patient discomfort, wound strength, size of the expander, and location. Typical areas that are more resistant to inflation include the lower leg, midline of the back, and areas of previous surgery, injury, or irradiation. The galea also shows an initial resistance to inflation. Within 3 to 10 days, the overlying skin becomes loose, and the implant becomes more freely movable within the underlying pocket. At this point, inflation is repeated at appropriate intervals until the desired expansion is obtained (Fig. 28–2). A second operation is then performed, during which the implant is deflated and removed; the final reconstructive procedure is completed using the expanded skin to close the defect (Fig. 28–3).

Disadvantages and Complications of Tissue Expansion

DISADVANTAGES

Unfortunately, there are some disadvantages associated with tissue expansion (Table 28–2). First, at least two operations are necessary, and multiple visits to the physician are often required during the 6 to 8 weeks of expansion. This may necessitate time away from work

TABLE 28–2. DISADVANTAGES OF TISSUE EXPANSION

Two surgical procedures required
Multiple visits required during expansion
Disfigurement occurs during expansion
Labor intensive
Modest pain at time of each expansion procedure

probably due to operator experience, location of the expander, and health of the tissue undergoing expansion. For example, complications are much lower for breast reconstruction than for head and neck reconstruction or lower leg reconstruction. Complication rates have also dropped significantly as surgeons have gained more experience with the procedure. Complication rates initially reported were much higher than those in more recent reports. Early leaders in tissue expansion now report complication rates as low as 3 to 7%. Expansion that occurs in previously scarred, irradiated, or burned tissue also has a higher rate of complications.[57]

Implant Extrusion

Implant extrusion usually occurs through necrosis of the overlying skin or through the original incision line. Most commonly this complication is a result of creation of an implant pocket that is too small. This places the implant in contact with the suture line. This complication can be prevented by slow expansion, waiting 2 to 3 weeks for appropriate healing of the initial incision, initial inflation only to the point of filling the dead space, and leaving sutures in place or securing with skin tape strips at the suture line. When implant exposure occurs,

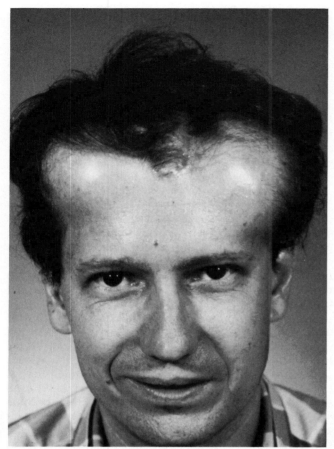

Figure 28–2. Bilateral forehead and scalp tissue expansion. (Courtesy of Michael Sullivan, M.D., Ohio State University, Columbus, OH.)

or school depending on how well the patient is able to emotionally cope with the temporary deformity, which is another disadvantage. Patient selection is very important, since each individual must be well informed, motivated, and mentally competent. Children can be an additional challenge, but successful expansion in children has been widely reported.[48–51]

COMPLICATIONS

Tissue expansion also has its complications.[17, 52–56] Fortunately, most complications are minor and can be resolved without interruption of the expansion procedure (Table 28–3). The overall rate of complications varies widely from 10 to 60%. This discrepancy is

TABLE 28–3. **COMPLICATIONS OF TISSUE EXPANSION**

Infection
Extrusion of implant
Seroma
Hematoma
Dehiscence
Bone erosion
Mechanical failure of expander
Tissue necrosis
Nerve dysfunction

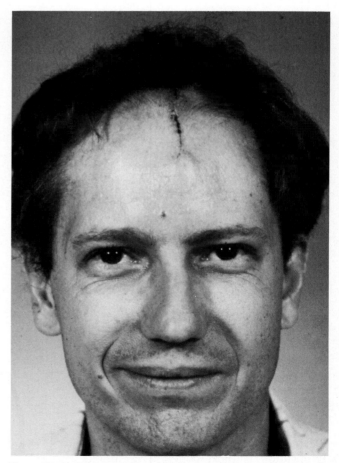

Figure 28–3. Clinical appearance after primary layered closure after removal of expanders. (Courtesy of Michael Sullivan, M.D., Ohio State University, Columbus, OH.)

expansion can sometimes be continued, with frequent inspection for evidence of infection or further extrusion. If the decision is made to continue expansion, the patient should be placed on antibiotics until expansion is fully completed.

Mechanical Failure

Mechanical failure is a rare complication. Two common causes are inadvertent needle perforation and breakage of the connecting tube. If implant failure occurs, the implant can be replaced. The new incision line should be allowed to mature and heal for 2 weeks before resuming inflation. At times, only a very minimal leak occurs, and expansion can sometimes be continued without removal of the implant.

Infection

Infection is a relatively uncommon complication, occurring in less than 1% of cases. Perioperative antibiotics are recommended to cover for possible staphylococcal or streptococcal infections. If a wound infection does not respond promptly to antibiotics, the expander should be removed.

Hematoma

Potential hematoma formation can be minimized by careful hemostasis at the time of surgery. Hematomas are treated by immediate evacuation, control of bleeding, and irrigation of the implant cavity. A drain should be used when necessary but removed as promptly as possible to eliminate any nidus for infection. Seromas around the implant are rarely a source of complications.

Nerve Dysfunction

Nerve dysfunction is uncommon despite placement of expanders at times over major nerves. In one study it occurred in only 3 of 76 expansions.[53] Rapid, large-volume expansion can cause nerve compression leading to neurapraxia. Symptoms usually resolve if the problem is recognized and treated before focal demyelination occurs.

Tissue Necrosis

Tisssue necrosis can occur from overzealous expansion with resultant tissue ischemia. However, pain and obvious blanching of tissue usually alert the physician to this potential complication. The risk of necrosis is greater in areas of previous irradiation or scar.

Bone Resorption

Bone resorption has been described but is quite rare; reported cases have involved the calvarium.[53, 57] This complication is most common in infants undergoing tissue expansion.

Expanded Skin and Soft Tissue Changes

Experimental studies in both animals and humans have provided information about soft tissue changes that occur during the process of expansion.[17, 58–64] Both light and electron microscopic studies have been reported. However, many unanswered questions remain about the histologic, physiologic, and biochemical changes that occur with expansion. In general, studies have shown that human and animal soft tissues respond almost identically during controlled tissue expansion.

Significant findings include the fact that only minimal changes occur in the epidermis. Most studies have shown no apparent change in the thickness of the epidermis during expansion. Electron microscopy reveals a more undulated basal lamina with somewhat larger bundles of tonofilaments in expanded tissue versus normal tissue. Intracellular spaces in all layers of the epidermis are reduced, which may be the result of increased epidermal mitotic activity.

Unlike the epidermis, significant changes occur in the dermis, with a marked decrease in the overall thickness. This reduction in thickness is most pronounced during the first several weeks of expansion and then continues at a slower rate. The papillary and reticular dermis becomes filled with thick bundles of collagen fibers, and fibroblasts increase in number. Myofibroblasts become evident in the deep dermis after several weeks of expansion. The presence of these myofibroblasts suggest that the dermis may be assuming a contractile function, possibly in response to the chronic tension from progressive expansion. In addition, elastic fibers become compact and thick and may form clusters. Although adnexal structures such as hair follicles and sweat glands are pushed apart, they remain unchanged in number and function. Hair growth continues in a normal pattern. Telogen effluvium after tissue expansion has not been reported.[23] Sweat glands are compacted but still secrete. No significant dermal inflammation has been noted.

Of all tissue types, adipose tissue appears to be the most intolerant of controlled expansion. There is a decreased thickness of the fatty layer and an absolute decrease in the number of adipocytes. This loss of fat apparently is permanent. Fat necrosis is usually not observed.

Much like fat, there is a decrease in muscle thickness and mass, but active function of the muscle is maintained. There is no functional loss of muscle strength nor decrease in the range of motion.

Within days, a dense fibrous capsule develops around the tissue expander and completely surrounds it. This capsule is composed of elongated fibroblasts and a few myofibroblasts, which lie between thick bundles of collagen fibers and are oriented parallel to the surface of the implant. The capsule is approximately 45 to 100 μ thick. Intracellular collagen fibers with normal periodicity are found within the cytoplasm of the fibroblast. The capsular membrane rapidly thins after removal of the expander, but an easily dissectable plane may remain for longer periods.

Rapid angiogenesis occurs in expanded tissue and is no doubt responsible for the increased viability of flaps created from expanded tissue.[10-13] The greatest increase in the number of vessels occurs at the junction between the capsule and the host tissue. The number of arterioles and venules increases within days after placement of the tissue expander. These vessels appear to communicate with smaller vessels in the papillary dermis overlying the implant. The exact mechanism of the physiologic stress that leads to neovascularization is uncertain, but it is thought that the resultant increase in capillary blood flow correlates well with the increased survival of these expanded flaps. Studies have postulated that mechanical tension or a hypoxic gradient is the stimulus for angiogenesis.

Mechanism of Tissue Expansion

There are several mechanisms that contribute to making tissue expansion successful, including the intrinsic or inherent stretch of elastic tissue, mechanical creep, and net gain in new tissue formation. Initially, tissue expansion stretches the skin as a result of the skin's inherent extensibility. The tensile strength of the skin is variable and depends on location, age, sex, and solar damage. The amount of stretch relates to the duration and intensity of the load; persistent tension will lead to irreversible changes and bonding between collagen fibers.[16] When skin is stretched beyond its elastic limit, it will not completely return to its original state. "Mechanical creep" refers to the skin being stretched beyond this inherent extensibility as tissue fluid is extruded out of the collagen network. When skin is stretched and held under a constant load, eventually the force required to keep the skin stretched at this distance gradually decreases. The stretching achieved from mechanical creep does not retract. Mechanical creep appears to have no effect on blood supply. Finally, expansion stimulates a net gain in tissue as evidenced by increases in collagen and fibroblast synthesis, myofilaments, mitotic activity, and neovascularization. The term biologic creep has been used for the generation of new tissue seen with expansion. Although inherent elastic stretch and mechanical creep are important, it is the stimulation of new tissue growth, the formation of a fibrous capsule, and angioneogenesis that allow successful expansion with resultant increase in size and improved flap viability.

Immediate Intraoperative Tissue Expansion

Immediate intraoperative tissue expansion (IITE), a modification of the conventional controlled tissue expansion technique, uses the skin's ability to immediately stretch and increase in surface area. Tissue expanders are placed at the time of surgery and undergo three or four expansion cycles. In a one-stage procedure, the expanders are removed, and the stretched skin is then used to close the surgical defect.[65] This technique was first reported in 1985 and again in 1987[58] using the term intraoperative sustained limited expansion (ISLE). This technique has also been known as rapid tissue expansion, immediate intraoperative tissue expansion, or intraoperative tissue expansion.[65-68]

The use of IITE should be considered when simpler alternative measures will result in distortion of surrounding structures or too tight a closure. This procedure may be performed without difficulty under local anesthesia using lidocaine (0.5 to 2%) with epinephrine (1:100,000 to 1:400,000). The planned location of the expander is about 2 to 6 cm from the surgical defect and is based on the expected tissue movement that will be used to reconstruct the defect. The expander may be placed and tissue expansion performed either before or after excision of the lesion.

Standard tissue expanders or Foley catheter balloons may be used for IITE. Expanders specifically designed for IITE with multiple shapes, designs, and sizes are also available. These consist of a silicone balloon connected to a valve by tubing, with volumes ranging from 1 to 100 ml. Foley catheter balloons may also be used for IITE. These balloons are available in sizes of 5, 10, 30, and 75 ml. The ease of availability and the relatively low cost make these balloons ideal for IITE. Foley catheter balloons generally can be inflated to two to three times their recommended volumes before rupturing.

When IITE is planned before excision of a lesion, a small incision is made, and a tunnel is created with blunt dissection to the area to be expanded. The level of this tunnel is based on the proper level of undermining for the location and planned depth of the defect. A Foley catheter and balloon are then inserted through the tunnel to a subcutaneous pocket under the skin to be expanded (Fig. 28–4).

When IITE is planned after excision of a lesion such as a Mohs surgical defect, the tunnel may be made from a distant site or from within the defect itself. The expander may then be inserted through the tunnel to the subcutaneous pocket under the skin to be expanded. When inserted from the defect, the catheter may be anchored to the wound edge with towel clamps or sutures to prevent migration of the balloon toward the defect during expansion (Fig. 28–5). Partial closure of the wound with sutures or clamps will also help to prevent migration of the expander.

With the expander in place, expansion proceeds with a series of three to four cycles of inflation for 3 to 10 minutes each, followed by a deflation period of 2 to 5 minutes (Fig. 28–6). The expander should be inflated enough that the skin overlying the expander becomes very tense and blanches. The use of multiple expanders may be used to facilitate the expansion process. Greater volumes of saline can usually be infused into the expander with each subsequent inflation cycle. After the final expansion cycle, the expander is removed, and the reconstructive procedure is performed in the usual manner (Fig. 28–7). Postoperative wound care and interval for suture removal are routine (Fig. 28–8).

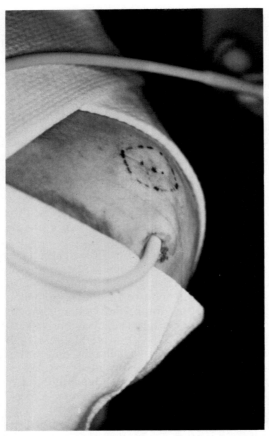

Figure 28–4. Foley catheter inserted through a small incision placed inferior to the planned excision. (From Johnson TM, Brown MD, Sullivan MJ, Swanson NA: Immediate intraoperative tissue expansion. J Am Acad Dermatol 22:283–287, 1990.)

Unlike conventional tissue expansion, minimal histologic and ultrastructural changes occur in the expanded skin after IITE. The ability of the skin to immediately stretch is partly explained by a mechanical tissue creep. As discussed earlier, tissue creep is defined as the gradual lengthening of skin that results when it is stretched under a constant load.[69, 70] An effective way to recruit extra skin is by this cyclic stretching. Mechanical tissue creep occurring during IITE may be secondary to a relative dehydration of tissue caused by displacement of ground substance and fluids, a parallel realignment of randomly positioned collagen fibers, elastic tissue microfragmentation, and adjacent tissue migration into the field owing to the stretching force.[69, 70] The tissue gain observed during IITE may be explained based on a three-dimensional mechanical force exerted by the tissue expander resulting in relative dehydration and adjacent migration of tissue into the field as a result of the stretching force. The amount of tissue gain during IITE is unknown. However, depending on the anatomic site, between 0.5 and 2.5 cm of tissue gain can be expected.[66] Forehead flaps can increase in width by up to 20%.[67]

No significant light microscopic changes have been demonstrated in the expanded skin of patients who underwent IITE.[66] The response of pig skin to IITE has

also been examined ultrastructurally, and no changes in expanded skin versus control skin were noted by light microscopy using hemotoxylin-and-eosin stains, collagen stains, and elastic tissue stains.[63] Immunofluorescent antibody studies, as well as electron microscopy, also failed to demonstrate any changes in collagen or elastic tissue in pig skin undergoing IITE. The only finding was the presence of greatly dilated superficial dermal capillaries seen by electron microscopy in expanded skin; this corresponds to the ecchymosis and vascular congestion seen clinically in immediately expanded skin.

Complications secondary to IITE are similar to those observed during conventional tissue expansion and are lowest in the head and neck region and highest on the distal lower extremities.[66] Scar spread may occur over time but has not been noted in most patients. The only way to truly evaluate scar spread is to compare the same wound and closure in a patient with and without expansion.

IITE is a procedure requiring careful surgical planning and technique, and many unanswered questions remain. Additional research is needed to determine the actual tissue gain, the complete ultrastructural changes, and the degree of scar spread in expanded human skin.

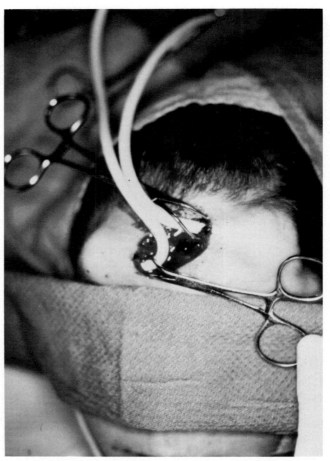

Figure 28–5. Bilateral Foley catheters held in place by hemostats. (From Johnson TM, Brown MD, Sullivan MJ, Swanson NA: Immediate intraoperative tissue expansion. J Am Acad Dermatol 22:283–287, 1990.)

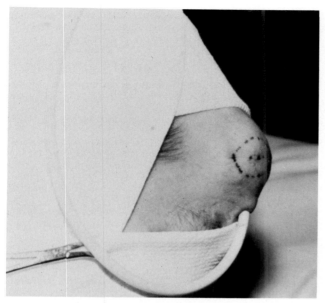

Figure 28–6. IITE with a 10-ml Foley catheter inserted through a 5-mm incision approximately 6 cm below the planned surgical site for re-excision of a 1.3-cm melanoma. (From Johnson TM, Brown MD, Sullivan MJ, Swanson NA: Immediate intraoperative tissue expansion. J Am Acad Dermatol 22:283–287, 1990.)

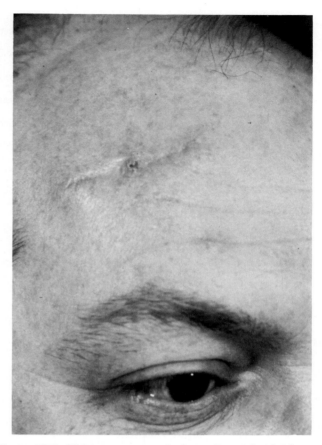

Figure 28–8. Clinical appearance 2 weeks after performing layered closure. (From Johnson TM, Brown MD, Sullivan MJ, Swanson NA: Immediate intraoperative tissue expansion. J Am Acad Dermatol 22:283–287, 1990.)

However, knowledge of the technique of IITE adds to the surgeon's armamentarium, allowing additional possibilities to provide the best reconstructive effort possible to the patient.

SUMMARY

Tissue expansion is a remarkable natural event in which human tissue adapts to intrinsic and extrinsic forces, leading to a net gain in surface area. The initial application of controlled tissue expansion for breast reconstruction has been greatly broadened to include expansion of almost any area of the body. Tissue expansion is currently being applied where reconstructive procedures are either impossible, require several procedures, or will give inferior cosmetic results. As more physicians become aware of tissue expansion, more patients will benefit from its potential uses. Although many cutaneous surgeons will never employ controlled tissue expansion, a basic knowledge of the technique will allow them to assist patients when expansion would be beneficial. Indications include traumatic and scarring alopecias, male-pattern alopecia, giant congenital nevi, giant cerebriform nevi, large tattoos, scar revisions, and reconstruction of large or anatomically difficult defects after removal of skin neoplasms. Certainly, intraoperative tissue expansion can be easily added to the surgical armamentarium of most cutaneous surgeons to assist in closing defects with less tension. Future studies and continued imaginative applications of controlled and intraoperative tissue expansion are certain to broaden even further the uses of this procedure.

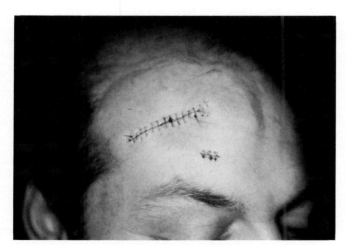

Figure 28–7. Immediate layered closure after three cycles of IITE of 20 ml each. (From Johnson TM, Brown MD, Sullivan MJ, Swanson NA: Immediate intraoperative tissue expansion. J Am Acad Dermatol 22:283–287, 1990.)

REFERENCES

1. Neumann CG: The expansion of an area of skin by progressive distention of the subcutaneous balloon. Plast Reconstr Surg 19:124–130, 1957.

2. Radovan C: Adjacent flap development using an expandable Silastic implant. Presented at the Annual Meeting of the American Society of Plastic and Reconstructive Surgeons, Boston, 1976.

3. Radovan C: Breast reconstruction after mastectomy using the temporary expander. Plast Reconstr Surg 69:195–208, 1982.

4. Radovan C: Tissue expansion in soft tissue reconstruction. Plast Reconstr Surg 74:482–490, 1984.

5. Austad ED, Rose GL: A self-inflating tissue expander. Plast Reconstr Surg 70:588–593, 1982.

6. Baker SR, Swanson NA: Clinical applications of tissue expansion in head and neck surgery. Laryngoscope 100:313–319, 1990.

7. Agris J: Tissue expansion—a new vista in reconstruction. Am J Cosmet Surg 4:301–308, 1987.

8. Marcus J, Horan DB, Robinson JK: Tissue expansion: past, present and future. J Am Acad Dermatol 23:813–825, 1990.

9. Swanson NA, Argenta LC: Tissue expansion. In: Roenigk RK, Roenigk HH (eds): Dermatologic Surgery: Principles and Practice. Marcel Dekker, New York, 1989, pp 347–354.

10. Cherry GW, Austad ED, Pasyk KA, et al: Increased survival and vascularity of random-pattern skin flaps elevated in controlled expanded skin. Plast Reconstr Surg 72:680–685, 1983.

11. Cummings CW, Goding GS, Trachy RE: Tissue expansion and cutaneous blood flow. Laryngoscope 98:919–922, 1988.

12. Marks MW, Burney RE, MacKenzie JR, Knight PR: Enhanced capillary blood flow in rapidly expanded random pattern flaps. J Trauma 26:913–915, 1986.

13. Saxby PJ: Survival of island flaps after tissue expansion: a pig model. Plast Reconstr Surg 81:30–34, 1988.

14. Van Rappend JH, Molenaar J, Van Doorn K, et al: Surface area increase in tissue expansion. Plast Reconstr Surg 82:833–839, 1988.

15. Austad ED, Thomas SB, Pasyk KA: Tissue expansion: dividend or loss? Plast Reconstr Surg 78:63–67, 1986.

16. Roenigk RK, Wheeland RG: Tissue expansion in dermatologic surgery. Dermatol Clin 5:429–436, 1987.

17. Argenta LC, Marks MW, Pasyk KA: Advances in tissue expansion. Clin Plast Surg 12:159–171, 1988.

18. Argenta LC, Marks MW, Grabb WC: Selective use of serial expansions in breast reconstruction. Ann Plast Surg 11:188–195, 1983.

19. Argenta LC: Reconstruction of the breast by tissue expansion. Clin Plast Surg 11:257–264, 1984.

20. Gibney J: Long term results of tissue expansion for breast reconstruction. Clin Plast Surg 14:509–518, 1987.

21. Versaci AD, Balkovich ME, Goldstein SA: Breast reconstruction by tissue expansion for congenital and burn deformities. Ann Plast Surg 16:20–31, 1986.

22. Russell IS, Collins JP, Holmes AD, Smith JA: The use of tissue expansion for immediate breast reconstruction after mastectomy. Med J Aust 152:632–635, 1990.

23. Roenigk RK, Wheeland RG: Tissue expansion in cicatricial alopecia. Arch Dermatol 123:641–646, 1987.

24. Vallis CP: Surgical treatment of cicatricial alopecia of the scalp. Clin Plast Surg 9:179–196, 1982.

25. Leonard AG, Small J: Tissue expansion in the treatment of alopecia. Br J Plast Surg 39:42–56, 1986.

26. Manders EK, Graham WP: Alopecia reduction by scalp expansion. J Dermatol Surg Oncol 10:967–969, 1984.

27. Pierce HE: Possible uses of the Radovan tissue expander in hair replacement surgery. J Dermatol Surg Oncol 11:413–417, 1985.

28. Nordstrom RE, Devine JW: Scalp stretching with a tissue expander for closure of scalp defects. Plast Reconstr Surg 75:578–581, 1988.

29. Adson MH, Anderson RD, Argenta LC: Scalp expansion in the treatment of male pattern baldness. Plast Reconstr Surg 79:906–914, 1987.

30. Argenta LC, Watanabe MJ, Grabb WC: The use of tissue expansion in head and neck reconstruction. Ann Plast Surg 11:31–37, 1983.

31. Adamson JE: Nasal reconstruction with the expanded forehead flap. Plast Reconstr Surg 81:12–20, 1988.

32. Muenker R: Nasal reconstruction with tissue expansion. Facial Plast Surg 5:328–337, 1988.

33. Kroll SS: Forehead flap nasal reconstruction with tissue expansion and delayed pedicle separation. Laryngoscope 99:448–452, 1989.

34. Spence RJ: Clinical use of a tissue expander–enhanced transposition flap for face and neck reconstruction. Ann Plast Surg 21:58–64, 1988.

35. Antonyshyn O, Gruss JS, Zuker R, Mackinnon SE: Tissue expansion in head and neck reconstruction. Plast Reconstr Surg 82:58–68, 1988.

36. Bauer BS: Role of tissue expansion in reconstruction of the ear. Clin Plast Surg 17:319–325, 1990.

37. Victor WH, Hurwitz JJ, Gruss JS: The development of a new tissue expander for use in ophthalmic plastic surgery. Ophthalmic Surg 17:661–665, 1986.

38. Manders EK, Oaks TE, An VK, et al: Soft tissue expansion in the lower extremities. Plast Reconstr Surg 81:208–219, 1988.

39. Hallock GG: Extremity tissue expansion. Orthop Rev 16:606–611, 1987.

40. Mackinnon SE, Gruss JS: Soft tissue expanders in upper limb surgery. J Hand Surg 10:749–753, 1985.

41. Sellers DS, Miller SH, Demuth RJ, et al: Repeated skin expansion to resurface a massive thigh wound. Plast Reconstr Surg 77:654–657, 1986.

42. Maves MD, Lask RP: Tissue expansion in the treatment of giant congenital melanocytic nevi. Arch Otolaryngol Head Neck Surg 113:987–991, 1987.

43. Hagerty RC, Zubowitz VW: Tissue expansion in the treatment of hypertrophic scars and scar contractures. South Med J 79:432–436, 1986.

44. Hallock GG: Tissue expansion. Contemp Surg 29:34–39, 1986.

45. Goldstein RD, Shuster SH: Methylene blue: a simple adjunct to aid in soft tissue expansion. Plast Reconstr Surg 80:452, 1987.

46. Marks MW, Argenta LC, Thorton JW: Rapid expansion: experimental and clinical experience. Clin Plast Surg 14:455–463, 1987.

47. Pietila JP, Nordstrom REA, Virkhunnen PJ, et al: Accelerated tissue expansion with the overfilling technique. Plast Reconstr Surg 81:204–207, 1988.

48. Zuker RM: Use of tissue expansion in pediatric scalp burn reconstruction. J Burn Care Rehabil 8:103–106, 1987.

49. Bauer BS, Johnson PE, Lovato G: Applications of soft tissue expansion in children. Pediatr Dermatol 3:281–290, 1986.

50. Cole WG, Bennett CS, Perks AG, et al: Tissue expansion in the lower limbs of children and young adults. J Bone Joint Surg 72:578–580, 1990.

51. Bauer BS, Vicari FA, Richard ME: The role of tissue expansion in pediatric plastic surgery. Clin Plast Surg 17:101–112, 1990.

52. Austad ED: Complications in tissue expansion. Clin Plast Surg 14:49–50, 1987.

53. Antonyshyn O, Gruss JS, Mackinnon SE, et al: Complications of soft tissue expansion. Br J Plast Surg 41:239–249, 1985.

54. Manders EK, Schenden MJ, Furrey JA, et al: Soft-tissue expansion: concepts and complications. Plast Reconstr Surg 74:493–507, 1984.

55. Masser MR: Tissue expansion: a reconstructive revolution or a cornucopia of complications? Br J Plast Surg 43:344–348, 1990.

56. Neale HW, High RM, Billmire DA, et al: Complications of controlled tissue expansion in the pediatric burn patient. Plast Reconstr Surg 82:840–848, 1988.

57. Fudern GM, Orgel MG: Full thickness erosion of the skull secondary to tissue expansion for scalp reconstruction. Plast Reconstr Surg 82:368–369, 1988.

58. Austad ED, Pasyk KA, McClatchey KD, et al: Histomorphologic evaluation of guinea pig skin and soft tissue after controlled tissue expansion. Plast Reconstr Surg 70:704–710, 1982.

59. Pasyk KA, Austad ED, McClatchey KD, Cherry GW: Electron microscopic evaluation of guinea pig skin and soft tissues expanded with a self-inflating silicone implant. Plast Reconstr Surg 70:37–45, 1982.

60. Pasyk KA, Austad ED, Cherry GW: Intracellular collagen fibers in the capsule around silicone expanders in guinea pig. J Surg Res 36:125–133, 1984.

61. Johnson PE, Kernahan DA, Bauer S: Dermal and epidermal response to soft tissue expansion in the pig. Plast Reconstr Surg 81:390–397, 1988.

62. Pasyk KA, Argenta LC, Hassett C: Quantitative analysis of the thickness of human skin and subcutaneous tissue following controlled expansion with a silicone implant. Plast Reconstr Surg 81:516–523, 1988.

63. Bartell TH, Mustoe TA: Animal models of human tissue expansion. Plast Reconstr Surg 83:681–686, 1989.

64. Sasaki GH, Pang CY: Pathophysiology of skin flaps raised on expanded pig skin. Plast Reconstr Surg 74:59–60, 1984.

65. Johnson TM, Brown MD, Sullivan MJ, Swanson NA: Immediate intraoperative tissue expansion. J Am Acad Dermatol 22:283–287, 1990.

66. Sasaki GH: Intraoperative sustained limited expansion (ISLE) as an immediate reconstructive technique. Clin Plast Surg 14:563–573, 1987.

67. Hoffman HT, Baker SR: Nasal reconstruction with the rapidly expanded forehead flap. Laryngoscope 99:1096–1098, 1989.

68. Greenbaum SS, Greenbaum CH: Intraoperative tissue expansion using a Foley catheter following expansion of a basal cell carcinoma. J Dermatol Surg Oncol 16:45–48, 1990.

69. Gibson T: The physical properties of skin. In: Converse JM (ed): Reconstructive Plastic Surgery. WB Saunders, Philadelphia, 1977, pp 70–77.

70. Gibson T, Kenedi RM, Craik JE: The mobile microarchitecture of dermal collagen: a bioengineering study. Br J Surg 52:764–769, 1965.

71. Guida RA, Johnson TM: Assessment survival and ultrastructural changes in immediate intraoperative expanded flaps in the porcine model. Arch Otolaryngol. In press.

CHAPTER 29

Lip Wedges

DONALD J. GRANDE and ALLAN C. HARRINGTON

The need to maintain the normal position and contour of the lip during reconstructive surgery is aesthetically and functionally critical. However, the freely movable nature of the vermilion and cutaneous lip makes this area highly susceptible to distortion. Wedge resection provides the cutaneous surgeon with an effective procedure that produces cosmetically gratifying results. The oral lips have important functions besides the obvious cosmetic ones. An intact lip is important for social interaction. Nonverbal communication can be initiated with the slightest of labial movements. A wide spectrum of emotions can be conveyed, from happiness with a smile to disappointment with a pout. The lips also participate in the expression of sensuality and sexuality. The full range of phonation with enunciation of sounds such as "b," "m," "p," "a," "w," and "v" requires normal functioning lips.[1] Finally, a competent oral seal is required to contain liquids and solids and is dependent on an intact sphincter mechanism, especially of the lower lip.

Superficial Lip Anatomy

An understanding of lip anatomy is important for optimal surgical results. The surface anatomy of the lip covers more area than the red margin or vermilion border. The area of the labial unit parallels the underlying orbicularis oris muscle, with extension superiorly to the nose and inferiorly to the chin.[2] It is helpful to think of the lip in terms of cutaneous lip, vermilion, and mucous membrane. Any surgical repair must take into account these subdivisions and the key surrounding contours such as the labiomental and nasolabial lines (Fig. 29–1). If possible, reconstruction should always attempt to restore these subunits and simultaneously place the scars within the contour lines. Other important topographic landmarks of the lip are the philtrum,

Cupid's bow, and the commissure or angle of the mouth (Fig. 29–1). The last-named serves as the general site of attachment for the circumoral muscle bundles. The midpoint of the upper cutaneous lip is highlighted by the two vertically oriented ridges of the philtrum. At the base of the philtrum is the characteristic concavity of Cupid's bow. Preservation of these two vital landmarks is always given a high priority in lip surgery.

Deep Lip Anatomy

The deep anatomy of the lip is structurally quite simple. It is best understood in terms of the muscle and submucosal layers, which are sandwiched between the external skin and the internal mucous membrane (Fig. 29–2). Histologically, the vermilion is distinguished from the cutaneous lip by lack of the pilosebaceous structures and thickening of the epidermis with prominent rete ridges.[3, 4] Between the rete ridges the thin epidermis

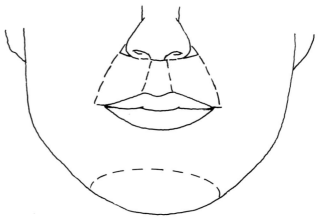

Figure 29–1. Superficial anatomy of the lip.

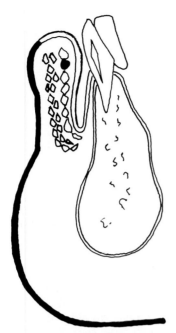

Figure 29–2. Cross-sectional view of the lip showing the muscular and submucosal layers sandwiched between the skin and the mucous membrane.

overlies richly vascularized dermal papillae. It is this anatomic finding that accounts for the bright pink or red lip color seen in Caucasians. Occasionally, an ectopically placed sebaceous gland, known as Fordyce's spot, may be observed on the vermilion.

The transition from keratinized vermilion to the stratified squamous parakeratotic epithelium of the mucosa occurs with loss of the stratum granulosum.[4] The frenulum linguae appears in the midline as a fold of mucous membrane and connects the mucous membrane of the lip with the floor of the mouth and gingiva.[5] The major muscle of the lip is the orbicularis oris. This circumferentially oriented muscle is responsible for the sphincter function of the mouth. There are also circumoral muscles that are intimately associated with the orbicularis oris (Fig. 29–3). These muscles help to elevate, depress,

and retract the lip, which produces the complex movement pattern associated with normal labial function.

Numerous salivary glands lie in the submucosa between the orbicularis oris and the mucosa. These glands empty directly into the vestibule of the mouth and provide the moisture for the labial mucosa. However, because the vermilion is not supplied by these salivary glands, its surface remains dry. The vascular supply of the upper and lower lip is provided by the superior and inferior labial arteries, respectively (Fig. 29–4). These vessels are branches of the facial artery and are found within the submucosa. Sensory innervation of the upper lip is a function of the infraorbital nerve (V2), while the mental nerve (V3) provides sensation to the lower lip (Fig. 29–4). The motor innervation of the orbicularis oris is provided by the buccal branch of the facial nerve. The circumoral muscles are innervated by either the buccal or the marginal mandibular branches of the facial nerve. Lymphatic drainage of the middle lower lip flows to the submental lymph nodes, while the lymphatics of the upper and lateral lower lip (Fig. 29–4) flow to the submandibular glands.[5]

Surgical Technique for Lip Wedge Resection

Wedge resection is an important procedure in the treatment of infiltrating lesions of the lower lip. The most frequent clinical indication for this procedure is the presence of squamous cell carcinoma. Other lip lesions that are encountered less commonly, such as keratoacanthomas, hemangiomas and basal cell carcinomas, are also amenable to treatment with this procedure. The need for clear surgical margins in treating squamous cell carcinomas is underscored by their potential seriousness. The incidence of metastasis in squamous cell cancers is 5 to 20% on the lower lip and as high as 50% on the upper lip.[6, 7] The 5-year control rate for lower lip squamous cell carcinomas in the absence of lymphadenopathy is 90%, but this optimistic figure is reduced to 45% when there is evidence of lymphadenopathy.

Figure 29–3. The arrangement of the orbicularis oris and the intimately associated circumoral muscles. The deeper muscle bundles are illustrated on the left and the more superficial muscles on the right.

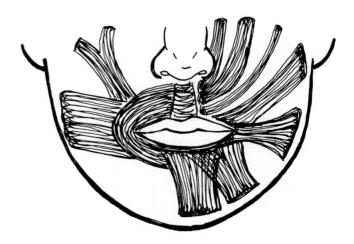

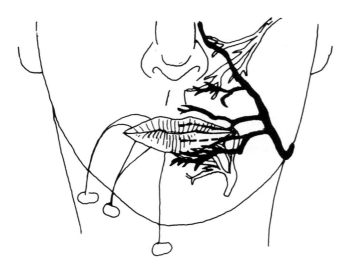

Figure 29–4. The arterial supply and the sensory innervation to the labial unit are shown on the right. The lymphatic flow with the middle lower lip draining to the submental lymph nodes, and the upper lip and the lateral lower lip draining to the submandibular lymph nodes, is illustrated on the left.

Wedge resection is an effective procedure that can be used to reconstruct defects of one third, and in some instances up to one half, of the diameter of the lower lip and one fourth of the diameter of the upper lip.[8–10] For larger defects, a lip-switch procedure, local or distant flap, is typically required for reconstruction.[11–13] Preoperative evaluation and planning is of paramount importance for the best results. The need for a lip shave or vermilionectomy in conjunction with wedge resection to treat severe or extensive actinic damage of the vermilion should be determined preoperatively. Malalignment of the labiocutaneous junction results in an undesirable and obvious asymmetry. Accurate reapproximation of the vermilion border is essential for satisfactory cosmetic results. Recommended methods to ensure matching of the vermilion borders include marking the junction with silk sutures, needle tattooing with methylene blue, and superficially nicking the skin with a scalpel.[9]

The standard wedge resection is a V-shaped excision (Figs. 29–5, 29–6). For larger defects, a pentagonal excision can be used to reduce the risk of notching (Fig. 29–7). For wider lesions, a sliding flap (Fig. 29–8), or an inferiorly based M-plasty (Fig. 29–9) may be designed.[1, 10, 14, 15] The initial incision should be made decisively using a No. 10 or 15 scalpel blade. Care must be taken to immediately identify the inferior labial artery so that it can be clamped with a hemostat and ligated

with 5–0 Vicryl or comparable absorbable suture material. It is important to recognize that a shorter incision is needed on the mucosal side of the resection. Many cutaneous surgeons have their assistant squeeze the lip to aid in hemostasis and better stabilize it while making the incisions. In addition, placement of a cotton dental roll between the labial mucosa and teeth improves the exposure of the lower lip and decreases the volume of blood in the surgical field. Suction may also be used to ensure a clear operative field.

Before suturing any defects located away from the midline, it is necessary to evaluate the lip for any asymmetry in the vermilion thickness when the red margins are brought together. If these are unequal in size, a triangular piece of mucosa must be removed from the wider side. The triangle is designed so that its base is adjacent to the defect (Fig. 29–10); this corrects any size discrepancy and helps to avoid significant notching of the vermilion line. Suturing the final defect is accomplished in layers (see Fig. 29–9B). The most common technique uses buried interrupted Vicryl or silk sutures to close the mucosa from the posterior triangle to the vermilion border. Next, the muscle is also closed with simple Vicryl interrupted sutures. Finally, the cutaneous lip is closed with interrupted synthetic nylon sutures, and the vermilion with silk or a soft braided suture. Postoperatively, antibacterial ointment is applied on the wound surface and a sterile dressing placed on

Figure 29–5. The basic design of the V-shaped wedge biopsy.

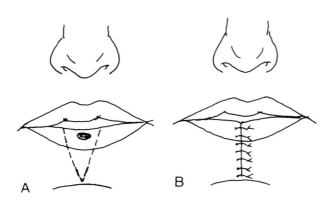

A   B

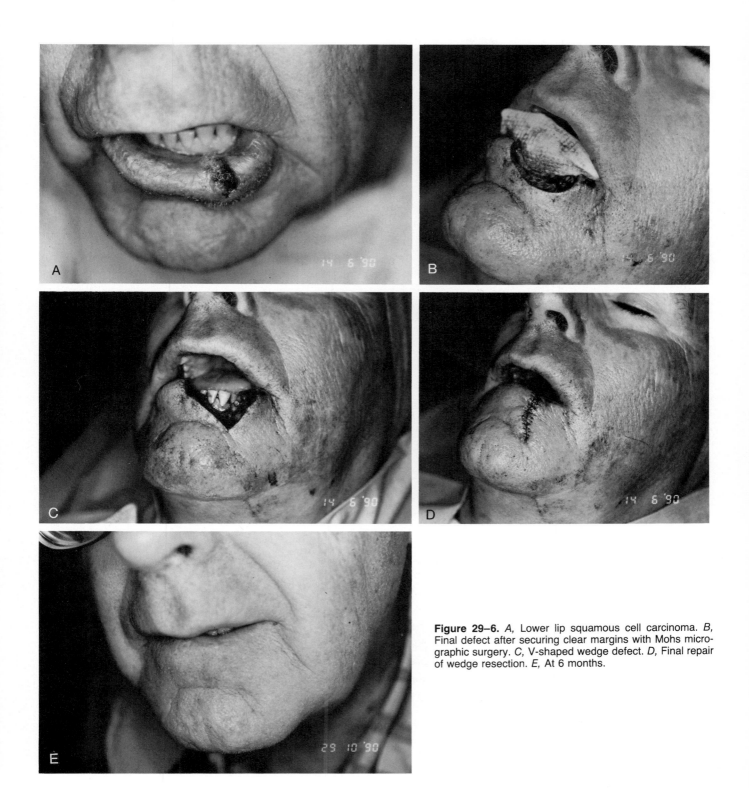

Figure 29-6. *A,* Lower lip squamous cell carcinoma. *B,* Final defect after securing clear margins with Mohs micrographic surgery. *C,* V-shaped wedge defect. *D,* Final repair of wedge resection. *E,* At 6 months.

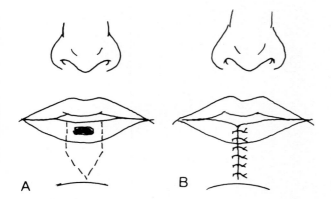

Figure 29–7. Pentagonal design.

Figure 29–8. Sliding flap.

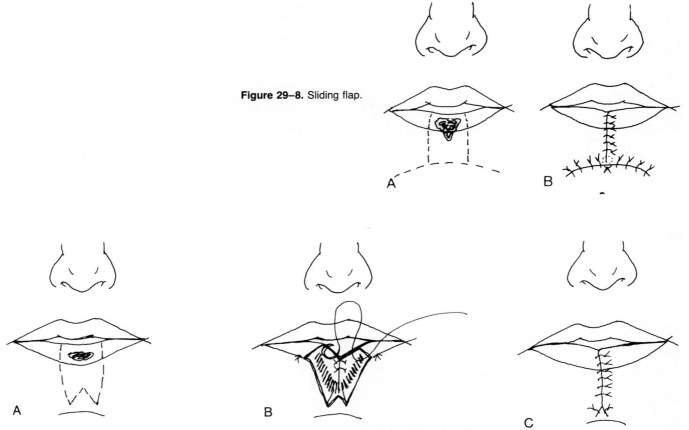

Figure 29–9. *A*, M-plasty design. *B*, Defect illustrating layer closure. *C*, Final repair.

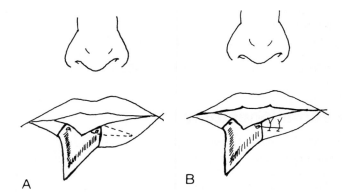

Figure 29–10. *A*, Triangular shape designed on the mucosal surface of the wider lip section. *B*, Correction in thickness.

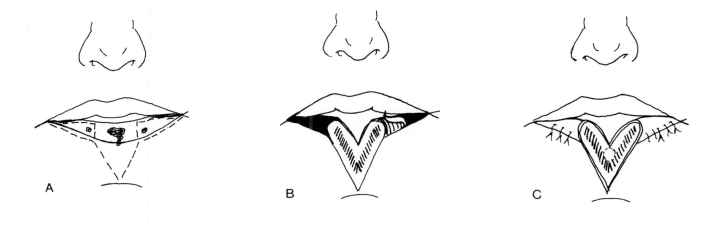

Figure 29–11. *A*, Design of the combination of wedge resection and vermilionectomy. *B*, Final wedge-shaped defect and stripping of the vermilion. *C*, Reapproximation of mucosal advancement followed by layered closure of the wedge defect. *D*, Final repair.

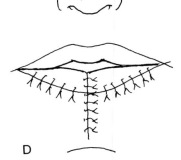

the involved cutaneous lip. Daily wound care involves cleaning the cutaneous excision with sterile saline or a solution of 3% hydrogen peroxide, followed by reapplication of the antibacterial ointment and a new dressing. The cutaneous sutures are typically removed in 5 to 7 days.

Vermilionectomy

Many patients who undergo wedge resections for squamous cell carcinomas also have severe actinic damage elsewhere on the lower lip. In these patients, a lip shave or vermilionectomy may be performed at the time of the wedge resection.[1, 10] This procedure involves excising the exposed vermilion border from the labiocutaneous junction to the point of contact of the upper lip (Fig. 29–11). The labial mucosa is then undermined and advanced to complete the reconstruction and 6–0 silk sutures are used to reapproximate the skin edges of the lower lip. These sutures are ususally removed in 5 to 7 days. If a mucosal advancement flap is required, it should be done before closure of the wedge excision.

SUMMARY

Wedge resection offers the cutaneous surgeon an effective technique to treat infiltrating lesions of the lower lip. An understanding of the basic surgical principles and the labial anatomy helps to ensure optimal cosmetic and functional results.

REFERENCES

1. Yarington CT Jr, Larrabee WF Jr: Reconstruction following lip resection. Otolaryngol Clin North Am 16:407–421, 1983.
2. Salasche SJ, Bernstein G (eds): In: Surgical Anatomy of the Skin. Appleton & Lange, Norwalk, CT, 1988, pp 223–240.
3. Liebgott B: The Anatomical Basis of Dentistry. BC Decker, Toronto, 1986, pp 144–147.
4. Ross MH, Reith EJ, Romrell LJ: Histology: A Text and Atlas. Williams & Wilkins, Baltimore, 1978, pp 44–47.
5. Woodburne RT, Burkel WE: Essentials of Human Anatomy. Oxford University Press, New York, 1988, pp 261–262.
6. Million RR, Cassisi NJ, Clark JR: Cancer of the head and neck. In: DeVita VT Jr (ed): Cancer, Principles & Practice of Oncology. JB Lippincott, Philadelphia, 1989, pp 448–598.
7. Calcaterra TC, Juillard GJ: Oral cavity and oropharynx. In: Haskell CM (ed): Cancer Treatment. 3rd ed. WB Saunders, Philadelphia, 1980, pp 373—378.
8. Davidson TM, Bartlow GA, Bone RC: Surgical excisions from and reconstructions of the oral lips. J Dermatol Surg Oncol 6:133-l42, 1980.
9. Stegman SJ, Tromovitch TA, Glogau RG: Basics of Dermatologic Surgery. Year Book, Chicago, 1982, pp 91–94.
10. Zide BM: Deformities of the lips and cheeks. In: McCarthy JG (ed): Plastic Surgery. Vol 3. The Face. WB Saunders, Philadelphia, 1990, pp 2009–2027.
11. Panje WR: Lip reconstruction. Otolaryngol Clin North Am 15:169-178, 1982.
12. Pelly AD, Tan EP: Lower lip reconstruction. Br J Plast Surg 34:83–86, 1981.
13. Salasche SJ, Grabski WJ: Flaps for the Central Face. Churchill Livingstone, New York, 1990, pp 61–87.
14. McGregor IA, McGregor FM: Cancer of the Face and Mouth. Churchill Livingstone, Edinburgh, 1986, pp 135–176.
15. Wheeland RG: Reconstruction of the lower lip and chin using local and random pattern flaps. J Dermatol Surg Oncol 17:605–615, 1991.

CHAPTER 30

Ear Wedges

GARY P. LASK

The ear is a frequent site of cutaneous carcinoma as a result of its prominence and subsequent exposure to the sun. Carcinomas of the external ear are common and constitute 5 to 8% of all skin cancers. Approximately 50 to 60% of malignancies of the external ear are squamous cell carcinomas, 30 to 40% are basal cell carcinomas, and 2 to 6% are malignant melanomas.[1]

When undertaking reconstruction of the ear, the complexity of the convolutions becomes readily apparent. In addition, the multiple convexities and concavities and varying degrees of cartilaginous thickness (Fig. 30–1) all influence the potential reconstructive possibilities.

The ear, unlike other anatomic structures, is seldom, if ever, referred to as beautiful, and the normal ear often goes relatively unnoticed. However, an unusual-appearing or abnormal ear *is* noticed. For this reason, the primary goal of reconstruction is to re-create a relatively normal and symmetric ear. There are two main methods used for correcting auricular defects in a single procedure. The first is by direct closure using an ear wedge that reduces the circumference of the ear. The second is by using local or distant tissue to preserve the original size of the ear. Ear wedges can be an effective method of surgical reconstruction if used in appropriate circumstances.

Anatomy of the External Ear

The skin on the anterior aspect of the ear is thin, pale, and closely adherent to the underlying cartilage, since little subcutaneous tissue is present. There is a thin fascial layer between the skin and perichondrium that contains blood vessels and nerves. The skin on the posterormedial aspect of the ear is loose, soft, and matlike in texture. It is also generally thicker and much less adherent to the cartilage and can wrinkle. There are two layers of fat divided by a neurovascular fascia containing the arteries, veins, lymphatics, and motor and sensory nerves. The amount of excess skin increases more inferiorly along the ear. The most inferior aspect of the ear is the earlobe, which is composed entirely of relatively thick skin and subcutaneous tissue and contains no cartilage.

The blood supply to the ear comes from the superficial temporal artery anteriorly and from the posterior auricular artery posteriorly. Both these blood vessels are branches of the external carotid artery. The posterior auricular artery supplies the majority of blood to the ear. Cutaneous sensory innervation of the ear is supplied by the greater auricular and lesser occipital nerves from the cervical plexus, the auriculotemporal branch of the mandibular nerve, and the auricular branch of the vagus nerve. Most ear sensation comes from the greater auricular nerve, with the superioanterior lateral auricular surface supplied by the auriculotemporal branch. The floor of the external auditory canal is supplied by the vagus nerve, the posterior wall by the auriculotemporal branch, and the inferior and superior walls by the greater auricular nerve. The mastoid region is supplied by the lesser occipital nerve.[2–5]

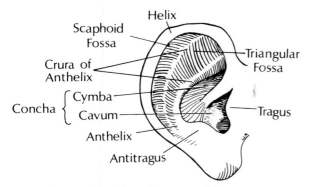

Figure 30–1. Normal anatomy of the ear.

The auricle continues to grow during the first decade of life. By 6 years of age, 85% of the growth has occurred. During adolescence there is continuous slow growth, followed by a rest period until approximately 50 years of age, when slow growth resumes under hormonal influences.[4] The average length of the auricle is 63.5 mm in men and 59 mm in women. The normal protrusion of the ear is about 30 degrees, or between 2 and 2.5 cm.[3, 4]

Anesthesia Techniques

Small defects of the ear can be anesthetized by local infiltration with lidocaine with or without epinephrine. When larger reconstructions are performed, an ear block is usually required to facilitate the procedure. The sensory innervation of the ear can be divided into three areas: innervation of the anterior aspect by the auriculotemporal nerve, innervation of the posterior half by the greater auricular and lesser occipital nerves, and innervation of the concha and ear canal by the auricular branch of the vagus nerve. There may also be some sensory innervation of the concha and the ear canal by the glossopharyngeal facial nerves.[1, 2, 6]

To perform an ear block, local anesthetic must be infiltrated from the base of the ear anteriorly along the preauricular border and then posteriorly around the postauricular sulcus. A solution of 1% lidocaine with epinephrine 1:100,000 is usually recommended. Because of the rich blood supply of the ear, secondary necrosis from epinephrine-induced vasoconstriction is not normally a problem. However, tissue necrosis can result from use of epinephrine in patients with arteriolar insufficiency.[5] Local infiltration of the concha and the external canal is also necessary to complete the anesthesia. This is performed by injecting anesthetic into the anterior aspect of the concha just posterior to its junction with the auditory meatus. With an ear nerve block, tissue distortion caused by extensive local infiltration can be avoided, but the beneficial local vasoconstrictive effects of epinephrine are lost.

Ear Wedge Techniques

Reducing the circumference of the ear by an ear wedge technique is often much simpler technically and causes less vascular compromise of the tissue than other methods. While wedges can provide good restoration of the anatomic landmarks of the ear, the disadvantages include a decrease in the circumference of the ear, a reduction in the vertical height of the auricle, some distortion of adjacent landmarks, and a failure to restore anatomic landmarks when very large defects are present.

The type of lesion that is ideally suited for wedge excision is a relatively small invasive tumor of the helix. If less than one fourth of the helix is removed, asymmetry will not be obvious, even though a measurable change in the height of the ear results from wedge excision. A 5-mm difference in length and a 3- to 4-mm

difference in width are not obvious under routine observation. True ear length cannot be judged visually. The size of the ear is estimated by the location of the upper and lower ear edges as it relates to various features of the upper and lower face. If an ear is narrower than normal but of normal length, it will appear longer than it really is.[4]

V-SHAPED WEDGE EXCISION

Sterile preparation of the ear and the surrounding skin with chlorhexidine before surgery and close adherence to sterile technique are advised to avoid any possible infection of the cartilage. For very small helical defects, a simple wedge in a V-shaped excision is ideal (Fig. 30–2). If this technique is attempted for larger lesions, significant notching will occur, and there will be marked lateral protrusion of the helix. The V-shaped wedge excision with approximately a 30-degree apex is drawn out with a surgical marking pen. The surgeon can also incise the skin at the apex of the wedge for an additional 1 cm to permit excision of the disc of cartilage. This maneuver can facilitate closure of the superior cartilage.

After the area has been excised, hemostasis is achieved with electrocautery. Extensive cauterization of the cartilage should not be used to avoid inducing cartilaginous necrosis. The cartilage is then reapproximated using 4-0 absorbable suture; during this procedure, the perichondrium must be included in the suture on both sides. If undermining is necessary to aid in tissue eversion, it should be done above the perichondrium.[1]

The skin is closed with 5-0 or 6-0 nonabsorbable suture by means of an interrupted or continuous suturing technique. A few vertical mattress sutures may be necessary to aid in tissue eversion. However, multiple simple interrupted sutures should be spaced between these,[7] as the vertical mattress sutures tend to constrict epidermal tissue and can cause noticeable suture scars. To avoid notching, some authors recommend stepping

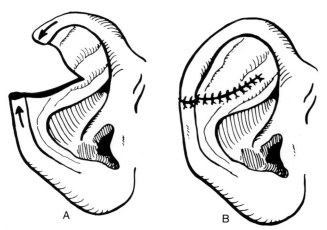

Figure 30–2. *A,* Appearance of the defect resulting from a V-shaped wedge excision. *B,* Appearance after linear closure.

up or down of the incision at the medial edge of the helix.[8–10]

W-SHAPED WEDGE EXCISION

When the size of the lesion causes the apex of the wedge to extend far enough to distort the architecture of the ear, a W-shaped wedge can be used. This shortens the length of the incision and allows for better preservation of normal architecture distant from the lesion. With a marking pen, the wedge excision is drawn out on the ear in the form of a W. The apex angles of the W-shaped wedge should be approximately 30 degrees. The tip of the wedge can be closed with simple sutures, or a tip stitch can be used. The resulting closure occurs in a "Y" configuration, giving a good cosmetic result with minimal distortion of the conchal area of the ear.

STELLATE WEDGE EXCISION

With larger helical defects or with lesions of the anthelix, a stellate excision can be used (Fig. 30–3). When dealing with lesions of the anthelix, this allows better preservation of the helix, which would normally be sacrificed if an ordinary wedge excision was used. In drawing out the stellate excision, V-shaped wedges (Burow's triangles) are placed near the center margin of the standard wedge with the long axis perpendicular to the margins of the primary excision.[1, 10] The base of the superior and inferior wedges should be approximately one third the size of the base of the standard wedge, with the length also approximately one third that of the standard wedge. If necessary, smaller wedges can be extended to facilitate closure.

WEDGE EXCISION ALONG THE HELICAL RIM

Another variation of the ear wedge is a wedge excision of the anthelix performed along the helical rim; this can be viewed as a type of advancement flap. The defect is

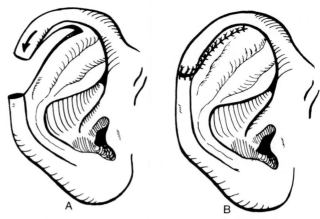

Figure 30–4. Appearance of the defect resulting from a wedge excision performed along the helical rim. *B,* Appearance after closure using an advancement flap.

simply closed in side-to-side fashion after advancing the helical rim (Fig. 30–4).

Postoperative Care

After surgery, adhesive tape strips are applied over the suture line and secured in place with Mastisol. A dressing is placed on the surface to provide protection. The outer aspect of the dressing can be changed as needed, but the tape strips are left in place until the sutures are removed in 7 days. If preferable, the entire dressing can be changed daily after cleaning the wound with 3% hydrogen peroxide and applying an antibiotic ointment. Some physicians recommend placing all patients on prophylactic oral antibiotic therapy for 5 to 7 days, but the merit of this procedure has not been clearly established.[7]

Recurrence Rates for Cancers on the Ear

In removing carcinomas, it is important to recognize that the recurrence rate, morbidity, and mortality are greater for malignant tumors of the ear than for other anatomic sites in general.[1, 7] In one series, squamous cell carcinomas of the external ear had a 14% recurrence rate.[11] An 8.3% recurrence rate was reported in another study on the ear compared with an overall recurrence rate of only 6%.[12] Squamous cell carcinomas of the external ear may also be more likely to metastasize,[13] with a 10% rate of metastasis reported.[14] Anatomic location also plays a role in the recurrence rate of basal cell carcinomas.[15] One series reported a 33.3% recurrence rate of basal cell carcinomas on the external ear, compared with a 6.8% rate overall.[16] Adequate margins must always be obtained; difficult lesions are appropriately treated with Mohs micrographic surgery.

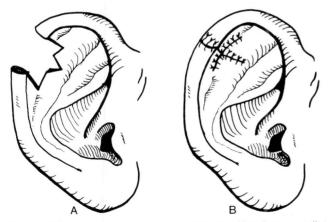

Figure 30–3. *A,* Appearance of the defect resulting from a stellate excision of the ear. *B,* Appearance after closure.

Complications of Ear Wedges

In all wedge excisions of the ear, the major limitation is the decrease in ear circumference. When the size of the defect exceeds one fourth of the auricular circumference, it can be quite noticeable and may be unacceptable to the patient. For these larger defects, an alternative method of reconstruction is advised. Even with smaller defects, some patients may not be satisfied with a smaller ear; this must be discussed with them before performing wedge reconstruction. If patients are reluctant to accept the possibility of a smaller ear, an alternative reconstructive procedure is advisable.

A potentially serious, though infrequent, complication is auricular perichondritis. Its occurrence is even less frequent than formerly with the availability of ciprofloxacin. However, if perichondritis does occur, the area usually must be drained, and intravenous antibiotics may be required. Malignant external otitis, a rare but possibly fatal complication,[17] is caused by *Pseudomonas aeruginosa* and occurs primarily in elderly diabetics. In elderly diabetic patients undergoing surgery of the ear in which cartilage is affected, meticulous preparation of the surgical site and strict adherence to sterile technique are required. Use of prophylactic antibiotics in patients at increased risk for wound infection is certainly appropriate. With good surgical technique, careful tissue handling, and adequate hemostasis, surgical complications such as hematoma, dehiscence, and necrosis should be extremely rare.

SUMMARY

If patient selection and anatomic location are carefully analyzed, ear wedges can yield very acceptable cosmetic results in reconstructing defects of the ear. For treatment of malignant tumors, the primary goal must be removal of the entire carcinoma, and the cosmetic result is of only secondary importance.

REFERENCES

1. Ceilley RI: Regional dermatologic surgery: ears. Semin Dermatol 6:187–202, 1987.
2. Salasche S, Bernstein G, Senkarik M: Surgical Anatomy of the Skin. Appleton and Lange, East Norwalk, CT, 1988.
3. Weerda H: Embryology and structural anatomy of the external ear. Facial Plast Surg 2:85–91, 1985.
4. Davis J: Aesthetic and Reconstructive Otoplasty. Springer-Verlag, New York, 1987.
5. Jackson IT: Ear reconstruction. In: Jackson IT (ed): Local Flaps in Head and Neck Reconstruction. CV Mosby, St. Louis, 1985, pp 251–271.
6. Auletta MJ, Grekin RC: Local anesthesia for dermatologic surgery. Churchill Livingstone, New York, 1991.
7. Bennett RG: Fundamentals of Cutaneous Surgery. CV Mosby, St. Louis, 1988.
8. Coleman W: Wedge excision. In: Coleman W, Colon G, Davis S (eds): Outpatient Surgery of the Skin. Medical Examination Publishers, New Hyde Park, NY, 1983, pp 43–52.
9. Grabb WC, Smith JW: Plastic Surgery. 3rd ed. Little, Brown, Boston, 1979.
10. Tromovitch TA, Stegman SJ, Glogau RG: Flaps and Grafts in Dermatologic Surgery. Year Book Medical, Chicago, 1989.
11. Byers R: Squamous carcinoma of the external ear. Am J Surg 146:447, 1983.
12. Mohs FE: Chemosurgery: Microscopically Controlled Surgery for Skin Cancer. Charles C Thomas, Springfield, IL, 1978.
13. Warren S, Hoerr SO: A study of pathologically verified epidermoid carcinoma of the skin. Surg Gynecol Obstet 69:726, 1939.
14. Freedlander E, Chung FF: Squamous cell carcinoma of the pinna. Br J Plast Surg 36:171–175, 1988.
15. Shanoff LB, Spira M, Hardy SB: Basal cell carcinoma: a statistical approach to rational management. Plast Reconstr Surg 39:619, 1967.
16. Bart RS: Scalpel excision of basal cell carcinomas. Arch Dermatol 114:739, 1978.
17. Zaky DA: Malignant external otitis: a severe form of otitis in diabetic patients. Am J Med 61:218, 1976.

CHAPTER 31

Nail Surgery

ROBERT E. CLARK and WHITNEY D. TOPE

Competent cutaneous surgical care requires a complete knowledge of the uniqueness of the response of the nail elements to various infectious and inflammatory disease processes, congenital abnormalities, tumors, and trauma. The nail plate serves a vital role in facilitating manual dexterity by functioning in the pincer grip and increasing the discriminatory ability of the acral pulp. This structure also protects the terminal phalanx and fingertips from trauma and facilitates the action of scratching. In humans, the nail plate also serves an aesthetic and cosmetic role when decorated with colorful polishes and other adornments.

The term nail unit is used to describe the nail and its surrounding structural components. The six components of the nail unit include the nail matrix, nailbed and phalangeal bone, nail plate, eponychium and hyponychium, anchoring portion of the nailbed, and the nail folds (Figs. 31–1, 31–2).[1–3] A thorough understanding of the functional and structural organization of the nail unit is necessary to correctly diagnose the clinical entities that may affect the nail plate. These diseases usually are expressed as a dysfunction of the nail plate and often require surgical intervention and reconstruction of the nail unit.

Embryology of the Nail Unit

The embryologic events that are involved in the development of the components of the nail unit (Fig. 31–3) progress in a cephalic to caudal direction. As a result, the fingernails start developing earlier in embryologic life than the toenails, a maturation sequence that is maintained throughout the period of embryogenesis.

Development of the nail unit begins in the ninth week of gestation with differentiation of the nail field. The nail field is a histologically distinguishable group of epithelial cells, known as the distal ridge, that are localized to the distal phalanx. Starting at the distal groove, the cells of the distal ridge undergo cephalic migration, giving rise to the nail bed. By the twelfth week of gestation the proximal nail groove is formed by an invagination of the migrating epithelial cells from the nail field. These migrating epithelial cells become the matrix primordium. The nail field undergoes orthokeratinization, forming the nailbed.

During the thirteenth week, the matrix primordium gives rise to the matrix proper, and nail plate formation commences. Bone, cartilage, and sweat gland development also begin at this time. The nail plate, a specialized product of the nail unit, is a unique, keratinized structure of the nail matrix.[1, 2, 4] After 20 weeks, the nail matrix is mature, with adult-type keratinization forming the nail plate. At this time, formation of the nail plate is completed as it becomes attached to the nailbed at the site of the distal ridge by way of the onycholemmal keratin of the solehorn. This attachment anchors the distal portion of the nail plate to the underlying mesenchymal structures.[5–7]

Anatomy of the Nail Unit

Surgical intervention and repair of the nail unit requires a thorough understanding of the topographic anatomy of the nail unit (Figs. 31–1, 31–2). These components include the proximal nail fold, distal matrix, nailbed, and cuticle or eponychium. The nail plate is a flat, rectangular, convex, translucent hard structure that rests on top of the digit and extends past the free edge of the finger.[8] The nail plate is bordered by the nail folds laterally and proximally. The ventral surface of the nail plate rests on the nailbed, and the cuticle spans all sides of the plate except the free margin.

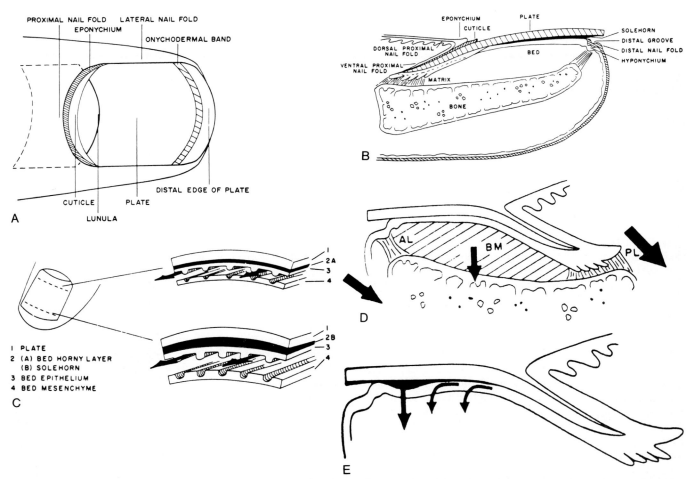

Figure 31–1. Dorsal *(A)* and sagittal *(B)* views of the normal nail unit anatomy. *C,* Cross section of the normal nail plate showing the interaction between the nailbed epithelium and the corrugated mesenchyme (superior = mid nailbed, inferior = distal nailbed). *D,* Sagittal view of the normal nail plate showing anchoring of the nail grooves and support of the nailbed. AL, Anterior ligament; BM, mesenchymal bed; PL, posterior ligament. *E,* Cross section of the normal nail plate showing the adherence of the plate provided by the solehorn and the nailbed horny layer. (From Scher RK, Daniel CR [eds]: Nails: Therapy, Diagnosis, Surgery. WB Saunders, Philadelphia, 1990, pp 13, 27–28.)

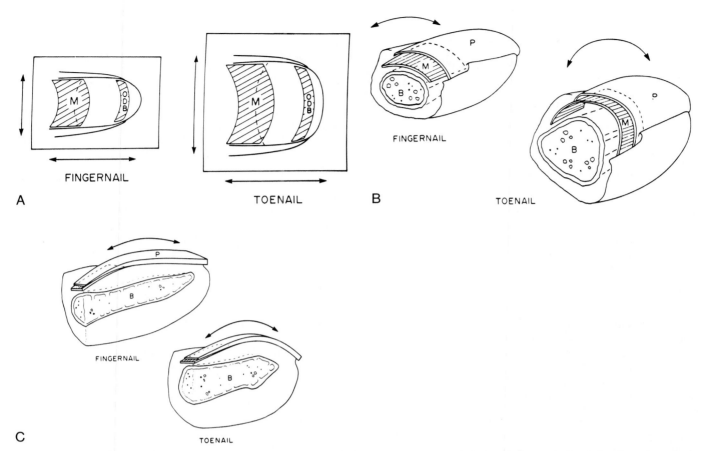

Figure 31–2. A, Shape of the nail plates. M, Matrix; ODB, onychodermal band. B, Transverse convexity of the nail plate and matrix. C, Longitudinal convexity of the nail plate and sloping of the nailbed. (From Scher RK, Daniel CR [eds]: Nails: Therapy, Diagnosis, Surgery. WB Saunders, Philadelphia, 1990, pp 22–23.)

BLOOD SUPPLY

The nail unit derives its blood supply from two arterial sources: the lateral digital arteries and branches from medium-sized vessels of the digital artery.[9, 10] The lateral digital arteries form superficial arcades that supply the proximal and distal portions of the nail unit. These arteries enter the distal phalanx near the volar surface of the bone and then form multiple, small dorsal branches in the pulp space of the distal phalanx. These

dorsal branches divide into proximal and distal arcades that supply the matrix and nailbed, respectively (Fig. 31–4).

The second blood supply to the nail unit is derived from medium-sized vessels that arise from the digital artery. These vessels branch from the digital artery at the midpoint of the middle phalanx. They remain on the dorsal surface of the digit and do not enter the pulp space. Superficial arcades derived from the medium-sized vessels of the digital artery anastomose with the

Figure 31–3. Proposed derivations of the adult structures of the nail unit. Thick arrows indicate epithelial derivatives of the matrix; thin arrows indicate the cornified products of the matrix. (From Scher RK, Daniel CR [eds]: Nails: Therapy, Diagnosis, Surgery. WB Saunders, Philadelphia, 1990, p 15.)

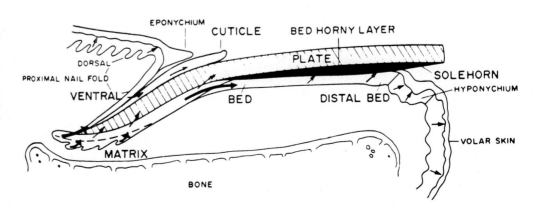

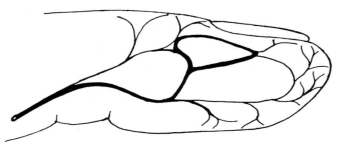

Figure 31–4. Lateral view showing the anastomosing arcade of blood vessels that arise from the lateral digital artery to supply the digit.

superficial arcades formed from the lateral digital arteries to provide a dual blood supply to the nail matrix. The vascular supply to the rete ridges of the nailbed is derived from the anastomotic arch arteries and the superficial terminal arteries of the digital arterial system.[11]

Venous drainage of the nail unit results from the combination of two proximally located veins on either side of the nail plate lying within the proximal nail fold.[7] Beneath the hyponychium, long, thin-walled, looped vessels with wide lumina are found. Rupture of these vessels allows blood to fill the longitudinal troughs of the nailbed, which results in the formation of splinter hemorrhages. Arteriovenous anastomoses are found throughout the arterial and deep venous circulation in all areas of the nail unit except the proximal nail fold. These anastomoses may be simple, unmodified anastomoses or complex associations of vessels.[11]

NERVE SUPPLY

The nerve supply to the nail unit parallels the arterial blood supply to this area (Fig. 31–5).

Patient Evaluation

Surgical procedures involving the nail unit should be accompanied by a thorough preoperative patient evaluation that includes a complete patient history and physical examination. The affected nail unit should be carefully inspected and the remaining integumentary structures examined as necessary. Physical findings from the skin examination will often assist the cutaneous

surgeon in deciding whether to perform a complete physical examination. The patient's medical history should include the present illness leading to the nail unit dysfunction; information regarding past nail unit surgical procedures, other previous surgeries, past medical problems, current medications, and drug allergies; and a review of systems. The preoperative patient evaluation may also require laboratory studies, including a complete blood cell count with platelets, prothrombin time (PT), partial thromboplastin time (PTT), and serum electrolyte and renal function tests. Preoperative radiograph studies are obtained when the condition suggests possible involvement of the bony structure of the phalanx.

Before surgery, the patient should be counseled about scarring and possible nail plate deformity, which may be temporary or permanent with functional or physical disfigurement of the nail unit. Because marked discomfort may follow surgery involving the nail unit, patients should also be informed of the potential for temporary incapacity to carry out their usual expected duties and that time away from work may be required. A standard operative consent form should be reviewed in detail with the patient by the surgeon. This consent should include permission to perform the anticipated surgical procedure, as well as permission to obtain photographic documentation. Pertinent risks, side effects, and possible complications that may result from the surgical procedure should be fully explained and documented on the consent form.

Instrumentation

Approximately 5 to 10% of new patient visits to cutaneous surgeons are for nail problems.[12] For this reason, it is important to be well equipped clinically and surgically to deal with nail disorders. Several relatively inexpensive specialized instruments can help to make nail surgery safer and easier to perform. Nail surgery kits can be prepackaged and sterilized so that the required special instruments are always available once surgery has begun.

Separation of the nail plate from the underlying nailbed and the overlying cuticle is greatly facilitated by the use of a dental spatula (Fig. 31–6) or a Freer septum elevator. The slim design of these instruments allows them to be easily advanced between the nailbed and nail plate to free the attachment between these structures. The dental spatula provides the mechanical advantage necessary for avulsing the lateral wings of the nail plate from the lateral nail horn. Nail avulsion can

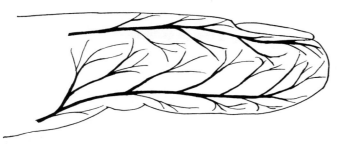

Figure 31–5. The nerve supply for the nail unit parallels the arterial blood supply.

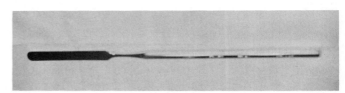

Figure 31–6. Dental spatula used to facilitate avulsion of the nail plate.

be performed remarkably easily with only minimal trauma by using these instruments.

The nail splitter is particularly useful when performing partial nail avulsion. The design of this instrument allows the wedge-shaped lower blade to separate the nail plate from the underlying nailbed. When the nail splitter is in position, the scissor-like upper blade is used to cut through the nail plate. The special design of this instrument provides a marked mechanical advantage for dealing with tough, thickened nails. Heavy nail nippers (Fig. 31–7) are also helpful in cutting thickened nail plates. At times, a nail grinder (Fig. 31–8) can be useful in treating markedly dystrophic nails. A Dremel Moto-Tool equipped with a drum-shaped sanding attachment is very effective in treating these types of nails. However, when using the grinder, all operating room personnel should wear face masks and protective eyewear. In addition, a smoke evacuator should also be used to remove the nail dust generated by the procedure.

Biopsy of the nail unit can be performed using a punch or a standard excisional technique. Punch biopsies of the nail unit can be easily performed using standard trephine punches. Surgical excisions can be performed using a standard No. 15 scalpel blade or a No. 67 Beaver blade. The No. 81 Beaver blade is an especially good chisel for splitting thick, friable nail plates.[13] Use of No. 2 and No. 3 Fox curettes are effective for curetting the nail matrix during matricectomy or for removing of other lesions involving the nail unit. Single- and double-pronged skin hooks are used to reflect the proximal and lateral nail folds and allow examination of the nail grooves during surgical procedures.

A ⅜-inch Penrose drain can be used as a tourniquet to provide hemostasis during surgical procedures involving the nail unit. The drain should be marked with two "X's" 27 mm apart. The drain is placed around the digit and held securely with a hemostat clamped at these two points. This technique prevents use of excess pressure that could cause strangulation of the digit during the surgical procedure. Trauma to the underlying digital nerves can be avoided by using 2″ × 2″ cotton gauze padding wrapped around the digit before application of the tourniquet. Depending on the surgeon's interest and

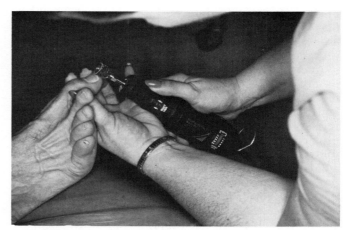

Figure 31–8. Dremel Moto-Tool with drum sanding attachment used for nail plate debridement.

skill, additional instrumentation may include electro-surgical instrumentation, chemical cauterants, and a carbon dioxide laser.

Anesthesia

The anticipation of pain from nail surgery frequently results in significant emotional distress and apprehension. The possible discomfort resulting from administration of local anesthesia is often of paramount concern. However, properly administered local anesthesia will significantly reduce patient anxiety and allow the procedure to be completed in a more efficient manner.

Because of possible vasovagal responses, local anesthesia should be administered while the patient is reclining or in a supine position. This positioning facilitates placing the patient in the Trendelenburg position if the need should arise. Use of a 30-gauge needle helps minimize the discomfort of the needle puncture, while slow, continuous infusion of the anesthetic reduces the burning or stinging sensation. The use of a Luer-Lok syringe to inject the local anesthetic agent reduces the possibility of the needle separating from the syringe as a result of the high injection pressure. Surgery should be delayed 10 minutes after infusion of the anesthesia to achieve maximal effectiveness.

A 1% or 2% solution of lidocaine provides excellent local anesthesia with a proven high safety record.[13, 14] Although the addition of epinephrine to the anesthetic solution is safe in nearly all patients, because of the possibility of unexpected localized ischemia, epinephrine-free anesthetics should be used. Bleeding can be adequately controlled by using a tourniquet or applying manual compression to the lateral digital arteries. Local anesthetics without epinephrine are always recommended for patients with diabetes, scleroderma, Raynaud's disease, or arterial vascular disease.

When prolonged anesthesia of 1 to 2 hours is desired, 0.25% bupivacaine (Marcaine) or a 1:1 combination of 0.5% bupivacaine and 1% prilocaine (Citanest) may be used. Postoperative pain can be minimized for a period

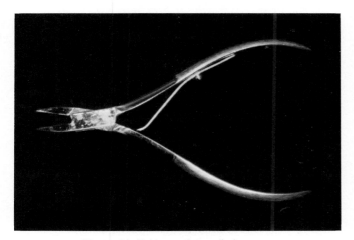

Figure 31–7. Heavy-duty nail nippers.

of 8 to 12 hours by injecting a mixture of 0.6 ml of 0.5% bupivacaine and 0.4 ml of 4 mg/ml dexamethasone[13] around the nail unit at the completion of the procedure.

Anesthesia of the nail unit may be achieved by distal or proximal digital nerve block. Distal digital nerve block anesthesia is effective for procedures involving the nail folds or the nail matrix. This nerve block is performed by injecting the anesthetic approximately 3 mm proximal to the junction of the proximal and lateral nail folds (Fig. 31–9). Complete anesthesia may require additional injections at 5-mm increments across the proximal nail fold. Each injection site is infused with 0.5 ml of 1% or 2% lidocaine. This small volume of anesthetic avoids vasospasm or tamponade, which could compromise the vascular supply of the distal digit.[14–17] The distal digital nerve block achieves anesthesia of the terminal transverse and descending branches of the digital nerve.

The proximal digital nerve block anesthetizes the dorsal and ventral digital sensory nerves distal to the metacarpophalangeal or metatarsophalangeal joints (Fig. 31–10). The anesthetic is infused beneath the dermis, starting midway between the dorsal and ventral aspects of the digit. Excellent anesthesia is achieved by injecting the anesthetic in radial fashion from the dorsal to the palmar aspect of the digit. The dorsal and palmar digital nerves on the medial and lateral aspects of the digit are anesthetized by injecting approximately 1 ml of anesthetic into each side of the digit. A combination of proximal and distal digital nerve blocks may be used to achieve prolonged anesthesia.

Postoperative Care and Dressings

Enhanced recovery rates and improved long-term results occur when patient compliance results in provid-

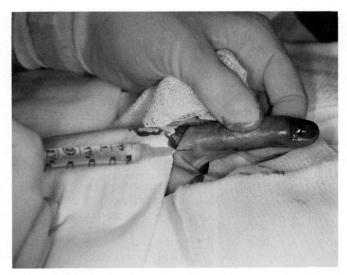

Figure 31–10. Injection site for proximal digital nerve block anesthesia.

ing proper postoperative care. Preprinted instructions help prevent avoidable problems and also assist patients in basic home care. Postoperative expectations can also be reviewed in the written instructions to reduce patient anxiety and provide information on to how to obtain assistance should problems arise after office hours. Postoperative nail unit wounds are subject to pain, spontaneous throbbing, easy traumatization, bleeding, exudation, and infection, and patient education can address these issues and help minimize their potential impact on wound healing and long-term results.

Minor nail unit surgical procedures such as evacuation of a subungual hematoma or punch biopsy of the nail unit may not require extensive dressings or analgesia. Routine wound cleansing using hydrogen peroxide followed by application of an antibiotic ointment and a simple adhesive bandage is usually sufficient for wound coverage and protection. For minor wounds, the dressings may be changed on a daily basis until healing is complete.

More extensive surgical procedures require application of an antibiotic ointment followed by placement of a nonstick Telfa dressing padded by the addition of several 2″ × 2″ cotton gauze pads. Paper tape may be positioned longitudinally over the padded dressing to hold it in place. Circumferential wrapping of the digit must be avoided, as it may cause venous congestion, swelling, pain, and possible digital necrosis. This bulky dressing is then supported by X-Span tubing or a Surgitube dressing (Fig. 31–11).[13, 15, 18, 19]

The ideal bulky postoperative dressing for nail unit surgical procedures should be sufficiently absorbent to collect the serosanguineous drainage, adequately elastic to accommodate the anticipated swelling of the digit, nonadherent, and satisfactorily bulky to protect the wound from minor trauma.[13, 15]

If there is significant bleeding after completion of the surgical procedure, oxidized cellulose (Gelfoam) or collagen matrix sponges (Instat or Helistat) can be added

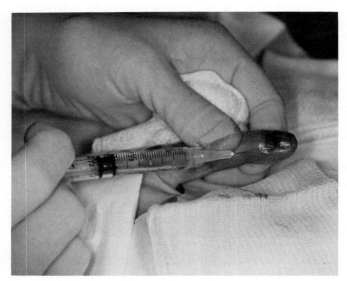

Figure 31–9. Injection site for distal digital nerve block anesthesia.

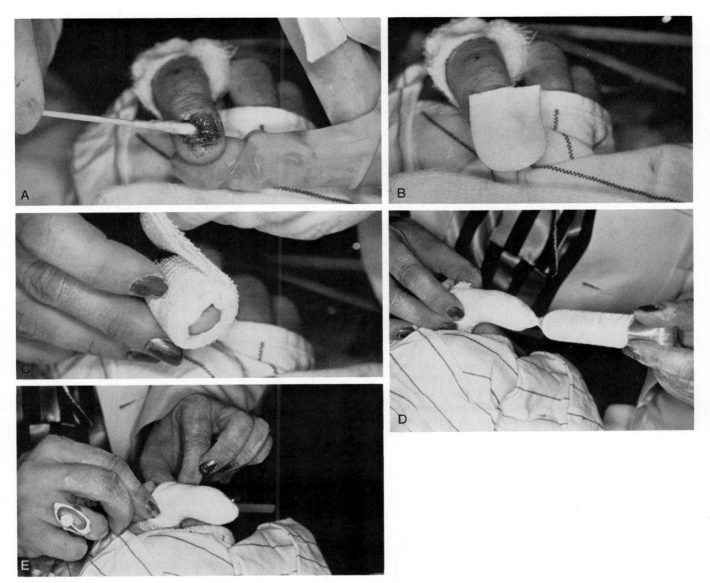

Figure 31–11. Components of the standard postoperative dressing after nail surgery. *A,* Application of antibiotic ointment to the surgical wound. *B,* Nonadherent dressing is applied to the wound. *C,* The nonadherent pad is loosely wrapped with gauze. *D,* Application of Surgitube dressing. *E,* The completed surgical dressing.

beneath the nonstick pad to help provide hemostasis.[13, 15] Monsel's solution, a chemical hemostatic agent, should be avoided, as it may result in tattooing of the healed wound, which can interfere with future histopathologic studies of tissue obtained from or near the nail unit surgical site.[16]

Immediate postoperative pain can be minimized by elevating the limb as much as possible during the first 48 hours after surgery. Use of acetaminophen with 30 mg of codeine, nonsteroidal anti-inflammatory drugs, or aspirin may occasionally be needed to control postoperative pain.[13, 20] If significant pain is anticipated after the surgical procedure, the patient can be premedicated 1 hour before surgery with an intramuscular injection of 60 mg of ketorolac tromethamine (Toradol). This po-

tent, non-narcotic, injectable, nonsteroidal anti-inflammatory analgesic agent produces no troublesome central nervous system side effects, and this dose is comparable to an intramuscular injection of 12 mg of morphine or 100 mg of meperidine.[21]

Unless significant hemorrhage or drainage occurs, the bulky dressing should be changed after 24 hours. The digit should then be soaked for 15 minutes in a solution of magnesium sulfate (Epsom salt)[22] or a 1.5% hydrogen peroxide solution.[13, 15] The digit should be carefully dried, followed by application of topical antibiotic ointment, a nonadherent pad, 2″ × 2″ gauze padding, and tube dressing. Alternatively, warm water soaks may be used once or twice daily, depending on the degree of exudation.[20] Dressing changes and soaks should be performed on a daily basis to minimize the formation of serosanguineous pockets of exudative material that serve as a potential site for colonization by microorganisms.

Patients scheduled for extensive nail unit surgical procedures of the toes should purchase an orthopedic Reese or Zimmer boot to wear postoperatively to provide additional protection and immobilization of the digit after surgery. An arm sling is also useful after surgical procedures involving the digits of the hand to elevate the extremity, immobilize the digit, and protect it from minor trauma. The use of postoperative antibiotics remains controversial and should be determined on an individual basis.

Biopsy of the Nail Unit

GENERAL CONSIDERATIONS

Removal of the nail plate, nailbed, nail matrix, proximal or lateral nail fold, hyponychium, or any combination of these structures may be necessary to obtain the proper biopsy specimen, depending on the clinical setting (Fig. 31–12). With appropriate attention paid to selection of the type of biopsy required and preoperative patient education, an accurate clinical diagnosis may be substantiated with the least possible discomfort and often without resultant deformity.[23] Nail biopsies may be indicated to diagnose chronic mycotic infections,[24, 25] to differentiate onychomycosis from psoriasis,[25] to di-

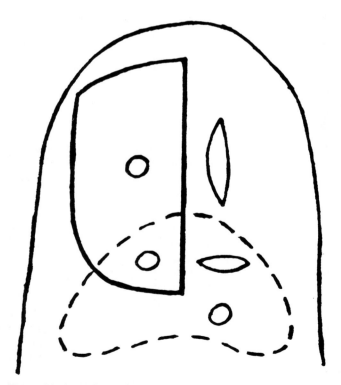

Figure 31–12. Nail unit biopsy techniques: through the nail plate *(left)* to the nailbed (distal) and to the matrix (proximal); after avulsion of the nail plate *(right):* longitudinal fusiform excision of the nailbed (distal), transverse fusiform excision of the matrix (middle), and punch biopsy of the matrix (proximal).

TABLE 31–1. PROPER APPROACH TO PERFORMING NAIL BIOPSIES

1. Always use the procedure with the highest benefit:risk ratio.
2. Limit the biopsy to a single anatomic unit.
3. Perform biopsy only on the tissue that will aid in making the correct diagnosis.
4. Remove the smallest amount of tissue possible to make the diagnosis.
5. Avoid scarring or deformity.
6. Always obtain a specimen from the nailbed rather than the nail matrix when possible.
7. Use fusiform excisions less than 3 mm wide, when possible.
8. Close excisions primarily after careful undermining.
9. Orient excisions transversely in the matrix and longitudinally in the nailbed.
10. Always incise the biopsy specimen down to the bone.

agnose dermatoses affecting the nail unit,[26, 27] to diagnose and potentially eradicate benign and malignant neoplasms,[28, 29] and to correct ingrown toenails.[29] Relative contraindications to nail unit biopsy include untreated bacterial or viral periungual infection, diabetes mellitus, scleroderma, peripheral vascular disease, and various immunocompromised states.[30, 31]

Before embarking on a nail biopsy, a thorough evaluation should be carried out to identify concurrent infection and any bony abnormality of the distal phalanx. The presence of marked tissue distortion or a firm tumor should prompt radiographic evaluation.[28] The biopsy may proceed once infections have been treated and bony causes ruled out. Adherence to recommendations[32] for selecting appropriate nail area biopsies will yield the best possible cosmetic result (Table 31–1) and still provide adequate tissue for examination.[13]

HISTOPATHOLOGIC AND LABORATORY CONSIDERATIONS

Structural alterations such as nail ridging or splitting can often be avoided by selecting the best biopsy technique. To ensure that the pathologist receives an adequate, well-preserved specimen, special attention must be given to proper tissue handling and processing.[31] Gentle manipulation of the specimen during its removal will prevent crush artifact and separation of normally contiguous structures. Histopathologic orientation is most easily lost when processing a cylindric piece of tissue obtained by a punch biopsy. For this reason, it may be best to submit a specimen that can be marked with sutures to assist the pathologist in orienting the specimen so that it may be properly sectioned to make an accurate pathologic diagnosis.

Accurate sectioning of specimens that also include the nail plate requires softening of the hardened nail keratin first. Otherwise, the nail plate will be shorn away from the underlying epithelium during sectioning. Many different softening or wetting techniques can be used for this purpose.[20, 33, 34] Biopsies are embedded in a paraffin wax and sectioned to create a flat surface. The cut surface may be immersed in 1% aqueous polysorbate 40 at 4°C for 1 hour before the final sections are cut,[34] or the specimen can be soaked overnight in a solution of calcium hydroxide, sodium thioglycolate, and calcium thioglycolate before paraffin embedding. This produces a more pliable surface that can be easily sectioned.

Each nail biopsy is routinely stained with hematoxylin and eosin (H&E), although special stains may be useful in some settings. For example, periodic acid–Schiff (PAS) or Gomori methenamine silver (GMS) stains are often helpful to demonstrate fungal elements in mycotic nails, and Giemsa and Masson-Goldner trichrome stains can be used to define altered or abnormal keratinization.[31]

TYPES OF BIOPSIES

Nail Plate Biopsy

A biopsy of the nail plate and a portion of the hyponychium is often performed to diagnose onychomycosis or psoriasis. After anesthesia is achieved, either a shave or punch technique may be used. In performing a shave biopsy, scissors, a bone rongeur, or a scalpel can be employed to remove a wedge of tissue that includes the distal hyponychium and overlying dystrophic nail plate.[24, 25, 31] Alternatively, a 3-mm punch biopsy may be taken through the nail plate down to the periosteum[16, 31] and fine scissors used to remove the specimen. Pressure or application of a small piece of oxidized cellulose is used to provide hemostasis.[28] The punch biopsy technique can be used on any area of the nail plate and subjacent nailbed, but the matrix must be avoided.

The biopsy specimen is submitted for routine H&E and PAS staining, as both psoriasis and onychomycosis may be manifested histologically as hyperkeratosis of the nailbed and may also show parakeratosis and neutrophils. In psoriatic nails, the parakeratotic cells are typically found in small mounds topped by neutrophils that are separated from one another by foci of orthokeratosis. The PAS stain will almost always demonstrate hyphae and spores in the keratinized portion of the nailbed or the lowest region of the nail plate.[35]

Nailbed Biopsy

Biopsy of the nailbed may be performed with or without avulsion of the overlying nail plate. Although avulsion of the nail plate may interfere with subsequent histologic examination,[16, 18] removal facilitates visualization of the biopsy site and also allows primary closure of the nailbed.[13] When possible, nailbed biopsies are preferable to nail matrix biopsies to avoid scarring and nail plate deformity.[36]

To most effectively biopsy the nailbed and avoid avulsion, thinning of the nail plate may be required. A sharp 3-mm punch is driven through the nail until the periosteum is met, and the specimen is then removed using fine curved iris scissors. A two-punch technique[36] may also be used. In this procedure, a larger punch is first used to remove the nail plate, and then a smaller punch excises the nailbed down to bone. Hemostasis is achieved using pressure, Monsel's solution, or oxidized cellulose, and the defect heals by second intention.

Alternately, the nail may be avulsed first to permit better visualization and positioning of the biopsy or to perform a larger nailbed biopsy. For most small lesions, the punch technique is carried out, but for larger lesions an elliptical or fusiform wedge excision will allow better orientation of the specimen and permit primary closure to reduce the risk of subsequent nail plate deformity.[13, 31, 36] Using a scalpel, a long, narrow ellipse is cut through the nailbed down to bone. The ellipse must be oriented longitudinally and should not exceed 3 mm in width,[13] with care taken to avoid the matrix. Fine iris scissors are then used to free the specimen, and a 30-gauge needle is used to skewer the specimen's distal end. The needle is bent after it passes through the tissue to provide a handle during scissor removal of the biopsy from the bone, prevent inadvertent crush artifact, and act as a ready point of orientation for the dermatopathologist. The ellipse is undermined and closed with fine, interrupted absorbable sutures. Making relaxing incisions at the lateral edges of the nailbed may be useful in permitting tensionless closure.[31]

Nail Matrix Biopsy

A nail matrix biopsy is used to evaluate nail abnormalities that originate in the nail matrix. These include suspicious melanonychia striata, tumors involving the matrix, and full-length nail plate malformations.[32] Small tumors of matrical origin can be excised using a 3-mm punch, but the biopsy must not bisect the matrix, or a permanently split nail will result.[29] Distal positioning of the punch, without violating the lunular edge, will place potential defects on the undersurface of the nail plate similar to those produced by subungual hematomas affecting the matrix.[37] As in nail biopsies, an elliptical excision oriented transversely in the matrix permits primary closure of the defect and superior cosmetic results. Again, the integrity of the distal lunular curve must be maintained to prevent distal onycholysis and abnormal curvature of the free edge of the nail plate. It is important to recognize that both types of biopsies will result in a thinned nail plate.

A nail matrix biopsy begins with exploration of the proximal nail groove. For accurate positioning of the biopsy, an indelible mark should be placed on the proximal nail fold aligned with the lesion. After the area is prepared and anesthetized, bilateral longitudinal incisions are made at the juncture of the proximal and lateral nail folds proximally to expose the matrix area. The Freer septum elevator is inserted beneath the proximal nail fold to guide the incision and prevent laceration of the matrix. The incision should not extend proximally more than 6 mm distal to the distal interphalangeal joint. The proximal nail fold is then reflected using either skin hooks or holding sutures.[15] Although dissection and removal of only the proximal one third of the nail plate—leaving the distal two thirds intact to protect the nailbed—is often recommended,[38] total avulsion can be performed atraumatically and provide rapid exposure.[13] A transverse elliptical excision can be used to remove all or part of the lesion. The distal edge of the ellipse should parallel the curve of the lunula. The specimen is freed from the periosteum with fine curved scissors. Undermining is followed by primary closure using fine absorbable suture, such as 5-0 polyglycolic acid or rapidly absorbed 6-0 surgical gut plain type A.[13] The proximal nail fold is repaired with sutures or sterile tape strips. A small piece of Xeroform gauze may be placed between the nail fold and matrix to prevent adhesion.

En Bloc Nail Unit Biopsy

A biopsy of the entire nail unit, often referred to as longitudinal biopsy or resection,[20, 29, 30] can provide the chronology of a given pathologic state as it is manifested in the nailbed and nail plate.[30] An en bloc biopsy can also be used to diagnose and ablate neoplastic processes, to treat ingrown toenails[29] (Fig. 31–13), and to provide a histologic diagnosis of several primary skin diseases, such as lichen planus[26] and Darier's disease,[27] that present as nail abnormalities. This technique is not restricted to lateral nail processes but may be employed in investigating lesions within the confines of perionychium. The risk of causing cosmetically significant nail plate abnormalities is greater after centrally located longitudinal biopsies. In any location this technique may decrease the width of the nail, fissure the nail plate, or scar the proximal nail fold.

In this technique a sterilized single-edge razor blade is used to make two parallel incisions from the proximal nail fold to the tip of the finger.[30] The distance between these incisions should never exceed 3 mm, or severe scarring will result. The tip of the blade should gently slide over the bony phalanx. The shorter sides of the rectangle are cut using a scalpel, while the outlined nail sample is dissected, beginning at the tip of the finger, with the aid of slightly curved pair of iris scissors. A longitudinal piece of tissue is removed, being careful to keep the tips of the scissors on the dorsal surface of the bony phalanx. No sutures are used, as they may disturb the normal shape of the nail and lead to ingrown toenails. One modification of this technique[29] first avulses the nail plate on either side of the specimen before excising the centrally located specimen. After removal of the biopsy, the defect is undermined and closed primarily with careful apposition of the proximal nail fold, matrix, and hyponychium using fine silk, nylon, or Dacron sutures, which are removed after 5 to 10 days.[23]

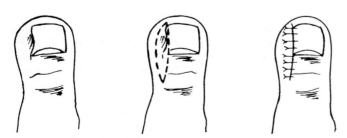

Figure 31–13. Longitudinal biopsy of the lateral nail fold at the site of chronic swelling and inflammation *(left)* and with planned fusiform excision outlined *(center)*. The repaired defect is shown on the right.

Previous avulsion of the lateral portions of the nail plate is not critical to successful en bloc biopsy. For removing small tumors that involve the matrix, total nail avulsion precedes removal of a longitudinal section carried proximally only as far into the matrix as is necessary to excise the tumor. Primary closure helps to avoid permanently split nails. The same technique may also be applied to the lateral nail fold with only a slight reduction in nail width and less risk of producing cosmetically unacceptable results. A more disfiguring variation has been advocated[20] in which the entire lateral nail fold is incorporated in the biopsy. However, excision of the lateral nail fold does not usually add to the diagnostic information derived from biopsies that exclude the lateral nail fold. Consequently, this variation should be avoided unless the lateral nail fold is clinically involved by the disease process being investigated.[31]

Surgical Nail Avulsion

Avulsion of the nail plate from its bed may occur as the result of a deliberate surgical procedure or from a traumatic shearing or crushing force applied to the nail unit. Either partial or total nail avulsion procedures may be employed in routine practice. In a partial avulsion procedure, thin longitudinal strips of the nail plate are removed from the underlying structures. The purpose of nail plate avulsion is to expose the nailbed, matrix, and proximal and lateral nail folds for examination and exploration as a prelude to chemical or physical matricectomy and nailbed and matrix biopsy or as an adjunct to the treatment of onychomycosis, chronic mucocutaneous candidiasis, or ingrown nails.[13, 31, 39] Nail avulsion alone is not curative of onychodystrophy caused by matrix disease, ingrown toenails, or large nailbed defects. If this procedure is repeated, it may cause onychauxis or overcurvature of the nails.[40]

The nail must be separated from its two points of attachment, the nailbed and proximal nail fold, to perform an avulsion. One of two different techniques for total nail avulsion (the distal or proximal approach) may be used depending on the clinical indication. Although the straight hemostat, dental spatula,[18, 39] nail elevator,[41] and Freer septum elevator[42] have all been recommended for performing these techniques, the Freer septum elevator is often superior for this particular task.[13] Nails with an intact distal free edge are avulsed using the distal technique by first separating the nail from the free edge proximally. Once the area is prepared and anesthetized, distal avulsion begins with loosening the proximal nail fold and the lateral horns from the plate using the Freer elevator. The elevator is then inserted in longitudinal fashion at the distal free edge between the nail plate and the nailbed. The initial resistance that is felt as the elevator slides over the nailbed "gives way" over the matrix. Once over the matrix, the elevator should be pushed gently until the proximal nail groove is met. Injury to the proximal groove from overzealous insertion results in prolonged healing time and potential nail dystrophy. This same maneuver is repeated using side-to-side longitudinal strokes (rather than moving the elevator horizontally under the nail plate) until the nail plate is completely detached. This method causes the least possible trauma to the nailbed and matrix.[13] The nail plate finally is grasped with a straight hemostat and removed with a rolling motion. There should be little, if any, hemorrhage from the nailbed or matrix. The exposed surface and surrounding folds should be gently cleared of debris using a gauze-wrapped hemostat or a small curette.[31]

Partial avulsion by the distal technique is most commonly used alone or before partial matricectomy for the treatment of ingrown toenails, overcurvature of the nails, or pincer nail deformity. A thin elevator or spatula is inserted in one longitudinal movement between the nail plate and bed on the involved site. The avulsion must continue proximally to separate the lateral horn from the matrix. In the critical maneuver, the unseparated nail is held in place to prevent inadvertent total nail avulsion, while gentle upward force is applied on the avulsed strip of nail. The nail plate with its lateral horn can be "flipped out" of the proximal and lateral nail folds. Finally, a 3- to 4-mm strip of the nail plate is cut away using nail splitters.

The proximal approach for nail avulsion initially was used for removing nails involved with distal subungual onychomycosis.[43, 44] However, it may also be helpful in any condition in which the distal free edge of the nail has become sufficiently dystrophic to obscure the potential cleavage plane between the nail plate and bed.[39] In this technique, the digit is firmly grasped and the proximal nail fold loosened with the Freer elevator. The elevator is then turned upside down so that its concave surface is directed away from the finger, inserted under the proximal nail fold to the proximal edge of the nail, rotated around this edge, and directed distally under the nail plate. In this position the elevator is oriented correctly, with its curve matching that of the underside of the nail. Once the tip of the elevator protrudes from beneath the dystrophic free edge, it is withdrawn, and the maneuver is repeated in side-to-side fashion until the nail is free of its attachments. A hemostat is then used to release the nail. The relative lack of attachments of the nail plate to the matrix enables this technique to be performed.[42]

Matricectomy

INDICATIONS

Matricectomy is among the most common and most useful surgical techniques in the management of nail unit disorders. This surgical procedure involves the partial or total destruction of the nail matrix. Partial or segmental matricectomy is the destruction of that portion of the nail matrix responsible for causing nail unit disease. This procedure affects only a portion of the matrix, so the uninvolved matrix remains viable and capable of producing a nail plate. Total matricectomy, or the complete removal of the nail matrix, completely destroys the ability of the nail unit to generate a nail

plate. Partial matricectomy is particularly helpful in the treatment of ingrown nails or onychocryptosis. Total matricectomy is also frequently used in the surgical management of pincer nail deformities, onychauxis or thickened nails, onychomycosis, and onychogryphosis.

SURGICAL TECHNIQUES

A variety of techniques have been employed for performing partial or total matricectomies. The most commonly used techniques include scalpel excision, electrodesiccation and curettage, laser ablation, and chemical destruction.

Scalpel Excision

Partial or total matricectomy may be achieved by surgical excision of the portion of the nail matrix that is responsible for producing the diseased nail plate. When performing a segmental matricectomy, the initial incision is made in a longitudinal fashion from the most proximal portion of the matrix to the distal portion of the exposed matrix. The incision is then extended to the lateral nail fold and proximally along the nail groove to the lateral horn. The incision is carried to the depth of the periosteum, and the wedge of tissue containing the matrix is removed using curved scissors.

Total scalpel excision matricectomy is performed by completely removing the matrix from the proximal nail groove to the distal portion of the lunula, allowing the surgical wound to heal by second intention. Postoperative care consists of elevation of the digit as much as possible for the first 48 hours, daily soaks to reduce inflammation, and cleansing with 3% hydrogen peroxide followed by application of an antibiotic ointment and a nonadherent dressing.

The chief disadvantage of scalpel excision matricectomy is the relatively high rate of nail plate regrowth in the lateral nail horn area,[45] which is due to incomplete excision of the matrix from this recessed area. Recurrence rates can be minimized by dorsally reflecting the proximal nail fold to provide better exposure of the lateral nail horn. After excision of the matrix, the proximal nail fold is repositioned and sutured at its junction with the lateral nail fold.

Electrodesiccation and Curettage

Partial or total matricectomy may be performed by vigorously curetting the matrix followed by electrodesiccation or electrocoagulation. This is a relatively simple yet effective technique in which the curette is used to displace the exposed matrix from the underlying dermis and the remaining matrix destroyed by electrosurgery. This is also helpful in providing excellent hemostasis after nail avulsion.

This matricectomy technique is performed by first avulsing the offending portion of the nail plate, ensuring its complete removal at the lateral nail horn area. A No. 2 Fox curette is used to remove the exposed portion of the matrix by vigorous curetting, particularly along the lateral nail horn area. This portion of the matrix is then treated by electrodesiccation or electrocoagulation to facilitate destruction of any remaining cells. Electrosurgical destruction of the matrix requires application of the electrical current to the treatment site for approximately 5 seconds. The tissue is then allowed to cool for 10 seconds, and the process is repeated for an additional 5 seconds. Care should be taken to avoid electrosurgical injury to the ventral surfaces of the proximal and lateral nail folds, as this may result in significant scarring.

Monopolar electrocoagulation using Teflon-coated probes is ideal for performing partial or total matricectomies. These probes have a flat surface with one side insulated by Teflon and the other side uninsulated to facilitate tissue destruction (Fig. 31–14). When using these specialized probes, the Teflon-coated side is placed against the ventral surface of the proximal nail fold, and the uninsulated side of the probe is slowly moved back and forth across the exposed portion of the matrix to produce the desired tissue destruction.[46] Total matricectomy is performed similarly, except that the entire nail plate is avulsed, and a larger Teflon-coated electrocoagulation probe is used.

The main advantages of electrocoagulation and curettage for matricectomy are the simplicity of the procedure, the excellent hemostasis that is provided, and the avoidance of making an incision to dorsally reflect the proximal nail fold. The main disadvantages of this technique are potential thermal damage to the underlying bony phalanx and the expense of purchasing the necessary equipment and accessories to perform the procedure.

Carbon Dioxide Laser Ablation

The carbon dioxide (CO_2) laser has been particularly useful in nail surgery, as this wavelength is precisely absorbed by water. Nearly total energy absorption occurs when energy from the mid-infrared CO_2 laser beam impacts the soft tissues and the inter- and intracellular water is instantly converted to steam at 100°C, resulting in immediate tissue destruction.[47, 48]

Partial or total matricectomy may be performed using CO_2 laser ablation in a method similar to that using traditional electrocoagulation and curettage. The offending portion of the nail plate is first removed, and the underlying matrix is exposed, either by lifting the proximal nail fold with a skin hook or by dorsally reflecting the proximal nail fold by incising at the junction of the proximal and lateral nail folds. Wet sponges, towels, or drapes are placed around the operative site to avoid injuring the adjacent normal tissue. All medical personnel and the patient must wear protective eyewear made of glass or wraparound plastic or polycarbonate lenses. The matrix is then vaporized using the CO_2 laser in a defocused mode with a 2- to 3-mm beam and an irradiance of 400 to 600 W/cm². This causes full-thickness coagulation of the matrix and the underlying superficial dermis. A smoke evacuator should be used to remove both the smoke and the noxious odors that are generated during the vaporization process. Alternately, the exposed matrix can first be curetted using a No. 2 Fox curette while the remaining fragments of the matrix are vaporized by the CO_2 laser.

Cutaneous surgeons who are unaccustomed to using the CO_2 laser should select the pulsed or discontinuous mode to minimize thermal damage to the deep dermis and underlying bony phalanx. With short pulse intervals of 0.2 to 0.5 seconds, the underlying dermis and bone can generally be spared from thermal damage. As with the other techniques, the surgical site is allowed to heal by second intention.

The main advantages of using the CO_2 laser include minimal postoperative edema and inflammation and

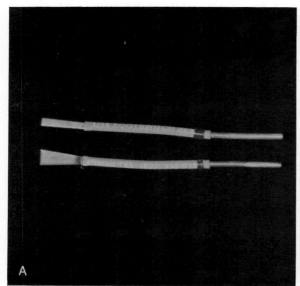
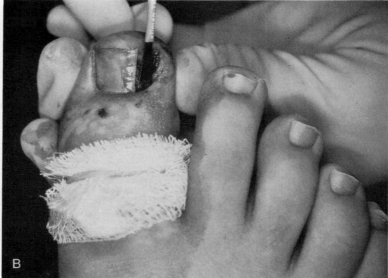

Figure 31–14. *A,* Teflon-coated electrodes used in performing electrosurgical matricectomy. *B,* The electrosurgical probe is inserted between the ventral surface of the proximal nail fold and the exposed matrix during electrosurgical matricectomy.

excellent hemostasis both during and after the procedure. The main disadvantages of CO_2 matricectomy include the costs of the laser and the smoke evacuation system and the potential for fire.[49, 50]

Chemical Cautery

Partial and total matricectomies can be effectively and efficiently performed by chemical destruction of the germinative epithelium of the nail matrix. Chemical matricectomy is an excellent alternative to surgical, electrosurgical, or laser techniques; the two most commonly employed agents are concentrated (88%) phenol[51–54] and 10% sodium hydroxide solution.[55, 56]

Phenol matricectomy is probably the most common chemical cautery method used.[51, 57] The affected digit is first anesthetized, and an exsanguinating tourniquet is applied to produce a bloodless operative field. The offending portion of the nail plate is then avulsed and the lateral horn areas inspected for residual nail plate and cuticle. A No. 2 Fox curette is used to physically debride the exposed matrix. Next, a thick layer of petrolatum is placed over the exposed nailbed and proximal and lateral nail folds. Concentrated phenol is then applied to the exposed matrix using a cotton-tipped applicator. The applicator is firmly advanced into the most lateral recesses of the lateral horn areas, using a firm twisting motion (Fig. 31–15). In a similar fashion, the applicator is moved along the surface of all exposed matrix adjacent to the lateral horn. The phenol is allowed to remain in contact with the matrix for a total of 90 seconds. Dilution of the phenol is accomplished using either boric acid[57] or 3 to 5% acetic acid.[56] The nail unit is then washed of all remaining phenol, an antibiotic ointment is applied, a nonadherent dressing is placed over the site, and a tube dressing is used to cover the digit. The concentrated phenol solution should

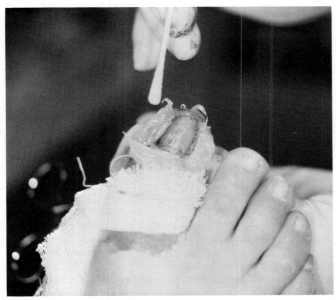

Figure 31–15. Application of concentrated phenol to the exposed matrix during chemical cautery matricectomy.

be discarded and replaced with fresh product every 6 months to avoid using outdated or contaminated products.[58] Pain, inflammation, and postoperative infection can be minimized by elevation of the affected site and application of a mixture of hydrocortisone 1%, polymyxin B sulfate, and neomycin sulfate solution twice daily for the first 2 weeks.[59]

Sodium hydroxide chemical cautery ablation of the nail matrix is performed in a similar fashion. The portion of the matrix to be destroyed is exposed after the surrounding tissues have been protected by applying a thick layer of petrolatum. A solution of 10% sodium hydroxide is then applied using a cotton-tipped applicator and a twisting motion to firmly advance the applicator into the recesses of the lateral horn area and along the exposed matrix. The solution is allowed to remain in contact with the matrix for 3 seconds to 3 minutes depending on the response of the affected tissues.[59] The matrix is allowed to undergo liquefactive necrosis until coagulation of the capillaries of the nail matrix is noted. The sodium hydroxide solution is then neutralized by the addition of 3 to 5% acetic acid.[55, 59] A standard wound dressing is applied at the completion of the procedure.

Chemical cautery matricectomy is relatively simple to perform and requires no specialized instruments. It has a very high success rate (98 to 100%)[50, 56] and low morbidity. The entire procedure can be completed in 20 minutes, making it an ideal technique for the management of certain nail disorders. The only contraindication to chemical cautery matricectomy is moderate or severe arterial disease of the hand or foot.

Paronychial Surgery

The paronychial region is made up of the proximal and lateral nail folds. Diseases affecting the paronychial area[56] that require surgical intervention include infectious disorders, inflammatory conditions, and benign and malignant tumors (Table 31–2). Surgical procedures commonly performed on the paronychial region of the nail unit include incisional biopsies, excisional biopsies, en bloc excisions of the proximal nail fold, and total nail unit excisions.

INCISIONAL BIOPSY OF THE PROXIMAL OR LATERAL NAIL FOLD

The incisional biopsy technique is most commonly used for diagnostic purposes and may be performed on the proximal or lateral nail fold areas of the nail unit. This technique permits removal of adequate tissue for histologic studies. Depending on the differential diagnoses, tissue may be submitted for staining with hematoxylin and eosin, periodic acid–Schiff,[60, 61] acid-fast, or Brown-Brenn. When infectious etiologies are suspected, tissue samples can also be submitted for culture of bacteria, deep fungi, or atypical mycobacteria.

The transverse incisional biopsy of the proximal nail fold is performed parallel to the relaxed skin tension

TABLE 31–2. **TUMORS INVOLVING THE NAIL UNIT**

Benign tumors
Acquired digital fibrokeratoma
Bone cysts
Enchondroma
Osteochondroma
Solitary bone cysts
Subungual exostosis
Fibromas of tuberous sclerosis
Glomus tumors
Keratoacanthoma
Myxoid cyst
Neurofibroma
Pigmented nevus
Pyogenic granuloma
Verruca vulgaris
Periungual
Subungual
Malignant tumors
Basal cell carcinoma
Bowen's disease
Malignant melanoma
Squamous cell carcinoma

lines. In the diseased area, a fusiform elliptical incision is made so that the angles of the incision measure approximately 30 degrees. This facilitates primary closure of the surgical incision without undermining. The site of the surgical incision[13] should be made at least 3 mm beyond the distal interphalangeal joint to avoid cutting the tendon of the extensor digitorum communis (Fig. 31–16). The extensor digitorum communis tendon inserts into the proximal dorsal portion of the terminal phalanx. This tendon may be subject to surgical trauma when procedures are carried out on the most proximal portion of the proximal nail fold. The incision should be carried down to the periosteum of the bony phalanx, and the nail fold is then removed using curved scissors or a scalpel blade.

Fusiform elliptical incisions may also be performed along the lateral nail fold. The incision is oriented in a longitudinal direction extending from the proximal to the distal portion of the lateral nail fold and is extended to the depth of the bony phalanx. The elliptical incision of the proximal or lateral nail fold area allows for primary closure with preservation of the normal nail fold anatomy. Closure is achieved without undermining using nonreactive simple interrupted nylon sutures, which should remain in place for at least 7 days. Postoperatively, the digit should be elevated as much as

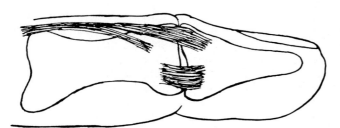

Figure 31–16. Attachment of the extensor digitorum communis tendon to the proximal end of the distal bony phalanx.

possible for 48 hours. Wound care consists of cleansing with hydrogen peroxide and application of an antibiotic ointment. Soaks with magnesium sulfate (Epsom salt) or 1.5% hydrogen peroxide solution once or twice daily will reduce inflammation and facilitate cleansing of the wound.

The incisional biopsy technique is particularly useful for diagnosing acute paronychia caused by bacteria or fungal organisms. Histologic confirmation of connective tissue disorders can also be facilitated by examination of tissue obtained using this technique.[60, 61] Chronic paronychia resulting from deep fungal infection, atypical mycobacterial infection, or foreign body granuloma can also be diagnosed using this method.

EXCISIONAL BIOPSY OF THE LATERAL AND PROXIMAL NAIL FOLD

Excision of cutaneous lesions involving the lateral or proximal nail fold area is performed in a fashion similar to that used for the incisional biopsy technique. However, the excisional technique involves complete removal of the cutaneous lesion followed by repair of the defect to restore the structural and functional integrity of the nail unit.

Excisional surgery involving the lateral nail fold is commonly indicated for removal of hypertrophic tissue that has developed in response to chronic onychocryptosis. Using a nail splitter, the offending portion of the ingrown nail plate is cut longitudinally from the free edge of the nail to the proximal portion of the plate beneath the proximal nail fold. This segment of nail plate is then grasped with a pair of hemostats and removed by slowly twisting the hemostat toward the lateral nail horn, making sure that no nail plate or cuticle is allowed to remain in this recess. A longitudinal incision is then made starting 3 mm distal to the nailbed and extending proximally to a point on the proximal nail fold 10 mm above the cuticle. The second incision is extended from the proximal nail fold through the hypertrophic lateral nail fold to a point that intersects the first incision on the tip of the digit. The incisions are extended to the level of the periosteum, and the wedge-shaped section of tissue including the hypertrophic lateral nail fold is removed with curved scissors. The excised tissue includes a portion of the nailbed, nail groove, proximal nail fold, and lateral nail wall (Fig. 31–17). The remaining lateral nail fold is reapproximated to the nail plate using 4-0 nylon sutures that are placed through the nail plate in a simple interrupted fashion with the knot positioned on the nail plate.[14]

An alternative method for repair of a hypertrophic lateral nail fold resulting from an ingrown nail plate is the fusiform excision of a wedge of the lateral nail with closure of the surgical defect. Repair of the defect results in retraction of the hypertrophic lateral nail fold from the edges of the ingrown nail plate. The offending portion of the nail plate is removed as a longitudinal segment using the nail splitter, and partial matricectomy is then performed. The surgical defect is repaired using

4-0 nylon sutures placed in a simple interrupted fashion. By debulking the lateral nail fold, the foreign body stimulus produced by the offending nail plate is removed, which allows resolution of the hypertrophic tissue with restoration of normal nail unit anatomy.

Excisional procedures involving the proximal nail fold are carried out in a fashion similar to that used for lateral nail fold excisions. However, the orientation of the elliptical excision is along the relaxed skin tension lines of the proximal nail fold. Caution must be exercised when placing the excision within 3 mm of the distal interphalangeal joint to avoid releasing the extensor digitorum communis tendon from its attachment to the proximal portion of the terminal phalanx. The excision should also avoid the distal free margin of the proximal nail fold to prevent notching. Primary closure of the excisional site involving the proximal nail fold can usually be accomplished, but undermining may be necessary.

Excisional procedures of the proximal nail fold are particularly useful in the treatment of myxoid cysts. These fluid-filled cysts appear to arise from the synovial lining of the distal interphalangeal joint,[62] but this remains controversial. There are reports that these cysts may arise from mucoid degeneration of the connective tissue of the proximal nail fold area[63] or from embryonic rests that form the periarticular tissue and synovial membranes.[64] Extensive pathologic studies have confirmed that a communication between the myxoid cyst and the joint space exists by way of a pedicle.[65-67]

Excision of a myxoid cyst requires meticulous dissection and separation of the cyst wall from the surrounding tissues and identification of its communicating pedicle. Caution should be taken to avoid cutting the extensor digitorum communis tendon during the dissection of the myxoid cyst. The pedicle should be carefully dissected as far as possible before the lumen of the stalk is destroyed by electrodesiccation. The excision site is usually closed primarily, but on occasion a local advancement flap may be necessary for repair.

If it is impossible to complete the dissection of the myxoid cyst, the capsule can be incised and the mucoid material drained. The cyst cavity should then be injected with triamcinolone (20 mg/ml).[68] Should the myxoid cyst recur after excision, an en bloc excision of the proximal nail fold is recommended.

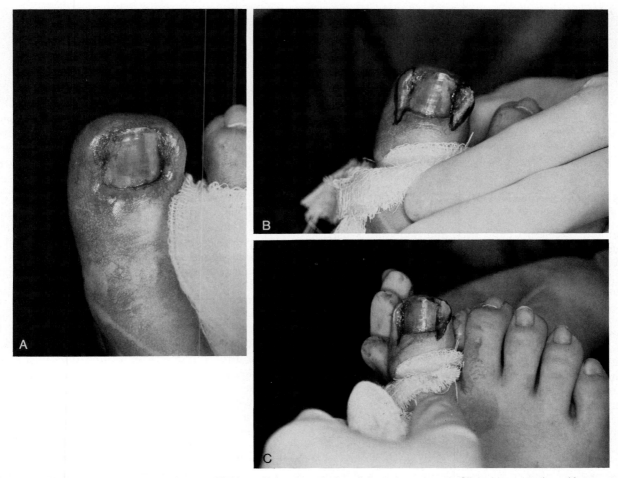

Figure 31–17. Excision of hypertrophic lateral nail folds and electrosurgical partial matricectomy. *A,* Clinical presentation with hypertrophy of the lateral nail folds owing to onychocryptosis. *B,* Outline of planned surgical excisions of the hypertrophic lateral nail folds. *C,* Appearance of the nail unit after excision.

Illustration continued on following page

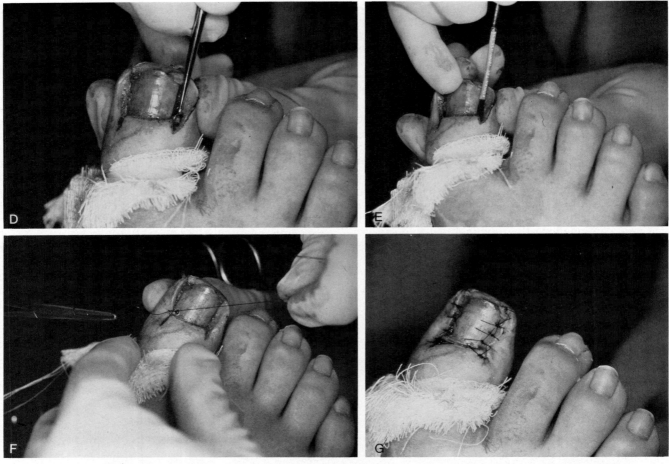

Figure 31–17 *Continued D,* Bilateral debridement of the exposed matrix with a Fox curette. *E,* Electrosurgical destruction of the remaining matrix with a Teflon-coated probe. *F,* Reapproximation of the lateral nail folds to the nail plate. *G,* Appearance of the digit at completion of surgery.

EN BLOC EXCISION OF THE PROXIMAL NAIL FOLD

Complete excision of the proximal nail fold is used for the treatment of chronic paronychia,[14, 69] recurrent myxoid cysts,[70] a number of benign and malignant tumors, and collagen vascular disorders.[60, 61] Using a surgical marker, a symmetric, crescent-shaped excision line is drawn, extending from the junction of the proximal and lateral nail folds to an identical site at the opposite proximal-lateral nail fold junction. Caution is again advised regarding the position of the extensor digitorum communis tendon, which attaches to the distal bony phalanx. This tendon can be inadvertently released from its insertion site on the phalanx when the sweep of the crescent-shaped excision extends within 2 to 3 mm of the distal interphalangeal joint.

En bloc excision of the proximal nail fold requires the digit to be anesthetized using a proximally based digital block. A tourniquet or manual compression of the digital arteries may be used to facilitate hemostasis. A dental spatula or Freer septum elevator is used to separate the nail plate from the cuticle. The instrument is carefully advanced to the proximal portion of the nail groove so that it is sandwiched between the ventral surface of the proximal nail fold and the dorsal surface of the nail plate. A scalpel, with the blade beveled toward the dental spatula, is used to excise the proximal nail fold. As the scalpel passes along the planned excision line, the spatula is moved in concert beneath the proximal nail fold, serving to protect the underlying nail plate and matrix (Fig. 31–18).

Hemostasis is obtained by selective electrocoagulation, and a standard wound dressing is applied. Postoperative care includes elevation of the digit for the first 48 hours after surgery, with wound dressings changed daily. Cleansing of the surgical site is performed with hydrogen peroxide followed by the application of an antibiotic ointment. Daily soaks in 1.5% hydrogen peroxide or a magnesium sulfate solution can reduce inflammation and remove serosanguineous exudate. En bloc excision of the proximal nail fold usually provides a cosmetically acceptable outcome, with healing occurring by second intention over a 6- to 10-week period.[68] However, the patient should be informed that the cuticle margin will be proximally displaced 5 mm from its previous location.

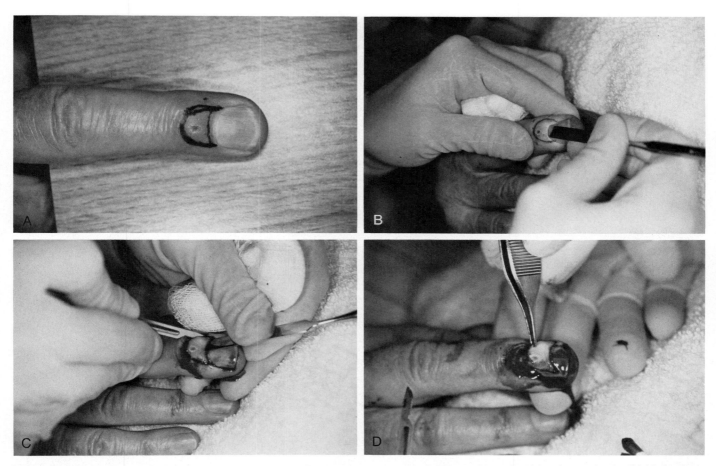

Figure 31–18. En bloc excision of the proximal nail fold. *A,* Clinical presentation of a digital myxoid cyst involving the proximal nail fold showing the anticipated en bloc excision of the proximal nail fold. *B,* Separation of the eponychium and ventral surface of the proximal nail fold from the nail plate is accomplished using a dental spatula. *C,* The dental spatula is sandwiched between the ventral surface of the proximal nail fold and the nail plate during excision of the proximal nail fold and is moved in concert with the scalpel to protect the underlying matrix. *D,* Beveled appearance of the proximal; nail fold following en bloc excision with hemostasis obtained by electrocoagulation and pressure. The surgical site is allowed to heal by second intention.

EXCISION OF THE NAIL UNIT

Excision of the nail unit involves the complete surgical removal of all the components of this structure, including the proximal and lateral nail folds, nail grooves, nail matrix, nailbed, nail plate, and hyponychium. This extensive procedure is justified when treating a malignant tumor of metastatic potential but would be considered a radical treatment for conditions such as onychogryphosis or onychocryptosis, which typically cause only limited morbidity.

Proximal and distal anesthesia of the affected digit is first achieved, and a padded tourniquet is applied for hemostasis. The surgical excision extends from the proximal nail fold transversely to the opposite lateral nail fold and distally along the lateral nail fold to a point 2 to 3 mm distal to the hyponychium. The excision is then carried across the tip of the digit to the opposite lateral nail fold and then proximally along the lateral nail fold to the starting point. The surgical excision is carried down to the level of the bony phalanx, and the entire nail unit is separated from the underlying bone by careful dissection with curved scissors (Fig. 31–19).

Hemostasis is achieved by electrocoagulation, and the surgical defect is repaired using a full-thickness skin graft harvested from the medial flexor aspect of the elbow or upper arm. A tie-over pressure dressing is applied and left in place for 7 to 10 days.

Postoperative wound care includes elevating the digit for the initial 48 hours after surgery and minimizing use of the affected extremity to reduce the possibility of dislodging the skin graft. The wound margins around the skin graft are cleansed daily with hydrogen peroxide followed by the application of antibiotic ointment, but daily soaks are not recommended.

Excision of the nail unit is an effective treatment modality when this structure is involved with basal cell carcinoma, squamous cell carcinoma, Bowen's disease, or malignant melanoma in situ.[71] However, if bony involvement is present, disarticulation at the distal interphalangeal joint is necessary to provide for adequate treatment. Evidence of lymphatic spread should be sought by physical examination, and lymph node biopsy should be performed when clinically indicated to avoid delays in initiating regional or systemic therapy.

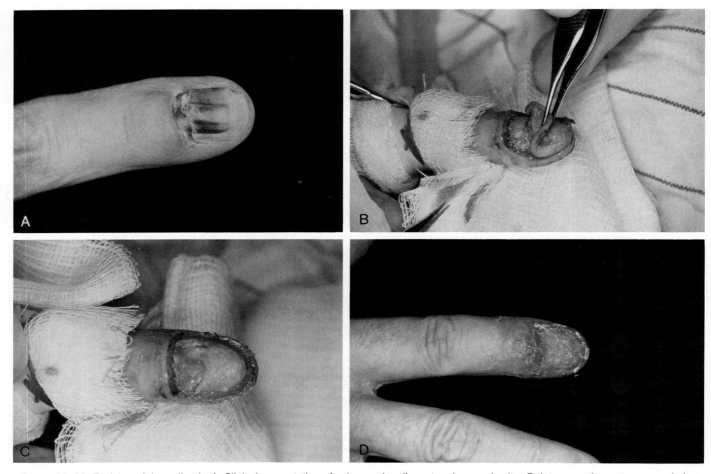

Figure 31–19. Excision of the nail unit. *A,* Clinical presentation of subungual malignant melanoma in situ. *B,* Intraoperative appearance during excision of the nail unit. *C,* Immediate postoperative appearance of the distal digit after nail unit excision. *D,* Clinical appearance 1 month after repair of the surgical defect using a full-thickness skin graft harvested from the flexor aspect of the elbow.

Malignant melanoma in situ of the nail matrix can be treated by total nail unit excision.[72] If dermal invasion is not identified histologically, nail unit excision is usually adequate treatment. However, invasion of the tumor into the dermis or evidence of bony involvement necessitates a minimum treatment of joint disarticulation or consideration of possible metacarpal or metatarsal ray amputation with or without regional node dissection.[73]

Mohs Micrographic Surgery for Tumors of the Nail Unit

Mohs micrographic surgery[74] is used to excise tumors involving cutaneous surfaces by microscopically mapping the subclinical extensions of tumor into adjacent tissue to spare as much uninvolved normal tissue as possible (see Chaps. 62 and 63). Squamous cell carcinoma, a slowly progressive and low-grade malignancy,[75, 76] is the most common malignancy involving the nail unit and is frequently treated using Mohs micrographic surgery. Although the reported rates of metastasis from squa-

mous cell carcinomas involving the nail unit are low, no comprehensive studies have accurately documented the rate of metastasis.[77]

The diagnosis of squamous cell carcinoma of the nail unit is frequently delayed for months or years, as patients are usually treated for a variety of acute and chronic conditions before a skin biopsy is finally obtained. Despite these delays in diagnosis, no significant difference in mortality rate has been noted. This supports the concept that squamous cell carcinoma of the nail unit is a slowly progressive lesion with low metastatic potential.

When the diagnosis of squamous cell carcinoma involving the nail unit is confirmed histologically, the patient should be evaluated by radiologic studies of the affected digit to ascertain whether there is bone involvement. If no involvement is noted, amputation is unwarranted, and Mohs micrographic surgery should be considered. However, when bone invasion is evident, amputation at or proximal to the distal interphalangeal joint should be performed.

Mohs micrographic surgery has an excellent cure rate for the treatment of squamous cell carcinoma involving the nail unit.[77, 78] Previously, the treatment of choice for squamous cell carcinoma of the nail unit was amputation,[79, 80] but considering the slow, progressive growth of this tumor, its low-grade malignancy, and very low rate of metastasis, such a radical surgical procedure is unwarranted. The importance of a conservative surgical approach when dealing with tumors of the nail unit is underscored by the fact that this tumor frequently involves the thumb. The thumb is responsible for 40% of the hand's normal function, and amputation at the distal interphalangeal joint results in 75% impairment of the normal function of the thumb and 30% hand disability.[81]

Squamous cell carcinoma in situ (Bowen's disease) of the nail unit can be treated by several surgical techniques. These include scalpel excision, electrodesiccation and curettage, Mohs micrographic surgery, and cryosurgery.[82, 83] However, invasive squamous cell carcinoma involving the nail unit is generally treated by electrosurgery, scalpel excision, Mohs micrographic surgery, or radiation therapy, but Mohs micrographic surgery has consistently demonstrated the highest cure rates for treatment of these cutaneous malignancies.[84]

The Mohs micrographic technique for removing squamous cell carcinoma involving the nail unit can be performed using either the fixed tissue or the fresh tissue technique. The surgical defect must be allowed to heal by second intention after use of the fixed tissue technique. However, after treatment using the fresh tissue technique, healing may proceed by second intention, or the wound may be repaired using a flap or skin graft technique (Fig. 31–20).

Traumatic Nail Injuries

The distal phalangeal apparatus provides a unique and important interface with the environment. Trauma to the distal phalanx pulp and nail unit endangers the normal structure and function of the distal digit. For this reason, the care of distal phalangeal injuries must be directed to the repair of viable tissues and reconstruction of tissue defects. Conservative management, or second-intention healing, is acceptable only when small amounts of soft tissue injury have occurred; virtually all nail apparatus injuries should be considered for surgical repair. Failure to repair these types of injury may lead to cosmetic and functional abnormalities of the nail unit (e.g., onychodystrophy, irregular distal onycholysis, pterygium, split nail deformity, misaligned nails, and hooked nail deformity)[31, 71, 85–87]; a painful, unstable distal phalanx from pseudarthrosis[88]; or impaired sensation from lost pulp or a lost fingertip.[31, 89–96]

Distal phalanx trauma occurs primarily in men, involving, in decreasing order of frequency, the middle, ring, index, and small fingers and the thumb.[95] These injuries are classified as simple (36%) or stellate (27%) lacerations, crush injuries (22%), or avulsions (15%). Distal phalangeal fractures are found in 51% of cases. As expected, patients with crush and avulsion injuries suffer significantly worse cosmetic and functional long-term results than do those with simple or stellate lacerations.

Accurate evaluation and management of lacerations and avulsion or crush injuries require both historical and radiographic data. The history should determine whether there has been possible contamination of the wound. Wounds are optimally treated within hours or days, but satisfactory repair may still be possible even after 1 to 2 weeks.[96, 97] Radiographic studies ascertain the presence and degree of fracture and also assist in wound exploration. Physical examination should evaluate joint mobility, distal sensation, level of amputation, exposure of bone, and the degree of soft tissue, nailbed, and nail matrix injury or loss.[92] Potentially contaminated open wounds such as crush injuries should be cultured and the specimen examined with Gram stain. Before exploration and repair, the involved digits should be prepared in sterile fashion, anesthetized, and subjected to saline irrigation. Tourniquet application ensures a bloodless field. A significant subungual hematoma (i.e., greater than 25% involvement) suggests the presence of a laceration requiring repair.[98] These hematomas should

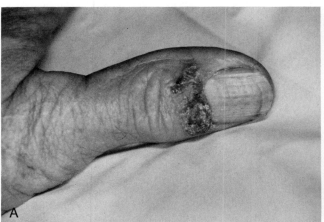 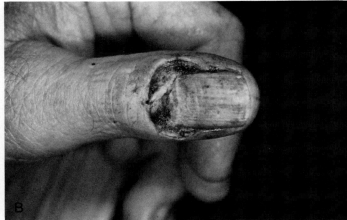

Figure 31–20. *A,* Preoperative appearance of squamous cell carcinoma of the proximal nail fold. *B,* Immediate postoperative appearance after Mohs micrographic surgery.

be drained and the nail avulsed. Avulsion of the plate from beneath the proximal nail fold with adherence of the nail plate to its bed distally is pathognomonic for nailbed laceration.[91] The use of magnification often enhances both the initial evaluation of the wound and the surgical repair.

SUBUNGUAL HEMATOMA

Hemorrhage under the nail, in the form of splinter hemorrhage or subungual hematoma, may occur from the extrusion of blood into the potential space that exists between the nail plate and nailbed or matrix. Although subungual hematoma usually forms because of trauma to the nail plate, splinter hemorrhages commonly arise in a number of conditions that presumably increase the fragility[31] of nailbed capillaries (Table 31–3) and do not often require surgical treatment. Subungual hematomas often are accompanied by exquisite pain, necessitating immediate evacuation for relief. Those subungual hematomas that result from significant crush injuries may indicate further surgical evaluation to rule out injury to underlying structures.

Splinter Hemorrhage

The linear nature of splinter hemorrhages directly relates to the anatomy of the nailbed–nail plate junction. The dermal rete ridges beneath the nail plate align in linear arrays or arcades that extend longitudinally from the lunula to the hyponychium, forming rigid grooves on the undersurface of the nail plate.[99] Bleeding from the capillaries present within the dermal ridges allows blood to flow into the potential space beneath the nail plate and along the grooved interface, resulting in the appearance of splinter hemorrhages.[31]

Splinter hemorrhages[100] may occur singly or multiply as red, purple, brown, or black streaks. Although normally located within the distal aspect of the nail plate, they may also occur proximally.[101, 102] These are usually asymptomatic but may occasionally be painful.[102] The distal position of the splinter hemorrhages corresponds to the location of the spiral capillaries, which are seen clinically as the pink line 3 to 4 mm proximal to the nail's free edge. Histologically, this correlates with the juncture of the nail plate and the termination of the stratum granulosum, an area protected by only a thin layer of hyponychium.[102, 103]

TABLE 31–3. DIFFERENTIAL DIAGNOSIS OF SUBUNGUAL HEMATOMAS

Basal cell carcinoma
Bowen's disease (squamous cell carcinoma)
Exostosis
Glomus tumor
Kaposi's sarcoma
Keratoacanthoma
Malignant melanoma
Melanonychia striata
Onychomycosis nigricans
Squamous cell carcinoma
Trauma

TABLE 31–4. CAUSES OF SPLINTER HEMORRHAGES

Infectious diseases	Drugs
Septicemia	Tetracycline
Onychomycosis	Acetylsalicylic acid
Subacute bacterial endocarditis	Ketoconazole
Trichinosis	Griseofulvin
Tetany	Cytostatic agents
Inflammatory disorders	Methoxsalen (phototoxic)
Rheumatoid arthritis	Benoxaprofen (phototoxic)
Rheumatic fever	Embolic phenomena
Beçhet's disease	Arterial emboli
Buerger's disease	Nutritional causes
Collagen vascular diseases	Scurvy
Raynaud's disease	Blood dyscrasias
Vasculitis	Severe anemia
Sarcoidosis	High-altitude purpura
Malignancies	Cryoglobulinemia
Leukemia	Hemophilia
Histiocytosis X	Primary cutaneous disorders
Endocrine disorders	Psoriasis
Thyrotoxicosis	Eczematous dermatitis
Hypoparathyroidism	Darier's disease
Iatrogenic causes	Pterygium
Brachial artery cannulation	Onychotillomania
Repetitive trauma	Miscellaneous conditions
Occupational hazard	Hypertension
Radial artery puncture	Renal disease
Hemodialysis	Peptic ulcer
Peritoneal dialysis	Pulmonary disease
	Idiopathic
	Atrophy of advanced age
	Heart disease
	Mitral stenosis
	Severe internal medical or
	surgical illnesses

There are many reported causes of splinter hemorrhages[31] (Table 31–4), but the pathogenic mechanisms in many of these conditions remains unclear. Embolic occlusion of terminal capillaries with subsequent hemorrhage may result from instrumentation of proximal arteries or infectious conditions such as subacute bacterial endocarditis,[100] sepsis, or trichinosis. In *Trichinella spiralis* infection, larvae are released into the circulation and lodge in capillaries. Hemorrhage results from rupture of the capillaries caused by larvae in the early invasive stage. Because the larvae develop synchronously, the hemorrhages all appear in similar stages of development, which may provide a differentiating point when comparing the hemorrhages produced in endocarditis.[3, 104]

Hemorrhage owing to inherent capillary fragility occurs with advanced age, steroid use, or vitamin C deficiency. It has also been reported to occur in hereditary fashion among healthy individuals.[101] Splinter hemorrhages presumably develop in other conditions on the basis of altered blood viscosity seen with some malignancies and blood dyscrasias, vasospastic phenomena, and immunologic processes leading to thromboses in inflammatory or autoimmune diseases. Tetracycline, griseofulvin, high-dose acetylsalicylic acid, and cytostatic drugs have also been implicated in splinter hemorrhages. Benoxaprofen and methoxsalen may produce these hemorrhages in phototoxic reactions. Bullous drug eruptions may manifest in the nails as splinter hemorrhages before onycholysis.[3, 105] Splinter hemorrhages are non-specific findings in many different disease states and may also occur in healthy individuals as a result of minor trauma. As clinically significant clues to pathologic states, splinter hemorrhages seem to be most helpful when they develop in otherwise healthy people[106] or in previously asymptomatic hospitalized patients.[101]

Subungual Hematoma

This most common injury of the distal phalanges begins with trauma to the nail plate. Red or blue discoloration beneath and within the nail plate, edema, and severe and pulsating pain rapidly ensue. With time, the area turns black, which signifies blood coagulation.[3] The hematoma may occupy only a small portion or involve the entire area of the nail and perionychium. Extensive hematomas may lift the nail plate and stretch the hyponychium.

A number of conditions must be considered in the differential diagnosis of subungual hematoma. A subungual melanoma can be misdiagnosed as a hematoma,[107–109] especially because almost half of such patients inaccurately report trauma as the cause of the lesion.[110] This demonstrates the propensity for bleeding in occult subungual melanoma. A history of acute trauma is helpful, but not infallible, in distinguishing subungual hematoma from melanoma. Other subungual tumors (e.g., glomus tumors, keratoacanthomas, and Kaposi's sarcoma) may also initially present as subungual hematoma. In general, it is possible to differentiate subungual hematoma by its rapid onset, uniform color, well-demarcated margins, and distal elimination at the free edge.[109] Conversely, subungual melanoma usually begins with pigmentation at the matrix and subsequently develops a halo of pigmentation at the proximal nail fold, a phenomenon known as Hutchinson's sign. This grows distally to form a band of pigmentation.[32, 107] Ulceration and loss of the nail plate without regrowth may follow. As a consequence of these diagnostic possibilities, any pigmented lesion of uncertain origin should undergo biopsy to rule out melanoma.

Appropriate management of subungual hematomas should be oriented toward relieving pain, recognizing any accompanying injuries, and preventing potential complications by promoting regrowth of a functionally and cosmetically acceptable nail. The subungual collection of blood produces pressure directly on the sensitive periosteum, which causes exquisite pain with each arterial pulsation. This pain is immediately relieved by release of this pressure on evacuation of the hematoma. Lacerations of the nailbed, sometimes involving the perionychium in fractures of the distal phalanx, frequently accompany hematomas. Unrepaired lacerations of the nailbed or matrix or compression of these structures by the hematoma can result in nail loss, prolonged regrowth, or permanent nail dystrophy.[85, 86, 98] Acute management of subungual hematoma should consist of rapid hematoma evacuation and repair of any laceration or fracture.

Evacuation of subungual hematoma is easily accomplished by trephination. Before arrival at an appropriate medical facility, patients may dramatically reduce bleeding and pressure by simple elevation of the affected nail as high as possible.[111] At the time of the initial evaluation, the size of the hematoma relative to the overall nail area should be noted. Small subungual hematomas may do well with simple observation, but larger or symptomatic hematomas with greater than 25% nail plate involvement require drainage. Various instruments and techniques have been advocated for nail trephination, including hot paper clip cautery, hot No. 18 needle, a Bell Hand Engine with a dental bur, a scalpel blade used as a drill, and hand-held cautery units.[31, 112–115] For extensive hematomas involving the free edge with consequent stretching of the hyponychium, the hyponychium may simply be incised. The most readily available method, a paper clip heated to red hot with any convenient flame source, works quite well, but multiple heatings may be required for thickened nails. The paper clip should be held with a large hemostat. Hand-held cautery units are expensive in comparison but have the advantage of maintaining constant temperatures up to 1232°C.[113] In either case, the trephine of choice is heated and directed perpendicularly to the nail over the hematoma. Although the hematoma may act as a cushion to prevent penetration of the nail bed,[112] caution requires use of slow, steady, light pressure with immediate removal of the instrument once the characteristic gush of blood occurs and there is immediate relief of pain. Complete evacuation of the hematoma, which may require more than one penetration, should be performed. Digital block anesthesia may be necessary before trephination to obtain proper evacuation.[116]

Further evaluation of the patient with subungual hematoma depends on the size of the hematoma and clinical judgment. In patients with subungual hematoma involving more than 25% of the nailbed, 94% of those with fractures of the distal phalanx also had nailbed lacerations, and 19% of those without fracture had significant lacerations.[25] Hematoma size did not correlate with the presence of a fracture. In patients with a hematoma involving more than half of the nailbed, 60% had a laceration requiring repair. For these reasons, subungual hematomas involving more than 50% of the nail should be evaluated radiographically and the nailbed explored if a fracture is discovered. The use of radiography in managing patients with subungual hematoma is frequently valuable,[116] as 19 to 25% of patients have a distal phalangeal fracture,[115, 117] and the hematoma size does not correlate well with the presence of a fracture.

The most commonly recommended approach to the management of subungual hematomas is evacuation by thermal transection of the nail plate. Because of the poor correlation of hematoma size and phalangeal fracture, radiographic examination is appropriate to ensure accurate diagnosis and documentation and informed management and follow-up. Fractures of the distal phalanx often are accompanied by partial or total avulsion of the nail and nailbed lacerations. Laceration repair and replacement of the nail in its anatomic position enable reduction of these fractures and natural external splinting. The presence of a distal phalangeal fracture, cleavage of the nail plate, a large hematoma, or persistent bleeding after hematoma evacuation requires exploration of the nailbed for significant lacerations. After appropriate anesthesia, the nail is atraumatically avulsed and simply lifted in "car hood" fashion[98] or removed. Lacerations of greater than 2 to 3 mm are then located and repaired using fine absorbable sutures.[98] The avulsed nail plate is cleaned, trimmed, and reattached by sutures to the lateral nail folds.[31] Nail plate preservation provides an even guide for the regrowing nail, acts as a natural splint to reduce and immobilize phalangeal fractures, and allows precise apposition of the edges of nailbed lacerations, which decreases healing time.[118, 119]

Dressings for the nail should be comfortable and bulky enough to protect the digit and should enable continued absorption of drainage. Application of a generous layer of zinc oxide ointment maintains the patency of trephination holes to assist in drainage.[114] Hematomas treated only with trephination require use of a dressing applied tightly enough to prevent free bleeding.[120] Artificial splints are unnecessary but may be helpful in protecting the injured finger from trauma.[112]

Other than nail loss (expected in a large proportion of patients)[116] and potential nail dystrophy, very few complications have been reported. Although local infection is uncommon,[112] it was seen in 4.2% of patients in one study but responded within days to antibiotic therapy.[116] The apparently low incidence of osteomyelitis contradicts the theoretical conversion of a closed terminal phalangeal fracture to an open fracture by trephination.[121] However, use of systemic antibiotics is advised after trephination over a fractured distal phalanx[90] or after crush injuries from potentially contaminated sources. Tetanus prophylaxis should be employed using recommended guidelines.

LACERATIONS

Simple

Simple lacerations, which are usually limited to the nailbed or lateral nail folds, most often result from cutting tools or sharp-edged implements. Simple superficial lacerations of the soft tissues heal well after the edges are apposed with tape strips or nylon sutures. Simple lacerations involving less than 3 mm of the nailbed usually do not require surgical repair.[98] It is generally believed that simple lacerations through the plate without matrix involvement will heal adequately as the nail grows.[71] However, larger nailbed lacerations are often associated with hematoma and fracture of the distal phalanx, and repair is advisable to achieve hemostasis, reduce the fracture, and prevent later nail dystrophy.

To properly repair simple nailbed lacerations, the nail plate should be avulsed distally for several millimeters proximal to the laceration. By leaving the nail plate intact proximally, the matrix is protected, which facilitates regrowth. Any remaining nailbed that is adherent to the nail plate should be left in place, as the plate will provide correct apposition once repositioned. Otherwise

the nail plate should be trimmed and scrubbed with antiseptic solution. Nail that is completely shorn away should be located, cleaned, and trimmed,[87, 119] as small fragments of nailbed may survive repair.[91] Any sharp debridement of nonviable tissue is directed toward the creation of linear borders, which may be closed primarily.[14] Nailbed lacerations are closed with 5-0 or 6-0 absorbable interrupted sutures. The involved hyponychium or lateral nail fold is closed with interrupted 5-0 or 6-0 nylon sutures.

Replacement of the cleaned and trimmed nail plate or a substitute protects the repaired laceration and provides a smooth guide for nail regrowth.[119] Suture holes are created laterally in the nail plate by trephination. The nail plate is then repositioned using nonabsorbable mattress sutures placed through the lateral nail folds; these are removed in 2 to 3 weeks. The prosthetic nail remains in place until it is pushed out after 1 to 3 months by the regenerating nail.[93] Completely avulsed and lost nails may be replaced by cadaveric nails stored in mercury antiseptic,[31] by a 0.5-mm-thick silicone sheet, or by nonadherent petrolatum gauze.[93–95] The cadaveric or silicone nail substitute must be positioned under the proximal nail groove to prevent adhesion of the ventral and dorsal aspects of the proximal nail fold. This is performed using 6-0 nylon mattress sutures, which are removed in 2 weeks.[119] No statistically significant difference could be demonstrated for any of these methods in one study.[95] The silicone sheet was found to be less easily maintained in position and extruded more quickly. If nonadherent gauze is selected, it should be carefully packed into the proximal nail groove and replaced at each dressing change.

Complex or Stellate

Complex or stellate lacerations involving the nail matrix and proximal nail fold[31, 71] most commonly result from a crushing force applied to the distal phalanx, causing the nail plate to be fragmented or partially or entirely avulsed. Subsequent nail deformities and dystrophies occur with greater frequency after these injuries. The guiding principle of surgical correction is careful reapposition of each anatomic unit by primary repair.

The nail plate must be completely avulsed for adequate visualization and closure of the matrix. Fragments of bone are removed through the laceration. Any necessary debridement is then performed, and the wounds are reapposed. Fine absorbable suture is used to close the nailbed and matrix, while the lateral nail folds and hyponychium are repaired with nylon sutures. The proximal groove may be reconstructed with interrupted 7-0 chromic gut sutures placed with knots positioned within the groove, not buried.[93, 94] The exterior of the proximal nail fold is repaired with nylon suture. A nail plate or substitute is sewn into the proximal nail fold with nonabsorbable mattress sutures. The proximal groove must not be left without a barrier to adhesion, or pterygium will result.[86]

Avulsive lacerations always result in tissue loss, which may obviate restoration of normal anatomy. Avulsion of small portions of the proximal nail fold may be repaired using a local rotation flap from the dorsal digital skin combined with a small split-thickness skin graft. The distal edge is trimmed to re-create the smooth curvature of the proximal fold. The flap is sewn into place with fine nylon sutures. To prevent adhesion of the underside of the flap to the nail matrix, a split-thickness skin graft is sewn to the underside, and the groove is packed with nonadherent gauze. The flap defect is filled with a split-thickness skin graft. Alternately, a split-thickness skin graft may be used to fill the entire defect, with its distal edge folded over on itself to re-create the proximal nail fold. More extensive tissue loss may require a cross-finger pedicle flap. Avulsion of the nailbed can be repaired with a reverse dermal graft,[86, 122] full-thickness nailbed graft,[123] split-thickness nailbed graft,[124] or split-thickness skin graft.[93]

Complex avulsive lacerations result in the loss of finger pulp, nailbed, and distal phalanx.[125] In these cases failure of second-intention healing within 6 weeks is followed by split-thickness skin grafting. Full-thickness grafts should be used over the ventral bony phalanx if pulp is lost. Depending on the degree and location of soft tissue loss, various pedicle flaps may be also employed to replace the missing tissue.

Although it is more serious in nature, even a nail matrix avulsion can be successfully corrected surgically. Partial matrical avulsion with adherence to the avulsed nail plate is best treated by reapproximating the nail plate and in so doing repositioning the lost matrix.[119] If the avulsed matrix is lost, a split-thickness skin graft[85, 94] or split-thickness nailbed graft[124] provides a good repair in many cases. Subsequent nail dystrophy may be corrected later in a clean wound with free nail grafts. A system of free nail grafts to reconstruct injuries resulting in total matrix and nailbed loss and variable loss of the surrounding tissues has been reported.[126] Partial nail grafts consist of a central section of the great toenail plate, nailbed, and matrix from one of the lesser toes. Composite nail grafts consist of the entire nail plate, nailbed, and matrix; proximal and lateral folds; and a shave of periosteum, again from a lesser toe. The final results appear to depend on the presence of a smooth, well-vascularized recipient site and firm fixation of the graft, which is held in place with mattress sutures. Cosmetically acceptable prosthetic nails can be fabricated for use after complete surgical or traumatic matricectomy.[127]

AMPUTATION OR GUILLOTINE INJURIES

Amputation or guillotine injuries usually result from inadvertent contact with tools, which typically leave a cleanly lacerated surface. Appropriate management is strictly individualized and depends on the level and plane of amputation, demands for distal interphalangeal joint function, the length of the distal phalanx, and the patient's age.[91] One classification[91] of amputations that assists in planning reconstruction considers the functional interdependence of the nail apparatus, distal phalanx, and pulp. Zone I amputations occur distal to the tip of the bony phalanx; zone II, distal to the lunula; and zone III, proximal to the distal aspect of the lunula. The planes of tissue loss are characterized as dorsal oblique, ventral oblique, transverse, axial oblique, and central or gouging.

In zone I amputations the bony phalanx and the proximal two thirds of the nailbed are preserved. These should be managed conservatively with second-intention healing assisted by topical application of antibiotic ointment and frequent dressing changes. The presence of fragmented edges or subsequent development of a pyogenic granuloma may require debridement. Although the significant loss of pulp in these injuries may cause a hooked nail deformity,[96] most patients achieve good functional results. Size guidelines for repairing zone I injuries can be misleading and may be inapplicable in persons with small hands. Skin grafts in small zone I amputations yield poorer results because they are anesthetic and the hyperpigmentation makes them cosmetically apparent.

Zone II amputations produce exposed bone and loss of support for the nailbed. These defects are repaired with local or remote pedicle flaps, which are oriented with respect to the plane of tissue loss. Bilateral[128] or single ventral[91] island pedicle flaps or V-Y flaps work well to reconstruct the fingertip. Adequate nail stability requires at least 5 mm of viable proximal nailbed. Judgment must be used to decide whether to ablate the remaining nail unit or enhance it with a free nail graft.[126] Use of the amputated digital tip as a free composite graft is useful only in young children with distal zone II defects.[129]

Loss of the entire nailbed and portions of the matrix, as well as bone exposure, occurs in zone III guillotine injuries. This irreparable damage commonly renders reconstruction impossible, and so any remaining matrix should be ablated. Again, reconstructive efforts must be tailored to the degree of injury and the needs of the patient. Distal interphalangeal joint preservation requires further shortening of the phalanx to allow pedicle flap coverage without tension.

FRACTURES

Distal phalangeal fractures occur commonly in digital injuries, most often as a result of crushing injuries.[90] Evaluation of subungual hematomas will reveal a fracture in 19 to 25% of cases. Fractures have been found in 51% of patients with lacerations, avulsions, or crush injuries.[95] Radiographic examination requires dorsoplantar, lateral, and oblique views. Treatment of digital fractures varies with the number and position of bony fragments and whether the fracture is closed or open.[88] Nondisplaced, stable fractures may simply require protection from the usual weight-bearing forces applied to the digit. Immobilization via external splinting is indicated for less stable, nondisplaced fractures. In lesser digital fractures, immobilization is accomplished by splinting the injured digit to its neighbor using tape and felt. Hallux fractures of this type must be externally and rigidly splinted to the foot or wrist and arm.

Displaced fractures must be reduced in closed or open fashion. At the distal phalanx, reduction depends on the surrounding soft tissues. In planning reduction, it should be remembered that soft tissue rupture will occur on the convex aspect of the fracture with preservation of the concave surface structures. Thus, reversal of the impinging force that caused the fracture often results in adequate reduction. Once reduced, fractures should be immobilized to enable the bony structures to withstand telescoping and oblique forces. Long oblique, spiral, and comminuted fractures are inherently unstable and require closed reduction and external fixation or open reduction and internal fixation.

The first concern must be to identify fractures that involve the distal interphalangeal joint or proximal phalanges so that appropriate orthopedic consultation can be obtained. Often, the fractures encountered are in the distal phalangeal shaft and tuft, which usually produce small bony fragments. These must be removed by irrigation and direct visualization, either through the accompanying nailbed laceration or a ventral longitudinal incision. Failure to remove these bony fragments will lead to healing with interspersed soft tissue pseudarthrosis manifested as a painful unstable fingertip.[88] This condition can be corrected by bone grafts placed over the ventral aspect of the tuft and cross-pinning with 1-mm Kirschner wires.[130]

Shaft fractures fall into three categories: single transverse, multiple, and open fractures that transgress the distal interphalangeal joint.[31] Single shaft fractures with little damage to the pulp are frequently accompanied by nailbed or matrix laceration. After avulsion of the nail plate, reapproximation and closure of the laceration reverses the fracture force and allows reduction of the fracture with appropriate alignment. Reapplication of the nail plate (or a substitute) to the nailbed then acts as a natural external splint.[93, 94, 119] To maintain closed reduction, Kirschner wires are placed percutaneously, under sterile conditions, along the axial plane into the distal phalanx,[131] using serial fluoroscopy to ensure proper placement.[88] Axial wires must not be positioned so as to transfix the distal interphalangeal joint, which may result in contracture.[71]

Crush injuries frequently present with multiple shaft fractures and soft tissue damage. Bone fragments must be removed and the remaining bones reapproximated if union is to occur. This is followed by appropriate fixation and soft tissue repair, which may cause a reduction in the length of the distal phalanx. Open fractures impinging on the distal interphalangeal joint are treated with amputation or joint fusion at a 180-degree angle.[131]

Postoperatively, the patient should elevate the affected digit for several days. External splints are removed after this time and replaced by external splinting only of the distal phalanx. Active motion of the distal interphalangeal joint is encouraged, and the internal fixation wires and external splints are removed after 4 weeks. Physical therapy for active range of motion will speed rehabilitation.[96]

Treatment of Verrucae

Benign tumors affecting the paronychial region can be treated by surgical methods other than scalpel excision. The most common techniques for treating these benign lesions include electrosurgery, CO_2 laser ablation, and cryosurgery. Periungual and subungual verrucae are the most common benign lesions affecting the paronychial region. These viral infections have a finite life span, with two thirds of the lesions resolving spontaneously within 2 years.[132] Generally, periungual warts are treated with keratolytic agents, cantharidin preparations, or cryosurgery. Warts that persist after routine treatment methods require the use of alternative physically destructive modalities such as electrosurgery or CO_2 laser ablation.

ELECTROSURGICAL TREATMENT

Electrosurgical procedures generally require distal digital anesthesia. However, tourniquets are not usually required, as hemostasis is maintained by manual compression of the lateral digital arteries combined with the electrocoagulation effect of electrosurgery. Treatment of periungual or subungual verrucae by electrosurgery can be facilitated by application of a saline-soaked dressing to the affected digit. Moisture from the dressing is allowed to hydrate the lesion for approximately 5 to 10 minutes. By increasing the moisture content of the hyperkeratotic lesion, tissue vaporization will be facilitated.[46] The tissue is vaporized by applying the tip of the electrosurgical device to the hyperkeratotic tissue until the lesion is noted to "bubble." Any resultant char is removed by curettage or scissor excision. Electrosurgery is continued until the entire wart has been vaporized. During this procedure, a smoke evacuator should be used to eliminate virus-laden smoke from the environment.

Subungual verrucae treated by electrosurgery require removal of the overlying nail plate by physical debridement. After the lesion is completely exposed, it is destroyed by electrosurgery. Thermal damage to the underlying bony phalanx and surrounding soft tissues is a potential complication of electrosurgery. This damage prolongs wound healing and increases the incidence of scarring. These potential complications should be discussed with the patient before electrosurgery.

CARBON DIOXIDE LASER TREATMENT

CO_2 laser ablation is frequently used to treat persistent periungual and subungual verrucae (see Chap. 73). This technique offers the advantages of precise control of the depth of tissue destruction, reduced postoperative pain, and decreased healing time. Under local or digital block anesthesia, the verruca is vaporized with the CO_2 laser adjusted to a power setting of 5 to 10 W and delivered with a 2-mm spot size. For warts in a subungual location, the nail plate can be debrided or vaporized directly with the CO_2 laser. Again, a smoke evacuator is again necessary to avoid dissemination of virus-laden smoke. The tissue char is removed by curettage or scissor excision, and laser ablation is continued until all gross evidence of the infected tissue is destroyed. Care must be taken to avoid thermal damage to the underlying bony phalanx and surrounding soft tissues. Postoperative care is identical to that used after electrosurgery.

CRYOSURGICAL TREATMENT

Cryosurgery is the most common method used for treating verrucae involving cutaneous surfaces (see Chap. 61). The parameters that affect the response are the type, diameter, depth, and location of the lesion.[133] Periungual and subungual verrucae are particularly resistent to freezing, probably because these lesions are often deep, of long duration, and hyperkeratotic.

Cryosurgery of warts causes significant discomfort, which often results in premature discontinuation of the freezing process. Digital anesthesia can be used to allow longer freeze times, which are necessary for the cryodestruction of the verruca. Cryosurgery of verrucae involving the nail unit can be facilitated by applying 10% salicylic acid ointment with occlusion to the wart daily for 3 days before cryotherapy. Subungual verrucae will require debridement of the overlying nail plate before application of the salicylic ointment.[134] Liquid nitrogen is then applied by spray freezing or application with a cotton-tipped applicator. The freeze-thaw time should be 30 to 45 seconds, with repeat freeze-thaw cycles for a total of two to three treatments. The advantages of cryosurgery include high cure rates, low cost, and few complications. Disadvantages include significant postoperative pain, blister formation, and open wounds that require 2 to 5 weeks to heal by second intention, depending on the size, location, and depth of freezing.

Nail Plate Debridement

CHEMICAL TECHNIQUES

Chemical or nonsurgical destruction of the nail plate followed by paring or avulsion was first described in Russia in the 1960s[135] and subsequently reported in the United States.[136, 137] This technique continues to have a role in the treatment of symptomatic dystrophic nails in patients who are at high risk for poor wound healing or infection after surgical correction.[138, 139] Painful nail dystrophies, mycotic nail infections, and onychauxis occur commonly in patients with diabetes mellitus, peripheral vascular disease, advanced age, and significant immunosuppression. Chemical debridement is indicated in this group of patients, as well as in those who decline surgical nail avulsion, for treatment of hypertrophic dystrophies (e.g., onychauxis and onychogryphosis), to relieve pain, and to treat post-traumatic bacterial or yeast infections of the nail plate and acral pustulosis. It is also useful in exposing the underlying normal nail plate or nailbed to therapeutic agents. Although *Trichophyton rubrum*–initiated onychomycosis is difficult to eradicate, other dermatophytes within the nailbed and lower nail plate are easily exposed for treatment with topical antifungal agents.[137] Hypertrophic psoriatic nails are also amenable to chemical debridement followed by application of potent topical steroid ointments or steroid-impregnated tape.[137]

A number of preparations containing urea, salicylic acid, or potassium iodide in combination with other ingredients may be compounded for use in dissolving dystrophic nails.[137, 138, 140, 141] Urea ointment, or "emplastrum urea," perhaps the most popular compound, contains 40% urea, 5% beeswax, 20% lanolin, 25% petrolatum, and 10% silica gel type H and has a shelf life of 4 months. Urea, which is a keratolytic, protein denaturant, and hydrating agent, appears to soften the dystrophic nail plate and dissolve its bonds to the nailbed.[137, 139] Urea only removes the dystrophic portion of the nail, leaving the normal nail intact.[137] A combination of salicylic acid and urea[141] is effective in the destruction of painful nondystrophic nails.[142] A salicylic acid and urea combination[141] and a preparation of salicylic acid combined with potassium iodide[138] may also be useful for less dystrophic nails.

Successful chemical debridement requires a method to occlude and hold the paste on the nail while sparing the surrounding skin. One method uses a sheet of adhesive felt that is folded in half and cut so that a hole outlines the nail plate.[138] The felt is then applied to the skin surrounding the nail plate. Several layers may be necessary to create a well deep enough to hold the debriding compound around the nail. Minimally thickened nails require a coating at least 3.13 mm thick, with more added for thicker nails. A waterproof, stretchable, hypoallergenic tape is applied to provide an adherent and occlusive dressing; finger cots are too tight for this dressing and should be avoided. Patients must keep the dressing dry by wearing plastic booties or gloves. After several days, the paste is removed, and the softened dystrophic nail is debrided down to a normal level using a nail elevator and heavy-duty nail nippers.[139] Alternately, the completely dystrophic nail may be avulsed painlessly and trimmed to just under the proximal nail fold and the exposed nailbed curetted of adherent nail plate.[137]

After chemical debridement, topical and intralesional medications may be used. Miconazole, clotrimazole, or ciclopirox olamine may be rubbed into the nailbed twice daily to treat onychomycotic nails. Treatment with 10- to 20-second phenolization of the nailbed followed by topical application of borotannic complex is quite effective in eradicating onychomycosis.[143] Psoriatic nailbeds are treated with topical triamcinolone or fluocinolone twice daily. Intralesional triamcinolone (2.5 mg/ml) injected into the proximal nail fold in small amounts (0.2 to 0.4 ml) may also be used.[144]

Several factors may cause failure of chemical debridement.[137] Thickened nail plates without significant dystrophy respond poorly to chemical debridement. Immersion of the dressing dilutes the debriding paste, and inadequate occlusion prevents adequate hydration of the nail plate. Potential complications include irritant or allergic contact dermatitis from urea, tincture of benzoin, or adhesives[145] and mild bleeding after curettage.

MECHANICAL TECHNIQUES

Mechanical debridement is an excellent palliative treatment for symptomatic onychauxis, onychogryphosis, or any other hypertrophic nail dystrophy.[31, 38, 146] Cutting markedly thickened nails with heavy-duty nail nippers is often successful but may be painful because of twisting and distortion of the nail plate. Double-action forceps, which dynamically conform to the shape of the nail, will cause less discomfort. Cautious rotary sanding can also yield good results with little discomfort using a dermabrasion Hand Engine, a hobby hand drill, or an air-powered drill.[147] A variable-speed drill that can operate at low speed should be used, as high speed will generate thermal energy that can injure the matrix or nailbed and cause pain. However, although lower speeds are more comfortable, they cause more vibration. The burs come in many shapes with different grades of sand or diamond dust on their surfaces and may be autoclaved. Because a great deal of nail dust is produced during rotary sanding, both the patient and the physician should wear masks and protective eye wear. Because the procedure can be repeated as needed, it should be remembered that the objective is to relieve pain by debulking, not extirpating, the hypertrophic nail.

SUMMARY

The nail plays a vital role in the normal function of the hand and also in the aesthetic appearance of both the hands and the feet. The number of internal and external disorders that can influence the qualitative appearance of the nails is enormous. A detailed understanding of the anatomy and physiology of the nail unit is required to determine the proper biopsy to perform to make a correct histologic diagnosis of an inflammatory, infectious, or neoplastic process without causing unnecessary nail dystrophy. Special modifications of standard surgical procedures—including excisions, skin grafts, and local flaps—are required in the surgical management of many disorders of the nail unit.

REFERENCES

1. Dauber RPR, Baran R: Structure, embryology, comparative anatomy, and physiology of the nail. In: Baran R, Dauber RPR (eds): Diseases of the Nails and Their Management. Blackwell Scientific Publications, Oxford, 1984, pp 1–24.
2. Samman PD: Anatomy and physiology. In: Samman PD, Fenton DA (eds): The Nails and Disease. Year Book Medical, Chicago, 1986, pp 1–19.
3. Pardo-Castello V, Pardo OA: Diseases of the Nails. Charles C Thomas, Springfield, IL, 1960, pp 74–77.
4. Norton LA: Nail disorders—a review. J Am Acad Dermatol 2:451–467, 1980.
5. Hashimoto K, Gross BG, Nelson R, et al: The ultrastructure of the skin of human embryos. The formation of the nail on sixteen to eighteen week old embryos. J Invest Dermatol 47:205–217, 1966.
6. Zaias N: Embryology of the human nail. Arch Dermatol 87:37–53, 1963.
7. Gonzalez-Serva A: Structure and function. In: Scher RK, Daniel CR (eds): Nails: Therapy, Diagnosis, Surgery. WB Saunders, Philadelphia, 1990, pp 11–30.
8. Brademas ME: Embryology. In: Scher RK, Daniel CR (eds): Nails: Therapy, Diagnosis, Surgery. WB Saunders, Philadelphia, 1990, pp 31–35.
9. Samman PD: The human toenail—its genesis and blood supply. Br J Dermatol 71:296–302, 1959.
10. Lewis BL: Microscopic studies of fetal and mature nail and surrounding soft tissue. Arch Dermatol Syphilol 70:732–747, 1954.
11. Hale AR, Burch GE: The arteriovenous anastomoses of the blood vessels of the human finger. Medicine 39:191–240, 1960.
12. Scher RK: Diseases of the nails. In: Rakel RE (ed): Conn's Current Therapy. WB Saunders, Philadelphia, 1984, pp 649–654.
13. Salasche SJ: Surgery. In: Scher RK, Daniel CR (eds): Nails: Therapy, Diagnosis, Surgery. WB Saunders, Philadelphia, 1990, pp 258–280.
14. Baran R: Surgery of the nail. Dermatol Clin 2:271–284, 1984.
15. Salasche SJ, Peters V: Tips on nail surgery. Cutis 35:428–438, 1984.
16. Scher RK: Punch biopsies of nails: a simple, valuable procedure. J Dermatol Surg Oncol 4:528–530, 1978.
17. Scher RK: Nail surgery. In: Epstein E (ed): Techniques in Skin Surgery. Lea & Febiger, Philadelphia, 1979, pp 164–170.
18. Albom MJ: Avulsion of a nail plate. J Dermatol Surg Oncol 3:34–35, 1977.
19. Scher RK: The nail. In: Roenigk RK, Roenigk HH (eds): Dermatologic Surgery—Principles and Practice. Marcel Dekker, New York, 1989, pp 509–526.
20. Bennett RG: Technique of biopsy of nails. J Dermatol Surg 2:325–326, 1976.
21. Arzeno S, Siegel J: Toradol (ketorolac tromethamine)—a product monograph. Syntex Laboratories, Palo Alto, CA, 1990, pp 1–47.
22. Dockery GL: Nails: fundamental conditions and procedures. In: McGlamry ED (ed): Comprehensive Text Book of Foot Surgery. Sanstache, Baltimore, 1987, pp 3–37.
23. Baran R, Sayag J: Nail biopsy—why, when, where, how? J Dermatol Surg 2:322–324, 1976.
24. Achten G: Histologie ungueale. Bol Ist Dermatol S Gallicano, 8:3–28, 1972.
25. Scher RK, Ackerman AB: The value of nail biopsy for demonstrating fungi not demonstrable by microbiologic techniques. Am J Dermatopathol 2:55–56, 1980.
26. Ronchese F: Nail in lichen planus. Arch Dermatol 91:347–350, 1965.
27. Zaias N, Ackerman AB: The nail in Darier-White disease. Arch Dermatol 107:193–199, 1973.
28. Stone OJ, Barr RJ, Herten RJ: Biopsy of the nail area. Cutis 21:257–260, 1978.
29. Scher RK: Longitudinal resection of the nails for purposes of biopsy and treatment. J Dermatol Surg Oncol 6:805–807, 1980.
30. Zaias N: The longitudinal nail biopsy. J Invest Dermatol 49:406–408, 1967.
31. Bureau H, Baran R, Haneke E: Nail surgery and traumatic abnormalities. In: Baran R, Dauber RPR (eds): Diseases of the Nail and Their Management. Blackwell Scientific, Oxford, 1984, pp 347–402.
32. Hutchinson J: Notes toward the information of clinical groups of tumor. Am J Med Sci 91:470, 1886.
33. Alvarez R, Zaias N: A modified polyethylene glycol-pyroxylin embedding method specially suited for nails. J Invest Dermatol 49:409–410, 1967.
34. Lewin K, DeWit SA, Lawson R: Softening techniques for nail biopsies. Arch Dermatol 107:223, 1973.
35. Scher RK, Ackerman AB: Histologic differential diagnosis of onychomycosis and psoriasis of the nail unit from cornified cells of the nail bed alone. Am J Dermatopathol 2:255–256, 1980.
36. Siegle RJ, Swanson NA: Nail surgery: a review. J Dermatol Surg Oncol 8:659–666, 1982.
37. Stone OJ, Mullins JF: The distal course of nail matrix hemorrhage. Arch Dermatol 88:186–187, 1963.
38. Fosnaugh RP: Surgery of the nail. In: Epstein E (ed): Skin Surgery. Charles C Thomas, Springfield, IL, 1982, pp 981–1007.

39. Scher RK: Surgical avulsion of nail plates by a proximal to distal technique. J Dermatol Surg Oncol 7:296–297, 1981.

40. Runne U: Operative Eingriffe an Nagelorgan: Indikationen und Kontraindikationen. Z Hautkr 58:324–332, 1983.

41. McKay I: Nail elevator. Lancet 1:864, 1973.

42. Baran R: More on avulsion of nail plates. J Dermatol Surg Oncol 7:854, 1981.

43. Cordero CFA: Ablacion ungueal. Su uso en la onicomicosis. Dermatol Int 14:21, 1965.

44. Linares JL: Ablacion ungueal. Evaluacion terapeutica de la teenica creada par el Dr. F.A. Cordero. Dermatol Revista Mex 11:161, 1967.

45. Murray WR, Bedi BS: The surgical management of ingrowing toenails. Br J Surg 62:409–412, 1975.

46. Pollack SV: Electrocoagulation. In: Pollack SV (ed): Electrosurgery of the Skin. Churchill Livingstone, New York, 1991, pp 37–50.

47. Milonni PW, Eberly JH: Atoms, molecules and solids. In: Milonni PW, Eberly JH (eds): Lasers. John Wiley & Sons, New York, 1988, pp 130–135.

48. Milonni PW, Eberly JH: Specific lasers and pumping mechanisms. In: Milonni PW, Eberly JH (eds): Lasers. John Wiley & Sons, New York, 1988, pp 437–439.

49. Ratz JL, Bailin PL: CO_2 laser. In: Roenigk RK, Roenigk HH (eds): Dermatologic Surgery—Principles and Practice. Marcel Dekker, New York, 1989, pp 865–880.

50. Labandter H, Kaplan I: Experience with a continuous laser in the treatment of suitable cutaneous conditions: preliminary report. J Dermatol Surg Oncol 3:527–530, 1977.

51. Siegle RJ, Harkness J, Swanson NA: Phenol alcohol technique for permanent matricectomy. Arch Dermatol 120:348–350, 1984.

52. Nyman SP: The phenol-alcohol technique for toenail excision. J NJ Chiropract Soc 5:4–6, 1956.

53. Suppan RJ, Ritchlin JD: A nondebilitating surgical procedure for ingrown toenail. J Am Podiatr Assoc 52:900–902, 1962.

54. Yale JF: Phenol alcohol technique for correction of infected ingrown toenail. J Am Podiatr Assoc 64:46–53, 1974.

55. Brown FC: Chemocautery for ingrown toenails. J Dermatol Surg Oncol 7:331–333, 1981.

56. Travers GR, Ammon RG: The sodium hydroxide chemical matricectomy procedure. J Am Podiatr Assoc 70:476–478, 1980.

57. Monheit GD: Nail surgery. Dermatol Clin 3:521–530, 1985.

58. Glick N: Prevention of recurrence in radical toenail procedures. Curr Podiatr 10:26–27, 1961.

59. Anton-Athens V, Ketai DL: Use of cortosporin otic solution in phenol nail surgery. J Am Podiatr Med Assoc 75:31–33, 1985.

60. Scher RK, Tom BWK, Lally EV: The clinical significance of periodic acid-Schiff-positive deposits in cuticle-proximal nail fold biopsy specimens. Arch Dermatol 121:1406–1409, 1985.

61. Schnitzler L, Baran R, Sivatte J, et al: Biopsy of the proximal nail fold in collagen diseases. J Dermatol Surg 2:313–315, 1976.

62. Nasca RJ, Gould JS. Mucous cysts of the digits. South Med J 76:1142–1144, 1983.

63. Gross RE: Recurring myxomatous, cutaneous cysts of the fingers and toes. Surg Gynecol Obstet 65:289–302, 1937.

64. Jensen DR: Ganglia and synovial cysts, their pathogenesis and treatment. Ann Surg 105:592–601, 1937.

65. King ESJ: Mucous cysts of the fingers. Aust NZ J Surg 21:121–129, 1951.

66. Kleinert HE, Kutz JE, Fishman AH, et al: Etiology and treatment of the so-called mucous cyst of the finger. J Bone Joint Surg 54A:1455–1458, 1972.

67. Eaton RG, Dobranski AI, Littler JW: Marginal osteophyte excision and treatment of mucous cysts. J Bone Joint Surg 55A:570–574, 1973.

68. Friden JS: Surgical treatment of diseases of the nail. Primary Care 13:447–463, 1986.

69. Baran R, Bureau H: Surgical treatment of recalcitrant chronic paronychia of the fingers. J Dermatol Surg Oncol 7:106–107, 1981.

70. Salasche SJ: Myxoid cysts of the proximal nail fold: a surgical approach. J Dermatol Surg Oncol 10:35–39, 1984.

71. Herndon JH, Myers SR, Akelman E: Advanced surgery. In: Scher RK, Daniel CR (eds): Nails: Therapy, Diagnosis, Surgery. WB Saunders, Philadelphia, 1990, pp 281–293.

72. McLeod GR: Management of melanoma in situ. In: Balch CM (ed): Pigment Cell: Surgical Approaches to Cutaneous Melanoma. Karger, Basel, 1985, pp 1–7.

73. Scher RK: Nail surgery. In: Epstein E, Epstein E Jr (eds): Techniques in Skin Surgery. Lea & Febiger, Philadelphia, 1979, pp 164–170.

74. Albom MJ: Squamous cell carcinoma of the finger and nail bed—a review of the literature and treatment by Mohs surgical technique. J Dermatol Surg 1:43–48, 1975.

75. Mineiro LEG, Salter JJ, Orduna CC: Squamous cell carcinoma of the nail bed: report of two cases. Arch Surg 100:6–7, 1970.

76. Nelson LM, Hamilton CF: Primary carcinoma of the nail bed. Arch Dermatol 101:63–67, 1970.

77. Mohs FE: Chemosurgery in Cancer, Gangrene, and Infections. Charles C Thomas, Springfield, IL, 1956, pp 96–110.

78. Mikhail GR: Bowen's disease and squamous cell carcinoma of the nail bed. Arch Dermatol 110:267–270, 1974.

79. Eichenholtz SN, DeAngelis C: Squamous cell carcinoma of the nail bed. JAMA 191:102–104, 1956.

80. Conway H, Hugo NE, Tulenko JF: Surgery of Tumors of the Skin. Charles C Thomas, Springfield, IL, 1966, pp 179–181.

81. Guides to the Evaluation of Permanent Impairment. Monograph. The American Medical Association, Chicago, 1971, pp 4–5.

82. Klein E, Stoll HL, Milgrom H, et al: Tumors of the skin XII: topical 5-fluorouracil. J Surg Oncol 3:331–349, 1971.

83. Goette DK: Erythroplasia of Queyrat: treatment with topically administered fluorouracil. Arch Dermatol 110:271–273, 1974.

84. Mohs FE: Chemosurgery for the microscopically controlled excision of skin cancer. J Surg Oncol 3:257–267, 1971.

85. Flatt AE: Nailbed injuries. Br J Plast Surg 8:34–37, 1955.

86. Ashbell T, Kleinert H: The deformed fingernail: a frequent result of failure to repair nailbed injuries. J Trauma 2:177–189, 1967.

87. Recht P: Fingertip injuries and a plea for the nail. J Dermatol Surg 2:327–328, 1976.

88. Downey M: Digital fractures. In: McGlamry ED (ed): Comprehensive Textbook of Foot Surgery. Williams & Wilkins, Baltimore, 1987, pp 852–859.

89. Massengill JB: Pitfalls in the management of fingertip injuries and hand lacerations. Primary Care 7:231–243, 1980.

90. Coyle MP, Leddy JP: Injuries of the distal finger. Primary Care 7:245–258, 1980.

91. Rosenthal EA: Treatment of fingertip and nail bed injuries. Orthop Clin North Am 14:675–697, 1983.

92. Zacher JB: Management of injuries of the distal phalanx. Surg Clin North Am 64:747–760, 1984.

93. Zook EG: Injuries of the fingernail. In: Green DP (ed): Operative Hand Surgery. Churchill Livingstone, New York, 1982, pp 895–914.

94. Zook EG: Fingernail injuries. In: Strickland JW, Steichen JB (eds): Difficult Problems in Hand Surgery. CV Mosby, St. Louis, 1982, pp 22–27.

95. Zook EG, Guy RJ, Russell RC: A study of nail bed injuries: causes, treatment, and prognosis. J Hand Surg 9A:247–252, 1984.

96. Melone CP, Grad JB: Primary care of fingernail injuries. Emerg Med Clin North Am 3:255–261, 1985.

97. Zook EG: The perionychium: anatomy, physiology and care of injuries. Clin Plast Surg 8:21–31, 1981.

98. Simon RR, Wolgin M: Subungual hematoma: association with occult laceration requiring repair. Am J Emerg Med 5:302–304, 1987.

99. Lewin K: The normal finger nail. Br J Dermatol 77:421–430, 1965.

100. Horder T: Discussion of the clinical significance and course of subacute bacterial endocarditis. Br Med J 2:301–304, 1920.

101. Miller A, Vaziri ND: Recurrent atraumatic subungual splinter hemorrhages in healthy individuals. South Med J 72:1418–1420, 1979.

102. Martin BF, Platts MM: A histological study of the nail region in normal human subjects and in those showing splinter haemorrhages of the nail. J Anat 93:323–330, 1959.

103. Heath D, Williams DR: Nail haemorrhages. Br Heart J 40:1300–1305, 1978.

104. Fitzpatrick TB, Eisen AZ, Wolff K, et al: Dermatology in General Medicine. McGraw-Hill, New York, 1987, p 2490.

105. Bork K, DeKornfeld TJ: Cutaneous Side Effects of Drugs. WB Saunders, Philadelphia, 1988, pp 266–267.

106. Monk BE: The prevalence of splinter haemorrhages. Br J Dermatol 103:183–185, 1980.

107. Hutchinson J: Melanosis often not black: melanotic whitlow. Br Med J 1:491, 1886.

108. Rushforth GF: Two cases of subungual malignant melanoma. Br J Surg 58:451–453, 1971.

109. Grisafi PJ, Lombardi CM, Sciarrino AL, et al: Three select subungual pathologies: subungual exostosis, osteochondroma, and subungual hematoma. Clin Podiatr Med Surg 6:355–364, 1989.

110. Pack GT, Oropeza R: Subungual melanoma. Surg Gynecol Obstet 124:571–582, 1967.

111. Rodbard S: Treatment of injury to the root of the nail. JAMA 205:940, 1968.

112. Wee GC, Shieber W: Painless evacuation of subungual hematoma. Surg Gynecol Obstet 131:531, 1970.

113. Palamarchuk HJ, Kerzner M: An improved approach to evacuation of subungual hematoma. J Am Podiatr Med Assoc 79:566–568, 1989.

114. Newmeyer WL, Kilgore ES: Common injuries of the fingernail and nailbed. Am Fam Phys 16:93–95, 1977.

115. Iselin M: Surgery of the Hand. Churchill Livingstone, London, 1940.

116. Farrington GH: Subungual haematoma—an evaluation of treatment. Br Med J 1:742–744, 1964.

117. Ranjan A: Subungual haematoma. J Ind Med Assoc 72:187–188, 1979.

118. Baran R, Bureau H: Surgical management of some conditions in and about the nails. J Dermatol Surg 2:308–312, 1976.

119. Schiller C: Nail replacement in fingertip injuries. Plast Reconstr Surg 19:521–530, 1957.

120. Stewart PJ: Blood under the nail. Lancet 1:518, 1982.

121. Hutchinson GH, David TJ: Is nail trephining safe? Arch Dis Child 55:321–325, 1980.

122. Clayburgh RH, Wood MB, Cooney WP: Nail bed repair and reconstruction by reverse dermal grafts. J Hand Surg 8:594–598, 1983.

123. Saito H, Suzuki Y, Fujino K, et al: Free nail bed graft for treatment of nail bed injuries of the hand. J Hand Surg 8:171–178, 1983.

124. Shepard GH: Treatment of nail bed avulsions with split-thickness nail bed grafts. J Hand Surg 8:49–54, 1983.

125. Engber WD, Clancy WG: Traumatic avulsion of the fingernail associated with injury to the phalangeal epiphyseal plate. J Bone Joint Surg 60B:713–714, 1978.

126. McCash CR: Free nail grafting. Br J Plast Surg 8:19–33, 1956.

127. Bautista BN, Nery EB: Replacement of a malformed fingernail with acrylic resin material. Plast Reconstr Surg 55:234–236, 1975.

128. Kutler W: A new method for finger tip amputation. JAMA 133:29–30, 1947.

129. Idler R, Strickland JW: Management of soft tissue injuries of the finger tips. Orthop Rev 11:25, 1982.

130. Itoh Y, Uchinishi K, Oka Y: Treatment of pseudoarthrosis of the distal phalanx with the palmar midline approach. J Hand Surg 8:80–84, 1983.

131. Green DP, Anderson JR: Closed reduction and percutaneous pin fixation of fractured phalanges. J Bone Joint Surg 55A:1651–1654, 1973.

132. Massing AM, Epstein WL: Natural history of warts. Arch Dermatol 87:306–310, 1963.

133. Dachow-Siwiec E: Technique of cryotherapy. Clin Dermatol 3:185–188, 1985.

134. Dachow-Siwiec E: Treatment of cryosurgery in the premalignant and benign lesions of the skin. Clin Dermatol 8:69–79, 1990.

135. Arievich AM, Vikhreva OV, Lebedev BM: Vestn Dermatol Venerol N5–N7, 1960.

136. Farber EM, South DA: Urea ointment in the non-surgical avulsion of nail dystrophies. Cutis 22:689–691, 1978.

137. South DA, Farber EM: Urea ointment in the non-surgical avulsion of nail dystrophies—a reappraisal. Cutis 25:609–612, 1980.

138. Averill RW, Scher RK: Simplified nail taping with urea ointment for nonsurgical nail avulsion. Cutis 38:231–233, 1986.

139. Hay RJ, Baran R: Fungal (onychomycosis) and other infections of the nail apparatus. In: Baran R, Dauber RPR (eds): Diseases of the Nails and Their Management. Blackwell Scientific, Oxford, 1984, pp 121–155.

140. Dorn M, Kienitz T, Ryckmanns F: Onychomycosis: experience with non-traumatic nail avulsion. Hautartz 31:30, 1980.

141. Buselmeier FJ: Combination urea and salicyclic acid ointment nail avulsion in non-dystrophic nails: follow up observation. Cutis 25:393, 1980.

142. Dockery CL: Nails: fundamental conditions and procedures. In: McGlamry ED (ed): Comprehensive Textbook of Foot Surgery. Williams & Wilkins, Baltimore, 1987, pp 3–37.

143. Harris L: A variation in the treatment concept of onychomycosis. J Am Podiatr Assoc 66:700, 1976.

144. Bedi TR: Intradermal triamcinolone treatment of psoriatic onychodystrophy. Dermatologica 155:24–25, 1977.

145. Fisher AA: Irritant reactions from topical urea preparations used for dry skin. Cutis 18:761, 1976.

146. Yale I: Podiatric Medicine. Williams & Wilkins, Baltimore, 1980, pp 193–214.

147. Cohen PR, Scher RK: Geriatric nail disorders: diagnosis and treatment. J Am Acad Dermatol 26:521–531, 1992.

PART THREE

Cosmetic Surgical Procedures

CHAPTER 32

Use of Cosmetics in Cutaneous Surgery

ZOE K. DRAELOS

A basic understanding of the use of cosmetics in camouflaging postsurgical wounds and erythema is valuable to the cutaneous surgeon. Cosmetics can also be used to camouflage pigmentation and contour abnormalities that cannot be optimally surgically corrected. To obtain the best results, proper selection of and application techniques for using cosmetics in the postsurgical patient must be fully understood. Knowledge of basic camouflage concepts for pigmentation and contour abnormalities is also useful in ideal patient management.

Postsurgical Cosmetic Selection

Cosmetics are important in postsurgical patients to restore a positive self-image and allow the most rapid return to normal public life. Female patients are especially self-conscious of surgical facial defects and will experience a faster emotional postsurgical recovery if appropriate cosmetic advice can be provided by the cutaneous surgeon or the surgeon's staff.[1-3] Facial cosmetics can be divided into four groups: facial foundations, colored facial cosmetics, eye cosmetics, and lip cosmetics.

FACIAL FOUNDATIONS

A facial foundation is a pigmented liquid, cream, or cake designed to conceal facial defects, add color, and blend uneven facial tones.[4] Products are available in oil-free, water-based, oil-based, and anhydrous formulations and come in a wide variety of colors to match virtually any complexion. Facial foundations are extremely valuable in postsurgical patients to cover erythema and camouflage incisional scarring. The ability of

a facial foundation to cover a defect is related to its thickness, color, and concentration of titanium dioxide. Thicker creams cover better than thinner liquids, darker colors cover better than lighter colors, and an increased concentration of titanium dioxide provides superior coverage.[5] The special needs of the postsurgical patient require a foundation that gives high coverage with minimal skin irritation and yet also permits easy removal while preserving a natural appearance.

Cake Foundations

Cake foundations, also known as cream/powder foundations, are composed of talc, kaolin, precipitated chalk, zinc oxide, titanium dioxide, and pigment compressed into a cake.[6] When the cake foundation is applied with a dry sponge, it functions as a powder. However, it becomes a cream when applied with a wet sponge, hence the name cream/powder foundation. Cake foundations can be formulated with a high concentration of titanium dioxide so that none of the underlying skin tones can be appreciated. Complete-coverage cake foundations are known as "pancake makeup." Water can be used to thin the foundation to obtain the desired amount of coverage. Unfortunately, because this foundation produces a somewhat flat facial appearance, other colored facial cosmetics must also usually be worn. Skin irritation is minimal, as no emulsifiers are required, and the foundation is easily removed with water.

Facial foundations should not be worn in the immediate postsurgical period until early reepithelialization has occurred or the sutures have been removed. No foundation will adhere to a wound with serous drainage. Furthermore, titanium dioxide and other particulate matter in the foundation could possibly enter an incisional site and create a granulomatous response. In the chemical peel or dermabrasion patient, titanium dioxide can increase the formation of milia.

Some patients may be tempted to purchase one of the high-coverage surgical anhydrous cream foundations. These products provide excellent coverage and are long lasting because of their waterproof characteristics, but they are best suited for patients who have long-standing pigment abnormalities. Forceful rubbing is required for application, and a special cleanser is necessary for removal; both of these can traumatize freshly epithelialized skin.

Undercover Cream

If superior coverage is required, either multiple layers of cake foundation can be applied or an undercover cream can be used. Undercover creams are color primers designed to be worn under a foundation. Green undercover creams can be used in postsurgical patients to cover erythema, since the mixing of green and red yields brown. Thus, the erythematous site is more easily camouflaged by a brown foundation once a green-colored primer has been used.[7]

Even though facial foundation can be applied with the fingertips or a sponge, a sponge is generally recommended for postsurgical patients. The sponge can be cleansed between uses with soap and water to reduce the risk of infection. The foundation should be gently dabbed and pushed into the surgical defect and then blended to the hairline, bilaterally around each tragus, and beneath the chin. It is best to apply the foundation to the rest of the face with broad downward strokes, as this will flatten facial vellus hairs and smooth skin scale, a most important factor in chemical peel and dermabrasion patients.

COLORED FACIAL COSMETICS

Colored facial cosmetics must be worn by postsurgical patients to restore a natural appearance if a high-coverage foundation has been chosen. The natural facial appearance is formed by subtle color variations, which are removed by high-coverage foundations. A valuable cosmetic to restore facial landmarks is known as "blush." Blush is a powder, cream, or gel in shades of pink or peach that is designed to add color to the upper cheeks. Postsurgical patients should select a compressed powder blush in a color suitable to the complexion. The blush should be lightly dusted over the upper cheeks, beginning at a point beneath the pupil on the fleshy portion of the cheek, and then swept upward beyond the lateral eye to restore the cheekbone landmark.[5] A small amount of blush should also be applied to the central forehead, the tip of the nose, and the chin to replace the natural shading of the face.

EYE COSMETICS

Postsurgical patients may elect to use camouflaging eye cosmetics if the surgical site is in the eye area. The most common cosmetic side effect of periorbital surgery is ecchymosis, resulting in skin discoloration. Eyelid discoloration can be camouflaged after reepithelialization has occurred or sutures have been removed by applying a cake facial foundation over the entire upper and lower eyelids. After the foundation has dried, powder eye shadow in the desired color can be applied. Eye shadows with a pearled or metallic shine should be avoided, since they may contain fish scale essence, mica, bismuth oxychloride, or metal particles that can be irritating to freshly healed skin.[8] Matte or dull finish eye shadows have less potential to be irritating. Other eye area cosmetics, such as eyeliner and mascara, can be worn as long as they are not of the waterproof variety. Waterproof eyeliner and mascara require a special petroleum-based solvent for removal, which can be extremely irritating to healing skin.

LIP COSMETICS

Adding color to the lips is one of the quickest ways to restore the appearance of well-being to a postsurgical patient. During the early phases of healing from facial surgery, most female patients can wear lipstick, even though the use of facial foundation, other colored facial cosmetics, or eye cosmetics must be delayed until reepithelialization has occurred. If the surgical site is on the lip, petrolatum-based lip creams can be used to simultaneously add color and keep the incision moist to facilitate healing. Firmer lipsticks or lip cosmetics with a pearled or metallic shine should be avoided until reepithelialization has occurred or the sutures have been removed.

Camouflaging Techniques

The cutaneous surgeon always attempts to design the procedure and its resultant scar with cosmetic considerations in mind in the hope that the patient will have an imperceptible or well-hidden scar that will not require long-term camouflaging. However, it is not always possible to produce an invisible scar, and long-term camouflaging techniques may sometimes be necessary to provide an acceptable appearance.

The two major types of abnormalities that require long-term camouflaging are pigmentation abnormalities and contour abnormalities. It is important to realize that cosmetics can cover only pigmentation abnormalities, not contour abnormalities.[9] As a matter of fact, cosmetics may actually accentuate contour abnormalities if inappropriate shading techniques are used.

PIGMENTATION ABNORMALITIES

Cosmetics can be effectively used to camouflage all pigmentation abnormalities, but the techniques employed depend on the color of the lesion. Pigmentation abnormalities can be divided into red, yellow, hyperpigmented and hypopigmented lesions (Table 32–1).

TABLE 32–1. **TECHNIQUES FOR CAMOUFLAGING PIGMENTED LESIONS**

Lesion Color	Sample Lesions	Undercover Cosmetic Color
Red	Port-wine stains Angiomas Telangiectases Scars	Green
Yellow	Solar elastosis Xanthelasma Sebaceous hyperplasia	Purple
Hyperpigmented lesions (brown/black)	Lentigines Nevi Seborrheic keratoses Chloasma Postinflammatory hyperpigmentation	White
Hypopigmented lesions (white/tan)	Vitiligo Pityriasis alba Postinflammatory hypopigmentation	Brown

Red Lesions

Some of the red skin lesions important to the cutaneous surgeon include port-wine stains (nevus flammeus), angiomas, immature scars, and telangiectases. In addition, dermatoses manifesting red facial lesions include systemic lupus erythematosus, psoriasis, rosacea, seborrheic dermatitis, and acne. The two methods used to cover red facial lesions are to combine a green undercover cosmetic with a facial foundation or to apply a complete coverage surgical foundation. It is generally agreed that the best method of concealing a red lesion is to combine a green undercover cosmetic with a facial foundation. The concept involves the layering of appropriate pigments to achieve a final brown color that is close to the natural complexion. If red and green colors are mixed, a brown color will result. Thus, a green undercover primer is applied to the red lesion initially, followed by use of a moderate- to heavy-coverage facial foundation, which is subsequently blended into the entire face. By using an undercover cosmetic, a more natural appearance can be obtained with a nonsurgical foundation, the application is easier and less time consuming, the cosmetics are less occlusive and more comfortable to wear, a special removal product is not required, and more fashion versatility is available.

Complete camouflaging can also be achieved through use of a full coverage surgical foundation. These products are waterproof and allow none of the underlying skin tones to be appreciated. They can also be custom blended to achieve an exact complexion color match. There is normal color variation on every face, but blending along the jawline is most important. Surgical foundations also tend to be quite occlusive, which can make them uncomfortable to wear in hot or humid conditions.

The application technique for all surgical foundations is similar. First, the required amount of the thick cream product should be removed from the jar and held in the palm of the hand. This warms and softens the cream to increase the ease of application and spreadability. A sponge or the fingertips can then be used to press the foundation into the skin; rubbing should be avoided, as this will result in uneven application. The foundation should first be applied over the red lesion and then blended into the rest of the face, including over the tragus bilaterally, beneath the chin, and about one-quarter inch into the hairline. Next, the nonpigmented finishing powder should be pressed into the foundation with a puff or the fingertips and any excess dusted away with a loose brush. A finishing powder must always be applied, as this keeps the foundation from rubbing off onto clothing and improves its waterproofing characteristics. Finally, other colored facial cosmetics must be applied to create a more natural appearance, since surgical foundations worn alone tend to produce a "masklike" face.

Because surgical foundations are waterproof, they cannot be removed with soap and water. Most come with a special removal solvent that is rubbed onto the face with a cotton ball. Some patients will be tempted to leave the cosmetic on the face overnight or for extended periods. This is not recommended, as the foundation is extremely occlusive and can cause perifollicular irritation and eccrine duct occlusion, resulting in an acneiform eruption.

Yellow Lesions

Yellow lesions of the face that may require cosmetic camouflaging include solar elastosis, xanthelasma, and sebaceous hyperplasia. Individuals who have renal failure or who are undergoing chemotherapy may have sallow complexion tones that require camouflaging. Again, the principles of color mixing are important. Because the combination of yellow and purple will yield brown, a purple undercover primer is used in conjunction with a medium- to heavy-coverage facial foundation. For individual lesions, the purple undercover may be applied selectively. However, if the whole face is to be corrected, the undercover cosmetic must be applied to the entire face. Full-coverage surgical foundations may also be used in a manner similar to that used for red lesions.

Hyperpigmented Lesions

Common brown or black lesions of the face include lentigines, nevi, seborrheic keratoses, chloasma, and

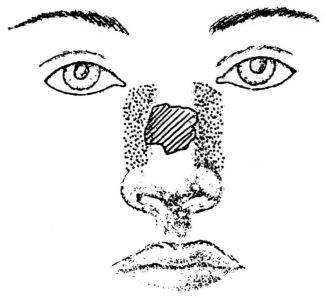

Figure 32–1. A schematic diagram demonstrating how shading techniques can be used to minimize a depressed scar. The stippled area represents darker shading; diagonal lines represent lighter shading.

postinflammatory hyperpigmentation. Lesions that are darker than the normal complexion are the hardest to camouflage, as it is cosmetically unacceptable to apply a dark enough foundation to allow blending of the lesions. Instead, a better camouflage is obtained by blocking out all facial pigmentation with a white undercover. The white undercover is applied to the entire face, not just the areas of hyperpigmentation, and then a suitable pigmented foundation is applied to the entire face for moderate to full coverage. Full-coverage surgical foundations may also be used separately.

Hypopigmented Lesions

In contrast to the hyperpigmented facial lesions, hypopigmented facial lesions are the easiest to camouflage. These include vitiligo, pityriasis alba, and postinflammatory hypopigmentation. Technically, vitiligo lesions are depigmented, not hypopigmented, but because the same camouflage methods apply, they will be discussed here. Areas that are lighter than the normal complexion can be corrected by applying a moderate- to full-coverage foundation to the involved areas only and then applying a second layer of foundation to the entire face. Brown undercover creams and surgical foundations can also be used for this purpose.[10] The camouflage product selected depends on the disparity in pigmentation.

CONTOUR ABNORMALITIES

Although facial pigmentation abnormalities can be relatively easily camouflaged with the appropriate foundation or undercover cosmetic, no such cosmetic exists to correct contour abnormalities. As a matter of fact, heavy or full-coverage facial foundations often accentuate contour abnormalities because of their thick, oc-

clusive character. Even the normally increased pore size over the nose will be accentuated with these cosmetics. Thus, contour abnormalities must be camouflaged with artistic shading to create the illusion of an even surface.

The shading of contour abnormalities is based on the premise that dark colors make surfaces recede, while light colors make surfaces come forward. Therefore, depressions are shaded with lighter colors, while protuberances are shaded with darker colors.[11] The cosmetic best suited for this purpose is a powder blush, buffer, or highlighter. A light pink blush with a pearled finish is required for shading depressions, while a darker rose highlighter with a matte finish is required for shading protuberances. If the complexion tones tend more toward orange, light peach and dark rust colors should be selected.

To camouflage a depressed scar following Mohs surgery for removal of a basal cell carcinoma on the nose (Fig. 32–1), the depressed scar is shaded with a light color, while the hypertrophied area surrounding the depression is shaded with a darker color. Other contour abnormalities can also be visually corrected in this same manner.

SUMMARY

Cosmetics can be extremely valuable in the management of the postsurgical patient who requires temporary camouflage until complete healing occurs or in the patient who requires more sophisticated camouflage techniques for permanent pigmentation or contour abnormalities. Cake facial foundations in combination with powder blush, matte-finish powder eye shadow, and nonwaterproof mascara or eyeliner can be safely used in the postsurgical patient to camouflage both the erythema and the incision site itself once early epithelialization or suture removal has occurred.

Permanent pigmentation abnormalities can be camouflaged by using the concept of color blending. Green primer can be added to red lesions, purple primer to yellow lesions, white primer to hyperpigmented lesions, and brown primer to hypopigmented lesions under a facial foundation to provide optimal coverage. Contour abnormalities require artistic shading, with lightening of depressions and darkening of protuberances, to create the illusion of a more uniform surface. By understanding these concepts and principles, the cutaneous surgeon can help return the patient to normal function as rapidly as possible after most surgical procedures.

REFERENCES

1. Stewart TW, Savage D: Cosmetic camouflage in dermatology. Br J Dermatol 86:530, 1972.
2. Theberge L, Kernaleguen A: Importance of cosmetics related to aspects of self. Precept Mot Skills 48:827, 1979.
3. Cash TF, Cash DW: Women's use of cosmetics: psychosocial correlates and consequences. Int J Cosmet Sci 4:1, 1982.
4. Lanzet M: Modern formulations of coloring agents: facial and eye. In: Frost P, Horwitz SN (eds): Principles of Cosmetics for the Dermatologist. CV Mosby, St. Louis, 1982, p 133.

5. Draelos ZK: Cosmetics in Dermatology. Churchill Livingstone, Edinburgh, 1990, pp 28, 147.
6. Wilkinson JB, Moore RJ: Harry's Cosmeticology. 7th ed. Chemical Publishing, New York, 1982, p 304.
7. Brauer EW: Coloring and corrective make-up preparations. Clin Dermatol 6:66, 1988.
8. Draelos ZK: Eye cosmetics. Dermatol Clin. In press.

9. Draelos ZK: Use of cover cosmetics for pigment abnormalities. Cosmet Dermatol 5:14, 1989.
10. Benmaman O, Sanchez JL: Treatment and camouflaging of pigmentary disorders. Clin Dermatol 6:50, 1988.
11. Hynds S: Classification of cosmetics and the art of self-adornment. In: Frost P, Horwitz SN (eds): Principles of Cosmetics for the Dermatologist. CV Mosby, St. Louis, 1982, p 349.

CHAPTER 33

Cosmetic Tattooing

DAVID J. GOLDBERG

By definition, tattooing is the introduction of various dyes and pigments into the skin after stabbing it with needles of various sizes. Whether tattooing is done for cosmetic or medical reasons, the pigments must be nontoxic, light stable, insoluble, nonirritating, and inert to immunologic destruction.

History of Tattooing

Evidence of tattooing has been documented archaeologically as first occurring in ancient Egypt around 4000 to 2000 BC. In ancient China, tattooing was first practiced in 1100 BC, but tattooing has also been performed in other eras for a variety of reasons. The Greeks and Romans used this technique to mark prisoners of war, criminals, and slaves. In the twentieth century, Nazi Germany marked concentration camp victims with tattoos. Such permanent personal "adornment" is still practiced for aesthetic, religious, and familial reasons, as well as for tribal marking in some parts of the world.

Cosmetic tattooing was first performed in the early second century AD by Galen, the Greek physician and prolific medical writer, who used tattooing to improve defects in "coloration." The first modern documented record of medical tattooing occurred in 1835, when tattooing was performed to color nevi, "congenital purple plaques," and other lesions of the skin.[1] Over the years, tattooing has been advocated to camouflage nevi,[2] for transplanted tattooed skin grafts,[3] and to change the contour of the lip vermilion.[4] Dufourmental described medical tattooing of wounds, scars, and burns.[5] In 1938, a tattooing technique was described not for cosmetic improvement but to relieve the symptoms of pruritus ani. The itching was relieved, and the texture of the skin returned to normal in each of 15 patients with primary pruritus ani treated by tattooing with mercuric sulfide. A similar method was also successfully used for pruritus vulvae and pruritus scroti.[5]

Despite the fact that the use of medical tattooing has grown rapidly, very few physicians have experience with this technique. There are six major areas in which cutaneous medical cosmetic tattooing has been used: flaps, grafts, and scars; port-wine stains; periareolar skin after mastectomy; margins of radiation treatment sites; lips and eyelids for improved cosmetic definition; and primary skin conditions such as vitiligo and alopecia areata.

Flaps, Grafts, and Scars

In 1934, the idea was first suggested to color skin grafts and scars to match the surrounding tissue through cosmetic tattooing.[6] Although some scars, flaps, and grafts often provide good color matches with the surrounding skin, sometimes there is such a striking contrast in color that the difference in pigmentation detracts from an otherwise good cosmetic result. While many women use makeup to hide these poor results, most men and some women prefer not to do so.

To understand the effectiveness of cosmetic tattooing for these types of problems, it is important to understand the two major factors involved in cutaneous pigmentation. Skin color is largely determined by two factors: the quantity of melanosome production in melanocytes and the volume of capillary blood flow through the skin. Scarred skin, flaps, and skin grafts taken from one part of the body and moved to another may be lighter or darker than the normal surrounding skin. The chief factor in the color contrast of adjacent skin is the absence of the red tone in the affected skin. Thus, it is very important to evaluate melanin pigmentation as well as subtle shades of red before performing cosmetic tattooing.[7]

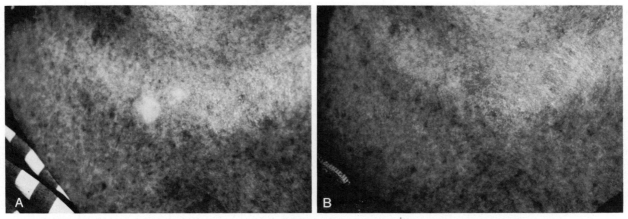

Figure 33–1. *A*, Hypopigmented scar before cosmetic tattooing. *B*, Normal pigmentation after cosmetic tattooing.

These concepts were first used in treating skin grafts and flaps.[6] Based on long experience, the following findings are usually true: firm or thick scars interfere with the insertion and distribution of tattoo pigment; soft white scars or areas lacking pigmentation are most amenable to tattooing; and old skin grafts are easier to tattoo than new grafts, because the skin is more relaxed, with the ideal graft being pure white in color. Yellow and brown tints in grafts are not serious drawbacks to tattooing, since they can be easily dealt with by blending the pigments. The most difficult grafts to treat with tattoos are those that are hyperpigmented or greenish-brown in color, since it is easier to darken a graft than to lighten one. Because flaps are more likely to be lighter than the surrounding skin, they are easier to improve with tattooing than grafts.

Although tattooing can be useful for scarring processes (Fig. 33–1), such processes can be more difficult to treat than flaps and grafts. Before treating a large scarred area, the proper choice of pigment color should be determined through repeat trials until an ideal color match is obtained (Fig. 33–2).

Port-wine Stains

Tattooing has been used to ameliorate the cosmetic deformity seen with port-wine stains.[8] A variety of techniques have previously been used to improve the cosmetic appearance of port-wine stains, including electrodesiccation, ultraviolet light therapy, and x-ray and radium therapy. Unfortunately, scarring, textural changes, and an increased risk of malignancy were the long-term results of the damaging effects of these modalities. Obviously, cosmetics could be used to cover many port-wine stains. However, people who perspired heavily, most men, and women who did not like the trouble and expense of extensive daily makeup application needed an alternative.

In an early published research paper on seven patients with facial port-wine stains treated with tattooing,[8] all were treated with mixtures of white, green, and red pigments and required 1 to 13 sessions of tattooing to obtain satisfactory improvement. All patients were improved, but one individual was noted to have some scarring. The definitive paper on cosmetic tattooing of patients with port-wine stains was presented in 1967.[9] These authors reviewed 1022 patients with port-wine stains treated with tattooing during a 20-year period. These patients required 5001 tattoo treatment sessions, and 996 patients finished their planned treatment. Of these, 836 (84%) were judged to have obtained a satisfactory result, but 160 patients (16%) were thought to have received an unsatisfactory result. An average number of five treatment sessions per patient was required. Of note, 14 patients had their treatment complicated by the onset of cellulitis after tattooing. In addition, 64 patients were noted to have developed "small cavernous hemangiomas," probably representing pyogenic granulomas, after tattoo treatment. Such a complication could follow the trauma of tattooing but has also been reported to occur spontaneously or after laser therapy in patients with port-wine stains.

Subdividing port-wine stains into the categories of subepidermal, dermal, and subdermal types, depending on the location of the blood vessels, it is thought that the dermal and subdermal lesions are most likely to respond favorably to tattoo treatment.[9] This is explained

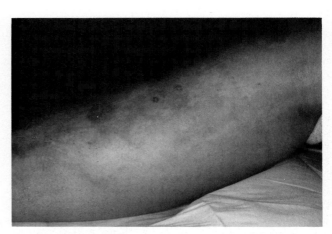

Figure 33–2. Attempts to determine appropriate pigment.

by the presence of a layer of uninvolved dermis overlying the abnormal vasculature that could accept the deposited tattoo pigment to provide a masking effect. The subepidermal variety often fails to show the same positive results, presumably because of the loss by desquamation of superficially deposited pigment. This type of portwine stain is often noted to show excessive bleeding after tattooing.

With the development of effective laser treatment for port-wine stains, cosmetic tattooing for this entity has fallen into disfavor. However, there are many port-wine stains that do not totally clear with laser treatments, and perhaps a renewed interest in tattooing by cutaneous surgeons could provide these patients with further improvement.

Periareolar Reconstruction

The extensive renewed interest in cosmetic tattooing since the 1980s has been responsible for a change in the substances used for tattoo pigments.[10] In the past, the base powder was usually barium sulfate, but currently titanium dioxide is most commonly used. Colored pigments, which once consisted of inorganic salts of metals, are now made from highly stable synthetic organic substances. Iron or ferrous oxides, however, continue to be used to obtain the brown shades and represent the majority of pigment used in modern cosmetic tattooing.[10] The suspensions are powders milled to a particle size of about 6 μ, similar to those found in modern cosmetics. This consistency in size provides the same uniform coloring from cosmetic tattooing as is seen in cosmetics.

The first reported reconstruction of the nipple-areola complex by intradermal tattooing occurred in 1986.[11] This technique allowed reconstruction without using the naturally pigmented skin of the labia or upper inner thigh for the nipple-areola unit. Tattooing is most helpful for older patients or those requiring bilateral reconstruction. By leaving a halo of clear skin around the newly created nipple margin, an illusion of projection can be created. The main advantages of the tattoo technique are that it is a minor procedure producing no scar at the donor site on the labia or upper inner thigh, and it provides an excellent cosmetic appearance of the areola that is often better than is possible with surgical re-creation by means of a skin graft.

Radiation Treatment Sites

To be effective, radiation therapy requires complete accuracy and reproducibility on a daily basis throughout the course of treatment. Treatment fields are often identified by use of small, permanent tattoo dots. These dots are usually administered with a 24-gauge needle and black India ink as the tattoo medium.[12] In fact, these radiation marks represent a type of amateur medical tattoo.

Lip Definition

As one ages, the definition around the lip margins is lost, and the lips lose color and become thinner. While dermabrasions, chemical peels, and injectable collagen can all help minimize the wrinkles, they do little to re-create a naturally pigmented lip line. Lip pigmentation can re-create fuller lips, adding youth and vitality to the aging lip. This technique was first described in 1987.[13] Because the tattoo technique is permanent, care must be taken in choosing ideal lip contours and shape. The pigment selected should also simulate the natural color of the vermilion border or be slightly darker.

Blepharopigmentation

Eyelid tattooing, known as blepharopigmentation, is the area of cosmetic tattooing most thoroughly investigated since the late 1980s.[14] Blepharopigmentation involves the introduction of ferrous oxide pigment into the dermis along the eyelash line in order to simulate

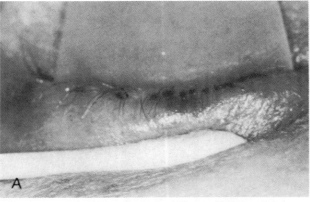 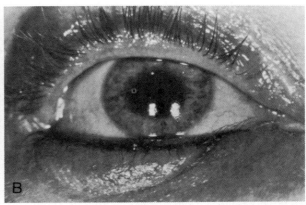

Figure 33–3. *A,* Several pigment dots have been implanted within the skin close to the eyelid edge. A slight oozing of blood indicates that the pigment has penetrated the dermis. *B,* Completed right lower eyelid blepharopigmentation. (From Patipa M: Eyelid tattooing. Dermatol Clin 5[2]:343, 1987.)

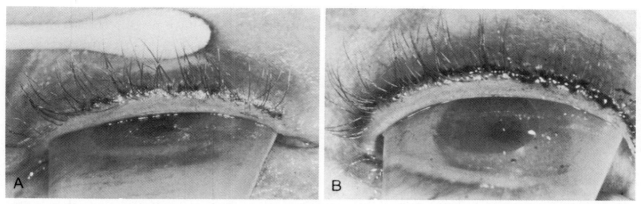

Figure 33–4. *A*, Several cardinal marking dots have been applied within the superior row of eyelashes of the upper eyelid. *B*, Upper eyelid blepharopigmentation has been completed. (From Patipa M: Eyelid tattooing. Dermatol Clin 5[2]:344, 1987.)

the appearance of cosmetic eyeliner (Figs. 33–3, 33–4). This technique makes the eyelid margin appear fuller and the eyelashes appear thicker. Any absent cilia can also be simulated with tattooing. Individuals interested in blepharopigmentation include those who cannot apply makeup because of physical difficulties, tremors, or visual problems. Women who wear contact lenses are also occasionally interested in this procedure. The technique can frequently be enormously helpful for women who are allergic to conventional eye makeup. However, women who merely like the cosmetic convenience of permanent eyelid and eyelash enhancement represent the largest group interested in this procedure. These patients are typically athletic or work outdoors. They may also have oily skin that causes their makeup to smear easily or may prefer to never be seen without makeup.

Because blepharopigmentation is often a purely cosmetic procedure, realistic patient expectations are very important to a successful outcome. Patients must be fully aware that the eyelid tattooing will be permanent. Although blepharopigmentation has become a very popular cosmetic procedure, there have been few documented complications.[14] The most common complication appears to be the result of improper technique. If the

ferrous oxide pigments are implanted too superficially, they will slough off as the epidermis desquamates. This complication is managed by simply repeating the treatment. A second complication is ocular injury, which occurs if the tattooing needle penetrates too deeply into the eyelid or the eyelid tissues are thin. This complication is preventable if a protective eye shield is used during blepharopigmentation. Finally, if the pigmenting procedure is too vigorous, dermal maceration and pigment fanning may occur. A similar procedure can also be used to simulate the appearance of eyebrows that have been lost as a result of disease or trauma (Fig. 33–5).

Vitiligo and Alopecia Areata Therapy

Use of cosmetic tattooing in the treatment of vitiligo and alopecia areata has very great appeal. Fourteen patients with vitiligo were treated with ferrous oxide pigment.[15] The tattoos were administered by means of a cluster of needles attached to a high-speed reciprocating apparatus manufactured by the Permark Division of

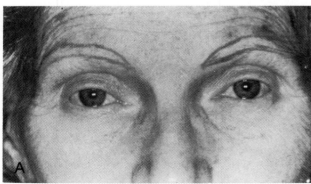
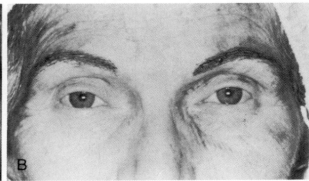

Figure 33–5. *A*, Marking the patient for eyebrow simulation. *B*, Immediately after eyebrow simulation. (From Patipa M: Eyelid tattooing. Dermatol Clin 5[2]:347, 1987.)

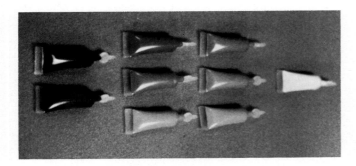

Figure 33–6. Various ferrous oxide pigments that can be used for cosmetic tattooing.

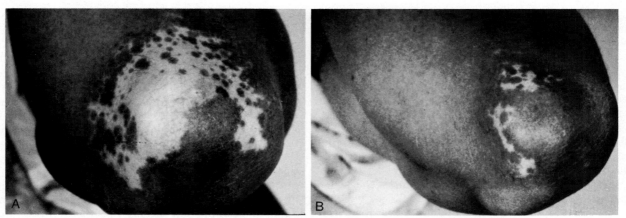

Figure 33–7. Vitiligo in black skin before *(A)* and after *(B)* cosmetic tattooing.

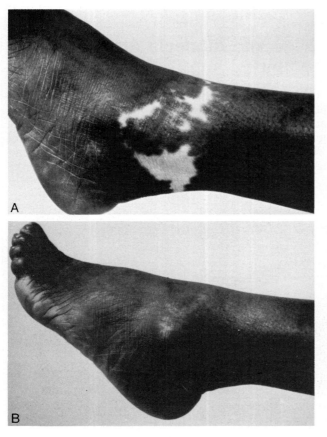

Figure 33–8. Vitiligo in black skin before *(A)* and after *(B)* cosmetic tattooing.

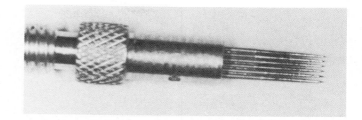

Figure 33–9. Permark Enhancer six-needle flat shading brush used for pigmenting wide areas. (From Patipa M: Eyelid tattooing. Dermatol Clin 5[2]:347, 1987.)

Micropigmentation Devices, Inc. The reported patients had a mean age of 40 and included blacks, whites, East Indians, and Asians; both sexes were represented. All patients were undergoing phototherapy with PUVA for the vitiligo, with variable results, at the time of medical tattooing.

INSTRUMENTATION

The tattooing apparatus, known as the Permark Enhancer II, consists of a main unit, a handpiece equipped with a needle holder tip, and a foot pedal that activates the handpiece. The handpiece is capable of variable speeds up to 9200 strokes per minute, and the depth of needle penetration is adjustable from 1 to 1.75 mm. The iron oxide pigments are available in more than 15 colors (Fig. 33–6).

In one study,[15] 21 fingertips, eight lips, four hands, and two axillae were treated with cosmetic tattooing. These are areas that do not often respond well to PUVA. The immediate post-tattoo results showed a dramatic aesthetic improvement. However, there was a moderate degree of fading in the majority of cases, most of which occurred within the first 6 weeks after treatment. After this time period, the remaining pigment usually persisted with minimal or no additional fading (Figs. 33–7 to 33–9). Of interest is the fact that results were similar in both blacks and whites. However, it is generally much more difficult to match colors in vitiliginous white skin than in vitiliginous black skin (Fig. 33–10).

Although there are very few published data relating to the use of medical tattooing in the cosmetic correction of alopecia areata, a woman with alopecia universalis has been reported who obtained an excellent result after permanent pigmentation of her eyebrows (Fig. 33–11).[14] The reason for the relative permanency of the results can be explained by the histologic site of the tattoo pigment, which is located primarily intracellularly within mononuclear cells.[16] When tattoo pigment is placed appropriately, there is no evidence of follicle damage, inflammation, or granuloma formation.

Complications

Complications from nonmedical tattoos have included a variety of infections and acquired sensitivities to tattoo pigments, as well as miscellaneous reactions such as keloid and granuloma formation and cutaneous malignancies arising at the tattoo site.[17] Although these are legitimate concerns when considering medical cosmetic tattooing, it should be noted that in more than 100,000 cases of ferrous oxide eyelid tattoo pigmentation, there have been no documented cases of allergic reactions (data on file, Permark Corporation).

SUMMARY

Medical tattooing is a fascinating although largely ignored aspect of cutaneous surgery. The procedure is safe and simple to perform, and the indications could

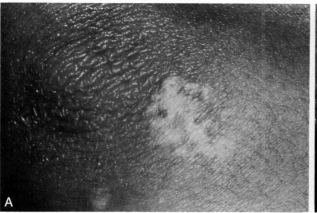
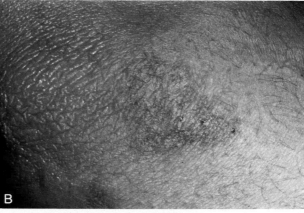

Figure 33–10. Vitiligo in white skin before *(A)* and after *(B)* cosmetic tattooing.

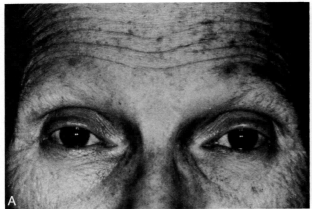
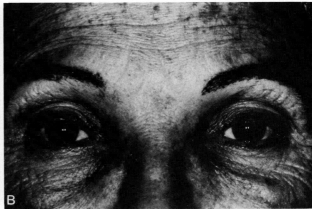
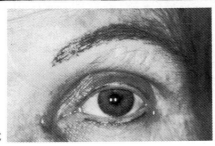

Figure 33–11. *A,* A woman with alopecia universalis before undergoing blephar-opigmentation and eyebrow pigmentation. *B,* Postoperative view. *C,* A close-up view showing left upper eyelid and left eyebrow. (From Patipa M: Eyelid tattooing. Dermatol Clin 5[2]:336, 1987.)

be almost limitless. One unsettled issue is the removal of undesired tattoo pigment. This may be necessary when a patient no longer wants the tattoo or when pigment has been errantly placed by the physician. Although black tattoos, such as those used in radiotherapy, can be expected to respond quite well to ruby laser treatment,[18, 19] it is unclear how ferrous oxide pigment will respond. A mixture of tannic acid in isopropyl alcohol has been used to repair misplaced pigment,[13] but this may not be a practical approach for certain anatomic sites or for treatment of large areas of the body. However, even with this reservation, it is clear that this highly neglected technique should be part of the armamentarium of the cutaneous surgeon.

The author gratefully acknowledges the photographic assistance of the Permark Division of Micropigmentation Devices, Inc., Edison, NJ.

REFERENCES

1. Pauli: Application de tatouage à la cyre des naevi materni. Siebold J 15:1, 1835.
2. Cordier: Cited by Lacassagne A, Magitot E: Dictionnaire Sci Med 95:103, 1886.
3. Schuh: Application de tatouage à la cheiloplastie. Wien Med Wochenschr 8:809, 1858.
4. Kolle, Ferdinand, Strange: Plastic and Cosmetic Surgery. D. Appleton & Co, New York, 1911.
5. Conway H: Tattooing of nevus flammeus for permanent camouflage. JAMA 152:666–669, 1953.
6. Hance G, Brown JB, Byars LT, et al: Color matching of skin grafts and flaps with permanent pigment injection. Surg Gynecol Obstet 79:624–628, 1944.
7. Byars LT: Tattooing of free skin grafts and pedicle flaps. Ann Surg 121:644–648, 1945.
8. Conway H, Docktor JP: Neutralization of color in capillary hemangiomas of the face by intradermal injection (tattooing) of permanent pigments. Surg Gynecol Obstet 84:866–869, 1947.
9. Conway H, McKinney P, Climo M: Permanent camouflage of vascular nevi of the face by intradermal injection of insoluble pigments (tattooing): experience through twenty years with 1022 cases. Plast Reconstr Surg 40:457–462, 1967.
10. Masser MC, Di Meo L, Hobby JA: Tattooing in reconstruction of the nipple and areola: a new method. Plast Reconstr Surg 84:677–681, 1989.
11. Becker H: Nipple-areola reconstruction using intradermal tattoo. Plast Reconstr Surg 81:450–453, 1986.
12. Uyeda LM: Permanent dots in radiation therapy. Radiol Technol 58:409–411, 1987.
13. Angres GG: Micropigmentation of the lips. Am J Cosmet Surg 4:179–185, 1987.
14. Patipa M: Eyelid tattooing. Dermatol Clin 5:335–347, 1987.
15. Halder RM, Pham HN, Breadon JY, et al: Micropigmentation for the treatment of vitiligo. J Dermatol Surg Oncol 15:1092–1098, 1989.
16. Wolfley DE, Flynn KJ, Cartwright J, et al: Eyelid pigment implantation: early and late histopathology. Plast Reconstr Surg 82:770–774, 1988.
17. Goldstein N: Complications from tattoos. J Dermatol Surg Oncol 5:869–878, 1979.
18. Taylor CR, Gange RW, Dover JS, et al: Treatment of tattoos by Q-switched ruby laser. Arch Dermatol 126:893–899, 1990.
19. Scheibner A, Kenny G, White W, Wheeland RG: A superior method of tattoo removal using the Q-switched ruby laser. J Dermatol Surg Oncol 16:1091–1098, 1990.

Topical Tretinoin for the Treatment of Photodamaged Skin

RICHARD B. ODOM

Until relatively recently, patients seeking treatment for a variety of skin conditions induced by sun exposure had only two choices of treatment: palliative topical applications or surgical intervention. In the past few years, however, treatment with topical tretinoin has emerged as a viable third choice.

For nearly 20 years, topical retinoic acid, or tretinoin, has been a valuable drug in the treatment of patients with acne vulgaris. More recently it has been observed that during topical tretinoin therapy, postadolescent females with persistent acne developed smoother, less wrinkled skin. This finding provided the impetus to study topical tretinoin for the treatment of photodamage.

Applied topically, tretinoin is the first drug to demonstrate reversal of many of the cutaneous clinical and structural abnormalities that result from chronic sun exposure. As a result, topical tretinoin has become the medical treatment of choice for initial repair of photodamaged skin. Its efficacy has generated much excitement, not only among cutaneous surgeons, but also among prospective patients, as well as the lay press. As with any new form of treatment, however, realistic goals have to be set, and both objective and subjective parameters must be established to determine the efficacy of treatment. Of course, surgical procedures can still be considered if the results achieved over time with topical tretinoin do not meet expectations. Furthermore, tretinoin should be considered an adjunct, not a substitute, for other cosmetic surgical procedures.

Photoaging

For many years it was believed that the process of photoaging was merely an acceleration of chronologic or intrinsic aging. However, it is now well known that the two processes are qualitatively different. The skin of elderly patients who have minimized their sun exposure remains smooth and unblemished, although it has some loss of elasticity and wrinkling. However, the skin of photodamaged patients exhibits various degrees of structural change, with both fine and coarse wrinkling, mottled hyperpigmentation, roughness, laxity, yellowing, lentigines, and telangiectasia.

These clinical observations reflect profound underlying histologic changes. The qualitative characteristic of intrinsic aging is atrophy: the epidermis is viable but thin, the dermal-epidermal junction becomes flattened, and there is a considerable decrease in dermal thickness.[1] In contrast, the primary characteristic of photodamage is hypertrophy: the skin seems to be in a state of chronic inflammation, and in the final stages of photodamage, the support matrix disintegrates (Table 34–1). Actinic keratoses, solar lentigines, keratoacanthomas, and basal cell and squamous cell carcinomas tend to develop almost exclusively in photodamaged skin.

EPIDERMAL CHANGES

Skin that has been exposed to the sun shows epidermal disorganization, and the epidermis may thicken up to twofold. Keratinocytes lose their typical alignment and develop progressive flattening with accumulation of excessive amounts of melanosome complexes. Melanocytes are also affected, as they enlarge, increase in number, and migrate to higher levels of the epidermis. Furthermore, ultraviolet light (UVL) alters the immunologic capability of epidermal Langerhans's cells by activating T-suppressor lymphocytes and evoking an inappropriate response.[2]

TABLE 34–1. COMPARISON OF INTRINSIC AGING AND PHOTODAMAGE

Feature	Intrinsic Aging	Photodamage
Clinical appearance	Smooth, unblemished surface; some deepening of surface markings; slight loss of elasticity	Nodular, leathery surface with hyperpigmented blotches and yellowing; deep wrinkles; significant loss of elasticity
Epidermis	Thin and viable	Marked acanthosis with cellular atypia
Elastic tissue	Slightly increased	Greatly increased, with degeneration into amorphous mass
Collagen	Thick, disoriented bundles	Marked decrease in bundles and fibers
Glycosaminoglycans, Proteoglycans	Slightly decreased	Markedly increased
Reticular dermis	Thinned; reduced number of inactive fibroblasts; mast cells decreased; no inflammation	Thickened, elastostic; increased, hyperactive fibroblasts; mast cells markedly increased; mixed inflammatory infiltrate
Papillary dermis	No grenz zone	Solar elastosis with grenz zone
Microvasculature	Moderate reduction	Great reduction, with abnormal, ectatic vessels

DERMAL-EPIDERMAL JUNCTION CHANGES

Photodamage results in the loss of rete ridges, which flattens the interface between the epidermis and dermis. This altered abutment is more susceptible to shearing forces than is the normal interlocked system of epidermal rete ridges and dermal papillae,[3] a change that is probably responsible for the characteristic laxity seen in photoaged skin and the easy bruising that occurs with minimal trauma.

DERMAL CHANGES

Photoaging produces the most profound changes in the dermis. Photodamage decreases the capability of dermal cells to divide.[4] Indeed, when cultured cells derived from paired biopsy specimens of sun-protected and sun-exposed skin sites were compared, the cell populations from sun-protected sites doubled in number and proliferated more rapidly than those from sun-exposed sites. In other studies on cutaneous aging,[5] the pathologic changes in actinically damaged skin included excessive depositions of elastotic materials, which appear as massive quantities of thickened, degraded elastic fibers extending into the midreticular dermis.

DERMAL BLOOD VESSEL CHANGES

Dermal vessels in UVL-exposed skin become dilated, twisted, and leaky. They thicken as a result of accumulation of excessive basement membrane–like material.[6]

EVOLUTION OF PHOTODAMAGED SKIN

Skin photoaging occurs very gradually over two to four decades of life, with little early clinical evidence. It is estimated that about 75% of the total lifetime UV radiation dose is accumulated before the age of 20, during a childhood spent outdoors.[7] Histologic deterioration begins with formation of thickened coils of abnormal elastic fibers and clumped aggregates of microfilaments and gradually leads to a breakdown of the connective tissue matrix (Table 34–2).

Assessment

In recent years, numerous studies have been carried out to determine the effect of topical tretinoin. The results obtained are fairly uniform and support the efficacy of this treatment modality. Parameters to assess therapeutic results fall into two categories: clinical and laboratory parameters. Clinical assessment of cutaneous changes focuses on fine and coarse wrinkling, telangiectasia, roughness, and overall skin appearance and is based on physician observations, parallel photographs comparing baseline appearance and treatment results, and patient impressions. Laboratory studies evaluate skin structure by image analysis of surface replicas and laser Doppler velocimetry to objectively measure treatment-induced changes.

LONG-TERM RESULTS

In an initial randomized 16-week double-blind study[8] of 40 patients with photodamage, 14 of the 15 evaluable patients showed global improvement in fine and coarse facial wrinkling, pinkness, and tactile roughness with the use of tretinoin cream. No vehicle-treated patients obtained statistically significant improvement, and neither group showed changes in telangiectasia or dermal edema.

TABLE 34–2. DEVELOPMENT OF PHOTODAMAGE

Stage I	Elastogenesis, hyperkeratosis, hypertrophy, acanthosis, increased blood flow
Stage II	Numerous cavities with dissolution of elastin matrix
Stage III	Dense aggregates of microfilaments with swollen, degenerated fibers
Stage IV	Chronic inflammation, massive dissolution of elastic fibers, loss of collagen, breakdown of connective tissue matrix

After completion of this study, 30 patients continued treatment in an open-label study,[9] using 0.1% or 0.05% tretinoin cream daily or every other day for a total of 22 months (21 patients continued for 10 months, 16 for 22 months). The same evaluation parameters were used, including a 4-mm full-thickness punch biopsy taken before treatment and again after 4, 10, and 22 months of therapy.

The results obtained in the initial 4-month study, particularly for fine and coarse wrinkling and skin texture, were sustained (Fig. 34–1). Most of the clinical changes occurred during the first 6 to 10 months of tretinoin therapy. After 6 months, 71% of discrete lentigines had disappeared. During tretinoin treatment, the skin typically increased in pinkness, causing a healthy, rosy glow in marked contrast to the sallow, yellow skin of untreated patients. Improvement in photodamaged skin initially treated with daily 0.1% tretinoin was effectively maintained with alternate-day 0.05% applications. This improvement persisted for at least 2 months after therapy was stopped and was followed by a gradual, partial regression of photodamage. Adverse effects consisted of episodic peeling, dryness, and erythema. This could be relieved by reducing the frequency of tretinoin use or avoiding application of the medication to the area of reaction for a few days.

Similar clinical effectiveness of topical tretinoin was achieved in a 6-month double-blind study comparing 0.05% tretinoin cream or vehicle cream.[10] The improvement, particularly of fine wrinkles, observed in the tretinoin-treated group was gradual and progressive (Fig. 34–2). Paired photographs taken before and after treatment showed fair to excellent improvement in 95% of patients. Adverse reactions were also similar: during the first 1 or 2 weeks of therapy, 70% of patients experienced mild, transient, patchy dermatitis sometimes associated with mild erythema.

Measurable Effects of Topical Tretinoin

IMAGE ANALYSIS OF SKIN SURFACE IMPRESSIONS

Pre- and post-treatment changes in skin surface topography were determined by a new technique that takes surface casts of the crow's-foot region with a silicone material.[11] Adhesive rings serve to delineate the site at which samples are taken, as well as to provide orientation. The impression material hardens several minutes after being lifted from the skin and is submitted for optical profiling by the Magiscan Image Analyzer, equipment developed by the National Aeronautics and

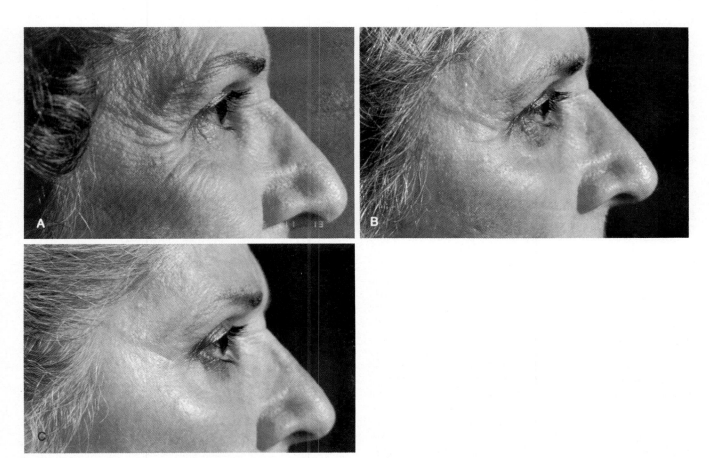

Figure 34–1. *A,* Before tretinoin therapy. *B,* After 6 months, and *C,* after 18 months of tretinoin therapy. (From Ellis CN, Weiss JS, Hamilton TA, et al: Sustained improvement with prolonged topical tretinoin [retinoic acid] for photoaged skin. J Am Acad Dermatol 23:629–637, 1990.)

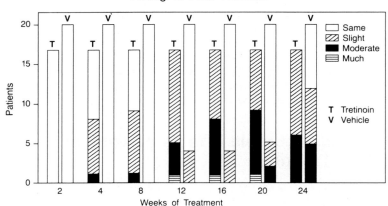

Figure 34–2. Degree of improvement in fine wrinkling as noted by the investigator at various observation points during the treatment period. (From Leyden JJ, Grove GL, Grove MJ, et al: Treatment of photodamaged facial skin with topical tretinoin. J Am Acad Dermatol 21:638–644, 1989.)

Space Administration (NASA) to study lunar landscaping. Three parameters are calculated:

1. Ra, the area of deviation above and below an average line through the center of the profile, which measures fine facial lines.
2. Rz, the average difference between maximal and minimal heights in each of five sections of the profile, which measures deep wrinkles.
3. Shadows, which is a measure of the area of dark shadows.

Application of this technique in a 6-month study[10] showed that the Ra and Shadows parameters were significantly improved in the tretinoin-treated group. This indicated that overall skin topography of tretinoin-treated patients had become smoother and less wrinkled than that of controls, which also correlated with clinical improvement. Improvement in Rz measurements, however, only barely approached significance, suggesting that tretinoin had less effect on major furrows and creases than on fine wrinkles (Fig. 34–3).

HISTOLOGIC EFFECTS

Topical tretinoin has been shown to exert its action on the skin's microscopic structures. In several studies of tretinoin-induced histopathologic changes in skin,[9] the woven pattern of stratum corneum became compacted[12] and homogeneous in appearance in nearly all the samples (Fig. 34–4). After 18 months, the stratum corneum returned to pretreatment conditions, probably signaling the skin's resumption of its function as a physiologic barrier against UVL radiation and water loss. In addition, the average number of cells in the granular layer doubled, and mean epidermal thickness increased by more than one third over the pretreatment value.

Another topical tretinoin study showed that a 14-month topical application abolished atypia and microscopic actinic keratoses.[13] After long-term treatment, the grenz zone was considerably widened and contained more active fibroblasts, a representation of reconstruc-

tion of the papillary dermis (Fig. 34–5). It was concluded that the more photodamaged the skin, the greater was the improvement with topical tretinoin application, resulting in an essentially normal, new epidermis in nearly all patients.

EFFECTS ON CUTANEOUS MICROCIRCULATION

Typically, patients undergoing topical tretinoin application develop a rosy, healthy glow. This finding has been attributed to drug-induced changes in the cutaneous microcirculation and has been supported histologically[13] by an increase in the number and uniformity of newly formed small blood vessels in the superficial dermis (Fig. 34–6). Cutaneous blood flow in the forearm has been measured[14] with laser Doppler velocimetry after a 6-month application of 0.05% topical tretinoin and a placebo. The instrument (Periflux PF3) propagates a helium-neon laser through a fiberoptic cable attached to the skin surface, illuminating a 1.2-mm² area of skin to a depth of 1 mm. The backscattered

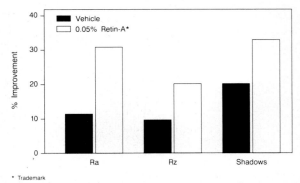

Figure 34–3. Results of computerized image analysis of skin surface impression for roughness and wrinkles. (From Leyden JJ, Grove GL, Grove MJ, et al: Treatment of photodamaged facial skin with topical tretinoin. J Am Acad Dermatol 21:638–644, 1989.)

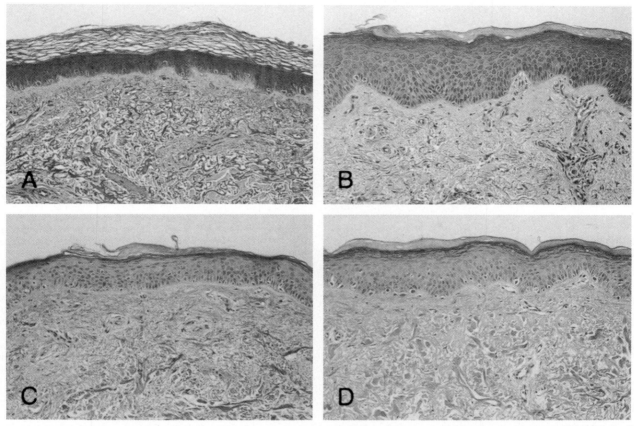

Figure 34–4. Representative photomicrographs of skin from the forearms. *A,* Before therapy, a woven stratum corneum with minimal cytologic atypia in epidermis normal in thickness for the forearm, and moderate elastosis in papillary dermis. *B,* After 4 months of tretinoin therapy, compaction of the stratum corneum, thicker epidermis without cytologic atypia, and slight elastosis in papillary dermis. *C,* After 10 months of tretinoin therapy, findings similar to those after 4 months: thickness of the epidermis greater than that before therapy but less than at 4 months, and slight dermal elastosis. *D,* After 22 months, similar to the 10-month picture but with moderate dermal elastosis. Variability in dermal elastosis is due to individual variation and not the result of therapy; there were no consistent changes in the dermis that could be observed by light microscopy. (H&E stain ×50.) (From Ellis CN, Weiss JS, Hamilton TA, et al: Sustained improvement with prolonged topical tretinoin [retinoic acid] for photoaged skin. J Am Acad Dermatol 23:629–637, 1990.)

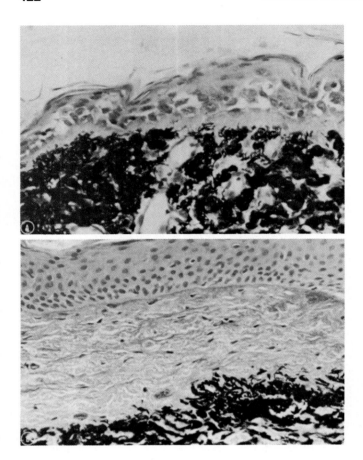

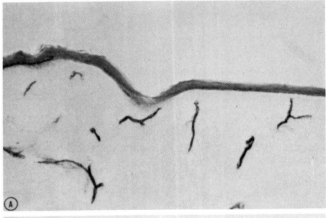

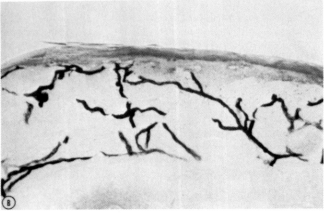

Figure 34–5. Induction of new collagen formation in severely photo-damaged facial skin (Luna stain, original magnification ×400). *A,* Pretreatment. The epidermis is severely dysplastic. Beneath it is a clear band consisting of fine collagen bundles, the so-called grenz zone. Below this, the dermis has been replaced by dense masses of elastotic material in which elastic fibers are in the final stages of degeneration. *B,* After 26 months of tretinoin. The grenz zone has expanded, pushing down the old elastotic material. This widened band of new collagen contains more fibroblasts and has a normal structure. The elastotic material appears unaltered. (From Kligman AM, Grove GL, Hirose R, Leyden JJ: Topical tretinoin for photoaged skin. J Am Acad Dermatol 15:836–859, 1986.)

Figure 34–6. Akaline phosphate staining for small blood vessels of severely photodamaged facial skin (original magnification ×650). *A,* Pretreatment. The vessels are sparse, thin, and irregular. *B,* After 14 months of tretinoin. The microvasculature has expanded greatly; the vessels are broad, branching, and in a more normal distribution. These are mainly venules. (From Kligman AM, Grove GL, Hirose R, Leyden JJ: Topical tretinoin for photoaged skin. J Am Acad Dermatol 15:836–859, 1986.)

light is integrated by a microprocessor into a voltage that corresponds to the motion of red blood cells. After topical tretinoin application, a fivefold increase (compared with the resting state) in the movement of red blood cells was measured. The peak response was also significantly greater than that of untreated skin. In the tretinoin-treated group, but not in the placebo group, the increased circulation was associated with improvement in overall clinical signs of photodamage.

It is believed that this tretinoin-induced increase in the movement of red blood cells is also associated with a greater responsiveness and vulnerability of the skin to other topical agents. Indeed, there is heightened frequency and severity of adverse reactions to substances that were previously well tolerated by some patients who undergo tretinoin therapy.[14]

Topical Tretinoin for Actinic Keratoses

Characterized as clones of anaplastic keratinocytes confined to the epidermis, actinic or solar keratoses occur commonly on sun-damaged skin of elderly people. Left untreated, these lesions may erode through the basement membrane of the epidermal-dermal junction and become invasive squamous cell carcinomas. Data from early studies at the National Cancer Institute indicated that topical tretinoin treatment yielded favorable results in some studies of actinic keratoses but not in others.[15]

More recently, the effect of 0.05% topical tretinoin in 30 patients with actinic keratoses was studied during a 3-month, double-blind study that was prolonged for an additional 12 months as an open study.[16] Punch biopsies of lesional and nonlesional sun-damaged skin were obtained before and after the 3-month treatment, as well as after 9 and 15 months. Three months of treatment proved inadequate to cause any changes in the number of lesions, but 6 months of therapy produced a statistically significant reduction in the number and size of actinic keratoses. After 15 months, the average number of actinic keratoses decreased to 40% of the pretreatment value, and the average lesion size and area decreased to 25%. Improvement was most marked in patients with early actinic keratoses, while those with advanced lesions responded poorly, and a few progressed to invasive squamous cell carcinoma. It is currently believed that topical tretinoin is effective for actinic keratoses in some patients, but further investigation is needed to ascertain its precise role.

Guidelines for the Management of Photodamage

Effective topical tretinoin therapy requires an individualized approach based on the extent of skin damage. Photodamage is estimated clinically by such parameters as fine and coarse wrinkling, skin yellowness and laxity, skin roughness, and lentigines.[7] In addition, skin sensi-

TABLE 34-3. GUIDELINES FOR INDIVIDUALIZATION OF TOPICAL TRETINOIN THERAPY

Patients with greatest sensitivity
1. Fair-skinned, freckled, blue-eyed, Celtic, Scotch, or Irish persons who sunburn easily and tan poorly
2. People with sensitive skin who report stinging after use of perfumes, sunscreens, or astringents
3. People whose faces turn red and feel hot ("flusher-burners") after embarrassment or consumption of alcoholic drinks
4. Middle-aged persons who have been heavy users of cosmetics, skin cleansers, and toiletries and commonly complain of dry skin
5. People with previous skin disorders such as eczema, rosacea, and seborrheic dermatitis

Patients with lowest sensitivity
1. Older persons with advanced photodamage
2. Darker, thick-skinned patients of Mediterranean descent, with larger pores and oilier skin

tivity and a history of exposure to the sun must be considered (Table 34-3).

APPLICATION OF TOPICAL TRETINOIN

Each patient must be carefully instructed in how to apply topical tretinoin effectively. Treatment may be initiated at a low dose of either 0.025% or 0.05%[7] or a higher dose of 0.1%.[17] On retiring at night, patients should be taught to wash their face with a mild soap, pat it dry, and then spread a thin layer of tretinoin over the areas of photodamage on the face, neck, and chest. Small amounts of tretinoin should also be applied with repeated gentle rubbing into wrinkles around the eyes and to the lips as well, particularly in patients with actinic cheilitis and other premalignant lip changes such as leukoplakia. Moisturizers should not be used simultaneously with the tretinoin application because of decreased efficacy. Furthermore, tretinoin's vitamin A acid component is an unstable compound that is incompatible with many fragrances and preservatives.

Patients with sensitive skin should apply tretinoin only every second or third night and gradually work up to daily use. As soon as tretinoin treatment is tolerated on a daily basis, generally within 3 to 4 weeks, the dose can be doubled. If a low tretinoin concentration was used initially, it can be increased. Also, by applying the medication thinly or thickly, patients can control the dosage themselves.

Every attempt should be made to reach the therapeutic dose of 0.1% tretinoin applied daily, as results have been shown to be dose related. All patients should be urged to adhere to an aggressive treatment regimen, adjusting the dose and frequency of application to their individual level of tolerance. Compliance can be checked simply by the frequency with which prescriptions are refilled. Because one tube lasts about 1 month, patients who refill their prescription every 3 or 4 months are not using the proper dose. Because patients can best determine their own level of tolerance, they should be encouraged to become active participants in the treatment program. Some strong-willed patients tend to go through the initial irritation period without dose reduction, while others need a more gradual adjustment with application every second or even every third night.

MAINTENANCE THERAPY

Maximal clinical benefit is usually obtained after 8 to 12 months of treatment at the highest tolerated dose. Thereafter, a maintenance schedule may be initiated with two or three applications a week and continued indefinitely, since skin changes progress inexorably with advancing years. Histologic improvement has occurred, especially after resorption of amorphous elastotic masses, and continues after 4 to 5 years, although cosmetic improvement seems to peak and level out after 2 to 3 years.[7]

SIDE EFFECTS

Patients must be carefully apprised of the side effects of tretinoin and at all times encouraged to continue treatment, despite the presence of such side effects. During the first few weeks, tretinoin causes a variable amount of irritation, which is felt as tightening of the skin and stinging. Irritation is also manifested as mild erythema with dryness and fine scaling that may last for a month or longer. Indeed, mild scaling is a sign that tretinoin is being effectively used.

On washing the face at night, patients who have started tretinoin treatment may find that sheets of stratum corneum, with the consistency of paste, will peel away. A washcloth can be gently used to help remove this scaling skin. When tretinoin is applied near the eyes and mouth, patients should be warned that the corners of the lips and the lateral canthi may become sore and reddened. If tretinoin enters the eye, there may be mucous discharge in the morning and occasionally blurred vision, which will disappear after blinking the eyes until the residue is cleared.[17] Because tretinoin is poorly absorbed, pregnant women need not fear congenital fetal malformation. In 20 years of tretinoin use for acne vulgaris, no fetal malformations have been reported.[7]

REALISTIC THERAPEUTIC EXPECTATIONS

Before beginning tretinoin treatment, patients should be asked about their therapeutic expectations so that realistic treatment goals can be set. This will also help to avoid later disillusionment or discontinuation of therapy. In general, patients with the greatest degree of photodamage can expect to see the greatest response. Most patients with yellow or sallow skin will rapidly develop a rosier glow, a result perceived as aesthetically pleasing. In time, fine wrinkling will disappear,[18] although coarse wrinkling may persist in some patients. Lentigines will also disappear, and the skin will become smoother and lose its initial laxity[18] as firmness increases. Parallel photographs taken before and after 3 or 6 months of therapy can help to provide objective comparisons.

THERAPEUTIC "DO'S" AND "DON'TS"

Tretinoin therapy should always be supplemented with daytime use of moisturizers and sunscreens. Because tretinoin dries the skin, a moisturizer should be applied every morning after washing the face. Greasy or heavy moisturizers such as petroleum jelly are often the most effective. Younger persons, however, may prefer lighter preparations (i.e., lotions rather than creams). Moisturizers that contain DNA, RNA, placenta extracts, or growth factors should be avoided, as should those with antiaging or skin-rejuvenating claims.

Sunscreens are recommended to protect the skin from further photodamage, particularly as tretinoin thins the stratum corneum, diminishing the physiologic barrier of the skin. Products with a sun protection factor (SPF) of at least 15 should be used and applied repeatedly when patients perspire, swim, or bathe. Those with fair skin and who burn easily and tan poorly should use a sunscreen with an SPF of 30, while patients living in tropical or subtropical areas should consider using a sunscreen with an SPF of 50.

Women who develop self-induced irritable skin as a result of long-term use of toiletries and cosmetics should be asked to discontinue all soaps and cosmetic treatments for at least 2 weeks before the start of topical tretinoin therapy. All harsh soaps, astringents, toners, peelers, and cleansers should be discontinued as well. Makeup used during tretinoin therapy may be removed only with warm water and by gently rubbing the fingers against the face.

Patients taking large doses of vitamins should be counseled to decrease this practice, since dry skin often results from large daily doses of vitamin A. Tretinoin is compatible with almost all oral drugs except photosensitizers such as thiazide, tetracycline, and chlorpromazine.[7]

RECOMMENDED DOSAGE AND FORMULATION

Tretinoin currently is supplied in numerous concentrations and formulations (Table 34–4). The type of vehicle is extremely important in predicting the likelihood of irritation. Gels are more irritating, because the vehicle is volatile and produces more dryness. For this reason, gels are best used in hot, humid areas, since they may prove too irritating to be used in dry northern climates.

Many younger patients prefer gels because they leave no residue and are compatible with almost any makeup.[7] Older persons with oily, thick, pigmented skin can typically tolerate both the gels and the solution. The

TABLE 34–4. TOPICAL TRETINOIN FORMULATIONS AND CONCENTRATIONS

Formulation	Concentration
Cream	0.025%, 0.05%, 0.1%
Solution	0.05%
Gel	0.01%, 0.025%

solution is most appropriate as spot therapy for focal lesions such as actinic keratoses. However, it is easiest to start treatment with creams, which provide a good compromise for most patients.

SUMMARY

Tretinoin is the first drug that has demonstrated the ability to reverse many of the clinical and structural cutaneous abnormalities caused by photodamage. Not only does tretinoin application improve the overall skin condition, it also tends to normalize the microscopic structures by measurably reducing wrinkle depths, mottled pigmentation, roughness, and laxity[18] and enhancing cutaneous microcirculation. It can also have a positive psychosocial effect.[19] Indeed, the more photodamaged the skin, the more apparent will be the tretinoin-induced changes. Topical tretinoin has also proved of value for some patients with actinic keratoses.

On the basis of these results, many cutaneous surgeons now routinely prescribe topical tretinoin for patients with photodamaged skin. The ensuing popular acceptance and endorsement of this medication have made it an important therapeutic approach to photodamaged skin. However, topical tretinoin does not preclude or eliminate the use of some surgical procedures employed for correcting the signs of aging or photodamage.

It is important to note that Retin-A, currently the only topical tretinoin available in the United States, is not approved by the Food and Drug Administration for treatment of photodamaged skin. Other products specifically designed and approved for treatment of photodamage, but with fewer side effects than Retin-A, are likely to become available in the relatively near future.

REFERENCES

1. Kligman AM, Lavker RM: Cutaneous aging: the differences between intrinsic aging and photoaging. J Cutan Aging Cosmet Dermatol 1:5–11, 1988.
2. Sunlight, ultraviolet radiation, and the skin: National Institutes of Health Consensus Development Conference Statement, May 8–10, 7:1–27, 1989.
3. Lavker RM: Structural alterations in exposed and unexposed skin. J Invest Dermatol 73:59–66, 1979.
4. Gilchrest BA: Prior chronic sun exposure decreases the life span of human skin fibroblasts in vitro. J Gerontol 35:537, 1980.
5. Uitto J, Fazio MJ, Olsen DR: Cutaneous aging: molecular alterations in elastic fibers. J Cutan Aging Cosmet Dermatol 1:13–26, 1988.
6. Lavker RM, Kligman AM: Chronic heliodermatitis: a morphologic evaluation of chronic actinic dermal damage with emphasis on the role of mast cells. J Invest Dermatol 90:325–330, 1988.
7. Kligman AM: Guidelines for the use of topical tretinoin (Retin-A) for photoaged skin. J Am Acad Dermatol 21:650–654, 1989.
8. Weiss JS, Ellis CN, Headington JT, et al: Topical tretinoin improves photoaged skin: a double-blind vehicle-controlled study. JAMA 259:527–532, 1988.
9. Ellis CN, Weiss JS, Hamilton TA, et al: Sustained improvement with prolonged topical tretinoin (retinoic acid) for photoaged skin. J Am Acad Dermatol 23:629–637, 1990.
10. Leyden JJ, Grove GL, Grove MJ, et al: Treatment of photodamaged facial skin with topical tretinoin. J Am Acad Dermatol 21:638–644, 1989.
11. Grove GL, Grove MJ, Leyden JJ: Optical profilometry: an objective methodology for quantification of facial wrinkles. J Am Acad Dermatol 21:631–637, 1989.
12. Bhawan J, Gonzalez-Serva A, Nehal K, et al: Effects of tretinoin on photoaged skin: a histologic study. Arch Dermatol 127:666–672, 1991.
13. Kligman AM, Grove GL, Hirose R, Leyden JJ: Topical tretinoin for photoaged skin. J Am Acad Dermatol 15:836–859, 1986.
14. Grove GL, Grove MJ, Zerweck CR, Leyden JJ: Determination of topical tretinoin effects on cutaneous microcirculation in photoaged skin by laser Doppler velocimetry. J Cutan Aging Cosmet Dermatol 1:27–32, 1988.
15. Peck GL: Topical tretinoin in actinic keratosis and basal cell carcinoma. J Am Acad Dermatol 15:829–835, 1986.
16. Balin AK, Lin AN, Pratt L: Actinic keratoses. J Cutan Aging Cosmet Dermatol 1:77–86, 1988
17. Goldfarb MT, Ellis CN, Weiss JS, Voorhees JJ: Topical tretinoin therapy: its use in photoaged skin. J Am Acad Dermatol 21:645–650, 1989.
18. Weinstein GD, Nigra TP, Pochi PE, et al: Topical tretinoin for treatment of photodamaged skin: a multicenter study. Arch Dermatol 127:659–665, 1991.
19. Gupta MA, Goldfarb MT, Schork NJ, et al: Treatment of mildly to moderately photoaged skin with topical tretinoin has a favorable psychosocial effect: a prospective study. J Am Acad Dermatol 24:780–781, 1991.

CHAPTER 35

Revision of Acne, Traumatic, and Surgical Scars

TIMOTHY J. ROSIO

Though with great difficulty I am got hither
to arrive where I am
My marks and scars I carry with me,
to be a witness for me . . .
JOHN BUNYAN, *THE PILGRIM'S PROGRESS*

Progress, man's distinctive mark alone,
Not God's and not the beasts':
God is, they are,
Man partly is and wholly hopes to be.
ROBERT BROWNING

S cars are the inevitable testimony of living and being injured, but the result of this reparative process is varied, individual, and full of contradictions. Depending on the culture, a scar may be regarded as a badge of courage, a source of pride, or an embarrassing blemish. Even though they are the natural consequence of living, scars are often viewed paradoxically, and because of this, many people have contradictory opinions of scars and may find difficulty in accepting them.[1] Robert Browning's poem,[2] "A Death in the Desert," accurately captures our dissatisfaction and hunger for perfection.

Ultimately, many patients and cutaneous surgeons alike are required to deal philosophically with those scars that cannot be effectively changed and revise those scars that can be improved. The basis of scar revision was adequately described by the theologian Archbishop Stephen Langton, who admonished his followers to "bend what is stiff, warm what is cold, guide what goes off the road."[3] In that light, cutaneous surgeons are often charged with the task of modifying scars to make them more aesthetically pleasing.[4]

At times unsatisfactory scars are not revised because the surgeon may be ignorant of new scar revision mo-dalities, there may be doubt as to the anticipated scar outcome, or it may be hoped that the patient will learn to accept the deformity, that gradual improvement will occur spontaneously as the scar matures, or that the patient will seek treatment elsewhere, since his or her expectations are greater than what the surgeon can expect to achieve.[5]

Approach to the Patient with a Scar

DEFINITION OF SCARS

The average patient may not be able to precisely define a scar but knows that it looks bad and has caused a change in his or her appearance. The patient's own subjective opinion will constitute the standard for judging success or failure of any procedure. It is important that the surgeon prepare the patient for the result of scar revision by describing the procedure as an attempt to modify, adjust, reposition, improve, or remedy the scar.

Scars are discerned by their size; their deviations in contour, tension, color, texture, pattern, and direction; and how well they blend in with the surrounding skin. Useful descriptive terms for the clinical analysis of scars should include location, direction with respect to the relaxed skin tension lines (RSTLs), level (elevated, depressed, or atrophic), maturation (mature, hypertrophic, or keloidal), color (hypo- or hyperpigmented), texture, shape (trapdoor, web, stellate, linear), length, and width.

BIOCHEMICAL CHANGES ASSOCIATED WITH SCARS

Histologically, a cutaneous scar is fibrous tissue (collagen) usually formed as a local response to traumatic, surgical, or inflammatory injury of the skin. Misconceptions about the nature of scar tissue are common. Some assume that all raised red scars are abnormal or that keloids simply represent excess scar tissue. However, it has been established that specific biochemical changes are associated with scar tissue production, breakdown, and maturation over time and are influenced by tension, genetics, and age.

Young normal scars have an increased proportion of type III collagen content relative to older normal scars, which have, in turn, slightly more type III content compared with normal skin. This young collagen is further characterized by hydroxyallysine cross-links similar to embryonic collagen. Normally this collagen matures with cross-linkages derived from allysine or is degraded. However, hypertrophic and keloid scars fail to follow the time-related maturation of normal scars, instead maintaining increased proportions and total content of embryonic collagen and fibronectin. This indicates a continued rapid turnover of the collagen.[6, 7]

Hypertrophic scars may exhibit mild to marked thickening indicative of a greater total amount of collagen. Differences in peptide and cross-linkages result in less extensibility.[8] Hypertrophic scars often improve without treatment, but this may require years. Two thirds of sternotomy scars in children remained hypertrophic at 1 year, and one fourth remained hypertrophic for a mean period of 5.5 years.[9] Keloids are also characterized by increased quantities of collagen. By definition, they extend beyond the wound margins and do not spontaneously resolve. Surgical cure rates are much poorer for keloids than hypertrophic scars, and the response varies markedly by anatomic location and from individual to individual.

Of vital importance is the interplay between local tissue tension, scar tissue formation, maturation, and scar tension production. Above a certain tension threshold, fibroblasts secrete more collagen and orient fibrils relative to the force placed on them.[10] Scar tissue creates additional tension because of the tendency for scars to condense and contract as they mature. This tension is associated with the elasticity of surrounding skin. Such tension may oppose scar maturation resulting in a hypertrophic scar. The contractile force may become directional in a scar with linear elements and is transmitted locally. These forces are equal on both sides of the scar, parallel to it, and gradually diminish with distance from the scar.[11] The net result can vary from a nearly invisible scar without local distortion to a prominent one with great deformity, depending on the degree and direction of these forces and the extensibility of the surrounding skin and local landmarks. Evaluation of these factors can help determine which surgical approach should be considered for scar revision to relieve tension and facilitate formation of a scar that will mature normally.

OBJECTIVES OF SCAR REVISION

The goal of scar revision is to obtain a more aesthetically pleasing and better functioning scar (Table 35–1). While this can be accomplished in some cases, in other instances the appearance of a scar may be partially sacrificed for an improvement in function. For example, this is often the case when extensive Z-plasties are performed to relieve a contracture, resulting in a greatly lengthened, more flexible, but more noticeable scar. The two major factors that are always beyond the surgeon's control in scar revision are the anatomic location and the amount of tissue that has been lost as a result of trauma or disease. However, two factors that can be controlled are the direction the scar follows in relation to the RSTLs and the uninterrupted straight length of the scar.[5]

The primary objectives in scar revision are to disguise incisions in hair-bearing areas whenever possible, improve scar direction in relation to both RSTLs and anatomic or cosmetic junctions, redirect tension to eliminate distortion of anatomic landmarks, lengthen or add elasticity in a particular direction, eliminate elevations and depressions, narrow widened scars, break scars into smaller components to make them less noticeable, and camouflage scars by surgical homogenization of color and texture through dermabrasion, planing, cross-hatching, or other adjunctive techniques. The techniques used to achieve these objectives must be atraumatic and aimed at maintaining an ideal wound healing environment.[12]

GENERAL APPROACH TO SCAR REVISION

A thorough evaluation is required to analyze the individual patient and scar, as well as to choose the most appropriate revision technique (Table 35–2).

Determining What Bothers the Patient

Understanding the patient's dissatisfaction with a scar will help develop a better relationship and allow a more efficient discussion of the treatment alternatives. It will also guide the cutaneous surgeon in assessing the patient's expectations and ability to comply with the required postoperative wound care, which is vital to obtaining a good result. Patients often have higher initial expectations for scar revision than commonly can be achieved.

TABLE 35–1. **SCAR REVISION OBJECTIVES**

Hide scar
Improve scar direction
Redirect tension
Level contours
Narrow scar width
Shorten linear components
Camouflage scar

TABLE 35–2. SCAR REVISION TECHNIQUES

Invasive surgical methods
  Fusiform scar revision (FSR) and serial excision
  Z-plasty
  W-plasty
  Geometric broken line excision
  Punch excision and elevation
  Punch excision and graft replacement
  Excision and flap coverage
  Dermabrasion or laserbrasion
  Laser (carbon dioxide, Nd:YAG) excision of keloids
  Skin grafts (full- or split-thickness)
  Planing
Noninvasive methods
  Laser photothermolysis of telangiectasia
  Dermal augmentation with filler substances
  Silicone gel sheeting
  Exogenous electric current
  Compression
  X-ray therapy
  Medications (see Table 35–6)

Psychological and Physical Considerations

To obtain a good result, the patient must be physically and psychologically capable of complying with the postoperative instructions. Factors such as skin texture, pigmentation, healing characteristics, age, health, and nutritional status all may influence the outcome. The patient must be aware of the influence of these factors before the operation. The patient should also be aware that fine skin texture with few adnexal structures often heals with a thinner, finer initial scar than thicker skin. However, thick skin with many adnexa will often improve far more than thin skin from camouflaging procedures such as dermabrasion. While hyperpigmentation usually improves over many months, hypopigmentation is more often a permanent side effect.

Categories of Scars

Although descriptive characteristics of scars often overlap, they remain very important in categorizing the cicatrix (Table 35–3). These characteristics include contour, color, shape, length, width, and direction. A fundamental task is to distinguish between mature and

TABLE 35–3. DESCRIPTIVE CATEGORIES OF SCARS

Contour
  Elevated
  Hypertrophic
  Keloid
  Atrophic or spread
  Depressed linear
Color
Shape
  Curved or trapdoor
  Web
  Stellate
  Linear
  Ice-pick or pitted
Length
Width
Direction

immature scars, hypertrophic and keloid scars.[13] While the age of the scar may be helpful, appearance and sensation are often more reliable indicators, since individual and local factors may sustain hypertrophic scars for years.

Contour. Elevated mature scar tissue (Fig. 35–1) typically results from healing of wounds under tension; bevelled or oblique incisions that contract diagonally to produce an overhang of tissue; apposition of skin with markedly different dermal thicknesses, resulting in a step-off deformity; and trapdoor scarring with an elevation of the central normal tissue surrounded by a semicircular scar.

Thickened scars caused by high wound tension (e.g., a large deltoid scar) are unlikely to be improved by surgical scar revision attempts.[14] A zigzag, thickened scar may be even more noticeable, and dermabrasion may produce a scar that is more irregular and larger than before surgery. Steroid injections are most often used to induce local atrophy in thickened scars. Scars that result from inadequate wound support, poor wound conditions, or inadequate postoperative care may be improved by scar revision.[9, 15, 16]

Poorly apposed wounds or those resulting from angled incisions normally develop contracture of the maturing

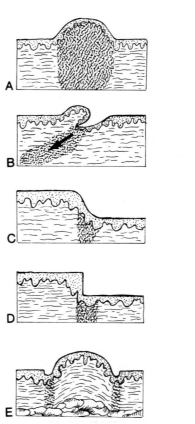

Figure 35–1. Cross section of elevated scars. *A,* Increased scar tissue from healing of wounds under tension. *B,* Elevated scar tissue shelf resulting from diagonal contracture of a bevelled or oblique incision. *C,* Elevated scar shelf from apposition of skin with markedly different dermal thickness. *D,* Scar step-off caused by apposition at different levels. *E,* Trapdoor scar effect in which an elevation of normal tissue is produced by a semicircular scar contracture.

Elevated Scars: Cross Sections

oblique scar, leading to an overhanging shelf of tissue and surface irregularities. These scars may be improved by dermabrasion or planing with a safety razor.[17–19] Dermabrasion or planing frequently results in central hypopigmentation, peripheral hyperpigmentation, telangiectasia, and pore pattern abnormalities when 1 mm or more of tissue is removed.[20] Excision with precise closure of elevated scars resulting from poor initial coaptation is indicated if such excision can be accomplished without excessively increasing wound tension.

Options used to correct marked differences in dermal thickness include running W-plasty or broken-line closure scar revision techniques to graduate the level differences. Incision and graduated thinning of the thicker wound edge for 1 cm away from the suture line may also help. Dermal filling substances or fat grafting to the thinner side are other potential solutions.

Trapdoor tissue elevations are caused primarily by circumferential wound contraction in semicircular incisions. Trapdoor scars can be greatly improved by performing Z- and W-plasties along the outer margin. The Z-plasty has a greater leveling effect than W-plasty, which provides a smoother broken line effect for longer incisions. Both may be combined in the same scar. The trapdoor scar can also be improved with wider peripheral undermining and thinning of the excess tissue at the margin.

Hypertrophic Scars. If a scar is hypertrophic, the cause must be evaluated.[13] The age of the scar is also very important. Because mildly thickened, young, normal scars will likely improve spontaneously in 6 to 12 months, they are often best left untreated or treated very cautiously with low concentrations of intralesional steroids. Correctable causes such as poor scar orientation can be improved with use of Z-plasties. If excision is contemplated, placement of permanent buried sutures to decrease wound tension can sometimes narrow the scar and decrease the risk of reformation. However, in areas of high tension such as the presternum and deltoid, revision is frequently unsuccessful.

Keloid Scars. Keloids are often treated with pressure, steroid injections, and infrared lasers such as the carbon dioxide and neodymium-yttrium-aluminum-garnet (Nd:YAG) lasers combined with periodic steroid injections and close follow-up for a minimum of 6 to 12 months.

Atrophic or Stretched Scars. Atrophic redundant skin caused by local or regional volume loss secondary to weight reduction, resolved hemangioma, or other cause may easily be revised using standard principles of excision and closure. Atrophic tissue resulting from second-intention wound healing under tension or hypertrophic scars previously injected with corticosteroids are at much greater risk for hypertrophic scar formation if excised.

Stretched or Spread Scars. Stretched scars are wide scars that often exhibit atrophy. They often form in mobile areas such as the chest, arm, back, and neck, as well as relatively fixed areas such as the scalp. Prolonged wound support during the critical period of scar maturation can result in narrower and less depressed scars. This may be accomplished with use of permanent buried sutures such as nylon or polypropylene. Scalp reduction scars were found to be 76% wider after 3 months in patients whose wounds were closed in layers using buried absorbable sutures compared with those whose wounds were closed with buried polypropylene sutures.[21] In a similar study, excisional scars on the upper arm were 37.5% narrower using buried nonabsorbable sutures. It was noted that 80% of the stretching occurred during the first 6 months after surgery.[22]

Permanent anchoring or tethering sutures should be placed at least 5 to 10 mm away from the wound margin and as deeply as possible. The advancing wound margin or flap is pulled into position with the suture, and the anchoring site is adjusted for some stretch relaxation. Fixation may be through both halves of the dermal incision or from one side tethered to the periosteum, perichondrium, or deeper scar layers (Fig. 35–2A). The suture is tied securely and the ends trimmed short. Additional temporary support may be provided with skin hooks (Fig. 35–2B) or temporary skin sutures while the final epidermal sutures are placed. This technique is also valuable in preventing landmark distortion, since deeper fixed structures support the tissue tension. Occasionally, permanent buried sutures will "spit" as they undergo transepidermal elimination. When the use of permanent buried sutures is judged inadvisable, a running mid-dermal subcuticular suture may be a useful

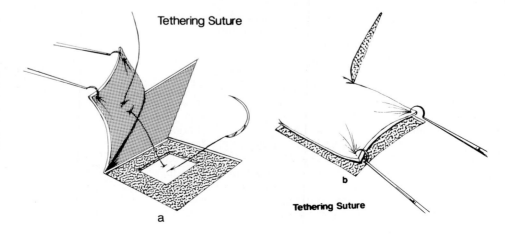

Figure 35–2. Tethering or anchoring suture. *A,* A tethering suture is placed at least 5 to 10 mm away from the wound margin. Fixation may be through both halves of the dermal incision or from one side tethered to the periosteum, perichondrium, or deeper scar layers. The suture is tied securely and the ends trimmed short. *B,* Additional temporary support may be provided with skin hooks or temporary skin sutures while final epidermal sutures are placed.

Depressed Scar Elevation by Advancement

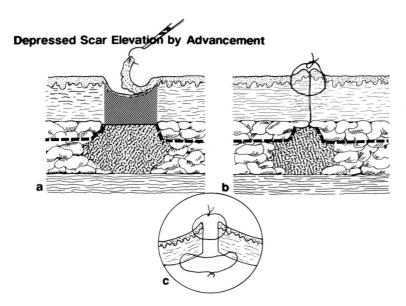

Figure 35–3. Revision techniques for depressed scars. *A,* Deepithelialization and removal of the superficial scar is followed by undermining *(dashed lines). B,* Advancement of two adjacent skin flaps over the residual scar bulk to correct depression. *C,* Prolonged tissue support is important to avoid stretched and depressed scar formation. (From Lewin ML, Keunen HF: Revision of the posttracheotomy scar. Correction of the depressed, retracted scar. Arch Otolaryngol 91:395–397, 1970. Copyright 1970, American Medical Association.)

alternative. If the suture is removed at 3 weeks, one study showed there was 25.7% greater narrowing of the scar, which compared favorably with techniques using absorbable layered closure or permanently buried suture.[22]

Depressed Linear Scars. Depressed linear or geometric scars may occur when early wound healing conditions are less than ideal (e.g., hematoma formation or wound infection). Recontouring may be achieved by tissue augmentation and dermabrasion, planing, or laser vaporization. Punch graft excision and transplantation, usually reserved for pitted scars and hair transplant revisions, have been described for depressed linear scars from flap and excisional surgery as well. Two sessions with 1- to 2-mm grafts spaced one graft apart are placed in the scar line and leveled 6 weeks after the last session.[23]

Moderate scar depression commonly results from antitension line scars or other incisions closed under tension. Use of the Z-plasty is a classic technique to elevate such depressed scars and release tension. However, this technique does produce some tissue irregularities, which tend to improve over time. Use of the W-plasty sacrifices some tissue but produces less irregularity. If there is an antitension line component to the depressed scar, either a Z- or W-plasty may be specifically indicated.[24]

Depressed scars may result from deep injuries with loss of subcutaneous fat. Contracted fibrous tissue may adhere to fascia, periosteum, or perichondrium. Innovative techniques (Fig. 35–3) for revising depressed scars include rotation of subcutaneous transposition Z-flaps beneath the suture line[25, 26]; overlapping leaves of directly advanced subcutaneous flaps[27]; and deepithelialization of the scar, followed by undermining and advancement of two adjacent skin flaps over the residual scar tissue for bulk.[28] Useful modifications to further raise the vertical height of the scar include tubing (Fig. 35–4) or trifolding (Fig. 35–5) the central scar,[29] plication of the scar island,[30] and undermining of the scar tissue

in two separate layers to allow offset of deep and superficial scar line closure.[31] Scar tissue plication (Fig. 35–6) may also benefit scar revision by reducing tension on the wound edges in a fashion similar to that used for fascial plication.[32] Contraction of the deep tissue by the suture reduces tissue drag and compression of the advancing superficial flaps without tension. This reduces stretching forces that can compromise the vascular supply and ultimately lead to spread and depressed scars.

Color. Immature scars generally become less red and

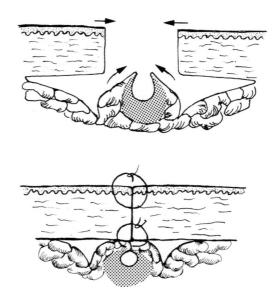

Depressed Scar Elevation by Tubing

Figure 35–4. Depressed scar elevation by scar tubing. A scar can be elevated by undermining the scar island laterally and tubing it. (From Lewin ML, Keunen HF: Revision of the posttracheotomy scar. Correction of the depressed, retracted scar. Arch Otolaryngol 91:395–397, 1970. Copyright 1970, American Medical Association.)

DEPRESSED SCAR ELEVATION BY SCAR FOLDING

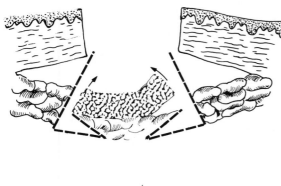

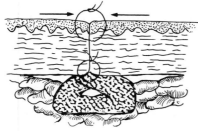

Figure 35–5. Depressed scar elevation by scar folding. A scar can be elevated by undermining the scar island laterally and folding it. (From Lewin ML, Keunen HF: Revision of the posttracheotomy scar. Correction of the depressed, retracted scar. Arch Otolaryngol 91:395–397, 1970. Copyright 1970, American Medical Association.)

Depressed Scar Elevation by Plication

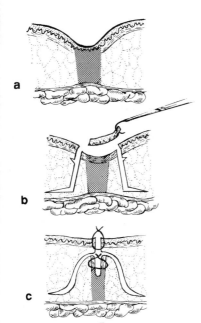

Figure 35–6. Depressed scar elevation by plication. *A*, Appearance of the initially depressed scar. *B*, Plication of the scar island is done with small incisions made within the dermis. *C*, Eversion of the wound edges is facilitated. (From Regnault P, Daniel RK: Depressed scars and soft tissues. Ann Plast Surg 10:427–436, 1983. Reprinted with permission.)

pale with maturation over 1 to 3 years. However, hypertrophic and keloid scars are exceptions because of continuing collagen turnover of embryonic type.[6] Older scars that are red in color may be caused by telangiectasia, epidermal atrophy, or both. Dye lasers, emitting 577 to 585 nm yellow light, can lighten these scars. A solitary blue line within a mature scar may represent an ectatic vein, which may be treated with sclerotherapy or laser photocoagulation.

Shape. The shape of a scar consists not only of its contour but also of other elements that create several different types of patterns. One of the more common patterns is caused by a pursestring effect on semicircular incisions resulting in contracture that causes a trapdoor scar (Fig. 35–7). Small trapdoor tissue elevations may sometimes be excised completely with fusiform scar revision. Otherwise, an optimum result is usually achieved with Z- or W-plasties (Fig. 35–8) performed along the outer margin.[33–36] A zigzag line in the form of darts added to the lateral portion of perioral full-thickness skin grafts have greatly reduced secondary pursestring deformity after burn scar revision.[37] Wider undermining peripheral to the trapdoor flap may also help oppose reformation of a trapdoor deformity. The proposed mechanism for this effect is an outward-pulling contraction force that offsets the inwardly directed forces. In treatment of trapdoor scars, Z-plasty has a greater leveling effect than W-plasty, while W-plasty accomplishes a smoother broken line effect for longer incisions. Both may be combined in the same scar to balance these features.

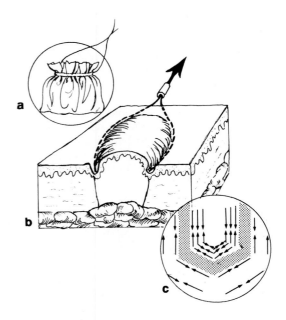

Trapdoor Scar Formation

Figure 35–7. Trapdoor scar formation. *A*, A pursestring effect causes trapdoor tissue elevation primarily by circumferential wound contraction in semicircular incisions. *B*, Linear contractive forces along numerous tangents are condensed within the confines of the circular flap, pulling tissue toward the center. *C*, Surgery interrupts and redirects these centrifugal forces.

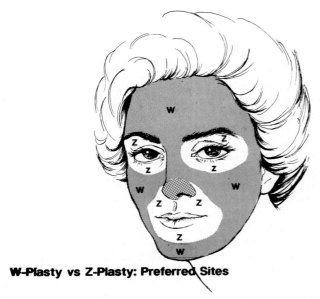

W-Plasty vs Z-Plasty: Preferred Sites

Figure 35–8. Preferred sites for W- or Z-plasty. Scars over broad concave expanses such as the forehead, chin, and cheek benefit from W-plasty, while the normal landmarks around the nose, eyelids, and lips are easily distorted by scars, and Z-plasties are the treatment of choice. (From Borges AF: Principles of scar camouflage. Facial Plast Surg 1:181–190, 1984.)

Scar Types

Web scars occur across concavities created by a bridge effect caused by scar contracture. The Z-plasty is most often the technique of choice for revision, as the additional tissue introduced will allow conformation to the anatomic depression. However, the W-plasty has been used advantageously for web scar revision in the narrow confines of the epicanthal area, with less scarring and canthal distortion encountered than with other techniques.[38]

Small stellate scars are often the result of a sharp, penetrating injury. These most often may be revised with a fusiform excision aligned with the RSTLs. Short linear scars, 2 cm or less in length and close to RSTLs, are usually best revised by fusiform excision. Moderate-length scars, however, are best treated with a zigzag

closure unless they closely parallel the RSTLs. The Z-plasty (Fig. 35–9) is optimum in areas of greater tension (Fig. 35–10) and when the scar's direction is up to 35 degrees from the RSTLs. Stairstep W-plasty is advised for scars 35 to 60 degrees off the RSTLs and the standard W-plasty for 60- to 90- degree inclined scars.

If ice-pick or pitted scars lie within a wrinkle line, punch removal is performed while applying traction perpendicular to RSTLs. On broad convexities such as the cheek, punch removal followed by punch graft transplantation from postauricular donor sites and dermabrasion is commonly recommended.[39, 40]

Length. Small scars are usually amenable to fusiform scar revision (FSR) with placement in RSTLs. This simple approach is preferable unless anatomic landmark distortion results. Medium-length scars may be broken into smaller components easily, without sacrifice of additional tissue, by Z-plasties, which relieve tension and achieve a leveling effect. Longer scars with minimal tension can be treated by any of the zigzag closures. However, the revision may be less noticeable after revision by W-plasties or geometric broken line (GBL) closure owing to fewer surface depressions and elevations. Longer scars with significant tension may require Z-plasties, perhaps in combination with a W-plasty or GBL closure, to avoid increased tension.

Width. Wide scars are usually an indication of significant tension in primarily closed wounds. A study comparing abdominal wounds closed with taping with those closed with regular skin sutures showed wider scars with taping alone.[41] If causation is attributable to unfavorable direction relative to RSTLs, zigzag scar revision may improve both the tension and the appearance of the scar. Prolonged dermal support after excision has been shown to produce narrower scars.[13, 21, 22] One method to minimize spread scars of the back is to narrowly excise the lesion and allow second-intention healing. This results in considerably smaller and narrower scars than traditional excision, undermining, and layered closure.[42] Wide scars that run close to the RSTLs or form as a result of significant tissue loss or muscle action are less likely to benefit from revision attempts and may even worsen.[14, 43]

Direction. Relatively linear scars that parallel RSTLs or lie close to cosmetic unit boundaries are usually best

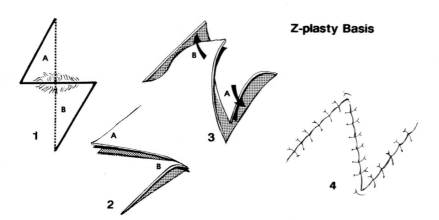

Z-plasty Basis

Figure 35–9. Z-plasty basis. The central limb defines the direction of lengthening and coincides with the long axis of the scar; the dashed line joining the equal lateral limbs defines the new central limb orientation; the equal limbs define two isoceles triangles (A and B), which are undermined; the transposed triangles are secured with interrupted and three-point sutures.

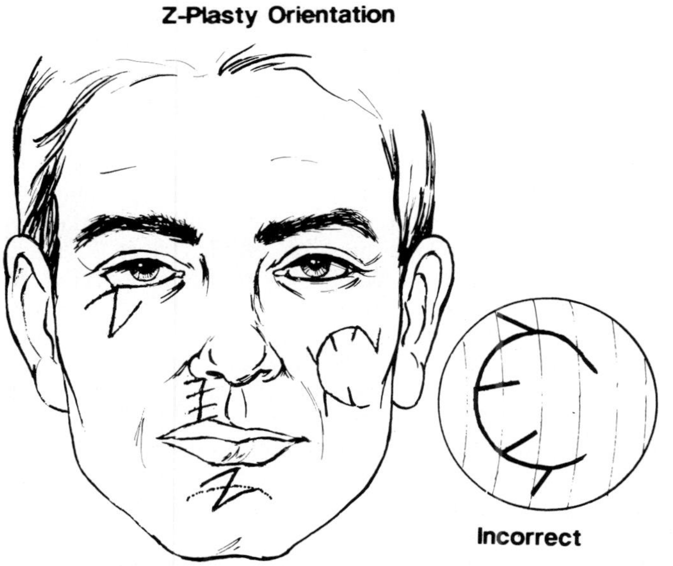

Z-Plasty Orientation

Figure 35–10. Z-plasty orientation. Two orientations are possible for the lateral limbs, with closest alignment to relaxed skin tension lines (RSTLs) being preferable. Note that the eyelid Z-plasty after transposition will place the central limb coincident with natural infraorbital crease. The chin Z-plasty will place the final central limb in the natural mentolabial crease. The upper lip serial Z-plasty places terminal incisions coincident with the vermilion border and the inferior alar-labial boundary crease.

treated by FSR, especially when the length is up to 2 cm or contraction is unlikely to distort important landmarks such as the eyelids, lip, or nose.[20] Scars that run perpendicular to RSTLs or in antitension lines (ATLs) are best revised with W-plasty. Oblique scars should be revised[4] with Z-plasty when inclined 35 degrees from the RSTLs, with stairstep W-plasty when inclined from 35 to 50 degrees, and with W-plasty when inclined from 60 to 90 degrees.

Regional and Local Factors Affecting Scar Revision

Location. Favored sites for less conspicuous scarring after revision include the eyelids, the preauricular area, and the forehead. Unfavorable sites include the distal nose, chin, chest, shoulders, back, and legs. Influences recognized as chiefly responsible for these local scarring differences are tension, skin thickness, and number of sebaceous glands.[44] The surgeon should also be aware of scar proximity to cosmetic units, anatomic boundaries, and adjacent available skin. Scars parallel to RSTLs that do not distort anatomic landmarks are usually best revised with linear techniques. ATL scars over broad concave expanses such as the forehead, chin, and cheek benefit from W-plasty and GBL closure. The nose, eyelids, and lips are easily subject to distortion from ATL scars and Z-plasties are usually the treatment of choice.[4] The lateral submandibular area is notable for its tendency to form hypertrophic scars, which may be difficult to treat even when applying proved scar revision principles.

Local Skin Tension. More than any other factor, wound tension influences the quantity and character of scar tissue.[10] The fact that mature scars are relatively unaffected by such stress provides the basis for scar revision and early scar management (from weeks to 12 months) with tension-relieving sutures and dressings, steroids, pressure, support, and immobilization.[45] By simply reducing wound tension, hypertrophic scar tissue will substantially convert to a normal scar, both chemically and histologically, within 14 days.[46]

RSTLs. Determining the best elective incision line is of paramount importance in scar revision. The likelihood of producing a thin, small scar is greatest when the incision line is parallel with respect to RSTLs, intermediate when oblique to RSTLs, and least when perpendicular to RSTLs. Simultaneously, the likelihood of hypertrophic scar formation is inversely related to the degree to which the incision line parallels the RSTLs.[47] When performing complex scar revisions with lines at varying angles, it is recommended to place as many of the incisions as possible within or close to RSTLs (Fig. 35–11).

Multiple investigators have proposed elective incision skin lines that deviate slightly from one another and the recognized RSTLs, including the best known ones variously derived by Langer, Cox, Rubin, Kraissl, Straith, and Bulacio. The cutaneous surgeon may therefore choose a natural wrinkle line or a muscle contraction line to orient a planned incision. RSTLs are defined by pinching relaxed skin and observing furrows and ridges that form on either side. These ridges and furrows extend for a greater distance when pinching at right angles to the RSTLs.[48]

Previous Treatment. Adjacent scars or radiation changes near the contemplated scar revision should

Figure 35–11. Nasolabial Z-plasty placement. A, The limbs of the Z-plasty are drawn so that lengthening will release the upper lip; the dashed line coincides with the nasolabial crease. B, The contracted scar elevating the right upper vermilion is incised, the flaps are undermined and transposed. C, The completed single Z-plasty releases the upper lip, and coincides with RSTLs. D, A running Z-plasty accomplishes same objective with smaller broken line.

Nasolabial Z-Plasty Placement, Serial Z-Plasty

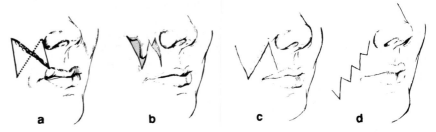

a   b   c   d

always be carefully considered. Extensive scars reduce both the vascularity and the ease of transposition and increase the chance of flap necrosis. The means of reducing tip necrosis include curving the angled limbs of the Z-plasty,[49] delaying the flaps,[50] and substituting tapes for sutures.[51]

Timing

The optimal time to revise a scar varies with the physician. Some advocate immediate revision, whereas others treat only fully mature scars unless there is a functional problem or landmark deformity. Proponents of the delayed revision technique point to the spontaneous softening, fading, and flattening that occur that often yield acceptable results.[52–55] Because children less than 7 years of age show slower scar maturation and a greater tendency for hypertrophic scars, a minimum delay of 6 months is strongly preferred in these patients.[4, 5] However, a study of sternotomy scars in very young children showed that the younger the child at operation, the better the scar result.[9] There is a trend toward earlier scar revision in adults and older children, with claims that a delay of only 4 to 8 weeks yields optimum results.[4, 56] Proponents of early scar revision note that reepithelialization over the scar is more uniform, and maturation may proceed more rapidly in the revised scar. It may also be better psychologically for some patients to have immediate revision performed so that their self-image may be restored to normal as soon as possible.

Scar Revision Techniques

HISTORICAL ASPECTS

While the first attempt at scar revision is unknown, significant progress has certainly occurred over a period of several hundred years. References to early transposition flaps usually document the early work performed by Hindus for nasal mutilation repair. The first published use of the Z-plasty was by Horner in l837.[57–59] Ombredanne is credited with explaining W-plasty excision and mobilization of tissue to treat constricting band scars in 1937. In 1969, Webster described a broken-line technique that he had been working on for many years. The technique randomly introduced triangles and rectangles to the W-plasty and has since been known as the GBL closure.[60]

In the 1950s and l960s, mathematical analysis and engineering models were used to obtain greater precision, predictability, and progress in surgical results.[11, 61–63] However, limitations in applying these nonextensile models have been demonstrated in experimental studies of human Z-plasty flaps in which measured variation in length gains were from 16% less to 27% greater than predicted.[64] Furthermore, in a Z-plasty study on dogs, actual gains in length were always less than mathematically predicted, ranging from 28 to 45% less than calculated.[65] Although Z-plasties and other flaps may provide a solution to a difficult closure,[66] they may also be a cause of a closure dilemma.

ZIGZAG SCAR REVISION TECHNIQUES

FSR and Serial Excision

Serial FSR takes advantage of the gradual expansion capabilities of skin and may be combined with other scar revision and camouflaging techniques.[67] Modifications to the standard fusiform excision can be regularly used in successful scar revision. Curvilinear variations of the fusiform shape may be employed to enhance incision placement in RSTLs or to better parallel an anatomic boundary. To narrow a scar and prevent depression, placement of permanent or absorbable sutures 1 cm away from the incision line will provide superior support and eversion. Unequal undermining and the use of a tethering suture can also be used to decrease wound tension and reduce anatomic distortion. Use of an M-plasty along with the FSR can spare additional normal tissue. More importantly, from an aesthetic standpoint the length of the continuous line is shortened, the more complex scar has a camouflaging effect, and the Y-V flap movement may also have a leveling effect.[68, 69]

Z-Plasty

The geometric basis of the Z-plasty is transference of available tissue to the central axis of a scar to lengthen it, leading to contraction in the lateral axis and a shifting of wound tension approximately 90 degrees (Fig. 35–9). A Z-plasty is accomplished by a transpositional exchange of two triangular flaps after undermining beyond the extent of the flaps to obtain closure with minimal tension. The triangles share a common central limb, which is generally equal to the length of their lateral limbs.[70] The position of the new central limb of the Z after flap transposition will coincide with an imaginary line that connects the two free ends of the Z. Tension-relieving interrupted sutures are placed along the sides of the transposed triangles before placing three-point (half-buried) tip stitches. With this technique, the scar tissue is divided longitudinally, and each half is relocated to a different position in the incision. This technique also provides a conservation of tissue and a reduction in tension. Although the scar line becomes three times longer after Z-plasty, the lengthening achieved with 60-degree angles may only approach 73%, the practical maximum for the technique.[62, 65, 71]

The design, planning, and placement of the incisions for performing a Z-shaped transposition flap require an understanding of the optimal direction and length of the central limb, the angles of the lateral limbs, the ideal length and number of the lateral limbs, the direction the lateral limbs should face, and whether the scar should be merely incised or excised.

Direction and Length of the Central Limb. The lengthening in a Z-plasty coincides with the direction of the central limb (see Fig. 35–9). The gain depends on both the length of the central limb and the angles of its lateral triangles. A linear scar or the direction of desired extensibility will define the direction of the central limb (see Fig. 35–11). In a broad scar, the central limb is placed in the ATL or perpendicular to the RSTLs. One example of applying Z-plasty for a narrowed orifice can be found in the gynecologic literature,[72] where patients with introital stenosis caused by lichen sclerosis et atrophicus were effectively treated with peripheral Z-plasties.[73] Note the similarity of this application to revision of a trapdoor scar (see Fig. 35–10).

In another sizing consideration, not only will the lengthening in a Z-plasty usually be less than calculated, but shorter Z-plasties will show even less than proportional lengthening compared with longer Z-plasties. For 60-degree Z-plasties in which 75% lengthening is calculated, actual values were closer to 50% gain for an 8-cm Z-plasty compared with a 30% gain for a 1-cm Z-plasty. As the lateral limb angles increase, so does central limb lengthening and tension of closure. For each increase of 15 degrees in both lateral limb angles, there is a theoretical increase in length of 25% along the central limb of the Z (Table 35–4). In practice, 60-degree triangle flaps are used as the common upper limit for Z-flap size as a result of both an exponential increase in tension with larger angles (seven to ten times that of smaller angles) and marked tissue distortion.[65] Angles of less than 30 degrees yield little lengthening and leveling benefits, although the scar may be broken up and made less noticeable.

Number and Size of Z-Plasties. Multiple Z-plasties may be combined serially to produce less tissue distortion and less tissue contraction and tension.[74] Also, because each lateral limb is shorter than a single large limb, serial Z-plasties may be used where a standard Z would run into an adjacent anatomic structure. Furthermore, smaller oblique limbs result in a less conspicuous broken-line scar. Smaller Z-plasties are preferred on the face for these reasons, with recommended central limb lengths ranging from 1 to 1.5 cm. Segments shorter than 1 cm may result in irregular furrows.[4] Nevertheless, segments as short as 5 mm are preferred to achieve a very narrow broken line in areas such as the upper lip. The main disadvantage to numerous smaller serial Z-plasties is the difficulty and loss of some lengthening

TABLE 35–4. Z-PLASTY LENGTHENING WITH CHANGING LIMB ANGLE

Lateral Limb Angles (degrees)	% Lengthening
30	25
45	50
60	75
75	100

compared with a single Z-plasty of the same central limb length.

Orientation. After drawing the central limb of the Z, two different orientations are possible for the lateral limbs. After transposition, the new lateral limbs will lie parallel to the old one and will extend from the opposite side of the reoriented central limb. Another way to visualize the position of the completed Z-plasty is to reverse the initial Z and rotate it 90 degrees. Because the lateral limbs will retain their orientation after transposition, the original limb incisions should be aligned as closely as possible with RSTLs or natural boundary lines (see Fig. 35–10). For precise planning, it should be realized that the real rotation is slightly less than 90 degrees and the end points and suture lines will be different than originally planned.[75] However, an improvement in incision line orientation with respect to the RSTLs may be obtained (Fig. 35–12) owing to the elastic properties of skin.

Incision or Excision of the Scar. The decision to excise or incise existing scar tissue depends both on the anticipated tension and the appearance of the original cicatrix. Excision of the scar will inevitably result in less lengthening and greater closure tension. This potentially reduces the planned flap length that may be transposed. Thickened scars will often show notable clinical and biochemical improvement once they are repositioned in RSTLs.[46, 76] This supports the concept of an incisional approach to Z-plasties whenever possible.

Variations on the Standard Z-Plasty. Several varia-

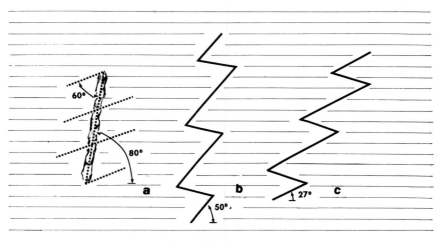

Figure 35–12. Running Z-plasty: calculated versus actual. Because of the elastic properties of skin, lateral limbs calculated to lie at 50 degrees to RSTLs actually assume a 27-degree orientation. (From Borges AF: Scar analysis and objectives of revision procedures. Clin Plast Surg 4:223–237, 1977.)

Running Z-Plasty: Calculated vs Actual

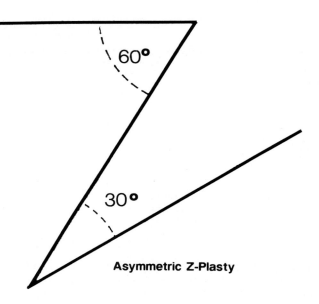

Asymmetric Z-Plasty

Figure 35–13. An asymmetric Z-plasty has unequal angles formed by its lateral limbs to the central trunk. This results in lengthening that is intermediate between 60-degree–60-degree and 30-degree–30-degree symmetric Z-plasties.

tions on the standard Z-plasty technique can be advantageously used in select circumstances to provide better results in scar revision.

Asymmetric Z-Plasty Flaps. Asymmetric Z-plasty flaps may be used to better fit a Z-plasty into restricted areas (Fig. 35–13). Lengthening is comparable to an average of two symmetric flap angles of similar sizes.

Z-Plasty Trunk-to-Limb Ratio. The most commonly described technique for performing Z-plasty specifies that the trunk and limbs should be of equal length.[49] However, the trunk of the Z can be made 22% or more longer than the limbs when treating a contracture.[63, 70] The rationale for this is that the incised contracture or trunk of the Z undergoes more shortening than the corresponding limbs. The relative lengthening of the trunk offsets this inequality and decreases the puckering and protrusion. If disproportionate shortening is not encountered, greater distortion will occur.

Planimetric Z-Plasty. This variation eliminates standing cones and depressions produced by the standard Z-plasty. The planimetric design utilizes a greatly shortened trunk-to-limb ratio and removal of triangles of skin before transposition of flaps (Fig. 35–14). The main advantages of this variation are plane adjustment to the body surface, shorter scars, removal of scarred skin areas, and 28% greater efficacy.[77, 78] The primary application is in the treatment of large planar surfaces where surface irregularities would be obvious after standard Z-plasty. The main disadvantage of this modification may be an increase in tension perpendicular to the long axis of the scar.

Double Z-Plasty of Spaeth. In this modification, two Z-plasties are joined at the ends of their central trunks, unlike the standard serial Z-plasty joining the lateral limbs (Fig. 35–15). This modification is primarily utilized for the repair of congenital epicanthal folds and for

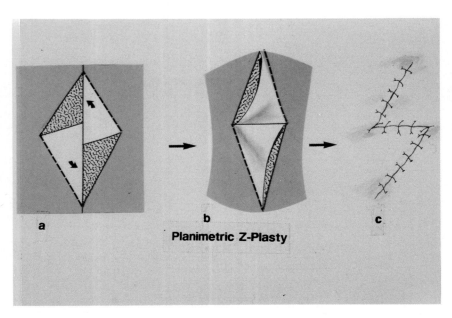

Planimetric Z-Plasty

Figure 35–14. The planimetric Z-plasty utilizes a greatly shortened trunk-to-limb ratio and removal of triangles of skin before transposition of flaps. This variation prevents surface elevations and depressions seen in the standard Z-plasty caused by flap traction and compression forces. (From Roggendorf E: The planimetric Z-plasty. Plast Reconstr Surg 71:834–842, 1983.)

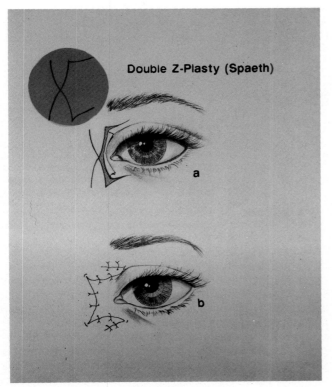

Figure 35-15. Double Z-plasty (Spaeth procedure). *A,* Two Z-plasties are joined at the ends of their central trunks. *B,* Two flaps of tissue from the nasal aspect are transferred closer to the canthus, thus inserting more tissue to line the concavity. (From Field LM: Repair of a cicatricial epicanthal fold by a double Z-plasty [Spaeth]. J Dermatol Surg Oncol 8:215–217, 1982. Reprinted by permission of the publisher. Copyright 1982 by Elsevier Science Publishing Co., Inc.)

revision of inner canthal scars. This dual Z-Plasty transfers two flaps of tissue from the nasal aspect closer to the canthus to flatten the raised fold of tissue.[79] A reduction in closure tension can be achieved by decreasing the medial limb angle. However, this will also narrow the medial flap pedicles. Use of a running W-plasty or Z-plasty should be considered before choosing this method for web scar revision.

Four-, Five-, and Six-Flap Z-Plasty. These variations are used for revision of web scars, especially those found on the hand and foot web spaces (Fig. 35–16). The original Z-plasty design was based on standard 90-degree–90-degree angles. In this modification, the 90-degree angles are bisected, which results in four 45-degree angle flaps. The six-flap variation has two additional 45-degree flaps added, one to each end of the zigzag incision line. These flaps are interdigitated and sewn into place. The main advantage is greater lengthening than is possible with the standard 60-degree–60-degree angle Z-plasty. The use of 45-degree angles also reduces tension compared with the 90-degree Z-plasty technique.[80, 81] The double-opposing Z-plasty is another modification sometimes used to relieve interdigital web scars.[82, 83] The V-W plasty, also known as the five-flap Z-plasty, is used to revise scars on concavities such as the neck, dorsum of the hand or antecubital or popliteal fossae. It is particularly useful when Y-V advancement is desired for relief of contracture. In addition, removal of considerable tissue is a possibility with this technique. In this technique, a Y-shaped incision is flanked by two triangular excisions, which results in three adjacent flaps straddling the forked limbs of the Y. All three flaps are advanced and closed.[49, 84]

W-Plasty

The geometric basis for the running W-plasty is a bilateral advancement flap with angulated leading edges. When used in scar revision, the scar tissue is excised with multiple juxtaposed triangles; this results in a zigzag line closure (Fig. 35–17). Undermining is performed 5 to 10 mm beyond the extent of the flaps as needed for closure with the least possible tension. For speed and simplicity, a continuous running, locked, chromic suturing technique sequentially secures all tips on one side of the incision to its corresponding groove. After crossing over to the opposite side, all contralateral tips are

Figure 35-16. Four-flap Z-plasty. The original design of Limberg is based on standard 90-degree–90-degree angles. *A,* The 90-degree angles are bisected at the dashed lines, which results in four 45-degree-angle flaps. *B,* These flaps are then interdigitated and sewn into place to provide greater lengthening and reduced tension. (From Woolf RM, Broadbent TR: The four-flap Z-plasty. Plast Reconstr Surg 49:48–51, 1972.)

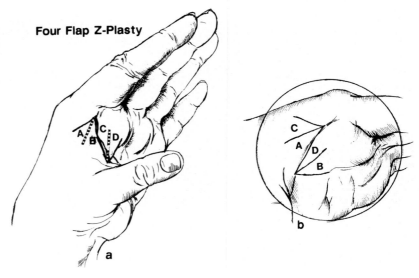

Running W-Plasty Basis

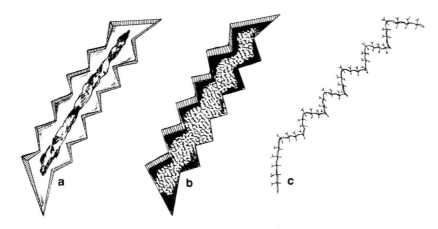

Figure 35–17. Running W-plasty basis is a bilateral advancement flap with angulated leading edges. *A,* Excision of the scar in the shape of multiple triangles. *B,* Repeating tip angles of 55 to 60 degrees are cut into both sides. *C,* The angles match and fit in a tongue-in-groove fashion, resulting in a zigzag line closure. (Adapted from Jackson IT: Local Flaps in Head and Neck Reconstruction. CV Mosby, St. Louis, 1985, p 28.)

likewise secured.[85] A more meticulous and time-consuming closure utilizes horizontal mattress sutures placed 1 cm or more away from the incision line. Then a running subcuticular suture is placed halfway between the tip and base of each individual triangle. Finally, individual three-point, half-buried, or simple interrupted sutures are used to secure the tips. The horizontal mattress and tip sutures are commonly removed at 5 days and the running subcuticular at 9 days.[86]

The functional basis for the W-plasty is the addition of multiple force vectors oblique to the original unfavorable ATL scar. The net contraction vector is greatly reduced, because it is perpendicular to the direction of the original scar (Fig. 35–18), which favors the creation of a satisfactory appearing scar.[87] Lateral tissue advancement provides modest lengthening of the original scar line through a Y-to-V movement and produces a leveling effect.

Another feature of the W-plasty is improvement that occurs as a result of disruption of the deeper scar tissue so that this deeper tissue no longer coincides with the superficial scar tissue. This displacement of the deep and superficial scar components has a leveling effect that improves scar depression. The zigzag line of the W-plasty is complex by virtue of its numerous shorter subunits, which bestows greater extensibility over the original linear scar.

Compared with Z-plasty, the W-plasty causes no tissue rotation but provides less lengthening and fewer leveling effects and results in additional tension perpendicular to the original scar line. Because the W-plasty does not cause tissue protrusion or depression typically seen with the Z-plasty, it may offer a smoother end result over broad planar surfaces such as the cheek and forehead. The W-plasty also produces a regular zigzag line that the eye recognizes with greater difficulty than a straight line.

Proper construction of a W-plasty requires an exact

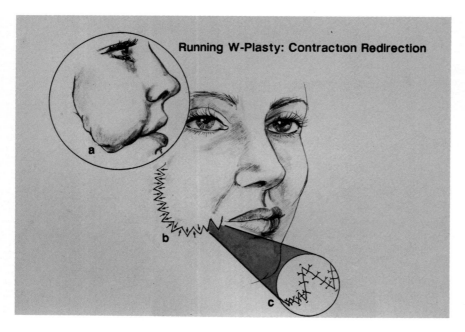

Running W-Plasty: Contraction Redirection

Figure 35–18. Running W-plasty. *A,* Multiple force vectors are substituted obliquely to the original unfavorable anti-tension line (ATL) scar. *B,* The net scar tissue contraction vector is greatly reduced and is perpendicular to the direction of the original scar. *C,* Z-plasties may be incorporated in a W-plasty wherever greater lengthening or leveling is desired.

determination of the limb size, angles, number of sub-units, and orientation. The direction and length of a W-plasty is usually determined by the scar that it encompasses. If only a portion of the scar needs revision, W-plasties may be performed only on the unsatisfactory segment. W-plasty limbs on the face should preferably be 4 to 7 mm in length and slightly larger elsewhere.[67, 86] Shorter segments may fail to accomplish the desired extensibility in the long axis of the scar but provide superior scar camouflage in critical areas such as the philtrum. Longer segments require sacrifice of greater amounts of skin with a concomitant increase in tension. A large W-plasty will also result in a greater tendency to produce dogear deformities at the poles of the incisions.

Cutting of the short angulated incisions of the W-plasty is aided by use of a No. 11 scalpel blade. The use of templates for drawing and measuring or pinking shears to eliminate sketching are often helpful.[88, 89] However, these templates may interfere with ideal incision placement in certain anatomic locations and the shears may produce segments that are too short to provide the necessary extensibility. Furthermore, the uniform 90-degree angles from shears may only be desirable in some stair plasties.[90]

In a standard W-plasty, repeating tip angles of 60 degrees are cut into both sides of the incision so that they will precisely match and fit together in a tongue-in-groove fashion. Lines bisecting these tip angles should remain perpendicular to the long axis of the original scar (Fig. 35–19). If one wound margin should mistakenly lack a triangular flap to equal its counterpart after the incisions have been completed, one flap may be bisected to compensate. Use of stair or step W-plasties for oblique scars inclined from 60 to 35 degrees have progressively larger tip angles up to 90 degrees. The sides of the triangles thus formed have one longer limb placed in the RSTL, and the shorter follows the ATL. A bowstring effect does not result from the many small, discontinuous ATLs.

The more acute the W-plasty angles, the greater will be the reduction in tension in the original scar line. The reduction of tension accomplished by W-plasty may be calculated by the following formula:

$$n = \cos \theta.$$

In this formula, n represents the force vector perpendicular to a side of the W-plasty triangle, and θ represents the angle between n and the spreading force of the original wound scar. An angle of 60 degrees accomplishes a 50% reduction in wound tension.[87] Use of more acute angles further decreases wound tension, but to avoid tip necrosis, these should never be much less than 55 to 60 degrees.

Variations on the standard W-plasty are employed to avoid dogears, obtain greater extension, improve application for curvilinear incisions, and blend better with RSTLs. At the ends of W-plasties, it is advisable to decrease the size of the triangles and make sure the terminal triangles have their bases perpendicular to the long axis of the scar line. Otherwise, an M-plasty or a fusiform excision may be performed at the poles of the W-plasty to reduce dogear formation. FSR at the poles of a W-plasty is advocated to excise the ATL scar created by closure of the distal triangles and to correct dogears.[86] This incision, which lies in the RSTLs, allows tissue movement similar to that of an A-to-T flap. An analogous treatment at the poles of a Z-plasty is used in excision of redundant neck skin that has been colorfully named the "turkey gobbler neck deformity."[91]

One or more Z-plasties may be incorporated in the incision at any point in a W-plasty wherever a greater lengthening or leveling effect is desired. For a mild lengthening effect, each groove of the W-plasty may be extended several millimeters. This enhances compression across the scar line and pushes the ends of the scar outward.[20] Curvilinear segments of scars undergoing W-plasty revision require that the incisions on the inner aspect be made slightly more acute than those on the corresponding outer aspect. Other variations of the W-plasty include the stair plasty and step plasty (Fig. 35–20). These are W-plasties that have one limb that coincides with an RSTL. The stair plasties are more uniform and, although parallel to wrinkles lines, may coincide with them by chance. Conversely, step plasties are made to coincide with active or passive wrinkle lines so as to be less regular and conspicuous in appearance.[88]

In considering scar revision, it should be remembered that scars perpendicular to RSTLs, or in ATLs, are best revised by standard W-plasty. However, a cicatrix up to 15 degrees from the RSTLs may be best treated with

Figure 35–19. Running W-plasty design. The standard W-plasty is used for nearly vertical (60- to 90-degree) scars. *A*, Terminal triangle bases are perpendicular to the long axis of the scar line. *B*, Lines bisecting standard 55- to 60-degree tip angles should remain perpendicular to the long axis of the original scar. *C*, At the ends of W-plasties the size of the limbs should be reduced to 30-degree angles to prevent dogear formation. (From Borges AF: Scar analysis and objectives of revision procedures. Clin Plast Surg 4:223–237, 1977.)

Running W-Plasty: Design

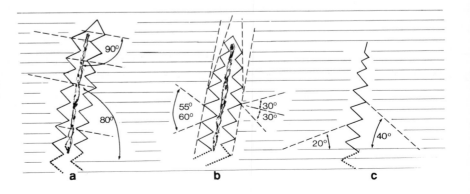

Stair/Step-Plasty Design

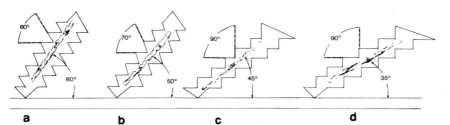

a b c d

Figure 35–20. The stairstep W-plasty is a modified W-plasty used for scars inclined from 35 to 60 degrees that have one limb that coincides with RSTLs. *A,* For scars inclined 60 degrees, the W angles are close to the standard 60 degrees. *B,* For scars inclined 50 degrees, the W angles increase to 70 degrees. *C,* For scars approaching 45 degrees, the W angles increase to the maximum of 90 degrees. *D,* The RSTL limb becomes proportionately longer than the ATL limb. (From Borges AF: Scar analysis and objectives of revision procedures. Clin Plast Surg 4:223–237, 1977.)

FSR, unless it closely borders the mouth, eyes, or nasal orifices. Mildly oblique scars may be revised with Z-plasty when inclined 35 degrees from the RSTLs. However, stairstep W-plasty is advantageous for scars inclined from 35 to 60 degrees and W-plasty for scars from 60 to 90 degrees.[4]

Other uses for W-plasty include performing cosmetic surgery of the glabellar rhytids,[92] removal of excess skin of the extremities,[93] treatment of hyperhydrosis,[94] revision of skin grafts, excision of angular tattoos, and provision of better exposure during surgery on the hand or other sites.[95]

Geometric Broken Line (GBL) Closure

GBL closure, like the W-plasty, is a bilateral advancement flap performed after excision of the scar it encompasses. This technique relies on the principles of zigzag scar revision for the same benefits. GBL closure can be considered a design extension of the W-plasty that can include random geometric shapes such as triangles, rectangles, and parallelograms and can be varied in size (Fig. 35–21). The random nature of the GBL provides better camouflage than the regularly repeating shapes of the W- and Z-plasties. Undermining is performed slightly beyond the base of the flaps to aid in tissue advancement and placement of tension-relieving buried sutures.

The size of various GBL elements varies depending on the shape. However, edges 6 mm long and longer are more readily apparent than edges 3 to 4 mm in length.[67] The smaller size creates less tension but also provides less extension and leveling benefit. The vertical or slightly beveled incisions are made with a No. 11 blade. The lines of GBL elements, known as crossbars, should be placed as parallel as possible to RSTLs. The parallelograms and triangles can have their long limbs placed close to RSTLs and the short limbs oblique to ATLs. Use of GBL templates can provide greater efficiency in planning[96] but may limit the degree of flexibility required to best fit the RSTLs.[97]

The angles of GBL elements follow the same constraints and benefits of W-plasty. Use of 45-degree tip angles produces greater contraction-reducing effects than a 60-degree flap but increases the risk of tip necrosis. When employing very small tips and angles, the extension benefits become minimal. Both Z-plasties and W-plasties may be combined with GBL to achieve the desired mixture of zigzag scar revision features (Table 35–5). For example, repeating triangular flaps are notably easier to use around a curve than rectangular flaps.[98] The terminations of GBL revision should include a 30-degree angle or M-plasty to minimize dogear formation.

Suturing techniques, as for W-plasty, depend on the body area and degree of tension. Permanent or absorbable buried sutures are recommended to relieve margin tension. For speed and simplicity a continuous running, locked 6–0 stitch may be used sequentially on the tips on one side of the incision; then the contralateral tips on the opposite side are likewise secured. A wound with greater tension may also require placement of horizontal mattress sutures 1 cm or more away from the incision line. Running subcuticular sutures are more difficult to place than in a W-plasty, since the very small irregular flap tips present are not especially suited for this suturing technique. Finally, individual three-point or half-buried and simple interrupted sutures may be used to approximate any remaining gaps. Horizontal mattress and any nonabsorbable tip sutures are typically removed at 5 to 7 days postoperatively, although some physicians employ running subcuticular sutures and leave them in place for as long as 21 days.[99]

TABLE 35–5. **SUMMARY OF FEATURES OF SCAR REVISION TECHNIQUES**

Technique	Lengthening	Tissue Sparing	Cosmesis	Distortion
Z-plasty	3+	3+	1+	3+
Planimetric Z-plasty	3+	1+	1+	1+
W-plasty	1+	1+	2+	1+
GBL closure	1+	1+	3+	1+

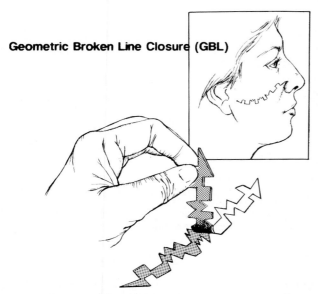

Geometric Broken Line Closure (GBL)

Figure 35–21. Geometric broken line (GBL) closure is a modified W-plasty that makes use of random geometric shapes such as triangles, rectangles, and parallelograms and variations in size of those shapes. The longer limbs of GBL incisions should be made as parallel as possible to RSTLs, the short limbs oblique to ATLs, to encourage favorable scar formation.

Punch Excision and Elevation

Revision of nongeometric, nonlinear, pitted scars resulting from acne, herpes zoster, or chickenpox, respond poorly to most scar revision techniques unless they are large and have soft contoured edges. Leveling procedures alone for deep pitted scars may produce even larger, more unsightly scars. Simple excision and suturing may be beneficial for pitted scars lying in wrinkle lines, but otherwise this technique will leave very noticeable scars.[100]

The technique of punch graft scar revision offers a unique and sound solution for the problem of depressed scars, especially on the face.[101] One modification[39] is based on the original punch elevation technique.[102] Punch transplantation scar revision has the benefit of elevating depressed scars without increasing tension, since full-thickness tissue from a distant site is exchanged for the completely removed pitted scar.[23] Furthermore, the transplanted tissue may be made slightly larger than the removed scar[40] to provide a snug fit. This further decreases tension and minimizes retraction of the graft. Two to 8 weeks following punch transplantation, dermabrasion is performed to blend the suface with the surrounding skin to make the graft clinically invisible or inconspicuous.

The procedure is performed with a simple tissue biopsy or hair transplant punch. The size of the punch is selected so that it is just large enough to encompass the entire pitted scar. The scar is excised completely and the subcutaneous pedicle is cut with scissors (Fig. 35–22). A full-thickness composite graft of nonscarred tissue is cut slightly larger than the defect to replace the scar plug and is held in place for 2 to 5 days with Steri-Strips. The donor plug should fit snugly within the recipient site and remain slightly elevated above the level of the surrounding skin (Fig. 35–23). The donor plug may be cut 0.25 to 2 mm larger than the punch used to remove the scar, depending on local tension. Thinner grafts may be taken from the posterior auricle, while thicker grafts are obtained from the mastoid areas.[103]

Transplanted grafts 4.5 to 5 mm in size may be secured by sutures, thin steel pins, or a small amount of cyanoacrylate glue, as is sometimes done for plugs in hair transplantation. Donor sites larger than 3 mm in size are sutured or allowed to heal secondarily. Sutures are removed after 2 to 5 days for small grafts or after 1 week for larger grafts in mobile areas.

Leveling any elevated grafts by dermabrasion to camouflage them with the surrounding skin can be done as early as 2 weeks after transplantation. Most cutaneous surgeons prefer to wait at least 4 weeks before perform-

Figure 35–22. Pitted scar removal. A biopsy or hair transplant punch large enough to remove the entire pitted scar is selected to narrowly excise it completely down to fat for removal.

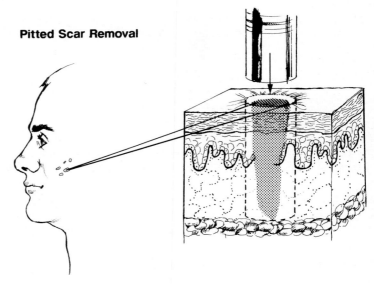

Pitted Scar Removal

Punch Graft Transplant

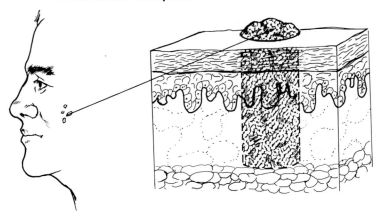

Figure 35–23. Punch graft transplant. A full-thickness composite graft of nonscarred tissue slightly larger than the defect replaces the scar plug, fitting snugly within the recipient site and slightly elevated above the level of the surrounding epidermis to prevent scar contraction.

ing dermabrasion to ensure that the grafts are securely positioned. Multiple approaches to leveling and blending have proven equally successful; these include dermabrasion with diamond fraises or a wire brush, carbon dioxide laser vaporization, and planing or shaving with blades (Fig. 35–24). New adjuncts and refinement of dermabrasion techniques may improve the results.[104] The superficial epidermis immediately around the grafts should be removed for a few millimeters along with the surface of the graft. Reepithelialization yields homogenous color and texture match along with a flat contour. According to one study, abrasion of the donor and recipient sites immediately before transplantation resulted in better healing and improved blending.[105] This is thought to be the result of a horizontal proliferation of keratinocytes that occurs before vertical differentiation and fibrosis of the graft can develop.[106]

Some ice-pick and depressed pitted scars on the face have been improved with pulsed and continuous vaporization using the carbon dioxide laser.[107] However, this technique is best performed only by expert laser surgeons and should be carried out cautiously. Scar, flap,

or graft scar revision by planing may be considered a variation of dermabrasion or carbon dioxide laserbrasion. Planing of scars with scalpels, shaving blades, or dermatomes can be a useful technique for functional or cosmetic reasons. Despite the likelihood of pigmentary and textural changes, planing offers improvement without the risk of producing wide "spread" scars from full-thickness scar removal. While greatly thickened scar tissue is unlikely to show improvement by planing alone, the application of split-thickness skin grafts (STSGs) to the planed scar tissue bed has been reported to provide rapid healing with better color, texture, and a more supple scar than before surgery.[108] Undesirable characteristics of the original hypertrophic scar return when nonmature scars are treated with planing and STSG. Benefits of planing compared with other methods of split-thickness tissue removal include relatively low cost, avoidance of blood aerosols from dermabrasion, ease and speed of setup, and greater uniformity in depth.[17–19, 109] Drawbacks include difficulties with small complex surfaces, visualization problems caused by bleeding, difficulty in blending over large surfaces, and

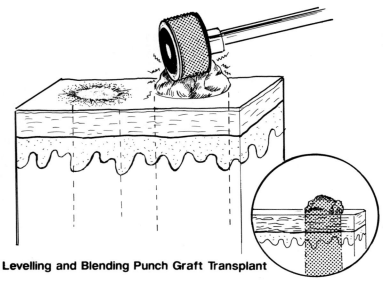

Levelling and Blending Punch Graft Transplant

Figure 35–24. Leveling and blending of the punch graft transplant can be performed with dermabrasion, carbon dioxide laser vaporization, or planing or shaving with blades to remove the superficial epidermis around the grafts down to the papillary dermis.

a high incidence of hypertrophic scarring on areas such as the chest, deltoid, and upper back.[110]

NONSURGICAL ADJUNCTS TO SCAR REVISION

Laser Photothermolysis

Surgically treated skin and some sclerotherapy sites may develop a persistent, cosmetically undesirable blush or matte telangiectasia, even though the scar is otherwise inconspicuous. Similarly, distinct dilated vessels commonly form over prominent scars or stretched skin. Laser photothermolysis of these vessels with the pulsed dye laser is most efficacious in resolving the bright red, indistinct, matte telangiectasia vessels. The larger distinct vessels over scars or stretched skin respond best to argon, tunable dye, and copper vapor lasers.[111]

Dermal Augmentation

Injectable collagen, fat, and silicone play a vital role in temporary and permanent improvement of certain types of scars.

Silicone Gel Sheeting

A silicone gel (Dow Corning X7–9119) has been successfully used in the management of hypertrophic scars. The gel results in softening and thinning of hypertrophic scars more quickly than pressure therapy. The mechanism is unknown but is unrelated to pressure, temperature, oxygen tension, or occlusion, and no silicone enters the tissue.[112–116]

Exogenous Electrical Current

Electrical current stimulation with negative polarity has been shown to stimulate and accelerate wound healing. Studies have confirmed in vivo reduction of scar thickness and hypertrophic scar formation.[117]

Compression and X-ray Therapy

Compression and x-ray therapy may be helpful in the management of keloid scars.

Antiscarring Pharmaceuticals

Many antiscarring pharmaceuticals have been used in research settings (Table 35–6), particularly for keloid management, but some may also prove useful in the future to control or prevent abnormal scar tissue formation.[118, 119] None are considered first-line therapy, and most remain experimental because of variable efficacy and toxicity. The mechanisms of action include nonspecific inhibition of rapidly proliferating cells by the antineoplastic agents; direct antagonism of fibroblast growth curves, as occurs with diphenhydramine[120]; inhibition of collagen production, as seen with colchicine; inhibition of both fibroblast proliferation and collagen production with tretinoin[121, 122]; increased breakdown of

TABLE 35–6. PHARMACEUTICALS THAT ALTER SCARS OR KELOIDS

Antineoplastic drugs
    Nitrogen mustard, thiotepa, methotrexate
Asiatic acid (medecassol)
BAPN
Colchicine
Intralesional corticosteroid injection
Diphenhydramine
Retinoic acid
Tetrahydroquinone
Zinc acid

collagen as a result of stimulated production of collagenase caused by colchicine; and impaired collagen cross-linking by lathyrogenic agents such as BAPN and penicillamine. Further work in this area promises to provide many new and effective alternatives in the surgical management of the healing wound and scar revision.[13, 123–127]

SUMMARY

Analysis of scars before and after surgery remains variable and largely subjective. Objective analytical tools have been slow to progress from the laboratory to the clinic. Examples include wound tonometry and ultrasonography,[128] tensiometry,[129, 130] measures of flexibility and pressure maintenance,[131] and a computerized optical analysis of the skin surface known as optical surfometry.[132] Such tools may help quantify and standardize scar revision results and improve the surgical approach in the future. Likewise, molecular biology is yielding new analytic and potential therapeutic options for the future. By increasing our understanding of scar revision techniques, it will be possible to improve function and simultaneously help patients obtain more aesthetically pleasing scars. Cutaneous surgeons must combine theoretical knowledge, individual patient assessment, experience, judgment, and learned skills to provide the best possible results.

REFERENCES

1. Orwell G: 1984. In: The Oxford Dictionary of Quotations. Book Club Associates, New York, 1984.
2. Browning R: A death in the desert. In: The Oxford Dictionary of Quotations. Book Club Associates, New York, 1980.
3. Langton AS: Quotation. In: The Oxford Dictionary of Quotations. Book Club Associates, New York, 1980.
4. Borges AF: Scar analysis and objectives of revision procedures. Clin Plast Surg 4:223–237, 1977.
5. Borges AF: Timing of scar revision techniques. Clin Plast Surg 17:71–76, 1990.
6. Bailey AJ: Characterization of the collagen of human hypertrophic and normal scars. Biochem Biophys Acta 405:412–421, 1975.
7. Nagata H, Ueki H, Moriguchi T: Fibronectin—localization in normal human skin, granulation tissue, hypertrophic scar, mature scar, progressive systemic sclerotic skin, and other fibrosing dermatoses. Arch Dermatol 121:995–999, 1985.
8. Dunn MG, Silver FH, Swann DA: Mechanical analysis of hypertrophic scar tissue: structural basis for apparent increased rigidity. J Invest Dermatol 84:9–13, 1985.

9. Lista FR, Thomson HG: The fate of sternotomy scars in children. Plast Reconstr Surg 81:35–39, 1988.

10. Weiss JB, Jayson MI (eds): Collagen in Health and Disease. Churchill Livingstone, New York, 1982.

11. Ju M: The physical basis of scar contraction. Plast Reconstr Surg 7:343, 1951.

12. Spicer TE: Techniques of facial lesion excision and closure. J Dermatol Surg Oncol 8:551–556, 1982.

13. Rudolph R: Wide spread scars, hypertrophic scars, and keloids. Clin Plast Surg 14:253–260, 1987.

14. Musgrave RM: The pitfall of surgical excision of vaccination scars in the deltoid area. Plast Reconstr Surg 51:198-199, 1973.

15. Arabi Y, Alexander WJ: Hypertrophic scarring after subcuticular polyglycolic-acid suture. Lancet 1:8066, 1978.

16. Pease R: The incidence of hypertrophic scar formation in wounds closed with subcuticular nylon or polyglycolic acid (Dexon). Br J Plast Surg 29:284–285, 1976.

17. Grabski WJ, Salasche SJ: Razor blade surgery. J Dermatol Surg Oncol 16:1121–1126, 1990.

18. Shelley WB: The razor blade in dermatologic practice. Cutis 16:843–845, 1975.

19. Shelley WB: Epidermal surgery. J Dermatol Surg 2:125–128, 1976.

20. Webster RC, Smith RC: Scar revision and camouflaging. Otolaryngol Clin North Am 15:55–68, 1982.

21. Nordstrm RE: Absorbable versus nonabsorbable sutures to prevent postoperative stretching of wound area. Plast Reconstr Surg 78:186–190, 1986.

22. Elliot D: The stretched scar: the benefit of prolonged dermal support. Br J Plast Surg 42:74–78, 1989.

23. Dzubow LM: Scar revision by punch-graft transplants. J Dermatol Surg Oncol 11:1200-1202, 1985.

24. Adamson PA, Smith OD: Revision of a vertical tracheotomy scar using the W-plasty technique. J Otolaryngol 18:362–364, 1989.

25. Vecchione TR, Pickering PP: The subcutaneous Z-plasty. Case report. Plast Reconstr Surg 56:579–580, 1975.

26. Lewis VJ, Manson PN, Stalnecker MC: Some ancillary procedures for correction of depressed adherent tracheostomy scars and associated tracheocutaneous fistulae. J Trauma 27:651–655, 1987.

27. Harahap M: Revision of a depressed scar. J Dermatol Surg Oncol 10:206–209, 1984.

28. Poulard A: Traitement de cicatrices faciales. Presse Med 26:221, 1918.

29. Lewin ML, Keunen HF: Revision of the posttracheotomy scar. Correction of the depressed, retracted scar. Arch Otolaryngol 91:395–397, 1970.

30. Regnault P, Daniel RK: Depressed scars and soft tissues. Ann Plast Surg 10:427–436, 1983.

31. Toomey JM: Practical suggestions on facial plastic surgery—How I do it. Revision of depressed scars of the head and neck. Laryngoscope 87:826–827, 1977.

32. Dzubow LM: The use of fascial plication to facilitate wound closure following microscopically controlled surgery. J Dermatol Surg Oncol 15:1063–1066, 1989.

33. Marino H: Leveling of linear scars with Z-plasties. Clin Plast Surg 4:239–245, 1977.

34. Webster R, Benjamin R, Smith R: Treatment of 'trap door deformity.' Laryngoscope 88:707–712, 1978.

35. McGregor I: The Z-plasty. In: Fundamental Techniques of Plastic Surgery. Churchill Livingstone, New York, 1980, p 51.

36. Koranda FC, Webster RC: Trapdoor effect in nasolabial flaps: causes and corrections. Arch Otolaryngol 111:421–424, 1985.

37. Neale HW, Billmire DA, Gregory RO: Management of perioral burn scarring in the child and adolescent. Ann Plast Surg 15:212–217, 1985.

38. Mulliken JB, Hoopes JE: W-epicanthoplasty. Plast Reconstr Surg 55:435–438, 1975.

39. Johnson WC: Treatment of pitted scars: punch transplant technique. J Dermatol Surg Oncol 12:260–265, 1986.

40. Solotoff SA: Treatment for pitted acne scarring: postauricular punch grafts followed by dermabrasion. J Dermatol Surg Oncol 12:1079–1084, 1986.

41. Webster DJ, Davis PW: Closure of abdominal wounds by adhesive strips: a clinical trial. Br Med J 3:696–698, 1975.

42. Barnett R, Stranc M: A method of producing improved scars following excision of small lesions of the back. Ann Plast Surg 3:391–394, 1979.

43. Borges AF: Principles of scar camouflage. Facial Plast Surg 1:181–190, 1984.

44. Gunter JP: Revision of scars of the head and neck. Otolaryngol Clin North Am 7:119–131, 1974.

45. Arem A, Kischer C: Effects of stress on healing wounds: intermittent noncyclical tension. J Surg Res 20:93–102, 1976.

46. Longacre JJ: The effects of Z plasty on hypertrophic scars. Scand J Plast Reconstr Surg 10:113–128, 1976.

47. Raju DR, Shaw TE: Results of simple scar excision and layered repair with elevation in facial scars. Surg Gynecol Obstet 148:699–702, 1979.

48. Borges AF: Relaxed skin tension lines (RSTL) versus other skin lines. Plast Reconstr Surg 73:144–150, 1984.

49. Smith JW, Aston SJ (eds.): Grabb and Smith's Plastic Surgery. Little, Brown, Boston, 1991, p 76.

50. Spina V: "Z" plasty. Rev Paul Med 36:347, 1950.

51. Wilkinson TS, Rybka RJ: Experimental study of prevention of tip necrosis in ischemic Z-plasties. Plast Reconstr Surg 47:37, 1971.

52. Lacy GM, Hemphill JE: Facial scar revision. Surg Clin North Am 49:1343–1350, 1969.

53. Farrior RT: Management of lacerations and scars. Laryngoscope 87:917–933, 1977.

54. Martin LW: Observations of the influence of age on wound healing. In: Longacre JJ (ed): The Ultrastructure of Collagen. Charles C Thomas, Springfield, IL, 1976, pp 10–19.

55. Marlowe FI: Early wound closure and late scar revision. Trans Pa Acad Ophthalmol Otolaryngol 31:49–52, 1978.

56. Yarborough J Jr: Ablation of facial scars by programmed dermabrasion. J Dermatol Surg Oncol 14:292–294, 1988.

57. Borges AF: The five single Z-plastics. Va Med 101:618–624, 1974.

58. Borges AF, Gibson T: The original "Z-plasty." Br J Plast Surg 26:237–246, 1973.

59. Borges AF: The enigma of Serre's "Z-plasty" technique. Plast Reconstr Surg 76:472–474, 1985.

60. Borges AF: Historical review of the Z- and W-plasty: revisions of linear scars. Int Surg 56:182–186, 1971.

61. McGregor I: The theoretical basis of the Z-plasty. Br J Plast Surg 9:256, 1957.

62. Limberg A: Planning of Local Plastic Operations on the Body Surface: Theory and Practice. Medgiz, Leningrad, 1963.

63. Limberg A: Design of local flaps. In: Gibson T (ed): Modern Trends in Plastic Surgery. Butterworth, London, 1966.

64. Gibson T, Kenedi R: Biomechanical properties of skin. Surg Clin North Am 47:279–294, 1967.

65. Furnas D, Fischer G: The Z-plasty: biomechanics and mathematics. Br J Plast Surg 24:144–160, 1971.

66. Mandy SH: The practical use of Z-plasty. J Dermatol Surg 1:57–60, 1975.

67. Webster RC: Cosmetic concepts in scar camouflaging—serial excisional and broken line techniques. Trans Am Acad Ophthalmol Otolaryngol 73:256–265, 1969.

68. Davidson T, Webster R, Gordon B: The principles and dynamics of local skin flaps. Am Acad Otolaryngol Head Neck Surg Foundation, Washington, DC, 1988, pp 25–53.

69. Webster RC, Davidson TM, Smith RC, et al: M-plasty techniques. J Dermatol Surg 2:393–396, 1976.

70. Yanai A, Nagata S, Okabe K: The Z in Z-plasty must have a long trunk. Br J Plast Surg 39:390–394, 1986.

71. Wolfe A: Z-plasty. N Engl J Med 292:319–320, 1975.

72. Rankin RJ: The use of Z-plasty in gynecologic operations: case reports. Am J Obstet Gynecol 117:231–232, 1973.

73. Pinkney R Jr: The use of Z-plasty in gynecologic operations: case reports. Am J Obstet Gynecol 117:231–232, 1973.

74. McGregor IA: The Z-plasty in hand surgery. J Bone Joint Surg 49:448–457, 1967.

75. Yanai A, Okabe K, Hirabayashi S: Direction of suture lines in Z-plasty scar revision. Aesthet Plast Surg 10:97–99, 1986.

76. Berry HK: Urinary excretion of collagen degradation products following Z-plasty to hypertrophic scars. In: Longacre JJ (ed): The Ultrastructure of Collagen. Charles C Thomas, Springfield, IL, 1976, pp 285–293.

77. Roggendorf E: Planimetric elongation of skin by Z-plasty. Plast Reconstr Surg 69:306–316, 1982.

78. Roggendorf E: The planimetric Z-plasty. Plast Reconstr Surg 71:834–842, 1983.

79. Field LM: Repair of a cicatricial epicanthal fold by a double Z-plasty (Spaeth). J Dermatol Surg Oncol 8:215–217, 1982.

80. Limberg A: Skin plastic with shifting triangle flaps. Leningrad Traum Inst 8:62, 1929.

81. Woolf RM, Broadbent TR: The four-flap Z-plasty. Plast Reconstr Surg 49:48–51, 1972.

82. Shaw DT: Interdigital butterfly flap (the double opposing Z-plasty). Handchirurgie 4:41–43, 1972.

83. Shaw DT: Interdigital butterfly flap in the hand (the double-opposing Z-plasty). J Bone Joint Surg 55:1677–1679, 1973.

84. Koyama H, Fujimori R: V-W plasty. Ann Plast Surg 9:216–220, 1982.

85. Wolfe D, Davidson TM: Scar revision. In: Roenigk RK, Roenigk HH Jr (eds): Dermatologic Surgery, Principles and Practice. Marcel Dekker, New York, 1988, pp 935–958.

86. Borges AF: W-plasty. Ann Plast Surg 3:153–159, 1979.

87. Fleming JH, Williams HE: Mathematical analysis of the W-plasty and related scar revisions. Clin Plast Surg 4:275–281, 1977.

88. Ship AG, Weiss PR: Colloquium: W-plasty. Ann Plast Surg 3:160–167, 1979.

89. Sokolowich D, Zimman O: W-plasty: make it easy. Plast Reconstr Surg 83:928–929, 1989.

90. Borges AF: W-plasty. Plast Reconstr Surg 83:929, 1989.

91. Cronin TD, Biggs TM: The T-Z-plasty for the male turkey gobbler neck. Plast Reconstr Surg 47:534–538, 1971.

92. Borges AF: W-plastic glabellar rhytidectomy. Br J Plast Surg 23:386–389, 1970.

93. Borges AF: W-plastic dermolipectomy to correct "bat-wing" deformity. Ann Plast Surg 9:498–501, 1970.

94. Borges AF: For axillary hyperhidrosis, W-plastic fusiform excision. Va Med 108:550–552, 1981.

95. Kelleher JC: W-plasty scar revision and its extended use. Clin Plast Surg 4:247–254, 1977.

96. Harnick DB: Broken geometrical pattern used for facial scar revision. Laryngoscope 94:841–842, 1984.

97. Marlowe FI: Broken geometrical pattern used for facial scar revision. Laryngoscope 94:1517, 1984.

98. Webster RC, Davidson TM, Smith RC: Broken line scar revision. Clin Plast Surg 4:263–274, 1977.

99. Wessberg GA, Hill SC: Revision of facial scars with geometric broken line closure. J Oral Maxillofac Surg 40:492–496, 1982.

100. Ellis DA, Michell MJ: Surgical treatment of acne scarring: non-linear scar revision. J Otolaryngol 16:116–119, 1987.

101. Arouete J: Correction of depressed scars on the face by a method of elevation. J Dermatol Surg 2:337–339, 1976.

102. Orentreich N, Durr NP: Rehabilitation of acne scarring. Dermatol Clin 1:405–413, 1983.

103. Stegman SJ Tromovitch TA: Cosmetic dermatologic surgery. Arch Dermatol 118:1013–1016, 1982.

104. Alt TH: Technical aids for dermabrasion. J Dermatol Surg Oncol 13:638–648, 1987.

105. Mancuso A, Farmer G: The abraded punch graft for pitted facial scars. J Dermatol Surg Oncol 17:32–34, 1991.

106. Woodley D, O'Keefe E, Prunieras E: Cutaneous wound healing: a model for cell-matrix interactions. J Am Acad Dermatol 12:420–433, 1985.

107. Garrett AB, Dufresne RG Jr, Ratz JL, Bailin PL: Carbon dioxide laser treatment of pitted acne scarring. J Dermatol Surg Oncol 16:737–740, 1990.

108. Hynes W: The treatment of scars by shaving and skin graft. Br J Plast Surg 10:1–10, 1957.

109. Stal S, Hamilton S, Spira M: Surgical treatment of acne scars. Clin Plast Surg 14:261–276, 1987.

110. Stegman SJ, Tromovitch TA: Benign facial lesions. In: Cosmetic Dermatologic Surgery. Year Book Medical, Chicago, 1984, pp 6–26.

111. Rosio TJ: Matte telangiectasias. In: Apfelberg DB (ed): Atlas of Cutaneous Laser Surgery. Raven Press, New York, 1992, pp 356–358.

112. Ahn ST, Monafo WW, Mustoe TA: Topical silicone gel: a new treatment for hypertrophic scars. Surgery 106:781–786, 1989.

113. Beranek JT: Why does topical silicone gel improve hypertrophic scars? A hypothesis. Surgery 108:122, 1990.

114. Kirn TF: Silicone gel appears inexplicably to flatten, lighten hypertrophic scars from burns. JAMA 261:2600, 1989.

115. Quinn KJ: Non-pressure treatment of hypertrophic scars. Burns Incl Therm Inj 12:102–108, 1985.

116. Quinn KJ: Silicone gel in scar treatment. Burns Incl Therm Inj 14:117–119, 1987.

117. Weiss DS, Eaglstein WH, Falanga V: Exogenous electric current can reduce the formation of hypertrophic scars. J Dermatol Surg Oncol 15:1272–1275, 1989.

118. Cohen IK: Can collagen metabolism be controlled: theoretical considerations. J Trauma 25:410–412, 1985.

119. Cohen IK, McCoy BJ: The biology and control of surface overhealing. World J Surg 4:289–295, 1980.

120. Topol BM, Lewis VJ, Benveniste K: The use of antihistamine to retard the growth of fibroblasts derived from human skin, scar, and keloid. Plast Reconstr Surg 68:227–232, 1981.

121. Daly TJ, Weston WL: Retinoid effects on fibroblast proliferation and collagen synthesis in vitro and on fibrotic disease in vivo. J Am Acad Dermatol 15:900–902, 1986.

122. Janssen de Limpens AM: The local treatment of hypertrophic scars and keloids with topical retinoic acid. Br J Dermatol 103:319–323, 1980.

123. Grierson I: Wound repair: the fibroblast and the inhibition of scar formation. Eye 1:135–148, 1988.

124. Chvapil M, Koopmann CJ: Scar formation: physiology and pathological states. Otolaryngol Clin North Am 17:265–272, 1984.

125. Hogan VM: Cutaneous scars and cosmetic surgery. Surg Clin North Am 51:491–500, 1971.

126. Peacock EJ: Pharmacologic control of surface scarring in human beings. Ann Surg 193:592–597, 1981.

127. Pollack SV: Wound healing: a review—systemic medications affecting wound healing. J Dermatol Surg Oncol 8:667–672, 1982.

128. Katz SM, Frank DH, Leopold GR, Wachtel TL: Objective measurement of hypertrophic burn scar: a preliminary study of tonometry and ultrasonography. Ann Plast Surg 14:121–127, 1985.

129. Wray RC: Force required for wound closure and scar appearance. Plast Reconstr Surg 72:380–382, 1983.

130. Bartell TH, Monafo WW, Mustoe TA: A new instrument for serial measurements of elasticity in hypertrophic scar. J Burn Care Rehabil 9:657–660, 1988.

131. Clark JA: Mechanical characterisation of human postburn hypertrophic skin during pressure therapy. J Biomech 20:397–406, 1987.

132. Gormley DE: Computer models and images of the cutaneous surface. Dermatol Clin 4:641–649, 1986.

CHAPTER 36

Soft Tissue Augmentation

GARY D. MONHEIT

The request for safe and effective filling agents for soft tissue and skin augmentation has been the pursuit of many cosmetic surgeons since the 1960s. The history of dermal filling substances includes reputable and useful agents, as well as agents such as oil, paraffin, and wax that have produced disastrous results. Only since the 1980s have tested and approved implants become available for general use, with U.S. Food and Drug Administration (FDA) approval of Zyderm collagen and, later, Fibrel.

The search for an ideal dermal filler that is safe, easily administered, permanent, and physiologic has also challenged investigators experimenting with wound healing and collagen synthesis. Techniques were developed using substances such as oils and paraffins to cause inflammation and stimulate new collagen deposition. These materials could enhance collagen synthesis in scars and beneath rhytides. However, problems developed such as prolonged inflammation and scarring.[1, 2] The silicone microdroplet technique was designed to stimulate an encapsulating ring of collagen that results in scar correction. Zyderm collagen implants were first thought to stimulate native collagen production, but subsequently this theory proved to be wrong. However, Fibrel injections have been shown to stimulate collagen production through reinjury and inflammation. Each of these techniques has attempted to re-create the body's natural method of wound repair, resulting in soft tissue augmentation.

Implant safety remains an important and controversial issue with many of these materials. Potential side effects and complications—including granulomatous reactions with scarring, allergy, infarction, and the possible induction or stimulation of systemic disease—have all been reported in association with the use of implant materials. In addition, emotional reports in the lay press have indicted some implant materials, with little solid scientific data to back up the allegations.[3]

None of the current implant materials is permanent; each has its own particular longevity based on the material used, the anatomic location, and the type of defect being treated. A thorough understanding of each of these variables is necessary to master the use of these materials for skin contour correction. The most commonly used implants are Zyderm collagen, Fibrel, silicone, and microlipoinjection. Since receiving FDA approval, the first two agents have become a mainstay in the correction of cutaneous scars and wrinkles. The indications and usage for each of these implants are dependent on the chemical nature of the implant, the characteristics of the individual patient, and the variations of the defect being treated. For these reasons, each patient should always have a thorough pretreatment consultation to evaluate the lesion to be treated and the patient's particular needs and demands. Before initiating treatment, the patient must understand the nature of the implant as well as the longevity, morbidity, and potential complications associated with it. At the time of the consultation, the cutaneous surgeon should strive to develop a good professional relationship with the patient that will serve to encourage cooperation both during and after treatment. Informed consent and operative permits should be reviewed with the patient at this time, as is done with other cosmetic surgical procedures. Preoperative photographs and allergy testing are also performed at the completion of the consultative appointment, if the patient wishes to pursue treatment and there are no contraindications. Taking this extra time and effort will also send an unspoken message of quality care and allow each patient to recognize that the problem is being given serious consideration.

Zyderm Collagen Implants (ZCI)

Zyderm collagen is prepared from bovine dermal collagen by purification, sterilization and depyrogenation producing 95% type I collagen and 5% type III collagen. The collagen is centrifuged and resuspended in buffered physiologic saline with 0.4% lidocaine (Table 36–1), producing collagen concentrations of 35% and 65% by volume.[4] At a refrigerated temperature of 0° to −4°C, the product is fluid, but at body temperature, the larger fibers swell and the implant congeals.

TYPES OF IMPLANTS

The three implant products currently available are Zyderm I, which is 35% collagen by volume; Zyderm II, which is 65% collagen; and Zyplast (Table 36–2). The most recently approved product, Zyplast, is cross-linked bovine collagen that is highly bound by glutaraldehyde. As a consequence of its greater resistance to physical pressure and proteolytic degradation, it may persist for a longer period of time. Initial animal studies predicted the implant would last longer than was demonstrated in subsequent clinical trials.

Many histologic studies have been performed to determine what happens to the implant after injection.[5] Sequential facial collagen injections in humans have been studied using biopsies and special stains. From these studies, it was discovered that the collagen implant disperses into smaller deposits by 3 months as a result of little fibroblastic activity. The implant deposits filter downward between 3 and 6 months, and by 9 months, no evidence of the implant remains. The downward migration of collagen into the dermis probably leads to extrusion into the subdermal spaces, which would partially explain the loss of correction seen clinically with time. Zyplast implant deposits histologically appear larger than normal host collagen and displace it downward. In 6 to 9 months, this implant also migrates deeper into the dermis and disappears without evidence of residual autologous collagen.[6] Both Zyderm and Zyplast appear to last longer in scars than in creases or furrows, which is probably a function of the greater mobility of expression lines compared with scars.

INDICATIONS

Collagen is used predominantly for the treatment of age and movement-related skin lines and wrinkles (Table 36–3). It is also useful for elevating the depressed scars that result from acne or trauma. Since its introduction, more than 400,000 patients have been treated with the product, firmly establishing the proper technique of administration.[7]

TABLE 36–1. COMPOSITION OF COLLAGEN IMPLANTS (ZYDERM)

95% Type I collagen
5% Type III collagen
Suspended in saline
0.4% Lidocaine
Small-diameter fibers

TABLE 36–2. TYPES OF COLLAGEN IMPLANTS (ZYDERM)

Zyderm I	35 mg/ml Type I collagen
Zyderm II	65 mg/ml Type I collagen
Zyplast	Glutaraldehyde cross-linked collagen

Zyderm I is an ideal product for the treatment of shallow wrinkles that are related to facial movement. The meilolabial and nasolabial creases, horizontal forehead creases, vertical glabellar creases, radial lines around the mouth, and other movement creases on the cheek and chin respond well to this treatment. Expression lines are best demonstrated with the patient in a seated position, as most of these lines disappear as the patient becomes supine. Tangential lighting is also important to demonstrate rhytides, which appear as a shadow along the depression. It is important for each patient, using a mirror, to demonstrate for the cutaneous surgeon which lines are to be corrected so that these lines can be marked before treatment. The depth of the crease should also be evaluated, as deeper creases and furrows may need Zyplast rather than Zyderm I, and some may not respond to the implants at all. Fine eyelid creases should probably not be treated, as the limited amount of dermis is insufficient to hold the collagen, resulting in a beaded white plaque that may remain for an extended period of time. However, crow's feet lines on the lateral canthus can be satisfactorily treated with small amounts of Zyderm I collagen.

Zyderm is used to correct depressed acne, postsurgical, and traumatic scars. Ovoid malleable scars that distend with manual stretching can be expected to respond best to collagen implants. Ice-pick and fibrotic scars do not elevate with injections and may even become more apparent, as the injection can cause a radial circle to form around the scar. All scars should first be tested by stretching the skin for scar elevation before performing implantation.

Each of the three Zyderm products have different physical properties and should be used individually for correcting different types of skin defects (Figs. 36–1 through 36–3). For example, fine wrinkle lines on the lips and glabella and crow's feet around the eyes are best treated with Zyderm I. Deeper creases and acne scars are often best treated with Zyderm II, while nasolabial furrows and deeper acne scars should be treated with Zyplast collagen.

TABLE 36–3. INDICATIONS FOR COLLAGEN IMPLANTATION

Zyderm I	Shallow lines of expression
	Fine wrinkles
	Superficial scars
Zyderm II	Moderately deep creases
	Deep scars
Zyplast	Nasolabial furrows
	Deeper scars

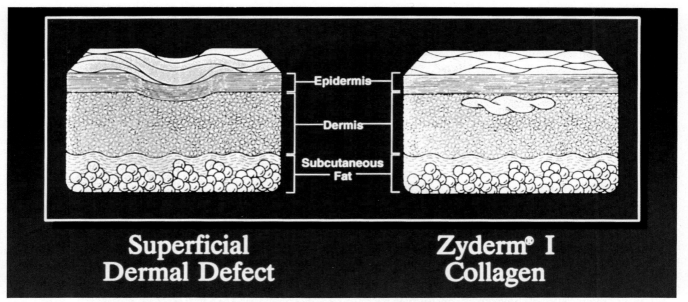

Figure 36–1. Schematic showing how Zyderm I is placed in the upper dermis for superficial defects.

PROPER INJECTION TECHNIQUE

The proper use of dermal fillers is extremely technique dependent and is best learned by direct observation. Variances in technique are based on the type of lesion being treated, the product used, and the quality of the tissue. Thick, sebaceous cheek skin requires more implant material placed superficially, while thinner lip skin should have less implant placed deeper. Zyplast, which forms a larger implant, is always positioned deeper[8] in the dermis than Zyderm I.

Treatment sessions should be scheduled to allow sufficient time to prepare the patient, inject the selected lesions, and provide detailed postoperative instructions.

Before treatment, all makeup should be removed by washing the face with soap and water. Rhytides and scars are then outlined with a marker while the patient observes the process in a mirror. Local anesthesia and sedation are not necessary for most patients, but the anxious patient can be given a preoperative dose of 5 mg diazepam orally. Topical anesthetic creams such as eutectic mixture of local anesthetics (EMLA) can be used on the injection site and occluded for 60 minutes before beginning the injections to reduce discomfort. Both scars and wrinkles should be treated vertically with the patient's head elevated 45 degrees. This allows the surgeon to see the actual depth of the defect and objectively evaluate the degree of filling.

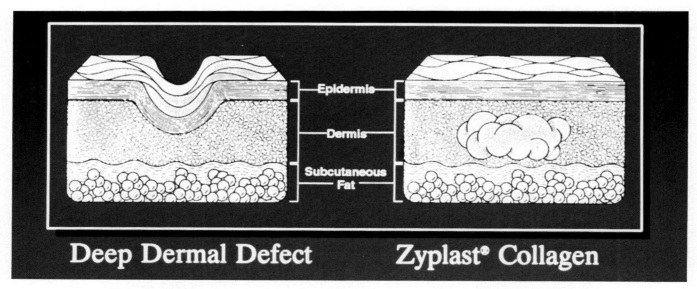

Figure 36–2. Schematic showing how Zyplast is injected in the deep dermis for deep dermal defects.

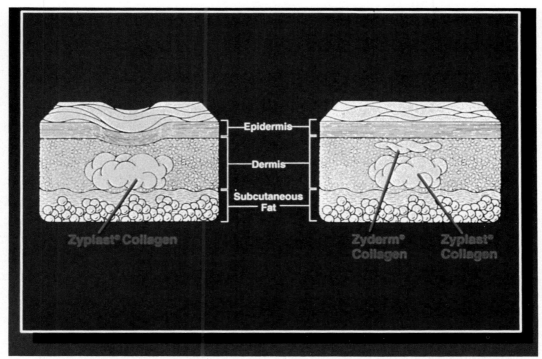

Figure 36–3. Schematic showing how layering of Zyderm I and Zyplast is used for combined defects.

Zyderm is supplied in a tuberculin syringe and injected through a 30-gauge needle. Whether the bevel is placed up or down when attempting to keep the material within the dermis is a matter of personal preference. The needle should pierce the skin at a 45-degree angle and then be advanced horizontally once within the dermis. As the filler is injected, the dermis balloons upward, and the upper dermis becomes distended. This produces blanching and a peau d'orange appearance when the injection of Zyderm I is properly placed in the upper dermis. Injection of Zyplast in the lower dermis produces induration of the dermis, which can be detected by palpation, but no blanching. It is important for the cutaneous surgeon to become familiar with these signs of dermal compartmental filling so as to be able to properly monitor the injection process.

The injection can be encumbered by leakage of implant material through follicular orifices or by inadvertent injection of implant material into the subcutaneous space. Either maneuver wastes the implant material, which is designed only for placement within the dermis. If the collagen extrudes from the pores, the needle should be repositioned before continuing the injection. Injection into the subcutaneous tissue can be recognized by visually monitoring the appearance of the skin as the collagen is implanted.

Correction to the level of the skin is an acceptable end point for the use of Zyplast, but Zyderm I or II should produce an elevation of 150 to 200% (Figs. 36–4, 36–5). This allows for the changes that occur as the saline and lidocaine components of the implant are absorbed shortly after injection. Various injection tech-

niques are used to position the implant within the dermis of the skin defect. The linear puncture and fanning techniques are best used for creases and shallow furrows (Fig. 36–6). The crease is stretched longitudinally, and the needle is inserted at one end. The needle is then advanced horizontally within the dermis as the necessary filling is achieved. Other injections are made at various intervals along the length of the crease (Figs. 36–7, 36–8). The fanning technique is a variation of this process that allows for changes in directions along irregular creases and furrows.

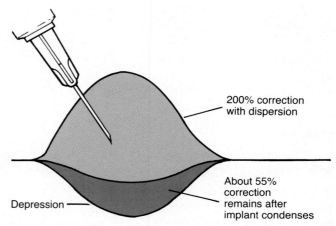

200% correction with dispersion

About 55% correction remains after implant condenses

Depression

Figure 36–4. Schematic showing how injection of Zyderm I produces scar elevation with a 200% correction. (Redrawn courtesy of Collagen Corporation, Palo Alto, CA.)

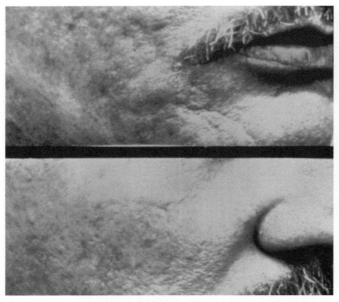

Figure 36–5. Distensible scars *(top)* corrected with Zyderm I collagen *(bottom)*.

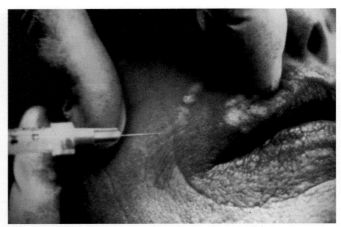

Figure 36–6. Multiple puncture technique with Zyderm I producing peau d'orange appearance.

The multiple-injection technique can be used to elevate depressed scars to ensure that the implant is placed only within or under the scar (Fig. 36–9). It is also useful for correcting vertical furrows on the lips and vermilion. The experienced cosmetic surgeon can place the implant just within the depressed dermal zone to maximally elevate the crease or scar. A two-layer technique is typically reserved for treating deeper furrows within thick, sebaceous skin. Zyplast is used to fill the bulk of the furrow within the deeper dermis, while the remainder of the defect is filled with a more superficially placed Zyderm I implant.[9]

Massaging the injection site immediately after treatment will help to mold the implant within the skin and smooth the edges. Gauze pressure and ice packs can also be used to provide stability and reduce inflammation.

Allergenicity and Adverse Reactions

SKIN TESTING

Skin testing is necessary because of the 3% incidence of pre-existing collagen allergy in the general population. Most positive reactions occur within the first 72 to 96 hours, but a smaller number can occur for up to 4 weeks after the procedure.[10] Typically, a 6-week waiting period is recommended before beginning treatment to

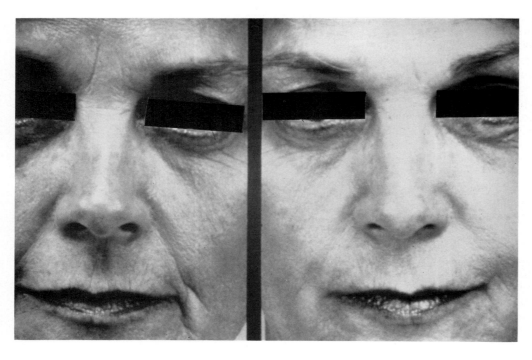

Figure 36–7. Glabella and lip-cheek groove furrows *(left)* corrected with Zyplast *(right)*.

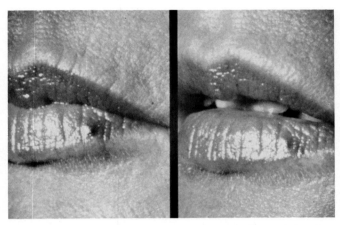

Figure 36–8. Lip rhytides *(left)* corrected with Zyderm I *(right)*.

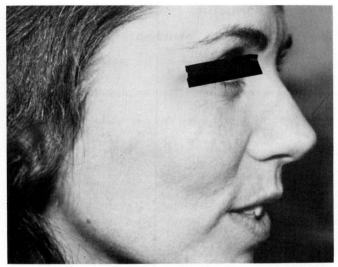

Figure 36–10. Allergic reaction to Zyderm I collagen in a patient who had a negative skin test after 1 month.

ensure that the patient does not develop a delayed reaction. Even with one negative skin test result, there is still a 2% chance that the patient will develop allergic sensitization to collagen during treatment. For this reason, some cutaneous surgeons recommend double skin testing to re-create the first treatment exposure during the second skin test (Fig. 36–10). Because most treatment reactions occur shortly after the first treatment, performance of a second skin test (Table 36–4) will reduce the incidence of this complication.[7]

The incidence of allergic treatment reaction increases with each collagen exposure. Consequently, any patient who presents for retreatment after an interval of 1 year or more should undergo a repeat skin test. This helps to prevent previously treated patients from having undesirable allergic reactions with touch-up treatments.

ADVERSE REACTIONS

Complications and undesirable effects can be subdivided into injection reactions, true allergic reactions, and mechanical complications. Injection reactions occur from mechanical trauma produced by the needle or from injection of the implant itself and include bruising,

intermittent swelling, purpura, and induration. Herpes simplex virus infection, acne nodules, and milia also may occur at the local injection site. These problems are transient and resolve spontaneously in a short period of time.

The allergic reaction to Zyderm collagen is identical at both the skin test site and the treatment site. It consists of a delayed, cell-mediated hypersensitivity reaction that may not appear for several weeks or months after the implant has been placed. The patient will notice acne-like nodules within the crease or scar lines that may initially wax or wane but eventually become persistent. All injected sites, including the skin test, usually react with nodule formation. These reactions gradually fade over the ensuing 6 to 12 months as the collagen is digested. No therapy seems to shorten the reaction time, although topical and local anti-inflammatory treatment may be needed for patient comfort. Use of intralesional or systemic steroids can provide temporary relief but may prolong the allergic reaction time.

Patients who develop an allergic reaction need to have detailed counseling and frequent follow-up treatment for as long as their reactions last. A pretreatment warning of potential allergenicity means much to these patients in sharing the responsibility for this untoward event. Immunologic studies on patients with hypersensitivity reactions have shown that 90% of them have

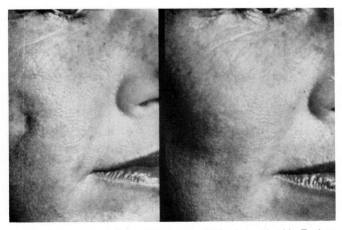

Figure 36–9. Deep distensible scars *(left)* elevated with Zyplast *(right)*. (Courtesy of Collagen Corporation, Palo Alto, CA.)

TABLE 36–4. **COLLAGEN SKIN TESTING**

First Test (Forearm)
    Inspect at 72 hours (60% of reactions)
    Recheck at 4 weeks
Second Test (Face)*
    Inspect at 72 hours
    Recheck at 2 to 4 weeks

*Double testing reduces the risk of adverse reactions.

immunoglobulin G (IgG) antibodies directed against bovine collagen. However, 8.4% of untreated patients also have circulating IgG antibodies to bovine collagen. Fortunately, these antibodies do not cross-react with other mammalian collagen or human collagen (Table 36–5). The antibody titers seem to persist longer than the treatment reactions.[11] A subgroup of these patients become persistent reactors and develop intermittent nodules for years; many have positive antibody titers. Although gradual improvement occurs with time, many of these patients may have allergic flares of nodules exacerbated by exercise, consumption of alcohol, or even the ingestion of beef.

A more severe allergic reaction characterized by draining nodules and cysts has also been reported. These reactions are more common with Zyplast collagen, but 80% of patients have antibodies directed against Zyderm collagen. Because these destructive cysts can result in scarring, early intervention is necessary to suppress the inflammation, drain the cysts, and prevent secondary infection.[12]

Physical problems can result from overcorrection or from collagen placed in the wrong tissue plane. Zyderm collagen placed in the high dermis of thin skin (e.g., the eyelid or lips) can produce white, pearly nodules that have an appearance similar to that of milia (Fig. 36–11). These can last 2 to 4 weeks but will resorb with time. When Zyplast, the most dense of the filling substances, is placed in the upper dermis, it can produce a significant white swelling that may last for months or even years.

Embolization of the implant material has also been reported with Zyplast collagen, especially in the glabellar area. Localized tissue necrosis occurs within the area injected, presumably because of artery obstruction and embolization. This is related to the heavy viscosity of the Zyplast collagen placed at the deeper dermal-subcutaneous junction.

SYSTEMIC REACTIONS

Systemic reactions to Zyderm collagen have been theorized but never proven. Flulike syndromes have been reported after collagen injection, but only sporadically. Dermatomyositis has been implicated temporally in random patients undergoing Zyderm collagen injections. The statistical and epidemiologic data have been reviewed, and no such link can be found between Zyderm collagen and collagen vascular diseases or autoimmune diseases in humans.[3] Although the lay press has reported sensational stories of collagen-related autoimmune diseases, the best medical experts affirm that no current data suggest a link between xenogeneic

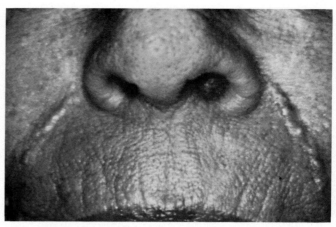

Figure 36–11. Injection of Zyplast in the upper dermis resulted in prolonged nodules in the meilolabial folds that remained for 9 months. (Courtesy of Collagen Corporation, Palo Alto, CA.)

dermal collagen and the precipitation of autoimmune disease.

Fibrel

Attempts to discover the ideal filling material intrigued researchers as early as 1944, when the results of a study were first published on the use of fibrin from pooled plasma to elevate cutaneous scars.[13] It was theorized that chemical agents in plasma initiate healing, resulting in collagen synthesis. This same mechanism was exploited in an attempt to produce excess collagen beneath depressed scars and wrinkles, an attempt that led to the development of Fibrel (Fig. 36–12).

The first report on the use of fibrin foam to successfully treat depressed scars in more than 7000 patients appeared in 1975.[13] This treatment was further refined by formalizing the ingredients and technique. It was renamed the GAP repair technique because it was made from a mixture of gelatin powder, aminocaproic acid, and plasma from the patient.[14] This material was injected under depressed scars to provide lasting cosmetic improvement in many patients. The GAP technique was further refined by mixing lyophilized gelatin powder with aminocaproic acid and fibrin moiety from the patient's serum. Clinical trials over 4 years resulted in FDA approval of this product in 1985 for the treatment of depressed cutaneous scars and wrinkles.[15]

MECHANISM OF ACTION

Fibrel utilizes the mechanisms of wound healing to re-create the necessary events for the production of collagen in a specific confined location. Normally, an injury to the skin results in the release of platelets and thromboplastic and thrombolytic factors. Fibrinogen, through the release of thrombin, is changed to fibrin, which then stimulates fibroblasts in and near capillaries to produce collagen.[16] Simultaneously, plasma profibrinolysin in the resultant clot is converted to fibrinolysin,

TABLE 36–5. IMMUNOLOGY OF COLLAGEN IMPLANT REACTIONS

90% of patients have circulating immunoglobulin G (IgG) to bovine collagen.
8.4% of untreated patients also have IgG to bovine collagen.
No cross-reaction with human collagen.

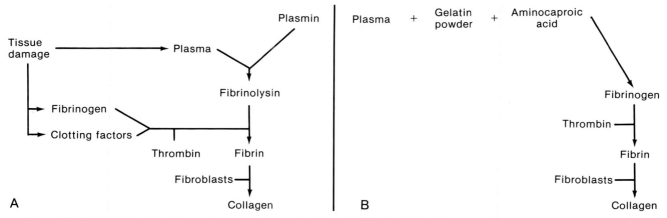

Figure 36–12. *A,* Mechanism of normal wound healing after injury. *B,* Effects of Fibrel in re-creating the wound healing mechanism.

which inhibits or destroys the fibrin clot, thus curtailing further collagen production.

Fibrel provides the necessary components to re-create these normal wound healing processes beneath scars and wrinkles. The absorbable gelatin powder provides a framework for the clot to form and remains stable under the scar. Plasma provides the necessary ingredients for collagen synthesis, while ε-aminocaproic acid (EACA) inhibits the production of fibrinolysin, stabilizes collagen, and stimulates the synthesis of new collagen within the clot.[17] Thus, treatment of depressed scars with Fibrel implantation results in the formation of a fibrin clot in which new collagen is created that will give lasting elevation of the scar.

PRODUCT COMPOSITION

Fibrel is composed of a lyophilized mixture of 100 mg absorbable gelatin powder with 125 mg EACA. The gelatin powder is a porcine derivative of low immunogenicity that is widely used as a hemostatic agent. It elevates the depression and provides a matrix to trap clotting factors for the deposition of new collagen. EACA has been shown to enhance collagen synthesis through a blockade of the fibrinolytic system.[17] Both the

gelatin and EACA components of Fibrel are routinely used as hemostatic agents. Blood plasma provides a supplemental source of fibrinogen and other clotting factors that enhance the collagen matrix and add to the efficacy of this product. Unlike collagen and silicone, which remain as foreign implants beneath the skin surface, Fibrel is absorbed as the new collagen is gradually incorporated into the skin.

Histologic and preclinical data suggest that within 90 days the implant is colonized by the patient's own normal connective tissue as cells and blood vessels grow into the implant.[18] Theoretically, Fibrel is a physiologic implant with little chance of allergenicity or foreign body reaction. The gelatin powder elevates the depression, provides a matrix to enhance blood clotting by entrapping the necessary clotting factors, and serves as a template for the subsequent deposition of new extracellular matrix, which is essential for wound healing. The antifibrinolytic action of EACA has a stabilizing effect on fibrin. In animals, EACA has been shown to enhance new collagen synthesis through blockage of the fibrinolytic system.[17]

Fibrel is supplied in a sterile kit that has a long shelf life and contains everything needed for treatment (Fig. 36–13). The mixture of lyophilized gelatin powder and

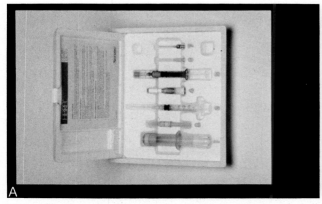
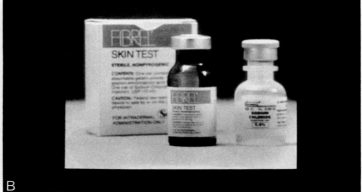

Figure 36–13. *A,* The Fibrel kit contains the gelatin powder, ε-aminocaproic acid, and the needles and syringes for phlebotomy, mixing, and injection. *B,* A skin test is given 6 weeks before injection by diluting the Fibrel suspension with saline.

EACA is contained within a syringe in the kit and is reconstituted with 0.5 ml of the patient's serum and 0.5 ml of 0.9% normal saline. The syringe with the gelatin mixture is connected with an adapter to the saline-serum syringe, and the two are slowly mixed by making 10 to 12 horizontal passes of the solution from one syringe to another, making the suspension ready for injection.[19]

SKIN TEST PROCEDURE

An intradermal skin test is injected into the patient's arm using 0.5 ml of the Fibrel suspension in a 1:1000 saline solution. A delay of 1 month is necessary to determine whether the patient is allergic to the implant. A positive reaction occurs in 1.9% of patients and is defined as induration and erythema that persist longer than 24 to 48 hours.[15]

INDICATIONS

Fibrel is indicated as a dermal implant for the correction of depressed cutaneous scars and wrinkles. A thorough consultation and examination of the patient's defects should be performed before treatment, and those scars or wrinkles that will likely respond are identified. Fibrel is used for correcting cutaneous scars that can be elevated by stretching the skin at the edges of the scar. Fibrotic or ice-pick scars do not normally elevate well and require special treatment. Deeper creases, furrows, and grooves may also be treated with Fibrel. However, fine creases on the eyelids or lips and photoaging rhytides on facial skin do not respond well to Fibrel injections because of the viscosity of the implant and the associated inflammation. During the consultation visit, lesions that will likely respond to treatment are identified, and a thorough explanation of the treatment technique, potential side effects, morbidity, and complications is given to the patient. Particular emphasis must be placed on the differences between this filling agent and Zyderm collagen, because the mechanism used to create collagen through wound healing requires an inflammatory reaction as a necessary component of the treatment with Fibrel. Because the patient will likely develop postoperative erythema, induration, and swelling lasting as long as 5 days, the necessary time for

recovery must be scheduled by the patient. Final collagen synthesis may take 6 to 8 weeks to develop. Patients must be informed of these consequences so they will fully understand the nature of healing and implant formation.

EXCLUSION CRITERIA

Patients who should be excluded from treatment with Fibrel are those with a history of keloid formation; those with a known sensitivity to gelatin or aminocaproic acid; those with bleeding disorders or a history of cardiac, renal, or autoimmune diseases; those with herpes; and women who are pregnant or lactating.

INJECTION TECHNIQUES

One month after skin testing, the patient returns for re-examination. If the skin test is negative, treatment may begin. Each scar or wrinkle to be treated is outlined (Fig. 36–14) and categorized as either distensible or fibrotic and bound down. Phlebotomy is then performed to remove approximately 10 ml of the patient's blood. This is centrifuged for 10 to 15 minutes, and the clear serum is drawn into the mixing syringe. This is connected to the syringe with the gelatin powder and mixed together using horizontal exchanges. The mixing exchanges should be performed slowly to avoid causing bubbling or frothing of the mixture. The process is completed with Fibrel in the delivery syringe. After the air bubbles have been expressed, the patient is ready for injection.

Distensible Scars

Distensible scars can be injected with a 30-gauge needle using a multiple puncture or fanning technique. These types of scars do not require preinjections of local anesthesia to place the implant directly into the middle or upper dermis. In this technique, the needle enters at a 35-degree angle (Fig. 36–15), and the injection produces blanching and a peau d'orange appearance. A correction of 150% is necessary owing to equalization of serum and fluids during clot resorption. Care must be taken to avoid both implant extrusion through pores

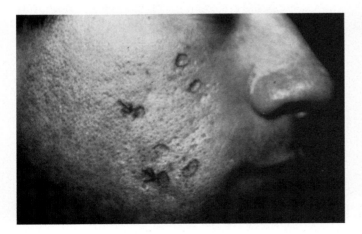

Figure 36–14. Scars are circled with the patient in a vertical position; an arrow indicates the fibrotic scars for the undermining technique.

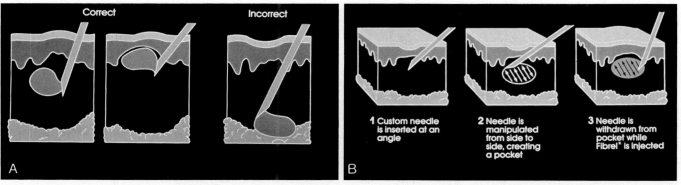

Figure 36–15. *A,* Schematic showing the proper position of bevel and needle to place the implant in the middle dermis. *B,* Schematic showing the fanning or threading technique used for correcting distensible scars.

or around the needle orifice and injection into the subcutaneous tissue. In the direct puncture technique, the needle is first placed at the edge of the scar and then is advanced into it so that the middle of the scar can be injected (Fig. 36–16*A*). In the fanning technique, an adaptation of the single puncture method, the needle is advanced in a circumferential pattern throughout the entire scar, and the filler substance is injected into the middle and upper dermis (Fig. 36–16*B*). Common to all of these techniques is the placement of Fibrel in the middle or upper dermis of the scar (Fig. 36–17).

Fibrotic Scars

The approach to fibrotic scars utilizes a customized undermining needle that is available in the kit (Fig. 36–18*A*). This device allows the cutaneous surgeon to create a dermal pocket for subsequent injection of the filler substance. This loosens the strands of scar tissue that hold the scar down and allows the upper dermis and epidermis to be elevated by injection of the implant (Fig. 36–18*B*). A field block using 1% lidocaine must be instilled around the scar before undermining is performed. The customized 18-gauge undermining needle is advanced at a 35-degree angle within the dermis in multiple passes to sever the bands of scar tissue and create a filling pocket. After undermining has released the upper portion of the scar and the pocket has been created, filling material is injected to elevate the scar (Fig. 36–19). Extrusion of the implant from the needle site is prevented by applying direct pressure after the injection. Implant molding is important for all treated scars, and ice packs are used on the treated area after the injection.

Wrinkles and Furrows

Wrinkle lines and furrows are treated with Fibrel in a similar fashion by placing the implant in the middle to upper dermis. Treatable wrinkles include glabellar furrows, forehead wrinkle lines, nasolabial and meilolabial wrinkles, and those at the lip commissure (Fig. 36–20) and cheek. Treatment of crow's feet and the smaller fine lines on the lips with Fibrel should be avoided, as it results in inflamed nodules that can last for a pro-

longed period of time. Most wrinkles are treated in a manner similar to that used for treating distensible scars (i.e., with a 30-gauge needle and intradermal filling). Using the linear injection technique, the needle is placed in the base of the furrow and advanced intradermally along and under the groove. The implant is then injected under the groove, resulting in elevation, a peau d'orange appearance, and blanching. The needle is then advanced farther up the groove, and the injection is continued until the full length of the crease has been elevated. Immediate molding and compression are performed before an ice pack is placed over the treatment site.

RESULTS

Postoperative erythema, inflammation, and induration occur with almost all Fibrel injections. This is a necessary requirement for scar correction, although the degree of inflammation is highly variable. Iced dressings placed over injection sites will help reduce the amount of inflammation, but anti-inflammatory agents should not be used, as they will reduce the amount of collagen formation and the degree of scar correction. Inflammation and induration usually last 48 to 72 hours, although occasionally they may persist for 4 to 5 days.

A multicenter study published in 1987 described the results in 321 patients treated with Fibrel.[15] These patients were evaluated for the degree of scar correction and longevity of correction over a two-year period using parameters of physician evaluation, patient evaluation, and photogrametric analysis (Fig. 36–21). The latter measurement used a scar mold that was analyzed using computer analysis to monitor the volume correction of the scar. This study showed that 60 to 75% of the scars were correctable with Fibrel. Of those correctable scars, 80% were found to have maintained their correction at the end of 2 years using all three evaluation parameters.[15] A 5-year subjective analysis of this group showed that 50% of the scars maintained their correction for that period of time.[20] This study strongly suggests that Fibrel does provide lasting scar correction for a greater period of time than that provided by Zyderm collagen implants. Similar studies on the effectiveness of this treatment for wrinkles are not yet available.

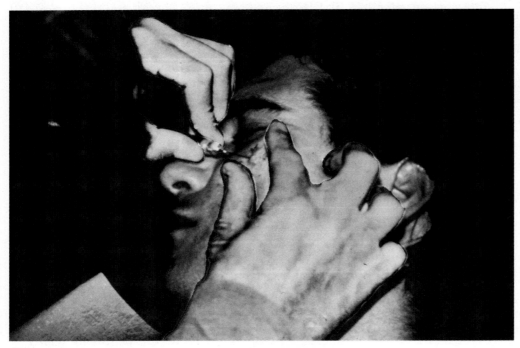

A

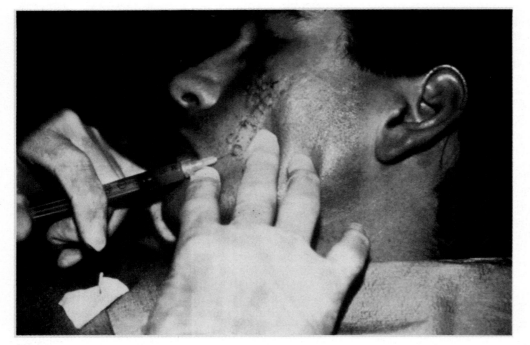

B

Figure 36–16. *A*, Injection of distensible scars with a 30-gauge needle. *B*, Undermining technique with a customized needle.

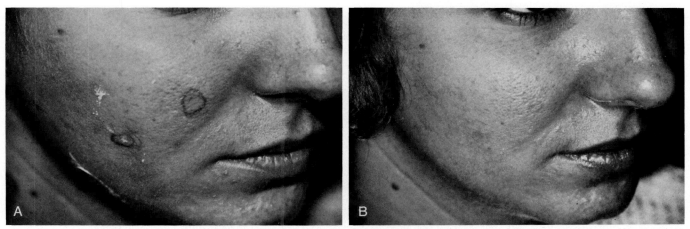

Figure 36–17. *A,* Distensible acne scars seen before injection with Fibrel. *B,* Postoperative appearance.

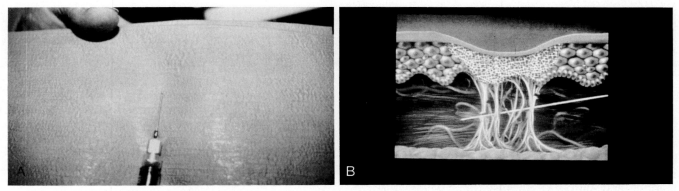

Figure 36–18. *A,* The customized needle used for fibrotic scars. *B,* Schematic showing how the cutting surface of the needle is used to sever the fibrotic bands to create a deep dermal pocket for implant injection.

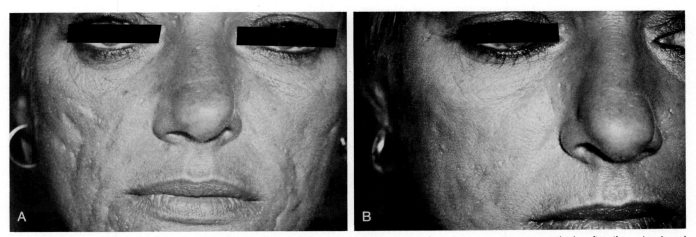

Figure 36–19. *A,* Multiple distensible and fibrotic scars seen preoperatively. *B,* Result seen 1 year postoperatively after three treatment sessions with Fibrel.

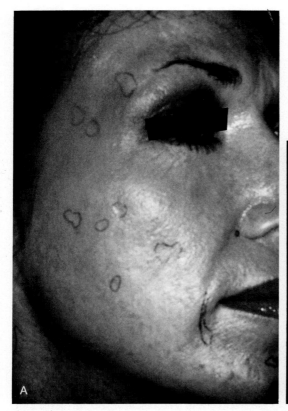

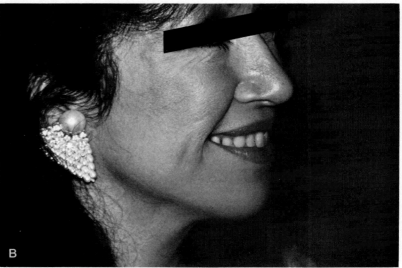

Figure 36–20. *A,* Preoperative appearance of a patient with both wrinkles and scars. *B,* Appearance 6 months after treatment with Fibrel.

SIDE EFFECTS AND COMPLICATIONS

Most side effects found with Fibrel have been localized and restricted to the trauma caused by the injection itself. These include pain, induration, erythema, inflammation, and purpura. Because the inflammatory response (Fig. 36–22) is a necessary part of the mechanism for collagen synthesis, it should not be considered a true side effect. Bruising and purpura can prolong the inflammatory response, and nodules may persist for 1 to 2 weeks. An exacerbation of acne at the site of injection and activation of herpes simplex virus infection have also been reported.[21]

As Fibrel usage has become more common, rare complications have been reported. One of these, a prolonged inflammatory response, has lasted as long as 4 to 6 weeks in some patients.[22] This is essentially an exaggeration of the normal inflammation and induration that typically resolve in 3 to 5 days. This response is not thought to be allergic in nature, but rather is considered an idiosyncratic exaggeration of the necessary inflam-

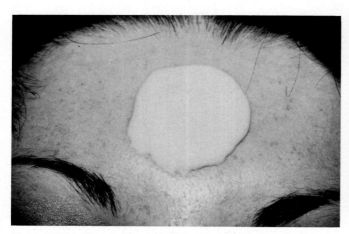

Figure 36–21. Scar mold used to determine photogrametric analysis.

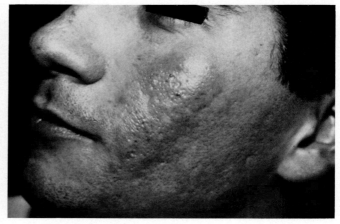

Figure 36–22. Significant inflammation can occur after Fibrel injections.

mation required for the full effect to be achieved. These patients have negative skin test results without evidence of allergy and also develop a similar response to the injection of serum alone. No antecedent factors have been identified that can accurately predict who will develop this prolonged inflammatory response.[22] However, it is more commonly seen with injection of the lips, glabella, and periorbital skin. This reaction resolves spontaneously, but ice compresses and pressure seem to help speed the resolution. Because of the time that is often required, however, patients will frequently need the physician's support and counseling during this period.

Embolization with cutaneous necrosis has also been reported when Fibrel is injected into the subcutaneous tissue. As with Zyplast collagen, the heavier suspension can cause infarction of larger subdermal vessels, which results in local tissue necrosis. One complication reported with Fibrel occurred when a rhinoplasty defect was corrected with injection, but treatment resulted in infarction and loss of skin over the nose. This was found to have been due to injection of the material into subcutaneous tissue and fascia, rather than skin.[23] Because Fibrel is a dermal filler substance, it should be used only to correct skin defects. Special care must be taken when treating the glabella or nose.

There has been little evidence of a true allergy to Fibrel. Although the possibility of an allergic reaction to porcine products in the gelatin must always be considered, thus far only a few cases have been reported. Most importantly, patients who have become allergic to Zyderm collagen have been successfully treated with Fibrel without difficulty. For this reason, there seems to be no cross-reactivity between the autoantibodies to collagen and allergic reactions to Fibrel. There has also been no association between the use of Fibrel and any collagen-vascular or autoimmune diseases or the precipitation of adverse systemic reactions.

Fibrel is a safe and useful physiologic material that causes the production of autologous collagen for the elevation of scars and wrinkles. The biggest disadvantage of this material is that it is more complicated to inject than Zyderm collagen, requiring mixing with the patient's serum and, in some instances, use of a local anesthetic. There is also increased morbidity postoperatively because of the development of inflammation, which is necessary for the subsequent creation of collagen. These differences must be understood by each patient to fully appreciate the nature of this implant material and to ensure total compliance during healing. Despite some problems, this product has many distinct advantages, including increased longevity, low allergenicity, and superior scar elevation.

Microlipoinjection

Autologous fat transplants to correct skin and soft tissue contour defects have been used in cosmetic surgery for a century. The early trials consisted of placing small pieces of sharply dissected bulk fat in subcutaneous pockets. These bulk fat grafts provided variable results and disappeared spontaneously in up to 50% of patients.[24, 25]

The goal of lipoinjection is the transplantation of living, autologous adipose tissue to provide a viable graft. The advent of liposuction surgery gave the cutaneous surgeon the necessary tools to harvest fat successfully. Whereas liposuction surgery is used to remove fat and contour the area of removal, lipoinjection uses fat to fill soft tissue defects. The methods of fat removal are different from those used for lipoinjection, since the procedure must not injure or kill the lipocytes. The extreme negative pressure created by most liposuction aspirators for traditional liposuction will damage lipocytes and probably kill the fat implant. For this reason, use of a 14-gauge needle attached to a syringe with limited negative pressure has been advocated as the best technique to harvest the grafts.[26] The lipoextraction systems for lipoinjection have been further modified by the use of a blunt cannula and a glass syringe for fat harvesting, washing, and injecting.[27]

INDICATIONS

The indications for fat replacement are soft tissue contour defects resulting from the loss or destruction of subcutaneous tissue. Lipoinjection is a fat replacement technique, and adipose tissue should not be used as a dermal filler or to rebuild a dermal defect. The defects that will most likely respond to microlipoinjection include facial aging defects resulting from senile fat atrophy of the cheeks, chin, and temples; deep grooves and furrows of the meilolabial fold that are accentuated by fat loss; fat atrophy after cystic acne, traumatic scarring, steroid atrophy, or lipodystrophies; and subcutaneous defects created by liposuction.

SURGICAL TECHNIQUE

Lipoinjection requires different techniques for harvesting the fat from the donor area and for injecting the soft tissue contour defects. The donor area should be accessible to the surgeon, contain enough viable fat for the procedure, and allow coverage by clothing to hide the postoperative bruising. The medial and lateral thigh, buttocks, and abdomen are the primary areas of choice.[7]

The patient is first treated with a surgical preparation solution and covered with a sterile drape. The area is then infiltrated with a diluted solution of 1% lidocaine with epinephrine. Using a syringe with an attached 16-gauge or lipoextraction tip needle (Fig. 36–23), the fat is atraumatically removed using gentle forward strokes while negative pressure is kept on the syringe. With this technique, only two or three 10- to 20-ml syringes of fat are necessary to correct most facial contour defects.

There is some controversy over the value of washing the fat or adding insulin, glucose, or saline and rinsing the fat in heparin.[28, 29] An individual technique should be developed for managing fat, based on a thorough evaluation of the arguments for and against each protocol.[28] There is general agreement among most cutaneous surgeons that the serum and blood should be drained and the fat cells washed with lactated Ringer's solution before injection (Fig. 36–24). This can be

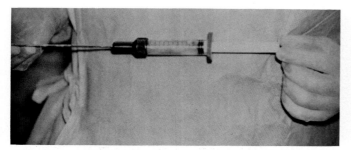

Figure 36–23. The fat is harvested using a blunt-tipped cannula.

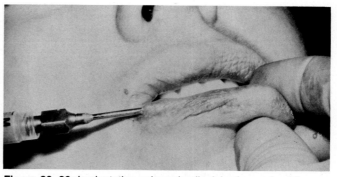

Figure 36–25. The cleaned fat is placed in an injection syringe.

accomplished by positioning the needle down so that the fat floats to the top of the syringe, allowing the blood and serum to be ejected. The cycle is repeated with saline or Ringer's solution until a suspension of pure, viable fat cells (Fig. 36–25) is produced for injection.[30]

Implantation injections are performed under local anesthesia (Fig. 36–26). The defect is first outlined with a surgical marker, and the patient is positioned so that the head is elevated at least 45 degrees. The skin is pricked with a No. 11 blade, and the needle is advanced into the subcutaneous tissue. The fat suspension is then infiltrated evenly throughout the defect to elevate the surface 100 to 150% (Fig. 36–27). The implant can be molded and secured in proper position with tape.

COMPLICATIONS

This technique is more complicated than injections utilizing either Zyderm collagen or Fibrel and requires the same surgical discipline and environment used in liposuction. Inherent in this procedure are the potential complications associated with more invasive surgical procedures. Donor area complications include hemor-

rhage and hematoma, excessive bruising, and potential contour defects. At the recipient site, excessive bruising, prolonged inflammation and induration, local infection, and hematoma formation have all been described. Each patient should be fully informed of these potential problems and given a realistic appraisal of the likely results obtainable with this technique.

GRAFT LONGEVITY

The major unresolved issue in lipoinjection is the longevity of the graft. One estimate has been made that 30 to 40% of the graft is retained after 1 year.[7] However, there has been little objective analysis of the long-term clinical results. Most cutaneous surgeons agree that the correction rarely lasts longer than 1 year, and 6 months is a more typical life span for the fat graft. Methods of prolonging graft survival are under active investigation and include techniques that separate autologous collagen from fat and biochemical methods for harvesting lipocytes. These exciting developments represent a new frontier in soft tissue augmentation that may eventually result in the development of an ideal skin and soft tissue implant.

Injectable Silicone

Injectable silicone theoretically seems to satisfy many of the established criteria for an ideal cutaneous implant. It is permanent and relatively inert and can be implanted relatively simply. However, it is also a foreign, non-

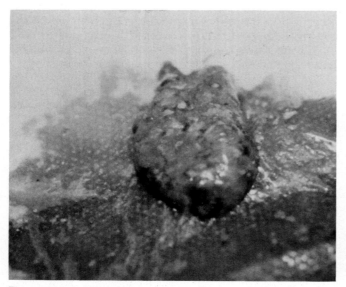

Figure 36–24. The fat is washed with saline to remove all blood products and contaminants.

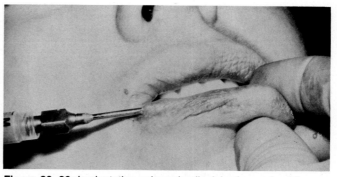

Figure 36–26. Implantation using microlipoinjection and a 16-gauge needle for lip augmentation after obtaining local anesthesia.

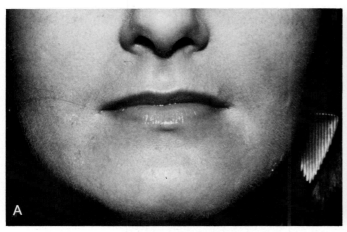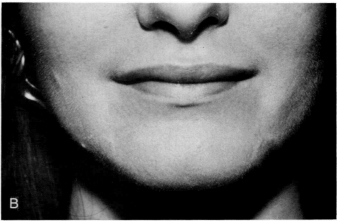

Figure 36–27. Clinical appearance before lip augmentation *(A)* and after microlipoinjection *(B)*.

physiologic material that has raised serious concerns about its safety. The FDA has also withheld approval for its use, distribution, and promotion. In fact, clinical trials on silicone use have never been completed. The recent disclosures concerning adverse reactions to breast silicone implants and the FDA's decision to place a moratorium on the use of silicone implants for cosmetic breast augmentation have also restricted further scientific investigation on its use for skin augmentation. For these reasons, this discussion will be limited to an historical perspective and an analytical review of data concerning the use of injectable silicone.

COMPOSITION

Silicone refers to a group of polymers based on the element silicon; medical-grade liquid silicone (Dow-Corning 360) is a dimethylsiloxane polymer (MDX4-4011). Its viscosity is dependent on the degree of polymerization, which also largely determines its clinical applicability as a dermal filler. Polydimethylsiloxane fluid of 35 centistokes appears to be the ideal silicone derivative for injection. It is a clear, colorless, oily material that maintains its viscosity at both room and body temperature. This material is capable of being steam sterilized, does not support bacterial growth, and has a long shelf life. Because it can be absorbed by various hydrocarbons, it should not be stored in rubber or plastic vials or syringes and should not be gas sterilized.[31]

MECHANISM OF ACTION

Silicone is injected into the dermis using a microdroplet technique. These small deposits of silicone induce a mild inflammatory reaction that slowly subsides within 6 months. The injected silicone then becomes encapsulated by an accumulation of autologous collagen, which produces the augmentation effect. The eventual tissue response to silicone is fibroblastic in nature, resulting in increased collagen deposition. This response is self-limited and without continual granulomatous or inflam-

matory reaction. Antibodies to silicone have not been demonstrated, and true autoimmune disease has not been scientifically demonstrated.[32]

TECHNIQUE AND INDICATIONS

Dermal implantation of silicone is performed using the microdroplet technique, utilizing a volume of 0.005 to 0.01 mg at each injection site.[33] The serial puncture technique utilizes a 30-gauge needle with a 1-ml tuberculin syringe. Microdroplets are placed in the middle or upper dermis, with multiple punctures beneath the scar or rhytide. Undertreatment is necessary, as the fibroblastic response will elevate the injection site during the ensuing 2- to 4-month period.

Microinjection of silicone has been found useful for augmenting distensible acne scars, furrows on the forehead and glabella, grooves at the lip-cheek junction and labial commissures, vertical lip grooves, and rhytides on the cheeks, skin, and periorbital creases.

Microinjection of silicone is very technique dependent, and proper use is necessary to obtain good cosmetic results without sequelae. Complications can arise if large volumes of silicone are injected or if the silicone is placed too superficially within the dermis. The depth of injection should be varied according to skin thickness and anatomic location. Thin skin (e.g., along the vermilion border or the eyelids) is prone to developing nodules, which produce a beaded effect.[34] The permanence of silicone is both an advantage and a detriment. While proper use of the product can give predictable results in skin augmentation, misplaced silicone will create nodules that are not absorbed and are very difficult to correct.

COMPLICATIONS

The majority of problems associated with silicone injections have actually been the result of the many adulterants that have been added to pure silicone products. These silicone mixtures have been used for soft tissue and skin augmentation, often with disastrous results. Paraffin and mineral oil have been used in the past for treating facial furrows by creating a foreign body inflammatory response characterized histologically as a paraffinoma. Other silicone additives have included animal and vegetable oils, fatty acids, beeswax, fish oils, and olive oil. The Sakuri formula, a mixture of silicone and olive oil, was used for breast augmentation in Japan, but the massive amounts of material injected caused tissue fibrosis and necrosis, with severe, mutilating complications.[31]

Because of these complications, the medical use of silicone has been severely restricted in the United States.[35] Clinical investigations have been suspended, and the FDA has refused to authorize additional scientific study of this material. Hopefully, silicone can soon be studied objectively without bias. Until then, the potential of this permanent, inert substance for skin augmentation will not be fully realized.

SUMMARY

For many patients with contour scars and certain types of deformities caused by aging, soft tissue augmentation can provide a satisfactory degree of improvement without requiring incisions or significant postoperative wound care or producing marked morbidity. By properly evaluating each individual patient and each particular type of problem, the most ideal filler substance can be selected. With the collagen-based products, once skin testing has been completed, sequential injections can be safely performed.[36] Although permanent correction is not possible with currently available materials, additional investigations hopefully will lead to the eventual development of more effective materials for the safe correction of cutaneous defects.

REFERENCES

1. Urbach F, Wine SS, Johnson WC, Davies RE: Generalized paraffinoma (sclerosing lipogranuloma). Arch Dermatol 103:277–285, 1971.
2. Klein JA, Cole G, Barr RJ, et al: Paraffinomas of the scalp. Arch Dermatol 121:382–385, 1985.
3. Klein AW: Bonfire of the wrinkles. J Dermatol Surg Oncol 17:543–544, 1991.
4. Stegman SJ, Tromovitch TA: Injectable collagen. In: Stegman SJ, Tromovitch TA (eds): Cosmetic Dermatologic Surgery. Year Book Medical, Chicago, 1984, pp 131–149.
5. Kligman AM, Armstrong RC: Histologic response to intradermal Zyderm and Zyplast (glutaraldehyde cross-linked) collagen in humans. J Dermatol Surg Oncol 12:351–357, 1986.
6. Stegman SJ, Cha S, Barsch K, et al: A light and electron microscopic evaluation of Zyderm collagen and Zyplast implants in aging human facial skin. Arch Dermatol 123:1644–1649, 1987.
7. Stegman SJ, Tromovitch TA: Filling agents. In: Stegman SJ, Tromovitch TA (eds): Cosmetic Dermatologic Surgery. Year Book Medical, Chicago, 1990, pp 148–160.
8. Monheit G: Surgical treatment of acne scars. Cosmet Dermatol 2:17–21, 1989.
9. Klein AW: Implantation techniques for injectable collagen. J Am Acad Dermatol 9:224–228, 1983.
10. Delustro F, MacKinnon V, Swanson NA: Immunology of injectable collagen in human subjects. J Dermatol Surg Oncol 7:49–55, 1988.
11. McCoy JP Jr, Schade W, Siegle RJ, et al: Immune responses to bovine collagen implants. J Am Acad Dermatol 16:955–960, 1987.
12. Hanke CW, Higley HR, Jolivette DM, et al: Abscess formation and local necrosis after treatment with Zyderm or Zyplast collagen implant. J Am Acad Dermatol 25:319–326, 1991.
13. Spangler AS: Treatment of depressed scars with Fibrin foam—seventeen years of experience. J Dermatol Surg 1:65–69, 1975.
14. Gottlieb S: GAP repair technique. Poster exhibit at the annual meeting of the American Academy of Dermatology, Dallas, TX, December, 1977.
15. Millikan L, Rosen T, Monheit G: Treatment of depressed cutaneous scars with gelatin matrix implant: a multicenter study. J Am Acad Dermatol 16:1155–1162, 1987.
16. Clark RAF: Cutaneous tissue repair: basic biologic considerations. J Am Acad Dermatol 13:701–725, 1985.
17. Nilsson IM, Sjoerdsam A, Walderstron J: Antifibrinolytic activity and metabolism of ε-aminocaproic acid in man. Lancet 1:1233–1236, 1960.
18. Postlethwaite AE, Seyer JM, Kang AH: Chemotactic reaction of human fibroblasts to type I, II and III collagens and collagen-derived peptides. Proc Natl Acad Sci USA 75:871–875, 1978.
19. Instruction Guide. Fibrel Technique Workshop, MEDED program for Serono Corporation, July 28, 1987.
20. Millikan L: Long term safety and efficacy with Fibrel in the treatment of cutaneous scars. J Dermatol Surg Oncol 15:837–844, 1989.
21. Rosen T: Fibrel, a new implant material. J Am Acad Dermatol 16:155–162, 1987.
22. Physicians reporting complications to the Mentor Corporation, private communication, 1990.
23. Physicians reporting complications to the Mentor Corporation, private communication, 1991.
24. Peer LA: Transplantation of Tissues: Transplantation of Fat. Williams & Wilkins, Baltimore, 1959.
25. Ellenbrogen R: Free autologous pearl fat grafts in face. Ann Plast Surg 16:179, 1986.
26. Fournier PF: Micro lipo extraction and micro lipo injection. 13th Annual Meeting, American Society of Dermatologic Surgery, Rancho Mirage, CA, April, 1986.
27. Asken S: Autologous fat transplantation. In: Roenigk RK, Roenigk HH Jr (eds): Dermatologic Surgery: Principles and Practice. Marcel Dekker, New York, 1989, pp 1179–1213.
28. Glogau RG: Micro lipoinjection: autologous fat grafting perspectives. Arch Dermatol 124:1340–1343, 1988.
29. Agris J: Autologous fat transplantation: a three year study. Am J Cosmet Surg 4:2, 1987.
30. Asken S: A Manual of Liposuction Surgery and Autologous Fat Transplantation Under Local Anesthesia. Keith C. Terry and Associates, Irvine, CA, 1986, pp 119–143.
31. Orentreich D, Orentreich N: Injectable fluid silicone. In: Roenigk RK, Roenigk HH Jr (eds): Dermatologic Surgery: Principles and Practice. Marcel Dekker, New York, 1989, pp 1349–1395.
32. Selmanowitz VJ, Orentreich N: Medical grade fluid silicone. J Dermatol Surg Oncol 3:597–611, 1977.
33. Fuleihan N, Webster R, Smith R: Injectable silicone. Aesthet Plast Surg 15:669–685, 1991.
34. Duffy D: Silicone: a critical review. In: Callen JK, Dahl MV, Golitz LE, et al (eds): Advances in Dermatology. Year Book Medical, Chicago, 1990, pp 93–110.
35. Schwartz RM: Action on silicone injection marks busy regulatory period for the FDA. Cosmet Dermatol 5:48–51, 1992.
36. Karam P, Kibbi A-G: Collagen injections. Int J Dermatol 31:467–470, 1992.

CHAPTER 37

Superficial Chemical Peels

LAWRENCE S. MOY, HOWARD MURAD, and RONALD L. MOY

A chemical peel is the application of a chemical agent that causes a controlled destruction of the outer layers of the skin. The treatment concept is to damage the skin deeply enough to cause exfoliation of some tissue layers while remaining superficial enough to allow regeneration from the appendiceal structures and papillary dermis.[1-3] The superficial damage to the skin takes advantage of wound healing to reduce scars, wrinkles, pigmentation abnormalities, and certain lesions such as actinic keratoses and lentigines.

The first reported use of chemicals to smooth and improve the skin was in Egypt when Cleopatra bathed in sour milk, probably for the lactic acid effect.[4] During the time of the French Revolution, the ladies of the court would apply old wine, which contained tartaric acid, to their faces. Gypsies in Europe applied various caustic chemicals to their skin. The first chemical peels in the United States were introduced by German dermatologists in the 1930s,[5] but it was during the early 1960s that phenol peels began being used extensively. Later, newer peeling agents such as trichloroacetic acid (TCA) were tried. Other peeling agents that have been used include formulations of resorcinol, plant enzymes, pancreatic enzymes, alpha-hydroxy acids, and salicylic acid.[5, 6]

There are three depths of peels that are commonly performed by the cutaneous surgeon. Deep peels, using phenol or pyruvic acid, penetrate to the depth of the midreticular dermis. Medium peels, using 40 to 50% TCA, penetrate to the deeper areas of the papillary dermis. Superficial peels[1] penetrate through the epidermis and to upper regions of the papillary dermis (Table 37-1). Superficial peels cause only superficial damage and thus can be repeated every few weeks. Repeated superficial peels may be as beneficial as deeper peels for some conditions.

More patients are candidates for superficial peels than

for deeper peels. Deep chemical peels are usually not recommended for olive- or dark-skinned patients[7] because of pigmentary side effects. Because of the potential cardiac toxicity of phenol,[8] cardiac monitoring and life support systems are required for greatest safety. Baker's phenol chemical peel solution is not recommended unless the patient is advised that hypopigmentation often occurs and accepts the fact that long-term use of makeup may be required.[2]

Although superficial peels can be repeated, they still cannot achieve the deeper changes that phenol or higher strength TCA peels achieve. Although repeated superficial peels are safer for a greater number of patients, deeper peels are more effective for deep wrinkles. Depending on the nature of the condition being treated and the skin type of the patient, deeper peels or dermabrasion may be recommended over repeated superficial chemical peels.

Indications for Superficial Chemical Peels

Superficial peels are very effective for many different skin conditions (Table 37-2). The most common conditions treated with superficial peels will be discussed individually.

TABLE 37-1. POPULAR SUPERFICIAL PEELING AGENTS

Glycolic acid in concentrations of 50% and 70%
Trichloroacetic acid in concentrations of 15%, 20%, 25%, and 35%
Jessner's solution
Resorcin
Retinoic acid

TABLE 37–2. INDICATIONS FOR SUPERFICIAL CHEMICAL PEELS

Actinic keratoses
Wrinkles
Melasma
Lentigines
Acne and acne scarring
Skin rejuvenation
Flat seborrheic keratoses
Verruca plana
Freckles
Postinflammatory hyperpigmentation
Hypertrophic scars
Tattoos

WRINKLES (RHYTIDES)

Wrinkled, sun-exposed skin shows an accumulation of elastotic material. This elastotic deposition is thought to lack structural support quality, which gives a sagging, nonelastic, wrinkled appearance to the skin. The precise nature of this elastotic deposition is not understood, but one theory is that the fibroblasts are damaged by ultraviolet radiation and produce altered collagen and elastin.[9]

The improvement of photoaged skin by chemical peels involves the deposition of new collagen on top or in place of the upper papillary zone of the elastotic depos-

its.[5, 10] Medium and deep peels are thought to function histologically like dermabrasions by causing similar scar formation in the upper papillary dermis.[11] Superficial peels may achieve satisfactory results by repeatedly stimulating new collagen growth without requiring the deeper wound healing associated with deep chemical peels.

For treating wrinkles, glycolic acid or TCA penetration can be enhanced by increasing the strength of the peel (Figs. 37–1, 37–2). Repeated applications of 70% glycolic acid and 35% TCA can be used but will require pretreatment with Jessner's solution or solid carbon dioxide (CO_2) slush to increase the depth of damage.[2]

ACTINIC KERATOSES

Superficial peels can be used to treat actinic keratoses that are not excessively hyperkeratotic. A tendency to produce hypopigmented scars is seen when individual actinic keratoses are treated with spot liquid nitrogen cryosurgery or electrocautery. Although 5-fluorouracil can effectively remove multiple lesions, it is very uncomfortable and causes a longer period of morbidity than a superficial chemical peel, and therefore many patients will not be compliant. Topical retinoic acid has been reported to be only minimally effective as a solitary agent for treating actinic keratoses, although it can complement the penetration of 5-fluorouracil for patients with thicker hyperkeratotic lesions.

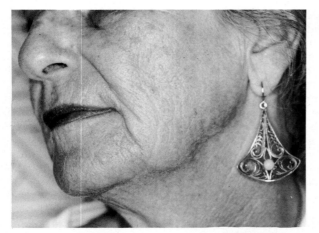

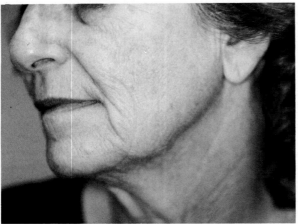

Figure 37–1. *A,* An older individual with multiple fine wrinkles caused by photodamage. *B,* Appearance after 2 years of therapy with glycolic acid.

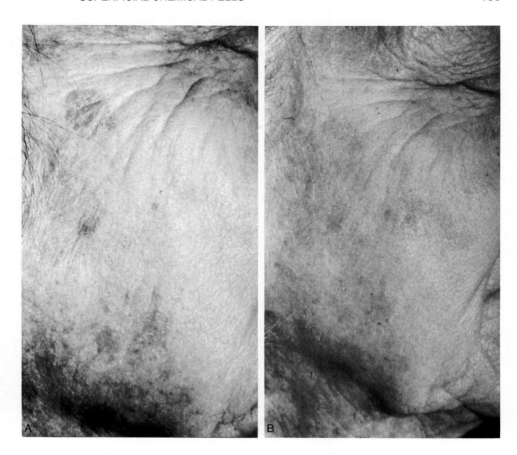

Figure 37–2. An 80-year-old female with wrinkles and keratoses before *(A)* and after *(B)* 5 months of twice-a-day application of 10 to 15% AHA creams. (Courtesy of Eugene Van Scott, M.D.)

A solution of 70% glycolic acid increases epidermolysis and discohesiveness of the cells, which thins actinic keratoses[12] and may cause some lesions to resolve completely (Figs. 37–3, 37–4). Even if the thicker actinic keratoses do not resolve, they are always thinner, making them easier to treat with 5-fluorouracil or other modalities. The advantages of pretreating with chemical peels before 5-fluorouracil are the decreased discomfort and reduction in application time.[13]

TCA in a concentration of 30 to 35% has also been found to be effective in treating actinic keratoses.[14] TCA is more effective in removing lentigines and wrinkles than 5-fluorouracil cream and is equally as effective in removing actinic keratosis. TCA can also be applied locally to specific individual lesions. However, thicker actinic keratoses may require liquid nitrogen cryosurgery or other therapy.

Another variation for actinic keratoses treatment is to treat with 5-fluorouracil for a short period (2 weeks) to bring out many previously subclinical lesions.[15] This is then followed with a peel induced by glycolic acid or TCA localized to the remaining inflamed lesions. Using repeated peels after this initial procedure has been completed may prevent or retard the appearance of new actinic keratoses.

ACNE

Although acne is not usually treated with superficial peels, chemical peeling may effectively reduce come-dones and pustules.[1] Glycolic acid has been reported to readily penetrate[12] into open and closed comedones. TCA may be successfully used as an acne exfoliant for active lesions and also to improve acne scarring.[1, 16]

The recommended application period for glycolic acid or TCA for acne and acne scarring is shorter than for other peel indications. Thus, 50% glycolic acid should be applied for only 1 to 2 minutes over the entire face. Often no redness is seen at the time the glycolic acid is neutralized. After one or two light peels, the acne may look the same or even worse. However, on close inspection, new comedones come to the surface after several peels, and after three to five peels have been performed at 3-week intervals, a majority of comedones and pustules are gone. If 10% glycolic acid is used thereafter, the peel effect may be maintained for at least 6 months. TCA in a concentration of 15 to 20% is applied for 30 to 45 seconds and then thoroughly neutralized. After a number of these very light peels, both acne and acne scars are improved.[17] These peeling agents can provide more effective keratolytic and comedolytic therapy than retinoic acid.

MELASMA

Melasma is a blotchy, irregular hyperpigmentation that typically appears on the forehead, upper cheeks, and upper lip,[18, 19] but other areas of the face can also be similarly affected. Two hormones, estrogen and progesterone, are thought to be partially responsible for

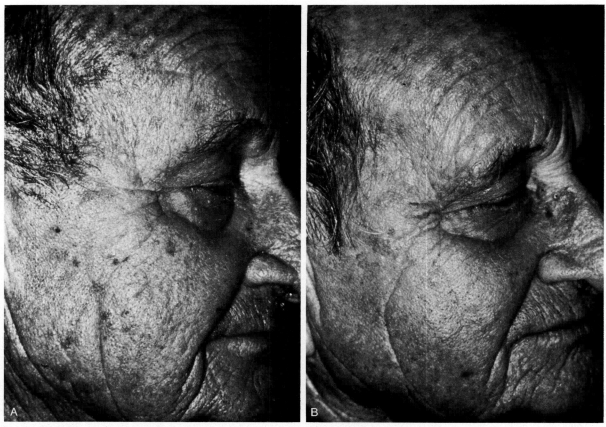

Figure 37–3. *A,* Patient with multiple actinic keratoses across the cheek and forehead. *B,* Resolution of many actinic keratoses after 4 months of glycolic acid therapy consisting of four 70% peels and daily application of 10% glycolic acid lotion.

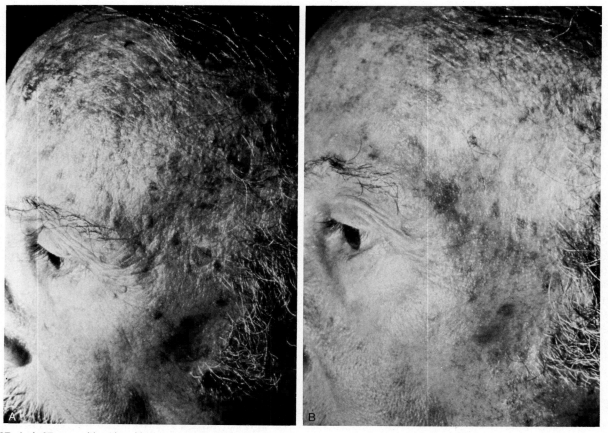

Figure 37–4. A 67-year-old male with numerous facial keratoses before *(A)* and after *(B)* 3 months of twice-a-day treatment with 10 to 20% AHA creams. (Courtesy of Eugene Van Scott, M.D.)

causing melasma, especially during pregnancy or with the use of oral contraceptives.

Much of the difficulty in treating melasma is that patients prone to having melasma also have a tendency to develop postinflammatory hyperpigmentation. Dermabrasions and deeper peels have been used, but results are inconsistent and have been associated with a higher incidence of side effects than superficial chemical peels.[6]

Patients can apply a mixture of either 10% glycolic acid and 2% hydroquine or topical tretinoin, with 4% hydroquinone and mild corticosteriods[19] twice a day before and after a series of peels. Chemical peels using 50% glycolic acid or 15 to 25% TCA peels are both helpful, although TCA peels may be less consistent in their response. Crusting should be avoided because of the risk of hyperpigmentation in patients with darker complexions. Usually four to five chemical peels are necessary before clear clinical improvement is seen (Fig. 37–5). Use of sunscreens with maximal ultraviolet radiation A and B coverage is strongly recommended postoperatively to prevent further darkening.[2, 5, 6]

The mechanism by which glycolic acid and TCA work on hyperpigmentation is not known. Glycolic acid, as with other alpha-hydroxy acids, is chemically related to ascorbic acid.[12] Some studies suggest that ascorbic acid has a direct inhibitory effect on melanocyte activity. Another possible benefit of glycolic acid and light TCA peels is that they allow better penetration of the hydroquinone to the melanocytes in the basal layer of the epidermis or upper papillary dermis. They may also directly damage and decrease the number of melanocytes.

LENTIGINES

Lentigines are flat brown macules that develop on the sun-exposed areas of the hands and face, especially the temples and upper cheeks (Fig. 37–6). Some cutaneous surgeons believe that lentigines may have a keratotic component[12] along with an increase in the number and activity of melanocytes in the epidermal basal layer. Chemical peels can be very effective in the treatment of lentigines. This is usually accomplished by repeated light peels using glycolic acid or 20 to 35% TCA (Figs. 37–7, 37–8, 37–9). Deeper peels are also very effective when applied to each individual lesion and are well tolerated on the hands, chest, and back. Jessner's formula is a good pre-peel adjunct to enhance the penetration of the chemical.[3] When treating lentigines, the patient should apply 10% glycolic acid or topical retinoic acid before and after the superficial chemical peels.

Histologic Findings of Chemical Peels

Histologic studies have been done to analyze the effects of chemical peels on the different layers of the skin. Both the wounding and healing have been noted to be identical to those caused by dermabrasion.[10] The initial reaction is epidermal coagulation[20] along with cellular and connective tissue destruction in the papillary dermis. A thin crust composed of keratin, necrotic keratinocytes, and a proteinaceous precipitate forms later. Epidermal regeneration typically occurs after 2 to

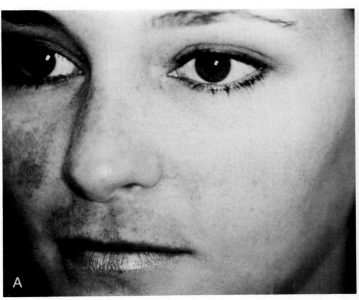

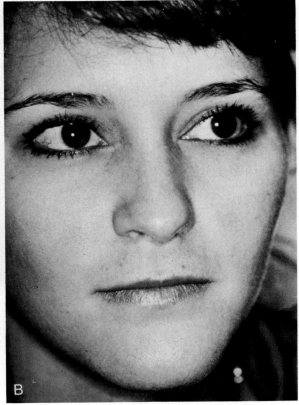

Figure 37–5. *A,* A young patient who had had melasma for several years related to oral contraceptive use. *B,* Melasma dramatically cleared with only two very superficial chemical peels of 50% glycolic acid and daily application of 10% glycolic acid and 2% hydroquinone lotion for 2 months.

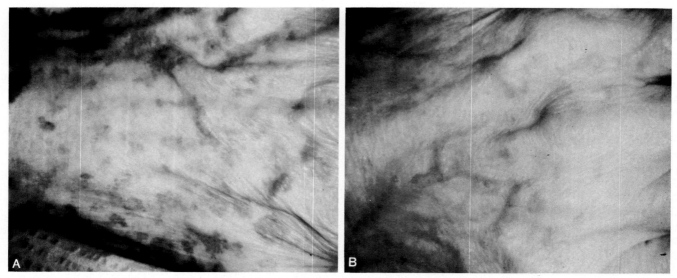

Figure 37–6. *A,* Multiple lentigines and superficial actinic keratoses of the dorsal hand. *B,* Clinical appearance 4 months after two treatments to each individual lesion with 25% trichloroacetic acid (TCA) during a 14-day interval. Once adequate treatment of the lesions was obtained, the entire back of the hand was peeled with a 25% solution of TCA to ensure an even pigmentation of the area. (Courtesy of Dr. Paul S. Collins, M.D.)

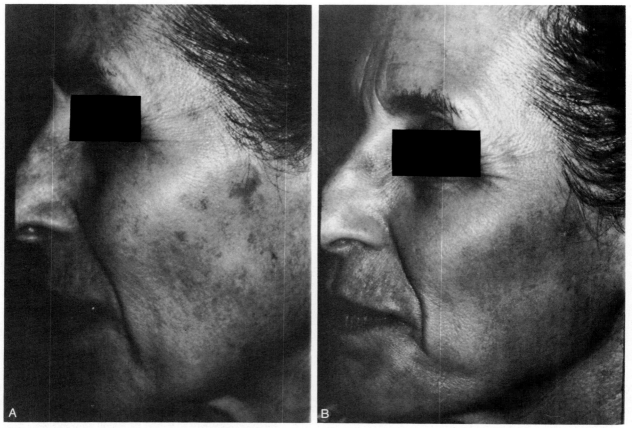

Figure 37–7. *A,* A female patient with multiple solar lentigines on the cheeks and temples. *B,* Photograph demonstrating clearing of the lentigines 1 month after a treatment with 35% TCA.

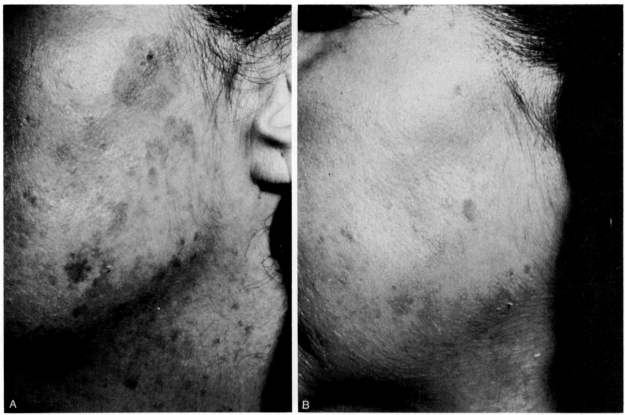

Figure 37–8. A 37-year-old female before *(A)* and after *(B)* 6 weeks of twice-a-day treatment with 15% glycolic acid cream, showing improvement of facial keratoses.

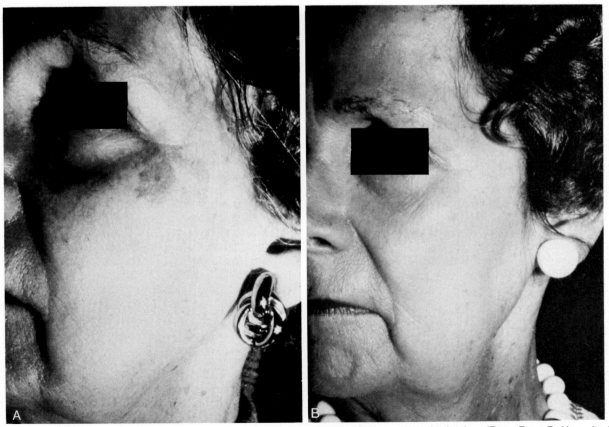

Figure 37–9. *A,* Large solar lentigo near the left eye. *B,* After glycolic acid therapy to remove the lentigo. (From Frost P, Horowitz S [eds]: Principles of cosmetics for the dermatologist. CV Mosby, St. Louis, 1982, p 73.)

7 days. After 2 weeks, the epidermis is completely healed with partially reformed rete ridges. In addition, dermal thickening with fibroblast proliferation and new collagen deposition has been observed in the papillary dermis.[5, 20] This new dermal collagen deposition probably accounts for most of the cosmetic improvement and rejuvenation of the skin.[5, 21]

Biopsies show horizontally arranged new collagen with a predominance of fibroblasts 2 to 3 weeks after chemical peels.[22–24] The sun-induced elastotic changes with basophilic degeneration and homogenization of collagen disappear, and the zone of new collagen remains for up to 1 year. Finely wrinkled, actinically damaged skin is benefited most by treatment with superficial peels. Subsequent biopsies performed after chemical peeling demonstrate both a reduction in the melanosis of the epidermis and fewer melanocytes at the dermal-epidermal junction.[25] A long-term histologic study on phenol peels showed the same new, horizontally arranged collagen deposits seen with superficial peels, but these collagen changes in the papillary dermis are maintained for at least 12 years[25] and may be permanent.[26]

In a study of the penetration of TCA, phenol, and Baker's solution into sun-damaged and sun-protected sites, the same proportional penetration was found in both areas. The zone of new collagen formation within the papillary dermis was also proportional to the depth of wounding. A series of postpeel biopsies on minipigs[27] demonstrated a similar zone of new papillary dermal collagen that was more prominent than in dermabraded skin.

A guinea pig model for dermabrasions and chemical peels has been developed to help understand the physiologic dynamics of peels and to standardize the different peeling agents.[28] Superficial TCA peels mostly affect the epidermis and upper papillary dermis but do not wound deeply enough to correct skin that is severely damaged. Epidermal regeneration begins within 1 day and is usually completed within 7 to 10 days. Deeper peels require epithelialization to occur from adnexal structures.[21] The actual changes from peels involving collagen and elastin regeneration in the dermis have not been studied. However, one study did measure the depth of tissue necrosis from various concentrations of TCA in a pig model.[29] It was found that higher concentrations of TCA caused deeper tissue necrosis. With 20% TCA, a common superficial peel concentration, only intraepidermal necrosis was noted. With 35% TCA, full-thickness epidermal necrosis with very superficial reticular dermal damage was seen.

Specific Superficial Chemical Peeling Agents

GLYCOLIC ACID

Alpha-hydroxy acids are a class of compounds derived from various fruits and foods and are therefore sometimes called "fruit acids." Glycolic acid comes from

TABLE 37–3. ALPHA-HYDROXY ACIDS WITH POTENTIAL FOR CLINICAL USE

Acetylmandelic acid
Glycolic acid
Lactic acid
Mandelic acid
Methylmandelic acid
Galacturonic acid
Pyruvic acid
Malic acid
Tartaric acid
Citric acid

sugar cane, malic acid comes from apples, tartaric acid comes from grapes, citric acid comes from citrus fruits, and lactic acid comes from sour milk.[30] Glycolic acid is the smallest alpha-hydroxy acid,[13] composed of a two-carbon molecule. Other alpha-hydroxy acids also have potential uses on the skin (Table 37–3).

Glycolic acid has been used extensively for treating various skin lesions,[29] including conditions associated with excessive corneocyte cohesion such as ichthyosis.[13] It is thought that alpha-hydroxy acids decrease corneocyte cohesion by interfering with ionic bonding. Many epidermal lesions, including seborrheic keratoses, verrucae vulgaris, acne, and actinic keratoses, have also been successfully treated with alpha-hydroxy acids.[30] In addition, definite resolution of wrinkles has been found using glycolic acid.

The mechanism by which glycolic acid exerts its influence on wrinkles and hyperpigmentation relates to its similarity to ascorbic acid. Ascorbic acid, a derivative of alpha-hydroxy acid, has been shown to stimulate collagen production[31] and decrease melanin production.[32, 33] Another possibility is that glycolic acid works on wrinkles by increasing the synthesis of glycosaminoglycans and other intercellular ground substances.[2] One laboratory study on fibroblasts suggests that glycolic acid may stimulate the production of collagen in fibroblasts.[34] This is in contrast to other peeling agents, such as TCA and phenol, that damage the skin and cause a thickened zone of papillary collagen to form. Crusting and sloughing of the skin are not the desired effects from chemical peels. In a minipig study, 12% lactic acid was shown to deposit as much new papillary collagen as 25% TCA or 25% phenol after 21 days. Histologic studies of topical retinoic acid have suggested a similar effect.

When 50 to 70% glycolic acid is left on the skin for 15 minutes, a depth of necrosis occurs that is between the depths caused by 35% and 50% TCA. With shorter exposures, 50% and 70% glycolic acid will cause less depth of damage than 35% TCA.[35]

TCA

TCA is a versatile peeling agent that is effective for light peels in 10 to 35% concentrations. TCA was first used as an alternative to phenol and can be modified to produce superficial or deep peeling without systemic toxicity.[36, 37] It has been used for many years because of its wide spectrum of applications over a range of different concentrations. For specific thick keratotic lesions, 70% TCA can be applied repeatedly using concentrations of 15 to 35%. The use of 25% TCA as a light peeling agent every 2 weeks can achieve a deeper peel effect without a substantial risk of scarring.[18] A progression of deeper effects is found with increasing concentrations, resulting in additional new collagen formation as the peels are repeated. Using this principle, even severe photodamage can be improved with TCA peels (Fig. 37–10).

A 35% TCA solution is made by mixing 35 gm TCA crystals with 100 ml distilled water. Solutions of 10%, 20%, and 30% TCA are made correspondingly in 100 ml of water. To maintain maximal stability of TCA, several recommendations have been made.[38] Dark glass bottles are more stable than plastic bottles, which degrade over time. Refrigerated samples maintain their concentration better than those kept at room temperature. The bottle should not be left open for an extended period of time, as evaporation will occur,[37] and crystals of TCA may form along the sides of the bottle. Instead, a small sample should be poured out of the stock bottle

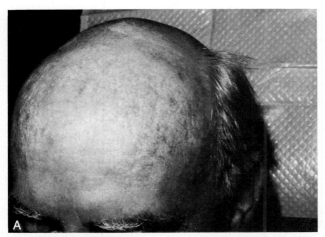

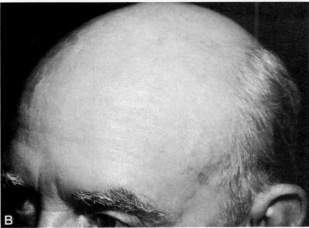

Figure 37–10. *A,* Widespread basophilic degeneration of collagen from actinic degeneration of the forehead and scalp. *B,* After two applications of TCA, first with a 45% solution and 6 weeks later with a 35% TCA solution, the actinic degenerative changes disappeared. (Courtesy of Paul S. Collins, M.D.)

before each use,[38–40] and a new stock solution should be made every 6 months.

Technique for Superficial Chemical Peels

PLANNING THE PEEL: CONSIDERATIONS BEFORE PROCEDURE

Before beginning a peel on a patient, it is important to assess factors that may affect the outcome. For instance, the previous use of topical retinoic acid, glycolic acid, or 5-fluorouracil, as well as oral 13-*cis*-retinoic acid may sensitize a patient's skin. While there is also a possible increased potential for scarring after dermabrasion[41, 42] for patients previously treated with 13-*cis*-retinoic acid, it is not clear whether oral or systemic retinoids increase the risk of scarring from chemical peels.[43] Other medications such as photosensitizing drugs or oral contraceptives may increase the risk of pigmentary problems. It has been speculated that previous dermabrasions or deep chemical peels may increase the potential for scarring,[2] and therefore caution should be used if the patient has had either procedure. Patients with atopy and fair skin may also be more sensitive than others to superficial peels.[17]

The physical characteristics of the skin are also very important to evaluate. Patients who tolerate stronger peeling agents tend to be older with more chronic sun exposure, solar lentigines, and deep wrinkles. This increased tolerance may be a result of the fact that the penetration of the peeling agent is partially blocked by the accumulation of solar elastosis in the upper papillary dermis. Conversely, patients with ruddy, telangiectatic skin or multiple actinic keratoses may be less tolerant, depending on how much erythema is present.

Thick, sebaceous skin may better tolerate superficial peels than thin, less sebaceous skin.[37] Part of the resistance to peels may be the quantity of oil that is present on the skin surface. Consequently, skin preparation with alcohol and acetone must be more vigorous in some areas, such as the nose, where scrubbing may be required to achieve an even peel.

It is always prudent to thoroughly document the peeling procedure[29] in the medical record. Procedural documentation is very important in providing consistency of technique. In addition, the skin condition being treated and the skin characteristics that may affect the peel should always be noted. A record sheet with anatomic drawings for superficial peels helps to keep track any of variations in the technique (Fig. 37–11). Records should emphasize skin preparation method, duration of the peel, and the type and concentration of the agent. Consistently good photographs can be difficult to take from the same angle and with the same lighting, but they can be very important documentation for the medical record. Relatively uniform pictures can be taken even without a special photography room. From the side view, the top of the ear should be lined up horizontally with the lateral canthus of the eye, and the tip of

Date: _____

Patient's name: _____

Age: _____

CLINICAL SKIN DESCRIPTION   ANATOMIC DRAWINGS

A. Pigment _____
B. Acne and acne scars _____
C. Photo-aging _____
D. Wrinkling _____

MEDICATION

Retin A _____
Accutane _____
Other _____

PREVIOUS HISTORY

Allergies _____
Eczema _____
Radiation _____

PHOTOGRAPHS TAKEN

_____ Yes _____ No

Date of first application: _____
Cleansing agent(s): _____
Agent(s) used after application: _____
Home care recommended: _____

Date of other applications and comments:
1. _____
2. _____
3. _____
4. _____
5. _____

Figure 37–11. Form for superficial peel procedure.

the nose should be lined up vertically with the edge of the contralateral cheek.

Pretreatment with daily topical retinoic acid or alpha-hydroxy acid may increase the efficacy of the peel.[3, 5] Many patients are given 10% glycolic acid to apply daily for 2 weeks as pretreatment before a chemical peel.

SKIN PREPARATION

The patient is instructed to remove all makeup or sunscreen lotion. This is followed by skin preparation with chlorhexidine, acetone, or Jessner's solution. The purpose of the preparation is to remove all surface debris and a variable amount of stratum corneum to enhance the effect of the peel. Jessner's solution will remove most of the stratum corneum, acetone removes some of the stratum corneum, and chlorhexidine probably only removes surface debris and oils. Often, two cleansings are performed to evenly remove surface oils, makeup, and debris. Degreasing is important, because even a small amount of oil remaining on the skin will increase the surface tension and permit less penetration of the peeling agent. If erythema occurs on sensitive skin after cleaning with acetone, use of a lower chemical concentration or a shorter application time is recommended. Some cutaneous surgeons will continue to gently scrub with alcohol and acetone until the dark film

of the keratin debris stops appearing on the gauze.[40] Skin preparation with acetone scrubbing will cause a much deeper peel than gentle cleaning with chlorhexidine solution.[44]

APPLYING GLYCOLIC ACID PEEL

The glycolic acid is applied using either cotton-tipped applicators or cotton balls. A simple tray is set up to do the peel (Fig. 37–12). A heavily soaked cotton ball works well, since the amount of glycolic acid is not as important as the length of time of application (Fig. 37–13). The glycolic acid is carefully applied to one cosmetic unit at a time to ensure even coverage. One hand is used to stretch out furrows and creases while applying the solution with the other hand. A cotton-tipped applicator is used to apply more of the glycolic acid into furrows or fine creases (e.g., nasolabial folds or perioral creases) to enhance the effect (Fig. 37–14). Thick keratotic areas will not respond as well and may require additional firm rubbing to react properly. Because 50 to 70% glycolic acid is a gel-like substance, some of the peeling agent may collect on certain anatomic areas. However, unlike TCA, glycolic acid does not produce a greater reaction if a greater amount of it is applied.

The area around the eyes should be treated separately, using a semimoist cotton applicator, to ensure

left on for a carefully timed 3 minutes. If the patient has repeated peels every 2 to 4 weeks, the time is increased by 30 seconds during each chemical peel procedure, or the concentration of the glycolic acid is increased to 70%. If the patient has very sensitive skin, the peel may be started at 2 to 2½ minutes. Eventually, some patients will tolerate peels lasting for up to 10 minutes, especially if they have severe chronic sun damage. In patients with acne, it appears that the peeling agent penetrates the pores and plugs more readily than the epidermis. When glycolic acid is used to treat acne, it is usually left on for only 1 to 2 minutes.

APPLYING TCA PEEL

TCA peels are applied in a manner similar to that used for glycolic acid, although some differences should be noted. Small variations in technique can cause larger variations in depths of peeling and possible scarring.[37] Such variations in technique are evident in reports that describe the use of TCA,[45–47] but any of the procedures, when used consistently, can be safely and effectively used. The skin preparations to remove oils and excess keratin debris are the same for TCA as for glycolic acid. TCA is applied evenly with several cotton-tipped appli-

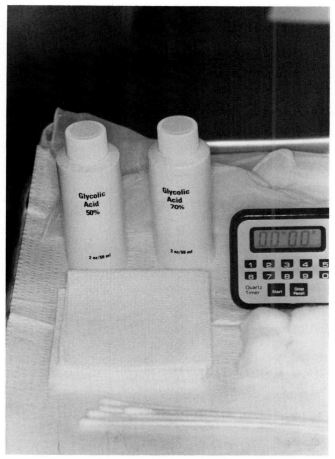

Figure 37–12. Standard tray for glycolic acid peels.

that the peeling agent does not get into the eyes. The patient is instructed to keep the eyes closed to minimize tearing. Tears are wiped dry to avoid capillary movement of the chemical agent into the eye. The application should be stopped 4 to 5 mm away from the eyelid ciliary margin. All types of peels should be feathered below the jaw and into the hairline to minimize the line of demarcation.[40] The glycolic acid is left on the skin for the prescribed amount of time by monitoring with either a stopwatch or a timer started at the time of initial contact of the glycolic acid. The skin is then neutralized twice very carefully with water-soaked gauze, followed by an application of a mild cleansing lotion such as Cetaphil or Aquanil. The patient then rinses the skin under cool running water. Occasionally, a patient will complain of stinging of the eyes even if no glycolic acid has actually entered them. This will resolve after the peel has been neutralized. A water-soaked gauze can be used to gently wipe the eyes, or a squeeze bottle with water can be kept at hand to rinse the eyes if needed. Patients with moderate to severe erythema are given a mild topical corticosteroid cream to apply twice daily to affected areas for 2 days after peeling.

Superficial chemical peels need to be repeated to provide the maximal benefit.[17] The initial application usually employs a 50% glycolic acid solution, which is

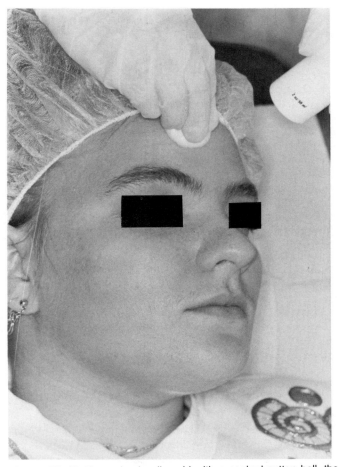

Figure 37–13. To apply glycolic acid with a soaked cotton ball, the forehead is covered first, followed by the cheeks, chin, and nose.

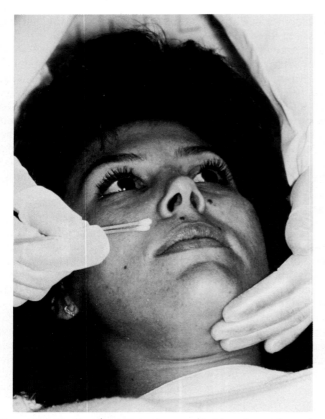

Figure 37–14. Glycolic acid can be reapplied into deeper furrows or to specific lentigines to maximize the local effects.

cators or cotton balls. The same basic pattern—starting on the forehead and continuing down one cheek and around the face to the other cheek—is recommended. TCA can be reapplied to furrows in a manner similar to that used for glycolic acid. However, keratotic lesions can be retreated with a cotton-tipped applicator, since keratoses can be more resistant to frosting. TCA should be drained at the side of the bottle, rather than poured, to decrease the chances of dripping. Unlike with glycolic acid, erythema develops very quickly with TCA application, and frosting appears within 1 to 2 minutes. It is important not to let the TCA drip or collect in a pool; otherwise, overreaction will occur. Because the discomfort with TCA can be more severe than with glycolic acid, having the patient fan the skin will provide some relief. If the discomfort is too great, the peel can be stopped for several minutes before proceeding to allow patients time to recover.

TCA may be applied evenly once or reapplied until frosting is achieved. Neutralization is usually performed with water or a 5% bicarbonate solution. Neutralization for superficial peels of TCA should be performed within 60 to 90 seconds or soon after frosting appears. Because the skin may neutralize the chemical itself, many cutaneous surgeons do not neutralize it at all.[40] Neutralization after frosting is probably not very helpful.

Usually the first application of TCA should be light, and TCA should not be reapplied to any areas. One useful approach is to apply a test dose of 10% or 15% TCA for 1 minute before neutralizing. The timer is started at initiation of TCA application, and at the end of 1 minute, the area is rinsed or wiped with water. The process is repeated once a week or biweekly and the time increased by 30 seconds to a maximum of 2 minutes. Depending on the results, the TCA concentration can then be increased to 25% or 30%. When the TCA concentration is increased, the time period before neutralization is again reduced to 1 minute.

Another technique is to use a 30% or 35% solution without progressing to higher concentration peels. After skin preparation, TCA is applied to all the peel areas. Without reapplication the skin is allowed to frost or blanch.[37, 41] The area is then neutralized immediately after blanching, although it may have little effect. Often, it is easier to section the face into anatomic units to apply TCA, then neutralize before moving on to the next facial area.

A number of different factors may influence the choice of the chemical used in performing a superficial peel (Table 37–4). The most important difference between applying TCA and applying glycolic acid is that glycolic acid reactivity is very dependent on the length of time that it stays on the skin, but the amount of glycolic acid applied is not critical as with TCA peels. On the other hand, TCA is very dependent on both the concentration and the amount of chemical used, as well as the application pressure. If a lower concentration of TCA is continuously applied several times or reapplied after the frost appears, the peel will be deeper. The time before neutralization makes a difference in the peel reaction only if neutralization occurs after 1 to 2 minutes and before frosting.[37]

COMBINATION PEELS

Topical retinoic acid has been used on a daily basis.[43] While several studies have advocated the use of topical retinoic acid for the treatment of actinic keratoses, wrinkles, and abnormal pigmentation, further investigation is needed to evaluate its effectiveness. Topical retinoic acid as a pre-peel treatment 2 weeks before dermabrasion has been shown to reduce healing time and decrease complications.[48] "Retinizing" the skin is thought to improve wound healing and speed reepithelialization. Topical retinoic acid can also be used in conjunction with a superficial peel to enhance the effects. Studies focusing on the use of the two modalities

**TABLE 37–4. FACTORS INFLUENCING THE
CHEMICAL PEELING TECHNIQUE**

Severity of skin damage
Type of cleansing agent to prepare skin
Concentration of chemical
Time in contact with peeling agent
Amount of chemical applied
Degree of rubbing
Quantity of reapplication
Extent of neutralization

together have not been performed, although the combination is commonly advocated.[37] One caution to be kept in mind when using retinoic acid is that it will deepen the effect of peels, probably by thinning the stratum corneum and upper stratum malpighian layers of the epidermis.

An alternative to topical retinoic acid as a pre-peel agent is 10% glycolic acid, which can be used for 2 weeks before performing a superficial peel with glycolic acid or TCA.[39] Although further studies are warranted, pre-peel use of 10% glycolic acid may enhance penetration of superficial peels in a similar fashion to topical tretinoin.

The principle behind combining peels is that one agent can enhance the penetration of another while decreasing some of the toxicity and morbidity of deeper peels. Use of 35% TCA alone does not consistently penetrate deeper than the papillary dermis. However, a 45 to 60% concentration of TCA has a significant risk of pigmentary alteration and scarring.[45] TCA in a 50 to 70% concentration has an even higher risk of uneven hypopigmentation and persistent erythema.

One study showed that solid CO_2 applied before use of 35% TCA created a wound that was similar in depth to that created by phenol without the risks of the higher strength TCA.[44] Solid CO_2 blocks are dipped into a 3:1 solution of acetone and alcohol, then applied directly to the skin for 3 to 10 seconds before applying several coats of TCA (Fig. 37–15). The use of Jessner's solution before applying 35% TCA has proven to be beneficial, as the combination of the two reduces the significant scarring risk associated with higher concentrations of TCA.[3] Jessner's solution is applied with moist cotton-tipped applicators and allowed to lightly frost. After several minutes, 35% TCA is applied evenly with several cotton-tipped applicators. The combination of these two peels is rated as a medium-depth peeling procedure. As designed, both peels are a substitute for deep phenol peels to improve deep wrinkles and darker hyperpigmentation with limited side effects.

Jessner's solution or 20% TCA can enhance the effects of 50% and 70% glycolic acid. These combinations allow for more accelerated peeling while producing only mild erythema and focal crusting. As with other superficial peels, these combinations can be repeated regularly every 2 to 4 weeks. Preliminary histologic studies suggest that the depth of penetration is enhanced when combinations with glycolic acid are used.[36]

The procedure for applying a pre-peel agent before glycolic acid is similiar to the regular peel procedure described for TCA. Jessner's solution may be (1) applied thinly and allowed to dry on the face for 2 minutes, (2) firmly rubbed into the skin, or (3) applied in multiple even coats. Next, the glycolic acid is applied and neu-

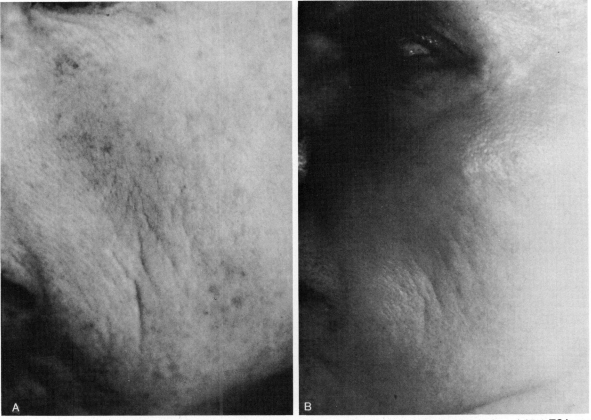

Figure 37–15. *A*, A 52-year-old patient with actinically damaged skin before medium-depth carbon dioxide slush and 35% TCA peel. *B*, The same patient 6 months later, with improvement in actinic rhytides and pigmentation. (Courtesy of Harold J. Brody, M.D.)

TABLE 37–5. **FORMULA FOR JESSNER'S SOLUTION**

14 gm resorcinol
14 gm salicylic acid
14 ml lactic acid
100 ml Q.S. ethanol

tralized.[3, 46] The skin is likely to develop more erythema and show more sloughing and crusting of the epidermis than when glycolic acid alone is used.

Other Peeling Agents

Jessner's solution, composed of resorcinol, salicylic acid, lactic acid, and ethanol (Table 37–5), is one of the light peels that has been used in facial salons as well as physicians' offices for many years.[17] Jessner's solution is applied lightly with a soaked cotton ball or cotton-tipped applicator. The solution is allowed to dry without neutralization. It can be applied several times to achieve deeper penetration.[46] Histologic studies have not been done to determine the differences in penetration depth that occur from layered applications of the solution. However, rubbing the solution more vigorously into the skin can deepen the effects of the peel. Improvements in pigmentation and fine wrinkles can be seen after using Jessner's solution (Fig. 37–16), but because of reports of systemic toxicity, the use of Jessner's solution is often limited to the face. Jessner's may enhance the effects of TCA and glycolic acid by allowing a more even and deeper penetration.[3]

Resorcin, a derivative of phenol,[47] has been used since it was first introduced in 1882. It has been shown to cause a separation in the epidermis at the level of the stratum granulosum while inducing a dense inflammatory response. Histologic studies have shown that resorcin causes an increase in glycosaminoglycans, elastic fibers, and fibroblasts and a thickening of the papillary dermis.[35] It can be effective for treating fine wrinkles, actinic damage, and abnormal pigmentation.[47] Formulations for superficial peeling vary from 10 to 50% (Table 37–6).

Rescorcin paste is applied as a mask and layered across the face using a tongue blade or small brush. After removal in 5 to 10 minutes, a "resorcin membrane" remains that persists for 4 to 5 days. Reepithelialized skin appears when the damaged tissue desquamates. Complications are usually minimal, with hyperpigmentation reported in less than 1% of treated patients in an Hispanic population.[47]

Postoperative Instructions

Patients are warned that crusting and erythema will persist for 3 to 7 days after any superficial chemical peel. Mild discomfort consisting of stinging and pruritus is

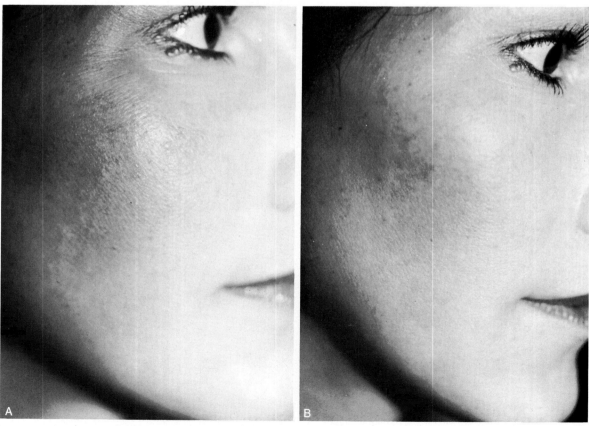

Figure 37–16. *A,* Light freckling before heavy Jessner's solution application with sable brush. *B,* Fading of freckling as a result of partial epidermal sloughing. (Courtesy of Harold J. Brody, M.D.)

TABLE 37–6. FORMULA FOR RESORCIN SUPERFICIAL PEELING SOLUTION

24.0% sulfur
24.0% resorcin
0.5% carboxymethyl cellulose
1.0% aluminum–magnesium silicate
2.5% sorbitol
2.5% glycerine
45.5% deionized water

usually present only during the procedure. Analgesics and oral steroids are usually not required afterward. However, mild topical cortisone creams can be used postoperatively if the inflammation and erythema are uncomfortable. The face can be rinsed, but the patient is told not to scrub. A noncleansing lotion can be used if necessary. For crusting, an antibiotic ointment is applied, but the crusts should not be mechanically removed.[2] To avoid deepening the reaction of the peel,[37] patients are advised not to apply alpha-hydroxy acids or topical retinoic acid for at least 4 to 5 days. Protection from sun exposure is strongly recommended for at least 2 weeks, especially when the treatment is being performed for pigmentary problems. It is important to provide patients with written information on the discomfort, crusting, and erythema along with instructions on the general care of the skin.

Complications

Hyperpigmentation is probably the most common side effect seen with chemical peels. Usually the deeper peels performed with phenol are more susceptible than superficial peels to postinflammatory hyperpigmentation and may occur in 67% of patients.[49] Patients with medium pigmentation or olive skin (e.g., Asians or Hispanics) can develop irregular pigmentation after peeling.[8, 50] If patients experience persistent hyperpigmentation 2 weeks after a peel, application of 10% glycolic acid with 2% hydroquinone lotion or 4% hydroquinone alone can help to lighten the affected areas. Hyperpigmentation can occur with TCA, even at concentrations of 10 to 35%, and may be persistent. Glycolic acid has not been reported to cause permanent hyperpigmentation. Even deeper peels using CO_2 and 35% TCA have caused very few complications.[2]

A line of demarcation can occur in patients with dark complexions. For this reason, the edges of anatomic areas such as under the angle of the jaw, around the eyebrows, and in the hairline should be feathered. Many pre-peel factors can influence the development of hyperpigmentation, including pregnancy, prolonged sun exposure, use of photosensitizing drugs, and oral contraceptives. Some anatomic areas, such as the jawline and perioral areas, are more susceptible to hyperpigmentation.

Persistent erythema occurs uncommonly with superficial peels[2] and should not last more than 2 to 3 months. Most patients will experience resolution within 2 to 3

weeks. Low-potency cortisone ointments can be applied for 2 days after the peel for patients with severe erythema. Erythema may represent a sensitivity to chemical peels resulting in persistent inflammation. Typically, TCA tends to cause more erythema than glycolic acid.

Infection has not been a problem with superficial peels. Both skin preparation and peeling agents are bactericidal, although the crust may harbor and colonize sufficient organisms to cause an infection. The crust found in superficial peels is thinner and less adherent than that found in deeper peels. Patients should apply an antibiotic ointment and gently wash the face daily to cause the crust to separate in 2 to 3 days.

Reactivation of herpes simplex infection can occur after light chemical peels, and hyperpigmentation and hypertrophic scarring are potential hazards.[18] Patients should be questioned about previous herpetic outbreaks and eliciting factors. Even though a patient may not have had an herpetic outbreak for years, postoperative herpetic flares and scarring can occur with chemical peels.[51] Susceptible patients should be started preoperatively on acyclovir, 200 mg orally three times/day.[2]

Hypertrophic scarring is very rare in superficial peels, since this type of scarring is largely a function of the depth of injury to the skin. Low-dose intralesional steroid injections are useful in the management of this complication. No allergies have been seen with TCA or glycolic acid, and renal, hepatic, or cardiac toxicities have not been reported.

SUMMARY

Superficial chemical peels can be safe and effective procedures for treating a variety of skin problems. Newer peeling agents such as glycolic acid and pyruvic acid make chemical peeling easier and safer to perform and allow for a wider selection of patients to tolerate the procedure.[52] Histologic studies have furthered our understanding of chemical peels and compared the effects of various peeling agents. These studies support the increased use of chemical peels in an even greater variety of skin conditions.

REFERENCES

1. Monheit GD: Chemexfoliation: a review. Cosmet Dermatol 1:16–19, 1988.
2. Brody HJ: Complications of chemical peeling. J Dermatol Surg Oncol 15:1010–1019, 1989.
3. Monheit GD: The Jessner's and TCA peel: a medium-depth chemical peel. J Dermatol Surg Oncol 15:945–950, 1989.
4. Murad H: Something old, something new. Dermascope April, 1989.
5. Stegman SJ, Tromovitch TA: Chemical peels in cosmetic dermatologic surgery. In: Stegman SS, Tromovitch TA, Glogau RG (eds): Cosmetic Dermatologic Surgery. Year Book, Chicago, 1984, pp 27–46.
6. Townshend R: Skin peeling: a master's tool in skin care. Aesthet World 12:16–22, 1984.
7. Truppman ES, Ellenberg JD: Major electrocardiographic changes during chemical face peeling. Plast Reconstr Surg 63:44–48, 1979.
8. Goldman PM, Freed MI: Aesthetic problems in chemical peeling. J Dermatol Surg Oncol 15:1020–1024, 1989.

9. Uitto J, Fazio MJ, Olsen DR: Cutaneous aging: molecular alterations in elastic fibers. J Cutan Aging Cosmet Dermatol 1:13–26, 1988.
10. Ayres S III: Superficial chemosurgery: its current status and its relation to dermabrasion. Arch Dermatol 89:395–403, 1964.
11. Ayres S III: Dermal changes following application of chemical cauterants to aging skin. Arch Dermatol 82:578, 1960.
12. Van Scott EJ, Yu RJ: Alpha hydroxy acids: procedures for use in clinical practice. Cutis 43:222–229, 1989.
13. Van Scott EJ, Yu RJ: Hyperkeratinization, corneocyte cohesion, and alpha hydorxy acids. J Am Acad Dermatol 5:867–879, 1984.
14. Brodland DG, Roenigk RK: Trichloroacetic acid chemoexfoliataion (chemical peel) for extensive premalignant actinic damage of the face and scalp. Mayo Clin Proc 63:887–897, 1988.
15. Van Scott EJ: Personal communication, March, 1990.
16. Stagnone JJ: Chemical peeling and dermabrasion. In: Epstein E, Epstein E Jr (eds): Skin Surgery. 6th ed. WB Saunders, Philadelphia, 1987, pp 412–422.
17. Stagnone JJ: Superficial peeling. J Dermatol Surg Oncol 15:924–930, 1989.
18. Collins PS: The chemical peel. Clin Dermatol 5:57–74, 1987.
19. Kligman AM, Willis I: A new formula for depigmenting human skin. Arch Dermatol 111:40, 1975.
20. Spira M, Dahl C, Freeman R, et al: Chemosurgery—a histological study. Plast Reconstr Surg 45:247–253, 1970.
21. Rees RD: Chemabrasion with special reference to rehabilitation of the aging face. Geriatrics 20:1039–1047, 1965.
22. Stegman SJ: A comparative histologic study of the effects of three peeling agents and dermabrasion on normal and sun damaged skin. Aesthetic Plast Surg 6:123–135, 1982.
23. Baker TJ, Gordon HL: Chemical face peeling and dermabrasion. Surg Clin North Am 51:387–401, 1971.
24. Mackee GM, Karp FL: The treatment of post-acne scars with phenol. Br J Dermatol 64:456–459, 1952.
25. Kligman AM, Baker TJ, Gordon HL: Long-term histologic follow-up of phenol face peels. Plast Reconstr Surg 75:652–659, 1985.
26. Baker T, Gordon H, Mosienko P, Seckinger DL: Long-term histological study of skin after chemical face peeling. Plast Reconstr Surg 53:522–525, 1974.
27. Behin F, Feverstein SS, Marovitz WF: Comparative histological study of mini-pig skin after chemical peel and dermabrasion. Arch Otolaryngol 103:271–277, 1977.
28. Stegman SJ: A study of dermabrasion and chemical peels in an animal model. J Dermatol Surg Oncol 6:490–497, 1980.
29. Brodland DG, Cullimore KC, Roenigk RK, Gibson LE: Depths of chemexfoliation induced by various concentrations and application techniques of trichloroacetic acid in a porcine model. J Dermatol Surg Oncol 15:967–971, 1989.
30. Van Scott EJ, Yu RJ: Substances that modify the stratum corneum by modulating its formation. In: Frost P, Horwitz SN (eds): Principles of Cosmetics for the Dermatologist. CV Mosby, St. Louis, 1982, pp 70–74.
31. Pinnell SR, Murad S, Darr D: Induction of collagen synthesis by ascorbic acid: a possible mechanism. Arch Dermatol 123:1684–1686, 1987.
32. Haas JE: The effect of ascorbic acid and potassium ferricyanide as melanogenesis inhibitors on the development of pigmentation in Mexican axolotols. Am Osteopath 73:674, 1974.
33. Lotter AM: Human pigment factors relative to chemical face peeling. Ann Plast Surg 3:231–239, 1979.
34. Moy LS, Murad H, Moy RL: Effect of glycolic acid on collagen production by human skin fibroblasts. In press.
35. Letessier SM: Chemical peel with resorcin. In: Roenigk RK, Roenigk HH (eds): Dermatologic Surgery: Principles and Practice. Marcel Dekker, New York, 1989, pp 1017–1024.
36. Moy LS, Piece S, Moy RL: Epidermal and dermal histologic effects of different peeling agents on the skin of guinea pigs and minipigs. In press.
37. Collins PS: Trichloroacetic acid peels revisited. J Dermatol Surg Oncol 15:933–940, 1989.
38. Spinowitz A, Rumsfield J: Stability time profile of trichloroacetic acid at various concentrations and storage time conditions. J Dermatol Surg Oncol 15:974–975, 1989.
39. Brody HJ: The art of chemical peeling. J Dermatol Surg Oncol 15:918–921, 1989.
40. Greenbaum SS, Lask GP: Facial peeling: trichloroacetic acid. In: Parish LC, Lask GP (eds): Aesthetic Dermatology. McGraw-Hill, New York, 1991, pp 139–143.
41. Roenigk HH Jr, Pinski JB, Robinson JK, Hanke CW: Acne, retinoids, and dermabrasion. J Dermatol Surg Oncol 11:396–398, 1985.
42. Alt TH: Therapeutic facial dermabrasion. In: Epstein E, Epstein E Jr (eds): Skin Surgery. WB Saunders, Philadelphia, 1987, pp 327–343.
43. Moy RL, Moy LS, Bennett RG, et al: Effects of systemic 13-cis-retinoic acid on dermal wound healing in rabbit ears in vivo. J Dermatol Surg Oncol. In press.
44. Stegman SJ: Chemical face peeling. J Dermatol Surg Oncol 12:432, 1986.
45. Resnick SS: Chemical peeling with trichloroacetic acid. J Dermtol Surg Oncol 10:549–550, 1984.
46. Brody HJ, Hailey CW: Variations and comparisons in medium-depth chemical peeling. J Dermatol Surg Oncol 15:953–963, 1989.
47. Perez EH: Different grades of chemical peels. Am J Cosmet Surg 7:67–60, 1990.
48. Mandy SH: Tretinoin in preoperative and postoperative management of dermabrasion. J Am Acad Dermatol 15:878–879, 1986.
49. Litton C, Trinidad G: Complications of chemical face peeling as evaluated by a questionnaire. Plast Reconstr Surg 67:739–743, 1981.
50. Pierce HE, Brown LA: Laminar dermal reticulotomy and chemical face peeling in a black patient. J Dermatol Surg Oncol 12:69–73, 1986.
51. Rappaport MJ, Kamer F: Exacerbation of facial herpes simplex after phenolic face peels. J Dermatol Surg Oncol 10:57–58, 1984.
52. Brody HJ: Medium depth peeling of the skin. J Dermatol Surg Oncol 12:1268–1275, 1986.

CHAPTER 38

Dermabrasion

R. STEVEN PADILLA

In 1905, Kromeyer, a German physician, reported on the use of a motor-powered rotating abrader on chilled skin.[1] However, because his method was considered to lack control, it was never truly accepted. In 1947, Iverson, a plastic surgeon from Philadelphia, described sandpaper abrasion for improving the appearance of traumatic facial tattoos.[2] Although the results were good, there were many drawbacks to the technique, including the need for hospital admission and administration of a general anesthetic. Most importantly, the technique lacked finesse and created a bloody field that obscured the natural lines of the face. In 1948, McEvitt was the first to apply this technique for the correction of acne scarring.[3] In 1953, Kurtin, a New York dermatologist, developed the modern technique of ambulatory dermabrasion.[4, 5] As originally described the procedure was called corrective surgical planing of the skin or plastic planing.[6] It was not until 1954 that the term dermabrasion was coined[7] by Blau, whose close collaborative work with Robbins resulted in the development of the modern equipment necessary to perform dermabrasion on an outpatient basis.

Equipment for Performing Dermabrasions

DERMABRADER

The choice of dermabrasion equipment is personal and depends primarily on the surgical technique. Various machines and dermabrading tips are available for performing dermabrasions.[8] The main factor in choosing a particular piece of equipment is the ability to abrade skin, which is a function of the rotational speed of the tip and the torque that is generated. The power source of the more widely used machines is either electricity or compressed nitrogen gas. The compressed gas units are capable of generating greater torque and rotating faster. However, the need to store and replenish the nitrogen gas cylinders is one drawback to their wide use.[1]

For years the electrically powered, cable-driven unit was the standard machine. In this system, the motor is attached to a cable, and the dermabrader tip is inserted into the handpiece at the opposite end. The machine is able to generate rotational speeds of 800 to 1200 revolutions per minute (rpm). One drawback to this unit is the potential for bending the cable, which creates friction and may result in burnout of the cable. The fast rotational speeds of these units also produce a high-pitched noise that can be distressing to both the surgeon and the patient.

Since the 1980s, smaller, electrically powered, hand-held machines have been developed and are now universally available. The hand-held abrader is easily maneuvered and is relatively quiet. The unit is compact and attached by an electrical cord to a handpiece. The rotational speed of the tip can be controlled by a foot switch. The speed varies with the machine type, but a range of 400 to 33,000 rpm is commonly available (Fig. 38–1). While the torque provided by these machines is only 80% or less of that provided by the older standard models, this is certainly satisfactory for dermabrading skin. The machine with the greatest speed and torque is the high-speed Schreuss (Derma III). This unit provides rotation speeds of 15,000 to 16,000 rpm, is manufactured in Germany, and is available in the United States through A. Schumann Precision Manufacturers, Concord, MA.

DIAMOND FRAISE

The actual cutting tools for performing dermabrasions are the diamond fraise, the wire brush, and the serrated wheel. The most widely used are the diamond fraise and the wire brush (Figs. 38–2 through 38–4). Fraises are

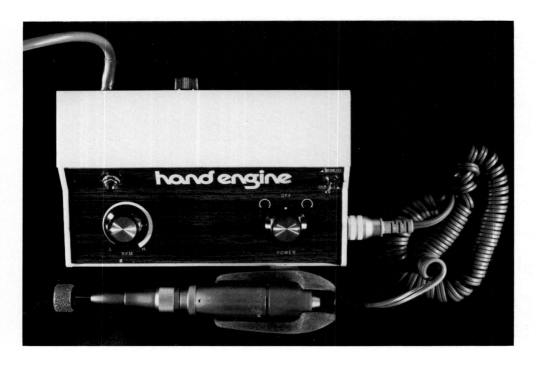

Figure 38–1. Dermabrasion equipment: Bell International hand engine unit with an operating range of 800 to 33,000 revolutions per minute (rpm).

usually stainless steel wheels with industrial-grade diamonds bonded to them.[8] They are graded according to the width of the barrel and the coarseness of the diamonds. In general, the more coarse or rough the cutting surface, the faster the speed of cutting and the greater the penetration into tissues. For the beginning cutaneous surgeon, a wide barrel with either a fine or moderately coarse diamond fraise is usually best, because it is easier to control and reduces the chance of tissue gouging. With experience, coarser diamond fraises with shorter barrels or wire brushes can be safely used.

SERRATED WHEEL

Serrated wheel tips are circular wheels with small surface spikes. Their action is similar to that of coarse diamond fraises, and they do not appear to provide any particular advantages. Because of the wider spacing of the notches, there is a greater likelihood of tissue gouging and a greater difficulty in controlling the depth

to ensure uniform tissue planing. This type of fraise should only be used by an experienced cutaneous surgeon.

WIRE BRUSH

The wire brush is thought by many to be the best cutting instrument[8] and was the standard tip used in the early development of the technique. Brushes are made of stainless steel and come with slightly angled or straight bristles. The slightly angled brush is more widely used, because it cuts more deeply and quickly into tissue and tends to thrust the small abraded tissue fragments away and out of the operating field. Some operators prefer the wire brush because it offers less friction and has a microlacerative effect.[9] However, it can cause deeper and more rapid tissue planing and has a greater potential for tissue damage.

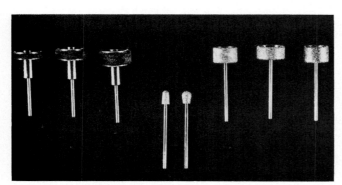

Figure 38–2. Representative sample of commonly used diamond fraises *(upper right)* and wire brushes *(upper left)* plus specialty cone- and pear-shaped fraises *(center).*

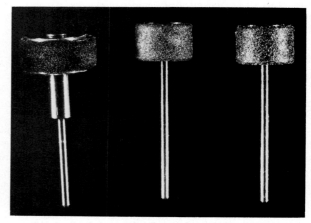

Figure 38–3. Close-up view of diamond fraises—fine *(center)*, extra-coarse *(right)*—and wide *(left)* wire brush.

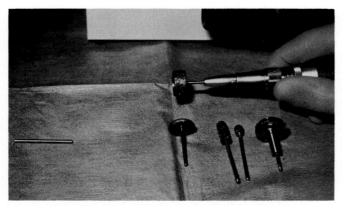

Figure 38–4. Final assembled unit with coarse diamond fraise.

Equipment Maintenance

All dermabrasion equipment should be carefully maintained. Depending on the machine, routine lubrication may be necessary to ensure smooth operation. The cable should be checked for any small particulate matter that could impede its free rotation. Electrical cords should be checked to make sure they are thoroughly insulated and free of crimping, cuts, or breaks. The tips, fraises, brushes, and wheels must be routinely inspected and manually cleaned. The cleaning of the wire brush usually necessitates the use of a special comb to remove entrapped particulate matter. After cleaning, all tips should be repackaged and sterilized, and tips should be periodically checked to ensure their sharpness, as they do wear out over time and may need to be replaced.

Patient Selection

Two of the main indications for performing facial dermabrasion are scarred and aged skin (Table 38–1). Scarring may be secondary to acne, trauma, or chickenpox or other infections. Photodamaged or aged skin is also amenable to treatment. Dermabrasion as a therapeutic tool for treating epidermal dysplasia and actinic keratoses can be very helpful both in preventing the development of skin cancers and in improving cosmetic appearance. Fine wrinkles associated with aged skin can also be improved or eliminated with dermabrasion.

CONSULTATION

The initial consultation with the patient is the time to thoroughly evaluate the patient and ascertain the appropriateness of the patient's expectations about the procedure.[10] During the consultation an explanation of the benefits that are anticipated by the surgeon should be discussed, as well as preoperative preparation, risks, complications, costs, alternative procedures, postoperative care and physical limitations, and need for follow-up visits. If both parties are agreeable, written informed consent should be obtained and the procedure scheduled.[11] Medicolegally, physicians performing cosmetic procedures are held to a higher standard of ensuring informed consent[12] than are physicians performing other types of procedures.

When obtaining the patient's medical history, specific information should be sought about previous exposure to any blood-borne infectious diseases such as hepatitis or human immunodeficiency virus. If seropositivity is present, it may contraindicate a cosmetic procedure,

---

TABLE 38–1. **CONDITIONS TREATED WITH DERMABRASION**

Acne rosacea	Linear epidermal nevus
Actinically damaged skin	Lupus erythematosus
Active acne	Mibelli's porokeratosis
Adenoma sebaceum	Molluscum contagiosum
Angiofibromas of tuberous sclerosis	Multiple pigmented nevi
Basal cell carcinomas (superficial type)	Multiple seborrheic keratoses
Blast tattoos (gunpowder)	Multiple trichoepitheliomas
Chloasma	Neurotic excoriations
Chronic radiation dermatitis	Nevus flammeus
Congenital pigmented nevi	Postacne scars
Darier's disease	Professionally applied tattoos
Dermatitis papillaris capillitii	Pseudofolliculitis barbae
Early operative scars	Rhinophyma
Facial wrinkle lines	Scleromyxedema
Favre-Racouchot syndrome	Smallpox or chickenpox scars
Fox-Fordyce disease	Striae distensae
Freckles	Syringocystadenoma papilliferum
Hair transplantation (elevated recipient sites)	Syringomas
Hemangiomas	Tattoos (amateur and professional)
Keloids	Telangiectasia
Keratoacanthomas	Traumatic scars
Leg ulcers	Verrucous nevus
Lentigines	Vitiligo
Lichen amyloidosis	Xanthelasma
Lichenified dermatoses	Xeroderma pigmentosum

since it has been documented that infectious and non-infectious particulate matter becomes aerosolized during a dermabrasion procedure,[13] and infection of the operating room personnel and the surgeon is a possible risk that must be considered.[14-16] These matters should be thoroughly understood by all patients before any procedure is performed. Blood tests for cryoglobinopathy should also be performed when warranted by historical findings.[17]

CONTRAINDICATIONS

Contraindications to performing dermabrasion should be carefully sought (Table 38–2). Questions about keloid formation, a tendency for irregular pigmentation with minor injuries, and a past history of chronic recurrent herpes simplex infections should be specifically asked. Some cutaneous surgeons consider herpes simplex infections a minor problem since the advent of oral acyclovir.[18] Use of this drug before and during the procedure has been shown to suppress the development of herpes infections in the dermabraded area.[18]

USE OF DERMABRASION TEST SPOTS

Test spot dermabrasion before performance of the full procedure may be helpful.[19] Opponents say that the results of a test spot in one area do not accurately predict the overall outcome, which is probably true. However, test spots can provide valuable additional information about the procedure for the patient as well as the surgeon. For example, the patient will have a clearer understanding of the procedure and the outcome and can better judge its potential value. In some instances, the patient may decide not to proceed with the procedure after evaluating the results of a test spot.

Surgical Technique

PREOPERATIVE CONSIDERATIONS

Several procedures have been shown to enhance the overall outcome of dermabrasion and should be considered preoperatively. The first is pretreatment of the face with topical application of tretinoin 0.05% cream. Use of this medication has been shown to shorten the re-epithelialization time and reduce the incidence of post-

TABLE 38–2. **DERMABRASION CONTRAINDICATIONS**

Burns
Deep thermal
Chemical
Congenital ectodermal defect
History of keloids
History of hypertrophic scars
Radiodermatitis
Pyoderma
Psychosis
Warts

operative milia formation and hyperpigmentation[20] if the drug is restarted within 1 week after the procedure. The second preoperative consideration is to remove the most prominent scars with previous excision followed by primary closure or punch grafting.[21, 22] Deep irregular scars, sinus tracts, or prominent deep pox marks are best improved by a combination of initial excision followed by dermabrasion. Punch grafting is most beneficial for ice-pick scars of 2 to 5 mm in size. If the scar removed by punch excision is only 2 mm in diameter, the defect can be simply sutured together. However, larger punch excisions must usually be grafted with postauricular, non–hair-bearing, full-thickness skin grafts cut 0.5 mm larger than the defect. These grafts are sutured in place with fast-absorbing gut. If this is not done in combination with dermabrasion, there may be small, prominent, linear scars; mild elevations in the punch grafts; or incomplete planing of the pox marks. When performed together, the two procedures maximize the camouflaging of facial scars. Injectable collagen has also been used to improve facial planing by gradually elevating soft, sloping furrows.[23] Collagen injections alone are of little value in hard, fixed, ice-pick scars.

MEDICATIONS AND ANESTHETICS

Before prescribing and administering preoperative medication, it is essential to determine what medications the patient has been taking and what medical problems, if any, are present by taking a detailed initial patient history. Prescription and nonprescription medication use, as well as illicit drug use, should be sought out. Many of these medications alter the desired effects of sedatives and general anesthetics or can exacerbate respiratory or cardiovascular illnesses. Of greatest importance are anticoagulants, antihypertensives, and central nervous system depressants.

The choice of anesthesia is a personal one.[24, 25] The procedure can be performed using general anesthesia, sedation, regional nerve block, or even topical anesthetics. Currently, most dermabrasions are performed in an outpatient setting using sedation only. Many cutaneous surgeons prescribe a mild sedating agent to be taken the night before the procedure. Use of oral dimenhydrinate (Dramamine) in a dose of 100 to 200 mg before retiring will ensure the patient has a good preoperative night. The day of the procedure the patient should be given an additional oral dose of dimenhydrinate or 100 mg of secobarbital sodium (Seconal). Intramuscular injections of meperidine hydrochloride (50 to 100 mg) are preferred by some surgeons, although it has been suggested that the first two medications have a wider margin of safety.[25] No matter what medication is used, the actions and side effects must be thoroughly understood. Before beginning the procedure, an intravenous drip is started with 5% dextrose in water. This is maintained throughout the procedure to allow administration of any additional medications, if needed. At the beginning of the procedure diazepam (5 mg), meperidine (50 mg), or both may be given as an intravenous bolus to provide additional sedation.

Injectable midazolam hydrochloride, a benzodiazepine with a quicker onset and shorter duration of action, has been used with success. The goal of sedation is to provide adequate pain relief and reduce anxiety. During the procedure the patient should remain responsive to verbal commands. Vital signs must be monitored throughout the duration of the procedure. At the beginning of the procedure, some surgeons also perform a regional facial block with an injection of 1% lidocaine either plain or with epinephrine 1:200,000, but this is not essential if adequate sedation and pain relief have been accomplished. The most commonly anesthetized nerves are in the periorbital and submental areas. It is important to remember to allow the skin to return to its normal contour before beginning the procedure if a local anesthetic has been used, for the anesthetic can distend and distort the normal topography. After completion of the procedure, monitoring should be continued until the patient is fully recovered.

Prophylactic antibiotics are not generally prescribed for dermabrasions. However, prophylactic antiviral agents have been shown to be effective in preventing dissemination of facial herpes simplex in individuals with a history of trauma-induced skin infection. Oral acyclovir has been effectively used to prevent recurrent herpes simplex in a dosage of 1 gm/day for 10 days, beginning 3 days preoperatively.[18]

STANDARD OPERATIVE PROCEDURE

Many technical variations have been described, and the choice of procedure is largely based on personal preference and the experience of the surgeon.[26] However, a relatively standard operating procedure with a simple operative tray (Fig. 38–5) can be described.[27–29]

After initiating sedation, about 30 minutes before beginning the procedure, the face is pre-chilled with direct application of ice packs (Fig. 38–6). This will enhance the effectiveness of the subsequent local spray anesthesia. The operating team should be properly outfitted with gloves, gowns, and plastic face masks. The assistant should probably wear cotton gloves on top of the rubber gloves to help grip the skin[30] and to serve as added protection against freezing. A sterile ointment, goggles, and gauze pads are used to cover and protect the patient's ears, eyes, and nose. Both the patient and the surgeon should be in a comfortable position.

The surgeon stands to the side of the patient corresponding to his or her dominant hand. The entire area of planned dermabrasion is painted with either gentian violet or methylene blue, generally extending 2 to 3 mm into the hairline and 10 to 12 mm below the jawline (Fig. 38–7). This helps to obtain a uniform, cosmetically symmetric, smooth surface. A topical refrigerant spray is used to freeze the site. Four-by-four gauze dressings or cotton towels border the area (Fig. 38–8A). The site is frozen by the surgeon or the assistant using a circular motion for 20 to 30 seconds until the skin is firm to the touch and covered with a white frost.[31] Care should be taken not to freeze the skin too deeply, particularly over bony prominences such as the mandibular ramus, zygomatic arch, chin, and forehead.

When dermabrading, the assistant's hands and the free hand of the surgeon apply tension to the skin by pulling horizontally (Fig. 38–8B). This helps to create a relatively stable and uniform planing surface. The depth of the abrasion is controlled by the scar depth but generally does not go deeper than the midreticular dermis, because the probability of scar formation is increased by going deeper (Fig. 38–8C). The gentian violet helps to provide uniformity and also guides the depth of the abrasion by revealing the correct depth

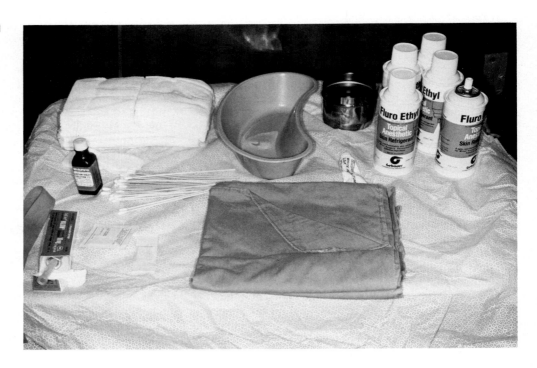

Figure 38–5. Equipment needed for standard dermabrasion.

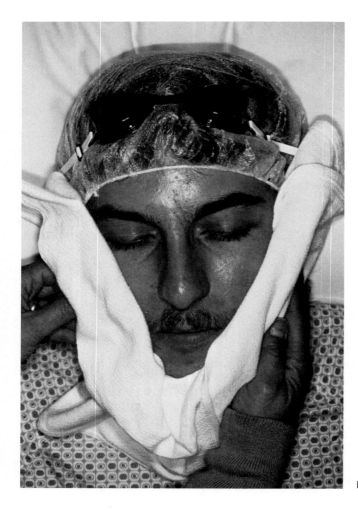

Figure 38–6. Preoperative chilling with application of ice packs.

necessary to remove particularly deep scars. When in doubt, it is better to be conservative, for additional planing procedures are preferable to coping with hypertrophic scarring created by an overzealous initial dermabrasion.

After an area has been planed, it should be covered with gauze or an absorbent cotton towel. Care should be taken not to greatly overlap adjacent areas, since this subjects them to refreezing, causing more tissue damage and scarring.[32] Pressure is applied by the assistant to the previous site to aid in hemostasis. If additional hemostasis is required, gauze pledgets soaked in a 1:1000 Adrenalin solution are very useful. The direction of the planing is perpendicular to the direction of rotation of the fraise or wire brush to help prevent tissue gouging and provide the surgeon with greater control.

Many different freezing agents are available.[33] Ethyl chloride was popular initially but is currently used only infrequently because of its flammable and explosive properties; it is also necessary to use a blowing fan to enhance its evaporation. The safest and most widely used and recommended agents are Frigiderm and Fluro-Ethyl.[33] These agents can cool the skin in about 25 seconds to a range of $-40°$ to $-42°C$. Two other agents, Cryosthesia ($-30°$ and $-60°C$) and Medi-Frig, appear to cause more tissue necrosis and possibly result in

excess scarring.[33–35] Freezing and planing should proceed in an orderly fashion, usually beginning on the forehead and then moving to the temples and cheeks, followed by the mandibular area, nose, and perioral and ocular areas. This particular order is not essential, but a definitive plan should be followed for the sake of efficiency of time, as well as surgeon and patient movement. After completion of the initial dermabrasion (Fig. 38–9A), areas of deeper scarring or persistent gentian violet are retreated using a bullet- or pear-shaped fraise (Fig. 38–9B, C) to obtain a uniform contour (Fig. 38–9D). One addition to this technique is to use a peripheral or periorbital chemical peel with 30 to 50% trichloroacetic acid to help achieve a more uniform degree of pigmentation in areas not in need of dermabrasion.[36]

Postoperative Care

PATIENT INSTRUCTIONS

Patient instructions regarding postoperative wound care should be given in both written and oral form. It is often beneficial to provide a written wound care instruction sheet to the patient at the time of initial consultation, which allows time for the patient to review

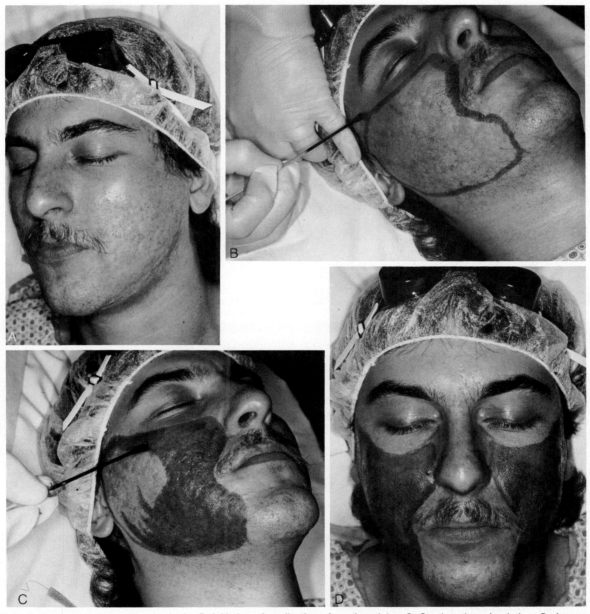

Figure 38–7. *A,* Acne scars seen preoperatively. *B,* Initiation of application of gentian violet. *C,* Continuation of painting. *D,* Appearance after completion of painting of gentian violet to both cheeks.

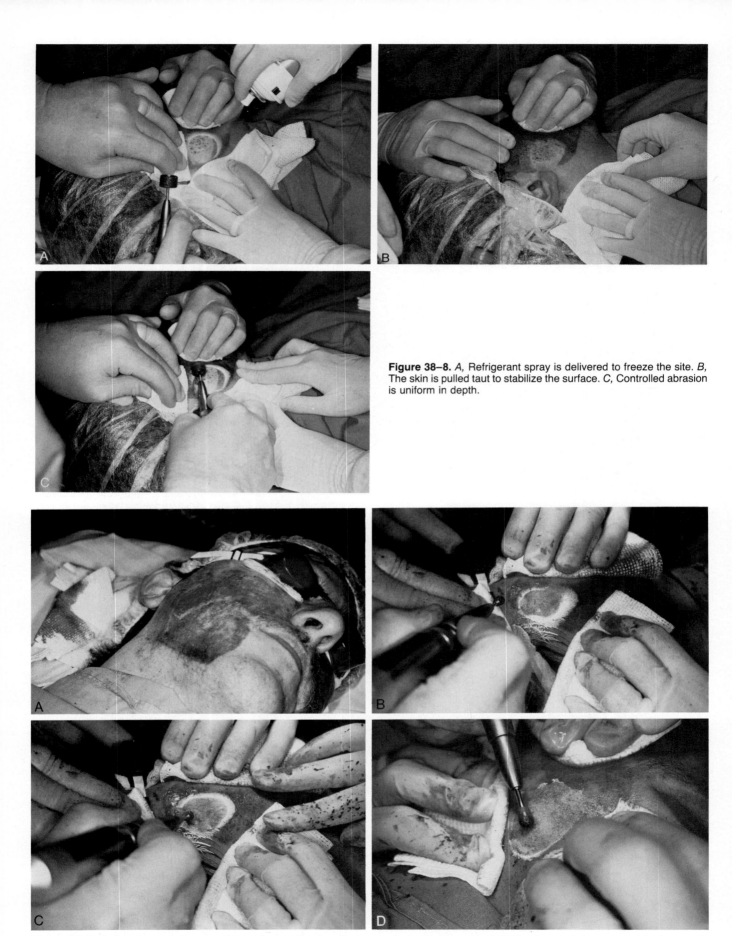

Figure 38–8. *A,* Refrigerant spray is delivered to freeze the site. *B,* The skin is pulled taut to stabilize the surface. *C,* Controlled abrasion is uniform in depth.

Figure 38–9. *A,* Appearance after completion of dermabrasion. *B,* A pear-shaped fraise is used. *C,* Treatment of deeper persistent scars. *D,* Final contours are smoothed.

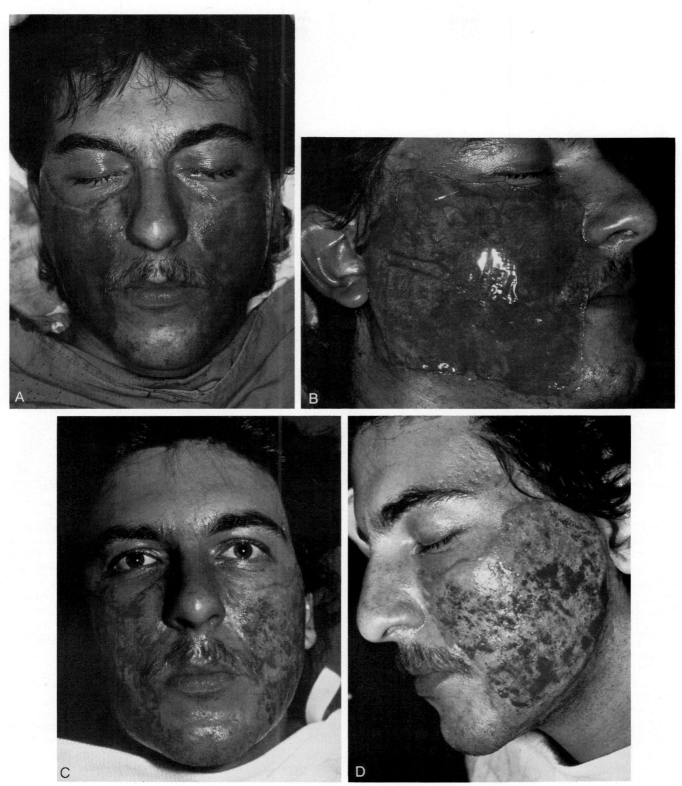

Figure 38–10. *A,* Final appearance immediately after completion of dermabrasion. *B,* Polyethylene oxide water hydrogel stops much of the postoperative discomfort. *C,* Frontal view 24 hours after dermabrasion with slight swelling of the cheeks. *D,* Lateral view 24 hours postoperatively showing moist, shallow wound.

Illustration continued on following page

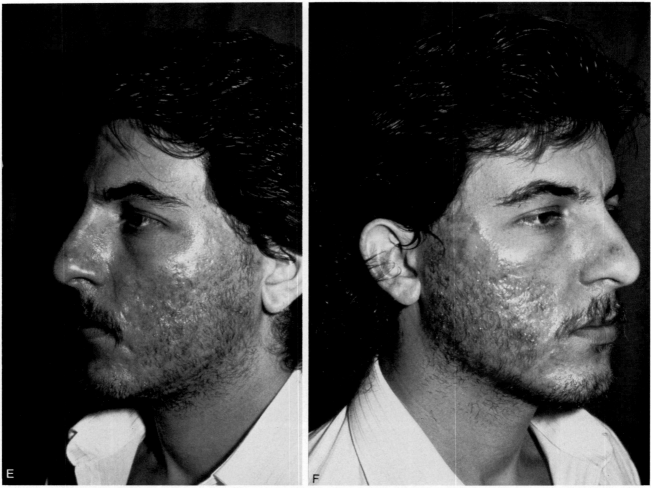

Figure 38–10 *Continued E,* Left profile view at 1 week showing complete reepithelialization. *F,* Right profile view at 1 week showing complete reepithelialization.

the information, ask additional questions, and purchase the necessary postoperative wound dressings. Wound care varies according to the surgeon but typically consists of wound cleansing, application of an emollient cream or topical antibiotic ointment, and an absorbent dressing.

BANDAGING AND CLEANSING TECHNIQUES

Immediately after completion of the procedure (Fig. 38–10A), a full-face dressing is applied with openings for the eyes, nose, and mouth.[37] This begins with application of an antibiotic ointment such as erythromycin ointment or a polyethylene oxide water hydrogel synthetic surgical dressing (Fig. 38–10B). This is followed by a layer of gauze squares and a Kerlix gauze wrap around the head to keep the bandages in place. After completion of the procedure, the wound tends to ooze a serosanguineous material, and a highly absorbent dressing is most useful. The patient returns the following morning for a dressing change (Fig. 38–10C, D). At this time the patient views the wound and is reassured and reinstructed on wound care. Depending on the amount of drainage, either a bulky dressing is reapplied or a

polyethylene oxide water hydrogel wound dressing is used.[38, 39] Biologic dressings are easy for the patient to handle, decrease pain, and promote faster wound healing.[40, 41] The patient is instructed to clean the wound once or twice daily with normal sterile saline or a 50:50 solution of water and 3% hydrogen peroxide, followed by reapplication of antibiotic ointment or emollient. The patient is generally seen 5 days later or sooner, depending on the patient's ability to care for the wound (Fig. 38–10E, F).

Complications

Untoward reactions associated with dermabrasion are uncommon but do occur (Table 38–3). However, a thorough understanding of the limits of skin planing and the depth of skin abrasion, an awareness of high-risk patients and anatomic regions, care in depth of freezing, and overall good surgical technique help decrease the possibility of adverse results and complications. Experienced cutaneous surgeons have found that certain agents may be associated with particular adverse effects. Atypical keloids occurring after dermabrasion have been

TABLE 38–3. **DERMABRASION COMPLICATIONS**

Milia formation
Cysts
Hypertrophic scarring
    Isotretinoin-associated scarring
    Scarring from excessive cold produced by skin refrigerants
Hyperpigmentation
Hypopigmentation
Infections
    Viral
    Bacterial
    Fungal
Persistent erythema
Edema

reported in individuals who had taken oral isotretinoin (Accutane).[42, 43] The mechanism leading to this abnormal scar formation is unknown. It is recommended that the procedure should be delayed for 6 months to 1 year after discontinuation of this medication to help minimize the risk of this potential problem. Whether the drug alone or in combination with some other aspect of the procedure, such as freezing, is responsible for this complication is unknown. One laboratory study[44] failed to implicate isotretinoin as the sole agent causing postdermabrasion scarring. If such scarring does form, in many instances it will respond to topical or intralesional corticosteroid treatment.

Milia are a relatively common problem after dermabrasion but have been reported to be lessened by pre- and postoperative use of topical tretinoin (Retin-A).[18] The mechanism of dermabrasion-associated milia is thought to be implantation of epidermal fragments in the healing wound that continue to keratinize.[45] It has been demonstrated that saline gauze washings performed after completion of the procedure help lessen the incidence of this problem.[45]

Herpes infection induced by dermabrasion has been rare since the introduction of acyclovir. Reports indicate that preoperative treatment with acyclovir can suppress the virus.[18] It is generally accepted that a previous history of traumatically induced herpes simplex reactivation is not a contraindication to performing dermabrasions.

Hyper-[46] and hypopigmentation[47] have both been reported after skin planing. Freezing is also known to affect melanocytes, resulting in hypopigmentation.[48] If this occurs, there is no effective treatment other than the use of cosmetics or possibly experimental melanocyte grafting. Hyperpigmentation is difficult to predict but is generally more likely to occur in those individuals who are likely to experience pigmentation after ultraviolet light exposure. Mottled skin pigmentation, or me-

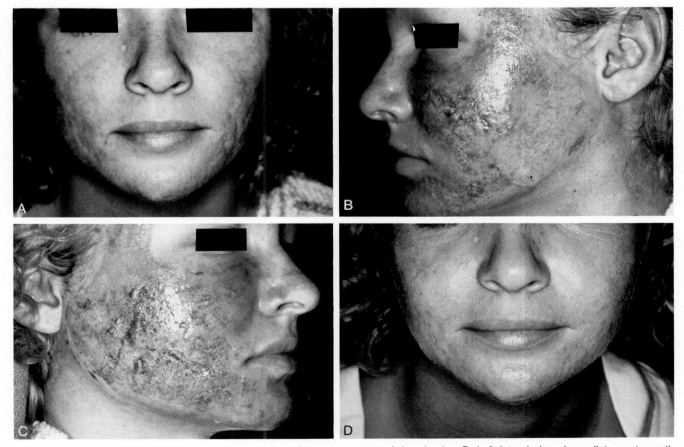

Figure 38–11. *A,* Preoperative view of a patient with prominent acne scars of the cheeks. *B,* Left lateral view, immediate postoperative appearance showing superficial abrasion and smooth contours. *C,* Right lateral view, immediate postoperative appearance showing superficial abrasion and smooth contours. *D,* Postoperative appearance showing improved contours and reduced prominence of scars.

lasma, may be a clinical clue to this potential problem. If this complication does occur, the use of sunscreens and the passage of time may allow it to resolve by itself. However, topical bleaching agents have been shown to be effective in returning the skin to a more normal appearance.[49, 50]

Bacterial and fungal[51] infections are relatively uncommon. If they develop, they should be treated by administration of an appropriate antibiotic after a culture has been performed and sensitivities have been determined.

SUMMARY

Despite the introduction of filler substances to correct certain types of scars and signs of aging, dermabrasions continue to be a useful procedure (Fig. 38–11). When the patient has been properly counseled and has appropriate expectations, this procedure can be successfully employed to correct certain types of traumatic or infectious scars, as well as some features of aging, including large numbers of actinic keratoses.

REFERENCES

1. Kromeyer E: Rotationsinstrumente: ein neues technisches Verfahren in der dermatologischen Kleinchirurgie. Dermatol Z 12:26–33, 1905.
2. Iverson PC: Surgical removal of traumatic tattoos of the face. Plast Reconstr Surg 2:427–432, 1947.
3. McEvitt WG: Acne pits. J Mich Med Soc 47:1243, 1948.
4. Robbins N: Dr. Abner Kurtin, father of ambulatory dermabrasion. J Dermatol Surg Oncol 14:425–431, 1988.
5. Kurtin SB: A look back at Abner Kurtin, M.D. J Dermatol Surg Oncol 13:602–603, 1987.
6. Kurtin A: Corrective surgical planing of skin. AMA Arch Dermatol Syphilol 68:389–397, 1953.
7. Blau S, Rein CR: Dermabrasion of the acne pit. AMA Arch Dermatol Syphilol 70:754–766, 1954.
8. Stegman SJ, Tromovitch TA: Dermabrasion equipment. In: Cosmetic Dermatologic Surgery. Year Book Medical, Chicago, 1984, pp 47–74.
9. Yarborough JM Jr: Personal communication. April, 1990.
10. Yarborough JM Jr: Preoperative evaluation of the patient for dermabrasion. J Dermatol Surg Oncol 13:652–653, 1987.
11. Duffy DM: Informed consent for chemical peels and dermabrasion. Dermatol Clin 7:183–185, 1989.
12. Hirsh BD: Informed consent applied more strictly to cosmetic procedures. Cosmet Dermatol 3:22–26, 1990.
13. Wentzell JM, Robinson JK, Wentzell JM Jr: Physical properties of aerosols produced by dermabrasion. Arch Dermatol 125:1637–1643, 1989.
14. Vaughn RY, Lesher JL Jr, Chaldker DK: HIV and the dermatologic surgeon. J Dermatol Surg Oncol 16:1107–1110, 1990.
15. Kemsley GM: Transmission of hepatitis B virus in dermabrasion. Plast Reconstr Surg 56:440, 1975.
16. Sawchuk WS: Infectious potential of aerosolized particles. Arch Dermatol 125:1689–1692, 1989.
17. Mahaffey P: AIDS and dermabrasion. Plast Reconstr Surg 80:757, 1987.
18. Yarborough JM Jr: Dermabrasion surgery: state of the art. Clin Dermatol 5:75–80, 1987.
19. Swinehart JM: Test spots in dermabrasion and chemical peeling. J Dermatol Surg Oncol 16:557–563, 1990.
20. Mandy SH: Tretinoin in the preoperative and postoperative management of dermabrasion. J Am Acad Dermatol 15:878–889, 1986.
21. Burks J: Dermabrasion and Chemical Peeling. Charles C Thomas, Springfield, IL, 1979.
22. Lowenthal L: Punch biopsy with autograft. Arch Dermatol Syphilol 67:629–631, 1953.
23. Ellis DA, Michell MJ: Surgical treatment of acne scarring: nonlinear scar revision. J Otolaryngol 16:116–119, 1987.
24. Orentreich D, Orentreich N: Acne scar revision update. Dermatol Clin 5:359–368, 1987.
25. Fulton JE: Modern dermabrasion techniques: a personal appraisal. J Dermatol Surg Oncol 13:780–789, 1987.
26. Alt TH: Technical aids for dermabrasion. J Dermatol Surg Oncol 13:638–648, 1987.
27. Roenigk HH Jr: Dermabrasion: state of the art. J Dermatol Surg Oncol 11:306–314, 1985.
28. Farrior RT: Dermabrasion in facial surgery. Laryngoscope 95:534–545, 1985.
29. McKinnon CC, Fulton JE Jr: Facial dermabrasion: modern techniques and protocols. AORN J 51:739–741, 744–745, 748–750, 1990.
30. Ayres S, Luikart T: Cotton glove in place of gauze for traction in surgical planing. Arch Dermatol 71:744–745, 1955.
31. Franekl EB: Use a palpating finger in dermabrasion. J Dermatol Surg Oncol 11:855, 1985.
32. Dzubow LM: Histologic and temperature alterations induced by skin refrigerants. J Am Acad Dermatol 12:796–810, 1985.
33. Hanke CW, O'Brian JJ, Solow EB: Laboratory evaluation of skin refrigerants used in dermabrasion. J Dermatol Surg Oncol 11:45–49, 1985.
34. Strick RA, Moy RL: Low skin temperatures produced by new skin refrigerants. J Dermatol Surg Oncol 11:1196–1198, 1985.
35. Hanke CW, O'Brian JJ: A histologic evaluation of the effects of skin refrigerants in an animal model. J Dermatol Surg Oncol 13:664–669, 1987.
36. Stagnone JJ: Chemabrasion. J Dermatol Surg Oncol 3:217–219, 1977.
37. Pinski JB: Dressings for dermabrasion: new aspects. J Dermatol Surg Oncol 13:673–677, 1987.
38. Cramers M: Wound dressing after skin planing. Acta Dermatol Venereol 69:453–454, 1989.
39. Fulton JE Jr: The stimulation of postdermabrasion wound healing with stabilized aloe vera gel–polyethylene oxide dressings. J Dermatol Surg Oncol 16:460–467, 1990.
40. Pinski JB: Dressings for dermabrasion: occlusive dressings and wound healing. Cutis 37:471–476, 1986.
41. Friedman SJ, Su WP, Doyle JA: Treatment of dermabrasion wounds with a hydrocolloid occlusive dressing. Arch Dermatol 121:1486–1487, 1985.
42. Rubenstein R, Roenigk HH Jr, Stegman SJ, Hanke CW: Atypical keloids after dermabrasion of patients taking isotretinoin. J Am Acad Dermatol 15:280–285, 1986.
43. Zachariae H: Delayed wound healing and keloid formation following argon laser treatment or dermabrasion during isotretinoin treatment. Br J Dermatol 118:703–706, 1988.
44. Moy RL, Moy LS, Bennett RG, et al: Systemic isotretinoin: effects on dermal wound healing in a rabbit car model in vivo. J Dermatol Surg Oncol 16:1142–1146, 1990.
45. Cohen BH: Prevention of postdermabrasion milia. J Dermatol Surg Oncol 14:1301, 1988.
46. Ship AG, Weiss PR: Pigmentation after dermabrasion: an avoidable complication. Plast Reconstr Surg 75:528–532, 1985.
47. Falabella R: Postdermabrasion leukoderma. J Dermatol Surg Oncol 13:44–48, 1987.
48. Taylor AC: Survival of rat skin and changes in hair pigmentation following freezing. J Exp Zool 110:77–111, 1949.
49. Gilchrest BA, Godwyn RM: Topical chemotherapy of pigment abnormalities in surgical patients. Plast Reconstr Surg 67:435–439, 1981.
50. Kligman AM, Willis I: A new formula for depigmenting human skin. Arch Dermatol 111:40–48, 1975.
51. Siegle RJ, Chiaramonti A, Knox DW, Pollack SV: Cutaneous candidosis as a complication of facial dermabrasion. J Dermatol Surg Oncol 10:891–895, 1984.

CHAPTER 39

Phenol Chemical Peels

SETH L. MATARASSO

The application of a caustic chemical to improve the appearance of the skin has been practiced for centuries. However, only with controlled experimentation, histologic corroboration, and defined safety parameters has chemical peeling using a variety of agents and methods evolved into a surgical science since the 1940s. Phenol has stood the test of time and retains its major role of importance in the armamentarium of peeling solutions.

History

Although MacKee[1] has been credited with using phenol in the treatment of acne scarring as early as 1903, the first published aesthetic use of phenol did not occur until 1941,[2] when a phenol lotion was used in the treatment of facial blemishes. Sporadic anecdotal reports[3, 4] of phenol usage appeared in the literature until the 1960s, when interest in peeling burgeoned.[5–7] Publications describing different formulas, techniques,[8] and indications were followed by reports of complications, durability, and histologic studies.

Phenolic Preparations

While there is little disagreement regarding the efficacy of phenol as a peeling agent, there remains much personal bias as to the best phenol concentration, composition, and technique to use. Concentrations of phenol ranging from 30 to 90% have been advocated. Additives to phenol have included croton oil, creosol, olive and sesame oils, sodium salicylate, camphor, anhydrous glycerin, and ethanol.[9] The amount of phenol, method of application and use, and type of occlusion dressing also vary tremendously. The two most popular phenol preparations are plain, full-strength 88% phenol and Baker's

saponified formula,[10] which consists of 3 ml phenol 88%, three drops of croton oil, eight drops of liquid hexachlorophene soap (Septisol), and 2 ml distilled water and is thus an emulsion with a phenol concentration of 45%. Despite having the same primary ingredient, the two preparations have remarkably different depths of penetration. Baker's peel, with or without occlusion, is a deep peel that penetrates down to the midreticular dermis.[11] Full-strength phenol, however, creates a medium-depth wound, since it penetrates only to the upper reticular dermis.

Pharmacology of Phenol

Phenol (C_6H_5OH), commonly known as carbolic acid, consists of a benzene ring with a hydroxyl group (Fig. 39–1). Although its formula does not contain the carboxyl group (—OH), which is characteristic of an organic acid, the hydroxyl group indicates that it is closer to being an organic base or an alcohol.[9] Pure phenol is a colorless solution with an aromatic odor and a burning taste. It can be produced from coal tar or manufactured synthetically from monochlorobenzene.[12] While there are few remaining uses for phenol as an antiseptic, it is bacteriostatic in a concentration of approximately 0.2%, bactericidal in concentrations of more than 1%, and fungicidal in concentrations of more than 1.3%. At a concentration of 5%, it can exert an anesthetic effect. Phenol is diffusible and can penetrate intact unabraded skin as well as mucous membranes.[13] The depth of penetration is contingent on, and inversely proportional to, the concentration, so that the more dilute the solution, the deeper is the penetration.

Full-strength 88% phenol produces immediate coagulation of epidermal keratin, which inhibits deep dermal penetration and makes the solution a medium-depth peeling agent. The more dilute phenol solutions (44 to

491

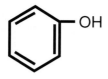

Phenol
(C₆H₅OH, Carbolic Acid)
Figure 39–1. The chemical structure of phenol.

55%), as found in Baker's formula, cause keratolysis, which disrupts rather than denatures the epidermal sulfur bridges, resulting in greater dermal exposure. The other components found in Baker's formula act to emulsify the solution. Liquid hexachlorophene soap (Septisol) inactivates phenol, decreases surface tension, and retards phenol penetration and absorption. Conversely, croton oil, an epidermal vesicant, acts as an irritant and thus facilitates phenol penetration.[14, 15]

Disruption of epidermal proteins is accompanied by dermal hyperemia and subsequent rapid absorption.[12] Absorption and toxicity are primarily influenced by the amount of skin exposed at one time, not by the concentration of the phenolic solution. Within 30 minutes of the application of 3 ml of 50% phenol, which is more than the amount used in a full-face peel, 70% of the phenol has been absorbed through the skin.[16] Blood levels of 0.68 mg/100 ml, 0.19 mg/100 ml, and 0.10 mg/100 ml have been observed 1, 2, and 4 hours, respectively, after application.[9] In experimental animal studies, 3% of absorbed phenol can still be found in the body after 24 hours. Most phenol is excreted in the urine, with only traces found in the feces.[12]

Excretion and Toxicity

Although little is known about the pharmacokinetics or pharmacodynamics of phenol, the detoxification and excretion of orally administered phenol has been studied.[17] Phenol is eliminated by three processes: excretion, oxidation, and conjugation. After absorption, 25% of phenol is metabolized to carbon dioxide and water. Before renal excretion, the remaining 75% of phenol can take one of three routes within the liver: it can be conjugated with glycuronic or sulfuric acids, oxidized to hydroquinone or pyrocatechin, or excreted unchanged.[9]

When consumed orally, phenol is extremely caustic to the gastrointestinal mucosa. However, even in these situations, toxic levels have not been accurately defined in humans. Although fatalities have been reported with oral doses ranging from 1 to 15 gm, survival has been reported with blood levels of 23 mg/ml.[9] Phenol is a protoplasmic protein that affects the cardiovascular and central nervous systems. After oral ingestion, the signs and symptoms of phenol poisoning are fulminant, consisting of central nervous system depression, progressive renal failure, and hepatic toxicity.[18] A direct effect on the myocardium and blood vessels occurs immediately, resulting in cardiac arrhythmias and a fall in blood pressure. Systemic toxicity, when it occurs, usually begins within a few minutes of application, and intractable cardiac depression, respiratory embarrassment, and death occur within 24 hours.

Therapeutic Indications

PHOTOAGING

Use of phenol is primarily indicated for the treatment of fine mosaic wrinkles, actinic damage, and irregular pigmentation associated with photoaging (Fig. 39–2). Subsequent wound repair produced by the controlled partial-thickness injury results in the creation of a new epidermis, as well as new dermal connective tissue. The clinical improvement results from a reduction in the amount of solar elastosis and collagenosis, which in turn enhances the quality and texture of the skin while also

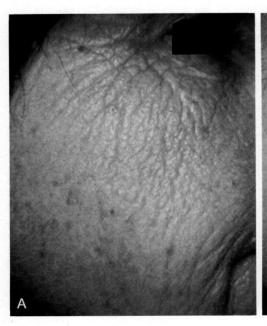
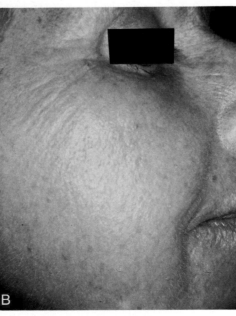

Figure 39–2. *A,* Fine mosaic wrinkles seen clinically before treatment. *B,* Clinical appearance 2 months after nonoccluded Baker's chemical peel.

improving the appearance of rhytidosis. Because rhytidosis is variable in its etiology and severity, its management should be individualized.

Rhytides associated with increased sun exposure are amenable to treatment with medium and deep peels, but dynamic, motion-associated creases, furrows, and folds are not. Surgical intervention with rhytidectomy, a coronal brow lift, or blepharoplasty is indicated to correct skin redundancy, muscular flaccidity, and alterations in the subcutaneous fat. Soft tissue augmentation with injectable filler substances such as collagen or autologous fat transplantation can be used to elevate subcutaneous depressions. In its purest form, phenol is ideally suited for patients who desire improvement in photoaged skin but wish to avoid invasive surgical procedures. A medium peel is indicated for patients with moderate elastosis without deep rhytides or for patients who want to avoid the longer postoperative morbidity associated with deep peels.[19]

Phenol as an Adjunct to Surgery for Photoaging

Treatment of the aging face often includes chemical peels as an adjunctive procedure. Excisional surgery addresses the structural deformity, while chemical peels improve the textural and pigmentary abnormalities of the skin. These procedures are not mutually exclusive, but rather are complementary in nature.[20] Advanced planning is extremely important when combining surgery with full-face chemical peels. If the surgical procedure involves a muscle-skin flap or extensive undermining, full-face phenol peeling should usually be postponed for 3 months; after blepharoplasties, peeling should be delayed for 6 months.[21] This delay is necessary because the blood supply of the flap is compromised by the surgery, and additional injury caused by a chemical peel could result in a full-thickness skin slough.[22-24] A perioral peel, however, may be safely performed simultaneously with rhytidectomy in most cases.

When surgery is insufficient to ablate perioral and periocular rhytides, regional phenol peels may be helpful (Fig. 39–3). In these cases, regional phenol peels should extend roughly 5 mm beyond the natural boundaries of the proposed aesthetic unit. To minimize the difference in contrast with the surrounding tissue,[14] the remainder of the face can be peeled with a second superficial peeling agent. A variation in the depth of the injury can also be accomplished with occlusion. Evaluation of rhytidosis requires an appreciation of the pathogenesis and the degree of the deformity followed by selection of the proper technique to correct it.

SCAR CORRECTION

The two methods most commonly used for removing layers of skin to improve soft tissue defects are chemical

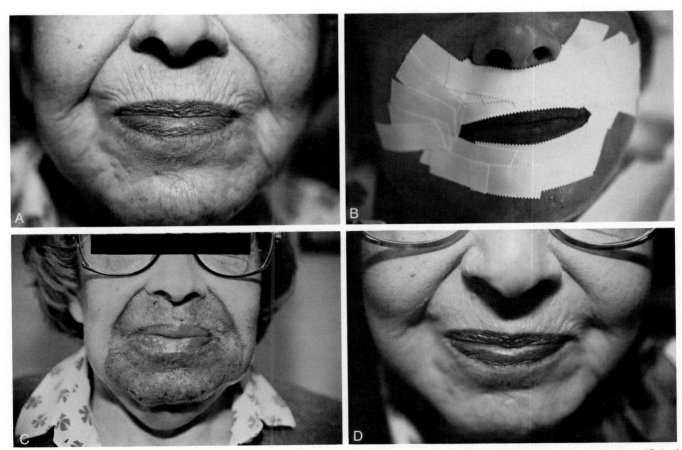

Figure 39–3. *A,* Preoperative frontal view of prominent perioral wrinkles. *B,* Appearance of a tape mask immediately after application of Baker's solution. *C,* Clinical appearance after 24 hours of occlusion. *D,* Two months postoperatively with marked softening of perioral rhagades.

peeling and dermabrasion.[15] While both can improve rhytides, peeling is not the best way to treat most depressed scars, as dermabrasion is generally more effective. While superficial acne scars can generally be improved with multiple light peels, phenol peeling for the treatment of deep scarring has given disappointing results.[25] Pitted acne scars and scars of dermal or fat atrophy will not respond to peeling and are best approached surgically with punch grafts before dermabrasion (see Chap. 35). In treating acne scars, care must be taken on the central cheek and chin to avoid sharp demarcation between dermabraded and nontreated skin. Feathering 88% phenol into the hairline, below the mandible and onto the unabraded skin will help to soften this contrast.

BENIGN LESIONS

Application of 88% phenol should be included in the list of localized destructive techniques such as cryotherapy, dermabrasion, hot cautery, and curettage used for the treatment of benign and superficial premalignant lesions such as seborrheic and actinic keratoses,[26] lentigines, sebaceous hyperplasia, xanthelasma, and viral infections such as verruca vulgaris, molluscum contagiosum, and condyloma acuminatum. As with other destructive techniques, factors such as location, pathology, and thickness of the lesion should be considered when applying the solution. Areas of thin skin and few adnexal structures, such as the eyelids, atrophic dorsal hand, neck, and mucous membranes, should be peeled with caution. Macular lesions may require a thin coat, while hypertrophic lesions are more recalcitrant, despite occlusion or more generous and repeated applications of phenol.

Peels performed on isolated lesions have the advantages of easy access, minimal equipment requirements, lack of need for anesthesia, capability of treating multiple lesions in a single session, minimal morbidity, and limited postoperative care. After degreasing the skin with acetone for better penetration, the solution is applied with a cotton-tipped applicator to the entire lesion and a tiny border of normal skin. After the appearance of a white frost and dusky erythema, the patient can be safely discharged. Standard wound care and healing are similar to those for full-face chemical peels.

Selected superficial pigmentary dyschromias may also respond well to chemical peeling. Because the response of a pigmented lesion is dependent on melanocyte depth, the degree of improvement is somewhat unpredictable. Lesions such as ephelides or lentigines are entirely epidermal and can be successfully removed with medium-depth or superficial peeling agents. However, because melasma and postinflammatory hyperpigmentation may vary in depth, they have a more unpredictable response to peeling. It might be prudent in these cases to attempt multiple superficial peels before proceeding with a medium or deep peel. However, in all cases, patients should be warned that any pigmentation abnormality may become worse with treatment (Table 39–1).

TABLE 39–1. **INDICATIONS FOR PHENOL PEELS**

Actinic damage
Rhytides, mild to moderate
Pigmentary abnormalities
    Lentigines
    Melasma
Epidermal lesions
    Seborrheic keratoses
    Verrucae
Superficial neoplasia
Premalignant lesions
    Actinic keratoses
Superficial scarring
Adjunct to aesthetic procedures
    Rhytidectomy
    Blepharoplasty
    Dermabrasion

Contraindications

PATIENT SELECTION CRITERIA

Proper patient selection will help reduce dissatisfaction. The ideal patient for a phenol peel is a woman with thin, dry skin; fair complexion; and fine wrinkles.[26] Because of the possibility of hypopigmentation, patients with skin types I to III are preferable so there will be less color contrast between treated and nontreated skin.[27] Care must be used when peeling patients with dark skin, but patients with skin types IV to VI can be successfully treated with phenol if they are willing to accept a 10 to 20% lighter skin color, a sharp demarcation between treated and untreated areas, and spotty pigmentary aberrations.[28, 29] Asian, Hispanic, and Indian patients with type V skin have the most unpredictable result with all types of peels.[30]

Although men can be successfully treated with phenol peels, they are not generally considered ideal candidates. This is because of their typical reluctance to use makeup postoperatively to camouflage the pigmentary abnormalities that follow phenol peeling and also because the thicker sebaceous skin of a man does not respond as well as the skin of a woman.[31]

ANATOMIC LOCATIONS AND SKIN APPENDAGES

Thick, coarsely textured sebaceous skin produces excess surface oil, which increases the probability of uneven penetration. Such skin may also require more diligent preparation with defatting agents before peeling and may require a greater volume of peeling solution to produce an adequate frosting. Patients with thin skin generally are preferable candidates for phenol peeling, but any patient with diminished or absent dermal appendages, as seen after radiation therapy, is a very poor candidate. Because epidermal regeneration is dependent on intact adnexa, the absence of such structures causes delayed wound healing and can result in abnormal color and texture. A demonstration of normal cutaneous architecture, either histologically or clinically by observing the number of vellus hairs present, is generally a good indication that the epidermis will be able to regenerate normally after a chemical peel.[12, 32] Probably because of the paucity of adnexal structures in the skin of the neck, the risk of hypertrophic scarring in this location is high.[14, 15] Although it is appropriate to feather over the mandibular line, phenol peels normally should not be extended onto the skin of the neck.

Systemic use of retinoids, including isotretinoin, has been shown to have a suppressive effect on both sebaceous gland size and activity, as well as a modulating effect on connective tissue metabolism. Because the pilosebaceous apparatus is an integral part of reepithelialization, it is theoretically possible that acute wound healing could be adversely affected by agents such as isotretinoin that suppress sebaceous gland activity.[33] Although the need for delay has not been scientifically documented, it is probably best to postpone phenol peels for 6 to 12 months after discontinuation of systemic retinoid therapy. Fortunately, this is not a frequent dilemma, as most patients presenting for phenol peels are not isotretinoin candidates.

An oil-free skin surface permits greater absorption of the peeling solution. Penetration can also be enhanced with preoperative use of topical retinoic acid cream, which is applied nightly for 1 to 2 weeks. Retinoic acid promotes shedding of corneocytes, thins the stratum corneum, and stimulates fibroplasia. Caution should be exercised, however, because over drying from overzealous use of retinoic acid can deepen the effects of a peel.[34–37]

INAPPROPRIATE USAGE

The types of wrinkles that patients most often find distressing are the perioral rhagades, periorbital "crow's feet," glabellar folds, horizontal rhytides on the forehead, and accentuated lines of facial expression around the nasolabial folds. However, only fine mosaic lines will be eliminated with phenol peels, while the deeper lines typically soften only as the skin contracts.[38] Deep peels can be viewed as a primary or adjunctive procedure but not as a substitute for facial rejuvenation surgery. For example, it would be inappropriate to equate chemical peels with the surgical effects that result from plication of the submusculoaponeurotic system (SMAS) and rhytidectomy.

INTERNAL MEDICAL DISORDERS

As phenol is absorbed, it can be toxic to the heart, kidneys, and liver. Therefore, patients should be in good health without significant underlying medical illnesses. A preoperative history plus a physical examination with a baseline electrocardiogram, complete blood cell count, electrolytes determination, and hepatorenal profile will help to exclude those patients with unrecognized medical problems. An internal medicine consultation should be obtained for patients with questionable medical histories. Caution should be exercised and the procedure modified as indicated for patients with certain types of internal diseases involving the heart, kidneys, or liver. Atopic individuals may also be particularly susceptible to certain problems as a result of xerosis as well as increased sensitivity to certain topical products.

INFECTIOUS DISEASES

Care should be exercised if a patient has a positive history of herpes simplex viral infection, since reactivation can occur during the postoperative period. This can be prevented with prophylactic use of acyclovir.[39] To avoid complications, the procedure should be postponed until any active herpetic lesions have completely healed.

CONCOMITANT MEDICATION USE

Estrogen and progesterone may exacerbate postoperative pigmentary changes. It is important that the patient abstain from hormonal replacement therapy or use of birth control pills for at least 6 months postoperatively (Table 39–2).[30, 40]

Preoperative Considerations

If the patient is an acceptable candidate, the procedure should be explained in detail. Printed information about the procedure and the perioperative period are helpful in assisting patients to prepare for the procedure. The preoperative discussion should focus on technique, discomfort, wound care, estimated healing time, and long-term care, with special emphasis on sun precautions. The patient should be made aware of potential complications, limitations, and alternative methods of treatment and informed that there may be some permanent alteration in the texture and color of the skin. The cutaneous surgeon should assess whether the patient's expectations are realistic and appropriate. Both the patient and the family should be aware of the likely appearance of the patient during the first few days after a chemical peel. Despite careful written and verbal

TABLE 39–2. **RELATIVE CONTRAINDICATIONS FOR PHENOL PEELS**

Cardiac disease
Renal disease
Hepatic disease
Herpes simplex infection
Hormonal therapy
    Estrogen
    Progesterone
Continuous or prolonged ultraviolet light exposure
Recent use of isotretinoin
Psychological problems
    Unreliability
    Unrealistic expectations
Previous ionizing radiation therapy
Skin type IV to VI
Predisposition to keloid formation
Anatomic locations with few adnexa
Recent extensive facial surgical undermining

explanations, the patient or family members may be shocked at the immediate postoperative appearance. It is often helpful to have a second follow-up consultation before the procedure to ensure complete understanding.

Information made available during the consultation should be accurately documented. The patient should be photographed both preoperatively and postoperatively with full-face, lateral or profile, and oblique or three-quarters views.[19] Areas of special concern, such as the perioral and periorbital areas, should be photographed at close range. It is also important to evaluate and document the skin pigmentation and texture, as well as previous injury sites or scars.

Surgical Technique

TESTING

If there are no contraindications, a small test spot of approximately 1 cm² is treated in an inconspicuous location, such as the hairline of the forehead, using the proposed chemical solution (Fig. 39–4). This should be examined for the development of possible abnormal pigmentary or textural changes in about 4 weeks. Although not absolutely predictive, the test results serve as an indication of the quality of wound healing, including pigmentation, textural changes, and scarring, as well as the time required for reepithelialization to occur. In addition, the test procedure also gives the cutaneous surgeon an opportunity to evaluate the patient's anxiety level, pain tolerance for the discomfort of the procedure, and ability to follow proper postoperative wound care instructions. The test procedure allows time to perform the indicated preoperative medical evaluation and to "prime" the skin with topical retinoic acid. It also permits the cutaneous surgeon to establish a good rapport with the patient and determine the patient's reliability. The test spot is a simple procedure that can help prevent potential medicolegal, psychological, and physical complications.[41, 42] The full-face chemical peeling

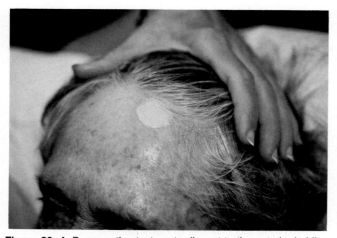

Figure 39–4. Preoperative test spot adjacent to the anterior hairline, to be observed for abnormal healing.

procedure is frequently performed in the fall or winter to reduce the risk of postoperative sun exposure.

Additionally, the patient should make arrangements for postoperative ancillary home care and transportation, as significant morbidity is associated with this procedure, the edema and dressings can impair vision, and the medications can alter the sensorium.

OPERATIVE TECHNIQUE

The chemical face peel is generally performed as an ambulatory procedure in an operating room that should be well ventilated to dissipate phenol fumes. First, intravenous access with a large-bore catheter is obtained. Hydration with 500 ml of Ringer's lactate solution given before the procedure and 1000 ml given during and after the procedure promotes diuresis and serves to protect the renal tubules from the toxic effects of phenol metabolites. Pulse oximetry and blood pressure and cardiac monitoring are also used during the procedure to observe for cardiac arrhythmias (Fig. 39–5).

Although phenol has anesthetic properties, the peel causes an exothermic reaction that can be quite painful and often requires additional analgesia. Numerous combinations of preoperative sedatives and analgesics have been recommended, but the ultimate selection is often dependent on the individual cutaneous surgeon's preferences. A combination of diazepam and meperidine hydrochloride, titrated to the patient's pain threshold, is most commonly used. Regional nerve blocks in the supraorbital, infraorbital, mental, superior alveolar, and preauricular areas can be supplemented with local infiltration anesthesia to diminish discomfort. Despite this, the skin does retain some sensation to the exfoliative insult. Epinephrine-containing local anesthetics, which could induce cardiac arrhythmias, should be avoided.

The patient is placed on the operating room table with the head slightly elevated to 30 degrees. Skin preparation ranges from simple removal of all makeup and facial oils with soap and water to vigorous degreasing with cotton or gauze using solvents such as ether, acetone, or alcohol.[32, 43] This reduces the epidermal barrier and provides deeper and more uniform phenol penetration. Phenol should cause the immediate development of a white frost. If the frost does not develop, facial oils probably have not been adequately removed, and the area should be recleansed.

Neck skin is unpredictable in its response and can be a dangerous area to peel with phenol solutions. For this reason, with the patient sitting, a line is drawn at the mandibular ramus where the neck and facial skin join. The solution should be feathered 1 to 2 cm beyond this inferior boundary but not onto neck skin. This maneuver anticipates a posterior shift with reclining and postoperative upward contraction of the skin, which should help hide the demarcation of treatment in the shadow of the mandibular ramus.

The extent of phenol absorption depends more on the total area of skin exposed than on the concentration of solution employed. For this reason, the face is divided

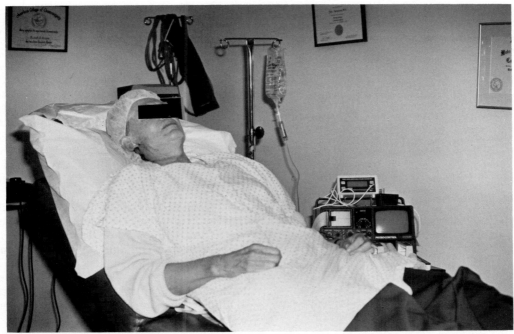

Figure 39–5. Phenol chemical peeling operating room. The intravenous line is attached to a large-bore catheter. A pulse oximeter and an electrocardiograph are used to monitor cardiac function.

into multiple aesthetic units: right and left halves of the forehead, right and left cheeks, perioral, perinasal, and periorbital areas (Fig. 39–6A). The solution is usually applied first to the least sensitive area, the forehead, and last to the most sensitive area, the eyelids (Fig. 39–6B). To minimize systemic toxicity, it is crucial to allow intervals of at least 15 minutes between treatment of each aesthetic unit. If there are many deep creases, which increase the surface area, the units may be further subdivided. With this regimen, a full-face peel will require 90 to 120 minutes, with the patient monitored for an additional 30 minutes after the conclusion of the procedure. A flow sheet indicating anatomic region and

time of application should be kept in the patient's chart (Table 39–3).

The solution is kept in a glass container and placed on a stand to the side of the patient's head. To avoid accidental exposure, a saturated applicator or solution-filled container should never pass directly over the patient. The phenol solution is applied with wooden cotton-tipped applicators. A fresh applicator should be used for each application. Depending on anatomic location, one or two applicator sticks can be used. On the cheeks and forehead, the solution can be applied with two applicators, but for areas that require precise control, such as the nose, mouth, and eyelids, one applicator

Figure 39–6. Aesthetic units of the face. *A,* Numbers indicating normal order of treatment. *B,* Feathering extends into the hairlines of the scalp, sideburns, and eyebrows as well as the tragus, earlobes, and mandibular ramus.

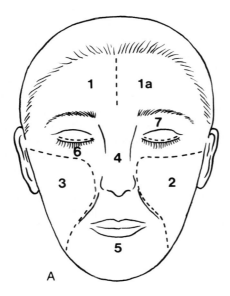

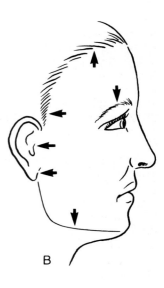

TABLE 39–3. SUGGESTED SEQUENCE FOR FULL-FACE PHENOL PEELS

8:30 AM	Preoperative preparation. Skin is cleansed, analgesia is provided, intravenous access is established, cardiac monitoring begins.
9:00 AM	Peeling solution is applied to the forehead to the level of the zygoma as two units that bisect the forehead at the midline.
9:15 AM	One cheek is treated from the lateral aspect of the nose to the tragus and from the infraorbital rim to the mandible. Peeling solution is applied over the mandibular margin, but not onto the neck.
9:30 AM	The contralateral cheek is treated in similar fashion.
9:45 AM	The nose and glabella are treated.
10:00 AM	The perioral area and vermilion are treated.
10:15 AM	The lower eyelids, with the eyes directed superiorly, are treated, preserving 1 to 3 mm at ciliary margins.
10:30 AM	The upper eyelids, with the eyes closed, are treated, maintaining a 1- to 3-mm zone at the ciliary margin and feathering into the eyebrows.
11:00 AM	The patient is observed and monitored during recovery for 30 minutes postoperatively; then the wounds are dressed and the patient is discharged.

is preferred. Proctology swabs generally are avoided, as they apply too much solution at one time.

When using Baker's formula (Fig. 39–7), the solution should be freshly prepared. The ingredients are measured with individual 3-ml syringes and mixed in a transparent glass cup. The formula provides 5 ml of solution, with only 1 to 1.5 ml actually used for the peel. The solution is an unstable emulsion, with the phenol and water tending to separate and form distinct layers. A transparent container helps to ensure that a uniform mixture is applied to each region, although agitation of the solution is necessary before each application.[38] After the solution has been stirred with the applicator, a semiwet applicator, used for most of the face, can be obtained by rolling an applicator against the edge of the glass container. A semidry applicator, used predominantly in the periocular area, is prepared by removing excess fluid by blotting the applicator against dry gauze (Fig. 39–8).

Whether a solitary unit or the entire face is being treated, the chemical is first applied to the base of the deepest wrinkles (Fig. 39–9). Using the pointed tip of a broken applicator and stretching the skin gently (Fig. 39–9D), the fluid is applied evenly to coat the depth of the wrinkle. The solution is then uniformly applied to the rest of the treatment area in a sweeping motion (Fig. 39–9E). As the solution comes in contact with the skin, it immediately turns white, and the patient experiences an uncomfortable burning sensation. This pain is transient, lasting only about 30 seconds, at which time the anesthetic quality of the phenol exerts its effect on the sensory nerve endings.[12] The white color is replaced by a dusky erythema (Fig. 39–9F), which is generally accompanied by a second, more intense pain, which can persist for up to 8 hours. The initial discomfort can be

alleviated with ice packs, cool compresses (Fig. 39–9F), and a fan directed at the patient (Fig. 39–8). The second, more intense postoperative pain requires analgesia and sedation.[44]

The forehead is generally treated first, because it is less sensitive to pain. The solution should be feathered into hair-bearing areas (Fig. 39–6) to prevent a sharp line of demarcation from developing.[26] Because it does not affect hair growth or color, the solution is carried into the scalp hairline, eyebrows, and sideburns. Fifteen minutes after the forehead application, one cheek is similarly treated. The solution is applied on the cheek up to the inferior orbital rim, to the lateral aspect of the nose, into the nasolabial lines, and to the lateral aspects of the chin, including the "marionette lines" that lead from the oral commissure to the ramus of the jaw. The treatment should extend roughly 1 cm below the mandibular margin. While the cheek is being treated, the solution should also be applied to both the earlobe and tragus. The same procedure can be performed on the contralateral cheek 15 minutes later. This is followed by similar peeling of the glabella and nose, including the nasal rim and columella.

Special Considerations for the Lips

Although similar principles are used when peeling the perioral area, two points require special emphasis. First, it is important not only to carry the peel onto the vermilion border but also to feather it 1 to 2 mm beyond that onto the lip. Folded gauze should be placed in the mouth to prevent accidental oral ingestion. Second, the rhytides perpendicular to the vermilion are of a different origin from those on the forehead but are usually of equal severity. Both areas require application of additional solution and should be manually stretched to expose the entire surface to the agent.

Special Considerations for the Eyes

Local anesthesia is difficult to obtain in the periorbital area without obliterating the wrinkles, so patients may require additional systemic analgesia. For this reason, and because of the extensive edema that is produced, it is usually best to treat this area last. Periorbital skin is very thin and requires only a small amount of solution, which can be applied with a semidry applicator. Elimination of all excess fluid also reduces the potential risk of retrograde reflux of solution into the patient's eye.

The lower eyelids are peeled first, followed by the upper lids, with about a 5-minute interval between each application. For treatment of the lower lids, the patient's eyes are kept open and directed superiorly as the solution is brushed on, away from the eye itself. For the upper lids, the eyes are kept closed and the peeling solution applied in upward strokes. The physician can greatly facilitate the positioning of the eyelids by manually retracting the skin. The solution is conservatively applied, preserving 1 to 3 mm of normal skin at the ciliary margin to avoid possible corneal or conjunctival burns.

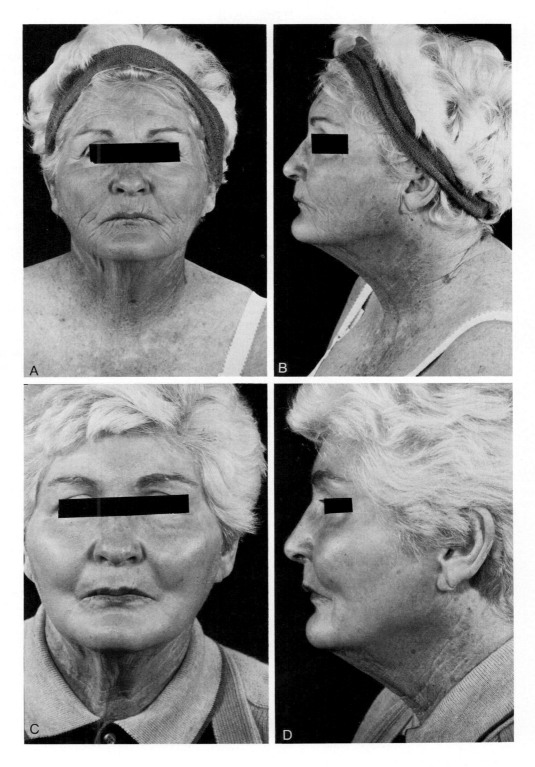

Figure 39–7. *A,* Frontal and *B,* lateral views showing the patient's preoperative appearance. *C,* Frontal and *D,* lateral appearance 2 months after Baker's chemical peel, showing marked improvement in both rhytides and abnormal pigmentation. (Photographs courtesy of Dr. Nicolajs Lapins.)

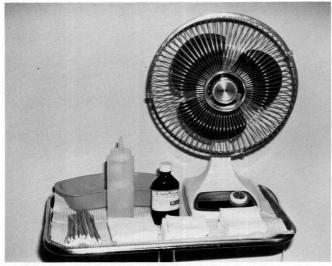

Figure 39–8. Phenol chemical peeling equipment: Mayo stand with cotton-tipped applicators, dry gauze, degreasing agent in a basin, squirt bottle filled with propylene glycol for possible ocular irrigation, and fan for cooling. Precut tape should be accessible for occluded peels.

Tears dilute the peeling solution, which can potentiate deeper penetration and convert a second-degree peel to a third-degree wound. It can also leave streaks of uneven pigmentation. To ensure a dry field, the physician should avoid the use of ophthalmic ointments and drops, which can initiate both tearing and excess moisture. In addition, an assistant should be ready with dry applicators at the medial and lateral canthi to absorb any tears.

FINAL CONSIDERATIONS

The sequence in which aesthetic units are peeled is not as crucial as the amount of time given between areas. Similarly, the standard anatomic or aesthetic divisions should not be considered absolute. To avoid missed areas, it is important to slightly overlap adjacent treatment areas. The final clinical effects of the peel are a function of wound depth, which is determined by skin preparation, amount and concentration of solution, and occlusion (Table 39–4). Correction of severe actinic damage requires a deeper peel, vigorous degreasing, and repeat application of the solution. Occlusion provided either by tape or ointment serves as a mechanical vapor barrier to prevent phenol evaporation. This increases absorption and maceration and provides deeper penetration.

POSTOPERATIVE DRESSING

The type of occlusive dressing used is largely determined by the surgeon's own personal bias. Generally, in patients having delicate, thin, fair skin with moderate wrinkling, the phenol should be allowed to partially evaporate before tape is applied. In patients with coarser rhytides, the occlusive dressing is applied as soon as the

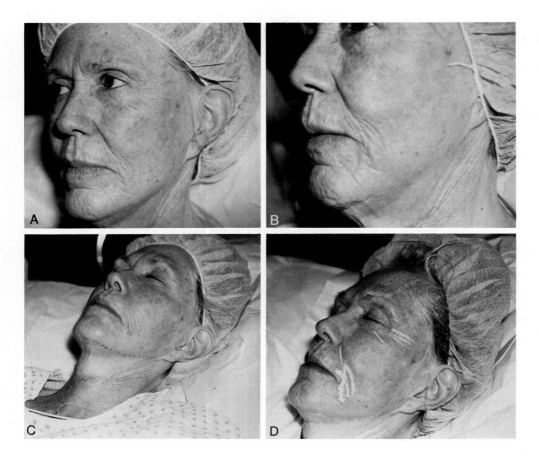

Figure 39–9. *A,* Lateral and *B,* close-up appearance of a patient before treatment. *C,* The patient is positioned with her head elevated at a 30-degree angle after having had her face scrubbed and mandibular border marked. *D,* Phenol is first applied to the deepest creases.

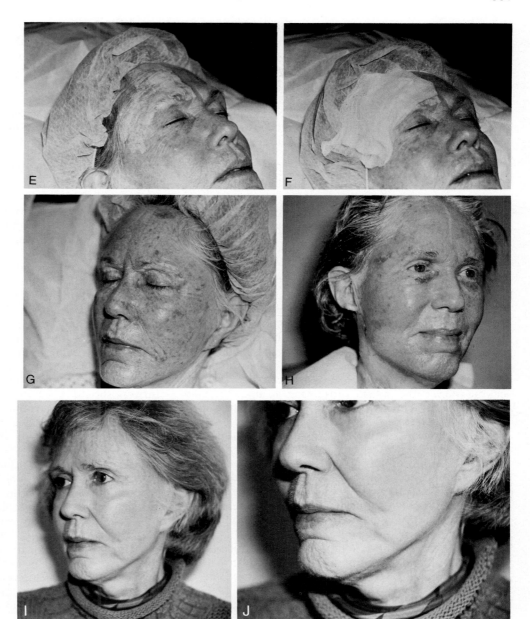

Figure 39–9 *Continued E,* Phenol is next painted on one aesthetic unit, which immediately results in a white frosted appearance. *F,* After the development of a dusky erythema, cool compresses can be applied to reduce pain without potentiating the penetration of the chemical. *G,* Immediate postoperative appearance showing marked edema and erythema. *H,* Clinical appearance after 1 week showing marked residual erythema and one "skip" area of the midforehead at a junction of two aesthetic units. *I,* Lateral and *J,* close-up views 4 months postoperatively.

aesthetic unit is painted. It can also be applied only to selected areas that require deeper wounding.[15] Taping should not go beyond the mandibular border and is never used when pigmentation is the primary indication for treatment.[45]

Commercially available 0.5-inch-wide waterproof or occlusive zinc oxide tape is cut in lengths of 1.5 to 4 cm before beginning the procedure. Tape sufficient to produce a mask of two or three layers should be readily available. For the first layer, strips of tape are applied edge to edge, in hingelike fashion, to adapt to facial contours and to permit any expansion resulting from edema. Shorter segments of tape are especially helpful in difficult areas such as the infraorbital rim, nose, and upper and lower lips. Longer strips may be used where there is less anatomic curvature (e.g., the central cheek

TABLE 39–4. FACTORS DETERMINING THE DEPTH OF A CHEMICAL PEEL

Agent
    Solution type
    Concentration
    Volume applied
Integrity of epidermal barrier
    Pretreatment with topical retinoic acid
    Skin cleansing
        Soap and water
        Alcohol
        Ether
        Acetone
Skin thickness
    Density of adnexa
    Anatomic location
Occlusion
    Duration

and forehead). The second and third layers provide additional reinforcement and help minimize missed areas. Missed areas and streaking can be minimized by using palmar pressure to flatten folds in the tape, maximizing contact between the skin and the tape. Uneven scalloping or saw-toothing of the tape at the margins gives a less noticeable, irregular line and softens the contrast between occluded and nonoccluded skin.[44] This is especially important at the infraorbital rim where the cheek and eyelid skin merges and at the mandibular margin. Taping of the earlobes, eyelids, nostrils, and hair-bearing areas is both unnecessary and undesirable. The tape mask can be left intact for 24 to 48 hours. There is controversy about any potential benefit that may result from leaving the tape in place for longer periods.

Postoperative Instructions

The intravenous line and cardiac monitoring are maintained for about 30 minutes after completion of the procedure. During this time, application of cool compresses can help to decrease discomfort and edema (Fig. 39–9F). When tape occlusion is used, care should be taken to prevent moisture from the compresses from leaking under the mask and lifting it up. A bulky dressing is not necessary, but a coat of ointment can be applied to unoccluded or open areas.

Postoperative pain typically lasts up to 8 hours and gradually subsides. Acetaminophen-codeine or hydrocodone (Vicodin) tablets may be taken orally every 3 to 4 hours as needed for pain relief. Use of oral diazepam in dosages of 5 to 10 mg twice daily may also be helpful. Discomfort is usually associated with edema, especially around the mouth and eyes. Use of analgesics while resting in a sitting or semireclining position is often helpful. During the first 24 hours, facial motion should be minimized, and all communication should be written. The diet should be restricted to foods that can be consumed with a straw.[31]

The first morning after treatment, the patient may experience some residual pain. The skin will be edematous and ashy gray in color. The first sign of desquamation may not become apparent until 24 to 48 hours later. At 24 hours, a serous exudation begins to appear in most cases. If a mask is present, it will become less adherent and can simply be removed in the shower. Despite this, patients frequently need reassurance during the immediate postoperative period to allay fears and avoid any possible confusion about wound care instructions. In most cases, it may be advisable to remove the mask in the office with the use of mild analgesics. This is done by slowly and gently lifting up the tape. Use of topical sterile saline or hydrogen peroxide compresses will help to remove the coagulum, revealing a weeping, exudative surface with spots of pinpoint bleeding similar to the appearance of a second-degree burn.

EARLY WOUND CARE

Formation of a thick crust with application of thymol iodine was previously common, but this technique has been discontinued.[46, 47] Currently, a wet technique is typically used to keep the wound free of crusts, speed healing, and reduce the risk of infection. For the first week, the patient is instructed to hydrate the skin at least three to five times a day with cool tap water supplemented with wet packs and an atomizer. Half-strength boric acid or antiseptic skin cleansers such as Betadine or Hibiclens can be used to help remove the exudate. This is followed by generous lubrication using bland noncomedogenic emollients such as petrolatum (Vaseline), vegetable shortening, or A & D Ointment, or antibiotic ointments such as Bacitracin or Polysporin. Lotions should be avoided because of their high alcohol content, which can irritate and desiccate the newly formed epidermis. A mild corticosteroid ointment may also be helpful to prevent desiccation and decrease both pruritus and inflammation. Potent topical and systemic steroids should be avoided, however, because they can significantly inhibit epithelial cell migration and retard dermal regeneration. Despite diligent hydration, some crusting may occur. In these situations, the adherent crusts should not be removed by the patient, as premature separation may cause scarring. Total avoidance of sunlight is necessary until reepithelialization is complete, which usually occurs by the tenth or twelfth postoperative day. After reepithelialization, generous use of moisturizers should be supplemented with cream-based sunscreens and topical tretinoin.

LATE WOUND CARE

Despite significant residual erythema, patients can generally resume a normal schedule within 2 to 3 weeks. Abnormal color and scaling can be camouflaged with a green-based, hypoallergenic makeup made by Dermage or Estee Lauder. The erythema gradually diminishes and is replaced within 3 to 5 months by skin that is slightly lighter in color than the untreated areas. By that time, light makeup is usually sufficient to camouflage the treated areas. Emphasis must be placed on continuous sunlight avoidance in addition to generous use of sunscreens with a high sun protection factor (SPF). This is important, because the newly formed tissue is very sensitive and susceptible to pigmentary changes, which

---

TABLE 39–5. **CHECKLIST FOR PHENOL PEELS**

Proper indications
Judicious patient selection
Preoperative work-up to rule out internal diseases
Signed consent form
Preoperative photographic documentation
Cardiac monitoring
Intravenous line for access and hydration
Tray with peeling solution, applicators, tape, gauze, flush bottle with glycerol or propylene glycol
Transparent glass container with fresh, constantly stirred, peeling solution kept away from possible contact with patient's eyes
Adequate skin preparation and analgesia
Application of solution to base of deep wrinkles
Sectional peeling with adequate pauses
Feather into hair-bearing skin and adjacent areas
Tape occlusion of two to three layers with scalloped edges
Meticulous postoperative wound and skin care
Complete ultraviolet light avoidance

can begin as early as 3 weeks postoperatively (Table 39–5).

Histologic Features

The major indication for phenol chemical face peels is treatment of the aging face, which is characterized by sallow color, lentigines, keratoses, telangiectasia, loss of translucency, reduced elasticity, and rhytides.[48] To appreciate the effect of phenol and its rejuvenative properties, the ultrastructural characteristics of the aging face must be understood.

NORMAL AGING

Even with minimal exposure to the physical elements, the skin ages with time. Even sun-protected skin will show epidermal atrophy, reduced organization of the basal and spinous cell layers, and a decreased and uneven distribution of melanocytes. The dermal-epidermal junction becomes flat, with loss of rete ridges and dermal papillae. The reticular dermis becomes thinned, with a reduction in both the amount and organization of collagen and elastic fibers. There is also a decrease in the number of fibroblasts, macrophages, and mast cells, along with a reduction in the amount of glycosaminoglycans. These changes become more pronounced in sun-exposed skin.

PHOTOAGED SKIN

Histologic analysis of photoaged skin shows a compact and laminated stratum corneum without a clear transition to the underlying stratum lucidum (Fig. 39–10*A*). Epidermal cells show dysplasia, atypia, vacuolization, necrosis, and loss of vertical polarity and cell alignment. Beneath the dermal-epidermal junction, there is a narrow zone of densely packed collagen. The papillary dermis is elastotic, with formation of amorphous masses as a result of homogenization of the ground substance and breakage of fibers. The elastic tissue eventually becomes densely matted and irregular in appearance.[49] Solar-induced changes are added to the changes that occur naturally with aging alone.

HISTOLOGIC APPEARANCE AFTER CHEMICAL PEELING

The few early attempts to describe the microscopic changes of chemical peels were very inconsistent in their findings. It was only relatively recently that the histologic appearance of treated skin was found to mirror the clinical improvement (Fig. 39–10*B*). In 1982, the depth of injury was reported to correlate with the concentration of the peeling agent and the degree of occlusion. This confirmed the clinical impression that Baker's formula was the strongest agent, comparable to dermabrasion, and produced deeper effects than phenol alone.[50, 51]

Histologically, Baker's solution was found to completely obliterate the epidermis by keratolysis and produce an inflammatory zone of cellular destruction that extended throughout the entire papillary dermis and into the upper half of the reticular dermis. This reaction was found to peak at 48 hours, at which time epidermal regeneration began. However, dermal thickening did not begin until about 2 weeks after treatment, as the

Figure 39–10. *A,* Histologic appearance of untreated sun-exposed skin showing a broad band of pale-staining amorphous elastotic material in the upper dermis. *B,* Histologic appearance of sun-exposed skin 90 days after treatment with full-strength phenol showing replacement of the elastotic dermis with a normal zone of collagen fibers immediately beneath the epidermis. (Original magnification 10×, colloidal iron stain.)

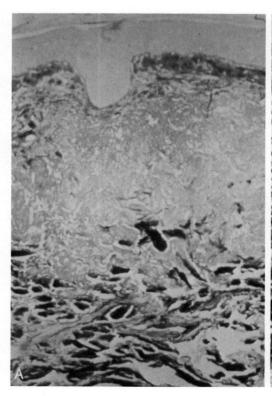
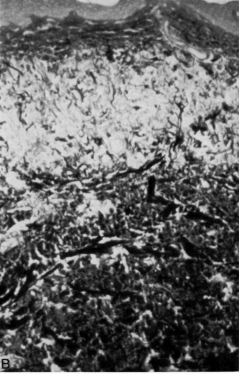

inflammatory reaction subsided.[45] Complete epidermal regeneration was not evident for 10 to 14 days, and dermal inflammation was found to persist for up to 3 months.

Long-term histologic studies of up to 13 years in duration have demonstrated that there are three histologic changes that are consistent, predictable, and apparently permanent with phenol peels. The most important of these, in terms of clinical benefit, is the homogenization of the upper dermal collagenous architecture.[52] The wavy papillary collagen is reorganized into a 0.2- to 0.3-mm-thick zone of straight fibers that stain normally and lie parallel to and just beneath the basement membrane of the epidermis. Replacement of the basophilic elastotic dermis is accompanied by an increase in the density of fibroblasts. Simultaneously, a "dermal scar" develops in the reticular dermis. This "scar" is composed of an increased amount of elastic tissue with thick, closely aligned fibers.[50, 53] In the epidermis, there is a marked decrease in melanosomes, accompanied by the return of normal polarity to the basal cell layer. Basal columnar cells are also more uniform in size, show no cytologic atypia or disarray, and stain more homogeneously.

Full-strength phenol has effects that are similar to, but less profound than, those produced by Baker's formula. Like Baker's solution, full-strength phenol necroses the epidermis and produces papillary edema. However, the denatured epidermal proteins caused by phenol limit its dermal penetration,[54] resulting in only minimal edema and inflammation of the upper reticular dermis. Occlusive dressings prevent evaporation and increase maceration, resulting in increased wound depth histologically and a broader and deeper zone of inflammation.[45, 50] Clearly, the degree of clinical change correlates with the depth of injury. Deep injury produces more complete clinical improvement up to the anatomic limit of the reticular dermis, where the healing response shifts from reorganization to the production of scar tissue with extensive fibroblast and collagen production. The most important considerations remain the selection of the appropriate chemical agent and use of the technique that can provide the desired clinical result without undesired or untoward effects.

Complications

The results of chemical peeling can be very gratifying, but as with any cutaneous surgical procedure, complications can occur. The risk and severity of complications increase with the depth of the cutaneous injury and the use of occlusion (Table 39–6).

PIGMENTARY CHANGES

By far the most common local complication of chemical peeling is the production of abnormal pigmentation,[55] which ranges from complete depigmentation to hyperpigmentation (Fig. 39–11). The risk increases with the depth of the peel. Patients with light complexions

TABLE 39–6. COMPLICATIONS FROM PHENOL PEELS

Cutaneous	Infectious
Pigmentary	Bacterial
Depigmentation	*Staphylococcus*
Hypopigmentation	*Streptococcus*
Hyperpigmentation	*Pseudomonas*
Irregular pigmentation	Toxic shock syndrome
Streaking	Viral
Mottled color	Herpes simplex
Blotchiness	Verruca
Lines of demarcation	Miscellaneous
Persistent flushing	Milia
Scarring	Pruritus
Hypertrophy	Textural changes
Atrophy	Follicular orifice enlargement
Keloids	Telangiectasia
Full-thickness necrosis	Temperature sensitivity
Structural	Neuropsychiatric disorders
Ectropion	Depression
Eclabium	Destabilization
Systemic	Laryngeal edema
Cardiac	
Renal	
Hepatic	
Hematologic	

(skin types I to III) have fewer problems with abnormal pigmentation than patients with dark pigmentation. Generally, lighter peels have been associated with hyperpigmentation and deeper peels with hypopigmentation.[40] The reduction in pigmentation, sometimes even complete depigmentation, seen with deep peels is actually not a complication but a normal sequela of phenol peels. The need for postoperative camouflage makeup should be anticipated in most cases. Hypopigmentation after phenol is directly proportional to the amount of solution applied and the degree of occlusion. Freckling, rather than tanning, occurs with sun exposure after phenol peels. Postinflammatory hyperpigmentation can be transient or permanent and can result in an irregular, streaked pattern.

Spotty hyperpigmentation can be caused by premature sun exposure or systemic hormonal therapy. Streaking

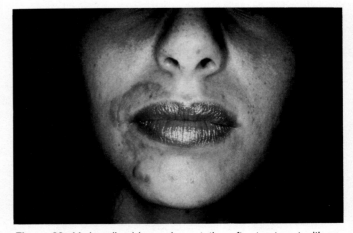

Figure 39–11. Localized hyperpigmentation after treatment with occluded Baker's peel.

can be caused by unequal application of the solution or dilution from tearing. Sun avoidance and postoperative use of retinoic acid and hydroquinone will help to minimize the risk of hyperpigmentation. Sunscreens should be applied as soon as healing is complete. However, retinoic acid and hydroquinone creams should not be applied to denuded skin that is still irritated, as they may interfere with wound healing and can induce pigmentary changes. Bleaching agents are usually applied at the first sign of darkening. However, some cutaneous surgeons incorporate it prophylactically as a standard part of postoperative care as soon as reepithelialization is complete.[26] Irregular pigmentation can be improved 3 to 4 months postoperatively with localized spot peeling.

An obvious line of demarcation can occur between treated and untreated areas. This is usually reduced by feathering into the surrounding skin using a cotton-tipped applicator or a less concentrated solution. Feathering is especially important when performing regional peels and along the mandible or adjacent to hair-bearing areas. Nevi can also become hyperpigmented postoperatively and should be considered for removal 1 to 2 weeks preoperatively.[22] Although it is impossible to predict when pigmentary problems will occur, they are most common in patients with dark complexions, those requiring systemic administration of estrogen or progesterone, patients who become pregnant within 6 months after treatment, and patients who use photosensitizing drugs or are exposed to excessive amounts of sunlight postoperatively.[30]

SCARRING

Hypertrophic scarring is one of the most common complications after chemical peels. In the absence of a positive family history of abnormal scarring, the cause cannot generally be determined, but facial movement or local tension may play a role. Unfortunately, test spots do not always accurately predict how a patient will react to full treatment, so scarring and pigmentary problems can arise despite a good test result. As with most complications, the frequency of scarring increases with occlusion and depth of peel (Table 39–7).

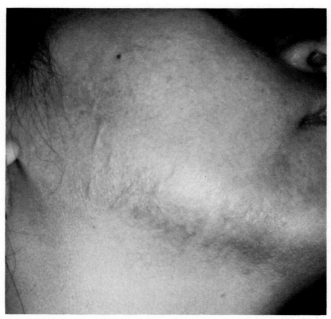

Figure 39–12. A hypertrophic scar has developed along the mandibular line after treatment with occluded Baker's peel.

Scars are initially manifested as indurated subcutaneous areas with variable amounts of erythema that usually appear within 3 months of the procedure. Fortunately, these areas are generally small and isolated, the greatest predilection being for the upper lip and inframandibular region (Fig. 39–12).[22, 55] Simply massaging the area can cause spontaneous resolution. However, because persistent localized erythema may portend a poor prognosis, early and aggressive treatment using potent steroids is often necessary. Triamcinolone acetonide administered intralesionally, topically, or in a tape vehicle can help reduce the size and thickness of scar tissue.[14] Daily application of fluocinonide-impregnated tape to an early scar may abort the scar's development. Infection may be a prelude to scarring, which is one reason to aggressively care for the postoperative wound.

Hypertrophic or contractural scar formation can impair normal facial function and movement. Surgical intervention with either simple excision or a tension-releasing procedure may be necessary. If a skin slough occurs as a result of simultaneous peeling and surgical undermining, the skin should be allowed to heal by second intention and then be surgically revised at a later date.[22]

INFECTION

Fortunately, despite the seemingly overwhelming insult produced by peeling agents, infection is rare (Fig. 39–13). Patients often become frightened or intimidated by their postoperative appearance, which may result in inadequate wound care. This results in secondary impetiginization, maceration, and accumulation of necrotic debris. Local wound care with antiseptic compresses and

TABLE 39–7. POTENTIAL RISK FACTORS FOR SCARRING WITH PHENOL PEELS

Undue facial motion
Disruption of wound reepithelialization
    Premature eschar removal
    Excoriation
    Delayed healing
    Infection
    Previous dermabrasion or chemical peel
    Isotretinoin therapy
Interference with lymphatic or vascular supply
    Edema
    Extensive recent subcutaneous undermining
Excessive depth of injury
    Occlusion
    Dilution
    Excess volume of peeling solution
Dark pigmentation
History of keloid formation

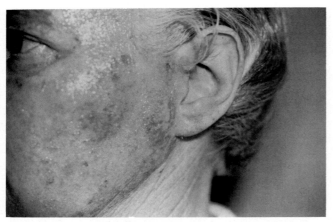

Figure 39–13. A green purulent exudate is indicative of infection by the gram-negative bacteria *Pseudomonas aeruginosa* 2 days after an open straight phenol peel.

topical antibiotics and an empiric course of broad-spectrum systemic antibiotics are advised until a specific organism can be identified. *Pseudomonas* is a common pathogen and may colonize the wound. Frequent showering, topical use of acetic acid soaks, and oral ciprofloxacin can prevent infection (Fig. 39–14). Secondary impetiginization is not always a sign of impending scarring, but steps should be taken to avoid this potential complication with frequent hydration of the skin postoperatively.[30] Streptococcal or staphylococcal folliculitis caused by occlusive dressings rapidly appears in the immediate postoperative period. These pustules respond readily to treatment with oral antibiotics and typically heal without scarring.

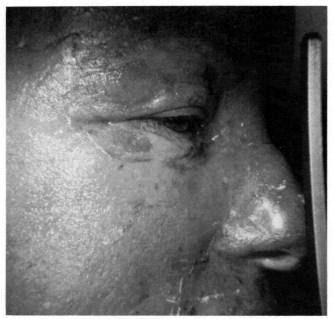

Figure 39–14. Widespread pustules on skin denuded by a chemical peel associated with a grapelike odor is suggestive of *Pseudomonas* infection. Scarring can be prevented by acetic acid soaks.

Chemical peels can reactivate infections caused by the herpes simplex virus.[39] Some cutaneous surgeons feel that a positive history of this infection may be an absolute contraindication for chemical peeling. Because many patients are unaware of their exposure to the herpes virus, the risk of reactivation can be reduced by treating all patients prophylactically with oral acyclovir (Zovirax) (200 mg) three times/day for 1 to 2 days before and 4 to 5 days after chemical peeling. Heralded by unusual and unexpected postoperative pain or intense pruritus, a herpetic flare is treated with oral acyclovir 400 mg four times a day. This regimen controls the infection and typically allows healing without scar formation.[26, 30, 56]

PERSISTENT ERYTHEMA

Although persistent erythema can be problematic and no specific treatment is available, time, combined with the meticulous use of sunscreens and topical and systemic corticosteroids, is frequently successful in resolving this problem.[23] Prolonged erythema (more than 60 days for medium-depth peels and 90 days for deep peels) may be a sign of contact dermatitis. The cause for this should be pursued.

MILIA

Milia typically appear 4 to 6 weeks after treatment as a result of occlusion of the pilosebaceous orifices. They can be easily removed with cautery, incision and drainage, abrasion, application of retinoic acid, or gentle manipulation by the cutaneous surgeon. They usually heal without scarring.

TEXTURE CHANGES

Atrophy manifested by translucency and loss of normal skin markings may follow application of the chemical solution to thin skin, such as that in the periorbital area, or after multiple deep peels.[30] Enlarged pores may result from removal of the stratum corneum. Although transient improvement in pore size may occur, permanent results are unlikely and are certainly unpredictable.[56, 57]

PSYCHOLOGICAL PROBLEMS

To prevent any misunderstanding, the patient must have realistic expectations and be completely prepared for the amount of postoperative wound care required. After an open peel or removal of the occlusive dressing, the patient's appearance can be quite frightening. The skin is macerated and covered with an exudate, and edema can distort the normal facial anatomy. Despite warnings, some patients may become anxious at this point. Assurance by the cutaneous surgeon is essential and often helps avoid psychological distress.

SYSTEMIC EFFECTS

Clearly the most profound and detrimental complication of phenol peels is the potential systemic effect.

Although absorbed rapidly through the skin, the potential for toxicity depends on the total area of skin treated at one time rather than on serum phenol levels. Because phenol is metabolized in the liver and excreted by the kidneys, possible hepatorenal complications have been anticipated. However, to date, none has been reported in the literature except from industrial or accidental cutaneous exposure.[25] Two additional (but fortunately uncommon) complications that have been reported with chemical peeling are toxic shock syndrome[58, 59] and laryngeal edema.[60] These two complications require that patients have a thorough understanding of the signs and symptoms of infection so that they can carefully monitor and report any changes that may occur as early as possible. They also underscore the need for diligent postoperative evaluation of chemical peel patients by the cutaneous surgeon to exclude the possible development of these and other serious potential complications.

A more common and significant complication is that of cardiotoxicity. Cardiac arrhythmias reported during phenol peels include premature ventricular contractions, ventricular bigeminy, ventricular tachycardia, and paroxysmal atrial tachycardia. Unfortunately, a normal preoperative electrocardiogram and a negative cardiac history do not preclude the development of cardiac toxicity. Also, there is no direct correlation with the administration of oxygen or the patient's age, sex, or serum phenol levels. However, this risk is greater in anxious patients or those extremely sensitive to pain, patients with a history of cardiac arrhythmias or mitral valve prolapse, and those who have more than one third of their face peeled in a period of 15 minutes or less. No cardiac changes have been reported when 50% or more of the face was peeled over a 60-minute period.[24, 61–64] Intravenous hydration also assists in clearing phenol from the circulation, which decreases the likelihood of toxicity. If arrhythmias do occur, the peeling procedure should be immediately stopped and restarted only when a normal sinus rhythm has returned and been maintained for 15 minutes.[30, 32, 63]

SUMMARY

There are many surgical modalities available to help reverse the effects of time and sun damage. Selection of the appropriate technique requires critical analysis so that therapy can be individualized to meet the needs of each patient.[20, 65] Ideally suited for fair-skinned women, phenol peels, alone or in conjunction with other facial rejuvenative procedures, have consistently proved valuable in improving actinic damage and rhytidosis. The risks of this procedure can be minimized if the indications are appropriate, patient selection is carefully performed, and patient expectations are realistic. It is important to obtain adequate training to achieve the best results. With meticulous attention to technique and a complete understanding of the management of both expected and unusual sequelae, an excellent outcome can be anticipated in most cases. Despite heightened public awareness of the harmful effects of ultraviolet light, actinically damaged skin is not restricted to the older patient population. This has increased the demand for chemical peels. Although it is rewarding to see years of aging and sun damage disappear with treatment, phenol should not be considered a "fountain of youth."[19]

REFERENCES

1. MacKee GM, Karp FL: The treatment of post-acne scars with phenol. Br J Dermatol 64:456–459, 1952.
2. Eller JJ, Wolff S: Skin peeling and scarification. JAMA 116:934–938, 1941.
3. Urkov JC: Surface defects of skin: Treatment by controlled exfoliation. IL Med J 89:75–81, 1946.
4. Winter L: Method of permanent removal of freckles. Br J Dermatol Syphilol 62:83–84, 1950.
5. Ayres S: Dermal changes following application of chemical cauterants to aging skin. Arch Dermatol 82:578–585, 1960.
6. Ayres S: Superficial chemosurgery in treating aging skin. Arch Dermatol 85:125–133, 1962.
7. Monash S: The uses of diluted trichloroacetic acid in dermatology. Urol Cutan Rev 49:119–120, 1949.
8. Brown AM, Kaplan LM, Brown MA: Phenol-induced histological skin changes: hazards, techniques, and uses. Br J Plast Surg 13:158, 1960.
9. Litton C: Chemical face lifting. Plast Reconstr Surg 29:371–380, 1962.
10. Baker TJ: Chemical face peeling and rhytidectomy. Plast Reconstr Surg 29:199–207, 1962.
11. Brody H: The art of chemical peeling. J Dermatol Surg Oncol 15:918–921, 1989.
12. Baker TJ, Gordon HL: Chemical peel with phenol. In: Epstein E, Epstein E Jr (eds): Skin Surgery. 6th ed. WB Saunders, Philadelphia, 1987, pp 423–438.
13. Goodman LS, Gilman AG: The Pharmacological Basis of Therapeutics. Macmillan, New York, 1980, p 968.
14. Asken S: Unoccluded Baker-Gordon phenol peels—review and update. J Dermatol Surg Oncol 15:998–1008, 1989.
15. Rees TD: Chemabrasion and Dermabrasion. WB Saunders, Philadelphia, 1980, pp 749–769.
16. Wixler J, Halon DA, Teitelbaum A, et al: The prevention of cardiac arrhythmias produced in an animal model by the topical application of a phenol preparation in common use for face peeling. Plast Reconstr Surg 75:595–598, 1984.
17. Reudeman R, Deichmann WB: Blood phenol level after the topical application of phenol-coating preparation. JAMA 152:506, 1953.
18. Gleason MD, Gosselin RE, Hodge HC, Smith RP: Clinical Toxicology of Commercial Products. Williams & Wilkins, Baltimore, 1969, pp 189–192.
19. Matarasso SL, Glogau RG: Chemical face peels. Dermatol Clin 9:132–149, 1991.
20. Matarasso SL, Salman SM, Glogau RG, Rogers GS: The role of chemical peeling in the treatment of photodamaged skin. J Dermatol Surg Oncol 16:945–954, 1990.
21. Litton C, Trinidad G: Chemosurgery of the eyelids. In: Aston SJ, Hornblass A, Meltzer MA, et al (eds): Third International Symposium of Plastic and Reconstructive Surgery. Williams & Wilkins, Baltimore, 1982, pp 341–345.
22. Spira M, Gerow FJ, Hardy SB: Complications of chemical face peeling. Plast Reconstr Surg 54:397–403, 1974.
23. Lober CW: Chemoexfoliation—indications and cautions. J Am Acad Dermatol 17:109–112, 1987.
24. Litton C, Fournier P, Capinpin A: A survey of chemical peeling of the face. Plast Reconstr Surg 51:645–649, 1973.
25. Stegman SJ, Tromovitch TA: Chemical peeling. In: Cosmetic Dermatologic Surgery. Year Book Medical, Chicago, 1984, pp 27–46.
26. Collins PS: The chemical peel. Clin Dermatol 5:57–74, 1987.
27. Fitzpatrick TB: The validity and practicality of sun-reactive skin types I through VI. Arch Dermatol 124:869–871, 1988.
28. Burks JW: Dermabrasion and Chemical Peeling. Charles C Thomas, Springfield, IL, 1979, pp 209–226.

29. Pierce HE, Brown LA: Laminar dermal reticulotomy and chemical face peeling in the black patient. J Dermatol Surg Oncol 12:69–73, 1989.

30. Brody HJ: Complications of chemical peeling. J Dermatol Surg Oncol 15:1010–1019, 1989.

31. Mosienko P, Baker JS: Chemical peel. Clin Plast Surg 5:79–80, 1978.

32. McCollough EG, Langston PR: Dermabrasion and Chemical Peel: A Guide for Facial Plastic Surgeons. Thieme, New York, 1988, pp 43–54.

33. Rubenstein R, Roenigk HH Jr, Stegman SJ, Hanke SW: Atypical keloids after dermabrasion of patients taking isotretinoin. J Am Acad Dermatol 15:280–285, 1986.

34. Weiss J, Ellis CN, Headington JT, et al: Topical tretinoin improves photoaged skin: a double-blind vehicle controlled study. JAMA 259:527–532, 1988.

35. Kligman AM, Grove GL, Hirose R, Leyden JJ: Topical tretinoin for photoaged skin. J Am Acad Dermatol 15:836–859, 1986.

36. Hung VC, Lee JY, Zitelli JA, Hebda PA: Topical tretinoin and epithelial wound healing. Arch Dermatol 125:65–69, 1989.

37. Mandy SH: Tretinoin in the preoperative and postoperative management of dermabrasion. J Am Acad Dermatol 15:878–879, 1986.

38. Alt TH: Occluded Baker-Gordon chemical peel: review and update. J Dermatol Surg Oncol 15:980–993, 1989.

39. Rapaport MJ, Kramer F: Exacerbation of facial herpes simplex after phenolic face peels. J Dermatol Surg Oncol 10:57–58, 1984.

40. McCollough EG, Hillman RA: Chemical face peel. Otolaryngol Clin Am 13:353–365, 1980.

41. Swinehart JM: Test spots in dermabrasion and chemical peeling. J Dermatol Surg Oncol 16:557–563, 1990.

42. Matarasso SL, Glogau RG: Chemical face peel. J Dermatol Surg Oncol 17:623–624, 1991.

43. McCollough EG, Langsdon PR: Chemical peeling with phenol. In: Roenigk RK, Roenigk HH Jr (eds): Dermatologic Surgery: Principles and Practice. Marcel Dekker, New York, 1989, pp 997–1016.

44. Stegman SJ, Tromovitch T, Glogau RG: Chemical peels. In: Stegman SJ, Tromovitch TA, Glogau RG (eds): Cosmetic Dermatologic Surgery. Year Book Medical, Chicago, 1990, pp 35–58.

45. Spira M, Dahl C, Freeman R, et al: Chemosurgery—histological study. Plast Reconstr Surg 45:247–253, 1976.

46. Stuzin JM, Baker TJ, Gordon HL: Chemical peel: a change in the routine. Ann Plast Surg 23:166–169, 1989.

47. Baker TJ, Gordon HL: Chemical face peeling. In: Baker TJ, Gordon HL (eds): Surgical Rejuvenation of the Face. CV Mosby, St. Louis, 1986, pp 37–100.

48. Balin A, Pratt L: Physiological consequences of human skin aging. Cutis 43:431–436, 1989.

49. Montagna W, Carlisle S: Epidermal and Dermal Histological Markers of Photodamaged Human Skin. Richardson-Vicks, Shelton, CT, 1988.

50. Stegman SJ: A comparative histologic study of the effects of three peeling agents and dermabrasion on normal and sundamaged skin. Aesthetic Plast Surg 6:123–135, 1982.

51. Stegman SJ: A study of dermabrasion and chemical peels in an animal model. J Dermatol Surg Oncol 6:490–497, 1980.

52. Kligman AM, Baker TJ, Gordon HL: Long-term histologic follow-up of phenol face peels. Plast Reconstr Surg 75:652–659, 1985.

53. Hayes DK, Berkland ME, Stambaugh KJ: Dermal healing after local skin flaps and chemical peel. Arch Otolaryngol Head Neck Surg 166:794–797, 1990.

54. Brody HJ, Hailey CW: Medium-depth chemical peeling of the skin: a variation of superficial chemosurgery. J Dermatol Surg Oncol 12:1268–1275, 1986.

55. Litton C, Trinidad G: Complications of chemical face peeling as evaluated by a questionnaire. Plast Reconstr Surg 67:738–743, 1981.

56. Brody HJ: Variations and comparisons in medium-depth chemical peeling. J Dermatol Surg Oncol 15:953–963, 1989.

57. Gross BG, Maschek MD: Phenol chemosurgery for removal of deep facial wrinkles. Int J Dermatol 19:159–164, 1980.

58. Dmytryshyn JR: Chemical face peel complicated by toxic shock syndrome. Arch Otolaryngol 109:170, 1983.

59. LoVerme WE: Toxic shock syndrome after chemical face peel. Plast Reconstr Surg 80:115–118, 1987.

60. Klein DR, Little JH: Laryngeal edema as a complication of chemical peel. Plast Reconstr Surg 71:419–420, 1983.

61. Gross D: Cardiac arrhythmia during phenol face peeling. Plast Reconstr Surg 73:590–594, 1984.

62. Truppman F, Ellenbery J: The major electrocardiographic changes during chemical face peeling. Plast Reconstr Surg 63:44, 1979.

63. Beeson WH: The importance of cardiac monitoring in superficial and deep chemical peeling. J Dermatol Surg Oncol 13:949–950, 1987.

64. Stagnone GJ, Orgel MG, Stagnone JJ: Cardiovascular effects of topical 50% trichloroacetic acid and Baker's phenol solution. J Dermatol Surg Oncol 13:999–1002, 1987.

65. Field LM, Farber G: Dermabrasion and chemical exfoliation. J Am Acad Dermatol 10:521–522, 1984.

CHAPTER 40

Indications for and Techniques of Hair Transplantation

S. TERI McGILLIS

Most men and many women experience some degree of hair loss during their lifetime. When the loss is permanent or extreme, it can be of social and cosmetic concern to those affected. This is in part because of a societal notion that "more hair is more desirable." Although this notion is not based on any fact, it has persisted over time. The Egyptian papyrus of 1500 BC records attempts to regrow hair, and certainly Samson of biblical times is famous for the masculine prowess associated with his long locks.[1] Efforts to restore or enhance one's original pelage will continue until the process of balding is fully accepted.

Historical Aspects

The earliest use of hair-bearing grafts to correct alopecia dates back to at least 1893.[2, 3] These early endeavors primarily consisted of free grafts intended for scalp coverage and not for cosmesis (Fig. 40–1). Japanese investigators were among the first to successfully use small-diameter hair-bearing tissue to correct alopecia of the scalp, eyebrows, and mustache areas.[4, 5] These original grafts were much like current hair transplantation grafts, and while Japanese investigators are said to have routinely performed transplant procedures on radiation victims after the atomic bombings, their work was virtually unknown to the Western world, presumably because of the war.

Credit for popularizing hair transplantation specifically for the correction of male-pattern baldness goes to Norman Orentreich, who in 1959 published an important treatise on this subject.[6] This work catapulted medical specialists into a new era of understanding of hair loss and presented an effective and more permanent solution to the many medicaments, potions, and camouflage techniques used in previous decades.

Physiologic Aspects

As a result of Orentreich's early work, the concept of donor dominance was discovered. Donor dominance refers to skin or hair-bearing grafts that preserve their characteristics regardless of the recipient site into which they are placed. In early works on androgenic alopecia, it was noted that when a small, hair-containing graft from the occiput was transplanted into a bald area of scalp such as the vertex, the character of the occipital hair was maintained and continued to grow indefinitely. Thus donor dominance became the major premise on which hair transplantation surgery was based.

Male-pattern baldness, or androgenetic alopecia, is now known to be a process by which terminal scalp hairs are gradually converted into vellus hairs. An autosomal dominant sex-linked gene appears to influence which follicles will enter this cycle and at what time. Although excess androgen production is not a feature of male-pattern baldness, follicles that have been genetically programmed to lose hair have increased levels of 5α-reductase.[7–9] This enzyme is responsible for the conversion of testosterone into dihydrotestosterone, which in turn may promote vellus conversion by inhibiting adenyl cyclase. Hair follicles most susceptible to vellus conversion are those in the frontal and crown regions of the scalp.[10] While this is a very natural process, it induces much anxiety in men, primarily because of the uncertainty as to when balding may begin and how far it may progress.

At present, hair replacement surgery is the most

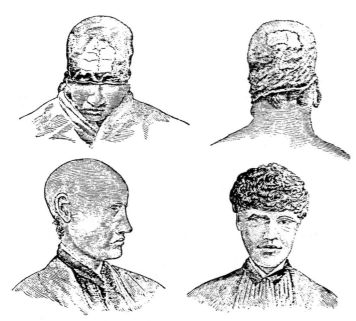

Figure 40–1. Early nineteenth century attempts to correct hair loss were crude at best. (From Gould & Pyle: Anomalies and curiosities of medicine. WB Saunders, Philadelphia, 1897, p 545.)

requested aesthetic surgical procedure by male patients. In 1984, approximately 12,000 patients were treated with transplantation in the United States alone.[11] Although the basic technique has remained unchanged, refinements and modifications continue to evolve and contribute to the ongoing success of the original autograft hair transplant technique.

Indications for Hair Transplantation

The most common cause of hair loss in both sexes is androgenetic alopecia,[12] the condition for which autograft transplantation is most frequently used.[13] However, reports have also emerged of its use in alopecia prematura, alopecia areata, alopecia cicatrisata, morphea, vitiligo, and lupus erythematosus, with varying degrees of success.[6] In 1976, the success rates for the punch autograft method were compared in patients with alopecia caused by chronic discoid lupus erythematosus (DLE), patients with traumatic alopecia, and patients with androgenic alopecia. The mean graft survival rates were 72%, 97%, and 104%, respectively.[14] Transplantation of hair into depigmented scars caused by DLE has resulted in repigmentation of these areas in addition to hair growth.[15] Transplantation may offer DLE patients some hope for improvement. However, it is essential that alopecia resulting from collagen vascular and autoimmune phenomena be quiescent for at least 6 months before transplantation is considered. The periphery of such localized alopecias often abuts normal or nearly normal vascularized scalp. Because these areas have a better chance at successful "take," they should undergo transplantation before the more scarred or

atrophic regions. Patients with extensive scars or severe atrophic alopecias are not ideally suited to transplantation, but transplantation has been successfully used to correct alopecia of the eyebrows resulting from leprosy and other conditions.[16-23] Transplantation of single hairs from the scalp to reconstruct eyelashes has also met with much success.[24, 25]

One technique uses epilation to induce scalp hairs to enter their catagen phase. As a result, catagen follicles migrate higher into the dermis, and thinner grafts can be harvested without sacrificing hair bulbs. These "thinner grafts" (up to 8 mm wide) are harvested from the mastoid region and used to resurface denuded areas of the beard.[26, 27]

Transplants have also been used to correct alopecia resulting from burns,[28, 29] trauma,[30, 31] congenital abnormalities,[32, 33] radiation defects,[34, 35] and the use of artificial hair implants.[36] The Japanese, who were early masters of hair transplantation, have used hair-bearing grafts to replenish pubic hair.[37] Occasionally, patients request fuller chest or pubic hair or ask for hair to be placed in unusual areas. While these solicitations are infrequent, they serve as reminders that transplantation is not strictly limited to androgenetic alopecia. Provided an active or reversible cause of alopecia is ruled out, any alopecic or minimal hair-bearing region is potentially amenable to transplantation. The basic requirement is a healthy donor source in conjunction with a well-vascularized recipient bed.

Preoperative Evaluation

All cosmetic surgery procedures require careful preoperative consultation, and hair transplantation is no exception. Time spent evaluating the patient and establishing realistic goals will lead to greater patient and physician satisfaction. The preoperative evaluation should include attention to original pattern and location of the hairline, classification of baldness, rate of hair loss, favored hair styles, color and texture of the hair, donor density, estimate of total grafts required, ultimate goals, and adjunctive procedures.

ORIGINAL PATTERN AND LOCATION OF THE HAIRLINE

A hands-on evaluation of the scalp and hair is important for two reasons. First, the patient is more likely to develop trust in a cutaneous surgeon who is willing to carefully consider the problem, and second, the surgeon can gain a more complete picture of the surgical candidate. The scalp should be assessed for primary cutaneous conditions, evidence of previous surgeries, and the presence of traumatic scars that may require additional hair transplants for full camouflage. Black patients should be assessed for keloids and hypopigmentation. Scalp laxity should be determined to help define patients who may benefit from scalp reduction procedures.

Most personal encounters in life are face to face, and loss of the frontal hairline is a particular concern to balding persons. Careful inspection of the frontal scalp will, in most cases, reveal persistent fine vellus hairs at the site of the original hairline, even in the baldest of men. It has been estimated that the rate of frontal hairline recession is approximately 1 cm per decade beginning at age 20.[38] The degree and amount of recession beyond the original hairline should be carefully noted. Patients are often anxious to reconstruct their childhood hairlines but should be discouraged from this, as such hairlines rarely look natural in a mature adult. Under no circumstances should a new hairline be planned anterior to the original hairline.

CLASSIFICATION OF BALDNESS

Several classification schemes for baldness exist, with the purpose of helping cutaneous surgeons predict the eventual outcome of thinning so that hair replacement procedures can be optimized. The first useful classification of male-pattern baldness was published in 1951[7] but was later modified.[39] This classification is a widely accepted standard and consists of seven categories of baldness, plus a variant. Other authors[40] have greatly simplified this original classification to reflect four typical balding patterns (Fig. 40–2) as follows:

Class I: Frontal baldness only, with or without an anterior tuft of hair
Class II: Frontal and midscalp thinning with no thinning of the crown
Class III: Frontal to occipital (crown) baldness
Class IV: Crown baldness only

Most men will develop a class III pattern if given enough time.[40] For this reason, it is imperative to assess the midscalp and crown for any signs of hair loss. If thinning is evident, especially in a young person, it is more likely that a patient with a clinically apparent class I pattern may evolve into a class III pattern. Consequently, the transplantation procedures should be planned to anticipate this future loss. The danger in initiating transplantation before a distinct pattern has become established is that the transplants may be more obvious with time should extensive hair loss occur. As a rule of thumb, older patients and those with extensive baldness make the best candidates, primarily because their loss is likely to be stable. Younger patients require very careful assessment. Because of this, some surgeons suggest waiting until age 30 before performing transplantation.[41, 42] Age, however, is not a limiting factor.

RATE OF HAIR LOSS

Normal hair loss occurs at a rate of approximately 100 hairs per day.[43, 44] As terminal hairs are replaced with vellus hair growth, a 50% reduction is needed for thinning to be clinically apparent, although most patients are aware of hair loss at the time it begins. With this information, the surgeon can get an idea of how stable or unstable the hair loss is before transplantation. Most patients have a driver's license or photograph that can substantiate the hair loss claim if the photograph is at least 1 year old. If patients do not undergo surgery within 18 months of the original consultation, it is best to re-evaluate them as extensive additional loss may have occurred, requiring a new surgical plan.

FAVORED HAIR STYLES

Many balding patients attempt to conceal their baldness with a particular hair style. A man with a low side

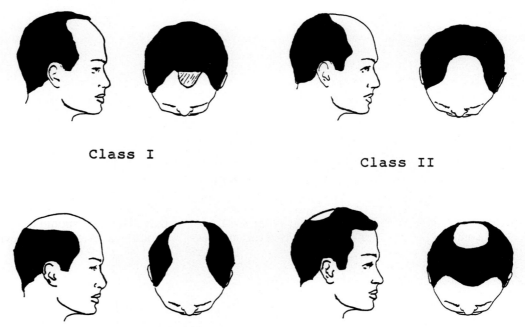

Figure 40–2. Mayer-Fleming classification of male-pattern baldness. (Adapted from Paparella MM, Shumrick DA, Gluckman JL, Meyerhoff WL: Otolaryngology. Vol IV. 3rd ed. WB Saunders, Philadelphia, 1991, p 2784.)

Class I   Class II

Class III   Class IV

part and a meticulous sweep of temporal hair meant to camouflage a thinning dome is a common site. Hair style says a lot about a person and to some extent correlates with the degree of concern and motivation a patient has for undergoing surgery. The consultation is an ideal time to broach the subject of hair grooming. Many styling modifications are available and are often necessary accompaniments to hair transplantation surgery. For instance, patients who comb their hair straight back will emphasize and expose the grafts along the frontal hairline, so alternative styles should be encouraged. By contrast, patients willing to consider a permanent wave after transplantation procedures will reap the rewards of a simulated increased density (Fig. 40–3). A permanent wave places curls into straight hair, which provides greater coverage. Ideally, the patient should be willing to wear a style incorporating a paramedian or side part so that hair can be styled over transplanted grafts. These factors become important when designing the hairline and should always be discussed with the patient in advance.

COLOR AND TEXTURE OF HAIR

It is important to assess the color and texture of the hair. Hair color is significant only when it provides sharp contrast with the skin tone. Black hair transplanted into a fair scalp will emphasize the tufted appearance of the grafts more than black hair transplanted into a dark scalp. Patients with "salt-and-pepper" graying are ideal candidates for hair transplantation, because the alternating colors blend the plugs more naturally with the skin. Hair color is of minor importance, however, and should not be an exclusionary factor for transplantation surgery, although it may be helpful in terms of predicting final results. For the same reason that permanent waves appear to give greater density, patients with naturally curly or kinky hair can generally achieve better results than those with fine, straight hair.

DONOR DENSITY

The donor region or fringe area of the scalp must be carefully evaluated, as this is the source from which hair is to be taken. Typical donor sites include the occiput, temple, and parietal hair. An average of at least 10 hairs per 4-mm-diameter area is needed for optimal results. If the patient has had or will undergo scalp reduction or tissue expansion before the transplantation, it should be remembered that these procedures may decrease absolute hair follicle density by gradually stretching the skin in the donor regions.

The available donor supply also obviously decreases as balding progresses. Therefore, it is important to estimate not only the number of hairs per graft, but also the surface area of the donor zone. Any thinning along the posterior crown should be carefully noted. Other options such as flaps or tissue expansion may give more satisfactory results in those with large balding recipient sites and small donor zones.

The density of hairs at the recipient area is of less importance, since much of this hair will ultimately be lost. Greater density will obviously provide some natural coverage while the new grafts are growing, but prema-

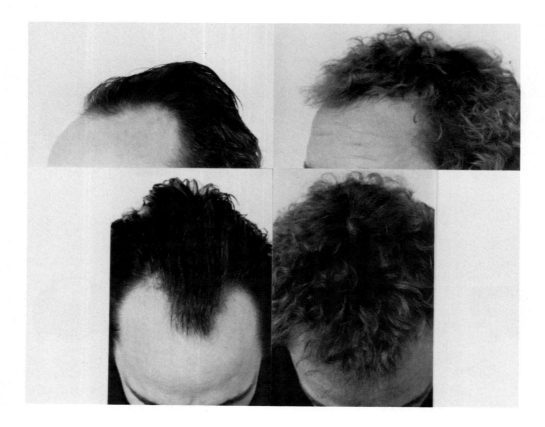

Figure 40–3. Same patient seen before (*left*) and after (*right*) a single transplant session followed by a permanent wave. Note the increased appearance of hair density. (Hair is slightly bleached from use of hydrogen peroxide.)

ture transplantation into a fairly dense recipient area may lead to accelerated hair loss.[45] This loss occurs because some hairs are mechanically removed when creating recipient sites and also because surrounding hairs may be traumatized, resulting in telogen effluvium. While these hairs will regrow, they may be progressively finer in caliber with each growth cycle.

ESTIMATE OF TOTAL GRAFTS REQUIRED

Most transplant surgeons estimate that at least four sessions of 50 to 60 4-mm grafts are required to build an adequate frontal hairline.[41, 46–48] Obviously, variation in size of plugs, hairline design, anticipated ancillary procedures, and refinement techniques will all affect this estimate. In any case, all hair transplant candidates must understand that surgery is not a "one shot–instant hair" event, but rather a dynamic, changing, multistage surgical process that is constantly being revised or modified to accommodate for future loss or thinning.

ULTIMATE GOALS

Realistic goals should be set, since every patient desires a full head of hair, even though this may not be achievable. Hair replacement surgery is actually a sophisticated form of camouflage. Although it is not possible to produce more hair, it is possible to move existing hair to create an illusion of more hair. Understanding this, the patient's expectations and motivations for surgery should be explored. Patients who desire perfection or are obsessed with their appearance will often be disappointed with even the best results. Patients should leave the consultation with a complete understanding of the procedure and its limitations. Some surgeons use a doll's head with silicone plugs to demonstrate results,[49] while others rely on before-and-after comparison photographs of other patients who have had hair transplantation. However, photographs can be misleading unless patients with similar hair color, density, and degree of loss are used for comparison. If any doubt remains in the physician's mind as to the patient's mental suitability and understanding of transplantation, surgery should be deferred.

ADJUNCTIVE PROCEDURES

Most hair transplant surgeons are well versed in a variety of hair replacement modalities. Scalp reductions, hair-bearing flaps, and tissue expansion techniques all play important roles in the treatment of male-pattern baldness. Scalp reduction was first used in conjunction with hair transplantation in 1977,[50] which demonstrates the relatively recent development of multimodality hair replacement surgery. It is currently the most frequent adjunctive procedure performed with hair transplantation.[51–53] In some individuals, primarily those with dense frontal hair and balding limited to the midscalp, one or more reduction operations will diminish or even possibly eliminate the need for the use of grafts by decreasing the size of the recipient area. With some artistic skill,

the surgeon can individualize the procedures to effectively meet each patient's individual hair replacement needs. As long as the patient has reasonable expectations, understands the nature of the procedures, and is given an estimate of the final results, satisfaction can be achieved in most cases.

Medical Evaluation

Careful inquiry into existing medical problems, current medications, and social habits will help to avert problems at the time of surgery. Any medical history of cardiovascular disease, hypertension, epilepsy, diabetes, bleeding diatheses, and drug allergies should be fully explored. These problems should be under control at the time of surgery and clearance obtained from an internist if necessary.

Drug or alcohol abuse is of particular concern, as such patients often require additional sedation preoperatively and more pain medication postoperatively. In addition, because intravenous drug abusers have an increased potential for human immunodeficiency virus (HIV) exposure, this risk should be carefully assessed. Patients who use marijuana socially have also experienced adverse effects on hair growth in their transplanted grafts.[38] These facts imply that a social drug history should be a prerequisite in the medical evaluation.

Preferred laboratory evaluations vary with the surgeon and should obviously be individualized according to each patient's medical history. Tests for HIV exposure, hepatitis antigen, prothrombin time (PT), and partial thromboplastin time; complete blood cell counts; and a chemistry profile are all routinely performed before the first transplantation. If all test results are normal and the initial procedure has no complications, the tests are not usually repeated for subsequent procedures.

Use of anticoagulants, aspirin, aspirin-containing medications, nonsteroidal anti-inflammatory medications, and vitamin E all increase bleeding, and the formation of a hematoma under any graft, including hair transplants, will impede its take. To avoid this risk, these medications are stopped 1 to 2 weeks before surgery (see Chap. 13). The use of alcohol should be discouraged for 24 hours before surgery because of its vasodilatory effects. Nicotine has also been shown to decrease circulation and affect graft take. As a consequence, if at all possible smoking should be stopped several weeks before surgery.[54–56]

The use of topical minoxidil is common in hair loss patients, and many are reluctant to discontinue its use. However, minoxidil promotes vasodilatation and can contribute to bleeding at the time of hair transplantation surgery. Its use is discouraged for 6 to 8 weeks before transplantation. Some early investigations have suggested that initiating its use postoperatively may decrease the postsurgical shedding of hair[57, 58] and encourage nutrient vessel formation and graft acceptance. While minoxidil may prove to be an important adjunct to transplantation, further studies are needed to confirm its benefits.

The use of prophylactic antibiotics remains controversial. The scalp is a highly vascular region with a concomitant low risk of infection. In one survey,[59] more than one third of the responding cutaneous surgeons reported an infection rate of slightly more than 1% when not using prophylactic antibiotics. Routine use of perioperative antibiotics beginning 2 to 24 hours before surgery has been reported to decrease the infection rate from 0.5% to 0.1%.[47] In any case, infection rates are extremely low, and the decision to use prophylactic antibiotics remains at the discretion of the surgeon. Antibiotics maximally suppress infection if given *before* surgery,[60] and to maintain a low rate of infection, erythromycin (333 mg tid) can be started the day before surgery and continued several days postoperatively.

One study has shown that immunizations or vaccinations occurring within 3 months of hair transplant surgery can lead to graft failure in patients who had previously undergone successful transplants.[38] While this may be coincidental, it should raise some concern for hair transplant surgeons in the United States who are treating foreign patients in whom immunizations may be necessary before a visa permit can be obtained.

Special Instrumentation

The trephine, or hand-held punch biopsy device, is similar to the punch tool designed for leather craftsman and is an elegantly simple instrument that plays an important role in hair transplantation surgery. Edward Keyes first published reports of its use in 1887.[61] Motorized punches were first introduced in 1951[62] and have become standard equipment among hair transplant surgeons. They have increased the overall quality of grafts and the efficiency of obtaining them. Several units are commercially available, including the Landow power unit and the more popular Bell hand engine (Fig. 40–4). Both systems consist of a rapidly rotating handpiece that can be adapted to accept a wide variety of punch sizes. Many different sizes and styles of punches are currently available. Punches range in diameter from 1 to 5.5 mm and are available in increments of 0.25 mm. The thin-walled, internally beveled punch[63] cuts a cylindrically shaped plug with a slightly wider bottom. The original punch was externally beveled and produced a plug with a tapered base. This punch has been modified over the years.[64, 65] The Australian punch is made of carbon steel, has both external and internal bevels, and is considered to be of superior quality. With time and experience, many surgeons develop a preference for a particular type of punch.

Power-driven punches are primarily used for harvesting plugs from the donor zone, while hand-held punches are preferred for creating the defects at the recipient site. This is because rotary punches can catch existing hair and pull it out, which can have a negative effect on previously transplanted plugs that are finally beginning to grow. Use of hand-held punches for the recipient area has the further possible advantage of creating a more conical opening into which the power-driven cylindrical grafts fit more precisely.[63]

It is often preferable to perform hair transplantation with the patient in a supine or prone position. To facilitate comfort, a specially designed head rest or face mask is used (Fig. 40–5). Other surgeons prefer to perform transplantation with the patient in a semireclining position. The upright patient, however, may be more prone to syncope. As long as patient comfort is maintained, there is little advantage to either position. Other

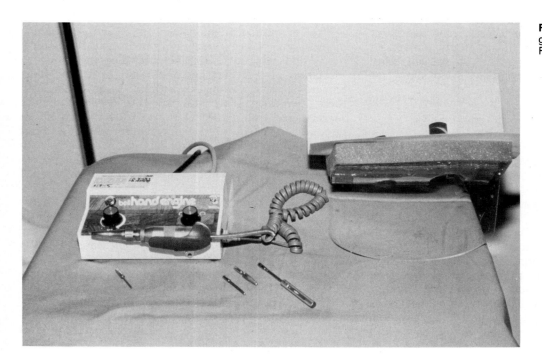

Figure 40–4. *Left,* Bell hand engine with various trephines. *Right,* Face mask for head stabilization.

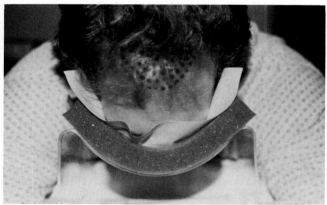

Figure 40–5. Close-up of face mask used while harvesting grafts from the occiput. This provides for patient comfort and head stabilization.

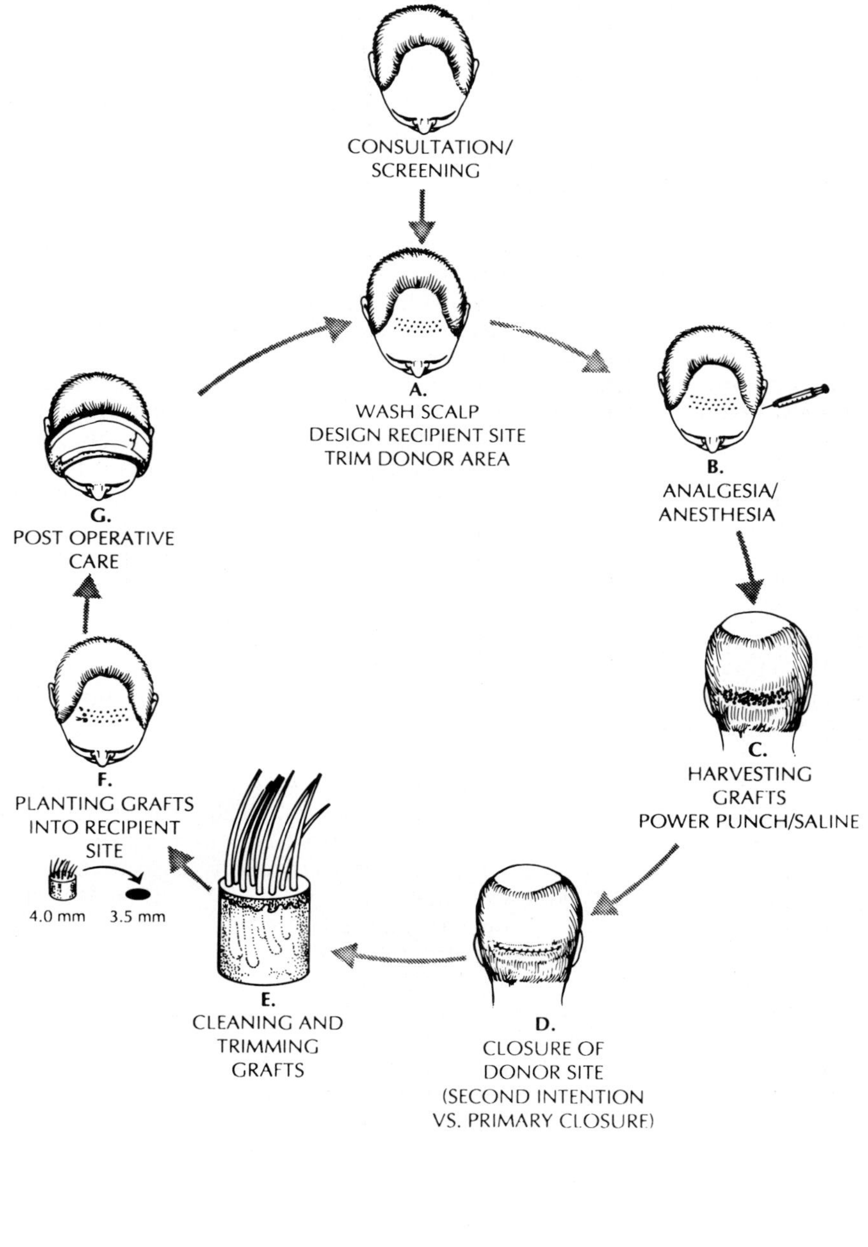

Figure 40–6. Flow diagram of the basic steps of hair transplantation. Each is described in detail in the text.

instruments used in hair transplantation are found on standard sterile surgical excision trays. A wire mesh strainer and a container with iced saline are added to the tray to hold the harvested plugs. It is also useful to have Petri dishes available for storing and grading the trimmed plugs.

Techniques of Transplantation

Most reports of hair transplantation have been dedicated to technical variations, planning methods, and final results, all with the intent of improving current methods. Despite individual variations in technique, the procedure consists of six important steps (Fig. 40–6): designing the recipient site, administering sedatives and local anesthesia, harvesting the grafts, closing the donor

HAIR TRANSPLANTATION TECHNIQUE

CONSULTATION/
SCREENING

A.
WASH SCALP
DESIGN RECIPIENT SITE
TRIM DONOR AREA

B.
ANALGESIA/
ANESTHESIA

C.
HARVESTING
GRAFTS
POWER PUNCH/SALINE

D.
CLOSURE OF
DONOR SITE
(SECOND INTENTION
VS. PRIMARY CLOSURE)

E.
CLEANING AND
TRIMMING
GRAFTS

F.
PLANTING GRAFTS
INTO RECIPIENT
SITE

4.0 mm   3.5 mm

G.
POST OPERATIVE
CARE

site, preparing and implanting the grafts, and providing postoperative care. These steps will be described individually.

STEP ONE: DESIGNING THE RECIPIENT SITE

The art of this procedure is in the design. Bad results stand out ominously, while good results should appear natural enough to go unnoticed. Good aesthetic results occur with careful assessment of the recipient site and detailed attention to hairline placement and configuration. For this reason, the most important decision is where to place the hairline. When in doubt, always err on the conservative side. Hairlines placed too high can be lowered at a later date by adding rows of grafts, but a hairline placed too low cannot be raised.

The great artist Leonardo da Vinci conceptualized the male human face as a square that could be divided into three main sections.[66] The first contained the region from the chin to the nasal spine; the second extended from the nasal spine to the glabella; and the third encompassed the area between the glabella and the hairline. The upper section should be approximately four fingerbreadths wide. One rule of aesthetics applicable to both artists and surgeons is that the hairline should be placed above the upper third of the face to create the most natural appearance.

The contour of the hairline is equally important to hairline placement. A properly placed hairline can look unnatural if its shape is poorly planned. The normal adult male has a slightly convex or U-shaped hairline when viewed posteriorly to anteriorly. There should always be an angle laterally where the frontal hairline meets the temporal hairline; this is often referred to as the temporal gulf. Blunted temporal gulfs, concave or straight frontal hairlines, and artificially created widow's peaks rarely look natural. If the patient is planning to wear a part, which should be encouraged, the frontal hairline should stop just medial to it. If this precaution is not observed, the grafts will be exposed whenever the patient parts the hair. For most men, a part line should ideally be worn somewhere above the midlateral portion of the eyebrow. Parts created more laterally are often necessary when baldness is extreme.

The crown area also requires careful planning. This area is generally fairly resilient, so when hair loss is extensive, scalp reduction procedures should be considered. If at all possible, scalp reduction should be done before grafting, because the anterior hairline may be moved posteriorly as a result of tissue excision. The natural pattern of hair growth at the crown is whorled, spiraled, or comma-shaped. Each graft must be carefully placed to maintain this natural configuration.

The intended hairline should be marked out and shown to the patient before initiating the procedure or sedation. Any discrepancies can thus be addressed preoperatively until agreement is reached. A standard cotton-tipped applicator dipped in gentian violet or brilliant green approximates the size of a 4-mm punch and is a useful marker. If plugs of more than one size are planned, more than one dye color can be used.

Most initial procedures are done using larger grafts of 4 or 4.5 mm. Larger grafts contain more hair and thus provide more coverage but are less natural in appearance. Subsequent sessions can be performed with smaller grafts, and ultimately mini- and micrografts can be used to further improve the appearance of the hairline.

There has been very little difference in hair yield per surface area between 4-mm and 4.5-mm grafts.[67] Rarely are grafts larger than 4.5 mm selected. The central follicles in graft sizes greater than 4.5 mm theoretically receive less blood supply and may be prone to central necrosis. Larger grafts are useful, however, in that they can be divided or sliced into semicircular segments and used in adjunctive procedures such as split grafting or minigrafting.

Placement of plugs should be designed so that a distance equal to or just slightly less than a plug's diameter surrounds each graft. This maximizes vascular nutrition and optimizes graft take. The standard technique of transplantation typically consists of four sessions. The first session establishes the frontal hairline as well as the third and possibly fifth rows with an empty row between that is approximately the same width as the graft diameter. The second procedure can be performed as soon as 4 to 6 weeks later to create second and fourth rows to fill in between the two or three rows placed during the first session. The third and fourth sessions, best delayed until growth begins to occur from the first two surgical sessions, provide additional fill-ins as needed. At the end of these four transplant sessions, the patient is left with a new hairline approximately four to five plug diameters wide (Figs. 40–7, 40–8) from front to back.

If the donor supply does not appear sufficient to cover the frontal region as planned (that is, less than approximately 250 4-mm grafts), alternative designs should be used. For example, grafted hair allowed to grow six inches long at the part line can be combed over, providing more ultimate coverage than similar sized grafts placed randomly and allowed to grow to only two inches (Fig. 40–9).

While the standard four-session hair transplantation procedure works, it is fraught with several problems that deserve special consideration.[63] Not all patients have the time, inclination, or income to undergo successive surgeries as frequently as suggested. Those who delay additional procedures may need adjustments in their surgical plan so that some initial coverage is provided between sessions. Some patients may benefit from placing the majority of plugs along the anticipated part line so that the hair can be combed over to the other side (Fig. 40–9). Other variations of the basic procedure exist, and planning should be individualized. Not all patients fit into a fixed pattern, and alternative designs must be used for patients without standard patterns of hair loss.[68]

Transplants to the central portions of the scalp often have the poorest growth. This is especially true with consecutive sessions and is thought to be a result of the fact that the blood supply is gradually reduced with each

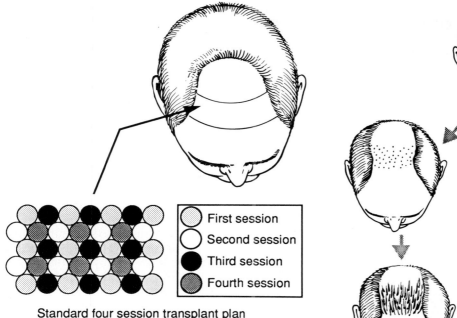

Standard four session transplant plan rebuilding the frontal hairline

Figure 40–7. Schematic showing the standard four-stage plan for hair transplantation surgery.

phase of transplant surgery. For this reason, this area might be transplanted first before the peripheral blood supply is reduced.[63] Once the plan is fully outlined and approved by the patient, the procedure can begin.

STEP TWO: ADMINISTERING SEDATIVES AND LOCAL ANESTHESIA

The patient should first be photographed and cleansed and recipient sites marked with the anticipated transplant plan. The patient may have some final questions regarding the procedure or the plan, and no sedatives should be given until these are addressed. It is not always necessary to administer preoperative sedatives

RANDOM PATTERN OF 50 GRAFTS   **ENHANCEMENT OF PARTLINE WITH 50 GRAFTS**

Figure 40–9. Comparison of random graft placement versus enhancement of the part line and use of hair growth for covering the remaining scalp.

for hair transplantation, and this should be done at the discretion of the surgeon. Diazepam (5 to 10 mg) is most routinely used and is administered either sublingually or intravenously over 3 to 5 minutes. Experience shows that diazepam greatly tapers anxiety and allows for ease of injecting the anesthetic. If sedatives are used, patients should come with a responsible person who can drive them home.

Figure 40–8. Photograph of a patient after partial rebuilding of the hairline. More grafts have been placed on the left side to enhance the patient's low-set part line. (Note the midline scar from previous scalp reduction procedures.)

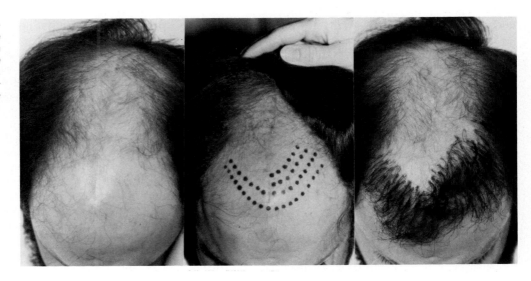

Lidocaine 1% with epinephrine 1:100,000 is the principal local anesthetic used in hair transplant surgery (see Chap. 9). This agent acts rapidly and will last several hours. Approximately 7 mg/kg or 50 mg of this concentration can be used before toxic levels of lidocaine are reached.[69] For this reason, it is important to keep track of the volume injected. Because saline is also used in transplant surgery, it is a good practice to use color-coded needle caps for each solution to avoid any miscounting of syringes or administration of the wrong agent.

Epinephrine is used primarily for hemostasis, and a full 15 to 20 minutes should be given to allow for maximal effectiveness. It has been reported that the vasoconstriction produced by epinephrine can cause a reduction in hair growth from grafts.[69] By using 1% lidocaine with a reduced concentration of epinephrine of 1:200,000, hemostasis can be maintained without compromising subsequent hair growth.[70] It must be remembered, however, that with less epinephrine, the absorption of lidocaine may be increased.

Injections into the subcuticular tissue plane are performed with a 30-gauge needle. The low pH of this solution can cause some pain on injection, but this discomfort can be attenuated by adding sodium bicarbonate as a buffer or by mixing the epinephrine with plain lidocaine just before use.[71–73] Warming the anesthetic agent to room temperature and injecting it slowly also eases discomfort somewhat.

If the transplantation is performed with the patient in the supine-prone position, it is customary for the recipient site to be anesthetized first. The patient is then turned over to have the donor site injected. This procedure results in less turning of the patient. Some surgeons prefer to delay anesthetizing the recipient site until the patient has returned to the supine position. By this time, however, much of the sedative effect will have been lost.

A peripheral or field block is advocated for both donor and recipient areas.[7] Peripheral blocks are accomplished by linear injections just anterior to the proposed hairline and 5 mm inferior and lateral to the donor site. The advantage of a peripheral block over a local block is that less anesthetic is generally required. Regional nerve blocks are also used but may require a field or local block to enhance the epinephrine effect.[74–76]

Experience has shown that the midline anterior portion of the scalp often requires additional anesthesia. This is because of the decussating nerve fibers that originate from the supraorbital and supratrochlear nerves that meet in this area. Reinjecting a second agent such as mepivacaine[63] or 4% lidocaine[47] greatly prolongs anesthesia in this area.[63] When injecting the frontal hairline, care must be taken to avoid intravascular injection into the temporal arteries. This is done by applying manual pressure anteriorly while anesthetizing and by aspirating from the syringe before injecting. Despite this, on rare occasions a rapid blanching of the forehead occurs, which is most often a result of rapid spread of the anesthetic down neurovascular bundles, rather than acute arterial spasm. Injecting close to this neurovascular area also provides satisfactory anesthesia

to the frontal portions of the scalp.[77] Nothing causes more anxiety in a patient than unexpected pain, so it is important to be sure that the patient is completely anesthetized before beginning the procedure.

STEP THREE: HARVESTING THE GRAFTS

The donor area is the residual fringe of hair that is not genetically programmed to go bald and can be used in accordance with the concept of donor dominance for hair transplantation. Before beginning harvesting, the donor regions must be carefully evaluated. It will become apparent that some areas, such as the upper part of the occiput, have a greater density of hair, while other areas have sparser growth.[45] Furthermore, hair superior to the ears and at the temporoparietal regions generally has a coarser texture than that at the occiput. The thickness of the scalp should be assessed and areas of scarring and contractures from previous surgeries identified. Approximately 40% of the population has a stork bite or nevus flammeus at the nape of the neck.[78, 79] Donor grafts from this area can fade but on occasion retain their red color when transplanted. This may necessitate final placement of these grafts to less noticeable recipient sites.

The donor site is identified and the hair trimmed so that it is about 2 mm long. This enables the surgeon to see clearly the direction of hair growth at the time of implantation. All surrounding hair is taped out of the field, and the area is anesthetized and cleansed with a standard skin preparation. Alternatively, the entire scalp can be shampooed with povidone-iodine soap (Betadine) at the start of the procedure to eliminate this step.

Many patterns of harvesting grafts have been described. These can be categorized by those that are left to close by granulation and those that are closed primarily. The original technique harvested plugs from a rectangular area with bridges of hair of approximately 3 mm remaining between each graft site. These bridges of hair provided enough tissue surrounding each graft site after contraction to adequately cover the donor site. In another harvesting method, grafts are taken from a single row as close together as possible. The bridges are then trimmed away and the remaining wound is closed primarily, interdigitating the scalloped edges.[80] Thus, the pattern selected for harvesting influences the final closure method. Since the early 1980s, the trend has been toward primary closure of the donor site. This trend has been supported with various primary closure techniques published by many hair transplant experts.[81–87]

The actual harvesting of the grafts is the most crucial technique in the entire procedure. The ideal graft should have the following characteristics: no transected follicles; walls that are smooth, even, and cylindrical in shape, lying parallel to the follicles; a round graft top without lipping or indentations; and no scarring in the graft from previous surgery. Two techniques that greatly assist in obtaining optimal grafts include the use of a power-driven punch and the use of saline edematization.[88] The power-driven punch quickly and uniformly cuts plugs that are more cylindrical and of better quality than those harvested by a hand-held punch. It is imperative, however, that the punch be very sharp. Sharpening the punch after each transplant procedure will ensure continued quality. A moderate speed of approximately 10,000 to 15,000 revolutions per minute (rpm) is used. Higher speeds make the punch difficult to control, and frictional heat damage to hair bulbs may occur.[41]

Saline edematization[89] is commonly performed immediately before harvesting plugs. This is done by injecting physiologic saline into the donor area until the area becomes very firm and the hair follicles stiffen somewhat. This provides some resistance to the punch, which results in much less distortion of the grafts, a phenomenon seen when harvesting from a soft, resilient scalp. Saline must be readministered after harvesting every 10 to 20 grafts because of its rapid absorption. Not only are the grafts of higher quality, but there is also an increased number of hairs per graft in patients who receive saline injections.[70]

The punch should cut through the epidermis perpendicular to the scalp and then be angled approximately 45 degrees to parallel the direction of the hair shafts (Fig. 40–10). This angle must be adjusted when harvesting grafts in black patients,[90] whose follicles are more curved; this is done by entering at an angle less than 45 degrees or by injecting enough saline so that follicles temporarily uncoil into a straight position. A slight "give" or loss of resistance will be felt as the punch reaches the level of the galea aponeurotica. Some surgeons do not feel that this depth is necessary and cut only to the subcutaneous layer.

If there is some doubt as to the quality of the grafts, one or two should be removed periodically and inspected so that any adjustments in the technique can be made. Bleeding is generally controlled by epinephrine, local pressure, and electrocautery. Hemostasis can be obtained with suture ligation in areas that continue to bleed. The cut grafts are left in place until harvesting is completed. Grafts are then removed from the donor

sites by gently grasping the epidermis with a pair of toothed forceps. If necessary, cutting may be required at the deepest fibrous component to free the graft. Grafts should not be traumatized by squeezing or grabbing at the base. Gauze and drapes should not be discarded until they have been fully inspected for any possible grafts that may have become dislodged.

Grafts are then placed in a Petri dish containing gauze soaked in physiologic saline and placed over ice. A frozen nontoxic gel can also be used. In theory, the iced environment may actually help reduce telogen effluvium.[67, 91] In any event, the grafts should not be allowed to dry out once they have been removed. Careful inspection of the grafts as they are removed may reveal one or two that have only minimal growth. These can easily be replaced by harvesting additional grafts while the patient is still anesthetized and in proper position.

STEP FOUR: CLOSING THE DONOR SITE

Once all grafts have been removed, the donor area of alternating holes and bridges of scalp will have a honeycombed appearance. The rows of bridges are trimmed and occasionally saved for micro- or minigrafting, leaving the scalloped edges to interdigitate as the wound is closed primarily. Very little undermining is generally needed to facilitate a tensionless closure. Absorbable 3-0 glycolic acid or polydioxanone suture is used as a subcuticular buried layer, and 3-0 prolene or polybutester completes the cutaneous closure. If the wound is well approximated, a running locked stitch is used; otherwise, interrupted sutures are placed. After placement of the final sutures, the patient is returned to a supine position. A towel-wrapped ice pack is placed under the donor site to help reduce edema while the grafts are implanted. The cutaneous sutures are removed approximately 10 to 14 days later. The advantage of closing the wound primarily is that there is less bleeding, postoperative wound care is simplified, the healing time is reduced, the harvest area is easily identified in successive procedures, and only a single linear scar is produced, rather than multiple round, white scars. Disadvantages are that it is time consuming, the patient may experience some discomfort postoperatively from the additional manipulations, and adverse sequelae, such as spitting of sutures, may occur.

STEP FIVE: PREPARING AND IMPLANTING THE GRAFTS

Grafts are prepared by removing hair fragments, foreign particles, or clots and by trimming the excess subfollicular fat. A well-illuminated area and magnification lenses greatly facilitate this task. It is essential *not* to trim off all of the fat, because the hair bulbs are often protected by a thin layer of fat and could be easily traumatized. However, excess fatty tissue can break down into irritating free fatty acids that impede graft acceptance. Because the frontal scalp is thinner than the occipital scalp, this debulking process allows for closer approximation of the grafts into their recipient sites. Most hair transplant surgeons use well-trained assistants

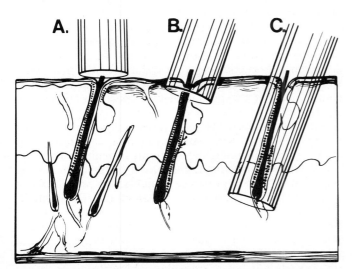

Figure 40–10. *A,* The trephine should pass through the epidermis at a 90-degree angle. *B,* The trephine is then angled approximately 30 to 45 degrees to parallel the hair shafts. *C,* This angle is continued to completion.

to trim and clean the grafts while the surgeon is preparing the recipient sites.

Once trimmed, the grafts are categorized according to quality. Those of similar hair density and graft quality are grouped together in a Petri dish (Fig. 40–11). It is convenient to assemble them into groups of five for easy counting. If donor grafts of more than one size have been harvested, these should be similarly sorted in separate dishes. The prime value of sorting is that it allows for ease of graft selection at the time of implanting. For instance, grafts with greater hair density may be needed in sparser areas or along the part line, while smaller and less dense grafts can be placed strategically between existing plugs for blending or normalizing the frontal hair line.

To prepare the recipient site, holes are cut at an angle of approximately 45 degrees to the scalp, using a hand punch for better control. This avoids the "pincushion" appearance that can result if 90-degree angle holes are made. Many patients have some vellus hair in the recipient area that will help direct proper orientation.

It is helpful to place the first graft into a central hole just above the glabella. This identifies the midline. This graft is placed with hairs angled at 45 degrees to the skin surface and pointed anteriorly toward the nasal bridge. The remaining grafts are implanted in radial fashion from this point. If the surgeon's thumbs are pointed anteriorly and oriented along the central graft, the remaining fingers will roughly indicate proper orientation of the lateral plugs.

Recipient holes are generally cut 0.25 to 0.75 mm smaller than the harvested grafts, with a hole 0.5 mm smaller being most common. Because the grafts shrink slightly on removal and the holes widen slightly, it is necessary to test several sizes until the best fit can be determined. The best fit is snug but not so tight that grafts require prodding for placement. Tight-fitting grafts are more likely to contract and result in trapdoor deformities or a cobblestoned appearance. A moistened cotton-tipped applicator can be used to gently push the graft into place so that it sits level with the surrounding scalp. If necessary, additional trimming can be done. Slight rotation is often required to obtain ideal orientation of the plugs. This is easily done after all of the grafts are placed to avoid further displacement as the implantation progresses.

When bleeding is encountered, gentle pressure generally stops it. Brisk bleeding should be controlled before the graft is placed, to avoid clot formation under it. A suture or a cotton-tipped applicator soaked in epinephrine can be inserted temporarily in the hole while the remaining plugs are placed to control bleeding. Once this is done, the final graft placement is performed.

Once the plugs have been implanted, firm, gentle pressure is applied to the entire recipient zone. Although not a standard procedure, some surgeons use cyanoacrylate adhesives to hold the plugs in place.[92, 93] This takes more time but may reduce the incidence of cobblestoning[93] and can eliminate the need for a bulky dressing.

STEP SIX: POSTOPERATIVE CARE

Postoperative care must always be discussed in detail with the patient. It is helpful to have a written sheet of instructions available for the patient to take home, as many patients do not always pay close attention. Topical care consists of gently cleaning the recipient sites with 3% hydrogen peroxide, followed by application of an antibacterial ointment such as Polysporin or Bacitracin. Telfa pads are used to prevent adherence to the bulky full-head dressing, which consists of woven cotton gauze and Coban elasticized wrapping. The patient leaves this dressing in place for 24 hours, so no wound care is required until after that time.

Immediately postoperatively, patients are given an intramuscular injection of 1 ml or 6 mg of betamethasone. Steroids have been shown to significantly reduce postoperative edema.[94] Patients are asked to sleep with their heads elevated and are provided with pertinent phone numbers should problems arise during the night. Nausea and vomiting are of particular concern, since increased venous pressure created by the Valsalva maneuver could theoretically dislodge the grafts.

The effect of the lidocaine anesthetic wears off approximately 2 to 4 hours later, and patients may then begin to feel some pain or discomfort. Generally, acetaminophen with codeine is prescribed for the first night. Long-acting local anesthetics such as bupivacaine (Marcaine) have been suggested as an alternative to oral pain medications.[70]

Patients are seen the day after surgery for a dressing change. At that time any grafts that are improperly oriented can be realigned without difficulty. After approximately 3 to 4 days, the grafts begin to heal, and realignment is not possible. Patients are seen again in 10 to 14 days for suture removal from the donor site.

After surgery the grafts form a crust on the surface. Many of the transplanted hairs convert into a resting phase and begin to shed about 6 weeks later. If not informed of this, patients become unduly concerned at the loss of their newly transplanted hair. Hair begins to regrow about 12 to 16 weeks later. Patients should also be told that the first cycle of hair growth is often different from that occurring in the original donor hair and may

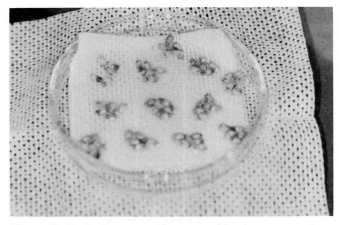

Figure 40–11. Grafts arranged in groups of five for easy counting.

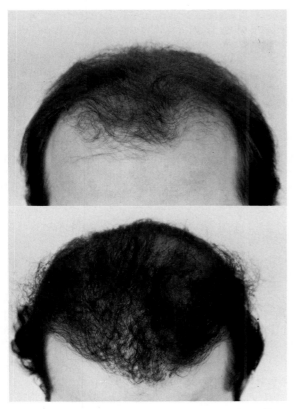

Figure 40–12. Patient seen between transplant sessions. Even with poor styling (e.g., combing the hair straight back), the patient has achieved good density. This is partly because of the coarse nature of his hair.

be straighter, curlier, or darker, but this generally corrects itself after a few anagen cycles.

Patients can proceed with the second transplant session in 6 to 8 weeks. A longer time is preferable, because the hair will be growing in from the grafts and the surgeon can better determine where more grafts are needed. Furthermore, the theoretical likelihood of removing grafts that have not grown hair is reduced (Fig. 40–12). In addition, this interval allows the vasculature time to recover, and the newly grown hair can help hide the acute phase of healing for the second procedure.

Complications

Hair transplantation is a safe and effective procedure with relatively few complications. Most complications can be divided into two types: medical and cosmetic (Table 40–1).

MEDICAL COMPLICATIONS

Bleeding

Bleeding during scalp surgery can be significant and tends to be most prolific in the donor area. Donor regions contain actively growing hair follicles that are nourished by branches of the posterior occipital artery.

Firm pressure and electrocoagulation are generally sufficient in providing hemostasis; however, any persistent arterial bleeding should be suture ligated. The recipient area generally stops bleeding when a graft is implanted. If this fails to ease bleeding, a suture can be placed or an epinephrine (1:10,000)–soaked cotton-tipped applicator can be held on the affected area for 3 to 5 minutes. Proper preoperative instructions regarding the use of aspirin, nonsteroidal anti-inflammatory agents, and alcohol will further reduce the incidence of bleeding.

Infection

Infection has rarely been reported after transplantation, occurring in only approximately 1% of patients. This is partially due to the highly vascular nature of the scalp, and because of this, the use of prophylactic antibiotics is controversial. If used, they should be administered before surgery. Some surgeons use a single injection of cephalosporin, while others use oral dicloxacillin, erythromycin, or tetracycline beginning the day before surgery. Fortunately, most postoperative infections respond to antibiotics and standard local care. If there is any doubt, appropriate cultures should be performed. For the most part, infection does not affect the ultimate outcome of the procedure.

Scarring

Donor site scars are inevitable. Wounds that are closed primarily can stretch on occasion. For the most part, because donor site scars are removed during subsequent phases of the procedure, they are not of particular concern. Donor sites that heal by second intention contract to form small, flat, hypopigmented scars. Again, these are of minimal cosmetic concern and are easily hidden by surrounding hair. Some surgeons have suggested doing "test grafts" to assess healing in both donor and recipient sites, but this is not standard procedure.

TABLE 40–1. **COMPLICATIONS OF HAIR TRANSPLANTATION**

Medical
Bleeding
Infection
Scarring or cobblestoning
Telogen effluvium
Osteomyelitis
Arteriovenous fistulas and aneurysms
Edema
Paresthesia
Folliculitis
Suture reactions
Postinflammatory pigmentary alterations
Inclusion cysts
Pyogenic granulomata
Syncope
Cosmetic
Poor hairline design
Hair growth in wrong direction
Poor hair growth
Patient dissatisfaction

Recipient site scars are potentially more visible and are of much greater concern. Cobblestoning, or persistent elevation of the grafts, results from circumferential retraction around the graft during healing, as well as from insufficient trimming of the grafts before implantation. This problem can be avoided by careful graft trimming and by stretching the recipient hole with normal saline before inserting the graft. It has also been suggested that using tissue adhesives after planting may help avoid cobblestoning.[91, 92] Should it occur, cobblestoning can be improved. Dermabrasion or electrocautery "blending" of graft edges into the surrounding scalp can be performed 12 weeks postoperatively. The reverse condition of sunken grafts is not as easily corrected and is best avoided by meticulous technique at the time of graft placement.

Telogen Effluvium

Telogen effluvium, a normal phenomenon, commonly follows transplantation, as the trauma of surgery causes many hairs to enter their resting phase. The transplanted hair falls out about 6 weeks postoperatively but resumes its growth in approximately 12 weeks. Hair grows at an average rate of 0.37 mm/day, so several months are required before coverage is appreciable. The trauma of surgery can also cause telogen effluvium in nontransplanted hairs, and this may be of particular concern to the patient. Although this is a disconcerting occurrence, it generally corrects itself spontaneously with time.

Osteomyelitis

A single case of osteomyelitis of the skull after scalp reduction and hair transplantation has been reported.[95] This is a rare and highly unusual complication. Awareness of this possibility will alert surgeons to early diagnosis, which should be considered in patients with infections that do not respond to routine treatment.

Arteriovenous Fistulas

Arteriovenous (AV) fistulas are a rare complication of hair transplantation and generally appear about 18 to 60 days after surgery. They present as a palpable, fluctuant nodule with a thrill-like murmur, most commonly in the donor area, and rarely resolve spontaneously. Treatment involves direct excision of the nodule[96, 97] or placement of a percutaneous suture in an attempt to tie off the lesion.

The nature of these fistulas has been studied using angiography.[98] Results suggest that most AV fistulas may actually be pseudoaneurysms. Aneurysms of the arterial or venous system occur much more frequently than AV fistulas and are also commonly present in the donor area. Aneurysms, however, tend to resolve spontaneously over several weeks.[99] Although arterial aneurysms may pulsate, they can be differentiated from fistulas by their lack of murmur.

Edema

Some patients experience painless facial swelling beginning on the second or third postoperative day. While this edema resolves spontaneously over time, it can be distressing to the patient. The use of methylprednisolone has been shown to alleviate this complication.[94] Some physicians administer this preoperatively, and others begin treatment postoperatively. Elevation of the head, especially at night, and reduction of physical activity will help to reduce this problem.

Paresthesia

A decrease in scalp sensation can occur after hair transplantation. The patient should be reassured that sensation will probably return to normal within 4 to 6 months.

Folliculitis

Occasionally a mild form of folliculitis develops around the recipient plugs a few weeks after surgery. This seems to be more common when micro- and minigrafts have been used and may be due in part to the occlusive nature of the antibiotic ointment. This condition does not appear to threaten the transplanted hairs and is easily treated with topical or oral antibiotics.

Suture Reactions

The donor site is often closed primarily and is subject to the same adverse reactions caused by sutures. Spitting of the buried suture can occur about 14 to 30 days after surgery and is generally of minimal concern. Suture granulomas can also occur as a result of contamination by talc from the surgeon's gloves or by the suture itself. Because most of these problems develop in the suture line, it is likely that they will be removed during a subsequent procedure, so patient reassurance is generally sufficient.

Postinflammatory Pigmentary Alterations

The melanocytes in grafts can regress, leaving a hypopigmented area. Migration into the graft from surrounding recipient skin may occur with ultraviolet light exposure. Transplanting from donor scalp that is rarely exposed to the sun may give a false appearance of hypopigmentation. This also generally corrects itself with time.

Inclusion Cysts

Accidental burying of composite grafts or failure to remove all harvested areas before closure can lead to subcutaneous hair growth,[100] cysts, or granulomatous reactions.[101] This can be avoided by careful counting and removal of plugs.

Pyogenic Granuloma

The appearance of multiple pyogenic granuloma-like lesions after hair transplantation has been reported.[102] These lesions can develop approximately 3 weeks after surgery and presumably result from trauma. They can be treated in a standard manner with electrodesiccation, excision, or argon laser irradiation.

Syncope

Intraoperative syncope has been reported, primarily in patients treated in the sitting position. This complication can be avoided altogether by performing transplantation with the patient in a supine/prone position.

COSMETIC COMPLICATIONS

Cosmetic complications are primarily the result of poor planning. A hairline that is poorly oriented or grafts that grow in the wrong direction need little more than foresight for prevention. Poor hair growth can be the result of several factors. First, if too many plugs are implanted closely together, the vascular supply may be compromised, and the quality of the hair growth from these grafts may be reduced. This has been most frequently seen in patients in whom 200 to 300 grafts are implanted in a single session. Second, if the grafts are not kept moist before placement, desiccation may result in decreased growth. Third, transplanting into scarred or atrophic areas with diminished vascularity may result in decreased growth. Fourth, overzealous defatting of grafts may destroy viable hair bulbs. Despite careful planning and good technique, patient dissatisfaction can occur and should be addressed individually.

Modifications and Refinements

Numerous modifications and refinements in hair transplantation surgery have resulted in improved cosmetic results. Perhaps the most important contribution to hair replacement surgery has been the success of using smaller mini- and micrografts to naturalize the appearance of the hairline. While the concept of using individual hairs for the repair of eyebrows was born many years ago, its use in hair transplant surgery for male-pattern baldness is relatively new. This development was due in part to the observation that the most anterior 2 to 3 cm of a transplanted frontal hairline is noticeable because of gaps and the abrupt transition to coarse terminal hair, giving it an unnatural appearance. A natural frontal hairline consists of a graduated coarsening of hairs as they merge into terminal hair growth. By using small grafts containing fine hair from the lower occiput, the gaps can be filled in to provide a less noticeable transition to terminal hairs. The primary indication for the use of smaller grafts is to soften or naturalize the hairline. Other promising modifications include square grafts, strip grafts, incisional slit grafts, and minireductions performed with the motorized punch.

MICROGRAFTS AND MINIGRAFTS

As their names suggest, micro- and minigrafts are smaller versions of traditional grafts and may contain only a single hair. The use of small grafts to soften the appearance of the reconstructed frontal line was originally conceived in 1977.[103] Currently, micro- and minigrafts are being used more frequently, and various methods for obtaining them have been reported.[104–108]

Micrografts

Micrografts are the smallest graft unit, often containing from one to five hairs. Various investigators have reported a unique array of techniques for harvesting these small hair-bearing units. Most typically, standard 4-mm grafts are harvested from the lower occipital region, which are then sliced longitudinally into approximately six smaller grafts, each containing approximately three follicles.[109] These grafts are trimmed of excess fat and epidermis. The recipient sites for micrografts are made as simple stab incisions created with a No. 11 or No. 15 scalpel blade into the frontal hairline between previously implanted grafts. The micrograft is then inserted using fine jeweler forceps. Because the procedure is quite tedious, several sessions are usually necessary to provide sufficient coverage.

Another technique for harvesting micrografts[110] uses the hair-bearing bridges that are left behind in the donor area at the conclusion of standard transplantation. In such instances micrografts consist of one or two hairs that are obtained by teasing the intact follicles from the periphery of the bridges or from the periphery of standard 4-mm hair transplant grafts. Generally a tongue blade is used to stabilize the tissue, while a scalpel or razor blade is used to obtain the grafts.

Minigrafts

Minigrafts generally contain more hairs than micrografts. Quartergrafts are minigrafts obtained by dividing a routine 4- or 4.5-mm punch graft into quarters. This method[111] routinely places approximately 240 to 320 such grafts, made from 60 to 80 full-size grafts, during a single procedure. In performing this technique, it is not essential that the four quarters be equal in size. Unequal quarters have the advantage of being less uniform and thus may appear more natural when implanted. Using punches smaller than 3 mm in a power-driven punch is one effective means of obtaining minigrafts.[105]

Stainless steel dilators[112] can be used to aid in the placement of micro- and minigrafts. Recipient sites are created with a stab incision using an 18-gauge needle into which a 16-gauge dilator is placed. While dilation is occurring, routine 4-mm plugs can be placed into other traditional recipient sites. The micro- or minigrafts are inserted one at a time as the dilators are removed. Dilators facilitate insertion and provide hemostasis, thus permitting larger numbers of micrografts to be placed quickly in a single session.

It is no longer necessary to wait until a frontal line has been completely established before beginning micro- and minigrafting. Simultaneous placement of both types of grafts can be done, ensuring a more aesthetically acceptable result, even after a single operating session. These techniques often require greater surgical skill, diligence, and patience to achieve effective results.

SQUARE GRAFTS

The use of square, rather than round, grafts is not a new innovation, as such grafts were first described in 1977.[113-117] With this technique, a square scalp graft, actually an oblique hexahedral plug, is placed into a square incision line. Square grafts are obtained by taking strips of hair from the donor site and sectioning them into 4-mm² grafts using the scalpel. Recipient sites are prepared by making square perforations in the scalp using a specially designed scalpel. The square graft provides an average of 25% more hair than a circular graft by virtue of its greater area for an equivalent diameter. Square grafts also have the advantage of producing a linear donor defect without any residual islands of hair; this can be easily closed without any excess donor tissue being lost. Because special instrumentation is required, this graft technique has not been as widely used by hair transplant surgeons as its potential benefits would suggest.

STRIP GRAFTS

As the name implies, strip grafting utilizes strips of hair-bearing skin, rather than small-diameter plug grafts, for implantation. In this procedure, strips of skin measuring approximately 6 to 8 mm in width and several centimeters in length are obtained from the parieto-occipital area.[118, 119] As with punch grafts, however, it is very important that the strip of hair be placed at an appropriate angle. This procedure requires much attention and experience. One author[120] reported an overall success rate of less than 60% with this technique, suggesting that more experience is needed before this procedure becomes the preferred choice in hair replacement surgery. Strip grafts may have a higher success rate when employed for replacement of eyebrows, mustaches, and sideburns.

INCISIONAL SLIT GRAFTING

Incisional slit grafting is a new and greatly improved technique in hair transplantation.[121, 122] Using a 4.75-mm punch to harvest round grafts from the donor area, grafts are halved or quartered using a No. 11 scalpel blade. The proportions of each size of graft are individualized for each patient. Incisional slits with a No. 15c blade are made for graft placement. This procedure differs from standard transplantation techniques in that no recipient tissue is removed before placement of the grafts. In addition, because the grafts are smaller, the technique can be used in combination with micro- and minigrafts. It is possible that this procedure may make standard transplantation techniques obsolete.

MINIREDUCTIONS

Minireductions can be used as adjuncts to traditional alopecia reductions.[123] Minireductions are achieved by using a power-driven 3- to 5-mm punch to excise a portion of the scalp. Instead of filling the hole with a graft, the hole is closed primarily. The purpose is to reduce the bald area rather than transplant hair into it. This is ideal for correcting the results of poor hair transplants and for patients who do not have enough donor grafts to fill in the gaps. The gaps can simply be removed to bring the existing grafts closer together. The disadvantage of this technique is that a small scar remains at the site of the excised tissue, which may limit the ability to deal effectively with large untransplanted areas. The benefits are that it is quick and easy and can be combined with standard transplantation methods. It also alleviates the need for larger scalp reduction procedures that require extensive undermining.

SUMMARY

Hair replacement surgery has undergone a substantial number of important evolutionary changes over the past 100 years. To most effectively manage patients with hair loss, a detailed and comprehensive plan must be developed, with substantial input from the patient. Constant re-evaluation and modification of the original plan is required to meet the changing needs of the patient that may occur during the period required for performance of the multiple surgical stages of this procedure.

REFERENCES

1. The Holy Bible. Judges 13:24–16:31.
2. Dunham T: A method for obtaining a skin flap from the scalp and a permanent buried vascular pedicle for covering defects of the face. Ann Surg 17:677, 1893.
3. Davis JS: Scalping accidents. Bull John Hopkins Hospital 16:257, 1911.
4. Okuda S: Clinical and experimental studies of transplantation of living hairs. Jpn J Dermatol Urol 46:135–138, 1939.
5. Sasagawa M: Hair transplantation. Jpn J Dermatol 30:493, 1930.
6. Orentreich N: Autografts in alopecias and other selected dermatologic conditions. Ann NY Acad Sci 83:463–479, 1959.
7. Bingham KD, Shaw DA: The metabolism of testosterone by human male scalp skin. J Endocrinol 57:111–121, 1973.
8. Schweikert HU, Wilson JD: Regulation of human hair growth by steroid hormones. Testosterone metabolism in isolated hairs. J Clin Endocrinol Metab 38:811–819, 1974.
9. Price VH: Hormonal control of baldness. Int J Dermatol 15:742, 1976.
10. Hamilton JB: Pattern loss of hair in man: types and incidence. Ann NY Acad Sci 53:708–728, 1951.
11. Coiffman F: Advancement in scalp grafts. Ann Plast Surg 18:421–428, 1987.
12. Orentreich N, Durr NP: Biology of scalp hair growth. Clin Plast Surg 9:197–205, 1982.
13. Orentreich N, Rizer RL: Medical treatment of androgenetic alopecia. In: Brown AC, Crouse RA (eds): Hair Trace Elements and Human Illness. Praeger, New York, 1980, pp 294–303.
14. Nordstrom RE: Hair transplantation. The use of hair-bearing compound grafts for correction of alopecia due to chronic discoid lupus erythematosus, traumatic alopecia, and male pattern baldness. Scand J Plast Reconstr Surg 14:1–37, 1976.
15. Lobuono P, Shatin H: Transplantation of hair bulbs and melanocytes into leukodermic scars. J Dermatol Surg 2:53–55, 1976.
16. Ranney DA: The role of punch grafting in eyebrow placement. Lepr Rev 45:153, 1974.
17. Yarchuk NI, Tertsionas PV: Reconstruction of eyebrows with free skin grafts. Acta Chir Plast 14:82–89, 1972.
18. Guerrero-Santos J, Casteneda A, Fernandez JM: Correction of

alopecia of eyebrows in leprous patients. Plast Reconstr Surg 52:183–184, 1973.

19. Limberg AA: Eyebrow reconstruction with free transplantation of small grafts of hairy skin with the subcutaneous fat layer. Vestn Khir 109:64–65, 1972.
20. Nordstrom RE: Eyebrow reconstruction by punch hair transplantation. Plast Reconstr Surg 60:74–76, 1977.
21. Arkawa I: Cosmetic evaluation of eyebrow surgery with transplants of single hairs. Jpn J Plast Reconstr Surg 10:1, 1967.
22. Fujita K: Reconstruction of the eyebrow. Leprosy 22:364, 1953.
23. Narita N: Free hair graft reconstruction of the eyebrow. Keisei-Geka Jpn J Plast Reconstr Surg 11:1–6, 1968.
24. Marritt E: Transplantations of single hairs from the scalp as eyelashes. J Dermatol Surg Oncol 6:271–273, 1980.
25. Unger WP: Eyelash transplantation. In: Unger WP, Nordstrom REA (eds): Hair Transplantation. 2nd ed. Marcel Dekker, New York, 1988, pp 316–317.
26. Clodius L, Smahel J: Resurfacing denuded areas of the beard with full thickness scalp grafts. Br J Plast Surg 32:295–299, 1979.
27. Clodius L, Smahel J: Precipitation of follicle atrophy before hair grafting. In: Unger WP, Norstrom REA (eds): Hair Transplantation. 2nd ed. Marcel Dekker, New York, 1988, pp 735–743.
28. Penaler JM, Dillon B, and Parry SW: Reconstruction of the eyebrow in the pediatric burn patient. Plast Reconstr Surg 76:434–440, 1985.
29. Savin RC: Hair transplants in burn scars and other alopecias. Conn Med 37:501–503, 1973.
30. Purita F: Hair transplants in accidental baldness. Hospital (Rio J) 77:1303–1305, 1970.
31. Muhlbauer WD: Hair transplantation in post-traumatic alopecia. Munch Med Wochenschr 112:1655–1659, 1970.
32. Bertolino AP: Hair transplantation between identical twins. J Am Acad Dermatol 19:418–421, 1988.
33. Pulg CJ, Haenschen RJ: Hair transplantation for congenital alopecia. J Am Osteopath Assoc 78:432–434, 1979.
34. Jacobs JB, Monell CM: Treatment of radiation induced alopecia. Head Neck Surg 2:154–159, 1979.
35. Nordstrom REA, Holsti L: Hair transplantation in alopecia due to radiation. Plast Reconstr Surg 72:454–458, 1983.
36. Monell CM: Repair of sequelae from artificial fiber hair implants with hair-bearing punch grafting. Head Neck Surg 7:332–335, 1985.
37. Tamura H: Pubic hair transplantation. Jpn J Dermatol 53:76, 1943.
38. Farber GA: The punch scalp graft. Clin Plast Surg 9:207–220, 1982.
39. Norwood OT: Hair Transplant Surgery. Charles C Thomas, Springfield IL, 1973, pp 45–49.
40. Mayer TG, Fleming RW: Aesthetic and reconstructive management of alopecia. In: Paparella MM, Shamrick DA, Gluckman JL, Meyerhoff WL (eds): Otolaryngology. Vol IV. 3rd ed. WB Saunders, Philadelphia, 1991, pp 2783–2797.
41. Knowles RW: Hair transplantation: a review. Dermatol Clin 5:515–530, 1987.
42. Nordstrom REA: The initial interview. Facial Plast Surg 2:179–187, 1985.
43. Kligman AM: The human hair cycle. J Invest Dermatol 33:307–316, 1959.
44. Kligman AM: Pathologic dynamics of human hair loss: telogen effluvium. Arch Dermatol 83:175–198, 1961.
45. Ayers S: Hair transplantation for male pattern baldness: aesthetic considerations and current status. Head Neck Surg 7:272–285, 1985.
46. Unger WP: Construction of the hairline in punch transplanting. Facial Plast Surg 2:221–230, 1985.
47. Unger WP, Nordstrom REA: Hair Transplantation. 2nd ed. Marcel Dekker, New York, 1987.
48. Pinski JB: Hair transplantation. In: Roenigk RK, Roenigk HH (eds): Dermatologic Surgery. Marcel Dekker, New York, 1988, pp 1047–1078.
49. Marritt E: The hair transplant model: a three-dimensional approach to the patient consultation. Cutis 24:159–161, 1979.
50. Blanchard G, Blanchard B: Obliteration of alopecia by hair lifting: a new concept and technique. J Natl Med Assoc 69:639–641, 1977.
51. Alt TH: Scalp reduction as an adjunct to hair transplantation, review of relevant literature, presentation of an improved technique. J Dermatol Surg Oncol 6:1011–1018, 1980.
52. Unger MG, Unger WP: Midline alopecia reduction combined with hair transplantation. Head Neck Surg 7:303–311, 1985.
53. Roenigk HH: Combined surgical treatment of male pattern alopecia. Cutis 35:570–577, 1985.
54. Sherwin MA, Gastwirth CM: Detrimental effects of cigarette smoking on lower extremity wound healing. J Foot Surg 29:84–87, 1990.
55. Lawrence WT, Murphy RC, Robson MC, et al: The detrimental effect of cigarette smoking on flap survival: an experimental study in the rat. Br J Plast Surg 37:216–219, 1984.
56. Rees TD, Liverett DM, Guy CL: The effect of cigarette smoking on skin-flap survival in the face lift patient. Plast Reconstr Surg 73:911–915, 1984.
57. Kassimir JJ: Use of topical minoxidil as a possible adjunct to hair transplant surgery. A pilot study. J Am Acad Dermatol 16:685–687, 1987.
58. Bouhanna P: Topical minoxidil used before and after hair transplantation. J Dermatol Surg Oncol 15:50–53, 1989.
59. Norwood O: Hair Transplantation Surgery. 2nd ed. Charles C Thomas, Springfield, IL, 1973, pp 150–151.
60. Burke JF: The effective period of preventive antibiotic action in experimental incisions and dermal lesions. Surgery 50:161–168, 1961.
61. Keyes EL: The cutaneous punch. J Cutan Genitourin Dis 5:98–101, 1887.
62. Urbach F, Shelley WB: A rapid and simple method for obtaining punch biopsies without anesthesia. J Invest Dermatol 17:131–134, 1951.
63. Stegman SJ, Tromovitch TA, Glogau RG: Cosmetic Dermatologic Surgery. 2nd ed. Year Book Medical, Chicago, 1990.
64. Stegman SJ: Commentary: the cutaneous punch. Arch Dermatol 118:943–944, 1982.
65. Hagerman D, Wilson JW: The skin biopsy punch: evaluation and modification. Cutis 6:1139–1143, 1970.
66. Wasserman J: Leonardo. Doubleday and Company, Garden City, NY, 1980, p 27.
67. Unger WP: Hair Transplantation. Marcel Dekker, New York, 1979, pp 77–78.
68. Norwood OT, Taylor BJ: Hair transplant surgery: innovative designs. J Dermatol Surg Oncol 16:50–54, 1990.
69. Moloney JM, Lertora JJ, Yarborough J, et al: Plasma concentrations of lidocaine during hair transplantation. J Dermatol Surg Oncol 8:950–954, 1982.
70. Sadick NS, Hitzig GS: Adjuvant techniques in punch graft hair transplantation. J Dermatol Surg Oncol 12:700–705, 1986.
71. McKay W, Morris R, Mushlin P: Sodium bicarbonate attenuates pain on skin infiltration with lidocaine, with or without epinephrine. Anesth Analg 66:572–574, 1987.
72. Christoph RA, Buchanan L, Begalla K, et al: Pain reduction in local anesthetic administration through pH buffering. Ann Emerg Med 17:117–120, 1988.
73. Stewart JH, Cole GW, Klein JA: Neutralized lidocaine with epinephrine for local anesthesia. J Dermatol Surg Oncol 15:1081–1083, 1989.
74. Frankel EB: Nerve block anesthesia for hair transplantation. J Dermatol Surg Oncol 7:73–75, 1981.
75. Monheit GD: Anesthesia. In: Unger WP, Nordstrom REA (eds): Hair Transplantation. 2nd ed. Marcel Dekker, New York, 1988, pp 133–143.
76. Kohn T: Regional anesthesia for hair transplantation. In: P. Robins (ed): Surgical Gems in Dermatology. Journal Publishing Group, New York, 1988, pp 81–82.
77. Sebben JE: A method of obtaining satisfactory anesthesia in the frontal portion of the scalp preliminary to hair transplantation. J Dermatol Surg Oncol 5:177, 1979.
78. Jacobs AH, Walton RG: The incidence of birthmarks in the neonate. Pediatrics 50:218, 1976.
79. Pratt AG: Birthmarks in infants. Arch Dermatol 67:302, 1953.
80. Pierce HE: An improved method of closure of donor sites in hair transplantation. J Dermatol Surg Oncol 5:475, 1979.
81. Hill TG: Closure of the donor site in hair transplantation by a cluster technique. J Dermatol Surg Oncol 6:190, 1980.

82. Morrison ID: An improved method of suturing the donor site in hair transplantation surgery. Plast Reconstr Surg 67:378–380, 1981.
83. Unger WP: A new method of donor site harvesting. J Dermatol Surg Oncol 10:524–529, 1984.
84. Alt TH: Evaluation of donor harvesting techniques in hair transplantation. J Dermatol Surg Oncol 10:799–806, 1984.
85. Sturm H: The benefit of donor site closure in hair transplantation. J Dermatol Surg Oncol 10:987, 1984.
86. Carrierao S, Lessa S: New techniques for closing punch graft donor sites. Plast Reconstr Surg 64:455, 1978.
87. Norwood OT: Single row donor site harvesting. J Dermatol Surg Oncol 16:453–455, 1990.
88. Pinski J: How to obtain the "perfect" plug. J Dermatol Surg Oncol 10:953, 1984.
89. Alt TH: The donor site. In: Unger WP, Nordstrom REA (eds): Hair Transplantation. 2nd ed. Marcel Dekker, New York, 1988.
90. Earles MR: Hair transplantation, scalp reduction, and flap rotation in black men. J Dermatol Surg Oncol 12:87–96, 1986.
91. Lepaw MI: Aids in cutaneous and hair transplant surgery. J Dermatol Surg Oncol 9:273–276, 1983.
92. Morrison ID: Tissue adhesives in hair transplant surgery. Plast Reconstr Surg 68:491–497, 1981.
93. Wilkinson TS, Iglesies J: Tissue adhesives as an adjunct in hair transplantation. South Med J 67:1408, 1974.
94. Nordstrom RE, Nordstrom RM: The effect of corticosteroids on postoperative edema. Plast Reconstr Surg 80:85–87, 1987.
95. Jones JW, Ignelzi RJ: Osteomyelitis of the skull following scalp reduction and hair plug transplantation. Ann Plast Surg 5:480–482, 1980.
96. Semashko DC, Schwartz ME, Kaynan A, et al: Arteriovenous fistula following punch-graft hair transplantation. J Dermatol Surg Oncol 15:754–755, 1989.
97. Williams LR, Robinson JK, Yao JS: Hair transplantation producing arteriovenous fistulization. Ann Vasc Surg 1:241–243, 1986.
98. Nordstrom REA, Totterman SMS: Iatrogenic false aneurysms following punch hair grafting. Plast Reconstr Surg 64:563–565, 1979.
99. Norwood OJ: Arteriovenous fistulae resulting from hair transplantation surgery. Cutis 8:263–264, 1971.
100. Nordstrom REA, Wahlstrom T: Hair growth in subcutaneously buried composite hair-bearing skin grafts. Scand J Plast Reconstr Surg 16:91, 1982.
101. Altchek DD, Pearlstein HH: Granulomatous reaction to autologous hairs incarcerated during hair transplantation. J Dermatol Surg Oncol 4:928–929, 1978.
102. Sarnoff DS, Goldberg DJ, Greenspan AH, et al: Multiple pyogenic granuloma-like lesions following hair transplantation. J Dermatol Surg Oncol 11:32–34, 1985.
103. Ayers S: Prevention and correction of unaesthetic results of hair transplantation for male pattern baldness. Cutis 19:117, 1977.
104. Nordstrom RE: "Micrografts" for improvement of the frontal hairline after hair transplantation surgery. Aesthetic Plast Surg 5:97, 1981.
105. Frechet P: Micro and mini grafting using the standard hair implantation procedure. J Dermatol Surg Oncol 15:533–536, 1989.
106. Lucas NW: The use of minigrafts in hair transplantation surgery. J Dermatol Surg Oncol 14:1389–1392, 1988.
107. Norwood OT: Micrografts and minigrafts for refining grafted hairlines. Dermatol Clin 3:545–552, 1987.
108. Brandy DA: Conventional grafting combined with minigrafting: a new approach. J Dermatol Surg Oncol 13:60–63, 1987.
109. Nordstrom REA: Minisurgery. In: Unger WP, Nordstrom REA (eds): Hair Transplantation. 2nd ed. Marcel Dekker, New York, 1988.
110. Cohen IS: Donor island harvesting for micro and minigrafting. J Dermatol Surg Oncol 15:384–385, 1989.
111. Bradshaw W: Quarter-grafts: a technique for minigrafts. In: Unger WP, Nordstrom REA (eds): Hair Transplantation. 2nd ed. Marcel Dekker, New York, 1988.
112. Marritt E: Micrograft dilators: in pursuit of the undetectable hairline. J Dermatol Surg Oncol 14:268–275, 1988.
113. Coiffman F: Use of square scalp grafts for male pattern baldness. Plast Reconstr Surg 60:228–232, 1977.
114. Coiffman F: Use of square scalp grafts for male pattern baldness. In: Unger WP (ed): Hair Transplantation. Marcel Dekker, New York, 1979, pp 159–162.
115. Coiffman F: Square scalp grafts. In: Vallis CP (ed): Hair Transplantation for the Treatment of Male Pattern Baldness. Charles C Thomas, Springfield, IL, 1982, pp 481–506.
116. Coiffman F: Square scalp grafts. Clin Plast Surg 9:221, 1982.
117. Coiffman F: Square grafting. In: Unger WP, Nordstrom REA (eds): Hair Transplantation. Marcel Dekker, New York, 1988.
118. Vallis CP: The strip graft method in hair replacement surgery. In: Ervin E, Ervin E Jr (eds): Skin Surgery. Charles C Thomas, Springfield, IL, 1982, pp 564–579.
119. Vallis CP: The strip scalp graft. Clin Plast Surg 2:229–240, 1982.
120. Pierce HE: Hairline replacement utilizing the strip graft technique. In: Unger WP, Nordstrom REA (eds): Hair Transplantation. Marcel Dekker, New York, 1988.
121. Stough DB IV, Nelson BR, Stough DB: Incisional slit grafting. J Dermatol Surg Oncol 17:53–60, 1991.
122. Swinehart JM, Griffin EI: Slit grafting: the use of serrated island grafts in male and female-pattern alopecia. J Dermatol Surg Oncol 17:243–253, 1991.
123. Unger WP: Concomitant mini reductions in punch hair transplanting. J Dermatol Surg Oncol 9:388–392, 1983.

CHAPTER 41

Scalp Reduction

LARRY LANDSMAN and STEPHEN H. MANDY

Almost 20 years after the first published description of autograft transplantation,[1] scalp reduction surgery was described as an important advance in the overall management of patients with male-pattern baldness. In the original 1977 report[2] of 100 patients, the fusiform excision of bald scalp with advancement of the hair-bearing skin was called "hair lifting." Subsequently, many surgeons modified the technique, which is now generally known as scalp reduction.[3–10]

Patient Selection

INITIAL EVALUATION

As with any surgical procedure, the physician must be certain that the patient understands and can withstand the physical and psychological stresses of the surgical procedure. A careful history and physical examination will usually indicate any underlying important medical conditions such as diabetes and hypertension, which must be controlled before surgery. A discussion with the patient's family physician or internist may also be indicated if there are any questions regarding the patient's medical status. A complete blood cell (CBC) count, platelet count, prothrombin time (PT), partial thromboplastin time (PTT), and bleeding time should be routinely ascertained in all patients to be certain that a bleeding disorder does not exist. Hepatitis screening and human immunodeficiency virus (HIV) status also might be considered worthwhile laboratory tests to obtain.

IDEAL CANDIDATES

Scalp reductions are most useful in the treatment of midline and vertex alopecia. As a consequence, patients with Hamilton[11] types 3 to 6 patterns of baldness are often appropriate candidates for scalp reductions (Fig. 41–1). In addition, patients with good scalp laxity (Bosley[12] class 3 or greater) are better candidates than those with Bosley class 1 or 2 (Fig. 41–2). However, with the aid of tissue expanders, even Bosley class 1 and 2 patients can be considered for scalp reduction.

TIMING OF PROCEDURES

In general, a delay of at least 3 months should be allowed between sequential reductions so sufficient scalp laxity can develop, permitting excision of a reasonable amount of tissue. The decision whether a patient undergoes scalp reduction before, during, or after hair transplantation is based on several factors. However, there are several advantages in doing scalp reductions before hair transplantation. First, it is easier to design the frontal hairline properly, since it will otherwise become higher and narrower after the reductions. Second, there is less concern about possible injury to grafts already in place. Preservation of vascular supply to the grafted area is essential when performing reductions first. Finally, undermining for scalp reductions is easier if it precedes hair transplantation.

One disadvantage of doing scalp reductions first is delayed patient gratification (i.e., seeing hair growth). In addition, scalp reductions stretch the donor area, which reduces the density of the number of hairs per graft for subsequent transplantation.

Keeping these factors in mind, some surgeons prefer to do the first scalp reduction before hair transplantation on patients who are candidates for both procedures. Four to 6 weeks later, the first hair transplant procedure is performed. The second hair transplant procedure is done 4 to 6 weeks after the first. At this point, approximately 3 months have passed since the first reduction, and it is possible to ascertain how well the first set of plugs are growing. The second reduction can be consid-

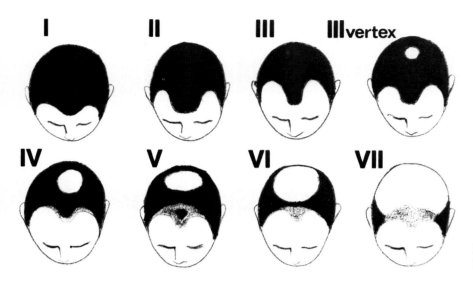

Figure 41–1. Hamilton categories of male-pattern baldness.

ered at that time, if the patient has redeveloped sufficient scalp laxity to make the procedure worthwhile. At the time of the second reduction, it is also possible to perform 20 to 30 standard punch grafts and 20 micro- and miniplugs simultaneously. Following a delay of 4 to 6 weeks after the second scalp reduction, a third hair transplant can be performed, if indicated. Additional transplants or reductions can be continued at appropriate intervals as required.

Alternatively, for the patient who psychologically needs the gratification of seeing hair grow as soon as possible, hair transplantation can be performed before scalp reduction surgery. Any necessary adjustments in the established hairline as a result of subsequent scalp reductions can be made at an appropriate later time.

PATTERNS OF EXCISION

Over the years, a variety of different excision patterns have been advocated (Fig. 41–3). However, the most commonly used patterns currently are the midline sagittal excision and the lateral crescentic excision, each of which has its own intrinsic set of advantages and disadvantages (Tables 41–1, 41–2).[7, 8]

Scalp Reduction Procedure

Preoperatively, the patient washes the hair with an antibacterial skin cleanser such as chlorhexidine or povidone-iodine both the night before and the morning of surgery. For anxious patients, a 10-mg dose of diazepam is administered orally 30 to 45 minutes preoperatively, or intravenous sedation (5 to 10 mg slow push) can be used immediately before injection of the local anesthetic.

The patient lies in a prone position with face resting on a Prōn-Pillō (Chattanooga Pharmaceutical Com-

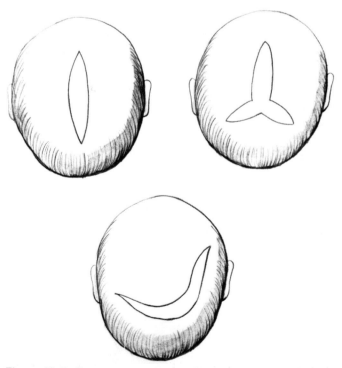

Figure 41–3. Common patterns of scalp reduction excision: simple midline fusiform *(upper left)*, trillium *(upper right)*, and lateral crescentic *(bottom)*.

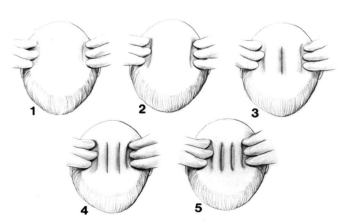

Figure 41–2. Bosley classification of the degree of scalp laxity, showing poor (1) to excellent (5) laxity.

TABLE 41–1. **SAGITTAL MIDLINE EXCISION: ADVANTAGES AND DISADVANTAGES**

Advantages
    Technically easier to perform
    More effectively uses lateral mobility and elasticity of the scalp
    Bleeding is reduced
    No postoperative hypoesthesia

Disadvantages
    Noticeable central scar
    Causes more distortion of bald area

pany). This positions the patient advantageously while supporting the forehead and cheeks. It also provides stability during surgery. A terry cloth headband is applied to the head to prevent any blood from running onto the patient's face. The scalp is prepped with chlorhexidine and draped with sterile towels, and only the area to be excised is shaved. Typically, anesthesia is obtained by deep dermal injection of 0.5 to 1.0% lidocaine containing epinephrine in a concentration of 1:100,000 to 1:200,000 as a ring block encircling the area of the planned procedure. For longer lasting anesthesia, bupivacaine 0.25% with epinephrine 1:200,000 can be injected at the completion of the procedure. Additional infiltration of local anesthetic can be performed along the planned incision lines to reduce any bleeding from the cut skin edges. The procedure is performed using full sterile technique with the surgeon wearing mask, gown, and gloves. The pattern of the scalp reduction used is normally based on the degree of alopecia and the surgeon's personal preference. It should be emphasized that the procedure begins with incising the skin on only one side of the planned excision. Next, hemostasis is achieved using electrocoagulation and occasionally suture ligatures. Dissection then begins and is continued down until the subgaleal plane is reached. This plane is avascular and is composed of loose areolar tissue. The use of a Shaw Optimatrix scalpel or a carbon dioxide laser[13] for incising the scalp is of great benefit in reducing the amount of bleeding.

Once the subgaleal plane has been reached and hemostasis achieved, the skin edges are elevated with a towel clamp, and Metzenbaum scissors are used to begin the dissection at the subgaleal plane so that the flap can be elevated from the periosteum. Once the proper plane

TABLE 41–2. **LATERAL EXCISION: ADVANTAGES AND DISADVANTAGES**

Advantages
    Less noticeable scar at fringe of bald area
    Less distortion of bald area
    Easier undermining and galeatomies
    Occipital hair is elevated

Disadvantages
    Technically more difficult to perform
    Hypoesthesia may occur in alopecic area
    Causes uneven elevation of one side of scalp until contralateral side is done
    Potential for decreased vascularity and poor graft growth in central scalp

of dissection has been established, further blunt dissection can easily be achieved by using an index finger or a periosteal elevator. Undermining should extend from ear to ear laterally, to the superior nuchal line posteriorly, and to the anterior tip of the incision. Galeatomies can also be performed to further increase the advancement of the flap. However, this is not done routinely, since there is an increased risk of bleeding and also a greater risk of injury to major neurovascular bundles with this technique. Galeatomies should probably be reserved for those rare occasions when some difficulty is encountered in closing a wound.

Once the flap has been undermined, the two skin edges are brought together and allowed to overlap. A series of transverse incisions are made in the flap that are equal to the amount of tissue overlap. This allows the surgeon to accurately determine the correct width of scalp that can be safely excised as the incision is completed (Fig. 41–4). The wound may be closed under some tension, and towel clamps may help to approximate and hold the wound margins together as the buried sutures are placed. Closure is achieved with two layers of sutures: 3-0 buried polyglycolic acid suture for the galea and staples or 4-0 nylon for the skin.

A thin layer of antibiotic ointment is placed along the incision line, and a polyethylene oxide water hydrogel occlusive dressing is held in place with a turban type cotton gauze bandage overnight. After 24 hours, the dressing is removed, the wound checked, and antibiotic ointment reapplied. This procedure is repeated daily until the staples or sutures are removed at 7 to 10 days. The patient is allowed to shampoo and get the wound wet after 48 hours. The patient is given prednisone (40 mg) and hydrochlorothiazide (50 mg) orally each day for 3 days after surgery to reduce swelling. Potent narcotic analgesics and sleep medications are often necessary for the first 24 hours postoperatively.

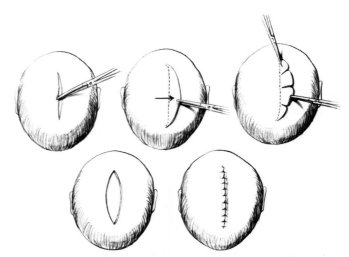

Figure 41–4. Schematic showing the stages of the traditional scalp reduction procedure after incision and undermining have been completed. The alopecic tissue is grasped with a clamp *(upper left)* and pulled over the incision line *(upper middle)*. Horizontal cross-cuts are made *(upper right)* to determine the correct width of the flap before completion of the excision *(bottom left)* and primary closure *(bottom right)*.

Complications

As with all surgical procedures, complications from the administered medications and infection are always possible but occur only infrequently. However, several other problems may be encountered with some regularity in scalp reductions.

EDEMA

Despite the postoperative use of systemic corticosteroids and diuretics, occasionally patients develop edema of the forehead and periorbital area that is so severe that the eyes become swollen shut. Although uncommon, the patient should be warned about this possibility and that it does not usually affect the ultimate result. Liberal application of ice packs during the first 12 to 24 hours postoperatively may also help to prevent edema.

BLEEDING

Bleeding can be avoided by meticulous hemostasis during the procedure. The tension under which the wound is closed and the pressure dressings that are applied also provide an extra measure of hemostasis after surgery. Even though hematomas form only rarely, if there is any question whether active bleeding is occurring postoperatively, the surgeon should open the incision and explore the wound to find and coagulate or tie any bleeding vessels.

STRETCH-BACK

"Stretch-back" occurs when the scar spreads after initial healing. This complication can generally be avoided by not closing the wound with undue tension. It is also less common with curvilinear incisions. If severe, it can be improved by performing a miniature scalp reduction and using careful layered closure.

WOUND NECROSIS

When the incision has been closed with undue tension, the edges of the flaps can become necrotic. When this occurs, the flaps are debrided and topical 3% hydrogen peroxide and Polysporin ointment are applied until the wound heals by second intention. This is not usually a major concern cosmetically, as the scar will likely be re-excised with a subsequent reduction at a future date.

TELOGEN EFFLUVIUM

Occasionally some patients develop telogen effluvium along the edge of the incision line. It is important to reassure the patient that this is a temporary problem that will resolve spontaneously with time.

Tissue Expander–Assisted Scalp Reduction

HISTORICAL ASPECTS OF TISSUE EXPANSION

In 1956, the use of an expandable balloon for auricular reconstruction was described,[14] and in 1976, an expand-

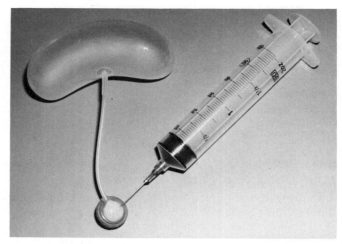

Figure 41–5. Silicone expander connected to a distant self-sealing injection port by tubing.

able Silastic implant was used for breast reconstruction.[15] In 1982, a self-inflating tissue expander that worked on the basis of an osmotic gradient was described.[16] Since that time, tissue expanders have been largely made of silicone and have buried self-sealing injection ports that connect to the prostheses by tubing so that they may be placed at a distance from the expander itself (Fig. 41–5).

CLINICAL FEATURES OF EXPANDED SKIN

Expanders come in various shapes and sizes depending on their purpose. Expander-assisted scalp reduction allows the development of excess hair-bearing scalp that provides a perfect match in the color and texture of hair to cover the defect created by the excision of an area of alopecia. Because the donor flap is "stretched skin," there is no secondary defect to repair. The expanders are inserted and removed through the same incision used for the reduction so that additional scars can be avoided. Increased vascularity from chronic expansion theoretically produces a flap with less chance of flap necrosis. Because more scalp can be excised and closed confidently at each procedure, the patient will generally require fewer operations to achieve maximal coverage. The technique can easily be incorporated by experienced surgeons into their standard surgical routine.[17–23]

HISTOLOGIC CHANGES SEEN WITH TISSUE EXPANSION

Studies in guinea pigs[24, 25] suggest that although the thickness of the epidermis does not appear to diminish significantly after tissue expansion, the intercellular spaces are decreased. Ultrastructurally, undulation of the basal lamina and larger bundles of tonofilaments in the cytoplasm of the epidermal cells are seen using the electron microscope. Increased epidermal mitosis combined with a lack of thinning of the epidermis suggests that there is a net gain of epidermal tissue during chronic tissue expansion.[26]

The dermal changes from tissue expansion are more

dramatic than those seen in the epidermis. While the dermal thickness is greatly decreased, the number of fibroblasts is increased, and there are thick bundles of collagen. Collagen synthesis and tissue vascularity are also increased[27] in the expanded tissue. Hair follicles and adnexal tissue, although reduced in density, remain unchanged after expansion. The subcutaneous fat becomes thinner, which is associated with a decrease in the number of cells and in the number of layers of fat. Fat necrosis is negligible, but any loss of fat is permanent.[17]

A dense fibrous capsule, which is composed of elongated fibroblasts and occasional myofibroblasts lying between thick bundles of collagen fibers and oriented parallel to the surface of the implant, forms within days after implantation of a tissue expander. Also seen within days after implantation is an increase in the number of arterioles and venules in the capsule. The increased viability of flaps created by tissue expansion may be due in large part to the increased neovascularization that occurs at the junction of the capsule and host tissue.[17]

TECHNIQUE OF CHRONIC EXPANSION

In chronic expansion the expander is placed under the hair-bearing scalp in a subgaleal pocket adjacent to the area of alopecia that is to be excised. It is important to be sure that the expander is placed at some distance from the bald scalp so that only the hair-bearing scalp is expanded. Multiple expanders may be placed around the area to be excised. The injection port is placed at some distance away from the expander in an area where it can be easily palpated through the skin. Generally, superior placement in the scalp is used, because with lateral placement, the patient may lie on the port while sleeping. After placement of the expander, the incision is closed in two layers as with standard scalp reduction surgery. These sutures are removed approximately 2 weeks later. The patient is seen at 1- to 2-week intervals, at which time saline is injected percutaneously through the port into the expanders. Often the scalp will become tense or the patient will complain of discomfort during inflation. If either occurs, the injection should be stopped. Usually the scalp will accommodate the added volume well, and over 2 to 3 days, the tension in the scalp decreases. The development of erythema of the overlying skin is thought to be due to an increase in the number of blood vessels. Over several months, enough hair-bearing scalp can be expanded with multiple injections that the patient can undergo the second phase of the procedure, which consists of removal of the tissue expander, excision of the alopecic skin, and primary closure of the defect.

INTRAOPERATIVE TISSUE EXPANSION FOR SCALP REDUCTION

Until recently, chronic tissue expansion for scalp reduction surgery has been the most commonly used surgical technique. However, intraoperative tissue expansion has also become an accepted alternative approach.[23, 28, 29] This technique eliminates many of the disadvantages of chronic expansion, as it is a one-stage procedure done at the time of the initial surgical procedure. With this technique, the patient does not have to live with the temporary deformity seen with chronic expansion. In addition, because the scalp expansion is performed under local anesthesia, there is no pain during the procedure. The procedure increases the standard operating time by only 15 to 30 minutes, but the amount of scalp that can be excised is 20 to 30% greater than possible with standard scalp reduction.[29] Total elimination of the area of alopecia cannot be accomplished in one session, but when compared with standard reduction, intraoperative tissue expansion makes it possible to correct chronic vertex alopecia in fewer sessions.

The technique employs an S-shaped incision beginning anteriorly at the front of the temporal resection and continuing posteriorly along the fringe to the opposite occipitoparietal area. The incision is extended through the galea to the subgaleal plane. It is important to angle the incision so that it is parallel to the hair follicles to minimize the transection of the follicles adjacent to the incision line. Hemostasis is achieved with electrocautery and occasionally with suture ligatures. The scalp is undermined widely under the hair-bearing flap but not under the bald area.

A 125- or 250-ml tissue expander is then inserted into the newly established subgaleal pocket (Figs. 41–6, 41–7). To prevent the expander from extruding through the incision line, towel clamps are used to hold the incision together. Sterile normal saline is used to fill the expander. A Meghan tissue fill kit is used to facilitate the inflation of the expander. It is possible to determine by tissue turgor, pallor, and resistance to injection when the end point of expansion has occurred (Fig. 41–8). At that point the expander is left inflated for ½ to 2 or 3 minutes. It is then deflated for 2 to 3 minutes to allow the expanded scalp to regain blood flow. This cyclic inflation and deflation of the expander is repeated sev-

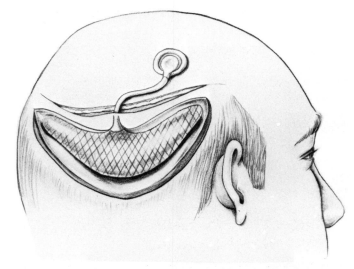

Figure 41–6. Schematic showing placement of a silicone expander for intraoperative expansion.

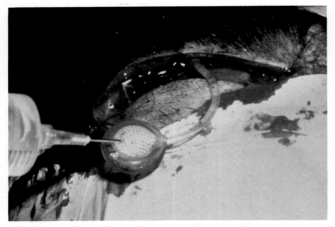

Figure 41–7. Photograph of intraoperative expansion carried out by injecting saline into the distant port.

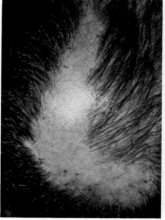
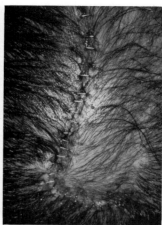

Figure 41–9. Clinical appearance before *(left)* and immediately after *(right)* scalp reduction using intraoperative tissue expansion.

eral times over a 15- to 30-minute period. On subsequent cycles, more saline is injected to produce maximum inflation, an indication that stretching of the flap is occurring. When the expander will no longer accept increasing amounts of saline, it can be assumed that maximal tissue stretch has been achieved. At this point the expander is deflated, the towel clamps are removed, and the expander is withdrawn. The bald tissue is then undermined in standard fashion, hemostasis is ensured, and excision completed (Fig. 41–9).

Complications

The complication rate in tissue expansion scalp surgery ranges from 3 to 7%[17, 20] and is highest with the chronic expansion technique.

INFECTION

The infection rate associated with tissue expansion is less than 1%.[19] While use of perioperative antibiotics

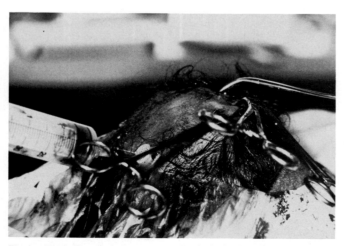

Figure 41–8. Towel clamps are used to hold the incision line together after maximum resistance has been reached.

helps to reduce the infection rate, long-term administration of antibiotics does not. Should an infection occur, irrigation, drainage, and antibiotic therapy should be tried before the expander is removed. Once the infection has resolved, a new expander can be inserted.

PAIN

Patients undergoing chronic expansion commonly complain of pain the first postoperative night and after each subsequent visit when maximal inflation has occurred. This discomfort typically diminishes in 4 to 6 hours.[17] The patient undergoing intraoperative tissue expander–assisted scalp reduction will report a feeling of pressure at the time of inflation, but pain does not occur because of the use of local anesthesia. Commonly, patients who have previously had standard scalp reduction will report less postoperative pain after tissue expansion surgery. This may be a result of neurapraxia of the pain fibers.[29]

HEMATOMA AND SEROMA

Hematomas and seromas are treated by drainage and irrigation of the implant cavity. Infection, capsule formation, and increased tension of expanded tissue can be avoided by early recognition and treatment. Meticulous hemostasis and use of drains, if necessary, at the time of surgery will help to minimize the risk of hematoma formation.

NECROSIS

Skin necrosis occurs when blood flow to the expanded skin is interrupted resulting in hypoxia. Overzealous inflation and prolonged inflation times are common causes of this complication. During chronic expansion, pain usually signals ischemia before the occurrence of necrosis. If this occurs, some of the injected saline should be withdrawn to allow the capillaries to refill.[23]

IMPLANT FAILURE AND EXTRUSION

Complications from implant failure or exposure are uncommon. While minor leakage from the expander may not require replacement, implant deflation will.[23] Exposure or extrusion of the expander is most often the result of creation of a pocket of insufficient size, which allows the expander to remain in contact with the suture line.[20] Other causes include manipulation by the patient, dehiscence of the incision, and erosion through the overlying tissue. These complications may be prevented by delaying tissue expansion for 2 weeks after insertion, externally supporting the skin with tape strips or wraps, and using a slow expansion technique. Bone resorption after forehead expansion has been reported in two patients,[30] and striae have been reported in one.[30] Use of intraoperative tissue expansion will help to reduce the risk of many of these complications.

SUMMARY

Scalp reduction with or without tissue expansion is an important part of the surgical approach to the patient with alopecia. When combined with the traditional hair replacement surgical techniques of plug autografts, minigrafts, and micrografts, these techniques have allowed a greater number of patients with extensive hair loss to be effectively treated. Knowledge of this procedure will provide better results in a shorter time than was previously possible.

REFERENCES

1. Orentreich N: Autografts in alopecia and other selected dermatological conditions. Ann NY Acad Sci 83:463–479, 1959.
2. Blanchard G, Blanchard B: Obliteration of alopecia by Lasi lifting: a new concept and technique. J Natl Med Assoc 69:639–664, 1977.
3. Stough DB, Webster RC: Esthetics and refinements in hair transplantation. The International Hair Transplant Symposium, Lucerne, Switzerland, February 4, 1978.
4. Sparkhul K: Scalp reduction: serial excision of the scalp with flap advancement. The International Hair Transplant Symposium, Lucerne, Switzerland, February 4, 1978.
5. Unger MG, Unger WP: Management of alopecia of the scalp with a combination of excisions and transplantations. J Dermatol Surg Oncol 4:670–672, 1978.
6. Alt TH: Scalp reduction as an adjunct to hair transplantation: review of relevant literature, presentation of an improved technique. J Dermatol Surg Oncol 6:1011–1018, 1980.
7. Norwood OT, Sheil RC: Scalp reductions. In: Norwood OT (ed): Hair Transplant Surgery. 2nd ed. Charles C Thomas, Springfield, IL, 1984, pp 163–200.
8. Unger MG: Alopecia Reduction. In: Unger WP, Nordstrom REA (eds): Hair Transplantation. Marcel Dekker, New York, 1988, pp 435–518.
9. Marzola M: An alternative hair replacement method. In: Norwood OT (ed): Hair Transplant Surgery. 2nd ed. Charles C Thomas, Springfield, IL, 1984, pp 315–342.
10. Brandy DA: The bilateral occipito-parietal flap. J Dermatol Surg Oncol 12:1062–1066, 1986.
11. Hamilton JB: Patterned loss of hair in men: types and incidence. Ann NY Acad Sci 53:708–728, 1951.
12. Bosley LL, Hope CR, Montroy RE, Straub PM: Reduction of male pattern baldness in multiple stages: a retrospective study. J Dermatol Surg Oncol 6:498–503, 1980.
13. Wheeland RG, Bailin PL: Scalp reduction surgery with the carbon dioxide (CO_2) laser. J Dermatol Surg Oncol 10:565–569, 1984.
14. Neumann CG: The expansion of an area of skin by progressive distention of a subcutaneous balloon. Plast Reconstr Surg 19:124, 1957.
15. Radovan C: Adjacent flap development using expandable Silastic implants. American Society of Plastic and Reconstructive Surgery Forum, Boston, MA, September 30, 1976.
16. Austad ED, Rose GL: A self inflating tissue expander. Plast Reconstr Surg 70:588, 1982.
17. Marcus J, Horan DB, Robinson JK: Tissue expansion: past, present and future. J Am Acad Dermatol 23:813–825, 1990.
18. Ryan TJ: Biomechanical consequences of mechanical forces generated by distention and distortion. J Am Acad Dermatol 21:115–130, 1989.
19. Swanson NA, Argenta LC: Tissue expansion advantages in dermatology. In: Callen JP (ed). Year Book of Dermatology. Year Book Medical, Chicago, 1988, pp 243–258.
20. Argenta LC: Advances in tissue expansion. Clin Plast Surg 12:159–171, 1985.
21. Sasaki GH: Scalp repair by tissue expansion. In: Burd B (ed): The Artistry of Reconstructive Surgery. Moody, St. Louis, 1987.
22. Manders EK: Scalp Expansion for the Treatment of Male Pattern Baldness. Dow Corning Wright, Arlington, TN, 1987.
23. Manders EK, Schenden MJ, Furrey JA, et al: Soft tissue expansion: concepts and complications. Plast Reconstr Surg 74:493–507, 1984.
24. Austad ED, Pasyk KA, McClatchey ED, et al: Histomorphological evaluation of guinea pig skin and soft tissue after controlled tissue expansion. Plast Reconstr Surg 70:704–710, 1982.
25. Pasyk KA, Austad ED, McClatchey ED, Cherry GW: Electron microscopic evaluation of guinea pig skin and soft tissue "expanded" with a self inflating silicone implant. Plast Reconstr Surg 70:37–45, 1982.
26. Austad ED, Thomas SB, Pasyk K: Tissue expansion: dividend or loan? Plast Reconstr Surg 78:63–67, 1986.
27. Argenta LC, Anderson RD: Tissue expansion for the treatment of alopecia. In: Unger WP, Nordstrom REA (eds): Hair Transplantation. Marcel Dekker, New York, 1988.
28. Sasaki GH: Intraoperative Tissue Expansion. Dow Corning Wright, Arlington, TN, 1987.
29. Mandy SH, Landsman L: Adjuncts to scalp reduction surgery intraoperative tissue expanders and hyaluronidase. J Dermatol Surg Oncol 17:670–672, 1991.
30. Antonyshyn O, Gruss JS, Mackinnon SE, et al: Complications of soft tissue expansion. J Plast Surg 41:239–249, 1988.

CHAPTER 42

Hair-bearing Flaps

THOMAS P. CHU, D. BLUFORD STOUGH III, and DOWLING B. STOUGH IV

Since the 1970s, the art of hair replacement surgery has evolved greatly, as evidenced by the development of minigrafts, micrografts, and slit grafting.[1] These advances have been applied to the frontal hairline, with great emphasis on more accurately reproducing a natural hairline pattern. This more natural appearance of the transplanted scalp has led to a growing interest in hair replacement techniques by patients with androgenic alopecia. Currently, punch autografting alone or in combination with scalp reduction is the most popular surgical treatment of male-pattern alopecia. However, hair-bearing flaps created by the office-based cutaneous surgeon to correct baldness are a viable treatment alternative in a certain subset of patients.

Anatomic Considerations

The scalp is a richly vascularized and innervated structure that can be divided into five layers: the skin, which consists of the dermis and epidermis; the subcutaneous layer of fat and connective tissue containing the major arteries, veins, nerves, and lymphatics; the galea aponeurotica, a thick, fibrous musculoaponeurotic sheath that is contiguous with the fasciae of the frontalis, temporalis, and occipitalis muscles; the subaponeurotic layer, a layer of loose areolar and fibrous tissue; and the pericranium or periosteum, which covers the calvaria.

The rich vascular supply of the scalp is almost certainly responsible for the high incidence of flap survival and low incidence of postoperative infection. The arterial system consists of five pairs of regional vessels. The frontal region is supplied by the supraorbital and supratrochlear arteries, as well as branches of the ophthalmic artery, which originates from the internal carotid artery. The preauricular region is supplied by the superficial temporal artery and the postauricular region by the posterior auricular and occipital arteries, all of which originate from the external carotid artery. These five pairs of arteries form intricate anastomoses within the scalp, deep in the subcutaneous tissue and just superficial to the galea aponeurotica.

The venous system of the scalp parallels the arterial system both anatomically and in its importance to scalp flap survival. It is apparent that scalp flap necrosis may result from venous stasis as often as arterial insufficiency.[2] This is most likely due to the care with which arteries are preserved and the relative impunity with which veins are ligated and transected during dissection. Another important venous consideration in scalp surgery is the possible intracranial spread of infection by the drainage of the supraorbital, supratrochlear, and emissary veins into intracranial sinuses. Fortunately, this is rare.

Certain principles of scalp surgery relate to this anatomic structure. To obtain local anesthesia and properly execute a ring block, the level of injection should be deep in the subcutaneous layer to reach the larger nerve trunks. When undermining the scalp, the dissection should be limited to the subgaleal space or subaponeurotic layer, as this affords a relatively bloodless plane with little risk of damage to major blood vessels and nerves. The approximation of the galea, the strongest layer of the scalp, helps to reduce tension and provides greater strength for wound closure than skin and subcutaneous closure alone.

Patient Selection

Proper patient selection is critical to the success of any cosmetic surgical procedure, including hair replacement surgery. The patient should be in good physical and mental health, possess realistic expectations, and exhibit a high degree of self-motivation. This selection process is even more important when evaluating the patient who seeks surgical correction of androgenic alopecia in view of the proliferation of various nonsurgical alternatives. These include camouflage techniques such as hair weaving and the use of hair pieces, as well as medical treatment with minoxidil. Once the patient decides to pursue hair replacement surgery, the various surgical modalities of hair transplantation, scalp reduction, and flap creation must be considered. It is the surgeon's responsibility to provide the patient with a complete discussion of the comparative risks and benefits of each procedure. Only with this understanding can the patient be truly informed and capable of selecting the most appropriate treatment for the individual problem.

In determining the relative benefits a patient will receive from punch autografting, scalp reduction, flap surgery, or a combination of any of the three, the hair replacement surgeon must combine strong aesthetic judgment with an objective evaluation of the individual characteristics of the patient. Considerations that are of paramount importance include the anticipated final pattern of alopecia, the texture and quality of the hair, the thickness and laxity of the scalp, and the patient's desired outcome.

ANTICIPATED FINAL PATTERN OF ALOPECIA

As male-pattern alopecia is solely predestined by genetic factors that are poorly defined by mendelian

TABLE 42–1. GRADES OF HAIR TEXTURE AND DENSITY

Grade	Texture	Density
A	Very coarse	Very dense
B	Medium coarse	Medium dense
C	Medium to fine	Medium to sparse
D	Very fine	Sparse

principles, the estimation of the final appearance is often based on the age of the patient at presentation, as well as the presence and degree of baldness in the family. Clinical clues are sometimes helpful in predicting the ultimate pattern of baldness for each patient. The presence of sparse hair of decreased caliber and length, resembling the vellus hair of prepubescence, is suggestive of future hair loss in the areas where it is seen. The presence of fine, curly "whisker" hair[3] in the periauricular region also usually portends eventual extensive alopecia. Figure 42–1 shows a commonly employed classification outlining the patterns and variations of male-pattern alopecia.[4]

TEXTURE AND QUALITY OF HAIR

The texture and density of the patient's hair[5] may be classified into four general grades (Table 42–1). Using these broad categories, it can be generally stated that patients with fine, sparse hair and advanced alopecia are less than ideal candidates for hair transplantation.

Figure 42–1. Norwood classification of the common types of male-pattern alopecia. (From Norwood OT, Shiell R: Hair Transplant Surgery. 2nd ed. 1984. Courtesy of Charles C Thomas, Publisher, Springfield, Illinois.)

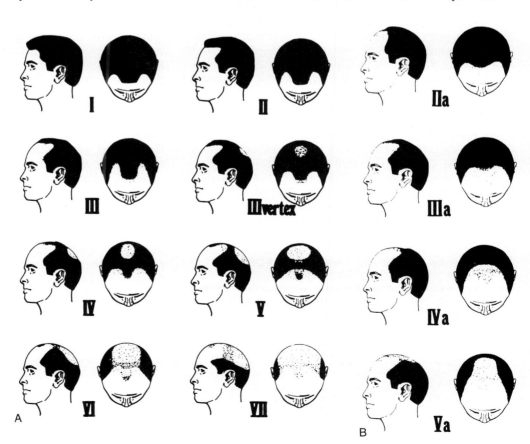

However, performing the procedure may depend solely on the attitude and motivation of the patient.

THICKNESS AND LAXITY OF SCALP

The thickness and laxity can be estimated by manually manipulating the patient's scalp. A thin and inelastic scalp usually limits or precludes scalp reductions and flap surgery. These patients are often better candidates for punch autografting.

PATIENT'S DESIRED OUTCOME

The outcome desired by the patient is obviously idiosyncratic and usually idealistic. This idealism must be tempered by objective analysis of the degree of alopecia correction that is technically possible. After a thorough discussion, the surgeon and patient should arrive at a mutually agreeable, realistic, and satisfactory individual goal before initiating any surgical procedures (Table 42–2).

Temporoparieto-occipital Flap

Transposition flaps of hair-bearing scalp for the treatment of alopecia can be traced to Passot[6] and, later, Lamont.[7] In 1975, Juri reported the use of a twice-delayed parieto-occipital flap, based on the superficial temporal artery, for the treatment of male-pattern alopecia.[8] The Juri flap attempted to create a complete anterior hairline by the transposition of a long flap traced along the distribution of the posterior branch of the superficial temporal artery to the distribution of the ipsilateral occipital artery. By design, this flap did not cross the midline of the occipital region, thus necessitating extensive undermining into the neck for closure of the donor site.

The search for a less formidable procedure with similar results led to the description of a once-delayed temporoparieto-occipital (TPO) flap whose pedicle was based on the posterior branch of the superficial temporal artery.[9] The TPO flap created a complete frontal hairline. The main advantage of this flap lay in its design, which followed the distribution of the ipsilateral occipital artery so that the distal portion of the flap could continue as a random flap into the distribution of the contralateral occipital artery. This change in the course of the flap obviated the need for undermining into the neck, which made closure of the donor site less arduous for patient and surgeon. This, in turn, allowed the entire procedure to be performed under local anesthesia, rendering it a practical office-based procedure.

The TPO flap consists of two operative stages performed 10 days apart. In the first stage, the recipient bed is prepared and the frontal hairline designed and its anterior margin incised. Release and undermining of the tip and incision of the anterior margin of the frontal hairline may be performed separately in an optional intermediate stage 5 days after completion of the first stage. The preparation of the flap begins with its design and subsequent incision, leaving an intact skin bridge as a method of delay. In the second stage, the bridge is severed, the tip is released, and the entire flap is transposed 180 degrees and aligned in its recipient bed. The donor region is closed, the recipient bed is modified, and the flap is secured.

SPECIAL POINTS OF EMPHASIS
Design of the Frontal Hairline

In hair replacement surgery, the design of the frontal hairline is fundamentally based on aesthetics. By effectively framing the face, a properly shaped and positioned hairline can restore aesthetic proportion to a face distorted by male-pattern alopecia. By definition, then, the design of the frontal hairline must incorporate several important features. The first is the shape of the face and head. The more round these features appear, the flatter the hairline should be designed. The less round these features are, the more angular the hairline should be. A second feature is the shape and quality of the temporal hair. The lower and more sparse this fringe appears, the more posterior the hairline should be placed and the more obtuse the frontotemporal angles should be designed. Finally, the height and contour of the forehead are also important.

Ideal aesthetic proportions incorporate three relatively equal subunits of the face: the hairline-to-glabella subunit, the glabella-to-columella subunit, and the columella-to-chin subunit. The hairline forms the upper boundary of the forehead as the upper one third of the face. The design of the hairline, therefore, should attempt to achieve these facial proportions in both the frontal and lateral views. These features, which are unique to each individual, should be considered in concert rather than separately. This will result in the design of a hairline that blends well with the rest of the face and is natural in appearance. However, because the transposed occipital hair is permanent as well as permanently dense, it must also remain natural in appearance as the patient matures. This is accomplished by the creation of a hairline whose position and bitemporal recession closely mimic those occurring naturally.

Design of the Flap

The design, outline, and incision of the flap within its donor bed are the most important factors in ensuring

TABLE 42–2. GENERAL GUIDELINES FOR HAIR REPLACEMENT SURGERY

Alopecia Type	Surgical Procedure(s) Required
I to III	Hair transplantation
III Vertex	Scalp reduction
	Rhomboid flaps
	Hair transplantation
IV to V	Scalp reduction
	Hair transplantation
	Temporoparieto-occipital flap
VI to VII	Hair transplantation
	Scalp reduction
	Diffuse minigrafting

the viability of the flap and success of the procedure. This procedure is initiated by tracing the path of the artery using a Doppler flowmeter, the importance of which cannot be overstated. Palpation of the pulse alone is insufficient to determine the tortuous anatomic course of the artery. Inadvertent exclusion of the artery in the pedicle will ensure necrosis of the flap.

Once the course of the artery has been identified, the width of the pedicle is outlined with the artery as its midline. The width of the pedicle is determined in such a way as to allow a 180-degree transposition with minimal torsion and minimal dogear formation as well as inclusion of the superficial temporal vein. Although the course of the superficial temporal vein usually mirrors that of its companion artery, it may occasionally be widely displaced. By scoring the galea aponeurotica during the incision of the flap in the first stage, the course of the vein may be identified and its incorporation into the pedicle ensured. If the vein is not seen within the margins of the pedicle, the design of the pedicle may be altered at that point to include the displaced vein. Failure to include the vein in the design of the pedicle may lead to venous engorgement and eventual necrosis of the flap.

The flap is initially an axial-pattern flap following the path of the superficial temporal artery and its posterior branch superiorly. However, at this point the course of the flap turns 90 degrees posteriorly and widens as it continues into the occipital region as a random-pattern flap. The length of the flap is calculated to complete the previously designed frontal hairline. The pivot point is determined by the presence and quality of the temporal hair, the ipsilateral frontotemporal angle, and the flow of the artery.

Use of a Delay

The rationale behind the 10-day delay and the use of a bridge method of delay[10] is to increase the viability of the flap by allowing it to establish its own autonomous circulation. This is thought to occur through the shunting of arteriovenous anastomoses.[11] Although unnecessary for an axial-pattern flap, this delay is crucial to the survival of the distal portion of the TPO flap. However, there is a more pragmatic reason for use of the bridge delay: if the distal portion of the flap is nonviable, this will become manifest while the flap is still in the occipital donor bed, before transposition. This allows the surgeon to excise and repair the nonviable portion and transpose a shortened viable flap into an altered recipient bed. A scar in the occipital region is greatly preferable to one in the frontal hairline, which occurs after transposition of a nonviable and eventual necrotic flap tip.

OPERATIVE TECHNIQUE

First Stage

Patient Preparation. The patient is instructed to use an antimicrobial skin cleanser as a shampoo the night before and the morning of the procedure. The patient is given diazepam (10 mg orally) as an anxiolytic agent 30 minutes before surgery. The hair is taped into braids to aid in visualization and marking of the scalp and to keep the surgical field free of stray hairs. A ring block of the scalp is initially performed using 0.5% lidocaine with 1:200,000 epinephrine buffered with sodium bicarbonate solution, followed by injection of 0.25% bupivacaine with 1:200,000 epinephrine. It should be noted that solutions containing epinephrine are not used in the pedicle region to avoid any possibility of vascular compromise to the flap. Complete sustained anesthesia is usually attained after the injection of only 45 to 50 ml of the anesthetic solutions.

Preparation of the Recipient Bed. The position and shape of the anterior margin of the new frontal hairline is designed so that the new frontal hairline is outlined to be 2.2 cm wide, which is two thirds the width of the flap in the occipital region. The margins are marked using a slide caliper. The anterior margin is incised at an acute angle to the superficial subcutaneous layer with a No. 10 scalpel blade (Fig. 42–2). The incision is then completed to the subaponeurotic layer using the Shaw Oximetrix scalpel, which simultaneously cuts and coagulates. The incision is then closed with skin staples alone.

Preparation of the Flap (Fig. 42–3). The superficial temporal artery is identified by using the Doppler flowmeter (Fig. 42–4). The margins of the pedicle are then outlined by drawing parallel lines on both sides of the course of the artery to create a pedicle that is 2.5 cm wide. The artery and its posterior branch is followed superiorly until it intersects the incised anterior margin of the frontal hairline. Here the flap is designed to turn posteriorly at a 90-degree angle, and its width increases to 3 cm. The width of the flap increases to 3.4 cm in the occipital region and maintains this width for the remainder of the flap. The flap continues across the sagittal midline to a point at which its length is sufficient to cover the previously designed frontal hairline when transposed. The distance from the pedicle to the tip must be equal to the distance from the pedicle to the end point of the incised frontal hairline.

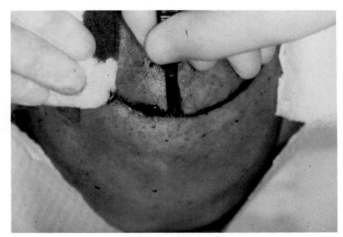

Figure 42–2. Preparation of the recipient bed. The anterior margin of the designed hairline is incised at an acute angle.

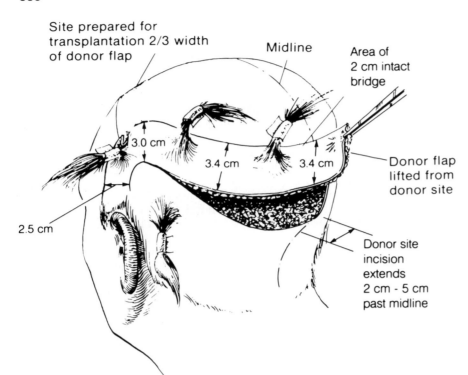

Figure 42–3. Design and preparation of the flap. (Reprinted with permission from Stough DB: Updating reduction and flap procedures for baldness. Ann Plast Surg 8:287–295, 1982.)

The margins of the flap are then incised to the subaponeurotic layer at an angle parallel to the hair follicles to minimize the number of transected follicles. This incision proceeds from pedicle to tip, leaving a 2-cm intact bridge at the superior margin of the tip. At the 90-degree-angle pivot point of the flap, the galea is scored to ensure inclusion of the superficial temporal vein into the pedicle. The base of the flap is then undermined in the subgaleal plane (Fig. 42–5), leaving the distal 5 cm of the flap intact. Hemostasis is achieved by ligation of transected vessels and electrocoagulation. The incision is then closed with skin staples alone.

Second Stage

Release and Transposition of the Flap. Ten days after the initial stage, all staples are removed, and the margins of the flap are dissected through the galea, including the previously intact bridge. The entire flap is undermined to the pivot point, raised, and transposed 180 degrees to the frontal recipient bed (Fig. 42–6). The anterior margin of the recipient bed is dissected at its acute angle, and the corresponding anterior edge of the flap is beveled at a complementary angle and positioned to encourage hair growth into the eventual scar.[12] The anterior margin of the flap is secured with skin staples, which leaves the posterior margin temporarily free, pending closure of the donor area.

Closure of the Donor Region. Extensive undermining of the entire scalp is performed in an effort to achieve a tensionless closure (Fig. 42–7). If this is not accomplished, a relaxing incision of the galea can be made 3

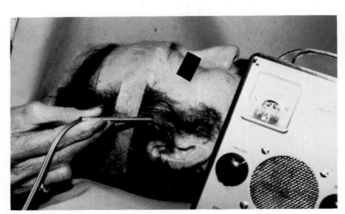

Figure 42–4. Use of the Doppler flowmeter to trace the course of the superficial temporal artery.

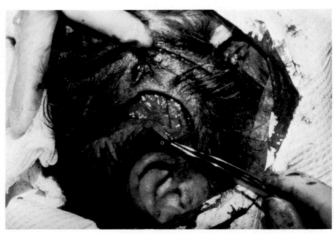

Figure 42–5. Incision and undermining of the base of the flap.

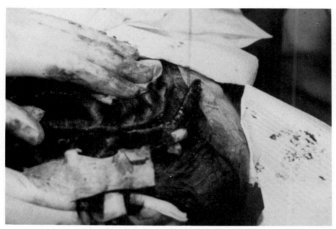

Figure 42–6. Placement of the flap in the frontal recipient bed after transposition.

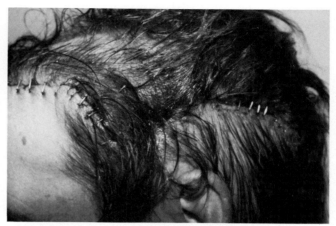

Figure 42–8. Lateral view after closure of the donor region.

cm superior and parallel to the line of closure. If this is still insufficient to approximate the edges of the wound without significant tension, a full-thickness skin graft from the soon-to-be-excised frontal scalp can be used, or the wound may be allowed to heal by second intention and the scar revised at a later date. Undermining alone is usually sufficient for tensionless closure, and the galea can then be approximated using polydioxanone absorbable sutures to provide prolonged strength. Skin closure is completed using skin staples (Fig. 42–8).

Completion of the Frontal Hairline. After the anterior margin of the flap has been secured, any excess skin posterior to the flap is draped over the posterior margin of the flap and excised. The surgery is completed by approximating the wound edges with skin staples (Figs. 42–9, 42–10).

Adjunctive Measures

The obvious advantages of the immediate dense frontal hairline created by the TPO flap are accompanied by

certain inherent features that may be perceived as disadvantageous. The first of these is that the direction of hair growth in the flap is anterior to posterior. This direction is opposite to that of natural hair growth in the frontal region and results from the natural direction of hair growth in the occipital donor region. The second is that the hairline is uniform in density. Although this is considered flattering by most patients, it may appear unnatural. Third, the hair of the flap has greater density and different texture than that of the adjacent parietal scalp. In some patients, this may lead to a perceptible zone of demarcation between the two regions. Finally, the frontotemporal angles may be asymmetric. This may occur even with flawless design as a function of the pivot point of the flap. When transposed, this point may create an ipsilateral frontotemporal angle that is less acute and lower than the contralateral angle formed by the tip of the flap (Fig. 42–11).

GROOMING AND STYLING

Proper attention to styling of the TPO flap will minimize the features noted above (Fig. 42–12). A curly permanent wave performed preoperatively can render

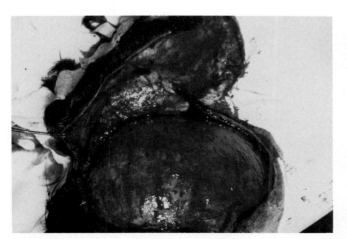

Figure 42–7. Extensive undermining of the entire scalp in preparation of closure of the donor region.

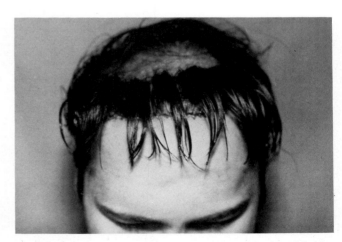

Figure 42–9. Clinical appearance after closure of the frontal hairline.

Donor flap
stapled in
position

Donor site
closed with
staples

Figure 42–10. Schematic of the scalp after completion of the procedure. (Reprinted with permission from Stough DB: Updating reduction and flap procedures for baldness. Ann Plast Surg 8:287–295, 1982.)

Figure 42–11. *A*, Frontal preoperative view before the temporo-parieto-occipital (TPO) flap. *B*, Lateral preoperative view. *C*, Frontal postoperative view after the TPO flap. *D*, Lateral postoperative view.

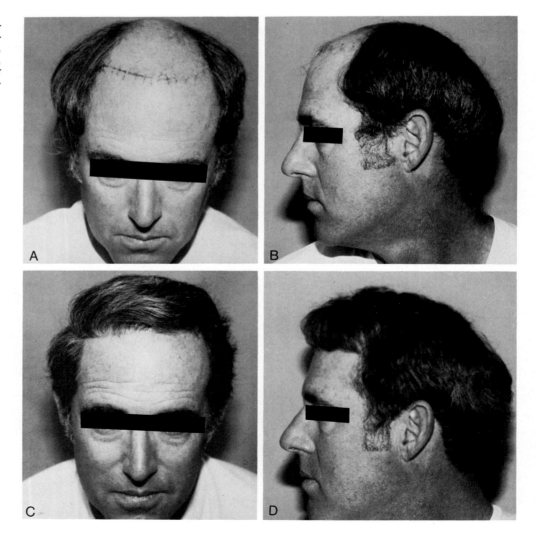

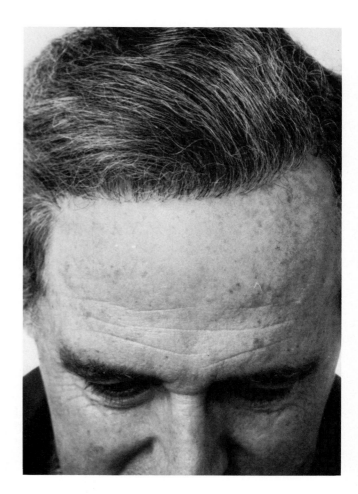

Figure 42–11 *Continued E,* Close-up of the frontal hairline showing blunting of the right frontotemporal angle.

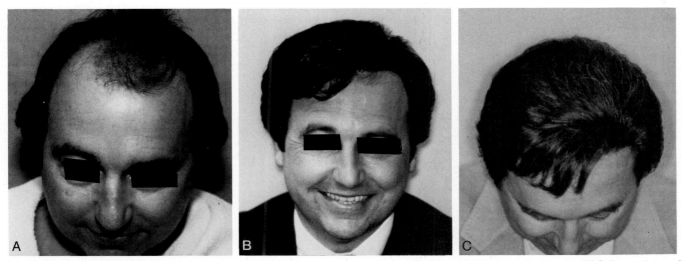

Figure 42–12. *A,* Clinical appearance before the TPO flap. *B,* Appearance after the TPO flap. *C,* Appearance after the TPO flap and use of proper styling so the hair of the flaps blends well with the hair of the adjacent regions.

the margins of the flap imperceptible and effectively camouflage the resultant scars of the procedure immediately after surgery.

HAIR TRANSPLANTATION BY PUNCH AUTOGRAFTS

Most patients find the dense hairline of the TPO flap to be too abrupt compared with the normal surrounding tissue. This can be remedied by transplanting micrografts containing one to two hairs each into the scalp directly anterior to the flap to create a feathering zone, or zone of transition. Larger punch autografts can likewise be used in the parietal scalp to lessen any visible difference in density of the two regions.

SCALP REDUCTION

Scalp reductions may be employed to augment the punch autografts in the less dense parietal region. Furthermore, a well-placed, small, elliptical scalp reduction can be used to correct an unsightly blunted or lowered frontotemporal angle. An excision of scalp superior to the flap elevates and sharpens the ipsilateral angle to mirror its opposing angle, which restores symmetry to the frontal hairline.

These imperfections are seen as flaws of the TPO flap procedure. However, to the informed and well-motivated patient who immediately gains a dense hairline, these are viewed as mere inconveniences. As illustrated earlier, proper grooming and styling are imperative to achieve optimal aesthetic outcome with the TPO flap procedure. This should be emphasized preoperatively and forcefully reiterated postoperatively.

The patient who is willing to undergo the rigors of the TPO procedure seeks an immediate frontal hairline of greater density than any achievable by punch autografting. Furthermore, he ideally exhibits stable Norwood type IV or V alopecia patterns (see Fig. 42–1B). The TPO flap remains a viable and valuable alternative in this subset of patients who are seeking correction of male-pattern alopecia.

Preauricular Flap

The preauricular flap is a hair-bearing transposition flap with a superiorly based pedicle. It is designed as a nondelayed, random-pattern flap with a 4:1 length-to-width ratio, which permits construction of a 2 × 8 cm flap in this region (Fig. 42–13). The preauricular flap has been used effectively in the correction of male-pattern baldness by re-creating a dense frontotemporal angle and partial frontal hairline (Fig. 42–14). Its advantages lie in its ease of execution and the natural direction of forward hair growth obtained when the flap is transposed. Its glaring disadvantage relates to its design as a random-pattern flap, which limits its length to only one third or one half of the length of the entire frontal hairline. This necessitates the use of another flap from the contralateral preauricular region or punch autografts for the creation of a complete hairline.

The current usefulness of the preauricular flap is for reconstruction of the frontal and preauricular regions of

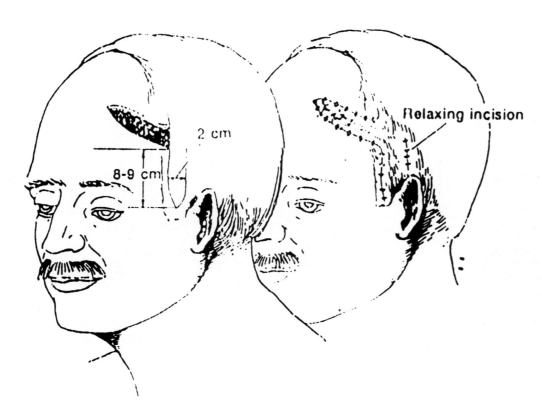

Figure 42–13. Design of the preauricular flap. (Reprinted with permission from Stough DB: Updating reduction and flap procedures for baldness. Ann Plast Surg 8:287–295, 1982.)

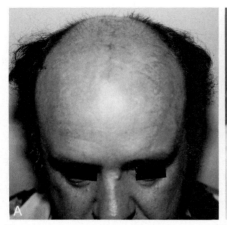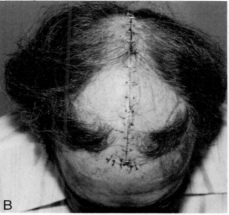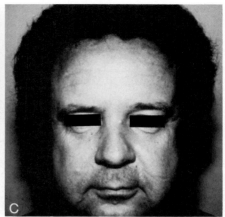

Figure 42–14. *A,* Patient with Norwood type VI alopecia pattern. *B,* Same patient after bilateral preauricular flaps and scalp reduction. *C,* Same patient after hair transplantation with punch autografts and a permanent wave.

the scalp for the correction of cicatricial alopecias caused by trauma, radiation (Fig. 42–15), or previous surgical procedures. Because the preauricular flap is simply a transposition flap performed without delay, its execution does not differ greatly from that performed in other regions. Occasionally, a through-and-through relaxing incision 3 cm posterior to the designed flap is needed to promote tensionless closure of the recipient region. With this one exception, the preauricular flap is one of the least demanding hair-bearing flaps to perform accurately.

Triple Rhomboid Flap

Patients with stable type III vertex alopecia present unique problems for the hair replacement surgeon. Correction of the normal hair growth pattern with a standard midline or paramedian scalp reduction requires several serial excisions. Furthermore, linear excisions

over this convex surface can lead to the formation of dogears and contour defects of the scalp.

The triple rhomboid flap has been used for reconstruction of the forehead and anterior scalp[13] and has been applied with success in the treatment of patients with well-demarcated vertex alopecia of limited size.[14] The ideal candidate for this procedure is a patient with stable Norwood type III vertex alopecia; dense, curly hair; and good scalp laxity.

The triple rhomboid flap is an extension of the classic Limberg flap, in which a rhomboid defect is created and adjacent tissue transposed in the form of a parallelogram to cover the defect. The triple rhomboid flap procedure consists of the creation of an hexagonal defect that is repaired with the transposition of three rhomboid flaps at alternating corners of the hexagon (Fig. 42–16). These points are selected from the six potential positions at each corner of the hexagon. This determination is made based on the relative mobility of the skin adjacent to each limb for ease of closure. For correction of vertex

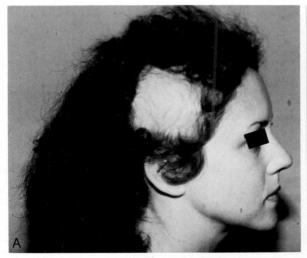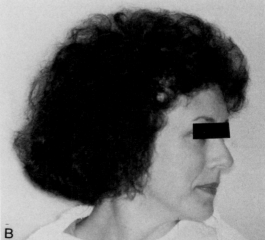

Figure 42–15. *A,* Patient with a well-demarcated area of alopecia at the site of radiation ports for an intracranial tumor. *B,* Same patient after a preauricular flap and a permanent wave.

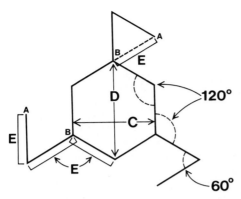

Figure 42–16. Design of the triple rhomboid flap so the three flaps are created at alternating corners from the six possible points on the hexagon.

alopecia, however, the hexagon should be oriented so that two of the three flaps are transposed from the inferior occipital region rather than the vertex (Fig. 42–17A). This is because the tissue in this region is lax and easily transposed, and the hair in this region is of greater density so as to provide more efficient camouflage of the resulting scars. Furthermore, the direction of transposition of the three rhomboid flaps is designed to re-create the patient's natural vertex swirl.

OPERATIVE TECHNIQUE

Initially, the entire circular or oval area of vertex alopecia is converted to a hexagon and outlined. Each transposed rhomboid flap is designed by drawing a line that bisects the 120-degree angles at a length equal to one side of the hexagon. From the end of this line, another line of corresponding length is drawn at a 60-degree angle parallel to the respective side of the hexagon (Fig. 42–17B).

The surrounding hair is either taped into braids or clipped to facilitate visualization and transposition of the three flaps. The entire surgical field, including a broad area of undermining, is first infiltrated with 0.5% lidocaine with 1:200,000 epinephrine, followed by infiltration of 0.25% bupivacaine with 1:200,000 epinephrine for sustained anesthesia, and the hexagonal defect is then created (Fig. 42–18). Extensive undermining is then performed. It should be noted that during the excision, branches of the occipital artery may be inadvertently transected. These may be ligated without fear of flap compromise because of the abundant anastomoses from the superficial temporal and posterior auricular arteries to this region.

The three designed flaps are then incised and released (Fig. 42–19), care being taken to angle the incisions parallel to the existing hair shafts. The flaps are then transposed sequentially in the same direction (Figs. 42–20, 42–21) over the entire defect. The key sutures of the three flaps are then placed (Fig. 42–22), and staples or sutures are used to complete the closure (Fig. 42–23). The scars at 1 month (Fig. 42–24) and at 1 year (Fig. 42–25) are quite acceptable.

This procedure offers several advantages over a conventional scalp reduction or punch autografting for patients with vertex alopecia. First, the area of alopecia can be generally corrected in one procedure, while this degree of correction would typically require serial scalp reductions or several sessions of punch autografting. In addition, the density of hair in the area of correction quite closely matches that of the surrounding areas. This density cannot be duplicated by the use of punch autografts alone. Finally, the design can be oriented so that the three transposed limbs re-create the natural swirling hair growth found in the vertex. For these reasons, the triple rhomboid flap should be considered in the patient with stable Norwood type III vertex alopecia.

Postoperative Care After Scalp Flap Surgery

After scalp flap surgery, antibiotic ointment should be applied to the incisions and the entire head bandaged

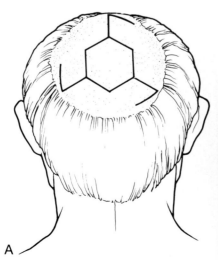

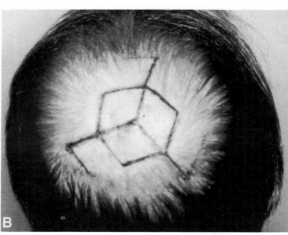

Figure 42–17. A, Schematic representation of the design of the triple rhomboid flap in the vertex region. B, The triple rhomboid flap designed in the vertex of a patient with Norwood type III vertex alopecia. (A reprinted by permission of the publisher from Stough DB IV, Stough DB III: Triple rhomboid flap for crown alopecia correction. J Dermatol Surg Oncol 16:543–548, 1990. Copyright 1990 by Elsevier Science Publishing Co., Inc.)

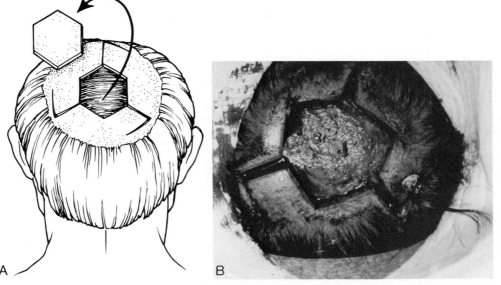

A

B

Figure 42–18. *A*, Schematic showing how the hexagonal defect is excised. *B*, Clinical appearance after removal of the central hexagon and incision of the flaps.

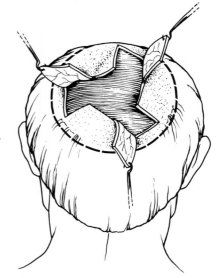

Figure 42–19. The three flaps are released.

Figure 42–20. The first flap is transposed.

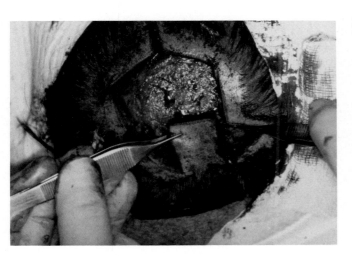

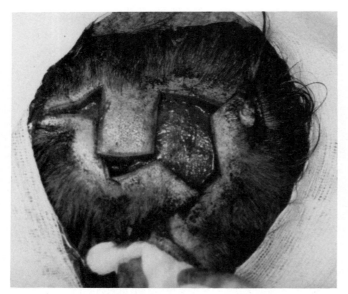

Figure 42–21. Appearance before transposition of the third flap.

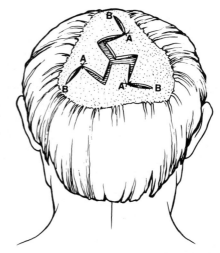

Figure 42–22. Key sutures of each flap are placed.

with nonadherent gauze and wrapped with an elastic bandage. Care should be taken not to apply undue pressure over the flap to avoid possible vascular compromise. The patient should be seen daily for the first week after surgery. Sutures and staples are routinely removed at 2 weeks.

Pain and edema are the most common problems encountered after scalp flap surgery. Pain in the immediate postoperative period can be greatly reduced by performing a ring block using 0.25% bupivacaine with 1:200,000 epinephrine at 4-hour intervals from the time of the initial preoperative ring block. Oral analgesics are prophylactically prescribed on discharge from the recovery area. Edema of the flap and the adjacent undermined scalp can be minimized by the use of intramuscular corticosteroids.

Complications

TIP NECROSIS

Up to 15% of patients who have undergone the TPO flap procedure will note that the distal 1 to 4 cm of the flap is darker in color after 24 hours. This may not herald eventual tip necrosis and should not be perceived as an emergency warranting immediate debridement. As many as 85 to 90% of these flaps will exhibit only a superficial slough and eventually have dense hair regrowth. The remaining flaps may manifest true necrosis and rapidly proceed to eschar formation. This undesirable but manageable outcome is almost invariably a result of exclusion of the superficial temporal artery or vein from the pedicle of the flap. Subsequent loss of the flap is a result of inadequate perfusion or venous engorgement. Flap necrosis can be minimized by routine use of the Doppler flowmeter to identify the true path

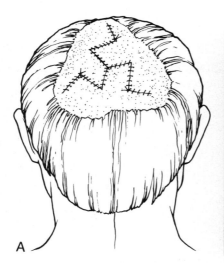

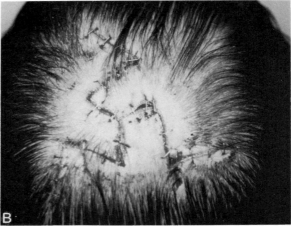

Figure 42–23. Staples or sutures are used to complete closure of the incision.

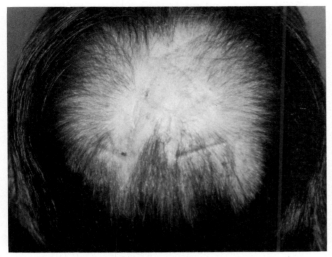

Figure 42–24. Appearance of the scars after 1 month.

of the artery and by scoring the galea at the pivot point of the flap to identify the vein.

The natural consequence of tip necrosis of the TPO flap is cicatricial alopecia of the contralateral frontotemporal angle. If this is large enough to be unsightly, small punch autografts can be transplanted into this area for camouflage and complete restoration of the frontal hairline. If disfiguring, this scar can be reconstructed by transposition of a hair-bearing flap from the ipsilateral preauricular region.

TELOGEN EFFLUVIUM

Some degree of telogen effluvium is common after extensive scalp procedures. Mild transient episodes of hair loss may occur postoperatively despite flawless execution of any scalp flap procedure. Broad areas of prolonged severe alopecia, on the other hand, may result from vascular compromise or direct trauma to the hair follicles. The most common cause of this is wound closure performed under tension or improper dissection at a level superficial to the galea aponeurotica.

HEMATOMA

The scalp is an extremely vascular structure that is difficult to bandage adequately without causing undue compression of the underlying flap. Because of this, postoperative bleeding and hematoma formation in scalp flap surgery can be more common than in surgery of other areas. These complications can be reduced by performing diligent preoperative screening to exclude the patient with a bleeding diathesis. Strict abstinence from ingestion of alcohol and compounds known to increase bleeding (e.g., vitamin E, aspirin, and nonsteroidal anti-inflammatory agents) for at least 2 weeks preoperatively is also of great importance. Lastly, meticulous hemostasis should always be maintained during the procedure. When a hematoma does occur, it should be promptly evacuated, the source of bleeding identified

and treated, and the use of a drain considered. These measures will minimize the risk of flap compromise.

INFECTION

Significant wound infection is rare in scalp flap surgery performed as an office procedure. This is undoubtedly due to strict adherence to aseptic technique.

WOUND DEHISCENCE

The dehiscence of an incision after scalp surgery is most commonly due to closing the wound under inordinate tension, poor flap design, or insufficient undermining. When dehiscence occurs, the wound may be allowed to heal by secondary intention or covered with a skin graft to be revised later once wound healing is complete.

SCARRING

Scars in the vertex and occipital regions are rarely noticeable, since they are readily covered by hair growing from the flap and adjacent tissue. A noticeable frontal hairline scar can be improved with the use of micrografts consisting of one to two hairs each that are inserted into the scar. This procedure can be concomitantly used to disrupt the uniform line of the anterior margin of the flap to provide a more natural appearance.

SUMMARY

Hair-bearing flaps for aesthetic correction of male-pattern alopecia were developed as alternatives to hair

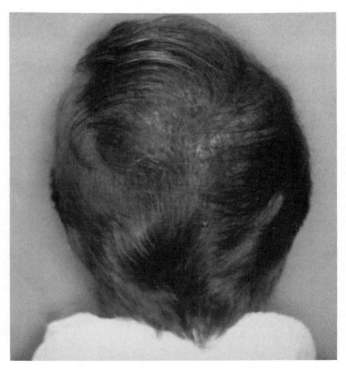

Figure 42–25. Appearance of the scars after 1 year.

transplantation by punch autografting. By employing a flap, uniformly dense hair can be transposed to cover an area of bald scalp without the requisite grace period and the unsightly and distinctive "doll's hair" appearance produced by transplanting large round grafts. The advent of micrografts, minigrafts, and slit grafting techniques has led to a more natural appearance of the transplanted scalp. Because of the benefits provided by the immediate dense hair coverage of a properly executed flap, this procedure is a viable option for a carefully selected subset of patients seeking correction of male-pattern alopecia and can be used in conjunction with the traditional plug autograft technique, as well as the newer techniques of micro- and minigrafts and slit grafting.

REFERENCES

1. Stough DB IV, Nelson BR, Stough DB III: Incisional slit grafting. J Dermatol Surg Oncol 17:53–60, 1991.
2. Stough DB III, Freilich IW: Hair bearing flaps for baldness. Facial Plast Surg 2:283, 1985.
3. Norwood OT: Whisker hair. Arch Dermatol 116:930–931, 1980.
4. Norwood OT, Shiell R: Hair Transplant Surgery. Charles C Thomas, Springfield, IL, 1984, pp 107–115.
5. Stough DB, Abramson LJ, Strange P: A contemporary approach to male pattern alopecia. J Dermatol Surg Oncol 13:756–759, 1987.
6. Passot R: Chirurgic Esthetique Pure. Doin & Cie, Paris, 1931.
7. Lamont ES: A plastic surgical transformation: a report of a case. West J Surg Obstet Gynecol 65:164, 1957.
8. Juri J: Use of parieto-occipital flaps in the surgical treatment of baldness. Plast Reconstr Surg 55:456–460, 1975.
9. Stough DB III, Cates JA: Transposition flaps for the correction of baldness: a practical office procedure. J Dermatol Surg Oncol 6:286–289, 1980.
10. Toomey JM, O'Neill JV, Snyder GG: Bridge method of skin-flap delay. Arch Otolaryngol 103:26–28, 1977.
11. Reinisch JF: The pathophysiology of skin flap circulation. Plast Reconstr Surg 54:591–594, 1974.
12. Elliott RA Jr: Lateral scalp flaps for instant results in male pattern baldness. Plast Reconstr Surg 60:699, 1977.
13. Jackson IT: Local Flaps in Head and Neck Reconstruction. CV Mosby, St. Louis, 1985, pp 66–67.
14. Stough DB IV, Stough DB III: Triple rhomboid flap for crown alopecia correction. J Dermatol Surg Oncol 16:543–548, 1990.

CHAPTER 43

Liposuction

WILLIAM P. COLEMAN III

During the twentieth century, interest in physical conditioning and a trim physique has increased. As a result, various surgical procedures have been devised to remove localized deposits of excess fat. Many early attempts ended in failure. The curettage approach of Dujarrier in the 1920s[1] resulted in seromas, infection, and even amputation. Dermatolipectomy, which involved removing the fatty deposits along with overlying skin,[2] became popular in the 1960s. Although this direct excision approach was successful in recontouring, its main drawback was the large surgical scar.

In the 1970s, Fischer and Fischer devised a blunt instrument that could be attached to a suction pump for removal of fat cells.[3] Although incorrectly described as curettes, their early instruments were blunt on the outside and contained a sharp edge within the shaft to facilitate expulsion of the extracted material.[4] The Fischers used a multiple incision approach to achieve crisscross tunneling throughout the treated areas.[5] Their pioneering work was quite successful and ushered in the modern era of liposuction.

Illouz in Paris observed the Fischers' work and adapted readily available abortion cannulas and suction pumps to replace the expensive devices invented by the Fischers.[6] Fournier observed both Illouz and the Fischers and then helped to further refine the liposuction procedure. Fournier and Illouz are primarily responsible for dissemination of the liposuction technique throughout North America and the rest of the world.[7]

American surgeons began visiting France in the late 1970s to learn about liposuction. Field was probably the first American to learn the technique.[8] By 1982, American interest accelerated, and liposuction was officially introduced to the United States by the American Academy of Cosmetic Surgery and the American Society of Plastic and Reconstructive Surgery.[9] Controversy soon developed over who was best trained to perform the procedure, but in reality, all American medical specialists learned liposuction from Illouz and Fournier at about the same time. The newly formed American Society of Liposuction Surgery held the first live symposium on liposuction in June, 1983.

This new procedure was rapidly assimilated by a number of specialities, including dermatology, otolaryngology, and plastic surgery. The American Society of Liposuction Surgery declared liposuction an interspecialty procedure and supported educational symposia for physicians of all specialities. Dermatologists were involved in the evolution of liposuction surgery from the earliest days of its introduction into the United States. As each specialty evolved its own unique style for performing this procedure, dermatologists led the way in developing techniques for outpatient liposuction surgery.[10] The outpatient environment best suited the experience and needs of many cutaneous surgeons, which meant developing approaches to broaden the use of local anesthetics to large tissue areas. Although a number of innovative techniques were proposed initially, these proved to be feasible only for low-volume liposuction procedures. In 1987, the tumescent local anesthetic technique, based on the use of large volumes of very low concentrations of lidocaine and epinephrine, was introduced.[11] The vastly decreased concentration of local anesthetic employed with this technique enabled the cutaneous surgeon to perform larger liposuction procedures under local anesthesia without the risk of lidocaine toxicity. The tumescent technique also obviated the need for intravenous sedation or general anesthesia for most liposuction procedures. In addition to these advances in safety, the tumescent technique resulted in a profound reduction in blood loss during liposuction.[12]

Meanwhile, dermatologists also pioneered techniques in fat transfer surgery. The concept of recycling the fat removed during liposuction was perfected into a straightforward technique of soft tissue augmentation known as microlipoinjection.[13–15] This became a natural extension of the other soft tissue augmentation techniques already being performed. The processing of extracted fat into autologous collagen has also become feasible, and its long-term benefit is currently being evaluated.[16]

The American Academy of Dermatology has developed practice guidelines for liposuction in addition to promoting education and training in this surgical technique. The American Society for Dermatologic Surgery has also been quite active in supporting educational endeavors in liposuction since the earliest days of its introduction into the United States. This procedure has now joined the long list of other techniques that comprise the specialty of cutaneous surgery.

Fat Cell Physiology

Most people eventually accumulate excess fat. The fat cell, or lipocyte (adipocyte), is the fundamental unit of fat storage. This active metabolic center stores triglycerides, which are metabolized into and from free fatty acids in the blood. A number of hormones exert effects on cell metabolism.[17]

Although it was originally thought that the number of fat cells remains static after puberty, it is now apparent that large increases in weight result in increased numbers of adipocytes.[18] These new fat cells develop from a stem cell, the preadipocyte, as a response to overfilling of the existing adipocytes. Small weight gains that result only in enlargement of the existing lipocytes are termed hypertrophic obesity. When enough fat storage is generated that new adipocytes are formed, this is referred to as hyperplastic obesity.[19]

Many individuals go through cycles of gaining 15 to 20 pounds and then gradually losing the extra weight, only to regain it later. Each time they return to their original baseline weight, they note an increased accumulation of fat. This is probably because of the development of new fat cells in response to overfilling of available adipocytes. The specific sites of excess fat accumulation are determined by hereditary influences. Women tend to accumulate excess fat in the thighs, over the buttocks, and in the lower abdomen in what is known as gynecoid obesity. Men tend to store excess fat in the abdomen and flank areas in what is known as android obesity. Gynecoid obesity results in a "pear" shape and is due primarily to fat storage in subcutaneous tissue. Android obesity results in an "apple" shape and usually represents intra-abdominal fat accumulation. Android obesity is associated with increased risk of cardiovascular disease.[19]

Human subcutaneous fat is distributed in two discrete layers: a superficial subdermal layer and a deep layer. The superficial layer remains approximately 1 cm thick throughout most of the body. The deeper layer, however, increases dramatically in size with weight gain, especially in specific anatomic areas. It is important for the liposuction surgeon to preserve the superficial fat, which provides a buffer zone for the overlying dermis. Liposuction surgery is intended to reduce the size of the deep fat layer in sites of localized fat excess.

Dietary manipulation of localized excess fat is often unsuccessful, because adipocytes in these locations tend to be the most resistant to fat deprivation. Animal studies have shown that fat cells can become as much as 20 times more active metabolically after dieting and during starvation. In this way, they are increasingly primed to store additional fat as soon as it becomes available.[20] Many individuals find that to reduce the size of swollen adipocytes in one area, it is often necessary to lose so much weight that they produce an unattractive gaunt appearance in other parts of the body. For instance, many women complain that losing enough weight to slim their thighs causes involution of the breasts and the face. Liposuction is a more successful alternative to localized fat reduction when the patient is near ideal body weight, because only the unwanted fat is removed.

Exercising the muscles under an adiposity will also fail to reduce the size of the overlying fat cells. Fat storage depends on systemic metabolic events and not on regional muscular development. In the abdominal area, firming the rectus muscles produces a more attractive appearance but does not decrease the size of the overlying subcutaneous layer. Only when enough exercise is performed to exert an overall systemic effect on caloric balance does exercise achieve reduction of adipocytes. Once again, liposuction is the only currently available method for removing fat cells in specific areas.

Liposuction is not, however, a treatment for generalized obesity. Liposuction may remove a few pounds of fat from a given area but does not replace the dieting and appropriate behavior modification that are needed to influence the course of obesity. Although serial liposuction has been used as an approach to removal of large volumes of fat, this application correctly remains an experimental procedure.[21]

Patient Selection

Although the liposuction literature often refers to the "ideal patient," no rigorous standard has been determined. Patients best suited for liposuction are those with localized adiposities. They should be in good physical health and free of infectious disease. The better the skin elasticity, the better the surgical results will be. Some older patients have much better skin elasticity than younger ones, especially in non–sun-exposed areas. However, poor quality, wavy skin cannot be expected to smooth out well after liposuction.

Certain patients are poor surgical risks. These include individuals on anticoagulant medications, including aspirin, as excess bleeding may seriously complicate the surgical outcome. As with any elective procedure, liposuction should be postponed if there is a doubt as to the patient's clotting ability, which should be verified preoperatively with appropriate laboratory tests. If the patient has a severe metabolic disorder such as diabetes mellitus, it may be wise for the cutaneous surgeon to consult with the patient's primary physician to obtain medical clearance. The same principle applies to patients with chronic infectious diseases such as hepatitis. Patients with active infectious diseases, including human immunodeficiency virus (HIV), should be deferred until they are better candidates for surgery and no longer pose a risk to the medical personnel performing the procedure.

Anatomic Variations

Any localized accumulation of excess fat is potentially correctable by liposuction. However, the obtainable results vary by anatomic site, and consequently, the areas most commonly treated by liposuction must be evaluated individually.

FACE

Liposuction can be used to remove excess fat from the jowls. This is usually performed in conjunction with a face lift and has largely replaced the sharp removal of fat during this procedure.[22] Liposuction has also been employed for the reduction of the medial cheeks at the nasolabial folds. The rationale for this approach is to decrease the transition between the fatter cheeks and the depressed furrow in patients with deep nasolabial folds.[23] However, this approach may cause skin surface irregularities and has not been widely accepted.[23]

NECK

Liposuction of the neck has become popular to reduce the thickness of the fat above the platysma muscle. This can be done independently or combined with a face lift. Patients with loose, inelastic neck skin usually require a lifting procedure to tighten the redundant tissue. However, liposuction can be employed in many individuals to reduce a "double chin." Even individuals in their sixties may have enough inherent elasticity to completely contract the neck skin after liposuction (Fig. 43–1).

Some individuals develop excess fat over the lower posterior neck. The most exaggerated expression of this is the "buffalo hump." This deformity is due to hyperfunction of the adrenal gland and is a feature of Cushing's syndrome. This unsightly and sometimes painful condition can be successfully treated by liposuction.[24]

BREASTS

Excess breast tissue in males is termed gynecomastia if the excess is entirely glandular. "Pseudogynecomastia" refers to male breast enlargement that is composed primarily of excess fat.[25] Enlarged breasts are quite disturbing cosmetically to men who develop this condition, and they often seek surgical help. True gynecomastia may require sharp removal of the excess breast

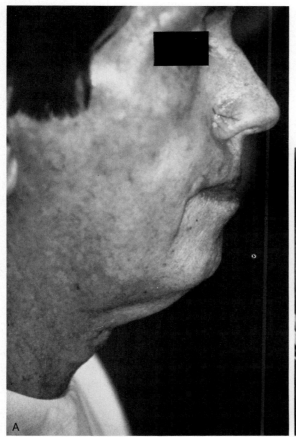
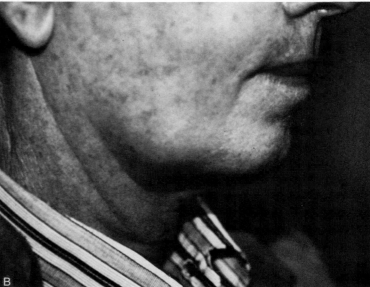

Figure 43–1. *A*, A 65-year-old patient with excess fat and loose skin of the neck. *B*, Three months after liposuction, excellent retraction of the neck skin is apparent.

tissue combined with liposuction. However, pseudogynecomastia is often treatable by liposuction alone.

ARMS

Excess fat accumulates in some individuals on the dorsal arms superior to the elbows. This deformity can be improved by liposuction if the patient has good elasticity of the skin in this area. In some patients the overlying skin fails to completely contract after liposuction, necessitating excision of the redundant tissue.

TRUNK

Accumulations of fat in the upper lateral back emanating from the posterior axillary fold can also be improved by liposuction. If there is severe redundancy of the overlying skin, liposuction alone may not dramatically improve the problem. The flanks are also a common problem area treatable by liposuction (Fig. 43–2). These so-called "love handles" are quite common in men in otherwise good physical condition. Liposuction is especially efficient at flattening out these troubling contour flaws. However, bleeding is much greater during liposuction of the flanks than during abdominal or thigh procedures, probably because of increased vascularity in male subcutaneous tissues. Passage of the cannula is also more difficult.[26]

ABDOMEN

The upper abdomen is a marginal area for liposuction intervention. The skin in the supraumbilical abdomen is quite thick compared with that in the lower abdomen and may not retract fully after liposuction. Liposuction in this area is usually performed in conjuction with lower abdominal fat removal.

The lower abdomen is one of the most frequently requested sites for fat removal (Fig. 43–3). Infraumbilical accumulations of excess fat are typically well defined and easily removed. If the patient has severe diastasis of the rectus muscles and loose overlying skin, an abdominoplasty may be necessary. However, this procedure carries a much greater risk of serious complications, especially when combined with liposuction. Increased problems with fat embolism, thrombophlebitis, and skin slough have been reported.[27-29] When muscle tone is fairly good, liposuction alone often achieves satisfying results, even though a perfectly flat stomach is not produced. The greater morbidity and risk associated with abdominoplasty can often be avoided by this conservative approach.

HIPS

Liposuction of the hips is often performed in conjunction with abdominal or outer thigh procedures. The fat over the iliac crests is usually quite soft, which facilitates liposuction. Many women despise their "violin-shaped" figures as fat accumulates over the hips and outer thighs, but this can be corrected by resculpting these adiposities.

BUTTOCKS

Women also commonly complain about excess fat of the buttocks area. Gravity produces a bowing of the outer thigh tissue, causing the appearance of a "saddlebag" deformity. These false "saddle bags" can be demonstrated by asking the patient to contract her buttock muscles. If the "saddle bags" disappear, liposuction should be confined to the outer buttocks and not directly performed over these areas (Fig. 43–4). Improperly treating the outer thighs instead of the buttocks may cause severe dimpling postoperatively. To avoid producing a flat derriere, the central buttocks should not be suctioned. It is also important to avoid the so-called "Bermuda triangle" over the medial buttocks during liposuction (Fig. 43–5), confining surgery to the lateral and superior buttocks instead.

LEGS

The posterior thighs often accumulate fat in a banana-shaped distribution just below the subgluteal fold. Removal of this defect is often executed in conjunction with liposuction of the lateral thighs. The lateral thigh, or "saddle bag," is the most commonly requested site for liposuction. Many women store excess fat in the

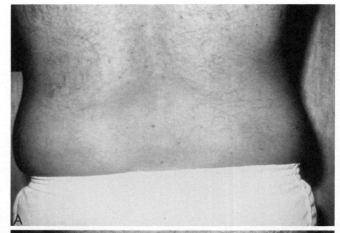
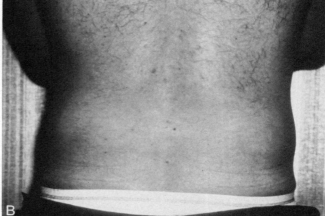

Figure 43–2. *A,* Excess fat in the "love handle" area of the flanks. *B,* After liposuction, better contours are seen.

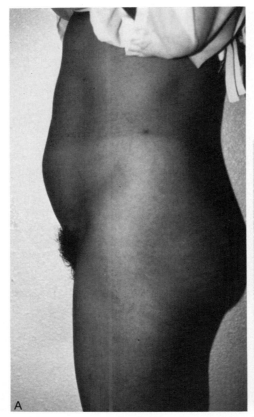
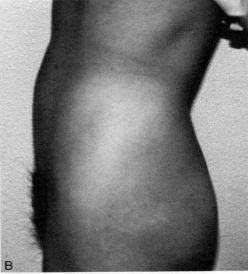

Figure 43–3. *A,* Lower abdominal fat excess before liposuction. *B,* Six months after liposuction, there has been dramatic improvement.

thighs in an unattractive pattern that is difficult to conceal with clothing. Liposuction of this area is often done in conjunction with that of the lateral buttocks, especially if the weight of the overhanging buttocks contributes to the saddle-bag defect (Fig. 43–6).

The inner thighs accumulate fat in an inverted triangle distribution. This fat is often diet resistant and may be covered by poor-quality, inelastic skin. For this reason, liposuction of the inner thigh often results in minor contour abnormalities, as the skin fails to contract completely after surgery. Despite this, a reduction in such an adiposity makes pants fit better and eliminates chafing from rubbing of the thighs.

Fat accumulates over the suprapatellar and medial aspects of the knees in many individuals. This is commonly seen in association with the saddle-bag deformity. Liposuction is quite effective at recontouring these adiposities (Fig. 43–7).

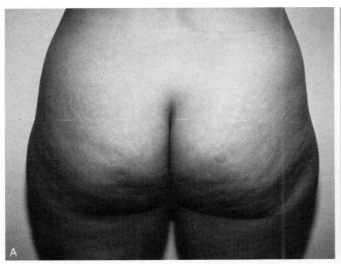
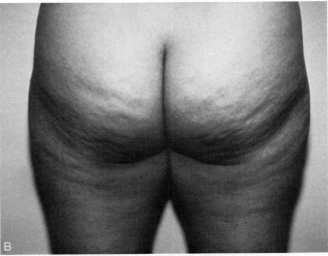

Figure 43–4. *A,* Apparent excess fat of the outer thigh. *B,* On tightening the buttocks, these false "saddle bags" disappear.

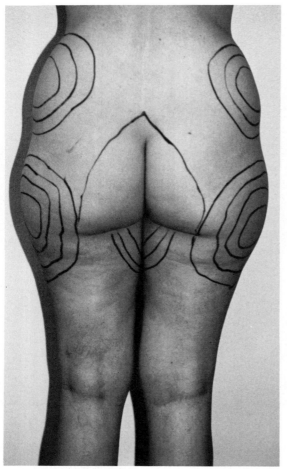

Figure 43–5. The central buttocks, or "Bermuda triangle," should be avoided during liposuction to prevent flattening.

Liposuction may be successfully used on the lower legs to recontour the calves and ankles. This is helpful in patients who have a "peg-leg" appearance as a result of excess fat storage inferior to the gastrocnemius muscle. It must be noted that all lower extremity surgery heals more slowly because of poorer vascular supply and

hydrostatic pressure. For this reason, liposuction in this area is fraught with more complications, such as surface irregularities or even skin necrosis, than other sites. This procedure should be limited to patients with true excess fat in these areas.[30]

Liposuction Consultation

The purpose of the consultation is to provide patients with enough information about the procedure to make an informed decision as to whether to undergo liposuction. The consultation also serves as an opportunity for the surgeon to decide whether the patient is intelligent enough to understand the nature of the surgery, as well as the risks, benefits, and possible complications. The surgeon may also be able to determine during the consultation if the patient is emotionally prepared for the cosmetic surgical procedure.

The initial part of the consultation includes a physical examination to ensure that the patient is an appropriate candidate medically for liposuction. The portions of the body being considered for liposuction should be carefully examined with the patient completely unclothed. The cutaneous surgeon should make detailed observations about the physical findings as the examination is completed so as to instruct the patient in what can and cannot be accomplished with liposuction.

Having the patient bend forward from the waist allows easier assessment of the thickness of abdominal fat. The patient should be asked to contract the muscles underlying the areas being considered for surgery. This allows the surgeon to adequately assess the thickness of the subcutaneous tissue. The "pinch test" is used to estimate the thickness of the fat. When the skin is pinched into a sandwich of two layers of skin and subcutaneous tissue, a thickness of 2 cm is considered normal. Thus if one can only "pinch an inch," then liposuction will not likely be helpful. Liposuction necessitates sparing a 1-cm buffer zone of fat immediately below the dermis to avoid dimpling or waviness. The pinch test can also be used to delineate where the areas for potential liposuction

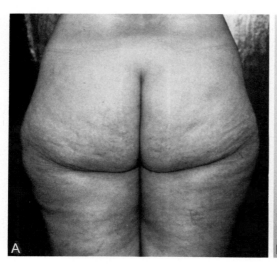
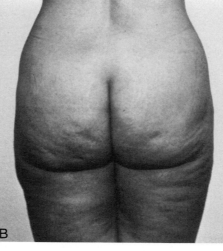

Figure 43–6. *A,* "Saddle bags" of the outer thighs. *B,* One year after liposuction, the buttocks and thigh contours are improved.

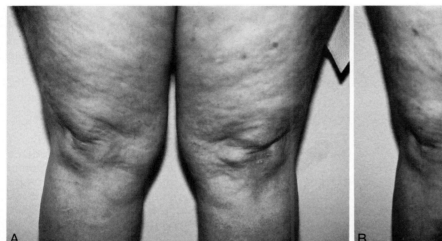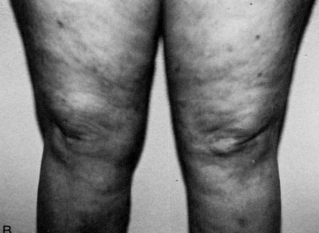

Figure 43–7. *A,* Excess fat of the medial and suprapatellar knees. *B,* After liposuction, a more pleasing contour is apparent.

should begin and end as they fade into normal surrounding tissue (Fig. 43–8).

The cutaneous surgeon should also gauge the elasticity of the skin overlying the potential liposuction sites. Although the dorsal hand skin is commonly used to measure elasticity, this sun-damaged tissue may not accurately predict the behavior of the abdominal or thigh skin. Elasticity can be estimated by the promptness with which the skin snaps back after it is stretched. Additionally, the examiner must evaluate the quality of the patient's skin. Cellulite or wavy skin will not be improved by liposuction. Patients must be told that if their skin quality is poor, a smooth result cannot be expected.

The examining surgeon should also look for scars from previous abdominal surgery. Some patients have had so many intra-abdominal procedures that access to the lower abdominal fat is very limited without suctioning through these incisions. This is associated with an increased risk of intraperitoneal penetration. Examination for hernias is also very important, especially in the

umbilical area. Any weakness in the muscle wall of the abdomen presents a danger of intra-abdominal penetration with the cannula. After the physical examination is completed, the patient can get dressed, and the verbal part of the consultation can begin.

Informed consent is both a legal requirement and a moral duty. Unless patients fully understand the nature of the liposuction procedure, they cannot make an informed decision as to whether they should undergo the procedure.[31, 32] Many individuals come to the consultation with misconceptions of what liposuction can accomplish. Many people wrongly believe that liposuction is an alternative to proper dieting, and others perceive it as a cure for generalized obesity. These erroneous ideas must be corrected, which may mean that the cutaneous surgeon convinces a potential patient not to have the procedure performed.

The liposuction procedure should be explained in depth, including the preoperative laboratory evaluation that is required, the cost involved, the payment policy of the practice, the anesthetic principles employed, the degree of sedation used during the procedure, the procedure itself, and the usual postoperative recovery. The surgeon must also warn the patient of both the most likely and the less common potential complications (Table 43–1). Finally, the surgeon must also discuss the usual sequelae that can be expected after liposuction that do not represent true complications (Table 43–2).

In addition to providing information to the patient, the surgeon should use the consultation to obtain infor-

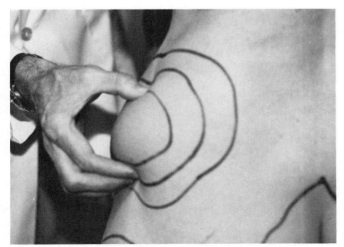

Figure 43–8. The pinch test is used to delineate the thickness of various areas for potential liposuction.

TABLE 43–1. **RARE COMPLICATIONS OF LIPOSUCTION**

Hematomas
Seromas
Infection
Fat emboli
Pulmonary thromboembolism
Tissue necrosis
Fluid and electrolyte imbalance
Nerve injury

TABLE 43–2. NORMAL SEQUELAE OF LIPOSUCTION

Skin dimpling
Bruising
Persistent edema
Paresthesias
Hyperpigmentation
Unsightly scars
Asymmetry

mation from the patient. The surgeon must be certain before agreeing to operate that the patient is a good candidate both emotionally and physically for liposuction. Patients may exhibit any of a number of psychiatric disorders, which may make them more liable to be unhappy with the surgeon or the results of the procedure.[33] Even mentally healthy individuals may go through periods (e.g., during times of marital discord) when they are ill-suited to undergo cosmetic surgical procedures. Furthermore, surgeons may find that they are incompatible with certain patients, which is certainly a poor basis from which to embark on an elective procedure such as liposuction.

If the surgeon is not satisfied with the patient's knowledge of the procedure and his or her emotional stability, a second preoperative visit may be advisable before deciding whether to schedule the surgery. Alternatively, the patient may wish to consult another surgeon, which may be an indication that the patient is uncertain about the procedure, and it probably should not be performed. A psychiatrist may help determine whether the patient is sufficiently emotionally sound to undergo liposuction. Because liposuction can always be delayed, it is important that cutaneous surgeons feel totally comfortable about each patient on whom they will operate.

Preoperative Preparations

After the patient and the surgeon are both thoroughly committed to performing the liposuction procedure, the surgery can be scheduled. It is wise to plan an additional preoperative visit 10 days or so before the procedure to be sure that all the preoperative preparations have been accomplished. This visit also affords another opportunity for the patient to ask any unanswered questions or to cancel the liposuction. It is customary in many surgical practices for the procedure to be paid for in advance to confirm the appointment time. At this visit, all preoperative and postoperative prescriptions for medications can also be written. These medications include antibiotics and sedatives that will be taken preoperatively and postoperative pain medications. It is wise to have all consent forms signed at this same visit so that these documents are valid. A sedated patient can not give full informed consent for any surgical procedure.

Preoperative blood tests can also be performed or ordered at this same visit. These may include a complete blood cell count, platelet determination, general blood chemistry, and bleeding studies such as prothrombin time and partial thromboplastin time. Some physicians order additional tests to exclude patients with hepatitis, HIV infection, and syphilis. Traditional preoperative studies such as urinalysis, chest radiograph, and electrocardiogram are generally unnecessary unless the patient has a medical history that suggests a need to evaluate these additional areas.

During this visit it is also prudent to review the postoperative instructions and emphasize that patients will require another person to drive them home, as well as a person to stay with them during the recovery day. If a surgical girdle is to be used postoperatively for compression, the appropriate garment can be ordered or reserved from the surgeon's inventory. If the patient lives some distance from the practice location, plans must be made for appropriate postoperative follow-up, including overnight stays in the vicinity after surgery.

Photography

Good quality photographs are an essential part of the medical record for cutaneous surgery.[34] This is especially true for liposuction. Both the patient and the physician quickly forget the original preoperative appearance, and photographs are necessary to judge the success of the procedure. It is customary to photograph the patient preoperatively and at every postoperative visit beginning 2 weeks after the procedure. This provides a way to measure the success of the procedure even for patients who fail to return for subsequent visits.

The preoperative photographs should be taken in duplicate to minimize the potential for error. The photographs should also be standardized to provide an accurate basis for comparison. Patients should be photographed standing and fully unclothed. Some modest individuals will object to this, but it is necessary, as clothing that has been pulled away from the operative site often finds its way into the photograph, which is distracting and may distort the adiposity.

Eight standard photographic positions are usually required: anterior, posterior, two lateral, and four oblique views. The background should be consistent and should provide sufficient contrast with the skin color. A personal approach to camera distance and lighting must be developed so that the photographs are consistent.

Although 35-mm slides are the usual photographic medium used for liposuction, prints and videotape are also alternatives. Instant Polaroid prints are particularly useful, because they can be shaded in to illustrate to the patient the contour changes that are achievable by liposuction. Using a marker of the same color as the background behind the patient, a "photographic liposuction" can be performed by shading out the areas to be treated (Fig. 43–9). The use of imaging devices can also illustrate the intended results of liposuction for the patient. The patient must be warned that these are only estimates of the contour changes achievable by surgery and individual healing variations will determine the final results of liposuction.

Because of the personal nature of liposuction photography, the surgeon must be certain to obtain proper informed consent for taking such photographs. This

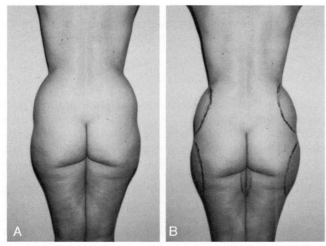

Figure 43–9. A "photographic liposuction" can be demonstrated by shading in Polaroid prints. *A*, Preoperative appearance. *B*, Postoperative appearance indicated by shading.

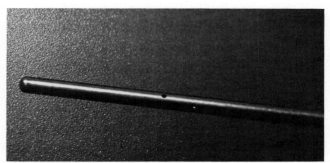

Figure 43–10. The Byron injection needle is blunt, with multiple small apertures arrayed 1 to 2 cm proximal to the tip.

consent must also include permission for any authorized use of the photographs, including publication and scientific or educational lectures. Like any part of the medical record, these photographs should not be released without the patient's permission.

Anesthesia for Liposuction

Although general anesthesia has been used for liposuction,[35] cutaneous surgeons have pioneered approaches to local anesthesia, which has proved safer and easier on the patient.[11, 12] The advent of tumescent anesthesia has eliminated the use of general anesthetics and intravenous sedation for most liposuction procedures.[36, 37] Furthermore, this approach has been shown to result in much less blood loss and allows removal of up to 2000 ml of fat without the need for blood transfusions.[38]

A typical approach to liposuction anesthesia begins with the patient taking 10 mg diazepam orally at bedtime the night before surgery and another 10 mg orally before arriving at the surgical facility. On arrival, vital signs are measured, and the patient is given 2.5 mg triazolam (Halcion) sublingually. At this time, 50 mg meperidine and 50 mg hydroxyzine are injected intramuscularly, allowing 30 minutes for these agents to achieve their sedative and analgesic effects before the injection of local anesthetics is begun.

After the patient has been prepped, a small wheal is raised using 1% lidocaine with epinephrine 1:100,000 at each planned entry site. A small stab incision is made, and a 14-gauge Byron injection needle is introduced into the subcutaneous layer. This needle has multiple injection ports arranged approximately 1 cm from the blunt tip (Fig. 43–10). Sterile intravenous (IV) tubing is attached to the needle and to an IV bag containing 1000 ml of the previously prepared tumescent fluid (Table 43–3).[39] Some cutaneous surgeons prefer a 0.1% concentration of lidocaine for tumescent anesthesia.[40]

Often, two needles are used to inject paired areas simultaneously. A mechanical blood pump or blood pressure cuff is placed around each IV bag, and the IV pole is then raised to its highest level and the pumps or cuffs inflated to accelerate the delivery of the anesthetic through the needles (Fig. 43–11). The needles are moved about the operative site after each portion becomes adequately tumescent, which is manifested when the area is nearly rock hard (Fig. 43–12).

Blanching of the overlying skin indicates intense vasoconstriction. If the flow of the anesthetic from the IV bag slows to a trickle, the needle should be repositioned. There is usually some backflow of the anesthetic fluid from the incision, and a sterile cloth towel can be used to absorb this drippage. An adequate amount of tumescent fluid can normally be injected into two paired areas in about 15 minutes. If the procedure involves multiple sites, additional tumescent anesthetic infiltration is repeated at each site. A peristaltic pump can also be used to inject the fluid, but several of these devices are required to infiltrate multiple sites at once. Using the tumescent technique, up to 35 mg/kg of lidocaine can be employed without causing systemic toxicity.[36]

Some pretunneling effects will result from using the Byron injection needle, which facilitates insertion of the liposuction cannula. Most liposuction procedures are performed in a criss-cross manner from two incisions superior and inferior to the adiposity. The Byron needle infiltration technique can also be used from each of these sites to thoroughly anesthetize tissue and to take maximal advantage of the pretunneling effect.

Once the areas are adequately anesthetized, liposuction can be performed easily with only the previously described preoperative medications. No intravenous sedatives are normally required. In difficult patients who have low pain thresholds, a small amount of intravenous midazolam can be administered. Because this agent is

TABLE 43–3. TUMESCENT LOCAL ANESTHETIC FORMULA*

1000 ml sodium chloride 0.9%
25 ml plain lidocaine 2.0%
2.5 ml sodium bicarbonate 84 mg/ml
1 ml epinephrine 1:1,000

*Concentration = 0.05% lidocaine, 1:1,000,000 epinephrine.

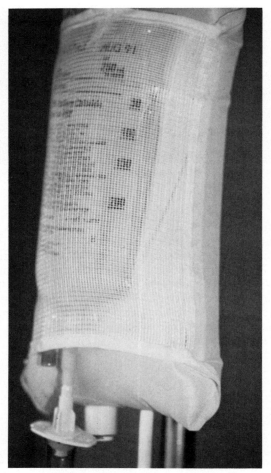

Figure 43–11. A blood pump is used to force tumescent fluid out through intravenous tubing and into the injection needle.

very potent and can cause respiratory depression even in small doses, it is advisable to administer it in 1-mg increments.[41] Midazolam is supplied as a 5 mg/ml mixture, and thus it is important to avoid an error in administration by using a tuberculin syringe, administering 0.2 ml or 1 mg at a time. This can be repeated every 15 minutes or so as needed. When the surgeon

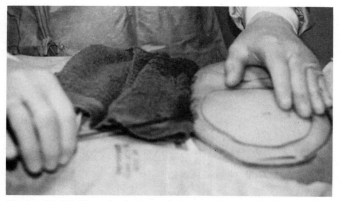

Figure 43–12. The injection needle is moved about in the operative site until it becomes rock hard and blanched.

chooses to use intravenous sedation, it is important to adequately monitor the patient's blood pressure, pulse, and blood oxygen saturation with a pulse oximeter.[42, 43]

Antiseptic Measures

Although infection was a feared complication of liposuction during the early days of its development, this complication is rare. The prospect of a large subcutaneous wound becoming infected is sobering to any surgeon. The use of preoperative antibiotics, although controversial for many procedures, has become common in liposuction surgery. Oral antibiotics should be administered one day before the procedure and continued for several days after liposuction. If parenteral antibiotics are used, adequate blood levels must be achieved before surgery.

Liposuction should be approached as a sterile procedure. Although drippage of fluids may compromise this, the surgeon and staff should take all precautions to minimize bacterial contamination.[44] All instruments should be properly sterilized and particular attention given to cleaning the cannulas, which may harbor pieces of aspirated material.[45] The use of disposable cannulas is becoming more prevalent and avoids this problem, although it creates an environmental burden.

Because the liposuction surgeon is often working around the perineal area, it is important to take extra cleansing measures. Patients can be given a vial of surgical cleanser such as chlorhexidine with which to perform an extensive perineal preparation before arrival at the surgical facility. Furthermore, it is convenient to have a shower near the surgical unit in which patients can again thoroughly clean the entire body just before the procedure, using a surgical scrub.

In the operating room, the patient should be prepped and draped with sterile sheets. Sterile towels placed underneath the patient help to absorb dripping fluids. After the patient is situated on the table, another prep is performed by the operating room personnel and extended well beyond the intended surgical sites. During the procedure, the surgeon and assistants should be garbed in full sterile operating gowns with head covers, masks, shoe covers, and sterile gloves. Every attempt should be made to avoid any break in sterile technique. A circulating nurse is required to facilitate this.

Preparing for Surgery

After the shower prep is complete, the patient is led into the operating room clothed in a surgical gown. Before the IV line is started and monitors are attached to the patient, photographs can be taken if this has not already been done. After taking the photographs, the surgeon can mark out the extent of the intended liposuction while the patient is standing. It is important not to do this marking on a reclining patient, because the effects of gravity must be taken into account when planning the procedure. An ordinary felt-tipped marking pen is suitable. The liposuction surgical sites can be

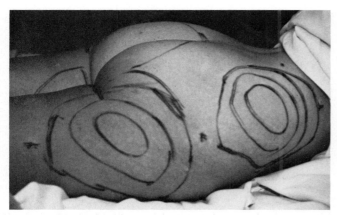

Figure 43–13. Concentric circles are used to indicate increasing thickness throughout an adiposity.

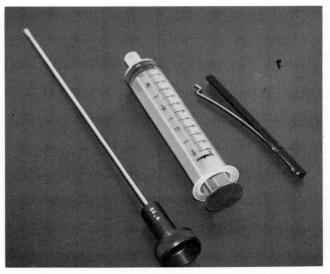

Figure 43–14. A syringe cannula suction apparatus with a spring device to hold the plunger out.

marked out topographically, with the predicted areas of largest fat excess represented by the smallest of a series of concentric circles (Fig. 43–13). The intended insertion points of the cannula should also be marked. It is important for the surgeon not to make an incision directly through this ink mark, as a tattoo may result. Some surgeons prefer to diagram the intended individual tunnels on the skin surface, but this is a matter of individual choice.

After the marking is complete, the patient is positioned on the operating room table and an IV line started. When the tumescent technique is employed, it is not necessary to replace fluids[46] or blood as when liposuction is performed under general anesthesia.[37, 38] Therefore, an open line using Ringer's lactate solution is all that is required.

Instruments

Liposuction requires negative pressure and a suction cannula. The suction source can be either a large-volume syringe or an electrical aspiration unit. A small minority of cutaneous surgeons, led by Fournier, prefer the syringe, because it is disposable, inexpensive, and sterile.[47, 48] However, the surgeon must retract the plunger and hold it back manually or with a spring device each time the syringe becomes full and the contents expelled (Fig. 43–14). Because the most efficient syringe size is 60 ml, the surgeon must constantly manipulate the syringe to maintain suction. Furthermore, during the procedure it is not uncommon for a loss of suction to occur if the aperture of the cannula is drawn too close to the insertion site. This means additional work for the surgeon. Liposuction for fat transfer is best performed with a 5- or 10-ml syringe attached to a 14-gauge minicannula. The same syringe can be used to reinject the fat (Fig. 43–15).

Most surgeons use an electrical aspiration device that consists of a pump to draw the aspirate into a reservoir bottle. These machines are easy to use and can rapidly achieve 1 atm of negative pressure. However, they are expensive and difficult to clean, and there is a slight risk

of vaporization of viral particles from the machine exhaust. A variety of syringe systems and aspiration machines are available from several different manufacturers.

Liposuction cannulas are available in myriad shapes, designs, widths, and lengths. After gaining experience, the surgeon will usually rely on two or three favorite cannulas. These can be attached directly to a syringe or through plastic tubing to an aspiration device. When choosing cannulas, there are several important parameters to consider. The length of the cannula affects the ability of the surgeon to reach the entire width of an adiposity from each incision site. However, long cannulas are more difficult to precisely control than short ones. Curved cannulas allow easier access around contoured areas. Flat cannulas, such as the spatula design, are ideal for liposuction of the neck (Fig. 43–16).

The location of the apertures on the cannula also affects the surgical efficiency. When the apertures are grouped well away from the distal end of the shaft, suction is lost more easily as the cannula is drawn close to the insertion site. The design of the cannula tip is also important. Blunt-tipped cannulas feature apertures located 1 cm or more back from the tip and are more gentle to the tissues. When the aperture is located in the tip, the cannula behaves more like a curette.[49] This is useful for difficult-to-suction areas such as the male

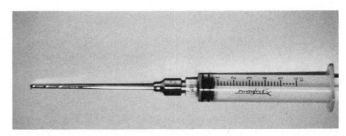

Figure 43–15. A small syringe with a 14 gauge minicannula attached.

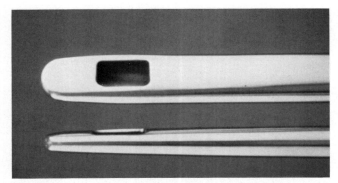

Figure 43–16. The spatula design is a flat cannula ideal for liposuctioning the neck. (Courtesy of Wells Johnson Company, Tucson, AZ.)

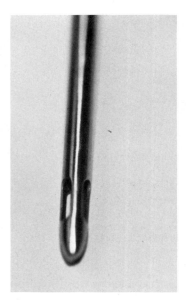

Figure 43–18. A 3.5-mm blunt cannula with three apertures is more gentle to the tissues.

breast or the flank (Fig. 43–17). However, such cannulas cause more bleeding and are a liability for liposuction of most other areas. Cannulas with more apertures remove fat more readily. These are sometimes designed in a series around the shaft or in groups down the length of the shaft (Fig. 43–18).

The diameter of the cannula is also very important. Cannulas larger than 6 mm create tunnels that may retract postoperatively into dents or waves that are visible on the skin surface. This was a common problem in the early days of liposuction, but as surgeons began using smaller diameter cannulas this problem has largely disappeared. The usual cannula for liposuction is 4 to 6 mm in size. Although the surgeon will have to make more than twice as many tunnels using a 4-mm cannula compared with a 6-mm one, the final result is usually smoother. For thicker adiposities, however, a 6-mm cannula will save time during the liposuction and will work quite well if used deeper in the fat. Minicannulas of 12 to 14 gauge are ideal for feathering around liposuction sites or under thin, fragile skin such as the medial thighs.

Surgical Technique

After the patient has been prepped and the tumescent anesthesia injected, liposuction can begin on the areas that were injected first. This usually requires 15 to 30 minutes from the time of the injection of the tumescent fluid to the onset of the suction procedure.

The incision site can be widened by spreading it with a pair of blunt scissors until it is large enough to permit passage of the appropriate size cannula. The 4- to 6-mm cannula, depending on the thickness of the adiposity, is gently inserted through the entire length of the adiposity and then, with the suction machine turned on, it is gently drawn back and forth through segments of the tunnel until no more resistance is felt. Usually 10 to 12 strokes through a tunnel are required. The tunnels should be designed parallel to the skin surface. The cannula must not be allowed to drift superficially within 1 cm of the dermis or too deeply where it will traumatize the underlying fascia. The surgeon's nondominant hand is used to assess the position of the cannula, as well as to gently "milk" fat cells and intracellular debris into the aperture of the cannula[50] (Fig. 43–19). If blood is detected in the clear tubing, suction in that tunnel should be abandoned (Fig. 43–20).

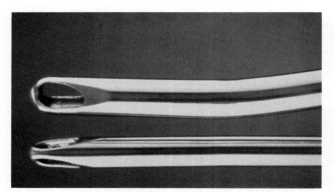

Figure 43–17. The cobra design features apertures in the tip and allows more aggressive liposuction. (Courtesy of Wells Johnson Company, Tucson, AZ.)

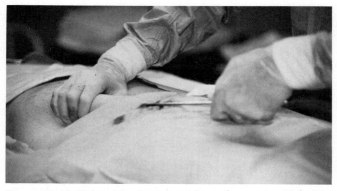

Figure 43–19. The nondominant hand is used to gently milk fat into the cannula.

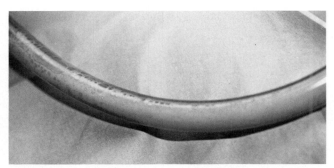

Figure 43–20. The clear tubing allows the surgeon to detect blood in the aspirate.

Suctioning continues in this fashion through a series of tunnels developed in a fan-shaped pattern from the original incision site. A side-to-side, windshield-wiper type motion should be avoided, because it creates a large area of dead space. After a series of tunnels have been developed from the original insertion site, an additional fan-shaped pattern is developed from a second insertion site, usually on the opposite side of the adiposity. These two overlapping fan-shaped patterns create a grid, or criss-cross, lipoplasty (Fig. 43–21).

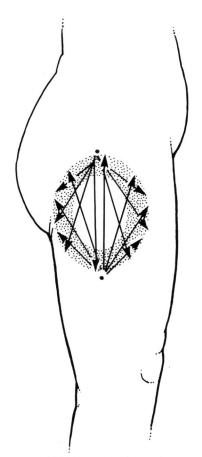

Figure 43–21. Two overlapping fan-shaped patterns of tunnels create a criss-cross lipoplasty. (From Coleman WP III, Hanke CW, Alt T, Asken S [eds]: Cosmetic Surgery of the Skin. BC Decker, Philadelphia, 1991.)

It is important that liposuction tunneling be limited to a cephalocaudal direction. When tunneling is performed in a horizontal direction, the effects of gravity may lead to draping of the suctioned tissue, resulting in visible folds.[4] It is impossible to suction only in a superoinferior direction without making numerous incisions. However, it is feasible to deviate from the vertical direction up to 45 degrees. Thus each insertion site results in the creation of a series of tunnels arrayed like a fan.

At all times, a 1-cm buffer zone must be maintained beneath the dermis to avoid injury to the superficial fat layer. If this fat is traumatized, surface dents may result.[51] Several layers of tunnels may be required for thick adiposities. Each of these layers is ideally positioned about one cannula width below the tunnel above. After liposuction the adiposity consequently has a "Swiss cheese" appearance. Subsequent retraction of the tunnels during healing exerts a two-dimensional tightening effect.

The fat is removed through a combination of suction and avulsion of fat cells. Certainly a large portion of the destroyed fat cells are not removed during the suction procedure but undergo subsequent necrosis during the healing stage. This explains why the benefits of liposuction are eventually much greater than would be anticipated by the amount of fat removed.

After the surgeon has finished tunneling throughout the adiposity from at least two different directions, the "pinch test" is used to determine the thickness of the remaining fat. Pinching the skin between the thumb and index finger allows the surgeon to compare the treated areas with the untreated surrounding tissue. If additional suctioning is required, it can then be immediately performed in the appropriate areas. One of the benefits of using local anesthesia is that the patient can also be asked to stand up to evaluate the effects of gravity on the liposuction areas. The pinch test is again used to determine the adequacy of suction.

Once the surgeon is satisfied that a thorough liposuction has been performed, it is appropriate to feather the operative site with a peripheral mesh dissection. This is done with the suction turned off, using a small cannula to free up a 1-cm peripheral zone around the liposuctioned areas.[52] This allows the skin to contract more easily and diminishes the otherwise abrupt transition between suctioned and nonsuctioned skin. An alternative way to achieve the same result is to design the fan-shaped tunnel pattern so that the most peripheral tunnels are just outside the adiposity. During the liposuction, these transitional tunnels are developed by making only one or two passes with the cannula.

After all suctioning is completed and before the incisions are closed, it is usually necessary to milk the treated sites of excess tumescent fluid. After use of the tumescent technique, drainage of a clear to pink fluid can be expected for up to 24 hours. If some of this fluid is expressed before suturing and bandaging the wounds, this annoying postoperative drainage can be minimized. It is also helpful to have the patient stand up for a few minutes to expedite the removal of this excess fluid before the surgeon sutures the incisions. This can be most efficiently done in the shower of the surgical unit and gives the nurse an opportunity to clean the patient before applying the bandages. Each surgical wound is usually closed with a single 5-0 nylon suture. Wounds excessively traumatized from the cannula passage may require surgical revision before closure.

Postoperative Instructions

After completion of the liposuction procedure, the incisions are closed, an antibiotic ointment is applied to the suture sites, and a nonstick dressing is applied. Over this a layer of gauze squares is added to absorb any leaking fluid. Next, elastic adhesive tape is used to secure the gauze. Finally, a splint is fashioned from strips of 4-inch elastic tape placed vertically over the suctioned areas with enough pressure to compress the underlying tunnels. A special surgical elastic garment can then be worn over this splint to complete the dressing.

Some cutaneous surgeons no longer use the tape splint, believing that enough compression can be achieved with the elastic garment alone. This eliminates the irritation caused by tape and the bathing restrictions that also result from its use. However, the proponents of tape use note that this splint ensures postoperative compression. Unreliable patients may remove the girdle postoperatively and may not follow instructions, which may compromise the result. Some surgeons prefer to use both tape and a compression garment to ensure maximal compression. The tape is removed after 1 week. A warm bath with oil added to the water will facilitate tape removal. Use of the compression garment is continued full time for another week, decreasing to 12 hours a day for an additional 2 weeks.

A number of surgical garments are available for postoperative compression after liposuction. These are made to fit the various parts of the body that are commonly treated by this procedure (Fig. 43–22). More recently, there has been a trend to employ ready-to-wear elastic garments, especially after liposuction of the abdomen and lower extremities. Spandex tights or exercise shorts provide excellent compression. However, unlike the surgical garments, they are not designed with Velcro fastenings to open on one side, and therefore tight-fitting garments may be difficult to put on. One option is to apply a loose-fitting Spandex garment first and then slide a tighter garment on over this. One advantage of using the tights rather than surgical girdles is that they are much more fashionable and allow the patient more clothing options postoperatively.

Postoperative compression should be continued for at least 2 weeks after surgery. The instruction to use the garment for 12 hours a day for the second 2 weeks is appreciated by most patients, since the support decreases residual sensitivity, which may continue for several weeks after the surgery. Other modalities have been recommended for postoperative liposuction care, including the use of ultrasound and massage.[53] Although these are comforting to the patient, scientific studies

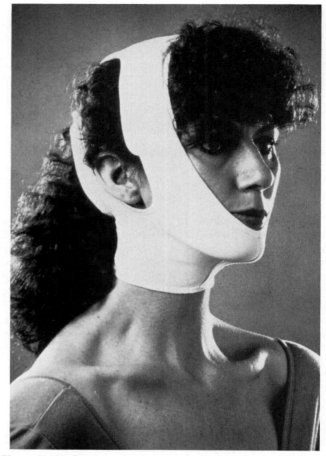

Figure 43–22. Postoperative compression garments are available for each anatomic site. (Courtesy of Wells Johnson Company, Tucson, AZ.)

have not shown that these improve the results of the procedure.

Liposuction patients are generally seen 2 to 3 days after the procedure and then again at 1, 2, 4, 8, and 12 weeks postoperatively. The purpose of these visits is to be sure that the patient is healing normally and to provide reassurance that everything is going well. The final results of liposuction are often not appreciable for at least 3 months after surgery, and it is important to continually remind the patient of this fact. As enthusiasm dwindles after 1 to 2 weeks postoperatively, patients often become uncertain of the success of the procedure. It is important to inform patients preoperatively that this feeling is likely to occur and to reassure them that swelling in the liposuction areas is normal and usually begins to fade after about 6 weeks.[54] This edema may be worse in some patients than in others. It is also important to note that some patients may obtain good results almost immediately; in such cases both the surgeon and the patient are pleased after only 1 week. However, other patients must wait until the edema subsides to appreciate the full benefit of the procedure.

The best results are often achieved in patients who undergo a "touch-up" procedure 1 year after the original liposuction. This affords the surgeon an opportunity to refine small imperfections and to reduce any new accumulations of fat in the surrounding areas. All patients should be notified in advance that this may be necessary. It is common to charge a fee for the "touch-up" procedure, although this fee is usually less than that charged for the original procedure. Patient should be informed of this in advance so that they are not surprised by any additional fee.

Important Axioms of Liposuction

Maximum Volume of Extracted Aspirate Is Limited by Blood and Fluid Loss. The more tissue the surgeon removes during liposuction the greater will be the blood loss. This loss is profoundly influenced by the type of anesthesia used. Liposuction performed under general anesthesia with minimal attention to infiltration with epinephrine is associated with far more bleeding than that performed using the tumescent technique.[12] When liposuction is performed using only local anesthesia, it is necessary for the surgeon to adequately infiltrate every portion of the surgical site. This thorough infiltration with lidocaine also delivers epinephrine to even the smallest of blood vessels, which results in profound vasoconstriction and dramatically decreases the amount of bleeding during the procedure.[38] When the tumescent technique is employed, it is common for the liposuction aspirate to be entirely yellow in color with only a trace of red (Fig. 43–23). When general anesthesia is used, some infiltration of local anesthetic is often employed, but this is usually done less thoroughly than in the tumescent technique, since it is not done for pain relief. Two liters of tumescent fluid are usually required to produce maximal vasoconstriction and anesthesia for liposuction of the abdomen. The injected fluid is also absorbed readily and automatically corrects the fluid losses from liposuction, which decreases the need for IV fluid replacement.[37]

Liposuction Should Be Performed Gently. Tissue preservation is an important component of all successful surgical procedures. Rough tissue handling is likely to result in more infections and greater bleeding. The firm, distorted tissue produced by the tumescent technique facilitates the penetration of the cannula. This allows a much more delicate technique and results in less trauma than when the procedure is performed under general anesthesia with little attention given to local infiltration.[46] Furthermore, patients who are awake will require the use of a more gentle technique to avoid any discomfort. A more refined liposuction technique with appropriate infiltration of the tumescent fluid and careful tunneling results in minimal bruising, less postoperative pain, and smoother results.

Men Bleed More Than Women. Even when the most advanced approaches to tumescent anesthesia are employed, men will show increased blood in the aspirate. This may well be due to the "hardness" of the male subcutaneous tissue.[46] Men also more commonly request liposuction of the flanks or breasts,[26] two areas with very firm fat that provides greater resistance to the cannula,

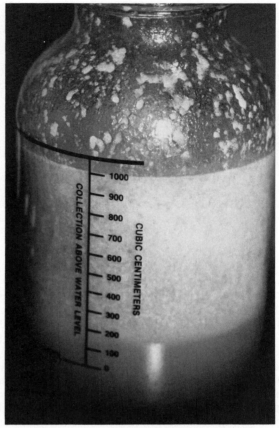

Figure 43–23. Typical liposuction aspirate when the tumescent technique is employed. (Note only a small amount of blood-tinged infranate fluid.)

which results in more trauma and more bleeding. Cannulas with a more distally placed aperture, such as the cobra cannula, are often required in areas where the fat is firm. These instruments act more like a curette than those with more proximally placed apertures. Consequently, they provide more efficient liposuction but also cause more bleeding.

Liposuction Must Be Performed With Caution in Certain Anatomic Areas. In the neck there is a risk of injury to the cervical and marginal mandibular branches of the facial nerve. Small, flat cannulas should be used in this area, and the level of dissection should be maintained in the subcutaneous tissue above the platysma muscle. It is unwise to attempt to tunnel over the mandible from a neck incision in an effort to flatten out the jowl fat. This subcutaneous tissue is better approached from a preauricular incision to avoid the superficially located fibers of the marginal mandibular nerve as they pass over the mandible. In the axilla, liposuction for hyperhidrosis (Fig. 43–24) should be performed in the upper subcutaneous tissue, taking care to avoid deeper dissection that might injure the brachial plexus.[55, 56]

The Smallest Cannula Possible Should Always Be Used. Although it is easier to remove fat with larger cannulas, there is also a greater risk of bleeding, pain,

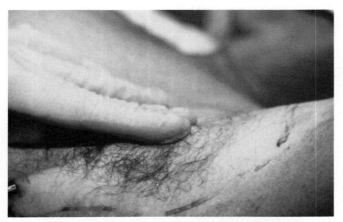

Figure 43–24. Liposuction of the axilla for hyperhidrosis must be confined to the superficial fat to avoid injury to underlying structures.

and subsequent surface dents or waffles. Smaller cannulas require more tunneling but are more precise and pass through the tissue much more easily. Microcannulas are appropriate in areas where the overlying skin is thin, such as the medial inner thigh (see Fig. 43–15). They are also useful for feathering or blending throughout the body.

Vertical Criss-Cross Tunneling Should Always Be Used. Horizontal tunneling may lead to skin waviness. Criss-cross tunneling gives a more thorough result and better utilizes the forces of wound contraction to tighten the skin postoperatively. In most situations the incisions for tunneling should be placed superior and inferior to the adiposity (see Fig. 43–21).

Patients With Loose Skin May Require Excision After Liposuction. Patients with loose skin overlying an area of fat excess may require skin excision to avoid sagging after the liposuction procedure. This is especially true in the neck, where inelastic skin may not fully retract, requiring a face lift. It is also true in the lower abdomen, where abdominoplasty may be needed to eliminate overhanging skin. In some cases only skin resection is required, especially if the loose skin is primarily below the umbilicus. However, other patients with diastasis of the rectus muscles will require a traditional abdominoplasty.[57]

The Infragluteal Fold Is an Important Buttress. Liposuction in the infragluteal fold destroys this compact fibroadipose area and may lead to ptosis of the buttocks.[58] The buttocks are usually approached from lateral incisions about 1 cm superior to the infragluteal fold. Liposuction of the posterior thighs is best approached from an incision 1 cm below the infragluteal fold. It is tempting to hide the incision site in the fold, but suctioning from this location destroys much of the support for the buttocks and often results in sagging.

The Central Buttocks Should Not Be Suctioned. The so-called "Bermuda triangle" is located over the central buttocks (see Fig. 43–5). This area provides buttocks projection, and suctioning here will flatten the derriere. Instead, buttocks suctioning should be confined to the lateral portions, where excess fat may cause bowing of the lateral thigh tissues. Often, treatment of the buttocks

alone solves a false saddle-bag problem, in which there is no true excess fat in the outer thigh.

Noncosmetic Applications for Liposuction

Although liposuction was primarily developed for cosmetic purposes, there are a number of medical conditions for which it can also be successfully used. In these situations, it is appropriate for the health insurance carrier to cover the expense of the liposuction procedure just as is done for any other noncosmetic procedure.[25]

FAT DEPOSITS THAT CAUSE FUNCTIONAL PROBLEMS

Liposuction is sometimes required for functional reasons. Fat distribution may impair movement or interfere with proper skin hygiene. Some older patients develop sufficient excess fat in the lower abdomen to create a fold that encourages intertriginous infection with yeast or bacteria. If dietary manipulation is not successful, conservative liposuction of this area can be used to ameliorate this problem. Of course, the patient must understand the limited cosmetic goals of this approach. A similar situation may also occur with excess fat of the upper medial thighs that causes chafing. Localized liposuction can be successful in improving this problem.

CORRECTING AREAS OF FAT NECROSIS

Traumatic injuries may result in areas of fat necrosis appearing as large skin depressions. Using liposuction to resculpt these areas by suctioning fat and then transplanting it into the atrophic sites can be successful in restoring these deformities to their previous contours.

LIPOMAS

Lipomas are tumors derived from adipocytes. Liposuction is a natural approach to removing these lesions.[59] The goal with liposuction is not to remove the whole lipoma, but rather to tunnel through it thoroughly so that scar contraction will reduce the growth sufficiently to normalize skin contours (Fig. 43–25). Because some large tumors may actually be liposarcomas, it is always wise to submit at least a portion of the tissue removed for pathologic examination.[25]

It is usually not advantageous to use liposuction to remove lipomas smaller than 2 to 3 cm in diameter. Small lipomas are best removed by direct excision. Even some large, firm lipomas are more efficiently removed by making a small incision, about one third the diameter of the lesion, and dissecting around the tumor with a pair of curved blunt scissors. These lesions can then be removed through the incision by circumferential manual compression. However, large, soft lipomas are usually best treated by liposuction, as smooth contours can be achieved by using feathering techniques, and only two tiny incisions are required.

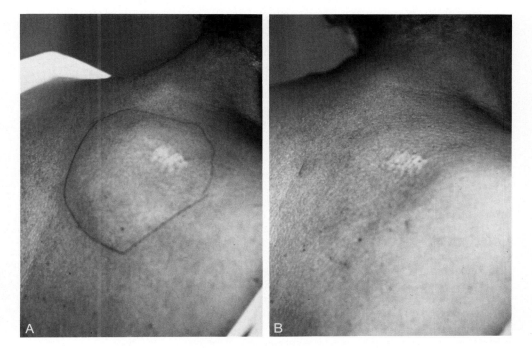

Figure 43–25. *A,* A large lipoma of the back with a scar from previous incomplete excision. *B,* After liposuction, the contours are flattened, with only two small scars.

Some lipomas contain a fibrous skeleton that must be removed to obtain adequate reduction of the tumor. After the tunneling has been completed, the surgeon can grasp and pull this material out through the same incisions using a hemostat. After liposuction of a lipoma, it is important to compress the operative site with elastic tape. This should remain in place for 1 week postoperatively. After removal of the tape, the contours of the treated areas initially are not smooth and may require several months to contract and achieve the best cosmetic appearance.

AXILLARY HYPERHIDROSIS

Axillary hyperhidrosis can often be helped by liposuction. This embarrassing problem is the result of excessive eccrine sweat production. Traditional approaches to treatment have included various topical antiperspirants and systemic anticholinergics. When these medical therapies fail, surgical excision of the axillary skin has traditionally been employed to remove the excess eccrine sweat glands.[55, 56]

Liposuction is successful in treating axillary hyperhidrosis, because these glands are deep in the dermis and upper subcutaneous tissue. The cannula is used with its aperture directed toward the skin surface in a plane just below the dermis (Fig. 43–24). This allows the surgeon to scrape the deeper dermis while removing superficial subcutaneous tissue. The plane of dissection must be kept well above the underlying brachial plexus. A bidirectional criss-cross procedure is performed from incisions in the most superior and inferior portions of the axillary vault.

The tumescent anesthetic technique has proved particularly valuable for this application of liposuction, because it allows the surgeon to easily maintain a proper plane of dissection. Engorgement from the anesthetic also creates a buffer zone from the underlying deep axillary structures. The superficial dissection plane may cause minor injury to the deeper dermis, but full thickness necrosis has not been a problem. Some bruising is apparent for 7 to 10 days postoperatively, but healing is typically uneventful. Preoperative antibiotics may decrease the potential for infection. It is usually wise to perform this procedure on one axilla at a time, with at least a 2-week interval between surgeries.

The results of liposuction for axillary hyperhidrosis are usually excellent. Patients typically note a complete absence of sweating for several weeks postoperatively, followed by a gradual return to a more normal degree of sweating. This procedure avoids the deforming scars associated with excisional approaches to hyperhidrosis. Because liposuction can be performed under local anesthesia in an outpatient ambulatory facility, it has become a relatively inexpensive way to control axillary hyperhidrosis.

RECONSTRUCTIVE SURGERY

Liposuction techniques have also been adapted for use in reconstructive surgery. Tunneling around a large cutaneous defect allows relatively bloodless undermining and good mobilization of the surrounding tissues.[60, 61] The blunt cannula, unlike sharp undermining instruments, usually avoids damage to neurovascular bundles. This is particularly useful for large cutaneous defects created after removal of tumors in the neck and lower face. This approach is a "spin-off" of the use of liposuction for facilitating face lift surgery.

Liposuction can also be used for debulking flaps. Large areas of transferred tissue may result in thick, poorly contoured masses of skin after the flap has become established. This is particularly true of myocutaneous flaps.[62] After about 3 months, the flap has usually become sufficiently revascularized and swelling has subsided, so liposuction can be used to recontour the flap. This debulking procedure is accomplished using standard liposuction techniques. It is often so successful that loose skin must be removed from the periphery of the flap after liposuction. It is wise to avoid the pedicle area of the flap so that the blood supply is not compromised.

SUMMARY

After a decade of universal acceptance, liposuction has become a refined, predictable technique. The most important advance in liposuction during the 1980s was the development of the tumescent anesthetic technique. In the 1990s, laser liposuction may become a reality. Already a few cases have been performed using a blunt-tipped cannula attached to a neodymium:yttrium-aluminum-garnet laser. Early reports describe a substantial reduction in bleeding compared with traditional suction approaches. Future research will determine what place this instrument will have in liposuction.

REFERENCES

1. Ottani F, Fournier P: A history and comparison of suction techniques until their debut in North America. In: Hetter G (ed): Lipoplasty: The Theory and Practice of Blunt Suction Lipectomy. Little, Brown, Boston, 1984, pp 19–23.
2. Pitanguy I: Trochanteric lipodystrophy. Plast Reconstr Surg 34:280–283, 1984.
3. Fischer A, Fischer G: First surgical treatment for molding body's cellulite with three 5 mm incisions. Bull Int Acad Cosmet Surg 3:35, 1976.
4. Fischer G: Liposculpture: the correct history of liposuction. Part I. J Dermatol Surg Oncol 16:1087–1089, 1990.
5. Fischer A, Fischer G: Revised techniques for cellulitis fat reduction in riding breeches deformity. Bull Int Acad Cosmet Surg 2:40–41, 1977.
6. Illouz Y: Body contouring by lipolysis: a 5 year experience with over 3000 cases. Plast Reconstr Surg 72:511–524, 1983.
7. Coleman WP III: The history of dermatologic liposuction. Dermatol Clin 8:381–383, 1990.
8. Field L: The dermatologist and liposuction—a history. J Dermatol Surg Oncol 13:1040–1041, 1987.
9. Newman J: Liposuction surgery: past, present, future. Am J Cosmet Surg 1:1–2, 1984.
10. Coleman WP III: The dermatologist as a liposuction surgeon. J Dermatol Surg Oncol 14:1057–1058, 1988.
11. Klein JA: The tumescent technique for liposuction surgery. Am J Cosmet Surg 4:263–267, 1987.
12. Lillis PJ: Liposuction surgery under local anesthesia: limited blood loss and minimal lidocaine absorption. J Dermatol Surg Oncol 14:1145–1148, 1988.
13. Asken S: Liposuction Surgery and Autologous Fat Transplantation. Appleton & Lange, East Norwalk, CT, 1988.
14. Glogau R: Microlipoinjection: autologous fat grafting. Arch Dermatol 124:1340–1343, 1988.
15. Skouge J: Autologous fat transplantation in facial surgery. In: Coleman WP III, Hanke CW, Alt T, Asken S (eds): Cosmetic Surgery of the Skin. BC Decker, Philadelphia, 1991, pp 239–250.
16. Hanke CW, Coleman WP III: Collagen filler substances. In: Coleman WP III, Hanke CW, Alt T, Asken S (eds): Cosmetic Surgery of the Skin. BC Decker, Philadelphia, 1991, pp 99–102.
17. Arner P: Human adipose function, development and metabolism. In: Hetter G (ed): Lipoplasty: The Theory and Practice of Blunt Suction Lipectomy. Little, Brown, Boston, 1984, pp 41–48.
18. Billings E, May J: Historical review and present status of free fat autotransplantation in plastic and reconstructive surgery. Plast Reconstr Surg 83:368–381, 1989.
19. Skouge J: Adipose tissue and the pathophysiology of obesity. Dermatol Clin 8:385–393, 1990.
20. Brownell K, Steen S: Modern methods for weight control: the physiology and psychology of dieting. Phys Sports Med 15:122–137, 1987.
21. Tobin HA: Large-volume liposuction. Planned staged treatment in the obese patient. Am J Cosmet Surg 4:61–66, 1987.
22. Mladick R: Lipoplasty: an ideal adjunctive procedure for the face lift. Clin Plast Surg 16:333–341, 1989.
23. Matarasso S: A regional approach to patient selection and evaluation for liposuction. Dermatol Clin 8:401–414, 1990.
24. Narins R: Liposuction surgery of a buffalo hump, secondary to Cushing's disease. J Am Acad Dermatol 21:307, 1989.
25. Coleman WP III: Non-cosmetic applications of liposuction. J Dermatol Surg Oncol 14:1085–1090, 1988.
26. Lewis C: Lipoplasty in males. Clin Plast Surg 16:355–360, 1989.
27. Teimourian B: Complications associated with suction lipectomy. Clin Plast Surg 16:385–394, 1989.
28. Teimourian B, Rogers WB: A national survery of complications associated with suction lipectomy: a comparative study. Plast Reconstr Surg 84:628–631, 1989.
29. Christman K: Death following suction lipectomy and abdominoplasty. Plast Reconstr Surg 78:428, 1986.
30. Reed C: Lipoplasty of the calves and ankles. Clin Plast Surg 16:365–368, 1989.
31. Coleman WP III, Coleman J: Liposuction and the law. Dermatol Clin 5:569–580, 1990.
32. Coleman WP III, Guice W: Office surgery and the law. Adv Dermatol 2:207–229, 1987.
33. Wright M: Psychological evaluation of a cosmetic surgery patient. In: Coleman WP III, Hanke CW, Alt T, Asken S (eds): Cosmetic Surgery of the Skin. BC Decker, Philadelphia, 1991, pp 373–379.
34. Sebben J: Photography for cosmetic surgery. In: Coleman WP III, Hanke CW, Alt T, Asken S (eds): Cosmetic Surgery of the Skin. BC Decker, Philadelphia, 1991, pp 13–28.
35. Coleman WP III: Liposuction and anesthesia. J Dermatol Surg Oncol 13:1295–1296, 1987.
36. Klein JA: Tumescent technique for regional anesthesia permits lidocaine doses of 35 mg/kg for liposuction: peak plasma lidocaine levels are diminished and delayed 12 hours. J Dermatol Surg Oncol 16:248–263, 1990.
37. Klein J: The tumescent technique. Anesthesia and modified liposuction technique. Dermatol Clin 8:425–437, 1990.
38. Lillis PJ: The tumescent technique for liposuction surgery. Dermatol Clin 8:439–450, 1990.
39. Coleman WP III, Bademe A, Phillips JH: A new technique for injection of tumescent anesthetic mixtures. J Dermatol Surg Oncol 17:535–537, 1991.
40. Narins R, Lillis P: Liposuction. Presented at the Annual Meeting of the American Society for Dermatologic Surgery, Orlando, FL, March, 1991.
41. Baker T, Gordon H: Midazolam (Versed) in ambulatory surgery. Plast Reconstr Surg 82:244–246, 1988.
42. Singer R, Thomas P: Pulse oximeter in the ambulatory aesthetic surgical facility. Plast Reconstr Surg 82:111–114, 1988.
43. Guidelines of Care for Liposuction (revised). American Academy of Dermatology, Chicago, IL, 1990.
44. Stegman S: Technique variations in liposuction surgery. Dermatol Clin 8:451–461, 1990.
45. Weber P, Wulc AE, Jaworsky C, Dzubow LM: Warning: traditional liposuction cannulas may be dangerous to your patient's health. J Dermatol Surg Oncol 14:1136–1138, 1988.
46. Chrisman B, Coleman WP III: Determining safe limits for untransfused outpatient liposuction. Personal experience and review of the literature. J Dermatol Surg Oncol 14:1095–1102, 1988.
47. Fournier P: Why the syringe and not the suction machine? J Dermatol Surg Oncol 14:1062–1069, 1988.
48. Fournier P: Reduction syringe undermining. Dermatol Clin 8:539–551, 1990.
49. Collins P: Selection and utilization of liposuction cannulas. J Dermatol Surg Oncol 14:1139–1143, 1988.
50. Collins P: The methodology of liposuction surgery. Dermatol Clin 8:395–400, 1990.
51. Coleman WP III: Liposuction. In: Coleman WP III, Hanke CW, Alt T, Asken S (eds): Cosmetic Surgery of the Skin. BC Decker, Philadelphia, 1991, pp 213–238.

52. Fournier P: Liposculpture: My Technique. Arnette, Paris, 1989, pp 269–279.
53. Lewis C, Pruitt M: Massage and ultrasound. In: Hetter G (ed): Lipoplasty: The Theory and Practice of Blunt Suction Lipectomy. Little, Brown, Boston, 1984, pp 175–178.
54. Coleman WP III: Liposuction surgery. In: Demis DJ, Burgdorf WHC, Smith EB, Thiers BH (eds): Clinical Dermatology. JB Lippincott, Philadelphia, 1988, 37–3, pp 1–9.
55. Coleman WP III: Liposuction for hyperhidrosis. In: Robins P (ed): Surgical Gems in Dermatology. Igaku-Shoin, New York, 1991, pp 100–102.
56. Lillis P, Coleman WP III: Liposuction for treatment of axillary hyperhidrosis. Dermatol Clin 8:479–482, 1990.
57. Matarasso A: Abdominoplasty. Clin Plast Surg 16:289–303, 1989.
58. Fischer G: Liposculpture: The "correct" history of liposuction. Part I. J Dermatol Surg Oncol 16:1087–1089, 1990.
59. Pinski K, Roenigk H Jr: Liposuction of lipomas. Dermatol Clin 8:483–492, 1990.
60. Field L, Skouge J, Anhalt T, et al: Blunt liposuction cannula dissection with and without suction assisted lipectomy in reconstructive surgery. J Dermatol Surg Oncol 14:1116–1122, 1988.
61. Field L, Spinowitz A: Flap elevation and mobilization by blunt liposuction cannula dissection in reconstructive surgery. Dermatol Clin 8:493–499, 1990.
62. Baird W, Naha F: The use of lipoplasty in contouring and debulking flaps. Clin Plast Surg 16:395–399, 1989.

CHAPTER 44

Blepharoplasty and Brow Lift

BRUCE B. CHRISMAN

Blepharoplasty and brow lift are complementary procedures, and for a given patient, either or both may be necessary. Although upper lid blepharoplasty can be learned relatively easily, the anatomy of the periocular zone and of the contiguous, interrelated forehead and temporal zones yields complexities that can tax the analytic and surgical abilities of even the most skilled cutaneous surgeon. Certainly the face can be greatly improved through blepharoplasty alone, but some of these patients are also candidates for a brow lift. The surgeon must analyze each patient carefully and consider what surgical techniques should be used to obtain the best result.

Patient Evaluation

The examination of the upper part of the face is begun by asking the patient to sit forward in a chair and look straight ahead with his or her back perpendicular to the floor. The surgeon must be seated at approximately the same eye level as the patient. It may be necessary to ask the patient to relax the face or even to manually smooth the brows downward, as anxiety, coupled with interest in the examination, often causes the patient to lift the brows or open the eyes more than usual. Both the lids and the brows must be in a resting position for proper evaluation. The surgeon then asks the patient to visually follow a finger left, right, up, and down so that the function of the extraocular and levator muscles can be evaluated. It is helpful to gently fix the patient's chin in position with one hand while asking him or her to follow the index finger of the other hand. This gentle contact also sets the stage for the next part of the examination, in which the patient is asked to close the eyes gently and not open them as the examiner, using the thumbtips, tries to lift the upper lids several millimeters to evaluate Bell's reflex. The function of Bell's

reflex is particularly important in the first several days after blepharoplasty, when the lids may not close well. The stronger this reflex, the better the cornea will be moistened by the incomplete blinking that occurs during the early healing period.

Next, the lower lids are lightly pinched and pulled outward and downward to evaluate their ability to snap back when released. The surgeon then evaluates the patient for the possible presence of malar bags just inferior to the lateral lower lid zone; lateral crow's feet rhytides; and infratarsal creases on the lower lids, including Denny's lines. Hypertrophy of the orbicular muscle in the pretarsal zone is determined by asking the patient to squint as if the sun were bright. These conditions, along with the lid-cheek groove (commonly seen just inferior to the medial portion and midportion of the lower lids) and other variables in the lower lid zone, are important factors to assess. They should be pointed out to the patient using a hand mirror, as they very well may not change after a lower lid blepharoplasty, which is primarily a fat removal procedure. The presence or absence of scleral show is best evaluated by direct examination as well as careful observation of the patient during the remainder of the consultation.

The upper lids are evaluated for the possible presence of an epicanthal fold, which is not exclusive to Asians; definition and symmetry of the supratarsal crease; any secondary creases that may be present on the pretarsal area; and the presence of a supracrease sulcus, more likely seen in thin-skinned and older patients. The presence of ptosis and pseudoptosis, which are caused by the weight of bulky upper lid tissues or low brows, is also evaluated. The globe is examined for exophthalmos or enophthalmos, keeping in mind that there is considerable normal variation in the set of the globe in its skeletal framework. Pterygia, conjunctival injection, and inadequate tear film should also be noted at this time. Lesions and scars in the periorbital region should also be observed. The presence of previous blepharoplasty scars should also be determined, because some patients may be reluctant to relate this history, and previous surgery can significantly complicate the blepharoplasty procedure and its possible results. Finally, it is important to observe whether the palpebral fissures and eye position are symmetric.

The position of the brows and the brow hair is also important. The surgeon should carefully observe the patient during the initial part of the periocular examination to check for asymmetry of brow position, often caused by habitual facial mimetics. However, one brow that sits at a higher position than the other some or all of the time may be the result of increased strength of the frontalis muscle on one side of the forehead or motor nerve weakness. Ideally, the male brow should lie over or only slightly below the superior orbital rim, while the arch of the female brow should lie above it.

If the brows are low, the patient should be shown this in a hand mirror held at eye level. Most female patients habitually look downward into their mirrors and hold their brows up while doing so. Consequently, they may not be aware of their ptotic brows. The surgeon can then lift up one or both brows by placing the fingertips on the patient's forehead to demonstrate the effect that brow lifting or forehead lifting will have on the appearance of the periorbital zone. In some instances, the upper lid area is perfectly fine, and the patient is quite surprised to find that he or she does not need upper lid surgery and would benefit more from some form of brow lifting. In other patients, the brows are moderately low, and brow lifting becomes an option that should be discussed during the consultation, as the patient may wish to have it performed concomitantly with blepharoplasty.

Evaluation of the forehead should be performed by having the patient squint, frown, and elevate the brows so that the action of the corrugator, procerus, and frontalis muscles can be observed. The examiner should also look for visible rhytides in the nasofrontal angle, glabella, and forehead. The height and density of the forehead and temporal hairlines should also be carefully observed.

Because of the increased prevalence of cosmetic tattooing (see Chap. 33), the examiner should look closely for tattooed brows. If the brows have been placed permanently in a relatively high position, it may not be possible to adequately lift them without creating a clownlike appearance.

Medical and Ocular History

The patient's medical and ocular history must also be carefully reviewed and should include specific questions about any bleeding tendency, thyroid disease, diabetes, high blood pressure, eye or eye zone trauma, blurred vision, cataracts, glaucoma, internal eye problems (e.g., detached retina or uveitis), and the use of glasses or contact lenses. Patients with contact lenses should be advised that they will need to cease using them for about 2 weeks after blepharoplasty and should have glasses available for use during this period. The patient should also be specifically asked about intake of aspirin and other nonsteroidal anti-inflammatory agents and carefully cautioned about the negative effects of their use as related to surgery; this is likewise true of vitamin E. Additional information should include dry eye symptoms, the use of eye drops, allergic symptoms, excess tearing, and any history of periorbital edema. A complete medical and surgical history should also be routinely reviewed.

Contraindications to Surgery

Brow and forehead lifting should be approached with caution in patients who have had permanent brow tattooing. Very heavy eyeliner tattooing, particularly as performed by some nonmedical personnel, may also be a relative contraindication to upper lid blepharoplasty, because after surgery the stretched and more visible pretarsal zone may make the tattooed areas appear obvious or even grotesque. The female patient with a high forehead and sparse temporal hair may also not be a good candidate for coronal forehead lifting unless she wears her hair forward in bangs or similar styling. Likewise, patients with relatively thin frontal hair or those who part their hair in the midline should be aware that the coronal lift scarline could be visible in this area. Males are seldom candidates for coronal lifting because of thinning of the hair, particularly bitemporal recession, which often extends close or into the coronal incision zone. The pretrichial variation of the coronal lift keeps the frontal hairline intact but presents its own relative contraindications because of scar visibility and paresthesias, particularly during the first few months of healing. Such patients must be willing to accept the possibility of a permanently visible scar and sensory deficits.

Patients who have tight upper lids, particularly those who have had previous upper blepharoplasty, should be asked to close their eyes gently while the examiner lifts the brows to check for lagophthalmos. In some instances, there is not enough skin remaining in the upper lid zone to permit satisfactory brow lifting. A history of dry eye syndrome or a result of less than 5 mm on a 5-minute Schirmer test should also make the surgeon quite cautious about performing blepharoplasty. In these cases, a more conservative technique should be considered, and the future possibility of increased dry eye symptoms with or without blepharoplasty should be discussed. Usually, uncontrolled thyroid disease and hypertension are also contraindications to cosmetic surgery, as is congenital stenosis of the lids. Glaucoma could also be a problem because of some of the medications used during surgery. These conditions should prompt a discussion with the patient's ophthalmologist.

Patients with unilateral blindness must consider very carefully whether they wish to have blepharoplasty performed because of the very rare occurrence of blindness with this procedure.[1-3] Another relative contraindication is the use of nonselective, beta-blocker medications, as these have been reported to cause severe, life-threatening hypertension and cardiac collapse with the use of epinephrine,[4] an agent ordinarily used in these cosmetic procedures. If so approved by the patient's primary care physician, beta-blocker dosage should be reduced by 50% for 2 days preoperatively. A history of intolerance to epinephrine is another contraindication.

One of the most important relative contraindications to performing blepharoplasty is the patient with thyroid-induced or congenital exophthalmos with or without a sallow or regressed upper cheek. In such patients, the lids have difficulty closing around the globe in their natural state; this condition is exacerbated after alteration by blepharoplasty. Several studies have documented that this anatomic feature is more important in the consideration of postoperative dry eye syndrome than the tear film and the results of the Schirmer test.[5, 6] Because these patients often have lagophthalmos on gentle closure, as well as scleral show on forward gaze, they need to be thoroughly counseled on the problems that may be encountered after blepharoplasty. The surgeon should plan a more conservative upper lid procedure for such patients and a possible lid shortening or tightening procedure for the lower lids.

Consultation with the Patient

It is remarkable how often patients seek correction of a relatively minor problem while allowing glaring cosmetic defects (at least in the eyes of the surgeon) to continue. A patient may have severely drooping brows and prominent crow's feet rhytides but desire correction of moderately bulging lower lids. Other patients may have such severe upper lid dermatochalasis that they have to tilt their heads slightly backward to see well, and yet they are primarily concerned about their transverse forehead creases. Thus, it is extremely important for the cutaneous surgeon to first find out what the patient wants and then, by using a hand mirror, gently guide them to consider other existing aesthetic problems. It is not necessary to point out all such problems, but demonstrating those that are related to the particular surgical site the patient is concerned about is an appropriate and necessary part of the consultation. It is often helpful to gently smooth down patients' brows while they look into a hand mirror so that they can see themselves as others see them in facial repose and also so that they can see the subconscious hyperactivity of their frontalis muscle. Often patients immediately realize why their forehead and brow area feel fatigued in the evenings or why they have especially droopy lids or headaches at such times.

This sets the stage for a discussion of brow lifting and its relationship to upper lid blepharoplasty. Conscious or manual relaxation of the brow may also clearly demonstrate the obstruction of the upper outer visual field caused by brow ptosis or dermatochalasis of the upper lids. In such instances, photographic documentation of this problem may allow patients to obtain partial insurance coverage for the desired corrective procedure. Unfortunately, visual field testing by some physicians is done with the patient consciously or unconsciously holding the brows up, which is inappropriate. If the patient has drooping tissue that extends down onto the pretarsal upper lids or touches the eyelashes with the frontalis muscle at rest, there is a danger of accidental injury from overhead objects, such as open cupboard doors or hanging light fixtures. This visual field defect should be corrected to reduce this risk.

It is particularly helpful to use drawings or to make sketches to help patients understand where and why incisions are placed, what tissues are removed, where fixation or surface sutures are placed, and other basic technical aspects of surgery; in this way they can comprehend both the possibilities and the limitations of these surgical procedures. It will also help lessen their anxiety as they begin to understand the procedures. Blepharoplasty and coronal lift frequently incorporate intravenous sedation plus local anesthesia, which should be explained to the patient. Direct and mid forehead brow lifts often can be completed with local anesthesia alone.

A discussion of the treatment options is particularly appropriate, because at least one third of patients who present for blepharoplasty consultation are candidates for brow lifting as well (Fig. 44–1). Perhaps 5% of such patients are not candidates for upper blepharoplasty at all, but instead are candidates for brow lifting (Fig. 44–2). Consultation regarding the periorbital and forehead region is somewhat complex because of the different number of procedures that can be utilized. However, such consultation helps the patient to recognize what options are available and to understand that the results can differ considerably as a result of the various anatomic and aging factors in this region.

Regarding the eyelids, the patient should understand that pretarsal rhytides or a prominent supracrease sulcus will probably not be altered by blepharoplasty surgery. Similarly, lower lid rhytides and crow's feet rhytides will also not be removed. For this reason, the subject of chemical peeling or long-term use of topical retinoic acid may be appropriately brought up during the consultation. Patients must understand, particularly if they are Asian or older, that upper lid creases may not be formed as precisely as desired and may even appear to "fall out" or redevelop over time, necessitating a possible second surgical procedure.

With the aid of a hand mirror, the patient can see what upper lid blepharoplasty alone may do as compared with a brow lift, forehead lift, or both. Some patients may need to have both procedures performed and should be shown in the mirror, in comparative fashion, why this is necessary. The direct brow lift procedure is explained to those patients who are brow lift candidates and do not have significant transverse forehead rhytides and glabellar creases, particularly if they have relatively smooth, dry skin. Patients with thicker, oily, more poral skin can also undergo direct brow lifting, but healing time is usually longer, and the scar is likely to be more visible. In addition, such patients may experience small acne-like inflammatory lesions along the healing scarline or difficulties with suture spitting. Patients with low hairlines, transverse forehead rhytides, glabellar creases,

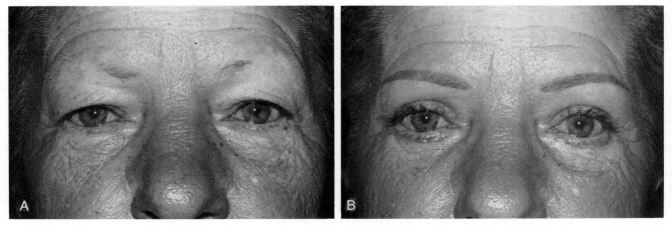

Figure 44–1. *A,* Patient who is candidate for either brow lifting or upper blepharoplasty. Note that forehead rhytides have resulted both from habitually lifting the brows and from the excess skin and fat of the upper lids. *B,* Ten weeks after upper and lower blepharoplasty (with brow makeup).

and low brows are ideal candidates for coronal lifting. This technique and what it can accomplish should also be explained using a mirror.

The mid forehead brow lift has its strong advocates[7] and is appropriate in some patients, particularly those with visible, nonsymmetric mid forehead rhytides. All brow lift and coronal lift patients should be told that the brow may appear overcorrected at first, which is purposely planned to allow for predictable stretchback. Women, who have smoother, drier, thinner skin, are generally better candidates for the direct brow lift procedure than men. In addition, women often brush their brows upward and use a brow pencil, which can substantially help to disguise the direct brow lift scar during healing. Glasses are also readily available in styles with high frames and tinted lenses, both of which can help camouflage the surgical area during the healing phase for both direct brow lift and blepharoplasty. However, many women are more likely to choose coronal lifting over direct brow lifting because of the hidden scarline. The complications of the appropriate procedures for each patient must also be discussed as a part of the consultation.

The Male Patient

Male patients comprise a special subset of cosmetic surgery patients, particularly with regard to very visible areas such as the eyelids and forehead, and they need to be specifically informed of the necessary recovery time related to these surgeries, as well as their expected appearance postoperatively. Men usually do not have sufficient hair length to allow for hair style changes that may help to cover coronal or even direct brow lifting. They also are not usually amenable to the use of makeup, brow brushing, tinted glasses, or other aids that could assist in hiding the wounds during healing. Male patients not only are more sensitive about others knowing they have had cosmetic surgery, but are also less accustomed to discomfort than female patients and usually have undergone fewer surgical procedures than their female counterparts. True to the "macho image," men often believe that they will be able to return to work and social contacts in only a day or two, despite the strongest admonitions by the surgeon to the contrary. Thus, it is important to make it very clear that severe bruising can occur after blepharoplasty or brow

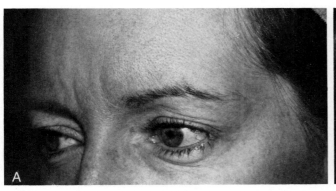
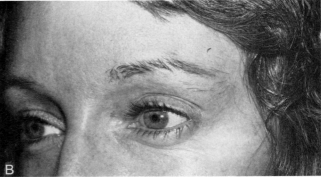

Figure 44–2. *A,* Patient who has glabellar frown lines and drooping brows, without excess skin or fat of the upper eyelid when the brow was lifted. *B,* Five months later, showing full correction of the upper lid zone after only a coronal forehead lift.

or forehead lifting. Scars may also be more apparent in the thick, sebaceous skin of men, which often seems to heal more slowly and with a greater inflammatory reaction. Again, a clear, detailed explanation is in order, and postoperative use of coverup makeup is advised, although seldom used. The direct, mid forehead, and coronal brow lift may be technically excellent procedures for some men but psychologically contraindicated in others.

Performing a Brow or Forehead Lift Simultaneously with Upper Lid Blepharoplasty

Many surgeons are very disinclined to perform a brow or forehead lift concomitantly with an upper blepharoplasty.[8–10] Both procedures can create lagophthalmos, particularly during the early postoperative phase. Furthermore, neither can be thoroughly completed when both procedures are done at the same time, even though some surgeons choose to combine the two procedures for expediency or perhaps monetary reasons.

On the other hand, lower lid blepharoplasty is an excellent accompaniment to brow or forehead lift. The overactive frontalis muscle will gradually relax, and both patient and surgeon can decide after approximately 6 weeks whether an adjunctive upper blepharoplasty is indicated. Surgeons who follow this principle will find that the forehead or brow lift will commonly correct the upper lid zone to such an extent that the patient does not desire upper blepharoplasty for some time thereafter, which is an obvious benefit for the patient. Upper blepharoplasty is not a difficult procedure, and there is no major reason not to defer it. However, if upper blepharoplasty is necessary or desirable after the results of the brow lift become apparent, a better planned and more complete procedure can then be performed. In this way, the results are gratifying to both surgeon and patient, and the surgical risks and complications are reduced by temporally separating the two procedures.

Another problem is trying to get the patient to understand and agree to appropriate staging of these procedures rather than have them performed simultaneously. For this reason, many cutaneous surgeons discount the fees for a staged secondary procedure in much the same way as a secondary procedure done at the same sitting is discounted. For secondary procedures, there are additional costs to the patient in the form of anesthesia and operating room fees, but there are also a number of significant benefits to both the patient and the surgeon. These primarily relate to a reduction in both the morbidity rate and the potential complications. The professional fees for the evaluation and discussion are also reduced when dealing with patients with whom the cutaneous surgeon is already familiar, as such patients are already informed about the procedure.

Anesthesia

Most blepharoplasty patients can be made much more comfortable if intravenous sedation is used along with local anesthesia. In these cases, the patient receives an antiemetic (usually droperidol [Inapsine]), which also serves as an antihistamine and enhancer for narcotic drugs. Butorphanol (Stadol) can be used for less uncomfortable procedures such as blepharoplasty, but meperidine (Demerol) or fentanyl (Sublimaze) are also commonly used. Butorphanol is more likely to elevate blood pressure initially and should be avoided in patients with a systolic blood pressure of more than 140 to 150 mm Hg. However, butorphanol is also less likely to provoke nausea. Intravenous sedation is often additionally titrated with a sedative agent such as diazepam (Valium) or midazolam (Versed).

Adequate preoperative consultation with the physician and staff can often take the place of medications in allaying patient anxiety. This allows the surgeon to take photographs and mark the surgical area with the patient upright, discuss any last-minute additions or changes in the surgery, and review surgical or postoperative information just before surgery. It also avoids one of the most common problems of surgery; the administration of standardized doses of medication to every patient. Patients vary enormously in their need for and tolerance of sedatives, and because only the minimal amount of medication necessary should be used, titrated intravenous sedation is often the best way to achieve this goal.

For blepharoplasty,[11–13] the local anesthetic consists of 2% lidocaine with 1:50,000 fresh-mixed epinephrine added from a snap-top glass vial. Fresh epinephrine provides much more reliable hemostasis than can be obtained from premixed solutions. Both upper lids are injected first, and then a small amount of anesthetic is infiltrated along the incision lines for the lower lid. The lower lids are injected later so that local anesthesia is obtained only 10 to 15 minutes before the lid surgery is begun. The second upper lid is also lightly reinjected about 10 minutes before completion of the first upper lid. This fresh application of anesthetic means that good vasoconstrictor effects are present at the time of surgery before each individual lid is begun. For the direct or mid forehead brow lift, injection of commercially prepared 2% lidocaine with 1:100,000 epinephrine is usually adequate.

More sedation is usually necessary for the coronal lift than for blepharoplasty. Occasionally, a patient may benefit from the injection of small amounts of dilute methohexital sodium (Brevital), particularly if uncomfortable areas are affected by the surgery (e.g., along the brow ridges). Local anesthesia for coronal lifting begins with injection of the premarked coronal incision line using a 1-inch 30-gauge needle containing about 5 ml of 1% lidocaine with fresh-mixed 1:100,000 epinephrine. Next, the linear wheal of injected solution is extended anteriorly from just above each ear, across the lower temporal-zygomatic zone, and to the lateral orbital rim to anesthetize the ascending sensory fibers. The needle is then directed along each brow ridge, continuing across to the medial side in the region of the supraorbital and supratrochlear nerve bundles. Some anesthetic is also infiltrated into the nasofrontal and uppermost nasal bridge areas to permit lysis of the procerus muscle during surgery.

Anesthesia is completed by injecting a linear wheal

across the mid forehead from temple to temple. Although this is not done by most cutaneous surgeons, it can be very helpful in anesthetizing sensory fibers ascending in the forehead that are not anesthetized by the routine brow ridge block, as well as the small perforating sensory nerves that often exit the skull on each side of the forehead at this level.

Last, the coronal incision zone is reinjected. This is extremely helpful, as the anesthetic and vasoconstrictive effects are rapidly lost as a result of the vascularity of the scalp. However, the residual anesthesia will allow the second injection to be performed relatively painlessly. If an additional 10 minutes are spent with other preparations for surgery, there will be much less bleeding. The injection of the forehead and incision zone will require approximately 20 ml of the anesthetic solution.

For better control of postoperative pain, the surgeon may wish to mix 1% lidocaine with 0.25% bupivacaine in a ratio of 1:1. Despite these efforts and the use of intravenous sedation, some patients may still need reinjection in certain areas, particularly the lower margins of the flap and beneath the brows. If a sensitive area is encountered while beginning dissection of this zone, it is best to stop immediately and reinject the brow ridge, as adequate dissection here is absolutely vital for a good result. Keep in mind that lidocaine is a rapid vasodilator, whereas epinephrine exerts its vasoconstrictor effect much more slowly.

"Sequencing" is an important part of this surgery. For example, the coronal lift should always be done first, because it is a more uncomfortable procedure than blepharoplasty. In addition, during the final stages of the coronal lift, the procedure is ceased briefly so that local anesthetic can be injected for blepharoplasty. Thus, adequate vasoconstriction and anesthesia will be present when the blepharoplasty phase of the procedure begins.

Surgical Anatomy and Its Importance

UPPER EYELID

For the upper lid, it should be kept in mind that dermatochalasis is always accompanied by equal attenuation and looseness of the underlying orbicularis oculi muscle. This attenuated muscle can be removed along with the excess skin, although it may be preferable to remove each layer separately. In Asians and some Polynesians or blacks, a considerable amount of submuscular fat may also be present, particularly in the lateral part of this surgical zone.[13] This fat should be trimmed away, at least in females, to the septal level. The submuscular fat extends beneath the muscle cephalad to the surgical zone and may also be trimmed away as necessary to sculpt this infrabrow area, taking care to avoid the relatively large veins that run in the subcutaneous fat. It should also be noted that a considerable number of patients have supraorbital notches in the orbital rim rather than foramina for the supraorbital and

supratrochlear nerve. For this reason, any dissection in the superior medial upper lid zone should be done with care.[14]

Some patients have relatively weak orbicularis oculi muscles, a condition that may seem accentuated in the postoperative period by swelling or the lingering physiologic effects of the local anesthetic. Thus, removal of fat and orbicularis muscle in the pretarsal zone, as advocated by some surgeons, should be done with particular caution, as this portion of the pretarsal muscle is primarily involved with upper lid closure.

A lateral fat pad, either totally separate or associated on its medial end with the middle fat pad, is very commonly found in Asians and in a relatively small percentage of whites.[12, 13, 15] Like the lateral fat pad of the lower lids, this fat pad is closer to the ciliary margin than the middle and medial pads. Because it adds significant bulk to the lateral upper lid area, attention to its removal is particularly important in women. It is found by performing delicate dissection, using the tips of small scissors, through the relatively thick septum at a point approximately 8 mm above the lateral canthus. This fat pad, if entirely separate, has a medial and lateral attachment on either side of the inferior pole of the lacrimal gland (Fig. 44-3). It can usually be plucked up easily with fine-toothed forceps. It is important to be sure that the similarly colored lacrimal gland is not inferiorly herniated and excised along with the fat pad. A significantly ptotic lacrimal gland can be carefully suspended back into place with one or two 6-0 nylon sutures.

In Asians and some obese individuals, the orbital septum may be particularly thick or even multilayered with fibrous tissue and fat.[16] Nonetheless, the middle fat pad is usually not difficult to dissect, whereas the medial fat pad is lighter in color and more difficult to find and to tease upward for trimming. As a variant, the middle pad sometimes extends medially to the zone above the medial canthus, even taking the place of the medial fat pad insofar as the excess fat that can be removed. It may also extend laterally to fill the zone anterior to the lacrimal gland.

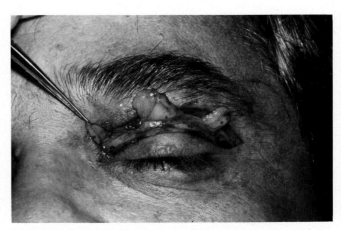

Figure 44-3. The forceps hold the medial fat pad, but dissection has also revealed *separate* middle and lateral fat pads.

LOWER EYELID

In the lower lid, particularly in patients with lax lids, it is wise to keep the lateral end of the incision over the orbital rim and at least several millimeters below the level of the lateral canthus so that the lateral canthal ligament and its inferior crus are left untouched. This ligament, its continuations of fibrous tissue across the ciliary zone of the lower lids, and the associated narrow tarsal plate and its overlying orbicularis muscle are the primary support structures for the lower lid. Medially, the punctum is readily apparent. Within the lid beneath it, the lacrimal duct extends about 2 mm inferiorly before turning rather sharply medially toward the lacrimal sac. The subciliary incision should stop just short of the punctum and several millimeters below it to reduce the risk of possible damage to the lacrimal duct.

In the lower lid, the lateral fat pad is often the most difficult to find surgically, being overlaid by a thicker septum similar to that of the upper lid. However, it is often the most visible herniated fat pad as patients turn their eyes from side to side. Light pressure on the upper lid will often push this pad sufficiently forward to make it visible for scissors dissection. Again, the middle pad is usually quite apparent, while the medial pad is lighter in color and more difficult to find. Caution is required when trimming the medial pads of both the upper and lower lids because of the occasional presence of large veins over and within these fat pads.

BROW

The anatomy of the brow region is somewhat complex. In most patients, the brows achieve their prominence by a conjunction of inferiorly and superiorly oriented hair growth in the medial portion and midportion of the brow, and the brow hairs generally grow outward and slightly downward in the lateral third of the brow. Recognition of this hair angle is very important in the direct brow lift procedure, because the incision over the medial and middle thirds of the brow must be beveled at an acute upward angle to avoid severing the follicles.

The brow hairs are also important in planning surgery for some patients, particularly Asians, because of very diffuse brow hairs that are more dense over the brow ridge. This is most important if a direct brow lift is being considered, because an excision superior to the main brow density will remove some of the fine hairs above it, creating an abrupt superior brow border and an artificial appearance when compared with the more diffuse nature of the inferior border. In addition, some brows are composed of hairs that all grow downward, making camouflaging of the direct brow lift scar more difficult in the early healing phase, because the brows cannot be brushed up. Fine hairs may also occur on the infrabrow skin as far down as the supratarsal crease in some patients, and removal of this skin during blepharoplasty may result in small cysts and even tiny ingrown hairs along the incision line.

The male brow tends to be horizontal and situated on or just slightly below the superior orbital rim. The arching female brow normally sits above the orbital rim with its peak about 1 cm above it. To be most aesthetically pleasing, the female brow should begin medially on a vertical line above the medial canthus or the lateral side of the ala and should end laterally on a line that starts at the lateral edge of the ala and passes through the lateral canthus as it ascends to the lateral brow ridge. The medial and lateral ends of the female brow should be on the same horizontal plane, and the peak or maximal arch of the brow should be between two tangential lines extended vertically from the lateral edge of the limbus as well as the lateral canthus.[7] Some patients may have plucked their brows into quite aesthetically unpleasing shapes. It is worthwhile to mention to these patients that after blepharoplasty or brow lift, the physician will evaluate their brows and suggest a more pleasing shape at that time. Nonetheless, it is difficult to convince some patients that their oddly arched or down-slanted brows are not representative of artistic perfection, as they may have come to believe them to be.

Just deep to the brow, the inferior limits of the deeper, thicker frontalis muscle interdigitate with the superior limits of the thin, superficial orbicularis muscle, and some of the frontalis fibers also insert more deeply into the superior orbital rim. Unfortunately, this is most true in the area of the bilateral nerve bundles, which makes dissection of this area more difficult. It also probably accounts for the relative lack of ptosis of this medial brow zone compared with the lateral brow area.

The normal course of the temporal or frontal branch of the facial nerve ascends on a line from just below the tragus of the ear through a point about 1.5 cm above the lateral end of the brow. However, the late bifurcation of this nerve and the thin tissues through which it passes to reach the forehead dictate that special care be taken when performing direct, mid forehead, and coronal brow lifting.[17, 18] The direct and mid forehead brow lifts take place in a subcutaneous plane and should not injure the motor nerve; however, traction, the injection of anesthetic, surgical trauma, and placement of fixation sutures all have the potential to temporarily or permanently injure the frontal nerve. With the coronal lift, the lateral portion of the dissection extends down along the temple. Because the deep fascia of the frontalis muscle is particularly thin in this critical area, delicate blunt dissection is required. A small sensory nerve may be found perforating the skull on one or both sides of the mid forehead region.

Removal of glabellar frown lines to improve a "worried" or "angry" look is commonly desired by many patients. The corrugator muscles may be particularly large in these patients. Unfortunately, these muscles lie over the medial brow ridge just superficial to the exiting supraorbital and supratrochlear nerve bundles, and delicate dissection is necessary to properly remove them in their entirety without injuring the nerves. The procerus muscle is of little importance in rejuvenating the forehead and glabellar zone and is adequately lysed by simple blunt scissors dissection at the nasal root.

Surgical trauma, severing of some fibers of the ascending forehead nerve bundles, the coronal incision itself, and probably the traction produced by the lifting commonly cause hypoesthesia, paresthesia, or anesthesia of the frontal scalp for at least a few months after a coronal lift. It is important to remember that the posterior branch of the superficial temporal vessels, usually encountered approximately 4 cm above the ear, is almost always severed by the inferior portions of the coronal lift incision and often requires cautery or even suture ligation. Also, consider that the scalp hairs in the upper portion and midportion of the coronal lift incision are angled forward at about a 45-degree angle, while the hairs in the lateral portions of the incision are angled downward. This is especially important when excising redundant scalp during coronal lifting, to preserve follicles adjacent to the incision line.

Surgical Instruments and Equipment

BLEPHAROPLASTY

Green marking forceps are quite helpful in pinching the upper lid skin for proper preoperative estimation of appropriate skin excision. For the lower lids, blunt-tipped tenotomy scissors are helpful in undermining the skin-muscle flap. For clamping the fat pads, a gently curved, fine-toothed hemostat is preferable. A 1-inch 30-gauge needle on a 3-ml syringe allows for the most delicate injection of the lids and the fat pads. An ordinary hyfrecator is a most convenient and excellent method for stopping pinpoint bleeding at the stump of resected fat pads. This method is superior to bipolar cautery and obviates the problem of electric current passing through the eye structures.[19]

DIRECT AND MID FOREHEAD BROW LIFT

Blunt tenotomy or small Metzenbaum scissors are useful for performing delicate dissection and for freeing the attachments of the orbicularis muscle to the frontalis muscle. Double skin hooks, with the paired hooks about 1 cm apart, are also useful.

CORONAL FOREHEAD LIFT

It is often helpful to obtain hemostasis during scalp incision through the use of a Shaw scalpel, a cutting-current spatula blade, or the "electric scalpel" with disposable No. 10 blades. Multihook Anderson rake retractors are also very helpful, as are Raney clips for incision line bleeders. Straight 7-inch face lift scissors with double-edged blades are also useful for blunt undermining, particularly at the lateral brow ridge and the nasofrontal angle.

Surgical Techniques

UPPER LID BLEPHAROPLASTY[7–10, 12, 13, 20–23]

The line of the superior incision generally parallels the arch of the brow. When joined to the inferior incision line, it should outline an excisional area that is significantly wider in its lateral third. Medially, the two incision lines need not come to a point but instead can be joined by an abrupt conjuncture whose dartlike point forms approximately a 60-degree angle (Fig. 44–4). The lid skin is so thin in this area that closure of this abrupt angle does not create a dogear. Once the submuscular fat has been thoroughly removed from the lateral one third of the excision area, persistent fullness of the septal zone just above the lateral canthus may suggest the presence of a lateral fat pad. Such a bulge will generally be lower and beneath a thicker septum than the rare ptotic lacrimal gland (Fig. 44–3).

If the septum is relatively thick, it can be opened side to side by simply removing a narrow strip of tissue with small curved scissors. This should always be done across the upper third of the excision zone to avoid trauma to the levator aponeurosis. Excess fibrofatty tissue should be delicately removed using fine forceps and scissors to allow better tissue fixation during healing and precise placement of temporary or permanent fixation sutures for the creation of the lid crease. Some surgeons prefer to leave the pretarsal zone of the eyelid alone, if possible. Removal of excess tissue bulkiness in this area or lysing of secondary lid creases across this zone tends not only to result in extended lid edema but can also make the placement of fixation sutures and the creation of bilateral symmetry difficult.

When removing orbital fat, slight pressure on the lower lid will reveal whether all the excess fat of the middle pad has been removed. The medial pad is removed conservatively so as not to create excess hollowing in this zone. After removal of the excess tissue, the stump of the medial pad is grasped with fine forceps before the clamp is released. This is done because significant bleeding is likely to occur from this pad, which may retract instantly when released, making hemostasis very difficult to obtain and risking hemorrhage into the deeper aspects of the orbit. Such hemorrhage calls for immediate opening of the tissues with scissors tips to allow the blood to escape while the bleeding vessel is sought.

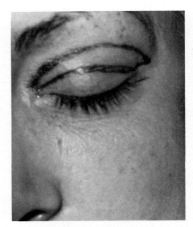

Figure 44–4. An area of upper blepharoplasty excision has been outlined with an abrupt medial end and enlarged lateral portion that extends well beyond the lateral canthus (for female patients).

In sculpting the upper lid zone, lids that are bulky in the infrabrow area should have at least some submuscular fat trimmed in a tapering fashion away from the inferior part of this area near the flap edge. However, patients with more hollow eyes who show some supracrease sulcus preoperatively should have this area left intact to avoid creating an even more hollow appearance and a "skeletonized" look as this fat layer regresses with aging. Buried tarsal fixation sutures, using 6-0 clear nylon, are usually three or four in number and confined to the central portion of the desired crease zone. The medial and lateral ends of the crease are allowed to form on their own during tissue retraction (Fig. 44–5). Surface sutures should penetrate and precisely appose both the skin and muscle layers to achieve a very fine scar line. If 6-0 nylon is used, the sutures are removed after 3 days. Temporary, externalized fixation sutures, if used, are removed after 7 days.

LOWER LIDS

The lateral fat pad should be treated first. It can most easily be found by piercing the somewhat thicker septum, often present at a point about 8 to 10 mm below the lateral canthus. In many whites this fat pad can readily be seen, but in Asians it may consist of many small, firm "granules" of fat overlaid by septal tissues, rather than a distinct soft pad that can be resected en bloc. The lateral fat pad excess should be removed aggressively, because this is the most likely area to show a recurrent bulge postoperatively. Again, the middle pad is excised to the septal level, checking for remnant excess with gentle pressure on the upper lid. As in the upper lid, the medial pad is excised conservatively with care.

It is often possible to use blunt scissors tips to free up the attachments of the orbicularis muscle to the lower orbital rim in seeking to diminish the lid-cheek grooves that are often clinically apparent. Such dissection may serve to create a very fine sheet of scar tissue in this area, which makes the lid slightly thicker and more opaque, causing these clinically visible grooves to appear less deep and less dusky in color. In some patients it may be possible to transpose small segments of more fibrous fat that still have some vascular supply into such a groove area and very delicately suturing them into place. Small free grafts will occasionally work for such an endeavor but can also bunch up into a visible papule beneath the skin or be resorbed.

The classic skin flap technique is of some value in patients whose primary problem is loose skin, but it can result in uneven lumpiness and very slow healing. It is also far more likely to generate patient complaints in the postoperative period than the more common skin-muscle flap. In addition, the skin-muscle flap allows thinning of the muscle along the upper edge of the flap if the patient has an orbicularis roll. The initial entry for this skin-muscle flap consists of a skin-only incision using just the tip of a Beaver miniblade (No. 6500) with its edge held upward. The muscle is then cut tangentially across the lid, using small scissors with the blades held at a downward angle so as to leave behind some of the muscle over the narrow tarsal zone. The tarsus and this narrow strip of muscle are the main support structures for the lower lid margin and help to prevent a round eye appearance and even ectropion.

Trimming of the lower lid flap excess is accomplished by having the lightly sedated patient open the mouth widely and look up. The lower lid skin-muscle flap is then draped very gently into place with no upward pull. Any excess tissue that extends above the subciliary incision line, which is usually only a small amount, is carefully trimmed off with small scissors, again beveling the cut downward to correspond with the angled initial entry. Closure is completed with spaced 6-0 silk sutures that pass through both skin and muscle for a precise closure; these are removed after 3 days. Close attention is paid to suturing the zone beneath the lateral canthus, where misalignment or slight grooving is more likely to occur during healing.

Malar bags (Fig. 44–6) that are present beneath the lower lids are best treated by making a small lateral crow's foot incision rather than the usual blepharoplasty incision. While pressing down on the zone of fullness

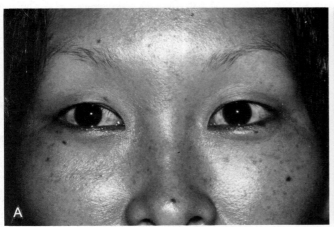
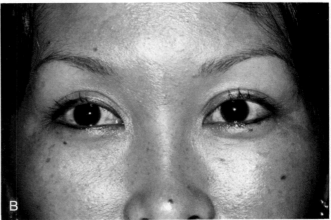

Figure 44–5. *A,* Asian woman before blepharoplasty without an eyelid crease. *B,* Three months after "double eyelid" blepharoplasty with only three fixation sutures above the central lid zone.

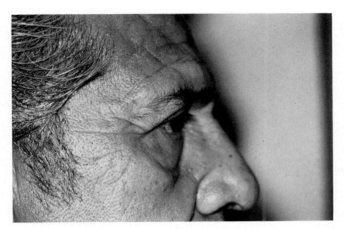

Figure 44–6. Man with remnant "malar bag" inferior to the middle and lateral lower lid, 7 months after blepharoplasty.

with the thumb of the opposite hand, the area is suctioned very delicately with a 14-gauge needle cannula on a 3- or 5-ml syringe.

DIRECT BROW LIFT

The direct brow lift procedure has not received the attention it should as a cosmetic procedure, largely because it was previously performed poorly or in too simplistic a fashion. However, when properly done, the direct brow lift almost always yields elegant and long-lasting results. Its advantage is that it is performed right where the problem is located, and the brow can be shaped with relative precision, even varying the lift from side to side to compensate for brow asymmetry. Another significant advantage is that it can be done with local anesthesia alone. Its drawbacks are visible overcorrection in the first week or two postoperatively and a slowly healing scar that may be visible for 6 months or more. Nonetheless, there is seldom the need for later dermabrasion or other scar camouflage, and patients who have accepted this procedure with the knowledge of its healing phase are usually very pleased with its results. Patients often wear bangs or large-framed glasses, in addition to makeup, during the early healing phase, with good effect.

The best candidate for a direct brow lift has smooth, thin skin; patients with thick, oily, poral skin do not do as well. To measure the amount of lift needed, the cutaneous surgeon holds a graduated rule vertically in the lateral canthal line with its base on the cheekbone while noting the level of the inferior brow margin with the patient's face at rest. The forehead is then manually elevated by the surgeon until the brow is at the desired position, and the height of the inferior brow border is again noted on the vertical rule. The amount of lift needed is usually about 7 or 8 mm. To mark the necessary area of excision, a line is first drawn directly along the superior margin of the brow from its medial to lateral end. At the lateral end, the line then extends outward and slightly upward for an additional 10 to 12 mm in a gentle "S" curve form. The superior line of the

incision begins at an acute angle with the medial end of the inferior line, arcing upward to peak vertically above the lateral limbus or lateral canthus, and then arcing slightly downward to meet the lateral end of the primary incision line. Thus, the amount of tissue removal in the lateral third of the excision is much more than in the medial third (Fig. 44–7). With meticulous closure, the temporal portion beyond the end of the brow is not a problem and heals very well.

After obtaining local anesthesia, the marked lines are carefully incised with a No. 15 blade to a depth of only 1 mm. This transepidermal cut merely allows the scalpel blade to follow the proper line as it is turned to a very steep angle of 45 to 60 degrees upward to follow the same angle as the brow hairs. A transcutaneous incision is completed from the medial end to a point about two thirds of the way across the brow, at which time the scalpel is gradually brought over an additional distance of about 1 cm to a vertical position once again in parallel with the brow hairs of the lateral third of the brow; in this way the incision of the inferior line is completed to its most lateral point. The superior line is incised in the same fashion so that it is again parallel to the hair follicles of the brow. Both upper and lower incisions repeat the same angle of beveling (Fig. 44–8). As the skin between the two incision lines is dissected free with the scalpel tip, care is taken to spare the underlying frontalis muscle with these incisions. Starting at the lateral end of the brow, where there is less decussation of frontalis and orbicularis muscle fibers, blunt tenotomy scissors are used to enter the zone beneath the brow and bluntly dissect beneath it from lateral to medial in a submuscular dissection deep to the brow.

The scissors are next used to transect the remnant narrow zone of interdigitating muscle fibers between the undermined brow and the area of resection just above the brow. This lysed strip represents the decussation between the orbicularis and frontalis fibers. At this point the brow itself is free to be easily lifted upward. The sharp, closed tips of iris scissors are then used to carefully pierce and spread the frontalis muscle in four

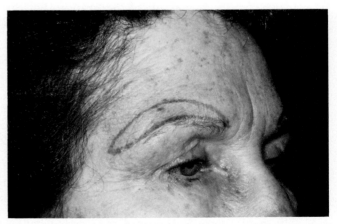

Figure 44–7. An area of direct brow lift excision has been outlined with a narrow medial end, a broad lateral portion, maximal width above the lateral canthus, and extension beyond the lateral end of the brow.

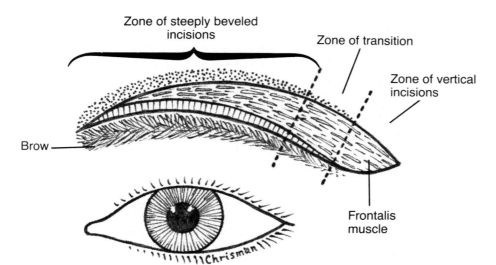

Figure 44–8. A schematic showing how the direct brow lift incisions parallel the brow hairs and gradually become perpendicular to the skin in the most lateral areas.

or five small areas about 1 to 1.5 cm apart along the superior margin of excision in the forehead. Using a small, curved needle, fixation sutures of 4-0 clear nylon are placed between the orbicularis muscle layer, just underneath the brow, and the periosteum deep to the small frontalis perforations. These perforations allow precise placement of the fixation sutures into the periosteum and provide visualization to ensure that the sutures are not encompassing any frontalis muscle fibers and therefore are not passing around one of the ascending sensory nerve fibers medially or motor nerve fibers laterally. The fixation sutures are then tied to lift the brow into the desired position. Significant inward puckering of the brow itself as a result of the fixation sutures must be avoided. The closure is completed with a series of precise 6-0 clear nylon subcuticular sutures and 6-0 nylon running surface sutures placed using very small bites to create slight eversion. A small dressing is applied once both brows have been finished. Surface sutures are removed after 4 to 5 days, and the lateral end of the lift zone beyond the brow is supported with adhesive tape strips. Immediately after surgery, the brow may seem to be slightly flattened and the forehead above it may be somewhat puffy as a result of the fixation, but this usually resolves spontaneously over a period of about 2 weeks.

MID FOREHEAD BROW LIFT

The advantages of the mid forehead brow lift lie in the fact that because the actual forehead rhytides can be used as entry zones, the closure lines may resemble rhytides and be less noticeable. The right and left excisions are at two different levels on the mid to upper forehead to make the closure lines asymmetric and therefore less obvious. The drawback is that the incision lines, even if placed asymmetrically as they should be, are quite visible, particularly in oily-skinned patients, especially men. Because this surgery is somewhat removed from the brow itself, if fixation sutures weaken or fail, stretch-back will occur as the skin between the incision and the brow relaxes and stretches, allowing

the brow to drop down more than is desired. Another potential problem is that bleeding from the muscle along the brow ridge area may be more difficult to manage, since the incision is 2 to 6 cm from the brow. Finally, there are fewer fixation sutures than in the direct brow lift, making the brow more difficult to shape and increasing the risk that the fixation sutures may pull out from the thin tissue beneath the brow.

Local anesthesia is again used with this procedure. A semi-ellipse of skin whose medial and lateral ends are on vertical lines above the medial and lateral brow ends is removed, with the widest part of the ellipse over the desired maximum arch of the brow. The skin between the excision zone and the brow is undermined, and at least two fixation sutures of 4-0 semipermanent or permanent material are used between the underside of the brow and the periosteum at the upper margin of the excision zone. Tightening these fixation sutures will lift the brow into its desired arched position so that careful layered closure can be completed.[7] A period of 6 months or more may be necessary for the scar to gradually mature and lose its discoloration.

CORONAL FOREHEAD LIFT

Since the 1980s, the coronal lift has enjoyed steadily increasing popularity because of both its hidden scar and its ability to simultaneously solve several cosmetic problems with only one procedure. It is ideal for the patient with a low or average hairline, transverse forehead rhytides, deep glabellar frown lines, and low brows (Fig. 44–9). In addition, drooping of the lower temple and lateral periocular areas, with accentuated crow's foot lines, is also usually helped by the coronal lift. The procedure's major drawbacks are that it is more extensive and thus subject to greater morbidity, and it requires significant sedation or general anesthesia for its completion. Patients should also understand that the frontal and temporal hairline will be elevated perhaps 2 cm initially and 1 cm permanently and that there will often be significant paresthesia or anesthesia of the frontal scalp for at least a few months after surgery.

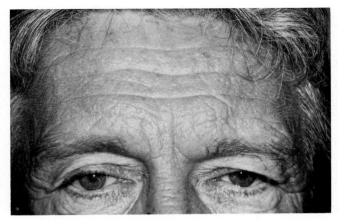

Figure 44–9. An ideal candidate for a coronal forehead lift with upper lid excess fat, drooping brows and temples with associated crow's-feet rhytides, glabellar frown lines, transverse forehead lines, and moderate hairline height.

They should also be aware that the forehead may be nearly inactive for 4 to 6 weeks postoperatively as a result of stretching of the frontal nerve and surgical edema, and that they will have little or no motion of the central forehead, as well as the glabellar frown area. Most patients are delighted to hear of the latter deficits.

After local anesthesia has been obtained and trimming of the hair in the zone of the anticipated scalp excision has been performed, the scalp is incised in perpendicular fashion. Because the hair angles forward in much of the coronal incision zone, this leaves follicles along the posterior edge of the cut which will later grow hair through the line of closure. The incision extends from side to side on a semicoronal line that starts about 2 cm above the ear on each side and runs more or less parallel to the hairline and approximately 6 to 7 cm posterior to it. This creates a gentle arch on each side that meets in a forward-facing angle of about 120 degrees at the superior midline. A cut is also made anteriorly for about 2 cm from the junction of the two incision arcs. Also, in anticipation of later resection, a back cut upward and forward about 2 cm long and using a 30-degree angle is created from the most inferior ends of the incision. All three of these cuts later become part of the scalp excision and aid in eversion of the forehead flap. Raney clips or an electrocautery are used to control bleeding along the incision line. Only occasionally are suture ligatures needed for the superficial temporal vessels.

A broad, paddle-shaped periosteal elevator with the edges ground off or a pair of face lift scissors are used to complete a subgaleal dissection of the mid and midlateral forehead. Great care is exercised for the lateral forehead and temporal portions of the dissection in the zone anterior to the hairline, as the frontal nerve is at risk in this area. Of special note is the fact that the galea becomes the deep frontalis fascia in this lateral area, and the fascia, as well as the muscle, is thin and attenuated in this zone. Also, the fascia in the midline tends to be adherent to the pericranium in the mid and lower forehead. Here the pericranium is adherent to the flap, and care should be taken to leave this protective layer intact as much as possible.

Utilizing palpation as well as direct vision, blunt-tipped scissors are used to carefully free the lateral and midlateral portions of the brow from the orbital rim. In the midline, the scissors tips also undermine the naso-frontal angle to lyse the attachments of the procerus muscle and also to dissect as far down on the nasal bridge as desired. Anderson rake retractors are used to fully evert the flap, placing tension on the exiting neurovascular bundles as well as the corrugator muscles in the medial and midmedial brow area. Careful dissection helps to preserve the ascending nerve fibers and to locate the corrugator supercilii muscles, which course from the medial aspect of the brow ridge near the midline upward and outward for a distance of about 2 cm to insert onto the lower aspects of the frontalis muscles where it meets the brow (Fig. 44–10). Because the corrugator muscles are only 2 to 3 mm thick and approximately 1 cm wide, surface dimpling is not a problem after their complete removal. Corrugator muscle function tends to recover rather easily, so it is important to try to remove all of the muscle under direct vision, cauterizing the medial and lateral stumps to avoid muscle bleeding and injury to the nerves. Electrodesiccation greatly reduces the incidence of periocular ecchymosis, hematoma formation, and postoperative pain caused by bleeding and swelling in the area of the supratrochlear and supraorbital nerves after coronal lifting. It may be useful to inject bupivacaine along the medial brow ridge area at the completion of the surgical procedure to help reduce postoperative pain.

Next, the thin fascia on the undersurface of the frontalis muscle is incised between the left and right midpupillary lines and along horizontal lines that correspond to the surface rhytides above them. This is easily done by placing the tip of the index finger on the surface rhytid and the thumb on the undersurface of the flap and then everting the flap enough to incise just the fascia beneath the rhytid, moving the fingers along as the cut is completed from side to side. Care should be taken to avoid the ascending nerves, which are often visible just beneath the fascia at about the midpupillary lines. These incisions allow a narrow sheet of scar tissue to form beneath each surface rhytid so that complete resection of the frontalis centrally or electrocautery cross-hatching (Fig. 44–11) are unnecessary.[24, 25]

Meanwhile, after completing the resection of the first corrugator muscle, the anticipated area of scalp excision is injected with local anesthetic. The forehead flap can be repositioned about 10 to 15 minutes later, after resecting the second corrugator, with greatly improved hemostasis. Closure is begun at the inferior ends of the coronal incision with staples, first closing the area of the back cut. Guided by stepwise skin-splitting incisions, the excess scalp is excised parallel to the follicles in segments 3 to 4 cm long. Each resected area is closed sequentially with staples so as to achieve a slight upward rotation of each side of the flap. More tissue is removed in the temporal part of the scalp, the maximum excision usually being 2 to 2.5 cm wide at about 6 cm above the ear.

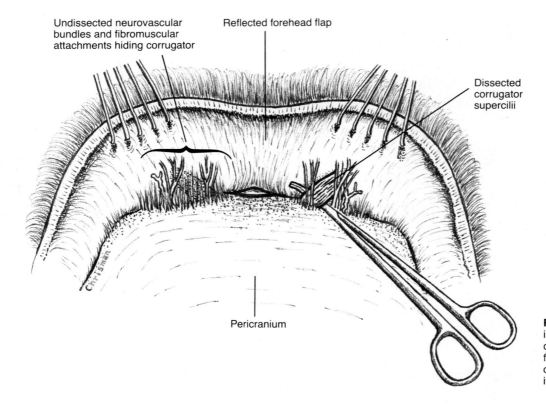

Undissected neurovascular bundles and fibromuscular attachments hiding corrugator

Reflected forehead flap

Dissected corrugator supercilii

Pericranium

Figure 44–10. A schematic showing the corrugator supercilii muscle dissected out, lying just superficial to the neurovascular bundles of the supratrochlear nerve and its primary branches.

Less scalp is removed superiorly, even though more could easily be taken, to avoid overlifting, which could result in the creation of a surprised look in the medial brow zone.

The goal is to move the lateral brows up as much as possible and the medial brows up only minimally. If there is no excess tension on the closure, there is no need to use galeal sutures. As the mildly up-rotating closure is completed, a relatively small dogear will result at the superior midline. To relieve this, a forward-pointing wedge is removed by excising the excess scalp on either side of the 2-cm forward cut that was made at the beginning of the procedure. This wedge is cut out

using inward beveling of both the right and left sides such that viable follicles will remain beneath the skin to later grow through the scar. Only enough scalp is removed to allow tensionless staple closure of this resected dogear, creating a V-to-Y juncture with the coronal line. Properly done, this closure site will heal almost invisibly.

Small rubberband drains are placed at the most inferior aspect of the incision lines only if there has been significant bleeding, which is rare. These drains, if used, are removed within 24 hours. A moderate head dressing is placed, extending well over the brow ridge so that greater pressure can be applied to this area than else-

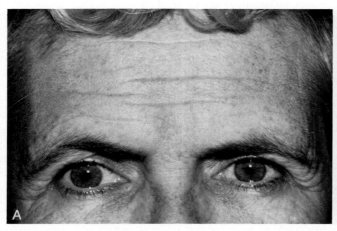

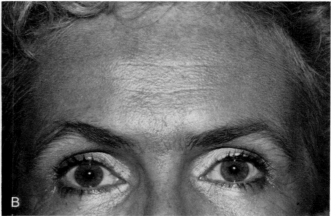

Figure 44–11. *A,* Preoperative appearance of a patient with transverse rhytides. *B,* Ten months after a coronal forehead lift, showing obliteration of transverse lines with the creation of a normal forehead after simple incision of the galea just beneath each rhytid.

where. The goal is to cause any blood in the brow zone to move upward rather than down into the periocular area. This dressing is left in place overnight. Only rarely do patients suffer radicular pain during the first 1 to 2 days postoperatively.

Complications and Adverse Sequelae

The complications of infection, scarring, skin slough, hematoma, and dehiscence—which are common with other surgical procedures—are very rare with blepharoplasty. However, patients should be aware that whenever bilateral surgery is done, healing may produce asymmetry. Also, poor healing or loose tissues can result in recurrent droop of the brow or supracrease lid tissues. Surgically created lid creases can also be asymmetric or dimpled. Lagophthalmos, common in the first few days after blepharoplasty, can cause a dry eye syndrome if persistent, as can lower lid retraction in the form of scleral show or ectropion. Persistent lagophthalmos, which may be caused by placing permanent fixation sutures too high on the levator aponeurosis, usually improves with time and lid exercises. Significant persistent scleral show or ectropion may occur in patients with lax lids. However, this is more often the result of excessive removal of lower lid skin and muscle in an attempt to correct the surface rhytides of the lower lid; such correction is better accomplished by a postblepharoplasty chemical peel. Excessive hollowing of the lower lid seldom occurs after blepharoplasty, but infrabrow hollowing of the upper lid may become obvious once dermatochalasis and excessive orbital fat have been removed, or it may occur as the result of overzealous removal of orbital or submuscular fat (Fig. 44–12).

Blindness, although rare, is obviously the most serious complication of blepharoplasty. All reported cases have apparently been associated with removal of orbital fat,[3] usually from the lower lids. For this reason, it is important to check the patient's visual acuity before and after blepharoplasty surgery and preferably the next day as well. Many cutaneous surgeons ask patients who are having lower lid blepharoplasty to get an ophthalmologic examination before surgery. Blindness seems to be most often associated with acute intra- or postoperative retrobulbar bleeding.[1, 2] Intraoperatively, such bleeding should be relieved as quickly as possible. A postoperative hematoma accompanied by acute increasing pain, particularly if there is any compromise of vision, calls for immediate decompression of the eye. This is accomplished by opening the incision line and possibly performing a lateral canthotomy, perhaps coupled with the use of intravenous acetazolamide (Diamox) and mannitol. Ophthalmologic consultation is always appropriate if there is any question of a visual problem postoperatively.

Direct and mid forehead brow lift carry little risk of complications other than relatively minor periocular ecchymosis, as long as the dissection is maintained in a plane above the frontalis muscle. However, the adverse sequelae of overcorrection and persistent scars may require secondary treatment after about 6 to 8 months of healing. Also, correction may be either less than expected or only temporary.

For the coronal lift, the main adverse sequelae are an expected anesthesia and dysesthesia of the frontal scalp anterior and posterior to the incision. There may be significant itching and tingling of this area for 3 to 6 months after surgery. Significant bleeding is very seldom a problem if the corrugator muscle stumps have been cauterized and hemostasis has been achieved along the incision lines. However, the patient should be forewarned of the possibility of a "black eye" or at least significant periocular ecchymosis. The most serious complication of coronal lifting is injury to the frontal branch of the facial nerve, which results in weakness or drooping of the forehead on one side. Additionally, coronal lifts do not always achieve the amount of brow lifting anticipated, and in some patients stretch-back of the forehead skin causes the brows to return almost to their former level over time. Patients should be aware that

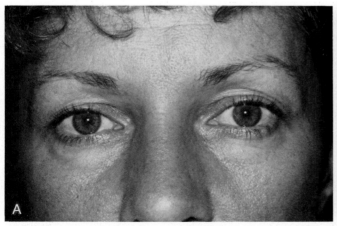 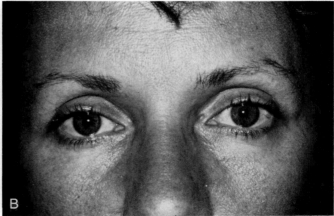

Figure 44–12. *A,* White patient with thin skin before upper blepharoplasty. *B,* Five months after conservative fat removal but with apparent "gaunt" eyelids due to anatomic factors.

temporary hair loss along the tension areas of the coronal lift closure is common for 3 to 6 months. Significant areas of permanent hair loss with scar width greater than 6 mm can be treated with full-sized hair transplants or minigrafts as necessary.

Long-Term Results

Blepharoplasty patients should be informed that rhytides, particularly those of the lower lids and the crow's feet area, will only be partially improved by the procedure. Also, the lower lids in particular require additional time for healing and resolution of edema. The results of lower lid surgery are best observed at least 4 to 6 months postoperatively, but upper lid results may be very rapidly apparent. Bulging of the lower lid lateral fat pad may recur despite efforts at thorough resection. Drooping of the upper lid tissues above the creaseline is especially likely to occur in low-browed patients who decline brow lift and in thin-skinned patients older than 40 years of age.

The results of direct brow lifting usually are maintained very well over time. This is the best method of permanent correction if the brows are the only cosmetic problem on the forehead (Fig. 44–13). After several months, coronal lift patients usually recover normal facial expression by using the lateral portions of the frontalis muscle, but the mid forehead usually remains pleasingly smooth. Surprisingly, some activity of the corrugator muscles may return despite thorough resection.

Variations on Standard Surgical Techniques

LASER BLEPHAROPLASTY

Laser blepharoplasty is gaining wide acceptance, as there is very little bleeding with this technique and therefore very little postoperative ecchymosis and swell-

ing.[26, 27] Transconjunctival lower lid laser blepharoplasty can also be done very rapidly. Patients experience minimal discomfort and show rapid and excellent cosmetic results. Unfortunately, much of the laser equipment is quite expensive to purchase and maintain, and the laser blepharoplasty procedure should only be performed by skilled and experienced laser surgeons. Nonetheless, it is very likely that more and more cosmetic surgery will be successfully performed with many of the currently available laser systems in the near future.

PRETRICHIAL FOREHEAD LIFT

The pretrichial forehead lift is simply a variation of the coronal lift in which the temporal incision lines arch forward more acutely, taking up a position along the frontal hairline until they meet in the midline.[9] The procedure takes longer than a coronal lift, because a very meticulous "stepped" incision is necessary along the frontal hairline to create a delicate and inconspicuous scar through which hairs will actually grow.[8] Patients with ruddy or dark complexions or severe sun damage should be aware that there may be a marked contrast between the lifted forehead skin and the pale scalp skin after healing. Although forehead dissection and brow zone surgery are easier to complete because of improved flap eversion, the pretrichial forehead lift carries an increased morbidity rate, because the ascending sensory nerves are severed several inches more proximally than with the coronal lift. These patients commonly have greater problems with both discomfort and dysesthesia in the frontal scalp that persists for a number of months after the procedure.

ADJUNCTIVE SCULPTING OF THE INFRABROW TISSUES

It is possible to delicately or aggressively remove the submuscular fat beneath the superior flap after routine upper lid blepharoplasty.[28] This fat can be removed all the way up to and beneath the brow, although care must be taken medially to avoid low-exiting supratrochlear

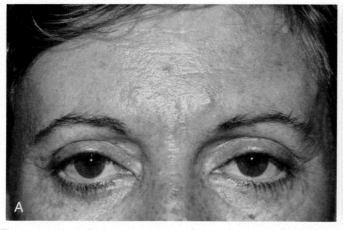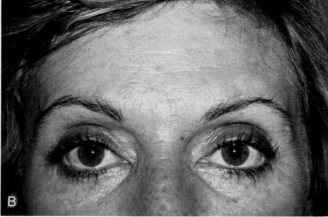

Figure 44–13. *A,* Patient who requested secondary upper lid blepharoplasty after previous surgery performed elsewhere gave poor results. *B,* Same patient wearing makeup 6 weeks after direct brow lift only, showing completely unhooded upper lids.

and supraorbital nerves. In addition, significant veins and small arteries course through this infrabrow fat, and meticulous use of the cautery is essential.

There may be diminished sensation at and above the brow for a few months after this more extensive version of blepharoplasty, but sculpting of the upper periocular region may be greatly improved, particularly in the patient with bulky infrabrow tissues. Adding this technique to upper blepharoplasty slightly increases the risk of hematoma.

INFRABROW LIFTING

In the infrabrow lifting technique, dissection takes place in the submuscular plane between the upper lid blepharoplasty zone and the middle and lateral third of the brow. This superior flap is then lifted with skin hooks, and permanent fixation sutures are placed between the inferior border of the brow and the more superior periosteum of the forehead. Adjustment in the number and position of these fixation sutures affects both the amount and type of brow lifting.[29, 30] This is a quick but somewhat less effective method of brow lifting. Because no tissue is removed above the brow, drooping of the brow would seem more likely to recur than with other methods of brow lifting.

LOWER LID TIGHTENING PROCEDURES

Pentagonal wedge resection and lateral canthopexy have been previously described in the blepharoplasty literature,[31-33] but more recently a simple technique of tightening the attenuated inferior crus of the lateral canthal ligament has been reported. In this technique, a routine skin-muscle flap blepharoplasty is done, but before closure, one or two permanent sutures are placed between the lateral end of the tarsal plate of the lower lid and the inner edge of the lateral orbital rim. These plicating sutures provide just the necessary support for the lower lid to prevent rounding or eversion of the lid during healing. This is a quick and simple technique[34] that certainly deserves attention.

TRANSCONJUNCTIVAL LOWER LID BLEPHAROPLASTY

Transconjunctival lower lid blepharoplasty utilizes topical anesthesia of the conjunctiva, a globe shield, and an electrocautery incision across the inferior aspect of the lower lid conjunctiva. This exposes the zone of the lateral, middle, and medial fat pads for relatively easy removal of the excess tissue. Closure is then accomplished with a single absorbable suture. With this technique, there is little risk of postoperative lid retraction or ectopion.[35] The main drawbacks are that there may not be much improvement in surface contour or rhytides, and it is impossible to remove excess lid tissue or sculpt an orbicularis roll. Nonetheless, this procedure is rapidly gaining acceptance for its speed and relative safety compared with the standard skin-muscle flap technique.

BLEPHAROPLASTY WITHOUT VIOLATING THE ORBITAL SEPTUM

With this technique, the fat pad bulges are identified, and the septum overlying them is cauterized and tightened by light, intermittent applications of electrodesiccation. No fat is removed, and the possibility of blindness is perhaps obviated.[19]

TISSUE-COMPATIBLE GLUES

Super-Glue does not provide ideal healing of tissues, but N-butyl-2-cyanoacrylate (Histoacryl) can be very useful for blepharoplasty, face lifts, and brow lifting.[36]

SUMMARY

Despite the fact that variations in anatomy and patient goals make blepharoplasty a challenging procedure, it can yield splendid results (Figs. 44–14, 44–15). However, blepharoplasty is so familiar to cosmetic surgeons and their patients that the ancillary procedures for the periocular and forehead zone are often not given appro-

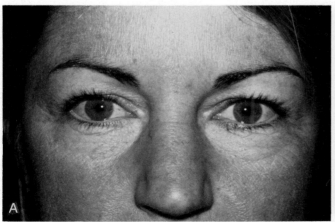
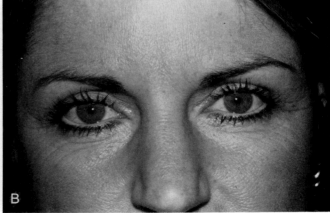

Figure 44–14. *A,* Preoperative appearance of a patient with dermatochalasis and blepharochalasis. *B,* Same patient wearing makeup 4 months after upper and lower blepharoplasty only.

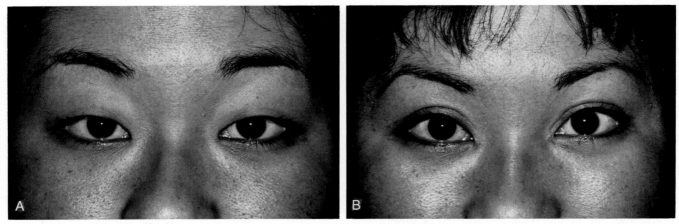

Figure 44–15. *A*, Preoperative appearance of an Asian woman, showing absence of lid creases. *B*, Seven months after double eyelid blepharoplasty, showing the effects of surgical sculpting and the creation of new lid creases.

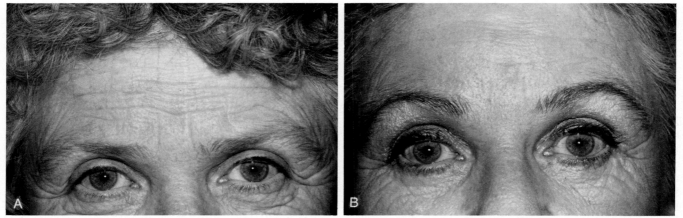

Figure 44–16. *A*, Preoperative appearance of a patient before a coronal forehead lift and lower blepharoplasty. *B*, Five months after these procedures, with improved brow height, forehead creases, and crow's-feet lines.

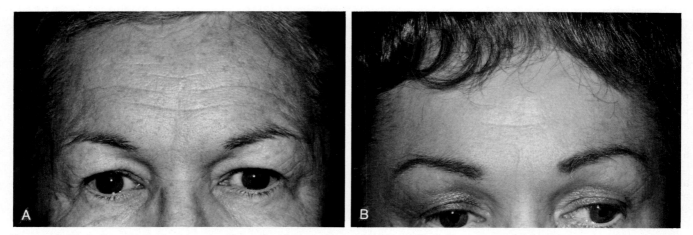

Figure 44–17. *A*, Preoperative appearance of a patient before a coronal forehead lift. *B*, Four years later, showing good results but that a simple secondary upper blepharoplasty is now indicated.

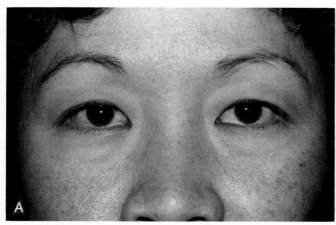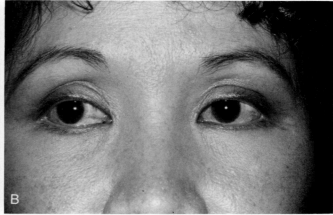

Figure 44–18. *A,* Asian patient before upper and lower blepharoplasty. *B,* Three months after aggressive surgery on the upper lids, yielding a high crease, a supracrease sulcus, and slight lowering of the lateral brows. Note that slight scleral show is also present, which may resolve with time.

priate consideration or recognition. At times, a patient may request blepharoplasty when the physical examination reveals that the upper lids are perfectly normal and the true problem is a ptotic brow and forehead tissues. Making the patient aware of these findings and performing an appropriate brow or forehead lifting procedure can yield extremely gratifying results (Figs. 44–16, 44–17) that are often much better than those a blepharoplasty alone could have achieved. Other patients obtain the best results by having a brow or coronal lift performed first, followed by a conservative upper lid blepharoplasty 6 weeks later when the frontalis muscle has relaxed. The simplicity of the procedure and the rapidity with which the incision lines of upper lid blepharoplasty heal often lead patients to pursue this procedure even if brow lift is indicated. However, these patients should be made aware that their choice may deny the possibility of brow or coronal lifting for 5 years or more until sufficient tissue laxity has occurred.

In some cases, patients who have had an aggressive upper lid blepharoplasty will have so little skin remaining that they may never be candidates for brow lifting. In addition, aggressive blepharoplasty may actually pull ptotic brows down even further as healing occurs (Fig. 44–18). Nonetheless, relatively aggressive upper lid blepharoplasty is quite acceptable in most cases, whereas lower lid blepharoplasty should involve conservative resection of excess tissue. Lower lid blepharoplasty, which is primarily a fat removal process, usually yields improvement only in surface contour, not rhytides.

Despite the interrelated complexities of the periorbital areas and scalp, cosmetic surgery of these areas can usually provide gratifying results with few complications and very little morbidity. These zones are the most important regions of facial animation and the first to show signs of aging, and the surgical techniques for treating these areas are numerous and are certain to undergo additional modifications and improvements in the future. As a consequence, surgery in these areas provides a great opportunity for cutaneous surgeons to demonstrate their significant knowledge and skills.

REFERENCES

1. Callahan M: Prevention of blindness after blepharoplasty. Ophthalmology 90:1047–1051, 1983.
2. Goldberg RA, Marmor RF, Shorr N, Christenbury JD: Blindness following blepharoplasty. Ophthalmol Surg 21:85–89, 1990.
3. Castillo GD: Management of blindness in the practice of cosmetic surgery. Otolaryngol Head Neck Surg 100:559–562, 1989.
4. Alexander GA, Roy RC, Ward CF: Letters to the Editor. Arch Otolaryngol Head Neck Surg 111:280–281, 1985.
5. Rees RD, La Trenta GD: The role of the Schirmer's test and orbital morphology in predicting dry eye syndrome after blepharoplasty. Plast Reconstr Surg 82:619–625, 1988.
6. McKinney P, Zukowski ML: The value of tear-film breakup and Schirmer's test in preoperative blepharoplasty evaluation. Plast Recontr Surg 84:572–576, 1989.
7. Cook TA, Brownrigg PS, Wang TD, Quatela VC: The versatile midforehead browlift. Arch Otolaryngol Head Neck Surg 115:163–168, 1989.
8. Kerth JD, Toriumi DM: Management of the aging forehead. Arch Otolaryngol Head Neck Surg 116:1137–1142, 1990.
9. Connel BF, Lambros VS, Neurohr GH: The forehead lift—techniques to avoid complications and produce optimal results. Aesthetic Plast Surg 13:217–237, 1989.
10. Bruck JC, Baker TJ, Gordon H: Facial mimics and the coronal brow lift. Aesthetic Plast Surg 11:199–201, 1987.
11. Chrisman B: Outpatient anaesthesia. J Dermatol Surg Oncol 14:939–946, 1988.
12. Chrisman BB: An overview of blepharoplasty. Cosmet Dermatol 2:28–31, 1989.
13. Chrisman BB: Blepharoplasty and browlift with surgical variations in non-white patients. J Dermatol Surg Oncol 12:58–66, 1986.
14. Webster RC: Supraorbital and supratrochlear notches and foramina: anatomical variations and surgical relevance. Laryngoscope 96:311–315, 1986.
15. Chrisman BB: The upper lateral fatpad in Oriental eyelids. Presented at the Plastic Surgery Section of the 17th Congress of the Pan Pacific Surgical Association, Sydney, Australia, 1984.
16. Chrisman BB: Oriental blepharoplasty. In: Coleman WP III, Hanke CW, Alt TH, Asken S (eds): Cosmetic Surgery of the Skin. BC Decker, Philadelphia, 1991, pp 303–315.
17. Pitanguy I, Ramos AS: The frontal branch of the facial nerve: the importance of its variation in face lifting. Plast Reconstr Surg 38:352–356, 1966.
18. Liebman EP: The frontalis nerve in the temporal brow lift. Arch Otolaryngol Head Neck Surg 108:232–235, 1982.
19. Bisaccia E, Scarborough DA, Swensen RD: A technique for blepharoplasty without incising or "puncturing" orbital septum. J Dermatol Surg Oncol 16:360–363, 1990.
20. Dedo DD: Rejuvenation of the forehead and brow. In: Dedo D (ed): The Atlas of Aesthetic Facial Surgery. Grune & Stratton, New York, 1984, pp 137–152.

21. Collins PS: Surgical procedures for correction of the ptotic brow. In: Coleman WP III, Hanke CW, Alt TH, Asken S (eds): Cosmetic Surgery of the Skin. BC Decker, Philadelphia, 1991, pp 317–333.

22. Brennan GH: The frontal lift. Arch Otolaryngol Head Neck Surg 104:26–30, 1978.

23. Asken S: Cosmetic eyelid surgery—blepharoplasty. In: Coleman WP III, Hanke CW, Alt TH, Asken S (eds): Cosmetic Surgery of the Skin. BC Decker, Philadelphia, 1991, pp 267–293.

24. Adamson PA: The forehead lift: a review. Arch Otolaryngol Head Neck Surg 111:325–329, 1985.

25. Fuleihan NS, Webster RC, Smith RC: The facelift and ancillary procedures. J Dermatol Surg Oncol 16:975–987, 1990.

26. David LA: The laser approach to blepharoplasty. J Dermatol Surg Oncol 14:741–746, 1989.

27. David LA, Abergel RP: CO_2 laser blepharoplasty. In: Coleman WP III, Hanke CW, Alt TH, Asken S (eds): Cosmetic Surgery of the Skin. BC Decker, Philadelphia, 1991, pp 295–301.

28. May JW Jr, Tearon J, Zingarelli P: Retro-orbicularis oculi (ROOF) resection in aesthetic blepharoplasty. Plast Reconstr Surg 86:682–689, 1990.

29. Paul MD: Surgical management of upper eyelid hooding. Aesthetic Plast Surg 13:183–187, 1989.

30. McCord CD, Doxanas MT: Browplasty and browpexy: an adjunct to blepharoplasty. Plast Reconstr Surg 86:248–254, 1990.

31. Anderson RL, Gordy DO: The tarsal strip procedure. Arch Ophthalmol 97:2191–2196, 1979.

32. Webster RC: A flap suspension technique in blepharoplasty on the lower lids. J Dermatol Surg Oncol 4:159, 1978.

33. Wolfley DE (ed): Blepharoplasty. (Monograph) Facial Plast Surg 1(Summer), 1984.

34. Jordan DR, Anderson RL: The tarsal tuck procedure: avoiding eyelid retraction after lower blepharoplasty. Plast Reconstr Surg 85:22–28, 1990.

35. Baylis HI, Long JA, Groth MJ: Transconjunctival lower eyelid blepharoplasty. Ophthalmology 96:1027–1032, 1989.

36. Ellis DA, Shaikh A: The ideal tissue adhesive in facial plastic and reconstructive surgery. J Otolaryngol 19:68–72, 1990.

CHAPTER 45

Cervicofacial Rhytidectomy

PAUL S. COLLINS

A face lift is a specific operative procedure that both removes and repositions facial tissue. Many different terms are used by authors to describe essentially the same procedure, and the terms face lift, cervicofacial rhytidectomy, facial rhytidectomy, and rhytidectomy are synonymous. Liposuction-assisted rhytidectomy signifies the same procedure performed with the assistance of liposuction and lipodissection using a liposuction cannula. The face lift procedure provides a "refreshed" or "rested" look, but it is not a "fountain of youth." A face lift treats the position and quantity of the skin by removing and tightening redundant, pendulous tissue and excess subcutaneous fat from the neck, jowls, and cheek. Thus it improves the aesthetic landmarks masked by the pendulous skin and deposition of fat. Demarca-

tion of the facial cheek and neck is accentuated, the submental chin is thinned and redefined, and redundant skin is eliminated.

A chemical peel treats the quality of skin by removing wrinkles, creases, lentigines, actinic keratoses, and pigmentary anomalies (Fig. 45–1). A phenol-based peel, such as Baker's or Litton's formula, will tighten facial skin but is not indicated for sagging skin. Furthermore, unlike for a face lift, the number of ideal candidates for a phenol peel is sharply limited. Patients with superficial fine rhytides and sagging skin may be best served by first performing a face lift and then, after an appropriate postoperative interval, proceeding with a nonphenolic chemical peel. The peel will brighten the skin tone and improve some of the fine rhytides present on the face and neck.

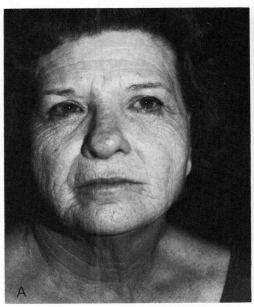 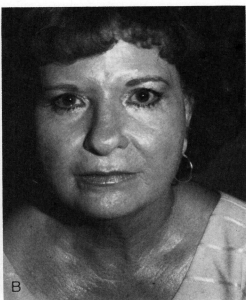

Figure 45–1. *A,* Preoperative appearance of a typical patient with wrinkles, creases, lentigines, actinic keratoses, and pigmentary anomalies that would benefit from a chemical peel. *B,* Postoperative view after a Litton's phenol formula chemical peel has dramatically improved the quality and texture of the skin. (Reprinted by permission of the publisher from Collins PS: The chemical peel. Clin Dermatol 5:66, 1987. Copyright 1987 by Elsevier Science Publishing Co., Inc.)

Preoperative Consultation

A thorough, complete consultation is imperative for obtaining a satisfactory outcome. The consultation should include the patient's desires and aspirations, evaluation of the appropriateness of the surgery desired, the patient's medical history, and a physical examination. It should establish the physician-patient relationship and result in selection of the most appropriate surgical course of action. No amount of surgical expertise can compensate for a poorly selected patient. When face lift candidates are properly informed and selected (both anatomically and psychologically), surgery designed to ensure effective rejuvenation is straightforward and fundamental. Patient inappropriateness or inattention or communication difficulties discovered before surgery are unlikely to improve after surgery, especially if there are any postoperative problems.

A cursory and superficial preoperative examination is an invitation for trouble. At the beginning of the consultation, inquiry should be made as to what features disturb the patient most. This information will assist in properly planning the surgical treatment[1] so that particular areas of concern can be appropriately managed. However, in some cases, it may be impossible to achieve the desired effect, and this should also be noted. Heavy jowls, a low hyoid bone, or prominent nasolabial folds may disturb the patient, but the experienced surgeon avoids overzealous attempts to correct them. The risk of complications is too great for the transient improvement gained; it is imperative that each patient realize this before surgery.

It is well documented that patients may have only limited retention of the details of a surgical consultation and may even repress a negative prediction by the surgeon in a mechanism of wish fulfillment. For this reason, the surgeon must thoroughly document in the medical record the specific details of the patient's problem areas and establish that the surgical limitations and expectations were conveyed to the patient.[2] During the initial interview, the patient must be allowed to indicate the anatomic areas of concern and express an understanding of what the anticipated surgical improvement should be. The surgeon must discuss each area in detail and explain the limitations of correction and the most common complications for each specific problem. Instructions should be provided as to the pre- and postoperative care and a list of medications to avoid should also be reviewed by the patient.

FACIAL EXAMINATION

All patients seeking facial surgery should be examined in great detail and the detailed physical findings recorded. The lower face should be examined for preexisting scars; prominent nasolabial folds; malar edema; adiposity of the cheeks; perioral rhytides; and skin qualities such as sebaceous gland activity, atrophy, actinic damage, degree of telangiectasia, porosity, pigmentary abnormalities, temporal hair line, herpetic lesions, and skin tumors. The neck is evaluated for the mento-hyoid angle, anterior platysmal folds or banding, submandibular gland ptosis, submental or diffuse adiposity, rhytides, and previous thyroid surgical scars.

Preoperative consultation and evaluation should include a detailed inquiry concerning previous facial nerve problems, especially a history of Bell's palsy. Because a postoperative seventh nerve deficit in a patient with a history of Bell's palsy is quite likely due to a recurrence of this disorder, a careful examination of the face for seventh nerve motor function is mandatory. Any facial asymmetry or facial muscle weakness noted during the preoperative examination should be pointed out to the patient and duly recorded before surgery.[3] The presence of any facial asymmetry during speaking and smiling should also be described. Patients rarely are aware of the presence of facial asymmetries and may later ascribe a pre-existing imperfection to the operative procedure.

The effects of aging on the ocular region—resulting in brow ptosis, dermatochalasis, and fat herniation—may compromise the results obtained by cervicofacial rhytidectomy. The effects of aging on the eyes are the most obvious, as the eyes are the commanding feature of the face, and any such effects will overshadow any improvement of the lower face and neck. This should be pointed out to the patient and discussed. The patient may be better served by performing another procedure such as a blepharoplasty, forehead lift, or a chemical peel in conjunction with, or in place of, a face lift (Fig. 45–1).

The patient should not be overweight, especially in the facial and cervical areas. An overweight patient, especially when there is excessive generalized facial fat, is at significant risk of obtaining an unfavorable result from a face lift. Loss of weight should be accomplished before surgery, as any marked loss of weight after the procedure will also compromise the results. Heavy nasolabial folds with deep creases, ptotic submandibular glands, retrognathia, and excessive jowls will also compromise a favorable face lift result. Deep facial rhytides, severe actinic damage, temporal hair thinning, and widened scars can also hamper results. Smokers, particularly heavy smokers, and alcohol abusers should be approached with caution because of a greater risk of complications.

MEDICAL EXAMINATION

Two general areas of assessment are critical in the preoperative evaluation: identification of risks relating to underlying medical disorders and evaluation for potential bleeding and coagulation problems. The most significant cardiac risk factors are uncompensated congestive heart failure and myocardial infarction within the preceding 6 months. Smoking, hypertension, stable exertional angina, mitral valve disease, cardiomegaly, and conducting system disease do not correlate with increased cardiac risk. Because of potential complications or aggravation of the underlying disease, elective surgery should be avoided in patients with congestive heart failure or recent myocardial infarction.[4]

The blood pressure should be taken during the initial

consultation and, if found to be elevated, treated and stabilized before scheduling surgery. Hypertension can increase bleeding, especially perioperatively. Any sudden increase in perioperative bleeding should prompt the physician to evaluate the patient's blood pressure and check for the presence of inadequate ventilation,which can also elevate blood pressure. In general, a complete physical examination, including an electrocardiogram, is necessary in patients older than 50 years and for patients with an abnormal medical history. The examining physician should be notified of the impending surgical procedure and the type of anesthesia to be used.

The potential for bleeding can be avoided by obtaining a detailed medical history and a history of recent drug ingestion. A previous history of postoperative, postdental (especially dental extraction), or postobstetric bleeding; a family history of coagulation disorders; and spontaneous bleeding or bruising require investigation and appropriate laboratory tests. Recent or chronic ingestion of aspirin, salicylate-containing medications, or nonsteroidal anti-inflammatory medications can cause excess and possibly severe perioperative and delayed postoperative bleeding. In sensitive individuals, these medications may cause prolonged bleeding for 2 or more weeks after cessation of ingestion. Alcohol can also result in prolonged bleeding and can be synergistic with aspirin and nonsteroidal anti-inflammatory medications.

It may be best to inform the patient that no medications should be taken before or immediately after surgery unless the surgeon is notified first. Patients often fail to list all the medications they are taking, especially if the medication is only occasionally used. At the initial interview, an extensive list of drugs that can cause excessive bleeding should be given to the patient (see Chapter 12, Table 12–1). This list reinforces the prevalence of medications that can interfere with clotting and stresses the importance of avoiding the use of any potentially complicating medication.

PSYCHOLOGICAL EVALUATION

The patient who seeks cosmetic surgery may erroneously expect that the surgery is without potential problems since it is elective in nature. The physician must be alert for any indications that the patient has unrealistic expectations. Many warning signs have been established[5] and should be well heeded. A positive self-image is important, and patients should want to look better for themselves, not to please others.

The surgeon must discuss the limitations of and alternatives to surgery and acknowledge that any surgery has inherent uncertainties. Complications should be discussed generally, not specifically. Most importantly, the surgeon should assure the patient that if a complication occurs, the surgeon will be available and willing to help the patient until the complication is resolved.[6] When a complication arises, patients are often afraid that the physician will be angry or abandon them, and too often the physician schedules visits less frequently than is prudent, in hopes that the problem will go away.

It is acceptable to state that most face lift patients may be back at work in 7 to 10 days, but the physician should also note that occasionally healing may take several weeks. Healing and recovery are individual functions and are largely unpredictable, so a delay in recovery should not be construed by the patient as related to inferior or improper surgical technique. Smokers should be informed that their healing process will be delayed.

While the cosmetic surgeon cannot be a master psychologist, it is important to be aware of psychic pathology.[6] It is the patient with a personality disorder who is most prone to sue the surgeon for malpractice. Such a disorder reveals symptoms of maladaptive behavior rather than of mental or emotional disturbances. Surgery cannot mend what is missing from this patient's personality, which is the ability to feel deeply or sincerely. These types of patients are potentially problematic, and surgery should be avoided, as any untoward effect, however trivial, will be met with displeasure.

PHOTOGRAPHS, INSTRUCTIONS, AND FEES

A complete set of photographs should be taken during the initial interview. It is often best for the photographs to be taken by the surgeon.[11] Standard and uniform views should be obtained, along with any additional photographs needed to document facial abnormalities. The photographing and posing provide an opportunity for more dialogue between the patient and surgeon with respect to specific facial features.

A full set of instructions for both preoperative and postoperative surgical care is given to the patient (Tables 45–1, 45–2). These should instruct the patient in what should be done the day before and the day of the surgery. A list of medications to avoid is reviewed to prevent inadvertent use of a potentially harmful drug. Consent forms that describe the surgery to be performed and possible complications must be discussed and then signed by the patient. Part of the consultation should be devoted to what the patient can expect from the surgery (e.g., bruising, swelling, discomfort, and dressing changes) as well as whom to contact at night or on weekends. This information is also reinforced in the instruction sheets. There should be a full discussion of the possible complications and how they are usually treated. This assures the patient that although complications can occur, the physician will be available for treatment. The patient should sign and be given copies of the risk and authorization forms delineating the discussion on complications and risks of face lift surgery (Table 45–3). Postoperative limitations on exercise and physical activities are also stressed.

Explicit postoperative instructions should include symptoms that require immediate care by the physician. It is important to remember that the surgical fee should include all postoperative care. Improper or inadequate postoperative care can compromise not only the surgery but also the doctor-patient relationship.

All financial aspects of the surgery are reviewed. The patient is given a list of the procedures to be performed and the fees. The patient is instructed that payment

TABLE 45–1. PREOPERATIVE INSTRUCTIONS FOR THE FACE LIFT SURGERY PATIENT

The surgical fee must be paid at least 1 week before the day of surgery. The quoted fee is applicable for 6 months from date of original consultation.

Laboratory tests are required for your surgery. Results must be either phoned in or sent to the office no later than 1 week before your surgery date.

The following is a complete list of instructions. It is very important that you read and follow these instructions carefully. If you are unclear about any of them, please contact the office.

1. **No aspirin or products containing aspirin or vitamin E should be taken 2 weeks before the surgery date.** Do not take any medications without informing the doctor, as they may be contraindicated for your surgery.
2. Do not eat or drink anything, including water, after midnight on the evening before surgery, unless instructed otherwise.
3. Shampoo your hair thoroughly the night before surgery. Do not use hairspray or setting lotion. Do not have your hair cut for 3 weeks before surgery.
4. Wash your face the morning of surgery, and do not apply any cosmetics or lotions. Men should shave closely on the day of surgery.
5. Women may wish to bring a scarf to wear home.
6. Wear minimal clothing that is easy to remove without having to be pulled off over the head.
7. DO NOT wear jewelry or bring valuables to the office.
8. Dentures, if worn, should remain in place during the procedure.
9. You may take a tranquilizer or sleeping pill the night before surgery.
10. Make plans to have someone transport you to the office and take you home after your surgery. **You MUST NOT drive yourself home after surgery.**

must be made before surgery. This eliminates financial pressures after the surgery, when the physician and patient should be concentrating on obtaining the most optimal surgical results. The fees should include any necessary follow-up visits and minor treatments. This is important, as some patients may avoid or delay necessary treatment because they do not wish to pay additional fees. Thus, a simple complication may become a complex one because of inappropriate delay.

Objectives of the Cervicofacial Rhytidectomy

Several fundamental points of the cervicofacial rhytidectomy procedure are key to maximizing the effects of the operation. By addressing these points with an effective operative technique, the surgeon can maximize the benefits of the face lift. Optimal benefits of the face lift

TABLE 45–2. HOME CARE AFTER FACE LIFT SURGERY

The healing process after face lift surgery requires both time and patience. **Your active participation in the postoperative care is as important as the surgery itself.** CALL IF YOU HAVE ANY QUESTIONS. WE ARE AVAILABLE 24 HOURS A DAY TO ANSWER YOUR QUESTIONS.

You will leave the operating room with a large mummy-like dressing covering your entire face except for your mouth, nose, and eyes. This dressing will feel snug, but do not attempt to remove or loosen it. The dressing is supposed to be snug to keep down swelling and prevent bleeding. The dressing will also help minimize head and neck movements, which can cause excess bleeding. If the dressing is too tight around the neck, it may be loosened by snipping the tape at the neck. The dressing will be removed after 48 hours in the office. At that time, additional directions will be given. You may eat soft food when you return home, but you should avoid foods that require excessive chewing.

There is very little pain associated with face lift surgery, but you may have some discomfort. Any discomfort you feel should be relieved by the prescribed pain medication. You should take only those medications prescribed by your physician. Do not take aspirin, medications containing aspirin, or anticoagulants. NOTIFY THE OFFICE IMMEDIATELY IF YOU ARE EXPERIENCING PAIN, AS IT MAY BE A SIGN OF EXCESS BLEEDING.

Please follow the instructions listed below. If you have questions, please do not hesitate to call the office. We are here to help you.

1. Should any sudden swelling, bleeding, or continuous discharge occur, report it to our office by telephone.
2. When you get home, stay in bed with your head elevated on at least two pillows, or sit in a comfortable chair with your legs up for the first 24 hours. **Keep your head still and avoid twisting your neck from side to side, which can cause bleeding and bruising.** After 10 days, you may resume most of your normal activities. However, you should avoid athletic and strenuous activities for 1 month.
3. You may wash your face and incisions **gently** with a mild soap and warm water after the bandage has been removed. The incisions should be kept moist with an antibiotic ointment at all times. Dry, crusted incisions will not heal as readily as those kept covered with an ointment.
4. Do not wash your hair for the first 4 days. It is important that you do **not** lean or bend forward to wash your hair in a sink for 3 weeks. Do not use hooded dryers, dyes, tints, or permanents for 1 month. Do not wear earrings for 6 weeks.
5. Avoid prolonged exposure to sunlight for 1 month, as it can adversely affect healing and also result in pigmentary problems.
6. You may begin to use makeup to cover bruises at the end of the first week. Be sure to remove the makeup thoroughly at the end of the day. Avoid placing makeup directly on the suture lines.
7. Avoid wearing pullover clothing until complete healing has occurred.
8. You may experience some numbness and stiffness of your face; this is considered normal and will subside with time.
9. It is natural to feel fatigued for several days after face lift surgery, and some individuals may also experience depression. You may be surprised at the initial appearance of your face, but remember to be patient, as swelling and bruising are normal. In general, the face and neck will have a socially acceptable appearance within 10 to 14 days.

TABLE 45–3. **FACE LIFT RISK FORM**

You and your doctor are considering a plastic surgical procedure to remove wrinkles and folds from your face. The operation is called a "rhytidectomy," also known as a "face lift." This type of operation is done by making surgical cuts at the temple, around the ears, and in the scalp. This surgery is elective; it is not required to improve or protect your physical health. It is possible that your appearance will be unlike your expectations and therefore less pleasing after the operation than it is now. Because of these facts, your doctor cannot guarantee a favorable result from the operation you are considering. Furthermore, even if the surgery is successful, the results will not be permanent because of natural aging. Although complications and adverse results are uncommon from this type of operation, they do sometimes occur. Your doctor will try to avoid possible complications, but it is impossible to guarantee that they will not occur.

Some of the possible complications of rhytidectomy surgery are:
Bleeding; abnormal collections of blood underneath the skin of the face and neck; discoloration of the face; nerve damage causing temporary or permanent loss of feeling in the face and weakness, distortion, and paralysis of portions or all of the face; abnormal contours of the face; distortion, and deformity of the ears; loss of skin and hair of the face and scalp; infection; prolonged pain and swelling of portions or all of the face; and insufficient or excessive amounts of wrinkle removal. Personality changes and mental difficulties also sometimes occur after surgery, even when the operation has been a cosmetic success. Allergic or other adverse reactions to one or more of the substances and medications used in the operation can also occur. Complications from this operation may result in a need for further surgery. Some of the complications can cause prolonged illness, draining wounds, the need for blood transfusions, unsightly and painful scars, and permanent deformity, and inconvenience. Allergic reactions have been known to cause death.
There are other rare complications from this operation in addition to the ones noted above. However, it is not possible to advise you of every conceivable complication. The purpose of this form is not to frighten or upset you. The complications stated above are very unlikely to occur. The purpose of this form is merely to ensure that your decision to have this operation is not made in ignorance of the risks of a rhytidectomy or face lift operation and that you fully realize that no promises can be made that complications will not occur.

I CERTIFY that I have read or have had read to me the contents of this form. I understand the risks involved in this operation. All blanks or statements requiring insertion or completion were filled in or crossed out before I signed. I will receive a copy of this form for my own personal records.

Patient Signature _____ Date _____

Witness _____

This is not a consent form. A consent form must also be signed by the patient.

are obtained by elevating and improving the pendulous skin in the jowl and neck regions. While extension of undermining in an effort to improve results in other areas may enhance the initial appearance, such improvement is often short-lived and is obtained at a cost of increased tissue insult, producing greater postoperative edema and discomfort and theoretically increasing the risk of significant complications.[7]

Liposuction and lipodissection of the neck have considerably improved the benefits of face lift surgery. Adequate lipectomy of the neck and occasionally of the face is essential for lasting improvement. Liposuction effectively removes excess neck fat rapidly and with minimal blood loss. The loosened and defatted neck skin flap can then be efficiently elevated. There is a decrease in the weight and tension of the elevated skin flaps that otherwise with time would negate the results.

The improvement offered by neck liposuction and lipodissection cannot be overemphasized. Adequate submandibular and submental lipectomy is essential to provide lasting results in the cervical region. Lipectomy contours the neck, defining the mandibular line and flattening the submental region. Even in those patients with minimal neck adiposity, lipodissection is a fast and efficient procedure that vastly improves the cervicomental angle and aids in the lifting and tightening of the neck tissues.[8]

The beneficial results of the face lift are as much a consequence of redistribution of facial and cervical tissues as of frank skin excision. A procedure that rotates and advances the skin flap while minimizing skin tension should enhance results while minimizing morbidity. The degree of tension that a skin flap can withstand is inversely related to the extent of undermining. Tissue insult secondary to tension can be minimized by redistributing the tension rather than concentrating it in several areas. The Webster procedure,[9] which uses a short flap and minimal undermining, can tolerate greater tension than a long flap with wide undermining.[10]

Anatomy

A precise understanding of the anatomy encountered during cervicofacial rhytidectomy is essential not only to avoid complications but also to obtain optimal surgical results.

FACIAL NERVE

The facial nerve supplies motor innervation to all the muscles of the face through its many branches (Fig. 45–2).[12–15] The main trunk is the most consistent portion of the nerve and usually has a bifurcation inside the parotid gland. Other variations include a bifurcation with the addition of a buccal branch, a quadruplet, or, rarely, a plexiform design of the branches. Considerable variation is seen in the arborization pattern of the facial nerve from one side to the other, even in the same individual. As the main trunk of the facial nerve and its divisions run anteriorly in the gland, they become more superficial. However, almost all the branching and connecting occurs within the parotid gland.[16] Injury to the facial nerve within the parenchyma of the parotid gland is uncommon, as the face lift dissection should not violate this area. It is the more distal branches that are at risk in a face lift.

Within the parotid, the facial nerve typically bifurcates

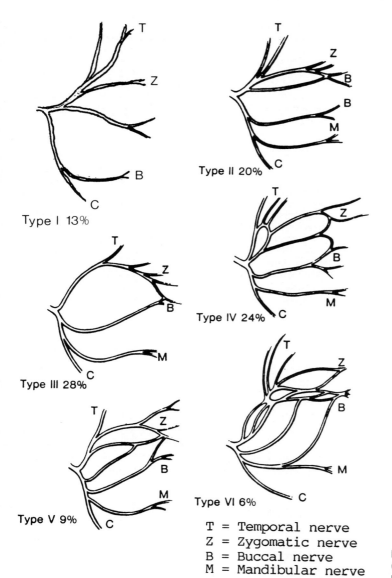

Type I 13%

Type II 20%

Type III 28%

Type IV 24%

Type V 9%

Type VI 6%

T = Temporal nerve
Z = Zygomatic nerve
B = Buccal nerve
M = Mandibular nerve
C = Cervical nerve

Figure 45–2. Variations in the branches of the facial nerve. (From Bernstein L, Nelson RH: Surgical anatomy of the extraparotid distribution of the facial nerve. Arch Otolaryngol 110:177, 1984. Copyright 1984, American Medical Association.)

Figure 45–3. Anatomic location of the temporal branch of the facial nerve. (Modified from Robbins TH: The protection of the frontal branch of the facial nerve in face-lift surgery. Br J Plast Surg 34:95, 1981.)

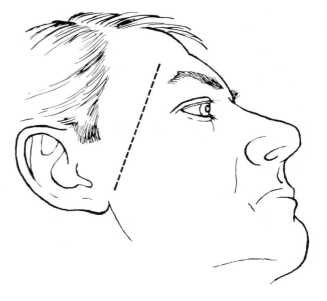

into the temporal and cervical divisions. The temporal division has many interconnections of its own branches as well as connections with other nerves in the face (Fig. 45–3). There are five to eight branches, usually consisting of one to the frontal area, two to the orbital area, three to the zygomatic area, and two to the buccal area. The zygomatic branch is the largest and most important, while the frontal branch has the smallest number of connections and is a terminal branch in 85 to 90% of patients. Based on experience[16] and corroborated by cadaver studies,[14, 15] connections between the major divisions are frequent, occurring in 70 to 90% of patients. Not only do each of the main divisions of the facial nerve (temporal, zygomatic, buccal, and mandibular) have multiple branches, but often the branches themselves have interconnections.[15] This accounts for the fact that partial and, in many instances, full recovery may occur with nerve injuries resulting from facial rhytidectomy.

The cervical division is almost always the smallest and usually has three to five branches: one buccal, three mandibular, and one cervical. All of these branches are approximately the same size and have frequent interconnections. The ramus mandibularis mandibulae is a delicate branch and connects with the other branches in only 10 to 15% of patients. This nerve branches anterior to the parotid gland and lies just beneath the superficial masseteric fascia, while the mandibular and cervical branches lie deep to the platysma muscle.

Temporal Branch

The temporal branch of the facial nerve is most vulnerable at the midpoint of the zygomatic arch (Fig. 45–3). As it emerges from the superior pole of the parotid gland, it crosses the zygomatic arch in the superficial temporal fascia. The superficial temporal fascia is a thin layer of fibrous fatty tissue that is in intimate contact with the overlying skin. While passing over the arch, it is usually a single branch and bifurcates only after it reaches the undersurface of the frontalis muscle via the temporalis fascia. The nerve is in particular jeopardy at this point in individuals who are thin and have little soft tissue covering the zygomatic arch. Hydrodissection by infiltration with a local anesthetic solution will help to separate the overlying skin from the underlying fascia, providing protection during surgical dissection.

The expected pathway of the temporal nerve can be estimated by several methods. The path of the frontal branch can be drawn on the skin by two diverging lines that start from the region of the earlobe and go to the lateral end of the eyebrow and to the highest frontal crease (Fig. 45–3).[17] Distal to this, the nerve branches become even more superficial, finally approaching the surface when the nerve enters the frontalis muscle at the bony supraorbital ridge above the lateral orbit. Another method to ascertain the pathway of the frontal branch is to draw its pathway on the skin as a line passing from the earlobe to a point 1.5 cm from the lateral border of the brow.[17, 18]

A stretched or traumatized temporal branch will usually recover within 6 months. However, complete transection will result in permanent paralysis or incomplete recovery of forehead movement, as fewer than 15% of the nerve fibers at the brow have any connection with other branches of the facial nerve. On the other hand, because of the multiple interconnections among the facial nerve branches to the orbicularis oculi, paralysis of the eyelids is most unusual after one of these branches is cut.[6]

Zygomatic Branch

Cadaveric studies[15] have demonstrated that the zygomatic branches that go toward the eye cross the zygomatic arch deep in the facial fat after exiting from the parotid gland. Other inferiorly directed branches go beneath the prominence of the zygoma, where they also lie protected deep in the fat. No nerves cross over the prominence of the zygoma. Exiting from the parotid gland, the nerve branches lie relatively deep in the subcutaneous fat, which explains the relative infrequency of injury to these nerve branches.

Buccal Branch

The buccal branches of the facial nerve are typically located in the buccal pocket, a space deep to the superficial musculoaponeurotic system (SMAS) just inferior to the zygoma, containing the fat pad of Bichat, Stensen's duct, and the buccal blood vessels. The buccal pocket can be found simply by pressing the tissues of the cheek with the tip of the index finger immediately inferior to the zygoma.[19] The lower buccal branches cross over the masseter muscle. In thin people, the nerves lying in the fascia of the masseter muscle are more exposed owing to less subcutaneous tissue. Considerable variation is found in the depth of the buccal branches. The more superior branches are protected by the fat underneath the zygoma, whereas the lower branches overlie the bulge of the masseter and are more exposed. Dissection above the SMAS should not endanger the nerves.

The buccal branches angle deep in the fat when they reach the anterior border of the masseter and enter the facial muscles. Excess skin and fat are found at the nasolabial fold. Because of their deep location in this region, there is less probability here of severing either the buccal or zygomatic nerve branches during dissection of the skin and fat.[17]

Mandibular Branch

Clinical experience[16] with parotidectomies and radical neck dissections has demonstrated that the mandibular branch of the facial nerve is located 1 to 2 cm below the lower border of the mandible in almost every instance (Fig. 45–4). The mandibular nerve does have multiple branches and variations. In some individuals with lax and atrophic tissues, the branches are 3 to 4 cm below the mandible. Where the nerve crosses the facial artery and vein, it is lifted more superficially, particularly in thin people.

While the descending cervical division innervates the main body of the platysma muscle, the mandibular division innervates the upper and anterior portion of this muscle in at least half the cases. Any surgical

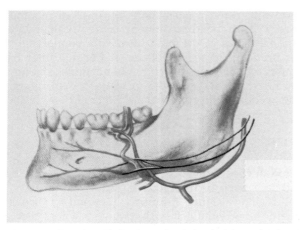

Figure 45–4. The mandibular branch of the facial nerve along or below the inferior border of the mandible. (From Dingman RO, Grabb WC: Surgical anatomy of the mandibular ramus of the facial nerve based on the dissection of 100 facial halves. Plast Reconstr Surg 29:266, 1962.)

intervention in this region or deep to the platysma muscle for the removal of fat can put this nerve in jeopardy.[20] Approximately 15% of patients have a connection between the mandibular division and the buccal division from the upper segment of the facial nerve. Consequently, function of the mandibular nerve may be recovered to some degree after the nerve is cut. In the remainder of cases, however, injury to this nerve may leave a permanent deficit. It may be a subtle deficit if only the platysma muscle branches are affected or a conspicuous deficit if the entire mandibular division is involved.

The possibility of injuring the mandibular and cervical branches during dissection of the submental skin and fat has been studied[17] through an incision in the cervical region. The anatomic pathway of the mandibular branch behind the facial artery is located above the lower border of the mandible in 80% of cases. In the remaining 20%, the pathway forms an arch beneath the lower border of this bone. Anterior to the facial artery, all the nerve branches to the muscles of the lower lip are situated above the lower mandibular border. The mandibular branch behind the facial artery always runs within or deep to the platysma muscle fibers, so there is almost no danger of injuring the nerve if the dissection is kept superficial to the platysma muscle.

Surgery superficial to the platysma muscle should not injure the nerve branches during elevation of the skin flap by scissors or lipodissection or during removal of excess subcutaneous fat with liposuction. However, development of this muscle varies, and the muscle may be extremely thin and atrophic in elderly patients. Although the mandibular nerve branches are relatively superficial for part of their course, they always enter the innervated muscles deeply on the lateral undersurface. Dissection of the skin near the border of the mandible is unlikely to cause injury to the mandibular branch, as the nerve has already penetrated the platysma muscle in this area.[17]

GREAT AURICULAR NERVE

The great auricular nerve, one of the nerves injured more frequently during rhytidectomy, is a purely sensory nerve derived from the second and third cervical roots and is the largest ascending branch of the cervical plexus. From the back of the neck and deep to the border of the sternocleidomastoid muscle, it sweeps cephalad and ventral at a 45-degree angle toward the corner of the jaw.[21, 22] As the nerve becomes more superficial, it emerges onto the sternocleidomastoid muscle, wraps around the belly of the muscle, gives off a small postauricular branch, and then pierces the parotid gland, from which it emerges to innervate the skin.[23] Transection of the nerve results in numbness of the lower two thirds of the ear and the preauricular and postauricular skin. A neuroma may also form, producing a mass in the middle neck that evokes Tinel's sign on palpation and can be painful on motion.

In dissections,[21] the main trunk of the nerve is found to consistently cross the sternocleidomastoid muscle at the same point (Fig. 45–5). With the head turned 45 degrees in the face lift position, the nerve always crosses the midtransverse belly of the sternocleidomastoid muscle 6.5 cm below the caudal edge of the bony external auditory canal. At this point, the external jugular vein is parallel and 0.5 cm ventral to the nerve.

The skin is adherent to the fascia in the mastoid area, and there is no distinct aponeurotic layer in the region caudal to the ear. An accurate subcutaneous dissection of the skin flap is necessary during rhytidectomy to prevent injury to the nerve. The nerve trunk should not be damaged when skin flaps are elevated if the subcutaneous plane is dissected. However, in the region where the main nerve trunk crosses over the sternocleidomastoid muscle, it is relatively easy to penetrate the superficial musculoaponeurotic system. By marking the proximate point where the nerve crosses the sternocleidomastoid muscle, the surgeon can take extra precautions to keep the dissection superficial.

The great auricular nerve is completely covered by the SMAS during its entire course. Although the nerve, SMAS, and skin are essentially adherent at the most superficial point, they become increasingly separated as the nerve starts its final deep course into the parotid gland. Therefore, at the anterior border of the sternocleidomastoid muscle, there is adequate separation between the nerve and the SMAS for a flap to be lifted, with preservation of the nerve.

POSTERIOR AURICULAR NERVE

The posterior auricular nerve crosses the mastoid region and attaches to the aponeurosis of the sternocleidomastoid muscle immediately below the superficial fascia to innervate the occipital belly of the occipitofrontalis muscle. Because it is sometimes deeper than the rest of the undermining, the nerve is at risk of being severed at the level of the incision line. Also, during retroauricular undermining of the neck lift, the superficial fascia containing the posterior auricular nerve may be included in the occipitomastoid flap.[23, 24]

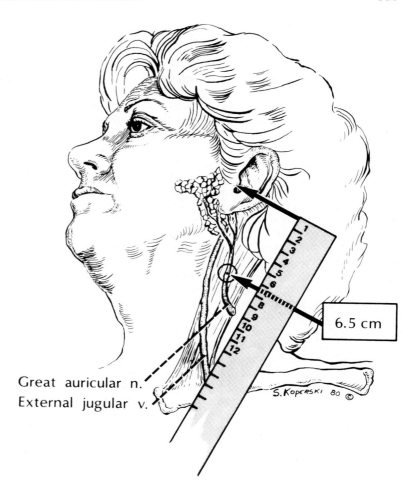

6.5 cm

Great auricular n.
External jugular v.

S. KOPERSKI 80 ©

Figure 45–5. Anatomic location of the great auricular nerve in the neck. (From McKinney P, Katrana DJ: Prevention of injury to the great auricular nerve during rhytidectomy. Plast Reconstr Surg 66:675, 1980.)

Severing the nerve will paralyze the occipital belly of the occipitofrontalis muscle. Tension on the scalp will be released, and the scalp will be drawn forward by the action of the frontal belly of the occipitofrontalis, corrugator supercilii, procerus, and orbicularis oculi muscles. This can cause additional wrinkling of the forehead, with drooping of the eyebrows. Superficial undermining in the occipital and mastoid regions will preserve the nerve.

SMAS

The SMAS can be divided into two broad segments: the parotid area and the cheek area.[24] The parotid area of the SMAS is a condensed mesh, distinct from the fascia of the parotid gland. It is adherent in the pretragal area for 1 to 2 cm and then becomes separate from the parotid sheet. Microscopic studies show that the SMAS can be composed of one to three layers lying between the parotid fascia proper and the skin. Sometimes the muscular fibers are obvious within the fibrous layer, hence the term musculoaponeurotic system. In the cheek, the SMAS becomes a thin, continuous fibrous net sending several extensions out to the dermis. This network constantly covers the facial muscles and comprises all of the attachments from these muscles to the dermis.

All the motor branches of the facial nerve lie deep to the SMAS. In the parotid area, only the sensory nerve branches of the anterior cervical plexus are located between the dermis and the SMAS. The facial nerve and its branches run deep in the parotid gland, where they are protected by the parotid fascia and the external lobe of the gland. In the cheek area, the facial motor nerves run deeper than the SMAS. Thus, the only nerves that go through the SMAS are the sensory nerves. The motor branches reach the superficial layer of the facial muscles through their deeper aspect. An important layer of fat is often located between the SMAS and the dermis and is completely separated from Bichat's fat pad by the SMAS.

The SMAS is kept tensed superiorly by the superficial temporal muscles, the external part of the frontalis muscle, and the orbicularis oculi muscles. It is kept tense inferiorly by the platysma muscle. It is attached posteriorly to the tragus and the mastoid area. The main vessels—the facial artery and vein—lie deep to the SMAS, but their perforating branches go through it, while the subdermal vascular network lies superficial to it. Thus, the SMAS forms the deep border of the neurovascular and muscular cutaneous complex.

Elevation of the SMAS Flap

Extreme caution is mandatory during any elevation of the SMAS or a platysma muscle flap. In patients with atrophy or hypoplasia of the platysma muscle, there is very little muscle or fascia over the marginal mandibular branch of the facial nerve. In secondary face lifts, there may be extensive subcutaneous fibrosis with adhesions of the skin to the underlying platysma muscle. This may distort the normal anatomy and make penetration of the muscle possible, endangering the underlying facial nerve branches. For this reason, extensive undermining must be done cautiously, preferably under direct vision.

Studies have demonstrated that dissection in a plane deep to the SMAS over the parotid can be efficacious in a rhytidectomy. In this region, the facial nerve is well protected by the overlying gland. However, anterior to the parotid area, the SMAS is thin, and surgical dissection of it in this area may be both dangerous and difficult. In patients with scant subcutaneous tissue or small parotid glands, the nerve branches do not have much protection.

In the pretragal area, the SMAS and the parotid fibrous fascia are united in a dense layer of connective tissue so that surgical dissection is safe. The dissection is begun anterior to the tragus by inserting Metzenbaum scissors between the SMAS and the parotid fascia. The SMAS is freed carefully from this fascia, and the dissection becomes easy once the proper plane is found. The dissection is not carried farther upward than 1 cm below the zygomatic arch or farther downward than 1 cm above the inferior margin of the mandible. Once the SMAS is freed from the parotid fascia, it is possible to lift the face much more easily and strongly than can be done with simple skin undermining. The SMAS generally becomes thinner or even discontinuous in the cheek area, especially in individuals older than 50 years.[24]

Distal to the parotid gland, nerve branches that become superficial are the distal temporal branches, the lower buccal branches, the upper mandibular branches over the masseter muscle, and the marginal mandibular branch as it crosses the facial artery. Some protection at these danger areas is provided by fascia, especially the superficial temporal and masseteric, while the platysma provides some protection for the mandibular branch. However, fascial and muscle protection is less in thin individuals. Face lift dissection can be rapid in areas where facial nerve branches are deep or absent (e.g., the postauricular area, the area inferior to the zygomatic prominence, and the area near the earlobe).[15]

In the temporozygomatic region, the SMAS crosses in front of the zygomatic arch and adheres to the periosteum by thin expansions. The temporal branch of the facial nerve lies deep to the SMAS, with the sensory nerve branches running between the SMAS and the dermis. However, the space overlying the external part of the zygomatic arch is very thin, making dissection of the SMAS difficult and dangerous. For this reason, a better plane of dissection is found superficial to the SMAS.

The SMAS is in close contact with the superficial fibers of the platysma in the mandibular region, but at the nasolabial fold, it is deep, thin, and separated from the dermis by a large amount of fat. Posteriorly at the mastoid area, the SMAS is intimately attached to the dermis and to the fibrous tissue around the insertions of the sternoclavicular muscles. It is rather difficult to isolate the SMAS around the ear, because the various fibrous layers are closely intertwined.

RETAINING LIGAMENTS OF THE FACE

There are two categories of retaining ligaments seen during face lift dissection.[25] One consists of condensations of the platysmal fascia that extend to the dermis; these are the platysmal auricular ligament and the anterior platysmal cutaneous ligament. The other type consists of ligaments that tether the skin to the facial muscle; these are the mandibular and zygomatic ligaments. These ligaments restrain the facial skin against gravitational forces and delineate the anterior border of the jowl area (Fig. 45–6).

Platysmal Auricular Ligament

The platysmal auricular ligament anchors the platysma to the dermis of the inferior auricular skin and lies over the lower parotid. During initial dissection of the infra-auricular area anterior to the sternocleidomastoid muscle, the ligament tends to force the direction of the dissection deep. However, an attempt to stay superficial in the subcutaneous layer may result in skin perforation owing to the intimate association of the dermis with the ligament.

Anterior Platysmal Cutaneous Ligaments

The anterior platysmal cutaneous ligaments are inconsistently present and connect the anterior platysma to the skin of the middle and anterior cheek. The ligaments may form a heavy, fibrous fascial investment of the platysma, with stout extensions to the skin of the cheek. The cutaneous insertions may cause striking dimpling of the skin when the skin flap is pulled up. Separating the SMAS from the dermis by severing this ligament will free the flap and eliminate dimpling.

Mandibular Ligaments

The mandibular ligaments originate from bone along a line about 1 cm above the mandibular border and extending along the anterior third of the mandibular body. These fibrous bundles interdigitate with the muscle fibers of the platysma, the triangularis muscles, and the skin. A sensory nerve and a cutaneous artery usually accompany these ligaments. They can be identified in some patients by applying a lifting force to the cheek flap, but this force is poorly transmitted to the submandibular or jowl area. As the skin flap is pulled, the skin may dimple and bunch at the anterior border of the jowls as a result of the ligamentous attachment. Severing this ligament will provide for a more effective, uniform lifting of the skin and jowls.

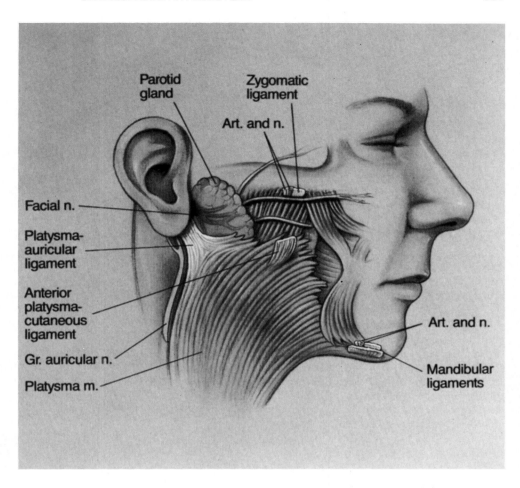

Parotid gland
Zygomatic ligament
Art. and n.
Facial n.
Platysma-auricular ligament
Anterior platysma-cutaneous ligament
Gr. auricular n.
Platysma m.
Art. and n.
Mandibular ligaments

Figure 45–6. Location of the four retaining ligaments of the face. (From Furnas DW: The retaining ligaments of the cheek. Plast Reconstr Surg 83:11, 1989.)

Zygomatic Ligament

The zygomatic ligament anchors the skin of the cheek to the inferior border of the zygoma just posterior to the origin of the zygomaticus minor muscle. Usually an artery and a sensory nerve course to the skin along with the ligament. Transection of the ligament will cause brisk bleeding as a result of injury to the artery. This must be completely controlled, as absolute hemostasis is necessary to avoid postoperative hematoma formation.

ANATOMIC DANGER AREAS

Areas where the nerve branches become more superficial and exposed are primarily those where the nerve has to cross an underlying convex structure. The more distal temporal branches are at risk for injury as they cross the zygoma. The lower buccal and upper mandibular branches lying over the bulge of the masseter are also superficial, particularly in thin individuals. In thin people, the main mandibular nerve branch is lifted more superficially as it crosses the facial artery.[15]

The danger areas (i.e., distal temporal branches, lower buccal and mandibular branches over the masseter, and the mandibular branches over the facial artery) are all distal to the main trunk of the nerve. At this level, multiple branches are found, and injury to a nerve branch would be expected to show some recovery be-

cause of both the distal location of the injury and the fact that there are multiple branches with interconnections. The temporal and mandibular branches are the most commonly injured motor nerves, but spontaneous recovery is common because of the numerous nerve interconnections. Both the zygomatic and the upper buccal branches are largely protected by their deeper placement within the fat of the midcheek.

Some protection for the more superficial nerve branches is provided by the superficial fascial layers of the face. In the temporal region, although the nerve branches are close to the dissected surface, portions of the anterior superficial temporal fascia lie between the nerve and the face lift plane. Dissection in a subcutaneous plane should be safe. In the masseter region, the lower buccal and upper mandibular branches are protected partly by the fascia overlying the masseter and partly by the overlying fatty fibrous tissue and the SMAS. In the area below the zygoma, the superficial fascia is a component of the fatty subcutaneous tissue, which protects the nerve branches in this region. Protection for the mandibular nerve branch as it crosses the facial artery is provided by the overlying platysma. In thin patients, the fascial layers are more tenuous and fragile. While no review has compared the risk of face lift facial nerve damage in thin and fat patients, atrophy of the SMAS and the subcutaneous fat may place thin patients at greater risk.

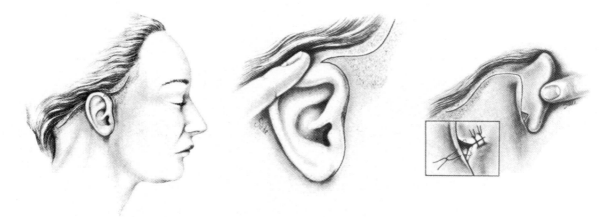

Figure 45–7. The face lift incisions. (From Johnson CM, Adamson PA, Anderson JR: The face-lift incision. Arch Otolaryngol 110:371, 1984. Copyright 1984, American Medical Association.)

Incisions

The incisions should produce a well-camouflaged scar while providing the surgeon with sufficient exposure to safely undermine the skin flap and perform the needed contouring and suspension. Minimal distortion of the surface anatomy, which includes the temporal hairline, tragus, earlobe, postauricular sulcus, and postauricular hairlines, is essential.[26, 27] Components of the incisions include temporal, preauricular, earlobe, postauricular, and masto-occipital sections (Fig. 45–7).[27, 28] The incisions should be marked precisely (Fig. 45–8), using specific reference points,[29] before anesthetic infiltration, which can distort the local anatomy (Fig. 45–9).

TEMPORAL INCISIONS

The temporal incision parallels the gentle curve of the hairline, starting at the otobasion superius and ending at the temporal hairline. The incision is oblique, parallel to the hair bulbs, and approximately 4 to 5 mm into the hair, where follicle density is sufficient to hide the scar. The prime advantage of this incision is that it preserves the important preauricular tuft of hair in the temporal region. An incision placed farther posteriorly may displace the hairline posteriorly and superiorly with flap suspension, producing an unnatural appearance. A second, later lift will further increase this distortion, producing temporal alopecia. A posterior incision may also jeopardize this hair owing to dissection at an improper level, excess flap tension, or both.

An incision along the hairline obviates the need to change the plane of dissection as one proceeds anteriorly from temporal hair to temporal glabrous skin. Because the temporal branch of the facial nerve is most vulnerable to injury in this region, a subcutaneous, single-level dissection is safest. An anteriorly placed curved incision also allows a shorter flap in the anteroposterior direction.

One disadvantage of the temporal incision is that the resulting anteriorly placed scar is potentially more obvious. However, the inferiorly directed hair growth

pattern in this region typically hides the scar and allows most patients to even wear the hair combed back. Careful wound closure in this area is essential to obtain the most optimal results.

At the otobasion superius, the temporal and preauricular incisions are carried posteriorly to form a "V." This will close from a "V" to "Y" by the downward tension created from anchoring the facial flap at this point. Any

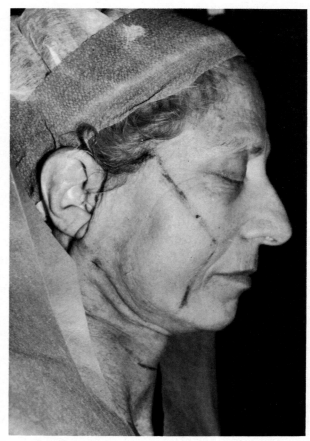

Figure 45–8. Preoperative markings delineate the extent of dissection of a long flap in a nonsmoking patient.

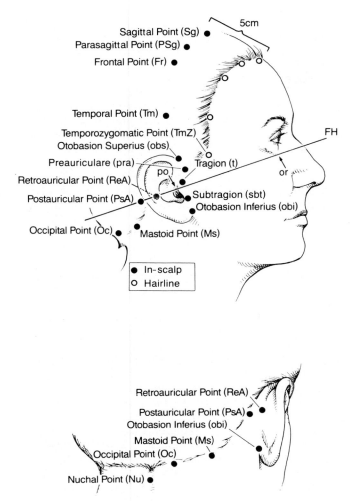

Sagittal Point (Sg) ●
Parasagittal Point (PSg) ●
Frontal Point (Fr) ●

Temporal Point (Tm) ●
Temporozygomatic Point (TmZ) ●
Otobasion Superius (obs) ●
Preauriculare (pra)
Retroauricular Point (ReA)
Postauricular Point (PsA) ●
Occipital Point (Oc) ●
Mastoid Point (Ms) ●

Tragion (t)
Subtragion (sbt)
Otobasion Inferius (obi)

5cm

FH

or

po

● In-scalp
○ Hairline

Retroauricular Point (ReA)
Postauricular Point (PsA) ●
Otobasion Inferius (obi)
Mastoid Point (Ms)
Occipital Point (Oc)
Nuchal Point (Nu) ●

Figure 45–9. Anthropometric landmarks used in making the face lift incisions. (From Furnas DW: Anthropometric landmarks for precision planning in rhytidectomy. Clin Plast Surg 14:639, 1987.)

bunching of the skin at the junction of the temporal and preauricular incisions is thus prevented. In men, the temporal and preauricular incisions meet just above the tragus to preserve the sideburns. A 1-cm strip of glabrous skin is left intact in front of the ear. This avoids bringing the beard close to the pinna, which would make shaving difficult.

PREAURICULAR INCISION

The preauricular incision simply follows the anatomic attachment of the pinna, producing a bilobed, curvilinear incision. The superior and inferior preauricular curvilinear incisions bisect at a point above the tragus. Thus, the incision curves to produce a surgical scar that will mimic the anterior border of the ear. A straight-line incision should be avoided, as it may result in scar contracture and a noticeable preauricular deformity. For minimal scarring, the wound in this area should be closed with little or no tension. Post-tragal incisions often are not used because of the tendency to pull the

tragus forward. The auditory meatus is uncovered and exposed with forward contraction of the tragus, giving an artificial, aesthetically unpleasing appearance to the ear.

EARLOBE INCISION

It is imperative that the earlobe incision line be marked precisely before infiltration of local anesthetic, which might distort the earlobe. The earlobe incision should follow the margins of the lobe closely. By staying close to the lobe posteriorly, the resultant scar is hidden from lateral view by the lobe.

POSTAURICULAR INCISION

In women, the postauricular incision immediately courses 0.5 cm onto the concha so that the resultant scar will be hidden by the pinna. With the incision kept on the concha, the resultant scar will fall into the conchal sulcus as it drifts posteriorly as a result of tension and stretch. Any excess bunching of tissue will also fall into the sulcus, where it will flatten over time. In men, however, the retroauricular incision is made in the postauricular sulcus. Posteroinferior migration after surgery places any beard-growing skin far enough from the ear to allow shaving.[30] In both sexes the incision extends superiorly above the plane of the external auditory canal before curving onto the mastoid.

MASTO-OCCIPITAL INCISION

The masto-occipital incision arcs off the concha onto the mastoid in a curved line at a level slightly higher than the inferior crus, which effectively hides the scar behind the ear. It then courses posteroinferiorly for 6 to 8 cm almost parallel to, but slightly above, the hairline. The incision ends posteriorly in the vicinity of the nuchal point with a slight upward turn that extends it 1.5 to 2.0 cm into the nape of the neck, where the hair is thicker.

The ideal masto-occipital incision is perpendicular to the direction of pull to be exerted on the submental and neck skin. The upward turn of the incision into the hairline is necessary to minimize a rumple or "dogear" deformity of the suspended skin flap at its posterior extent of attachment. A masto-occipital incision positioned more horizontally does not permit this ideal direction of pull. The flap shifts posteriorly during suspension and excision, resulting in a "windswept" appearance to the face. A horizontal incision may prevent accurate apposition of the flap to the scalp at the junction of the hair-bearing and non–hair-bearing skin. This results in an irregular, notched hairline, or "step deformity."[27, 28] In patients with noticeably lax neck skin, an incision that follows the posterior hairline facilitates removal of this laxity, as the surgeon does not have to deal with the difficulty of realigning the hairline to avoid a step deformity.[5]

Lipodissection and Liposuction of the Neck

The most important advance made in the face lift procedure since the introduction of the SMAS suspension technique has been the development of lipodissection and liposuction of the neck. These result in dramatic, long-lived improvement of the neck and mental area,[8, 31, 32] as they efficiently remove excess adipose tissue from the chin and neck that would normally be lifted onto the mandibular area, without the risk of excessive hemorrhaging. Eliminating this excess tissue weight also decreases any subsequent sagging of the tissues at the mandible. The cervicomental angle is simultaneously restored, which is an important feature of the improvement obtained with the face lift. Lipodissection loosens the entire neck area, aiding in the lift. It also dissects and frees the skin and subcutaneous fat off the platysmal bands. Although not all bands are eliminated, there is usually marked improvement.

The neck liposuction and lipodissection may be done either before or after elevating the facial flaps. Furthermore, the use of neck liposuction and lipodissection is an ideal way to correct early aging deformities of the chin and neck.[33] In many patients, the first sign of aging is an accumulation of fat in the cervicomental region (the "jowls"), with mild sagging. Laxity of the facial skin has not usually occurred at this point, and thus a face lift is not essential for correction.

SURGICAL TECHNIQUE

A 1-cm incision is made in the submental crease.[34] Blunt scissors create a pocket in the subcutaneous fat for easy access by the flat 4-mm cannula, which is used initially to create tunnels (Fig. 45–10). This will facilitate entry of a round 6-mm cannula, which is optimal for fat removal. Liposuction is carried out in a back-and-forth motion, maintaining the cannula in the superficial fat layer above the platysma. Suctioning is carried out from the suprasternal notch inferiorly to the sternocleidomastoid muscles laterally. During this time it is important to keep the opening of the cannula pointed downward in thinner patients. However, in patients with thicker skin and a large amount of fat in the neck, the cannula opening may need to be turned upward to face the underside of the neck flap. This is important, as a large amount of fat can otherwise be missed, producing surgical results that are less than expected. After liposuction of the neck is completed, the flat 4-mm cannula is reinserted, and any small septa that inhibit the free sweep of the spatula cannula across the neck are dissected. This is an extremely important step, as suspending a completely freed skin flap is necessary for a good result.

After the anterior neck skin is completely freed, the 4 mm cannula is directed toward the mandibular rim to dissect and suction any excess fat in the area. It is important to be especially careful in this region and to keep the tip of the cannula in a superficial plane. Deep penetration or too-vigorous suctioning can injure the submandibular branch of the facial nerve, which lies in this region. If the nerve is injured, the result is a temporary paralysis of the depressor anguli oris and depressor labii inferioris muscles, causing deformity of the mouth during animation. This paralysis has been reported to be temporary, with full recovery expected.[34]

Finally, the subplatysmal deep midline fat is extracted.

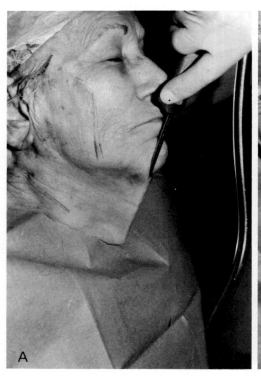
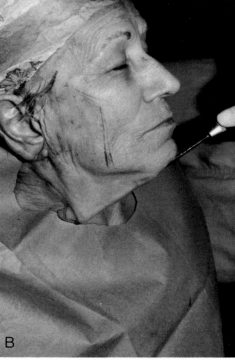

Figure 45–10. *A,* The liposuction cannula is inserted through a small submental incision so that liposuction can be completed from the submental region down to the area just superior to the sternal notch and laterally to the border of the sternocleidomastoid muscle. *B,* Lipodissection frees the entire neck flap and separates the platysmal bands from the skin with a flat cannula, allowing it to be lifted as a unit.

A

B

The round 6-mm cannula is pressed between the fibers of the platysma with the hand, and short back-and-forth strokes are used to suction any subplatysmal fat in the submental region. It is important to stay in the midline to avoid damaging any structures in this region. Any fat present at the incisional opening is removed by carefully turning up the cannula aperture to suction the fat off the skin flap. After liposuction is completed, both sides of the neck are carefully examined to ensure symmetric fat removal. It is imperative that no residual fat pockets are left in the submandibular area. Bunching or puckering of the neck skin flap is corrected by lipodissection.

PLATYSMAL BANDS

Platysmal cords are caused by stretching and loss of contractility of the skin and fat overlying the anterior platysma muscles. This is a result of aging and the many contractions the platysmal muscles undergo; these selectively stretch the overlying tissues.[35] In addition, the SMAS, which in youth holds the muscle strongly and closely to the confines of the concavity of the neck, stretches so that the muscle webs more easily out of the concavity when contracted and returns to normal less completely on relaxation.

Platysmal cords or bands are the folds of excess skin, fat, and, at times, muscle that persist even when the muscle is relaxed.[35] These muscles are part of the SMAS. Treatment should be directed toward tightening the skin and the SMAS and supporting the muscle in its reverted, more youthful position. A posterosuperior motion placed on the skin, superficial fascia, and platysma muscles will flatten the skin excesses and draw the platysma back into the concavity of the neck. This can be accomplished more successfully when excess neck fat has been removed by liposuction.

Flap Undermining

Facial skin flaps are undermined at a level slightly below the subdermal plexus of vessels, but not so deep as to threaten the deeper vascular arcade or facial nerve branches (Fig. 45–11). Thus, the skin flaps are relatively thin, having only 2 to 3 mm of fat on their undersurface. The thickness of the flap is carefully controlled by evaluating the intensity of the overhead operating lights shining through the underside of the flap.[10] By noting the intensity of light penetrating the skin flap, the surgeon can determine the thickness of the flap being created. Traction by the surgeon and countertraction by the assistant can provide the necessary flap tension at the subcutaneous fat and dermal junction for proper dissection. By tenting the skin and raising the subcutaneous fat junction perpendicular to the skin flap, a parallel, rather than an oblique, dissection can be accomplished.

The initial dissection is best accomplished via sharp dissection with a scalpel or a pair of 5-inch Jabaley straight scissors. Eight-inch Metzenbaum scissors are then employed to complete the flap elevation, using gentle scissor dissection done under direct visualization. Forceful spreading of the scissors may injure flap vasculature or even "fracture" the dermis, creating striae as a result of the thinness of the flap. Because the facial nerve branches are all deep to the plane of dissection, no injury will occur if the proper plane of dissection is maintained.

Dissection produces two flaps that are superiorly separate but inferiorly contiguous. The anterior flap is the facial cheek flap anterior to the ear. The posterior flap is created from the neck posterior to both the ear and sternocleidomastoid muscle. Both flaps blend into one below the level of the ear. The long flap procedure relies on restructuring and suspension, rather than tension, for its effect. Tightening of the SMAS and the use of two anchoring points provide all the tension required to adequately suspend the flaps.

ANTERIOR FLAP DISSECTION

Once the incisions are made, the anterior flap is usually developed first. As noted earlier, initial dissection may be performed using a scalpel or sharp scissors. The skin is more loosely applied to the underlying structures anterior to the parotid gland and the sternocleidomastoid muscle. The tendency is to descend deeper during dissection in these areas, so a conscious effort must be made to stay in the proper superficial plane. Again, countertension provided by the surgical assistant is important to allow the surgeon to maintain a thin flap. The tension also exposes the edge of the scissor dissection in the subcutaneous fat, preventing the plane of dissection from dipping deeply. Any bleeding is controlled by bipolar electrocoagulation.

POSTERIOR FLAP DISSECTION

Sharp dissection is necessary to initially free the posterior flap. The subcutaneous dissection of the skin flap over the mastoid and the region caudal to the ear must be accurate. The skin over the mastoid area is very adherent, and no distinct aponeurotic layer is present to separate the subcutaneous layer from the underlying muscle. In the region of the main trunk of the sternocleidomastoid muscle, it is relatively easy to penetrate the superficial musculoaponeurotic system. Here the surgeon must stay in a subcutaneous plane, not only because of the adherence of the dermis to the superficial muscloaponeurotic system but also because tensing the sternocleidomastoid muscle forces the great auricular nerve closer to the surface. Skin flaps developed in a subcutaneous plane superficial to the SMAS should not endanger the great auricular nerve or any deeper neck structure.

Dissection is completed when the posterior flap connects with the border of the anterior flap and the neck lipodissection and extends inferiorly to the presurgical markings. Absolute hemostasis is mandatory over the areas of the anterior and posterior flaps. This is in stark contrast to the neck flap raised by lipodissection, in which hemostasis is a result of the ability of the cannula

Text continued on page 608

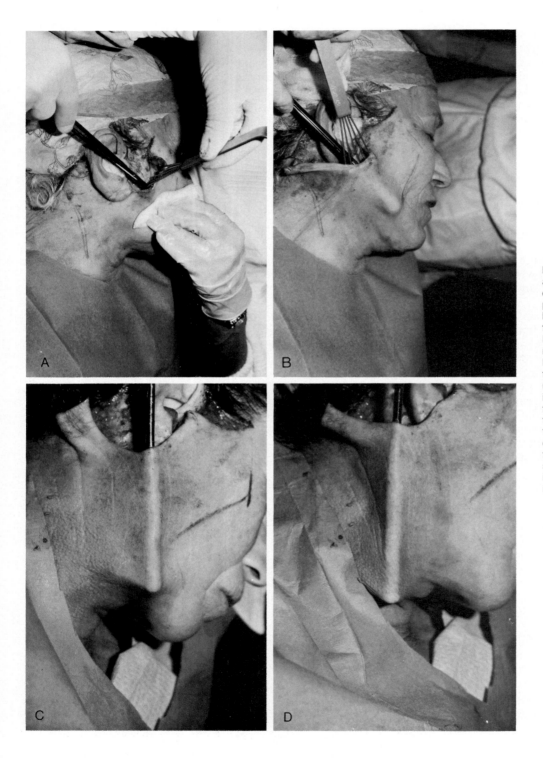

Figure 45–11. *A,* Counteraction applied by the assistant facilitates dissection in the correct surgical plane while the flap is tensed up by the surgeon with an Anderson five-prong face lift retractor. *B,* Dissection of the flap in a subdermal plane is accomplished with long Metzenbaum scissors, the tips of which can easily be noted under the skin flap. *C,* Undermining is extended to the designated facial border carrying the dissection just short of the nasolabial fold in the long flap. *D,* Scissor dissection at the neck extends to the neck flap created by lipodissection to allow unrestrained lifting of the redundant skin in the neck.

Figure 45–11 *Continued E,* The brightness of the overhead operating light penetrating through the undersurface of the flap is carefully observed to determine and maintain the correct thickness of the flap. *F,* The skin flaps are reflected to expose the SMAS and to obtain meticulous hemostasis so that excess fat can be suctioned from the cheek area under direct observation. *G,* The postauricular incision arcs over the ear concha before curving into and parallel to the mastoid hair line. *H,* A lazy "S" incision in the SMAS extends from a point inferior to the zygomatic arch to the anterior border of the sternocleidomastoid muscle so that scissor dissection can be used to raise the SMAS flap.

Illustration continued on following page

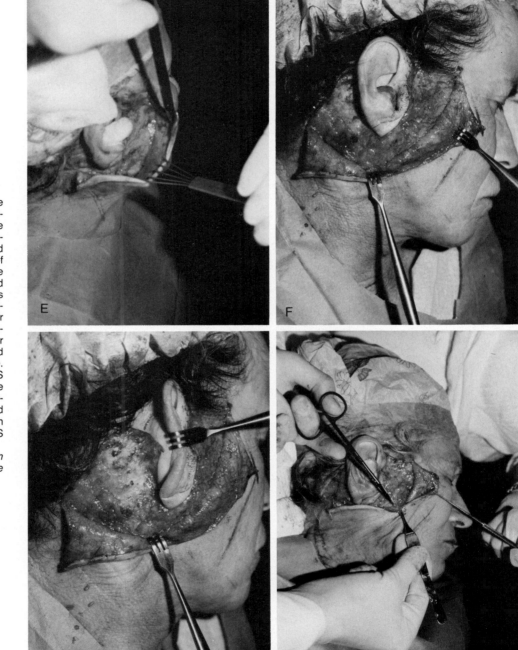

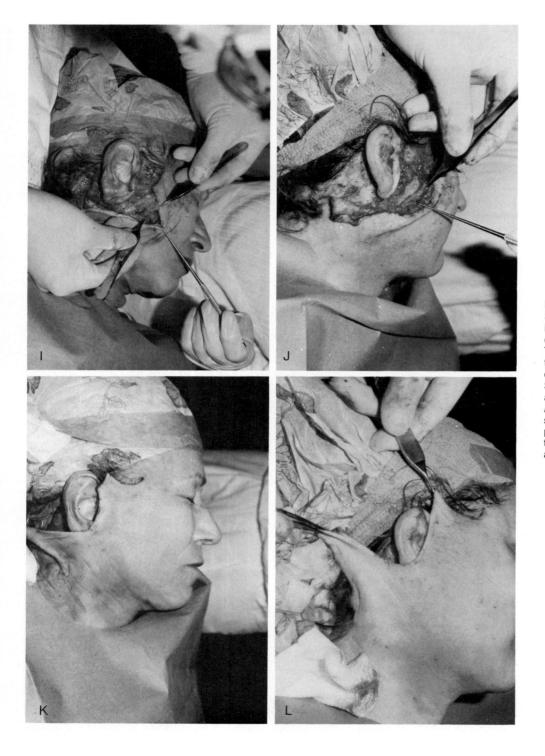

Figure 45–11 *Continued I,* The SMAS is carefully elevated, avoiding penetration through the underlying parotid gland fascia. *J,* The SMAS flap is lifted, revealing the underlying parotid gland fascial envelope. *K,* Plication of the SMAS flap pulls the skin flap up and over the lower part of the ear. *L,* The facial flaps are gently stretched several times in a superior and posterior vector to obtain optimal lift along the mandible and neck.

Figure 45–11 *Continued M,* The anterior flap is pulled and stretched in a superior and posterior direction and a No. 15 scalpel blade stab wound is made in the flap so that the incision will be parallel to the temporal incision. *N,* The scalpel blade is then turned and the flap bisected. *O,* The flap is pulled up with tension in preparation for anchoring to the temporal incision line. *P,* The anterior flap is again stretched to ensure that the correct line of pull has been obtained. Note the flap elevation at the submental as well as the lower and lateral periorbital regions.

Illustration continued on following page

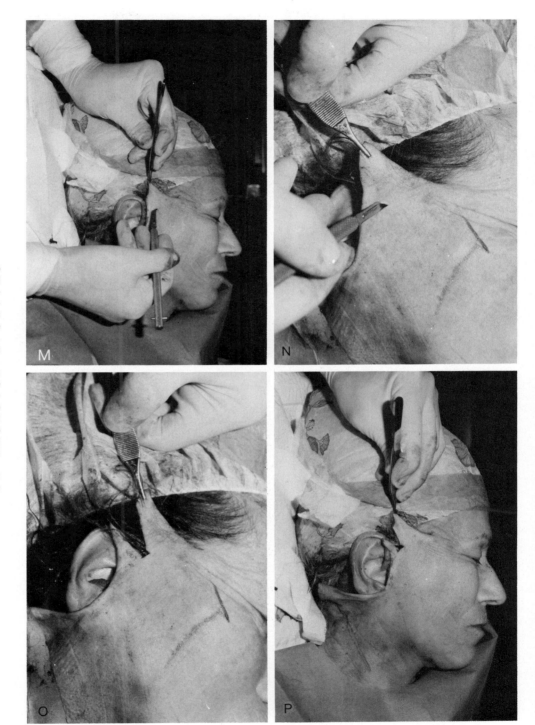

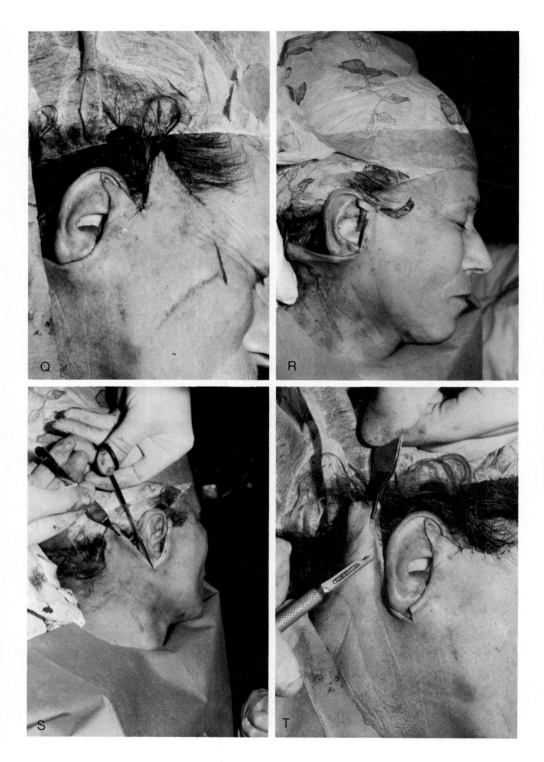

Figure 45–11 *Continued Q,* A suspending suture is placed above the ear at the otobasion superius to place moderate tension on the anterior flap. *R,* The temporal skin is trimmed from the anterior flap, leaving an elliptical gap. The skin can now be anastomosed with stainless steel staples along the temporal incision. *S,* The scissor blades parallel the posterior edge of the ear while separating the anterior and posterior flaps so that the earlobe can be lifted from behind the flap. *T,* A stab wound is made in the posterior flap for placement of the second anchoring suture.

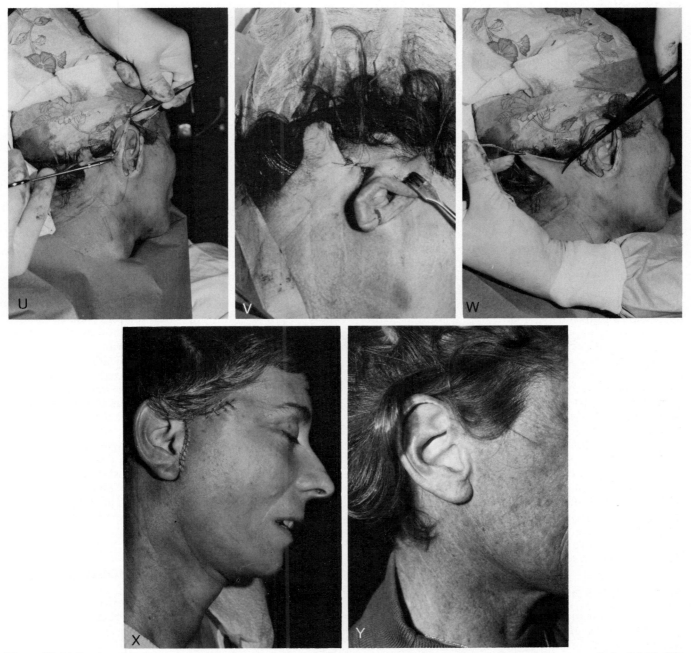

Figure 45–11 *Continued U,* The posterior flap is anchored just posterior to the retroauricular sulcus in the mastoid area so that relatively little skin is excised from the immediate postauricular region. The skin will lie within the auriculomastoid sulcus to preserve, rather than blunt, this natural angle. *V,* A tense postauricular suspension holds the posterior flap in its new position. *W,* The posterior flap is trimmed before closure with stainless steel staples. *X,* Final appearance after excess skin has been removed from the preauricular area and all incisions have been closed. *Y,* Lack of tension at the temporal and preauricular incisions results in a barely perceptible scar after 3 months.

to minimize vascular disruption during dissection and suctioning. Once hemostasis is assured and the neck has been suctioned and dissected, the surgeon is ready to suspend the superficial fascia of the cheeks or SMAS.

SMAS SUSPENSION

There are many surgical options for suspending the SMAS. Suspending the SMAS lifts it to a new position so that it can be sutured into place. This procedure is not to be confused with "suspending sutures," which are defined as sutures running from sites located at a distance to other sites in the SMAS or around it. Suspending the SMAS tightens some of the pendulous tissues responsible for the sagging jowls and drooping corners of the mouth. SMAS suspension is not a substitute for adequate skin resection or adequate fat removal. All three maneuvers should be performed and, when there is no offending fat, the other two are advisable in face lifting.[36, 37]

Dissection beneath the SMAS must be done very carefully to avoid damaging the branches of the facial nerve or the parotid gland. Injury can occur during a retrofascial dissection when the SMAS is thin, when the superficial lobe of the parotid is short and does not protect the nerves, when the retrofascial dissection is carried too far forward beyond the anterior border of the parotid gland, or when dissection proceeds to the mandible or onto the zygomatic arch. Careful palpation of the underlying structures while elevating the SMAS flap will help delineate the extent of dissection.

Two different approaches can be used for suspending the SMAS. The approach chosen is dependent on the facial anatomy and the quality of the SMAS exposed after the skin flaps have been elevated. When there is a well-developed SMAS, especially in the presence of a round face, imbrication is performed. During SMAS imbrication, a flap or edge of SMAS tissues overlaps deeper structures and other SMAS elements. The SMAS is incised and dissected to perform the imbrication. In the presence of marked gauntness of the cheeks or an underdeveloped and atrophied SMAS, plication is preferred. Plication causes the sutures to fold the SMAS layer on itself without incising or dissecting the SMAS.[36] This is a less time-consuming procedure, with minimal risk of damage to the underlying nerves and structures.

SMAS IMBRICATION

SMAS imbrication and suspension require only a limited amount of undermining of the SMAS. The dissection curves from the anterior border of the parotid, posterior to the angle of the mandible, to the anterior border of the sternocleidomastoid approximately 2 cm below the mandible. This limited dissection avoids the facial branches of the seventh cranial nerve and provides an adequate flap for deep tissue tightening. In creating the flap, it is important to avoid undermining to the angle of the mandible, as dissection here will place the marginal mandibular branch of the facial nerve at risk.[28]

The inferior border of the zygomatic arch is palpated to ascertain the superior limit of SMAS incision. A scalpel incision is carefully made into the SMAS, starting from the lower border of the zygomatic arch and curving posteriorly to the anterior border of the sternocleidomastoid muscle. The SMAS is then separated from the underlying parotid fascia. The flap created is 2 to 3 cm wide at its greatest width on the cheek. Once dissection is complete, a crescent, approximately 1.5 to 2 cm, is trimmed from the flap, producing a gap in the SMAS layer.

This gap is then closed with six to ten buried 4–0 or 3–0 monofilament polypropylene sutures. The flap is pulled and suspended in a posterosuperior direction. The suture needle should enter the incised nondissected border in the direction of the underlying nerves to avoid their entrapment. Because the great auricular nerve and its branches run inferiorly on the sternocleidomastoid muscle, the suture needle should also enter and exit the SMAS overlying the muscle in a posterosuperior direction.

SMAS PLICATION

Plication is a quick, noninvasive, and less hazardous procedure for suspending the SMAS. The SMAS is folded on itself in a curved line starting just below the prominence of the zygomatic arch and extending to the neck anterior to and on the sternocleidomastoid muscle. Again, six to ten buried 4–0 or 3–0 monofilament polypropylene sutures are used to secure the suspended SMAS. Folding of the SMAS in the hollow of the cheek will improve the gaunt cheek appearance demonstrated by some patients. Conversely, the plicated SMAS in the lower preauricular and upper neck region may produce an unsightly bulge. This bulge of fat and SMAS can be carefully scissor trimmed and flattened after plication. Any bulkiness caused by fat may also be improved by liposuction.

Both imbrication and plication tighten some of the pendulous tissues responsible for the jowls and drooping of the corners of the mouth. SMAS suspension also has a "hammock effect" on platysmal cording by pulling the platysma up and under the chin. The suspended flap will also form a solid, stable base over which the skin can be draped.

Flap Suspension and Closure

The skin is redraped in two superiorly separate but inferiorly contiguous flaps. Closure of these two flaps is based around two anchoring points. The anterior flap is anchored at the superior preauricular angle where the preauricular incision dissects the temporal incision (otobasion superius). The anchoring point of the posterior flap is at the height of the masto-occipital angle just posterior to the postauricular sulcus. The flaps are pulled in a superoposterior direction perpendicular to the temporal and masto-occipital incisions.

Care must be taken not to pull the flap in a posterior direction, which will create an unnatural windswept appearance. The surgeon is especially likely to pull the posterior neck flap in an inferior and superior direction, as this actually facilitates the removal of excess skin. However, the object is not to remove maximum excess skin, but to suspend the pendulous skin in the most aesthetic position possible. Both anchoring points must be snug, and the flaps pulled firmly over the face and neck without any skin laxity. These are the only two points where any tension should be applied to the flaps.

The tension applied to these long flaps is less than that associated with the short-flap rhytidectomy.[37] This more extensive procedure relies on restructuring and suspension, rather than tension, for its effect. Any significant degree of widespread tension on these long flaps may collapse the already compromised blood supply to the skin, resulting in skin slough. Tightening of the SMAS and the use of two anchoring points provide all the tension necessary to adequately suspend the flaps. Avoiding excess tension on the flaps is facilitated by turning the patient's head to anchor the flaps.

Upon completion of flap dissection, neck lipodissection and liposuction, and SMAS suspension, the entire flap is gently but firmly pulled and stretched in a posterior and superior direction several times. This lengthens the flap and allows greater tissue removal. While stretching the flap, the surgeon should observe the facial skin and neck for skin puckers, which may occur along the edge of the flap dissection, so that they can be corrected before attachment of the flaps. Simple but careful dissection will loosen the flap edge, releasing the pucker. The area should then be carefully observed for any bleeding. The skin flaps are then drawn superiorly and posteriorly to their new position and secured with two heavy anchoring sutures of 3–0 nylon. Adjusting the placement of these two sutures regulates the tension on the flap. It is difficult to describe the degree of tension applied to the flap during the closure to ensure optimal lift without compromising the circulation. Furthermore, this tension is not the same in both areas. The temple may be closed under considerable tension with relative impunity from skin necrosis, while even moderate tension on the posterior flap may cause serious circulatory problems. It is always better to apply less tension than to risk circulation compromise and tissue necrosis, especially if the patient may be prone to circulatory compromise from atherosclerosis or smoking.

FLAP SUSPENSION

The anterior flap is anchored before the posterior flap. The initial anchoring is in the region of the otobasion superius at the intersection of the temporal and preauricular incisions. The anterior flap, pulled in a superoposterior direction, is stretched to its limit and then only enough to accommodate the downward mobility of the temporal skin.[10]

An initial stab incision is made with a No. 15 or No. 11 blade parallel to the temporal incision. This stab incision should be located at the lower border of the temporal incision line. If it is not, a new, lower stab incision must be made. The blade is then turned perpendicular to the stab incision, and the flap is divided posteriorly. A 3–0 nylon suture attaches the stab incision

of the anterior flap to the temporal skin at the otobasion superius. The tension on the secured flap is then carefully assessed to ensure its proper direction.

The anterior flap is then pulled perpendicular to the temporal incision. A curved incision is made parallel to the temporal incision, resulting in a crescent-shaped gap between it and the anterior flap. The gap, measuring approximately 1 to 1.5 cm, is carefully closed, using stainless steel staples to slightly evert the wound edges. Supplemental 4–0 nylon sutures may be used as necessary between the stainless steel staples.

Attention is next directed to anchoring the posterior flap at the postauricular point. The flap is pulled over the ear while it is being anchored and again is gently but firmly stretched several times. With the flap held in a posterosuperior direction, a stab incision is made parallel and just inferior to the masto-occipital incision. The blade is then turned perpendicular to the masto-occipital stab incision, and the flap is separated posteriorly. The flap is then anchored in place with a 3–0 nylon suture.

The posterior flap, once anchored behind the ear, is then attached along the masto-occipital incision. Pulling the flap perpendicular to the masto-occipital incision, the surgeon makes a curved incision, starting at the occipital area. Beginning the incision at the occipital region prevents formation of a noticeable dogear on the neck. There should be a crescent-shaped gap between the edge of the flap and the masto-occipital incision on completion of the curved incision. This gap is closed utilizing stainless steel staples.

EARLOBE IMPLANTATION AND FINAL SKIN CLOSURE

Correct reimplantation of the earlobe is necessary to make the face lift surgery inconspicuous. No tension should be placed on the earlobe at the time of closure, as this structure is apt to be pulled inferiorly with healing, creating a "devil's ear" deformity. There should be a slight upward push of the earlobe at the conclusion of the surgery to counter this downward pull.[27, 28] This will allow for some correction during postoperative tissue settling. The earlobe, when positioned obliquely backward, will increase the horizontal length of the jaw, which helps balance the facial features. The earlobe should never be directed obliquely forward.

Once the temporal and masto-occipital portions of the flaps have been anastomosed, the flap has to be cut for proper positioning of the ear and earlobe. The flap, which partially covers the ear, is cut along a line parallel to the postauricular sulcus. This incision extends to the level of the subtragion (intertragal notch) just superior to the earlobe. The cartilaginous framework of the ear at this point is sturdy and quite immobile, providing a fixed anatomic point. The earlobe is then pulled out from under the skin flap and suspended at the lower border of the incision between the anterior and posterior flaps.

The preauricular incision is next anastomosed using a 6–0 nylon locking suture closure. Starting at the otobasion superius, the flap is trimmed to curve in slightly above the tragus and then to curve out and around the tragus to the base of the earlobe. A small gap is allowable, but tension should be minimal to minimize scar formation. The posterior flap is trimmed to lie within the postauricular sulcus. The earlobe is held within the sling formed by the anterior and posterior flaps.

The earlobe may be overdeveloped in some aging faces. A flabby and mobile lobe can easily be distorted during surgery and must be handled with great care. The overdeveloped lobe must be carefully positioned obliquely backward within the sling created by the flaps. Careless reattachment will result in the lobe being pulled down, producing a deformity. During the operation the lobe may be reduced in size before repositioning.[23] However, it is more appropriate to have a slightly larger lobe that hangs freely and can accept earrings than a lobe that is too small and attached to the neck.

Finally, the postauricular gap is closed with nylon sutures. Closure is loose so that the flap will fall into the sulcus as the head is repositioned forward. This will also allow any accumulation of blood to leak out onto the dressing. After the opposite side is closed, the submental incision is sutured. A final suctioning through the submental incision with a 4-mm cannula may be performed to remove any blood that may have accumulated in the lower neck.

Postoperative Care

The immediate postoperative plan is to minimize swelling and edema and prevent hematoma formation and infection. The use of steroids peri- or postoperatively will decrease edema and reduce the tension on the flap. (C. M. Johnson, verbal communication, 1986).[32, 38] Intramuscular betamethasone (1.0 to 1.5 ml) can be given at the conclusion of the procedure to effectively reduce or limit postoperative edema. During the procedure, corticosteroids can be given by intravenous drip, along with antibiotics. Some cutaneous surgeons prefer to routinely administer antibiotics intramuscularly at both initiation and completion of the procedure and then continue oral antibiotics for an additional 4 days.

DRESSING AND SUTURE REMOVAL

The cervicofacial rhytidectomy dressing serves several purposes. It is a circumferential, supportive bulky dressing that should be applied snugly but without constrictive pressure on the flaps. Its theoretical purpose is not to prevent a hematoma, but to apply even pressure. This will disperse the expected minimal oozing of blood, thus not allowing it to pool and form a small hematoma. The dressing also protects the flaps from trauma and immobilizes the head and neck. Frequently the patient is exhilarated postoperatively and does not understand that major surgery has been performed. Failure to restrict postoperative activities will increase the inci-

dence of hematoma and the strain on the incisions. A bulky dressing helps to limit movement of the head.

The patient is seated upright on completion of the surgery. The incisions are cleansed of all blood. Antibiotic ointment is applied abundantly to the incisions, especially behind the ear. A nonstick Telfa gauze pad (8x3 inches) is slit longitudinally down the middle. The gauze is placed around the ear with the slit up, covering the incisions made in front and behind the ear. Two equal lengths of cotton fluffs are cut so that they cover the distance from the top of the head to the opposite hairline, thereby overlapping the lower face. A cotton gauze roll secures the cotton fluffs snugly but without tension over the anterior and posterior flaps. The ability to slip several fingers under the dressing ensures that excess tension has not been exerted by the dressing (Fig. 45–12). If the dressing becomes restrictive, the patient is instructed to loosen it at the neck by cutting the border with scissors.

The dressing is not removed until the second postoperative day. The incisions are then cleansed with 3% hydrogen peroxide, and an antibiotic ointment is reapplied. The preauricular incision sutures are removed on the fourth or fifth day, and tape strips are applied to the wound. Half of the temple staples are also removed at this time. The remaining sutures and staples are removed on the ninth or tenth postoperative day. All wounds are continuously covered with an antibiotic ointment until completely healed.

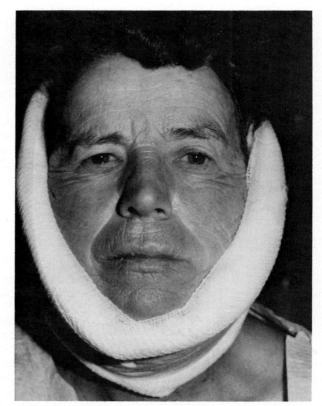

Figure 45–12. Upon completion of the face lift, a bulky dressing of Telfa, cotton fluff, and Kerlex provides support to the newly repositioned skin, stabilizes the neck, and minimizes movement.

POSTOPERATIVE ACTIVITY

Attentive and sympathetic care is as important as the operation itself.[39] It is not uncommon for the patient to experience mild postoperative depression. This may be due to the anesthesia, the normal psychological letdown after the completion of surgery, the postsurgical appearance, or the physical restrictions the patient must endure.

Patients must severely restrict activities for the first 48 hours; complete bed rest is appropriate. The first 24 to 48 hours of the postoperative period are critical to avoid formation of a hematoma, the most common face lift complication. The head and neck should remain immobile, because even minimal movement could place tension on the flaps. The head of the bed is elevated, but not enough to cause flexion of the neck, which can compromise circulation. Talking, especially telephone conversations, should also be minimized. During the first 24 hours, a responsible individual should aid the patient in all activities, including bathroom visits, to prevent any slips or falls. The patient is placed on a soft or liquid diet until the dressing is removed. An appropriate sedative is prescribed for the first 2 days, especially for anxious patients, to prevent elevations in blood pressure and maximize bed rest.

Antibiotic ointment must be applied several times daily once the dressing has been removed. This moistens the incisions, prevents crusting and hastens healing. Gentle washing of the face and the incisions, using lukewarm water, is permissible. Avoidance of alcohol and any medications that can cause bleeding is mandatory for the first week.

After the dressing is removed, patients are allowed to move about the house but must not perform any lifting or strenuous activity that may increase the blood pressure or heart rate. The patient is advised to avoid excessive head turning for the first 2 weeks. Light activity such as walking is acceptable when the first sutures are removed, and routine activities may be slowly resumed after 2 weeks. Excess sun exposure, especially in the presence of bruising, may result in persistent pigmentary changes.

After 4 days, and just before initial suture removal, patients may gently wash their hair for the first time, using a mild shampoo. This is done in the shower; washing the hair in the sink, in which the patient has to bend over and strain, must be avoided. The patient may wash the hair regularly beginning 2 days after the initial sutures are removed. The face and scalp should be handled or massaged gently during shampooing to prevent injury. Hair permanents must be avoided until all the incisions are healed and no longer exhibit irritation. The hairdresser should use only mild chemicals during the initial postoperative visit to minimize the risk of injury to the incisions and flaps. The patient is requested to return every 2 weeks for the first month to ensure that healing is progressing as expected. A 2-month visit is also scheduled, and the patient is instructed to call at any time if there are any questions concerning the surgery. If the patient is compliant in these postoperative instructions, good results can be anticipated (Figs. 45–13 through 45–20).

Complications

Most litigation suits arise when the doctor-patient relationship goes awry.[6] The cutaneous surgeon must learn to be secure enough not to take a patient's hostility personally. It is imperative to resist the temptation to reason or argue with the patient; instead, the physician should try to understand the patient and also make himself or herself understood. With time, most face lift complications can be expected to improve or resolve. Frequent office visits, with the physician demonstrating an understanding and concerned attitude, will help the patient through this trying time. Consultation with a physician of the surgeon's choice may also be reassuring.

A surgical procedure is not fully comprehended until the surgeon is well versed in its complications. Knowledge not only of how to treat complications but also of why they occur will often enable the surgeon to avoid them. Furthermore, by recognizing a potential or early complication, appropriate corrective action can be initiated so that the potential impact can be modified or avoided. Complications may be the result of inadequate preoperative surgical planning, the surgical procedure, inappropriate postoperative care, or patient error or may even be unrelated to any mismanagement by the surgeon or the patient.

The surgeon who recognizes a potential complication preoperatively can discuss and record this information with the patient to help minimize liability. Informing the patient of the potential hazards shares the burden of risk. The surgeon promises to the best of his or her ability to avoid the hazard. The patient understands and is willing to undertake the risk so that the surgery can be performed. If the risk is unacceptable to either the patient or the physician, the surgery should be delayed or canceled. Alternatively, by mutual consent, both may opt for a modification of the surgical procedure that produces inferior results but carries minimal risks.

All surgical procedures produce some undesirable effects. Some are the result of the procedure and of normal variance in surgical technique. In contrast, a complication is an unexpected condition resulting from inappropriate surgical technique. An extensive procedure such as a rhytidectomy can be expected to have its share of undesirable effects (Table 45–4). It may be wise to limit the extent and number of other procedures to be performed in conjunction with the cervicofacial rhytidectomy to minimize the risk.

HEMATOMA

The most frequent and troublesome complication of rhytidectomy is a hematoma.[40–42] It can result in discomfort and pain, prolonged ecchymosis, skin pigmentation, subcutaneous nodules, puckering of the skin, subcutaneous scar contraction, (especially at the neck), skin necrosis, infection, alopecia, and increased difficulty in the event of a second operation. Hematomas can be

Text continued on page 618

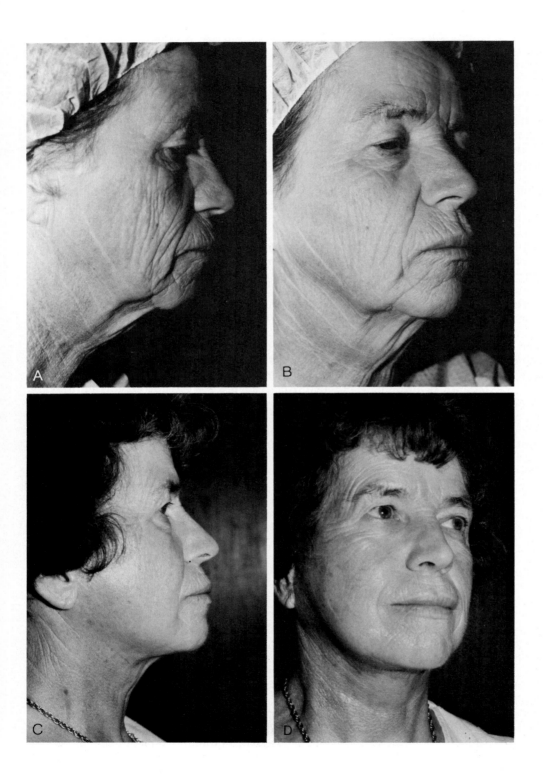

Figure 45–13. *A*, Preoperative profile view. *B*, Preoperative oblique view. *C*, Postoperative profile and *D*, oblique appearance 3 months after cervicofacial rhytidectomy.

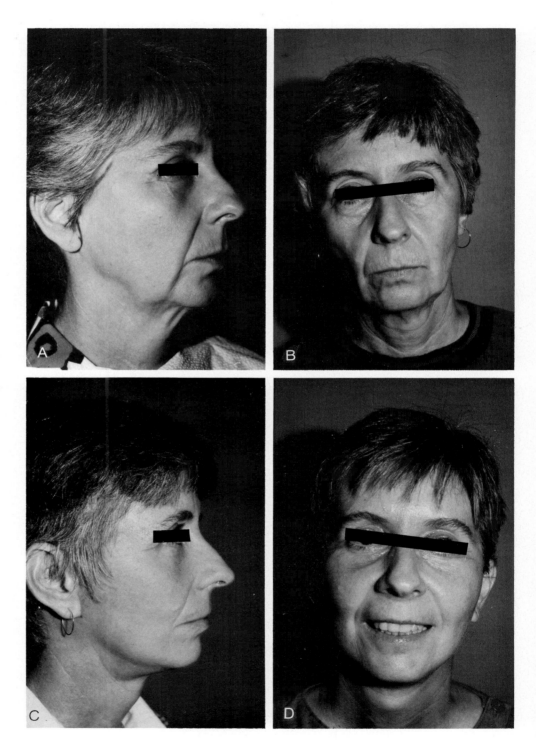

Figure 45–14. *A,* Preoperative profile and *B,* frontal views. *C,* Postoperative profile and *D,* frontal appearance 3 months after cervicofacial rhytidectomy.

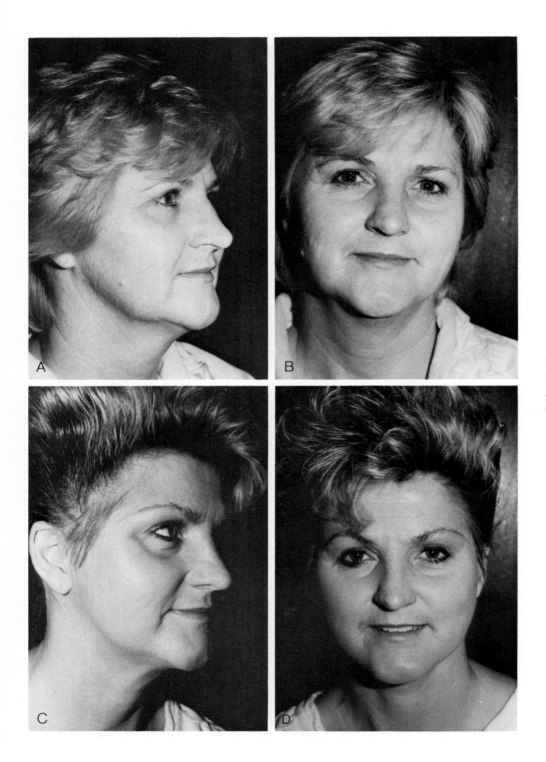

Figure 45–15. *A,* Preoperative profile and *B,* frontal views. *C,* Postoperative profile and *D,* frontal appearance 3 months after cervicofacial rhytidectomy.

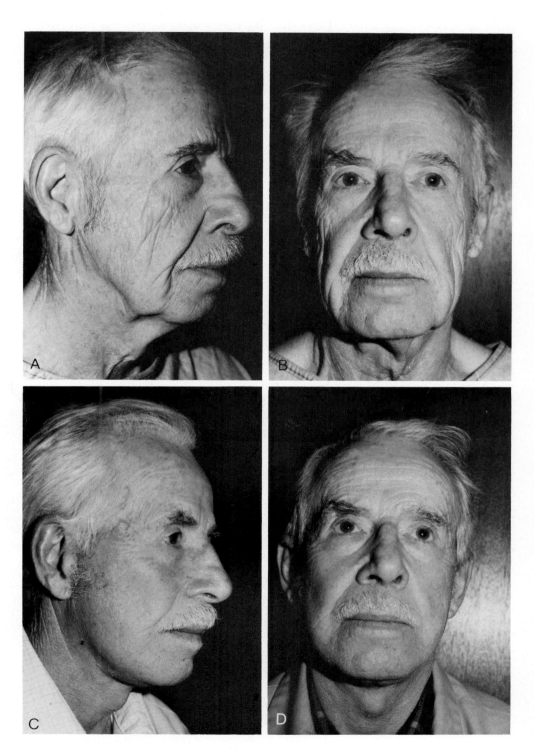

Figure 45–16. *A,* Preoperative profile and *B,* frontal views. *C,* Postoperative profile and *D,* frontal appearance 3 months after cervicofacial rhytidectomy.

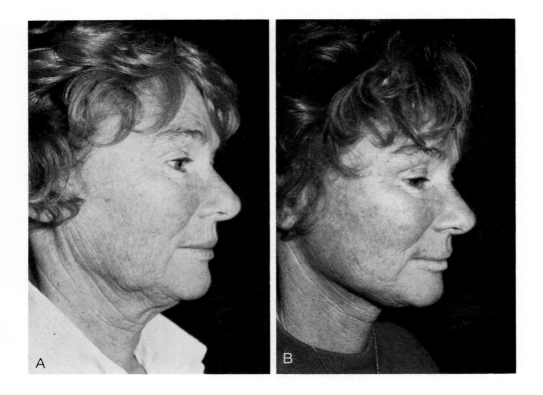

Figure 45–17. *A,* Preoperative profile view. *B,* Appearance 3 months after cervicofacial rhytidectomy.

Figure 45–18. *A,* Preoperative profile view. *B,* Appearance 3 months after cervicofacial rhytidectomy.

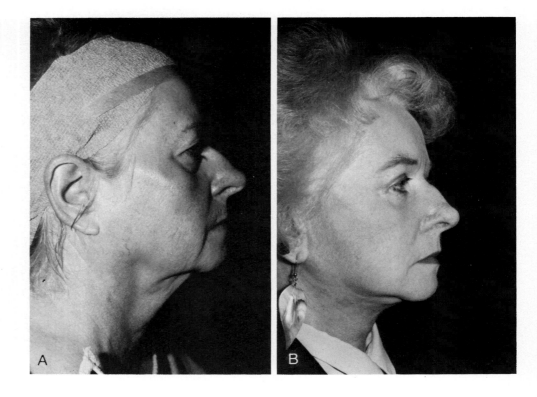

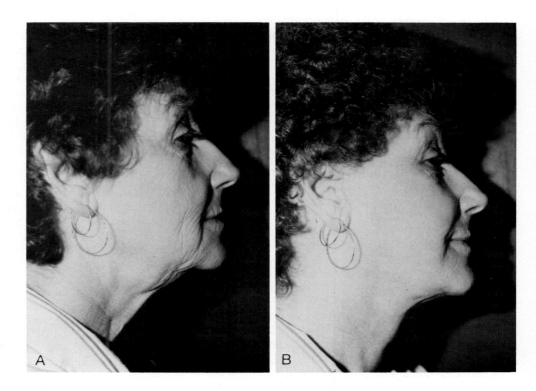

Figure 45–19. *A,* Preoperative profile view. *B,* Appearance 3 months after cervicofacial rhytidectomy.

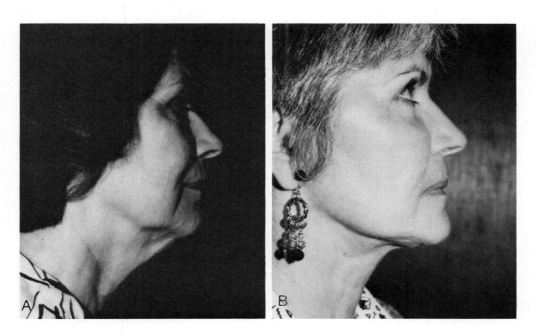

Figure 45–20. *A,* Preoperative profile view. *B,* Appearance 3 months after cervicofacial rhytidectomy.

TABLE 45–4. **COMPLICATIONS ASSOCIATED WITH CERVICOFACIAL RHYTIDECTOMY**

Hematoma	Pain
Prolonged ecchymosis	Infection
Skin slough	Scarring
Flap tip necrosis	Visible scars
Nerve injury	Hypertrophic scars
Anesthesia	Contractive scars
Paralysis	Alopecia
Hypoesthesia	Liposuction ridging
Skin flap buttonholing	SMAS irregularities
Earlobe deformity	Persistent platysmal bands
Anesthetic allergy	Psychological depression
Hypertension	Increased difficulty with
Pigmentary abnormality	subsequent second procedure
Telangiectasia	

either expansive (requiring reoperation for evacuation) or small (requiring simple incision and drainage). Small hematomas are relatively common, with reported quoted rates of 8.9 to 15.4%.[40] The incidence of expanding hematomas ranges from 0.78 to 2.6%, and the overall hematoma rate is approximately 4.8%. Males have a greater tendency for bleeding at the time of surgery and a higher incidence of postoperative hematomas.[3]

Most hematomas occur within the first 24 hours postoperatively. However, they also can occur many days after the operation. Any exertional activity that elevates blood pressure can cause bleeding and should be avoided until healing is complete. Large expanding hematomas are the most common serious face lift complication demanding immediate attention. Onset is almost always heralded by sudden and acute pain, usually followed by unilateral swelling and ecchymosis. Failure or delay in evacuating a large hematoma may lead to venous engorgement and circulatory compromise of the flap with eventual sloughing and necrosis.

Most patients have minimal discomfort after a face lift operation. Excessive pain warrants removal of the dressing for a complete inspection of the surgical site. A hematoma should be evacuated immediately by removing the sutures and evacuating all clots to relieve tension on the skin flaps. After the clot is removed, the wound should be irrigated and any bleeding vessels electrocoagulated. Removal of the hematoma results in prompt relief of pain and usually a drop in blood pressure, which is typically elevated when expanding hematomas are present.[2] Extensive ecchymosis and prolonged edema generally follow treatment of a hematoma, and the patient should be instructed to expect this. Close patient observation is recommended until healing is complete. The final result should not be compromised unless skin sloughing and necrosis occur.

Minute hematomas are absorbed spontaneously within a few weeks and usually leave no sequelae. Small hematomas often form discrete nodules that may not be detected until the initial generalized edema subsides. They can appear as an area of firmness, an ecchymosis, a subcutaneous nodule, or a skin surface irregularity. An effort should be made to evacuate or aspirate these small hematomas when they liquefy, usually between the seventh and fourteenth days. A small hematoma

located near a suture line may be "milked out" after several sutures have been removed. A clot located distant from the nearest suture line may be expressed from a small stab incision made in a natural skin crease overlying the hematoma.

After the fourteenth day, the clot becomes firm and fibrotic and will result in a puckering or minor contour deformity of the skin that can take several months to resolve. Low-dose intralesional steroids may help to minimize or hasten resolution of this deformity, but dilute doses are recommended to minimize the occurrence of subcutaneous atrophy at the injection site.

The most common causes for hematoma are medications, high blood pressure, inadequate operative coagulation, and postoperative patient noncompliance. In general, the more extensive the undermining, the greater the chance for a postoperative hematoma. Coughing and vomiting were formerly common causes but are now relatively rare.[42]

Numerous prescription and nonprescription medications can affect coagulation, and such medications are probably the most common cause of postsurgical bleeding. Taking a careful history; performing hematologic screening with prothrombin, partial thromboplastin, and bleeding times; and providing the patient with a list of medications to avoid all will help to prevent this complication. Aspirin-containing medications and nonsteroidal anti-inflammatory drugs (NSAIDs) must be avoided for a minimum of 2 weeks and preferably for 4 weeks before surgery. These should not be resumed until the tenth to fourteenth postoperative day.

Patients prone to high blood pressure must have their blood pressure under complete control before surgery is performed. It is better to delay surgery until hypertension is controlled, rather than risk bleeding, hematoma, and complications. Nonselective beta-adrenergic blockers may cause uncontrolled hypertension and bleeding when the patient is treated with epinephrine.[43–45]

SKIN SLOUGH AND NECROSIS

Skin slough and necrosis, two of the most feared complications of rhytidectomy, are due to a diminished blood supply to the flap. Skin slough usually occurs in direct proportion to the amount of tension placed on the skin. Increased tension causes a decrease in blood supply to the area, leading to blistering and necrosis (Fig. 45–21A). Skin necrosis and slough are first recognized by a pallor, caused by arteriole compromise, or by a bluish tinge resulting from venous congestion.[3] This is usually noted within the first 48 hours but can develop days later. A superficial slough may resemble a second-degree burn with blistering and desquamation. Although healing is generally satisfactory (Fig. 45–21B), there may be residual pigmentation, telangiectasia, or superficial scarring of the skin.

The incidence of skin slough has been reported as 1.1 to 3.0%.[41, 46] Vascular compromise can be caused by many factors, including delayed recognition of a hematoma, superficial dissection of the flap, trauma to the

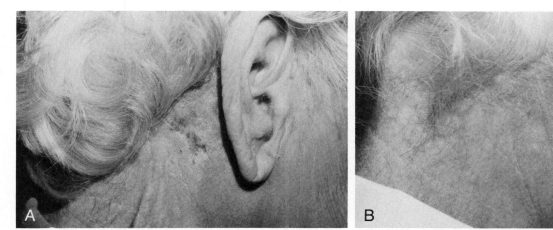

Figure 45–21. *A,* A minor skin slough is present in the retroauricular area where the skin flap is thinnest, the tension greatest, and the blood supply most tenuous. *B,* These sloughs are rarely extensive and usually are superficial with only epidermal sloughing, so that a cosmetically acceptable result can usually be anticipated within 2 weeks.

flap from retractors, tension on the skin flap, excess pressure from a tight dressing, extensive undermining, impaired circulation from previous scars, infection, and heavy smoking. It has been shown that 80% of patients who developed sloughs smoked at least one pack of cigarettes per day.[47] It has been postulated that nicotine slows the rate of wound healing and decreases the cutaneous blood flow. A conservative face lift procedure has been recommended in smokers to minimize the incidence of complications.[48] Because the physician cannot control whether the patient smokes, a conservative lift, with a reduction in the length of the flap, helps to minimize the risk of a slough (Fig. 45–22).

Minor losses of skin adjacent to the suture line are not uncommon. These typically occur in the retroauricular area and especially at the mastoid. The mastoid

area has the greatest occurrence of sloughs, as this is where the skin flap is thinnest, the tension greatest, and the blood supply of the flap most tenuous. Fortunately, these sloughs are rarely extensive and usually are superficial, with only epidermal sloughing. The resulting scar is also behind the ear, where it can be easily hidden by appropriate hair styling.

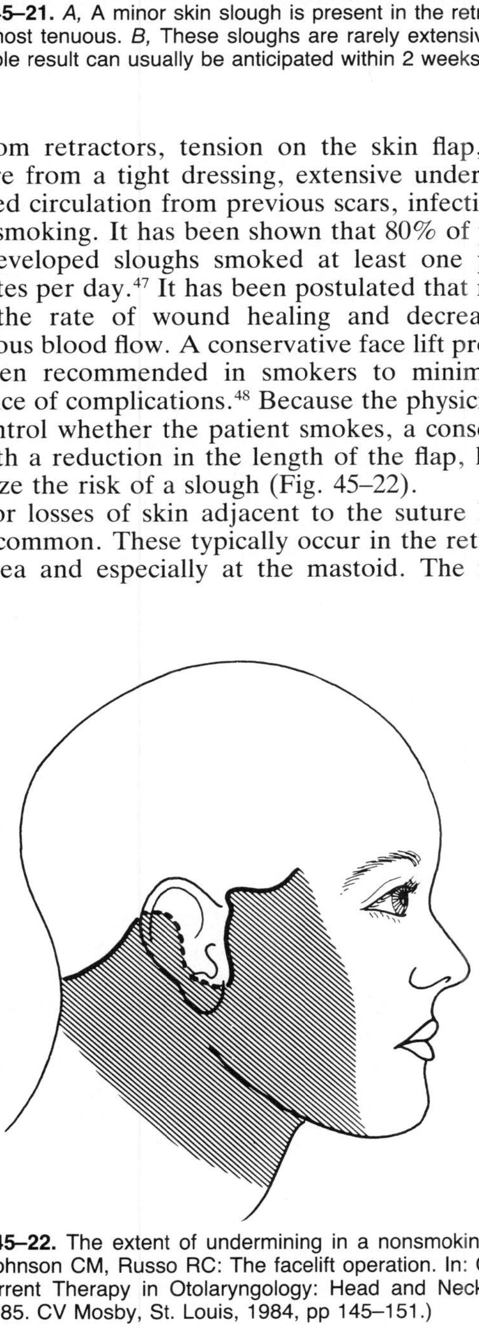

All sloughs should be treated conservatively, as they often heal with minimal scarring if the area involved is small. Superficial sloughing may produce only an area of oozing and superficial ulceration. An eschar eventually develops where full-thickness loss has occurred, and healing takes place by second intention. Those patients understandably require much reassurance during the healing period, which may be as long as several weeks or months.

Covering the wound with an antibiotic ointment or a synthetic surgical dressing or biologic membrane will provide moisture, prevent drying, aid healing, and minimize scarring. Eschar formation also acts as a biologic dressing and therefore should be treated conservatively, unless signs of infection appear, by debriding only the eschar edge as it separates from the underlying healthy skin. If infection appears, immediate debridement is warranted. Major full-thickness skin sloughs rarely occur and usually are secondary to a massive hematoma that has been neglected. In such cases, the resulting scar may be unsightly and require excision and repair or skin grafting if the area is large.

Hypertrophic scars that follow skin sloughs will respond to small, repetitive doses of intralesional steroids. Early recognition and treatment will produce optimal results with minimal side effects. Obviously, skin sloughs that produce atrophic scars are poor candidates for this treatment. The best treatment of skin slough is prevention, which requires gentle handling of tissue, avoidance of excess flap tension, and meticulous hemostasis.

NERVE INJURIES

Injuries to sensory nerves are more common than injuries to motor nerves and may cause prolonged

Figure 45–22. The extent of undermining in a nonsmoking patient. (From Johnson CM, Russo RC: The facelift operation. In: Gates GA [ed]: Current Therapy in Otolaryngology: Head and Neck Surgery 1984–1985. CV Mosby, St. Louis, 1984, pp 145–151.)

numbness or even neuralgia when a major branch of the cervical plexus has been damaged. Motor injuries to the facial nerve have been reported to occur in approximately 1% of all face lift patients, with only 0.1% being permanent.[3, 41] Most injuries to the facial nerves usually resolve spontaneously, and function returns to normal after a period of time. In more than 80% of facial nerve injuries, spontaneous recovery occurs within 6 months, so waiting is usually the most prudent course of action. Before surgery, it is important to inquire about previous facial nerve problems (e.g., Bell's palsy), because a recurrence of nerve palsies in the postoperative period may erroneously be attributed to nerve injury from the operation.

Facial nerve injury after rhytidectomy includes many reversible causes.[49] These are preoperative palsy, coincidental Bell's palsy, and other concomitant neuropathology; normal facial asymmetry hidden by pendulous tissue that is uncovered by the surgery; trauma from the heat of electrocoagulation; injection of local anesthetics directly into the nerve; nerve entrapment by deep ligatures or plication sutures; crushing by forceps or clamps; excessive traction or undue stretching; transection of a nerve during deep dissection; hematoma or edema within the nerve sheath; inflammation and infection; and distortion of normal anatomy caused by adhesions from previous trauma, face lifts, or other surgery.

The nerves most frequently injured are the temporal and marginal mandibular motor nerves and the great auricular sensory nerve. Paralysis of the orbicularis oculi muscle is almost impossible because of its multiplicity of branches. Injury to the buccal branch of the facial nerve is also uncommon. The marginal mandibular nerve, because of its superficial location and the surgical intervention in this region, is commonly injured. The temporal nerve is less vulnerable when a pretemporal hair incision is used.

A marginal mandibular palsy results in an inability to draw the upper lip downward and laterally or to evert the vermilion border. The deformity is due to an inability of the depressor anguli oris and depressor labii inferioris on that side to draw that half of the lower lip downward and laterally. This deformity is not apparent in repose, because the other muscle depressors are not functioning.[16]

The marginal mandibular nerve normally consists of two or three branches, so injury to only one branch may cause only slight weakness, which commonly improves spontaneously over time. The mandibular branch of the facial nerve is located 1 to 2 cm below the lower border of the mandible. In some individuals with lax or atrophic tissues, the branches may be located 3 to 4 cm below the mandible. It is also important to recognize that when the surgeon extends the neck of the patient on the operating table, this draws the nerve even lower. The nerve is covered by the platysma muscle, which can be thin and atrophic, providing minimal protection. Anterior to the facial artery, all the branches of the nerve are above the inferior border of the mandible.[50] While liposuction should not cause permanent damage, temporary dysfunction can result from stretching or bruising the nerve. Because dissection of the SMAS below the

mandible and anterior to the angle of the mandible can unnecessarily place this nerve in jeopardy, such dissection should be avoided.

A stretched or minimally traumatized temporal branch of the facial nerve usually recovers within 6 months. However, complete transection will result in permanent paralysis or incomplete recovery of forehead movement, because fewer than 15% of the nerve fibers in the brow have any connection with other branches. This causes flattening of the forehead and an inability to wrinkle the forehead or elevate the eyebrow. With time, the ensuing muscle atrophy leads to eyebrow ptosis, which, coupled with redundant upper eyelid skin, can obscure the upper visual field. Compensatory wrinkling of the forehead and elevation of the eyebrow on the opposite nonparalyzed side may produce an asymmetric puzzled or quizzical appearance.[12]

The surgeon can help avoid injury to the frontal branches by infiltrating the superficial layer overlying the nerve with local anesthetic, which aids in dissection. The area at risk can be determined by palpating the frontal branch of the superficial temporal artery, since the nerve branches typically penetrate the muscle just below the arterial branches.[17] Another method to ascertain the pathway of the frontal branch is to draw its pathway as a line that passes from a point 0.5 cm below the tragus of the ear to an area 1.5 cm from the lateral border of the brow.[18]

The great auricular nerve is frequently injured because it is the most superficial nerve encountered during rhytidectomy. Many patients may experience transient numbness in the preauricular area and the lower portion of the ear secondary to transection of small sensory nerves. Transient numbness in and around the ear is so common after rhytidectomy that it is considered to be a sequela rather than complication. Although anesthesia of the earlobe usually improves over a period of several weeks or months, the patient should be cautioned that during this recovery period, the earlobe may be injured unknowingly. Earrings, frigid temperatures, and hair treatments can be hazardous to an anesthetized earlobe. In contrast, transection of the great auricular nerve can produce permanent loss of sensation in a wider area, with resulting paresthesias and even severe pain. There is loss of sensation in the preauricular and postauricular skin and the lower two thirds of the ear.

Injury to the great auricular nerve is best prevented by plotting the area of greatest danger before performing the dissection. With the patient's head turned 45 degrees in the face lift position, the nerve crosses the midtransverse belly of the sternocleidomastoid muscle 6.5 cm below the caudal edge of the bony external auditory canal. At this point, the external jugular vein is also parallel and 0.5 cm ventral to the nerve.[51] In this area, dissection of the skin overlying the sternocleidomastoid muscle should be meticulously performed very superficially to prevent penetration through the protective fibroaponeurotic layer.

When an injury to the nerve is recognized during surgery, it should be repaired immediately. In most instances, the sensory loss from these nerves is minimal and accepted by most patients. However, severe persistent pain may occur rarely.[3, 41] Under these circumstances, re-exploration to search for a neuroma or suture transfixion may be justified.

SKIN FLAP BUTTONHOLING

Buttonholing of the skin flap is a frequent complication for the inexperienced surgeon. It commonly occurs immediately inferior to the earlobe at the attachment of the platysma-auricular ligament and over the mastoid and sternocleidomastoid muscle where the dermis is adherent to the underlying fascia. Any defect should be closed primarily with fine sutures, which are removed in 3 to 4 days.

EARLOBE DEFORMITIES

Incorrect positioning of the lower portion of the earlobe is an obvious defect (Fig. 45–23). When the dropped facial tissues are returned to their original location in the face, the earlobe may be positioned incorrectly. An earlobe positioned obliquely forward will be stretched downward, creating a "devil's ear" or "pixie-like" deformity (Fig. 45–24), thereby compromising the surgical results.[23]

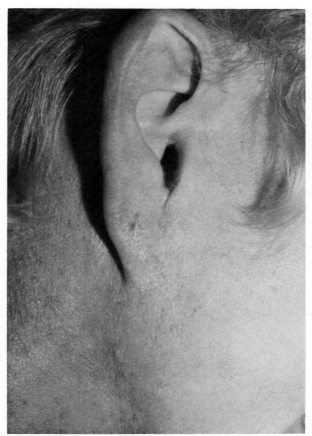

Figure 45–24. Incorrect positioning of the earlobe after a face lift will result in a "devil's ear" or pixie-like deformity as scar contraction occurs.

COMPLICATIONS CAUSED BY LOCAL ANESTHETICS

Nonselective beta-adrenergic blockers may cause uncontrolled hypertension when the patient is treated with epinephrine.[43-45] Selective beta-adrenergic blockers, however, will not result in a hypertensive crisis when epinephrine is administered (Table 45–5). Nonselective beta-adrenergic blockers include propranolol hydrochloride, nadolol, pindolol, timolol maleate, alprenolol hydrochloride, oxyprenolol hydrochloride, and sotalol. Selective beta-adrenergic blockers include metoprolol tartrate, atenolol, and acebutolol. The use of beta-adrenergic drugs by patients undergoing cervicofacial rhytidectomy should be discontinued at least 3 days before administration of an epinephrine-containing anesthetic.

PIGMENTATION ABNORMALITIES

Any pigmentary abnormalities that exist before surgery may be aggravated by the resolving ecchymoses; patients with a history of easy bruising are most susceptible. The dissolving blood produces iron pigments that can tattoo the skin. This pigmentary change is more likely to occur at the neck, where blood gravitates. Lipodissection and liposuction have a tendency to cause traumatic neck ecchymoses. Excessive sun exposure to the ecchymotic skin can stimulate additional pigmentation and consequently should be strictly avoided.

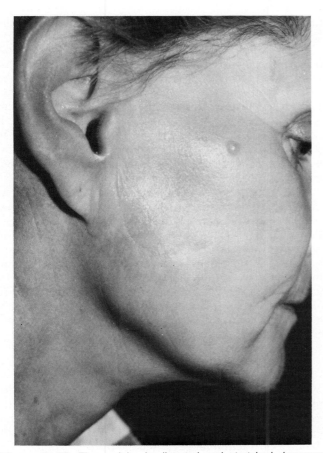

Figure 45–23. The earlobe is distorted and stretched downward owing to improper placement, and the incision has been placed too far forward, resulting in an exposed suture scar line around the earlobe.

TABLE 45–5. **NONSELECTIVE BETA-ADRENERGIC BLOCKERS THAT INTERACT WITH EPINEPHRINE**

Propranolol hydrochloride	Alprenolol hydrochloride
Nadolol	Oxyprenolol hydrochloride
Pindolol	Sotalol
Timolol maleate	

Hyperpigmentation can occur at areas of ecchymoses or minute hematomas. The degree of pigmentation is related more to skin type than to the amount of ecchymosis, and patients with dark complexions can be anticipated to develop greater degrees of pigmentation.[3] Larger hematomas that are amenable to drainage should be evacuated to help minimize this possible sequela.

TELANGIECTASIA

Telangiectasia can be the result of skin undermining, liposuction, undue tension on the skin flap, a resolving hematoma, or a superficial skin slough. Preoperative telangiectasia may also be exacerbated by the procedure. Telangiectases present on the neck may be lifted onto the face, where they may be more prominent. Although they are difficult to treat when widespread, small lesions can be improved with laser photocoagulation or covered with cosmetics.

CUTANEOUS ANESTHESIA

Hypoesthesia is common but usually temporary. Although some patients may note persistence in localized areas, this is usually not of significant concern. Permanent, annoying anesthesia of the ear will occur if the great auricular nerve is severed. If this nerve is severed, the cut ends should be anastomosed immediately to help correct this complication.[51]

PAIN

Postoperative soreness and mild discomfort are not uncommon complaints. Pain is distinctly unusual and must be regarded and investigated immediately as a possible sign of a developing hematoma. Discomfort in the neck may result from a restrictive dressing aggravated by postoperative edema. Patients seldom complain about the dressing pressing against the stainless steel staples at the neck and temple. However, during the early postoperative period, an assortment of complaints of minor concern may be voiced. Discomfort in the neck, evidenced by a feeling of tightness when turning the head, is not uncommon during the first few days or weeks. Localized soreness over the cheeks may occur for several weeks and be quite uncomfortable to pressure. This may be due to entrapped sensory nerves within the SMAS-tightening sutures. The use of intralesional steroids may hasten recovery but also carries a risk of atrophy. Anesthesia or hypoesthesia of the face, neck, or earlobes may last several months. The loss of feeling at the ear is always temporary unless the great auricular nerve was sectioned during surgery and left unrepaired.

In the neck, small neuromas may occur along the cervical sympathetic nerves or at the free ends of a transected great auricular nerve. This discomfort occurs during the late postoperative period along the area of the sensory nerve distribution and usually disappears by the third postoperative month. Repeated frequent regional nerve blocks are often helpful in reducing the pain. In general, chronic pain after rhytidectomy should encourage the cutaneous surgeon to investigate possible psychological causes.[41]

INFECTION

Infection after rhytidectomy is uncommon because of the rich blood supply of the face. However, the presence of a hematoma is a major contributing factor to infection. Diabetic patients are prone not only to infection but also to delayed wound healing.[52]

VISIBLE SCARS

The preauricular skin should have a gap of only 3 to 4 mm before suturing and should be closed without tension. A larger gap can lead to increased wound tension and scarring. An aesthetically pleasing scar is unlikely to result when a straight, preauricular vertical incision is made, as contracture develops, and the scar becomes very noticeable. The preauricular scar should be curvilinear and placed to split, or go behind, the tragus. After scar contracture develops, distortion of the tragus occurs.[53]

Excess tension in the region of the earlobe will produce noticeable suture lines as well as hypertrophic scars. The inferior incision should first delineate the earlobe and then proceed onto the posterior concha. Failure to place it on the ear will result in subsequent migration of the scar onto the posterior neck, where it can easily be seen. Bunching of the skin may occur in the postauricular sulcus and initially be mistaken for hypertrophic scarring but will resolve without treatment in 1 to 2 months.

An incision that does not arc through the retroauricular sulcus when passing from the concha to the mastoid scalp will produce a tethered hypertrophic scar across the concave surface. Along the posterior neck incision line, hypertrophic scarring can result from suture tension. If the incision is placed within the hairline and made parallel to the hair bulbs, the scar will not be noticeable. Destruction of the hair bulbs will result in alopecia and conspicuous scars, but with time, even if left untreated, these scars will soften and become acceptable in appearance.

ALOPECIA

Hair loss in the temporal region is associated with placement of the incision in the temporal hair rather than anterior to it. Permanent hair loss may be due either to superficial dissection with resultant hair bulb damage or traction alopecia secondary to tension on the suture line.[3, 41] The same mechanism that causes skin slough can also produce permanent loss of the hair bulbs. Telogen effluvium may occur along the incision line, requiring 3 months for the hair to regrow. Temporal alopecia can occur when the hairline is displaced by either hair excision or surgical elevation of the temporal hairline. If no hair growth occurs, a scalp flap can be transposed into the site of alopecia.

The occipital incision should traverse parallel within the hairline to help avoid a step deformity.[1] The knife should be held parallel to the hair follicles; otherwise, an area of alopecia separating the hairline from the scar will occur, and the resulting scar will be conspicuous.

LIPOSUCTION IMPERFECTIONS

Liposuction has immensely improved the results of the face lift without significant untoward effects.[54, 55] However, several annoying blemishes may result if the surgeon is not discriminating in the use of the adjunctive procedure. Lipodissection may be used as the method of dissection of the lower face; ridging can result if the cannula is too large or the dissection is not uniform. If suctioning is done simultaneously, the cannula must not be allowed to rest in one position, as excessive fat removal at that area can produce a depression.

At the neck, the skin should be pinched around the cannula tip to control penetration and direct fat into the lumen. However, pinching will traumatize fragile skin and produce multiple ecchymoses that become noticeable during the operation. Although these ecchymoses may be alarming, they do resolve simultaneously without sequelae. More troublesome is the cording or banding that may develop as a consequence of neck liposuction, simulating a platysmal band. Hematoma formation and dermal injury from the cannula aperture have also been implicated as causes of banding. During suctioning, it is often necessary to squeeze the skin around the aperture in an attempt to remove troublesome fat deposits. During this attempt, the dermis may inadvertently be pushed into the aperture, producing injury and cording for up to 4 weeks after the procedure. Aggressive and early use of both intramuscular and intralesional corticosteroids will help to resolve this complication.

SMAS IRREGULARITIES

It is not unusual to notice some fullness just anterior and inferior to the earlobe after surgery; this is due to edema from the plicated SMAS. Such edema is less common when the SMAS is trimmed and imbricated and will usually disappear over a period of several weeks. However, if inadequate operative defatting was performed, residual fullness will remain. By careful and meticulous trimming or suctioning any excess fat from the plicated SMAS, permanent irregularity can be avoided. Extrusion or spitting of SMAS sutures has been blamed on failure to bury the knot and on the use of absorbable suture materials. Correctly buried permanent sutures (e.g., polypropylene) do not seem to cause this problem.

NECK IMPERFECTIONS

Platysmal bands may not be completely eliminated by surgery. Many operations have been devised to correct banding, including transection of the platysma muscle, with posterior attachment to the sternocleidomastoid muscle, or creation of a platysma sling. Unfortunately, any surgical procedure that interrupts the platysma muscle carries an increased risk of damage to the facial nerve that lies deep to it. Platysma surgery can also result in ptosis of the submandibular gland and an asymmetric or irregular neckline.

Persistence of platysma banding may be the result of inadequate placement of plication sutures, which allows the platysma to "cord up" medially and become prominent. Hematomas over the anterior neck that are unrecognized or left untreated may produce fibrosis and retraction and mimic platysmal banding. However, the use of local or systemic corticosteroids will hasten resolution of the retraction.

A pre-existing unilateral or bilateral submandibular ptosis may become obvious once the neck has been defatted and tightened. This should be noted during the original consultation so that the patient will not attribute it to the surgery.

DEPRESSION

It is not clear why many patients experience a period of depression after highly successful cosmetic surgery. Postoperative depression occurs frequently and should always be anticipated by the surgeon.[55] Medications such as narcotics and sedatives administered during the procedure may contribute to development of depression, which may last weeks before resolving. A depressed patient often will express concern over minor complications, and gentle reassurance and frequent office visits may be necessary.

SUMMARY

Every intricate surgical procedure has complications, and face lifts are no exception. Because the operation is completely elective, the ultimate goal is to achieve good results with only minimal risk. The final outcome is affected by many factors, including the surgeon's experience and skill; the patient's psychological profile, life style, and habits; and the unpredictable qualities of the tissues.[40, 41] Each patient must be aware of these facts in advance. In addition, the patient must realize that all face lifts will eventually deteriorate over time because of the inexorable pull of gravity and the inevitable decrease in skin elasticity and tone that occurs with aging. Early recurrence of the aging deformity is more likely when the first rhytidectomy is undertaken at an older age than when done early, such as in the third and fourth decade of life. Patients with severe sagging and wrinkling are more likely to need an early revision of their rhytidectomies because of the inherent laxity of their skin. Any weight loss that occurs after rhytidectomy will also increase the laxity of the skin, so any planned weight loss should be achieved before surgery. The patient should also be aware that the skin will become more lax in the first 6 to 12 months after the operation.

Results can be less than optimal because of many intrinsic patient factors. Obesity, a low hyoid bone, retrognathia, marked skin flaccidity, platysmal banding, poor tissue elasticity, a square face, ptosis or hypertrophy of the submandibular glands, and the basic skeletal structure of the face are a few of the factors that may lead to an unfavorable result. The personal habits of a patient (e.g., smoking, alcohol abuse), exposure to solar radiation, weight fluctuations, and other environmental insults occurring after surgery can also affect the final result or reduce the duration of the lift. These compromising factors should be noted and explained to the patient before surgery. It is also important to point out to the patient any pre-existing facial asymmetries, skin abnormalities, and scars that will not be corrected by the procedure and may actually detract from the outcome. Occasionally, such an abnormality may actually become more evident after cervicofacial rhytidectomy.

In many patients, the results can be enhanced by performing ancillary surgical procedures specifically designed to correct regional manifestations of aging. Because the face lift operation is designed only to tighten the sagging jowl and cervical skin, it will not improve perioral rhytides or prominent nasolabial folds. Furthermore, features of orbital and brow aging may overshadow most of the positive effects of the face lift because of the incongruity of the facial features. Treating associated manifestations of aging with ancillary procedures will often help to balance the facial features, placing the total face in synchronous harmony. Nothing can stop or reverse the aging process, and regardless of the technique employed, gravity and facial aging will inexorably resume. At best, the cutaneous surgeon can only slow the process. With a complete understanding of these important issues, appropriate expectations can be fulfilled in most patients.

REFERENCES

1. Fredericks S: Rhytidectomy. In: Courtiss EH (ed): Aesthetic Surgery: Trouble, How to Avoid It and How to Treat It. CV Mosby, St. Louis, 1978, pp 118–131.
2. Owsley JQ Jr: The unfavorable result following face- and neck-lift. In: Goldwyn RM (ed): The Unfavorable Result in Plastic Surgery. Little, Brown, Boston, 1984, pp 591–609.
3. Rees TD, Aston SJ: Complications of rhytidectomy. Clin Plast Surg 5:109–119, 1978.
4. Goldman L, Caldera DL, Nussbaum SR, et al: Multifactorial index of cardiac risk in non cardiac surgical procedures. N Engl J Med 297:845–850, 1977.
5. Baker TJ, Gordon HL: Surgical Rejuvenation of the Face. CV Mosby, St. Louis, 1986, pp 103–104.
6. Wright MR: The problem patient: prevention and treatment. Am J Cosmet Surg 2:10, 1985.
7. McCurdy JA Jr: An approach to face-lift surgery. Head Neck Surg 5:211–217, 1983.
8. Chrisman BB: Liposuction with facelift surgery. Dermatol Clin 8:501–522, 1990.
9. Webster RC, Davidson TM, White MF, et al: Conservative face lift surgery. Arch Otolaryngol 102:657–662, 1976.
10. Anderson JR, Johnson CM Jr: Some tips on face-lifting. Otolaryngol Head Neck Surg 87:522–532, 1979.
11. Cook TA, Musgrave-Zwetsch J: Adjuncts to face lifting procedures. Otolaryngol Clin North Am 13:321–335, 1980.
12. Salasche SJ, Bernstein G, Senkarik M: Surgical Anatomy of the Skin. Appleton & Lange, Norwalk, CT, 1988, pp 99–109.
13. Bernstein L, Nelson RH: Surgical anatomy of the extraparotid distribution of the facial nerve. Arch Otolaryngol 110:177–183, 1984.
14. Davis BA, Anson BJ, Budinger JM, et al: Surgical anatomy of the facial nerve and the parotid gland based upon a study of 350 cervicofacial halves. Surg Gynecol Obstet 102:385, 1956.
15. Rudolph R: Depth of the facial nerve in face lift dissections. Plast Reconstr Surg 85:537, 1990.
16. Baker DC, Conley J: Avoiding facial nerve injuries in rhytidectomy. Plast Reconstr Surg 64:781–795, 1979.
17. Corereia P, Zani R: Surgical anatomy of the facial nerve as related to ancillary operations in rhytidoplasty. Plast Reconstr Surg 52:549, 1973.
18. Pitanguy I, Silveira RA: The frontal branch of the facial nerve: the importance of its variations in face lifting. Plast Reconstr Surg 38:352, 1966.
19. Peterson RA, Johnston DL: Facile identification of the facial nerve branches. Clin Plast Surg 14:785–788, 1987.
20. Nelson DW, Gingrass RP: Anatomy of the mandibular branches of the facial nerve. Plast Reconstr Surg 64:479–482, 1979.
21. McKinney P, Katrana DJ: Prevention of injury to the great auricular nerve during rhytidectomy. Plast Reconstr Surg 66:675–679, 1980.
22. McKinney P, Gottlieb J: The relationship of the great auricular nerve to the superficial musculoaponeurotic system. Ann Plast Surg 14:310–314, 1985.
23. Loeb R: Posterior auricular nerve preservation, double chin leveling, and earlobe reimplantation during neck lifts. Clin Plast Surg 10:405–422, 1983.
24. Mitz V, Peyronie M: The superficial musculo-aponeurotic system (SMAS) in the parotid and cheek area. Plast Reconstr Surg 58:80–88, 1976.
25. Furnas, DW: The retaining ligaments of the cheek. Plast Reconstr Surg 83:11–16, 1989.
26. Johnson CM, Russo RC: The facelift operation. In: Gates GA (ed): Current Therapy in Otolaryngology: Head and Neck Surgery, 1984–1985. CV Mosby, St. Louis, 1984, pp 145–151.
27. Johnson CM, Adamson PA, Anderson JR: The face-lift incision. Arch Otolaryngol 110:371–373, 1984.
28. Shire JR, Johnson CM Jr, Orr JB: The large flap sculptured facelift. J Dermatol Surg Oncol 14:1352–1356, 1988.
29. Furnas DW: Anthropometric landmarks for precision planning in rhytidectomy. Clin Plast Surg 14:639–661, 1987.
30. Webster RC, Fanous N, Smith RC: Male and female face-lift incisions. Arch Otolaryngol 108:299–302, 1982.
31. Newman J, Fallick H: Lipo-suction tunneling in conjunction with rhytidectomy. Am J Cosmet Surg 1:19–20, 1984.
32. Chrisman BB, Field LM: Facelift surgery update: suction-assisted rhytidectomy and other improvements. J Dermatol Surg Oncol 10:544–548, 1984.
33. Newman J, Nambiar M, Deleon A: The closed neck lift. Am J Cosmet Surg 6:4, 1989.
34. Collins PS: The methodology of liposuction surgery. Dermatol Clin 8:395–400, 1990.
35. Webster RC, Smith RC, Smith KF: Face lift: etiology of platysmal cording and its relationship to treatment. Head Neck Surg 6:590–595, 1983.
36. Webster RC, Smith RC, Smith KF: Face lift: plication of the superficial musculoaponeurotic system. Head Neck Surg 6:696–701, 1983.
37. Webster R: Facelift. Videos Part I and II, San Diego Classics in Soft Tissue and Cosmetic Surgery, San Diego, CA, 1976. American Academy of Facial Plastic and Reconstructive Surgery, Washington, DC.
38. Nordstrom REA, Nordstrom RM: The effect of corticosteroids on postoperative edema. Plast Reconstr Surg 80:85–87, 1987.
39. Tardy EM Jr, Klingensmith M: Face-lift surgery: principles and variations. In: Roenigk RK, Roenigk HH Jr (eds): Dermatologic Surgery: Principles and Practice. Marcel Dekker, New York, 1989, pp 1239–1288.

40. Kridel RWH, Aguilar EA III, Wright WK: Complications of rhytidectomy. Ear Nose Throat J 64:584–592, 1985.
41. Baker DC: Complications of cervicofacial rhytidectomy. Clin Plast Surg 10:543–562, 1983.
42. Rees TD, Lee YC, Coburn RJ: Expanding hematoma after rhytidectomy. Plast Reconstr Surg 51:149, 1973.
43. Hansten PD: Beta-adrenergic blockers and epinephrine. Drug Interact Newslett 3:41–43, 1983.
44. Brummett RE: Warning to otolaryngologists using local anesthetics containing epinephrine. Arch Otolaryngol 110:561, 1984.
45. Foster CA, Aston SJ: Propranolol-epinephrine interaction: a potential disaster. Plast Reconstr Surg 72:74–78, 1983.
46. McGregor MW, Greenberg RL: Rhytidectomy. In: Goldwyn RM (ed): The Unfavorable Result in Plastic Surgery: Avoidance and Treatment. Little, Brown, Boston, 1972, pp 338–340.
47. Rees TD, Liverett DM, Guiy CL: The effect of cigarette smoking on skin-flap survival in the face lift patient. Plast Reconstr Surg 73:911–915, 1984.
48. Webster RC, Kazda G, Hamdam US, et al: Cigarette smoking and face lift: conservative versus wide undermining. Plast Reconstr Surg 77:596–602, 1986.
49. Castañares S: Facial nerve paralysis coincident with, or subsequent to, rhytidectomy. Plast Reconstr Surg 59:24, 1974.
50. Dingman RO, Grabb WC: Surgical anatomy of the mandibular ramus of the facial nerve based on the dissection of 100 facial halves. Plast Reconstr Surg 29:266–272, 1962.
51. Lewin ML, Tsur H: Injuries of the great auricular nerve in rhytidectomy. Aesthet Plast Surg 1:409–417, 1978.
52. Guyuron B, Raszewski R: Undetected diabetes and the plastic surgeon. Plast Reconstr Surg 86:471–474, 1990.
53. Fodor PB, Liverett DM: Sideburn reconstruction for postrhytidectomy deformity. Plast Reconstr Surg 74:430–434, 1984.
54. Newman J, Dolsky RL: Complications and pitfalls of facial liposuction surgery. Am J Cosmet Surg 2:8, 1985.
55. Rees TD: Aesthetic Plastic Surgery. Vol II. WB Saunders, Philadelphia, 1980.

CHAPTER 46

Chin Implants

J. MICHAEL CARNEY

A glance through any current fashionable magazine or catalog will show that image makers believe that a strong chin is part of the ideal "look." What they may not know is that they are following in the path of DaVinci, Michelangelo, and other great artists who through the ages believed that a strong chin was part of the ideally proportioned face. In fact, artists and sculptors throughout history portray stronger chins than actually exist in our population[1] (Fig. 46–1).

A "weak" chin often conveys many negative attributes such as weakness. However, a strong chin is considered a desirable quality, giving the impression of power, confidence, intelligence, determination, dominance, and assertiveness. This is supported by a study[2] of 250 women who were asked to judge photographs of men, scoring features they felt were attractive. A large chin was considered one of the top three most attractive features, along with big eyes and prominent cheekbones.

Chin augmentation with implants is often considered a minor operation, but the technique is not widely presented at medical meetings or in professional journals or discussed by the media and the public. However, this adjunctive procedure has a major role in bringing harmony and balance to the face, either independently or as part of other surgical procedures. If performed properly, with appropriate preoperative planning and operative skill, chin augmentation with alloplastic implants can enhance surgical results in proportions exceeding its degree of difficulty while creating an attractive feature, the strong chin.

Aesthetic Facial Proportions and Landmarks

A thorough understanding of aesthetically pleasing facial proportions is required when the cutaneous surgeon considers augmenting the structural framework of the face. Commonly used soft tissue landmarks[3] (Fig. 46–2) include the trichion, or the midpoint at the hairline; the glabella, the most prominent point in the midline between the brows; the nasion, or the deepest depression at the root of the nose; the subnasale, the point under the nose where the columella merges with the upper lip; the stomion, the interval between the lips; the pogonion, the most anterior soft tissue point on the chin; the menton, the lowest contour point of the chin; the cervical point, the innermost point between the submental area and the neck, located at the intersection of lines drawn tangentially to the neck and submental areas; the porion, the highest point on the external auditory meatus; the orbitale, the lowest point on the inferior orbital rim; and the Frankfort horizontal plane, or the horizontal line extending from the porion to the orbitale.

A series of articles[4-6] has described a method of studying the profile based on extensive research into classical standards of beauty developed by artists and sculptors, anthropologists, and orthodontists. Albrecht Dürer,[4] a sixteenth century German artist, is responsible for developing the generally accepted concept[3, 7] that the face is divided into thirds: from the hairline (trichion) to the eyebrow (glabella); from the eyebrow (glabella) to the base of the nose (subnasale); and from the subnasale to the lowest part on the chin (menton). The lower third can be further subdivided, with the upper one third occurring from the subnasale to the stomion and the lower two thirds occurring from stomion to menton.

In 1962, the quantitative principle for studying the profile using two reference lines was introduced.[4] The first line was the Frankfort plane, a horizontal line extending from the porion to the orbitale. The second was a vertical line dropped downward from the nasion, the deepest part of the root of the nose. This vertical line, called the zero meridian,[5] crossed the Frankfort

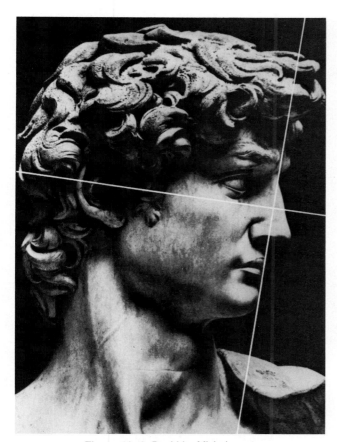

Figure 46–1. David by Michelangelo.

horizontal line at a right angle. These lines created an axis for evaluating defects of the profile. The facial plane was defined as the line from the nasion to the most anterior soft tissue point on the chin, the pogonion. In several classic articles, various works of art and the theories of artists through the ages were reviewed to define parameters and relative proportions of beauty. It was concluded that in the "beautiful" faces throughout history, the relationship of the facial plane to the Frankfort horizontal line was very close to 90 degrees, and the chin was tangential to the zero meridian (Fig. 46–1).

When the chin falls behind the zero meridian,[5, 6] this indicates a chin deficiency and a possible benefit that could result from chin augmentation. The difference between the chin and the ideal vertical or zero meridian serves as a guide to the required correction.

Many authors have described variations on this description of the location of the ideal vertical line, using the glabella instead of the nasion to give a slightly larger chin.[3] Others[8, 9] drop a vertical line from the lower lip. If the chin and lower lip line up on a vertical line perpendicular to the Frankfort plane, the patient's chin has ideal projection. The projection in women should fall somewhat behind that in men, about 1 to 2 mm posterior to that line[10] to 2 to 5 mm posterior to a line dropped vertically from the vermilion border.[11] The chin projection should remain 1 to 2 mm posterior to the

lower lip projection,[12] since it is rarely attractive if it projects anterior to the lower lip.

In addition to chin projection, there are several other more complex methods of evaluating the ideal profile. For surgeons who also perform contouring procedures affecting the neck (e.g., submental liposuction and face lift), the mentocervical angle[3] helps define the ideal. A line from the glabella through the pogonion is transected by a line from the cervical point to the menton. The optimal angle is considered to be 80 to 95 degrees. The hyomandibular angle[13] is formed by the submenton and anterior cervical line and should be approximately 90 degrees.

The goal in augmentation mentoplasty is to provide better balance to the face. Many factors, such as the nose, forehead, midface, lip posture, and frontal view, as well as ethnic differences, also play a role in deciding how far anteriorly and laterally to augment. The judgment and experience of the cutaneous surgeon, along with the desires of the patient, combine to arrive at an optimal surgical plan.

Anatomy

The mental symphysis is the ridge formed by the junction of the two halves of the mandible; it divides to form the mental protuberance[9] (Fig. 46–3). The mental

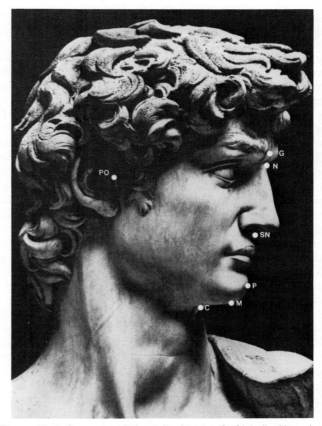

Figure 46–2. Common soft tissue landmarks. G, Glabella; N, nasion; SN, subnasale; P, pogonion; M, menton; C, cervical point; PO, porion.

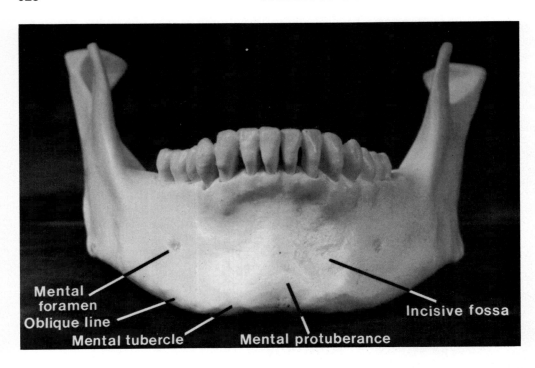

Mental foramen
Oblique line
Mental tubercle
Mental protuberance
Incisive fossa

Figure 46–3. Skeletal anatomy of the chin.

tubercles are raised areas on either side of the mental symphysis. The oblique line is a ridge extending posteriorly from each tubercle. While the mental foramen is generally found below the second premolar tooth, its position is not constant. It has been described below and slightly anterior to the second premolar tooth.[7] The mental foramen may vary from 27 to 37 mm from the midline[11] and has been variably described as being (1) halfway between the upper and lower edges of the mandible, below the apex of the second premolar in the midpupillary line and approximately 2.5 cm from the midline[14]; (2) lateral on the mandible, approximately on a vertical line drawn downward from the lateral border of the supraorbital notch[15]; and (3) at the base of the second premolar or between the second premolar and the first molar. It may also occasionally be double.[16] An anatomic study of 100 mandibles[17] revealed that in 50% of cases the mental foramen is at the level of the second premolar, in 20 to 25% it is found between the first and second premolars, and in 24% it is posterior to the second premolar. It is as anterior as the first premolar or as posterior as the first molar in 1 to 2% of people. Its position is affected by age, so that in children, it is lower on the mandible and more anterior, while in older edentulous patients, because of atrophy of the alveolar ridge, its relative position is higher.[14]

The muscles of the chin are the depressor anguli oris (triangularis), the depressor labii inferioris (quadratus), and the mentalis. The two depressors originate on the oblique line. The triangularis inserts partly into the skin and is partly continuous with the upper part of the orbicularis oris near the lateral part of the lip. The quadratus travels upward in front of the mental foramen, passing among fibers of the lower portion of the orbicularis oris and inserting into the skin and mucosa of the lower lip. The mentalis muscle arises from the mandible in the incisive fossa at the level of the root of the lower lateral incisor and passes downward to insert into the skin of the chin, mostly lying deep to the quadratus.

The marginal mandibular branch of the facial nerve is the motor nerve to these three muscles, and it enters them deeply on the lateral undersurface.[18] The mentalis nerve, a branch of the mandibular nerve of the third division of the trigeminal nerve, supplies sensation to the skin of the chin and lower lip as it emerges from the mental foramen and before breaking up into small slips. The mentalis[18] draws the skin of the lip upward and helps force the lower lip against gums and teeth. The depressors pull their respective portions of the lip downward and laterally. The depressor labii inferioris also everts the vermilion border.

The anatomy of this area has been re-examined,[19] and both bony and soft tissue changes have been noted with aging.[19] The anterior mandibular groove, or geniomandibular, develops on the bone under the prejowl sulcus, a soft tissue depression between the chin and jowl. Atrophy of the mentalis and depressor muscles also contributes to the aging chin.[20]

Microgenia, or a small chin, occurs as a result of underdevelopment of the mandibular symphysis.[7] It must be distinguished from micrognathia, which is hypoplasia of various parts of the jaw. Chin augmentation is appropriate for individuals with microgenia who have normal dental occlusion. (Malocclusion is commonly seen with microgenia.) Occlusion may be evaluated by the Angle classification,[3, 7] which is based on the anteroposterior relationship of the first upper and lower molar teeth. There are three classes in this scheme: in class I, or orthognathic, the mesobuccal cusp of the upper first molar occludes with the buccal groove of the lower first molar, which is normal occlusion; in class II, or retrognathic, the buccal groove of the lower first molar is posterior to the mesobuccal cusp of the upper first molar, and the upper teeth may be protruded or retruded; in class III, or prognathic, the buccal groove of the lower first molar is anterior to the mesobuccal cusp of the upper first molar, and the lower teeth protrude anterior to the upper teeth.

These occlusion patterns are generally reflected in the patient's profile. A patient with class I occlusion usually has a relatively normal profile, though microgenia may exist. In class II, a retrognathic or micrognathic patient may have a very weak-appearing chin. A class III prognathic patient will have a protruding lower jaw. Microgenia may exist with class I or II occlusion. Chin augmentation using alloplastic implants is a reasonable approach for patients with microgenia with normal, class I, or mild class II occlusion or in patients whose micrognathia has been corrected surgically or orthodontically, but in whom there is still a chin deficiency.[21] Patients with class II or III occlusion should be offered an opportunity to deal with the malocclusion orthodontically or surgically.[8] If they elect to accept a mild class II occlusion, chin implantation may help to improve the profile.

Preoperative Evaluation

Because public awareness of chin augmentation is not high, there is little likelihood that individuals with microgenia are aware of or concerned about their problem. The identification of a weak chin is often brought out during consultation for rhinoplasty, face lift, or submental liposuction. The surgeon often mentions it first, including a weak chin in the deficiencies that can possibly be corrected to add balance and harmony to the face. Many patients are unaware of the important role that the lower third of their face (particularly chin projection and definition) plays in defining and placing into relative proportion other parts of the face. Also, many surgeons overlook the possible benefits of chin augmentation, since training in this technique is somewhat uncommon.

One reason chin deficiencies go unrecognized is the very common habit of projecting the chin and extending the neck so as to place the facial plane at the zero meridian of Gonzalez-Ulloa, so that the chin lines up with a vertical line dropped from the nasion or lower lip (Fig. 46–4). This can only be done by positioning the head in violation of the Frankfort horizontal plane. If this posture goes unrecognized by the surgeon, results of other procedures for defects, when combined with the compensatory head posture, will not be optimal.

Polaroid photographs taken during the examination with the head in the Frankfort horizontal plane can be of great use in pointing out the deficiency to patients, since many have never seen or studied their profile. Often when the patient is posing for photographs, the head, even when it has been properly positioned, will drift up out of habit, breaking the horizontal plane. It is uncommon for a patient with microgenia to voluntarily drop the chin, placing the head in the Frankfort plane,

as this accentuates chin deficiency and neck skin and fat deformities. Slouching also contributes to this anterior positioning of the chin and neck extension.

The use of mirrors, Polaroid photographs, or computer imaging is essential to point out a chin deficiency in the profile. With a Polaroid photograph taken with the head in the Frankfort plane (Fig. 46–5), the vertical lines from the nasion or lower lip may be demonstrated with any straight object. Computer imaging (Fig. 46–6) is an excellent way to demonstrate profile abnormalities and the ability of chin augmentation to correct them. The computer images can be used to show sequentially projected results of submental liposuction alone, then adding the augmented chin to demonstrate how the appearance is enhanced.

In evaluating preoperative patients from their profile, the deficiency from the vertical line is noted. A slight pinch forward can give the patient and surgeon an idea of what the degree of correction would look like. On the frontal examination, vertical height, symmetry, and occlusion must be noted. Good candidates have adequate vertical height, symmetry, and normal or nearly normal occlusion. If the distance from the mentolabial crease to the menton is less than one third of the subnasale-menton distance, there may not be adequate vertical height for an implant. To correct vertical deficiency and asymmetry, a sliding horizontal osteotomy should be suggested. Significant malocclusion should be corrected by orthognathic surgery or orthodontia, but an implant may be appropriate either during or after that process if any chin deficiency remains.[21]

Inspection and palpation of the position of the hyoid bone is helpful in predicting what can be achieved with neck contouring procedures. A low-lying or anteriorly placed hyoid limits improvement. However, if microgenia exists, a chin implant may improve the angle between the submentum and the anterior cervical line as an illusion.[13] The physical examination should also note the presence of scars, especially submental scars, since many patients have such scars but may be unaware of them. If these are present, they may influence the choice of approach, either intraoral or extraoral. The thickness of skin should also be noted, as the edges of an implant may be more palpable in a thin-skinned patient. This may favor selection of a smaller implant or one of softer consistency or placement in a subperiosteal location.

The intraoral examination should make note of the presence or absence of dentures, height of the alveolar ridge, palpation of the mental foramen, and evaluation of dental hygiene. Testing of chin sensation and muscle function should also be carried out. Photographs demonstrating various facial expressions, especially lip depressor function, are important for documentation.

History taking should include routine medical and surgical history. Careful evaluation and preoperative counseling regarding bleeding tendencies and the role of anticoagulants and hypertension in hemostasis are important. Other points pertinent to chin augmentation are a history of dental infections or herpes labialis. Prophylactic acyclovir may be warranted to prevent a stress-induced outbreak in the operative field.

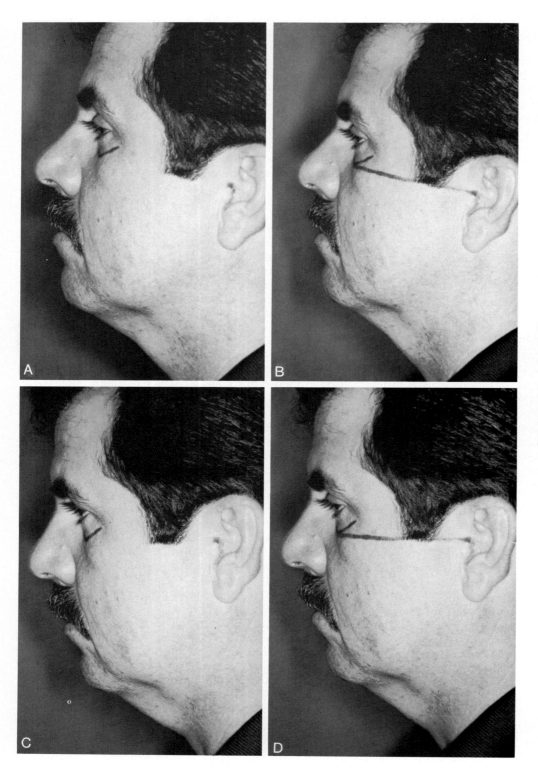

Figure 46–4. *A,* Normal head position, with the chin extended to compensate for the deficiency, which is not readily apparent. *B,* The Frankfort plane is not horizontal in this compensatory position. *C,* The deficiency becomes readily apparent with proper positioning. *D,* With the Frankfort plane horizontal, the chin deficiency is obvious.

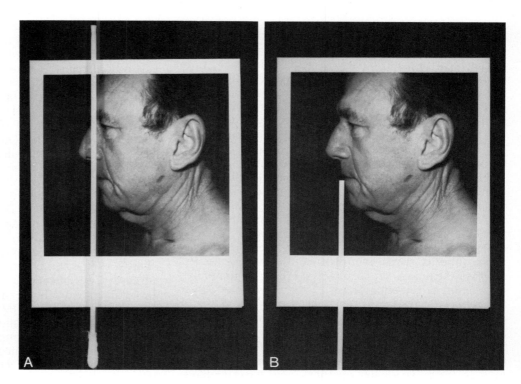

Figure 46–5. *A,* Polaroid taken with the head held in the Frankfort horizontal plane. The vertical or zero meridian is made with a cotton-tipped applicator. *B,* Same photo with the vertical line dropped from the lower lip, showing the estimate of the required augmentation.

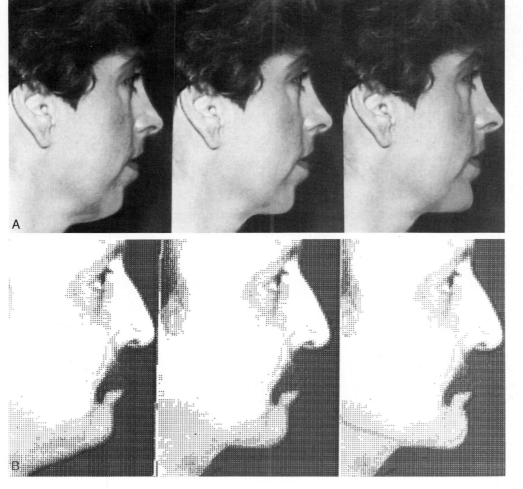

Figure 46–6. *A,* Preimaging (*left*), with simulated results of a submental liposuction and face lift (*middle*), and improved profile by chin augmentation (*right*). *B,* Preimaging (*left*), with simulated results of a submental liposuction and face lift (*middle*), and improved profile by chin augmentation (*right*). (Note that the relative prominence of the nose is reduced without rhinoplasty in both *A* and *B.*)

Implant Selection

The ideal implant should be a natural-feeling, non-carcinogenic substance that is well tolerated; resists resorption; is stable, with little or no movement; and is easily removable, if necessary. Numerous substances such as gold, silver, paraffin, and ivory have been used for this purpose in the past.[22] However, these substances had an unnatural consistency and frequently showed a tendency to extrude. Grafts of bone, cartilage, dermis, and fat have also been used,[23] with the principal problem being resorption. With newer technologic advances, alloplastic implants have replaced grafts.

Plastic polymers offered new options in implant materials. Polyamide[24-26] mesh is an organopolymer that is chemically related to nylon and dacron. It is porous, allows fibrous tissue ingrowth, and conforms to the shape of the mandible. However, it is difficult to remove if infection or rejection occurs. There have been only a few reports of untoward reactions, mostly consisting of extrusion after infection and shrinkage or "disappearance" of correction.

Proplast is a derivative of polytetrafluoroethylene (Teflon),[23] a highly porous compound with pore sizes ranging from 50 to 400 microns. This porosity lends itself to fibrous tissue ingrowth, minimizes displacement, and maximizes conformity to underlying bone. However, porosity makes this material slightly less resistant to infection. Because it has a unique ability to fix to bone, if placed subperiosteally it may be very difficult to remove. Proplast also may be unpredictable, with shrinkage leading to asymmetry, puckering, and alteration of profile.[24]

Mersilene mesh is favored by some cutaneous surgeons for its tissue ingrowth ability, stability, and pliability.[22] A custom fit is possible, since the mesh can be rolled and tailored at the time of surgery.[22] Tissue ingrowth makes it resistant to dislocation but also may make it difficult to remove. Sterile abscesses have developed after trauma several years postoperatively, believed to result from an inflammatory reaction.

Acrylic (polymethylmethacrylate) implants are hard.[24-29] They are well tolerated but do not conform to underlying bone, so any asymmetry leads to palpable edges. A bone rongeur and file or a special cone burr attached to a hand-held electric drill are necessary to alter the shape. A larger incision is required than for softer implants. Suture fixation is not an option because of the hardness, and trauma may displace the hard implant.

Silicone, the most commonly used material for chin augmentation, is supplied in fluid, sponge, gel, and rubber (elastomer) forms. However, the fluid form has not been approved by the U.S. Food and Drug Administration. The sponge is easy to carve and insert but has unpredictable resorption problems and higher infection rates[25] and has been taken off the market.[29]

Silicone gel–filled implants have been used with good results.[30] However, suture fixation is not possible, because the implant would rupture. A Dacron patch[31] may be placed on the back of the implant to create stability for suture or tissue fixation, but this patch can cause tissue reactivity and may make removal difficult.[31] Tissue reaction to the backing has been associated with bone resorption when the backing was placed subperiosteally on the bone.[32] Scar contracture may distort gel-filled implants, producing an unnatural shape.[33]

Silicone elastomer or rubber is an organosilicone polymer. The length of the polymer chain determines the firmness of the implant, with longer chains forming firmer implants.[23] Thus silicone fluid has a short polymer chain, while silicone elastomer has a longer one. Silicone elastomer is very well accepted by tissues and resists absorption or changes in shape. A thin fibrous capsule forms around the implant, but the implant's firmness resists distortion from capsular contraction. There is no fibrous tissue ingrowth, so removal is easy. Silicone elastomer may be supplied in prefabricated sizes and shapes, carved from blocks to custom shapes, or ordered to custom specifications. Preformed implants may also be trimmed with a blade or modified with a dermabrader fraise. For example, wedges may be carved in the back of a firm implant to allow better conformity to the mandibular margin.[34] Some companies currently supply this as a preformed "articulated" implant.

There are many other variables in the type of implants supplied (Fig. 46–7), including feathered or rounded edges, notches for a dimple, holes for suture fixation or tissue ingrowth,[35] midline markers, and flat or concave backs. Firmness varies by manufacturer from extra soft to firm. Softer implants are easier to insert through smaller incisions and the edges are less palpable and more conforming to the angle of mandible and may also cause less bone resorption.

Custom designs are generally available. For example, a midline hole or two may be placed inferiorly for suture fixation to the periosteum or soft tissue of the menton. Implants of the exact dimensions requested may be fashioned by some manufacturers. Dimensions vary from supplier to supplier so that a medium-sized implant from one company may differ in length, width, or anterior projection from a medium-sized implant made by another company. Dimensions of central or standard curvilinear silicone elastomeric implants range from 3.1 (horizontal) × 1.1 (vertical) × 0.4 cm (anterior projection) to 5.1 × 1.7 × 0.8 cm. These implants will

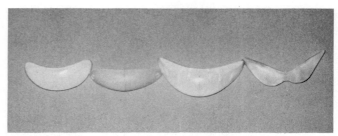

Figure 46–7. Four variations of size and shape of standard or central chin implants: *left,* a firm silicone implant with blunt edges; *left center,* a less firm silicone implant with midline marker and holes at the ends for tissue ingrowth; *right center,* a soft silicone implant with pronounced anterior projection, midline marker, and holes for tissue ingrowth; *right,* a hard acrylic implant with a central dimple.

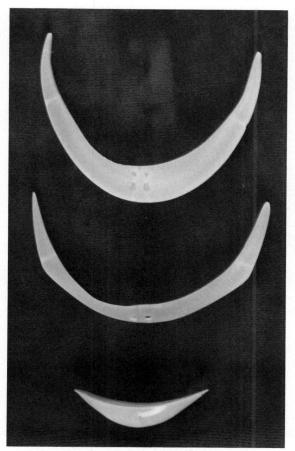

Figure 46–8. Relative differences between extended Pre Jowl-Chin implant (*top*), Pre Jowl implant (*middle*), and standard or central curvilinear implant (*bottom*). (Note that a lack of anterior projection (0.1 cm) is seen in the Pre Jowl implant and that there are lateral thickenings in the Pre Jowl area.)

generally fit between the mental foramina to augment the chin centrally.

Many authors[12, 19, 33] have recognized the need for implants larger than the central or standard curvilinear type (Fig. 46–8). This is due to the fact that, in certain individuals, the smaller implants may be too narrow, may not augment enough laterally, or may sit on the point of the chin and create a pointed chin, a "button" chin,[22] or a "pharaonic" look.[36] In others, they may sufficiently augment anteriorly, but accentuate the prejowl sulcus. These extended or anatomic prejowl/chin implants are larger horizontally, approximately 6 cm from tip to tip, with a wrap-around, inner concave arch distance of from 6 to 12 cm, with anterior projections ranging from 0.4 to 1.4 cm. These require placement under and laterally beyond the mental nerve to augment the chin, broaden the mandible, and fill in the anterior mandibular groove and prejowl sulcus.

A relatively recent addition is the Mittleman Pre Jowl Implant[19] (Fig. 46–8). It is only 0.1 cm thick anteriorly but gradually thickens to 0.4 to 0.6 cm laterally in a position to augment the anterior mandibular groove and prejowl sulcus in those patients who do not require anterior chin augmentation. This prefabricated implant

is available in graduated sizes. The chin implants are valuable in face lift surgery, since it is often difficult to completely eliminate the prejowl sulcus, even with superficial musculoaponeurotic system (SMAS) plication or imbrication. Chin implants can prolong face lift improvement by at least 2 years, because they provide better definition.[37] Thus, with the Pre Jowl-Chin or Pre Jowl implant, a smooth, more youthful, jawline can be created with or without chin augmentation. The cutaneous surgeon should become familiar with the various products provided by the many different distributors.

Surgical Technique

Preoperatively, patients are given oral lorazepam in a dose of 1 to 2 mg the night before surgery, and an oral broad-spectrum antibiotic is begun 24 hours before surgery, if there is no history of allergy, and continued for 6 days after surgery.

The morning of surgery, the patient is given 10 to 15 mg diazepam sublingually, 50 to 75 mg meperidine intramuscularly, and 0.125 mg droperidol (Inapsine) intramuscularly. A bilateral mental nerve block is accomplished by injecting 1 to 2 ml of 0.5% lidocaine with 1:200,000 epinephrine to obtain anesthesia of the chin and lower lip. After the regional block but before prepping the skin and injecting local anesthetic, skin markings (Fig. 46–9) are made in the midline from the lower lip to neck, at the incision site, and at the mental foramen. A submental crease or scar is used for the planned incision site. If a crease is difficult to find, a "pinch-and-push" test anteriorly on the submental skin and fat will usually help to reveal it. The mental foramen is then marked. Usually the notch can be felt intraorally along the alveolar ridge at the base of or anterior to the second lower premolar. A cotton-tipped applicator can then be placed on the foramen and the mouth closed. This can be palpated through the skin to precisely indicate the position of the mental foramen, which is then marked with a surgical marking pen. This distance

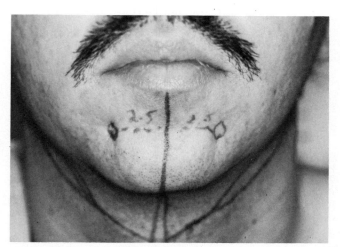

Figure 46–9. Skin markings at the midline and mental foramina, with indicated measurements from the midline.

is then measured from the midline and lined up with the midpupillary line for confirmation, if the foramen is difficult to locate.

The surgical field includes the entire face and neck, which is next prepped with povidone-iodine solution. Local infiltration with 1.0% lidocaine with 1:100,000 epinephrine is used to provide additional anesthesia and improve hemostasis. A 1-inch, 30-gauge needle is used and advanced directly down to the bone. The injection is begun subperiosteally and continued for a few millimeters on withdrawal to infiltrate just above the periosteum and into the deeper muscle fibers. Care is taken not to inject too much so that distortion of tissue will not occur. This is continued until the area of proposed dissection, including the incision and slightly below it, has been infiltrated. The operative field is prepped and draped with sterile towels.

It may be helpful to the surgeon beginning this procedure to trace around the implant or sizer on the skin with a sterile skin marker to help accurately estimate the size of the pocket. The true pocket must extend beyond these markings for the implant to fit properly. The implant should also be visually examined for symmetry, as the midline marker may not truly be in the midline. If this is not recognized, the implant will be placed in the pocket and appear asymmetric. If no midline marker is present, a small notch can be placed. After the implant is inspected, it is placed in a bowl of gentamicin antibiotic solution.

SUBMENTAL APPROACH

An incision through the submental skin is advantageous when a scar is already present, when large implants are used, when another procedure such as liposuction requires a submental scar, when the patient has poor dental hygiene or dentures, and possibly when using porous implants to reduce the risk of infection. The 1- to 2.5-cm scar in this area is usually inconspicuous after several months.

Before making the initial incision, the talc should be washed from the gloves of the surgical team. The incision is then carried through skin, fat, and muscle to the lower border of the mandible (Fig. 46–10). The soft tissue above is retracted with a rake or Desmarres retractor to expose the periosteum of the mandible. The dissection at this point can proceed above or below the

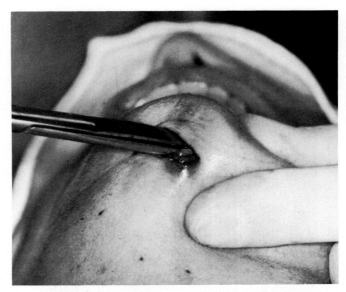

Figure 46–11. A supraperiosteal pocket is being developed with blunt scissors while the opposite hand guides dissection.

periosteum. A supraperiosteal pocket is developed with Metzenbaum scissors. As the pocket is being developed, the fingers of the opposite hand should guide the dissecting instrument (Fig. 46–11), protecting the marked mental foramen above and staying above the inferior border of the mandible. Utmost care must be taken to avoid the mental nerve. Dissection also must be limited superiorly so as not to extend higher than the labiomental sulcus.

The pocket should be only large enough to accommodate the implant without buckling. A pocket that is too large leaves dead space and may allow for later malposition or shifting. A pocket that is too small may cause malposition or later extrusion. If the plane is to be subperiosteal, then the periosteum is incised horizontally, and a periosteal elevator (Fig. 46–12) is carefully advanced under it to the full extent of the predetermined

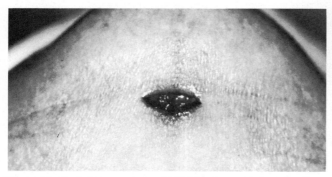

Figure 46–10. A 1.5-cm submental incision for a standard curvilinear implant.

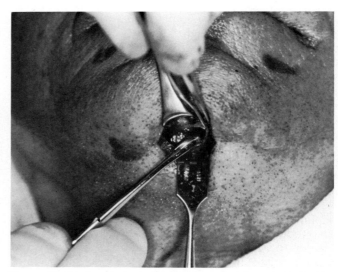

Figure 46–12. A periosteal elevator is inserted through the incision for subperiosteal dissection.

pocket. The thumb and forefinger of the opposite hand are useful to help remain in the proper space.

The less vascular[38] subperiosteal plane (Fig. 46–13) permits easy dissection,[7] holds the edges of implants down, and provides greater stability. Disadvantages include greater risk of bone resorption and a theoretically greater risk of infection because of the avascular plane under the implant. After hemostasis has been obtained by electrocautery, the pocket is irrigated with an antibiotic solution.

Sizers are available from several companies that can be cleaned, resterilized, and used again to properly estimate size.[9] Sizers inserted before placement of the actual implant can give a good estimate of the proper implant size to use. The surgeon should always have more than one size of implant available. It is always safest to be conservative and use the smaller implant.

Before insertion of the implant, the surgeon may loop two 5-0 polydioxanone or polyglycolic acid sutures on either side of the midline of the implant, just at the inferior edge. These will be placed once the implant is in the pocket to fixate it in the bed. The implant is removed from the antibiotic solution with forceps or a hemostat. One end is inserted in the incision as the opposite hand guides the insertion into the full extent of one side of the pocket (Fig. 46–14). Once this has been positioned, the other end is then grasped with forceps and the implant folded to insert it into the opposite end of the pocket (Fig. 46–15). A periosteal elevator may help to ensure that the limbs of the longer and softer implants are not folded or buckled.

Once the implant has been inserted, the edges are palpated for proper positioning within the premarked pocket, just above the inferior border of the mandible. The midline marker is inspected to ensure that it is in line with the midline marked on the skin. Sitting the patient up to evaluate the frontal and profile views gives an idea of the amount of correction attained.[9] If not, lifting the jaw so that the teeth are in occlusion will also help to visualize the upright profile. When satisfied with

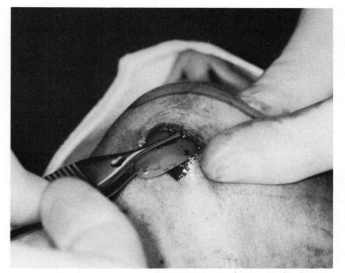

Figure 46–14. Inserting a standard implant into the pocket.

the size and position of the implant, sutures are placed in the periosteum or the soft tissue of the menton. The periosteum, muscle, and subcutaneous layers are closed with 5-0 polydioxanone, and then the skin is carefully approximated using 5-0 polypropylene (Fig. 46–16).

Postoperatively, a hammock or sling type dressing is lightly applied under very little tension, using 1-inch elasticized tape above and below the implant (Fig. 46–17) for compression to prevent hematoma and impart stability during the early postoperative phase. The patient is instructed to eat a soft diet for the first 3 days. The dressing and sutures are removed on the fifth postoperative day.

The proper position is over the thick, dense, cortical bone of the lower mental symphysis,[7] over the bony pogonion. If placed higher on the suprapogonion, the

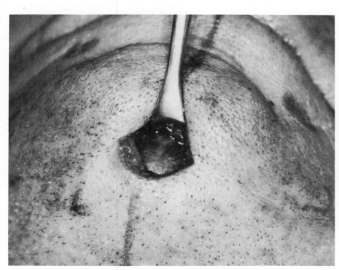

Figure 46–13. Mandibular bone is visible with the periosteum reflected.

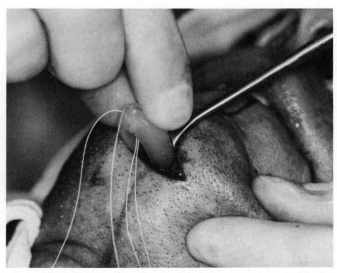

Figure 46–15. An extended Pre Jowl-Chin implant is folded while the second limb is inserted into the pocket. (Note that fixation sutures have been looped through the inferior holes of the implant.)

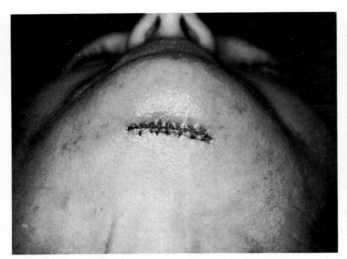

Figure 46–16. Final appearance of the closed incision used for inserting an extended 2.5-cm implant.

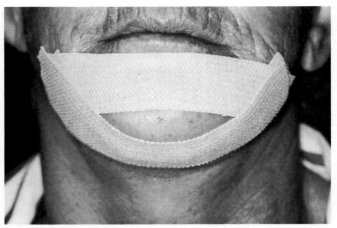

Figure 46–17. Application of 1-inch elastic tape above and below the implant postoperatively.

thin cortex poorly resists the pressure of the implant and can lead to erosion into the softer cancellous bone, damaging the roots of the incisors.

INTRAORAL APPROACH

In the intraoral approach,[12, 39] a 1- to 1.5-cm incision is made on the labial side of the gingivolabial sulcus, leaving at least a 1-cm cuff anterior to the sulcus to provide enough mucosa for closure. The incision is carried down to bone, and a pocket is developed down to the inferior border of the mandible. The dissection may be performed above or below the periosteum.

Dissection is carried out laterally in a similar fashion, taking care to avoid the mental nerve. The lateral pockets caudally along the mandibular margin are dis-

sected before additional dissection is carried out cephalad toward the mental foramen. The implant is inserted as described for the submental approach and the wound closed in layers with chromic gut suture. Rolled gauze is placed in the sulcus for 24 hours postoperatively.

Results

Chin augmentation can be subtle or dramatic. Versatility derives from a technique that blends many options for the type of implant used with the potential for enhancing other complementary procedures. In the properly selected patient, chin augmentation with implants gives satisfying results as an independent procedure (Fig. 46–18), with submental liposuction (Fig. 46–19), with rhinoplasty (Fig. 46–20), and with a face lift (Fig. 46–21).

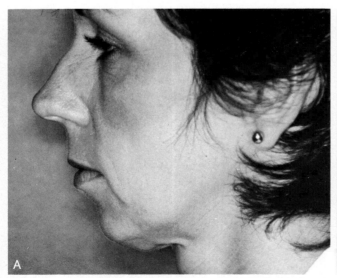
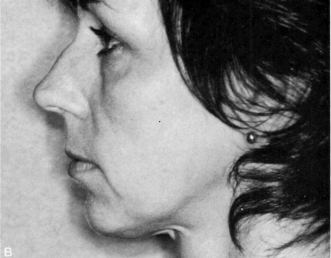

Figure 46–18. *A,* Preoperative profile view demonstrates microgenia and loose skin in the submental area. *B,* Postoperative view after a chin implant showing improved facial balance and reduction of loose skin after redraping.

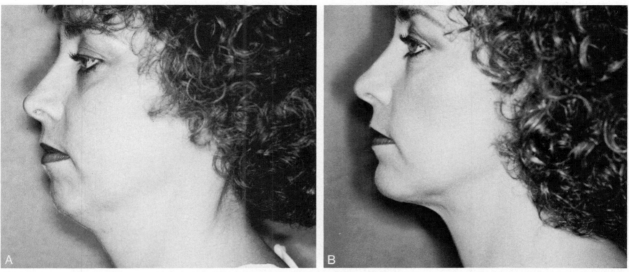

Figure 46–19. *A,* Preoperative profile view displays microgenia and a small amount of submental fat. *B,* Postoperative view after chin augmentation and submental liposuction with improvement of both the mentocervical and hyomandibular angles.

Figure 46–20. *A,* Preoperative view of a patient with microgenia and nasal deformity. *B,* Postoperative view after a chin implant and rhinoplasty with improvement in facial balance.

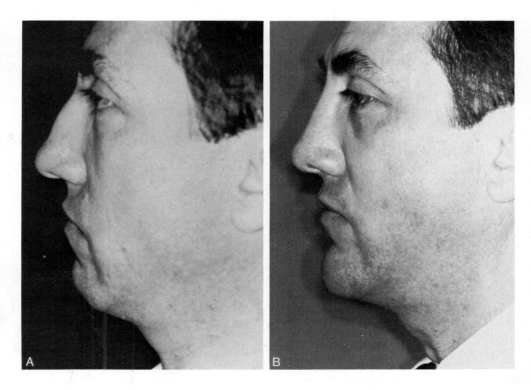

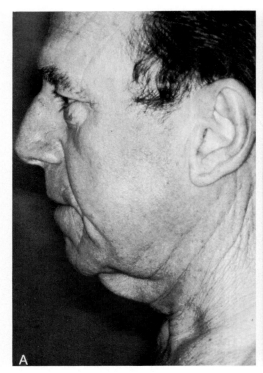
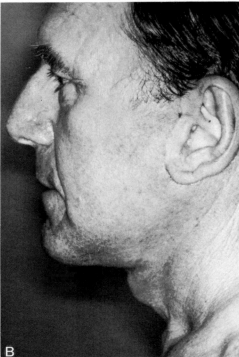

Figure 46–21. *A,* Preoperative view of microgenia, prejowl sulcus, jowls, and excess neck skin. *B,* Postoperative view 6 days after a Pre Jowl-Chin implant and face lift, showing enhanced aesthetic planes of the face, including a smoother, more youthful jawline with augmented prejowl sulcus.

Complications

INFECTION

Infection is rare, and the rates of infection are similar whether the implant is introduced through the submental or the intraoral route.[22, 40] There has been one report[25] of a slightly higher rate of infection and extrusion with the silicone elastomer implant inserted intraorally compared with a methyl methacrylate implant. Poor oral hygiene, however, would be a contraindication to the intraoral route because of this possibility. Prophylactic oral antibiotics, use of an antibiotic solution to soak the implant and irrigate the pocket, meticulous hemostasis, and adherence to sterile technique all serve to keep the infection rate low. Infection may occur at any time postoperatively, and dental infection[41] or trauma[16] is a likely causative factor. If infection is apparent, the implant should be removed to avoid complications such as osteomyelitis, Ludwig's angina, or skin necrosis[9]; the surgeon has the option of replacing it 6 to 12 months later.

HEMATOMA

Hematoma is also unusual,[42] since there are no major blood vessels traversing the proper plane of dissection, whether supraperiosteal or subperiosteal. The mental artery, a terminal branch of the inferior alveolar artery, exits the mental foramen along with the mental nerve,[43] both of which are carefully avoided. There may be more ecchymosis laterally when using an extended implant such as the Pre Jowl or the Pre Jowl-Chin implant,

because the dissection extends under the loose, thin prejowl sulcus. Providing careful preoperative instructions on avoiding anticoagulants and controlling hypertension, dissecting in the proper plane, and infiltrating epinephrine as a hemostatic agent will contribute to a dry field. A tape compression dressing will also help prevent postoperative bleeding. A large hematoma requires opening of the wound to control bleeding. One case of postoperative hemorrhage from a pseudoaneurysm of the inferior labial artery deep to the orbicularis oris has been reported after mentoplasty through an intraoral approach.[44]

ASYMMETRY

Early postoperative asymmetry may be due to swelling,[9] hematoma, operative misplacement or displacement, an asymmetric implant, or unrecognized natural asymmetry; a small hematoma may cause asymmetry for several months.[40] These may be differentiated by visual examination and palpation. Advancing a 30-gauge, 1-inch needle into the area under local anesthesia can help determine the consistency of the swelling, unless a gel-filled implant was used. Malposition may be corrected by removing the implant, dissecting the pocket to the proper size, and fixing the implant in place with suture.

Preoperative asymmetry must be appreciated and pointed out to the patient. To correct minor asymmetry, individualized silicone implants may be carved,[42] or a precise custom fit can be fashioned out of mesh. Patients with preoperative asymmetry should be given the option of a sliding osteotomy.

VISUAL OR PALPABLE PROJECTIONS

Occasionally the edges of an implant may be evident through the skin[42] (Fig. 46–22). This may occur with the use of too large an implant, with nonconforming hard acrylic or firm silicone implants, when there is thin skin laterally, or with asymmetric placement. The implant pocket may have been created too superficially (usually laterally), and the implant edge may show.[40] Total or lateral[10, 11, 45] subperiosteal placement has been recommended to avoid this problem. A sharp edge on a carved implant may also be more visible and may tend to extrude. A manufacturer error (i.e., producing an asymmetric implant or one with the midline marker off center) may also produce asymmetry with one edge showing. Careful inspection of prefabricated implants should be routinely performed.

REACTION TO COLD

Hard implants may feel cold in the skin or against the bone when exposed to cold temperatures.[24]

OVERCORRECTION

The use of intraoperative sizers and preoperative appreciation of harmonious facial proportions, along with a conservative surgical approach, should help avoid overcorrection. When in doubt, it is always safer to undercorrect. Allowing a patient being treated under local anesthesia to sit up and evaluate the profile and frontal views with the sizer or implant placed may also be helpful in achieving the desired correction.[9] If done in conjunction with rhinoplasty or submental liposuction, the changes in other aspects of the profile must be taken into account so as not to overdo the correction. That is, for a given size implant, its relative impact on the balance of the profile is greater if other procedures are done to change the facial balance or angles. A smaller nose makes a chin appear larger, and lifting or suctioning the neck also changes the cervicomental angle. This must be taken into account when planning the order of cosmetic procedures.

Postoperative swelling or hematoma will also make an implant appear larger. There is more prolonged swelling with extended implants, because there is more lateral dissection. Patience and reassurance may be necessary, as spontaneous resolution can take up to 6 months.

REMOVAL OF IMPLANTS

Some or all of the increase in projection persists after removal of an implant secondary to scar fibrosis and periprosthetic capsule formation.[9, 31, 39, 42, 46] The soft tissue chin pad may become deformed after removal.[7]

SENSORY ALTERATION

Transient postoperative change in sensation is not uncommon[9] and is probably secondary to swelling affecting the mental nerve. Men should be cautioned about this, for shaving the chin may result in painless but bloody cuts. Extended implants increase the risk of damage to the mental nerve, as the dissection must be carried out underneath the mental foramen (Fig. 46–23). This is in contrast to the shorter standard or central type of implants that generally lie between, not beyond, the foramina. Extreme care must be taken to keep the dissection low and along the inferior border of the mandible. A microgenic mandible may present more difficulty than a normal one in avoiding the mental nerve, as the distance between the lower border of the mandible and the mental foramen is often decreased.[7]

Stretch and cautery injury to the nerve, displacement of the implant, and hematoma are other possible causes of injury to the mental nerve and resultant hypoesthesia or anesthesia of the chin and lower lip. This is usually temporary but may persist for several weeks or months. Permanent anesthesia results if the nerve is cut during surgery.

MIGRATION OR MALPOSITION

Solid silicone prostheses, more than any other type of implant, tend to become malpositioned.[21] Upward mi-

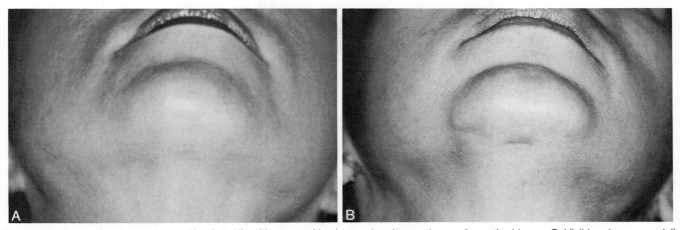

Figure 46–22. *A,* Normal smooth transition laterally with a central implant and an inconspicuous 6-month-old scar. *B,* Visible edges, especially when stretched, of a central silicone elastomer implant that was too large and did not conform to the mandible.

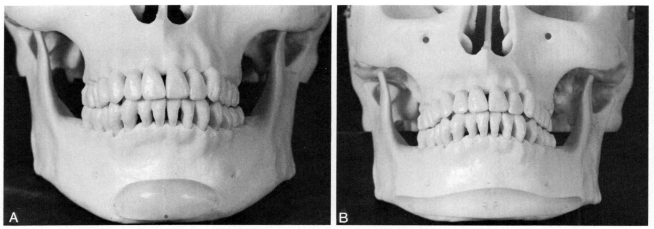

Figure 46–23. *A,* Standard implant positioned over the mental protuberance at the inferior margin of the mandible, between the mental foramina. *B,* Pre Jowl-Chin implant wrapping around the lower mandible under and beyond the mental foramina.

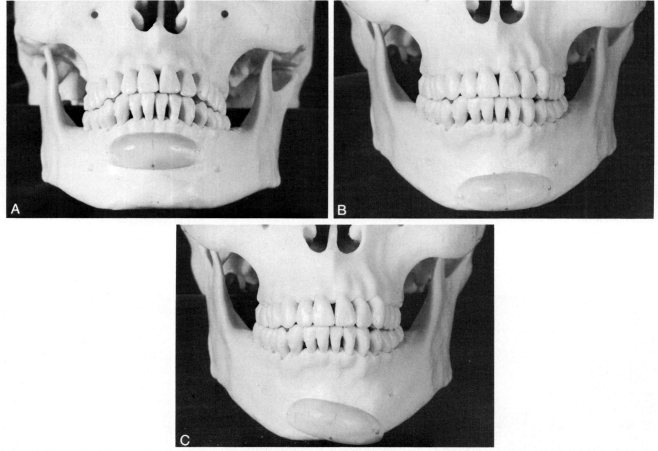

Figure 46–24. *A,* Superior placement of an implant at the level of the roots of the incisor teeth. *B,* Asymmetry from an implant positioned to one side of the midline. *C,* Asymmetry results in a visible and palpable edge.

gration (Fig. 46–24) occurs most often with the intraoral approach,[10] resulting in fullness or obliteration of the mentolabial sulcus or bone resorption and sensory changes in the incisor teeth. This occurs either because of inadequate inferior dissection of the pocket to the inferior border of the mandible or capsular contraction toward the plane of superior dissection.

Inferior displacement is more common with the submental approach,[10] and a "witch's chin" may result.[9] Suture fixation to periosteum or soft tissue is helpful to keep the implant in place (Fig. 46–25). It is also important to close the wound in layers, beginning with the periosteum, followed by the muscle, subcutaneous tissue, and finally the skin. A single suture will hold the implant at the midline but not prevent it from rocking, and therefore two fixation sutures should be used to stabilize the implant. Use of a pocket that is just large enough for the implant is also important. A pocket that is too small may force an implant to buckle or dislocate, and a pocket that is too large, without the use of suture fixation, may allow migration.

Subperiosteal placement is said to provide more implant stability than periosteal placement.[11, 47] Lateral subperiosteal placement[10, 11, 45] may help prevent migration of an implant placed supraperiosteally in the center. Displacement may also occur secondary to hyperfunction of the chin muscles in patients with severe retrusion of the mental symphysis. Taping the chin for 3 to 10 days postoperatively may also help hold the implant in place.[7, 47] Surgeons who place the dacron patch on the back of silicone gel implants do so to achieve a soft

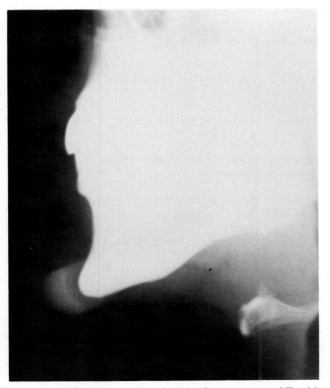

Figure 46–25. Radiograph of an implant that was not stabilized by suture fixation and shows both anterior and inferior displacement.

supraperiosteal implant with fixation. However, acute and chronic reaction around the Dacron backing has been shown to contribute to bone resorption.[32]

EXTRUSION

Any implant may extrude, usually through the incision.[9] This is often the result of a pressure point on the skin or oral mucosa. A pocket that is too tight or an implant that is too large, especially one inserted intraorally,[7] may cause tension on the closure and result in subsequent extrusion. It can be replaced later, paying attention to proper pocket size and fixation of the implant, although there may be enough fibrosis remaining to satisfy the patient cosmetically. Extrusion may also be related to hematoma[9] or infection.[41] A delayed reaction may be heralded by granuloma, draining sinus tracts, or persistent pain.[24] Trauma[46] also has been reported to lead to extrusion. Extrusion should be treated by removal of the implant and culture of the wound, with possible later reinsertion.

SKIN NECROSIS

A compression dressing placed too tightly over a hard acrylic implant has been reported to cause ischemia and necrosis of the skin.[48] Therefore, tape should be applied with minimal tension,[47] leaving the central part of the chin uncovered to avoid pressure.

BONE RESORPTION

Bone resorption under chin implants was first reported in 1969, with demonstrable radiographic evidence of absorption occurring in 12 of 14 patients.[49] In another study,[38] 47 of 85 patients had evidence of bone resorption. Two factors related to positioning were implicated. First, all but two of these implants were placed subperiosteally. Animal studies[50] have confirmed that bone resorption is greater when silicone implants are placed subperiosteally. However, there is also evidence of resorption when implants are placed above or below the periosteum. Second, implants placed too high, over the suprapogonion, eroded more easily through the thin cortex over the alveolar and cancellous bone than when properly placed over the thick cortical bone of the mental protuberance, the pogonion.[7, 10, 31] Erosion through the softer alveolar and cancellous bone can lead to possible damage to the roots of the teeth and possible premature loss of the central incisors. Any local symptoms, such as incisor toothache, should be evaluated radiologically.[9] If the apices of the teeth are involved, the implant should be removed.

Other implicated factors have been the size and hardness of the implants, which may be related to the pressure applied by muscular action. More severe microgenia or mandibular retrusion has been related to a greater amount of bone resorption. This may be the result of a greater degree of tensing of the mentalis muscle to obtain a good lip seal.[38]

Erosion over the thick cortical bone of the mental

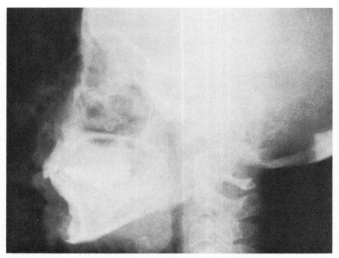

Figure 46–26. An implant has "settled" into the mandible by bone resorption. (From Coburn RJ, Rees TD, Horowitz S: Mentoplasty. In: Rees TD [ed]: Aesthetic Plastic Surgery. WB Saunders, Philadelphia, 1980.)

symphysis appears to take place within the first 6 to 12 months and is self-limiting[9, 38, 39, 51] if the implant is properly positioned over the mental protuberance or pogonion (Fig. 46–26) so that it "settles" into place without additional bone absorption. This may even help to stabilize the implant. It has been noted that the soft tissue profile often remains unchanged during this process. Resorption does not cause pain or discomfort unless the teeth are involved.[52] Complete regeneration of bone occurs 5 to 9 months after removal of the implants.[53] In the past, much had been written about bone resorption. Unless the implant is placed too high and damages the teeth, this does not seem to be harmful, and it does not appear that removal is necessary.[9, 38, 47, 51]

ALTERATION OF SMILE

The consequences of swelling and stiffness of the lower lip may be evident on smiling. The central portion of the lower lip may appear weak by not retracting inferiorly as much as the lateral lip. This alteration of smile may persist for the first few months postoperatively and may occur more often with the intraoral approach.[12]

POOR PLANNING

Chin augmentation with alloplastic implants may not always be the best procedure to perform. Asymmetry, increased or decreased vertical height, or severe microgenia requiring a very large implant are best corrected by osteotomy or orthodontic management. A Pre Jowl or extended type implant may be preferable to a central chin implant. Augmentation mentoplasty, however, may improve excess vertical height by causing the illusion of additional forward and lateral projection.[12]

SPEECH IMPEDIMENT

In a small percentage of patients, a temporary speech impairment may exist secondary to the depressor muscles being affected by swelling or dissection or by superior displacement of the implant into the labial sulcus.[9, 54]

PROBLEMS WITH THE EXTRAORAL OR SUBMENTAL INCISION

An external scar results from this approach, but these scars usually heal well and are easily hidden,[22] although they may become hypertrophic or atrophic. Any misplacement or subsequent displacement usually occurs inferiorly because of insufficient superior dissection or contraction of the capsule downward in the plane of dissection. The implant may migrate inferiorly with trauma if it has not been stabilized by suture fixation in the dissected pocket, and a "witch's chin" may result.

PROBLEMS WITH THE INTRAORAL INCISION

The healing wounds may become disrupted if a large implant causes too much tension or if it is so close to the gingiva that it is difficult to suture.[9] If the dissection is not inferior enough, the implant will be placed too high and may erode through the thinner suprapogonial bone and damage the roots of the incisors. It may bulge into the gingivolabial sulcus, obliterate the labiomental angle, or even cause drooling and slurring of speech.[54] If there is sufficient upward pressure, the implant may even extrude.

MOTOR NERVE DAMAGE

The marginal mandibular nerve innervates the muscles of the chin from their lateral undersurfaces.[18] Injury can be avoided by keeping the dissection deep, either subperiosteally or in the plane just above the periosteum, and not within the muscles.

CHANGE IN PRE-EXISTING CHARACTERISTICS

Patients should be carefully informed that dimples or clefts may change after surgery.[12] If the patient strongly desires to preserve a dimple, a nonabsorbable suture reinforcement from the periosteum to the dermis may be necessary.

CONSIDERATIONS FOR DENTURE WEARERS

Denture wearers may have a shorter vertical mandible height. Custom-designed implants with shorter vertical height may be necessary so that the edge of the dentures will not rest on the implant in the labial sulcus.[12] The intraoral approach may also create a problem in denture wearers,[22, 31] as the edge of the dentures may disrupt the incision.

SUMMARY

The role of the chin is very important in determining cosmetic symmetry and proper balance of the face. When chin implantation is performed using proper indications and precautions, it is one of the few cosmetic surgery procedures in which almost 100% of treated patients are satisfied with the results.[55]

REFERENCES

1. Farkas LG: Inclinations of the facial profile: art versus reality. Plast Reconstr Surg 75:509–579, 1985
2. Cunningham MR, Barbee AP, Pike CL: What do women want? Facialmetric assessment of multiple motives in the perception of male facial physical attractiveness. J Personality Soc Psychol 59:61–72, 1990.
3. Powell N, Humphreys B: Proportions of the Aesthetic Face. Thieme-Stratton, New York, 1984.
4. Gonzalez-Ulloa M: Quantitative principles in cosmetic surgery of the face. Plast Reconstr Surg 29:186–198, 1962.
5. Gonzalez-Ulloa M: A quantum method for the appreciation of the morphology of the face. Plast Reconstr Surg 34:241–246, 1964.
6. Gonzalez-Ulloa M, Stevens E: The role of chin correction in profile-plasty. Plast Reconstr Surg 41:477–486, 1968.
7. McCarthy JG, Kawamoto H, Grayson BH, et al: Surgery of the Jaws. In: McCarthy JG (ed): Plastic Surgery. WB Saunders, Philadelphia, 1990, pp 1188–1474.
8. Spear SL, Kassan M: Genioplasty. Clin Plast Surg 16:695–706, 1989.
9. Snyder GB: Augmentation mentoplasty. In: Goldwyn RM (ed): The Unfavorable Result in Plastic Surgery—Avoidance and Treatment. Little, Brown, Boston, 1984, pp 651–471.
10. Szachowicz E, Kridel RWH: Adjunctive measures to rhinoplasty. Otolaryngol Clin North Am 20:895–912, 1987.
11. Webster RC: Chin augmentation: subperiosteal and supraperiosteal implants. Aesthetic Plast Surg 1:149–160, 1977.
12. Flowers RS: Alloplastic augmentation of the anterior mandible. Clin Plast Surg 18:107–138, 1991.
13. Brennan GH, Parkes ML: Submentoplasty, classification and theoretical outline of management. Arch Otolaryngol 95:24–29, 1972.
14. Auletta MJ, Grekin R: Local Anesthesia for Dermatologic Surgery. Churchill Livingstone, New York, 1990, pp 62–63.
15. Hollinshead WH: Anatomy for Surgeons. Vol 1: The Head and Neck. Harper & Row, Philadelphia, 1982, p 294.
16. Wolfe AS: Aesthetic Procedures on the Chin. In: Regnault P, Daniel RK (eds): Aesthetic Plastic Surgery, Principles and Techniques. Little, Brown, Boston, 1984, pp 221–244.
17. Tebo HG, Telford IR: An analysis of the relative positions of the mental foramina. Anat Rec 106:254–255, 1950.
18. Baker DC, Conley J: Avoiding facial nerve injuries in rhytidectomy. Plast Reconstr Surg 69:781–775, 1979.
19. Mittleman H: Product information. Distributed by Implant Tech, Sepulveda, CA, and McGhan Medical Corp, Santa Barbara, CA.
20. Parkes ML, Kanodia R: "How I do it." Helpful hints in augmentation mentoplasty. Laryngoscope 90:1740–1743, 1980.
21. Mallen RW: Mentoplasty. Fac Plast Surg 4:197–201, 1987.
22. McCullough EG: Augmentation mentoplasty using Mersiline mesh. Arch Otolaryngol Head Neck Surg 116:1154–1158, 1990.
23. Adams JS: Grafts and implants in nasal and chin augmentation: a rational approach to material selection. Otolaryngol Clin North Am 20:913–930, 1987.
24. Binder WJ, Kamer FM, Parker ML: Mentoplasty—a clinical analysis of alloplastic implants. Laryngoscope 91:383–391, 1981.
25. Beekhuis GJ: "How I do it." Augmentation mentoplasty using polyamide mesh. Laryngoscope 86:1600–1605, 1976.
26. Beekhuis J: Augmentation mentoplasty with polyamide mesh—update. Arch Otolaryngol 110:364–367, 1984.
27. Novamed Inc: Product information. Houston, TX.
28. Newman J, Dolsky RL, Mai ST: Submental liposuction extraction with hard chin augmentation. Arch Otolaryngol 110:454–459, 1984.
29. Davis PKB: Chin augmentation with rhinoplasty: a tutorial dissertation. Br J Plast Surg 36:204–209, 1983.
30. Parkes ML, Kamer F, Bassilios M: Experience with gel-filled implants in augmentation mentoplasty. Arch Otolaryngol 103:292–293, 1977.
31. Snyder G: A new chin implant for microgenia. Plast Reconstr Surg 61:854–861, 1978.
32. Lilla JA, Vistnes LM, Jobe RP: The long-term effects of hard alloplastic implants when put on bone. Plast Reconstr Surg 58:14–18, 1976.
33. Toranto IR: Mentoplasty: a new approach. Plast Reconstr Surg 69:875–878, 1982.
34. Mahler D: Chin augmentation—a retrospective study. Ann Plast Surg 8:468–473, 1982.
35. Feuerstein SS: Intraoral augmentation mentoplasty with a hinged Silastic implant. Arch Otolaryngol 104:383–387, 1978.
36. Goldwyn RM: Comments on augmentation mentoplasty. In: Goldwyn RM (ed): The Unfavorable Result in Plastic Surgery—Avoidance and Treatment. Little, Brown, Boston, 1984, p 670.
37. Kunes E: The face-lift of the nineties. Longevity 50–55, May, 1990.
38. Friedland JA, Coccaro PJ, Converse JM: Retrospective cephalometric analysis of mandibular bone absorption under silicone rubber chin implants. Plast Reconstr Surg 57:144–151, 1976.
39. Coburn RJ, Rees TD, Horowitz S: Mentoplasty. In: Rees TD (ed): Aesthetic Plastic Surgery. WB Saunders, Philadelphia, 1980, pp 770–832.
40. Millard DR Jr: Augmentation mentoplasty. Surg Clin North Am 51:333–390, 1971.
41. Hoffman S: Loss of a Silastic chin implant following a dental infection. Ann Plast Surg 7:484–486, 1981.
42. Rees TD, Baker DC: Complications of aesthetic facial surgery. In: Conley JJ (ed): Complications of Head and Neck Surgery. WB Saunders, Philadelphia, 1979, pp 401–447.
43. Salashe SJ, Bernstein G, Senkarik M: Surgical Anatomy of the Skin. Appleton & Lange, Norwalk, CT, 1988, p 245.
44. Miller SH, Petro JA, Latshaw RF: Postmentoplasty hemorrhage from pseudoaneurysm of the inferior labial artery. Plast Reconstr Surg 65:353–355, 1980.
45. Dmythryshyn JR: Mentoplasty. J Otolaryngol 10:181–184, 1981.
46. Pitanguy I: Augmentation mentoplasty. Plast Reconstr Surg 42:460–464, 1968.
47. Kaye BL: Mentoplasty. In: Courtiss EH (ed): Aesthetic Surgery, Trouble—How to Avoid It and How to Treat It. CV Mosby, St. Louis, 1978, pp 97–106.
48. Gonzalez-Ulloa M, Stevens E: Implants in the face. Plast Reconstr Surg 33:532–541, 1964.
49. Robinson M, Shuken R: Bone absorption under plastic chin implants. J Oral Surg 27:116–118, 1969.
50. Jobe R, Iverson R, Vistnes L: Bone deformation beneath alloplastic implants. Plast Reconstr Surg 51:169–173, 1973.
51. Spira M: Editorial addenda. Plast Reconstr Surg 51:174, 1973.
52. Robinson M: Bone resorption under plastic chin implants: follow-up of a preliminary report. Arch Otolaryngol 95:30–32, 1972.
53. Peled IJ: Mandibular resorption from silicone chin implants in children. J Oral Maxillofac Surg 44:346–348, 1986.
54. Pitanguy I: Augmentation mentoplasty: a critical analysis. Aesthetic Plast Surg 10:161–167, 1986.
55. Rees TD: Editorial addenda. Plast Reconstr Surg 51:174–175, 1973.

PART FOUR

Special Surgical Procedures

CHAPTER 47

Management of Cutaneous Cysts

HARRY L. PARLETTE III

Cutaneous cysts are so common that they are not generally given the consideration they deserve. While it is true that epidermoid cysts constitute about 80% of all cutaneous cysts,[1] the clinical variables of location, number, size, mobility, and symptoms should elicit from the cutaneous surgeon a long list of differential diagnostic possibilities. In addition, a profusion of epidermoid cysts, frequently accompanied by lipomas, fibrous tissue tumors, and osteomas, may be the first clinical sign of Gardner's syndrome with its associated premalignant colonic polyposis. Furthermore, it should be recognized that failure to evaluate a dermoid cyst with appropriate studies and consultation may result in the creation of a wound with intracranial communication. In addition, a cyst should never be simply discarded without histopathologic examination, since it has been suggested that 1%[2] of epithelial cysts may have a basal or squamous cell carcinoma in their wall. For all of these reasons, knowledge of the different types of cutaneous cysts is extremely important.

Origin of Cysts

The origin of cutaneous cysts is a rather mixed heritage. Some predominantly arise from the epidermis or attached adnexal structures (e.g., epidermoid cysts, trichilemmal cysts, and milia). Some, such as myxoid cysts, ganglions, and mucous cysts, develop from dermal depositions but are, in fact, pseudocysts, since the cyst cavity does not possess an epithelial lining. Many of the less common cysts are the result of embryologic developmental defects (e.g., dermoid cysts, median raphe cysts, and thyroglossal duct cysts). Still others, such as cutaneous ciliated cysts, have no determined cause or, like the pseudocyst of the auricle, are in a class by themselves.

Epidermoid Cysts

The epidermoid cyst is also known as an epidermoid inclusion cyst, epidermal cyst, epithelial cyst, keratinous cyst, and keratin cyst. While they often arise as sequelae of an inflamed, ruptured pilosebaceous follicle in association with acne vulgaris, they may also form as a developmental defect, from squamous metaplasia of a sebaceous duct, or from the traumatic implantation of surface epidermis. Recent work from Japan indicates that the human papillomavirus is linked to plantar epidermoid cysts in humans, just as Shope's papillomavirus induces cystic papillomas in rabbits.[3]

HISTOPATHOLOGY

These unilocular, intradermal, or subcutaneous cysts, which are composed of laminated keratin admixed with epidermal lipid, are enclosed by a wall of true keratinizing epidermis. The consistency and odor of the contents are dependent on the relative amounts of keratin and lipid, the presence or absence of bacterial infection, and decomposition. A connection with the surface epidermis is sometimes evident. The nature of the epithelial lining is consistent with an origin from the surface epidermis, the pilosebaceous infundibulum, or the sebaceous duct. Rupture of the cyst, whether initiated by trauma or infection, generates a foreign body reaction. Pseudocarcinomatous proliferation of the cyst wall remnants may also develop in rare cases.

CLINICAL APPEARANCE

Epidermoid cysts are asymptomatic, slowly enlarging, firm to fluctuant, dome-shaped, flesh-colored, yellowish or whitish growths that are not erythematous or tender unless inflamed or infected. Occasionally a small, usually

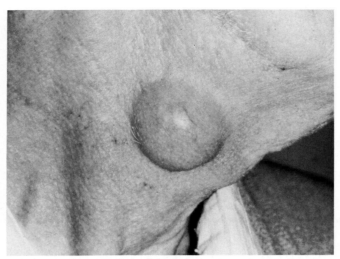

Figure 47–1. Solitary, large epidermoid cyst of the neck with thinned telangiectatic skin of the dome.

central, punctum connecting with the cyst cavity can be appreciated. The size of the cyst may vary from several millimeters to more than 5 cm. The cyst is mobile within the skin unless fibrosed down by previous inflammation. Pilar cysts have an identical clinical appearance, and milia are distinguishable only by their smaller size (1 to 2 mm).

Most epidermoid cysts are found in the acne-prone areas of the face, neck, and upper trunk, although they can occur anywhere, including the palms, soles, and digits (Figs. 47–1 to 47–3). They are also common on the scrotum but are rarely present before puberty. Because the cyst wall constitutes keratinizing epidermis, a potential exists for developing tumors of epidermal origin. Fortunately, malignant transformation is quite rare. However, squamous cell carcinoma, Bowen's disease, and basal cell carcinoma have all been reported.[2, 4–6] In addition, proliferating epidermoid cysts at one time were considered to be malignant.[7]

The differential diagnosis of epidermoid cysts could be expanded to include a host of other cutaneous cysts and tumors, but pilar cysts, lipomas, and steatocystomas are routinely considered. The rare fixed dermoid cyst, parotid tumors, and Gardner's syndrome with multiple cutaneous cysts and tumors must also be considered because of their potential importance.

TREATMENT

Therapeutic options for epidermoid cysts include cold steel removal, laser excision, cryosurgery, electrosurgical drainage, and the use of chemical irritants. Cold steel approaches include excision, which is always appropriate, punch removal, and several specialized procedures. When a specimen is produced by the procedure, it is important to send it for histopathologic examination.

Preparations for Surgery

The skin is prepared in a sterile manner. Gentian violet is used to mark the planned incision lines before

distorting the tissue by the infiltration of the local anesthetic agent. Unless the cyst is on the digit, local anesthesia is routinely obtained by injecting 1% lidocaine with 1:100,000 epinephrine around the cyst. If local anesthetic can be injected in the plane surrounding the cyst wall, it will often help dissect out the cyst at the time of surgery. While desirable, this is not often possible. No attempt should be made to inject into the cyst itself, as this will increase the likelihood of cystic rupture during surgical removal. In addition to gloves, eye protection should also be used.

Punch Removal Technique

Punch removal is fast and easy, and cysts up to 1 cm in diameter are easily removed using only a 2- to 4-mm skin punch.[8] The punch is positioned over the visible central punctum. With the skin held taut perpendicular to the relaxed skin tension lines (RSTLs), the punch is advanced through the overlying skin into the cyst cavity. The contents are then evacuated with firm lateral pressure, being careful to remove all the keratinous debris and the entire cyst wall. The edge of the wall usually presents itself at the wound margin as the contents are evacuated. Once the cyst has been emptied, a small regular or burred curette may be used to impale and

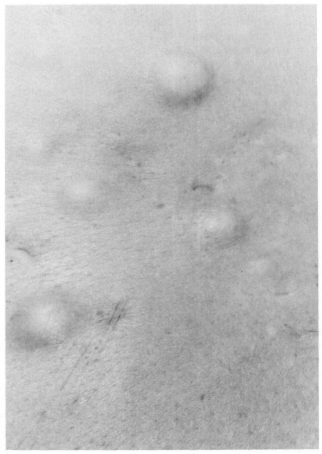

Figure 47–2. Multiple epidermoid cysts and old acne scars on the chest.

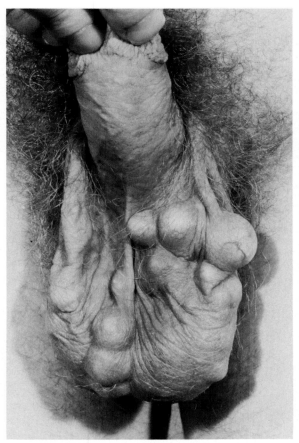

Figure 47–3. Multiple epidermoid cysts of the scrotum.

extract the cyst wall with gentle traction. Alternatively, small, curved, preferably blunt-tipped scissors such as tenotomy scissors or baby Metzenbaum scissors can be used to bluntly dissect around the cyst wall, with the curvature of the blades conforming to the curve of the cyst. By applying traction with Adson forceps or a hemostat, the cyst wall can generally be removed intact.

Larger punches, of course, can also be used to remove even larger cysts but are more likely to leave defects requiring a "dogear" correction on closure. When the lateral tension on the wound edges is released, the circular punch defect will tend to form an ellipse that is properly oriented in the RSTL, thus facilitating a cosmetic closure. The punch technique is best used on smaller cysts and untreated nonfibrosed cysts. The site of trephining may be sutured or allowed to heal secondarily. Suturing reduces the wound care requirements for the patient and may also give a superior cosmetic result. Healing by second intention usually requires 2 weeks but reduces the incidence of postoperative hematoma, infection,[9] and possibly recurrence while still leaving a nearly imperceptible scar in most cases. Larger cysts and fibrosed cysts are more difficult to treat with the punch method, and there is a greater chance of complications, including retained wall fragments, excessive tissue handling, or a large dead space that may result in hematoma formation.

Incisional Surgical Technique

An optional approach for small- to medium-sized cysts is to make a single linear incision aligned in the RSTLs or existing wrinkles over the cyst. The incision may be stopped at the level of the glistening white cyst wall; the cyst is then dissected out bluntly. Conversely, the incision may be carried into the cyst cavity, which is then evacuated before removal of the wall. The length of the incision can be made considerably shorter than the diameter of the cyst, since removal of the evacuated cyst is possible through a smaller wound, with the added benefit of a smaller scar. It is perfectly acceptable to empty the cyst's contents before removal as long as care is taken to prevent portions of the wall or the keratinous debris from remaining behind. Retained residual portions of the wall could be the focus for the development of a new epidermoid cyst or a proliferating epidermal cyst. Retained keratin debris can generate a foreign body response. To prevent that possibility, the wound should be irrigated with sterile saline before closure.

Technique of Fusiform Excision

Medium- to large-sized cysts are best handled by excising a fusiform of overlying skin to include the punctum, a site of potential recurrence (Fig. 47–4). Removing this segment of skin will help keep the convex deformity caused by the cyst from becoming a concave deformity of redundant skin after closure. Furthermore, some larger epidermoid cysts will show such thinning and telangiectasia of the overlying skin that it is cosmetically unacceptable to leave it. In the case of a giant epidermoid cyst,[10] the amount of excised skin should comprise only a small part of the skin overlying the cyst. The remaining amount is dissected free from the cyst and used to cover the excision site.

Laser Surgical Technique

The carbon dioxide laser has been used as a relatively bloodless alternative for incising the skin over epidermoid or pilar cysts[11]; a focused superpulsed laser beam at 18 W power is used. The need for this approach would seem rather limited but could perhaps be useful in a patient on anticoagulant medication or with a bleeding diathesis. In addition, the carbon dioxide laser has also been successfully used to vaporize small vellus hair cysts. Based on this experience, it has been hypothesized that a similar approach might be successful for small epidermoid cysts, small lesions of steatocystoma multiplex, and hidrocytomas.[12]

Excision and Second-Intention Healing Technique

A special but not uncommon problem is the male patient with an acne diathesis who presents with numerous small epidermoid cysts of the lower posterior auricular skin, the lobe, the posterior auricular sulcus, and the posterior auricular scalp skin over the mastoid. The small size and large number of these cysts frequently

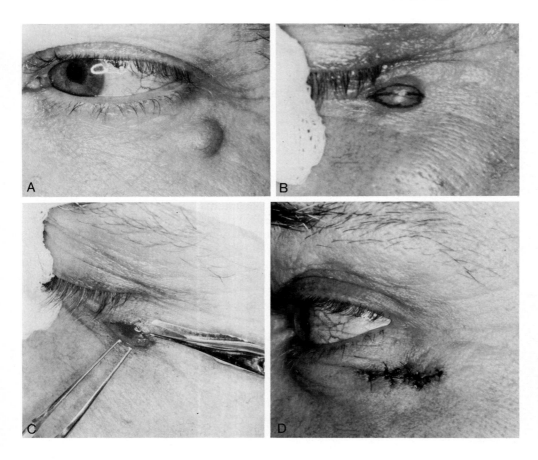

Figure 47–4. *A,* Epidermoid cyst of the lower lid. *B,* Lines of excision marked in relaxed skin tension lines before local anesthesia. *C,* Stevens tenotomy scissors (blunt, curved) and Adson forceps. *D,* Sutured wound.

make selective incision and drainage, isolated excisions, or observation the usual treatment choices. A more aggressive method of treatment has been described[13] in which excision to the deep subcutaneous level, almost to the periosteum or perichondrium in places, is performed. The resulting wounds are allowed to heal by second intention over a 1- to 2-month period utilizing daily hydrogen peroxide cleansing followed by application of a standard nonadherent antibiotic ointment dressing. Because concave areas favor second-intention healing, the cosmetic result should be good to excellent. Discomfort after surgery is minimal in most cases. If the excision site is carried too far onto the posterior surface of the lobe, fibrosis may cause a deformity in some cases. Only well-informed and well-motivated patients are candidates for this approach.

Electrosurgical Technique

Electrosurgery[14, 15] offers a less dramatic and less definitive approach to the treatment of retroauricular epidermoid cysts. The technique can, of course, be applied elsewhere as well. Under local anesthesia, a small needle electrode utilizing a low-current flow is introduced into the skin and through the cyst wall. This will decompress the cyst either immediately, if the contents are under pressure, or over the ensuing several days as the devitalized central core sloughs. Immediate forceful extrusion is not needed. Both infected and quiescent epidermoid cysts can be treated in this man-

ner. However, because the cyst wall is not removed with this technique, the recurrence rate is higher than with other procedures.

Cryosurgery Techniques

Cryotherapy has been described as a means of therapy for cutaneous cysts but cannot be routinely recommended because of the marked local tissue reaction and long time required for healing compared with alternative techniques.[16]

Chemical Irritant Techniques

An older method with limited applicability consists of the insertion of a silver nitrate crystal into the cyst cavity through a puncture wound. On the subsequent day the cyst wall may be extracted.[17] Injection of chemical irritants has also been described.[18]

Infected or Inflamed Cysts

An epidermoid cyst can usually be removed easily providing the cyst wall has not become fibrosed to the adjacent tissue after previous manipulation, surgery, or infection. If a cyst is acutely inflamed or infected, the margins are often indistinct, the cyst wall is more friable and likely to fragment, and the wound edges are likely to heal less favorably. It is often preferable to treat inflamed cysts empirically with an oral antibiotic appropriate for *Staphylococcus aureus,* to instill a small amount (5 mg/ml) of intralesional triamcinolone acetonide into the cyst cavity, and to have the patient apply warm, moist compresses. If the cyst is fluctuant, incision and drainage should be performed and the draining material cultured for bacteria. Routinely, a stab incision is made through the dome of the fluctuant cyst, and the contents are drained before inserting gauze packing. Inflamed or infected skin provides an acidic medium that impairs the effectiveness of local anesthetics. For this reason, the stab incision is often made after first lightly freezing the skin with a topical freezing agent. The punch approach may also be used to drain a cyst before performing the final excision. Gauze packing should be continued for several days after incision and drainage. The definitive excision is planned for 6 to 8 weeks later.

Excisional Surgical Technique

Only a few simple instruments are requrred for cold steel cyst removal. These include a No. 3 scalpel handle; a No. 15 scalpel blade; small curved blunt-tipped scissors, such as Stevens tenotomy scissors or baby Metzenbaum scissors, to avoid inadvertently rupturing the cyst; Halstead straight hemostats or Adson tissue forceps for grasping the cyst; Webster needle holders; and suture scissors. Standard fusiform excision is performed in the usual fashion. In most cases, wound closure is simple. Tissue handling should be gentle and kept to a minimum, as with all cutaneous surgery, as excessive handling will crush the tissue and render the damaged skin more prone to infection. If the defect left by cyst removal is small, only skin sutures may be required. Depending on the location of the cyst, the suture material may be a 4-0 to 6-0 monofilament such as nylon. If the defect is larger, buried sutures will be required to obliterate the dead space and reduce the risk of developing a hematoma or seroma and subsequent infection. Depending on the size of the surgical opening and the size of the cyst cavity, three types of deep sutures should be considered: routine buried sutures with a buried knot, pursestring sutures, and deep sutures that plicate the bottom of the cyst cavity along with the sides.

The most common extracolonic manifestation of Gardner's syndrome is the occurrence of multiple cutaneous epidermoid cysts. In patients with many epidermoid cysts, optimal cosmetic results can often be achieved by making the excision narrow but aligned in such a way as to permit extensive undermining in the superficial subcutaneous tissue.[19] Similarly, when epidermoid cysts develop on the fingers, surgical excision is often effective, even if the cyst has eroded into the bone of the distal phalanx.[20]

Milia

Milia are miniature epidermoid cysts that develop spontaneously in susceptible individuals, especially after superficial dermal injury. The injury can be associated with subepidermal blistering diseases such as porphyria

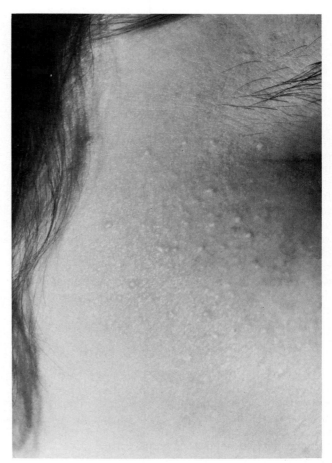

Figure 47–5. Facial milia in a female. (Courtesy of Dr. K. E. Greer.)

cutanea tarda, bullous pemphigoid, and epidermolysis bullosa or trauma such as burns and dermabrasion.

HISTOPATHOLOGY

Milia are classified as either primary or secondary.[21] Primary milia arise spontaneously from the external root sheath of vellus hair follicles at the level of the sebaceous duct. Secondary milia derive from injured epithelial structures such as sweat ducts, pilosebaceous follicles, or the epidermis itself, with subsequent proliferation at the site.

CLINICAL APPEARANCE

These cysts appear as tiny, 1- to 2-mm, white to yellowish, spheroid, keratin-filled papules with no visible opening lying superficially in the dermis (Fig. 47–5). Seen in patients of all ages, they are most common in middle-aged to older women. They may occur anywhere, although the spontaneous variety is noted primarily in the central facial area, especially on the eyelids. Diagnostically a milium causes little confusion; however, a fibrous papule, sebaceous hyperplasia, or a small basal cell carcinoma can be considered.

TREATMENT

Milia may resolve spontaneously either by rupturing to the surface or after topical application of tretinoin. Surgical evacuation using a small, sharp, sterile device such as a stylet or No. 11 blade in conjunction with a comedone extractor quickly and almost painlessly clears the problem. A fine-tipped cautery can be very briefly and lightly touched to the top of the milium to produce resolution without scarring or postinflammatory hyperpigmentation.[22] Very low current electrodesiccation using an epilating needle or electrode can accomplish the same result without subjecting the patient to heat from the cautery. Using this technique, a number of milia can be treated quickly and easily without local anesthetic. While the milia that form after dermabrasion are a common occurrence, they generally resolve without intervention. Their incidence has been significantly reduced by scrubbing with a gauze pad and irrigating with copious amounts of normal saline immediately after dermabrasion to dislodge small trapped fragments of epithelium.[23]

Trichilemmal Cyst

The trichilemmal cyst is also known as a pilar cyst, sebaceous cyst, or wen. It is a common form of keratinizing cyst usually found on the scalp and inherited as an autosomal dominant trait. The term sebaceous cyst is generally considered a misnomer, because the cyst wall contains no true sebaceous gland cells.[24]

HISTOPATHOLOGY

These cysts show trichilemmal keratinization characterized by an absent granular layer but demonstrate swollen palisaded epithelial cells that swell before undergoing abrupt keratinization and shedding. The margination of the cyst wall from its contents is indistinct. The contents are composed of a homogeneous eosinophilic material that appears amorphous and without lamination. Focal calcification, absent in epidermoid cysts, is seen in about 25% of pilar cysts. Trichilemmal keratinization occurs in the outer root sheath or trichilemma of the hair.[21]

CLINICAL APPEARANCE

Clinically, pilar cysts are often indistinguishable from epidermoid cysts. They account for most cysts on the scalp and rarely occur elsewhere (Fig. 47–6). They are multiple in 70% of cases,[25] and the typical patient is a young to middle-aged woman. Malignant degeneration is very rare.[2] Trichilemmal cysts have a thicker, firmer wall that allows much easier removal than an epidermoid cyst. However, their contents are commonly less solid than is found with epidermoid cysts.

TREATMENT

The therapeutic possibilities for trichilemmal cysts are the same as for epidermoid cysts. Incision followed by

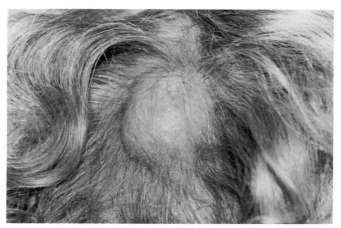

Figure 47–6. Solitary trichilemmal cyst of the scalp.

curette removal of the sac is one good approach (Fig. 47–7). However, the punch excision method is particularly well suited for trichilemmal cysts. Because they have a tougher wall, are less likely to fragment, and have a greater tendency to pop out easily, pilar cysts readily lend themselves to trephining. Once the contents are evacuated with finger pressure on both sides of the punctured cyst, the cyst wall often is extruded spontaneously, although sometimes traction with a hemostat or forceps is needed. Use of the punch technique requires no clipping of hair, since the surrounding hair may be combed down and removed from the operative field with paper tape, or it may be thoroughly moistened with water before combing it out of the way.

Large cysts may be more satisfactorily trephined on the scalp than elsewhere, and larger punches may be used if required. Wounds may be allowed to heal by second intention, since cosmetic considerations are usually less significant in this location. If the wound is closed, suturing with a large needle will often completely obliterate the dead space. Staples are also excellent on the scalp, as they do not entangle the hair and can be easily located for removal. However, staples do not eliminate dead space in large defects. With either punch or routine excision, the wound can usually be managed without a dressing. Flexible collodion applied to the surface of the repaired wound at the end of surgery or the daily application of an antibiotic ointment will suffice.

Solcoderm, a solution of organic acids and copper ions in moderately strong nitric acid, has been reported to be successful in the management of a single case.[26] However, the technique was not described in exact detail.

Proliferating Trichilemmal Tumor

The proliferating trichilemmal tumor is also known as a proliferating pilar tumor, proliferating epidermoid cyst, pilar tumor of the scalp, and proliferating trichilemmal cyst. Rupture of a trichilemmal cyst, whether from excessive growth or trauma, can initiate a proliferative

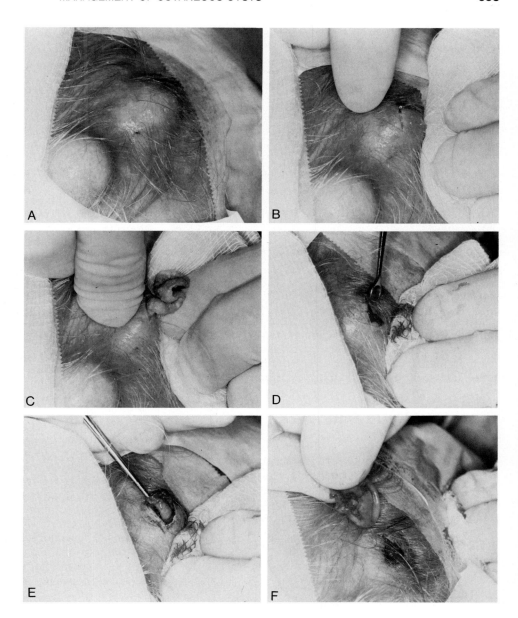

Figure 47–7. *A,* Pilar cysts. *B,* Incision through the skin into the cyst cavity. *C,* Expression of caseous, malodorous contents with lateral finger pressure. *D,* Curette ready to remove the cyst wall. *E,* Entwined cyst wall beginning to deliver. *F,* Cyst wall delivered in toto. (Courtesy of Dr. K. E. Greer.)

response, rather than destruction of the cyst wall as seen with epidermoid cysts. The proliferative response may be so progressive that it may mimic squamous cell carcinoma both clinically and histologically.[7] Rarely, a proliferating trichilemmal tumor may develop in an organoid nevus.[27]

HISTOPATHOLOGY

This tumor is typically well demarcated and shows trichilemmal keratinization, foci of individual cell keratinization, cellular atypia, and calcification. The sharp margination and abrupt keratinization help to distinguish it from squamous cell carcinoma.[21, 28] Within the squamous epithelial-lined cystic spaces, there are trabeculae and lobules of squamous epithelium that are suggestive of squamous cell carcinoma.[21, 28–30]

CLINICAL APPEARANCE

The typical patient is an elderly woman with a large, slowly growing, ulcerated, fungating, foul-smelling tumor of the scalp. These tumors typically begin as a small subepidermal nodule that slowly enlarges inexorably over several years or even decades to reach enormous size (10 to 25 cm). These tumors rarely occur at sites other than the scalp or posterior neck. This tumor may occur in association with one or more normal trichilemmal cysts. Carcinomatous transformation and distant metastases have occurred in several cases.[31, 32]

TREATMENT

Excision is usually performed in these cases with an adequate margin to prevent recurrence.[29, 30, 33] The large size of these tumors often necessitates use of a flap or

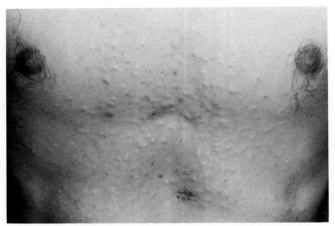

Figure 47–8. Steatocystoma multiplex. Multiple small lesions of the anterior chest. (Courtesy of Dr. K. E. Greer.)

graft for wound closure. Faced with the histologic diagnosis of a proliferating trichilemmal tumor in a cyst that has been drained, the recommended approach is to excise around the scar down to periosteum with 1- to 2-cm margins.[33, 34] This is because of the high local recurrence rate seen after inadequate excision.

Steatocystoma Multiplex

Steatocystoma multiplex is also known as generalized steatoma, sebocystomatosis, trichosebaceous cystic nevus, and hereditary epidermal polycystic epidermal disease. This is an autosomal dominant condition that is manifested as multiple cutaneous cysts. Steatocystoma multiplex suppurativum is a clinical variant with multiple inflammatory, suppurative lesions that resemble cystic acne. Steatocystoma simplex[35] is a nonhereditary solitary tumor of similar histology.

HISTOPATHOLOGY

These cysts have a thin, folded wall that contains lobules of sebaceous glands and other adnexal structures. Keratinization is of the trichilemmal type as seen with trichilemmal cysts. Occasionally lanugo and immature hairs may be found within the cyst contents.[21]

CLINICAL APPEARANCE

Steatocystoma multiplex usually becomes clinically evident in adolescence. The soft, flesh-colored or yellowish cysts show a special predilection for the sternum, proximal extremities, axillae, and scrotum, although the torso may also be involved (Fig. 47–8). The cysts often measure several millimeters to several centimeters in diameter. There is a tendency for some of the lesions to become inflamed or infected, and they may heal with scarring that is reminiscent of conglobate acne. The contents of the cysts range from caseous material to a yellowish-brown, oily liquid. Patients who have dozens or even hundreds of these cysts are often faced with a combination of cosmetic, medical, and psychosocial problems.[36]

TREATMENT

A patient with a limited number of cysts in noncritical areas may be managed easily. However, patients with a very large number of cysts often present a therapeutic dilemma. Unfortunately, there are no unique surgical procedures for treating steatocystomas. The therapeutic options remain the same as for treatment of epidermoid cysts. The main challenge is in choosing the proper method or combination of methods that will give the patient the most improvement with the least amount of scarring and lowest operative risk.[36] These cysts have an epithelial wall, and if this is not removed or destroyed, the cysts are apt to recur.

Cryosurgery has also been used by freezing the surface of the cyst to $-160°C$ (probe temperature).[16] The patient returns after 3 or 4 days to have the necrotic roof of the cyst debrided. The contents and wall are then extruded through the resulting wound with firm lateral digital pressure. The wound is allowed to heal by second intention, which produces a scar that becomes more acceptable with time. This somewhat uncomfortable and inconvenient therapy can produce acceptable cosmetic results. For the patient with a small number of lesions, removal of the cyst through a small incision or with punch excision is often very satisfactory in terms of ease, cosmesis, and cure.

One nonsurgical option for the treatment of steatocystoma multiplex is the use of isotretinoin (13-*cis*-retinoic acid). However, it seems to be beneficial only in cases of steatocystoma multiplex suppurativum, as it reduces the number of inflamed and suppurative lesions but exerts no apparent effect on noninflamed lesions.[37, 38] In addition, one report questions whether isotretinoin could have aggravated steatocystoma multiplex,[39] and another reported patient showed a response to isotretinoin only after it had been discontinued.[40]

Eruptive Vellus Hair Cysts

Eruptive vellus hair cysts, an abnormality[41] of vellus hair follicles, probably evolve from a keratinous plug that blocks the follicular infundibulum, resulting in subsequent proximal dilation of the follicle.

HISTOPATHOLOGY

A mid-dermal keratinous cyst containing multiple vellus hairs is found on biopsy.

CLINICAL APPEARANCE

Eruptive vellus hair cysts have a predilection for the anterior chest and extremities, especially the extensor surfaces of the upper extremities. While involvement of many other anatomic sites has also been recorded, facial involvement creates the most concern. These relatively common, small, flesh-colored to yellow-brown or even blue, smooth or slightly rough, 1- to 2-mm, asymptomatic papules usually occur as an isolated finding, although autosomal dominant inheritance has been described.[42, 43] Most frequently described in children and adolescents, they can occur at any age.[44] While spontaneous resolution may occur after several years, persistence is the rule. Transepidermal elimination is one means of resolution.[45] Clinical differential diagnoses include keratosis pilaris, steatocystoma multiplex, papular acne, and perforating papular dermatoses.[44]

TREATMENT

These cysts represent a benign, asymptomatic, occasionally self-limited problem that is generally of only minor cosmetic significance. Common sense suggests that the treatment should not be worse than the problem. Emollients, keratolytics, epidermabrasion with a Buf Puf, and topical tretinoin have all been tried, with only limited success.[46] The most significant therapeutic success has been reported with the carbon dioxide laser.[12] With this technique, hundreds of 1- to 4-mm papules can be successfully ablated under local anesthesia by individually vaporizing the lesions at 160 W/cm^2 using 5 W of power (reduced to 3 W for the eyelids), 0.2-second pulses, and a 2-mm beam and then lightly curetting the base to identify any deeper extensions. This may prove to be the method of choice for lesions that require treatment.

Hidrocystoma

A hidrocystoma, or sweat apparatus cyst, may be of either eccrine or apocrine origin. In both cases, the cyst is small (1 to 3 mm), slightly blue in color, and almost exclusively facial, especially periocular, in location. Apocrine lesions are usually solitary, but the eccrine lesions may be solitary or multiple and can be initiated by warm surroundings. Apocrine hidrocystomas or apocrine cystadenomas sometimes reach 1 cm in size. Apocrine hidrocystomas are regarded as an adenomatous glandular proliferation, while eccrine hidrocystomas are viewed as retention cysts. An epithelial cell wall is present in each case.[21] Treatment consists of simple excision if the cyst is bothersome. Topical 1% atropine ointment can be effective for treating multiple eccrine hidrocystomas.[47] Because hidrocystomas will recur after simple drainage and electrosurgery may leave an unacceptable scar, CO_2 laser vaporization may be a satisfactory form of treatment for small lesions.[12]

Bartholin's Duct Cyst

Bartholin's duct extends for a length of approximately 1½ inches and empties into the posterior vaginal vestibule just distal to the hymenal ring. Obstruction of this duct leads to a retention cyst, a common gynecologic disease.[48-52] Should the cause of obstruction be gonorrhea or some other infection, an abscess will result.

Routinely this problem is diagnosed and managed by a gynecologist. However, since cutaneous surgeons may also rarely be faced with a tender cystic swelling of the posterolateral introitus, they should be aware of this condition, as well as the therapeutic options available. Incision and drainage, excision, marsupialization, fistulization with a catheter, and CO_2 laser management are the usual options, although complications can be seen with each. Incision and drainage are associated with a high recurrence rate. Hemorrhage has been a problem with excision. Marsupialization is generally satisfactory, although long-term dyspareunia may develop. Currently the most favored methods of management are fistulization and CO_2 laser ablation. Fistulization, done by placing a Word catheter into the cyst through a stab incision, is quick, easy, inexpensive, and effective. During the 4 to 6 weeks the catheter is in place, an epithelialized fistula will form. The CO_2 laser can be used to minimize bleeding and scarring while incising the cyst and destroying the cyst capsule. A low rate of recurrence and normal postoperative function are the main advantages of the laser method.

Myxoid Cyst

The myxoid cyst is also known as a mucous cyst, mucoid cyst, myxomatous cyst, focal mucinosis, synovial cyst, and periungual ganglion. There are divergent opinions regarding the etiology of these cysts. They may develop from a localized mucinous change in the dermis[53] or from a connection to the joint space.[54] These two types of myxoid cysts may be periungual or, rarely, subungual in distribution.

HISTOPATHOLOGY

Focal accumulations of hyaluronic acid from proliferating fibroblasts coalesce to form a cystic space. Collagen is compressed at the periphery, so a true cyst wall is not present. Thus the myxoid cyst is actually a pseudocyst.[55]

CLINICAL APPEARANCE

A myxoid cyst is usually a solitary tense or slightly fluctuant, clear or flesh-colored, smooth, semitranslucent nodule usually located on the dorsal digits between the distal interphalangeal joint and the proximal nail fold (Fig. 47–9). The fingers are affected more often than the toes. The cysts may range in size from several millimeters to more than 1 cm. These cysts are chronic and occasionally tender, and spontaneous resolution is rare. If the cyst overlies the nail matrix, pressure may result in a longitudinally grooved nail. When the cyst is punctured, the clear, thick, gelatinous contents may be expressed with pressure. Osteoarthritis of the adjacent joint is a common associated finding that may be an initiating factor. The typical patient is 40 to 70 years of age.

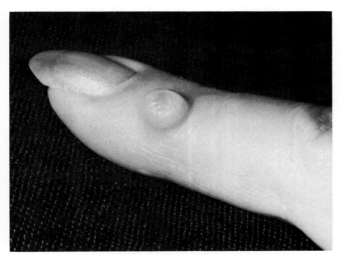

Figure 47–9. Typical myxoid cyst.

TREATMENT

Myxoid cysts are prone to recur after various treatment methods. Expressing the contents through a puncture wound made with a 20-gauge needle, followed by injection of 5 mg/ml triamcinolone acetonide into the base to fill the cavity may be helpful in about 30% of cases. This treatment may be repeated at 3- to 4-week intervals for several sessions. Cure rates as high as 70% have been reported with the repeat puncture and content expression technique.[56] Patients can be instructed in how to puncture the cyst themselves with a 26-gauge needle and express the contents whenever the cyst becomes noticeable, since local anesthesia is not required. However, for the procedure to be performed correctly, patient selection and education are important. Most commonly, two to five such procedures will result in resolution, although considerable variation is noted.

Evacuation of the cyst followed by electrosurgical destruction or electrosurgical destruction coupled with curettage has also been advocated. The cyst may be unroofed, and a variety of caustic chemicals such as 89% phenol, trichloroacetic acid, or bichloracetic acid may be applied. The latter two approaches require local anesthesia. Complete healing takes 3 to 4 weeks, and significant scarring is likely to result.

Cryotherapy has demonstrated impressive results in some series. In this procedure, after aseptically puncturing the cyst and emptying the contents, a direct, intermittent, open-spray technique is used without anesthesia in a single freeze-thaw cycle.[57] The spray is directed at the center of the lesion, and the freeze is continued until a 2-mm frost halo forms beyond the cyst margin. Freezing time is dependent on the size of the cyst but ranges from 15 to 20 seconds; thaw time varies from 50 to 90 seconds. Using routine local wound care, healing is complete in 4 weeks, with good cosmetic results. Notching of the proximal nail fold can follow cryosurgery of cysts that extend onto the nail fold. Because of an appreciable recurrence rate with the single freeze-thaw cycle technique,[58, 59] a double freeze-thaw cycle technique has been used, with greater success.[58, 60]

A different approach to myxoid cysts of the proximal nail fold has also been described.[61] After local infiltration of lidocaine without epinephrine, a symmetric, crescentic, en bloc, beveled excision of the proximal nail fold is performed, and the wound is allowed to heal by second intention. Second-intention healing proceeds better with a beveled edge than with a vertical wound edge. During excision, a Freer elevator is placed under the proximal nail fold to guard against cutting the matrix or the extensor tendon. Routine postoperative care consists of application of an antibiotic ointment and a nonadherent dressing. Wound healing is usually complete in 8 to 10 weeks. The use of chemical hemostatics and electrosurgery will cause more postoperative pain and will also prolong wound healing, so Gelfoam should be used for hemostasis. Cure rates are excellent, and cosmesis is very satisfactory with this approach.

Long-term cures have been reported after carbon dioxide laser vaporization.[62] A power setting of 5 W in a defocused mode is used under local anesthesia. Presumably because the CO_2 laser is very precise in its effect, there is less morbidity with this technique than with cryosurgery.

Sclerotherapy has also been reported to be effective in managing myxoid cysts.[63] One to three injections with sodium tetradecyl sulfate provided complete healing without pain, and no damage to the nail matrix was noted. The risk of necrosis and anaphylaxis must be considered, even though such risk appears to be small.

If these methods fail, excision of the distal interphalangeal joint ganglion may be required.[64] In this technique, the cyst is mobilized, traced to its origin at the adjacent joint space, and excised with a portion of the joint capsule. Some residual limitation of joint mobility may be an unfortunate sequela of this procedure.

Ganglion

The origin of the ganglion is much debated. One theory that has been advanced is that a ganglion represents the end product of myxoid change in collagen after metaplasia or trauma.[65] Others have held that a ganglion is a herniation of the synovial lining of a joint or a retention cyst after rupture of a synovial membrane.

HISTOPATHOLOGY

The wall of the cyst is composed of compressed collagen fibers without an epithelial or synovial lining.[64]

CLINICAL APPEARANCE

The ganglion is the most common soft tissue tumor of the hand and wrist.[64] It presents as a firm or fluctuant, well-defined nodule with clear viscous contents. Four types of ganglions have been described. Dorsal wrist ganglions (Fig. 47–10) account for approximately 70% of the total, with the volar wrist ganglion next at 20%. Third is the volar retinacular ganglion, which is derived from the flexor sheath of the fingers and appears as a

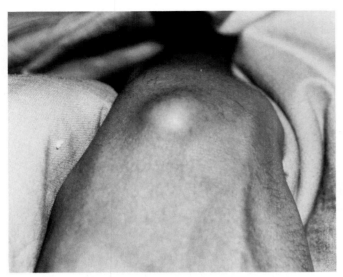

Figure 47–10. The most common type of myxoid cyst, the dorsal wrist ganglion. (Courtesy of Dr. K. E. Greer.)

firm, tender nodule distal to the metacarpophalangeal joint. Least common is the previously described distal interphalangeal joint ganglion, or myxoid cyst, which is frequently associated with degenerative arthritis and bone spurs. Spontaneous disappearance will be noted in 38 to 58% of patients[64, 66] with ganglia.

TREATMENT

Excision of the nodule along with any connections to the joint or tendon sheath is the definitive surgical approach and provides an 85 to 95% cure rate.[64] Nonoperative therapy[64, 67] includes closed rupture with a blunt object (e.g., the finger), aspiration followed by steroid instillation, sclerotherapy (which can be dangerous[66]), and needling using a large-bore needle and thumb pressure.[68] The cure rate is only slightly more than 50% with this last technique, but the procedure is trivial compared with surgery.

Mucous Cysts

A mucous cyst is also known as a mucocele or mucous retention cyst. Traumatic rupture of a mucous duct with localized extravasation of sialomucin within the tissue accounts for the development of most mucous cysts.[69] A few may result from the blockage of an excretory duct and represent a type of retention cyst.

HISTOPATHOLOGY

Mucin and inflammatory cells lie within tissue spaces surrounded by granulation tissue. The extravasation type of cyst is not lined by epithelium but may show a well-defined wall of compressed connective tissue.[69]

CLINICAL APPEARANCE

Mucous cysts occur predominantly on the mucosa of the lower lip but can also occur elsewhere on the oral mucosa (Fig. 47–11). A lesion located on the floor of the mouth is referred to as a ranula. Adolescents and young adults, perhaps because they are prone to trauma, are most commonly affected,[69] but no age group is spared. Varying in size from several millimeters to more than 1 cm, the cysts are fluctuant or tense, translucent, whitish to bluish, dome-shaped lesions. On rupture, the cyst exudes a clear, sticky, viscous fluid. A parotid duct cyst (when on the buccal mucosa) or a dermoid cyst (when on the floor of the mouth) must be considered in the differential diagnosis.[70]

TREATMENT

Excision[69] has been the standard approach, with the surgeon taking care to orient the excision and closure so as not to alter the appearance of the vermilion. Simply incising and draining the cyst are often not enough to prevent recurrences if the "feeding" mucous gland is left behind.[71] After incising the mucous membrane, the underlying mucous or minor salivary glands must be removed down to the orbicularis oris muscle beneath. The wound is then closed with chromic suture material so that suture removal is not required. The ranula, a mucocele arising from the submandibular gland, may require removal of the "feeding" gland. An attempt to dissect out the cyst usually results in rupture

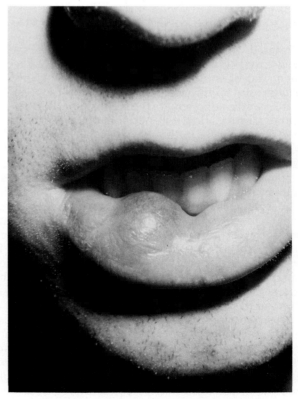

Figure 47–11. Large mucous cyst of the lower lip.

of the cyst, as there is no distinct cyst wall, only compressed adjacent connective tissue.

Spontaneous rupture or induced rupture, as with biting, is often followed by fibrosis and resolution. Fibrosis induced by the application of caustic chemicals, electrosurgery, or laser surgery can produce similar results. A cure rate of nearly 100% has been obtained using an intermittent open-spray technique with liquid nitrogen.[72] The cyst contents are not evacuated in this technique as is usually done before treating digital myxoid cysts. Liquid nitrogen is applied in a single freeze-thaw cycle to the center of the cyst until a visible ice ball reaches 2 mm beyond the edge of the lesion, which often requires a freezing time of 15 to 30 seconds. A cryoprobe can be used in place of an open spray.[73]

Dermoid Cyst

Dermoid cysts are an example of heterotopia, in which normal tissue occurs in an abnormal location. In this case, they are caused by sequestration of epithelium along embryonic closure lines.

HISTOPATHOLOGY

The dermoid cyst appears as a unilocular cyst lined with keratinizing stratified squamous epithelium. The wall contains hair follicles and sebaceous glands and often eccrine or apocrine glands. The lumen shows hair shafts mixed with the yellow, petrolatum-like contents of the cyst.[74]

CLINICAL APPEARANCE

Dermoids are 1 to 4 cm in size, asymptomatic, spongy to tense, and cystic. They are evident at birth or become evident during early childhood. These slowly growing subcutaneous lesions are not attached to the skin but are frequently adherent to the periosteum below. The predominant location for dermoid cysts is the head (80%),[74] principally in the region of the lateral third of the eyebrow (Fig. 47–12). They appear as a regular epidermoid or pilar cyst. In infants and children, a dermoid cyst is the most common periorbital mass.[75] Nasal dermoids may occur from the glabella to the base of the columella and may appear as a pit or a small papule. Dorsally, the occipital scalp may be involved. Other locations have been reported but are uncommon. With growth and pressure the dermoid may cause an indentation in the outer table of the skull. While less common than periorbital dermoids,[75] nasal and occipital dermoids demand attention because of the increased likelihood of deep or intracranial extension.[76–78]

The differential diagnosis for dermoids of the lateral brow includes epidermoid cysts, pilar cysts, and lipomas. These other cysts are not fixed to the periosteum. Included in the differential diagnostic possibilities for a nasal dermoid are extranasal glioma and encephalocele. Dermoids of the neck may resemble thyroglossal duct, branchial cleft, or bronchogenic cysts. A dermoid of the

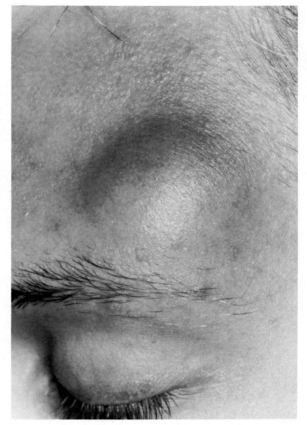

Figure 47–12. Dermoid cyst of the lateral brow present since early childhood in a young man.

floor of the mouth must be distinguished from a ranula and an occipital dermoid must be differentiated from a lipoma.

TREATMENT

Therapy consists of complete surgical excision. Skull films, computed tomographic (CT) scans, and magnetic resonance imaging (MRI) can be used to evaluate the dermoid and its potential intracranial extensions before surgery. Lateral orbital dermoids frequently may be removed under local anesthesia. An incision can be made directly over the cyst or through a lateral eyelid crease approach.[75] The cyst usually dissects easily from the surrounding soft tissue, but a periosteal elevator or sharp dissection may be needed to separate it from the adherent underlying periosteum. Care must be taken to avoid damaging critical structures in the area. Nasal, occipital, and most other dermoids may require excision under general anesthesia.

Median Raphe Cyst of the Penis

Median raphe cysts of the penis, which are uncommon, represent an error in embryologic development. Epithelial rests incident to incomplete closure of the urogenital folds in utero are believed to be the source of these cysts.[21, 79]

HISTOPATHOLOGY

Empty, intradermal cystic spaces are lined by pseudostratified columnar epithelium of entodermal origin. Mucin-containing cells are not common. Some cases previously reported as apocrine cystadenoma may actually have been median raphe cysts.[80, 81]

CLINICAL APPEARANCE

A cyst on the ventral surface of the penile shaft or glans should raise the suspicion of a median raphe cyst. Other diagnostic considerations include epidermoid cysts, steatocystoma, trichilemmal cysts, dermoid cysts, urethral diverticulum, and possibly apocrine cystadenomas. The median raphe cyst usually presents before age 30 as a symptomatic flesh-colored or translucent nodule that contains a clear watery fluid. The cyst may be tender and inflamed if secondarily infected with gonorrhea or other microbes.[82] There is no connection to the surface epithelium,[79] and unlike urethral diverticula, median raphe cysts do not connect to the urethra.

TREATMENT

Excision and primary closure are the recommended treatment after a urethral diverticulum has been excluded.

Pilonidal Sinus and Cyst

Pilonidal (nest of hair) disease may be classified as acute, chronic, or complex.[83] Pathogenesis is best explained by a combination of congenital and acquired factors. A congenital sinus tract derived from embryonal epithelial remnants in the region of natal (intergluteal) cleft predisposes to pilonidal disease. Heat, perspiration, and friction may result in hairs entering or possibly causing this sinus to form. This generates a foreign body reaction and results in infection. The classic intergluteal variety must be differentiated from the pure foreign body implantation variety reported in the interdigital webs of barbers, as well as in the umbilicus, axilla, scalp, and perineum and on amputation stumps.[84] The preferred treatment of the pure foreign body variety consists of first controlling the infection, then removing the hair and excising the sinus tract.

The classic intergluteal variety is found predominantly (71%) in males, particularly hirsute Mediterranean males. Approximately 80% of patients are younger than 35 years.[83] An acute pilonidal abscess, characterized by pain, swelling, and discharge, is managed like any other abscess. Incision and drainage should be coupled with appropriate local care and systemic antibiotics. Despite these measures, 85% of patients require additional surgery within 12 months.[83]

Pilonidal disease is characterized by recurrent acute flares and remissions, with a chronic sinus or cyst that may or may not be draining. Chronic pilonidal disease is the stage at which to attempt surgical cure. Of the various techniques applied in the past, there are essentially three methods from which to choose: fistulotomy with marsupialization, excision and second-intention healing, and excision with primary closure.[83] Fistulotomy with marsupialization has a recurrence rate of 4 to 8% and currently is the favored approach. However, it is a compromise between primary closure, which has a recurrence rate of 38%, and pure second-intention healing. Second-intention healing usually provides a high cure rate but requires about 8 weeks for healing. The surgery can be done in ambulatory surgery setting, often under local anesthesia. By passing a probe or grooved director into the sinus tract and cutting down on the probe, the devitalized tissue and overhanging walls can be excised. This is done with the patient in a prone jackknife position. Older methods such as incision and evacuation of the cyst followed by chemical cautery with silver nitrate crystals are still used.[85] Patients are able to ambulate and return to work within a week in most cases, but local wound care is still required. Complex pilonidal disease often requires more extensive surgery and closure using flaps.

Preauricular Sinus and Cyst

Preauricular cysts represent an embryologic malfusion involving elements of the first or second branchial arch. They are relatively common, affect 1% of the population, and are inherited as an autosomal dominant trait.[86] The affected individual is often unaware of the asymptomatic preauricular pit unless it becomes infected. These sinuses are usually bilateral but generally remain asymptomatic in most cases and require no treatment. If recurrent infection or chronic drainage poses a problem, excision and primary closure are indicated once any infection has been cleared. Epidermoid cysts have been reported to originate from a preauricular sinus.[87] The sinuses may extend deeply toward the mandibular condyle or middle ear.[87–89]

Cutaneous Ciliated Cyst

Cutaneous ciliated cysts, a rare type of skin cyst, are lined with ciliated epithelium.[90–93] They are generally asymptomatic and occur primarily on the buttocks or lower extremities of adolescent or young women. Cutaneous ciliated cysts have been reported in visceral organs as well. The etiology is unclear but probably represents a developmental anomaly of embryogenesis with displacement of müllerian duct–type epithelium (heterotopia). Specific ciliated cysts occurring in the skin, rather than the generic "cutaneous ciliated cysts," include mucinous cysts of the vulva, endometriosis, thyroglossal duct cysts, branchial cleft cysts, and bronchogenic cysts. A discussion of the differentiating histologic findings of these entities is beyond the scope of this chapter. There are no clinical characteristics that

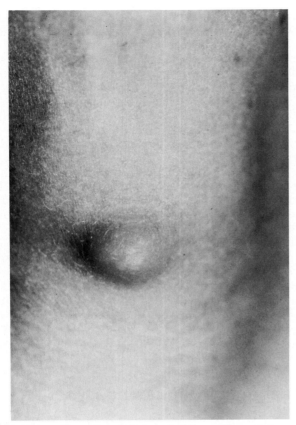

Figure 47–13. Thyroglossal duct cyst of the midline anterior neck. (Courtesy of Dr. K. E. Greer.)

distinguish this subcutaneous or deep dermal located cyst. Routine excision may be performed if the clinical situation dictates removal.

Thyroglossal Duct Cyst

The thyroglossal duct cyst, a relatively common cyst, is another example of a developmental anomaly.[94] The clinical presentation is that of a soft midline mass inferior to the hyoid bone (Fig. 47–13). Because of a persistent connection (thyroglossal duct remnant) with the hyoid bone and the root of the tongue (foramen cecum), the cyst moves upward when the patient protrudes the tongue or swallows. Although these are present since birth, decades may pass before the problem is brought to the attention of the physician out of curiosity, concern for cosmesis, discomfort, or infection. Should surgery be indicated, it is essential to establish preoperatively that the mass is a thyroglossal duct cyst and not an ectopic thyroid gland. If the cyst is infected, this should be treated before performing definitive surgery.

Branchial Cleft Cyst

The classic theory teaches that the branchial cleft cyst[94] or sinus originates from remnants of the branchial

apparatus, but a lymphoid origin has been more recently proposed. These are seen most often in adolescents or young adults. They are typically a unilateral, soft, painless swelling in the neck along the upper anterior (deep) border of the sternocleidomastoid muscle. They cause concern by their presence, especially if an increase occurs in the size or symptoms, at which time surgical removal is indicated.

Bronchogenic Cyst

The bronchogenic cyst is a rare cystic lesion that arises from a bud off the primitive foregut during development of the tracheobronchial tree.[94–97] While these tumors are usually found in the chest or mediastinum, they may also be found in the skin of the lower anterior neck, suprasternal notch, sternum, or shoulders. Treatment is usually by excision.

Cystic Hygroma

The cystic hygroma, a mass of lymphatic tissue also known as hygroma colli, involves the root of the neck and upper mediastinum.[94] It is generally present at birth and may be of such size as to cause problems with breathing or swallowing. Surgical removal may be ex-

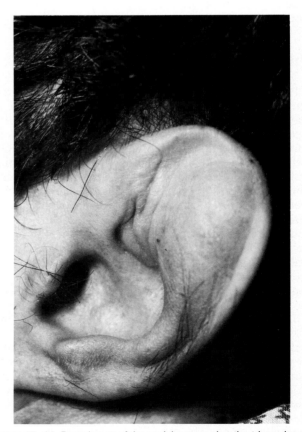

Figure 47–14. Pseudocyst of the auricle occupying the triangular and upper scaphoid fossae. (Courtesy of Dr. K. E. Greer.)

tremely difficult to perform, since these soft, compressible tumors often insinuate with the adjacent tissues. Cystic hygromas occurring in other areas such as the axilla, groin, or popliteal fossa may also present a difficult management problem.

Pseudocyst of the Auricle

The origin of auricular pseudocysts is uncertain; they may represent nontraumatic lysosomal enzyme-induced cartilaginous degeneration[98] or ischemic necrosis precipitated by trauma.[99]

HISTOPATHOLOGY

This lesion has a distinctive microscopic picture consisting of localized degeneration of cartilage with replacement by granulation tissue and fibrovascular tissue. The intracartilaginous cystic space does not have an epithelial lining.

CLINICAL APPEARANCE

This bulging, fluctuant, nontender cystic swelling of the ear is noninflammatory. It is characteristically on the upper half of the ear and often involves the scaphoid or triangular fossa (Fig. 47–14). The patient commonly presents shortly after the development of the cyst with a history of swelling that developed over a period of several days or weeks. Questioning may reveal only subtle trauma[99] or a blatant injury.[100] Trauma from hard pillows, a motorcycle helmet, or stereo headphones may be the cause. A viscous, yellowish fluid rich in albumin is contained within the cyst,[101] which suggests a lymphatic origin. Differential diagnosis should include hematoma, relapsing polychondritis, and cellulitis. A subperichondral hematoma is typically painful and associated with a history of trauma. The other two diagnoses usually are also painful but should be easily distinguishable by history and physical examination. A deformed auricle, or cauliflower ear, can result from either a hematoma or pseudocyst.

TREATMENT

Treatment is usually sought because of anxiety or cosmetic appearance but not often because of discomfort. Because the malady may spontaneously resolve with elimination of the repetitive trauma, it is important not to be too aggressive in treatment. Aspiration is usually rapidly followed by recurrence. The intralesional instillation of steroid and the insertion of a drain have both been followed by degrees of deformity.[99] Unroofing the conchal pseudocyst and removing the fractured cartilage down to the posterior perichondrium followed by packing the defect with an absorbable collagen hemostatic sponge have been reported to be successful.[100] The wound is allowed to heal secondarily, and an excellent cosmetic result can be expected. The treatment of choice, however, may be aspirating the cyst's contents followed by suturing a bolster in place and leaving it for at least a week.[102]

SUMMARY

Because of the multitude of different types of cysts that may be encountered in the skin, it is important that the cutaneous surgeon be familiar with both the common and uncommon types. Only in this way can appropriate steps be taken to carefully evaluate each cyst preoperatively and choose the most effective form of treatment for the individual patient.

REFERENCES

1. McGavran MH, Binnington B: Keratinous cysts of the skin. Arch Dermatol 94:499–508, 1966.
2. McDonald LW: Carcinomatous change in cysts of skin. Arch Dermatol 87:208–211, 1963.
3. Egawa K, Inaba Y, Ono T, Arao T: "Cystic papilloma" in humans? Demonstration of human papillomavirus in plantar epidermoid cysts. Arch Dermatol 126:1599–1603, 1990.
4. Shelley WB, Wood ME: Occult Bowen's disease in keratinous cysts. Br J Dermatol 105:105–108, 1981.
5. Delacrétaz J: Keratotic basal cell carcinoma arising from an epidermoid cyst. J Dermatol Surg Oncol 3:310–311, 1977.
6. Miller JM: Squamous cell carcinoma arising in an epidermal cyst. Arch Dermatol 117:683, 1981.
7. Jones EW: Proliferating epidermoid cysts. Arch Dermatol 94:11–19, 1966.
8. Lieblich LM, Geronemus RG, Gibbs RC: Use of a biopsy punch for removal of epithelial cysts. J Dermatol Surg Oncol 8:1059–1062, 1982.
9. Richards MA: Trephining large sebaceous cysts. Br J Plast Surg 38:583–585, 1985.
10. Arizpe SR, Candiani JO: Giant epidermoid cyst: clinical aspect and surgical management. J Dermatol Surg Oncol 12:734–736, 1986.
11. Dover JS, Arndt KA: Illustrated Cutaneous Laser Surgery. Appleton & Lange, Norwalk, CT, 1990, pp 27–28.
12. Huerter CJ, Wheeland RG: Multiple eruptive vellus hair cysts treated with carbon dioxide laser vaporization. J Dermatol Surg Oncol 13:260–263, 1987.
13. Mevorah B, Bovet R: Treatment of retroauricular keratinous cysts. J Dermatol Surg Oncol 10:40–44, 1984.
14. Davis WE, Templer JW, Renner GJ: Postauricular epidermoid cysts: treatment with electric current. Laryngoscope 94:124, 1984.
15. Danna J: A simple treatment for sebaceous cysts. N Orleans Med Sci J 98:5–8, 1945.
16. Notowicz A: Treatment of lesions of steatocystoma multiplex and other epidermal cysts by cryosurgery. J Dermatol Surg Oncol 6:98–99, 1980.
17. Robertson TM: Treatment of sebaceous cysts. Practitioner 233:700–701, 1989.
18. Kelly E: Treatment of sebaceous cysts. NY State J Med 50:679–680, 1956.
19. Marshall KA: Excision of multiple epidermal facial cysts in Gardner's syndrome. Am J Surg 150:615–616, 1985.
20. Baran R, Broutart JC: Epidermoid cyst of the thumb presenting as pincer nail. J Am Acad Dermatol 19:143–144, 1988.
21. Lever WF, Schaumburg-Lever G: Histopathology of the Skin. JB Lippincott, Philadelphia, 1983, pp 484–488, 532–534, 542–551.
22. Stegman SJ, Tromovitch TA, Glogau RC: Cosmetic Dermatologic Surgery. Year Book Medical, Chicago, 1990, pp 20–21.
23. Cohen BH: Prevention of postdermabrasion milia. J Dermatol Surg Oncol 14:1301, 1988.
24. Kligman AM: The myth of the sebaceous cyst. Arch Dermatol 89:253–256, 1964.

25. Leppard BJ, Sanderson KJ: The natural history of trichilemmal cysts. Br J Dermatol 94:379–390, 1976.
26. Brenner S: Treatment of pilar cysts with Solcoderm solution. J Am Acad Dermatol 14:145, 1986.
27. Rahbari H, Mehregan AH: Development of proliferating trichilemmal cyst in organoid nevus. J Am Acad Dermatol 14:123–126, 1986.
28. Carlin MC, Bailin PL, Bergfeld WF: Enlarging, painful scalp nodule. Arch Dermatol 124:935–940, 1988.
29. Foroughi D, Britton P: When is a "wen" a "wen"? A diagnostic dilemma. Br J Plast Surg 37:379–382, 1984.
30. Moreland ME: Pathology quiz. Arch Dermatol 117:440–442, 1981.
31. Holmes EJ: Tumors of the lower hair sheath: common histogenesis of certain so-called "sebaceous cysts," adenomas and "sebaceous carcinomas." Cancer 21:234–248, 1968.
32. Amaral ALMP, Naseimento AG, Goellner JR: Proliferating pilar (trichilemmal) cyst: report of two cases, one with carcinomatous transformation and one with distant metastases. Arch Pathol Lab Med 108:808–810, 1984.
33. Chait GE, Shemen LJ, Robbins KT, et al: Pilar tumor of the scalp. Otolaryngol Head Neck Surg 93:116–119, 1985.
34. Morgan RF, Dellon AL, Hoopes JE: Pilar tumors. Plast Reconstr Surg 63:520–524, 1979.
35. Brownstein MH: Steatocystoma simplex. A solitary steatocystoma. Arch Dermatol 118:409–411, 1982.
36. Egbert BM, Price NM, Segal RJ: Steatocystoma multiplex: report of a florid case and a review. Arch Dermatol 115:334–335, 1979.
37. Statham BN, Cunliffe WJ: The treatment of steatocystoma multiplex suppurativum with isotretinoin. Br J Dermatol 111:246, 1984.
38. Friedman SJ: Treatment of steatocystoma multiplex and pseudofolliculitis barbae with isotretinoin. Cutis 39:506–507, 1987.
39. Rosen BL, Bradkin RH: Isotretinoin in the treatment of steatocystoma multiplex: a possible adverse reaction. Cutis 37:115–120, 1986.
40. Moritz DL, Silverman RA: Steatocystoma multiplex treated with isotretinoin: a delayed response. Cutis 42:437–439, 1988.
41. Esterly NB, Fretzen DF, Pinkus H: Eruptive vellus hair cysts. Arch Dermatol 113:500–503, 1977.
42. Stiefler RE, Bergfeld WF: Eruptive vellus hair cysts: an inherited disorder. J Am Acad Dermatol 3:425–429, 1980.
43. Haynie LS, Taylor RM: Blue papules on the chest. Arch Dermatol 124:1101–1106, 1988.
44. Lee S, Kim J, Kang JS: Eruptive vellus hair cysts. Arch Dermatol 120:1191–1195, 1984.
45. Bovenmyer DA: Eruptive vellus hair cysts. Arch Dermatol 115:338–339, 1979.
46. Fisher DA: Retinoic acid in the treatment of eruptive vellus hair cysts. J Am Acad Dermatol 5:221–222, 1981.
47. Sperling LC, Sakas EL: Eccrine hidrocystomas. J Am Acad Dermatol 7:763–770, 1982.
48. Lashgari M, Keene M: Excision of Bartholin duct cysts using the CO$_2$ laser. Obstet Gynecol 67:735–737, 1986.
49. Davis GD: Management of Bartholin duct cysts with the carbon dioxide laser. Obstet Gynecol 65:279–280, 1985.
50. Kovar WR, Scott JC Jr: A practical, inexpensive office management of Bartholin's cyst and abscess. Nebr Med J 68:254–255, 1983.
51. Yavetz H, Lessing JB, Jaffa AJ, Peyser MR: Fistulization: an effective treatment for Bartholin's abscesses and cysts. Acta Obstet Gynecol Scand 66:63–64, 1987.
52. Downs MC, Randall HW: The ambulatory surgical management of Bartholin duct cysts. J Emerg Med 7:623–626, 1989.
53. Johnson WC, Graham JH, Helwig EB: Cutaneous myxoid cyst: a clinicopathological and histochemical study. JAMA 191:15–20, 1965.
54. Newmeyer WL, Kilgore ES, Graham WP III: Mucous cysts: the dorsal distal interphalangeal joint ganglion. Plast Reconstr Surg 53:313–315, 1974.
55. Goldman JA, Goldman L, Furray SJ, et al. Digital mucinous pseudocysts. Arthritis Rheum 20:997–1002, 1977.
56. Epstein E: A simple technique for managing digital mucous cysts. Arch Dermatol 115:1315–1316, 1979.
57. Bardach HG: Managing digital mucoid cysts by cryosurgery with liquid nitrogen: preliminary report. J Dermatol Surg Oncol 9:455–458, 1983.
58. Böhler-Sommeregger K, Kutschera-Hienert G: Cryosurgical management of myxoid cysts. J Dermatol Surg Oncol 14:1405–1408, 1988.
59. Sonnex TS, Dawber RPR: Cryosurgery for digital mucoid cysts. J Dermatol Surg Oncol 9:714, 1983.
60. Dawber RP, Sonnex T, Leonard J, et al: Myxoid cysts of the finger: treatment by liquid nitrogen spray cryosurgery. Clin Exp Dermatol 8:153–157, 1983.
61. Salasche SJ: Myxoid cyst of the proximal nail fold, a surgical approach. J Dermatol Surg Oncol 10:35–39, 1984.
62. Huerter CJ, Wheeland RG, Bailin PL, Ratz JL: Treatment of digital myxoid cysts with carbon dioxide laser vaporization. J Dermatol Surg Oncol 13:723–727, 1987.
63. Audebert C: Treatment of mucoid cysts of the fingers and toes by injection of sclerosant. Dermatol Clin 7:179–181, 1989.
64. Young L, Bartell T, Logan SE: Ganglions of the hand and wrist. South Med J 81:751–760, 1988.
65. Soren A: Pathogenesis and treatment of ganglion. Clin Orthop 48:173–179, 1966.
66. Mackie IG, Howard CB, Wilkins P: The dangers of sclerotherapy in the treatment of ganglia. J Hand Surg 9B:181–184, 1984.
67. Muddu BN, Morris MA, Fahmy NRM: The treatment of ganglia. J Bone Joint Surg 72:147, 1990.
68. O'Rourke DA: Ganglion—to cut or needle? Med J Aust 143:321–322, 1985.
69. Lattanand A, Johnson WC, Graham JH: Mucous cyst (mucocele): a clinicopathologic and histochemical study. Arch Dermatol 101:673–678, 1970.
70. Arnold HL, Odom RB, James WD: Diseases of the Skin. WB Saunders, Philadelphia, 1990, p 936.
71. Laskin DM: Surgery of the oral cavity. In: Epstein E, Epstein E Jr (eds): Skin Surgery. 6th ed. WB Saunders, Philadelphia, 1987, p 505.
72. Böhler-Sommeregger K, Kutschera-Hienert G: Cryosurgical management of myxoid cysts. J Dermatol Surg Oncol 14:1405–1408, 1988.
73. Kuflik EG, Lubritz RR, Torre D: Cryosurgery. Dermatol Clin 2:324, 1984.
74. Brownstein MH, Helwig EB: Subcutaneous dermoid cysts. Arch Dermatol 107:237–239, 1973.
75. Kersten RC: The eyelid crease approach to superficial lateral dermoid cysts. J Pediatr Ophthalmol 25:48–51, 1988.
76. Pollock RA: Surgical approaches to the nasal dermoid cyst. Ann Plast Surg 10:498–501, 1983.
77. Pensler JM, Bauer BS, Naidich TP: Craniofacial dermoids. Plast Reconstr Surg 82:953–958, 1988.
78. Wiemer DR: An occipital dermoid tumor and sinus. Ann Plast Surg 21:465–467, 1988.
79. Asarch RG, Golitz LE, Sausker WF, Kreye GM: Medium raphe cysts of the penis. Arch Dermatol 115:1084–1086, 1979.
80. Ahmed A, Jones AW: Apocrine cystadenoma. Br J Dermatol 1:899–901, 1969.
81. Powell RF, Palmer CH, Smith EB: Apocrine cystadenoma of the penile shaft. Arch Dermatol 113:1250–1251, 1977.
82. Sowmini CN, Vijayalakshmi K, Chellamuthiah C, et al: Infections of the median raphe of the penis. Br J Vener Dis 49:469–474, 1973.
83. Solla JA, Rothenberger DA: Chronic pilonidal disease. Dis Col Rectum 33:758–761, 1990.
84. Froidevaux H: Pilonidal sinus. In: Marti M-C, Givel J-C (eds): Surgery of Anorectal Disease. Springer-Verlag, Berlin, 1990, pp 99–101.
85. Hoehn GH: A simple solution to the therapeutic dilemma of pilonidal cysts. J Dermatol Surg Oncol 8:56–57, 1982.
86. Atherton DJ, Rook A: Naevi and other developmental defects. In: Rook A, Wilkinson DS, Ebling FJG, et al. (eds): Textbook of Dermatology. 4th ed. Blackwell Scientific Publications, Oxford, 1986, pp 218–219.
87. Yanai A, Okaba K, Nakamura Y: Epidermal cyst originating from the periauricular sinus. Plast Reconstr Surg 79:265–266, 1987.
88. Randall P, Royster HP: First branchial cleft anomalities. Plast Reconstr Surg 31:497–506, 1963.
89. Gaisford JC, Anderson VS: First branchial cleft cysts and sinuses. Plast Reconstr Surg 55:299–304, 1975.

90. Varma SK, Rayner SS, Brown LJR: Cutaneous ciliated cyst. Plast Reconstr Surg 86:344–346, 1990.
91. Farmer ER, Helwig EB: Cutaneous ciliated cysts. Arch Dermatol 114:70–73, 1978.
92. True L, Golitz LE: Ciliated plantar cyst. Arch Dermatol 116:1066–1067, 1980.
93. Leonforte JF: Cutaneous ciliated cystadenoma in man. Arch Dermatol 118:1010–1012, 1982.
94. Cruz AB Jr, Aust JB: The neck. In: Nora PF (ed): Operative Surgery: Principles and Techniques. 3rd ed. WB Saunders, Philadelphia, 1990, pp 131–154.
95. Fraga S, Helwig EB, Rosen SH: Bronchogenic cysts in the skin and subcutaneous tissue. Am J Clin Pathol 56:230–238, 1971.
96. Ambiavagar PC, Rosen Y: Cutaneous ciliated cyst of the chin: probable bronchogenic cyst. Arch Dermatol 115:895–896, 1979.

97. Muramatsu T, Shirai T, Sakamoto K: Cutaneous bronchogenic cyst. Int J Dermatol 29:143–144, 1990.
98. Engel D: Pseudocyst of the auricle in Chinese. Arch Otolaryngol 83:29–34, 1966.
99. Glamb R, Kim R: Pseudocyst of the auricle. J Am Acad Dermatol 11:58–63, 1984.
100. Grabski WJ, Salasche SJ, McCollough ML, Angeloni VL: Pseudocyst of the auricle associated with trauma. Arch Dermatol 125:528–530, 1989.
101. Fukamizu H, Imaizumi S: Bilateral pseudocysts of the auricles. Arch Dermatol 120:1238–1239, 1984.
102. Karakashian GV, Lutz-Nagey LL, Anderson R: Pseudocyst of the auricle: compression suture therapy. J Dermatol Surg Oncol 13:74–75, 1987.

CHAPTER 48

Management of Dysplastic and Congenital Nevi

DARREL L. ELLIS

Dysplastic Nevus Syndrome

DEFINITION

The dysplastic nevus syndrome (DNS) was originally described as the "atypical moles syndrome,"[1] "B-K mole syndrome,"[2] and "familial atypical multiple mole-melanoma syndrome."[3, 4] The name dysplastic nevus syndrome was proposed to standardize the nomenclature in the literature,[5] although discussions continue over whether "dysplastic" is an appropriate descriptive term for the atypical nevi found in these patients.

Familial dysplastic nevus syndrome (FDNS) is defined as an autosomal dominant inherited syndrome of melanocytic lesions with distinct clinical and histologic characteristics that identify patients at risk to develop melanomas. A second population of patients with non-familial malignant melanoma in association with the dysplastic nevus phenotype or sporadic dysplastic nevus syndrome (SDNS)[6] has also been identified.

DNS is defined by combined clinical and histopathologic criteria. Clinically, patients can have nevi that appear normal in distribution, shape, number, and size and also have dysplastic nevi as well. The dysplastic nevi have borders that are irregular, with indistinct margins (Fig. 48–1). These lesions are also predominantly macular, although there may be a central papule (Fig. 48–2), and the fine skin markings are retained. Loss of fine skin markings indicates possible melanoma and increased depth of the lesion. Although dysplastic nevi occur predominantly on sun-exposed surfaces such as the back, chest, abdomen, and arms, they also are found in sun protected areas such as the scalp, buttocks, genitalia, and female breasts, unlike normal nevi.[7] Lesions may vary tremendously in appearance within a given patient (Figs. 48–3, 48–4). Dysplastic nevi exhibit

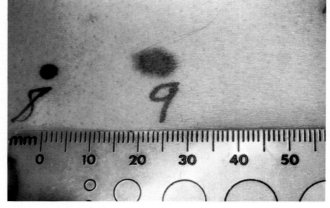

Figure 48–1. Nevi from a patient with dysplastic nevus syndrome, demonstrating interlesional variation, border irregularity, and indistinct margins on the lesion on the right.

great color variegation, with haphazard mixtures of tan, brown, and pink.[7] Any focal black area within a nevus suggests melanoma, and requires prompt excision. Dysplastic nevi are often larger in size (Fig. 48–4) than normal nevi, frequently ranging from 6 to 5 mm in diameter.[7] However, appearance is a more critical factor than size when making the clinical diagnosis of a dysplastic nevus. Since even melanomas may have diameters of 2 mm or less, it should be emphasized that the diameter of a lesion is not necessarily predictive of its malignant potential. Most DNS patients have a large number of nevi (Fig. 48–5), frequently more than 100.[7] However, families have been identified as having FDNS and a high incidence of melanoma but only a few nevi associated with the DNS phenotype. These patients must also be identified to permit close clinical monitoring.

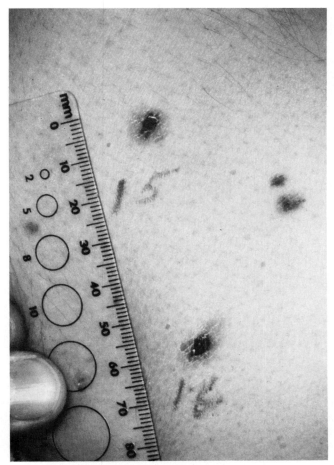

Figure 48–2. Dysplastic nevi with central papules.

HISTOLOGIC CRITERIA

The histologic criteria for diagnosing a dysplastic nevus are also still widely debated. Most dermatopathologists agree that dysplastic nevi represent a distinct pathologic entity, although this concept is not universally accepted.[8, 9] Controversy also exists regarding the clinical relevance of histologic dysplastic nevi.[10] A consensus

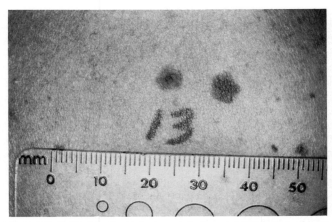

Figure 48–3. Dysplastic nevi, demonstrating variable lesion appearance and pigment variegation.

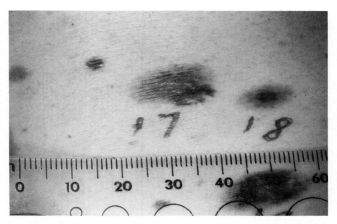

Figure 48–4. Dysplastic nevi that are more than 10 mm in diameter and show variable lesion appearance with border irregularity and pigment variegation.

conference[11] with dermatopathologists and pathologists was held in 1990 to identify the criteria used for the diagnosis of dysplastic nevi. The panel recommended that the diagnosis of a dysplastic nevus require the

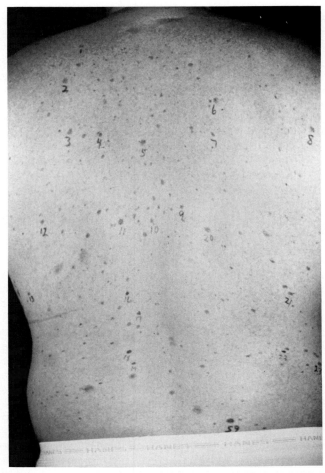

Figure 48–5. The back of a DNS patient, demonstrating multiple nevi and the photographic method used to document normal and involved skin.

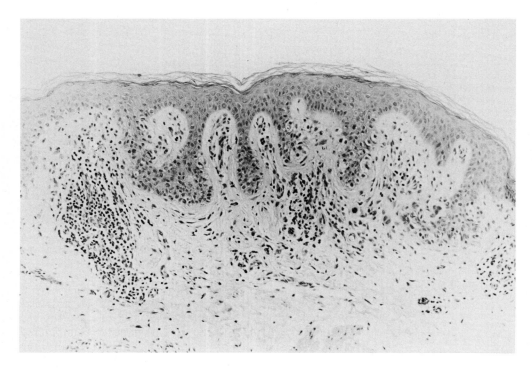

Figure 48–6. Histologic section of a dysplastic nevus.

fulfillment of two criteria: (1) *an architectural disorder* (bridging or lateral extension of melanocytes within the epidermis; concentric or lamellar fibroplasia; and irregular distribution or increased number of melanocytes at the dermal-epidermal junction) and (2) *easily identifiable melanocytic atypia* (melanocytes with abnormalities related to enlarged size, irregular shape or hyperchromasia of the nucleus, or abnormal cytoplasmic features). These histologic criteria for the diagnosis of a dysplastic nevus are similar to those previously published (Fig. 48–6).[12]

As defined, the dysplastic nevus must exhibit melanocytic atypia. A nevus exhibiting architectural disorder but not melanocytic atypia should be termed a nevus with an architectural disorder.[11] Whether nevi with architectural disorders show a clinical association with DNS or melanoma is unknown.

In treating DNS patients, the clinician must understand how the dermatopathologist defines a dysplastic nevus. If the criteria for melanocytic atypia are not used in the definition of a dysplastic nevus, many nevi with architectural disorders may be interpreted as dysplastic nevi. This will obviously lead to overdiagnosis of DNS in patients who may not have increased melanoma risk.[13] This overdiagnosis of DNS with resultant dilution of the percentage of patients with melanoma risk may be responsible for creating some of the confusion seen in the literature regarding the significance of the diagnosis of DNS by histologic examination.[13]

If possible, the clinician should always attempt to review the slides of the biopsy specimen with the dermatopathologist in order to obtain the best clinicopathologic correlation for the diagnosis of DNS and to ensure that representative sectioning of the nevus was done. Multiple sections through the nevus may be needed to demonstrate focal areas of early melanoma in nevi that

show marked clinical atypia. Better biochemical and histologic methods of diagnosing dysplastic nevi, as well as better biochemical or molecular biology methods for defining patients at the highest melanoma risk, are needed to resolve the current clinicopathologic difficulties in defining DNS patients. Hopefully, additional studies linking the DNS gene to chromosome 1p[14] will lead to use of diagnostic techniques such as RFLP (restriction fragment–linked polymorphisms) to diagnose FDNS patients who are at increased melanoma risk. Such a screening tool would be especially valuable in identifying children in FDNS families who will develop the DNS phenotype before their nevi actually begin to change.

Clinicopathologic correlation is currently required in dealing with pigmented lesions in patients with no family history of melanoma or DNS and who have clinically normal appearing nevi and that show mildly atypical histologic features. The clinical criteria for diagnosis of DNS are not met in these cases, assuming the clinician has performed a complete cutaneous examination and identified no atypical nevi. Patients with normal appearing nevi and no melanoma risk factors but with histologically mildly atypical nevi are probably not at an increased melanoma risk and do not require extensive clinical monitoring, although controlled long term studies of these patients have not been done. On the other hand, patients who clinically appear to have the DNS phenotype may not have histologically dysplastic nevi on initial biopsy. These patients should be classified as potential DNS patients and followed closely. They may later develop a changing nevus shown to be dysplastic histologically, thus making the diagnosis.

Patients with DNS are further classified as having the familial (FDNS) or sporadic (SDNS) type, depending on their family history.[5] Estimates of the incidence of SDNS run as high as 5% of the United States population.[15] There may also be more than 30,000 patients in the United States with FDNS.[16] Studies have shown that a patient's family history is often inaccurate, leading to an incorrect diagnosis of SDNS if first-degree family members are not carefully screened.[17] For families with FDNS in association with melanoma, screening is also crucial, because the incidence of new melanomas has been reported to be 14%.[1]

RISK FACTORS

The melanoma risk of FDNS patients with at least two family members who have had a melanoma is high. Preliminary data suggest a 100% lifetime risk,[16] but extended studies are required to confirm this observation. The lifetime risk of developing melanoma in other DNS patients has been estimated to be 18%.[16] Recent reports also suggest that patients who have SDNS may have a higher melanoma risk than would be anticipated.[18]

All patients with FDNS and a family history of melanoma are not at equal risk for the development of melanoma. Patients with greater than 100 nevi have a 19-fold greater risk of developing melanoma than those with fewer than 100 nevi.[19, 20] Patients with FDNS and "congenital-like" nevi have an 8.5-fold increased melanoma risk.[19, 20] Patients with DNS who sunburn easily and tan poorly also are at increased risk of melanoma.[20]

Ultraviolet light, both in the form of natural sunlight[21] and from tanning beds,[22] has been linked to melanoma development. Intermittent sun exposure, particularly blistering sunburns, has been associated with increased melanoma risk.[23] Childhood sunburns also lead to an increased melanoma risk.[24] Since the DNS phenotype cannot be identified in children, it is currently impossible to identify which children should be especially careful to use sunscreens and limit their sun exposure. Therefore, patients with FDNS should be advised to have all of their children use sunscreens.

Melanoma has been reported in association with multiple therapies for psoriasis.[25] Cytologically atypical melanocytes have been reported in patients treated with psoralens and ultraviolet light A (PUVA).[26] Patients with both FDNS and psoriasis may have an increased melanoma risk, as they often receive ultraviolet light therapy, including PUVA therapy, for their psoriasis.

Other factors may also cause DNS patients to be at increased melanoma risk. One of these is immunosuppression, as occurs in renal transplant patients,[27] patients with Hodgkin's disease,[28] or patients infected with the human immunodeficiency virus.[29] Dysplastic nevi have also been seen in patients after topical use of mechlorethamine.[30] Occupational contact with polychlorinated biphenyls[31] and possibly other petrochemicals[32] may increase the risk of melanoma in the general population. Whether DNS patients are particularly at increased melanoma risk when exposed to these and other chemicals is unknown.

Pregnancy and steroid hormones have also been reported to change dysplastic nevi.[1, 3] Pregnancy has been associated with clinical nevus change in up to one third of normal patients.[34] Long-term longitudinal studies need to be conducted on how pregnancy, oral contraceptives, and oral steroid hormones affect nevus change in DNS patients. Preliminary data indicate that pregnancy is associated with an increased rate of nevus change in DNS patients, but oral contraceptives are not.[33] Identifying all risk factors associated with an increase in changing dysplastic nevi is important, for close clinical evaluation is indicated during periods of increased risk of nevus change. In addition, modifying alterable risk factors (e.g., decreasing sun exposure) theoretically should be expected to decrease the incidence of melanoma.

CLINICAL MANAGEMENT

The clinical management of DNS patients is based on identification of patients with DNS, application of appropriate methods to identify early lesion changes, and surgical intervention to remove changing nevi. Identification of nevus change coupled with early surgical intervention should allow removal of melanomas when they are curable by simple cutaneous surgery, thus preventing invasive melanoma. A possible exception is in nodular melanoma, where no radial growth phase precedes the vertical growth phase, and so invasion may occur in even small lesions. Treatment of dysplastic nevi with such agents as topical 5-fluorouracil[35] or retinoic acid[36, 37] should be considered experimental at present.

At the initial evaluation of a DNS patient, a complete cutaneous examination should be performed. If the patient refuses a complete examination, this should be documented in the patient's records. Education about the possible danger of melanoma usually promotes compliance with the complete examination. Any lesions that clinically appear to be melanomas should undergo biopsy. If the patient has not had a previous diagnosis of a dysplastic nevus, one or two of the most atypical lesions should undergo biopsy to establish the diagnosis. Biopsy is best accomplished by either elliptical excision or punch biopsy, depending on the lesion size. A 2-mm clinical margin of excision is desirable to prevent recurrence. Shave biopsy is not recommended because of the possibility of the patient developing a nevus recurrens, which may clinically and microscopically be indistinguishable from a melanoma.[38, 39] Although it is benign, a nevus recurrens with atypia usually leads to a recommendation for large re-excision because of uncertainty as to whether the initial lesion was an incompletely excised melanoma.

Patients who are documented to have DNS by clinical and histologic criteria should be managed with family screening, education, physical examination, and follow-up of the nevi for evidence of change. Family screening is crucial, and a family history taken during the examination is usually inadequate. More complete family histories may be obtained by having patients complete a family history form at home that includes the extended first-degree relatives, grandparents, parents, aunts, uncles, siblings, and children. All family members in the extended first-degree pedigree should undergo a cutaneous examination by a dermatologist, if possible, to identify other patients with DNS or melanoma. Good family screening also provides a sound basis for genetic counseling.

Education is important for the patient and all first-degree relatives. They should be educated in melanoma recognition, conduction of monthly cutaneous examinations, sunscreen use, and risk factors for developing melanoma. Educational material (e.g., handouts, videotapes, or slide sets) is often a useful way to provide this information. Trained personnel (usually the physician) should discuss these materials with patients and their families. Education is the best aid in risk factor reduction and early melanoma identification by the patient.

Sunscreens with a sun protection factor (SPF) of 15 or greater are recommended for patient use. For patients with type I skin or multiple nevi, a sunscreen with an SPF of 30 or greater may be best.[40] Waterproof sunscreens are especially useful for children, patients involved in water sports, or those individuals who perspire heavily.

Patients should have a complete mucocutaneous examination as well as a complete physical examination. An ophthalmic examination is also recommended because of the small incidence of ocular melanomas in FDNS and SDNS patients.[41–43] Melanomas of the eye may be asymptomatic, precluding early treatment unless detected by a routine eye examination. Although one report found no significant increase in nonmelanoma cancers in FDNS patients,[45] general cancer screening should also be done, as patients may come from cancer-prone families.[3, 4, 44]

Monitoring nevi is best accomplished by a method of permanently recording the nevi. Serial photography is useful for documenting nevi and allowing early identification of melanomas.[46–49] The method used at some clinics is to number the most atypical nevi and then photograph these lesions at close range using a macro lens with a ring flash (Figs. 48–1 through 48–4). The cutaneous surface is then documented by pictures taken from a distance (Fig. 48–5). This not only records where nevi are present, but also where the skin appears clinically normal. Documenting the normal as well as clinically involved cutaneous surfaces is important, because melanomas may arise in clinically normal skin. DNS patients also may acquire new nevi during long-term follow-up, and these can be easily identified by referring to the photographs taken of the cutaneous surface. Patients should also record the numbers and diameters of their numbered nevi on a cutaneous chart given to them for use in their monthly cutaneous self examinations. This enables patients to identify those nevi that have the most atypical appearance and provides a baseline for monthly observations.

Other methods for documenting and following nevi have been proposed, but no long-term studies have been published comparing these techniques to the serial photography method. The photographic method is theoret-

ically applicable by any physician with adequate equipment and training. However, the time and expense involved have led to the evolution of pigmented lesion clinics at referral centers. Pigmented lesion clinics also provide sources of information for DNS patients and establish a clinical base of patients for epidemiologic studies required to further define risk factors for development of melanoma in DNS patients.

After documentation of the patient's nevi, long-term follow-up is instituted. Those patients with FDNS and a family history of melanoma, DNS patients with a personal history of melanoma, and DNS patients with other risk factors such as immunosuppression or pregnancy should be followed at 3-month intervals. Other DNS patients should be followed at 6-month intervals. The rationale behind these follow-up intervals is based on the approximate 6-month radial growth phase of superficial spreading melanomas. Thus the recommended intervals theoretically give the clinician two opportunities to observe nevus changes in high-risk patients and one opportunity in lower risk patients.

Children of DNS patients should be examined annually for development of the DNS cutaneous phenotype from the time they become at risk for development of atypical nevi (about 8 to 10 years old) until at least adulthood (20 years old).[50] Nevi in the scalp,[51] palmar, and plantar areas are often the first to change in children and should be closely monitored during puberty. Although children with DNS are not at markedly increased risk for the development of melanoma until their teenage years, education about sunscreens and melanoma risk factors is best done with younger patients, as studies have linked melanoma with childhood sunburns.[24] While patients usually develop the DNS phenotype before the age of 20, this is not universally true. In families with an extremely high incidence of melanoma, yearly cutaneous examination of family members without the obvious DNS phenotype should be conducted indefinitely.

Patients who discover a changing nevus during their monthly cutaneous self-examination should be seen immediately. Comparison of the nevus in question to the clinical photographs will confirm whether significant changes have occurred. Significant clinical changes may be defined as enlargement (>2 mm); development of inflammation (erythema); increased border irregularity; increased variegation of color, especially development of a black or dark brown spot; sustained new symptoms of more than 2 weeks duration of tenderness or pruritus within a nevus; and development of a new nevus showing any of these changes.[33] Two or more of these criteria are usually present in lesions requiring biopsy. Lesions that show only slight changes in color or border may be best managed with additional photographs and clinical follow-up.

Lesions exhibiting significant clinical change when compared with previous photographs should be removed by excisional biopsy. Because of anatomic difficulties in following scalp lesions, atypical scalp nevi may be electively excised, even though they are not changing. Biopsy with 2 mm clinical margins should be adequate for removing dysplastic nevi. However, when the histologic examination shows severe dysplasia, raising the

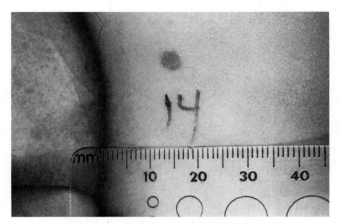

Figure 48–7. Small congenital nevus (less than 1.5 cm in diameter) that does not exhibit the classic clinical characteristics of a congenital nevus. This makes differentiating such a lesion from an acquired nevus difficult.

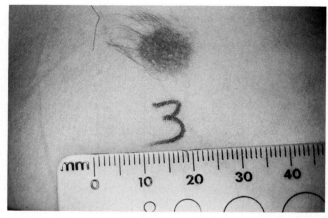

Figure 48–8. Small congenital nevus (less than 1.5 cm) that shows hypertrichosis and a pebbly appearance often associated with congenital nevi.

question of early melanoma, re-excision with conservative 0.5- to 1- cm margins may be indicated. Clinically dysplastic nevi that show frank melanoma histologically should be excised according to established criteria based on the depth of the lesion.[52–55] SDNS patients who develop melanoma during the course of longitudinal follow-up should be treated as high-risk patients and followed at 3-month intervals.

Congenital Nevi

DEFINITION

Congenital nevomelanocytic nevi are pigmented lesions composed of nevus cells in the epidermis or dermis that are present at birth. The history of the congenital nature of a nevus is often difficult to obtain. Baby pictures, hospital and pediatric newborn records, or parental or older sibling statements or records are needed to document that a nevus is congenital. This is especially true for small congenital nevi, which may not show "classic" clinical features of a congenital nevus (Fig. 48–7). Nevi that are not present at birth but develop within the first 2 years of life and clinically appear similar to congenital nevi are known as tardive congenital nevi.[56] The incidence of melanocytic nevi in newborn infants has been reported to be approximately 1%.[57, 58] Approximately 2.5% of adults have been reported to have "congenital nevus–like nevi" by clinical criteria.[59] Therefore, by relying on clinical criteria alone, a clinician will correctly identify less than 50% of cases of congenital nevi. Whether tardive congenital nevi or other acquired, congenital nevus–like nevi have an increased risk for developing melanoma is unknown.

The size of congenital nevi has been reported in various ways. Giant congenital nevi are variously defined as those not removable by surgery with primary closure, lesions the size of the patient's palm on the face or neck or twice that size on other anatomic areas,[60] lesions

covering 30% of the body surface area,[61] lesions covering 930 cm² in adults (or smaller in major anatomic areas),[62] or lesions larger than 20 cm.[63] Because surgical skills vary, defining "giant" according to the ease of surgical removal is imprecise. In one useful measurement method,[63] small congenital nevi (Figs. 48–7, 48–8) are defined as lesions less than 1.5 cm in diameter that may not always have the clinical features associated with congenital nevi. Medium-sized congenital nevi are defined as being 1.5 to 19.9 cm in diameter (Fig. 48–9), and giant-sized congenital nevi (Fig. 48–10) are ≥20 cm in diameter. However, measurement criteria are limited, because the size of a congenital nevus changes with the growth of the child. Congenital nevi show up to a ninefold increase in size, depending on anatomic location, by the time a child becomes an adult.[64] Despite this, classification of congenital nevi by diameter measurement allows objective classification of these lesions for clinical studies that are needed to obtain statistics for predicting the melanoma risk of congenital nevi, particularly smaller lesions.

Clinical features of congenital nevi include (1) a tendency to be larger in diameter than acquired nevi,

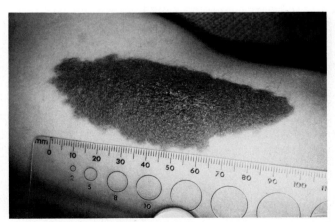

Figure 48–9. Medium-sized congenital nevus (1.5 to 19.9 cm) with even pigmentation and a mild pebbly surface.

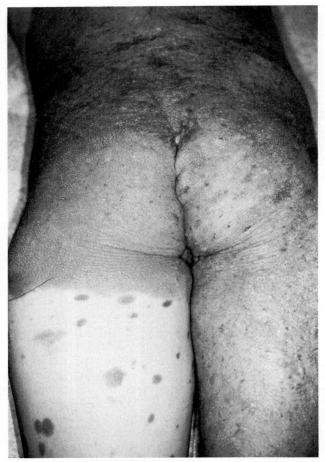

Figure 48–10. Giant congenital nevus of the garment or "bathing trunk" type. Note the multiple small congenital nevi, which are often associated with these giant nevi, and the variation in pigmentation seen in the giant lesion.

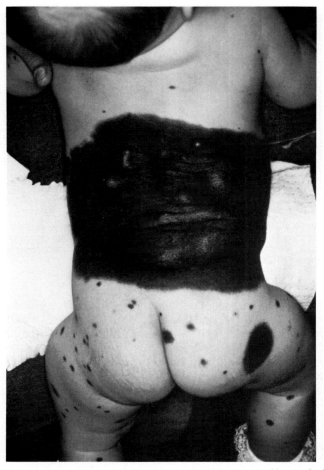

Figure 48–12. Giant "dysplastic" congenital nevus with atypical features of color (black), border irregularity, and multiple dermal nodules. The color and nodules make clinical follow-up difficult.

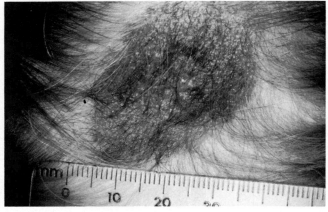

Figure 48–11. Medium-sized congenital nevus with two irregular dark macules within the lesion that are atypical, or "dysplastic" clinically.

and (2) development of thickening, verrucosity, and hirsutism with aging. The lesion surface may be smooth, pebbly, rugose, verrucous, cerebriform, or lobular.[56] Coarse, darkly pigmented hair or fine lanugo type hair may develop within the first 2 years of life. Most congenital nevi have a bland, even, tan or brown pigmentation (Figs. 48–7 to 48–9). However, a few lesions have irregular pigmentation, with areas of dark brown, black, or blue colors; uneven borders; or nodules ("dysplastic" congenital nevi) (Figs. 48–11, 48–12). When congenital nevi undergo biopsy, approximately 9% have atypia of intraepidermal melanocytes.[65] How these clinically and histologically "dysplastic" congenital nevi relate to each other and to the melanoma risk of "dysplastic" congenital nevus as compared with the regular congenital nevus is unknown. These data are difficult to obtain and interpret, because physicians are likely to remove atypical-appearing congenital nevi.

Congenital nevi may be associated with a number of anomalies,[56] including ear deformities, preauricular appendages, and angiomas.[66] Giant congenital nevi have been associated with ocular malformation,[67] elephantiasis of the affected extremities,[68] asymmetry of the trunk,[68] club foot, underlying bony atrophy, spina bifida occulta,[69] and meningocele. Associated tumors include neurofibromas,[69–71] neuroblastoma of the adrenal gland,[69] Wilms' tumor,[68] and leptomeningeal melanocytosis.[68, 72–78] Some patients with congenital nevi have multiple lesions, and in some families congenital nevi appear to be hereditary.[79–82] The inheritance is either autosomal dominant with incomplete penetrance or multifactorial, as identical twins with discordance for giant congenital nevi have been reported.[83,84]

Although histology has been cited as useful in the diagnosis of congenital versus acquired nevi,[65, 85, 86] no histologic features have proven to be diagnostic for congenital nevi,[64, 65] even when nevus cells are identified by techniques such as S-100 antibody and myelin basic protein immunohistochemistry.[64] Nevus cells have S-100 antigen but not myelin basic protein. Consequently, the diagnosis of a congenital nevus is primarily a clinical one, with histologic analysis being most useful to identify atypia or frank melanoma. Congenital nevi have been classified[87] into four histologic types depending on the distribution of nevus cells: the upper dermal diffuse type, upper dermal patchy type, upper and lower dermal diffuse type, and upper and lower dermal patchy type. Whether these classifications of congenital nevi will be able to differentiate congenital nevi with different clinical features, such as melanoma risk, remains to be determined. In addition to melanoma, other tumors associated with congenital nevi and seen histologically include schwannomas, neuroid tumors, neurofibromas, sebaceous nevi, blue nevi, spindle and epithelial cell nevi, and hemangiomas.[66, 67, 88, 89]

MELANOMA RISK FACTORS

Studies suggest that the risk of a giant congenital nevus developing a melanoma are between 2 and 31%,[63] with 5 to 10% being the most reported value. The melanoma risk of a small- or medium-sized congenital nevus is probably around 5%, with values reported from 3 to 21% depending on the method used to establish the congenital status of the nevus associated with the melanoma.[90] Studies examining the melanoma risk of "dysplastic congenital nevi" and the different histologic types of congenital nevi need to be done. The melanoma risk of a tardive congenital nevus is unknown.

Children with giant congenital nevi show melanoma susceptibility primarily between birth and 10 years of age; more than 60% of the melanomas occur during this period.[91] Patients have been reported who were born with melanoma in large congenital nevi,[92] although this is rare. On the other hand, small congenital nevi have an increased melanoma susceptibility at puberty[86] or after the age of 10.

MANAGEMENT

Key to the management of congenital nevi is education of nursery health care workers to identify and document the presence of congenital nevi, with referral to dermatologists for follow-up. This is crucial, because the only current method of diagnosing a congenital nevus is documenting its presence at birth. Education regarding congenital nevi also must be provided to the parents of the affected child. They should be informed of the potential risk of melanoma and the management

alternatives. Because of the possibility of familial inheritance of congenital nevi, a family history should also be obtained. When the family history is positive for familial congenital nevi, genetic counseling regarding the risks of inheritance is appropriate. Since most parents experience some guilt along with a feeling of responsibility for the presence of a congenital nevus in their child, education and counseling is also often required.

All congenital nevi should be followed closely clinically or excised; the preferred method continues to be debated in the literature.[90, 93–96] In clinically dysplastic congenital nevi, the dysplastic component should undergo biopsy to rule out intraepidermal melanocytic atypia, or frank melanoma.

Small congenital nevi are not a major surgical problem as they are easily excised, and their melanoma risk is not significant until puberty. Therefore, a reasonable approach is to initially monitor the nevus with photography and then electively excise the lesion under local anesthesia before puberty, when the child is capable of tolerating local anesthesia. The nevus could be indefinitely followed clinically, although the time and expense involved may justify elective excision. Excision also removes any potential melanoma risk of the lesion, another argument in favor of having small congenital nevi excised. On the other hand, the exact melanoma risk of a small congenital nevus is unknown, making surgery for all lesions unwarranted at the present. Management of medium-sized congenital nevi is similar. They may also be excised or clinically monitored if the lesion is in an anatomically unfavorable area for excision.

The giant congenital nevus is a dilemma due to its malignant potential and the technical difficulties associated with surgical removal. Monitoring these lesions with photography and close clinical examination is crucial. Clinical examination should include palpation of the lesion for new nodules. Any change in the lesion warrants an excisional biopsy of the changing area. Some giant congenital nevi may be removed by a combination of surgical techniques, such as tissue expansion and skin grafts[97] or epithelial autografts.[98] Cutaneous surgeons with special training in reconstructive procedures may remove these lesions.

Children with giant congenital nevi often have multiple small congenital nevi, all of which should be monitored for the possibility of melanoma development. Clinical photography using the method described for dysplastic nevi is useful for following these patients. Patients with "dysplastic"-appearing congenital nevi or patients who have shown recent nevus change should be followed at 3-month intervals, while other patients should be followed at 6- to 12-month intervals. Any changing area within the nevus should undergo biopsy. Biopsies should be done using the excision or punch technique. Because of the depth of congenital nevi, the shave biopsy technique is usually not appropriate.

Because giant congenital nevi of the head, neck, and lumbosacral area may have associated leptomeningeal melanocytosis and may develop melanoma or obstructive hydrocephalus, seizures, and focal neurologic deficits,[78] a neurologic evaluation with appropriate radiologic scans (e.g., computed tomography with contrast[75] or a more sensitive technique such as magnetic resonance imaging with gadolinium contrast[78]) may be indicated. Appropriate work-up and referral may also be required for any of the other associated abnormalities that may occur with congenital nevi.

Other difficult clinical management problems are the congenital nevus–like nevi. There have been no studies documenting an increase in melanoma risk for these lesions; therefore, prophylactic removal of these lesions, found in 1 to 2% of the population, is currently not medically indicated. It is probably best to photographically document the lesion, educate the patient in monthly cutaneous self-examination of the nevus, and perform clinical follow-up examinations every 6 to 12 months. Any change in the nevus warrants biopsy, just as for dysplastic nevi and congenital nevi.

SUMMARY

A thorough medical history and a meticulous physical examination are required to manage patients with dysplastic and congenital nevi most effectively. In addition, clinicopathologic correlation is necessary in evaluating those individuals with clinically normal-appearing nevi that show mildly atypical histologic features. Patient education, self-examination, appropriate photography, and routine examinations by a knowledgeable cutaneous surgeon will give patients with dysplastic or congenital pigmented nevi the best opportunity for early diagnosis of changes that may require surgical removal.

REFERENCES

1. Reimer RR, Clark WH Jr, Greene MH, et al: Precursor lesions in familial melanoma: a new genetic preneoplastic syndrome. JAMA 239:744–746, 1978.
2. Clark WH Jr, Reimer RR, Greene MH, et al: Origin of familial malignant melanomas from heritable melanocytic lesions: the BK mole syndrome. Arch Dermatol 114:732–738, 1978.
3. Frichot BC III, Lynch HT, Guirgis HA, et al: New cutaneous phenotype in familial malignant melanoma. Lancet 1:864–865, 1977.
4. Lynch HT, Fusaro RM, Pester J, Lynch JF: Familial atypical multiple mole melanoma (FAMMM) syndrome: genetic heterogeneity and malignant melanoma. Br J Cancer 42:58–70, 1980.
5. Greene MH, Clark WH Jr, Tucker MA, et al: Precursor naevi in cutaneous malignant melanoma: a proposed nomenclature. Lancet 2:1024, 1980.
6. Elder DE, Goldman LI, Goldman SC, et al: Dysplastic nevus syndrome: a phenotypic association of sporadic cutaneous melanoma. Cancer 46:1787–1794, 1980.
7. Greene MH, Clark WH Jr, Tucker MA, et al: Acquired precursors of cutaneous malignant melanoma: the familial dysplastic nevus syndrome. N Engl J Med 312:91–116, 1985.
8. Klein LJ, Barr RJ: Histologic atypia in clinically benign nevi. J Am Acad Dermatol 22:275–282, 1990.
9. Piepkorn M: A hypothesis incorporating the histologic characteristics of dysplastic nevi into the normal biological development of melanocytic nevi. Arch Dermatol 126:514–518, 1990.
10. Piepkorn M, Meyer LJ, Goldgar D, et al: The dysplastic melanocytic nevus: a prevalent lesion that correlates poorly with clinical phenotype. J Am Acad Dermatol 20:407–415, 1989.
11. NIH Consensus Conference. September 1990, Bethesda, MD.
12. Elder DE, Green MH, Guerry DP III, et al: The dysplastic nevus syndrome: our definition. Am J Dermatopathol 4:455–460, 1982.
13. Murphy GF, Halpern A: Dysplastic melanocytic nevi: normal variants or melanoma precursors? Arch Dermatol 126:519–522, 1990.
14. Bale SJ, Dracopoli NC, Tucker MA, et al: Mapping the gene for hereditary cutaneous malignant melanoma-dysplastic nevus to chromosome 1p. N Engl J Med 320:1367–1372, 1989.
15. Crutcher WA, Sagebiel RW: Prevalence of dysplastic naevi in a community practice. Lancet 1:729, 1984.
16. Kraemer KH, Greene MH, Tarone R, et al: Dysplastic naevi and cutaneous melanoma risk. Lancet 2:1076–1077, 1983.
17. Albert LS, Rhodes AR, Sober AJ: Dysplastic melanocytic nevi and cutaneous melanoma: markers of increased melanoma risk for affected persons and blood relatives. J Am Acad Dermatol 22:69–75, 1990.
18. Rigel DS, Rivers JK, Kopf AW, et al: Dysplastic nevi: markers for increased risk for melanoma. Cancer 63:386–389, 1989.
19. Greene MH, Clark WH Jr, Tucker MA, et al: Melanoma risk in familial dysplastic nevus syndrome. Abstract. J Invest Dermatol 82:424–425, 1984.
20. Kraemer KH, Greene MH: Dysplastic nevus syndrome: familial and sporadic precursors of cutaneous melanoma. Dermatol Clin 3:225–237, 1985.
21. Assessing the risks of stratospheric ozone depletion. In: Longstreth JD (ed): Ultraviolet Radiation and Melanoma. Vol IV. United States Environmental Protection Agency, Washington, DC, EPA400/1-87/001D 9, 1987, pp 8-1–8-12.
22. Swerdlow AJ, English JSC, MacKie RM, et al: Fluorescent lights, ultraviolet lamps, and risk of cutaneous melanoma. Br Med J 297:647–50, 1988.
23. MacKie RM, Aitchinson T: Severe sunburn and subsequent risk of primary cutaneous melanoma in Scotland. Br J Cancer 46:955–960, 1982.
24. Elwood JM, Gallagher RP, Davison J, Hill GB: Sunburn, suntan and the risk of cutaneous malignant melanoma—the Western Canada melanoma study. Br J Cancer 51:543–549, 1985.
25. Barnhill RL, Wiles JC: Malignant melanoma associated with multiple therapies for psoriasis. J Am Acad Dermatol 21:148–150, 1989.
26. Rhodes AR, Harrist TJ, Momtaz-T K: The PUVA-induced pigmented macule: a lentiginous proliferation of large, sometimes cytologically atypical, melanocytes. J Am Acad Dermatol 9:47–58, 1983.
27. Greene MH, Young TI, Clark WH Jr: Malignant melanoma in renal-transplant patients. Lancet 1:1196–1199, 1981.
28. Tucker MA, Misfeldt D, Coleman CN, et al: Cutaneous malignant melanoma after Hodgkin's disease. Ann Intern Med 102:37–41, 1985.
29. Duvic M, Lowe L, Rapini RP, et al: Eruptive dysplastic nevi associated with human immunodeficiency virus infection. Arch Dermatol 125:397–401, 1989.
30. Cosnes A, Revuz J, Wechsler J, Touraine R: Melanoma and dysplastic naevi after eight years of topical mechlorethamine. Ann Dermatol Venereol 111:127–132, 1984.
31. Bahn AK, Rosenwaike I, Herrmann N, et al: Melanoma after exposure to PCB's. N Engl J Med 295:450, 1976.
32. Blot WJ, Brinton LA, Fraumeni JF Jr, et al: Cancer mortality in US countries with petroleum industries. Science 198:51–53, 1977.
33. Ellis DL: Pregnancy and sex steroid hormone effects on nevi of dysplastic nevus syndrome patients. J Am Acad Dermatol 25:467–482, 1991.
34. Foucar E, Bentley TJ, Laube DW, et al: A histopathologic evaluation of nevocellular nevi in pregnancy. Arch Dermatol 121:350–354, 1985.
35. Bondi EE, Clark WH Jr, Elder D, et al: Topical chemotherapy of dysplastic melanocytic nevi with 5% fluorouracil. Arch Dermatol 117:89–92, 1981.
36. Meyskens FL, Edwards L, Levine NS: Role of topical tretinoin in melanoma and dysplastic nevi. J Am Acad Dermatol 15:822–825, 1986.
37. Edwards L, Jaffe P: The effect of topical tretinoin on dysplastic nevi: a preliminary trial. Arch Dermatol 126:494–499, 1990.
38. Kornberg R, Ackerman AB: Pseudomelanoma. Arch Dermatol 111:1588–1590, 1975.

Early melanoma histologic terms. Am J Dermatopathol 13:579–582, 1991.

39. Park HK, Leonard DD, Arrington JH III, Lund HZ: Recurrent melanocytic nevi: clinical and histologic review of 175 cases. J Am Acad Dermatol 17:285–292, 1987.

40. Kaidbey KH: The photoprotective potential of the new superpotent sunscreens. J Am Acad Dermatol 22:449–452, 1990.

41. Bellet RE, Shields JA, Soll DB, Bernadino EA: Primary choroidal and cutaneous melanomas occurring in a patient with the B-K mole syndrome phenotype. Am J Ophthalmol 89:567–570, 1980.

42. Vink J, Crijns MB, Mooy CM, et al: Ocular melanoma in families with dysplastic nevus syndrome. J Am Acad Dermatol 23:858–862, 1990.

43. Friedman RJ, Rodriguez-Sains R, Jakobiec F: Ophthalmologic oncology: conjunctival malignant melanoma in association with sporadic dysplastic nevus syndrome. J Dermatol Surg Oncol 13:31–34, 1987.

44. Bergman W, Watson P, de Jong J, et al: Systemic cancer and the FAMMM syndrome. Br J Cancer 61:932–936, 1990.

45. Greene MH, Tucker MA, Clark WH Jr, et al: Hereditary melanoma and the dysplastic nevus syndrome: the risk of cancers other than melanoma. J Am Acad Dermatol 16:792- 797, 1987.

46. Vasen HFA, Bergman W, Van Haeringen A, et al: The familial dysplastic naevus syndrome: natural history and the impact of screening on prognosis—a study of nine families in the Netherlands. Eur J Cancer Clin Oncol 25:337–341, 1989.

47. Rigel DS, Rivers JK, Kopf AW, et al: Dysplastic nevi: markers for increased risk for melanoma. Cancer 63:386–389, 1989.

48. Rivers JK, Kopf AW, Vinokur AF, et al: Clinical characteristics of malignant melanomas developing in persons with dysplastic nevi. Cancer 65:1232–1236,1990.

49. Masri GD, Clark WH Jr, Guerry DP IV, et al: Screening and surveillance of patients at high risk for malignant melanoma result in detection of earlier disease. J Am Acad Dermatol 22:1042–1048, 1990.

50. Greene MH, Clark WH Jr, Tucker MA, et al: The prospective diagnosis of malignant melanoma in a population at high risk: hereditary melanoma and the dysplastic nevus syndrome. Ann Int Med 102:458–465, 1985.

51. Tucker MA, Greene MH, Clark WH Jr, et al: Dysplastic nevi on the scalp of prepubertal children from melanoma-prone families. J Pediatr 103:65–69, 1983.

52. Veronesi U, Cascinelli N, Adamus J, et al: Thin stage I primary cutaneous malignant melanoma: comparison of excision with margins of 1 or 3 cm. N Engl J Med 318:1159–1162, 1988.

53. Shafir R, Hiss J, Tsur H, Bubis JJ: The thin malignant melanoma: changing patterns of epidemiology and treatment. Cancer 50:817–819, 1982.

54. Day CL, Mihm MC Jr, Sober AJ, et al: Narrower margins for clinical stage I malignant melanoma. N Engl J Med 306:479–482, 1982.

55. Cosimi AB, Sober AJ, Mihm MC Jr, Fitzpatrick TB: Conservative surgical management of superficially invasive cutaneous melanoma. Cancer 53:1256–1259, 1984.

56. Rhodes AR: Neoplasms: benign neoplasias, hyperplasias, and dysplasias of melanocytes. In: Fitzpatrick TB, Eisen AZ, Wolff K, et al (eds): Dermatology in General Medicine. 3rd ed. McGraw-Hill, New York, 1987, pp 877–946.

57. Walten RG, Jacobs AH, Cox AJ: Pigmented lesions in newborn infants. Br J Dermatol 95:389–396, 1976.

58. Alper J, Holmes LB, Mihm MC: Birthmarks with serious medical significance: nevocellular nevi, sebaceous nevi, and multiple cafe-au-lait spots. J Pediatr 95:696–700, 1979.

59. Kopf AW, Levine LJ, Rigel DS, et al: Prevalence of congenital-nevus-like nevi, nevi spili, and cafe au lait spots. Arch Dermatol 121:766–769, 1985.

60. Lorentzen M, Pers M, Bretteville-Jensen G: The incidence of malignant transformation in giant pigmented nevi. Scand J Plast Reconstr Surg 11:163–167, 1977.

61. Lanier VC, Pickrell KL, Georgiade NG: Congenital giant nevi: clinical and pathological considerations. Plast Reconstr Surg 58:48–54, 1976.

62. Greeley PW, Middleton AG, Curtin JW: Incidence of malignancy in giant pigmented nevi. Plast Reconstr Surg 36:26–37, 1965.

63. Kopf AW, Bart RS, Hennessey P: Congenital nevocytic nevi and malignant melanomas. J Am Acad Dermatol 1:123–130, 1979.

64. Nickoloff BJ, Walton R, Pregerson-Rodan K, et al: Immunohistologic patterns of congenital nevocellular nevi. Arch Dermatol 122:1263–1268, 1986.

65. Rhodes AR, Silverman RA, Harrist TJ, Melski JW: A histologic comparison of congenital and acquired nevomelanocytic nevi. Arch Dermatol 121:1266–1273, 1985.

66. Castilla EE, da Graca Dutra M, Orioli-Parreiras IM: Epidemiology of congenital pigmented naevi. I. Incidence rates and relative frequencies. Br J Dermatol 104:307–315, 1981.

67. De Anda G, Vignale RA, Pous M, et al: Nevo congenito pigmentado piloso gigante con tumores hamarto matosos multiples: una neurocristo pathia compleja. Rev Argent Dermatol 64:208–213, 1983.

68. Pack, GT, Davis J: Nevus giganticus pigmentosus with malignant transformation. Surgery 49:347–354, 1961.

69. Reed WB, Becker SW Sr, Becker SW Jr, Nickel WR: Giant pigmented nevi, melanoma, and leptomeningeal melanocytosis: a clinical and histopathological study. Arch Dermatol 91:100–119, 1965.

70. Conway H: Bathing trunk nevus. Surgery 6:585–597, 1939.

71. Crowe FW, Schull WH, Neel JV: A Clinical, Pathological and Genetic Study of Multiple Neurofibromatosis. Charles C Thomas, Springfield, IL, 1956, pp 1–181.

72. Fox H, Emery JL, Goodbody RA, Yates PO: Neuro-cutaneous melanosis. Arch Dis Child 39:508–516, 1964.

73. Savitz MH, Anderson PJ: Primary melanoma of the leptomeninges: a review. Mt Sinai J Med 41:774–791, 1974.

74. Lamas E, Lobato RD, Sotelo T, et al: Neurocutaneous melanosis: report of a case and review of the literature. Acta Neurochir 36:93–105, 1977.

75. Kudel TA, Bingham WT, Tubman DE: Computed tomographic findings of primary malignant leptomeningeal melanoma in neurocutaneous melanosis. Am J Radiol 133:950–951, 1979.

76. Kaplan AM, Itabashi HH, Hanelin LG, Lu AT: Neurocutaneous melanosis with malignant leptomeningeal melanoma. Arch Neurol 32:669–671, 1975.

77. Hoffman HJ, Freeman A: Primary malignant leptomeningeal melanoma in association with giant hairy nevi: report of two cases. J Neurosurg 26:62–71, 1967.

78. Kadonaga JN, Frieden IJ: Neurocutaneous melanosis: definition and review of the literature. J Am Acad Dermatol 24:747–755, 1991.

79. Rhodes AR, Slifman NR, Korf BR: Familial aggregation of small congenital nevomelanocytic nevi. Am J Med Genet 22:315–326, 1985.

80. Pickrell KL, Clay RC: Giant nevus of the thigh successfully treated by complete excision and primary grafting. Arch Surg 48:319–324, 1944.

81. Hecht F, LaCanne KM, Carroll DB: Inheritance of giant pigmented hairy nevus of the scalp. Am J Med Genet 9:177–178, 1981.

82. Miller TR, Pack GT: The familial aspects of malignant melanoma. Arch Dermatol 86:35–39, 1962.

83. Cantu JM, Urrusti J, Hernandez A, et al: Discordance for giant pigmented nevi in monozygotic twins. Ann Genet 16:289–292, 1973.

84. Amir J, Metzker A, Nitzan M: Giant pigmented nevus occurring in one identical twin. Arch Dermatol 118:188–189, 1982.

85. Mark GT, Mihm MC, Liteplo MG, et al: Congenital melanocytic nevi of the small and garment type. Hum Pathol 4:395–418, 1973.

86. Illig L, Weidner F, Hundeiker M, et al: Congenital nevi ≤ 10 cm as precursors to melanoma: 52 cases, a review, and a new conception. Arch Dermatol 121:1274–1281, 1985.

87. Stenn KS, Arons M, Hurwitz S: Patterns of congenital nevocellular nevi. J Am Acad Dermatol 9:388–393, 1983.

88. Solomon LM, Eng AM, Bene M, Loeffel ED: Giant congenital neuroid melanocytic nevus. Arch Dermatol 116:318–320, 1980.

89. Weidner N, Flanders DJ, Jochimsen PR, Stamler FW: Neurosarcomatous malignant melanoma arising in a nevoid giant congenital melanocytic nevus. Arch Dermatol 121:1302–1306, 1985.

90 Rhodes AR: Congenital nevomelanocytic nevi: histologic patterns in the first year of life and evolution during childhood. Arch Dermatol 122:1257–1262, 1986.

91. Rhodes AR: Pigmented birthmarks and precursor melanocytic lesions of cutaneous melanoma identifiable in childhood. Pediatr Clin North Am 30:435–463, 1983.

92. Schneiderman H, Wu AY-Y, Campbell WA, et al: Congenital melanoma with multiple prenatal metastases. Cancer 60:1371–1377, 1987.

93. Solomon LM: The management of congenital melanocytic nevi. Arch Dermatol 116:117, 1980.
94. Kirschenbaum MB: Congenital melanocytic nevi. Arch Dermatol 117:379–380, 1981.
95. Alper JC: Congenital nevi: the controversy rages on. Arch Dermatol 121:734–735, 1985.
96. Elder DE: The blind men and the elephant: different views of small congenital nevi. Arch Dermatol 121:1263–1265, 1985.
97. Bauer BS, Vicari FA: An approach to excision of congenital giant pigmented nevi in infancy and early childhood. Plast Reconstr Surg 82:1012–1021, 1988.
98. Gallico GG III, O'Connor NE, Compton CC, et al: Cultured epithelial autografts for giant congenital nevi. Plast Reconstr Surg 84:1–9, 1989.

CHAPTER 49

Management of Lipomas

ALLISON T. VIDIMOS

Introduction

Lipomas are probably the most common benign soft tissue tumor presenting to the cutaneous surgeon. Their variable clinical presentations prompt the clinician to consider a spectrum of treatment options ranging from observation or relatively simple incisional surgery to complicated excision with microdissection or even liposuction.

Clinical Description

Lipomas are benign tumors of adipose tissue that may arise throughout the body in visceral, inter- or intramuscular, or subdermal locations, with the last location being most frequent. Deeply invasive lipomas may involve nerves, fascia, muscle, and bone. These mesenchymally derived tumors usually present as asymptomatic, solitary, encapsulated, round or oval, subcutaneous nodules. On palpation they typically have a rubbery, compressible consistency and often have a lobulated configuration.

Sites of predilection include the trunk, shoulder, posterior neck, forearms, thighs, and axillae. Rarely, lipomas are found on the scalp (Fig. 49–1), face, sternum, inguinal skin, and lower legs.[1–4] Unusual sites include the orbit,[5] tongue,[6] palm,[7, 8] sole,[9] toe,[10] and vulva.[11]

Lipomas may range in size from a few millimeters to several centimeters. A study of 428 nonvisceral lipomas noted that the majority of solitary lipomas measured less than 5 cm in diameter, while subfascial lipomas averaged 6 cm in size.[2] The subfascial lipomas tend to be slow growing and asymptomatic and may not exhibit the encapsulated architecture of their more superficial counterpart.

Lipomas may appear at any age, although they generally arise in early adulthood and are rare in infancy and childhood. In general, solitary lipomas predominate in women, and multiple lipomas occur more frequently in men. Multiple lipomas are extremely rare in children. Women exhibit lipomas most commonly on the shoulder and thigh, while the head, neck, and chest are the most prevalent sites in males.[2] The precise origin of lipomas remains unknown. Multiple lipomas may be associated with a familial tendency, an underlying hereditary hyperlipidemia,[12] or diabetes mellitus.[13] Trauma is probably responsible for the discovery of lipomas, rather than being an actual cause of them.

Classification of Lipomas

Of the many variants of lipomas, most are solitary and encapsulated. Lipomas may be multiple and fall into one of the classes of lipomatosis: diffuse congenital lipomatosis, benign symmetric lipomatosis, familial multiple lipomatosis, angiolipomas, or miscellaneous variants.

SOLITARY LIPOMAS

Most solitary lipomas are superficial in location and small in size. Although solitary lipomas may develop in individuals concomitant with weight gain, they generally undergo little decrease in size with weight loss.

DIFFUSE CONGENITAL LIPOMATOSIS

Diffuse congenital lipomatosis is a nonhereditary clinical entity characterized by diffuse, poorly demarcated lipomas localized mainly to the trunk. These lipomas may infiltrate through muscle fibers and extend to the retroperitoneal space. For obvious reasons, they are notoriously recalcitrant to surgical excision.[14]

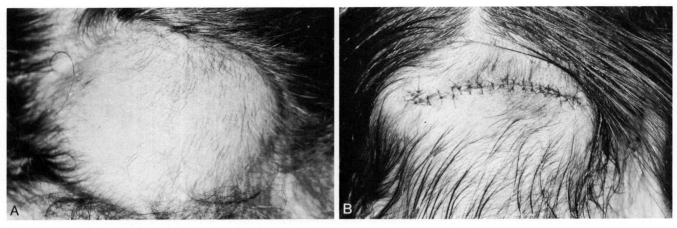

Figure 49–1. *A,* Large posterior occiput lipoma. *B,* Scalp wound after excision of an encapsulated 6 × 7 cm lipoma.

BENIGN SYMMETRIC LIPOMATOSIS

Benign symmetric lipomatosis (BSL) in adults, initially described by Madelung in 1888, is characterized by lipomatous involvement of the head, neck, shoulders, and proximal upper extremities. Males are affected four times more frequently than females, and there is often a history of heavy alcohol consumption. Other conditions associated with BSL include glucose intolerance, malignant tumors of the upper airways, hyperuricemia, obesity, renal tubular acidosis, peripheral neuropathy, and hepatopathy.[15, 16] These lipomas generally appear in middle age, and there may be a family history of similar lipomatous deposition.[17] Enhanced activity of lipoprotein lipase has been measured in the lipomatous tissue.[12] The differential diagnosis of benign symmetrical lipomatosis includes obesity, sialadenitis, goiter, or lymphatic tumor.[18]

FAMILIAL MULTIPLE LIPOMATOSIS

Familial multiple lipomatosis (FML) is a distinct clinical entity characterized by variable numbers of small, well-dermarcated, encapsulated lipomas involving the extremities, primarily the upper limbs, and trunk (Fig. 49–2). These lipomas generally appear during or soon after adolescence and commonly exhibit a symmetric distribution. There is frequently a family history of multiple lipomas, and an autosomal dominant mode of inheritance has been noted.[2] In contrast to BSL, the neck and shoulders are generally spared in FML.[17] Large subcutaneous masses in these patients may actually represent small, discrete, grouped, encapsulated lipomas.[19]

ANGIOLIPOMAS

Angiolipomas[20] present around adolescence as well-demarcated, soft subcutaneous nodules that are frequently painful. They are most prevalent on the trunk and extremities. On palpation they are frequently lobulated and may be firmer than lipomas. The pain associated with angiolipomas is generally vague in nature and may be spontaneous or associated with pressure. It rarely has a sharp or radiating character, unlike pain associated with glomus tumors. Increased vascularity has been associated with the degree of pain,[20] although no consistent correlation has been seen.[21] The pain from angiolipomas in one study, however, could not be reproduced by injection of vascular mediators, by vascular

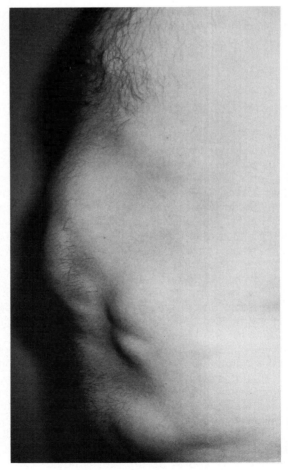

Figure 49–2. Multiple truncal lipomas.

occlusion, or by heat or cold application.[21] The origin of angiolipomas is unknown, although some authors propose trauma as an instigating factor.[20, 22]

Infiltrating angiolipomas generally present as deep, painless, slow-growing, nonencapsulated masses. They may infiltrate muscle but only rarely cause muscle dysfunction or sensory changes.[23–26] While these infiltrating angiolipomas are difficult to excise completely because of their diffuse muscular infiltration, malignant transformation has not been reported.

A variant of angiolipoma, the cellular angiolipoma,[27] has been described as part of a clinical picture of nonhereditary multiple, sometimes painful, subcutaneous nodules occurring on the trunk and extremities of otherwise healthy men. These encapsulated nodules exhibit dense cellular angiomatous tissue, frequently with prominent spindle cells, and may also be present along with more typical angiolipomas. This variant must be distinguished from Kaposi's sarcoma, spindle cell lipoma, and other vascular tumors.

MISCELLANEOUS VARIANTS

Two other variants of lipomas are the spindle cell lipoma and pleomorphic lipoma. Spindle cell lipomas generally occur in males during the fourth through seventh decades of life as painless subcutaneous slow-growing nodules on the neck, shoulder, or back.[28, 29] They are rarely found on the extremities, head, or in the oral cavity.[30] Pathologically, spindle cell lipomas may be distinguished from liposarcomas by the presence of mature fat cells and uniform spindle cells embedded in a mucinous matrix, with no lipoblasts. Pleomorphic lipomas occur predominantly in males during the fifth to seventh decades of life and are most commonly found in the subcutaneous tissues of the posterior neck, shoulder, and back[31] and rarely on the scalp.[32] As with the spindle cell lipoma, pleomorphic lipomas exhibit a benign biologic behavior, but histologically they, too, must be distinguished from liposarcomas. Pathologically, pleomorphic lipomas exhibit variable-sized fat cells, and bizarre multinucleated giant cells with characteristic floret giant cells. The absence of mitotic activity and the presence of pyknotic nuclei further help to distinguish pleomorphic lipomas from liposarcomas.[31, 32]

Dercum's disease, or adiposis dolorosa, initially described in 1892,[33] is a syndrome characterized by marked obesity and the insidious development of painful subcutaneous lipomas involving the shoulders, arms, forearms, trunk, legs, and rarely, the face and hands. Onset is generally in middle age, and women are affected five times more frequently than men. Males generally exhibit a less severe form of the syndrome.[34] Some patients exhibit a family history with an autosomal dominant mode of inheritance and variable expressivity.[34, 35] The cause of this syndrome is unknown, and pathologically the lipomas are most often of the common encapsulated type, although some may represent angiolipomas.

Multiple lipomas of the skin and internal organs may also be seen in patients with Gardner's syndrome. These patients exhibit polyposis of the colon and may have multiple epidermal cysts, osteomas, and desmoid tumors. An autosomal dominant inheritance with variable expressivity has been demonstrated. It is important to recognize these patients, because prognosis is greatly improved with early diagnosis and removal of the colon, as malignant degeneration often occurs before 30 years of age.

Histopathology

Lipomas are composed of a thin connective tissue capsule encasing a mass of normal-appearing fat cells, frequently with a fine interlacing connective tissue network. In contrast, an angiolipoma contains proportionately more blood vessels and fibrous septae, thereby giving it its firmer consistency and more reddish color on gross examination. Mast cells were noted in 50% of 248 angiolipomas examined in one study,[20] in addition to intravascular fibrin thrombi. No neural elements, fat necrosis, inflammation, or other histologic evidence indicative of the source of pain in angiolipomas was noted.

Differential Diagnosis

Soft tissue tumors that should be included in the clinical differential diagnosis of lipomas include hibernomas, lipoblastomas, liposarcomas, and neurofibromas. Large lipomas of the axillae must be differentiated from polymastia. Hibernomas generally present as solitary, well-circumscribed, asymptomatic, subcutaneous nodules in the interscapular region, although they may also be found in the axillae, on the neck, and in the mediastinum. Histologically, they are composed of embryonic brown lipoblasts.[36]

Lipoblastomas present in infants and young children as asymptomatic, subcutaneous nodules occurring predominantly on the lower extremities.[37–40] Two forms have been described: a superficial, well-encapsulated type and a deep, poorly circumscribed variety.[39] Boys are generally more often affected, and the benign course of these lesions warrants only complete local excision. Histologically, lipoblastomas are composed of a mixture of lipoblasts, fibroblasts, stellate myxoid cells, undifferentiated mesenchymal cells, lipocytes, and other intermediate cell forms. The cytoplasmic ultrastructure of these cells suggests a relationship to fetal white fat.[41]

Liposarcomas present as slowly enlarging, subcutaneous masses occurring predominantly on the popliteal fossa, medial thigh, and shoulder.[42, 43] They have rarely been described in the oral cavity.[44] Middle-aged or elderly men are most commonly affected. This rare tumor of lipoblasts is generally classified histologically into one of four groups: round cell, pleomorphic cell, myxoid cell, or well-differentiated cell type. The last two types have the best overall prognosis. Trauma has been cited as a possible triggering factor in the development of liposarcomas,[42] but there is much disagreement on this issue.[43] Liposarcomas probably arise de novo, but, a few case reports question their possible evolution from a benign lipoma.[20, 43] Lipomatous tumors larger than 5 cm in diameter,[2] and particularly those larger than 10 cm,[45] have a statistically greater chance of being liposarcomas, as do fatty tumors on the thigh or those found deep in soft tissue.

Treatment

Patients present for surgical removal of lipomas probably more often than for any other benign soft tissue tumor, usually because of symptomatic changes or cosmetic and functional concerns. The preoperative clinical diagnosis of lipomas may be accurately ascertained in most cases by the history, clinical appearance, consistency on palpation, and site. Infiltrating lipomas may be more difficult to accurately diagnose preoperatively and to remove. This is because of their tendency to be nonencapsulated and their ability to develop in intra- or intermuscular locations with infiltration of tendon, bone, and nerve.[46-52] Contraction of the involved musculature may allow better definition of these lipomas.

Surgical removal of a superficial encapsulated lipoma is generally a relatively simple procedure. However, careful consideration and evaluation should be given before removal of the more infiltrating lipomas, as interference with function or circulation of the involved limb may follow wide excision of the involved musculature and tumor. Careful microdissection may be required to preserve neural and vascular structures as much as possible.

In cases of suspected liposarcoma, fine needle aspiration[53, 54] and computed tomography (CT)[55, 56] may be valuable preoperative tools in planning an appropriate therapeutic procedure. It has been shown that CT scans may be useful in distinguishing between lipomas and liposarcomas, in addition to assessing the location and extent of the fatty tumors.[55, 56] In general, a lipoma appears as a well-delineated mass of homogeneous density and with attenuation values similar to those of normal fat. Liposarcomas show poor delineation, multilobulation, and less homogeneity and have higher attenuation values, generally between those of fat and muscle. Liposarcomas exhibit contrast enhancement, whereas lipomas do not.[55] In addition, magnetic resonance imaging (MRI) is helpful in ascertaining the location and extent of fatty tumors, but it is unable to distinguish benign from malignant tissue.[56]

Surgical Technique

"SQUEEZE" PROCEDURE

Small, superficial, encapsulated lipomas may be removed by way of a single linear stab incision that may be as short as one fourth to one third of the palpable diameter of the lipoma (Fig. 49–3). Pressure on the lateral aspects of the incision may be adequate to express the entire unit or multilobulated tumor, although gentle dissection with a curette; small, blunt undermining scissors; or a periosteal elevator[57] may be necessary to disrupt the fibrous tethers between the capsule and surrounding subcutaneous tissue. Normal saline may

also be injected preoperatively into the subcutaneous tissue immediately surrounding the lipoma to facilitate enucleation. Forceps or a curette[58] may then be used to extract the lipoma. The wound is closed with subcutaneous and surface sutures, and a pressure dressing may be applied. The ease and low morbidity rate of this technique have been frequently demonstrated.[58-60] However, it may not be adequate to remove lipomas located on the neck,[61] as many of these may be fibrolipomas, thus necessitating removal by sharp dissection. It is also suggested that the "squeeze" technique not be used for suspected lipomas located on the breast; instead, rather sharp dissection to the level of the deep fascia should be employed to diagnose a possible carcinoma that may lie deep to the lipoma.

DISTANT INCISION TECHNIQUE

When removing benign subcutaneous lesions on areas such as the forehead, lower eyelids, cheeks, lips, and sternal areas, a superior cosmetic result may be obtained by making the incision at a somewhat distant site.[62] It may be hidden in the scalp, eyelid or nasolabial folds, preauricular skin, oral mucosa, or inframammary folds. After local anesthesia is instilled, an incision with a length approximately equal to the distance between the lesion and the incision is made, and after gentle undermining, the lipoma is carefully dissected and removed through the newly created tract. Hemostasis is achieved, the wound is sutured, and a pressure dressing is applied for 24 to 48 hours. Knowledge of the local anatomy and careful tissue handling are imperative to avoid possible nerve injury and prevent excessive bleeding.

SURGICAL EXCISION

Larger lipomas are commonly removed with simple surgical excision. The palpable borders of the lipomas are marked on the skin before obtaining local anesthesia (Fig. 49–4). The skin is incised down to the capsule of the lipoma, and the lipomatous mass is gently dissected free from the surrounding tissue. Because lipomas commonly occupy large volumes, the dead space that results after their removal may be extensive. Therefore, meticulous hemostasis must be obtained, and buried absorbable sutures should be used to close this space as much as possible. As subcutaneous lipomas may act as natural tissue expanders, some of the excess overlying skin may need to be removed for proper wound closure. After suturing of the wound, a pressure dressing should be applied for 24 to 48 hours to prevent hematoma or seroma formation. Surgical drains may also be placed in wounds that are thought to be potential candidates for hematoma formation.

LIPOSUCTION

Liposuction has also proved to be a reliable method for the removal of large lipomas,[63-65] multiple lipomas or angiolipomas,[19, 66, 67] congenital infiltrating lipomatosis of the face,[68, 69] and benign symmetric lipomatosis, or Madelung's disease.[70-72] In a 1984 survey of complication

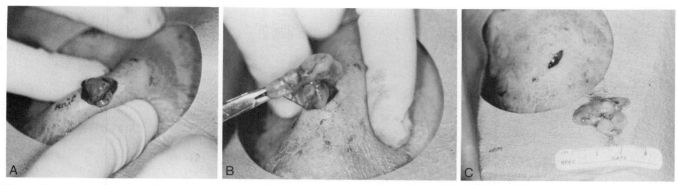

Figure 49–3. Enucleation of a lipoma on the forearm. *A,* After placement of a small incision in the center of the palpated subcutaneous nodule, pressure is applied around the wound, causing a lobule of the lipoma to mushroom out of the wound. *B,* With continued pressure, the multilobulated lipoma is easily removed from the wound with gentle traction. *C,* Multilobulated, encapsulated lipoma removed intact from a single incision.

rates associated with liposuction surgery, only 83 of the 5458 cases reported were lipoma extraction cases. None resulted in the surveyed complications of hematoma, paraesthesia, infection, or permanent skin irregularities.[73]

The removal of lipomas by liposuction utilizes a technique similar to that employed to treat areas of localized adiposity. After local anesthesia is obtained, a small incision is made into the skin adjacent to the lipoma, and a small suction cannula is inserted into the incision and tunneled in spokelike fashion through the lipoma. In contrast to surgical excision, all of the lipoma is not removed because of the tenacious fibrous supporting network traversing the lipoma. Liposuction is continued only until the area is flat, and then an elasticized pressure dressing is applied. In these cases, the

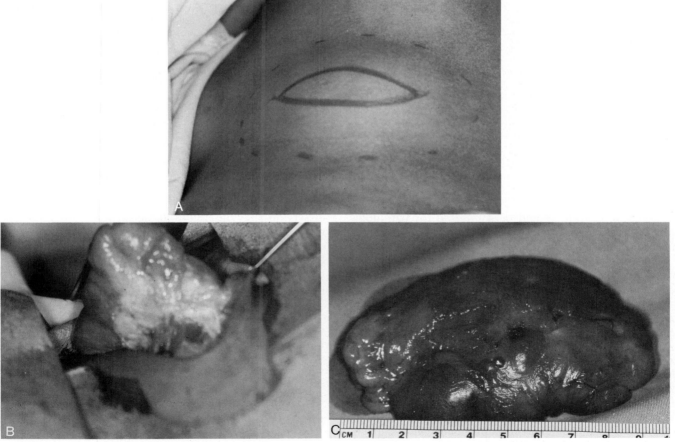

Figure 49–4. *A,* Large flank lipoma with palpable margins and planned excision drawn on the skin. *B,* A large intermuscular lipoma was found, necessitating sharp dissection off the latissimus dorsi musculature. *C,* Well-encapsulated, large lipoma.

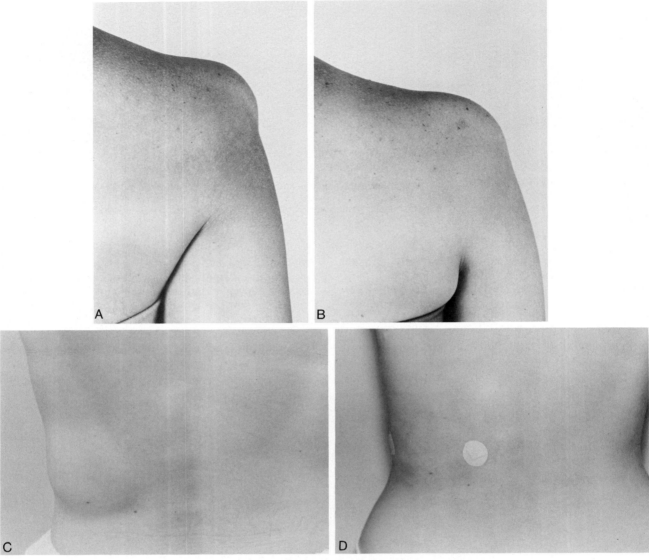

Figure 49–5. *A,* Large lipoma overlying the deltoid muscle. *B,* After liposuction. *C,* Flank lipoma. *D,* After liposuction.

liposuction aspirate should be submitted for pathologic testing to confirm the benign nature of the tissue removed.

Advantages of liposuction for the treatment of lipomas include reduced operating time and smaller, more cosmetically acceptable surgical incisions that may be strategically placed so as to be unobtrusive. In addition, multiple lipomas may be suctioned through a single cannula insertion site. In general, less bleeding may be encountered compared with conventional surgical excision, thereby decreasing the morbidity associated with hematoma formation. In addition, by carefully suctioning at the periphery of the lipoma, it is possible to blend the treated area into the surrounding tissue, thereby avoiding a depression in the skin overlying the lipoma (Fig. 49–5), a problem commonly seen with conventional surgical excision.[64, 74] In more fibrous lipomas, suction lipectomy may be more difficult, and sharp

dissection may be required to facilitate adequate removal.[63, 74, 75]

Benign symmetric lipomatosis, or Madelung's disease, has been treated by both excision lipectomy (Fig. 49–6)[15, 16, 18] and liposuction.[70–72] Liposuction is a favored initial as well as maintenance treatment for this notoriously recurrent and progressive condition, as it allows debulking of the lipomatous masses via a small surgical incision, produces less scarring, and results in less laborious dissection of the lipomatous tissue. In addition to the standard postoperative pressure dressing and wound care, patients should be encouraged to exercise, refrain from alcoholic beverage consumption, and follow a low-fat diet.[70]

SUMMARY

To most effectively manage patients with lipomas, it is important to be able to diagnose accurately both the

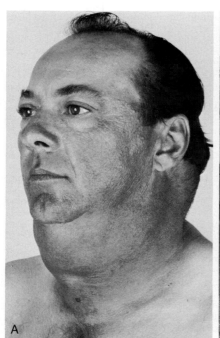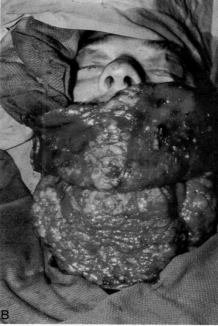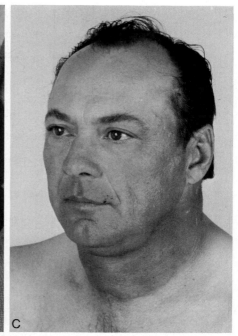

Figure 49–6. *A,* Middle-aged man with benign symmetric lipomatosis (Madelung's disease). *B,* Patient shown intraoperatively with exposed massive nodules of benign adipose tissue, which were subsequently sharply dissected from the underlying tissues. A similar procedure was later performed on the posterior neck. *C,* Patient after two lipectomy operations.

common and unusual variants, as well as to recognize the inherited syndromes that are sometimes seen in association with them.

REFERENCES

1. Adair FE, Pack GT, Farrior JH: Lipomas. Am J Cancer 16:1104–1120, 1932.
2. Rydholm A, Berg NO: Size, site, and clinical incidence of lipoma: factors in the differential diagnosis of lipoma and sarcoma. Acta Orthop Scand 54:929–934, 1983.
3. Salasche SJ, McCullough ML, Angeloni VL, Grabski WJ: Frontalis associated lipoma of the forehead. J Am Acad Dermatol 20:462–468, 1989.
4. Grosshans EM: Subfascial lipoma of the forehead. J Am Acad Dermatol 23:153–154, 1990.
5. Feinfield RE, Hesse RJ, Scharfenberg JC: Orbital angiolipoma. Arch Ophthalmol 106:1093–1095, 1988.
6. Van Steensel CJ, Wereldsma JCJ: Lipoma of the tongue. Neth J Surg 38:128, 1986.
7. Froimson AI: Benign solid tumors. Hand Clin 3:213–217, 1987.
8. Hoehn JG, Farber HF: Massive lipoma of the palm. Ann Plast Surg 11:431–433, 1983.
9. Feldman M, Healey K, Nach W, et al: Plantar approach for excision of bilateral soft tissue masses in a child. J Foot Surg 28:60–63, 1989.
10. Erichsen B, Medgyesi S: Congenital lipoma imitating gigantism of a toe: case report. Scand J Plast Reconstr Surg 17:77–78, 1983.
11. Fukamizu H, Matsumoto K, Inoue K, Moriguchi T: Large vulvar lipoma. Arch Dermatol 118:447, 1982.
12. Rubinstein A, Goor Y, Gazit E, Cabili S: Non-symmetric subcutaneous lipomatosis associated with familial combined hyperlipidemia. Br J Dermatol 120:689–694, 1989.
13. Feldman M: An appraisal of associated conditions occurring in autopsied cases of lipoma of the gastrointestinal tract. Am J Gastroenterol 36:413, 1961.
14. Carlsen A, Thomsen M: Different types of lipomatosis: case report. Scand J Plast Reconstr Surg 12:75–79, 1978.
15. Ruzicka T, Vieluf D, Landthaler M, Braun-Falco O: Benign symmetric lipomatosis Launois-Bensaude: report of ten cases and review of the literature. J Am Acad Dermatol 17:663–674, 1987.
16. Economides NG, Liddell HT: Benign symmetric lipomatosis (Madelung's disease). South Med J 79:1023–1025, 1986.
17. Leffell DJ, Braverman IM: Familial multiple lipomatosis: report of a case and review of the literature. J Am Acad Dermatol 15:275–279, 1986.
18. Luscher NJ, Prein J, Spiessl B: Lipomatosis of the neck (Madelung's neck). Ann Plast Surg 16:502–508, 1986.
19. Ersek RA, Lele E, Surak GS, et al: Hereditary progressive nodular lipomatosis: a report and selective review of a new syndrome. Ann Plast Surg 23:450–455, 1989.
20. Howard WR, Helwig EB: Angiolipoma. Arch Dermatol 82:924–931, 1960.
21. Belcher RW, Czarnetzki BM, Carney JF, Gardner E: Multiple (subcutaneous) angiolipomas: clinical, pathologic, and pharmacologic studies. Arch Dermatol 110:583–585, 1974.
22. Rasanen O, Nohteri H, Dammert K: Angiolipoma and lipoma. Acta Chir Scand 133:461–465, 1967.
23. Austin RM, Mack GR, Townsend CM, Lack EE: Infiltrating (intramuscular) lipomas and angiolipomas. Arch Surg 115:281–284, 1980.
24. Dionne GP, Seemayer TA: Infiltrating lipomas and angiolipomas revisited. Cancer 33:732–738, 1974.
25. Puig L, Moreno A, DeMoragas JM: Infiltrating angiolipoma: report of two cases and review of the literature. J Dermatol Surg Oncol 12:617–619, 1986.
26. Lin JJ, Lin F: Two entities in angiolipoma: a study of 459 cases of lipoma with review of literature on infiltrating angiolipoma. Cancer 34:720–727, 1974.
27. Hunt SJ, Santa Cruz DJ, Barr RJ: Cellular angiolipoma. Am J Surg Pathol 14:75–81, 1990.
28. Enzinger FM, Harvey DA: Spindle cell lipoma. Cancer 36:1852–1859, 1975.
29. Brody HJ, Meltzer HD, Someren A: Spindle cell lipoma. Arch Dermatol 114:1065–1066, 1978.
30. Levy FE, Goding GS: Spindle-cell lipoma: an unusual oral presentation. Otolaryngol Head Neck Surg 101:601–603, 1989.
31. Shmookler BM, Enzinger FM: Pleomorphic lipoma: a benign tumor simulating liposarcoma. Cancer 47:126–133, 1981.

32. Bryant J: A pleomorphic lipoma in the scalp. J Dermatol Surg Oncol 7:323–325, 1981.
33. Dercum FX: Three cases of a hitherto unclassified affection resembling in its grosser aspects obesity, but associated with special nervous symptoms—adiposis dolorosa. Am J Med Sci 104:521–535, 1892.
34. Lynch HT, Harlan WL: Hereditary factors in adiposis dolorosa (Dercum's disease). Am J Hum Genet 15:184–190, 1963.
35. Held JL, Andrew JA, Kohn SR: Surgical amelioration of Dercum's disease: a report and review. J Dermatol Surg Oncol 15:1294–1296, 1989.
36. Sutherland JC, Callahan WP, Campbell GL: Hibernoma: a tumor of brown fat. Cancer 5:364–368, 1952.
37. Vellios F, Baez J, Shumacker HB: Lipoblastomatosis: a tumor of fetal fat different from hibernoma. Am J Pathol 34:1149–1159, 1958.
38. Kauffman SL, Stout AP: Lipoblastic tumors of children. Cancer 12:912–925, 1959.
39. Chung EB, Enzinger FM: Benign lipoblastomatosis. Cancer 32:482–492, 1973.
40. Mahour GH, Bryan BJ, Isaacs H: Lipoblastoma and lipoblastomatosis—a report of six cases. Surgery 104:577–579, 1988.
41. Greco MA, Garcia RL, Vuletin JC: Benign lipoblastomatosis: ultrastructure and histogenesis. Cancer 45:511–515, 1980.
42. Enzinger FM, Winslow DJ: Liposarcoma: a study of 103 cases. Virchows Arch Pathol Anat 335:367–388, 1962.
43. Sampson CC, Saunders EH, Green WE, Laurey JR: Liposarcoma developing in a lipoma. Arch Pathol Lab Med 69:506–510, 1960.
44. Eidinger G, Katsikeris N, Gullane P: Liposarcoma: report of a case and review of the literature. J Oral Maxillofac Surg 48:984–988, 1990.
45. Brasfield RD, Das Gupta TK: Liposarcoma. Cancer 20:29, 1970.
46. Regan JM, Bickel WH, Broders AC: Infiltrating benign lipomas of the extremities. West J Surg Obstet Gynecol 54:87–93, 1946.
47. Kindblom LG, Angervall L, Stener B, Wickbom I: Intermuscular and intramuscular lipomas and hibernomas. Cancer 33:754–762, 1974.
48. Slavin SA, Baker DC, McCarthy JG, Mufarrij A: Congenital infiltrating lipomatosis of the face: clinicopathologic evaluation and treatment. Plast Reconstr Surg 72:158–164, 1983.
49. Kalisman M, Dolich BH: Infiltrating lipoma of the proper digital nerves. J Hand Surg 7:401–403, 1982.
50. Paletta FX, Senay LC: Lipofibromatous hamartoma of median nerve and ulnar nerve: surgical treatment. Plast Reconstr Surg 68:915–921, 1981.
51. Warner JJ, Madsen N, Gerber C: Intramuscular lipoma of the deltoid causing shoulder pain. Report of two cases. Clin Orthop 253:110–112, 1990.
52. Scherl MP, Som PM, Biller HF, Shah K: Recurrent infiltrating lipoma of the head and neck. Case report and literature review. Arch Otolaryngol Head Neck Surg 112:1210–1212, 1986.
53. Rydholm A, Akerman M, Idvall I, Persson BM: Aspiration cytology of soft tissue tumours: a prospective study of its influence on choice of surgical procedure. Int Orthop 6:209–214, 1982.
54. Akerman M, Idvall I, Rydbolm A: Cytodiagnosis of soft tissue tumours and tumour-like conditions by means of fine needle aspiration. Arch Orthop Trauma Surg 96:61–69, 1980.
55. Halldorsdottir A, Ekelund L, Rydholm A: CT-diagnosis of lipomatous tumors of the soft tissues. Arch Orthop Trauma Surg 100:211–216, 1982.
56. Wolfe SW, Bansal M, Healey JH, Ghelman B: Computed tomographic evaluation of fatty neoplasms of the extremities: a clinical radiographic and histologic review of cases. Orthopedics 12:1351–1358, 1989.
57. Fabri PJ, Adams JR: Simplified excision of lipomas. Surg Gynecol Obstet 165:173–174, 1987.
58. Hardin FF: A simple technique for removing lipomas. J Dermatol Surg Oncol 8:316–317, 1982.
59. Shelley ED, Shelley WB: Piezosurgery: a conservative approach to encapsulated skin lesions. Cutis 38:123–126, 1986.
60. Powell B, McLean NR: The treatment of lipomas by the "squeeze" technique. J R Coll Surg Edinb 30:391–392, 1985.
61. Harris WG: The treatment of lipomas by the "squeeze" technique. Letter. J R Coll Surg Edinb 31:258, 1986.
62. Peinert RA, Courtiss EH: Excision from a distance: a technique for removal of benign subcutaneous lesions. Plast Reconstr Surg 72:94–96, 1983.
63. Rubenstein R, Roenigk HH, Garden JM, et al: Liposuction for lipomas. J Dermatol Surg Oncol 11:1070–1074, 1985.
64. Pinski KS, Roenigk HH: Liposuction of lipomas. Dermatol Clin 8:483–492, 1990.
65. Hallock GG: Suction extraction of lipomas. Ann Plast Surg 18:517–519, 1987.
66. Kanter WR, Wolfort FG: Multiple familial angiolipomatosis: treatment of liposuction. Ann Plast Surg 20:277–279, 1988.
67. Spinowitz AL: The treatment of multiple lipomas by liposuction surgery. J Dermatol Surg Oncol 15:538–540, 1989.
68. Van Wingerden JJ, Erlank JD, Becker JH: Liposuction for congenital infiltrating lipomatosis of the face. Plast Reconstr Surg 81:989, 1988.
69. Slavin SA: Congenital infiltrating lipomatosis. Plast Reconstr Surg 83:929, 1989.
70. Serra JM: Treatment of cervicofacial lipomatosis with the suction-dissection technique. Facial Plast Surg 4:11–18, 1986.
71. Field LM: Liposuction surgery (suction-assisted lipectomy) for symmetric lipomatosis. J Am Acad Dermatol 18:1370, 1988.
72. Carlin MC, Ratz JL: Multiple symmetric lipomatosis: treatment with liposuction. J Am Acad Dermatol 18:359–362, 1988.
73. Newman J, Dolsky RL: Evaluation of 5,458 cases of liposuction surgery. Am J Cosmet Surg 1:25–28, 1984.
74. Coleman WP: Noncosmetic applications of liposuction. J Dermatol Surg Oncol 14:1085–1090, 1988.
75. Field L: Liposuction: a review. J Dermatol Surg Oncol 10:530–538, 1984.

CHAPTER 50

Management of Epidermal Tumors

EDWARD L. PARRY

Because a large number of entities make up epidermal tumors, an understanding of the broad clinical and histologic spectrum of these entities is necessary for the cutaneous surgeon to choose the most effective form of treatment. For some of the benign epidermal tumors, patient reassurance may be all that is required. Removal or biopsy may be necessary for other epidermal tumors because of the potential to develop malignancies. Systemic effects associated with some of the epidermal tumors may require a team approach involving a cutaneous surgeon, neurologist, pediatrician, cardiologist, ophthalmologist, dermatologist, and plastic and oral surgeons. An appreciation of the clinical entities and the methods of treatment will allow the clinician to maximize the effectiveness of treatment while minimizing morbidity.

Epidermal Nevi

Epidermal nevi are classified as hamartomas. As hamartomas, they consist of a malformation of normal tissue (i.e., normal tissue in a poorly organized or faulty form). The term nevus refers to a tumor of differentiated structures and does not indicate the presence of nevocellular nevus cells. Epidermal nevi occur in up to 3 out of every 1000 births. Lesions are usually present at birth but may evolve during adolescence or even in adulthood, and there is no particular racial or sexual prevalence.

Histologically, epidermal nevi are characterized by epidermal hyperplasia, acanthosis, hyperkeratosis, and papillomatosis. They are known by a large number of descriptive names and can occur in both a localized form and a more diffuse, systematized manner involving other organs. Clinically, they exhibit a papular, scaly,

verrucous, or warty surface. They may be dark gray, brown, or black and may form keratotic spines. Epidermal nevi are usually small (2 to 5 cm). Solitary lesions are referred to as localized nevus verrucosis. The lesions are most common on the extremities, especially the flexor aspects. When they occur in a linear or streaklike manner, they may be referred to as nevus unius lateris. When the linear nevi are psoriatic or inflammatory, they are called inflammatory linear verrucose epidermal nevi (ILVEN).[1] ILVEN may appear commonly on the lower extremity as a band of psoriasis or an eczematous process. Epidermal nevi that extend beyond a localized distribution to involve larger areas of the body are referred to as systemic epidermal nevi or ichthyosis hystrix (hystrix = porcupine) and may be found in irregular geometric patterns.

Abnormalities of other organ systems may occur in individuals with extensive epidermal nevi or epidermal nevi involving the head. These abnormalities are classified as part of the epidermal nevus syndrome (ENS)[2, 3] and include neurologic anomalies such as seizures or mental retardation (50% of patients), cerebral vascular malformations, skeletal abnormalities, ocular manifestations (up to 50% of patients), mucous membrane and oral cavity involvement, and cardiovascular and renal malformations (Table 50–1).

It has been theorized that epidermal nevi result from an abnormal induction of mesoderm and ectoderm, or possibly neuroectoderm, in early gestation. The establishment of this epidermal-dermal relationship may dictate the effectiveness of the various treatment modalities. If epidermal nevi are left untreated, the typical prognosis is persistence. Shortly after development, new lesions may continue to arise, and established lesions may increase in size. There appears to be no embryo-

TABLE 50–1. FEATURES OF EPIDERMAL NEVUS SYNDROME

Seizures
Mental retardation (50% of patients)
Cerebral vascular malformations
Skeletal abnormalities
Cardiovascular malformations
Renal abnormalities
Oral cavity involvement
Ocular abnormalities (50% of patients)

logic or anatomic rationale for the distribution of epidermal nevi.

A thorough evaluation should be carried out in any patient suspected of having ENS. The work-up should include a thorough history and physical examination, as well as an electroencephalogram (EEG); computed tomographic (CT) scan of the head; intravenous pyelogram (IVP); chest, skull, and long-bone radiographs; urinalysis; and an electrocardiogram (ECG). Noncutaneous systemic malignancies have been reported in increased frequency in patients with ENS.

Nevus Comedonicus

Nevus comedonicus (NC) is characterized by a linear or oval grouping of dilated follicular openings with keratin plugs. Although they are most commonly on the face and scalp, widespread distribution is also possible, and oral involvement has been reported. Because the follicular openings are plugged with keratin, the lesions can become pustular and simulate acne. Possibly a variant of epidermal nevus, NC is less common than either epidermal nevi or nevus sebaceous.

Nevus Sebaceus

Nevus sebaceus of Jadassohn (NSJ), or organoid nevus, occurs most commonly on the scalp or face and may have an oval or linear configuration similar to that of epidermal nevi. Before puberty, the sebaceous glands and hair follicles are hypoplastic, and NSJ typically appears as a hairless yellowish-to-brown patch on the scalp with a waxy, smooth surface. At puberty the lesion becomes warty and thickened as the epidermis becomes acanthotic and papillomatous and the sebaceous glands become hyperplastic. The hair follicles remain hypoplastic. Later in life, some NSJ lesions become ulcerated or develop nodular proliferations, which may signal the onset of a cutaneous malignancy. The likelihood of this is reported to be from 10 to 20%. Basal cell, squamous cell, and sebaceous carcinomas, syringocystadenoma papilliferum, hidrocystoma, and sebaceous adenoma have all been reported to occur.[4] Sebaceous nevi may be found as localized isolated lesions, lesions adjoining an epidermal nevus, or lesions occurring in a linear form with systemic implications. As such, they can be considered part of the epidermal nevus syndrome. The work-up for patients with extensive NSJ is similar to that for patients with ENS.

Treatment of Epidermal Nevi, Nevus Comedonicus, or Nevus Sebaceus

The treatment of epidermal nevi, nevus comedonicus, and nevus sebaceus is similar for all three conditions and is indicated for more than just cosmetic reasons. Large or extensive lesions can cause psychological as well as functional problems, and hyperkeratotic lesions can become odoriferous; with treatment, the development of cutaneous malignancies can also be prevented.

The plethora of topical therapies attests to their relative ineffectiveness. Topical steroids have been reported to be temporarily effective in reducing hyperkeratosis, erythema, and pruritus. Topical 5-fluorouracil has been unsuccessfully tried. Topical application of retinoic acid is helpful but must be continued to be effective. Topical ammonium lactate can be used to help control the hyperkeratosis, and alpha-hydroxy[5, 6] and alpha-keto acids may be similarly effective for some lesions. Other treatments include anthralin, coal tar, and ultraviolet light therapy. The long-term effectiveness of the topical therapies is limited by their inability to adequately deal with the dermal component of these nevoid conditions. Systemic aromatic retinoids have also been used, but their success is dependent on continued use.[7]

Because topical and medical therapies have failed to provide long-term successful management of these problems (Table 50–2), various surgical modalities have been tried.[8] Deep shave excision has been reported to be successful in treating ILVEN. Dermabrasion has been used,[9] but recurrences are commonly seen when a superficial technique is used. Only use of a deep dermabrasion technique, one that penetrates to the reticular dermis, has resulted in eradication of the lesions. How-

TABLE 50–2. MANAGEMENT OF EPIDERMAL NEVI, NEVUS COMEDONICUS, AND NEVUS SEBACEUS

Medical techniques
  Topical treatment
    5-Fluorouracil
    Retinoic acid
    Ammonium lactate
    Corticosteroids
    Anthralin
    Crude coal tar
    Alpha-hydroxy acids
    Alpha-keto acids
  Systemic treatment
    Aromatic retinoids
Surgical techniques
  Deep shave removal
  Dermabrasion
  Liquid nitrogen cryosurgery
  Carbon dioxide laser vaporization
  Excision
  Tissue expansion

ever, scarring as well as irregular pigmentation may result from the more aggressive technique. Cryotherapy using liquid nitrogen with a double freeze cycle and a 1- to 2-minute thaw time has been reported to be successful. Generally, quarter-sized areas are treated in this fashion. Long-term follow-up after cryosurgery has shown no recurrences.

Carbon dioxide laser vaporization has also been reported to produce good results.[10] Treatment parameters consisted of an incident power of 5 W, a 2-mm defocused spot, and an irradiance of 160 W/cm^2. This was delivered in the continuous discharge mode of operation. The depth of vaporization was continued until visual inspection revealed no evidence of the epidermal nevus. Scarring with any of the destructive or surgical modalities is both technique and site dependent. Experience is essential to be able to predict the type and extent of scarring, and properly selected treatment sites may also help in determining the quality of wound healing. Surgical excision resulting in a thin-line type of scar may afford the best cosmetic result along with long-term control. However, the anatomic location and extent of the lesion may preclude such an approach in some cases. Complete surgical removal of sebaceous nevi should be attempted whenever possible, since incomplete ablative treatment or partial removal will not eliminate the potential for malignant degeneration. New surgical techniques involving tissue expanders have been used in the management of giant congenital nevi and may be utilized in the future to allow total excision of larger epidermal nevi than was previously possible.[11, 12]

Porokeratosis

Another process that may be considered within the realm of epithelial nevi is porokeratosis. These lesions have a variable clinical presentation but are all characterized by a distinct histologic feature: the coronoid lamella. The coronoid lamella is a parakeratotic column that occurs clinically in the middle of the raised hyperkeratotic border, giving the lesions a furrowed raised border. The coronoid lamella represents the border between the expanding abnormal mutant clone of epidermal cells and the normal cells.

The clinical forms include the classic Mibelli type; the most common type, disseminated superficial actinic porokeratosis (DSAP)[13]; and linear porokeratosis.[14] Linear porokeratosis may occur in a unilateral systematized form like the linear epidermal nevus. The exact relationship of the different forms of porokeratosis is unclear, but the common form of autosomal dominant inheritance and the presence of the coronoid lamella suggest that the diseases may be different phenotypic expressions of a similar genetic defect. Males are affected two to three times more commonly than females. The lesions first appear as slightly pigmented keratotic papules that slowly enlarge to form irregular annular plaques with hyperkeratotic and well-demarcated borders. The center of the lesions is atrophic, variably pigmented, hairless, and anhidrotic.

The lesions can be found anywhere on the body, including the palms, soles, and face and even in the mouth. They are usually asymptomatic. They continue to enlarge slowly over time and are not known to spontaneously resolve, although they may be exacerbated during immunosuppressed states. Epithelial neoplasm or malignant degeneration has been reported in 7% of cases. Squamous cell carcinoma[15, 16] is the most common form of carcinoma found in lesions of porokeratosis, but basal cell carcinoma and Bowen's disease have also been reported.

Treatment of porokeratosis is indicated for cosmetic reasons as well as for cancer prevention. Medical management may include topical keratolytics to control the hyperkeratosis. Topical 5-fluorouracil[17] has been used successfully, but oral retinoids have given mixed results. Where successful, the retinoids must be continued, or relapses will occur. Surgical treatments, including electrocautery, cryosurgery, and excision, have also been used effectively. Carbon dioxide laser vaporization[18] with healing by second intention has been reported to clear porokeratotic lesions with less pain than other surgical modalities. Dermabrasion down to the midreticular dermis using a diamond fraise and a 15-second freeze has also been reported to clear these lesions.[19] In any of the surgical or destructive modalities, the procedure should first be performed on test sites, which are then evaluated for abnormal scarring, pigmentary changes, and effectiveness before widespread treatment is undertaken. Recurrences are common after inadequate destructive modalities. The location and extent of the lesions must also be considered when choosing the best method of treatment.

Seborrheic Keratosis

Seborrheic keratoses are the most common tumor in the older age group.[20] A dominant mode of inheritance is implicated, and although it is inconsistent, there is a definite familial tendency. The lesions are often located bilaterally and symmetrically on the face, extremities, and trunk but not on the palms or soles. The pathogenesis is unclear, but the growth and depth of pigmentation bear a direct relationship to sun exposure. The lesions exhibit a distinct "stuck-on" appearance and may vary in color from light tan or yellowish to dark black. Irritation may stimulate growth. The smooth-to-keratotic surface may show follicular plugging and exhibit a friable consistency. Histologically, seborrheic keratoses exhibit a benign epithelial proliferative process. If left untreated, they slowly enlarge and increase in thickness but do not spontaneously resolve.

CLINICAL APPEARANCE

Although these lesions are usually asymptomatic, their presence can be of cosmetic concern. Variably pigmented lesions may be confused with malignant melanoma. Cutaneous malignancies, including squamous cell carcinoma, basal cell carcinoma, and malignant melanoma, have been reported within seborrheic keratoses. Sudden appearance of a lesion with a rapid increase in size and number, known as the sign of Leser-Trelat, should suggest an internal malignancy, especially of the gastrointestinal tract. Even though these lesions have a distinctive clinical appearance, any suspicious lesion or reported change in pigmentation should prompt immediate biopsy.[21]

CLINICAL VARIANT

Black and Asian patients may develop a variant of seborrheic keratosis called dermatosis papulosa nigra.[22] These lesions may appear at adolescence and typically occur in the malar, upper cheek, and orbital areas. They consist of small, heavily pigmented papules that may become pedunculated. Cosmetic concern may necessitate treatment.

TREATMENT

Treatment of seborrheic keratosis and dermatosis papulosa nigra is most commonly performed for cosmetic reasons or because of irritation from clothing or jewelry. If there is concern about malignant degeneration, then a biopsy should be performed; curetted fragments of a lesion are inadequate for histologic evaluation. An excisional biopsy should be done in pigmented lesions if malignant melanoma is suspected. For the routine removal of typical seborrheic keratoses, treatment can be accomplished in many ways. The topical application of alpha-hydroxy acids[5, 6] has been reported to remove seborrheic keratosis when applied in either a concentrated form as an office procedure or using a lower strength formulation at home.

Liquid nitrogen cryosurgery can be used to treat multiple lesions without anesthesia. The lesion can be frozen with either a cotton-tipped applicator or a spray for approximately 30 seconds. Thicker or hyperkeratotic lesions may take 10 to 14 days to fall off. If there is residual growth after treatment, a shorter reapplication of liquid nitrogen can be done. Aggressive treatment can result in hypo- or hyperpigmentation. After freezing, a curette can be used to scrape off the seborrheic keratosis.[23] A rapid pronation or supination movement is used to "flick" off the lesion while it remains frozen. Use of a hemostatic agent such as Monsel's solution or aluminium chloride (for use on the face) may be applied after curettage.

Dermabrasion has been used for multiple and large seborrheic keratoses.[24] Light electrofulguration and electrodesiccation under local anesthesia can also successfully remove seborrheic keratosis. Scarring and pigmentary alterations are possible with more aggressive techniques.

Acrochordon

Acrochordons, skin tags, or fibroepithelial polyps are common on the neck, axilla, and major flexural areas of middle-aged to elderly persons. These are soft, fleshy,

yellowish to brown, 1- to 3-mm pedunculated papules. They are most common in women. They may become symptomatic as a result of external irritation or if they become necrotic from being twisted on their pedicle. They may be part of the normal aging process of the skin or the end stage of involution for pedunculated nevocellular nevi. They are not reported to have any malignant potential, but disputed reports have been made concerning a possible association with colonic polyps.

Many successful methods have been employed to destroy or remove acrochordons.[25] In some patients it is possible to snip acrochordons off at their base without anesthesia, thereby allowing multiple lesions to be treated in a single session. In other situations, infiltration of a small amount of local anesthetic at the base of the lesions is sufficient to allow the lesions to be snipped off, fulgurated, or electrodesiccated, or to have the pedunculated stalk crushed with a mosquito hemostat. Lesions twisted on their stalk may become necrotic and fall off on their own. A small thread or ligature can be tied around the base of the lesion with similar results. Any suspicious or atypical lesions should be routinely submitted for histologic examination.

Cutaneous Horn

A cutaneous horn is a hyperkeratotic, exophytic, white or pigmented lesion that usually occurs on the sun-exposed surfaces of the skin. These lesions are usually found on the hands, face, or ears of elderly men. The horn is made up of compact keratin and represents a reaction to some underlying process. A number of different pathologic processes can be found at the base of these excrescences. Fifty to eighty per cent of the underlying conditions are benign (e.g., actinic keratosis, seborrheic keratoses, and warts). The most common malignancy underlying a cutaneous horn is a squamous cell carcinoma.[26] The larger the cutaneous horn, the greater the possibility that it is associated with an underlying malignancy. Other pathologic processes have also been reported to give rise to cutaneous horns; these include basal cell carcinoma and angiomas. Performance of an adequate biopsy to evaluate the base is necessary to make an accurate histologic diagnosis.

A shave biopsy of a cutaneous horn that is deep enough to include the base can be done with either a scalpel blade or a horizontally oriented razor blade held between the thumb and index finger. All such specimens should be submitted for histopathologic examination. For many of the benign causes of cutaneous horns, biopsy may prove to be adequate treatment. Excisional biopsy of appropriate lesions can also be curative. Destructive methods of therapy in which an adequate specimen cannot be obtained for examination should be avoided.

Calluses and Corns

A callus is a thickening of the skin that is caused by pressure; these may occur on the hands or the feet. On the hands, they are usually well circumscribed and can result from occupational or recreational activities. On the feet, they are often poorly demarcated and may be caused by shoes or a depressed metatarsal head. Corns are better defined than a callus and are caused by greater direct pressure exerted on a smaller area. At the center of a corn is a cone-shaped hyperkeratotic wedge. Corns usually affect the feet. Unlike a callus, they lack papillary ridges and are typically painful. Soft corns occur between the toes and are caused by bony projections from the phalanges. Hard corns occur on the exposed surfaces of the feet.

Calluses can be treated with topical keratolytics such as salicylic acid or the alpha-hydroxy acids. They can be scraped off with a pumice stone or an emory board after first being soaked for 15 to 20 minutes in warm water. Paring with a razor blade or a scalpel can reduce the thickness of the lesion temporarily.[27] Calluses induced by occupational or recreational activities can be treated by padding and taping or use of gloves where appropriate. When corns or calluses are on the feet, pressure from ill-fitting shoes should be eliminated. Padding or corrective footwear may also be helpful. Hard corns can be enucleated by shelling out the central cone or wedge and then paring down the surrounding callosity. Hammer-toe deformities and underlying bony abnormalities such as exostoses or spurs may need to be surgically corrected. If surgical intervention for these underlying problems is not possible, temporary relief can be provided with lamb's wool padding or periodic paring of the lesion.

SUMMARY

The sheer variety of epidermal tumors, their frequency, and their variability in clinical appearance necessitate a thorough understanding of the main differences in the pathogenesis, prognosis, and available forms of treatment of each. Many of these conditions can be treated simply and easily and provide the patient with a good cosmetic and functional result. However, some of these lesions can be associated with malignant degeneration, and recognition of this potential is vital to obtaining a satisfactory outcome.

REFERENCES

1. Altman J, Mihregan AH: Inflammatory linear verrucose epidermal nevus. Arch Dermatol 104:385–389, 1971.
2. Solomon LM: The epidermal nevus syndrome. Arch Dermatol 97:273–285, 1968.
3. Hodge JA: The epidermal nevus syndrome. Int J Dermatol 30:91–98, 1991.
4. Goldstein GD: Basal cell carcinoma arising in a sebaceous nevus during childhood. J Am Acad Dermatol 18:429–430, 1988.
5. Van Scott EJ: Alpha hydroxy acids: procedures for use in clinical practice. Cutis 43:222–228, 1989.
6. Van Scott EJ: Alpha hydroxy acids: therapy potentials. Can J Dermatol 1:108–112, 1989.
7. Abdel-Aal MAM: Treatment of systematized verrucous epidermal nevus by aromatic retinoid (Ro 10-9359). Clin Exp Dermatol 8:647–650, 1983.
8. Fox BJ, Lapins NA: Comparison of treatment modalities for epidermal nevus: a case report and review. J Dermatol Surg Oncol 9:879–885, 1983.
9. Roenigk HH Jr: Dermabrasion for miscellaneous cutaneous lesions. J Dermatol Surg Oncol 3:322–328, 1977.
10. Ratz JL, Bailin PL, Wheeland RG: Carbon dioxide laser treatment of epidermal nevi. J Dermatol Surg Oncol 12:576–570, 1986.
11. Bauer BS: An approach to excision of congenital giant pigmented nevi in infancy and early childhood. J Pediatr Surg 23:509–514, 1988.
12. Wiltz H: Excision of the large congenital melanocytic nevus facilitated by the use of the tissue expanders. J Surg Oncol 38:104–107, 1988.
13. Marschalko M: Porokeratosis plantaris, palmaris et disseminata. Arch Dermatol 22:890–891, 1986.
14. Cox GF: Linear porokeratosis and other linear cutaneous eruptions of childhood. Am J Dis Child 133:1258–1259, 1979.
15. Loginsky AZ: Metastatic squamous cell carcinoma in linear porokeratosis of Mibelli. J Am Acad Dermatol 16:448–451, 1987.
16. James WD: Squamous cell carcinoma arising in porokeratosis of Mibelli. Int J Dermatol 25:389–391, 1986.
17. Goncalves JC: Fluorouracil ointment treatment of porokeratosis of Mibelli. Arch Dermatol 108:131–132, 1973.
18. Barnett JH: Linear porokeratosis: treatment with the carbon dioxide laser. J Am Acad Dermatol 14:902–904, 1986.
19. Cohen PR: Linear porokeratosis: successful treatment with diamond fraise dermabrasion. J Am Acad Dermatol 23:975–977, 1990.
20. Zimmerman MC: Seborrheic keratoses. J Dermatol Surg Oncol 10:586, 1984.
21. Lieblich LM: Use of a biopsy punch for removal of epithelial cysts. J Dermatol Surg Oncol 8:1059–1062, 1982.
22. Kauh YC: A surgical approach for dermatosis papulosa nigra. Int J Dermatol 22:590–592, 1983.
23. Krull EA: Surgical gems—the little curet. J Dermatol Surg Oncol 4:656–657, 1978.
24. Pepper E: Dermabrasion for the treatment of a giant seborrheic keratosis. J Dermatol Surg Oncol 11:646–647, 1985.
25. Rathbun ED: A method for removing the acrochordon (skin tag). Kans Med 91:11–12, 1990.
26. Bart RS: Cutaneous horns: a clinical and histopathological study. Acta Dermatol Venereol 48:507–515, 1968.
27. Sucullion PG: Dermatologic review: scalpel technique in removing heloma and hyperkeratosis. J Foot Surg 23:344–349, 1984.

CHAPTER 51

Management of Keloids

SHELDON V. POLLACK

K eloids occur as firm, variably pruritic or tender tumors that form after local skin trauma such as lacerations, tattoos, burns, injections, ear piercing, bites, vaccinations, or surgery.[1] They are distinct from hypertrophic scars in that they encompass skin sites beyond those involved in the original injury.[2] Although most common in dark-skinned races and Asians,[3] keloids also occur with a much lower incidence in whites. There is often a familial predilection for the development of keloids, particularly when multiple lesions are present.[4] These benign tumors frequently occur in anatomic sites where the skin is under increased tension, such as overlying the bony prominence of the shoulders, upper arms, sternum, and mandible.[5] Less often, they may involve the lower extremities or neck. Rarely, keloids may affect the eyelids, genitalia, palms, soles,[6] cornea,[7] or mucous membranes.[4] The lesions tend to persist and enlarge with time, but regression has been seen in older individuals.[1] While malignant degeneration has been reported, it is exceedingly rare.[8]

Pathogenesis

The pathogenesis of keloid formation has not been entirely elucidated. It is known, however, that keloids are more cellular than normal dermis,[9] and keloid fibroblasts secrete abnormally high levels of collagen[10] and glycosaminoglycans.[11] There is no evidence to suggest a deficiency of collagenase activity in keloids.[10, 12] However, the accumulation of α_2-macroglobulin and α_1-antitrypsin, two substances that inhibit collagenase, have been demonstrated in keloid tissue.[13] It has been theorized that these two substances, in addition to abundant proteoglycans,[14] may protect collagen deposited in keloids from enzymatic degradation. Increased levels of histamine have also been demonstrated in keloids,[10] which may contribute to the pruritus often associated

with these tumors. It has also been suggested that histamine plays a role in wound healing by stimulating fibroblasts[15] and may perhaps contribute to keloid growth.

Medical Therapy

Keloids are among the most perplexing of disorders treated by cutaneous surgeons. Patients often present for cosmetic reasons, but the discomfort frequently associated with these skin growths may also prompt them to seek medical attention. Many patients suffer some degree of pruritus, particularly when lesions are actively growing,[1] and others report significant tenderness with even light pressure on the tumor.

A variety of therapeutic tools have been used to treat keloids, including pressure, radiation therapy, pharmacotherapy, conventional excisional surgery, cryosurgery, and laser surgery. The treatments that have proved most effective are those that combine one or more of these approaches.

PRESSURE THERAPY

Constant compression of keloid tissue has proved beneficial in preventing regrowth after surgical excision of keloids.[16] To be effective, this pressure must be maintained for 4 to 6 months after surgery. Pressure garments can be custom made preoperatively from elasticized materials such as cervical collars, thoracolumbosacral garments, or elastic ski masks. Spring-pressure earring devices are used by some surgeons after earlobe keloidectomy.[17]

RADIATION THERAPY

Radiation therapy has been used both alone and as an adjunct to surgery in the management of keloids.

Adjunctive radiotherapy in the early postoperative period has often been used with good results to prevent keloid regrowth.[4, 18–20] It has been found that keloids greater than 2 cm in size, those that have received previous therapy, and those occurring in men have the greatest recurrence rate after combined surgery and radiation therapy.[20] The finding that males did poorly may be a reflection of the fact that 74% of the keloids studied involved the earlobe, an area that tends to do well with therapy, and most of these are presumably present in women.

Various types of radiotherapy have been used successfully for treating keloids, including kilovoltage irradiation (including superficial x-ray),[21–23] electron beam,[24, 25] and interstitial radiotherapy.[26] A total of 76.5% of 501 patients treated with 400 rads of superficial x-rays in single monthly doses, five times or less, with or without surgery, demonstrated disappearance of symptoms and keloid regression with improved cosmesis.[21] Approximately 15% had symptomatic relief only, while 8.4% failed to respond at all. The total dose of kilovoltage irradiation given to prevent the regrowth of an excised keloid appears to be more important than the time when irradiation is begun, the size of the largest fraction given, whether the irradiation is completed in 1 or 3 weeks, or the anatomic location.[23] In another study of postoperative superficial x-ray therapy, more favorable outcomes were achieved with smaller keloids and those on the head and neck area.[27]

Electron beam therapy alone has been reported to be successful in 26.3% of treated keloids, and 74.1% of keloids resolved when surgery was combined with this modality.[24] With interstitial radiotherapy, a thin plastic tube is incorporated into the sutured wound at the time of keloidectomy so that it emerges from the ends of the scar. Later, a radioactive iridium-192 wire is inserted into the plastic tubing and left in place for a sufficient time to deliver a dose of 2000 rads to the wound bed. Only a 20% recurrence rate has been reported during a 2-year follow-up period after this form of treatment in 31 keloids.[26]

Over the years, there has been some degree of hesitation in using potentially harmful radiation therapy to manage benign lesions such as keloids.[2] However, there has been a recent resurgence of interest in this modality, perhaps because therapists have been able to demonstrate good clinical responses in the absence of significant untoward effects.[25, 27–30]

PHARMACOTHERAPY

Various clinical and laboratory reports have suggested that certain agents, including vitamin A acid cream,[31, 32] adhesive zinc tape,[33] silicone gel,[34, 35] bacterial collagenase,[36] pentoxifylline,[37] and interferons gamma[38, 39] and alfa–2b,[40] may be useful in the treatment of keloids. However, for the most part, these accounts have been anecdotal and have not been subjected to rigorous scientific evaluation. Further studies will be required to determine whether any of these substances can yield consistently beneficial results in the therapy of keloids.

Some work has been done in which keloids are treated by inducing a state of lathyrism in the patient. This condition, produced by certain nitriles, was first observed in cattle that consumed the sweet pea, *Lathyrus odoratus*. In lathyritic animals, collagen fiber formation is decreased and healing wounds demonstrate significantly reduced tensile strength.[41] Beta-aminopropionitrile (BAPN) is an experimental drug that induces lathyrism by interfering with covalent cross-linking of collagen through the inhibition of the enzyme lysyl oxidase.[42] Another less potent lathyrogen is penicillamine,[43] a drug that exerts its effect by chelating collagen cross-linking sites. This poorly cross-linked collagen is more susceptible to digestion by tissue collagenase than normal cross-linked collagen.[44] The postoperative use of beta-aminopropionitrile fumarate and penicillamine[45] in combination with colchicine, a stimulator of tissue collagenase activity,[46] has been investigated in relation to the treatment of ten massive keloids. A measurable beneficial effect was noted in all patients. Unfortunately, BAPN has potential toxicity that may limit its long-term use, and keloid regrowth may be expected to accompany discontinuation of this drug.

Some investigators have recommended the use of cytotoxic or immunosuppressive drugs in combating keloids. A mixture of lidocaine, triamcinolone acetonide, mustine hydrochloride or nitrogen mustard, and hyaluronidase has been recommended for intralesional injection of keloids.[47] In a 3-year follow-up study, the cure rates exceeded those achieved with steroids alone. However, the occurrence of ulceration, which was noted in the keloids of eight patients, may limit the usefulness of this therapeutic approach. The effective use of keloidectomy combined with methotrexate therapy has also been reported.[48] Oral or parenteral methotrexate was begun a week before surgery and continued for approximately 4 months in a single dose of 15 to 20 mg repeated at 4-day intervals.

Of the various pharmacotherapeutic agents proposed for treating keloids, glucocorticosteroids are the most widely accepted and used. Intralesional steroids have proved effective in managing keloids both alone[49] and as an adjunct to keloidectomy.[3, 50, 51] Triamcinolone acetonide in a strength of 40 mg/ml is most often used.[52] In addition to exerting an inhibitory effect on collagen synthesis,[53] glucocorticoids may cause enhanced collagen breakdown in keloids.[13]

Small lesions can often be treated solely with intralesional injections (Fig. 51–1), administered directly into the bulk of the keloid mass. Such treatment may initially be difficult to perform because of the dense nature of untreated keloids. This task can be simplified by pretreating the lesion with cryosurgery,[54] which causes the lesion to swell, thus decreasing the density. The freezing itself may also have a therapeutic effect.

Injections can also be facilitated by use of a pressure jet apparatus[55] or a spring-loaded intraligamental dental syringe (Fig. 51–2).[56] When a standard syringe and needle is used, the Luer-Lok type is required in order to prevent separation of the needle from the syringe during the course of injection into firm lesions. Keloids

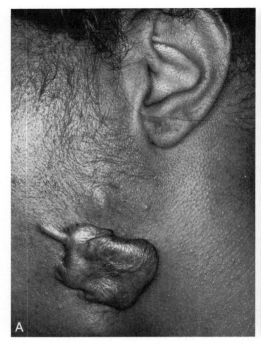
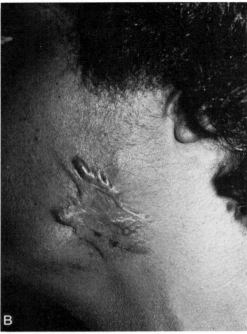

Figure 51–1. *A,* Facial keloid overlying the angle of the mandible in a young woman before treatment. *B,* Same lesion as it appeared after several intralesional injections of triamcinolone acetonide, 40 mg/ml.

progressively soften with each additional treatment, making successive intralesional injections less difficult to administer.

When used as an adjunct to surgical keloidectomy, steroids are injected into the operative site at the completion of surgery.[57] A high local concentration of triamcinolone acetonide can be expected to impair the normal wound healing process, requiring the sutures to be left in place for at least 10 to 14 days. The operative site is reinjected at the time of suture removal and at monthly intervals thereafter to prevent keloid regrowth. After 3 to 4 months, depending on the response, intervals between intralesional injections can be gradually increased to 2, 3, 4, 6, or even 12 months. It is essential that patients be made aware of the necessity for this very stringent schedule of postoperative injections. If at any time pruritus, swelling, or tumor regrowth becomes evident, the patient must immediately return for evaluation. In such cases, a monthly injection schedule should be re-established for several months until stabilization permits further attempts to increase the time interval between treatments.

Intralesional triamcinolone acetonide is not without potential hazards and the cutaneous surgeon should anticipate hypopigmentation as a likely complication (Fig. 51–3). This can be minimized by injecting the steroid directly into the keloidal mass rather than into the overlying or surrounding skin. This problem generally reverses itself over several months but patients should be warned of this complication before surgery. Skin thinning and the appearance of telangiectases may also occur with intralesional steroids. Necrosis, ulceration, and cushingoid features are other less commonly reported adverse effects.[1]

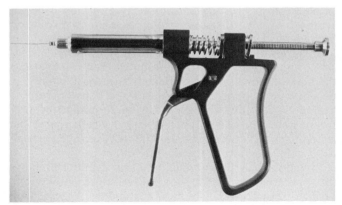

Figure 51–2. The Ligmaject is a dental syringe designed for intraligamental infiltration of local anesthesia. The device uses very sharp 30-gauge needles and is calibrated to deliver 0.2 ml of liquid per squeeze of the handle, under high pressure.

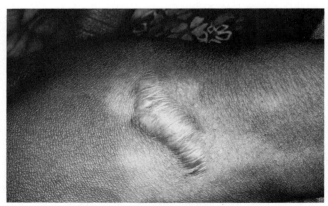

Figure 51–3. A common complication of intralesional steroid injection is hypopigmentation.

Surgical Therapy

The major difficulty with surgical treatment of keloids is the tendency for tumors to recur after otherwise unsupplemented surgical removal. Essentially 100% of keloids can be expected to recur within 4 years of such therapy.[1] For this reason, maintenance of an extended remission after keloidectomy is a formidable challenge that cutaneous surgeons treating keloids must face. Surgical treatment may involve the use of cryosurgery, laser surgery, electrosurgery, or simple conventional scalpel surgical excision, skin grafts, and skin flaps.

In dealing with keloids, some factors must be kept in mind to help predict the surgical outcome. First, certain locations are associated with a higher rate of recurrence after surgical excision. These include areas of high tension, particularly those overlying bony prominences, such as the presternum and shoulders. Areas of minimal tension, such as the earlobes, may carry less risk of recurrence after surgery. Remissions tend to be prolonged only when supplemental therapies, such as intralesional injections of steroids, are combined with surgical keloidectomy.

Second, some keloids exhibit a greater degree of clinical activity, and those lesions characterized by claw-like peripheral extensions, often with dumbbell shapes, are among the most resistant to therapy (Fig. 51–4). These tend to be in anatomic sites of high tension, such as the presternal area, and exhibit the greatest likelihood of recurrence, even when supplemental therapy is administered. Because of the high failure rate, surgery is best avoided in these particular lesions.

CRYOSURGERY

Cryosurgery has been used alone[58, 59] and in combination with glucocorticoids[60] to treat keloids. Once healing has occurred after deep cryosurgery, the operative site is injected with triamcinolone acetonide, 40 mg/ml at monthly intervals, to prevent regrowth. Injections are maintained at monthly intervals for several months to prevent relapse. Superficial cryosurgery before intralesional injection of keloids may cause the keloid tissue to swell, which decreases the relative bulk of the lesion and makes injections easier.[54]

LASER SURGERY

Early enthusiastic reports suggested that the carbon dioxide (CO_2)[61–63] and argon[62, 63] lasers provided a more effective permanent removal of keloids than did conventional surgery. Unfortunately, subsequent studies have failed to show significant advantage for CO_2[64, 65] or argon[66] lasers over conventional surgery. Investigations with the neodymium:YAG laser[67–70] have yielded promising results with demonstrated softening and flattening of the keloids, but this treatment remains investigational at present.

ELECTROSURGERY

Electrosurgical devices that include a cutting current may be used for removing keloids. When a combined cutting-coagulation current is available, electrosurgery can result in a near-bloodless excision (Fig. 51–5). This modality must be supplemented with intralesional steroids or other adjunctive measures. When using electrosurgery, it is important to note that the thermal damage that occurred adjacent to the incision line can act as a stimulus for renewed keloid formation.

CONVENTIONAL SCALPEL SURGERY

Conventional scalpel surgery is commonly used in combination with other adjunctive measures for treating keloids. This may take the form of simple excisions, skin grafts, or skin flaps.[71] In choosing a specific surgical method, one must consider the size and location and the anticipated resultant skin tension. Whenever possible, simple excision is probably the best alternative. However, this is possible only for relatively small lesions in areas where skin tension is minimal. An excess amount of tension on the suture line will act as a stimulus to fibroblast activity, resulting in increased fibrosis and a greater likelihood of recurrence.

SKIN GRAFTS AND FLAPS

When simple excision and closure is not possible, tension-relieving procedures such as skin grafts or skin flaps may be required. Unfortunately, keloid formation occurs at skin graft donor sites in approximately 50% of cases (Fig. 51–6). One way to avoid this complication is to harvest the skin graft from the skin overlying the keloid, thus avoiding an additional site of skin trauma.[72] This technique is particularly useful for treatment of very large keloids (Fig. 51–7).

Skin flaps are very useful[73] for smaller lesions and are frequently employed on the earlobes. In this location, it is best to attempt to preserve the epidermis and some dermis overlying the keloid, remove the bulk of the lesion, and then suture the skin back into its original site to repair the defect (Fig. 51–8). Alternatively, for anteroposterior earlobe keloids, in which keloidal

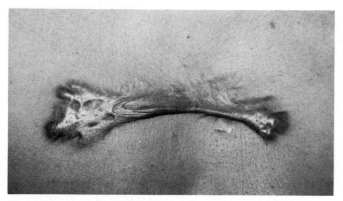

Figure 51–4. Dumbbell-shaped keloids in anatomic sites of high tension, such as the presternal area, are among the most resistant to therapy.

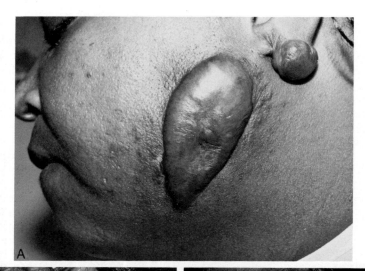

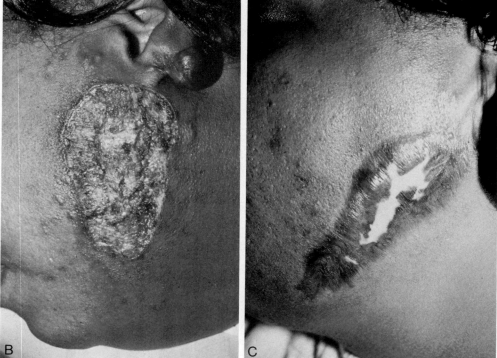

Figure 51–5. *A,* A keloid at the mandibular rim of a young woman before carbon dioxide (CO_2) laser surgery. *B,* Same patient immediately after CO_2 laser excision of the lesion (note the relatively bloodless field). *C,* Several months later the wound is well healed and remains flat, although there is slight hypopigmentation.

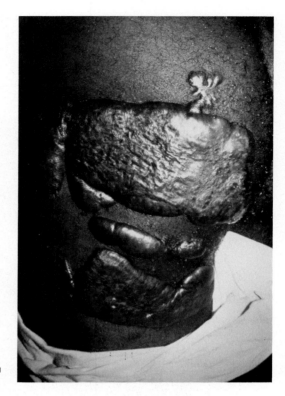

Figure 51–6. A keloid has developed within a split-thickness skin graft donor site on the posterior thigh of a middle-aged man.

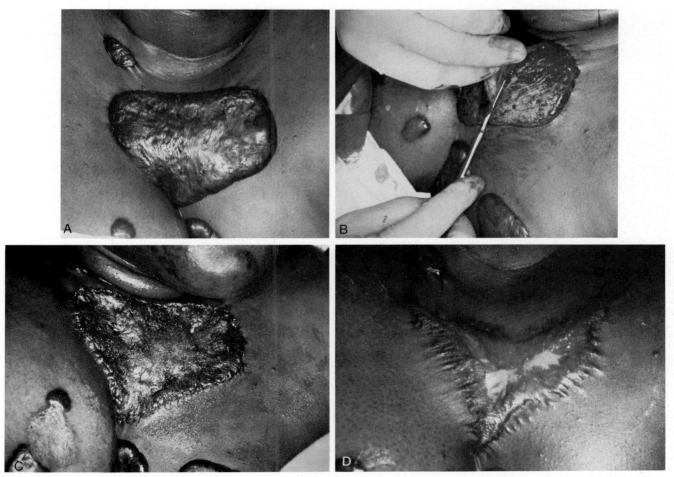

Figure 51–7. *A,* A large, tender keloid on the presternal area in a middle-aged woman. *B,* The skin overlying the keloid is harvested for use as a full-thickness skin graft to cover the defect after keloidectomy. *C,* After excision of the keloid mass, the skin graft is sutured in place. *D,* The postoperative result several months later shows minimal cosmetic improvement, but symptoms were significantly alleviated.

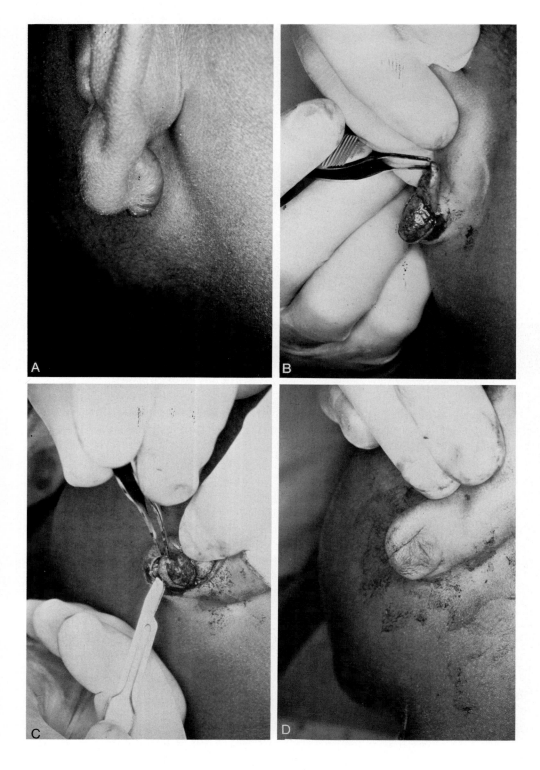

Figure 51–8. *A,* Posterior earlobe keloid in a young woman after ear piercing. *B,* The skin overlying the keloid is used to create a small skin flap. *C,* The flap is reflected upward while the keloid mass is surgically removed. *D,* The skin flap is returned to its original location, trimmed to fit the defect, and sutured in place. The wound bed is immediately injected with triamcinolone acetonide, 40 mg/ml.

growths are evident on both sides of the earlobe, the creation of through-and-through incisions has yielded excellent results.[74] In general, such lesions form at both ends of an epithelialized tract that occurs after ear piercing. This tract, thought to act as a nidus for keloid growth, can be easily removed with a sharp dermal punch (Fig. 51–9).

During any of these procedures, care should be taken to minimize tissue damage and limit the number of sutures used. Inflammation resulting from foreign body reactions is thereby reduced, which decreases the likelihood of recurrent keloidal growth. Hemostasis should

be obtained, as much as possible, by use of external pressure in order to limit the thermal damage that can accompany electrocoagulation. When possible, particularly on the earlobes, only nonabsorbable skin sutures of low reactivity, such as nylon, should be used instead of buried absorbable sutures, which can give rise to foreign body reaction and serve as a nidus for keloid regrowth. Pressure dressings are helpful in avoiding the complications of seroma and hematoma formation (Fig. 51–10).

On occasion, a keloid may be so extensive that total removal of the lesion will result in a significant degree

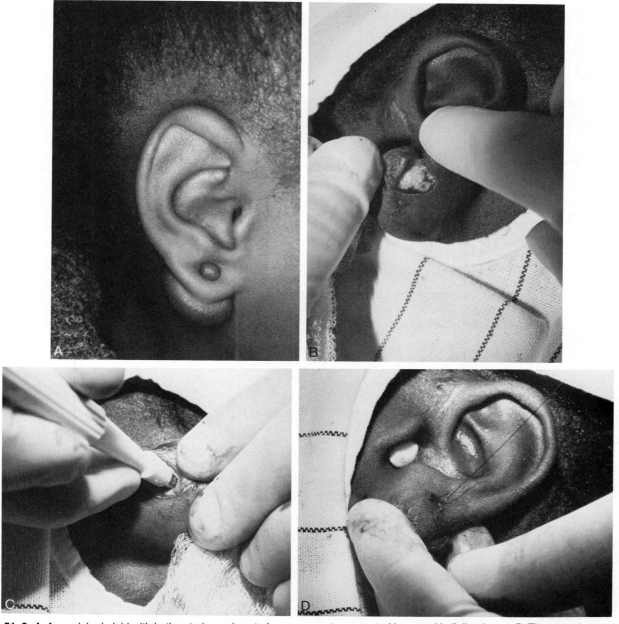

Figure 51–9. *A,* An earlobe keloid with both anterior and posterior components connected by an epithelialized tract. *B,* The posterior component of the keloid has been removed, exposing the epithelialized tract. *C,* A dermal punch is used to remove the tract, creating a through-and-through defect. *D,* The anterior and posterior defects are repaired, the wound bed is injected with the steroid solution, and a pressure dressing is applied.

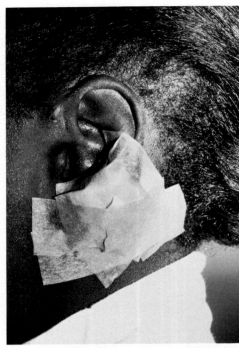

Figure 51–10. A pressure dressing is applied and left in place for 24 hours after earlobe keloid surgery to minimize the possibility of hematoma or seroma formation.

of deformity. This is particularly true in instances of previous unsuccessful surgery. Subtotal excision of a keloid may be performed without a greater likelihood of its recurring. In this way, portions of a keloid may

be left undisturbed for purposes of contouring or support.

Adjunctive Therapy

Adjunctive therapy is generally required to prevent recurrences of keloids after most surgical procedures. Although radiotherapy, pressure therapy, and a variety of systemic pharmacotherapies have been reported to be helpful, supplemental postoperative therapy most often takes the form of intralesional injections of corticosteroids (Fig. 51–11).

Depending on the size of the defect, 0.2 to 1.0 ml of triamcinolone acetonide, 40 mg/ml, is instilled into the operative bed at the completion of keloidectomy, after the placement of sutures. Lower concentrations of triamcinolone are ineffective in preventing keloid regrowth. Moreover, if the postoperative injection regimen is not strictly maintained, keloids usually recur within a few months. Most recurrent earlobe keloids are noted in patients who fail to present for adjunctive postoperative therapy. Patients should therefore be required to make a commitment to this regimen before undergoing keloidectomy. The success of a single intraoperative injection of betamethasone sodium phosphate and betamethasone acetate suspension in preventing regrowth of keloids in a pediatric population has been described.[75] If this observation is confirmed by other studies, keloid management may become much simpler in the future.

Although the mechanism of action remains unknown, an improvement in the texture, color, and thickness of

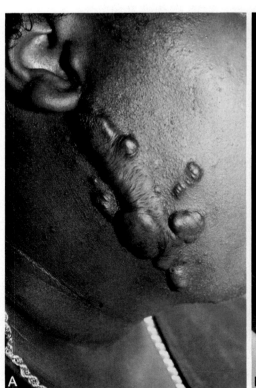
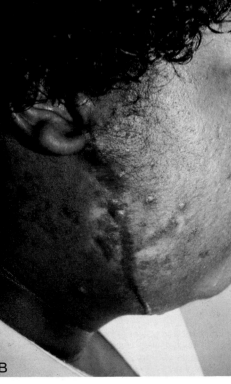

Figure 51–11. *A,* Preoperative appearance of a mandibular keloid in a young woman. *B,* Four months after surgical excision the keloid has not recurred, and monthly intralesional injections continue to be performed. Some hypopigmentation secondary to steroid injection is evident.

keloids and hypertrophic scars has been reported with use of a topical silicone gel sheeting for several hours a day.[76-80] Application of 20% silicone oil followed by coverage with an occlusive dressing has also proved useful in flattening keloids and hypertrophic scars.[81]

SUMMARY

The effective management of keloids requires that the cutaneous surgeon have a complete understanding of the biologic activity, the pathogenesis, and adjunctive forms of medical and surgical treatments available. Despite common recurrences at certain anatomic locations, many patients can obtain a significant cosmetic and functional improvement with treatment. New laser surgical and medical therapies are likely to further improve the success rate in managing patients with this difficult problem.

REFERENCES

1. Murray JC, Pollack SV, Pinnell SR: Keloids: a review. J Am Acad Dermatol 4:461–470, 1981.
2. Peacock EE Jr, Madden JW, Trier WC: Biologic basis of treatment of keloid and hypertrophic scars. South Med J 63:755–760, 1970.
3. Ketchum LD, Cohen IK, Masters FW: Hypertrophic scars and keloids: a collective review. Plast Reconstr Surg 53:140–154, 1974.
4. Cosman B, Crikelair GF, Ju DMC, et al: The surgical treatment of keloids. Plast Reconstr Surg 27:335–358, 1961.
5. Crockett DJ: Regional keloid susceptibility. Br J Plast Surg 17:245–253, 1964.
6. Kamin AJ: The etiology of keloids: a review of the literature and a new hypothesis. S Afr Med J 38:913–916, 1964.
7. O'Grady RB, Kirk HQ: Corneal keloids. Am J Ophthalmol 73:206–213, 1972.
8. Hayrati E, Hoomand A: The keloidal diathesis: a resistant state to malignancies. Plast Reconstr Surg 59:555–559, 1977.
9. Hoopes JE, Su C-T, Im MJ: Enzyme activities in hypertrophic scars. Plast Reconstr Surg 47:132–137, 1971.
10. Cohen IK, Diegelmann RF, Keiser HR: Collagen metabolism in keloid and hypertrophic scar. In: Longacre JJ (ed): The Ultrastructure of Collagen. Charles C Thomas, Springfield, IL, 1973, pp 199–212.
11. Bazin S, Nicoletis C, Delaunay A: Intercellular matrix of hypertrophic scars and keloids. In: Kulonen E, Pikkarainen J (eds): Biology of Fibroblast. Academic Press, London, 1973, pp 571–578.
12. Milsom JP, Craig RDP: Collagen degradation in cultured keloid and hypertrophic scar tissue. Br J Dermatol 89:635–643, 1973.
13. Diegelmann RF, Bryant CP, Cohen IK: Tissue alpha-globulins in keloid formation. Plast Reconstr Surg 59:418–423, 1977.
14. Linares HA, Larson DL: Proteoglycans and collagenase in hypertrophic scar tissue. Plast Reconstr Surg 62:589–593, 1978.
15. Russell JD, Russell SB, Trupin KM: The effect of histamine on the growth of cultured fibroblasts isolated from normal and keloid tissue. J Cell Physiol 93:389–393, 1977.
16. Kischer CW, Shetlar MR, Shetlar CL: Alteration of hypertrophic scars induced by mechanical pressure. Arch Dermatol 111:60–64, 1975.
17. Brent B: The role of pressure therapy in management of earlobe keloids: preliminary report of a controlled study. Ann Plast Surg 1:579–581, 1978.
18. Craig RDP, Pearson D: Early post-operative irradiation of keloid scars. Br J Plast Surg 18:369–376, 1965.
19. Sallstrom KO, Larson O, Heden P, et al: Treatment of keloids with surgical excision and postoperative x-ray radiation. Scand J Plast Reconstr Surg Hand Surg 23:211–215, 1989.
20. Kovalic JJ, Perez CA: Radiation therapy following keloidectomy: a 20-year experience. Int J Radiat Oncol Biol Phys 17:77–80, 1989.
21. Inalsingh CHA: An experience in treating five hundred and one patients with keloids. Johns Hopkins Med J 134:284–290, 1974.
22. Levy DS, Salter MM, Roth RE: Postoperative irradiation in the prevention of keloids. Am J Roentgenol 127:509–510, 1976.
23. Doornbos JF, Stoffel TJ, Hass AC, et al: The role of kilovoltage irradiation in the treatment of keloids. Int J Radiat Oncol Biol Phys 18:833–839, 1990.
24. King GD, Salzman FA: Keloid scars: analysis of 89 patients. Surg Clin North Am 50:595–598, 1970.
25. Nicolai JP, Bos MY, Bronkhorst FB, Smale CE: A protocol for the treatment of hypertrophic scars and keloids. Aesthetic Plast Surg 11:29–32, 1987.
26. Malaker K, Ellis F, Paine CH: Keloid scars: a new method of treatment combining surgery with interstitial radiotherapy. Clin Radiol 27:179–183, 1976.
27. Enhamre A, Hammar H: Treatment of keloids with excision and postoperative x-ray irradiation. Dermatologica 167:90–93, 1983.
28. Editorial: Keloids and x-rays. Br Med J 3:592, 1974.
29. Lukacs S, Braun-Falco O, Goldschmidt H: Radiotherapy of benign dermatoses: indications, practice, and results. J Dermatol Surg Oncol 4:620–625, 1978.
30. Borok TL, Bray M, Sinclair I, et al: Role of ionizing irradiation for 393 keloids. Int J Radiat Oncol Biol Phys 15:865–870, 1988.
31. Janssen de Limpens AM: The local treatment of hypertrophic scars and keloids with topical retinoic acid. Br J Dermatol 103:319–323, 1980.
32. Panabiere-Castaings MH: Retinoic acid in the treatment of keloids. J Dermatol Surg Oncol 14:1275–1276, 1988.
33. Soderberg T, Hallmans G, Bartholdson L: Treatment of keloids and hypertrophic scars with adhesive zinc tape. Scand J Plast Reconstr Surg 16:261–266, 1982.
34. Mercer NS: Silicone gel in the treatment of keloid scars. Br J Plast Surg 42:83–87, 1989.
35. Swanda Y, Sone K: Treatment of scars and keloids with a cream containing silicone oil. Br J Plast Surg 43:683–688, 1990.
36. Mandl I: Bacterial collagenases and their clinical applications. Arzneimittelforschung 32:1381–1384, 1982.
37. Berman B, Duncan MR: Pentoxifylline inhibits the proliferation of human fibroblasts derived from keloid, scleroderma, and morphoea skin and their production of collagen, glycosamino-glycans and fibronectin. Br J Dermatol 123:339–346, 1990.
38. Granstein RD, Rook A, Flotte TJ, et al: A controlled trial of intralesional recombinant interferon-gamma in the treatment of keloidal scarring. Clinical and histologic findings. Arch Dermatol 126:1295–1302, 1990.
39. Larrabee WF Jr, East CA, Jaffe HS, et al: Intralesional interferon gamma treatment for keloids and hypertrophic scars. Arch Otolaryngol Head Neck Surg 116:1159–1162, 1990.
40. Berman B, Duncan MR: Short-term keloid treatment in vivo with human interferon alfa-2b results in a selective and persistent normalization of keloidal fibroblast collagen, glycosaminoglycan, and collagenase production in vitro. J Am Acad Dermatol 21:694–702, 1989.
41. Gillespie JA, Burns JK: The strength and histology of skin wounds in lathyrism. Br J Surg 46:642–644, 1959.
42. Page RC, Benditt EP: Interaction of the lathyrogen, B-aminopropionitrile (BAPN) with a copper-containing amine oxidase. Proc Soc Exp Biol Med 124:454–459, 1967.
43. Youssef SA, Geever EF, Levenson SM: Penicillamine effect on wound healing. Surg Forum 17:89–90, 1966.
44. Harris ED, Farrell ME: Resistance to collagenase: a characteristic of collagen fibrils cross-linked by formaldehyde. Biochem Biophys Acta 278:133–141, 1972.
45. Peacock EE Jr: Pharmacological control of surface scarring in human beings. Ann Surg 193:592–597, 1981.
46. Chvapil M, Peacock EE Jr, Carlson EC, et al: Colchicine and wound healing. J Surg Res 28:49–56, 1980.
47. Oluwasanmi JO: Keloids in the African. Clin Plast Surg 1:179–195, 1974.
48. Onwukwe MF: Surgery and methotrexate for keloids. Schoch Letter 28:4, 1978.
49. Maguire HC: Treatment of keloids with triamcinolone acetonide injected intralesionally. JAMA 192:325–327, 1965.

50. Minkowitz F: Regression of massive keloid following partial excision and post-operative intralesional administration of triamcinolone. Br J Plast Surg 20:432–435, 1967.
51. Griffith BH, Monroe CW, McKinney P: A follow-up study on the treatment of keloids with triamcinolone acetonide. Plast Reconstr Surg 46:145–150, 1970.
52. Rudolph R: Wide spread scars, hypertrophic scars, and keloids. Clin Plast Surg 14:253–260, 1987.
53. Oikarinen AI, Uitto J, Oikarinen J: Glucocorticoid action on connective tissue: from molecular mechanisms to clinical practice. Med Biol 64:221–230, 1986.
54. Ceiley RI, Babin RW: The combined use of cryosurgery and intralesional injections of suspensions of fluorinated adrenocorticosteroids for reducing keloids and hypertrophic scars. J Dermatol Surg Oncol 5:54–56, 1979.
55. Vallis CP: Intralesional injection of keloids and hypertrophic scars with the Dermo-Jet. Plast Reconstr Surg 40:255–262, 1967.
56. Sagher U: The intraligamental dental syringe facilitates steroid injection into hypertrophic scars and keloids. Plast Reconstr Surg 84:542, 1989.
57. Pollack S: Keloids. In: Provost TT, Farmer ER (eds): Current Therapy in Dermatology 1985–1986. BC Decker, Philadelphia, 1985, pp 255–258.
58. Shepherd JP, Dawber RP: The response of keloid scars to cryosurgery. Plast Reconstr Surg 70:677–682, 1982.
59. Cirne de Castro JL, dos Santos AP, Cardoso JP, Ribeiro R: Cryosurgical treatment of a large keloid. J Dermatol Surg Oncol 12:740–742, 1986.
60. Hirshowitz B, Lerner D, Moscona AR: Treatment of keloid scars by combined cryosurgery and intralesional corticosteroids. Aesthetic Plast Surg 6:153–158, 1982.
61. Kantor GR, Wheeland RG, Bailin PL, et al: Treatment of earlobe keloids with carbon dioxide laser excision: a report of 16 cases. J Dermatol Surg Oncol 11:1063–1067, 1985.
62. Apfelberg DB, Maser MR, Lash H, et al: Preliminary results of argon and carbon dioxide laser treatment of keloid scars. Lasers Surg Med 4:283–290, 1984.
63. Henderson DL, Cromwell TA, Mes LG: Argon and carbon dioxide laser treatment of hypertrophic and keloid scars. Lasers Surg Med 3:271–277, 1984.
64. Stern JC, Lucente FE: Carbon dioxide laser excision of earlobe keloids. A prospective study and critical analysis of existing data. Arch Otolaryngol Head Neck Surg 115:1107–1111, 1989.
65. Apfelberg DB, Maser MR, White DN, Lash H: Failure of carbon dioxide laser excision of keloids. Lasers Surg Med 9:382–388, 1989.
66. Hulsbergen-Henning JP, Roskam Y, van Gemert MJ: Treatment of keloids and hypertrophic scars with an argon laser. Lasers Surg Med 6:72–75, 1986.
67. Abergel RP, Dwyer RM, Meeker CA, et al: Laser treatment of keloids: a clinical trial and an in vitro study with Nd:YAG laser. Lasers Surg Med 4:291–295, 1984.
68. Sherman R, Rosenfeld H: Experience with the Nd:YAG laser in the treatment of keloid scars. Ann Plast Surg 21:231–235, 1988.
69. Castro DJ, Saxton RE, Fetterman HR, et al: Bioinhibition of human fibroblast cultures sensitized to Q-switch II dye and treated with the Nd:YAG laser: a new technique of photodynamic therapy with lasers. Laryngoscope 99:421–428, 1989.
70. Apfelberg DB, Smith T, Lash H, et al: Preliminary report on use of the neodymium-YAG laser in plastic surgery. Lasers Surg Med 7:189–198, 1987.
71. Pollack SV, Goslen JB: The surgical treatment of keloids. J Dermatol Surg Oncol 8:1045–1049, 1982.
72. Apfelberg DB, Maser MR, Lash H: The use of epidermis over a keloid as an autograft after resection of the keloid. J Dermatol Surg Oncol 2:409–411, 1976.
73. Weimer VM, Ceiley RI: Treatment of keloids on earlobes. J Dermatol Surg Oncol 5:522–523, 1979.
74. Salasche SJ, Grabski WJ: Keloids of the earlobes: a surgical technique. J Dermatol Surg Oncol 9:552–556, 1983.
75. Golladay ES: Treatment of keloids by single intraoperative perilesional injection of repository steroid. South Med J 81:736–738, 1988.
76. Quinn KJ: Silicone gel in scar treatment. Burns 13:S33–S40, 1987.
77. Ohmori S: Effectiveness of Silastic sheet coverage in the treatment of scar keloid (hypertrophic scar). Aesthetic Plast Surg 12:95–99, 1988.
78. Ahn ST, Monafo WW, Mustoe TA: Topical silicone gel: A new treatment for hypertrophic scars. Surgery 106:781–787, 1989.
79. Mercer NS: Silicone gel in the treatment of keloid scars. Br J Plast Surg 42:83–87, 1989.
80. Murdoch ME, Salisbury JA, Gibson JR: Silicone gel in the treatment of keloids. Acta Derm Venereol (Stockh) 70:181–183, 1990.
81. Sawada Y, Sone K: Treatment of scars and keloids with a cream containing silicone oil. Br J Plast Surg 43:683–688, 1990.

CHAPTER 52

Management of Hyperhidrosis and Bromhidrosis

JOHN R. WEST

A xillary hyperhidrosis is a distressing disorder characterized by marked axillary eccrine hypersecretion that may handicap those affected both socially and in the work place. Secretion rates of up to 13 ml in 30 minutes from each axilla, or ten times the normal rate, have been documented.[1] Soaking, staining, and rotting of clothing, saturation of articles carried in shirt pockets, and social stigmatization are among the afflictions these patients must endure.[2, 3] For these reasons, the disorder cannot be regarded as merely a cosmetic problem.

Epidemiology

Axillary hyperhidrosis is a common condition, having a reported incidence of 0.6 to 1.0% among young people,[4] with no racial or sexual predilection.[2] The disorder never occurs before adolescence and is rare among the aged. While males generally exhibit higher axillary sweating rates, females are more likely to seek treatment. A family history of axillary hyperhidrosis, consistent with autosomal dominant transmission, is present in 45 to 89% of patients.[2, 5]

Clinical Characteristics

Axillary sweating is usually episodic, occurring in response to specific stimuli, although some patients may report continuous excessive sweating throughout the day. The problem usually remits during sleep.[6] Inciting factors include emotional stimuli such as anxiety, anger, or fear, which are reported by 98% of patients; thermal stimuli, seen in 92%; execution of fine manual tasks, reported by 76%; physical exercise, seen in 56%; inges-

tion of hot or spicy foods and alcohol, reported by 15%[4]; and pain.[7] Affected individuals do not appear unduly anxious,[3] however, and few have psychiatric disturbances apart from concern over their symptoms.[8]

Most patients deny any seasonal variation in the condition, although some report improvement during the summer when lightweight, cooler clothing affords increased evaporation of sweat.[9] Bromhidrosis rarely occurs in association with axillary hyperhidrosis, perhaps because the apocrine-derived precursors that yield odoriferous products through bacterial action are washed away by the flow of eccrine sweat.[2, 10, 11] In addition, concomitant palmar or plantar hyperhidrosis is reported in only 22 to 25% of patients,[5, 10] and axillary eczema occurs in about 20% of patients.

Diagnosis

Axillary hyperhidrosis is most commonly idiopathic in nature and occurs as a manifestation of primary or essential hyperhidrosis (Fig. 52–1). This process is usually symmetric and limited to the palms, soles, or axillae or some combination of these sites.[12] The diagnosis is usually evident on the basis of clinical findings: symmetric, localized, excessive, episodic sweating in response to specific stimuli; onset at or following puberty; a positive family history in many cases; minimal or no seasonal variation; and no associated bromhidrosis.

If unusual patterns of sharply focal or unilateral sweating are present, the physician must rule out localized hyperhidrosis caused by trauma or injury of the central or peripheral nervous system, including entities such as paresis, tabes dorsalis, neuritis, myelitis, or syringomyelia; conditions of the vasculature, such as

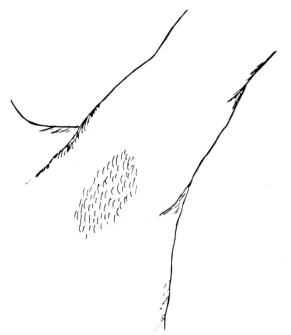

Figure 52–1. Schematic of a normal axilla.

cold injury, erythrocyanosis, arteriovenous defect, Raynaud's syndrome, or rheumatoid arthritis; or an hereditary syndrome such as recessive epidermolysis bullosa, blue rubber bleb nevus syndrome, Jadassohn-Lewandowsky syndrome, and Gopalan's syndrome.[7]

If generalized hyperhidrosis is present, underlying systemic causes should also be ruled out. These include febrile illnesses; metabolic or endocrine diseases such as alcohol intoxication, gout, diabetes mellitus, hyperthyroidism, hyperpituitarism, menopause, or pathologic obesity; vasomotor dysfunction resulting from shock or congestive heart failure; internal malignancy; disorders of the central nervous system such as tumors, trauma, or inflammation of the hypothalamus or its tracts; and certain hereditary syndromes, including intermittent hyperhidrosis, phenylketonuria, and Chédiak-Higashi syndrome.[7]

Pathophysiology

While the precise etiology of axillary hyperhidrosis remains unknown, much is understood about the anatomy, physiology, and regulation of eccrine sweat gland activity.

The eccrine gland consists of a simple tubular epithelial structure comprised of a duct and a secretory portion. The secretory portion is tightly coiled into a ball and is located either at the border between the dermis and the subcutaneous fat or in the lower third of the dermis, where it is surrounded by fatty tissue that connects with the subcutis.[13] The duct opens directly onto the skin surface, where it delivers a dilute electrolyte solution of sodium chloride, potassium, and bicarbonate and lesser amounts of lactate, urea, ammonia,

and proteolytic enzymes.[14] This watery secretion accounts for most axillary sweat production, as the apocrine glands produce only very limited quantities of a thick, viscid secretion, which is rendered odoriferous by bacterial action.[11]

While the lumen of the secretory portion of the eccrine gland measures approximately 20 microns in diameter, the secretory lumen of the apocrine gland may be ten times that size, or up to 200 microns in diameter.[13] A new type of sweat gland has also been identified that is intermediate in size between the apocrine and eccrine glands.[14] These glands, called apoeccrine glands, possess irregular dilatations of their secretory tubules, causing them to resemble apocrine glands; however, when stimulated, they produce extremely copious amounts of an eccrine-like serous secretion. Apoeccrine glands probably develop during puberty from the eccrine glands or eccrine-like precursor glands. They are found only in the adult axilla, where they may account for as much as 45% of all axillary glands and may significantly contribute to axillary sweating.

Eccrine glands are distributed over the entire body surface, with the exception of the vermilion border of the lips, external ear canal, nailbeds, clitoris, and labia minora.[13, 14] Each axillary vault contains about 25,000 eccrine glands.[6] Both eccrine and apocrine glands are most heavily concentrated within the central portion, or dome, of the vault. These central eccrine glands account for approximately 70 to 80% of axillary sweat secretion.[11] Eccrine gland density and responsiveness to emotional stimuli decrease toward the periphery of the axilla, while thermal responsiveness is maintained.[2]

Eccrine glands are richly innervated by sympathetic postganglionic cholinergic fibers, but sympathetic adrenergic innervation has also been demonstrated.[14]

Studies of the axillary eccrine glands of patients with axillary hyperhidrosis have failed to reveal any significant differences from those of normal individuals with respect to their number, histologic appearance, sympathetic innervation, and acetylcholinesterase levels.[2, 5, 6]

The efferent central sudomotor pathway consists of the cerebral cortex, hypothalamus, medulla, spinal cord, sympathetic ganglia, and postganglionic fibers. The hypothalamus regulates sweating to maintain a constant core temperature. Eccrine glands of the palms, soles, and axillae are unique in that they are activated predominantly by emotional stimuli.[10] Axillary eccrine glands, however, also respond to thermal stimuli to a variable extent. It has been postulated that in primary hyperhidrosis, the hypothalamic sweat center, which controls sweating of the palms, soles, and axillae in some patients, is under the exclusive control of the cerebral cortex, without thermoregulatory input. This would explain the episodic sweating that occurs in response to emotional stimuli and its cessation during sleep or sedation seen in some patients.[10]

Evidence suggests that primary palmar hyperhidrosis is mediated by hyperactivity of the sympathetic nervous system, resulting in excessive sympathetic outflow through the T2-3 ganglia that innervate the palmar sweat glands.[10] A similar process, under cortical control, may also occur in axillary hyperhidrosis, resulting in enhanced sympathetic outflow through the T4 ganglia that supply axillary sweat glands.

Nonsurgical Therapeutic Methods

Numerous treatments have been devised to control axillary hyperhidrosis. These include both topical and systemic medical and surgical approaches. All have some limitations because of side effects, lack of efficacy, or both. Clearly, those therapies that possess the lowest risk of significant side effects should be employed first, followed by more aggressive medical or surgical measures if initial treatment is ineffective or poorly tolerated.

TOPICAL THERAPY

Aluminum chloride hexahydrate 20% in anhydrous ethyl alcohol (Drysol) is the safest and most effective topical agent presently available and is considered the first line of therapy in most patients.[15] This solution is applied nightly to the dry, unshaved axillae, with or without occlusion, and washed off the following morning before the onset of daytime sweating. The mechanism of action of this agent appears to be occlusion of the intraepidermal eccrine duct below the level of the stratum corneum.[6] If moisture is present, hydrochloric acid will form, and skin irritation will result. Topical hydrocortisone cream is used to control this problem, which occurs to some extent in most patients and is the most common cause of treatment failure. Once sweating is controlled, usually after 1 to 2 weeks, the solution may be applied only once every week or as often as required to control symptoms. If tolerated, this treatment has a very high rate of efficacy and patient satisfaction (83 to 98%).[3, 15–17] However, one group of investigators reported that 26 of their 38 patients did not respond to this treatment and chose to undergo surgery.[18]

Topical anticholinergic agents have shown only limited success because of both inefficacy and systemic side effects. However, a 0.025% solution of benzoyl scopolamine hydrobromide applied to the axillae twice daily has been reported to reduce axillary sweating by 85% without causing systemic or local side effects.[19]

Tanning agents such as glutaraldehyde and formaldehyde may also be effective, but side effects limit their usefulness.[20] Glutaraldehyde causes a brown staining of the skin that is unacceptable to most patients. Formaldehyde carries a significant risk of inducing allergic sensitivity. Methenamine, which releases formaldehyde when exposed to aqueous solutions, has not been shown to be sensitizing or even reactive in patients with known formaldehyde sensitivity.[21] These agents act through eccrine ductal occlusion at the level of the stratum corneum.[22]

RADIATION

Radiotherapy, which has been shown to be effective only at high doses, cannot be considered a satisfactory alternative.[6]

IONTOPHORESIS

Iontophoresis is the passage of direct electrical current through the patient's palms, soles, or axillae while the patient is in contact with an aqueous ionic solution. The electric current introduces ions from the solution into the patient's skin and appears to inhibit sweating by occluding the eccrine ducts at the level of the stratum corneum.[3] A battery-powered unit for home use (Drionic) is available with special electrodes designed to treat the axillae.[23, 24] A 50% or greater reduction in axillary sweating has been reported in most patients treated for 3 weeks.[22] Most reports, however, describe a lower efficacy rate and indicate that the axillae are more difficult to treat by iontophoresis than are the palms and soles, which generally respond quite favorably.[15, 24, 25]

SYSTEMIC THERAPY

Anticholinergic agents and tranquilizers can be helpful as adjuncts to topical therapy,[20] particularly when reserved for use during brief periods when the need for control is greatest. Minor tranquilizers of the benzodiazepine class can be employed to induce a degree of indifference to emotional stimuli, thereby suppressing sympathetic discharge and reducing emotion-related sweating.[6] The tendency of these agents to induce drug tolerance and dependence must certainly always be considered.

Anticholinergic drugs are effective, at least transiently, in most patients, but unpleasant side effects limit their potential usefulness.[15] Glycopyrrolate (Robinul) or a combination of this drug and phenobarbital (Robinul PH Forte) has been recommended for patients whose condition has a significant emotional component.[20]

BIOFEEDBACK AND PSYCHOTHERAPY

Both biofeedback and psychotherapy have also been reported to be effective in certain patients.[20]

Surgical Treatment

For patients who fail to respond to the previous types of medical therapy, a variety of surgical approaches are available. Before the 1960s, upper thoracic sympathectomy was the only surgical technique available for the treatment of primary hyperhidrosis of the palms and axillae. While excellent results were reported,[20] the procedure carried a significant risk of potentially serious side effects, including Horner's syndrome, pneumothorax, postsympathetic neuralgia, phrenic nerve paralysis, dorsal scapular neuralgia, compensatory hyperhidrosis in other parts of the body, and chronic nasal congestion.[10] Nevertheless, sympathectomy is still indicated on occasion for palmar hyperhidrosis that is refractory to all nonsurgical therapies. However, with the development of safe and effective local surgical procedures for the treatment of axillary hyperhidrosis, sympathectomy cannot be justified any longer for isolated axillary involvement.

AXILLARY ANATOMY

Before discussing local surgical approaches to axillary hyperhidrosis, a brief review of pertinent axillary anatomy is in order. Beneath the skin and subcutaneous fat of the axillary vault lies the deep axillary fascia. Under this fascial layer are the lateral cutaneous branches of the upper intercostal nerves and the large axillary vein. Below the axillary vein are the nerves of the brachial plexus and the axillary artery,[26] the pulsations of which can be palpated from the skin surface when the upper extremity is abducted. Care must be taken to avoid injuring these structures when operating in the axilla. When using general anesthesia, the upper extremity should not be abducted more than 90 to 120 degrees from the lateral chest wall to avoid injuring the motor nerves to the muscles of the shoulder girdle that arise from C5 and C6.[27, 28] Such injury is caused by prolonged stretching of these nerves around the head of the humerus. While this precaution may not be necessary with the use of local anesthesia, the vulnerability of these structures should be kept in mind.

SURGICAL TECHNIQUES

Cryosurgery

Cryosurgery has been recommended for treating axillary hyperhidrosis but is very painful[29] and poorly tolerated.

Electrosurgery

Electroelimination of axillary sweat glands by means of insulated H-type electrosurgical needles inserted parallel to the skin surface into the uppermost subcutis at 50 to 70 different points in each axilla has been described.[30] Thirty watts of high-frequency current are applied for 1-second intervals at each insertion point. Five to six treatments at 1- to 3-month intervals are typically required. The technique is somewhat more effective for bromhidrosis than for hyperhidrosis: 75% of patients with bromhidrosis and 67% of those with hyperhidrosis experienced excellent to moderate clinical improvement. Alopecia, slight scarring, transient arm pain, and slight contracture were the only complications.

Surgical Resection of Axillary Glands

Many methods have been developed to surgically remove the hypersecreting glands from the axillae of patients with axillary hyperhidrosis. Most of these methods fall into one of three categories: (1) those that remove only subcutaneous tissue; (2) those that remove skin and underlying subcutaneous tissue by excision; and (3) those that combine excision of skin and underlying subcutis with undermining and removal of adjacent subcutaneous tissue.

Sweat Pattern Mapping. Preoperative mapping of axillary sweat gland activity allows the surgeon to confirm the presence of hyperhidrosis, determine its severity, and locate foci of greatest sweat secretion that must be removed if surgery is to be effective. Several methods have been described. The simplest involve pressing a single sheet of colored crepe paper,[31] facial tissue paper,[6] or toilet paper[32] flat against the skin of the dry, shaved axilla until sweat droplets create a visible wet spot on the paper, indicating the location of the most active hyperhidrotic area. This area can be marked on the skin by piercing the paper at several points along the border of the wet spot with a pointed wooden applicator stick dipped in waterproof ink or with a waterproof ink pen.

Greater accuracy can be achieved with Minor's method, described in 1927.[33] First, a solution of 3% iodine and 3% potassium iodide in 95% ethyl alcohol is painted on the dry, shaved axilla; two or more applications may improve results. Povidone-iodine antiseptic solution may be substituted for convenience and sterility.[34] When the iodine solution has dried thoroughly, which may be hastened by use of a blowdryer or by blotting with gauze, corn starch powder is dusted or patted over the area. If sterile starch is desired, it is available in the form of Biosorb glove powder.[34] Wherever sweat droplets are secreted, a blue-black dot appears from the reaction of the starch and iodine. Sites of greatest secretion are indicated by dark patches that result from confluence of these individual dots. These areas can then be outlined with waterproof ink before additional sweating washes the colored material away.

If significant sweating is not seen, the patient is asked to perform mental arithmetic, or an 18-gauge needle may be inserted into the patient's palm to induce a painful stimulus and cause the sweating response.[35] A one-step method in which pre-iodinated starch powder is sprayed on the skin using a simple, homemade atomizer has also been described.[36]

Usually, a single major focus of sweating is found that is roughly circular in shape, with a diameter of 3.5 to 4.5 cm and located in the apex of the axilla (Fig. 52–2). In some cases, one or two additional minor foci may be present, and less commonly, two nearly equal zones or diffuse axillary sweating may be seen. Interestingly, individual sweating patterns are remarkably stable and reproducible over time.[2] For this reason, limited excision of just the hyperhidrotic foci can produce permanent symptomatic relief.

Sweat patterns should be determined and photographed or drawn at the time of the initial examination of the patient. This allows the surgeon to discuss with the patient the expected outcomes of the surgical alternatives based on the patient's particular sweat patterns and to select the most appropriate method with regard to the patient's desires and expectations. Sweat pattern mapping should be repeated at the time of surgery to precisely delineate the sites to be treated.

Preoperative Considerations. Before surgery, axillary hair should be shaved and the axillae cleansed thoroughly with an appropriate germicidal soap. Prophylactic antibiotics are not recommended, since they have been shown to have no effect on the clinical course or complication rate of patients undergoing surgery for

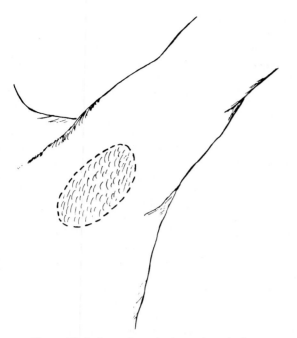

Figure 52–2. Area of greatest sweat production.

axillary hyperhidrosis.[37] Preoperative sedatives and anticholinergic agents must be avoided until the axillary sweat patterns have been determined, as these medications can dramatically alter the pattern and volume of axillary sweating. Local anesthesia (lidocaine with epinephrine 1:100,000) is usually employed. Many surgeons prefer concentrations of lidocaine ranging from 0.1 to 0.5%, which allows the infiltration of larger volumes of anesthetic solution. One technique uses an injection of 40 to 60 ml of a 0.25% lidocaine solution[32] or 30 ml of a 0.5% lidocaine solution[38] into the cleavage plane between the dermis and subcutaneous tissue of each axilla to induce tissue expansion to facilitate dissection.[32]

Methods That Remove Subcutaneous Tissue Only. Surgical methods of treating axillary hyperhidrosis that rely upon the removal of subcutaneous tissue only are effective for two reasons. First, the secretory portion of the eccrine gland is either at the junction of the dermis and the subcutaneous fat or in the lower third of the dermis, where it is surrounded by fatty tissue that connects with the subcutis.[13] Therefore, removal of the subcutaneous tissue will remove the secretory portion of many of these glands,[39] resulting in a reduction in axillary sweating.

Second, eccrine secretory activity is dependent on sympathetic nervous stimulation. Surgical removal of subcutaneous tissue disrupts the sympathetic innervation, resulting in complete but transient anhidrosis of the treated area. Secretory activity resumes when sympathetic innervation is restored. Studies on full-thickness skin grafts and flaps have shown that sympathetic reinnervation takes about 3 months[40] and coincides with the return of sensory function.[41] Postoperative studies of hyperhidrotic patients treated with surgical resection of axillary subcutaneous tissue have demonstrated a return of sweating after 1 to 3 months.[2, 39, 42] Usually, however,

the rate of sweat production is significantly diminished from preoperative levels.

The first and technically the most demanding operation of this type was described in 1962.[39] Without preoperative mapping of the sweat pattern, the hair-bearing axillary skin is incised down to the fascial layer to create four flaps (Fig. 52–3A). The flaps are extensively undermined beyond the border of the hair-bearing skin and reflected to expose the reddish-brown or gray apocrine glandular tissue, within which are interspersed innumerable eccrine secretory tubules. This tissue is then trimmed away from the deep dermis with curved scissors in the same way a full-thickness skin graft is prepared, until all glandular tissue is removed. An attempt should be made to preserve the vessels of the deep dermal plexus. After careful hemostasis and placement of a small rubber tube for drainage, the wound is closed with interrupted buried and vertical mattress sutures, with the latter fixed to the underlying fascia. A pressure dressing is applied for 1 week, and the drain is removed after 24 hours.

With this procedure, patients experience total anhidrosis for 2 to 3 months, followed by a resumption of sweating at a significantly diminished and clinically acceptable level. The result is considered good to excellent in all patients, and the only complications that have been reported are one wound infection and two hematomas. While most patients experience diminished axillary hair growth, none have developed scar contraction. In subsequent reports, skin loss as a result of necrosis was found to be insignificant.[28, 43]

The use of a simple housed razor (e.g., Schick adjustable) has been recommended as a way to facilitate the procedure.[44] However, care should be exercised to avoid undue thinning of the dermis, resulting in vascular compromise. The outcome of this method depends, to a great extent, on the surgeon's skill in handling the

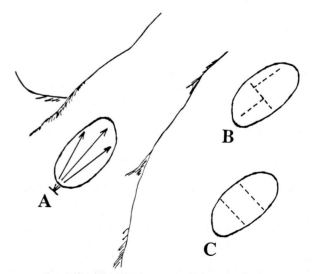

Figure 52–3. Subcutaneous resection techniques.
A, Roller ball excision.
B, Four-flap excision.
C, Dual parallel transverse incision technique.

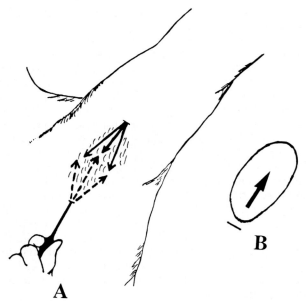

Figure 52–4. Subcutaneous resection technique using liposuction *(A)* or a curette *(B)*.

skin flaps atraumatically to avoid necrosis and subsequent contraction.

A simplified technique has been described using one or two parallel incisions made transversely across the hairy axilla[43] (Fig. 52–3*B, C*). The skin is undermined, reflected, and defatted as previously described. Wounds are closed after obtaining careful hemostasis with 6–0 nylon, and a pressure dressing is applied for 1 week. No drain is employed. Using this technique, sweating was reduced to a "normal" level 3 months after surgery. A subsequent report of 30 patients[45] operated on with this method showed similar results. Complications included one hematoma, two partial skin necroses, and two abscesses. These authors felt this technique was more reliable and produced less scarring and skin necrosis than previously described techniques.[39]

In 1975, a technique of subcutaneous curettage was described[46] (Fig. 52–4). After mapping the axillary sweat pattern, a 1- to 1.5-cm incision was made at the proximal margin of the hair-bearing axillary skin; through this incision extensive undermining with scissors was performed. The subcutaneous fat and lower dermis of the hair-bearing skin was removed with a curette, with special attention paid to the most active sweating foci. The appearance of petechiae on the skin surface was one indication of the adequacy of treatment. A suction drain was inserted, the wound closed with nylon sutures, and a simple dressing applied. The drain was removed on about the third postoperative day and the sutures were removed after 7 to 10 days. In a 1978 follow-up study of 161 patients,[47] 54% of patients were totally satisfied; and 10% were partially satisfied after one operation. Further improvement was achieved by repeating the procedure when unacceptable sweating persisted. In 322 separate axillary surgeries, complications

totaled seven hematomas; six cases of skin necrosis, one of which required reconstruction using a skin graft; and 5 infections. Another report described total relapse in 7 of 12 patients operated on using this method with only 2 patients satisfied with their result.[48] A subcutaneous tissue shaver was subsequently developed to expedite this procedure, which was reported to give excellent results in 2000 cases.[49]

Liposuction has also been recommended as a means of removing glandular tissue in the treatment of axillary hyperhidrosis (Fig. 52–4).[15, 50, 51] This is accomplished by first applying the liposuction cannula to the undersurface of the dermis in a manner similar to that used for the subcutaneous curettage technique[46] and then suctioning out the subcutaneous fat in the usual fashion. Advocates of this technique claim that axillary sweating is reduced to normal levels, trauma and axillary hair loss are minimized, and minor skin necrosis is the only complication.[15]

Methods That Excise Skin and Underlying Subcutaneous Tissue. In 1963, Hurley and Shelley were the first to describe local cutaneous excision for the treatment of axillary hyperhidrosis.[11] The technique was discovered serendipitously when a generous excisional skin biopsy from the axilla of a young man with axillary hyperhidrosis so relieved his symptoms that he insisted the physicians perform a biopsy on the other axilla. This technique is simple and consists of identifying the major sweating focus and excising an ellipse of tissue from the center of that focus, oriented transversely across the axilla, which measures 1 to 1.5 cm × 4 to 5 cm (Fig. 52–5). The incisions are carried to the level of the axillary fascia to ensure removal of both skin and subcutaneous tissue. The wound is closed with buried interrupted and vertical mattress sutures and covered with a bulky pressure dressing for the first 24 to 48 hours. Axillary sweating is reduced to normal levels in

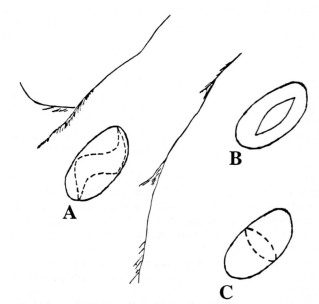

Figure 52–5. Subcutaneous and skin resection techniques using an S-shaped excision *(A)*, a longitudinal fusiform excision *(B)*, and a transverse excision *(C)*.

all patients, and no complications have been reported. Other authors have confirmed the ease and efficacy of this procedure.[34] In one series of 50 patients[48] treated by this method, 47 were pleased with the result, but three patients experienced no improvement. Seven were unhappy with the appearance of their scars, and three reported some limitation of arm movement.

This procedure was modified by placing the excision longitudinally in the axilla,[52] which permitted an increase in its width to 3 cm, thereby allowing more complete excision of the hyperhidrotic focus (Fig. 52–5). No patients experienced limitation of arm movement, and the cosmetic result was considered superior, as the entire scar could be contained within the axillary fossa. Excellent results or substantial improvement were obtained in 19 of 24 patients treated. The procedure was also effective in one patient treated for bromhidrosis. All patients experienced minor delays in wound healing, one patient developed recurrent infection, and one wound dehisced and subsequently healed by secondary intention.

In some cases, more complete excision of axillary glandular tissue may be necessary to reduce sweating to an acceptable level. Two methods of accomplishing this have been described. The simplest technique consists of mapping the axillary sweat pattern[32] and planning an excision that is oriented longitudinally in the axillary fossa to include at least 90% of the hyperhidrotic area. For this technique, 40 to 50 ml of a 0.25% solution of lidocaine with epinephrine should be infiltrated into each axilla and the excision carried down to the fascial layer. If a definite sweat pattern cannot be determined, at least 90% of the hairy axilla is taken. The outline of the excision is broken by a small triangular flap at the midpoint of the superior edge and by a corresponding incision at the lower edge, thereby forming an M- or bat-shaped wound measuring approximately 4 cm × 10 cm (Fig. 52–6). This pattern may also, of course, be inverted to form a W-shaped excision. After careful hemostasis, the wound is closed without undermining. The three flap tips are approximated with half-buried mattress sutures anchored to the axillary fascia, and the wound edges are closed with a combination of figure-of-eight or vertical mattress and simple interrupted sutures. No drains are required, and a small compression dressing is applied.

The mattress sutures are removed at 1 week and the remaining sutures at 2 weeks. This convalescent period is particularly recommended for individuals with jobs requiring heavy labor. With this technique, an excellent result has been obtained in 82% of patients, with no cases of hematoma, wound infection, or scar tightness. Significant scar spreading is common, however.[31] The angulated shape of the closed wound is designed to prevent excessive longitudinal scar contraction that might limit upper arm movement. The procedure is straightforward and does not require extensive training with the Z-plasty technique or in the management of flaps.

When complete anhidrosis of the axilla is desired and loss of all axillary hair is cosmetically acceptable, excision of the entire sweat gland-–bearing area has been

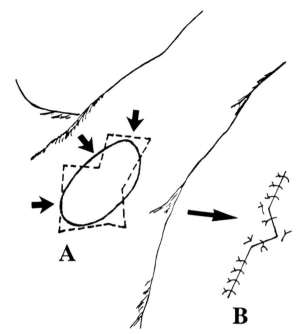

Figure 52–6. Subcutaneous and skin resection techniques using a geometric excision (A), which yields a V-shaped closure (B).

advocated.[5, 38, 53–55] Because this area corresponds closely to the hairy portion of the axilla, the procedure results in a large defect in a region where there is a relative deficiency of skin. Primary closure of such wounds leads to considerable tension, with a resultant detrimental impact on wound healing. To minimize this problem, incorporation of a Z-plasty in the closure has been recommended.[5, 38, 53, 54] A complete discussion of this advanced surgical technique is beyond the scope of this chapter, but its application in the treatment of axillary hyperhidrosis will be briefly described.

After mapping the axillary sweat pattern, the entire hyperhidrotic area, including all hair-bearing skin, is excised along with the underlying glandular tissue. The excision usually consists of an ellipse measuring 4 to 5 cm × 10 to 12 cm and situated longitudinally in the axillary fossa. The design of the Z-plasty is similar to that described for treatment of chronic hidradenitis suppurativa,[56] with the limbs of the Z measuring about half the length of the primary excision, and positioned no less than 60 degrees to its longitudinal axis. Viewing the patient in the anatomic position with the arm fully abducted to the vertical position, the incision forming the posterior flap meets the primary excision at a point superior to the corresponding point for the anterior flap. The incision forming the anterior flap should not extend beyond the anterior axillary fold where the scar could be seen.[38] A modified Z-plasty technique in which the arms of the Z curve to run parallel to the long axis of the excision (Fig. 52–7) has also been proposed.[54] As always, careful hemostasis is critical. A small, soft rubber drain is left in the wound for 2 to 7 days, and a light compression bandage is applied. The drain may be advanced 3 to 5 cm every other day with the dressing

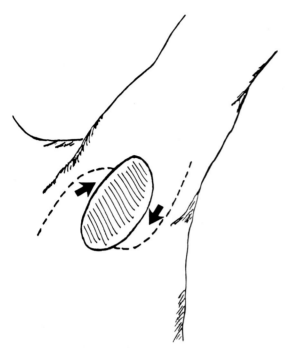

Figure 52–7. Excision using two rotation flaps.

change. The patient is instructed to avoid abduction of the arm until complete healing has occurred.

In a report of 123 patients operated on using this technique, 57% of patients experienced a 75 to 100% reduction of axillary sweating; 36% reported a 50 to 75% reduction.[5] Complications included six hematomas, five cases of limited flap necrosis, and ten minor complications such as seromas, suture abscesses, and sweat cysts. There were no cases of keloid formation or restricted arm movement from wound contracture, although scar widening did occur. While all patients healed satisfactorily (most in 2 weeks), healing was delayed in four cases for 3 to 8 weeks.[53]

Methods That Combine Cutaneous Excision and Resection of Subcutaneous Tissue. Perhaps the most practical techniques are those that combine the benefits of excising skin and subcutaneous tissue with the advantages of removing subcutaneous tissue only by incorporating the two approaches in one procedure. In 1966, Hurley and Shelley[2] described a modification of their original technique.[11] They suggested that, in addition to removing a single, transverse portion from the major sweating focus, one or two smaller specimens should be excised from the minor foci in a given axilla, followed by subcutaneous resection of sweat glands adjacent to each excision site. The dimensions of the primary excision are 4 to 5 cm × 1 to 1.5 cm and those of the secondary excisions are 2.5 to 3.5 cm × 0.3 to 0.8 cm. Resection of adjacent glands is accomplished by first undermining the remaining skin of the primary sweating focus at the level of the upper subcutaneous fat. The skin edge on each side of the excision is then reflected over the surgeon's index finger and the sweat glands trimmed away with curved scissors. Hair follicles should not be taken, and the dermis should not be trimmed so

cleanly that the cutaneous blood supply is compromised. A similar but less extensive procedure is performed on the skin surrounding the secondary excision sites, with the surgeon making sure that some nonundermined skin has been left between the excisions to maintain sufficient blood supply. Again, careful hemostasis, application of a substantial pressure dressing for 3 to 4 days, and limitation of arm abduction for about 2 weeks are crucial for a good outcome.

Patients who underwent quantitative studies of axillary sweating before and after this surgery demonstrated reductions in sweating ranging from 55% to 95% after surgery. Complications included one hematoma and three cases of retrograde lymphangitis that resolved spontaneously and without sequelae. A few patients experienced transient tightness of the skin, but none developed any permanent limitation of arm movement. Patients who felt their condition was not sufficiently improved were treated again with the same method to achieve an additional reduction in sweating. One interesting side effect was a significant increase in axillary odor in virtually all patients treated, which was easily controlled with aluminum-containing deodorant products. A slightly modified version of this technique confirmed its efficacy[57] in 1970. This procedure results in the removal of only one, larger, transverse portion, measuring 3 cm × 7 cm, from the primary sweating focus.

An additional modification of the technique was reported in 1977.[9] The transverse excision measured 5 to 6 cm × 2 to 3 cm, with undermining carried to 4 to 5 cm beyond the skin edges depending on the extent of the primary sweating focus. The undermined skin was then thinned aggressively, as in the preparation of a split-thickness skin graft, resulting in the removal of all glands, hair follicles, and blood vessels. This method produced permanent alopecia and virtual anhidrosis of the treated skin. In the treated patients, 16% developed hematoma and partial skin necrosis, 4% had wound dehiscence, 8% had superficial vein thrombosis, and one unsatisfactory scar required revision. However, 87% of patients available for follow-up reported very satisfactory results.

In another report,[58] the use of simple, transverse excisions through the primary sweating focus, as previously described,[22, 23] combined with wide undermining but without trimming the sweat glands from the undersurface of the dermis, also gave good results. Over an 8- to 24-month follow-up period, 90% of the patients were considered to be as dry or drier than "normal," and all were free from the limitations and embarrassment produced by their condition before surgery. It is doubtful, however, that wide undermining contributes more than a temporary reduction in sweating resulting from transient sympathetic denervation.

Excision of the posterior portion of the hairy axilla with a longitudinally oriented incision has also been advocated.[59] In this procedure the skin is undermined and the glands resected from the anterior portion only, and the wound is closed primarily. More than 70% of patients treated by this method were completely satisfied with the outcome. Only 13% of patients reported no improvement in one or both axillae, while 12% were unhappy with the appearance of their scars, and two patients developed limitation of arm movement from scar contracture. The advantage of this method is that only one side of the excision must be undermined, thereby simplifying the procedure and minimizing vascular compromise.

Use of an S-shaped excision (see Fig. 52–5) has also been described.[60] This is placed longitudinally in the axilla to remove a little more than one third of the hair-bearing skin. The resulting flaps are then undermined and reflected, and the subcutaneous tissue and glands are removed. The extent of the excision is determined by drawing an "S" on the area of sweating. Two additional curved lines are drawn so that the width of the excision is about 3 cm at its widest point. Although no numeric data were provided in this study, almost total elimination of axillary sweating was achieved while avoiding cutaneous necrosis in all cases. The curved shape of the excision reduces scar contracture and subsequent limitation of arm movement.

Postoperative Considerations

Meticulous hemostasis is critical to the success of this procedure, regardless of the surgical technique employed, to minimize the risk of hematoma formation with its associated complications of infection, cutaneous necrosis, and delayed wound healing. If significant undermining is performed or considerable serous drainage is noted, a drain of soft rubber tubing, such as a Penrose drain, should be left in the wound for a few days until drainage subsides. A pressure dressing that provides adequate upward pressure on the axillary vault should also be applied for the first few days to help prevent the development of a hematoma or seroma. The patient should be advised to limit arm abduction for several weeks to minimize tension across the wound. Sutures are generally removed 1 to 2 weeks after surgery. Because sympathetic reinnervation augments axillary sweating, the adequacy of surgery should not be assessed for approximately 6 to 12 weeks, when sensory and sympathetic reinnervation has occurred.

SUMMARY

Selection of a surgical procedure should be based on individual patients' sweating patterns, the severity of the hyperhidrosis, the degree of reduction in axillary sweating desired by patients, and their preferences regarding scarring and loss of axillary hair. For patients who are concerned about scarring and who will tolerate some residual sweating, removal of subcutaneous tissue through a small incision[46] or by modified liposuction is indicated. Patients with more severe disease who do not mind a scar but consider a hairless axilla cosmetically unacceptable should be treated with partial excision of the hyperhidrotic area, with or without undermining and resection of adjacent subcutaneous tissue. Aggressive resection of subcutaneous tissue will result in partial or

complete axillary alopecia if hair follicles are destroyed. Patients who desire total axillary anhidrosis and do not mind a hairless axilla and a wide scar are appropriately treated with one of the more extensive excision techniques, such as the bat-shaped excision,[32] double rotation flaps (Fig. 52–7), or total excision of the hairy axilla followed by Z-plasty repair.[5, 38, 53, 54] Of course, if there is any question as to which surgical approach is best for a given patient, the simplest and least disfiguring procedure that is likely to control the symptoms should be selected first. If the patient is not satisfied with the resulting reduction in axillary sweating, additional improvement may be achieved by repeating the previous procedure or substituting a more aggressive technique.

REFERENCES

1. Munro DM, Verbov JL, O'Gorman DJ, Du Vivier A: Axillary hyperhidrosis. Br J Dermatol 90:325–329, 1974.
2. Hurley HJ, Shelley WB: Axillary hyperhidrosis—clinical features and local surgical management. Br J Dermatol 78:127–140, 1966.
3. White JW: Treatment of primary hyperhidrosis. Mayo Clin Proc 61:951–956, 1986.
4. Adar R, Kurchin A, Zweig A, Mozes M: Palmar hyperhidrosis and its surgical treatment: a report of 100 cases. Ann Surg 186:34–41, 1977.
5. Bretteville-Jensen G, Mossing N, Albrechtsen R: Surgical treatment of axillary hyperhidrosis in 123 patients. Acta Dermatol Venereol 55:73–78, 1975.
6. Shelly WB, Hurley HJ Jr: Studies on topical antiperspirant control of axillary hyperhidrosis. Acta Dermatol Venereol 55:241–260, 1975.
7. Demis DJ, Thiers BH, Smith EB, Burgdorf WHC (eds): Clinical Dermatology. Vol 2, unit 9–3. JB Lippincott, Philadelphia, 1990, pp 1–5.
8. Savin JA: Excessive sweating of the palms and armpits. Br Med J 1:581–582, 1983.
9. Rigg BM: Axillary hyperhidrosis. Plast Reconstr Surg 59:334, 1977.
10. Sato K, Kang WH, Sato KT: Biology of sweat glands and their disorders. II. Disorders of sweat gland function. J Am Acad Dermatol 20:713–726, 1989.
11. Hurley HJ, Shelley WB: A simple surgical approach to the management of axillary hyperhidrosis. JAMA 186:109–112, 1963.
12. Rook A, Wilkinson DS, Ebling FJG, et al (eds): Textbook of Dermatology. Blackwell Scientific, Oxford, England, 1986, p 1887.
13. Lever WF, Schaumburg-Lever G: Histopathology of the Skin. JB Lippincott, Philadelphia, 1990, p 21.
14. Sato K, Kang WH, Saga K, Sato KH: Biology of sweat glands and their disorders. I. Normal sweat gland function. J Am Acad Dermatol 20:537–563, 1989.
15. Lillis PJ, Coleman WP III: Liposuction for treatment of axillary hyperhidrosis. Dermatol Clin 8:479–482, 1990.
16. Ellis H, Scurr JH: Axillary hyperhidrosis—topical treatment with aluminum chloride hexahydrate. Postgrad Med J 55:868–869, 1979.
17. Scholes K, Crow K, Willis JP, et al: Axillary hyperhidrosis treated with alcoholic solution of aluminum chloride hexahydrate. Br Med J 2:84–85, 1978.
18. Rayner CRW, Ritchie ID, Stark GP: Axillary hyperhidrosis, 20% aluminum chloride hexahydrate, and surgery. Br Med J 280:1168, 1980.
19. MacMillan FS, Feller HH, Snyder FH: The antiperspirant action of topically applied anticholinergic. J Invest Dermatol 43:363–377, 1964.
20. White JW: Treatment of primary hyperhidrosis. Mayo Clin Proc 61:951–956, 1986.
21. Cullen SJ: Topical methenamine therapy for hyperhidrosis. Arch Dermatol 111:1158, 1975.

22. Sato K, Dobson RL: Mechanism of the antiperspirant effect of topical glutaraldehyde. Arch Dermatol 100:564–569, 1969.

23. Akins DL, Meisenheimer JL, Dobson RL: Efficacy of the Drionic unit in the treatment of hyperhidrosis. J Am Acad Dermatol 16:828–832, 1987.

24. Elgart M, Fuchs G: Tapwater iontophoresis in the treatment of hyperhidrosis—use of the Drionic device. Int J Dermatol 26:194, 1987.

25. Midtgaard K: A new device for the treatment of hyperhidrosis by iontophoresis. Br J Dermatol 114:485–488, 1986.

26. Healy JE, Seybold WD: A Synopsis of Clinical Anatomy. WB Saunders, Philadelphia, 1969, pp 42–45.

27. Shaw MH: A serious complication of an operation for axillary hyperhidrosis. Br J Plast Surg 27:196–197, 1974.

28. Sabatier H, Picaud AJ: The surgical treatment of axillary hyperhidrosis. J Dermatol Surg 2:331–332, 1976.

29. Grice K: Treatment of hyperhidrosis. Clin Exp Dermatol 7:183–188, 1982.

30. Kobayashi T: Electrosurgery using insulated needles: treatment of axillary bromhidrosis and hyperhidrosis. J Dermatol Surg Oncol 14:749–752, 1988.

31. Stenquist B: Axillary hyperhidrosis: a simple surgical procedure. J Dermatol Surg Oncol 11:388–391, 1985.

32. Eldh J, Fogdestam I: Surgical treatment of hyperhidrosis axillae. Scand J Plast Reconstr Surg 10:227–229, 1976.

33. Minor V: Ein neues Verfahren zu der klinischen Untersuchung der Schweissabsonderung. Dtsche Z Nervenheil 101:302–306, 1927.

34. Davis EKB: Surgical treatment of axillary hyperhidrosis. Br J Plast Surg 24:99, 1971.

35. Hurley HJ: Local surgical treatment of axillary hyperhidrosis. In: Epstein E, Epstein E Jr (eds): Skin Surgery. 6th ed. WB Saunders, Philadelphia, 1987, pp 598–606.

36. Sato KT, Richardson A, Timm DE, Sato K: One-step iodine starch method for direct visualization of sweating. Am J Med Sci 295:528–531, 1988.

37. Ma S, Chiang SS, Fang RH: Prophylactic antibiotics in surgical treatment of axillary hyperhidrosis. Ann Plast Surg 22:436–439, 1989.

38. Bretteville-Jensen G: Radical sweat gland ablation for axillary hyperhidrosis. Br J Plast Surg 26:158–162, 1973.

39. Skoog T, Thyresson N: Hyperhidrosis of the axillae: a method of surgical treatment. Acta Chir Scand 123:531–538, 1962.

40. Conway H: Sweating function of transplanted skin. Surg Gynecol Obstet 69:756, 1939.

41. Ponten B: Grafted skin—observations on innervation and other qualities. Acta Chir Scand Suppl 257:1–78, 1960.

42. Harahap M: Management of hyperhidrosis axillaris. J Dermatol Surg Oncol 5:223–225, 1979.

43. Skoog T, Thyresson N: The surgical treatment of axillary hyperhidrosis. Br J Dermatol 78:551, 1966.

44. Kappesser HJ: The use of a housed razor blade in the surgical management of axillary hyperhidrosis. J Dermatol Surg Oncol 5:288–289, 1979.

45. Yoshikata R, Yanai T, Shionome H: Surgical treatment of axillary osmidrosis. Br J Plast Surg 43:483–485, 1990.

46. Jamec B: Abrasio-axillae in hyperhidrosis. Scand J Plast Reconstr Surg 9:44, 1975.

47. Jamec B, Hansen BH: Follow-up of patients operated on for axillary hyperhidrosis by subcutaneous curettage. Scand J Plast Reconstr Surg 12:65–67, 1978.

48. Ellis H: Axillary hyperhidrosis: failure of subcutaneous curettage. Br Med J 2:301–302, 1977.

49. Inaba M, Ezaki T: New instrument for hircismus and hyperhidrosis operation. Subcutaneous tissue shaver. Plast Reconstr Surg 59:864–866, 1977.

50. Shenag SM, Spira M: Treatment of bilateral axillary hyperhidrosis by suction assisted lipolysis technique. Ann Plast Surg 19:548–551, 1987.

51. Coleman WP III: Non-cosmetic applications of liposuction. J Dermatol Surg Oncol 14:1085–1090, 1988.

52. Gillespie JA, Kane SP: Evaluation of a simple surgical treatment of axillary hyperhidrosis. Br J Dermatol 83:684–689, 1970.

53. Taylor GD: Axillary skin excision for the treatment of axillary hyperhidrosis. Aust NZ J Surg 52:56–59, 1982.

54. Hill TG: Radical excision and reconstruction of axillary skin. J Dermatol Surg Oncol 9:299–303, 1983.

55. Hartmann M, Petres J: Operative therapie der hyperhidrosis axillaris. Hautarzt 29:82–85, 1978.

56. Greeley PW: Surgical treatment of chronic suppurative hidradenitis. Arch Surg 61:193–198, 1950.

57. Weaver PC: Axillary hyperhidrosis. Br Med J 1:48, 1970.

58. Tipton JB: Axillary hyperhidrosis and its surgical treatment. Plast Reconstr Surg 42:137–140, 1968.

59. Bergkvist L, Engevik L: The surgical treatment of axillary hyperhidrosis. Br J Surg 66:482–484, 1979.

60. Bisbal J, Cacho C, Casalots J: Surgical treatment of axillary hyperhidrosis. Ann Plast Surg 18:429, 1987.

CHAPTER 53

Management of Leg Ulcers

THEODORA M. MAURO

Lower extremity ulcers are a common affliction, affecting approximately 1% of the adult population.[1] Because the incidence of leg ulcers increases with age,[2] the frequency of this problem is also likely to increase as the United States' population ages.

Diagnosis

In approaching the patient with leg ulcers, the morphology, location, and associated internal diseases are all important. Most leg ulcers are caused by some combination of venous stasis, arterial insufficiency, or neurotropism, but less common causes (Table 53–1) can also produce leg ulcers. For this reason, it is necessary not only to carefully examine each patient but also to take a detailed history.

Physical Examination

The physical examination can help differentiate venous, arterial, or neurotropic ulcers. Ulcers resulting from venous stasis disease often occur on the lower third of the leg, especially around the lateral or medial malleolus. In contrast, ulcers caused by arterial or neurotropic disease most often occur on the toes or distal feet. Ulcers resulting from venous disease tend to be shallow, and when they undergo biopsy, they often bleed profusely, an indication of adequate blood supply to that area of the leg. Arterial ulcers tend to be deeper and often are very painful. Neurotropic ulcers may also be deep; however, they may be painless because of the underlying neuropathy. Other less common causes of ulcerations can produce distinctive clinical appearances. Vasculitic ulcers often display geographic borders. Pyoderma gangrenosum typically begins as a purple nodule that rapidly breaks down to form an ulcer with under-

mined bluish borders. Neoplasms such as squamous cell carcinomas may arise in chronic leg ulcers and will often show heaped-up borders and be associated with enlarged lymph nodes.

TABLE 53–1. ETIOLOGY OF LEG ULCERS

Vascular causes	Infectious causes
Venous insufficiency	Bacterial
Ischemic causes	*Mycobacteria*
Arteriosclerosis	Ecthyma
Arteriovenous fistula	*Pseudomonas*
Raynaud's disease	Diphtheria
Thromboangiitis obliterans	Anthrax
(Buerger's disease)	Tularemia
Malignant atrophic	Fungal
papulosis (Degos'	Sporotrichosis
disease)	Coccidioidomycosis
Embolic causes	Histoplasmosis
Subacute bacterial	Blastomycosis
endocarditis	"Madura foot"
Meningococcemia	(actinomycetes,
Vasculitic causes	Eumycetes)
Rheumatoid arthritis	Other
Systemic lupus	Syphilis (tertiary)
erythematosus	Yaws
Scleroderma	Leishmaniasis
Dermatomyositis	Neoplastic causes
Periarteritis nodosa	Squamous cell carcinoma
Livedoid vasculitis	Basal cell carcinoma
Neurologic causes	Cutaneous lymphoma
Peripheral neuropathy	Kaposi's sarcoma
Tabes dorsalis	Miscellaneous causes
Hereditary sensory neuropathy	Sickle cell anemia
Metabolic causes	Thalassemia
Diabetes mellitus	Cryoglobulinemia
Calcinosis cutis	Pyoderma gangrenosum
Gout	Lichen planus
	Epidermolysis bullosa
	Werner's syndrome
	Prolidase deficiency
	Sarcoidosis

709

Laboratory Evaluation

Laboratory studies are often helpful in differentiating the possible causes of lower extremity ulcers. In a patient whose pedal pulses are decreased, Doppler ultrasound is a noninvasive study that can provide information on the arterial supply to the lower extremity. In Doppler studies the systolic blood pressure of the ankle is compared with that of the arm. In normal individuals the ankle-to-arm Doppler index is 1; an index below 0.9 is indicative of arterial disease.[3] An index of less than 0.5 is associated with absent pedal pulses and is predictive of poor ulcer healing.[4, 5] The Doppler index can be falsely elevated in patients with small vessel disease such as diabetes. In this condition the vessels become calcified and a falsely high index results.[6]

A technique known as transcutaneous partial oxygen pressure ($TcPO_2$) determination is used to measure oxygen delivery to the tissues.[7-9] In this technique, the partial pressure of oxygen in the skin next to the ulcer is measured and compared with that at another reference point, usually the skin on the chest. This technique has the advantage of being a direct measurement of oxygen delivery to tissues. In patients with noncompressible blood vessels (e.g., diabetics), this technique produces a more accurate assessment of tissue oxygenation than the Doppler study. If the patient is thought to have evidence of arterial disease by physical examination and this is confirmed by Doppler examination, arteriography can often determine whether there is a surgically correctable lesion.

In patients with diabetes or other causes of peripheral neuropathy, measurements of sensory perception have been performed using a variety of techniques. The most common measurements use deformable monofilaments. However, much more sophisticated systems, such as those using current perception thresholds, have been used to measure the degree of neuropathy in these patients.[10]

In patients with leg ulcers, laboratory studies that may prove valuable in elucidating the cause include measurements of rheumatoid factor and antinuclear antibody levels; CH_{50} assay; and determination of cryoglobulin, serum protein electrophoresis, and anticardiolipin antibody levels. Skin biopsy is helpful to rule out primary or supervening carcinoma and to diagnose mycobacterial or fungal infections; it may also be valuable in identifying vasculitic lesions.[11]

Causes: Specific Clinical Entities

VENOUS STASIS ULCERS

Venous stasis ulcers are the most common type of leg ulcers, affecting between 0.3 and 1% of the population[2, 12, 13] and costing up to $40,000 per ulcer to treat.[14] As noted earlier, venous stasis ulcers are usually located on the ankle and tibial area (Fig. 53–1). The patient with venous stasis ulcerations typically has palpable pulses, varying degrees of pitting edema, and hyperpigmentation of the involved skin (Fig. 53–2). The ulcers often

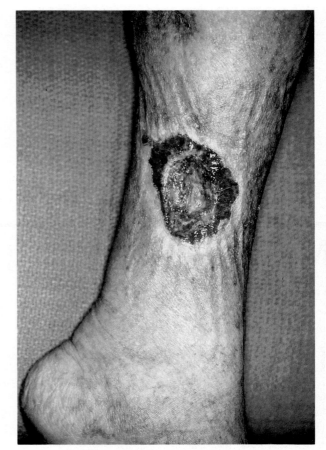

Figure 53–1. Venous stasis ulcer.

heal with white atrophic scars, which must be differentiated from similar scars found in livedoid vasculitis. Histologic features on skin biopsy include an increased number of dermal capillaries, and using the special stain phosphotungstic acid hematoxylin (PTAH), a collar of pericapillary fibrin can be seen around the dermal capillaries.[15] Doppler flow velocity studies demonstrate normal perfusion of the legs in patients whose venous disease is not complicated by arterial insufficiency.[16]

Although it is known that an inadequate venous return is necessary for the development of stasis dermatitis and ulcers, the etiology of incompetent venous valves remains unclear, and the link between venous stasis and skin ulcerations has been disputed. It was originally assumed that thrombophlebitis was the precipitating factor in almost all venous stasis ulcers. However, venograms performed on patients with chronic venous stasis have shown that only half of the patients have demonstrable changes of thrombophlebitis, implying that incompetent deep or superficial venous valves are the primary cause of venous stasis.[17]

How does venous stasis lead to ulcerations? Available evidence points to the deposition of fibrin around capillaries as the primary etiologic factor.[18] This fibrin acts as a barrier to oxygen diffusion, resulting in tissue anoxia and secondary ulceration.[15, 18] Studies of venous ulceration using positron emission tomography showed in-

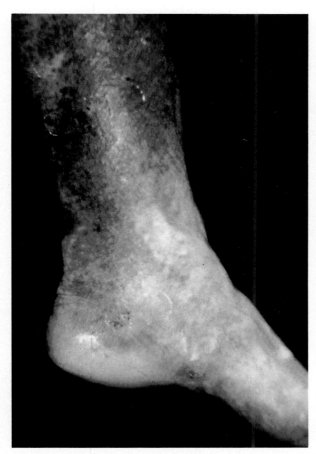

Figure 53–2. Hyperpigmentation and edema associated with stasis dermatitis.

creased blood flow but decreased fractional oxygen extraction in the legs of patients with venous stasis ulcers.[19] This finding could result from increased blood flow through the greater number of dermal capillaries,[15] with a barrier around the capillaries preventing oxygen diffusion into the interstitial tissues. This sheet of fibrin has been shown to allow carbon dioxide but not oxygen diffusion.[15] The syndrome characterized by clinical signs of venous stasis and histologic findings of pericapillary fibrin has been termed lipodermatosclerosis.[15, 18] Support for this theory comes from several studies that have shown that venous hypertension produced experimentally in canine hindlimbs results in a 600% increase in the net transport of fibrinogen into the interstitial tissue.[20] Interestingly, patients with venous stasis ulcers have been demonstrated to have decreased fibrolytic activity not only in the leg but also in hand veins,[21] as well as decreased plasma levels of protein C and protein S-32. These findings imply that a primary defect in fibrinolysis also contributes to the development of these ulcers.[22]

ARTERIAL DISEASE

Leg ulcers caused primarily by arterial insufficiency may be associated with ischemic heart disease, cerebral vascular disease, diabetes, hypertension, and smoking. It is important to remember that arterial disease can also complicate venous stasis ulcers. In a study of 94 patients with venous stasis disease, 15 patients also had coexistent arterial disease.[16] In patients with risk factors for arterial disease and ulcers in appropriate locations such as the toes, dorsal foot, or heel, palpation of pedal pulses often provides important information about the prognosis for ulcer healing. The presence of pedal pulses in both feet was found to correlate with an arm-to-ankle Doppler index of more than 0.5 and toe systolic pressures above 40 mm Hg, which are predictive of arterial healing.[4] Because patients with arterial ulcers often require surgical intervention, a referral to a vascular surgeon is usually indicated.

NEUROTROPIC ULCERATIONS

The most common cause of neurotropic ulcerations is long-standing diabetes mellitus. Neurotropic ulcers are usually located at points of pressure, especially the plantar surfaces of the foot. The ulcer often begins at a site of minor trauma. Characteristically, neurotropic ulcers are painless and are often surrounded by a thick callus. Debridement of these ulcers may reveal a much larger ulcer than was initially seen before callus removal. Ulcer infection is common and typically polymicrobial in nature.[23, 24] The ulcers frequently extend deeply into joint spaces or underlying bones. A grading system (Table 53–2) for diabetic ulcers has been described.[25] Feet with intact skin are labeled as grade 0. An ulcer that involves only skin or subcutaneous tissue is classified as grade 1, while ulcers that extend to underlying tendon or bone without osteomyelitis are classified as grade 2. Ulcers that extend to tendon, bone, or joint capsules with associated osteomyelitis are classified as grade 3. An ulcer associated with gangrene of the toes or distal forefoot is classified as grade 4, while an ulcer with gangrene of the midfoot or hindfoot is classified as a grade 5.

Neuropathy in patients with long-standing diabetes is extremely common. Its prevalence approaches 100% for patients who have had diabetes for more than 20 years.[25] Polyneuropathy with a stocking distribution with loss of pain and temperature sensation is the most common pattern. The associated autonomic neuropathy is often indicated by loss of sweating in the area of the ulcer.

TABLE 53–2. GRADING SYSTEM FOR DIABETIC ULCERS

Grade	Description
0	Intact skin
1	Involvement of skin and subcutaneous tissue
2	Extension to tendon or bone without osteomyelitis
3	Extension to tendon, bone, or joint capsule with osteomyelitis
4	Ulcer associated with gangrene of toes or distal forefoot
5	Ulcer associated with gangrene of mid- or hindfoot

Data from Wagner FW Jr: The dysvascular foot: a system of diagnosis and treatment. Foot Ankle 2:64–122, 1981.

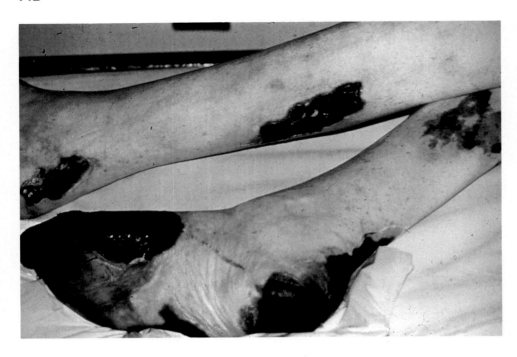

Figure 53–3. Rheumatoid arthritis: necrotizing vasculitis.

Diabetics with sensory neuropathy lose both the sensory and vasodilatory responses of the C fibers in their feet.[26] For this reason, peripheral neuropathy may be important because it increases the risk of trauma and decreases the wound healing response. Doppler measurements are often inaccurate in patients with diabetes, since the arterial walls of these patients become calcified. Patients with an ulcer that extends into a tendon or joint space require radiologic evaluation to rule out osteomyelitis.

VASCULITIC ULCERS

In the lower extremity, chronic indolent ulceration of the dorsal aspect of the toes or over the lower leg is the most common vasculitic ulcer.[27] This is associated with circulating immune complexes and reduced complement levels. Digital vasculitis presenting as small infarcts or gangrene in patients with rheumatoid arthritis is the result of an obliterative endarteritis.[28] Necrotizing vasculitis commonly presents with extensive areas of gangrene of the digits and well-defined geographic ulcers on the lower limb[27] (Fig. 53–3). This form of ulceration most often occurs in association with rheumatoid arthritis, particularly when there is deforming joint disease. Successful management requires early intervention with immunosuppressive therapy.

Vasculitis can involve both small and large vessels in rheumatic disease. However, with the exception of cutaneous periarteritis nodosa, the postcapillary venules are usually the vessels involved in cutaneous ulcers. Thus, foot pulses are usually preserved in patients with ulcerations caused by vasculitis.[27] Vasculitic ulcers are typically well demarcated, have a "punched out" appearance (Fig. 53–4), and are seen on the dorsum of the foot or lower leg. Vasculitic ulcerations are most commonly seen in rheumatoid arthritis but can also be seen in other entities such as systemic lupus erythe-matosus[29, 30] with or without anticardiolipin antibodies,[32] Sjögren's syndrome,[27] scleroderma,[32] and Behçet's syndrome.[33] Rare entities that also may present with leg ulcers include multifocal fibrosclerosis[34] and Takayasu's arteritis.[35]

Rheumatoid Arthritis

Patients with rheumatoid arthritis have been shown to have roughly double the number of leg or foot ulcers compared with age- and sex-matched controls.[36] It has been reported that up to 10% of rheumatoid arthritis patients will suffer from a leg ulcer at some point in their disease.[36] Lesions are most often found on the ankle or lower leg and occur less commonly on the toes. Ulcers tend to be "punched out" and extremely painful. Leukocytoclastic vasculitis is usually seen on histologic

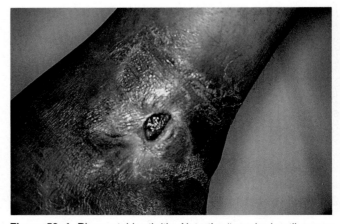

Figure 53–4. Rheumatoid arthritis. Note the "punched out" appearance of the ulcer.

examination, but its absence does not rule out vasculitic disease.[11]

Systemic Lupus Erythematosus

In one study, leg ulcers were found in 5% of patients with systemic lupus erythematosus.[31] These ulcers were noted to occur in the malleolar and pretibial areas and were associated with leukocytoclastic vasculitis or necrotizing arteritis on biopsy. Small and large vessel vasculitis may coexist and manifest as digital infarcts, skin ulcers, or peripheral gangrene. Patients with systemic lupus erythematosus who have circulating anticardiolipin antibodies are at high risk for leg ulcers.[30] Originally described as the "lupus anticoagulant," this antibody is found in patients with a syndrome of recurrent venous thrombosis, spontaneous abortions, livedoid vasculitis, thrombocytopenia, hemolytic anemia,[30, 37] pyoderma gangrenosum, and digital infarcts.[29]

Livedoid Vasculitis

This disorder, named by Bard and Winklemann,[38] is an uncommon cause of leg ulcers. Livedoid vasculitis and stasis dermatitis share the clinical findings of chronic leg ulcers that heal with white atrophic scars or atrophic blanche. Livedoid vasculitis is a separate entity, however, with a distinctive clinical picture of mottled telangiectasis or livedo reticularis (Fig. 53–5) and histologic findings of perivascular lymphocytic infiltration with occlusion and segmental hyalinization of dermal vessels.[38, 39] Livedoid vasculitis differs from the vasculides in that its cellular infiltrate is lymphocytic rather than neutrophilic in nature. Livedoid vasculitis can be idiopathic or associated with connective tissue diseases such as rheumatoid arthritis or systemic lupus erythematosus.

Miscellaneous Causes

Pyoderma gangrenosum usually begins as a purple pustule or nodule that rapidly spreads, with necrosis and ulceration at the center. Typically, an elevated overhanging border with a violaceous rim is seen. This lesion, seen more commonly in women, is associated with a variety of diseases, most often ulcerative colitis.[40] Other conditions associated with this entity are Crohn's disease,[41] chronic active hepatitis,[42] rheumatoid arthritis,[41] and leukemia.[43] Idiopathic pyoderma gangrenosum has been reported in 20[40] to 50%[41] of patients. Lesions of pyoderma gangrenosum heal with atrophic and irregular scars. Biopsies of these lesions show massive numbers of polymorphonuclear cells and vasculitis on histologic examination.

Necrobiosis lipoidica diabeticorum is a chronic disease characterized by ill-defined, yellow-brown plaques that may ulcerate. This condition is usually seen on the pretibial area in diabetics.[44] Histologic findings on biopsy include a dermal granuloma with central necrobiosis, peripheral palisading histocytes, and a decreased number of dermal nerves.

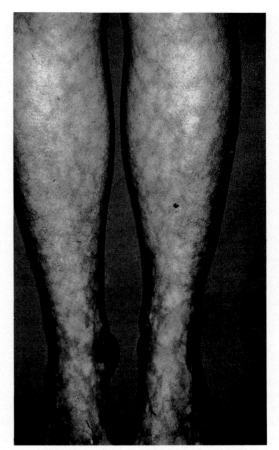

Figure 53–5. Livedoid vasculitis with livedo reticularis.

Infections may also be an important cause of leg ulcers, particularly in immunocompromised patients. *Mycobacterium tuberculosis* (Fig. 53–6), *Mycobacterium leprae*, as well as atypical mycobacterial and deep fungal infections are reported causes of leg ulcerations.[45–47] Barbiturates, ergotism, halogen ingestion, and coumarin have also been reported to cause leg ulcers. Thromboangiitis obliterans, or Buerger's disease, usually seen in men who are cigarette smokers, is an uncommon cause of leg ulcers. Histologic findings on biopsy of these lesions include thrombi in intermediate and small arteries. These lesions are indolent but will not remit until the patient stops smoking.

Leg ulcers seen in infants and children are caused by a different set of diseases. Hereditary sensory neuropathies[48, 49] are seen in infancy or childhood and can manifest as ulcers of the lower extremity. Werner's syndrome[50] and inherited forms of epidermolysis bullosa[51] present with leg or foot ulcerations. Other uncommon syndromes that begin with cutaneous ulcerations in childhood are prolidase deficiency[52] and "Georgian ulcers."[53]

General Treatment Considerations

In treating an ulcer, the physician must first recognize and treat any systemic condition that may inhibit

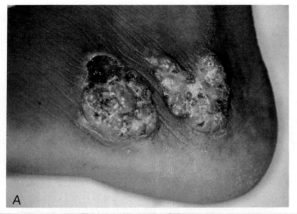

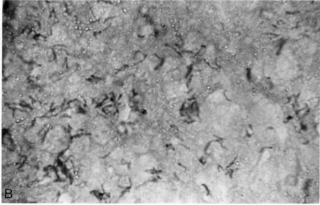

Figure 53–6. *A,* Ulcer caused by *Mycobacterium tuberculosis. B,* Acid-fast stain demonstrates bacilli in biopsy specimen.

wound healing. Systemic diseases, particularly malignant tumors[54] and diabetes mellitus, nutritional deficiencies, and some medications can decrease the rate of wound healing. In addition, deficiencies of vitamin C, zinc, iron, and protein can also retard wound healing, since these nutrients are needed to synthesize collagen. Some medications, such as systemic glucocorticosteriods, decrease the inflammatory response, thus blunting the stimulation of fibroblast collagen production and resulting in impaired wound healing. Other drugs, particularly cytotoxic drugs and nonsteroidal anti-inflammatory drugs, have also been reported to decrease the rate of wound healing.

INFECTION

Infection also slows ulcer healing and should be treated with appropriate antibiotics. Oral agents such as dicloxacillin are appropriate treatment for gram-positive infections, while amoxicillin-clavulanate (Augmentin) will extend bacterial coverage to some gram-negative organisms and anaerobes[23] but not to *Pseudomonas,* which can be effectively treated with ciprofloxacin. New topical agents, such as metronidazole and mupirocin (Bactroban), may prove important in treating some infected ulcers.

SURGICAL DRESSINGS

In recent years new topical dressings[55] have gained wide acceptance (see Chap. 11) in the treatment of leg ulcers (Table 53–3). These products can optimize wound healing by providing a moist environment, which aids keratinocyte migration over the surface of a wound. Some hydrocolloid dressings act to debride the ulcers, while some of the polyurethane and polyethylene dressings allow visualization of the ulcers. All these dressings have the advantage that they decrease pain in the ulcers on application. This is helpful in treating painful ulcers such as those seen in scleroderma. These dressings do not increase the risk of infection in ulcers colonized with bacteria. A problem has arisen when these dressings, particularly the adherent ones, are used on exudative ulcers, as the resultant periulcer skin maceration can actually cause the ulcers to enlarge.

VASOACTIVE MEDICATIONS

Some vasoactive agents have been reported to be effective in a variety of conditions. Nifedipine is effective in Raynaud's disease as a result of its ability to restore blood flow to the digits.[56] Ketanserin, an S-serotoninergic blocker, is helpful in treating ischemic ulcers, livedoid vasculitis, and stasis ulcers.[57, 58] Pentoxifylline (Trental) is effective in treatment of the above conditions[59, 60] and also in necrobiosis lipoidica diabeticorum[61] and ulcers caused by sickle cell anemia. The mechanism of action for pentoxifylline was originally thought to be a result of its ability to increase red blood cell deformity. However, it may also act by stimulating prostacyclin synthesis, decreasing platelet aggregation, and increasing fibrinolysis. Other physical modalities of treatment, such as transcutaneous electrical nerve stimulation,[62] may also act by increasing blood flow, in addition to possible direct effects on the skin.

Treatment of Specific Causes of Leg Ulcers

VENOUS STASIS ULCERS

Specific treatment of venous stasis disease must first be directed toward reducing the venous hypertension. The simplest method for achieving this is the use of support hose, either custom or ready made. Patients with venous stasis disease should wear support hose even when they do not have active ulcers, as this treatment will help prevent recurrences.

For patients with ulcers who cannot wear support hose, treatment with Unna boots has shown to help heal venous stasis ulcers. These boots, introduced in 1896, consist of a mixture of zinc oxide, calamine lotion, and glycerin used to wrap the extremity from the foot to the knee; this is covered with an elastic bandage and changed weekly. This form of treatment is often not well accepted by patients, as the boot must be kept dry, and it is inconvenient to use. However, studies comparing Unna boots to other treatments for venous stasis

TABLE 53–3. **SYNTHETIC SURGICAL DRESSINGS**

Dressing Type	Characteristics			
	Adhesive	Transparent	Absorbent	Gas Permeable
Polyurethane				
Op-Site	+	+	−	+
Tegaderm	+	+	−	+
Bioclusive	+	+	−	+
Ensure	+	+	−	+
Polyethylene oxide/water (Hydrogel)				
Vigilon	−	Partially	+	+
Spenco second skin	−	Partially	+	+
Hydrocolloid				
DuoDerm	+	−	+	−
Comfeel Ulcus	+	−	+	−

ulcers have shown them to be superior to both support hose and hydrocolloid dressings.[63, 64]

A third means of reducing venous hypertension is through the use of intermittent pneumatic compression. Devices that intermittently apply graded pressure to the ulcerated leg have been reported to improve the partial pressure of the oxygen in the skin adjacent to venous stasis ulcers,[8] although this effect has been disputed.[9]

For stasis ulcers that are refractory to these treatments, some of the surgical approaches include excision of incompetent valves, leg valve reconstruction, or transplantation of a competent brachial vein valve to leg veins.[65–67] Treatment of ulcers with hyperbaric oxygen has become less common, as it has been shown that this modality causes endothelial cell toxicity.[68]

Two avenues that have great potential therapeutic benefits are the topical use of growth factors and transplantation of cultured keratinocytes as skin grafts to cover these wounds. In clinical trials, treatment with epidermal growth factor has been shown to hasten healing at skin graft sites.[69] In addition, application of platelet-derived wound healing factor has been reported to optimize wound healing in patients with chronic ulcers.[70] Treating ulcers with a sheet of keratinocytes grown from either autologous[71] or allogeneic[72] cells has the advantage of requiring only a small amount of donor tissue, which can then be expanded by culturing the cells in a tissue culture laboratory. Allogeneic skin grafts using neonatal keratinocytes have the additional advantage of faster growth, better response to mitogens, and increased production of growth factors[73] (see Chap. 76). These new treatments can be used alone, in combination with topical agents, or with conventional grafting procedures.

Patients with ulcers caused by arterial disease are best managed with vascular surgery. However, ketanserin has also been reported to improve the profusion of skin in arterial ulcers.[57]

NEUROPATHIC ULCERS

The treatment of neuropathic ulcers focuses on relieving external pressure and treating concomitant infection. Relief of pressure requires avoidance of all weight-bearing activities on the affected area. This can be obtained with the use of crutches, a wheelchair, or total contact casting. Most patients with grade 1 or 2 neuropathic ulcers can be effectively managed with simple outpatient care. Patients with grade 3 ulcerations associated with osteomyelitis require hospitalization for treatment with intravenous antibiotics and surgical debridement. If these methods are ineffective, amputation is usually required.[5] It is important to note that even after effective treatment of an acute ulcer has resulted in healing, the patient must be carefully managed to prevent recurrences. This usually requires the use of special fitted shoes and careful attention to pedicures. All patients should be fully educated to note any small break in the skin and bring it to the rapid attention of a physician.

VASCULITIC ULCERS

Treatment of vasculitic ulcers can be difficult, as the medications that suppress the underlying condition often retard wound healing. General measures such as elevation of the leg and topical treatment can facilitate healing. Systemic suppression of the rheumatologic disease underlying the ulcers is often required. The mainstay of systemic therapy is corticosteroid treatment, usually in the form of oral prednisone. For rheumatoid arthritis, D-penicillamine, colchicine, dapsone, and cyclophosphamide have also been advocated in treating this type of ulcer. For ulcers associated with systemic lupus erythematosus, both azathioprine and cyclophosphamide have been reported to aid healing. It should be noted that clinical improvement in patients with anticardiolipin antibodies does not necessarily correlate with a decrease in antibody titers.[30] The mainstay of therapy in managing patients with livedoid vasculitis has been anticoagulation using aspirin, ticlopidine, or dipyridamole,[74] but newer drugs such as ketanserin[58] and pentoxifylline[60] have also been reported to improve this condition.

MISCELLANEOUS CONDITIONS

Pyoderma gangrenosum has generally been treated with corticosteroids (intralesional triamcinolone or oral prednisone) or pulse therapy.[75] Other regimens reported to be effective include a 2% topical solution of sodium cromoglycolate[76] and immunosuppressive agents such as cyclophosphamide and cyclosporine.[77-79] Antimicrobial agents such as clofazimine,[80] minocycline,[81] and vancomycin with mezlocillin[82] have also been reported to be effective.

Topical occlusive dressings are helpful in treating ulcers caused by epidermolysis bullosa acquisita and scleroderma.[83] Oral cyclosporine is effective in treating severe epidermolysis bullosa acquisita.[78] Ulcerative necrobiosis lipoidica diabeticorum may respond to topical clobetasol proprionate (Temovate), intralesional corticosteroids, or oral pentoxifylline.[61]

SUMMARY

Leg ulcers are a common condition, with most occurring in patients with venous stasis. Other diagnoses must be considered, particularly in patients with extremely painful ulcers, ulcers on the feet, or pre-existing diabetes or connective tissue disease. Surgical treatment includes biopsy,[11] debridement,[24] amputation,[5] correction of arterial insufficiency,[16] removal of incompetent venous valves,[65, 66] autologous skin grafts,[71, 72] and even simple pinch grafting techniques.[84] If success is to be achieved in treating a patient with a leg ulcer, the physician must recognize and treat secondary infection, immunosuppression,[85] underlying systemic or vascular disease, and other concurrent conditions that may interfere with wound healing.

REFERENCES

1. Callam MJ, Ruckley CV, Harper DR, Dale JJ: Chronic ulceration of the leg: extent of the problem and provision of care. Br Med J 290:1855–1856, 1985.
2. Hansson C: Studies on leg and foot ulcers. Acta Derm Venereol 136(S):1–28, 1988.
3. Prineas RJ, Harland WR, Janzon L, et al: Recommendations for use of non-invasive methods to detect atherosclerotic peripheral arterial disease in population studies. Circulation 65:1561A–1566A, 1982.
4. Christensen JH, Freundlich M, Jacobsen BA, Falstie-Jensen N: Clinical relevance of pedal pulse palpation in patients suspected of peripheral arterial insufficiency. J Intern Med 226:95–99, 1989.
5. Wagner FW Jr: Amputations at the foot and ankle: current status. Clin Orthop 122:62–69, 1977.
6. Harrelson JM: Management of the diabetic foot. Orthop Clin North Am 20:605–619, 1989.
7. White RA, Nolan L, Harley D, et al: Non-invasive evaluation of peripheral vascular disease using transcutaneous oxygen tension. Am J Surg 144:68–74, 1982.
8. Pertti JK, Pekanmaki K, Pohjola RT: Transcutaneous oxygen tension in patients with post-thrombotic leg ulcers: treatment with intermittent pneumatic compression. Cardiovasc Res 22:138–141, 1988.
9. Nemeth AJ, Falanga V, Alstadt SP, Eaglstein WH: Ulcerated edematous limbs: effect of edema removal on transcutaneous oxygen measurements. J Am Acad Dermatol 20:191–197, 1989.
10. Masson EA, Veves A, Fernando D, Boulton AJM: Current perception thresholds: a new, quick, and reproducible method for the assessment of peripheral neuropathy in diabetes mellitus. Diabetologia 32:724–728, 1989.
11. Scott DGI, Bacon PA, Tribe CR: Systemic rheumatoid vasculitis: a clinic and laboratory study of 50 cases. Medicine 60:288–297, 1981.
12. Dolen JE, Paraskos JA, Ockene IS, et al: Venous thromboembolism: scope of the problem. Chest 89(S):370–373, 1986.
13. Immelman EJ, Jeffery PC: The post-phlebitic syndrome: patho-
14. O'Donnell TF, Browse NL, Burnand KG: The socioeconomic effects of iliofemoral venous thrombosis. J Surg Res 22:483–487, 1977.
15. Burnand KG, Whimster I, Nardov A, Browse NL: Pericapillary fibrin in the ulcer bearing skin of the leg: the cause of lipodermatosclerosis and venous ulceration. Br Med J 285:1071–1072, 1982.
16. Sundrup JH, Groth S, Arnstrop C, et al: Coexistence of obstructive arterial disease and chronic venous stasis in leg ulcer patients. Clin Exp Dermatol 12:410–412, 1987.
17. Train JS, Schanzer H, Peirce C, et al: Radiological evaluation of the chronic venous stasis syndrome. JAMA 258:941–944, 1987.
18. Browse NL: The pathogenesis of venous ulceration: a hypothesis. J Vasc Surg 7:468–472, 1988.
19. Hopkins FG, Spinks TJ, Rhodes CG, et al: Positron emission tomography in venous ulceration and liposclerosis: study of regional tissue function. Br Med J 286:333–336, 1983.
20. Leach R, Browse NL: Effect of venous hypertension on canine hind limb lymph. Br J Surg 72:275–278, 1985.
21. Browse NL, Gray L, Jarrett PEM, Morland M: Blood and vein-wall fibrinolytic activity in health and vascular disease. Br Med J 1:478–481, 1977.
22. Wolfe JHN, Morland M, Browse NL: The fibrinolytic activity of varicose veins. Br J Surg 66:185–187, 1979.
23. Neu H: β-Lactamase, β-lactamase inhibitors, and skin and skin-structure infections. J Am Acad Dermatol 22:896–904, 1990.
24. Lipsky BA: Outpatient management of uncomplicated lower extremity infections in diabetic patients. Arch Intern Med 150:790–797, 1990.
25. Wagner FW Jr: The dysvascular foot: a system for diagnosis and treatment. Foot Ankle 2:64–122, 1981.
26. Parkhouse N, LeQuesne PM: Impaired neurogenic vascular response in patients with diabetes and neuropathic foot lesions. N Engl J Med 318:1306–1309, 1988.
27. Cawley M: Vasculitis and ulceration in rheumatic diseases of the foot. Clin Rheumatol 1:315–333, 1987.
28. Golding JR, Hamilton MG, Gill RS: Arteritis of rheumatoid arthritis. Br J Dermatol 77:207–210, 1965.
29. Grob J-J, Bonerandi J-J: Cutaneous manifestations associated with the presence of the lupus anticoagulant. J Am Acad Dermatol 15:211–219, 1986.
30. Alarcòn-Segovia D, Delez M, Oria C, et al: Antiphospholipid syndrome in systemic lupus erythematosus. Medicine 68:353–365, 1989.
31. Wallace DJ, Dubois EL: Dubois' Lupus Erythematosus. 3rd ed. Lea & Febiger, Philadelphia, 1987.
32. Tuffanelli DL, Winklemann RK: Systemic scleroderma: a clinical study of 727 cases. Arch Dermatol 84:359–371, 1961.
33. Lee SH, Chung KY, Lee WS, Lee SL: Behçet's syndrome associated with bullous necrotizing vasculitis. J Am Acad Dermatol 21:327–330, 1989.
34. Fisher GO, Delaney WE: Multifocal fibrosclerosis: cutaneous associations. Aust J Dermatol 27:19–26, 1986.
35. Perniciaro CV, Winkelmann RK, Hunder GG: Cutaneous manifestations of Takayasu's arteritis. J Am Acad Dermatol 17:998–1005, 1987.
36. Thurtle OA, Cawley M: The frequency of leg ulceration in rheumatoid arthritis: a survey. J Rheumatol 10:507–509, 1983.
37. Grattan CEH, Burton JL, Boon AP: Sneddon's syndrome (livedo reticularis and cerebral thrombosis) with livedo vasculitis and anticardiolipin antibodies. Br J Dermatol 120:441–447, 1989.
38. Bard JW, Winklemann RK: Livedoid vasculitis: segmental hyalinizing vasculitis of the dermis. Arch Dermatol 96:489–499, 1967.
39. Gray HR, Graham JH, Johnson W, et al: Atrophie blanche: periodic painful ulcers of the lower extremities: a clinical and histopathologic entity. Arch Dermatol 93:187–193, 1966.
40. Perry HO: Pyoderma gangrenosum. South Med J 62:899–908, 1969.
41. Hickman JG, Lazarus GS: Pyoderma gangrenosum: a reappraisal of associated systemic diseases. Br J Dermatol 102:135–137, 1980.
42. Byrne JP, Hewitt M, Summerly R: Pyoderma gangrenosum associated with chronic active hepatitis. Arch Dermatol 112:1297–1301, 1976.
43. Perry HO, Winkelmann RK: Bullous pyoderma gangrenosum and leukemia. Arch Dermatol 106:901–905, 1972.

13. physiology, prevention and management. Clin Chest Med 5:537–550, 1984.

44. Huntley AC: The cutaneous manifestations of diabetes mellitus. J Am Acad Dermatol 6:427–455, 1982.

45. Brown FS, Anderson RH, Burnett JW: Cutaneous tuberculosis. J Am Acad Dermatol 6:101–106, 1982.

46. Massa MC, Doyle JA: Cutaneous cryptococcosis simulating pyoderma gangrenosum. J Am Acad Dermatol 5:32–36, 1981.

47. Wilson JW, Cawley EP, Weidman FD, et al: Primary cutaneous North American blastomycosis. Arch Dermatol 71:39–45, 1955.

48. Dyck PJ, Mellinger JF, Reagan TJ, et al: Not indifference to pain but varieties of hereditary sensory and autonomic neuropathy. Brain 106:373–390, 1983.

49. Böckers M, Benes P, Bork K: Persistent skin ulcers, mutilations and acro-osteolysis in hereditary sensory and autonomic neuropathy with phospholipid excretion. J Am Acad Dermatol 21:736–739, l989.

50. Salk D: Werner's syndrome: a review of recent research with an analysis of connective tissue metabolism, growth control of cultured cells, and chromosomal aberrations. Hum Genet 62:1–15, 1982.

51. Fine JD, Johnson L: Efficacy of systemic phenytoin in the treatment of junctional epidermolysis bullosa. Arch Dermatol 124:1402–1406, 1988.

52. Pierard GE, Cornil F, Lapiere CM: Pathogenesis of ulcerations in deficiency of prolidase: the role of angiopathy and deposits of amyloid. Am J Dermatopathol 6:491–497, 1984.

53. Suster S, Ronnen M, Bubis JJ, Schewach-Millet M: Familial atrophie blanche–like lesions with subcutaneous fibrinoid vasculitis: the Georgian ulcers. Am J Dermatopathol 8:386–391, 1986.

54. Tan IB, Drexhage HA, Scheper RJ, et al: Defective monocyte chemostasis in patients with head and neck cancer. Arch Otolaryngol Head Neck Surg 112:541–544, 1986.

55. Wheeland RG: The newer surgical dressings and wound healing. Dermatol Clin 5:393–407, 1987.

56. Kahan A, Weber S, Amor B, et al: Nifedipine and Raynaud's phenomenon. Letter. Ann Intern Med 94:546, 1981.

57. Janssen PAJ, Janssen H, Cauwenbergh G, et al: Use of topical ketanserin in the treatment of skin ulcers: a double-blind study. J Am Acad Dermatol 21:85–90, 1989.

58. Rustin MHA, Bunker CB, Dowd PM: Chronic leg ulceration with livedoid vasculitis, and response to oral ketanserin. Br J Dermatol 120:101–105, 1989.

59. Sauer GC: Pentoxifylline (Trental) therapy for the vasculitis of atrophie blanche. Arch Dermatol 122:380–381, 1986.

60. Ely H, Bard JW: Therapy of livedo vasculitis with pentoxifylline. Cutis 42:448–453, 1988.

61. Littler CM, Tschen EH: Pentoxifylline for necrobiosis lipoidica diabeticorum. Letter. J Am Acad Dermatol 17: 314–315, 1987.

62. Ely H: Shocking therapy: uses of transcutaneous electric nerve stimulation in dermatology. Dermatol Clin 9:1–9, 1991.

63. Kikta MJ, Schuler JJ, Meyer JP, et al: A prospective, randomized trial of Unna's boots vs hydroactive dressing in the treatment of venous stasis ulcers. J Vasc Surg 7:478–483, 1988.

64. Hendricks WM, Swallow RT: Management of stasis leg ulcers with Unna's boots vs elastic support stockings. J Am Acad Dermatol 12:90–98, 1985.

65. Eriksson I: Reconstructive venous surgery. Acta Chir Scand Suppl 544:69–74, 1988.

66. Cikrit DF, Nichols WK, Silver D: Surgical management of refractory venous stasis ulceration. J Vasc Surg 7:473–477, 1988.

67. Taheri SA, Lazer L, Elias S, et al: Surgical treatment of postphlebitic syndrome with vein valve transplant. Am J Surg 144:221–224, 1982.

68. Heng MC, Kloss SG: Endothelial cell toxicity in leg ulcers treated with topical hyperbaric O_2. Am J Dermatopathol 8:403–410, 1986.

69. Brown GL, Nanney LB, Griffein J, et al: Enhancement of wound healing by topical treatment with epidermal growth factor. N Engl J Med 321:76–79, 1989.

70. Knighton DR, Fiegel VD, Austin LL, et al: Classification and treatment of chronic non-healing wounds: successful treatment of autologous platelet derived wound healing factor (PDWHF). Ann Surg 204:322–330, 1986.

71. Helton JM, Caldwell D, Biozes B, et al: Grafting of skin ulcers with cultured autologous epidermal cells. J Am Acad Dermatol 14:399–405, 1986.

72. Phillips TJ, Kehinde O, Green H, Gilchrest BA: Treatment of skin ulcers with cultured epidermal allografts. J Am Acad Dermatol 21:191–199, 1989.

73. Stanulis-Praeger BM, Gilchrest BA: Growth factor responsiveness declines during adulthood for human skin-derived cells. Mech Ageing Dev 35:185–198, 1986.

74. Yamamoto M, Danno K, Shio H, Imamura S: Antithrombotic treatment in livedo vasculitis. J Am Acad Dermatol 18:57–62, 1988.

75. Johnson RB, Lazarus GS: Pulse therapy: therapeutic efficacy in the treatment of pyoderma gangrenosum. Arch Dermatol 118:76–84, 1982.

76. De Cock KM, Thorne MG: The treatment of pyoderma gangrenosum with sodium cromoglycolate. Br J Dermatol 102:231–233, 1980.

77. Newell LM, Malkinson FD: Pyoderma gangrenosum: response to cyclophosphamide therapy. Arch Dermatol 119:495–497, 1983.

78. Gupta A, Ellis C, Nickoloff B, et al: Oral cyclosporine in the treatment of inflammatory and non-inflammatory dermatoses. Arch Dermatol 126:339–350, 1990.

79. Shelley ED, Shelley WE: Cyclosporine therapy for pyoderma gangrenosum associated with sclerosing cholangitis and ulcerative colitis. J Am Acad Dermatol 18:l084–1088, 1988.

80. Michaëlsson G, Molin L, Ohman S, et al: Clofazimine. A new agent for the treatment of pyoderma gangrenosum. Arch Dermatol 112:344–349, 1976.

81. Lynch WS, Bergfeld WF: Pyoderma gangrenosum responsive to minocycline hydrochloride. Cutis 21:535–538, 1978.

82. Kang S, Dover JS: Successful treatment of eruptive pyoderma gangrenosum with intravenous vancomycin and mezlocillin. Br J Dermatol 123:389–393, 1990.

83. Milburn PB, Singer JZ, Milburn MA: Treatment of scleroderma skin ulcers with a hydrocolloid membrane. J Am Acad Dermatol 21:200–204, 1989.

84. Wheeland RG: The technique and current status of pinch grafting. J Dermatol Surg Oncol 13:873–880, 1987.

85. Hotter AN: Wound healing and immunocompromise. Nurs Clin North Am 25:193–203, 1990.

CHAPTER 54

Management of Actinic Keratoses

SORREL S. RESNIK and BARRY I. RESNIK

Many modalities have been considered in the treatment of actinic keratoses, including simple surgical excision, electrosurgery, and dermabrasion; cryosurgery and lasers; and topical chemotherapy, including 5-fluorouracil alone or in various combinations with retinoids, trichloroacetic acid, or phenol.

Pathogenesis of Actinic Keratoses

Actinic keratoses (AKs) are mainly caused by ultraviolet light B (UVB) radiation in the wavelengths of 290 to 320 nm, which are implicated as the most carcinogenic, with augmentation by ultraviolet light A (UVA) radiation. AKs are most often seen on sun-exposed areas such as the extensor surfaces of the arms, dorsum of the hands, face, ears, scalp, neck, shoulders, and upper chest. The typical patient is most often a male in his fifties, with fair skin and a history of unprotected sun exposure. However, younger people, both male and female, are also currently presenting with AKs, a result of the inaccurate assumption that being tanned is related to being fit. Although tanning and sunbathing both continue to be problems, public education by way of television, radio, and newspapers has dramatically improved the awareness of the dangers of skin cancer. However, educating the pediatric and teen populations about these hazards is a most difficult problem. Sun damage early in life results in the premature appearance of AKs and skin cancers in individuals as young as 20, 30, and 40 years old. This damage may also be accelerated by the use of tanning parlors that cause artificial tanning, a practice that has dramatically increased since the mid-1980s. As a result, there are numerous reports of cutaneous burns and ocular damage consisting of both corneal and retinal injuries.[1]

Although the harmful skin effects from prolonged exposure with these devices is not fully known at this time, medical professionals should be prepared to treat the anticipated increased incidence of AKs and skin cancers that could result from this popular but dangerous activity.[2]

The importance of preserving the stratospheric ozone shield is an environmental issue of increasing debate. This ozone layer protects our skin from the damaging short-wavelength ultraviolet C (UVC) rays. Ozone is produced by the effect of ultraviolet light, which splits oxygen molecules in two. One of these atoms then combines with another oxygen molecule, forming the three-oxygen-atom molecule known as ozone. Chlorine removes ozone from the stratosphere and accumulates as a result of the production and release of man-made propellant and coolant gases such as chlorofluorocarbons.[3]

Clinical Features

Most AKs are less than 1 cm in diameter and occur as flat or slightly raised erythematous lesions with adherent epidermal scales on the surface. AKs are palpable as dry, rough, flesh-colored or whitish-yellow papules or nodules. Some lesions clinically show considerable hyperplasia (Fig. 54–1) and may require biopsy and histologic examination to rule out possible malignant degeneration. In addition, pigmented lesions also exist, which at times makes differentiation from lentigo maligna melanoma difficult.

Microscopic Features

There are five recognized histologic types of AKs: hypertrophic, atrophic, bowenoid, acantholytic, and pig-

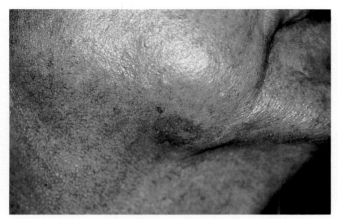

Figure 54–1. Clinical appearance of a hyperplastic type of actinic keratosis.

mented. The shared characteristic feature of all AKs is evidence of actinic damage. This includes moderate to severe elastosis of dermal collagen and a chronic inflammatory infiltrate of lymphocytes, histiocytes, and plasma cells. Parakeratosis, hyperkeratosis, hypergranulosis, atrophy, and acanthosis can all be found in both the epidermis and mucous membrane epithelium. Atypical keratinocytes begin to replace the basal layer of the epidermis above the sebaceous gland layer and are sometimes accompanied by liquefactive degeneration or acantholysis. Atypical keratinocytes are characterized by hyperchromatic nuclei, prominent nucleoli, abundant mitoses, and malignant dyskeratosis.

In the hypertrophic form, hyperkeratosis is a prominent feature, causing a build-up of scale. Atrophic AKs, on the other hand, show a thin, atrophic epidermis with dermoepidermal liquefaction degeneration. Bowenoid AKs, unlike the lesions in Bowen's disease, spare the outer root sheath of the hair follicle.

The distinction between an actinic keratosis and squamous cell carcinoma (SCC) may be difficult. Some dermatopathologists feel that AKs are SCCs in situ because of the morphologically anaplastic cells that are present.[4] One recent report has suggested that as many as 20% of patients with AKs will develop SCC in one or more lesions.[5] Microscopically, these lesions invade through the dermoepidermal junction with atypical keratinocytes that penetrate to various depths in the dermis.

Prognosis

Although there are reports of spontaneous disappearance of AKs[6] with reappearance weeks to months later, a percentage of AKs can be anticipated to develop into squamous cell carcinomas.[7, 8] Fortunately, the types of SCC that develop from AKs are less aggressive and usually do not metastasize. Therefore, it is best to consider AK lesions premalignant and institute treatment in all cases. For large, indurated, or atypical lesions, pathologic examination should be performed.

Treatment

The type of treatment required will vary depending on the size, duration, location, and aggressiveness of the lesion. The two main methods of treatment of AKs are surgical removal and topical chemotherapy (Table 54–1).

SURGICAL TREATMENT

Cryosurgery

The use of liquid nitrogen (LN_2) to destroy AKs is the most prevalent form of treatment (see Chap. 61). A cotton-tipped applicator is saturated by dipping into a thermos or a small steel cup containing LN_2 and applied for 5 to 15 seconds with contact pressure.[9] A cryostat spray apparatus can be used in place of cotton-tipped applicators. If a biopsy specimen is desired, the lesion can be removed by shaving with a scalpel to the desired depth and treating the resultant defect with cryosurgery. The main complication with LN_2 is the resultant permanent depigmentation. This can be most upsetting to patients when the upper chest and face are involved. Patients must be told of this possible permanent change before treatment. If the freeze is of short duration, usually less pigmentary alteration will occur.

Curettage and Electrodesiccation

If the lesion has indistinct borders, treatment with curettage and electrodesiccation is preferred. In this way, the lesion can be submitted for histologic examination. Electrodesiccation reduces the size of the surgical site but can also result in permanent depigmentation or hypopigmentation in some patients. Curettage allows the cutaneous surgeon to determine the depth of invasion into the underlying tissue. If the center is soft,

TABLE 54–1. **TREATMENT METHODS FOR ACTINIC KERATOSES**

Surgical removal methods
    Cryosurgery (liquid nitrogen)
    Curettage and electrosurgery
    Dermabrasion
    Excision
Topical chemotherapy methods
    5-fluorouracil (5-FU)
    5-FU plus tretinoin
    Tretinoin plus 5-FU and trichloroacetic acid (TCA)
    5-FU plus cryosurgery
    TCA
    Phenol
    Alpha-hydroxy acids
    Topical arotinoid
    Interferon
    Deoxycoformycin

more tissue can be removed to help differentiate neoplastic tissue from precancerous tissue.

Dermabrasion

Dermabrasion can be used if there is extensive skin damage from actinic degeneration and many AKs are present. This treatment is not recommended for the neck, arms, hands, or chest. This is an excellent treatment for lesions of the scalp, as they are often more inflamed, thicker and less responsive to treatment. Dermabrasion of scalp lesions with a coarse diamond fraise in patients age 61 to 71 years can result in eradication of AKs, improvement in both the color and texture of the skin, and a simultaneous reduction in the superficial telangiectasia.[10] Healing occurs in about 6 days, with erythema and a line of demarcation persisting for 6 to 8 weeks. Facial dermabrasion for widespread keratoses can also result in a more youthful, wrinkle-free appearance.[11] For both the scalp and face, the depth of dermabrasion is important when removing the epidermis and a portion of the papillary dermis. Dermabrasion that is too deep can result in permanent hypopigmentation and hypertrophic scarring.

Excision

AKs can be surgically excised and sutured. However, the resultant scar is larger and more disfiguring than with other techniques. Therefore, this procedure should be reserved for large or markedly anaplastic lesions, which are likely to show early evidence of SCC on histopathologic examination.

TOPICAL CHEMOTHERAPY

5-Fluorouracil

Topical 5-fluorouracil (5-FU) cream has been effectively used in treatment of AKs that involve large areas such as the face (Fig. 54–2 A), arms, dorsum of the hands, and chest.[12] The duration of treatment typically ranges from 4 to 8 weeks, but for more keratotic lesions, 12 weeks may be needed. Studies have shown that 1% and 5% creams are equally effective.[13] The 5-FU cream is applied twice daily, in the morning and at bedtime, to affected areas. The patient should be seen at weekly intervals, as after 1 to 2 weeks of treatment, many previously invisible or "silent" lesions will often become clinically apparent (Fig. 54–2B). Depending on skin type and lesion activity, cutaneous inflammatory reactions may be insignificant or severe. Patient reassurance may often be needed, especially if the reaction is severe. Marked inflammation can be treated with simultaneous application of topical steroid ointment, since this does not interfere with the desired antineoplastic effect. Inadequate treatment is usually a result of poor patient compliance secondary to discomfort or disfigurement. Other systemic chemotherapeutic drugs have also been shown to produce inflammation of pre-existing AKs[14] similar to that seen with 5-FU.[15] New topical agents for

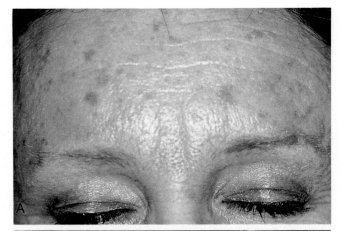

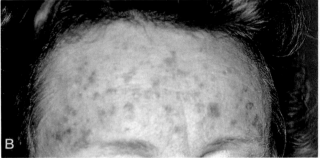

Figure 54–2. *A,* After 1 week of topical use of 1% 5-fluorouracil cream, a few actinic keratoses have become inflamed. *B,* Numerous actinic keratoses have become visible in the same patient after 2 weeks of treatment with topical 5-fluorouracil cream.

the treatment of AKs that cause less local irritation may soon be developed.

Topical 5-FU Cream and Tretinoin

Facial involvement with AKs normally can be treated with topical 5-FU cream alone. However, the reaction can be intensified by stripping off the statum corneum with the use of topical tretinoin cream at a concentration of 0.05%.[16, 17] The 5-FU cream is applied in the morning and evening, while the tretinoin cream is applied only at midday. This treatment program is continued for 4 weeks.

Treatment of the arms, hands, and scalp is invariably improved with tretinoin pretreatment or tretinoin used in conjunction with 5-FU cream.[18, 19] For pretreatment, tretinoin is applied every morning and evening for 2 weeks. At that time, tretinoin is replaced by 1% 5-FU cream. The inflammatory reaction is much more rapid, which reduces the treatment course to 4 weeks.

Combined Tretinoin and 5-FU Cream Plus Trichloroacetic Acid

This treatment program consists of application of 0.05% tretinoin cream in the morning and 5-FU cream at night. Application of 20 to 35% trichloroacetic acid (TCA) is done weekly in the physician's office to the involved areas.[20] TCA induces chemoexfoliation[21] with-

TABLE 54–2. TRICHLOROACETIC ACID FORMULAS

50% Formula		
TCA (USP) crystals	50 gm	
Distilled water qs ad	100 ml	
20% Formula		
TCA (USP) crystals	20 gm	
Distilled water qs ad	100 ml	

out resulting in systemic absorption.[22] A more intense reaction is produced in both normal skin and AKs with the combined treatment.[23] The length of treatment is reduced to 4 weeks with this combination. The intensity of the reaction can be reduced with brief cessation of treatment for 1 week followed by resumption of therapy.

Combined Topical 5-FU Cream and Cryosurgery

After 5-FU cream has been applied morning and night for a 2-week period, the AKs become highlighted by inflammation. This permits individual treatment with liquid nitrogen.[24] No additional topical therapy is required, and the treatment process is reduced by 2 to 4 weeks.

Trichloroacetic Acid

TCA alone can be applied to individual AKs in a manner similar to that used for LN$_2$. The strength of TCA used (Table 54–2) varies from 20 to 50%, with treatment always initiated at the lowest concentration (Fig. 54–3). If a lesion recurs after one treatment, it can be retreated using the next highest concentration. Hypopigmentation can occur but is a problem much less often than with either LN$_2$ or phenol treatment. In this technique, TCA is applied until the area becomes whitened, which indicates coagulation of the stratum corneum and epidermis and penetration into the upper dermis. If 20% TCA does not produce immediate whitening, it can be reapplied to the individual lesion to accelerate the reaction. Both 35% and 50% TCA precipitate whitening of the treatment area within seconds of application. The lesions begin to desquamate in 2 to 5 days, leaving normal-appearing skin. Incompletely removed lesions can be retreated in 2 to 3 weeks. Use of 50% TCA can cause hypo- or hyperpigmentation, depending on the treated area.

Phenol

The Baker-Gordon phenol formula (Table 54–3) can be used in the same manner as 20 to 50% TCA on individual lesions and is applied with cotton-tipped applicators. Because of reports of cardiac arrhythmias,[25] presumably because of the rapid absorption of phenol, treatment should be limited to only ten lesions per session. The common occurrences of de- and hypopigmentation are probably a result of the deep penetration

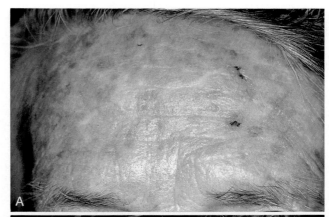
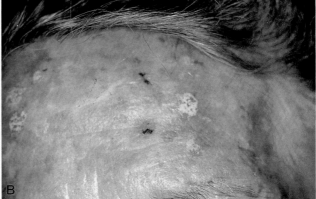

Figure 54–3. *A,* Clinical appearance of a patient with multiple actinic keratoses before treatment. *B,* Whitening or "frosting" of the skin surface is seen immediately after treatment with 50% trichloroacetic acid.

and the destructive effects of phenol on epidermal melanocytes.[26]

OTHER THERAPEUTIC MODALITIES

Alpha-hydroxy Acids

The alpha-hydroxy acids (AHA)—glycolic, pyruvic, and lactic acids—act to reduce corneocyte cohesion,[27] resulting in epidermolysis. They can be used in conjunction with 5-FU, similar to the procedure using topical tretinoin. The depth of wounding increases as alpha-hydroxy acid concentrations approach 12%.

Topical Arotinoid

It has been shown that topical arotinoid methyl sulfone 0.05% cream unmasks AKs, similar to 5-FU.

TABLE 54–3. BAKER-GORDON PHENOL FORMULA

USP phenol	3 ml	
Tap water	2 ml	
Septisol Liquid Soap	9 gtt	
Croton oil	3 gtt	

However, this agent causes much less erythema, scaling, and discomfort than 5-FU or tretinoin.[28]

Interferon and Deoxycoformycin

Systemic chemotherapy with interferon[29] and 21-deoxycoformycin[30] have been shown to cause inflammation of pre-existing AKs, in the same manner as systemic administration of 5-FU. Interferon can be injected intralesionally into AKs with clinical improvement. Although histologic studies revealed the persistence of AKs, there was evidence of reduced cell activity.[29] A regimen of three injections per week for 2 consecutive weeks gave the best results.

SUMMARY

The effective management of actinic keratoses requires that the cutaneous surgeon have a complete understanding of the pathogenesis of AKs, the patient prognosis, and the treatment options available for this common clinical entity. In addition, the number, distribution, and clinical features of the lesions must be considered to select the most appropriate form of treatment for each individual patient. Because a number of excellent treatment options are available, patients must be given detailed information so that they can help the physician choose the best form of treatment to ensure maximal patient compliance.

REFERENCES

1. Food and Drug Administration. The darker side of indoor tanning: skin cancer, eye damage, skin aging, allergic reactions. HHS publication No. (FDA) 87–8270. US Department of Health and Human Services, Public Health Service, Rockville, MD, 1987.
2. Council on Scientific Affairs. Harmful effects of ultraviolet radiation. JAMA 262:380–384, 1989.
3. Weinstock MA: The epidemic of squamous cell carcinoma. JAMA 262:2138–2140, 1989.
4. Lever WF, Schaumburg-Lever G: Histopathology of the Skin. 7th ed. JB Lippincott, Philadelphia, 1990, pp 542–546.
5. Marks R, Kennie G, Selwood TS: Malignant transformation of solar keratoses to squamous cell carcinoma. Lancet 1:795–797, 1988.
6. Marks R, Foley P, Goodman G, et al: Spontaneous remission of solar keratoses. Br J Dermatol 115:649–655, 1986.
7. Gross DJ, Waner M, Schosser RH, Dinehart SM: Squamous cell carcinoma of the lower lip involving a large cutaneous surface. Arch Dermatol 126:1148–1150, 1990.
8. Goldes JA, Kao GF: Premalignant lesions of the skin. In: Roenigk RK, Roenigk HH Jr (eds): Dermatologic Surgery—Principles and Practice. Marcel Dekker. New York, 1989, pp 563–590.
9. Kuflick, EG, Gage AA (eds): Cryosurgical Treatment for Skin Cancer. Igaku-Shoin Medical Publishers, New York, 1990.
10. Winton GB, Salasche SJ: Dermabrasion of the scalp as a treatment for actinic damage. J Am Acad Dermatol 14:661–668, 1986.
11. Field LM: Dermabrasion vs 5-FU for actinic damage. J Am Acad Dermatol 6:269–270, 1982.
12. Jansen TG: Use of topical fluorouracil. Arch Dermatol 119:784–785, 1983.
13. Simmonds WL: Double-blind investigation comparing a 1% vs. 5% 5-fluorouracil topical cream in patients with multiple actinic keratoses. Cutis 12:615–617, 1973.
14. Johnson TM, Rapini RP, Duvic M: Inflammation of actinic keratoses from systemic chemotherapy. J Am Acad Dermatol 17:192–197, 1987.
15. Flakson G, Schulz EJ: Skin changes in patients treated with 5-fluorouracil. Br J Dermatol 74:229–236, 1962.
16. Kligman AM, Grove GL, Hirase R, Leyden, JL: Topical tretinoin for photoaged skin. J Am Acad Dermatol 15:836–859, 1986.
17. Peck GL: Topical tretinoin in actinic keratosis and basal cell carcinoma. J Am Acad Dermatol 15:829–835, 1986.
18. Robinson TA, Kligman AM: Treatment of solar keratoses with retinoic acid and fluorouracil. Br J Dermatol 92:703–706, 1975.
19. Epstein JH: All trans-retinoic acid and cutaneous cancers. J Am Acad Dermatol 15:772–778, 1986.
20. Lober CW: Chemexfoliation—indications and cautions. J Am Acad Dermatol 17:109–112, 1987.
21. Resnik SS, Lewis LA, Cohen BH: Trichloroacetic acid and peeling. Cutis 17:127–129, 1976.
22. Resnik SS: Chemical peeling with trichloroacetic acid. J Dermatol Surg Oncol 10:549–550, 1984.
23. Resnik SS: Chemical peel with trichloroacetic acid. In: Roenigk RK, Roenigk HH Jr (eds): Dermatologic Surgery—Principles and Practice. Marcel Dekker, New York, 1989, pp 979–995.
24. Abadir DM: Combination of topical fluorouracil with cryotherapy for treatment of actinic keratoses. J Dermatol Surg Oncol 9:403–404. 1983.
25. Truppman ES, Ellenberg JD: Major electro-cardiographic changes during chemical face peeling. Plast Reconstr Surg 53:522–525, 1974.
26. Stegman SJ: Histologic changes on normal and sundamaged skin produced by various chemical peeling agents. Aesthet Plast Surg 6:123–135, 1982.
27. Van Scott EJ, Yu RJ: Alpha hydroxyacids: therapeutic potentials. Can J Dermatol 1:108–112, 1989.
28. Misiewicz J, Sendagorta E, Golebiowska A, et al: Topical treatment of multiple actinic keratoses of the face with arotinoid methyl sulfone. (Ro 14-9706) cream versus tretinoin cream: a double-blind comparative study. J Am Acad Dermatol 24:448–451, 1991.
29. Wickramasinghe MB, Hindson TC, Wacks H: Treatment of neoplastic skin lesions with intralesional interferon. J Am Acad Dermatol 20:71–74, 1989.
30. Camisa C, Grever MR, Bouronde B: Deoxycoformycin: a new chemotherapeutic agent of interest to dermatologists. J Am Acad Dermatol 12:1108–1109, 1985.

CHAPTER 55

Management of Keratoacanthomas

J. BLAKE GOSLEN

Keratoacanthoma (KA) is a common, distinctive, squamous cutaneous neoplasm typified by rapid growth that is often followed by spontaneous regression. It occurs most frequently on the sun-exposed skin of fair-complexioned elderly patients. This tumor is thought to arise from hair follicles and has been variably described as benign, premalignant, or pseudomalignant. It has been termed an abortive malignancy, implying a capacity to behave as a malignancy only in selected circumstances.[1] While most of these neoplasms behave in a banal fashion, a disturbing number invade deeply or metastasize in a fashion mimicking squamous cell carcinoma (SCC).[2-5] In such cases either SCC was misdiagnosed as a KA in the beginning or there was evidence of histologic progression during the clinical follow-up periods.[2, 6, 7]

The ambiguity regarding the biology of KAs has been the cause of many management problems. The clinician is confronted with the question of whether to allow the tumor to regress spontaneously or to treat it aggressively, sacrificing, in certain instances, an optimal cosmetic or functional result. For that reason, it is important for the cutaneous surgeon to be aware of the options currently available for the management of the typical KA and its clinical variants. To thoroughly understand this neoplasm, a knowledge of certain clinical and histopathologic aspects is necessary.

Typical Clinical Features

KAs occur primarily on sun-exposed, hair-bearing skin, although lesions on mucous membranes, palms, soles, and subungual areas have been reported. In general, elderly whites are affected most frequently, and males predominate in a ratio of 2:1.[8, 9]

The usual early clinical presentation of KA is a red, dome-shaped papule, occasionally with overlying, superficial scale. The tumor grows rapidly and achieves an average size of 10 to 25 mm within 6 to 8 weeks. At this point, it develops a characteristic central keratinous core (Fig. 55–1). The growth rate then stabilizes for 2 to 8 weeks as the tumor enters a maturation phase. Subsequently, as it typically undergoes spontaneous regression over an additional 2- to 8-week period, the keratinous core is extruded, and the tumor mass shrinks, leaving behind an atrophic scar.[10] For large lesions this regression may result in significant tissue destruction, especially when cartilaginous tissue is in the affected site.[8]

Variants With Multiple Lesions

Although a solitary lesion that spontaneously regresses constitutes the classic description of KA, it is important to realize that numerous clinical variants of this tumor also exist that do not follow the usual pattern of clinical behavior (Table 55–1).[10] In outlining a management strategy, it is important to recognize these variants so that the most effective treatment plan can be designed. Several conditions manifesting multiple KAs have been described.[11]

FERGUSON SMITH SYNDROME

The Ferguson Smith, or "self-healing," lesion is familial in nature and has its onset in adolescence or early adulthood. Numerous lesions occur in both exposed and nonexposed areas.[12]

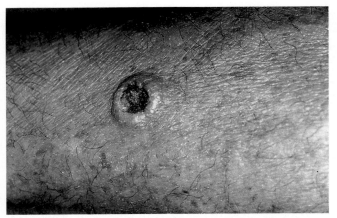

Figure 55–1. Typical keratoacanthoma with central keratinous core and dome-shaped side walls.

GRZYBOWSKI LESIONS

The Grzybowski, or eruptive, lesion occurs later in life and is characterized by hundreds of small, pruritic, follicular papules.[13] Mucous membranes are commonly affected, and spontaneous healing seldom occurs.

WITTEN AND ZAK VARIANT

The Witten and Zak variant combines features of both the Ferguson Smith and Grzybowski types.[14]

MISCELLANEOUS CAUSES

In addition, multiple KAs have been seen in xeroderma pigmentosum,[15] in the Muir-Torre syndrome,[16] and as a manifestation of an underlying internal malignancy.[17, 18] In these settings, spontaneous resolution is not a reliable feature.[19]

Unusual Clinical Variants

GIANT TUMORS

Giant KAs are defined as morphologically typical KAs that are greater than 3 cm in size (Fig. 55–2). These lesions often occur on the middle face, are extremely destructive, and may be relatively refractory to therapy.[20, 21]

KERATOACANTHOMA CENTRIFUGUM MARGINATUM

Keratoacanthoma centrifugum marginatum, or multinodular keratoacanthoma, is characterized by progressive peripheral growth with simultaneous central healing (Fig. 55–3A). These lesions can attain a large size, do not show signs of spontaneous regression, and may be very resistant to treatment.[22]

SUBUNGUAL LESIONS

Subungual keratoacanthoma is an important, frequently misdiagnosed KA variant[23] that typically presents with pain, swelling, and erythema of both the fingertip and the periungual tissues. It is especially common on the thumb or index finger of male patients. It has little or no tendency to spontaneously regress and can destroy both the nail plate and the distal bony phalanx by a pressure effect rather than by direct invasion. Radiographic changes are characteristic and show a crescent-shaped lytic defect without the accompanying periosteal thickening or reactive sclerosis of the underlying bone typically seen with SCC.[24, 25] These lesions are best treated conservatively with curettage or conservative excision. Amputation should be reserved as a therapy of last resort.[26]

Pattern of Behavior

KAs may be extremely aggressive, causing local tissue destruction; they may be refractory to therapy and recur frequently. In this setting, the clinician must consider factors that might predispose the patient to this pattern of behavior (Table 55–1). Aggressive or multiple KAs have been reported in association with visceral malignancies or compromised host immunologic defense mechanisms.[17, 27] The transformation of KA to SCC under the influence of polychemotherapy has been reported in a patient with Hodgkin's disease.[7] Other cases exist in which KAs maintain their histologic integrity but take on an atypical clinical appearance.[28]

Clearly, an important aspect of the management of KAs is the recognition of situations in which tumors are behaving in an atypical manner, either by their aggressive nature or by their eruptive or atypical appearance. The cutaneous surgeon should personally review the available histologic data in these cases and perform a second biopsy, as indicated, to be certain that SCC has not developed or been misdiagnosed. Furthermore, a search for underlying factors such as immunosuppression, concomitant hematologic or visceral malignancy, or an underlying syndrome should be undertaken to explain the atypical clinical picture. This evaluation is vitally important, as knowledge of these underlying factors or associations is critical in determining the most efficacious form of therapy.

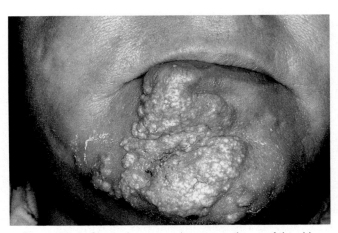

Figure 55–2. Giant, plaque-type keratoacanthoma of the chin.

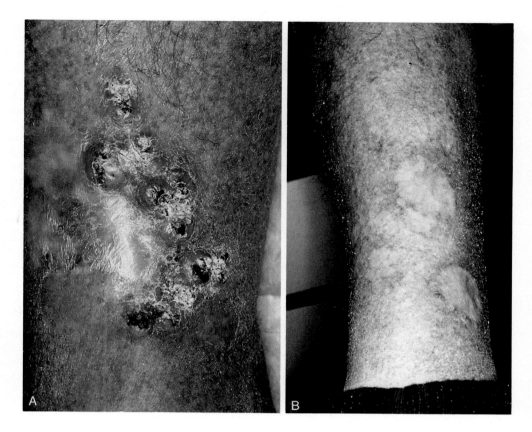

Figure 55–3. *A,* Multinodular keratoacanthoma of the lower leg showing peripheral extension and central scarring before treatment. *B,* Resolution of multinodular keratoacanthoma after treatment with etretinate (1 mg/kg/day) for 8 weeks.

Pathologic Features

One of the major sources of confusion in the KA literature is the problem that exists in distinguishing this neoplasm from SCC. In fact, such a separation is often considered to be artificial, and KAs may be classified as part of the spectrum of well-differentiated SCC.[6] This is a convenient way to explain the apparent transformation from KA to SCC in experimental animals as well as in certain clinical situations. Nevertheless, most dermatopathologists do make a distinction between these two

TABLE 55–1. **CLINICAL VARIANTS OF KERATOACANTHOMA**

Multiple keratoacanthomas
  Ferguson Smith type
  Grzybowski type
  Witten and Zak type
  Associated with Torre's syndrome, xeroderma pigmentosum, or internal malignancy
  Associated with aromatic hydrocarbon exposure
  Associated with benign dermatoses
Giant keratoacanthomas
Keratoacanthoma centrifugum marginatum (multinodular keratoacanthoma)
Keratoacanthoma dyskeratoticum and segregans
Subungual type
Verrucous type
Aggressive types
  Associated with visceral malignancy
  Associated with immunosuppression

lesions and feel they can be clearly separated from one another if adequate biopsy material is available.[29]

Although the best biopsy technique consists of complete excision of the entire lesion, including the deep margin, in some cases the lesions are so large that this is not practical. In such cases an elliptical incisional biopsy through the entire center of the lesion is recommended, being careful to include the deep margin and to maintain the integrity of the keratinous core.[30] Clearly, a simple punch biopsy from the rim of the lesion or a superficial shave excision in which the deep margin is not included is inadequate and frequently compounds the problem of excluding SCC.

The classic histopathologic appearance of a keratoacanthoma is an endoexophytic, dome-shaped tumor with a central crater that is filled with keratinous material. Epithelial lipping occurs with proliferation at both the lateral and deep margins (Fig. 55–4). The tumor cells have an abundant, "glassy" cytoplasm with a variable degree of cytologic atypia. One important characteristic is a neutrophilic infiltrate at the base of the tumor that often forms microabscesses within the tumor lobules. The deep margin of the tumor is expansive rather than invasive and usually does not extend below the level of the eccrine glands.[31, 32] A few reports exist in which KAs have demonstrated striking perineural or even vascular invasion. However, these changes do not appear to adversely affect either patient prognosis or response to therapy.[33, 34]

In contrast, SCCs are usually ulcerative, endophytic, and more invasive and lack the epithelial lipping and keratinous core. Both lesions can demonstrate dysker-

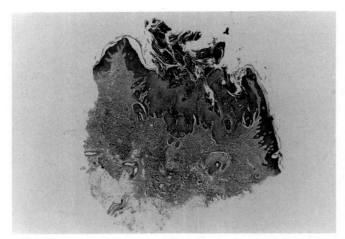

Figure 55–4. Characteristic low-power histologic appearance showing overhanging epithelial lips and central keratinous core (original magnification ×15; H&E stain).

atotic cells, acantholysis, and atypical keratinocytes with pleomorphic nuclei. However, SCCs are more frequently associated with a desmoplastic stromal response.[31, 32] Despite the criteria that have been used to differentiate these two tumors, much confusion still exists. In one histopathologic study examining the reproducibility of the pathologic diagnosis of KA versus that of SCC, the original diagnosis was reversed in 19% of KA diagnoses and 14% of SCC diagnoses.[32]

Management

EVALUATING THE PATIENT

After an adequate diagnostic biopsy has established the diagnosis of KA, the cutaneous surgeon must select the most appropriate form of therapy by using some general considerations. Several initial questions are important to ask. First, is the tumor simply a typical solitary KA, or is there evidence of one of the multiple-KA syndromes? A careful history will usually determine whether the patient has had other tumors in the past. If multiple tumors are present on a complete examination of the skin, it is likely that a pure surgical approach directed toward each lesion will be both a frustrating and a difficult undertaking. Therapies that incorporate intralesional agents or systemic therapy should be considered. In addition, a work-up to exclude a systemic malignancy or syndromes that have been associated with multiple KAs should be undertaken (Table 55–1).

Second, does the tumor have an atypical clinical presentation with nodular, plaquelike, giant, or aggressive KA patterns, despite a rather typical histologic appearance? In this setting, a careful evaluation for underlying diseases associated with immunosuppression (e.g., hematologic or visceral malignancies), concomitant immunosuppressive therapy, or older age should be undertaken.[11] Efforts to control the underlying disease process should be incorporated into the treatment plan in these cases. When immunosuppressive agents are being utilized for other reasons such as organ transplantation or collagen vascular disorders, efforts to minimize the effects of these drugs by dose reduction or substitution with other agents should be considered. This is not possible in many cases, and surgical, intralesional, or radiotherapeutic approaches must be combined with systemic prophylactic measures such as oral retinoid therapy.

Another important general consideration, in view of the propensity for many KAs to regress spontaneously, is whether to intervene at all. Although KAs do resolve spontaneously in a high percentage of cases, this process may be associated with significant scarring and tissue destruction that might be avoided if the tumor is treated early in the course of the disease.[8] Furthermore, certain of the rarer clinical variants of KA are statistically not as likely to regress spontaneously, a fact that should be kept in mind when confronted with this situation (Table 55–1).

DECIDING ON THERAPY

Many general arguments have been used to help make the decision to proceed with therapeutic intervention.[9, 10] Two of these are to hasten resolution for cosmetic reasons or to prevent impingement on vital structures that may result in a more acceptable cosmetic result. When the diagnosis is ambiguous or SCC cannot be excluded, surgical intervention is also often indicated. If the ultimate size of the lesion cannot be predicted but the treatment is usually thought to be safe and effective, intervention is appropriate. When the incidence of recurrence is likely to be less after therapeutic intervention or the statistical likelihood of spontaneous regression is remote, (e.g., with subungual KA, multinodular KA, the multiple-KA syndromes, or KAs associated with immunosuppression), one of several different types of therapy may be indicated.

CHOOSING THE FORM OF TREATMENT

Several different types of acceptable therapy are available for treating KAs, including excisional surgery, curettage and electrodesiccation, radiation therapy, intralesional or topical therapy, and systemic therapy with retinoids or methotrexate. Regardless of the method used, the average recurrence rate in most large series ranges from 3 to 8%,[8, 35] with most recurring within the first 6 months after treatment.[36]

Surgical Excision

Surgical excision remains the treatment of choice for most KAs. While margins should be clear of residual disease, they do not have to be large. Margins of 2 to 4 mm of normal-appearing skin are considered adequate in most circumstances. If a positive margin is encountered, most clinicians recommend conservative re-excision, although reports exist of nonrecurrence despite histologic evidence of residual disease.[37] The main advantages of surgical excision are that it provides an optimal specimen for diagnostic purposes and has a high cure rate.[2, 6, 38] One report described no recurrences in 57 consecutive KA patients treated with conservative excision.[39]

This procedure is indicated in most solitary KAs that are either small or intermediate in size. This is especially true when a diagnostic biopsy is unavailable or when some question exists in differentiating the lesion from an SCC.[37]

One potential problem with this method of treatment is marginal recurrence. Such recurrences have been noted and attributed to incomplete or inadequate removal or to an expression of the Koebnerization response, which is sometimes seen with this neoplasm.[40] An example of this phenomenon has been reported when a skin graft was used to resurface a defect resulting from excision of a KA. Subsequently, recurrences were found not only in the recipient site, but also in the skin graft donor area.[41] Another limitation of this technique occurs when many tumors exist. Here, surgical excision of each tumor with layered closure would be inefficient or impractical in most instances.

One modification of the standard surgical full-thickness excision with sutured closure is saucerization excision followed by second-intention healing.[42] This may be useful when multiple tumors are present and cosmetic appearance is of less concern. Mohs micrographic surgery has also been used to treat KAs. In the largest series reported of KAs treated with Mohs surgery, only one recurrence was seen in 43 treated lesions after a follow-up period varying from 6 months to 2 years.[43]

Curettage

Curettage, with or without electrodesiccation, has been used successfully to treat KAs. In the largest series reported[44] of KA patients treated with curettage only (no electrosurgery), only one recurrence was observed in 47 patients. Other authors report similarly encouraging results with a modification of this technique[45] that consisted of blunt dissection.

The advantages of this approach are its relative simplicity and speed, both of which are particularly important when numerous lesions are present. Problems include scars that are frequently wide, depressed, and hypopigmented.

Curettage is probably the initial treatment of choice for subungual KAs as an attempt to avoid the more aggressive treatment option of amputation typically reported in the hand surgery literature. A review of the literature found an overall cure rate after curettage of 86%.[26] A second curettage procedure may be appropriate in cases of recurrence. If lesions are multiply recurrent, despite two adequate curettage treatments, amputation is usually the next step. Although there are minimal data to support the use of other modalities, the potential effectiveness of intralesional 5-FU, oral retinoid therapy, or even radiotherapy might suggest a trial of these agents before performing amputation. According to one report, one patient with subungual KAs responded to oral etretinate therapy.[46]

Radiotherapy

Since many KAs are radiosensitive, the indications for radiotherapy might include patients who refuse surgery, patients with giant lesions in which surgery would be highly destructive or mutilating, and patients with lesions in cosmetically sensitive areas where surgery or spontaneous regression would result in significant tissue destruction or deformity. Several reports describe the merits of radiotherapy for KA.[47–50] Dosage regimens have differed somewhat but usually range between 2500 and 5600 cGy in 15 to 28 fractions, respectively. If cartilage destruction is present before radiotherapy, the potential cosmetic advantages offered by this treatment are reduced.[47] Although not emphasized in the radiotherapy literature, there are recurrences after radiotherapy that can be problematic.[21] Furthermore, radiotherapy may not be the treatment of choice for young patients, as the later cosmetic results are suboptimal, and secondary malignancies can develop in the radiation sites.

Intralesional Agents

A variety of drugs have been injected intralesionally to treat KAs, and responses have been surprisingly good in many instances. Use of intralesional corticosteroids has been reported in a series of 17 patients with KAs 2 cm or less in size.[51] These lesions were injected with triamcinolone diacetate (25 mg/ml) two to four times at 1- or 2-week intervals, and resolution occurred in all patients. A giant KA was reported to resolve with use of intralesional steroids after failing to respond to previous excision with adequate margins.[40] Unfortunately, not all lesions have regressed with this form of therapy, leading to a gradual abandonment of intralesional steroid treatment. Furthermore, it is conceptually difficult to rationalize the use of an anti-inflammatory agent to treat a neoplastic process.

As a consequence of this, clinical research has been directed at drugs with antineoplastic effects. The initial use of the antimetabolite fluorouracil occurred in 1962,[52] but since then has been reported by multiple authors.[53–56] The largest series reported 41 typical KAs in 30 patients who were treated with intralesional 5-FU (50 mg/ml).[53] Forty of these lesions cleared after an average of 3.4 weekly injections. A 27- or 30-gauge needle was used to inject 0.1 to 0.3 ml of fluorouracil tangentially and circumferentially into the base of the lesion, and an additional 0.1 to 0.2 ml was injected sublesionally.

Other authors have utilized intralesional 5-FU in conjunction with surgical debulking for multiple, relatively large, recurrent lesions.[55, 56] Success rates equivalent to those seen with smaller, more typical KAs have been observed. Cosmetic results have been superior to those obtained when similar lesions were treated with surgical methods. Therefore, intralesional 5-FU therapy should be considered in the following situations: solitary lesions, multiple lesions, lesions in relatively inaccessible sites where surgery might lead to a poor functional or cosmetic result, and large lesions on the head and neck in cosmetically sensitive locations.[56]

An important potential disadvantage of this technique exists when there is no histologic confirmation of the diagnosis before therapy. If a biopsy is not routinely performed before intralesional 5-FU therapy and this approach becomes universally adopted, treatment of a misdiagnosed SCC might be inappropriately delayed. The following guidelines for 5-FU treatment have been recommended for occasions when the diagnosis has not been confirmed by previous biopsy: the growth pattern of the lesion should be typical, the lesion should have a typical morphologic appearance, and any lesion that does not regress at least 60 to 80% after five injections during a period of 1 month should be excised and examined pathologically.[53, 54]

In addition to fluorouracil, bleomycin has also been successfully used intralesionally to treat KAs. In one report, six patients had typical, small KAs that resolved within 2 to 6 weeks after one injection of 0.2 to 0.4 ml of bleomycin (1 mg/ml) into each lesion, depending on size.[57]

Intralesional recombinant interferon alfa-2 has also been used successfully in one patient. The regimen consisted of 0.9×10^6 IU three times per week for 4 weeks.[58] More data are needed before this form of treatment can be advocated routinely.

Topical Agents

Topical fluorouracil, in a concentration of 5 to 20%, has also been used to treat KAs.[59–61] Fourteen of 15 patients treated topically with 5% 5-FU three times per day without occlusion cleared within 1 to 6 weeks. There was a 60 to 70% involution within 2 weeks.[60] Good results were similarly obtained using 20% 5-FU ointment with occlusion. In this concentration, however, a significant adjacent contact dermatitis developed in approximately 14% of patients.[61] In addition, care must be exercised when using topical 5-FU, as it may mask an underlying or misdiagnosed SCC. One patient has been reported who had an initial 75% flattening of a "KA" with topical 5-FU, only to have the lesion to recur 3 weeks after discontinuation of therapy. Excisional biopsy at that time revealed a poorly differentiated SCC on histopathologic examination.[62]

Podophyllin has also been reported to be a useful topical form of therapy[63] when a 25 to 50% solution was applied on a weekly basis. These data are hard to interpret, as the number of patients treated was small, and podophyllin was often used as an adjunct to surgical debulking or radiation therapy.

Finally, for multiple KAs of relatively small size, topical tretinoin (Retin-A), with or without concomitant topical 5-FU, has been reported as useful.[64]

Systemic Chemotherapy

Since the synthetic retinoids became available in the late 1970s, they have been used in the management of KAs many times.[65–67] These agents are modulators of epithelial cell differentiation and can suppress carcinogenesis in a number of epithelial tissues. The precise mechanism of these anticarcinogenic effects is unknown but it may work through a regulation of gene expression.[68, 69]

One of the earliest reports of retinoid therapy used isotretinoin in relatively large doses (2 to 6 mg/kg/day).[70] A response was noted within 3 weeks as older lesions regressed and new lesions were inhibited. However, maintenance therapy was required to continue this degree of improvement. Subsequent reports have used smaller dosages (0.5 to 1.5 mg/kg/day) with a maintenance dosage of 0.25 mg/kg/day. Both solitary and multiple lesions have been successfully treated with this technique.[62, 71]

Eretinate, in a starting dosage of 1 mg/kg/day has been similarly effective (see Fig. 55–3).[72–74] In one series, this dosage was continued for 8 weeks and then tapered by 0.25 mg/kg/day every week, eventually achieving a maintenance dosage of 0.5 to 0.75 mg/kg daily or every other day.[46] Unfortunately, retinoid therapy is invariably associated with many dose-related adverse effects, including mucocutaneous and musculoskeletal effects, elevation of serum cholesterol and triglyceride levels, and abnormal liver function studies. Indications for retinoid therapy include multiple lesions, lesions that recur after other forms of therapy, aggressive variants such as giant or multinodular KAs in cases where surgery would be deforming or excessive, and lesions that require conjunctive surgical treatment to reduce the risk of recurrence.

Systemic methotrexate has also been used to treat KAs in a dosage equivalent to that recommended for psoriasis. This form of therapy should probably be reserved for multiple larger or more aggressive lesions that are unresponsive to retinoid therapy and when adequate biopsy material is available for histologic evaluation.[75, 76]

SUMMARY

Proper management of patients with KAs requires that the cutaneous surgeon have a complete understanding of their biologic activity, histologic and clinical appearance, and occasional association with certain inheritable disorders and underlying internal malignancies and immunologic conditions. By thorough evaluation of each patient with this information in mind, the best form of medical or surgical intervention can be chosen to provide the patient with the best result.

REFERENCES

1. Schwartz RA: The keratocanthoma: a review. J Surg Oncol 12:305–317, 1979.
2. Jackson IT: Diagnostic problem of keratoacanthoma. Lancet 1:490–492, 1969.
3. Iverson RE, Vistnes LM: Keratoacanthoma is frequently a dangerous diagnosis. Am J Surg 126:359–365, 1973.
4. Schnur PL, Bozzo P: Metastasizing keratoacanthoma. Plast Reconstr Surg 62:258–262, 1978.
5. Requena L, Romero E, Sánchez M, et al: Aggressive keratoacanthoma of the eyelid: "malignant" keratoacanthoma or squamous cell carcinoma? J Dermatol Surg Oncol 16:564–568, 1990.
6. Goldenhersh MA, Olsen TG: Invasive squamous cell carcinoma

initially diagnosed as a giant keratoacanthoma. J Am Acad Dermatol 10:372–378, 1984.

7. Poleksic S, Yeung K-Y: Rapid development of keratoacanthoma and accelerated transformation into squamous cell carcinoma of the skin: a mutagenic effect of polychemotherapy in a patient with Hodgkin's disease? Cancer 41:12–16, 1978.

8. Kingman J, Callen JP: Keratoacanthoma: a clinical study. Arch Dermatol 120:736–740, 1984.

9. Ghadially FN: Keratoacanthoma. In: Fitzpatrick TB, Eisen AZ, Wolff K, et al (eds): Dermatology in General Medicine. McGraw-Hill, New York, 1987, pp 766–772.

10. Straka BF, Grant-Kels JM: Keratoacanthoma. In: Friedman RJ, Rigel DS, Kopf AW, et al (eds): Cancer of the Skin. WB Saunders, Philadelphia, 1991, pp 390–407.

11. Ahmed AR: Multiple keratoacanthoma. Int J Dermatol 19:496–499, 1980.

12. Lloyd KM, Hall JH: Ferguson Smith syndrome of multiple keratoacanthomata. Cutis 5:1093–1097, 1969.

13. Grzybowski M: A case of peculiar generalized epithelial tumours of the skin. Br J Dermatol 62:310–313, 1950.

14. Witten VH, Zak FG: Multiple, primary, self-healing prickle-cell epithelioma of the skin. Cancer 5:539–550, 1952.

15. Stevanovic DV: Keratoacanthoma in xeroderma pigmentosum. Arch Dermatol 84:53–54, 1961.

16. Descalzi ME, Rosenthal S: Sebaceous adenomas and keratoacanthomas in a patient with malignant lymphoma: a new form of Torre's syndrome. Cutis 28:169–170, 1981.

17. Snider BL, Benjamin DR: Eruptive keratoacanthoma with an internal malignant neoplasm. Arch Dermatol 117:788–790, 1981.

18. Inoshita T, Youngberg GA: Keratoacanthomas associated with cervical squamous cell carcinoma. Arch Dermatol 120:123–124, 1984.

19. Kopf AW: Multiple keratoacanthomas. Arch Dermatol 103:543–544, 1971.

20. Lo JS, Bergfeld WF, Taylor JS, et al: Multiple erythematous plaques with infiltrated borders on the forearms. Multiple keratoacanthomas. Arch Dermatol 126:103, 105–106, 1990.

21. Rapaport J: Giant keratoacanthoma of the nose. Arch Dermatol 111:73–75, 1975.

22. Eliezri YD, Libow L: Multinodular keratoacanthoma. J Am Acad Dermatol 19:826–830, 1988.

23. Stoll DM, Ackerman AB: Subungual keratoacanthoma. Am J Dermatopathol 2:265–271, 1980.

24. Keeney GL, Banks PM, Linscheid RL: Subungual keratoacanthoma: report of a case and review of the literature. Arch Dermatol 124:1074–1076, 1988.

25. Patel MR, Desai SS: Subungual keratoacanthomas in the hand. J Hand Surg 14A:139–142, 1989.

26. Pelligrini VD, Tompkins A: Management of subungual keratoacanthoma. J Hand Surg 11A:718–724, 1986.

27. Fathizadeh A, Medenica MM, Soltani K, et al: Aggressive keratoacanthoma and internal malignant neoplasm. Arch Dermatol 118:112–114, 1982.

28. Washington CV, Mikhail GR: Eruptive keratoacanthoma en plaque in an immunosuppressed patient. J Dermatol Surg Oncol 13:1357–1360, 1987.

29. Chalet MD, Conners RC, Ackerman AB: Squamous cell carcinoma versus keratoacanthoma: criteria for histologic differentiation. J Dermatol Surg Oncol 4:498, 1978.

30. Popkin GL, Brodie SJ, Hyman AB, et al: A technique of biopsy recommended for keratoacanthomas. Arch Dermatol 94:191–193, 1966.

31. McKee PH: Pathology of the Skin with Clinical Correlations. JB Lippincott, Philadelphia, 1989, pp 1420–1422.

32. Kern WH, McCray MK: The histopathologic differentiation of keratoacanthoma and squamous cell carcinoma of the skin. J Cutan Pathol 7:318–325, 1980.

33. Janecka IP, Wolff M, Crikelair GF, et al: Aggressive histological features of keratoacanthoma. J Cutan Pathol 4:342–348, 1978.

34. Lapins NA, Helwig EB: Perineural invasion by keratoacanthoma. Arch Dermatol 116:791–793, 1980.

35. Rook A, Whimster I: Keratoacanthoma—A thirty year retrospect. Br J Dermatol 100:41–47, 1979.

36. Stevanovic DV: Récidives du kérato-acanthome: reformation, exacerbation, recroissance, keratoacanthomata duplex. Ann Derm Syph (Paris) 96:415–420, 1969.

37. Pagani WA, Lorenzi G, Lorusso D: Surgical treatment for aggressive giant keratoacanthoma of the face. J Dermatol Surg Oncol 12:282–284, 1986.

38. Middleton AG, Curtin JW: Keratoacanthoma or squamous cell carcinoma? A surgeon's dilemma. Plast Reconstr Surg 38:56–59, 1966.

39. Cohen N, Plaschkes Y, Pevzner S, et al: Review of 57 cases of keratoacanthoma. Plast Reconstr Surg 49:138–143, 1972.

40. Epstein EH Jr, Epstein EH: Keratoacanthoma recurrent after surgical excision. J Dermatol Surg Oncol 4:524–525, 1978.

41. Dibden FA, Fowler M: The multiple growth of molluscum sebaceum in donor and recipient sites of skin graft. Aust NZ J Surg 25:157–162, 1955.

42. Johannesson A: Razor blade surgery of keratoacanthoma. J Dermatol Surg Oncol 12:1056–1057, 1986.

43. Larson PO: Keratoacanthomas treated with Mohs' micrographic surgery (chemosurgery): a review of forty-three cases. J Am Acad Dermatol 16:1040–1044, 1987.

44. Reymann, F. Treatment of keratoacanthomas with curettage. Dermatologica 155:90–96, 1977.

45. Habif TP: Extirpation of keratoacanthomas by blunt dissection. J Dermatol Surg Oncol 6:652–654, 1980.

46. Benoldi D, Alinovi A: Multiple persistent keratoacanthomas: treatment with oral etretinate. J Am Acad Dermatol 10:1035–1038, 1984.

47. Donahue B, Cooper JS, Rush S: Treatment of aggressive keratoacanthomas by radiotherapy. J Am Acad Dermatol 23:489–493, 1990.

48. Caccialanza M, Sopelana N: Radiation therapy of keratoacanthomas: results in 55 patients. Int J Radiat Oncol Biol Phys 16:475–477, 1989.

49. Shimm DS, Duttenhaver JR, Doucette J, et al: Radiation therapy of keratoacanthoma. Int J Radiat Oncol Biol Phys 9:759–761, 1983.

50. Farina A, Leider M, Newall J, et al: Radiotherapy for aggressive and destructive keratoacanthomas. J Dermatol Surg Oncol 3:177–180, 1977.

51. McNairy DJ: Intradermal triamcinolone therapy of keratoacanthomas. Arch Dermatol 89:136–140, 1964.

52. Klein E, Helm F, Milgrom H, et al: Keratoacanthoma: local effect of 5-fluorouracil. Skin 1:153–156, 1962.

53. Goette DK, Odom RB: Successful treatment of keratoacanthoma with intralesional fluorouracil. J Am Acad Dermatol 2:212–216, 1980.

54. Odom RB, Goette DK: Treatment of keratoacanthomas with intralesional fluorouracil. Arch Dermatol 114:1779–1783, 1978.

55. Eubanks SW, Gentry RH, Patterson JW, et al: Treatment of multiple keratoacanthomas with intralesional fluorouracil. J Am Acad Dermatol 7:126–129, 1982.

56. Parker CM, Hanke CW: Large keratoacanthomas in different locations treated with intralesional 5-fluorouracil. J Am Acad Dermatol 14:770–777, 1986.

57. Sayama S, Tagami H. Treatment of keratoacanthoma with intralesional bleomycin. Br J Dermatol 109:449–452, 1983.

58. Wickramasinghe L: Treatment of neoplastic skin lesions with intralesional interferon. J Am Acad Dermatol 20:71–74, 1989.

59. Grupper C: Treatment of keratoacanthomas by local applications of the 5-flourouracil (5-FU) ointment. Dermatologica 40S:127–132, 1970.

60. Goette DK: Treatment of keratoacanthomas with topical fluorouracil. Arch Dermatol 119:951–953, 1983.

61. Goette DK, Odom RB, Arrott JW, et al: Treatment of keratoacanthoma with topical application of fluorouracil. Arch Dermatol 118:309–311, 1982.

62. Cobb MW, Pellegrini AE: Squamous cell carcinoma following fluorouracil-responsive "keratoacanthoma." Arch Dermatol 123:987–988, 1987.

63. Cipollaro VA: The use of podophyllin in the treatment of keratoacanthoma. Int J Dermatol 22:436–440, 1983.

64. Winkelmann RK, Brown J: Generalized eruptive keratoacanthoma: report of cases. Arch Dermatol 97:615–623, 1968.

65. Levine N, Miller RC, Meyskens FL Jr: Oral isotretinoin therapy: use in a patient with multiple cutaneous squamous cell carcinomas and keratoacanthomas. Arch Dermatol 120:1215–1217, 1984.

66. Shaw JC, White CR: Treatment of multiple keratoacanthomas with oral isotretinoin. J Am Acad Dermatol 15:1079–1082, 1986.

67. Street ML, White JW Jr, Gibson LE: Multiple keratoacanthomas treated with oral retinoids. J Am Acad Dermatol 23:862–866, 1990.

68. Lippman SM, Kessler JF, Meyskens FL Jr: Retinoids as preventive and therapeutic anticancer agents. Cancer Treat Rep 71:391–405, 493–515, 1987.

69. Hong WK, Lippman SM, Itri LM, et al: Prevention of second primary tumors with isotretinoin in squamous-cell carcinoma of the head and neck. N Engl J Med 323:795–801, 1990.

70. Haydey RP, Reed ML, Dzubow LM, et al: Treatment of keratoacanthomas with oral 13-cis-retinoic acid. N Engl J Med 303:560–562, 1980.

71. Goldberg LH, Rosen T, Becker J, et al: Treatment of solitary keratoacanthomas with oral isotretinoin. J Am Acad Dermatol 23:934–936, 1990.

72. Fanti PA, Tosti A, Peluso AM, et al: Multiple keratoacanthoma in discoid lupus erythematosus. J Am Acad Dermatol 21:809–810, 1989.

73. Blitstein-Willinger E, Haas N, Nurnberger F, et al: Immunological findings during treatment of multiple keratoacanthoma with etretinate. Br J Dermatol 114:109–116, 1986.

74. Yoshikawa K, Hirano S, Kato T, et al: A case of eruptive keratoacanthoma treated by oral etretinate. Br J Dermatol 112:579–583, 1985.

75. Tarnowski WM: Multiple keratoacanthomata: response of a case to systemic chemotherapy. Arch Dermatol 94:74–80, 1966.

76. Kestel JL Jr, Blair DS: Keratoacanthoma treated with methotrexate. Arch Dermatol 108:723–724, 1973.

CHAPTER 56

Management of Basal Cell Carcinomas

JAMES Q. DEL ROSSO and RONALD J. SIEGLE

The nonmelanoma skin cancers (i.e., basal and squamous cell carcinomas) comprise approximately 50% of all new cases of cancer diagnosed in the United States each year.[1] Approximately 65 to 75% of all skin cancers in whites are basal cell carcinomas (BCCs), with the ratio of BCCs to squamous cell carcinomas (SCCs) increasing as latitude increases.[1-3] The true incidence of BCC, however, is difficult to ascertain because of the lack of organized cancer registries for ambulatory care. However, the number of cases occurring each year appears to be increasing.[4] In the 1970s, surveys by the National Cancer Institute suggested a 15 to 20% increase over a 6-year period.[5, 6] A more recent epidemiologic study evaluating BCC incidence in British Columbia from 1973 to 1987 demonstrated a 60% increase of BCC in men and a 48% increase in women.[7]

BCC is primarily seen in whites, especially those with fair complexions. It has a low incidence in the black population.[8-10] Regardless of race, the head and neck is affected in 80 to 90% of cases, with more than 65% of all BCCs involving facial sites.[11-13] The high frequency of facial BCC results in frequent involvement of sites that are functionally and cosmetically significant. While typically slow growing and indolent, BCC possesses the potential to produce significant morbidity if not adequately treated early in its course.[12, 14, 15] Destruction of skin structures occurs visibly or insidiously as neoplastic extensions progressively replace local tissues. Although metastasis is rare, both lymphatic and hematogenous spread can occur.[15-17]

In evaluating the effective management of BCC, interpretation of the literature is complex, because many studies analyze data retrospectively, and good prospective, comparative studies are largely lacking. Because BCC treatment involves practitioners in multiple disciplines, the medical literature includes the observations and biases of dermatologists, Mohs micrographic surgeons, cryosurgeons, plastic surgeons, otolaryngologists, ophthalmologists, and radiation oncologists. Nevertheless, enough data exist to substantiate some specific indications and relative contraindications regarding the management of BCC.

Many factors need to be considered when devising a treatment plan for the patient with BCC. The influences of various risk factors on the management plan must be thoroughly reviewed before choosing any form of treatment. Furthermore, an understanding of the clinical parameters, histopathologic variables, and individual treatment modalities available must be completely understood by the cutaneous surgeon to provide an individual patient with the most appropriate therapy.

The major goals of BCC treatment are to cure the cancer while preserving maximal function and allowing the most optimal cosmetic result after the cancer has been adequately treated.[4, 18] Proper management consists of thorough patient education, including self-examination for early detection of new and recurrent BCCs, and periodic follow-up examinations. Ultimately, the cutaneous surgeon must coordinate the overall treatment program with the needs and desires of the individual patient.

Risk Factors in Patients With BCC

Assessment of environmental, occupational, medical, and congenital risk factors is an integral part of patient management. Behavior modification may significantly decrease the future development of BCCs. Treatment and follow-up recommendations may also vary with specific clinical circumstances and risk categories, especially when multiple BCCs are expected to develop over time (e.g., in the basal cell nevus syndrome patient or the patient who has had previous ionizing radiation exposure).

ULTRAVIOLET EXPOSURE AND SKIN TYPE

Cumulative exposure to ultraviolet light (UVL) increases the risk for development of BCC.[11, 19, 20] Individuals who tan poorly, burn easily, or have a fair complexion are at greatest risk.[19, 21, 22] The long latency for BCC development resulting from cumulative UVL exposure underscores the need for periodic self-examination and follow-up in patients with a history of significant UVL exposure.[4, 21] Thorough education regarding sun protection guidelines and sunscreen use is imperative. Recommendations should be practical and tailored to the degree of risk and the life style of each patient.

RADIATION EXPOSURE

Both x-ray exposure and grenz ray exposure have been associated with BCC and SCC development.[2, 4, 23–27] The latency period of several years warrants periodic follow-up,[25, 28, 29] as multiple BCCs are frequently encountered.[24, 25, 28] BCC may occur even when clinical evidence of radiation dermatitis is subtle or not present.[4, 28] When present, radiation dermatitis may obscure the clinical presentation of BCC, thus requiring more careful and more frequent physical examinations by the physician.

ARSENIC EXPOSURE

Chronic arsenism has been associated with nonmelanoma skin cancers, including BCC.[4, 23] Exposures may be medicinal, occupational, or dietary, which is usually through ingestion of contaminated water supplies.[2, 30] Arsenic-related BCCs are usually multiple and tend to occur on sun-protected sites, especially the trunk.[2, 4] Affected patients require close follow-up with total body skin examination. Fortunately, chronic arsenism has decreased as a result of improved quality of water supplies and the discontinuation of arsenic as a medication and pesticide.

IMMUNOSUPPRESSION

Immunologic suppression, often drug induced, increases the risk for development of nonmelanoma skin cancers, with the risk for development of SCC much greater than that for BCC.[4, 23, 31–34] Sun-exposed sites are predominantly affected.[2, 31, 34] Patients in this category require careful follow-up and probably more aggressive therapy.[32]

OTHER MEDICINAL EXPOSURES

Topical nitrogen mustard (mechlorethamine), used in the treatment of cutaneous T-cell lymphoma (mycosis fungoides), has been associated with skin malignancies, including BCC.[35–38] Psoralen and ultraviolet A (PUVA) phototherapy, used to treat psoriasis and other dermatoses, has been associated with a modest increase in the risk of BCC and a significant increase in the risk of SCC, especially in patients on long-term therapy.[39–41] Periodic total-body skin examination is important in patients treated with topical nitrogen mustard or PUVA, as extensive body surface areas are exposed to treatment.

TRAUMA

BCC has been sporadically reported to occur in chickenpox scars,[42] vaccination sites,[43, 44] venous stasis ulcers,[45] burn scars,[46] hair transplant scars,[45] and tattoos.[45]

GENETIC/CONGENITAL FACTORS

Inherited syndromes associated with development of BCC includes xeroderma pigmentosum,[47, 48] basal cell nevus syndrome (Gorlin's syndrome),[48, 49] Bazex's syndrome[50, 51] albinism,[2, 4] and epidermolysis bullosa dystrophica.[52] Development of BCC in childhood or early adolescence should raise suspicion that an inherited disorder may be present.[45]

The development of BCC and other neoplasms within Jadassohn's nevus sebaceus is well documented.[53] Clinically apparent BCC, usually developing in adulthood, is seen in 5 to 7% of cases.[2] However, BCC may be present only on histologic examination.[53]

PAST HISTORY OF BCC

Patients with a history of previous BCC are at increased risk for development of new primary BCCs.[54] The possibility of recurrent BCC must also be considered, thus warranting evaluation of previously treated sites.

Factors Affecting the Management of BCC

It is important to recognize that not all BCCs are alike, and tumor aggressiveness varies significantly from one BCC to another.[14, 15] Clinical and histologic variables, which reflect tumor biology, should be used to select the most appropriate treatment. It is the cutaneous surgeon's responsibility to comprehensively evaluate all of the factors present in a given patient and ultimately work with the patient to select the most appropriate form of treatment for him or her (Table 56–1).

CLINICAL APPEARANCE

Most cutaneous surgeons are very familiar with the classic morphologic descriptions of primary BCC, although in practice they encounter several clinical variations. Histologic correlations, although sometimes pre-

TABLE 56–1. CHECKLIST FOR DETERMINING INDIVIDUAL TREATMENT OF BCC

- What risk factors relate to the cause of BCC in this patient?
- Is the BCC primary or recurrent?
- Are the clinical borders discrete?
- Where is the BCC located?
- How long has the lesion been present?
- What is the clinical size of the lesion?
- What histologic pattern is present in the pretreatment biopsy specimen?
- What individual patient-related factors affect the treatment selection?
- What follow-up plan is indicated?

dictable based on clinical appearance, vary significantly in individual cases. Close inspection of a suspicious lesion, under good lighting and with stretching of adjacent skin, often reveals inconspicuous marginal extensions.[55] Palpation may also demonstrate textural changes beyond the obvious clinical borders, possibly indicative of subclinical extension or scar formation related to previous therapy.

Nodular primary BCC typically presents as an opalescent papule or nodule.[56] Surface telangiectasia and ulceration may also be present. A nodular BCC usually exhibits discrete clinical margins that reflect the circumscribed microscopic growth of the tumor.[4] Such lesions, when less than 1 cm in diameter, usually exhibit subclinical extensions that are less than 3 mm.[55, 57] Unfortunately, nodular BCCs with associated aggressive histologic features, such as sclerosis or an infiltrative pattern, do not always demonstrate features that, by clinical examination alone, will distinguish them from purely nodular BCCs.[58] The histologic presence of aggressive features associated with nodular BCC may further increase the likelihood of tumor extension beyond the clinical borders of the lesion.[58–60] This may result in undertreatment, as the clinician anticipates a more discrete and cohesive tumor mass. Indurated plaques, with shades of erythema, an ivory color, or a yellowish hue, are typical of morpheaform BCC.[56, 57] Morpheaform BCCs have nondiscrete clinical margins as a result of aggressive microscopic growth that is often associated with asymmetric and marked subclinical extension.[4, 57, 61] Infiltrative and micronodular BCCs are aggressive histologic subtypes that do not exhibit characteristic clinical morphology. They often do not have discrete clinical borders,[4] and like morpheaform BCC, they demonstrate aggressive behavior through significant extension beyond their clinical borders.[4, 62] The more elusive and aggressive nature of morpheaform, infiltrative, and micronodular BCC results in a greater likelihood of recurrence after treatment.[57, 58, 60, 62–65]

Superficial basal cell carcinoma (SBCC) is a distinct category of BCC. This condition typically presents as a red scaly patch or plaque[2, 56] and may simulate psoriasis, eczema, or Bowen's disease.[56] Although not histologically diffuse in depth, SBCC typically extends radially beyond the physical borders of the lesion, which are usually well marginated.[4, 66] Deeper tumor foci may also bud from follicles without changing the clinical appearance of the lesion.[4] The presence of pigment, most often noted within the nodular or superficial BCC,[67] does not influence the biologic behavior or the degree of subclinical extension.

Assessing the probability of an aggressive microscopic growth pattern and subclinical extension is the cornerstone of the clinical examination of BCC. Ill-defined clinical borders complicate therapy by not allowing the physician to confidently select clinical margins for treatment. Correlation with other clinical variables and histologic examination is mandatory before treatment selection.[62]

ANATOMIC LOCATION

The anatomic location of BCC is one of the most significant variables affecting treatment selection.[68–71] It is important for cutaneous surgeons to recognize the "H zone" of the head, as this zone includes anatomic sites with a high propensity for subclinical extension and recurrence (Fig. 56–1).[72–78] Probable reasons for this enhanced biologic aggressiveness include embryologic fusion planes, irregular contours, and variations in microanatomy.[74–76]

Significant functional and cosmetic deformity may result from treatment in these areas, because the nose, eyes, ears, lips, and eyelids are included in the H zone. Unfortunately, in an attempt to prevent such problems, it is common to reduce recommended surgical margins, which also leads to increased recurrence rates.[70, 77, 78] The primary goal of therapy is complete cancer removal, and this goal must supersede the prejudice of surgical conservatism, which is designed to enhance cosmesis or maintain function. There is an unacceptably high rate of residual BCC after curettage and electrodesiccation of the midface, especially the nose and nasolabial sites.[79, 80] The high density of pilosebaceous units in the firm dermal stroma of the nose allows nests of tumor to elude even the smallest curette.[79] Although the scalp is not a part of the H zone, extensive BCC of the scalp is well documented.[81–83] These are usually large lesions with extensive subclinical spread. They require careful selection of treatment to permit optimal margin evaluation.

In general, primary BCCs of the trunk and extremities are less challenging therapeutically, since tissue conservation is usually not important. Most truncal lesions behave nonaggressively, probably because of increased dermal thickness, the lack of embryologic fusion planes, and greater incidence of SBCC below the neck. The incidence of recurrent BCC of the trunk and extremities is very low.[12, 70, 84] Occasional exceptions include large BCCs and those with aggressive histologic features.

SIZE

Discrete BCCs that are smaller than 2 cm in size tend to exhibit minimal subclinical spread and are amenable to treatment using a variety of modalities.[4, 12, 85] Larger BCCs are more difficult to cure and require more aggressive therapy.[4, 61, 85, 86] The unifying theme appears to be that the longer the period of growth, the larger

SKIN CANCER RECURRENCE RATES

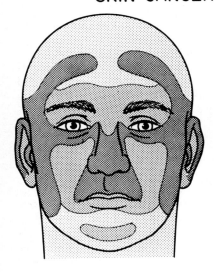
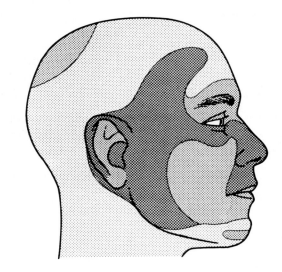

■ HIGHEST

▨ INTERMEDIATE

□ LOWEST

Figure 56–1. Correlations of skin cancer recurrence rates with anatomic location. (From Lambert DR, Siegle RJ: Skin cancer: a review with consideration of treatment options including Mohs micrographic surgery. Ohio Med 86:745, 1990.)

the tumor and the greater the probability of subclinical and asymmetric spread.[85] However, even for small BCCs, size alone should not be used as an independent variable in treatment selection. Small tumors with indiscrete borders, aggressive histologic features, or involvement of the H zone are likely to exhibit considerable subclinical extension and higher rates of recurrence.[4, 60, 69, 72, 84] Clinical estimates of actual tumor size and depth are apt to be inaccurate. Thus, size should be correlated with other factors when selecting treatment type (Fig. 56–2).[69]

LESION DURATION

The longer a given BCC is present, the greater the potential for deep and wide invasion.[12, 79, 87–89] BCC is a slow-growing neoplasm, and lesions that have been present for several years often require more aggressive treatment.

LESION NUMBER

There is a tendency to spare patients with multiple BCCs time, expense, and morbidity by using simpler modalities such as curettage and electrodesiccation. However, it is important to use selective judgment based primarily on histologic pattern and anatomic location to more accurately determine how to treat potentially aggressive BCCs most definitively.

EXTENUATING CIRCUMSTANCES

Specific circumstances may result in the selection of a nonstandard or nontraditional treatment choice.[90, 91] One example of this is the presence of another serious medical disorder producing poor general health and marked disability. Advanced, extensive BCC may result in the patient choosing a more tolerable palliative approach rather than a curative attempt involving more extensive surgery.[91] A given patient may also decide to stop treatment at a specific point. A decision to preserve an eye rather than undergo surgical ablation to remove the orbital extension of a tumor is an excellent example.

RECURRENT BCC

It is well documented that the best chance of cure for BCC exists at the time of initial treatment.[4, 92–94] Recurrent BCC represents a more difficult challenge for several reasons. First, the presence of scarring obscures clinical assessment of the extent of tumor.[63, 95, 96] BCC may be located within or below the cicatrix and extend a considerable distance from the site that is clinically suspicious for recurrence.[92, 94–97] Additionally, the clinical focus of recurrence may only be a small part of the actual tumor, as is seen with deep recurrences that later reach the skin surface.[63, 94] Also, foci of recurrent BCC may be multiple and noncontiguous within scar tissue.[97] As a result, removal of the entire scar associated with the initial treatment has been recommended.[94, 97]

When initial therapy has involved undermining or

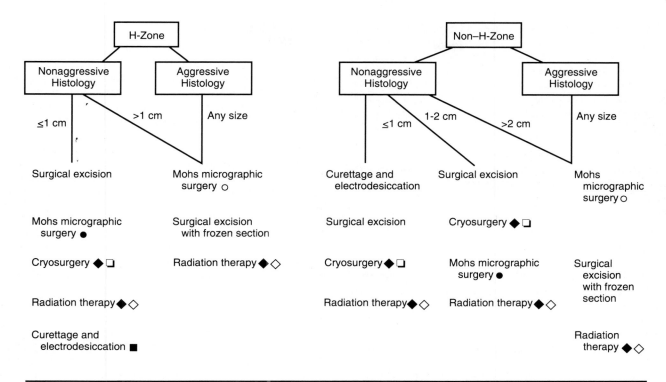

Figure 56–2. Treatment options for primary basal cell carcinoma (BCC) of the face and head region.

○ Treatment of choice

● Preferred if clinical borders are not discrete or if not possible to excise recommended margins without sacrificing functionally or cosmetically important structures

◇ Considered in patients who are poor surgical candidates; not indicated in patients <50 years of age

◆ Best avoided in hair-bearing areas because of resultant alopecia

❑ Tissue monitoring indicated

■ Applicable only for BCC with purely nodular histology <0.5 cm in size (excluding lesions on lower half of nose, nasolabial folds, and medial canthus)

tissue transfer with flaps or grafts, recurrent BCC may track under the site of repair.[94, 95] In these cases, the entire surgical field may need to be removed to successfully extirpate the tumor.[91, 94, 98, 99] Recurrent BCC presents additional challenges that may limit the treatment options.[63, 92, 94] A large body of evidence supports Mohs micrographic surgery (MMS) as the treatment of choice for recurrent BCC.[92, 93, 100–103] Cure rates achieved by curettage and electrodesiccation, conventional surgical excision, radiation therapy, and cryosurgery are significantly lower than those obtained with MMS.[4, 92, 93]

Pathologic Variables

The determination of the most ideal form of treatment of BCC is often dependent on a properly performed biopsy. Correlation of the clinical and histologic factors involved in each case is mandatory.[62]

PRETREATMENT BIOPSY

A pretreatment biopsy allows for confirmation of diagnosis and assessment of histologic growth pattern.[2, 4, 11, 88, 99] Saucerization is an effective biopsy method for suspected primary or recurrent BCC, as it allows for evaluation of the microscopic growth pattern.[63, 88, 99, 104]

The punch technique should be avoided for biopsy of suspected nodular or superficial BCC when treatment by curettage and electrodesiccation is anticipated,[105–107] as the punch penetrates the "dermal sling" that supports curettage and may allow the curette to artifactually penetrate into the subcutaneous fat.[63, 99, 105] However, lesions suspicious for recurrent BCC or primary BCC with an aggressive growth pattern may be biopsied by the punch technique, as evaluation of lesion depth and architecture is beneficial.[2, 4] In some cases of suspected recurrent BCC, multiple biopsy specimens taken from different sites may be beneficial, especially when noncontiguous foci are clinically suspicious.

When a pretreatment biopsy is considered impractical,

the physician must select treatment based on clinical assessment alone. In such cases a tissue sample should still be taken and submitted for histopathologic evaluation.[4, 99, 108] If histologic examination later indicates a high probability of inadequate therapy (e.g., aggressive features or involved excision margins), the patient can then be appropriately treated using a second definitive method.[4]

Most clinicians rely heavily on the pathologist for an accurate diagnosis. The clinician should expect the pathologist to indicate the histologic subtype or growth pattern of the BCC when such information is interpretable.[58, 66, 109, 110]

LESION HISTOLOGY

The microscopic growth pattern of BCC significantly affects the likelihood of treatment success (Fig. 56–3). Aggressive histologic patterns are commonly more refractory to treatment as a result of diffuse microscopic growth or the presence of sclerosis.[58, 60, 62, 66, 84, 109–112] Regardless of location, aggressive histologic features increase the risk of inadequate treatment.

There are several distinct histologic subtypes demonstrating aggressive behavior.[4, 15] Morpheaform BCC is recognized for its ability to subclinically extend large distances.[57, 58, 61, 70, 71, 112] The sclerotic nature of the stroma precludes treatment by curettage and electrodesiccation.[58, 107, 113, 114] As clinical borders are not clearly demarcated, zones of treatment for surgical excision, radiation therapy, and cryosurgery are also more difficult to determine.[4, 111, 115, 116] Unfortunately, the histologic subtypes of infiltrative and micronodular BCCs have not received the recognition they deserve among physicians who treat BCC. Both types are notably aggressive, with a propensity for wide or deep subclinical spread.[60, 62, 66, 84, 104, 110] Although their stroma is usually not sclerotic, the relatively sparse cellularity and depth of extension defies the benefits of curettage and electrodesiccation.[59, 87, 104] Like morpheaform BCC, micronodular and infiltrative BCCs usually exhibit ill-defined clinical borders and are apt to extend beyond recommended margins for surgical excision, cryosurgery, and radiation therapy.[4, 60, 104, 110] Although nodular BCC is recognized as a relatively nonaggressive pattern, recurrence of nodular BCC is well documented.[62, 84, 109, 117] The importance of sclerosis associated with nodular BCC has been emphasized as a factor increasing the risk of recurrence.[58, 109] Nodular BCC may sometimes contain foci associated with aggressive microscopic growth (e.g., infiltrative and micronodular patterns).[59, 60, 62, 66] These adjacent patterns may be located along the deeper aspect of the tumor, thus eluding detection by a superficial biopsy.[58, 59, 87]

Basosquamous (metatypical) carcinoma is thought by some to be a more aggressive histologic subtype of BCC[2, 71, 84, 91, 118–121] that may involve local invasion and a greater potential for metastasis. Other less common forms of BCC that have been reported to be more locally aggressive are eccrine epithelioma[122–125] and adenoid basal cell carcinoma.[2, 11, 112]

SURGICAL SPECIMEN

A major advantage of excisional modalities is the production of a surgical specimen that can be evaluated for the presence of tumor at the margins of the specimen.[126, 127] The method of margin evaluation used when processing the surgical specimen critically influences the value of the surgical pathology report.[128–130] The value of surgical excision as a treatment modality for basal cell carcinoma is directly proportional to the accuracy of specimen preparation by the histotechnician, the completeness of the processing method used to examine the margins of the specimen, and the ability of the pathologist to interpret the histologic sections provided.

The various terms used to refer to margins have been clearly described, and their significance has also been stressed.[129] The *clinical margin* refers to the visible or palpable border of the lesion. The *surgical margin* refers to the border of normal skin around the lesion that the surgeon removes along with the BCC. The *cut surgical margin* is the entire three-dimensional edge of the excised specimen, including both the lateral and deep faces. The cut surgical margin differs significantly from the *pathologic margins,* which are limited to those segments of the cut surgical margin that are actually examined histologically by the pathologist. The pathologic margins depend on the processing technique used by the laboratory.[129, 130] For example, the breadloaf method sections the specimen vertically in a stepwise fashion, providing a pathologic margin for evaluation at fixed intervals. Intervening segments of the specimen are not evaluated, leaving a significant fraction of the cut surgical margin unexamined histologically (Fig. 56–4).[129, 130] Other conventional processing methods commonly used by pathology laboratories include the cross-sectioning method and the breadloaf–cross-sectioning (combined) method. These methods, as well as most other standard histologic sectioning techniques, also allow only a fraction of the cut surgical margins to be evaluated microscopically.[62, 84, 129–132]

Several alternative methods have been suggested to improve the completeness of pathologic margin examination.[129, 130, 133–140] Some include the use of peripheral and horizontal sections, and a few methods can ideally approach complete pathologic evaluation of the cut surgical margin. However, these methods may be limited by some technical difficulties such as specimen type and size.[18, 129] Additionally, there can be difficulties in achieving proper anatomic orientation of tissues with irregular shape or inconsistent integrity (e.g., fat, muscle, and fascia).[141] In addition, in an attempt to provide complete peripheral or deep sections, the histotechnician may cut too deeply into the block, thus producing a false-positive pathologic margin that does not correlate with the true cut surgical margin.

The use of alternative methods of specimen evaluation may also be restricted by the ability of the pathology laboratory to provide the necessary processing method on a routine basis, as such methods are very time intensive and technically difficult.[129, 131, 142] In addition, the pathology laboratory is usually remote from the

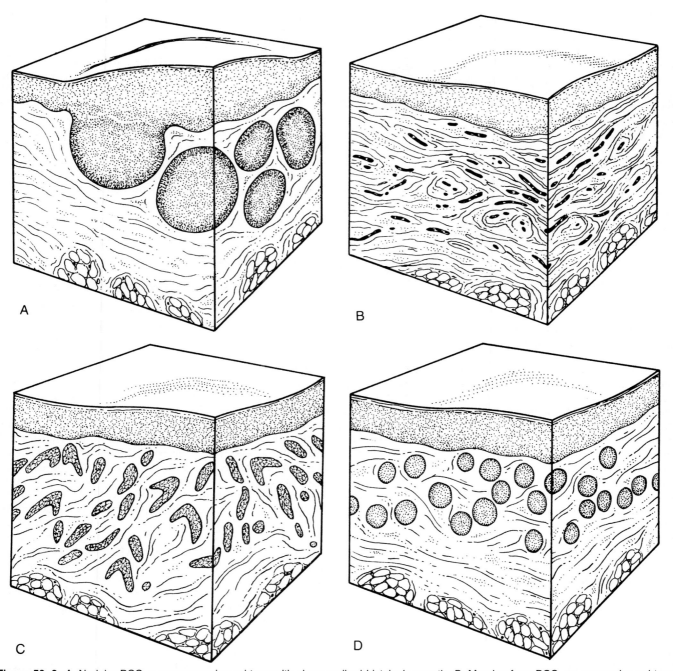

Figure 56–3. *A,* Nodular BCC, a nonaggressive subtype with circumscribed histologic growth. *B,* Morpheaform BCC, an aggressive subtype with poorly defined borders and fine invasive strands of tumor embedded in a sclerotic stroma. *C,* Infiltrative BCC, an aggressive subtype with poorly defined borders and ribbons and cords of tumor spreading in a nonsclerotic stroma. *D,* Micronodular BCC, an aggressive subtype with poorly defined tumor margins and round, relatively uniform, small, banal-appearing islands of tumor in a nonsclerotic stroma. (Courtesy of Nancy Sally.)

operatory, requiring an extremely compatible relationship between the surgeon and the pathologist to accurately understand tissue orientation and the terminology used by both physicians.[128, 129, 143] It is important to recognize that the various methods of sectioning designed to evaluate the complete cut surgical margins are not equivalent to the MMS technique,[4, 18] and most have not been studied as thoroughly as MMS.[18, 133] However,

despite these limitations, they may improve the quality and adequacy of conventional methods of surgical excision. The use of frozen sections at the time of conventional surgical excision to enhance the probability of clear pathologic margins can also help to improve the chance of cure.[11, 137, 144] However, frozen sections are subject to the limitations of the pathologic processing method used.

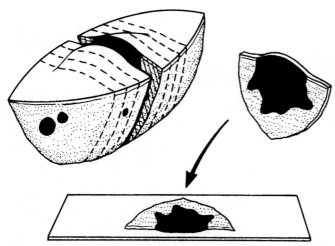

Figure 56–4. Conventional tissue processing of surgical excision specimen using the "breadloaf" technique, showing margins that would be reported as "tumor free" yet are actually involved with cancer. (Courtesy of Nancy Sally.)

PERINEURAL, PERIOSTEAL, AND PERICHONDRIAL INVOLVEMENT

Perineural invasion significantly influences the potential for subclinical extension by BCC. Once perineural invasion occurs, the tumor uses the nerve as a pathway of extension, potentially spreading in an antegrade or retrograde fashion.[145–147] Subclinical spread may track over large distances, potentially involving intracranial

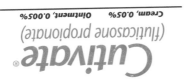

INCOMPLETELY EXCISED BCC ("POSITIVE MARGINS")

Studies performed in the 1960s propagated the notion that BCCs shown on pathologic examination to be incompletely excised do not need to be immediately re-excised, as only 30 to 40% will recur.[150, 151] In addition, immediate re-excision often failed to demonstrate any evidence of residual tumor, further supporting a "wait-and-see" approach.[90, 117, 127, 150, 152]

Controversy brewed as additional data supported the concept of immediate re-excision of incompletely ex-

cised BCCs.[12, 70] Later it was emphasized that incompletely excised BCCs exhibiting aggressive histologic features or involving the H zone recur in a large percentage of cases.[100, 153, 154] Several authors recommended immediate re-excision of BCCs shown by histologic examination to be incompletely excised.[4, 11, 12, 62, 70, 84, 94, 155–158] Because recurrent BCC may take years to manifest clinically, recognition of the recurrence depends on strict patient compliance with follow-up recommendations.[78] By the time recurrent BCC is clinically apparent, subclinical spread within and adjacent to the site of previous surgery is often extensive.[4, 62, 95] MMS is the preferred treatment for incompletely excised BCCs, as residual subclinical foci of tumor can be traced and selectively removed.[100, 140]

Treatment Alternatives

CURETTAGE AND ELECTRODESICCATION

Curettage and electrodesiccation (C&E) is a time-honored and effective modality for the treatment of some BCCs. The literature supports overall cure rates of greater than 90% for low-risk tumors.[113, 159–162] The success of C&E is maximized by the use of proper technique and by appropriate and careful patient selection.[80, 107, 113, 160–163] However, despite documentation of high cure rates, a uniformly agreed on protocol for the technique of C&E for BCC removal has not been firmly established.[59, 87, 164] Authors variably emphasize proper perilesional traction, vigorous curettage followed by delicate electrodesiccation, sequential use of smaller curettes to dislodge residual foci of tumor, repetition until complete tumor removal is sensed by the surgeon, and removal of a 2- to 4-mm rim of tissue around the curetted BCC.[87, 105, 107, 113, 114, 163] The use of curettage alone has been suggested but lacks extensive support.[113, 165–168] The use of electrodesiccation before curettage is discouraged, as normal tissue beyond the BCC is destroyed, diminishing the value of curettage.[105, 107] The value of proper training and experience has been documented[161, 162, 164] in reducing the risk of recurrence after C&E.

Penetration of the curette into pockets, creating a shelf of tissue, or into subcutaneous fat confirms extensive invasion of BCC.[79, 87, 99] Once this occurs, C&E should be abandoned in favor of an alternative approach.[79, 99, 107] Deep pockets or pits that create a "honeycomb" appearance of the lesion base are also indicative of deeper penetration warranting alternative therapy.[87] Surgical excision or MMS should be recommended in such circumstances.[99, 107]

Proper patient selection has always been the foundation of successful treatment with C&E. The procedure is most beneficial when limited to primary BCCs with discrete clinical borders.[4, 59, 69, 79, 92, 93, 113, 164] Other important parameters include site, size, histologic characteristics, and previous therapy.

Site. Histologic persistence of BCC after C&E is more frequent on the head, especially the nose and nasolabial folds, than on the trunk.[69, 79, 80, 162] This correlates with clinical experience implicating H-zone locations as sites that are prone to recurrence after C&E. Other regional considerations also merit discussion. C&E should not be used on locations with thin skin and minimal dermis (e.g., medial canthus, eyelids, and ears), as the skin is easily torn.[11, 87] Free margins such as the eyelids, lips, and nasal ala are difficult to immobilize and are subject to contracture during second-intention healing.[11, 79, 87] Distal lower extremities must be approached with caution, especially in elderly patients, diabetics, and patients with peripheral vascular compromise, as long delays in healing can be expected.[113] Therefore, C&E is most applicable for BCCs of the head and neck that do not involve the H zone and BCCs of the trunk and extremities.

Size. Recommendations regarding the maximum size of BCC of the head and neck that may be treated with C&E vary from 1 to 2 cm.[4, 12, 79, 106, 113, 160, 162] Based on literature review and clinical impression, it is suggested that C&E be limited to non–H-zone head and neck BCCs that are less than 1 cm in size and truncal or extremity BCCs (excluding superficial BCC) measuring less than 2 cm. Although not generally recommended, the use of C&E for BCCs involving the H zone may be applicable in special clinical circumstances. In such cases, C&E should be utilized only for discrete nodular BCCs less than 0.5 cm.[62, 160]

Histologic Characteristics. C&E is only indicated for nodular BCCs with discrete clinical borders and superficial BCC without clinical or histologic signs of deeper invasion.[4, 79, 107, 113] Aggressive histologic patterns (e.g., as seen in morpheaform, infiltrative, and micronodular BCCs) are usually less responsive to C&E, as small tumor islands and strands cannot be felt by the curette.[4, 59, 62, 107, 113] The presence of sclerosis also reduces the likelihood of cure by C&E, as the ability to feel tumor with the curette is eliminated.[58, 107, 113, 114]

Previous Therapy. The lack of efficacy of C&E for treatment of recurrent basal cell carcinoma is well documented, with cure rates of 40 to 59% reported.[92, 93, 164] The presence of scar from previous surgery and discontinuous foci of BCC within scar tissue decrease the efficacy of C&E.[92, 97, 107, 113]

Advantages

The C&E technique has the important advantage of being a time-efficient and technically simple surgical procedure that can be performed in the ambulatory setting under local anesthesia[106, 113, 163] for a large percentage of low-risk BCCs.[160, 162] It is usually less expensive than excision with advanced repair, MMS, and radiation therapy,[132] and postoperative pain is minimal and wound infection uncommon.

Disadvantages

The disadvantages of C&E are also important to consider. C&E is a "blind" technique, as no specimen for margin evaluation is generated.[4, 62] The procedure is not indicated for BCCs with high-risk features.[107, 113] The end point of treatment is determined subjectively based on tumor characteristics and operator experience. Healing is always by second intention and takes several weeks,[106, 113] resulting in a hypopigmented scar.[4, 106] Potential complications include stellate and hypertrophic scarring, persistent erythema, and unsightly wound contraction.[79, 106, 162–164]

SURGICAL EXCISION

A popular modality among all surgical specialties that treat BCC is surgical excision (SE). Overall cure rates of greater than 90% have been documented for primary BCC.[12, 126, 159] The generation of a pathology specimen allows objective pathologic evaluation of treatment adequacy.[126, 129] However, as with all modalities, specific advantages and possible pitfalls must be considered. In addition to variables such as site, size, histologic characteristics, and previous treatment, factors affecting the potential benefit of SE include surgical margins, pathologic margins, and "positive" margins after excision.

Site. SE is appropriate treatment for all low-risk BCCs and some high-risk BCCs.[126] The risk of recurrence after SE is increased in the H zone, where wider and deeper margins are often needed.[12, 68–72, 90, 127, 155, 169–171] Frozen section control is suggested in anatomic locations such as the H zone[11, 144, 156] that are more likely to develop recurrence.

Size. When evaluating size parameters, SE has been shown to be most effective for primary BCCs smaller than 2 cm.[4, 11, 12, 69, 94] The risk of recurrence increases with larger BCCs because of unpredictable increases in subclinical spread of tumor.[61, 85] When SE is used, frozen section control has been recommended[11] for BCCs larger than 2 cm on the face and larger than 4 cm on the trunk.

The generally acceptable cut-off value of less than 2 cm in size for SE is only applicable for locations that can accommodate sacrifice of significant amounts of normal tissue. If 4 mm are added to the surgical margins around a 2-cm lesion, the minimum diameter of excision is 2.8 cm. A wound of this size may be difficult to close effectively, especially in the H zone, without unnecessarily sacrificing structures important for function or cosmesis.

Histologic Characteristics. There are no specific histologic subtypes of BCC that are contraindications for the use of SE. BCCs with well-circumscribed growth patterns are most amenable to SE.[60, 62, 111, 131] Aggressive histologic subtypes of BCC have been shown to decrease the likelihood of complete surgical excision.[60, 62, 66, 70, 110–112, 170] In one large series, incomplete surgical excision was found in 18% of micronodular BCCs and 26% of infiltrative BCCs.[60] Mixed BCCs exhibiting both nodular and aggressive features demonstrate a behavior pattern similar to the aggressive pattern that is present.[60] The high percentages of incomplete excision may be accounted for by the frequent combination of indistinct clinical margins and greater subclinical extension.[57, 61, 62, 104] When using SE for a BCC with aggressive histologic features, wider surgical margins or frozen section control may be required to provide a greater chance of complete excision.[4, 11, 156]

Surgical Margins. Clinical judgment is extremely important when deciding on the proper surgical margins for an excision. The surgeon is encouraged to maximize complete tumor removal by carefully choosing surgical margins based on the size, histologic features, and location of BCC and by not decreasing the margins of excision necessary for cure to maximize the cosmetic result. The use of curettage before the final determination of surgical margins is strongly recommended. This helps to better delineate the size and direction of spread of BCC before determining surgical margins.[107, 111, 140, 172] Excision lines are drawn after curettage is completed.[88, 140]

Recommendations regarding surgical margins for BCC excision have ranged from 2 to 5 mm for low-risk BCCs less than 2 cm in size and 8 to 10 mm or more for BCCs over 2 cm in size, morpheaform BCCs, recurrent BCCs, and BCCs involving the auricular region.[4, 85, 88, 94, 126, 157, 170, 173] This wide range is mostly based on retrospective analysis and clinical impressions. Important guidelines for SE of BCC have been established.[85] Using a 4-mm surgical margin will allow for complete excision of a clinically discrete primary BCC smaller than 2 cm in 98% of cases. Lesser margins, even for BCCs 3 to 6 mm in size, may be expected to decrease the chance of total excision to approximately 80%.[133] Various authors have suggested 10-mm surgical margins for SE of discrete BCCs greater than 2 cm in size.[4, 88] Unfortunately, although this is likely to be curative, a large amount of normal tissue is often sacrificed.

At present, no studies have adequately addressed the issue of depth of excision.[4, 85] When invasion of the subcutis is not clinically apparent, it is reasonable to excise to the level of midsubcutaneous fat, provided a well-developed layer of adipose tissue is present and critical structures, such as motor nerves, that are not involved with tumor are not sacrificed. In locations where the subcutaneous fat is scant, excision to the fascial layer is appropriate. When there is uncertainty regarding tumor involvement of important deep structures (e.g., bone, cartilage, motor nerves, or blood vessels) or when tissue conservation is critical, MMS is far superior to SE.

Well-documented surgical margin recommendations for recurrent BCCs are nonexistent. The cutaneous surgeon cannot confidently assess the clinical margins of a recurrent tumor and must be suspicious of wide and deep invasion.[63, 94, 95] As a result, 1- to 3-cm surgical margins and the use of frozen section control have been suggested.[4, 11, 94, 156, 170, 173, 174] Again, MMS is clearly superior to SE for treatment of recurrent BCC.[69, 92–94, 126]

Advantages

SE of BCC offers several advantages. Most patients can be treated in an ambulatory setting using local anesthesia. A pathology specimen allows for some evaluation of the treatment adequacy.[126, 137, 140] Healing time is short,[88, 126] and the cosmetic results are generally very good.[126, 156]

Disadvantages

SE requires more time and experience than C&E. The procedure is most effective for BCCs with clinically discrete borders, depending on clinical judgment of surgical margins.[88, 140] The recommended excision margins require sacrifice of unknown amounts of normal tissues.[85, 126, 169] The results are affected by the limitations of tissue processing.[129] When frozen section control is added, time and expense are both increased.[132, 143]

RADIATION THERAPY

Radiation therapy (RT) has long been recognized as an effective modality for the treatment of BCC, with overall cure rates reported to be greater than 90%.[126, 159, 175, 176] Unfortunately, complications associated with older treatment protocols, inadequate safety protection, and the limitations of equipment available in past years diminished the popularity of RT as a treatment option.[177, 178] Currently, RT for skin cancer is primarily practiced at medical centers by specialists in radiation oncology.[88, 176] The noninvasive nature of most RT techniques is well tolerated by patients who are poor candidates for surgery.[178, 179] RT may also be used as adjunctive therapy, providing palliation in patients with inoperable BCC.[94, 180]

Various forms of RT—including soft x-ray,[177, 179] superficial x-ray,[177, 179] electron beam,[181–184] and iridium wire implants[185]—may be used to treat BCC depending on the specific clinical circumstances. In addition, grenz ray may be used to treat SBCC.[177, 179] While BCC responds to a variety of treatment schedules,[176, 178] fractionation of the total dose over the course of several days to weeks has generally replaced single-dose schedules, allowing deliverance of higher total doses with better tolerance by normal tissue.[176–179, 186, 187] The daily radiation doses used in specific protocols are dependent on tumor size, the number of treatments given, and the interval between treatments (time-dose relationship).[178, 179, 186]

Site and Size. RT has been recommended for the treatment of clinically discrete, medium-sized, primary BCCs involving the nose, lips, ears, and periorbital region. The following sizes have been suggested as most appropriate: nose, 1 to 3 cm; periorbital region, 0.5 to 1.5 cm; ear, 2 to 3 cm; and lips, 1 to 2 cm.[188] Smaller BCCs are best treated by surgical techniques.[178, 179, 189] Larger lesions are likely to heal with an undesirable functional or cosmetic result that will often require surgical revision at a later date.[188] BCCs involving cartilage or bone are best treated surgically but may also be treated using specialized radiologic techniques when surgery is contraindicated.[178, 188–190]

RT is discouraged for BCCs of the trunk or extremities because of delayed healing, poor cosmetic results, and sensitivity of treated sites to trauma.[176, 178, 186, 191]

Histologic Characteristics. All histologic subtypes of BCC are thought to be sensitive to RT, provided an adequate dose of the radiation is delivered to the entire tumor.[178] This is most easily accomplished with discrete nodular BCCs.[88] Histologic patterns exhibiting significant subclinical extension require increased zones of treatment.[4, 115, 176–179, 186] The presence of sclerosis has been associated with a decreased cure rate.[178]

Zones of Treatment. RT is a "blind" technique that does not produce a pathology specimen to evaluate treatment adequacy.[4, 62, 176] A pretreatment biopsy is critical to assist the radiation therapist in evaluating the histologic pattern and anticipating the depth of invasion.[177, 179] Careful clinical examination is also important, as the field of treatment is dependent on delineation of clinical borders of the BCC.[191] When borders are discrete and histologic features are nonaggressive, a margin of 0.5 to 1 cm is recommended.[176, 179, 190] An additional margin of at least 0.5 cm is treated when borders are not discrete or when biopsy reveals an aggressive pattern.[115, 176, 177, 179] Allowances for greater penetration of the beam are made when sites known to facilitate deeper extension (e.g., the nasolabial folds and retroauricular sulcus) are involved.[188] Tissues involved with BCC preferentially undergo necrosis after RT. It is important to recognize that all tissues included in the zone of treatment are exposed to radiation and thus are subject to potential acute and chronic complications.

Previous Treatment. RT has also been recommended for recurrent BCC; however, overall cure rates of 73% make it a less than optimal technique.[4, 92, 93, 174, 178] Difficulty in determining the exact location of recurrent tumor further decreases the likelihood of encompassing the entire lesion in the three-dimensional field of treatment.[4] Thus, RT is recommended only when surgery is absolutely contraindicated or refused by the patient.[92] The use of RT in the treatment of incompletely excised BCCs is also discouraged, as margin involvement indicates subclinical extension beyond the clinical judgment of the cutaneous surgeon, and localization of residual tumor cannot be determined with confidence.[41, 91, 190]

RT should not be used for recurrent BCC treated initially with radiation.[88, 94, 174, 178, 186, 190] The accumulation of additional radiation may cause severe chronic radiation dermatitis and increase the risk of cutaneous carcinogenesis.[88, 186] In addition, when radiation dermatitis is clinically present, it is more difficult to delineate clinical borders of a new BCC. It has also been noted that BCC recurring after initial radiation treatment behaves more aggressively than recurrences after other treatment modalities.[155, 192–194]

Treatment Sequelae and Complications

RT for BCC is followed by an expected reaction pattern of acute radiation dermatitis,[178, 191] which consists initially of erythema and edema followed by erosion and exudation.[28] Burning or pruritus also frequently accompanies the acute dermatitis. Healing occurs over an average of 4 to 8 weeks, depending on the size and depth of the lesion treated.[28, 191]

The initial cosmetic appearance after healing is usually very good for several months.[28, 179] Unfortunately, cosmesis worsens progressively over time,[177, 179] with many patients demonstrating atrophy, hypopigmentation, hyperpigmentation, and telangiectasia within 3 months to 2 years after completing radiation therapy.[28] Increased

sensitivity to minor trauma also occurs, and when hair-bearing areas have been treated, permanent alopecia occurs.[178, 188]

If healing of the eroded phase is delayed or necrosis is unexpectedly massive, the possibility of tumor penetration beyond the treatment field must be considered, and a biopsy of the deep tissue is indicated.[4] Other side effects of RT include transient comedone formation,[178] pseudorecidivism,[178, 195] and delayed postradiation ulceration or late radiation necrosis.[178, 179] The last reaction may develop several months or years after RT and usually resolves spontaneously over several months.[196] The lesions appear erosive or ulcerative and may suggest recurrent BCC.[179] Persistent delayed ulceration may require surgical excision.[177, 191] Current techniques using modern equipment are associated with a much lower incidence of untoward reactions involving deeper structures (e.g., bone or cartilage necrosis, postradiation chondritis, and impairment of the lacrimal system).[176, 188, 189, 195] The development of complications such as cataracts and thyroid cancer has also been significantly reduced as a result of proper placement of safety shields.[179, 197]

There is a well-established association between the development of BCC and SCC and the repeated use of small doses of RT over long periods of time.[28, 178, 198] Such radiation therapy regimens were used in the past to treat benign dermatoses such as acne, dermatophytosis, and hirsutism.[94] However, studies have indicated that the risk of cutaneous carcinogenesis is minimal when high-dose regimens used to treat BCC and SCC are administered over a short period of time.[28, 177] Most cases of radiation-induced skin malignancy have occurred in patients with clinical and histologic evidence of chronic radiation dermatitis.[28] Importantly, although clinical features of chronic radiation dermatitis may be subtle in these patients, the clinical appearance of radiogenic skin cancers does not differ from that of naturally occurring lesions.[28]

Contraindications

RT should be strongly discouraged in patients younger than 50 years old because of the long latency of cutaneous oncogenesis (average, 24 years) and less favorable cosmetic results in younger patients.[28, 88, 94] Younger patients will also be exposed to greater quantities of natural UVL over the ensuing years, further enhancing the risk of BCC induced by previous RT.[25, 178] RT is contraindicated in patients with xeroderma pigmentosum and is also not recommended in patients with basal cell nevus syndrome.[23, 178]

Advantages

RT is an excellent modality for the treatment of BCC in properly selected cases. It is most applicable for primary BCCs in patients who are not surgical candidates.[88, 179] RT may also be beneficial as palliative therapy to reduce pain or tumor bulk in patients with advanced lesions or inoperable tumors.[186, 191] Treatment is painless and generally well tolerated.[179]

Disadvantages

RT requires consultation with a physician who is highly skilled in the selection and delivery of appropriate therapeutic radiation techniques. Fractionation of total dosage over several visits is inconvenient because of the increased time, travel, and expense required.[176] Prolonged wound care is necessary, as healing takes several weeks. RT is more expensive than simpler modalities such as C&E and cryosurgery and may even exceed SE and MMS in cost.

CRYOSURGERY

Since the 1970s, cryosurgery has evolved into an effective modality for the treatment of BCC.[199] A better understanding of cryobiology, advanced delivery systems, improved treatment protocols, and careful patient selection has increased the efficacy of cryosurgery, with overall cure rates of greater than 90% reported for selected BCCs.[159, 200–202]

Available techniques for cryogen delivery include open spray, restricted spray using neoprene cones, and cryoprobes.[203, 204] Cotton-tipped applicators, although acceptable for some benign lesions, are not appropriate for treatment of skin malignancies.[202] Ultimately, successful treatment of BCC depends on the experience of the cryosurgeon and requires a complete understanding of the variables that affect outcome, such as freeze time, thaw time, halo thaw time, and the use of monitoring needles and measuring devices.[88, 201, 203]

The use of a device that monitors the breadth and depth of freeze is generally recommended, especially when treating BCCs located within the high-risk H zone.[4, 201] Available monitoring systems include units that measure electrical impedance or thermocouples linked to a pyrometer for tissue temperature measurements.[205] Appropriate placement of monitoring needles is critical, but unfortunately very subjective. Treatment of SBCC does not require a tissue-monitoring device.

Cryosurgery is a "blind" technique, since it does not generate a pathologic specimen.[4, 62] Therefore, adequate treatment depends on the cryosurgeon's ability and experience in determining a proper field of treatment. Initial debulking and curettage is recommended before determining the field of treatment. This technique helps to define microscopic tumor extension, allowing for improved delineation of the treatment field and presumably improved cure rates.[206–208] If curettage extends into subcutaneous fat, cryosurgery should be abandoned; SE or MMS is then recommended.[207] Patient selection is based on tumor appearance, location, size, and histologic features.[207] Cryosurgery works best when limited to primary BCCs with discrete clinical borders.[208–211] It is most effective for nodular BCC and SBCC and less effective for tumors with aggressive histologic features.[88, 116, 201, 207, 209–211]

Size. Cryosurgery has been shown to be effective for BCCs up to 2 to 3 cm in size.[4, 116, 207, 209] However, a maximal size of 1 cm is appropriate when the H zone is involved.[116, 211] BCCs involving cartilage or bone should not be treated by cryosurgery.[116]

Site. The use of cryosurgery at specific sites warrants some additional detailed considerations. Treatment of eyelid BCC with cryosurgery must be performed with caution and only by experienced cryosurgeons.[212, 213] When cryosurgery is properly applied for eyelid BCCs, complications such as ectropion, lacrimal occlusion, and lid notching are uncommon, and cure rates are excellent.[211–215] Unless the underlying cartilage or lacrimal apparatus is involved with tumor, these structures are usually spared, and cosmetic results are typically very good. Importantly, only clinically discrete primary BCCs measuring smaller than 1 cm should be considered for cryosurgery. A decrease in cure rates for eyelid lesions larger than 1 cm has been documented.[213, 214]

Other site-related problems can complicate cryosurgery. Notching may also occur on the alar rim and helix, especially if the underlying cartilage is involved by tumor.[116, 202, 216] Perforation of the nose, ears, and eyelids may sometimes occur.[202, 217] Contracted scars may result in an unsightly pulling that causes asymmetry after treatment of BCC involving the nasal ala, upper lip, mouth corners, and eyelids.[218] Treatment of distal extremity lesions with cryosurgery results in delayed healing.[201, 208, 209]

Previous Treatment. Cryosurgery is not recommended for the treatment of recurrent BCC or incompletely excised BCC.[92, 209] This is because the surgeon is unable to accurately determine the proper zone of treatment, as tumor foci are clinically imperceptible. Data supporting the use of cryosurgery for both recurrent BCC and incompletely excised BCC are significantly lacking.[92]

Treatment Sequelae and Complications

Cryosurgery for BCC is followed by an expected sequence of tissue reactions.[218] Erythema, urtication, and edema occur initially, followed by vesiculation and serous exudation after 12 to 24 hours. Postcryosurgical edema typically peaks at 24 to 36 hours after surgery and is likely to be most severe after treatment of periorbital or forehead BCCs.[217, 218]

Cryosurgery is also associated with other potential complications. Patients may become febrile for 24 to 48 hours after treatment.[116, 217] A migraine-like cephalgia lasting several hours often follows treatment of forehead, scalp, and temple BCCs.[116] Transient neuropathy, usually characterized by paresthesia or anesthesia, may develop and takes several months to resolve.[116, 219] The lateral digits, neck, arms, legs, and periauricular area are especially prone to neuropathy.[219, 220] After 1 to 2 weeks healing begins, and the eschar finally lifts after 5 to 6 weeks.[218] Because healing is by second intention, the postoperative course is longer than with procedures that allow for surgical repair.

Cosmetic results after cryosurgery vary with skin type, tumor characteristics, and tumor location. The resultant scar from cryosurgery is usually flat, slightly atrophic, and hypopigmented, especially when patients with darker skin are treated.[201, 217] Hypertrophic scarring may occur,[116, 202, 216] but healing with depression may also result, especially after treatment of larger or deeper tumors with associated tissue loss.[218] Loss of adnexa usually causes permanent alopecia when hair-bearing sites are treated.[202, 216, 217] Treatment of sebaceous skin may result in permanent, obvious, and unsightly changes in tissue texture after healing.[216]

Advantages

Cryosurgery is an excellent modality for the treatment of selected primary BCCs, especially for patients who are poor surgical candidates.[88, 209] It is a time-efficient and relatively inexpensive technique.[213, 221] While it may be used to treat patients of any age, patients older than 40 tend to heal with a more acceptable cosmetic result.[218] The procedure can be performed in an ambulatory setting or at the bedside in a hospital or nursing home, with or without local anesthesia.[202] It may also be used as palliative therapy for inoperable BCCs to decrease tumor bulk associated with pain, infection, or odor.[208]

Disadvantages

Cryosurgery is primarily limited to low-risk BCCs, because a pathologic specimen for evaluation of treatment adequacy is not generated. BCCs involving the H zone and those with aggressive histologic features are best treated by other modalities.[116, 201, 209] Treatment of eyelid BCCs should be limited to lesions smaller than 1 cm.[213] Training and specialized equipment are required. Healing is prolonged, and cosmetic results are variable.[202]

Contraindications

Cryosurgery is contraindicated in patients with cold sensitivity (e.g., those with cryoglobulinemia, cryofibrinogenemia, cold urticaria, Raynaud's disease, and collagen vascular disease).[116, 216, 219]

MOHS MICROGRAPHIC SURGERY

MMS is a type of SE combined with immediate frozen section analysis of the excised tissue to provide the highest cure rates for BCC and SCC.[92, 100, 159] In this technique, the Mohs micrographic surgeon serves as both surgeon and pathologist.[18, 222] The technique involves excision of thin disks of tissue around the cancer that are frozen, sectioned horizontally, and microscopically mapped. This allows for anatomic localization of all subclinical tumor extensions. Areas involved with tumor extension are subsequently excised as guided by the maps, and the process is repeated until a tumor-free plane is reached (Fig. 56–5).[103, 223–226]

Advantages

The advantages of this technique are significant. First, histologic evaluation of the cut surgical margins involves nearly 100% of the tissue,[103, 129, 132] compared with traditional vertical sectioning techniques that examine less than 1%.[132, 227, 228] Second, this complete margin analysis

allows identification and tracking of all foci of residual tumor, regardless of whether the tissue layer involved is skin, subcutaneous tissue, muscle, fascia, perineural tissue, cartilage, or bone.[132] Third, resection of only tumor-positive areas offers a tissue-sparing advantage (i.e., minimizing tissue loss and also often sparing functionally or cosmetically important structures).[91, 95, 169, 229] Factors that limit the success of SE, C&E, cryosurgery, and RT (e.g., nondiscrete clinical borders, aggressive histologic features, subclinical extensions, or scar tissue from previous therapy) do not alter the value of MMS, as tumor foci are traced microscopically and selectively removed.[4, 100, 132, 229]

The efficacy of MMS for the treatment of BCC has been heavily documented. While it offers the highest cure rate for all BCCs, it can be considered the treatment of choice for recurrent BCC,[92, 100, 222] including SBCC; BCCs with nondiscrete clinical borders[88, 91, 132]; histologically aggressive BCCs[91, 100, 229]; BCCs in anatomic locations associated with higher recurrence rates with non-Mohs techniques[4, 68, 91, 132] (e.g., the nose,[222, 230] perinasal region,[95] auricular region,[170, 231, 232] lips,[233] temple,[73, 234] and periocular area, including the medial canthus)[235–237]; primary BCCs in locations where tissue conservation is critical[132]; large BCCs (i.e., greater than 2 cm)[91, 229]; and incompletely excised BCCs,[100, 222] especially on the head and neck. Overall long-term cure rates with MMS are 98 to 99% for primary BCC and 95 to 96% for recurrent BCC.[92, 101, 102, 159]

In addition to offering high cure rates and sparing of normal tissues, MMS has several other advantages. The procedure is performed in an ambulatory setting using only local anesthesia.[91] In most cases, MMS can be completed in 1 day or less,[225] and reconstructive surgery can follow immediately.[132] Some defects produced by MMS may heal satisfactorily by second intention.[238–240] MMS is cost effective when used for properly selected tumors, especially when compared with RT or conventional SE performed in a hospital setting. However, because MMS is more expensive than cryosurgery and C&E, it may not be cost effective when used for small, low-risk BCCs that can be effectively treated by less expensive modalities.[91, 132]

Disadvantages

The disadvantage of MMS is that it requires specialized physician training and a laboratory staffed with a trained histotechnician.[91] It is a more costly technique than C&E and cryosurgery.

5-FLUOROURACIL

Topical application of 5-fluorouracil (5-FU) has been recommended for a variety of premalignant and malignant cutaneous conditions.[241] Unfortunately, the value of topical 5-FU in the treatment of BCC is very limited. Topical 5-FU 5% has been approved by the FDA for the treatment of SBCC, yet long-term cure rates have not been established.[242] Topical 5-FU is not indicated for other types of primary BCC or recurrent BCC, including recurrent SBCC.[241, 242]

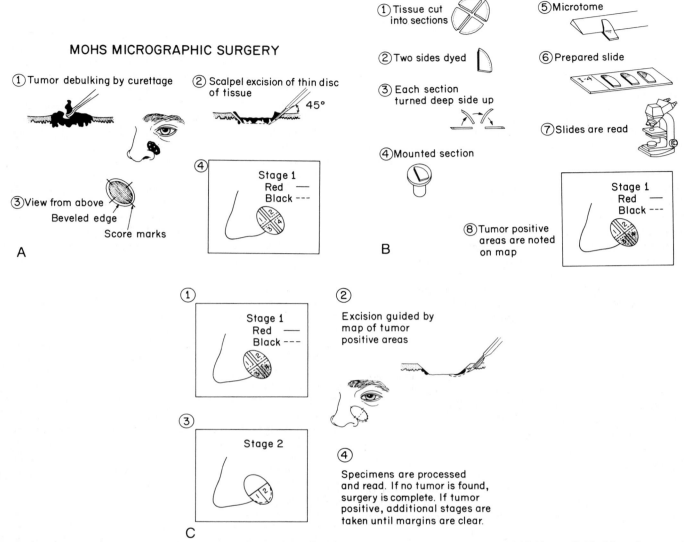

Figure 56–5. *A,* Excision of an initial Mohs surgical layer. *B,* Tissue preparation and interpretation of the initial layer. *C,* Excision of a second layer guided by a map of tumor-positive areas. (From Lambert DR, Siegle RJ: Skin cancer: a review with consideration of treatment options including Mohs micrographic surgery. Ohio Med 86:745, 1990.)

Unfortunately, the major drawback associated with 5-FU treatment is potential elimination of only the superficial component of the SBCC, with persistence of deeper subclinical foci.[243]

It has been suggested that topical 5-FU may be of prophylactic benefit in patients with basal cell nevus syndrome[241, 244] and that intralesional 5-FU may be effective for BCC.[245] Both of these require additional study and cannot be recommended as effective forms of treatment at present.[246]

INVESTIGATIONAL TREATMENTS

Retinoids

Systemic retinoids are being evaluated for chemotherapy in patients with BCC. Both isotretinoin and etretinate have been studied, primarily in patients with multiple tumors caused by basal cell nevus syndrome and xeroderma pigmentosum.[247, 248]

Chemotherapeutic dosage regimens inducing complete or partial regression of BCC have required the use of very high doses of systemic retinoids (isotretinoin greater than 2 mg/kg/day or etretinate 1 mg/kg/day),[249, 250] which are often limited by retinoid toxicity. Complete regression of even small BCCs less than 1 cm in size is seen in fewer than 10% of patients.[249]

Chemoprevention of BCC with systemic retinoids, however, appears to be more promising. Lower doses are required than are used to achieve a chemotherapeutic effect.[249–251] Studies have confirmed a significant reduction in new tumor formation during therapy, but discontinuation results in a return to the baseline rate of tumor formation.[249, 252, 253] The role of systemic retinoids in chemoprevention of and chemotherapy for BCC hopefully will be better defined by additional study, as well as by the development of newer agents.

Both topical retinoic acid (tretinoin)[252, 254] and topical isotretinoin[255, 256] have been studied in the treatment of BCC, but the responses have proven to be less than adequate, preventing recommendation of these agents for treatment of BCC.

Interferon

The interferons are a family of glycoproteins that exhibit antineoplastic, antiviral, and immunomodulatory effects.[257] Their ability to influence cell proliferation and differentiation has led researchers to study their effects on epidermal malignancies, including BCC.[258] Preliminary data indicate that intralesional interferon therapy may induce complete regression in up to 80% of primary nodular BCCs smaller than 2 cm and primary SBCCs smaller than 3 cm.[258-263] Both interferon alfa and high-dose interferon gamma have been found to be effective when administered three times per week over a 3-week period.[258-261] A sustained-release form of interferon alfa-2b that reduces the frequency of injections has also been developed.[262] At present, long-term cure rates are not available. Reported side effects include a flulike syndrome, transient leukopenia, and mild increases in hepatic enzymes.[259, 261, 262] Additional study is needed to define optimal dosages and treatment protocols.

Photodynamic Therapy

Photodynamic therapy (PDT) of BCC involves administration of a photosensitizing agent, usually by intravenous injection, followed in 48 to 72 hours by initial exposure to laser light of 400 nm. This results in fluorescence of tumor cells to help identify tumor location and is followed by exposure to laser light of 610–740 nm for tumor destruction.[264-266] The photosensitizing agents are concentrated by malignant cells such as those found in BCC, thereby allowing selective treatment of cancers.[264-266] Hematoporphyrin derivative and dihematoporphyrin ether are currently the most commonly used photosensitizers.[264] The argon-pumped tunable dye laser is the usual source of 630 nm red light for tumor destruction.[265]

One problem associated with systemic photosensitizers is prolonged generalized cutaneous photosensitivity that lasts several weeks.[264, 267] Topical agents have been studied and appear to be of benefit only for superficial lesions.[268] PDT is a promising experimental technique that will hopefully be refined for more routine application, especially in patients with multiple BCCs.

Advanced and Metastatic BCC

Large and deeply invasive primary or recurrent BCCs are sometimes not amenable to treatment using a single conventional modality. Patients with advanced BCCs may be poor candidates for extensive surgery, have an unresectable tumor, or require surgery that will result in marked disfigurement and loss of function because of tumor location or size. At times, palliation and improved quality of life may be the only achievable goals. Management warrants consultation with physicians from multiple disciplines so that treatment can be individualized based on the likelihood for cure or palliation and the desires of the patient and the family.

SE,[269, 270] MMS,[269, 271] RT,[180, 189] cryosurgery,[272] and chemotherapy[180, 270, 273, 274] may play a role in selected cases of advanced BCC. Combinations of these modalities may be utilized with success. For patients who are surgical candidates, combined surgical approaches utilizing MMS and traditional surgical techniques have been advocated by several authors.[82, 91, 95, 230, 232, 269, 275]

Fortunately, metastatic BCC is rare, with an incidence ranging from 0.028 to 0.1%.[15, 276] Most metastatic BCCs have developed in patients with extensive primary BCC or multiply recurrent BCCs.[276, 277] No correlation exists between methods of treatment of either the primary or recurrent lesion and development of metastasis. Metastatic BCC has originated in most cases on the head and neck; however, metastasis has also been reported from BCCs of the trunk, extremities, and genitalia.[16, 17, 277, 278, 279] There are no histologic criteria that help to predict which BCCs will metastasize. Solid (nodular) BCC, sclerotic BCC, adenoid BCC, and basosquamous (metatypical) BCC have all been associated with metastasic disease.[16, 277]

Metastasis of BCC may occur by either lymphatic or hematogenous spread.[16, 17] While metastases most often develop in a single site, diffuse spread to multiple sites occurs in approximately 30% of cases.[277] Regional lymph nodes are the most common site of involvement (60 to 70%), followed by the lungs (20 to 30%), bones (20 to 25%), and liver (18%).[16, 17, 279] When only one site is involved, the lymph nodes are affected in more than 50% of cases, followed by the lungs in 10%, and the bones in 10%.[16, 276] Diffuse metastasis of BCC has also been reported to involve the kidney, pancreas, diaphragm, adrenal gland, spleen, and dura.[17, 279, 280]

In most cases, an average of 9 to 11 years elapses between the onset of primary BCC and the discovery of metastasis.[16, 17] However, once metastasis occurs, the average duration of survival is 8 to 10 months.[16, 276] Patients with isolated lymph node metastasis appear to have a better prognosis, with an average survival of 3.6 years.[276]

There are no large prospective or comparative studies evaluating the treatment of metastatic BCC. Treatment recommendations are based on case reports and small series. MMS is recommended for the cutaneous component of the recurrent BCC. Surgery is recommended for removal of regional lymph node metastases, especially when nodes are the only site of involvement. A patient with metastatic BCC to regional lymph nodes should undergo radiologic evaluation of the chest, skeletal system, and liver to exclude other foci of metastasis before therapeutic lymph node dissection is initiated.[276] Radiation therapy and chemotherapy may be used to treat diffuse metastatic involvement, but experience with systemic chemotherapy for metastatic BCC is limited. Various drugs have been used either alone or in combination, with varied results.[278, 281] Although no specific chemotherapy protocol has been determined as optimal therapy for metastatic BCC, cisplatin and doxorubicin appear to be the most successful agents.

Follow-up Examination

Self-examination and regular follow-up by a cutaneous surgeon skilled in skin evaluation are integral parts of BCC management. Such follow-up is indicated to detect new primary BCCs and recurrent BCC early in their development.[88, 282–284] Patients with a history of BCC are at an increased risk for development of a new BCC.[54, 282, 284] It is common for patients to be unaware of new BCCs until they are detected during a screening examination.[282] Recurrences of BCC are generally detected within 2 to 5 years, but approximately 20% of recurrences occur between 6 and 10 years after treatment.[159] BCCs recurring more than 10 years after primary treatment have been reported.[151, 159, 161]

Lifelong follow-up is recommended after treatment of BCC. The frequency of visits varies with the needs of the individual patient. Most patients require evaluation only once or twice a year. High-risk patients (e.g., those with multiple BCCs, xeroderma pigmentosum, basal cell nevus syndrome, chronic radiation dermatitis, and immunosuppression) may require more frequent examinations.

SUMMARY

The prevalence of BCC and its multiplicity of clinical, histologic, and biologic features make it an extremely important cancer, and all cutaneous surgeons should have detailed knowledge of and expertise in treating BCC. Appropriate management often requires meticulous and frequent skin examinations with early biopsy of suspicious lesions in high-risk anatomic locations. Once BCC has been diagnosed, the cutaneous surgeon, with significant input from the patient, must thoroughly evaluate and determine the most appropriate form of treatment to satisfactorily manage each individual cancer. In this way, a very high cure rate with the least cosmetic and functional impairment can be achieved.

REFERENCES

1. Bickers DR, Harber LC, Kopf A: Non-melanoma skin cancer and melanoma. In: Harber LC, Bickers DR (eds): Photosensitivity Diseases. BC Decker, Toronto, 1989, pp 315–330.
2. Diwan R, Skouge JW: Basal cell carcinoma. Curr Prob Dermatol 2:67–91, 1990.
3. Gordon D, Silverstone H: Worldwide epidemiology of premalignant and malignant cutaneous lesions. In: Andrade R (ed): Cancer of the Skin. WB Saunders, Philadelphia, 1976, pp 405–434.
4. Lang PG, Maize JC: Basal cell carcinoma. In: Friedman RJ (ed): Cancer of the Skin. WB Saunders, Philadelphia, 1991, pp 35–73.
5. Scotto J, Kopf AW, Urbach F: Non-melanoma skin cancer among caucasians in four areas of the United States. Cancer 34:1333–1338, 1974.
6. Scotto J, Fears TR, Fraumeni JF: Incidence of nonmelanoma skin cancer in the United States 1981. Publication #(NIH) 82-2433. National Cancer Institute, Bethesda, MD, 1982.
7. Gallagher RP, Ma B, McLean DI, et al: Trends in basal cell carcinoma, squamous cell carcinoma and melanoma of the skin from 1973 through 1987. J Am Acad Dermatol 23:413–421, 1990.
8. Altman A, Rosen T, Tschen JA, et al: Basal cell epithelioma in black patients. J Am Acad Dermatol 17:741–745, 1987.
9. Mora RG: Surgical and aesthetic considerations of cancer of the skin in the black American. J Dermatol Surg Oncol 12:24–31, 1986.
10. Mora RT, Burris R: Cancer of the skin in blacks: a review of 128 patients with basal cell carcinoma. Cancer 47:1436–1438, 1981.
11. Bennett RG (ed): Non-melanoma skin cancers. In: Fundamentals of Cutaneous Surgery. CV Mosby, St. Louis, 1988, pp 619–659.
12. Shanoff LB, Spira M, Hardy SB: Basal cell carcinoma: a statistical approach to rational management. Plast Reconstr Surg 39:619–624, 1967.
13. Roenigk RK, Ratz JL, Bailin PL, et al: Trends in the presentation and treatment of basal cell carcinomas. J Dermatol Surg Oncol 12:860–865, 1986.
14. Pollack SV, Goslen JB, Sheretz EF, et al: The biology of basal cell carcinoma: a review. J Am Acad Dermatol 7:569–577, 1982.
15. Miller SJ: Biology of basal cell carcinoma (part I). J Am Acad Dermatol 24:1–13, 1991.
16. Domarus H, Stevens PJ: Metastatic basal cell carcinoma: report of five cases and review of 170 cases in the literature. J Am Acad Dermatol 10:1043–1060, 1984.
17. Mikhail GR, Nims LP, Kelly AP, et al: Metastatic basal cell carcinoma: review, pathogenesis and report of two cases. Arch Dermatol 113;1261–1269, 1977.
18. Braun M: Being certain the cancer is out. J Dermatol Surg Oncol 13:1058–1060, 1987.
19. Epstein JH, Ormsby A, Adams RM: Occupational skin cancer. In: Adams RM (ed): Occupational Skin Disease. WB Saunders, Philadelphia, 1990, pp 136–159.
20. Zaynoun S, Lina AA, Shaib J, et al: The relationship of sun exposure and solar elastosis to basal cell carcinoma. J Am Acad Dermatol 12:522–525, 1985.
21. Vitaliano PP, Urbach F: The relative importance of risk factors in nonmelanoma carcinoma. Arch Dermatol 116:454–456, 1980.
22. Vitasa BC, Taylor HR, Strickland PT, et al: Association of nonmelanoma skin cancer and actinic keratosis with cumulative solar ultraviolet exposure in Maryland watermen. Cancer 65:2811–2817, 1990.
23. Miller SJ: Biology of basal cell carcinoma (part II). J Am Acad Dermatol 24:161–175, 1991.
24. Burns FJ: Cancer risk associated with therapeutic irradiation of the skin. Arch Dermatol 25:979–981, 1989.
25. Davis MM, Hanke CW, Zollinger TW, et al: Skin cancer in patients with chronic radiation dermatitis. J Am Acad Dermatol 20:608–616, 1989.
26. Frentz G: Grenz ray-induced nonmelanoma skin cancer. J Am Acad Dermatol 21:475–478, 1989.
27. Lindelof B, Eklund G: Incidence of malignant skin tumors in 14,140 patients after grenz ray treatment for benign skin disorders. Arch Dermatol 122:1391–1395, 1986.
28. Panizzon RG, Goldschmidt H: Radiation reactions and sequelae. In: Goldschmidt H, Panizzon RG (eds): Modern Dermatologic Radiation Therapy. Springer-Verlag, New York, 1991, pp 25–35.
29. Martin H, Strong E, Spiro RH: Radiation-induced skin cancer of the head and neck. Cancer 25:61–71, 1970.
30. Wagner SL, Maliner JS, Morton WE, et al: Skin cancer and arsenical intoxication from well water. Arch Dermatol 115:1205–1207, 1979.
31. Hoxtell EO, Mandel JS, Murray SS, et al: Incidence of skin carcinoma after renal transplantation. Arch Dermatol 113:436–438, 1977.
32. Parnes R, Safai B, Myskowski PL: Basal cell carcinomas and lymphoma: biologic behavior and associated factors in sixty-three patients. J Am Acad Dermatol 19:1017–1023, 1988.
33. Gupta AK, Cardella CJ, Haberman L: Cutaneous malignant neoplasms in patients with renal transplants. Arch Dermatol 122:1288–1293, 1986.
34. Callen JP: Skin cancer in transplant patients. In: Scher RK (ed): Dialogues in Dermatology. Vol 27 [audio cassette]. American Academy of Dermatology, Evanston, IL, 1990.
35. Vonderheid EC: Topical mechlorethamine chemotherapy. Int J Dermatol 23:180–186, 1984.
36. Lee LA, Fritz KA, Golitz L, et al: Second cutaneous malignancies in patients with mycosis fungoides treated with topical nitrogen mustard. J Am Acad Dermatol 7:590–598, 1982.

37. DuVivier A, Vonderheid EC, Van Scott EJ, et al: Mycosis fungoides, nitrogen mustard and skin cancer. Br J Dermatol 99:61–63, 1978.

38. Kravitz PH, McDonald CJ: Topical nitrogen mustard induced carcinogenesis. Acta Derm Venereol 58:421–425, 1978.

39. Morrison W: Risks of therapy. In: Morrison W (ed): Phototherapy and Photochemotherapy of Skin Disease. Raven Press, New York, 1991, pp 197–213.

40. Abdullah AN, Keczkes K: Cutaneous and ocular side effects of PUVA photochemotherapy—a 10 year follow-up study. Clin Exp Dermatol 14:421–424, 1989.

41. Stern RS, Lange R: Nonmelanoma skin cancer occurring in patients treated with PUVA five to 10 years after first treatment. J Invest Dermatol 91:120–124, 1988.

42. Hendricks WM: Basal cell carcinoma arising in a chicken pox scar. Arch Dermatol 116:1304–1305, 1980.

43. Marzelmat WL: Malignant tumors in smallpox vaccination scars—a report of 24 cases. Arch Dermatol 97:400–406, 1968.

44. Hazelrigg DE: Basal cell epithelioma in a vaccination scar. Int J Dermatol 17:723–725, 1978.

45. McGibbon DH: Malignant epidermal tumors. J Cutan Pathol 12:224–238, 1985.

46. White SW: Basal cell carcinoma arising in a burn scar: case report. J Dermatol Surg Oncol 9:159–160, 1983.

47. Jung EG: Xeroderma pigmentosum. Int J Dermatol 25:629–633, 1986.

48. Worobec-Victor SM, Bene-Bain MA, Shaker DG, et al: Genodermatoses. In: Schachner LA, Hansen RC (eds): Pediatric Dermatoloy. Churchill Livingstone, New York, 1988, pp 311–387.

49. Hurwitz S: Neurocutaneous disorders. In: Hurwitz S (ed): The Skin and Systemic Disease in Children. Year Book, Chicago, 1985, pp 220–249.

50. Plosila M, Kiistala R, Niemi KM: The Bazex syndrome: follicular atrophoderma with multiple basal cell carcinomas, hypotrichosis and hypohidrosis. Clin Exp Dermatol 6:31–41, 1981.

51. Viksnins P, Berlin A: Follicular atrophoderma and basal cell carcinomas: The Bazex syndrome. Arch Dermatol 113:948–951, 1977.

52. Edwards L, Bangert JL, Goldberg GN, et al: Benign neoplasms, premalignant conditions and malignancy. In: Schachner LA, Hansen RC (eds): Pediatric Dermatology. Churchill Livingstone, New York, 1988, pp 1055–1083.

53. Morioka S: The natural history of nevus sebaceus. J Cutan Pathol 12:200–213, 1985.

54. Schreiber MM, Moon TE, Fox SH, et al: The risk of developing nonmelanoma skin cancers. J Am Acad Dermatol 23:1114–1118, 1990.

55. Epstein E: How accurate is the visual assessment of basal cell carcinoma margins? Br J Dermatol 89:37–42, 1973.

56. Habif TP: Premalignant and malignant skin tumors. In: Habif TP (ed): Clinical Dermatology—A Color Guide to Diagnosis and Therapy. CV Mosby, St. Louis, 1990, pp 519–550.

57. Salasche SJ, Amonette RA: Morpheaform basal cell epitheliomas—a study of subclinical extensions in a series of 51 cases. J Dermatol Surg Oncol 7:387–394, 1981.

58. Freeman RG: Histopathologic considerations in the management of skin cancer. J Dermatol Surgy Oncol 2:215–219, 1976.

59. Edens BL, Bartlow GA, Haghighi P, et al: Effectiveness of curettage and electrodesiccation in the removal of basal cell carcinoma. J Am Acad Dermatol 9:383–388, 1983.

60. Sexton M, Jones DB, Maloney ME: Histologic pattern analysis of basal cell carcinoma: study of a series of 1039 consecutve neoplasms. J Am Acad Dermatol 23:1118–1126, 1990.

61. Burg G, Hirsch RD, Konz B, et al: Histographic surgery: accuracy of visual assessment of the margins of basal cell epithelioma. J Dermatol Surg 1:21–24, 1975.

62. Lang PG, Maize JC: Histologic evolution of recurrent basal cell carcinoma and treatment implications. J Am Acad Dermatol 14:186–196, 1986.

63. Goldberg L, Stal S, Spira M: Recognition and treatment of recurrent basal cell carcinoma. Ann Plast Surg 11:313–318, 1983.

64. MacFarlane AW, Curley RK, Graham RM: Recurrence rates of basal cell carcinomas according to site, method of removal, histological type and adequacy of excision. Br J Dermatol 115(suppl 30):23, 1986.

65. Richman T, Penneys NS: Analysis of morpheaform basal cell carcinoma. J Cutan Pathol 15:359–362, 1988.

66. Sloane JP: The value of typing basal cell carcinomas in predicting recurrence after surgical excision. Br J Dermatol 96:127–132, 1977.

67. Maize JC, Ackerman AB: Nonmelanocytic clinical simulators of proliferations of melanocytes. In: Maize JC, Ackerman AB (eds): Pigmented Lesions of the Skin—Clinicopathologic Correlations. Lea & Febiger, Philadelphia, 1987, pp 271–320.

68. Mohs FE, Zitelli JA: Microscopically controlled surgery in the treatment of carcinoma of the scalp. Arch Dermatol 117:764–769, 1981.

69. Dubin N, Kopf AW: Multivariate risk score for recurrence of cutaneous basal cell carcinomas. Arch Dermatol 119:373–377, 1983.

70. Koplin L, Zarem HA: Recurrent basal cell carcinoma: a review concerning the incidence, behavior, and management of recurrent basal cell carcinoma with emphasis on the incompletely excised lesion. Plast Reconstr Surg 65:656–664, 1980.

71. Levine HL, Bailin PL: Basal cell carcinoma of the head and neck: identification of the high risk patient. Laryngoscope 90:955–961, 1980.

72. Mora GG, Robins P: Basal cell carcinoma in the center of the face: special diagnostic, prognostic and therapeutic considerations. J Dermatol Oncol 4:315–321, 1978.

73. Carruthers JA, Stegman SJ, Tromovitch TA, et al: Basal cell carcinomas of the temple. J Dermatol Surg Oncol 9:759–762, 1983.

74. Bailin PL, Levine HL, Wood BJ, et al: Cutaneous carcinoma of the auricular and periauricular region. Arch Otolaryngol 106:692–696, 1980.

75. Granstrom G, Aldenborg F, Jeppsson PH: Influence of embryonal fusion lines for recurrence of basal cell carcinomas in the head and neck. Otolaryngol Head Neck Surg 95:76–82, 1986.

76. Wentzell JM, Robinson JK: Embryologic fusion planes and the spread of cutaneous carcinoma: a review and reassessment. J Dermatol Surg Oncol 16:1000–1006, 1990.

77. Robins P, Albom MJ: Recurrent basal cell carcinoma in young women. J Dermatol Surg 1:49–52, 1975.

78. Lauritzen RE, Johnson RE, Spratt JS: Pattern of recurrence in basal cell carcinoma. Surgery 57:813–816, 1965.

79. Salasche SJ: Curettage and electrodesiccation in the treatment of midfacial basal cell carcinoma. J Am Acad Dermatol 8:496–503, 1983.

80. d'Aubermont PCS, Bennett RG: Failure of curettage and electrodesiccation for removal of basal cell carcinoma. Arch Dermatol 120:1456–1460, 1984.

81. Binstock JH, Stegman SJ, Tromovitch TA: Large aggressive basal cell carcinomas of the scalp. J Dermatol Surg Oncol 7:565–569, 1981.

82. Peters CR, Dinner MI, Dolsky RL: The combined multidisciplinary approach to invasive basal cell carcinoma of the scalp. Ann Plast Surg 4:199–204, 1979.

83. Hanke CW, Weisberger EC, Lingeman RE: Cancer of the scalp. Dermatol Clin 7:797–814, 1989.

84. Dixon AY, Lee SH, McGregor DH: Factors predictive of recurrence of basal cell carcinoma. Am J Dermatopathol 11:222–232, 1989.

85. Wolf DJ, Zitelli JA: Surgical margins for basal cell carcinoma. Arch Dermatol 123:340–344, 1987.

86. Rigel DS, Robins P, Friedman RJ: Predicting recurrence of basal cell carcinomas treated by microscopically controlled excision—a recurrence index score. J Dermatol Surg Oncol 7:807–810, 1981.

87. Salasche SJ: Status of curettage and desiccation in the treatment of primary basal cell carcinoma. J Am Acad Dermatol 10:285–287, 1984.

88. Albright SD: Treatment of skin cancer using multiple modalities. J Am Acad Dermatol 7:143–171, 1982.

89. Robinson JK, Pollack SV, Robins P: Invasion of cartilage by basal cell carcinoma. J Am Acad Dermatol 2:499–505, 1980.

90. Wiggs EO: Incompletely excised basal cell carcinoma of the ocular adnexa. Ophthalmol Surg 12:891–896, 1981.

91. Lang PG, Osguthorpe JD: Indications and limitations of Mohs micrographic surgery. Dermatol Clin 7:627–644, 1989.

92. Rowe DE, Carroll RJ, Day CL: Mohs surgery is the treatment

of choice for recurrent (previously treated) basal cell carcinoma. J Dermatol Surg Oncol 15:424–431, 1989.

93. Menn H, Robins P, Kopf AW, et al: The recurrent basal cell epithelioma—a study of 100 cases of recurrent retreated basal cell epitheliomas. Arch Dermatol 103:623–631, 1971.

94. Casson PC: Basal cell carcinoma. Clin Plast Surg 7:301–311, 1980.

95. Siegle RJ, Schuller DE: Multidisciplinary surgical approach to the treatment of perinasal nonmelanoma skin cancer. Dermatol Clin 7:711–731, 1989.

96. Skouge JW, Tromovitch TA: Basal cell and squamous cell carcinoma. In: Provost TT, Farmer ER (eds): Current Therapy in Dermatology II. BC Decker, Toronto, 1988, pp 71–73.

97. Wagner RG, Cottel WI: Multifocal recurrent basal cell carcinoma following primary tumor treatment by electrodesiccation and curettage. J Am Acad Dermatol 17:1047–1049, 1987.

98. Wagner RF: New primary basal cell carcinomas arising in skin flaps following Mohs micrographic surgery for primary and recurrent basal cell carcinoma. J Dermatol Surg Oncol 16:1044–1047, 1990.

99. Krull EA, Mitchell A: Squamous and basal cell carcinoma. In: Provost TT, Farmer ER (eds): Current Therapy in Dermatology 1985–1986. BC Decker/CV Mosby, Toronto, 1985, pp 76–78.

100. Swanson N: Mohs surgery—technique, indications, applications, and the future. Arch Dermatol 119:761–773, 1983.

101. Mohs FE: Carcinoma of the skin: a summary of therapeutic results. In: Chemosurgery: Microscopically Controlled Surgery for Skin Cancer. Charles C Thomas, Springfield, IL, 1978, pp 153–164.

102. Robins P: Chemosurgery: my 15 years of experience. J Dermatol Surg Oncol 7:779–789, 1981.

103. Tromvitch TA, Stegman SJ: Microscopic-controlled excision of cutaneous tumors by chemosurgery, fresh tissue technique. Cancer 41:653–658, 1978.

104. Siegel RJ, MacMillan J, Pollack SV: Infiltrative basal cell carcinoma: a nonsclerosing subtype. J Dermatol Surg Oncol 12:830–836, 1986.

105. Krull EA: The "little curet." J Dermatol Surg Oncol 4:656–657, 1978.

106. Jackson R, Laughlin S: Electrodesiccation and curettage. In: Schwartz RA (ed): Skin Cancer: Recognition and Management. Springer-Verlag, New York, 1988, pp 292–295.

107. Salasche SJ: Therapeutic curettage and electrodesiccation. In: Friedman RJ, Rigel DS, Kopf AW, et al (eds): Cancer of the Skin. WB Saunders, Philadelphia, 1991, pp 434–450.

108. Harrison PV: Therapy of basal cell carcinoma—treatment in 1980–81 compared with 1985–86 and advantages of shave excision for smaller tumors. Br J Dermatol 117:349–357, 1987.

109. Freeman RG, Duncan WC: Recurrent skin cancer. Arch Dermatol 107:395–399, 1973.

110. Jacobs GH, Rippey JJ, Altini M: Prediction of aggressive behavior in basal cell carcinoma. Cancer 49:533–537, 1982.

111. Johnson TM, Tromovitch TA, Swanson NA: Combined curettage and excision: a treatment method for primary basal cell carcinoma. J Am Acad Dermatol 24:613–617, 1991.

112. Hauben DJ, Zirkin H, Mahler D, et al: The biologic behavior of basal cell carcinoma. Plast Reconstr Surg 69:103–109, 1982.

113. Knox JM, Lyles TW, Shapiro EM: Curettage and electrodesiccation in the treatment of skin cancer. Arch Dermatol 82:197–204, 1960.

114. Sturm HM, Leider M: An editorial on curettage. J Dermatol Surg Oncol 5:532–533, 1979.

115. Bart RS, Kopf AW, Gladstein AH: Treatment of morpheaform basal cell carcinomas with radiation therapy. Arch Dermatol 113:783–786, 1977.

116. Zacarian SA: Complications, indications and contraindications in cryosurgery. In: Cryosurgery for Skin Cancer and Cutaneous Disorders. CV Mosby, St. Louis, 1985, pp 283–297.

117. Hauben DJ, Zirkin H, Mahler D, et al: The biologic behavior of basal cell carcinoma: analysis of recurrence in excised basal cell carcinoma (part II). Plast Reconstr Surg 69:110–116, 1982.

118. Borel DM: Cutaneous basosquamous carcinoma. Arch Pathol 85:293–297, 1973.

119. Farmer ER, Helwig EB: Metastatic basal cell carcinoma: a clinicopathologic study of seventeen cases. Cancer 46:748–757, 1980.

120. Schuller DE, Berg JW, Sherman G, et al: Cutaneous basosquamous carcinoma of the head and neck: a comparative analysis. Otolaryngol Head Neck Surg 87:420–427, 1979.

121. Rena YM, Bason MM, Grant-Kels JM: Basosquamous cell carcinoma with leptomeningeal carcinomatosis. Arch Dermatol 126:195–198, 1990.

122. Hanke CW, Temofeew RK: Basal cell carcinoma with eccrine differentiation (eccrine epithelioma). J Dermatol Surg Oncol 12:820–824, 1986.

123. Sanchez NP, Winkelman RK: Basal cell tumor with eccrine differentiation (eccrine epithelioma). J Am Acad Dermatol 6:514–518, 1982.

124. Cottel W: Eccrine epithelioma. J Dermatol Surg Oncol 8:610–611, 1982.

125. Freeman RG, Winkelmann RK: Basal cell tumor with eccrine differentiation (eccrine epithelioma). Arch Dermatol 100:234–242, 1969.

126. Bart RS, Schrager D, Kopf AW, et al: Scalpel excision of basal cell carcinomas. Arch Dermatol 114:739–742, 1978.

127. Taylor GA, Barisoni D: Ten years' experience in the surgical treatment of basal cell carcinoma. Br J Surg 60:522–525, 1973.

128. Abide JM, Nahai F, Bennett RG: The meaning of surgical margins. Plast Reconstr Surg 73:492–496, 1984.

129. Bennett RG: The meaning and significance of tissue margins. Adv Dermatol 4:343–357, 1989.

130. Rapini RP: Comparison of methods for checking surgical margins. J Am Acad Dermatol 23:288–294, 1990.

131. Barton FE, Cottel WI, Walker B: The principle of chemosurgery and delayed primary reconstruction in the management of difficult basal cell carcinomas. Plast Reconstr Surg 68:746–752, 1981.

132. Zitelli J: Mohs surgery—conceptions and misconceptions. Int J Dermatol 24:541–548, 1985.

133. Breuninger H: Histologic control of excised tissue edges in the operative treatment of basal cell carcinoma. J Dermatol Surg Oncol 10:724–728, 1984.

134. Schultz BC, Roenigk HH: The double scalpel and double punch excision of skin tumors. J Am Acad Dermatol 7:495–499, 1982.

135. Cott RE, Wood MG, Johnson BL: Use of curettage and shave excision in office practice—microscopic confirmation of removal. J Am Acad Dermatol 16:1243–1251, 1990.

136. Brooks NA: Curettage and shave excision. J Am Acad Dermatol 10:279–284, 1984.

137. Gross DA, Field LM: Cooperative frozen section surgery. J Dermatol Surg Oncol 13:1085–1088, 1987.

138. Swanson NA, Tromovitch TA, Stegman SJ, et al: A novel method of re-excising incompletely excised basal cell carcinomas. J Dermatol Surg Oncol 6:438–439, 1980.

139. Woods JE, Farrow GM: Peripheral tissue examination for malignant lesions of the skin. Mayo Clin Proc 66:207–209, 1991.

140. Sidell C: Excision of skin cancer. In: Schwartz RA (ed): Skin Cancer: Recognition and Management. Springer-Verlag, New York, 1988, pp 311–320.

141. Stegman SJ: The meaning and significant of tissue margins—editor's comments. Adv Dermatol 4:356–357, 1989.

142. Epstein E: Evaluation of excision margins for lentigo maligna and lentigo maligna melanoma. Pract Rev Dermatol Vol 3 [audio cassette], 1991.

143. Hanke CW: Cooperative frozen section surgery in perspective. J Dermatol Surg Oncol 13:1065, 1987.

144. Frank HJ: Frozen section control of excision of eyelid basal cell carcinomas: 8½ years experience. Br J Ophthalmol 73:328–332, 1989.

145. Mohs FE: Modes of spread of cancer. In: Chemosurgery: Microscopically Controlled Surgery for Skin Cancer. Charles C Thomas, Springfield, IL, 1978, pp 256–273.

146. Hanke CW, Wolf RL, Hochman SA, et al: Chemosurgical reports: perineural spread of basal cell carcinoma. J Dermatol Surg Oncol 9:742–747, 1983.

147. Carlson KC, Roenigk RK: Know your anatomy: perineural involvement of basal and squamous cell carcinoma of the face. J Dermatol Surg Oncol 16:827–833, 1990.

148. Mark GJ: Basal cell carcinoma with intraneural invasion. Cancer 40:2181–2187, 1977.

149. Levine HL, Kinney SE, Bailin PL, et al: Cancer of the preauricular region. Dermatol Clin 7:781–795, 1989.

150. Gooding CA, White G, Yatsuhashi M: Significance of marginal

extension in excised basal cell carcinoma. N Engl J Med 273:923–924, 1965.

151. Pascal RR, Hobby LW, Rafaelle L, et al: Prognosis of "incompletely excised" versus "completely excised" basal cell carcinoma. Plast Reconstr Surg 41:328–332, 1968.

152. Sarma DP, Griffing CC, Weilbaecher TG: Observations on inadequately excised basal cell carcinomas. J Surg Oncol 25:78–80, 1984.

153. Dellon AL, DeSilva S, Connolly M, et al: Prediction of recurrence in incompletely excised basal cell carcinoma. Plast Reconstr Surg 75:860–871, 1985.

154. Thomas P: Treatment of basal cell carcinomas of the head and neck. Rev Surg 27:293–294, 1970.

155. Richmond JD, Davie RM: The significance of incomplete excision in patients with basal cell carcinoma. Br J Plast Surg 40:63–67, 1987.

156. Marchac D, Papadopoulos O, Duport G: Curative and aesthetic results of surgical treatment of 138 basal cell carcinomas. J Dermatol Surg Oncol 8:379–387, 1982.

157. Blomquist G, Eriksson E, Laurtizen C: Surgical results in 477 basal cell carcinomas. Scand J Plast Surg 16:283–285, 1982.

158. DeSilva SP, Dellon AL: Recurrence rate of positive margin basal cell carcinoma: results of a five-year prospective study. J Surg Oncol 28:72–74, 1985.

159. Rowe DE, Carroll RJ, Day CL: Long term recurrence rates on previously untreated (primary) basal cell carcinoma: implications for patient follow-up. J Dermatol Surg Oncol 15:315–328, 1989.

160. Silverman MK, Kopf AW, Grin CM, et al: Recurrence rates of treated basal cell carcinomas: Part II: curettage and electrodesiccation. J Dermatol Surg Oncol 17:720–726, 1991.

161. Reymann F: Basal cell carcinoma of the skin: recurrence rates after different types of treatment. Dermatologica 161:217–226, 1980.

162. Spiller WF, Spiller RF: Treatment of basal cell epithelioma by curettage and electrodesiccation. J Am Acad Dermatol 11:808–814, 1984.

163. Jackson R: The treatment of skin cancer by electrodesiccation and curettage. J Surg Oncol 22:100, 1983.

164. Kopf AW, Bart RS, Schrager D: Curettage-electrodesiccation treatment of basal cell carcinomas. Arch Dermatol 113:439–443, 1977.

165. McDaniel WE: Surgical therapy for basal cell epitheliomas by curettage alone. Arch Dermatol 114:1491–1492, 1978.

166. Reymann F: Treatment of basal cell carcinoma of the skin with curettage. Arch Dermatol 103:623–627, 1971.

167. Reymann F: Multiple basal cell carcinomas of the skin—treatment with curettage. Arch Dermatol 111:877–879, 1975.

168. McDaniel WE: Therapy for basal cell epitheliomas by curettage only: further study. Arch Dermatol 119:901–903, 1983.

169. Bumsted RM, Ceilly RI: Auricular malignant neoplasms: identification of high-risk lesions and selection of method of reconstruction. Arch Otolaryngol 108:225–231, 1982.

170. Bumsted RM, Ceilly RI, Panje WR, et al: Auricular malignant neoplasms. Arch Otolaryngol 107:721–724, 1981.

171. Panje WR, Ceilly RI: The influence of embryology of the midface on the spread of epithelial malignancies. Laryngoscope 89:1914–1920, 1979.

172. Robins P, Cohen RW: Curettage followed by excisional surgery. In: Robins P (ed): Surgical Gems in Dermatology. Journal Publishing Group, New York, 1988, pp 18–21.

173. Pless J: Carcinoma of the external ear. Scand J Plast Reconstr Surg 10:147–151, 1976.

174. Sakura CY, Calamel PM: Comparison of treatment modalities for recurrent basal cell carcinoma. Plast Reconstr Surg 63:492–495, 1979.

175. Fitzpatrick PJ, Thompson GA, Easterbrook WM, et al: Basal and squamous cell carcinoma of the eyelids and their treatment by radiotherapy. Radiat Oncol Biol Phys 10:449–454, 1984.

176. Cooper JS: Radiotherapy in the treatment of skin cancer. In: Friedman RJ, Rigel DS, Kopf AW, et al (eds): Cancer of the Skin. WB Saunders, Philadelphia, 1991, pp 553–568.

177. Goldschmidt HG, Sherwin WK: Office radiotherapy of cutaneous carcinomas I. Radiation techniques, dose schedules and radiation protection. J Dermatol Surg Oncol 9:31–46, 1983.

178. Goldschmidt H: Radiation therapy of cutaneous carcinomas: Radiation techniques and dosage schedules. In: Goldschmidt H, Panizzon RG (eds): Modern Dermatologic Radiation Therapy. Springer-Verlag, New York, 1991, pp 65–85.

179. Helm F, Helm TN, Schwartz RA: Treatment of cutaneous cancers by radiotherapy. In: Schwartz RA (ed): Skin Cancer: Recognition and Management. Springer-Verlag, New York, 1988, pp 353–362.

180. Robinson JK: Use of a combination of chemotherapy and radiation therapy in the management of advanced basal cell carcinoma of the head and neck. J Am Acad Dermatol 17:770–774, 1987.

181. Viravathana T, Prempree T, Sewchand W, et al: Technique and dosimetry in the management of extensive basal cell carcinomas of the head and neck region by irradiation with electron beams. J Dermatol Surg Oncol 6:290–297, 1980.

182. Miller RA, Spittle MF: Electron beam therapy for difficult cutaneous basal and squamous cell carcinomas. Br J Dermatol 106:429–436, 1982.

183. Hunter RD, Pereira H: Megavoltage electron beam therapy in the treatment of basal and squamous cell carcinoma of the pinna. Clin Radiol 33:341–345, 1982.

184. Breneman JC: Electron beam therapy. In: Goldschmidt H, Pannizon RG (eds): Modern Dermatologic Radiation Therapy. Springer-Verlag, New York, 1991, pp 147–153.

185. Daly NJ, de Lafontan B, Combes PF: Results of the treatment of 165 lid carcinomas by iridium wire implant. Int J Oncol Biol Phys 10:455–459, 1984.

186. Farina AT: Current concepts in the use of radiotherapy for malignant epitheliomas of the skin. In: Robins P, Bennett RG (eds): Current Concepts in the Management of Skin Cancer. Clinicom, New York, 1986, pp 24–25.

187. Hliniak A, Maciejewski B, Trott KR: The influence of the number of fractions, overall treatment time and field size on the local control of cancer of the skin. Br J Radiol 56:596–598, 1983.

188. Goldschmidt H, Sherwin WK: Office radiotherapy of cutaneous carcinomas II. Indications in specific anatomic regions. J Dermatol Surg Oncol 9:47–76, 1983.

189. Petrovich Z, Kuisk H, Langholz B: Treatment of carcinoma of the skin with bone and/or cartilage involvement. Am J Clin Oncol 11:110–113, 1988.

190. Brady LW, Binnick SA, Fitzpatrick PJ: Skin cancer. In: Perez CA, Brady LW (eds): Principles and Practice of Radiation Oncology. JB Lippincott, Philadelphia, 1987, pp 377–394.

191. Hunter RD: Skin. In: Easson EC, Pointon RCS (eds): The Radiotherapy of Malignant Disease. Springer-Verlag, New York, 1985, pp 135–151.

192. Rodriguez-Sains RS, Robins P, Smith B, et al: Radiotherapy of periocular basal cell carcinomas: recurrence rates and treatment with special attention to the medial canthus. Br J Ophthalmol 72:134–138, 1988.

193. Smith SP, Foley EH, Grande DJ: Use of Mohs micrographic surgery to establish quantitative proof of heightened tumor spread in basal cell carcinoma recurrent following radiotherapy. J Dermatol Surg Oncol 16:1012–1016, 1990.

194. Smith SP, Grande DJ: Basal cell carcinoma recurring after radiotherapy: a unique, difficult treatment subclass of recurrent basal cell carcinoma. J Dermatol Surg Oncol 17:26–30, 1991.

195. Arnold HL, Odom RB, James WD (eds): Basal cell carcinoma: In: Andrews' Diseases of the Skin. 8th ed. WB Saunders, Philadelphia, 1990, pp 763–775.

196. Fischback AJ, Sause WT, Plenk HP: Radiation therapy for skin cancer. West J Med 133:379–382, 1980.

197. Goldschmidt H: Chronic radiation effects and radiation protection. In: Golschmidt H, Panizzon RG (eds): Modern Dermatologic Radiation Therapy. Springer-Verlag, New York, 1991, pp 37–48.

198. Walther RR, Grossman ME, Troy JL: Basal cell carcinomas on the scalp of a black patient many years after epilation by x-rays. J Dermatol Surg Oncol 7:570–571, 1981.

199. Torre D: Cutaneous cryosurgery: current state of the art. J Dermatol Surg Oncol 11:292–293, 1985.

200. Graham GF: Statistical data on malignant tumors in cryosurgery: 1982. J Dermatol Surg Oncol 9:238–239, 1983.

201. Zacarian SA: Cryosurgery of cutaneous carcinomas man 18 year study of 3,022 patients with 4,228 carcinomas. J Dermatol Surg Oncol 9:947–956, 1983.

202. Crutcher WA: Cryotherapy of cutaneous malignancies. In: Schwartz RA (ed): Skin Cancer: Recognition and Management. Springer-Verlag, New York, 1988, pp 299–310.

203. Torre D: Cryosurgery of basal cell carcinoma. J Am Acad Dermatol 15:917–929, 1986.

204. Torre D, Lubritz R, Kuflik E: Equipping an office for cryosurgery. In: Torre D (ed): Practical Cutaneous Cryosurgery. Appleton-Lange, Norwalk, CT, 1988, pp 25–41.

205. Torre D: Cryosurgical instrumentation and depth dose monitoring. Clin Dermatol 8:48–60, 1990.

206. Kuflik EG: Learning the basics. II. Debulking the lesion before cryosurgery. J Dermatol Surg Oncol 12:321, 1986.

207. Graham GF, Clark LC: Statistical analysis in cryosurgery of skin cancer. Clin Dermatol 8:101–107, 1990.

208. Torre D, Lubritz R, Kuflik E: Treatment of malignant lesions. In: Torre D (ed): Practical Cutaneous Cryosurgery. Appleton-Lange, Norwalk, CT, 1988, pp 87–119.

209. Dachow-Siwiec E: Cryosurgery in the treatment of skin cancers: indications and management. Clin Dermatol 8:80–85, 1990.

210. Kuflik EG, Gage AA: Skin cancer: characteristics and indications for cryosurgery. In: Cryosurgical Treatment for Skin Cancer. Igaku-Shoin, New York, 1990, pp 15–31.

211. Fraunfelder FT, Zacarian SA, Limmer BL, et al: Cryosurgery for malignancies of the eyelid. Ophthalmology 87:461–465, 1980.

212. Biro L, Price E, Brand A: Cryosurgery for basal cell carcinoma of the eyelids and nose. J Am Acad Dermatol 6:1042–1047, 1982.

213. Fraunfelder FT, Zacarian SA, Wingfield DL, et al: Results of cryotherapy for eyelid malignancy. Am J Ophthalmol 97:18–88, 1984.

214. Biro L, Price E: Cryosurgical management of basal cell carcinoma of the eyelid: a 10 year experience. J Am Acad Dermatol 23:316–317, 1990.

215. Kuflik EG: Cryosurgery for carcinoma of the eyelids: a 12 year experience. J Dermatol Surg Oncol 11:243–246, 1985.

216. Dawber RPR: Cryosurgery: complications and contraindications. Clin Dermatol 8:108–114, 1990.

217. Torre D, Lubritz R, Kuflik E: Morbidity and complications. In: Torre D (ed): Practical Cutaneous Cryosurgery. Appleton-Lange, Norwalk, CT, 1988, pp 51–60.

218. Kuflik EG, Gage AA: Tissue response and wound healing after cryosurgery. In: Cryosurgical Treatment for Skin Cancer. Igaku-Shoin, New York, 1990, pp 113–128.

219. Elton RF: Complications of cutaneous cryosurgery. J Am Acad Dermatol 8:513–519, 1983.

220. Faber WR, Naafs B, Smitt JHS: Sensory loss following cryosurgery of skin lesions. Br J Dermatol 117:343–347, 1987.

221. Hindson C, Lawlor F, Taylor AE: Liquid nitrogen cryotherapy of basal cell carcinomata. Irish Med J 75:418, 1982.

222. Albom MJ, Swanson NA: Mohs micrographic surgery for the treatment of cutaneous neoplasms. In: Friedman RJ, Rigel DS, Kopf AW, et al (eds): Cancer of the Skin. WB Saunders, Philadelphia, 1991, pp 484–529.

223. Lang PG: Mohs micrographic surgery: fresh tissue technique. Dermatol Clin 7:613–626, 1989.

224. Cottell WI, Proper S: Mohs surgery: fresh tissue technique: our technique with a review. J Dermatol Surg Oncol 8:576–587, 1982.

225. Stegman SJ, Tromovitch TA: Modern chemosurgery—microscopically controlled excision. West J Med 132:7–12, 1980.

226. Mohs FE: Chemosurgical techniques. In: Chemosurgery: Microscopically Controlled Surgery for Skin Cancer. Charles C Thomas, Springfield, IL, 1978, pp 7–29.

227. Davidson TM, Nahum AM, Haghibi P, et al: The biology of head and neck cancer. Arch Otolaryngol 110:193–196, 1984.

228. Lambert DR, Siegle RJ: Skin cancer: a review with consideration of treatment options including Mohs micrographic surgery. Ohio Med 86:745–747, 1990.

229. Roenigk RK: Mohs micrographic surgery. Mayo Clin Proc 63:175–183, 1988.

230. Baker SR, Swanson NA: Management of nasal cutaneous malignant neoplasms—an interdisciplinary approach. Arch Otolaryngol 109:473–479, 1983.

231. Mohs FE, Larson P, Iriondo M: Micrographic surgery for the microscopically controlled excision of carcinoma of the external ear. J Am Acad Dermatol 19:729–737, 1988.

232. Hanke CW, Temofew RK, Miyamoto RT, et al: Chemosurgical report: basal call carcinoma involving the external auditory canal—treatment with Mohs micrographic surgery. J Dermatol Surg Oncol 11:1189–1194, 1985.

233. Goslen JB, Thomas JR: Cancer of the perioral region. Dermatol Clin 7:733–749, 1989.

234. Grekin RC, Schaler RE, Crumley RL: Cancer of the forehead and temple. Dermatol Clin 7:699–710, 1989.

235. Robins P, Rodriguez-Sains R, Rabinovitz H, et al: Mohs surgery for periocular basal cell carcinomas. J Dermatol Surg Oncol 11:1203–1207, 1985.

236. Callahan MA, Monheit G, Callahan A: Twelve years experience with the Mohs-Tromovitch techniques of skin cancer removal. Int Ophthalmol Clin 29:247–251, 1989.

237. Monheit GD, Callahan MA, Callahan A: Mohs micrographic surgery for periorbital skin cancer. Dermatol Clin 7:677–697, 1989.

238. Bernstein G: Healing by secondary intention. Dermatol Clin 7:645–660, 1989.

239. Diwan R, Tromovitch TA, Glogau RG: Secondary intention after healing. Arch Otolaryngol Head Neck Surg 115:1248–1249, 1989.

240. Moscona R, Pnini A, Hirshowitz B: In favor of healing by secondary intention after excision of medial canthal basal cell carcinoma. Plast Reconstr Surg 71:189–195, 1983.

241. Goette J: 5-Fluorouracil. J Assoc Milit Dermatol 15:22–24, 1989.

242. Epstein E: Fluorouracil paste treatment of thin basal cell carcinomas. Arch Dermatol 121:207–213, 1985.

243. Auerbach R: Topical chemotherapy in treatment of skin cancer. In: Friedman RJ, Rigel DS, Kopf AW, et al (eds): Cancer of the Skin. WB Saunders, Philadelphia, 1991, pp 466–469.

244. Camisa C: The nevoid basal-cell carcinoma syndrome—simultaneous extirpation of numerous basal cell carcinomas on the face by curettage and electrodesiccation under general anesthesia. J Dermatol Surg Oncol 7:893–895, 1981.

245. Kurtis B, Rosen T: Treatment of cutaneous neoplasms by intralesional injections of 5-Fluorouracil. J Dermatol Surg Oncol 6:122–127, 1980.

246. Hazen PG, Tauv SJ: Basal cell nevus syndrome—unresponsiveness of early cutaneous lesions to topical 5-fluorouracil or dinitrochlorobenzene. Dermatologica 168:287–289, 1984.

247. Kraemer KH, DiGiovanna JJ, Moshell AN, et al: Prevention of skin cancer in xeroderma pigmentosum with the use of oral isotretinoin. N Engl J Med 318:1633–1637, 1988.

248. Peck GL, Gross EG, Butkus D, et al: Chemoprevention of basal cell carcinoma with isotretinoin. J Am Acad Dermatol 6:815–823, 1982.

249. Peck GL, DiGiovanna JJ, Sarnoff DS, et al: Treatment and prevention of basal cell carcinoma with oral isotretinoin. J Am Acad Dermatol 19:176–185, 1988.

250. Hodak E, Ginzburg A, David M, et al: Etretinate treatment of the nevoid basal cell carcinoma syndrome—therapeutic and chemopreventive effect. Int J Dermatol 26:606–609, 1987.

251. Goldberg LH, Hsu SH, Alcalay J: Effectiveness of isotretinoin in preventing the appearance of basal cell carcinomas in basal cell nevus syndrome. J Am Acad Dermatol 21:144–145, 1989.

252. Lippman SM, Kessler JF, Neyskens FL: Retinoids as preventative and therapeutic anticancer agents (part II). Cancer Treat Rep 71:493–515, 1987.

253. Peck GL: Long-term retinoid therapy is needed for maintenance of cancer chemopreventive effect. Dermatologica 175 (suppl):138–144, 1987.

254. Peck G: Topical tretinoin in actinic keratosis and basal cell carcinoma. J Am Acad Dermatol 15:829–835, 1986.

255. Sankowski A, Janik P, Gogacka-Zatorska E: Treatment of basal cell carcinoma with 13-cis retinoic acid. Neoplasma 31:615–618, 1984.

256. Sankowksi A, Janik P, Jeziorska M: The results of topical application of 13-cis retinoic acid on basal cell carcinoma. Neoplasma 34:485–489, 1987.

257. Dabski K, Helm F: Immunotherapy. In: Schwartz RA (ed): Skin Cancer: Recognition and Management. Springer-Verlag, New York, 1988, pp 363–377.

258. Boneschi V, Brambilla L, Chiappino G, et al: Intralesional alpha-2B recombinant interferon for basal cell carcinomas. Int J Dermatol 30:220–224, 1991.

259. Cornell RC, Greenway HT, Tucker SB, et al: Intralesional interferon therapy for basal cell carcinoma. J Am Acad Dermatol 23:694–670, 1990.

260. Greenway HT, Cornell RC, Tanner DJ, et al: Treatment of

basal cell carcinoma with intralesional interferon. J Am Acad Dermatol 15:437–443, 1986.

261. Edwards L, Whiting D, Rogers D, et al: The effect of intralesional interferon gamma on basal cell carcinomas. J Am Acad Dermatol 22:496–500, 1990.

262. Edwards L, Tucker SB, Perednia D, et al: The effect of an intralesional sustained-release formulation of interferon alfa-2b on basal cell carcinoma. Arch Dermatol 126:1029–1032, 1990.

263. Tank B, Habets JMW, Naafs B, et al: Intralesional treatment of basal cell carcinoma with low-dose recombinant interferon gamma. J Am Acad Dermatol 21:734–735, 1989.

264. Dover JS, Arndt KA, Geronemus RG, et al: Photodynamic therapy. In: Illustrated Cutaneous Laser Surgery: A Practitioner's Guide. Appleton-Lange, Norwalk, CT, 1990, pp 134–136.

265. Waldow SM, Lobraico RV, Kohler IK, et al: Photodynamic therapy for treatment of malignant cutaneous lesions. Lasers Surg Med 7:451–456, 1987.

266. Parrish JA: Laser medicine and laser dermatology. J Dermatol 17:587–594, 1990.

267. Geronemus RG, Reyes B: Laser surgery in the treatment of skin cancer. In: Friedman RJ, Rigel DS, Kopf AW, et al (eds): Cancer of the Skin. WB Saunders, Philadelphia, 1991, pp 470–483.

268. Sacchini V, Melloni E, Marchesini R, et al: Preliminary clinical studies with PDT by topical TPPS administration in neoplastic skin lesions. Lasers Surg Med 7:6–11, 1987.

269. Levine H: Cutaneous carcinoma of the head and neck: management of massive and previously uncontrollable lesions. Laryngoscope 93:87–105, 1983.

270. Chawla SP, Benjamin RS, Ayala AG, et al: Advanced basal cell carcinoma and successful treatment with chemotherapy. J Surg Oncol 40:68–72, 1989.

271. Wood BG, Levine HL, Tucker HM, et al: Principles of surgical management of midfacial carcinoma. Laryngoscope 92:1154–1156, 1982.

272. Gage AA: Cryosurgery of advanced tumors. Clin Dermatol 8:86–95, 1990.

273. Guthrie TH, McElveen LJ, Porubsky ES, et al: Cisplatin and doxorubicin man effective chemotherapy combination in the treatment of advanced basal cell and squamous cell carcinoma of the skin. Cancer 55:1629–1632, 1985.

274. Luxenberg MN, Guthrie TH: Chemotherapy of basal cell and squamous cell carcinoma of the eyelids and periorbital tissues. Ophthalmology 93:504–510, 1986.

275. Stanely RB, Burres SA, Jacobs JR, et al: Hazards encountered in management of basal cell carcinoma of the midface. Laryngoscope 94:378–385, 1984.

276. Riefkohl R, Wittels B, McCarty K: Metastatic basal cell carcinoma. Ann Plast Surg 13:525–528, 1984.

277. Amonette RA, Salasche SJ, Chesney TM, et al: Metastatic basal cell carcinoma. J Dermatol Surg Oncol 7:397–400, 1981.

278. Cieplinski W: Combination chemotherapy for the treatment of metastatic basal cell carcinoma of the scrotum. Clin Oncol 10:267–272, 1984.

279. Safai B, Good RA: Basal cell carcinoma with metastasis—review of the literature. Arch Pathol Lab Med 101:327–331, 1977.

280. Howat AJ, Lewick PL: Metastatic basal cell carcinoma. Dermatologica 174:132–134, 1987.

281. Coker DD, Elias G, Viravathana T, et al: Chemotherapy for metastatic basal cell carcinoma. Arch Dermatol 119:44–50, 1983.

282. Epstein E: Value of follow up after treatment of basal cell carcinoma. Arch Dermatol 108:798–800, 1973.

283. Robinson JK: What are adequate treatment and follow-up care for nonmelanoma cutaneous cancer? Arch Dermatol 123:331–333, 1987.

284. Robinson JK: Risk of developing another basal cell carcinoma: a 5-year prospective study. Cancer 60:118–120, 1987.

CHAPTER 57

Management of Squamous Cell Carcinomas and Lymph Node Evaluation

PEARON G. LANG, JR.

Squamous cell carcinoma (SCC) is a malignant neoplasm that may arise from any stratified squamous epithelium. In the skin it most commonly arises from the epidermis, but on occasion it may also originate from appendigeal epithelium. It is the second most common malignancy affecting the skin. In contrast to basal cell carcinoma (BCC), SCC of the skin and mucous membranes exhibits a significant propensity to metastasize.

Incidence and Epidemiology

Each year, between 400,000 and 500,000 people in the United States develop nonmelanoma skin cancers. Although the majority of these cancers are BCCs, 20% are SCCs, making it the second most common malignancy arising in the skin.[1] As with malignant melanoma (MM), there has been an alarming increase in the incidence of nonmelanoma skin cancer in recent decades.[2, 3] The depletion of the ozone layer, which normally filters out the harmful and carcinogenic ultraviolet light, has been suggested as playing a major role in this increase. In reality, this has contributed probably only minimally to the rapid rise in the incidence of skin cancer. Nevertheless, the ozone layer loss that has already occurred will almost certainly contribute significantly to the development of skin cancers in future generations.[4–6] Fortunately, the chlorofluorocarbons found in refrigerants and aerosol sprays, which have been indicted as a primary cause of the destruction of the ozone layer, are now being carefully regulated in many countries.[7, 8]

The most likely explanation for the relatively recent increase in skin cancer is the changes in dress and life styles resulting in greater sun exposure. This also probably explains why skin cancer now occurs at a younger age and is found more commonly in women than in the past.[3] Because of the increasing emphasis on personal appearance and the desire to maintain a "beautiful year 'round tan," tanning parlors have flourished. This additional source of excess ultraviolet light (UVL) is also expected to contribute to future increases in the incidence of skin cancer.[9]

Although people of any age may be affected, SCC of the skin and lip occurs most commonly in patients older than 60 years of age. It is also significantly more common in men than in women.[10–13] The typical patient has a fair complexion, burns easily, tans poorly, and shows evidence of chronic sun exposure, which may be manifested by coexisting BCCs and actinic keratoses (AKs). Patients with SCC of the lip frequently work outdoors and smoke. SCCs are most frequently located on the lower lip, while BCCs are more common on the upper lip.[14, 15] Eighty percent of SCCs occur on the head and neck,[16] and 90% affect sun-exposed areas.[13] Most SCCs occur on the head, neck, and upper extremities. Because of the protective effects of melanin, SCCs are rarely seen in black individuals.[17–19] Compared with those in whites, a significantly greater proportion of SCCs in blacks arise in association with pre-existing conditions such as chronic leg ulcers, burn scars, and lesions of discoid lupus erythematosus (DLE). Because of this, SCCs of the skin in blacks are often associated with significant morbidity and mortality.

Pathogenesis

SCCs in the skin most commonly arise from the epidermis but may also occasionally originate from appendigeal epithelium. It is likely that the malignant transforming events occur in the uncommitted basal cell layer of the epidermis that subsequently differentiates to form keratinocytes. It has been suggested that BCC and SCC are derived from the same pluripotential epithelial cell and that other factors, such as stromal interaction, ultimately determine whether a BCC or SCC develops.[20]

Growth, Development, and Tumor Biology

Despite differences in histologic features and sites of origin, SCCs show very similar cellular kinetics.[21–25] Although cellular proliferation is one facet of tumor growth, it is not the only important factor in determining how fast a cancer grows, which explains why clinical findings do not always correlate with the predicted cellular kinetics. Tumor cell death is probably one of several factors that ultimately determine the actual growth rate of cancers. When the actual growth rates of SCCs and BCCs were compared, it was found that SCCs grow at a rate of 1.85 mm per month, compared with 0.51 mm per month for BCCs.[26] However, changes in the growth rate during the life cycle of an individual SCC are also known to occur[21] and are probably caused by changes in the length of the cell cycle and reductions in the tumor cell death rate.[22, 27] This may be confirmed clinically, as a recurrent SCC often grows more rapidly than the original lesion. This may be a result of a shortening of the cell cycle and an increased rate of tumor cell production.[28–30]

One reason SCC behaves more aggressively and has a higher incidence of metastases relates to its stromal independence. Electron microscopic studies of SCCs suggest that this biologic aggression may also be partially due to a significant decrease in desmosomes and gap junctions.[31–34] Gap junctions chemically link adjoining cells and provide for intercellular communication. A decrease in gap junctions would likely result in a loss of control over cellular growth and differentiation.[34] At the periphery of some SCCs, desmosomes may actually be totally absent, which allows tumor cells to appear to "float free" in their stroma.[31] This could allow tumor cells to be implanted into lymphatics, blood vessels, or adjacent normal tissue during a surgical procedure. Furthermore, the extent of gap junction loss may determine the degree of differentiation of the SCC and how fast it can grow.

Microfilaments are important for cell mobility and are most numerous in tumor cells at the advancing edge of a cancer and in metastatic lesions. They are more numerous in SCCs than in BCCs, which may explain some of the differences observed in the biologic behaviors of these two neoplasms.[33] During evolution from a precancerous lesion into a fully developed invasive SCC, a progressive decline in desmosomes and gap junctions and an increase in microfilaments can be demonstrated.[32]

An increased level of collagenase has also been found in SCCs. These tumors appear to induce the production of collagenase by the contiguous fibroblasts.[35–38] The role this enzyme plays in tumor invasion remains unknown at present. SCCs also produce an angiogenic factor that can stimulate angiogenesis, which is necessary for both tumor growth and tumor survival.[39] Another sign of rapid tissue growth is the observation that polyamine biosynthesis is increased in SCCs,[40] although the significance of this finding is unclear.

Modes of Local Spread

Like BCCs, SCCs follow the "path of least resistance" as they spread through tissue along the perichondrium,[41–46] periosteum,[42, 44, 45] or tarsal plate.[45, 46] This type of spread can result in an "iceberg" phenomenon with substantial subclinical spread. However, in contrast to BCCs, SCCs are more apt to invade bone, cartilage, and muscle. These observations help to partially explain the difficulty in treating SCCs of the periocular area,[45–48] ear,[43–45] nose,[45, 46, 49] and scalp.[50, 51]

Embryonal fusion planes, vestiges of embryogenesis, appear to offer little resistance to the penetration and spread of this tumor. Because of this, areas at high risk of recurrence include the inner canthus, philtrum, nasolabial sulcus, preauricular area, and retroauricular sulcus.[42, 43, 46, 52–57] SCCs located in these areas are often more difficult to treat and have a high rate of recurrence because of extensive subclinical spread of tumor. Extensive subclinical dermal spread may rarely occur.[57] However, in areas such as the trunk, the thick, compact dermis may actually serve as a barrier to the penetration of tumor.[45] SCC also commonly spreads along fascial planes such as on the temple and in the neck. While SCC does not readily invade muscle, when it does, the spread is often parallel to the muscle fibers.[45, 48] SCCs may occasionally spread along blood vessels, but the extent of the spread is usually limited. Of much greater importance is its invasion of blood vessels and lymphatics, which portends systemic and regional metastases and may result in satellite lesions.[45]

Perineural spread (Figs. 57–1, 57–2) is much more common in SCC than in BCC.[45, 58, 59] In one series, perineural spread was observed in 2.4% of the SCCs but only 0.92% of the BCCs.[58] Another study reported an incidence of 4.9%,[60] while a third found an incidence of 14%.[61] The reason for this high rate of perineural spread is unclear, but the perineural space appears to offer little resistance to the tumor.[45, 61] Tumors that exhibit perineural involvement histologically are often poorly differentiated, adenosquamous or spindle cell SCCs.[45, 61] However, some authors feel that the histologic subtyping is not an important determinant in perineural involvement.[59, 62]

The fifth and seventh cranial nerves (CN V and CN VII) are commonly affected by cutaneous SCC.[61, 63–65] Tumors affecting these nerves may spread in a centrip-

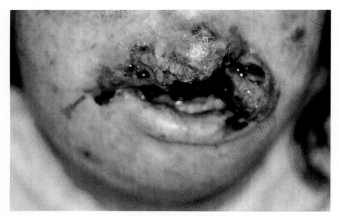

Figure 57–1. Patient with recurrent perineural squamous cell carcinoma (SCC) of the upper lip who subsequently developed metastases and died.

etal or centrifugal direction and may travel a considerable distance, sometimes even entering foramina, leading to diffuse intracranial spread.[59, 64, 66, 67] Tumor may be confined to the involved nerve without affecting the surrounding tissue, involve only the major nerve trunk, or affect numerous branches.[59, 61]

Perineural involvement may be present for years before neurologic signs and symptoms signal that the tumor has recurred.[59, 62, 63] Most patients with perineural involvement are asymptomatic at the time of presentation.[61, 64] However, when present, neurologic signs and symptoms include "crawling" sensations, burning, stinging, numbness, shooting pains, and motor deficits.[59, 61, 63–65] The size of the tumor is an unreliable predictor of perineural involvement, as even small tumors may exhibit extensive perineural spread.[62] Patients with perineural SCC are not only at high risk for local recurrence, but also are at significant risk for the development of regional and distant metastases.[61, 64–66, 68] However, metastases often occur only late in the course of the disease.[59, 60, 62]

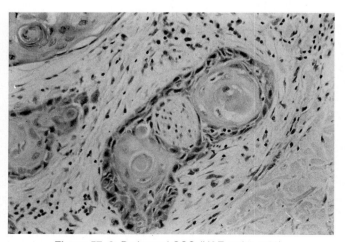

Figure 57–2. Perineural SCC (H&E stain; ×80).

Metastases and the Management of Regional Lymph Nodes

Unlike BCC, SCC of the skin and mucous membranes metastasizes with a significant degree of frequency. Thus, a patient who has been rendered locally tumor free by surgery may later succumb to metastatic disease. To prevent this, patients who are at high risk for regional and distal spread must be identified and adjunctive therapy administered. Unfortunately, very little research has been conducted on how to accurately identify patients at high risk for metastases and how to best manage their disease.

GENERAL LYMPH NODE MANAGEMENT

Regardless of the original lesion's size, depth of invasion, and anatomic location and the presence or absence of predisposing factors for perineural involvement, every patient with a previous history of SCC should be checked at each follow-up visit for possible regional node metastases. Just as with melanoma, the smallest, thinnest, and most innocuous SCC will occasionally metastasize. The frequency of follow-up for a patient with a previous history of SCC will depend on the likelihood that the patient will develop a metastasis, a recurrence, or a new lesion. In general, patients should be examined every 3 months during the first postoperative year, every 3 to 6 months for the next 2 years, and then yearly thereafter.

Typically, metastatic nodes are very firm on palpation and are generally described as being "rock hard." They may be matted together or fixed to the deeper structures. SCC usually first spreads to the regional nodes before spreading distally. However, on occasion distal spread will occur in the absence of regional spread or be present at the time that regional nodal disease is discovered. For this reason, the typical laboratory and radiologic evaluation of a patient with SCC should consist of a complete blood cell count with differential white blood cell count, a chemistry profile to evaluate liver function, and a chest radiograph. The chest radiograph is originally obtained at the time the primary lesion is treated and is then repeated periodically thereafter. These tests are usually done every 3 to 12 months, depending on the level of concern for potential metastatic disease. The more time that has passed since the initial treatment, the less frequently these studies need to be obtained. These studies are not routinely obtained for in situ SCCs or for small, superficially invasive SCCs, but rather are reserved for those patients with large, recurrent, deeply invasive, or perineural SCCs.

If regional lymph nodes are enlarged at the time of initial presentation, particularly if the SCC is ulcerated or clinically infected, a trial of antibiotic therapy may be indicated to determine whether the lymphadenopathy is reactive. Similarly, if the nodes enlarge immediately after surgery but do not resolve after several weeks of antibiotic therapy, a biopsy is indicated. Needle aspiration is typically used to perform a biopsy on a suspicious node, as some studies suggest that an open node biopsy may adversely affect the course of the patient's disease if tumor is present.[69–72] However, if needle aspiration is unsuccessful or results are inconclusive and metastases are strongly suspected, an open biopsy is indicated. This is usually performed in a setting where lymph node dissection can be immediately performed if the biopsy reveals SCC.[73–75]

If a patient has clinically palpable regional nodes, a sign of possible metastasis, the treatment of choice is lymph node dissection followed by postoperative irradiation.[76–84] Depending on the patient's age and health status and anticipated surgical morbidity, modification of this approach may be required after consultation with the radiation therapist, the head and neck surgeon, the cutaneous surgeon, the family, and the patient. Although effective for subclinical or minimal node disease (only one enlarged node, which is less than 1 cm in size), irradiation alone should not be expected to cure a patient with advanced nodal disease.

Controversy still surrounds the role of elective lymph node dissection (ELND) in the management of SCC patients without obvious nodal disease. While ELND does allow proper staging of a patient,[83] no large well-controlled prospective studies have addressed the value of this procedure. Moreover, much of the available data has been derived largely from noncutaneous SCCs of the head and neck or from SCCs that may behave differently than the typical SCC arising on sun-damaged skin. Currently, fewer ELNDs are being performed while criteria are being developed to help determine those candidates who most likely will benefit from the procedure and which nodes should be removed.[85]

One alternative to ELND is postoperative irradiation delivered to the area of lymphatic drainage. This treatment has been shown to be as effective as an ELND in patients at high risk for regional metastases.[86–89] However, use of specific criteria for selecting patients for this adjunctive therapy is mandatory. Postoperative irradiation is usually begun once the surgical site has healed, or approximately 4 to 6 weeks after surgery.[81, 86] The irradiation is delivered over a 6- to 8-week interval for a total dose of 6000 to 8000 rads (60 to 70 Gy) to the operative site, intervening lymphatics, and regional nodes.[80, 81]

COMPUTED TOMOGRAPHY AND MAGNETIC RESONANCE IMAGING

The role of computed tomography (CT) and magnetic resonance imaging (MRI) in detecting occult nodal metastases requires additional investigation. One study has reported that when physical examination was combined with CT and MRI scans, subclinical nodal metastases could be detected in all but 12% of patients at high risk for metastatic disease. Physical examination alone was unable to detect 39% of occult metastases.[90] Although CT and MRI scans may prove useful in selecting patients for ELND, in patients with palpable nodes, these studies are incapable of distinguishing between reactive nodes and those containing SCC.[91]

Patterns of Metastases

SCC usually first metastasizes to regional nodes, and distal spread in the absence of node involvement is rare.[92] The incidence of distal metastases is variable and appears to correlate with the anatomic location of the tumor, the presence or absence of predisposing factors, and the size and biologic aggressiveness of the tumor. Regional metastases usually occur within 3 years from the time of treatment of the primary tumor and often within the first year.[76–78, 81, 82, 92–97] A poor patient prognosis is usually associated with involvement of multiple nodes,[97] nodes in the lower neck and posterior cervical triangle,[97–100] and when there is extracapsular spread.[101, 102]

Unusual and atypical metastatic spread also occasionally occurs. In-transit metastases or satellite lesions may also be seen,[45, 103] which indicates that tumor emboli have gained access to the lymphatics, increasing the likelihood of regional node involvement. In this situation, ELND is justifiable, even without clinical involvement of the regional nodes.[45] If multiple tumor emboli are present, simple excision of the primary lesion and the satellites followed by extended-field irradiation probably offers a good chance of cure.[104]

On rare occasions, a metastatic SCC may demonstrate sufficient epidermotropism to be mistaken for a primary lesion.[105, 106] Management of such lesions may be difficult, but when feasible, simple excision with extended-field irradiation is probably the treatment of choice. Appropriate treatment of the primary lesion, if still present, is also important. Distant metastases to nonregional nodes or extranodal sites in the absence of regional node metastases are unusual,[92] with a reported incidence of 0 to 18.5%.[76, 107] The mortality rate in patients with regional metastatic SCC varies from 18.6% in unselected patients[76] to 100% in patients with SCC arising in scars.[108] The most frequent sites for distant metastases are the lungs, skin, bones, and parotid gland.[103, 109, 110]

Factors Determining Metastatic Spread

A number of variables have been found to influence the tendency of SCCs to metastasize. Unfortunately, multivariate analysis has not been utilized to determine which factors independently influence the tendency for metastases.

LOCATION

Certain anatomic locations are associated with a greater predilection for metastases by SCC. However, most studies have not attempted to match other variables that could influence metastatic spread (e.g., depth of invasion, degree of differentiation, or development within a pre-existing scar). Consequently, it is difficult to determine how important location is in determining metastatic spread. However, it is generally accepted that

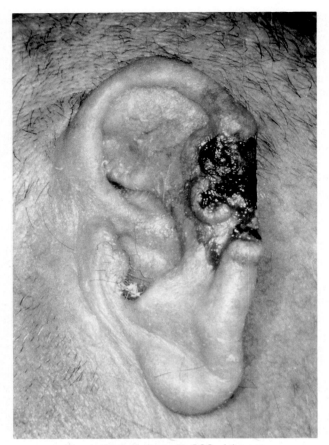

Figure 57–3. Patient with SCC of the ear.

SCC of the lip has a greater tendency to metastasize than SCCs that arise on actinically damaged skin. The incidence varies between 6.8[11, 77] and 15.8%.[76] Other high-risk areas include the temple (36.4%),[76] dorsal hand (16 to 20%),[76, 102] forehead (11.6%),[76] ear (10.2 to 14%)[76, 111–113] (Fig. 57–3), preauricular area (9.1%),[76] leg (12.6%),[16] trunk (14%),[16] arm (8 to 30%),[16, 112] and nose (8 to 27%).[112, 114] No satisfactory explanation has been offered as to why SCCs in these areas are more likely to metastasize.

SIZE

Although invasive SCCs that are less than 1 cm in diameter may metastasize,[81] most lesions that metastasize are greater than 2 cm in diameter.[13, 76, 78, 81, 94, 97, 114–116] Because large tumors invade deeply, it may be that the depth of invasion is actually more important than size in determining the tendency for metastases.

DEGREE OF DIFFERENTIATION

It has been suggested that metastatic SCCs are commonly of the poorly differentiated histologic subtype.[13, 103, 107, 114, 117, 118] However, there are many reports of well-differentiated or moderately well differentiated metastatic SCCs.[76, 85, 96, 119, 120]

RADIATION DERMATITIS

SCCs arising in areas of previous radiation demonstrate a significant propensity for metastases[92, 93, 121] (Fig. 57–4). The incidence of metastases in radiation-induced SCCs has been reported to be 10 to 30%[92, 121] with a mortality rate of greater than 12%.[122] Most commonly, the radiation was administered for treatment of a benign condition such as acne or hirsutism. However, SCCs may also arise in a cutaneous port through which deep radiation was delivered. Patients who develop radiation-induced SCCs may not demonstrate significant evidence of radiation dermatitis. The SCC may present as an ulceration or as a typical hyperkeratotic nodule. Because it may be misdiagnosed as radiation necrosis, any ulceration that occurs in an area of previous radiation should undergo biopsy if it does not respond promptly to conservative management.

SCAR CARCINOMA (MARJOLIN'S ULCER, BURN SCAR CARCINOMA)

SCCs arising in scars from burns, osteomyelitis, and chronic stasis ulcers (Figs. 57–5, 57–6) have a poor patient prognosis because of high recurrence rates and a risk of regional and distant metastases that varies from 10 to 30%.[85, 92–94, 103, 108, 109, 123, 124] However, it is difficult

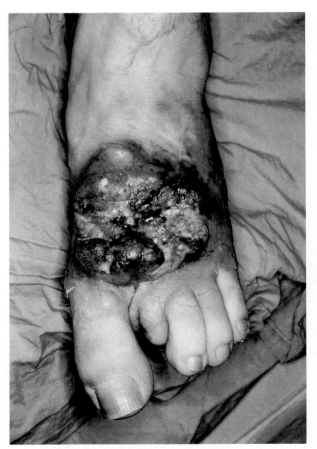

Figure 57–4. Patient with SCC arising in an area of previous irradiation of a wart.

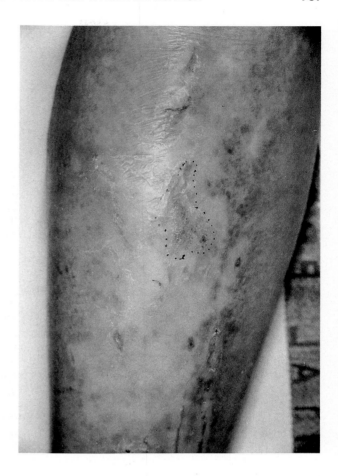

Figure 57–5. Clinical appearance of a patient with scarring from dystrophic epidermolysis bullosa and a superficial SCC (*outlined*).

to know if these cancers are biologically more aggressive or are associated with a poorer prognosis because delays in diagnosis allow them to become advanced.[94, 103, 109, 123] Positive staining for vimentin may serve as a marker for burn scar carcinomas that behave aggressively.[125] At the time of diagnosis, these tumors are often quite large and have infiltrated other tissue extensively, even muscle

and bone. The latent period for development of these SCCs is usually more than 20 years[103, 108, 109, 120, 123] but may be less than 2 years.[108, 126] The 5-year survival rate in these patients is 31 to 71%.[94, 103, 108, 109, 123, 126] Once metastases occur, patient prognosis is extremely poor, with reported mortality rates of 75 to 100%.[108] Distant metastases occur in up to 17% of patients.[109] In chronic

Figure 57–6. Patient with extensive scarring from lupus erythematosus and a previous burn who developed a rapidly growing SCC of the forearm that subsequently metastasized to the epitrochlear nodes.

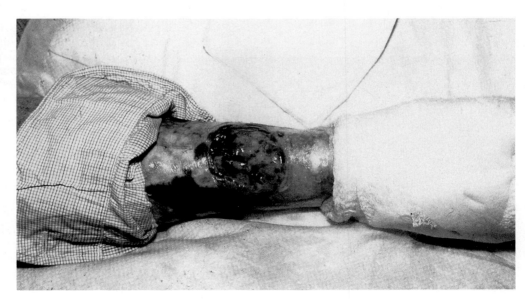

osteomyelitis, 85% of the SCCs arise on the leg in the epithelium that lines the sinus tracts.

DEPTH OF INVASION

SCCs that exhibit extensive and deep infiltration of the skin and underlying structures are more likely to metastasize. In an attempt to determine the critical level of invasion that is associated with metastases (Figs. 57–7, 57–8), Clark's levels of invasion and tumor thickness have been examined, as has been done in the staging of melanomas.[76, 107, 117] It has been shown that SCCs that invade to Clark's levels I, II, and III are not typically associated with recurrences or metastases.[107] While depth alone[76] cannot be used to predict metastatic potential, SCCs that metastasize have been found to invade more deeply (greater than 7.9 mm) than those that do not (4.2 mm). Conversely, patients with SCCs that were less than 4 mm thick usually did not develop metastases or have recurrence of their disease.[117] Even patients with tumors greater than 4 mm but less than 8 mm thick did well. However, patients with SCCs greater than 10 mm in thickness usually did poorly. Tumor thickness correlated better with prognosis than did depth of invasion or degree of differentiation. However, well-differentiated SCCs had a 6% recurrence rate and no mortality, while moderately differentiated tumors had a 10% recurrence rate and a 7% mortality rate, and poorly differentiated SCCs were associated with a 60% mortality rate. Furthermore, if tumor involved the deep dermis, a 10% recurrence rate was seen without fatalities, but if the tumor invaded the fat or deeper structures, the mortality rate was 67%. For this reason, it has been suggested that ELND be performed for SCCs more than 8 mm thick or when invasion of the subcutaneous fat or deeper structures occurs.

PREVIOUS TREATMENT

Metastatic SCCs are more likely to be recurrent than primary tumors.[13, 76, 81, 94, 96, 120]

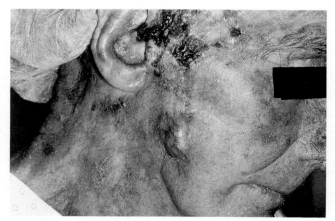

Figure 57–7. Patient with extensive recurrent basal cell carcinoma (BCC) and SCC.

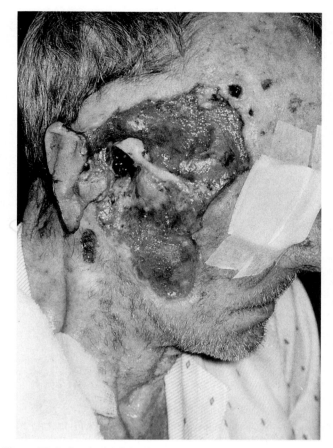

Figure 57–8. Surgical defect after Mohs surgery. Despite being locally cured, the patient presented three years later with regional metastases.

PRE-EXISTING ACTINIC DAMAGE

SCCs arising in sun-damaged skin or in pre-existing actinic keratoses tend to behave in relatively benign fashion.[127–131] Unfortunately, these data have been often misinterpreted to mean that an SCC arising on sun-damaged skin does not need to be treated with the same aggressiveness as an SCC occurring elsewhere. However, SCCs arising in sun-damaged skin can behave as aggressively as those occurring in other locations (Fig. 57–9), and they should be managed accordingly.[76, 93, 95, 112–119, 129, 132] The incidence of metastases in SCCs arising in actinically damaged skin varies from 0.5 to 10%.[119, 127]

HISTOLOGY

Histologic features that may be associated with an increased risk of metastatic spread include perineural involvement and the presence of tumor within lymphatic vessels.[45] For this reason, these patients should be treated with ELND followed by postoperative irradiation to the surgical site and the regional lymph nodes. SCCs characterized by infiltrating strands of tumor cells (Figs. 57–10, 57–11), "Indian filing," and single-cell invasion (Fig. 57–12) are more likely to recur and metastasize than are those tumors characterized by

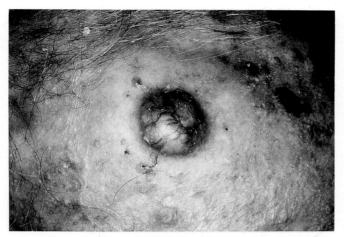

Figure 57–9. Elderly white male with extensive actinic damage who developed a rapidly growing SCC of the forehead and subsequent widespread metastases.

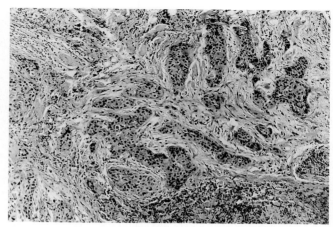

Figure 57–11. Higher power view of tumor strands (H&E stain; × 80).

islands of well-differentiated, tightly adhesive cells that have rounded borders (Figs. 57–13, 57–14).[133–135]

DE NOVO SCCS

Interestingly, SCCs that have no obvious predisposing cause appear to have a high metastatic potential. A 17% incidence of metastases has been reported for de novo SCCs,[136] but few details were provided, and no explanations for this phenomenon have been offered.

IMMUNE STATUS

Not only is the incidence of SCCs increased in immunosuppressed patients, but these tumors also behave in a very aggressive fashion on occasion. A significant incidence of metastases (6.45%) and mortality (5.4%) from SCC has been found in transplantation patients. Patients with lymphocytic lymphoma also have an increased incidence of SCCs, which are usually poorly

differentiated and extremely invasive in the absence of cellular pleomorphism or atypical mitoses. These tumors recur at a rate of 37 to 50%, with half of the patients developing metastases and 25% dying of the disease. Other types of lymphomas are also associated with an increased incidence of SCC,[137] and 22.9% of patients with metastatic SCC have been found to be immunocompromised.[138]

Histologic and Clinical Variants of SCC

A number of clinical and histologic variants of SCC have been described. Some of these are common, while others are rare.

SCC IN SITU (BOWEN'S DISEASE, QUEYRAT'S ERYTHROPLASIA)

Although SCC in situ is often considered to be synonymous with Bowen's disease,[139, 140] many believe two

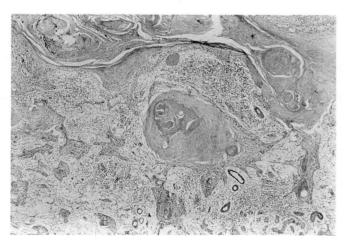

Figure 57–10. In addition to larger islands of tumor cells, there are infiltrating strands of tumor cells (H&E stain; × 40). (Courtesy of John C. Maize, M.D.)

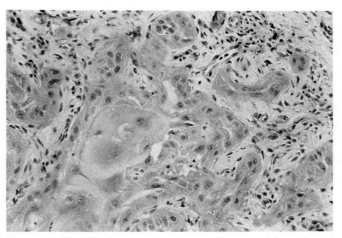

Figure 57–12. SCC demonstrating loose adherence of the cells and individual cell invasion of the dermis (H&E stain; × 100).

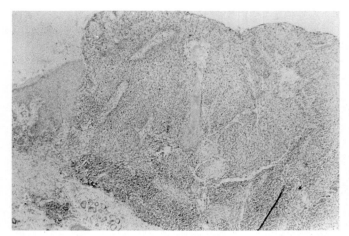

Figure 57–13. Superficially invasive SCC showing broad pushing border (H&E stain; × 40).

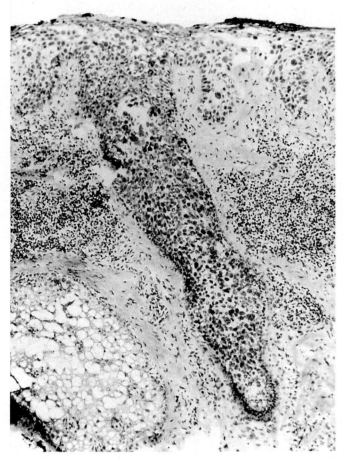

Figure 57–15. Biopsy specimen of patient with Bowen's disease with deep follicular involvement (H&E stain; × 40).

different forms of SCC in situ exist. The first is Bowen's disease (BD), and the second is noninvasive SCC arising within an AK. The primary reason for distinguishing between these two is that BD can show deep follicular involvement and may not be amenable to superficial forms of destruction (Fig. 57–15).

When an SCC in situ arises in an AK, the microscopic appearance is often that of a coexisting AK and SCC (Fig. 57–16). However, with time the SCC may entirely replace the AK. In contrast to an AK, the SCC shows marked dyskeratosis and epidermal disarray along with widespread cytologic atypia and pleomorphism. Compared with BD, SCC in situ arising in an AK will always show solar or basophilic degeneration of the upper dermis, characterized by clumps of pale blue–staining, actinically damaged collagen fibers. In time, in situ SCC may become invasive (Figs. 57–17, 57–18). Clinically, SCC arising in an AK may be indistinguishable from a hypertrophic AK.

In BD, the acanthotic epidermis causes elongation and thickening of the rete ridges[141] that may reduce the dermal papillae to thin strands. The stratum corneum is thickened and consists primarily of parakeratotic cells. The epidermal cells are large, atypical, and often multinucleate; the disarray gives them a "windswept" appearance. Individual cell keratinization, or malignant dyskeratosis, and occasional horn pearls may also be present (Fig. 57–19). If marked vacuolization occurs,

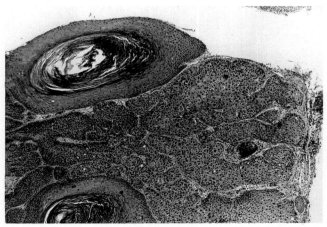

Figure 57–14. More deeply invasive SCC showing broad pushing borders (H&E stain; × 40).

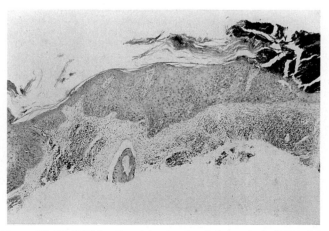

Figure 57–16. SCC in situ arising in an actinic keratosis (H&E stain; × 40).

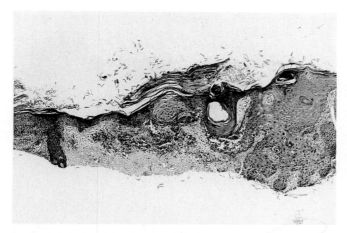

Figure 57–17. Superficially invasive SCC arising in an actinic keratosis (H&E stain; × 40).

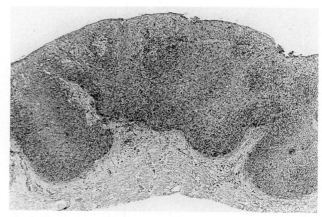

Figure 57–19. Biopsy of Bowen's disease (H&E stain; × 40). (Courtesy of John C. Maize, M.D.)

immunohistochemical staining for cytokeratin, carcinoembryonic antigen (CEA) and S–100 protein will allow differentiation of BD from extramammary Paget's disease and melanoma.[142] The demarcation between dermis and epidermis is distinct, and the basement membrane is intact. Clinically, BD may appear as a dry, scaling, dull red plaque that may resemble psoriasis, eczema, superficial multicentric BCC, or AKs (Fig. 57–20).

INVASIVE SCC

The term invasive is used as a means of distinguishing the "common form" of SCC from its other variants, such as verrucous carcinoma and acantholytic SCC, that will be discussed separately.

Histologically, in a typical invasive SCC, masses of epidermal cells proliferate downward and invade the dermis. The tumor consists of varying proportions of normal and atypical squamous cells. Depending on the proportion of atypical cells, the depth of invasion, and the amount of differentiation, the tumor may be graded into one of four categories (Figs. 57–21, 57–22). In grade I, the SCC has not penetrated below the level of the sweat glands. In some areas, the basal layer may be intact, whereas in other areas it will be disorganized or absent. The tumor masses consist primarily of differentiated squamous cells with well-developed intercellular bridges. Some of the cells have atypical nuclei, and horn pearls with incomplete or complete keratinization are common. Sheets of partially keratinized cells may be present, and there is often a marked inflammatory response.

In grade II, the invading cell masses are poorly demarcated from the stroma. Many of the nuclei are atypical, and only a few incompletely keratinized horn pearls are present.

In grade III, keratinization is absent in many areas, and horn pearls are not present. When keratinization is present, it is seen only in small groups of cells. Malignant dyskeratosis is observed, and many of the nuclei are atypical. The frequent mitotic figures are often atypical.

In grade IV SCC, keratinization is almost nonexistent, almost all of the nuclei are atypical, and the cells lack intercellular bridges. These tumors may be difficult to distinguish from amelanotic melanoma, atypical fibro-

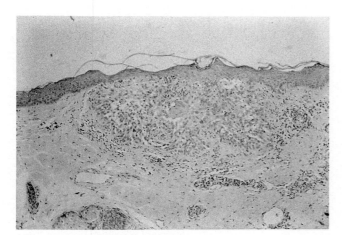

Figure 57–18. Advanced superficial SCC arising from an actinic keratosis (H&E stain; × 40).

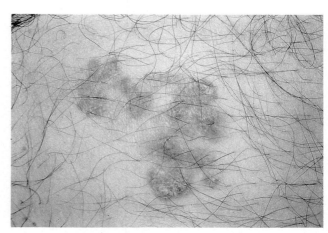

Figure 57–20. Lesion of Bowen's disease.

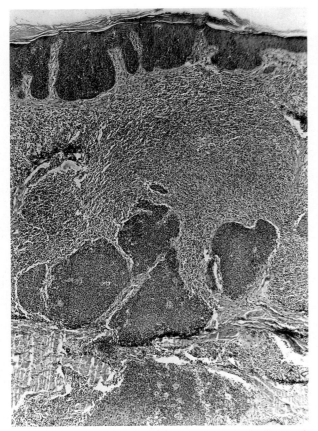

Figure 57–21. Biopsy specimen of Bowen's disease that has evolved into invasive SCC (H&E stain; ×40). (Courtesy of John C. Maize, M.D.)

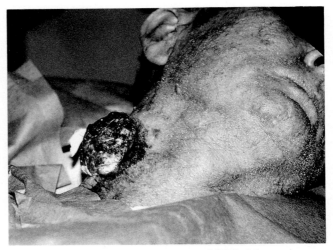

Figure 57–23. Clinical appearance of SCC of the neck.

differentiation. These features influence the biologic behavior of the tumor and may be helpful in planning the proper treatment.

It is important to note that on occasion, Merkel cell carcinoma may coexist with SCC.[143, 144] The explanation for this finding remains unknown, although it has been suggested that chronic UVL exposure is responsible for causing both lesions.[143]

Clinically, the appearance of invasive SCC is variable and may be indistinguishable from a hypertrophic AK or keratoacanthoma (KA). It may appear as a verrucous or hyperkeratotic papule, nodule, or plaque. Rapidly growing, aggressive SCCs may present as smooth vascular nodules (Figs. 57–23, 57–24), while slowly infiltrating tumors often present as an ulceration.

ADENOIDAL, ACANTHOLYTIC, OR PSEUDOGLANDULAR SCC

This variant of SCC is almost exclusively found on the sun-damaged skin of elderly patients, especially the

xanthoma, or malignant fibrous histiocytoma; immunohistochemical staining for cytokeratin, S–100 protein, and vimentin or electron microscopy studies may be required to make an accurate diagnosis.

Different areas within an SCC may show different histologic features. For that reason, it is always advisable to microscopically examine multiple areas of the tumor to determine the extent of invasion and the degree of

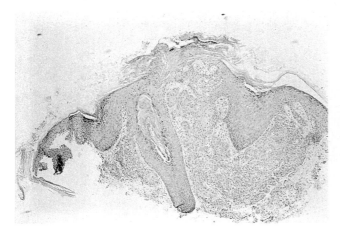

Figure 57–22. Biopsy of a moderately invasive SCC (H&E stain; ×40).

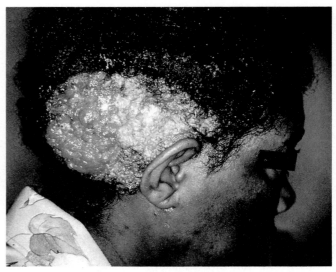

Figure 57–24. Clinical appearance of SCC of the scalp.

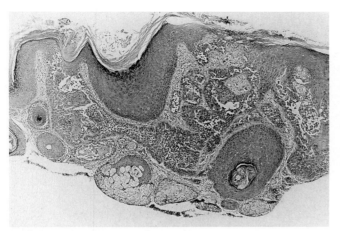

Figure 57–25. Low-power view of acantholytic SCC (H&E stain; ×40).

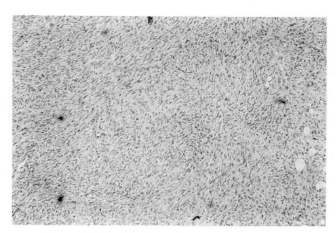

Figure 57–27. Spindle cell SCC (H&E stain; ×80).

face and ears. Occasionally it will occur on the vermillion border of the lower lip and it may arise de novo or from a pre-existing AK. Usually there is nothing distinctive about its clinical appearance, but on occasion it may resemble a KA.

Histopathologically, the adenoidal changes may be present throughout the lesion or may be focal (Figs. 57–25, 57–26). Frequently, a coexisting acantholytic AK is also present. On low-power magnification, the tumor appears nodular or cup-shaped. The tubular and alveolar lumina are lined by one or several layers of epithelium. When lined by a single layer of cells, the lumina resemble glands. However, in areas where several layers of epithelium line the lumina, squamous and partially keratinized cells form the inner lining. The lumina are filled with many desquamated acantholytic cells, which may be partially or fully keratinized. The tumor cells may be very atypical, and mitoses are common. In some instances, eccrine ducts at the periphery of these tumors show signs of dilatation and proliferation. The tumor often begins in the upper part of a hair follicle and adjacent epidermis but does not exhibit follicular extension.

There is some controversy regarding the biologic behavior of this tumor. The rate of metastases has been reported to vary from 1.5[136] to 14%[145] in tumors greater than 1.5 cm in size.

SPINDLE CELL SCC

In spindle cell SCC,[139, 140, 146] a poorly differentiated variant, the tumor cells are elongated or spindle shaped, are often pleomorphic, and have atypical nuclei (Fig. 57–27). Mitoses are common, and pleomorphic giant cells may be seen. The cells are intermingled with collagen fibers and may be arranged in whorls. If routine light microscopy does not allow spindle cell SCC to be differentiated from spindle cell melanoma, atypical fibroxanthoma, malignant fibrous histiocytoma, postradiation sarcomas, leiomyosarcoma, or dermatofibrosarcoma, the immunohistochemical staining for S–100 protein, vimentin, desmin, and cytokeratin or electron microscopy studies may be utilized to establish the correct diagnosis.[147–150]

These tumors usually present as an ulceration but may appear as an exophytic mass.[147] Regional and distal metastases occur in 25% of patients. Clark's levels of invasion correlate better with the biologic behavior than does tumor thickness.[146] This variant of SCC may arise in areas of previous radiation[146, 151] and has shown a predilection for perineural spread.[61]

VERRUCOUS CARCINOMA (GIANT CONDYLOMA, EPITHELIOMA CUNICULATUM, OR ORAL FLORID PAPILLOMATOSIS)

Microscopic examination of verrucous carcinoma reveals an exophytic tumor with marked papillomatous hyperplasia of the epidermis, as well as hyperkeratosis and parakeratosis (Fig. 57–28). The rete are blunt and bulbous and extend deeply into the underlying connective tissue, compressing and pushing the collagen bundles aside. Muscle and bone may be invaded (Fig. 57–29). Often, keratin-filled cysts can be found with the epithelial proliferation. Nuclear atypia, malignant dyskeratosis, and horn pearls are unusual. When occurring

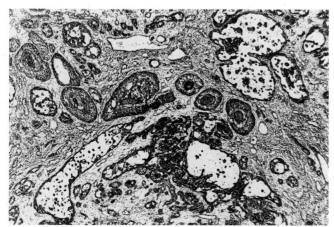

Figure 57–26. High-power view of acantholytic SCC (H&E stain; ×40). (Courtesy of John C. Maize, M.D.)

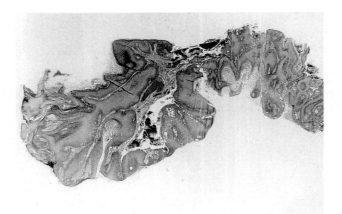

Figure 57–28. Low-power view of a verrucous carcinoma (H&E stain; ×10). (Courtesy of John C. Maize, M.D.)

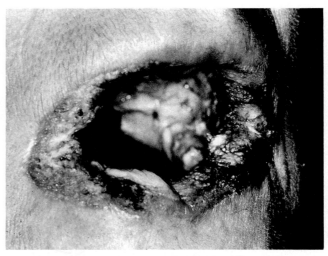

Figure 57–30. Patient with oral florid papillomatosis.

in the mouth (Fig. 57–30) and on the genitalia (Fig. 57–31), the lesions tend to be more exophytic and wartlike, while on the plantar surface they are more endophytic (Fig. 57–32). Marked sinus formation and islands of tumor with keratin-filled centers may be present, but the basement membrane is commonly intact. The inflammatory response may be intense, and microabscesses may form within either the stroma or the tumor. Rarely, perineural infiltration is seen.

Verrucous carcinoma is a low-grade SCC that may affect both the skin and mucous membranes, including the larynx and vagina.[139, 140, 152, 153] It typically occurs in the oral cavity, in the anogenital area, and on the plantar surface. In the mouth it appears as a white, cauliflower-like lesion and is known as oral florid papillomatosis. In the anogenital region it most commonly occurs on the glans penis and foreskin of uncircumcised males but can also affect the perianal area and vulva. Because of its resemblance to a large wart, it has been called the giant condyloma of Buschke and Löwenstein. On the plantar surface, verrucous carcinoma may mimic an intractable plantar wart and is known as epithelioma cuniculatum.[154] The deeply penetrating, keratin-filled cysts may pene-

trate the plantar fascia, destroy bones, and even invade the skin of the dorsum of the foot.[155, 156]

ADENOSQUAMOUS CARCINOMA OF THE SKIN (MUCIN-PRODUCING SCC, MUCOEPIDERMOID SCC)

This rare SCC variant usually occurs on the head or neck and appears to arise from the epidermis.[140, 157–159] However, a dermal origin from a pluripotential epithelial cell of the acrosyringium with secondary involvement of the epidermis has also been considered. These tumors are frequently deeply invasive and commonly metastasize even when less than 1 cm in size. Perineural involvement may occur, and multiple recurrences are common. The tumor may grow quickly, resulting in rapid death, or the patient may live for years. Histologically, infiltrating strands of squamous cells intermingle with glandular structures in a desmoplastic stroma. Some of the glandular structures resemble distorted eccrine ducts and stain positively for CEA. The material in the lumina of the glandular structures, as well as the mucin-producing cells lining these structures, demonstrate the staining characteristics of sialomucin. Consequently, these tumors must be differentiated from mucin-producing metastatic visceral and salivary gland neoplasms.

CLEAR CELL CARCINOMA

Clear cell carcinoma,[160] a rare variant of SCC, behaves in a very aggressive fashion and has a significant incidence of perineural involvement and metastatic spread. There appear to be three variants of this tumor. In one variant, numerous clear cells are intermingled with areas of typical keratinizing SCC. In a second variant, the tumor presents as a subcutaneous mass without connection to the epidermis, and anastomosing cords of focally necrotic tumor cells without foci of keratinization are seen microscopically. The third variant consists of numerous pleomorphic and clear cells that show areas of squamous differentiation, as well as areas of pseudo-

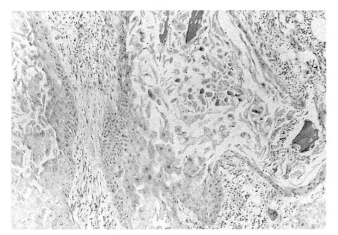

Figure 57–29. Verrucous carcinoma containing sequestered bone (H&E stain; ×80). (Courtesy of John C. Maize, M.D.)

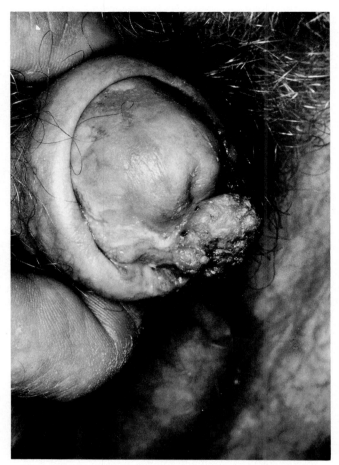

Figure 57–31. Patient with verrucous carcinoma of the penis.

glandular formation and acantholysis. The nature of these clear cells is unknown.

SIGNET RING SCC

Signet ring SCC is an unusual variant of SCC that is very aggressive in its biologic behavior.[161] These tumors

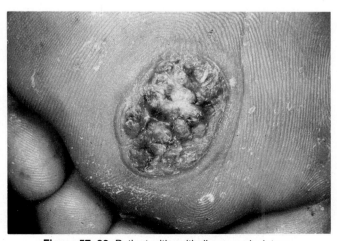

Figure 57–32. Patient with epithelioma cuniculatum.

are poorly differentiated, invade deeply, and frequently recur multiple times before eventually metastasizing. Signet ring cells, formed by tonofilaments arranged about the nucleus in concentric rings that create a paranuclear clear space, are found within the affected lymph nodes.

PSEUDOCARCINOMATOUS HYPERPLASIA

Pseudocarcinomatous or pseudoepitheliomatous hyperplasia (PEH)[140] is a reactive proliferation of the epidermis that is often mistaken for SCC. It may be a forerunner of SCC and may be seen in association with certain inflammatory or infectious processes such as bromoderma, blastomycosis, and hidradenitis suppurativa; chronic ulcerative processes such as pyoderma gangrenosum; stasis ulcers; osteomyelitis with sinus tract formation; burn scar ulcers[108, 162, 163] at the edge of ulcerating BCCs, overlying granular cell tumors, and at the edge of some surgical wounds.[164, 165]

To avoid an error in diagnosis, an incisional biopsy specimen should be submitted for pathologic examination. This specimen should include the subcutaneous tissue and be large enough to demonstrate the architectural pattern of the lesion and detect any primary process that has caused the reactive proliferation.

Histologically, PEH often resembles grade I or II SCC, and at times the two may be indistinguishable from one another.[108, 140, 162, 163] PEH shows irregular invasion of the dermis by uneven, jagged, often sharply pointed epidermal cell masses and strands with horn pearls and numerous mitotic figures. These downward proliferations may extend below the level of the sweat glands, where they may appear as isolated islands of epidermal tissue. The cells are usually well differentiated and lack individual cell keratinization, nuclear hyperplasia, and hyperchromasia. The epithelial proliferations are often invaded by leukocytes, resulting in epidermal cell necrosis, which may help in distinguishing it from SCC.[140] It has been proposed that PEH originates from the sweat ducts and follicular infundibula.[166] Indeed, at times the sweat ducts will proliferate in response to injury and form nests and strands of squamous cells that mimic SCC.[167]

PROLIFERATING TRICHILEMMAL CYSTS

Another entity that may be confused with SCC is the proliferating trichilemmal cyst.[140, 168] This tumor primarily occurs on the scalp of elderly women. As the cyst grows it may ulcerate, erode, bleed, or periodically become inflamed, causing the patient to seek medical treatment. Clinically, the most common diagnosis is a cyst. Histopathologic examination demonstrates lobules of squamous epithelium of variable size. The epithelium in the center of the lobules changes into an amorphous eosinophilic keratinous substance that is typical of trichilemmal cysts. The tumor may show slight cellular anaplasia, individual cell keratinization reminiscent of SCC, and horn pearls. However, the lack of origin from the epidermis, focal calcification, and retained remnants of the trichilemmal cyst help distinguish it from an SCC.

Many previously reported SCCs that arose in cysts were probably examples of this entity.

KERATOACANTHOMA

Of all the conditions that must be distinguished from SCC, keratoacanthomas (KAs) are the most common and the most difficult to differentiate.[139, 140] The clinical or histologic appearance, rapid growth rate, or response to intralesional therapy does not guarantee accuracy in distinguishing these two entities from one another (Fig. 57–33). When performing a biopsy on suspected KAs, excisional, incisional, or deep shave biopsy techniques that remove the entire tumor should be employed so that the overall architectural pattern and base of the tumor can be evaluated, as mitotic figures, dyskeratosis, and nuclear atypia are not unusual. An incisional biopsy should include the central crateriform portion of the tumor, as well as its shoulders. Microscopically, a typical KA will show a central cup-shaped keratin-filled crater, with the adjacent epidermis forming a buttress or lip at the edges of this crater. At the base of the crater, irregular epidermal proliferations extend both upward into the crater and downward away from it. The cells are eosinophilic and glassy in appearance, and horn pearls are common. In fully developed KAs, the base is reasonably well demarcated from the dermis and usually does not extend below the level of the sweat glands. A dense inflammatory infiltrate is often present at the base of the lesion, and microabscesses are sometimes present within the epithelial proliferations, which helps to distinguish this lesion from an SCC. Early KAs may be especially difficult to distinguish histologically from SCCs. It has been estimated that a firm histologic distinction between KA and SCC can be attained in only 81 to 86% of cases.[169] Although ancillary histologic techniques can help distinguish between these two tumors,[170–172] in borderline cases the results may still not be clear.[173]

Finally, it should be noted that there have been numerous reports of KAs transforming into SCCs or behaving in a biologically aggressive manner with deep

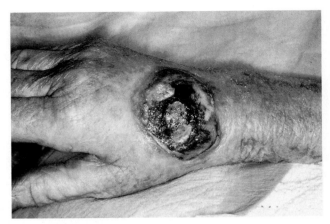

Figure 57–34. Elderly white woman with recurrent SCC of the hand that metastasized and resulted in her death 1 year later.

tissue invasion and even metastases. This has been particularly true of giant KAs.[174–179] Although these tumors were probably SCCs from the time of onset, these reports emphasize the need for extreme caution when managing these tumors.

Philosophy and Goals of Treatment

PHILOSOPHY

In managing patients with SCCs, it is important to totally remove or destroy the tumor while preserving function and minimizing the amount of normal tissue removed so as to provide the most optimal cosmetic result. Obviously, the most important goal must be to rid the patient of the tumor, for if this goal is not met, the other goals will ultimately not be achieved.[180]

In managing patients with skin cancer, preventive treatment is as important as removal of the cancer. Patients must be educated in the proper use of sunscreens to minimize sunlight exposure. Although some reports suggest that many AKs will spontaneously regress and only a few evolve to SCC,[181] most cutaneous surgeons still prefer to proceed with therapy of these lesions, because it is impossible to determine if or when malignant degeneration will happen (Fig. 57–34).[182]

TREATMENT PRINCIPLES

The type of treatment used for any SCC is largely a reflection of the lesion's anatomic location, etiology, size, and histologic appearance. However, before choosing any modality of treatment, certain important principles of management must be fully understood.

Biopsy

As with all skin cancers, it is often preferable to first biopsy the lesion and review the histologic results before deciding on the most appropriate form of treatment.

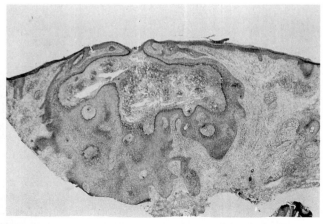

Figure 57–33. This recurrent lesion has the architectural appearance suggestive of a keratoacanthoma but showed SCC on deeper sections (H&E stain; ×40).

The biopsy should be of adequate size and depth so that there is sufficient material for the pathologist to make the correct diagnosis, as well as to identify any unusual features such as perineural spread. This is also important to help distinguish between an SCC and a KA or PEH. If the lesion is exophytic, removal of the entire lesion plus a 2-mm rim of surrounding tissue using a shave technique will often be satisfactory. This technique provides adequate tissue for pathologic diagnosis and causes minimal scarring if the lesion does not require additional treatment. If the lesion is flat, an alternative approach is to use an incisional or punch biopsy technique. If the lesion is large and bulky, an incisional biopsy helps avoid the sampling errors associated with a punch biopsy or the difficulties that will subsequently be encountered if curettage is chosen for treatment.[118, 183, 184]

Although there are times when a pretreatment biopsy need not be performed, if there is any question regarding the diagnosis, the extent of the tumor, or the presence of features such as perineural spread, a biopsy is mandatory.

Seeding and Implantation

Because of the potential risk of implantation of SCC when using the biopsy technique, it is important not to inject local anesthetic agents into the tumor itself, but instead to perform a field block around it. This same principle is applicable to Mohs surgery as well, where the scalpel blade should be changed and the instruments cleaned between layers to reduce the risk of implanting tumor cells in the wound bed.

Variables in the Selection of a Treatment Modality

AGE AND COSMESIS

It has been suggested in the past that elderly patients with SCCs should be treated with radiation instead of surgery (Table 57–1). However, people are currently living longer and enjoying a better quality of life than they did previously. As a consequence, there is no valid reason to deny a reasonably healthy elderly patient a definitive surgical procedure. Radiation therapy should be reserved for individuals who are older than 55 years of age, because the cosmetic results may deteriorate with time, there is a potential for carcinogenesis, and the risk of radiation necrosis increases with time. However, age and cosmesis are often interrelated, and many older patients are often more accepting of the hypopigmented scars that result from cryosurgery or curettage and electrodesiccation (C&D) than younger patients. The skin of elderly patients is also more "forgiving," so a reasonably good cosmetic result can usually be anticipated in most cases.

NUMBER OF LESIONS

The number of lesions may also determine the best form of treatment (Fig. 57–35). For example, a patient with multiple lesions of Bowen's disease of the trunk might be best managed with use of topical 5-fluorouracil (5-FU), cryosurgery, CO_2 laser vaporization, or C&D.

TUMOR SIZE

The size of the tumor is important in determining its metastatic potential as well as its tendency to recur. In general, invasive tumors that are greater than 2 cm in size are more likely to recur and metastasize. For that reason, it might be best to treat them with excisional surgery or Mohs micrographic surgery (MMS). However, for superficial SCCs that are less than 1 cm in size, management with "blind" techniques such as C&D or cryosurgery is appropriate. Radiation therapy may be used for SCCs that are greater than 1 cm in size if there are no contraindications for its use.

TUMOR BORDERS

Invasive SCCs with indistinct margins should not be managed by blind techniques such as cryosurgery and C&D. These tumors require surgical excision with good histologic control. If radiation is used to treat these lesions, a larger margin of normal skin should be included in the irradiation field.

PRIMARY VERSUS RECURRENT SCC

Although a number of modalities can be used to treat a primary lesion, a recurrent SCC is best managed by surgical excision using the MMS technique. It is important to recognize that recurrent SCCs are potentially lethal, because they often have perineural involvement and can metastasize. For that reason, they are unsuitable for C&D, because the curette cannot identify and effectively remove tumor nests that are embedded in scar tissue. Therefore, a more aggressive surgical approach (i.e., MMS), is usually required.

HISTOLOGY

Histologic parameters that influence the choice of treatment include the architectural pattern, degree of differentiation, presence of perineural spread or lymphatic invasion, depth of invasion, and tumor thickness.

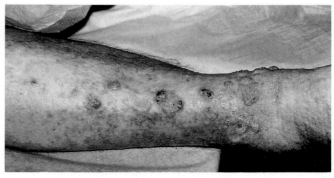

Figure 57–35. Patient with multiple SCCs of the leg.

TABLE 57–1. **MANAGEMENT OF SCC**

Variant	Location	Size	Degree of Differentiation	Treatment Modality
In situ non-Bowen's	Sun-exposed areas	—	—	Cryosurgery C&D Topical 5-FU Excision Radiation CO_2 laser Mohs surgery (recurrent lesion or lesion in high-risk area) ? Interferon ? PDT
Bowen's without deep follicular involvement	Sun-exposed or sun-protected areas	—	—	As above
Bowen's with deep follicular involvement	Sun-exposed or sun-protected areas	—	—	Excision Mohs surgery
Invasive	Sun-exposed or sun-protected areas (not lip or genitalia)	≤ 1 cm	Well-differentiated	C&D } If not deeply invasive Cryosurgery CO_2 laser Radiation Excision Mohs surgery (recurrent lesion or lesion in high-risk area)
Invasive	Sun-exposed or sun-protected areas (not lip or genitalia)	≤1 cm	Moderately or poorly differentiated	Excision } Preferable Mohs surgery Radiation
Invasive	Sun-exposed or sun-protected areas (not lip or genitalia)	>1 cm	All degrees of differentiation	Excision } Preferable, especially if not well differentiated Mohs surgery Radiation May want to consider postoperative radiation to surgical site and regional nodes if lesion >2 cm, deeply invasive, and/or moderately to poorly differentiated Multidisciplinary approach may be necessary
Burn scar carcinoma (Marjolin's ulcer)	All locations	All sizes	All degrees of differentiation	Excision Mohs surgery Amputation (for tumor invading muscle or bone in which cure by local excision is unlikely) Multi-disciplinary approach may be necessary Elective node dissection may be indicated in tumors that are not well differentiated and are large or deeply invasive
Radiation-induced	All locations	All sizes	All degrees of differentiation	Excision Mohs surgery (preferable) Wound management should be conservative, with graft or healing by second intention May require multidisciplinary approach
Perineural	All locations	All sizes	All degrees of differentiation	Mohs surgery (preferable) Excision Patient should receive postoperative radiation to surgical site and regional nodes May require multidisciplinary approach

TABLE 57–1. **MANAGEMENT OF SCC** *Continued*

Variant	Location	Size	Degree of Differentiation	Treatment Modality
Verrucous	All locations	All sizes	—	Excision Mohs surgery (preferable) May require multidisciplinary approach Amputation (if far advanced with bone invasion) Radiation (probably ineffective for skin lesions and may cause anaplastic transformation)
Subcutaneous	All locations	All sizes	All degrees of differentiation	Must rule out epidermotropic metastatic SCC Excision Mohs surgery (preferable) Extensive tumors and those with perineural spread may require multidisciplinary approach and postoperative radiation
Periungual/subungual	—	All sizes	All degrees of differentiation	Mohs surgery (preferable) Excision Amputation if significant bone or joint involvement (C&D, cryosurgery, CO_2 laser, radiation rarely are suitable)
Bowenoid papulosis*	Genitalia	—	—	C&D Cryosurgery CO_2 laser Topical 5-FU Excision ⎤ Mohs surgery ⎬ If lesion can't be distinguished from SCC in situ, especially if recurrent ?Interferon ⎦ ? PDT
Bowen's disease of the genitalia (in situ SCC, Queyrat's erythroplasia)*	—	—	—	CO_2 laser ⎤ If no deep follicular involvement ? C&D if ≤1 cm ⎬ Radiation ⎦ Topical 5-FU Cryosurgery Excision Mohs surgery ⎤ If deep follicular involvement or recurrent ? Interferon ⎬ ? PDT ⎦
Penile (invasive)*	—	Any size	Any degree of differentiation	Excision Mohs surgery (may require multidisciplinary approach) Radiation (only in young men with superficial, distal lesions < 3 cm) Amputation (partial or total) if tumor >3 cm, poorly differentiated, and deeply invasive Consider elective node dissection for deep disease of corpora or proximal penis
Vulvar (invasive)*	—	Any size	Any degree of differentiation	Excision Mohs surgery (may require multidisciplinary approach) Vulvectomy (may be necessary for extensive or multicentric lesion) Consider elective node dissection if tumor >2 cm, infiltrative, poorly differentiated, and >3 mm in depth

Table continued on following page

TABLE 57–1. **MANAGEMENT OF SCC** *Continued*

Variant	Location	Size	Degree of Differentiation	Treatment Modality	
Lip	—	≤1 cm	Well-differentiated	CO_2 laser C&D Cryosurgery	Only for SCC in situ or lesions ≤1 mm thick
				Excision Mohs surgery Radiation	
	—	>1 cm and <4 cm	All types	CO_2 laser Cryosurgery	In situ, or minimally invasive, well-differentiated lesions
				Excision Mohs surgery (may require multidisciplinary approach)	Preferable
				Radiation (superficial tumors, for palliation, or for lesions of commissures)	
				Consider postoperative radiation to operative site and regional nodes or elective node dissection if lesion is >2 cm, moderately or poorly differentiated, and ≥6 mm in thickness	
SCC with nodal metastases	All locations	—	—	Appropriate node dissection with postoperative radiation; patient should be evaluated for systemic spread with chest radiograph and blood tests	

*Screen patients for evidence of additional SCCs of the lower genital tract; sexual partners should be screened for similar lesions.

Tumors that show deep and extensive invasion or histologic features that correlate with a significant risk of recurrence and metastases (e.g., perineural spread) should not be managed by blind techniques.

PRE-EXISTING CONDITIONS

SCCs that arise in pre-existing lesions such as burn scars or areas of radiation dermatitis are generally best managed by surgical excision or MMS.

ANATOMIC LOCATION

Invasive SCCs that are located in high-risk areas for recurrence should be managed by surgical excision with histologic control or MMS. Depending on other variables, such as age and previous treatment, radiation therapy may be used if the chance for cure is good and the patient can be spared reconstructive surgery. The anatomic location may influence the treatment selection in that a patient might prefer a linear scar, such as that produced by excisional surgery, on the face as opposed to the round hypopigmented scar produced by C&D or cryosurgery. Effective curettage may be difficult to perform on some anatomic locations (e.g., the penis, eyelids, and lips),[185] and an alternative form of treatment may be required.

Cryosurgery is not commonly used to treat invasive carcinomas of the scalp, because of the difficulty in obtaining an adequate freeze,[186] or on the lower leg, because the healing time is prolonged, there is a significant risk of infection, and the cosmetic result is usually poor.[186] Although SCCs on the trunk can be excised, the procedure commonly results in the creation of scar spread or hypertrophy. In general, the trunk and extremities tolerate radiation poorly, and the cosmetic results may be inferior to those obtained with other equally effective modalities.[187, 188]

MANAGEMENT OF RECURRENT SCCS IN FLAPS AND GRAFTS

When an SCC recurs in a flap or graft, a decision must be made whether to remove the entire graft or flap so that any disconnected foci will not be missed. This decision is based on the depth, histology, size, and biologic behavior of the tumor and whether there have been multiple recurrences in different locations around the graft or flap. Often, as the cancer is traced out microscopically, it may involve the graft or flap, or there may be evidence of disconnected tumor foci, which would require removal of the entire graft or flap. By approaching patients with flaps and grafts and recurrent

SCCs in this manner, the cure rates are not compromised, and unnecessary large defects can be avoided.

MANAGEMENT OF SUBCLINICAL ACTINIC KERATOSES AFTER REMOVAL OF SCC

Patients with SCC often have severe actinic damage and numerous AKs. Not surprisingly, many of these patients demonstrate very dysplastic AKs on microscopic examination that are inapparent clinically. Although the likelihood of these evolving into SCC is unknown, it may be prudent to use topical 5-FU on and around the SCC scar to eliminate these lesions and prevent their evolution into another SCC.

Management of the Surgical Defect

Because SCCs can behave quite aggressively, their treatment may require the creation of a large surgical defect. Choosing the proper type of surgical repair requires evaluation of many factors, including the ability of the patient to deal with the cosmetic aspects of a temporary repair, the need to cover vital structures, the necessity of restoring function, and the plans for possible adjunctive therapy. However, when dealing with extensive, recurrent, or aggressive SCCs, it is often best to adopt a conservative approach to repairing the defect. If the patient is thought to be at significant risk for recurrence, it may be best to cover the defect with a thin split-thickness skin graft or let the wound heal by second intention and then follow the patient for a year before definitive reconstruction is performed.[108, 114, 189, 190] Some patients may choose to wear a prosthetic device as a temporary or permanent solution to their cosmetic deformity.

Even when tumor persistence or risk of recurrence is not a primary concern or limiting factor, some patients will not desire reconstruction with a graft or flap. In these instances, alternatives in wound management include healing by second intention,[191–193] use of guiding sutures,[193, 194] or a partial closure,[195] all of which may yield good cosmetic and functional results.

Treatment Modalities

In managing SCCs, great care must be used to properly determine the most ideal form of treatment. If inadequately treated, not only can an SCC recur, but with recurrence the risk of metastasis and mortality increases.[115, 190] The mortality rate associated with recurrent SCC has been reported to be as high as 24%.[190] In patients with perineural involvement and in those with large, extensive, and deeply invasive tumors, a CT or MRI scan may be helpful in determining the extent of both the neoplasm and the required resection.

CURETTAGE AND ELECTRODESICCATION

Although simple to learn and relatively easy to perform, C&D must be done properly to be effective.[196, 197]

Although some authors have suggested that C&D must be repeated a certain number of times,[196–198] this is not necessary. The C&D need be repeated only until a firm healthy base is achieved. Unnecessary repetition will only increase the likelihood of a poor cosmetic result without improving the chances of cure.[199] To achieve a high cure rate with C&D, the technique must be skillfully employed, and only appropriate lesions should be selected for treatment.[185, 196–198, 200–202] C&D is ineffective for treatment of recurrent tumors; for tumors enmeshed in a sclerotic stroma; for invasive tumors with deep involvement of the dermis, subcutaneous tissue, perichondrium, periosteum, or perineural tissue; for tumors in anatomic areas that are not firm or cannot be immobilized, such as the lips or eyelids; and for large invasive tumors that are greater than 1 cm in size.

Extreme caution must be exercised if C&D is used to treat tumors in areas at high risk for recurrence (e.g., embryonal fusion planes, scalp, ears, lips, eyelids, nose, and temples). In fact, blind techniques should not generally be used to manage tumors in these locations unless an adequate pretreatment biopsy specimen has been obtained, allowing the clinician to determine the growth pattern, degree of differentiation, depth of penetration, and other important histologic features. If a firm base cannot be achieved with curettage, the lesion should be managed by routine surgical excision or MMS, since a soft base indicates subclinical tumor spread.

The initial curettage can be done with a medium curette, but the final curettage should be done with a small curette to remove any residual small nests of tumor.[196, 198, 200, 203] If a biopsy is performed before C&D, a shave biopsy technique, not a punch biopsy, should be used. This is because the curette will "fall" into the hole created by the punch and render the procedure unreliable.[118, 183, 184] Most authors recommend that a 2- to 5-mm margin of clinically normal tissue be included in the area of treatment to destroy subclinical foci of tumor.[183, 185, 198, 200]

Although some guidance is offered by the feel of the curette when performing C&D, it is still considered a blind technique, since tissue cannot be submitted for a margin check. In an effort to make C&D less of a blind procedure and to increase its reliability, some cutaneous surgeons perform a "chemo check" at the completion of the procedure.[204–206] This is done by performing a shave excision that encompasses the entire periphery and depth of the C&D wound. A map is created, the tissue is subdivided into smaller specimens, the edges are color coded, and the specimens are submitted for horizontal sectioning and then examined microscopically to determine the adequacy of the procedure. Although this concept may be valuable, it is somewhat limited, because it is difficult to maintain the proper orientation of the specimens with the number of different individuals handling the specimens and the lack of experience most pathologists have in interpreting horizontal sections.[206]

Five-year cure rates as high as 100% have been reported for C&D in the treatment of primary SCCs of the skin.[10, 198, 200, 207–209] Most of these treated tumors were on sun-damaged skin. It is generally agreed that C&D should be used for small, well-differentiated, superficially invasive, nonrecurrent SCCs (see Figs. 57–16 through 57–18).[200, 207, 209, 210]

The primary advantages of C&D are that it is a simple technique that is fast and easy to learn and to perform, which makes it ideal for treating patients with multiple lesions. Its major disadvantages are that it may lead to unsightly hypopigmented and hypertrophic scars, especially in young adults; it can cause ectropion or notching if performed near mucocutaneous junctions such as the eyelid or lip; and residual tumor may be buried under scar tissue, delaying subsequent clinical diagnosis and making treatment more difficult.[211]

EXCISION

Surgical excision may be used to manage the smallest and simplest of lesions or the largest and most difficult of lesions, regardless of location. It offers the advantages of histologic control, rapid healing, and optimal cosmesis. Unfortunately, it is time consuming, sacrifices normal tissue, is less suitable for multiple lesions, requires a significant amount of training and skill, and may necessitate reconstructive surgery to correct the resultant cosmetic and functional defect.[184, 212] Furthermore, the histologic control it offers in the management of recurrent tumors is inferior to that achieved with MMS.[201, 212, 213] Nevertheless, when MMS is unavailable, excisional surgery is the treatment of choice for such lesions.

In an effort to improve the histologic control of excisional surgery, modifications in the surgical technique have been made to provide specimens that can be processed pathologically in a manner somewhat similar to that used for MMS specimens.[214, 215] Although they provide better margin control, these modifications require careful mapping of the surgical wound, maintenance of proper orientation of the specimen during tissue embedding, and effective communication between the surgeon and pathologist. These techniques should not be used in place of MMS when the latter is clearly the treatment of choice.[216, 217] For example, although excision of BD lesions has a 95% cure rate,[218] the large size of these lesions and their lack of follicular involvement may make another form of treatment, such as MMS, more suitable.

The recommended excisional margins for SCCs varies from 2 to 10 mm[115, 190, 210, 219, 220] according to the size, location, histologic features, and primary or recurrent nature of the tumor. All of these factors must be taken into account, as they can influence the tendency for subclinical spread. MMS has been used to determine the ideal margin for excising an SCC.[220] For well-differentiated tumors less than 2 cm in size; not occurring on the scalp, ears, eyelids, lip, or nose; and not involving the subcutaneous fat, 4-mm margins of clinically normal skin were found to be adequate. However, for poorly differentiated lesions greater than 2 cm in size that invaded subcutaneous fat, 6-mm margins were necessary. The depth of the excision is determined by the depth of invasion of the tumor. However, for superficially invasive, well-demarcated, primary tumors smaller than 2 cm and occurring in sun-exposed areas, incising

into the subcutaneous fat will usually yield clear, deep margins. Using the preceding guidelines for surgical margins, 5-year cure rates as high as 98.9% have been reported.[207, 208, 210]

Complications of excisional surgery include hematoma formation, wound dehiscence, bruising, swelling, pain, infection, hyperpigmentation, hypopigmentation, and cosmetic deformity. Fortunately, the cosmetic result typically improves with time, and scar revision is generally possible.[212]

MOHS MICROGRAPHIC SURGERY

MMS (see Chaps. 62 and 63) offers the best histologic control of tumor margins during surgery and also provides maximal preservation of normal tissue.[221–225] It remains the treatment of choice for poorly differentiated, large, ill-defined, infiltrative or deeply invasive, recurrent or incompletely excised SCCs and for tumors found in areas with a known high risk of recurrence (e.g., the nose, ear, periocular area, and embryonal fusion planes).[226] MMS is also the treatment of choice for lesions occurring in areas where maximal preservation of tissue is mandatory (e.g., the fingers or penis). MMS has the added advantage of being cost effective, since it is usually done under local anesthesia in an outpatient setting. It also extends operability to patients who are considered poor risks for general anesthesia.

Unfortunately, MMS has the disadvantage of not always being readily available, since it requires special training, equipment, and personnel. Also, MMS is both tedious and time consuming for the patient and the physician. Sometimes it must be performed using a multidisciplinary team approach to rid the patient of deep tumor, to preserve a vital structure such as the facial nerve, or to optimally reconstruct the surgical defect.[54, 57, 60, 227–229] Both the fixed and fresh tissue techniques of MMS can be utilized in the management of SCC with great success[221] (i.e., greater than 98% 5-year cure rate in patients without metastases). However, the fixed tissue technique currently is only rarely utilized, because it is painful for the patient, spares less tissue, often prolongs the surgery, causes difficulty in interpreting the histology, and limits the reconstructive options.

As with any modality, certain parameters are correlated with an increased risk of recurrence. If a disconnected focus of tumor exists from previous treatment, there is an increased likelihood of treatment failure.[221] It has been shown that males younger than 60 years with SCCs on the leg that required more than five MMS procedures were at increased risk of recurrence. The 5-year cure rate for this group of patients was 86.5%, compared with 97.2% for other patients with SCC.[230] In another series,[221] the lesion size, previous treatment, histologic grade, anatomic site of origin, and presence or absence of metastases also influenced the cure rate. These same variables also have been shown to influence outcome when radiation therapy or traditional surgical excision is employed. Lesions of the ear, because of their propensity for metastases, had the highest recurrence rate (8.3%).

For lesions less than 1 cm in size, the cure rate was 99.5%; for those between 1 and 2 cm in size, the cure rate was 98%; for those 2 to 3 cm in size, it was 83.3%; and for those greater than 3 cm in size, the cure rate was 59%. The lower cure rates for the larger lesions reflect the tendency of these tumors to invade deeply and metastasize. Previously treated lesions were cured only 76.3% of the time, while 97.3% of the patients with primary lesions were cured.

The effect of cellular differentiation on the cure rate has also been evaluated. For Broders' grade I lesions, the cure rate was 98.9%; for grade II, 94.2%; for grade III, 73.8%; and for grade IV, 45.2%. These data reflect the tendency of less differentiated lesions to invade vital structures and metastasize. Metastases, which occurred in 3.7% of the MMS patients, had a profound impact on the cure rate, with only 16.4% of these patients being cured, compared with a cure rate of 98.2% in those who did not have metastases. From this information, it can be concluded that if an SCC is operable and does not metastasize, there is a 98% or greater chance of cure with MMS. Although the operability of an SCC cannot be controlled, adjunctive treatment with radiation can be administered to those patients considered at high risk for metastases to hopefully improve the cure rate for this subset of patients with SCCs.

CRYOSURGERY

Cryosurgery is a relatively new modality that requires proper equipment and skill to be used effectively in the treatment of SCC (see Chap. 61). Discs and cotton-tipped applicators dipped in liquid nitrogen should not be used to manage SCCs. A thermocouple and liquid nitrogen spray unit are usually necessary to manage an SCC with cryosurgery. Tumors overlying bone may be frozen down to periosteum, at which point the tumor becomes fixed. If the tumor overlies cartilage, freezing can be continued until the cartilage is frozen through to the other side.[186] To produce an adequate tumor kill, a double freeze-thaw cycle with a tissue temperature of $-50°C$ is necessary.[231] Exophytic tumors may be debulked with curettage and then treated with cryosurgery to improve the results.[186, 210, 232, 233]

Because cryosurgery is a blind procedure, great care must be exercised when using this modality to treat SCCs. Ideally, pretreatment biopsies should be performed to determine follicular involvement, depth of invasion, histologic growth pattern, and degree of differentiation.[232] As with other modalities, cryosurgery may leave behind buried residual foci of tumor that may result in significant subclinical spread. Because of the scalp's vascularity and the difficulty in achieving the tissue temperatures necessary to kill tumor cells, cryosurgery is generally not used for SCCs of the scalp.[234] When used to treat SCCs of the lower leg, the resultant wound heals extremely slowly, the cosmetic result is often poor, and there is an increased risk of infection.[234] Hypertrophic scars may appear 4 to 6 weeks after cryosurgery, most often on the back and chest. Hypopigmented scars are common and most pronounced in individuals with dark complexions. Hyperpigmentation can also occur but usually resolves within a year.[234]

Cryosurgery is contraindicated in patients with cold intolerance, blood dyscrasias, dysglobulinemia, autoimmune disease, and pyoderma gangrenosum and in those on renal dialysis or immunosuppressive therapy.[234] When used to treat eyelid lesions, alopecia, hypopigmentation, atrophy, and notching with ectropion and lacrimal duct damage may occur.[86, 235, 236]

A single freeze-thaw cycle with a freezing time of 30 seconds has been found adequate for treatment of BD.[237] A 97.1% cure rate was reported after treating 128 lesions of BD and 34 SCCs.[238] A 95% cure rate was reported after treating SCCs using cryosurgery, but few details were given.[239] In treating in situ and superficial SCCs, a single freeze-thaw cycle provided a cure rate of 97.8%.[240]

In summary, cryosurgery is most suited for treating primary, well-differentiated, superficially invasive (Clark's level III or upper reticular dermis), well-demarcated tumors that are less than 2 cm in size and not in anatomic areas associated with a high risk for recurrence.

TOPICAL 5-FLUOROURACIL THERAPY

Topical 5-fluorouracil (5-FU) has limited usefulness in the management of SCC. It should be used only for treating SCC in situ without deep follicular involvement. Of the commercially available products, only the 5% concentration is suitable for this application, because the penetration of 5-FU is both variable and limited.[241-244] When used to treat invasive carcinoma, it may eliminate the superficial component, but the deep component may continue to grow beneath the scar, forming a subdermal mass with extensive subclinical spread.[243-246] In an effort to shorten the duration of treatment as well as increase the penetration and the potential effectiveness, both occlusion and curettage have been used before application of topical 5-FU.[241, 242, 245, 247, 248] Even with these modifications, topical 5-FU is still ineffective for treating invasive carcinoma,[210, 241, 242, 244, 245, 249] even when the depth of invasion is less than 1 mm.[242] One report detailed a 14% failure rate with topical 5-FU used to treat BD,[218] but another study reported a 92% cure rate.[250] Prolonged treatment for 6 to 16 weeks is required to achieve a high cure rate.[244, 250]

Sequelae from the use of 5-FU include hyperpigmentation, hypopigmentation, scarring, prolonged redness, onychodystrophy, onycholysis, and telangiectasia.[241, 242, 244, 247] After using topical 5-FU, 17% of patients have a positive reaction to it on a patch test,[251] and 3% of patients develop a contact dermatitis with continued or repeated exposure.[242]

RADIATION THERAPY

Currently radiation therapy is used only infrequently in the management of certain cutaneous and mucosal neoplasms. For radiation to be effective, the physician giving the treatments must be knowledgeable in the principles of therapy and thoroughly acquainted with the clinical and pathologic aspects of the tumor being treated. The major advantage of radiation therapy is that it spares normal tissue, thus possibly avoiding the deformity seen with surgical procedures. Consequently, radiation therapy is often advocated as the treatment of choice for tumors of the nose, ear, and periocular area, because it obviates the need for reconstructive surgery and spares the lacrimal apparatus.[187, 188, 252, 253] Another indication for radiation therapy is the treatment of skin cancers in elderly patients or patients who are unable to undergo surgery because of poor health.[188] Radiation therapy also can be used as palliation therapy in patients with inoperable tumors.[254]

Radiation therapy should not generally be used in young or middle-aged patients because of the presumably small risk of inducing another cancer in the area. In addition, the cosmetic results obtained from radiation therapy can be expected to deteriorate over time, while the risk of radiation necrosis increases.[187, 188, 201, 252-255] Although the immediate cosmetic result may be excellent, only 50% of patients still have a good cosmetic result 9 to 12 years after radiation therapy. The treated site is often atrophic, hypopigmented, and covered with telangiectases. Fractionation provides better cosmetic results, reduces the risk of radiation necrosis, and is especially important to use when treating tumors overlying bone or cartilage to prevent osteonecrosis, chondritis, and chondral necrosis.[187, 188, 252, 253, 255]

All tumors should undergo biopsy before being irradiated to confirm the clinical diagnosis and ascertain the degree of tumor differentiation. Biopsies also give the radiation therapist an idea of the depth of penetration of the tumor and may permit detection of other important features such as neural involvement. Well-differentiated SCCs require a larger dose of radiation than less differentiated SCCs.[80] Radiation therapy can result in a hidden, buried tumor that may grow for an extended interval before it becomes clinically detectable. Moreover, an area that has been irradiated is more predisposed to wound healing complications.

Complications of radiation include scarring; notching of free margins such as the eyelids, lips, or alar rim; and ectropion. Although radiation therapy usually spares the lacrimal duct, if there is marked involvement by tumor, fibrosis with resultant epiphora may occur.[255] Approximately 1 to 5% of patients will develop radiation necrosis,[188, 254, 255] which may occur 1 to 20 years after treatment. Areas of chronic irritation and those exposed to cold or sunlight are more predisposed to necrosis.[188, 254] Lesions that involve bone should not be irradiated, since the chances of cure are minimal and the risk for osteonecrosis is high.[80, 114, 115, 188] Tumor control has been claimed in 83% of patients with bone or cartilage involvement,[256] but it is unclear whether these patients were actually disease free. Treatment of periocular tumors may be complicated by keratitis, cataracts, or perforation of the globe,[187, 188] and 10% of patients will develop leukoplakic plaques of the conjunctiva secondary to backscatter radiation. These plaques usually resolve spontaneously,[188] but permanent loss of the eyelashes can be anticipated.[188] When treating periocular tumors, proper shielding of the eyes is mandatory.[188, 253] A transient mucositis may occur when

tumors of the nose or lips are treated,[188] so a lead shield should be placed behind the lip or in the nostril to protect the gingiva and nasal septum.[257]

Currently radiation therapists primarily use electrons and photons and orthovoltage x-rays to manage skin cancers. A high-energy electron beam is useful for treating lesions overlying bone or cartilage, because the radiation can be delivered in a more homogenous manner and the dose falls off rapidly, so there is less risk of damage to underlying structures. Mild scarring and patchy pigmentary changes are usually the only sequelae.[257, 258]

Bowen's disease, including lesions on the fingers, also may be managed by radiation therapy. Soft x-rays and grenz rays have also been used to treat this lesion.[187, 188, 259-261] Because the half-depth dose of grenz rays is 0.9 mm, proper lesion selection requires that a pretreatment biopsy be performed to determine the thickness of the lesion.[260] If the lesion is thick or if follicular involvement is present, grenz ray treatment is unsuitable.

Cure rates for radiation therapy for SCC of the skin have been reported to be 73 to 85% for tumors between 2 cm and 3 cm in size[187, 207] and 85 to 93% for tumors less than 2 cm in size.[201, 207] If the lesion is recurrent, the cure rate varies from 85 to 88%.[262, 263] A 94% 5-year control rate and an 88% 10-year control rate have been reported for both primary and recurrent SCCs.[256] Generally, tumors larger than 5 cm in diameter should not be treated by radiation therapy because of the high failure rate.[188, 256, 257] Radiation therapy should also not be used to treat tumors arising in areas of radiation dermatitis or scar carcinoma.[188]

In summary, radiation therapy offers the advantages of sparing normal tissue, thereby obviating the need for reconstructive surgery, and providing effective therapy for those patients who are too frail or unwilling to undergo surgery. However, it is a blind technique whose success rate depends on the skill and experience of the therapist. A significant failure rate is seen with recurrent tumors, tumors larger than 2 cm in size, poorly differentiated tumors, tumors with ill-defined borders, deeply invasive tumors, tumors with an infiltrating growth pattern, and tumors located in areas at high risk for recurrence. The key to success lies in careful patient selection. The inconvenience, expense, need for multiple treatments, and a cosmetic result that deteriorates over time are all disadvantages of this technique.

LASER THERAPY

Over the years, a variety of laser systems have been used in cutaneous surgery (see Chap. 73). The carbon dioxide (CO_2) laser has proven most useful in the management of skin cancers. It can be used in its focused or incisional mode to excise a tumor in relatively bloodless fashion and to create flaps in appropriate vascular anatomic locations to repair the resultant defects without significant bleeding. Unlike electrosurgery, which causes excessive tissue destruction, the CO_2 laser allows histopathologic examination of the specimen to determine whether the margins of excision are adequate. The CO_2 laser can also be used to remove cartilage or bone involved with tumor.[264] It is also useful in excising very vascular tumors,[264, 265] as it seals small blood vessels and lymphatics, which serves theoretically to decrease the dissemination of tumor cells. The CO_2 laser may also be used in the defocused mode to treat superficial lesions and may also be combined with curettage.[266, 267] In theory, it could be used in place of electrodesiccation to treat in situ SCC without deep follicular involvement. The control of tissue destruction is much finer with the CO_2 laser than with electrodesiccation, and thus the cosmetic results in general should be superior to those achievable with C&D.

The argon laser has only limited usefulness in the management of SCC. It has been reported to eradicate the red or pigmented lesions of SCC in situ.[267]

There have been a number of reports on the use of the neodymium:yttrium-aluminum-garnet (Nd:YAG) laser in the management of skin cancer. Because of its deep (5-mm) penetration and excellent hemostatic properties, it has proven useful in the treatment of deeply invasive tumors.[267–269] As in other treatment modalities, a pretreatment biopsy is mandatory to confirm the clinical diagnosis and to assess other histologic parameters that may influence the method of treatment.

Although the CO_2 laser may be useful in the management of certain skin cancers, it has the disadvantages of additional cost, increased safety hazards,[270–272] and decreased efficiency because of the awkward articulated-arm delivery system. Much more work needs to be done to determine what role lasers will play in the management of skin cancer.

PHOTODYNAMIC THERAPY

Photodynamic therapy (PDT), considered an experimental form of treatment, is still in its infancy (see Chap. 79). A photosensitizing agent, usually hematoporphyrin or one of its derivatives, is administered intravenously,[273, 274] topically,[275] or intralesionally.[274] Experimental studies that use a photosensitizer linked to a monoclonal antibody to prevent the generalized photosensitivity that normally accompanies PDT are currently being conducted.[276, 277] Once administered, the photosensitizer is activated by a 630-nm red laser light from a gold vapor or argon-pumped tunable dye laser, which causes tumor necrosis through the formation of singlet oxygen. Topical application of the photosensitizer results in such limited penetration that only superficial tumors can be treated.[275]

A cationic photosensitizer has also been used that preferentially concentrates in the tumor so that no damage is done to the adjacent tissue.[264] PDT can also be used in conjunction with a 400-nm light source to help determine the subclinical extent of a tumor, as a red fluorescence is emitted by the photosensitizer at this wavelength.[274]

BD and invasive SCC have been treated with PDT with encouraging results.[274, 276–280] However, there are many drawbacks to PDT, and much work needs to be done before it can play a major role in the routine management of skin cancer.

INTERFERON

Interferon has been used to treat SCCs in patients with and without epidermodysplasia verruciformis (EDV).[281–283] Intralesional therapy appears to be more effective than systemic administration.[281] Leukocyte-derived interferon (100,000 U administered every other day for 31 days), has achieved complete resolution of all the tumors so treated.[281] Interferon alfa-2b, administered at a dosage of 1.5 million U intralesionally three times a week for 3 weeks, achieved clinical and histologic tumor regression in 95.8% of the 24 SCC and SCC in situ lesions treated.[282] The only side effects were mild flulike symptoms and a hypopigmented macule.

Recombinant leukocyte interferon, in a dosage of 900,000 U three times a week for 3 weeks, was used to clinically and histologically cure patients with SCCs.[283] Local discomfort at the injection site was the only side effect. Although these preliminary results are encouraging, it should be remembered that this is a blind technique and patient selection is very important in obtaining the best results with this form of management of skin cancer.

CHEMOTHERAPY

Although chemotherapy plays only a minor role in the management of SCC, it may be quite helpful at times. The administration of cisplatin and intralesional bleomycin has been reported to treat SCC successfully.[284, 285] However, repeated injections are necessary, and scarring occurs when the lesion resolves.

For advanced and unresectable SCC, cisplatin and doxorubicin used alone or in combination with radiation therapy may be useful for palliation.[286] The response may be rapid, the regimen is usually well tolerated, and prolonged disease control is sometimes achieved. Systemic 5-FU therapy has been used in conjunction with cisplatin for advanced local disease and metastatic disease,[287] with encouraging results.

RETINOIDS

Retinoids may be useful in the prevention and palliation of SCC (see Chap. 58). The two retinoids that have been employed in the treatment of SCC are isotretinoin and etretinate. Isotretinoin is often preferred because of its shorter half-life and its theoretical lack of a harmful effect on organ transplant survival. Retinoids have proven beneficial in the prevention of new tumors in immunosuppressed patients, organ transplant patients, and patients with xeroderma pigmentosum (XP) and EDV.[288–290] A daily dose of 1 mg/kg of isotretinoin is usually necessary for chemoprevention, although daily doses as low as 0.25 mg/kg have also been reported to be effective.[289] This dose is usually well tolerated, except in older individuals, who often experience a significant increase in serum triglyceride levels. Fortunately this elevation in triglyceride levels can usually be controlled with either diet or medication. Unfortunately, once the retinoid is discontinued, the patient will begin to develop new tumors in a few months.[288, 289] Retinoids have been used to treat advanced recurrent and metastatic SCCs of the skin that were not considered manageable by any other means.[290, 291] A 71% response rate in these patients has been reported,[290] with approximately 20% having complete and sustained remissions. Doses larger than 1 mg/kg daily may be necessary when trying to rid patients of SCCs and KAs.[292, 293] Unfortunately, these higher doses are poorly tolerated, often resulting in subsequent reduction in dosage or discontinuation of treatment.[288] Well-differentiated SCCs may respond better than less well differentiated tumors.[291]

Management of Special Variants of SCC

PERINEURAL SCC

It is impossible to accurately diagnose perineural spread based on clinical symptoms. Even patients with extensive disease may be asymptomatic, and many patients with complaints of pain or discomfort do not have neural involvement. The size of the tumor is also not a reliable indicator of perineural disease, for even small tumors may demonstrate extensive subclinical perineural spread. If neural involvement is suspected, an incisional or excisional biopsy should be performed.

Two different types of perineural spread have been observed. The first is a limited form in which only a short segment of an isolated nerve is involved and that often presents as an incidental finding. Whether this variant might develop additional perineural spread with time is unclear. The second type is the classic form of perineural spread in which numerous nerve branches are involved and the tumor tracks along a major nerve trunk for great distances, even into a foramen. Although the first variant behaves no differently than an SCC without this finding and therefore is managed no differently, the second variant is a much more serious problem that can result in considerable morbidity and even death. This variant often requires an interdisciplinary surgical team approach for proper management, as these patients are at high risk for recurrence and regional metastases. Because histologic control is needed to trace out the microscopic extensions of these tumors, MMS is often the treatment of choice.[45, 58, 60] However, since numerous nerve branches may be involved and the tumor may change its direction of spread, a less conservative approach is often required, with an additional layer being removed with MMS if there is concern that tumor may have been missed.[294]

Although useful as an adjunct, radiation therapy alone is unlikely to cure patients with perineural SCC.[64, 66] However, according to one report, one patient with a perineural SCC was apparently cured by a combination of radiation therapy and chemotherapy consisting of cisplatin, bleomycin, and methotrexate.[68]

SCAR CARCINOMA (MARJOLIN'S ULCER)

Although a review of the literature would suggest that scar carcinoma almost always has a poor patient prog-

nosis, in reality, patient prognosis covers a wide spectrum. Often, the cancer may be relatively small and superficial and under these circumstances has an excellent prognosis. Despite this, good histologic control remains crucially important in managing these lesions. Many of the reported cases of scar carcinoma represent a more serious form of the disease and are associated with significant morbidity and mortality. These lesions are often far advanced by the time they are diagnosed because of either neglect or a delay in diagnosis.[94, 103, 109] For this reason repeat biopsies should be done in patients with scars of various origins and in whom recalcitrant ulceration develops. These biopsies should be incisional and should include a portion of the ulcer as well as its edge and should extend deeply into the subcutaneous fat.[108] This will help the pathologist discern between PEH and SCC. Moreover, a scar should not be allowed to go through multiple cycles of breakdown and healing but should be excised and grafted, because it is on this background that Marjolin's ulcer develops.[103, 108, 123]

MMS is the ideal way to manage those tumors amenable to surgical resection, although an interdisciplinary team approach may be needed. If MMS is not available, routine surgical excision is the treatment of choice. In addition to the cancer, the surrounding abnormal skin should be excised whenever possible to prevent another tumor from occurring in the area.[109] Radiation should not generally be used to manage these tumors because of (1) extensive subclinical spread,[123] (2) the fact that these tumors often occur on the extremities in unhealthy tissue that might predispose to radiation necrosis, and (3) the fact that radiation might add to the existing predisposition for development of cancer. If the chance for a cure with MMS or surgical excision appears unlikely or if there is bone or joint involvement, the affected extremity will often require amputation.[108]

Patients with deeply invasive scar carcinoma are at high risk for regional metastases. Unfortunately, no controlled studies have been done on the benefits of postoperative radiation or ELND. However, in patients with advanced but curable disease, especially if the tumor is not well differentiated, consultation with a radiotherapist and surgical oncologist is certainly appropriate.[85, 120, 126]

Patients with tumors smaller than 5 cm, without deep dermal involvement, and without regional metastases have the best chance of survival (71% vs. 57% after 5 years).[103] Invasion of muscle or bone and the presence of a poorly differentiated tumor carry a worse patient prognosis. Patients with nodal metastases had a worse outcome when the size and number of the affected nodes increased and when multiple node groups were involved. If the nodes are larger than 3 cm or there is extracapsular spread, the survival rate is worse (67% vs. 25%).[99] A strong correlation between survival and the degree of differentiation has also been found with SCC.[126] There was only a 6% mortality rate in patients with well-differentiated tumors, but a 63% mortality rate was found in patients with poorly differentiated tumors.

RADIATION-INDUCED CARCINOMA

Patients with radiation-induced SCCs[121, 122] suffer significant morbidity and mortality, with a 20% incidence of metastases and a 12% mortality rate. The previous radiation may also impair wound healing, making the repair of defects more difficult. Proper management of these patients requires close follow-up at least once every 3 months, at which time a biopsy is performed of any ulcer that does not respond to conservative treatment. If an SCC is diagnosed in this setting, it should be managed either with excision or MMS. If the resulting defect requires surgical reconstruction, random-pattern flaps should not be taken from the radiation-damaged area for fear of transferring occult tumor. Furthermore, if the disease is deep or extensive, reconstruction with flaps is contraindicated for fear of concealing tumor. Because of this, most defects should be grafted or allowed to heal by second intention.

UNUSUAL VARIANTS OF SCC

The unusual variants of SCC,[139, 140, 145, 148-151, 157-161] including acantholytic SCC, clear cell SCC, signet ring SCC, spindle cell SCC, and adenosquamous SCC, may behave in an aggressive manner with perineural spread and a significant risk of recurrence and metastases. Such lesions should be treated with MMS or routine surgical excision and not blind techniques. Adjunctive therapies such as ELND and postoperative radiation may be appropriate at times, but the decision to use these must be based on the depth and extent of local disease.

DE NOVO SCC

By definition, a de novo SCC does not arise in an ulcer, scar, area of previous radiation, or pre-existing lesion or on sun-damaged skin.[94, 117, 127] These cancers behave in an aggressive manner and have a significant incidence of metastases (61%).[94] In fact, it has been suggested that ELND should be performed in patients with de novo SCCs that are larger than 4 cm.

SUBCUTANEOUS SCC

Another unusual variant of SCC is the subcutaneous type[295] (Figs. 57-36, 57-37). Initial histopathologic examination of the tumors may fail to show a connection to the epidermis. However, in most cancers a focal connection with the epidermis can be demonstrated with multiple histologic sections. All reported patients with subcutaneous SCC have done well, except one who subsequently developed a coincidental intraorbital hemangiopericytoma and died without evidence of SCC at the time of death.

BOWEN'S DISEASE

If a blind technique or superficial means of destruction is used in the treatment of BD, a pretreatment biopsy is mandatory to look for both deep follicular involvement and invasive SCC. If deep invasion or follicular

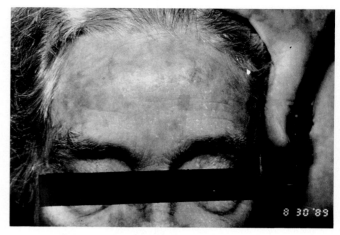

Figure 57–36. Patient with subcutaneous SCC.

involvement is present, the lesion should be excised. Because BD may be mistaken for an AK or patch of eczema, any keratotic lesion or eczematous patch that does not respond to appropriate standard therapy should undergo biopsy to rule out BD.[296]

The natural history of BD is one of slow centrifugal spread over a period of years until the lesion becomes quite large. However, 4 to 11% of patients will eventually develop areas of invasive SCC.[218, 297, 298] Once invasion occurs, the incidence of metastases has been reported to be 13 to 57%.[297-300] When invasive SCC develops, it usually shows basaloid or squamoid differentiation. However, if it demonstrates sebaceous or glandular differentiation, it may be mistaken for sebaceous gland carcinoma, sweat gland carcinoma, or metastatic adenocarcinoma.[298]

A long-standing controversy exists regarding BD, its relationship to arsenic, and its association with internal malignancy (Fig. 57–38). One study found that only 2%

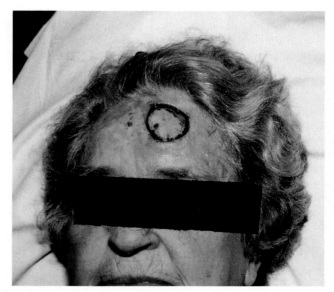

Figure 57–37. Mohs surgical defect after removal of a tumor involving the periosteum.

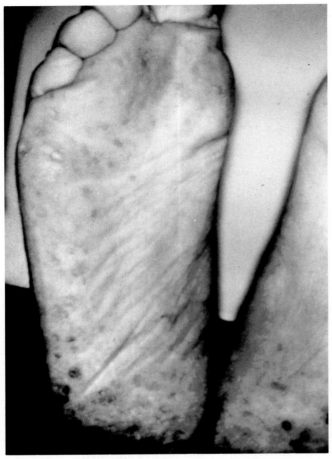

Figure 57–38. Patient with multiple lesions of Bowen's disease, superficial BCCs, and arsenical keratoses of the soles.

of patients with BD had arsenical keratoses.[218] However, increased levels of arsenic have been found in the lesions of BD and in the adjacent skin in 82% of patients, but increased lesional arsenic levels were also found in 59% of patients with senile keratoses.[301] Miki et al.[300] reported on a group of patients with increased levels of arsenic in their hair, palmar keratoses and pigmentary changes consistent with arsenic exposure, and multiple lesions of BD. Of these patients, 22.6% developed lung cancer. The authors suggested that the arsenic was responsible for both the BD and lung cancer.

Although other authors have also reported an increased incidence of internal malignancy in association with BD, adequate controls were lacking, and the results were variable. An association with internal malignancy was reported in patients with BD only on sun-protected skin,[299] and another report has suggested that both Bowen's and non-Bowen's squamous cell carcinoma in situ were markers for internal malignancy.[302] Other, more recent studies,[303–306] as well as an analysis of the literature,[307] have failed to confirm an association between BD and internal malignancy. However, there may be a subset of BD that is arsenic related and associated with internal neoplasms[304, 305, 308] and a non–arsenic-related subset of BD that is not a marker for internal malignancy. The best practical approach to this dilemma is to assess the patient with BD for other stigmata of arsenic ingestion. If these are not present and there are no signs or symptoms of internal neoplasia, no further evaluation is indicated. However, if there are signs of arsenic exposure or signs and symptoms of internal malignancy, additional work-up is both appropriate and indicated.[208]

Although the relationship of BD to internal malignancy is controversial, there is little question that females with BD of the vulva and perianal area are at high risk for the development of SCC of the vagina and cervix. Therefore, any woman presenting with BD of the vulva should have a complete gynecologic examination, including a Papanicolaou smear. Close follow-up in such patients is necessary, because they may develop other lesions of BD of the vulva, as well as SCC of the cervix or vagina. The tendency for multicentric BD of the vulva and associated SCC of the cervix and vagina is perhaps a reflection that human papillomavirus (HPV) infection caused by HPV types 16, 18, 31, and 33 may play an important role in the pathogenesis of these neoplasms.[309–329]

VERRUCOUS CARCINOMA

Verrucous carcinoma is a low-grade SCC that can be locally quite invasive and destructive but has a low propensity for metastasis. It may also be mistaken clinically for a large or recalcitrant wart. For this reason, any large, atypical, or recalcitrant warts should be sent for pathologic examination at the time of removal.

Verrucous carcinoma of the oral cavity may be associated with tobacco chewing, poor dental hygiene, snuff dipping, and poorly fitting dentures.[330, 331] Verrucous carcinoma of the genitalia appears to be associated with HPV infection, most commonly HPV types 6 and 11.[332, 333] HPV infection may also play a role in the pathogenesis of some verrucous carcinomas in extragenital sites.[334] Most males with verrucous carcinoma of the penis are uncircumcised, and the carcinoma occurs primarily on the glans and prepuce,[330, 332, 335] although the urethra may also be involved.[332, 335] Perineural spread may occur with verrucous carcinoma but is rare.[331, 336] Metastases are also rare and appear to be more common in patients in whom foci of typical SCC coexist with the verrucous carcinoma.[330, 332, 335, 337–340] When regional lymphadenopathy occurs in conjunction with verrucous carcinoma, it is most likely reactive.[330, 332]

When performing a biopsy on a suspected verrucous carcinoma, an incisional, excisional, or deep shave technique is preferable to a punch biopsy so that the overall architecture of the lesion is available for microscopic examination. The pathologist should also be alerted to the possibility of verrucous carcinoma so that appropriate clinicopathologic correlation will occur. By following these guidelines, a misdiagnosis of wart or PEH will not be made.[330]

Although superficial destruction with C&D, cryosurgery, or the CO_2 laser may be successful in the treatment of early, small, and superficially invasive lesions,[332] verrucous carcinomas should generally be managed by

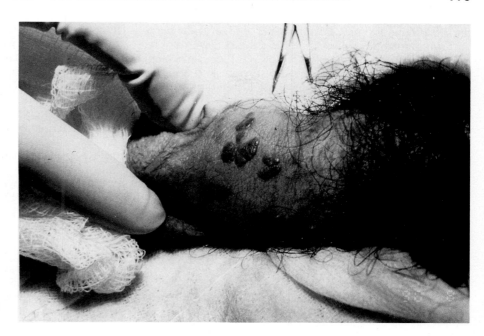

Figure 57–39. Patient with multiple lesions of bowenoid papulosis.

surgical excision or MMS.[332, 335, 336, 339, 340] Because these lesions are often far advanced, occur in areas where tissue conservation is important (e.g., the penis), and exhibit a significant rate of recurrence with routine surgical excision,[330, 331, 338, 341, 342] some authors believe these neoplasms should be managed by MMS.[335, 336, 339, 340] In some instances, the tumor may be so invasive and extensive that amputation is required.[336, 337, 340, 341]

The role of radiation therapy in the management of verrucous carcinoma is controversial.[330–332, 338, 339, 341, 343] Although some authors have suggested that radiation is a safe and effective way to manage this variant of SCC,[344] many disagree. There have been a number of reports in which the verrucous carcinoma initially appeared to respond to radiation therapy but subsequently recurred and exhibited rapid growth with ulceration and metastases.[330, 331, 338, 343] Biopsy of these recurrent tumors revealed anaplastic transformation.

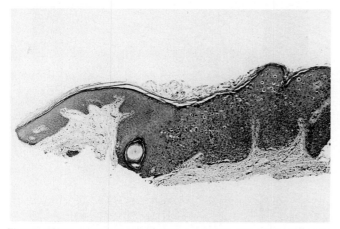

Figure 57–40. Biopsy specimen from a patient with bowenoid papulosis (H&E stain; ×40).

BOWENOID PAPULOSIS

Although bowenoid papulosis (BP) was first identified in 1978,[345, 346] a review of the literature suggests that this disease previously was often misdiagnosed as multicentric BD.[347–349] The disease appears to be associated with HPV infection, especially HPV types 16, 18, and 34, and many of these patients may have coexisting condylomata.[315, 316, 323, 328, 346, 350–353] One grave concern in this entity is carcinoma in situ of the cervix occurring in the consorts of patients with BP.[323] As with BD of the anogenital region, there is a significant association of BP with SCC of the lower genital tract.[309, 323] For this reason, female patients with BP need to be screened and followed closely. Sexual partners of patients with BP also need to be screened and followed closely for possible development of SCC.[347, 353]

The lesions of BP are often multiple, smaller than 1 cm, and red to brown in color; they may be velvety in appearance and may be pruritic. They may also appear as violaceous, pigmented, lichenoid, verrucoid, or leukoplakic (Fig. 57–39) coalescent plaques. They may resemble SCC in situ, flat condylomata, lichen planus, psoriasis, and leukoplakia. Typically, they occur on the vulva in young women and on the glans and shaft of the penis in young men.[316, 345, 346–351, 354–356] The perianal area[347, 349, 351, 355] and the lower abdomen may also be involved.[355] On occasion, BP may be seen in young children or the elderly.[355, 357]

Histologically, BP may be indistinguishable from SCC in situ.[355] In BP, the overall epidermis is normal in appearance but contains scattered atypical cells that spare the hair follicles but involve the sweat ducts (Fig. 57–40).

In young, healthy, immunocompetent males and females, BP appears benign, and spontaneous regression has been reported.[309, 323, 350, 351, 354–358] Conversely, the lesions may also persist for years.[355] Lesions that develop during pregnancy may resolve after delivery. In older and immunocompromised patients, the disease may be recalcitrant or progress to SCC.[323, 351, 356,359-361] It has been suggested that BP usually does not progress to invasive SCC, because the HPV is episomally located rather than genomically integrated.[320, 352, 362]

In performing a biopsy on patients with suspected BP, it must be recognized that warts treated with podophyllin may show histologic changes suggestive of SCC in situ.[316, 345, 363] Because BP generally appears to be a benign condition, conservative treatment is indicated.[345, 346, 349, 355, 358-360, 364] Topical 5-FU may be used, but 3 to 4 months of occlusive treatment may be necessary.[244, 309, 364] Cryosurgery, C&D, simple excision, and CO_2 laser surgery also have been used with success.[267, 309, 364] Preliminary studies with recombinant interferon suggest that it may also be an effective form of treatment for BP when given subcutaneously three times weekly in doses of 4 x 10^6 IU for 13 weeks.[365]

QUEYRAT'S ERYTHROPLASIA

Queyrat first coined the term erythroplasia to describe SCC in situ occurring on the glans penis.[366] Typically, the lesion is an asymptomatic, red, moist, velvety plaque located on the glans or prepuce of the penis in uncircumcised males[366, 367]; it may also encroach on the urethral orifice.[368] In one series,[367] 6% of patients had carcinoma of the genitourinary tract, which suggests a possible carcinogenic field effect. Although sometimes used to describe SCC in situ on any mucous membrane, Queyrat's erythroplasia (QE) is the preferred term only for SCC occurring on the penis. The term erythroplakia should be used for lesions of the oral cavity.[367, 369-372] Although QE histologically resembles BD, there is never follicular involvement, because there are no follicles on mucous membranes.[367] For this reason, many superficial techniques can be utilized to successfully treat QE. Like BD, QE may evolve into an invasive SCC in 10 to 32% of cases[335, 367]; this is often heralded by the onset of ulceration. Once invasion occurs, metastases have been observed in up to 20% of patients.[350] Mucous membrane QE evolves into invasive SCC and metastasizes more frequently than BD occurring on the skin.[370, 371]

QE may be managed by surgical excision, topical 5-FU,[244, 373, 374] C&D, cryosurgery,[375] MMS,[335, 372] laser surgery,[376] or radiation therapy.[257, 261] Several courses of topical 5-FU are often necessary to be effective. A review of the literature has demonstrated a high recurrence rate with C&D[367] but a low recurrence rate with surgical excision.[368] Cryosurgery with single and double freeze-thaw cycles of 30 seconds has also been used to treat QE.[375]

SCC in Selected Anatomic Locations

PERIUNGUAL SCC

Both invasive SCC and SCC in situ may occur in a periungual or subungual location (Fig. 57-41), with the

fingers being much more commonly affected than the toes. It may resemble granulation tissue or an ingrown toenail and appear as an ulceration or a verrucous plaque. The nail plate may be destroyed[377-381] and more than one digit may be affected.[382] Most commonly, the SCC begins in the lateral nailfold.[379, 382]

To accurately diagnose this condition, the biopsy performed must be of adequate depth and size. This usually requires an incisional, excisional, or deep shave biopsy. A superficial shave or punch biopsy is often inadequate.

Except for anogenital SCC, most studies have not linked SCC with HPV infection. The exception to this is SCC occurring in a periungual or subungual location. As in the anogenital area,[310, 312, 316, 328, 377, 380] there has been a strong association with HPV-16 infection. Consequently, it has been suggested that genital contact may explain this association.[310, 328, 380] HPV-34 has also been reported in patients with periungual SCC.[313] Trauma and previous radiation also appear to play a role in the pathogenesis of this disease in some patients.[380-382] Typically, these SCCs grow very slowly, and the diagnosis may be delayed for years. Even when there is invasion of bone, the incidence of metastases is less than 2%,[381, 383] but no explanation for this observation has been offered.

Although radiation, C&D, simple excision, CO_2 laser surgery, and cryosurgery may all cure some patients with early, small, superficial lesions, MMS is considered the treatment of choice.[379, 381, 382, 384] The surgical defects resulting from MMS usually are allowed to heal by second intention, since this method yields excellent cosmetic and functional results. If bone or a joint is involved, the fixed tissue technique of MMS may be used to eradicate the tumor.[381] However, because persistence of disease could result in metastases, under

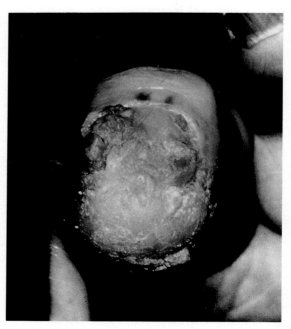

Figure 57-41. Patient with SCC of the nailbed.

these circumstances it is often best to amputate the digit, especially if the involved digit is not the thumb or index finger.[379, 381]

SCC of the Penis

SCC of the penis occurs primarily in uncircumcised males and is common in underdeveloped countries.[385] The presence of smegma in uncircumcised males is thought to play a role in pathogenesis, which may explain why circumcision in later life does not protect against its development.[385] Radical circumcision, which results in severe scarring, does not prevent the development of SCC. However, in these cases, SCC probably represents a variant of scar carcinoma.[386] Circumcision protects only against the development of SCC on the glans, not on the shaft.[387]

HPV infection has also been associated with penile carcinoma.[315, 316, 320, 328, 388–391] HPV types 6, 10, 11, 16, 18, and 33 have been found to be associated with SCC of the penis. SCC in situ of the penis is seen in consorts of patients with carcinoma in situ (CIS) of the cervix.[389] Some condylomata may evolve into invasive SCC,[391–393] and patients with anogenital warts need to be followed closely for the development of this complication.

It is often impossible to differentiate clinically between QE, BP, and BD. However, distinguishing among these diseases is crucial to select the most proper form of therapy. The management of SCC of the penis is somewhat controversial, and urologic consultation may be necessary to manage the more advanced and difficult tumors. For noninvasive lesions of the foreskin, simple circumcision and observation may be all that is required.[385, 394] However, a 2-cm margin of normal skin has also been recommended when doing a circumcision in this situation.[395]

For noninvasive or superficially invasive SCCs of the distal penis in young patients, some urologists prefer radiation therapy if the lesion is smaller than 3 cm. If this treatment fails, a distal amputation is performed.[394–396] For superficially invasive lesions of the shaft, surgical excision or MMS is recommended.[394] For invasive lesions of the glans and distal shaft, treatment consists of a partial penectomy, including 1.5 to 2 cm of normal proximal skin as a surgical margin. For invasive lesions of the proximal penis, a total penectomy is usually performed.[385, 394, 395] For in situ lesions, surgical excision is recommended, and partial penectomy is suggested for well-differentiated or small, moderately to poorly differentiated tumors. Total penectomy is recommended for large and poorly differentiated tumors.[397]

The role of radiation therapy is controversial, and many feel it should be limited to noninvasive lesions in young men,[394–396] while others think it has no role in the management of the primary lesion or nodes.[397] A few authors believe that radiation therapy is an effective way to manage penile carcinoma,[398, 399] while preserving fertility and sexual function. If radiation fails, many cases can still be salvaged by surgery. Between 14 and 20% of patients will ultimately require amputation because of either recurrent disease or complications of treatment (e.g., urethral necrosis, which occurs in 10%

of patients, or urethral stricture, which occurs in 16 to 47% of patients).[394, 395, 398]

MMS has also been used to manage SCC of the penis,[385, 400] with an overall 5-year cure rate of 68% reported in 29 patients with penile carcinoma. However, while the local cure rate was 92%, 21% of patients developed metastatic spread. This high local cure rate with MMS is impressive when one considers that a local recurrence rate of 40% has been reported with routine surgical excision.[385] MMS was used to treat 11 patients with invasive SCC of the penis with an average lesion size of 2.3 × 1.8 cm.[385] In this series, only one patient developed a local recurrence, but four patients developed metastases that appeared within a year of the treatment. Using cryosurgery, a 100% cure rate has been reported for SCCs of the glans and sulcus invading less than 2 cm in depth.[401] Although these data are impressive, additional studies are needed to confirm these results before cryosurgery can be recommended for the management of invasive SCC of the penis.

Management of regional lymph nodes in penile SCC is also controversial. A conservative approach to ELND is based on the depth of invasion, size, extent, and histology of the lesion.[396] Clinical evaluation is unreliable in predicting lymph node involvement, and even after a 6-week course of antibiotics, up to 35% of patients will still have lymphadenopathy, even though only 45% of these will have evidence of metastatic disease.[385, 396, 402–405]

Because the lymphatic drainage from the penis is bilateral to the inguinal and iliac nodes, a bilateral node dissection is necessary if an ELND is carried out. If a bilateral superficial and deep node dissection is carried out, 50% of patients will develop lymphedema of the genitalia and legs, with an associated 3% mortality rate.[403, 406] Other complications include lymphoceles, elephantiasis, phlebitis, pulmonary emboli, and poor healing on the affected extremity.[402, 404]

Radiation therapy appears to be ineffective for occult nodal disease and may make subsequent node evaluation more difficult.[397, 406] As might be anticipated, regional node metastasis has a significant impact on survival, with most studies showing only a 30 to 66% 5-year survival rate.[385, 396, 397, 405] Thus, local recurrence is not the problem in managing SCC of the penis; instead, regional spread is responsible for the significant surgical failure rate in this disease. If the sentinel nodes are negative, the 5-year survival rate is 90%; however, if the nodes are positive, the survival rate falls to 70%. If the inguinal nodes are also involved, the survival rate decreases to 50%, and if the iliac nodes are positive, the survival rate falls to 20%. Distant metastases occur in 10% of patients and occur late in the course.[385]

Based on this information, a number of important recommendations can be made regarding management of SCC of the penis. First, the primary lesion should be managed by surgical excision or MMS; radiation therapy should be reserved for patients with early superficial disease who refuse surgery; and penectomies and amputations should be reserved for those with large advanced lesions and those in whom it is not possible to preserve a functional penis. Second, in patients with

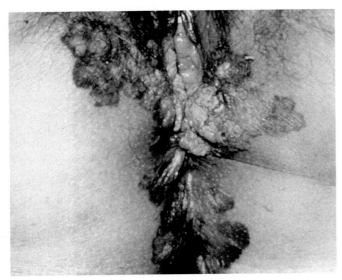

Figure 57–42. Patient with extensive pigmented Bowen's disease of the anogenital area.

palpable nodes, a 6-week course of antibiotics should first be prescribed, and if the lymphadenopathy persists, a node aspirate should be performed; if the aspirate is positive, a node dissection is indicated, with ilioinguinal dissection on the positive side and superficial dissection on the nonpositive side. If the inguinal nodes are positive, the iliac nodes should also be removed; if the node aspirate is negative and the patient is considered at significant risk for metastases, either a sentinel node dissection or a superficial lymphadenectomy should be done. If the result is negative, no further treatment is indicated; however, if the result is positive, a complete node dissection is indicated. Third, in the absence of palpable nodes, patients considered at low risk for metastases can simply be followed closely; however, if the risk for spread is significant, then a sentinel node biopsy or dissection should be done; any patient being followed for penile SCC should have node aspiration or superficial node dissection if lymphadenopathy develops. Fourth, for patients without palpable nodes, ELND is generally not indicated for disease of the distal penis but is recommended for deep invasive disease of the corpora or proximal penis; patients with nodal metastases who undergo node dissections should consult a radiation therapist with regard to postoperative radiation.

SCC of the Vulva

As with other anogenital SCCs, infection by HPV types 6/11, 16, and 18 has been associated with invasive SCC, BD, and BP of the vulva (Fig. 57–42).[309, 314, 315, 319, 320, 322, 324, 326–329, 407, 408] SCC of the vulva is also associated with carcinoma of the cervix and vagina. For this reason, a woman with vulvar SCC should be screened for lower genital tract carcinoma, and her sexual partner should be assessed for penile SCC. Probably because HPV plays a role in the development of these carcinomas, it

is not unusual to see the coexistence of condyloma and SCC in a biopsy specimen of the vulva.[409]

One common question relates to the malignant potential of lichen sclerosis et atrophicus (LS&A) of the vulva. It has been reported[410] that SCC develops in no more than 3% of women with LS&A. Presumably, the hyperplastic dystrophy or intraepithelial atypia that is seen in association with hyperplasia of the epithelium may predispose the patient to the development of SCC.[321]

To determine the most effective management of vulvar SCC, close attention must be paid to the age of the patient, whether the disease is unicentric or multicentric, and the nature of the lesion itself. Many patients less than 40 years of age should be managed conservatively and should not be subjected to procedures such as radical vulvectomies, since HPV infection is common in these patients and the disease is often rapid in onset, with spontaneous regression also being reported. These lesions appear to have little tendency to evolve into invasive SCC. Older women (i.e., more than 45 years of age) and immunosuppressed patients are more likely to develop invasive SCC and should be followed especially closely.[321, 322, 326, 329, 407, 408, 411, 412] Patients with one or two plaques instead of multiple papules may also be at higher risk for the development of invasive SCC and should be managed accordingly.

When evaluating or treating patients with suspicious lesions of the vulva or any other mucous membrane, the toluidine blue test may be helpful in selecting the most appropriate lesions for biopsy and to detect subclinical or early recurrent disease. However, false-positive and false-negative results may occur.[321, 326, 413] Acetowhitening may also be useful in detecting the subclinical spread of SCC in situ.[414]

Although women with SCC in situ of the vulva have undergone various types of vulvectomies,[314, 321] most clinicians consider this disease to be relatively benign, and more conservative management has been advocated.[322, 326, 329, 408] If only a few lesions are present, excision with 5 mm margins may be successful. For multiple lesions, cryosurgery or C&D may be used. Topical 5% 5-FU also may be used, but only a 50% response rate has been reported.[321] Severe irritation may limit its usefulness,[322] and if follicular involvement is present, 5-FU will not eradicate the disease.[415] The CO_2 laser[321, 322, 416] has also become popular in the management of this problem. When used in the vaporizing mode to treat the lesion, maintaining 5-mm margin of clinically normal skin,[416] a success rate of 91 to 94% has been reported.[329, 407, 416]

The current management recommendation for invasive SCCs of the vulva that are less than 1.5 cm in size and less than 5 mm in depth is to proceed with excision of the primary lesion, using 3-cm margins of clinically normal skin, and following this with an ipsilateral inguinal node dissection.[417, 418] If the nodes contain tumor, a bilateral inguinal and pelvic node dissection is performed.

The management of the regional nodes is based on the depth of penetration of the tumor and its histology. If infiltrating strands of SCC are present or the tumor

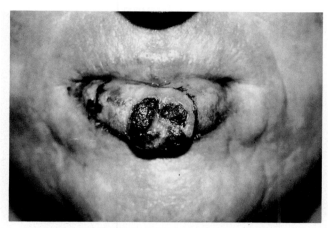

Figure 57–43. SCC of the lip in a renal transplant patient.

invades the tissue as single cells, there is an increased risk of metastases.[419, 420] In contrast, verrucous SCC and tumors with broad pushing borders are unlikely to metastasize.[420] Also, ELND is not indicated for tumors that are less than 3 mm deep since only 4.9% of these have nodal involvement.[419, 421]

Tumors less than 5 mm deep have a relatively low incidence of metastases (13%).[422, 423] However, poorly differentiated SCCs[321] are more likely to metastasize, regardless of their depth.[422, 423] Vascular invasion[422] and tumors larger than 2 cm are also more likely to metastasize.[321, 422, 423] Based on this information, ELND should be considered for patients with extremely poorly differentiated tumors larger than 2 cm that show invasion more than 3 mm in depth by single cells or strands of tumor cells.[424] Because SCC of the vulva is associated with a significant risk of metastases and may be associated with other malignancies of the genital tract, it is suggested that a gynecologic consultation be obtained and a multidisciplinary team approach employed in managing these individuals.

SCC of the Lip

SCC of the lip (Fig. 57–43) most commonly occurs on the lower lip of older white men. It is also common in alcoholics, smokers, immunosuppressed individuals, patients with poor dental hygiene, and those with an outdoor occupation.[11–15] Less than 1% of the SCCs arise in the commissures, and only 2 to 8% of cases involve the upper lip.[12, 425] Clinically, the lesion may present as an exophytic, verrucous, or ulcerated lesion.

Poor histologic differentiation is associated with an increased risk of metastases and a worse patient prognosis.[12] Only 5% of lip SCCs are of the poorly differentiated or spindle cell type. These tumors are often perineural and metastasize early. SCCs occurring on the upper lip and commissures tend to grow faster and to metastasize earlier than SCCs of the lower lip.[12, 80, 425] Less than 10% of patients with SCC of the lower lip have clinical metastases to the regional nodes at the time of presentation. However, more than 10% of patients with SCC of the upper lip and up to 20% of

those with SCC involving the commissures will have nodal metastases at the time of initial presentation. The 5-year survival rate for patients with commissural lesions is 34%; for those with upper lip lesions, it is 40 to 60%.[12, 425] SCCs that are larger than 2 cm are also more likely to metastasize. Involvement of the mandible is associated with a high incidence of metastases and a poor 3-year survival rate (33%). Most regional metastases develop within 6 to 36 months from the time of treatment of the primary lesion.[12, 77, 78, 425] Lesions of the lateral lower lip metastasize to the nodes of the submandibular triangle, whereas lesions of the upper lip usually metastasize to the preauricular or parotid nodes. Although metastases to the cervical nodes usually occur in patients with deeply invasive, large tumors (i.e., >2 cm), small, superficial tumors (<1 cm) metastasize in 3% of cases.[12, 78, 425] Up to 18.5% of patients will develop cervical node involvement,[78] and 15% of patients develop visceral metastases.

The incidence of metastases for SCC of the lip has been reported to be between 6.7[11, 77] and 15%[78, 79, 84, 426, 427] but can be as high as 33 to 100% with advanced lesions.[428] While cure rates as high as 96.7% have been reported for SCC of the lip,[11] once metastases occur, the 5-year survival rate falls to 56% or less.[11, 12, 79, 80, 84, 425–428] SCCs showing a KA-like or verrucous growth pattern usually behave in a relatively benign fashion, while deeply invasive tumors and those that grow in haphazard manner have a 77% incidence of metastases. Tumors more than 6 mm thick, tumors growing as infiltrating strands, tumors in which individual cells invade the tissues or muscle, and poorly differentiated tumors with marked nuclear atypia are most likely to metastasize.

In managing SCC of the lip, great care should be taken in selecting the appropriate treatment modality, since this disease is potentially lethal. Blind techniques such as cryosurgery and C&D have only a limited role in the management of small, well-differentiated lesions that are confined to the epithelium or are less than 1 mm thick. Excisional surgery, MMS, and radiation therapy are the treatments of choice for SCC of the lip. For small, superficial lesions, radiation and excisional surgery yield comparable cure rates.[12, 84, 426, 429] Radiation therapy may be administered as electron beam therapy,[12, 84, 344] contact x-ray,[12] or interstitial implants.[12] Orthovoltage and superficial x-rays also may be used.[344]

Although wedge excision of the lip is the traditional surgical procedure used to treat SCC of the lower lip, this method should be reserved for deeply invasive tumors. Many superficially invasive tumors can be excised[84] and the wound allowed to heal by second intention, or simple mucosal advancement can be employed to repair the defect. More advanced or invasive lesions may require wedge excision or more extensive and complex reconstructive procedures.

MMS has also been employed to treat SCC of the lip.[427, 430] In a report of 41 patients with SCC of the lip treated with MMS,[430] none of the 37 patients available for follow-up developed a recurrence or metastasis. Another report described a 94.1% cure rate after a 5-year follow-up period for 952 lesions of the lower lip treated with MMS.[427] Of the 56 treatment failures, 52 were a result of metastatic disease. This points to the need for adjunctive therapy for high-risk lesions. Tumor size is an important prognosticator, with cure rates of 98.3% for tumors smaller than 1 cm, 96.3% for tumors between 1 and 2 cm, 89.3% for 2- to 3-cm tumors, and only 58% for tumors larger than 3 cm. In addition, there is a reduced cure rate for recurrent lesions (87.4% compared with 95.4% for primary lesions). Poorly differentiated invasive SCCs showed cure rates of only 40% compared with 98.5% for well-differentiated superficial tumors. Patients who developed metastases showed a 5-year survival rate of 28% compared with 99.5% for those patients who did not develop metastases. In patients with nodal disease, a neck dissection with postoperative irradiation is usually recommended.[11, 78–80, 84, 428] However, no consensus exists regarding the management of clinically negative nodes in the patient with SCC of the lip.[11, 12, 80, 84, 133, 426, 428]

ELND is not indicated for SCC of the lower lip because of the low yield of tumor-positive nodes (less than 10%), and because ELND is no more effective than a therapeutic node dissection. However, ELND may be indicated for large or undifferentiated tumors of the commissure or upper lip.[11, 12, 84, 428] Patients are at high risk for recurrence and metastases if they have deeply invasive, poorly differentiated tumors that are larger than 2 cm in diameter, more than 6 mm thick, or show perineural involvement. These patients should receive postoperative radiation to the surgical site as well as the intervening lymphatics and regional nodes. Because SCC of the lip is a potentially serious disease, its treatment should not be undertaken lightly, and consultation with a radiation therapist and head and neck surgeon should be sought when managing patients at high risk for recurrence and metastatic spread. Also, because many of these patients have a background of actinic cheilitis and are at significant risk for developing a second SCC of the lip, the actinic cheilitis should be treated once the primary surgical site has healed.[429] Although a number of methods can be used to do this,

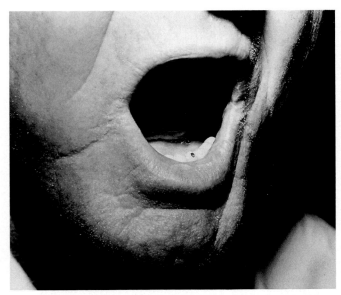

Figure 57–45. Clinical appearance of the healed lip 6 weeks later.

the CO_2 laser (Figs. 57–44, 57–45) is a well-tolerated and effective technique that gives good cosmetic results.[431–433]

Prevention of SCC

Patients with SCCs of the skin usually have had an excessive amount of solar damage and are at significant risk for developing additional SCCs, BCCs, and AKs. For this reason, close follow-up of these patients is important, not only for detecting recurrences, but also for diagnosing and treating new lesions as early in their evolution as possible. The use of sunscreens coupled with maximal avoidance of sunlight exposure is strongly suggested to help minimize the risk associated with additional sun damage.

SUMMARY

For the proper treatment of patients with SCC, the cutaneous surgeon must thoroughly evaluate the biologic behavior of the various histologic subtypes and individualize the therapy based on the lesion's location, size, and previous treatment, as well as the age of the patient and the desired cosmetic result. At times, an interdisciplinary team approach is required when managing large or deeply invasive tumors in high-risk locations.

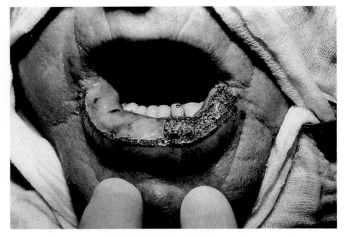

Figure 57–44. Patient with actinic cheilitis, half of which has been vaporized with a carbon dioxide laser.

REFERENCES

1. Scotto J, Fears TR, Faumeni JF Jr: Incidence of nonmelanoma skin cancer in the United States. NIH Publication no. 83–2433. National Institutes of Health, Bethesda, MD, 1983.
2. Scotto J, Kopf AW, Urbach F: Non-melanoma skin cancer among Caucasians in four areas of the United States. Cancer 34:1333–1338, 1974.
3. Glass AG, Hoover RN: The emerging epidemic of melanoma and squamous cell carcinoma. JAMA 262:2097–2100, 1989.

4. Jones RR: Ozone depletion and cancer risk. Lancet 2:443–446, 1987.
5. Rasmussen RA, Kahlil MA: Atmospheric trace gases: trends and distributions over the last decade. Science 232:1623–1624, 1986.
6. Cicerone RJ: Changes in stratospheric ozone. Science 237:35–42, 1987.
7. Fitzpatrick TB, Parrish JA, Haynes HA, et al: Ozone depletion and skin cancer. Dermatol Caps Comm 4:10–11, 1982.
8. Titus JG: Effects of changes in stratospheric ozone and global climate. US Environmental Protection Agency, Washington, DC, 1986.
9. Gus HP, Roy CR, Elliott G: Artificial sun tanning spectral irradiance and hazard evaluation of ultraviolet sources. Health Phys 50:691–703, 1986.
10. Honeycutt WM, Jansen T: Treatment of squamous cell carcinoma of the skin. Arch Dermatol 108:670–672, 1973.
11. Jorgensen K, Elbrond O, Andersen AP: Carcinoma of the lip. A series of 1869 patients. Acta Otolaryngol 75:302–313, 1973.
12. Baker SR: Cancer of the lip. In: Myers EN, Suen JY (eds): Cancer of the Head and Neck. Churchill Livingstone, New York, 1989, pp 383–415.
13. Warren S, Hoerr SO: A study of pathologically verified epidermoid carcinoma of the skin. Surg Gynecol Obstet 69:726–737, 1939.
14. Keller AZ: Cellular types, survival, race, nativity, occupations, habits, and associated diseases in the pathogenesis of lip cancers. Am J Epidemiol 91:486–499, 1970.
15. Ju DMC: On the etiology of cancer of the lower lip. Plast Reconstr Surg 52:151–154, 1973.
16. Swanbeck G, Hillstrom L: Analysis of etiological factors of squamous cell skin cancer of different locations. Acta Dermatol Venerol 51:151–156, 1971.
17. Oeltle AG: Skin cancer in Africa. Natl Cancer Inst Monogr 10:197–214, 1963.
18. Fleming ID, Barnwell JR, Burleson PE, et al: Skin cancer in black patients. Cancer 55:600–605, 1975.
19. Mora RG, Perniciaro C: Cancer of the skin in blacks: a review of 163 black patients with cutaneous squamous cell carcinoma. J Am Acad Dermatol 5:535–543, 1981.
20. Pinkus H: Premalignant fibroepithelial tumors of the skin. Arch Dermatol Syphilol 67:598–615, 1953.
21. Bresciani F, Paluzi R, Benasse M, et al: Cell kinetics and growth of squamous cell carcinomas in man. Cancer Res 34:2405–2415, 1974.
22. Chopra DP, Forbes PD: Analysis of cell kinetics during ultraviolet light–induced epidermal carcinogenesis in hairless mice. Cancer Res 34:454–457, 1974.
23. Friedland AN, Weinstein GD: Cell proliferation in human cutaneous squamous cell carcinoma. J Natl Cancer Inst 59:3–6, 1977.
24. Frindel E, Malaise F, Rubiana M: Cell proliferation kinetic in five human solid tumors. Cancer 22:611–620, 1968.
25. Weinstein GD, Frost P: Cell proliferation kinetics in benign and malignant skin diseases in humans. Natl Cancer Inst Monogr 30:225–246, 1969.
26. Schrek R: Cutaneous carcinoma: a statistical analysis with respect to measures of innate and clinical malignancy. Arch Pathol 31:422–433, 1941.
27. Chopra DP: Ultraviolet light carcinogenesis in hairless mice. Cell kinetics during induction and progression of squamous cell carcinoma as estimated by the double labeling method. J Invest Dermatol 66:242–247, 1976.
28. Griswold DP, Schabel FM, Wilcox WS, et al: Success and failure in the treatment of solid tumors. Cancer Chemother Rep 52:345–387, 1968.
29. Hermenus AF, Barendsen GW: Changes of cell proliferative characteristics in rat rhabdomyosarcoma before and after x-irradiation. Eur J Cancer 5:173–189, 1969.
30. Tubiana M: The kinetics of tumour cell proliferation and radiotherapy. Br J Radiol 44:325–347, 1971.
31. Montandon D, Kocher O, Gabbiani G: Cancer invasiveness: immunofluorescent and ultrastructure methods of assessment. Plast Reconstr Surg 69:365–371, 1982.
32. Kocher O, Amandruz M, Schindler AM, et al: Desmosomes and gap junctions in precarcinomatous and carcinomatous conditions of squamous epithelia. An electron microscopic and morphimetric study. J Submicrosc Cytol Pathol 13:267–281, 1981.
33. Gabbiani G, Csank-Brassert J, Schneeberger J-C, et al: Contractile proteins in human cancer cells: immunofluorescent and electron microscopic study. Am J Pathol 83:457–474, 1976.
34. Posalaky Z, McGinley D, Cutler B, et al: Intercellular junctional specializations in human basal cell carcinoma. A freeze-fracture study. Virchows Arch Pathol Anat 384:53–63, 1979.
35. Bauer EA, Gordon JM, Reddick ME, et al: Quantitation and immunocytochemical localization of human skin collagenase in basal cell carcinoma. J Invest Dermatol 69:363–367, 1977.
36. Hashimoto K, Yamanishi Y, Malepers E, et al: Collagenolytic activities of squamous cell carcinoma of the skin. Cancer Res 33:2790–2801, 1973.
37. Hashimoto K, Yamanishi Y, Dabbus MK: Electron microscopic observations of collagenolytic activity of basal cell epithelioma of the skin in vivo and in vitro. Cancer Res 32:2561–2567, 1972.
38. Bauer EA, Uitto J, Walters RC, et al: Enhanced collagenase production by fibroblasts derived from human basal cell carcinomas. Cancer Res 39:4594–4599, 1979
39. Wolf JE, Hubler WR: Tumor angiogenic factor and human skin tumors. Arch Dermatol 111:321–327, 1975.
40. Scalabrino G, Pigatto P, Ferioli ME, et al: Levels of activity of the polyamine biosynthetic decarboxylases as indicators of degree of malignancy of human cutaneous epitheliomas. J Invest Dermatol 74:122–124, 1980.
41. Robinson JK, Pollack SV, Robins P: Invasion of cartilage by basal cell carcinoma. J Am Acad Dermatol 2:499–505, 1980.
42. Levine HL, Bailin PL: Basal cell carcinoma of the head and neck. Identification of the high risk patient. Laryngoscope 90:955–961, 1980.
43. Ceilly RI, Bumsted RM, Smith WH: Malignancies on the external ear: methods of ablation and reconstruction of defects. J Dermatol Surg Oncol 5:762–767, 1979.
44. Bailin PL, Levine HL, Wood BG, et al: Cutaneous carcinoma of the auricular and periauricular region. Arch Otolaryngol 106:692–700, 1980.
45. Mohs FE: Modes of spread of cancer. In: Chemosurgery: Microscopically Controlled Surgery for Skin Cancer. Charles C Thomas, Springfield, IL, 1978, pp 256–273.
46. Mora RG, Robins P: Basal cell carcinoma in the center of the face. Special diagnostic prognostic and therapeutic considerations. J Dermatol Surg Oncol 4:315–321, 1978.
47. Ceilly RI, Anderson RL: Microscopically controlled excision of malignant neoplasms on and around eyelids followed by immediate surgical reconstruction. J Dermatol Surg Oncol 4:55–62, 1978.
48. Rosen HM: Periorbital basal cell carcinoma requiring ablative craniofacial surgery. Arch Dermatol 123:376–378, 1987.
49. Roenigk RK, Ratz JL, Bailin PL, Wheeland RG: Trends in the presentation and treatment of basal cell carcinomas. J Dermatol Surg Oncol 12:860–865, 1986.
50. Gormley DE, Hirsch P: Aggressive basal cell carcinoma of the scalp. Arch Dermatol 114:782–783, 1978.
51. Binstock JH, Stegman SF, Tromovitch TA: Large aggressive basal cell carcinomas of the scalp. J Dermatol Surg Oncol 7:565–569, 1981.
52. Gullane PG: Extensive facial malignancies. Concepts and management. J Otolaryngol 15:44–48 1986.
53. Granstrom G, Aldenburg F, Jeppsson RH: Influence of embryonal fusion lines for recurrence of basal cell carcinoma in the head and neck. Otolaryngol Head Neck Surg 95:76–82, 1986.
54. Levine H, Bailin P, Wood B, et al: Tissue conservation in the treatment of cutaneous neoplasms of the head and neck. Combined use of Mohs chemosurgical and conventional surgical techniques. Arch Otolaryngol 105:140–144, 1979.
55. Panje WR, Ceilly RI: The influence of embryology of the midface on the spread of epithelial malignancies. Laryngoscope 89:1914–1920, 1979.
56. Panje WR, Ceilly RI: Nasal skin cancer: hazard to a unique exposed structure. Postgrad Med 66:75–82, 1979.
57. Levine H: Cutaneous carcinoma of the head and neck: management of massive and previously uncontrolled lesions. Laryngoscope 93:87–105, 1983.
58. Mohs FE, Lathrop TG: Modes of spread of cancer of skin. Arch Dermatol Syphilol 66:427–439, 1952.

59. Ballantyne AJ, McCarten AB, Ibanez ML: The extension of cancer of the head and neck through peripheral nerves. Am J Surg 106:651–667, 1963.

60. Cottel WI: Perineural invasion by squamous cell carcinoma. J Dermatol Surg Oncol 8:589–600, 1982.

61. Goepfert H, Dichtel WJ, Medina JE, et al: Perineural invasion in squamous cell carcinoma of the head and neck. Am J Surg 148:542–547, 1984.

62. Koo KC, Carter RL, O'Brien CJ, et al: Prognostic implications of perineural spread in squamous carcinomas of the head and neck. Laryngoscope 96:1145–1148, 1986.

63. Morris JGL, Jaffe R: Perineural spread of cutaneous basal and squamous cell carcinomas. The clinical appearance of spread into the trigeminal and facial nerves. Arch Neurol 40:424–449, 1983.

64. Mendenhall WM, Parsons JT, Mendenhall NP, et al: Carcinoma of the skin of the head and neck with perineural invasion. Head Neck 11:301–308, 1989.

65. Mickalites CJ, Rappaport I: Perineural invasion by squamous cell carcinoma of the lower lip. Review of the literature and report of a case. Oral Surg Med Pathol 46:74–78, 1978.

66. Green N, Landman M: Perineural metastases from squamous cell carcinoma of the face. Therapeutic considerations. Ann Otolaryngol 90:183–185, 1981.

67. Carter RL, Pittam MR, Tanner NSB: Pain and dysphagia in patients with squamous carcinomas of the head and neck. The role of perineural spread. J R Soc Med 75:598–606, 1982.

68. Loeffler JS, Larson DA, Clark JR, et al: Treatment of perineural metastases from squamous carcinoma of the skin with aggressive combination chemotherapy and irradiation. J Surg Oncol 29:181–183, 1985.

69. McGuirt WF, McCabe BF: Significance of node biopsy before definitive treatment of cervical metastatic carcinoma. Laryngoscope 88:594–597, 1978.

70. Young JE, Archibald SD, Shier KJ: Needle aspiration cytologic biopsy in head and neck masses. Am J Surg 142:484–489, 1981.

71. Gooder P, Palmer M: Cervical lymph node biopsy—a study of its morbidity. J Laryngol Otol 98:1031–1040, 1984.

72. Rozack MS, Sako K, Marchetta FC: Influence of initial neck node biopsy on the incidence of recurrence in the neck and survival of patients who subsequently undergo curative resectional surgery. J Surg Oncol 9:347–352, 1977.

73. Jesse RH: Management of a suspicious cervical lymph node. Postgrad Med 48:99–102, 1970.

74. Martin H, Morfit HM: Cervical lymph node metastases as the first symptom of cancer. Surg Gynecol Obstet 78:133–159, 1944.

75. Martin H: Untimely lymph node biopsy. Am J Surg 102:17–18, 1961.

76. Dinehart SM, Pollack SV: Metastases from squamous cell carcinoma of the skin and lip. An analysis of twenty-seven cases. J Am Acad Dermatol 21:241–248, 1989.

77. Durkovsky J, Krajce M, Michalikova B: To the problem of lip cancer metastases. Neoplasm 19:653–659, 1972.

78. Sack JG, Ford CN: Metastatic squamous cell carcinoma of the lip. Arch Otolaryngol 104:282–285, 1978.

79. Petrovich Z, Kuisk H, Tobochnik N, et al: Carcinoma of the lip. Arch Otolaryngol 105:187–191, 1979.

80. Wang CC: Head and neck neoplasms. In: Mansfield CM (ed): Therapeutic Radiology. Elsevier, New York, 1989, pp 199–222.

81. Mendenhall NP, Million RR, Cassisi NJ: Parotid area lymph node metastases from carcinoma of the skin. Int J Radiat Oncol Biol Phys 11:707–714, 1985.

82. Shimm DS: Parotid lymph node metastases from squamous cell carcinoma of the skin. J Surg Oncol 37:56–59, 1988.

83. O'Brien CJ, Urist MM: Current status of neck dissection in the management of squamous cell carcinoma of the head and neck. Aust NZ J Surg 57:501–509, 1987.

84. Baker SR: Malignant neoplasms of the oral cavity. In: Cummings CS, Fredrickson JM, Harker LA, et al (eds). Otolaryngology—Head and Neck Surgery. CV Mosby, St. Louis, 1986, pp 1311–1313.

85. Wilson SM, Phillips JM, Hawk JC III: Metastases from squamous cell carcinoma of the skin. J SC Med Assoc 86:311–314, 1990.

86. Withers HR: Rationale for radiotherapy in subclinical nodal disease. In: Moloy PG, Nicolson GL (eds): Occult Nodal Metastases in Solid Cellular Carcinomata. Second International Symposium on Cellular Oncology. Cancer Research Monograph. Praeger, New York, 1987, pp 68–72.

87. Byers RM: The use of postoperative irradiation—its goals and 1978 attainments. Laryngoscope 89:567–572, 1979.

88. Chow JM, Levin BC, Krivit JS, et al: Radiotherapy or surgery for subclinical cervical node metastases. Arch Otolaryngol Head Neck Surg 115:981–984, 1989.

89. Weissler MC, Weigel MT, Rosenman JG, et al: Treatment of the clinically negative neck in advanced cancer of the head and neck. Arch Otolaryngol Head Neck Surg 115:691–694, 1989.

90. Friedman M, Mafee MF, Pacella BL, et al: Rationale for elective node dissection in 1990. Laryngoscope 100:54–59, 1990.

91. Harnsberger HR: CT and MRI of masses of the deep face. Curr Probl Diagn Radiol 16:141–173, 1987.

92. Moller R, Reymann F, Hori-Jensen K: Metastases in dermatological patients with squamous cell carcinoma. Arch Dermatol 115:703–705, 1979.

93. Epstein E, Epstein NN, Bragg K, et al: Metastases from squamous cell carcinoma of the skin. Arch Dermatol 97:245–251, 1968.

94. Glass RL, Spratt JS Jr, Perez-Mesa C: Epidermoid carcinomas of lower extremities. An analysis of 35 cases. Arch Surg 89:955–960, 1964.

95. Katz AD, Urbach F, Lilienfeld AM: The frequency and risk of metastases in squamous cell carcinoma of the skin. Cancer 10:1162–1166, 1957.

96. Ames FC, Hickey RC: Metastases from squamous cell carcinoma of the extremities. South Med J 75:920–923, 1982.

97. Ridenhour CE, Spratt JS Jr: Epidermoid carcinoma of the skin involving the parotid gland. Am J Surg 112:504–507, 1966.

98. Johnson J, Newman RK: The anatomic location of neck metastases from occult squamous cell carcinoma. Otolaryngol Head Neck Surg 89:54–58, 1981.

99. Stell PM, Morton RP, Singh SD: Cervical lymph node metastasis: the significance of the level of the lymph node. Clin Oncol 9:101–107, 1983.

100. Schuller DE, McGuirt WF, McCabe BF, et al: The prognostic significance of metastatic cervical lymph nodes. Laryngoscope 90:557–570, 1980.

101. Johnson JT, Myers EN, Bedetti CD, et al: Cervical lymph node metastases. Incidence and implications of extracapsular carcinoma. Arch Otolaryngol 111:534–537, 1985.

102. Snow GB, Annyas AA, VanSkooten EA, et al: Prognostic factors of neck node metastases. Clin Otolaryngol 7:185–192, 1982.

103. Shiu MH, Chu F, Fortner JG: Treatment of regionally advanced epidermal carcinoma of the extremity and trunk. Surg Gynecol Obstet 150:558–562, 1980.

104. Burkett FE, Jernstrom PH: Low-grade keratinizing squamous cell carcinoma recurrent in same extremity three times in nine years via local embolic interstitial dermal metastases. J Surg Oncol 21:117–120, 1982.

105. Weidner N, Elliott F: Epidermotropic metastatic squamous cell carcinoma. Report of two cases showing histologic continuity between epidermis and metastases. Arch Dermatol 121:1041–1043, 1985.

106. Saruk M, Olsen TG, Lucky PA: Metastatic epidermotropic squamous cell carcinoma of the vagina. J Am Acad Dermatol 11:353–356, 1984.

107. Immerman SC, Scanlon EF, Christ M, et al: Recurrent squamous cell carcinoma of the skin. Cancer 5:1537–1540, 1983.

108. Arons MS, Lynch JB, Lewis SR, et al: Scar tissue carcinoma. Part I. A clinical study with special reference to burn scar carcinoma. Ann Surg 161:170–188, 1965.

109. Edward MJ, Hirsch RM, Broadwater JR, et al: Squamous cell carcinoma arising in previously burned or irradiated skin. Arch Surg 124:115–117, 1989.

110. Storm FK, Eilber FR, Sparks FC, et al: A prospective study of parotid metastases from head and neck cancer. Am J Surg 134:115–119, 1977.

111. Wetmore SJ, Mattox DE: Cancer of the ear and temporal bone. In: Myers EN, Suen JY (eds): Cancer of the Head and Neck. Churchill Livingstone, New York, 1989, pp 691–709.

112. Schrek R: Cutaneous carcinomas: a statistical analysis with respect to site, sex, and pre-existing scars. Arch Pathol 31:434–448, 1941.

113. Binder SC, Cady B, Cathen D: Epidermal carcinoma of the skin of the nose. Am J Surg 116:506–512, 1968.

114. Blake GB, Wilson JSP: Malignant tumours of the ear and their treatment. Tumours of the auricle. Br J Plast Surg 27:67–76, 1974.

115. Modulin JJ: Cancer of the skin: surgical treatment. Mo Med 51:364–367, 1954.

116. Shiffman NJ: Squamous cell carcinoma of the skin of the pinna. Can J Surg 18:279–283, 1975.

117. Friedman HI, Cooper PH, Wanebo J: Prognostic and therapeutic use of microstaging of cutaneous squamous cell carcinoma of trunk and extremities. Cancer 56:1099–1105, 1985.

118. Freeman RG, Duncan WC: Recurrent skin cancer. Arch Dermatol 107:395–399, 1973.

119. Rueckert F: The malignant potential of face cancer. A study of seven cases of squamous cell carcinoma of the skin. Plast Reconstr Surg 32:21–29, 1963.

120. Lifeso RM, Bull CA: Squamous cell carcinoma of the extremities. Cancer 55:2862–2867, 1985.

121. Martin H, Strong E, Spiro RH: Radiation induced skin cancer of the head and neck. Cancer 25:61–71, 1970.

122. Pack GT, Davis J: Radiation cancer of the skin. Radiology 84:436–442, 1965.

123. Treves N, Pack GT: The development of cancer in burn scars. An analysis and report of thirty-four cases. Surg Gynecol Obstet 51:749–782, 1930.

124. Sedlin Ed, Fleming JL: Epidermoid carcinoma arising in chronic osteomyelitic foci. J Bone Joint Surg 45A:827–838, 1963.

125. Ikegawa S, Saida T, Takizawa Y, et al: Vimentin positive squamous cell carcinoma arising in a burn scar. A highly malignant neoplasm comprised of acantholytic round keratinocytes. Arch Dermatol 125:1672–1676, 1989.

126. Stromberg BV, Keiter JE, Wray RC, et al: Scar carcinoma: Prognosis and treatment. South Med J 70:821–822, 1977.

127. Lund HZ: How often does squamous cell carcinoma of the skin metastasize. Arch Dermatol 92:635–637, 1965.

128. Graham JH, Bendle BJ, Johnson WC: Solar keratosis with squamous cell carcinoma. A new biologic concept. Am J Pathol 55:26a, 1969.

129. Epstein E: Metastases of sun-induced squamous cell carcinoma. J Dermatol Surg Oncol 10:418, 1984.

130. Bendl BJ, Graham JH: In: New Concepts on the Origin of Squamous Cell Carcinoma. A Clinicopathologic and Histochemical study. Proceedings of the Sixth National Cancer Conference. JB Lippincott, Philadelphia, 1970, pp 471–488.

131. Graham JH, Helwig EB: Premalignant cutaneous and mucocutaneous disease. In: Graham JH, Johnson WC, Helwig EB (eds): Dermal Pathology. Harper & Row, Hagerstown, MD, 1972, pp 561–581.

132. Fukamizu H, Inoue K, Matsumoto K, et al: Metastatic squamous cell carcinoma derived from solar keratoses. J Dermatol Surg Oncol 11:518–522, 1985.

133. Frierson HF Jr, Cooper PH: Prognostic factors in squamous cell carcinoma of the lower lip. Hum Pathol 17:346–354, 1986.

134. Husseinzadeh N, Zaino R, Nahhas WA, et al: The significance of histologic findings in predicting nodal metastases in invasive squamous cell carcinoma of the vulva. Gynecol Oncol 16:105–111, 1983.

135. Barnes AE, Crissman JD, Schellhas HF, et al: Microinvasive carcinoma of the vulva: a clinicopathologic evaluation. Obstet Gynecol 56:234–238, 1980.

136. Johnson WC, Helwig EB: Adenoid squamous cell carcinoma (adenoacanthoma). A clinicopathologic study of 155 patients. Cancer 19:1639–1650, 1966.

137. Penn I: Principles of tumor immunity: immunocompromised patients. AIDS Update 3:1–14, 1990.

138. Dinehart SM, Chu DZJ, Maners AW, et al: Immunosuppression in patients with metastatic squamous cell carcinoma from the skin. J Dermatol Surg Oncol 16:271–274, 1990.

139. Wade TR, Ackerman AB: The many faces of squamous cell carcinomas. J Dermatol Surg Oncol 4:291–294, 1978.

140. Lever WF, Schaumburg-Lever G: Tumors and cysts of the epidermis. In: Histopathology of the Skin. JB Lippincott, Philadelphia, 1990, pp 523–577.

141. Bowen JT: Precancerous dermatosis. J Cutan Dis 30:241–255, 1912.

142. Rosen L, Amazon K, Frank B: Bowen's disease, Paget's disease and malignant melanoma in situ. South Med J 79:410–413, 1986.

143. Jones CS, Tyring SK, Lee PC, et al: Development of neuroendocrine (Merkel cell) carcinoma mixed with squamous cell carcinoma in erythema ab igne. Arch Dermatol 124:110–113, 1988.

144. Gomez LE, Maio SD, Silva EG, et al: Association between neuroendocrine (Merkel cell) carcinoma and squamous carcinoma of the skin. Am J Surg Pathol 7:171–177, 1983.

145. Wick MR, Pettinato G, Nappi O: Adenoid (acantholytic) squamous carcinoma of the skin. J Cutan Pathol 15:351, 1988.

146. Silvin NG, Swanson PE, Manivel JC, et al: Spindle cell and pleomorphic neoplasms of the skin. A clinicopathologic and immunohistochemical study of 30 cases with emphasis on "atypical fibroxanthoma." Am J Dermatopathol 10:9–19, 1988.

147. Evans HL, Smith JL: Spindle squamous carcinomas and sarcoma-like tumor of the skin. A comparative study of 38 cases. Cancer 45:2687–2697, 1980.

148. Battifora H: Spindle cell carcinoma: ultrastructural evidence of squamous origin and collagen production by the tumor cells. Cancer 37:2275–2282, 1976.

149. Feldman PS, Barr RJ: Ultrastructure of spindle cell squamous carcinoma. J Cutan Pathol 3:17–24, 1976.

150. Woyke S, Domagala W, Olszewski W, et al: Pseudosarcoma of the skin. An electron microscopic study and comparison with the fine structure of the spindle-cell variant of squamous carcinoma. Cancer 33:970–980, 1974.

151. Cade S: Radiation induced cancer in man. Br J Radiol 30:393–402, 1957.

152. Headington JT: Verrucous carcinoma. Cutis 2:207–211, 1978.

153. Ackerman LV: Verrucous carcinoma of the oral cavity. Surgery 23:670–678, 1948.

154. Aird I, Johnson HD, Lennox B, et al: Epithelioma cuniculatum. A variety of squamous carcinoma peculiar to the foot. Br J Surg 42:245–250, 1954.

155. Brown SM, Freeman RG: Epithelioma cuniculatum. Arch Dermatol 112:1295–1296, 1976.

156. Reingold IM, Smith BP, Graham JH: Epithelioma cuniculatum pedis, a variant of squamous cell carcinoma. Am J Clin Pathol 69:561–565, 1978.

157. Friedman KJ: Low-grade primary cutaneous adenosquamous (mucoepidermoid) carcinoma. Am J Dermatopathol 11:43–50, 1989.

158. Gallagher HS, Miller GV, Grampa G: Primary mucoepidermoid carcinoma of the skin. Cancer 12:286–288, 1959.

159. Weidner N, Foucar E: Adenosquamous carcinoma of the skin. An aggressive mucin- and gland-forming carcinoma. Arch Dermatol 121:775–779, 1985.

160. Kuo T: Clear cell carcinoma of the skin. A variant of the squamous cell carcinoma that simulates sebaceous carcinoma. Am J Surg Pathol 4:573–583, 1980.

161. Cramer SF, Heggeness LM: Signet-ring squamous cell carcinoma. Am J Clin Pathol 91:488–491, 1989.

162. Wagner RF, Grande DJ: Pseudoepitheliomatous hyperplasia vs squamous cell carcinoma arising from chronic osteomyelitis of the humerus. J Dermatol Surg Oncol 12:632–635, 1986.

163. Ju DMC: Pseudoepitheliomatous hyperplasia of the skin. Dermatol Int 6:82–92, 1967.

164. Armin AR, Eng AM, Warpeka RL: Infiltrating squamous metaplasia in debrided skin. J Assoc Milit Dermatol 12:18–21, 1986.

165. Weber PJ, Johnson BL, Dzubow LM: Pseudoepitheliomatous hyperplasia following Mohs micrographic surgery. J Dermatol Surg Oncol 15:557–560, 1989.

166. Grunwald MH, Lee JYY, Ackerman AB: Pseudocarcinomatous hyperplasia. Am J Dermatopathol 10:95–103, 1988.

167. Metcalf JS, Maize JC: Squamous syringometaplasia in lobular panniculitis and pyoderma gangrenosum. Am J Dermatopathol 12:141–149, 1990.

168. Brownstein MH, Arluk DJ: Proliferating trichilemmal cyst: a simulant of squamous cell carcinoma. Cancer 48:1207–1214, 1981.

169. Kern WH, McGray MK: The histopathologic differentiation of keratoacanthoma and squamous cell carcinoma of the skin. J Cutan Pathol 7:318–325, 1980.

170. Schaumberg-Lever G, Alroy J, Gavris V, et al: Cell surface carbohydrates in proliferative epidermal lesions. Distribution of AB and H blood group antigens in benign and malignant lesions. Am J Dermatopathol 6:583–589, 1984.

171. Ariano MC, Wiley EL, Ariano L, et al: H1 peanut lectin receptor

and carcinoembryonic antigen distribution in keratoacanthomas, squamous dysplasias, and carcinomas of the skin. J Dermatol Surg Oncol 11:1076–1083, 1985.

172. Schaumberg-Lever G, Alroy J, Ucci A, et al: Cell surface carbohydrates in proliferative epidermal lesions. Masking of peanut agglutin (PNA) binding sites in solar keratoses, Bowen's disease, and squamous cell carcinoma by neuraminic acid. J Cutan Pathol 13:163–171, 1986.

173. Smoller BR, Kwan TH, Said JW, Banks-Schlegel S: Keratoacanthoma and squamous cell carcinoma of the skin. Immunohistochemical localization of involucrin and keratin proteins. J Am Acad Dermatol 14:226–234, 1986.

174. Belisario JC: Brief review of keratoacanthoma and description of keratoacanthoma centrifugum marginatum. Aust J Dermatol 8:65–72, 1965.

175. Rook A, Whimster IW: Le keratoacanthome. Arch Belg Dermatol Syphilol 6:137–146, 1950.

176. Poleksic S, Yeung KY: Rapid development of keratoacanthoma and accelerated transformation into squamous cell carcinoma of the skin. Cancer 41:12–16, 1978.

177. Sullivan JJ, Colditz GA: Keratoacanthoma in a subtropical climate. Aust J Dermatol 20:34–42, 1979.

178. Piscoli F, Boi S, Zumiani G, et al: A gigantic metastasizing keratoacanthoma. Am J Dermatopathol 6:123–129, 1984.

179. Goldenhersh MA, Olsen TC: Invasive squamous cell carcinoma initially diagnosed as giant keratoacanthoma. J Am Acad Dermatol 10:372–378, 1984.

180. Robins P, Albom MJ: Recurrent basal cell carcinoma in young woman. J Dermatol Surg Oncol. 1:49–51, 1975.

181. Marks R, Foley P, Goodman G, et al: Spontaneous remission of solar keratoses: the case for conservative management. Br J Dermatol 115:649–655, 1986.

182. Marks R, Rennie G, Selwood T: The relationship of basal cell carcinomas and squamous cell carcinomas to solar keratoses. Arch Dermatol 124:1039–1042, 1988.

183. Popkin GL: Curettage and electrodesiccation. NY State J Med 68:866–868, 1968.

184. Popkin GL, Bart RS: Excision versus curettage and electrodesiccation as dermatologic office procedures for the treatment of basal cell carcinomas. J Dermatol Surg Oncol 1:33–35, 1975.

185. Salasche SJ: Curettage and electrodesiccation in the treatment of midfacial basal cell epithelioma. J Am Acad Dermatol 8:496–503, 1983.

186. Zacarian SA: Cryosurgery for cancer of the skin. In: Zacarian SA (ed): Cryosurgery for Skin Cancer and Cutaneous Disorders. CV Mosby, St. Louis, 1985, pp 96–98.

187. Braun-Falco O, Lukacs S, Goldschmidt H: In: Dermatologic Radiotherapy. Springer-Verlag, New York, 1976, pp 69–111.

188. Gladstein AH, Kopf AW, Bart RS: Radiotherapy of cutaneous malignancies. In: Goldschmidt H (ed): Physical Modalities in Dermatologic Therapy, Radiotherapy, Electrosurgery, Phototherapy, Cryosurgery. Springer-Verlag, New York, 1978, pp 95–121.

189. Albom MJ: The management of recurrent basal cell carcinoma. Please no grafts or flaps at once. J Dermatol Surg Oncol 3:382–384, 1977.

190. Glass RL, Spratt JS, Perez-Mesa C: The fate of inadequately excised epidermoid carcinoma of the skin. Surg Gynecol Obstet 122:245–248, 1966.

191. Lawrence CM, Comaish JS, Dahl MGC: Excision of skin tumours without wound closure. Br J Dermatol 115:563–571, 1986.

192. Muscona R, Pnini A, Hirshowitz B: In favor of the healing by secondary intention after excision of medial canthal basal cell carcinoma. Plast Reconstr Surg 71:189–195, 1983.

193. Zitelli JA: Wound healing by secondary intention. J Am Acad Dermatol 9:407–415, 1983.

194. Albright SD: Placement of "guiding sutures" to counteract undesirable retraction of tissues in and around functionally and cosmetically important structures. J Dermatol Surg Oncol 7:446–449, 1981.

195. Lang PG Jr: The partial closure. J Dermatol Surg Oncol 11:966–969, 1985.

196. Knox JM, Freeman RG, Heaton CL: Curettage and electrodesiccation in the treatment of skin cancer. South Med J 55:1212–1215, 1962.

197. Kopf AW, Bart RS, Schrager D, et al: Curettage-electrodesic-

198. Tromovitch TA: Skin cancer treatment by curettage and desiccation. Calif Med 103:107, 1965.

199. Spiller WF, Spiller RF: Treatment of basal cell epithelioma by curettage and electrodesiccation. J Am Acad Dermatol 11:808–814, 1984.

200. Knox J, Lyles TW, Shapiro EM, et al: Curettage and electrodesiccation in the treatment of skin cancer. Arch Dermatol 82:197–204, 1960.

201. Dubin N, Kopf AW: Multivariate risk score for recurrence of cutaneous basal cell carcinomas. Arch Dermatol 119:373–377, 1983.

202. Williamson GS, Jackson R: Treatment of basal cell carcinoma by electrodesiccation and curettage. Can Med Assoc J 86:855–862, 1962.

203. Krull EA: The "little" curet. J Dermatol Surg Oncol 4:656–657, 1978.

204. Tromovitch TA: The C&D check for skin cancer. Cutis 11:210–212, 1973.

205. Cott RE, Wood MG, Johnson BL Jr: Use of curettage and shave excision in office practice. Microscopic confirmation of removal. J Am Acad Dermatol 16:1243–1251, 1987.

206. Brooks NA: Curettage and shave excision: a tissue saving technic for primary cutaneous carcinoma worthy of inclusion in graduate training programs. J Am Acad Dermatol 10:279–284, 1984.

207. Freeman RJ, Knox, JM, Heaton CL: The treatment of skin cancer. A statistical study of 1,341 skin tumors comparing results obtained with irradiation, surgery, and curettage followed by electrodesiccation. Cancer 17:535–538, 1964.

208. Chernosky ME: Squamous cell and basal cell carcinomas. Preliminary study of 3,817 primary skin cancers. South Med J 7:802–803, 1978.

209. Williamson GS, Jackson R: Treatment of squamous cell carcinoma of the skin by electrodesiccation and curettage. Can Med Assoc J 90:408–413, 1964.

210. Albright SD III: Treatment of skin cancer using multiple modalities. J Am Acad Dermatol 7:143–171, 1982.

211. Grande DJ, Whitaker DC, Koranda FC: Subdermal basal-cell carcinoma. J Dermatol Surg Oncol 8:779–781, 1982.

212. Bart RS, Schrager D, Kopf AW, et al: Scalpel excision of basal cell carcinomas. Arch Dermatol 114:739–742, 1978.

213. Menn H, Robins P, Kopf AW, et al: The recurrent basal cell epithelioma. A study of 100 cases of recurrent, retreated basal cell epitheliomas. Arch Dermatol 103:628–631, 1971.

214. Gross PA, Field LM: Cooperative frozen section surgery. J Dermatol Surg Oncol 13:1085–1088, 1987.

215. Schultz BC, Roenigk HH Jr: The double scalpel and double punch excision of skin tumors. J Am Acad Dermatol 7:495–499, 1982.

216. Braun M III: Being certain the cancer is out. J Dermatol Surg Oncol 13:1058–1060, 1987.

217. Hanke CW: Cooperative frozen section surgery in perspective. J Dermatol Surg Oncol 13:1065, 1987.

218. Thestrup-Pedersen K, Ravnborg L, Flemming R: Morbus Bowen. A description of the disease in 617 patients. Acta Dermatol Venereol 68:236–239, 1988.

219. Beirne GA, Beirne CG: Observations in the critical margin for the complete excision of carcinoma of the skin. Arch Dermatol 80:344–345, 1959.

220. Brodland DG: Surgical margins for excision of primary cutaneous squamous cell carcinoma. Presented at the Annual Meeting of the American Society for Dermatologic Surgery. Lake Buena Vista, FL, March 13–17, 1991.

221. Mohs FE: Carcinoma of the skin. A summary of therapeutic results. In: Chemosurgery—Microscopically Controlled Surgery for Skin Cancer. Charles C Thomas, Springfield, IL, 1978, pp 153–164.

222. Robins P: Chemosurgery: my 15 years of experience. J Dermatol Surg Oncol 7:779–789, 1981.

223. Tromovitch TA, Stegman SJ: Microscopic-controlled excision of cutaneous tumors. Chemosurgery fresh tissue technique. Cancer 41:653–658, 1978.

224. Tromovitch TA, Stegman SJ: Microscopically controlled excision of skin tumors. Chemosurgery (Mohs) fresh tissue technique. Arch Dermatol 110:231–232, 1974.

225. Cottel WI, Proper S: Mohs surgery fresh tissue technique. Our technique with a review. J Dermatol Surg Oncol 8:576–587, 1982.

226. Abide JM, Nahoi F, Bennett RG: The meaning of surgical margins. Plast Reconstr Surg 73:492–496, 1984.

227. Lang PG Jr, Osguthorpe JD: Mohs micrographic surgery of the head and neck: a multidisciplinary approach. Dermatol Clin 7, 1989.

228. Baker SR, Swanson NA, Grekin RC: An interdisciplinary approach to the management of basal cell carcinoma of the head and neck. J Dermatol Surg Oncol 13:1095–1106, 1987.

229. Riefkohl R, Pollack S, Gerogiade GS: A rationale for the treatment of difficult basal cell and squamous cell carcinoma of the skin. Ann Plast Surg 15:99–104, 1985.

230. Dzubow LM, Rigel DS, Robins P: Risk factors for local recurrence of primary cutaneous squamous cell carcinomas. Treatment by microscopically controlled excision. Arch Dermatol 118:900–902, 1982.

231. Zacarian SA: Cryogenics: the cryolesion and the pathogenesis of cryonecrosis. In: Zacarian SA (ed): Cryosurgery for Skin Cancer and Cutaneous Disorders. CV Mosby, St. Louis, 1985, pp 1–30.

232. Gage AA: Cryosurgery of advanced tumors of the head and neck. In: Zacarian SA (ed): Cryosurgery for Skin Cancer and Cutaneous Disorders. CV Mosby, St. Louis, 1985, pp 163–186.

233. Spiller WF, Spiller RF: Cryosurgery and adjuvant surgical techniques for cutaneous carcinomas. In: Zacarian SA (ed): Cryosurgery for Skin Cancer and Cutaneous Disorders. CV Mosby, St. Louis, 1985, pp 187–198.

234. Zacarian SA: Complications, indications and contraindications in cryosurgery. In: Zacarian SA (ed): Cryosurgery for Skin Cancer and Cutaneous Disorders. CV Mosby, St. Louis, 1985, pp 283–297.

235. Fraunfelder FT: Cryosurgery of eyelid, conjunctival and intraocular tumors. In: Zacarian SA (ed): Cryosurgery for Skin Cancer and Cutaneous Disorders. CV Mosby, St. Louis, 1985, pp 259–273.

236. Kuflik EG: Cryosurgery for carcinoma of the eyelids. A 12 year experience. J Dermatol Surg Oncol 11:243–246, 1985.

237. DeLanza MP, Ralfs I, Dawber R: Cryosurgery for Bowen's disease of the skin. Br J Dermatol 103S:14, 1980.

238. Holt PGA: Cryotherapy for skin cancer: results over a 5 year period using liquid nitrogen spray cryosurgery. Br J Dermatol 119:231–240, 1988.

239. Kingston TP, Hartley A, August PJ: Cryotherapy for skin cancer. Br J Dermatol 119S:39, 1988.

240. Graham GF: Statistical data on malignant tumors in cryosurgery: 1982. J Dermatol Surg Oncol 9:238–239, 1983.

241. Ebner H: Treatment of skin epitheliomas with 5-fluorouracil (5FU) ointment. Influence of therapeutic design on recurrence of tumor. Dermatologica 140S:42–46, 1970.

242. Epstein E: Fluorouracil paste treatment of basal cell carcinoma. Arch Dermatol 121:207–213, 1985.

243. Klostermann GG: Effects of 5-fluorouracil (5FU) ointment on normal and diseased skin. Histological findings and deep action. Dermatologica 140S:47–54, 1970.

244. Goette DK: Topical chemotherapy with 5-fluorouracil. A review. J Am Acad Dermatol 4:633–649, 1981.

245. Klein E, Stoll HL, Miller, et al: The effects of 5-fluorouracil (5FU) ointment in the treatment of neoplastic dermatoses. Dermatologica 140S:21–33, 1970.

246. Mohs FE, Jones DL, Bloom RF: Tendency of fluorouracil to conceal deep foci of invasive basal cell carcinoma. Arch Dermatol 114:1021–1022, 1978.

247. Klein E, Stoll HL Jr, Milgrom H, et al: Tumors of the skin. Topical 5-fluorouracil for epidermal neoplasms. J Surg Oncol 3:331–349, 1971.

248. Reyman F: A follow-up study of treatment of basal cell carcinoma with 5-fluorouracil ointment. Dermatologica 144:205–208, 1972.

249. Jansen GT: Use of topical fluorouracil. Arch Dermatol 119:784–785, 1983.

250. Sturm HM: Bowen's disease and 5-fluorouracil. J Am Acad Dermatol 1:513–522, 1979.

251. Goette DK, Odom RB: Allergic contact dermatitis to topical fluorouracil. Arch Dermatol 113:1058–1061, 1977.

252. Chahbazian CM, Brown GS: Radiation therapy for carcinoma of the skin of the face and neck. Special considerations. JAMA 244:1135–1137, 1980.

253. Chahbazian CM, Brown GS: Skin cancer. In: Gilbert HA (ed): Modern Radiation Oncology. Classic Literature and Current Management. Harper & Row, Philadelphia, 1984, pp 152–163.

254. Hunter RD: Skin. In: Easson EC, Pointon RCS (eds): The Radiotherapy of Malignant Disease. Springer-Verlag, New York, 1985, pp 135–151.

255. Brady LW, Binnick SA, Fitzpatrick PJ: Skin cancer. In: Perez CA, Brady LW (eds): Principles and Practice of Radiation Oncology. JB Lippincott, Philadelphia, 1987, pp 377–400.

256. Petrovich Z, Kuisk H, Langhilz B, et al: Treatment results and patterns of failure in 646 patients with carcinoma of the eyelids, pinna and nose. Am J Surg 154:447–450, 1987.

257. Helm F, Helm TN, Schwartz RA: Treatment of cutaneous cancers by radiotherapy. In: Schwartz RA (ed): Skin Cancer Recognition and Management. Springer-Verlag, New York, 1988, pp 353–362.

258. Miller RA, Spittle MF: Electron beam therapy for difficult cutaneous basal and squamous cell carcinomas. Br J Dermatol 106:429–436, 1982.

259. Hauss H, Proppe A, Goldschmidt H: Radiotherapy of lentigo malignant and Bowen's disease. In: Goldschmidt H (ed): Physical Modalities in Dermatology Therapy. Radiotherapy, Electrosurgery, Phototherapy, Cryosurgery. Springer-Verlag, New York, 1978, pp 122–138.

260. Stevens DM, Kopf AW, Gladstein A, et al: Treatment of Bowen's disease with grenz rays. Int J Dermatol 16:329–339, 1977.

261. Blank AA, Schnyder UW: Soft x-ray therapy in Bowen's disease and erythroplasia of Queyrat. Dermatologica 171:89–94, 1985.

262. Fishback AJ, Sause WT, Plenk HR: Radiation therapy for skin cancer. West J Med 133:379–382, 1980.

263. von Essen CF: Roentgen therapy of skin and lip carcinoma. Factors influencing success and failure. Am J Roentgenol 83:556–570, 1960.

264. Bailin PL, Ratz JL, Lutz-Nagey L: CO_2 laser modification of Mohs surgery. J Dermatol Surg Oncol 7:621–623, 1981.

265. Sacchini V, Loro GF, Avioli N: Carbon dioxide laser in scalp tumor surgery. Lasers Surg Med 4:261–269, 1984.

266. Wheeland RG, Bailin PL, Ratz JL, et al: Carbon dioxide laser vaporization and curettage in the treatment of large or multiple superficial basal cell carcinomas. J Dermatol Surg Oncol 13:119–125, 1987.

267. Landthaler M, Haina D, Brunner R, et al: Laser therapy of Bowenoid papulosis and Bowen's disease. J Dermatol Surg Oncol 12:1253–1257, 1986.

268. Brunner R, Landthaler M, Haina D, et al: Treatment of benign, semi-malignant and malignant skin tumors with the Nd:YAG laser. Lasers Surg Med 5:105–110, 1985.

269. Kozlov AP, Moskalek KG: Pulsed laser radiation therapy of skin tumors. Cancer 46:2172–2178, 1980.

270. Sawdrak WS, Weber PJ, Lowy DR, et al: Infectious papillomavirus in the vapor of warts treated with carbon dioxide laser or electrocoagulation. Detection and protection. J Am Acad Dermatol 21:41–49, 1990.

271. Smith JP, Moss E, Bryan GJ, et al: Evaluation of a smoke evacuator used for laser surgery. Lasers Surg Med 9:276–281, 1989.

272. Garden JM, O'Banion K, Stelnitz LS, et al: Papillomavirus in the vapor of carbon dioxide laser-treated verrucae. JAMA 259:1199–1202, 1988.

273. Tse DT, Keisten RC, Anderson RL: Hematoporphyrin-derivative photoradiation therapy in managing nevoid basal cell carcinoma syndrome. A preliminary report. Arch Ophthalmol 102:990–994, 1984.

274. Waldow SM, Lobraico RV, Kohler IK, et al: Photodynamic therapy for treatment of malignant cutaneous lesions. Lasers Surg Med 7:451–456, 1987.

275. Sacchini V, Melloni E, Marchesini R, et al: Preliminary clinical studies with PDT by topical TPPS. Administration in neoplastic skin lesions. Lasers Surg Med 7:6–11, 1987.

276. Berns MW, McCullough JL: Porphyrin sensitized phototherapy. Arch Dermatol 122:871–874, 1986.

277. Wooten RS, Smith KC, Ahlquist DA, et al: Prospective study

of cutaneous phototoxicity after systemic hematoporphyrin derivative. Lasers Surg Med 8:294–300, 1988.

278. Goldman L, Gregory RO, LaPlant M: Preliminary investigative studies with PDT in dermatologic and plastic surgery. Lasers Surg Med 5:453–456, 1985.

279. Oseroff AR, Ohuoha D, Ara G, et al: Selective photochemotherapy of melanoma and human squamous cell carcinoma using cationic photosensitizers. Clin Res 35:708A, 1987.

280. Robinson PJ, Carruth JAS, Fairris GM: Photodynamic therapy: a better treatment for widespread Bowen's disease. Br J Dermatol 119:59–61, 1988.

281. Blanchet-Bardon C, Ruissant A, Lutzner M, et al: Interferon treatment of skin cancer in patients with epidermodysplasia verruciformis. Lancet 1:274, 1981.

282. Berman B, Whiting DA, Edwards L, et al: Efficacy of interferon alpha–2b for cutaneous squamous cell carcinoma. J Invest Dermatol 93:541, 1989.

283. Wickramasinghe L, Hindson TC, Wacks H: Treatment of neoplastic skin lesions with intralesional interferon. J Am Acad Dermatol 20:71–74, 1989.

284. Agani JA, Burgess MA: Multiple squamous cell carcinomas treated with intraarterial cisplatin in a patient with rheumatoid arthritis. Cancer Treat Rep 66:1987–1989, 1982.

285. Tanigaki T, Endo H: A case of squamous cell carcinoma treated by intralesional injection of oil bleomycin. Dermatologica 170:302–305, 1985.

286. Guthrie TH Jr, McElveen LJ, Porubsky ES, et al: Cisplatin and doxorubicin. An effective chemotherapy combination in the treatment of advanced basal cell and squamous cell carcinoma of the skin. Cancer 55:1629–1632, 1985.

287. Khansur T, Kennedy A: Cisplatin and 5-fluorouracil for advanced locoregional and metastatic squamous cell carcinoma of the skin. Cancer 67:2030–2032, 1991.

288. Kraemer KH, DiGiovanna JJ, Moshell AN, et al: Prevention of skin cancer in xeroderma pigmentosum with the use of oral isotretinoin. N Engl J Med 318:1633–1637, 1988.

289. Peck GL: Long term retinoid therapy is needed for maintenance of cancer chemopreventive effect. Dermatologica 175S:138–144, 1987.

290. Lippman SM, Kessler JF, Meyskins FL Jr: Retinoids as preventive and therapeutic anticancer agents (part II). Cancer Treat Rep 71:493–515, 1987.

291. Lippman SM, Meyskins FL Jr: Treatment of advanced squamous cell carcinoma of the skin with isotretinoin. Ann Intern Med 107:499–501, 1987.

292. Levine N, Miller RC, Meyskins FL Jr: Oral isotretinoin therapy. Use in a patient with multiple cutaneous squamous cell carcinoma and keratoacanthomas. Arch Dermatol 120:1215–1217, 1984.

293. Haydey RP, Reed ML, Dzubow LM, et al: Treatment of keratoacanthomas with oral 13-cis retinoic acid. N Engl J Med 303:560–562, 1980.

294. Robins P, Dzubow LM, Rigel DS: Squamous cell carcinoma treated by Mohs surgery. An experience with 414 cases in a period of 15 years. J Dermatol Surg Oncol 7:800–801, 1981.

295. Howe NR, Lang PG Jr: Squamous cell carcinoma presenting as subcutaneous nodules. J Dermatol Surg Oncol 17:779–783, 1991.

296. Gottlieb B, Newman BA: Bowenoid squamous cell carcinoma of the digits. Cutis 16:108–112, 1975.

297. Graham JH, Helwig EB: Bowen's disease and its relationship to systemic cancer. Arch Dermatol 80:133–159, 1959.

298. Kao GE: Carcinoma arising in Bowen's disease. Arch Dermatol 122:1124–1126, 1986.

299. Peterka ES, Lynch FW, Goltz RW: An association between Bowen's disease and internal cancer. Arch Dermatol 84:139–145, 1961.

300. Miki Y, Kawatsu T, Matsuda K, et al: Cutaneous and pulmonary cancers associated with Bowen's disease. J Am Acad Dermatol 6:26–31, 1982.

301. Graham J, Mazzante GR, Helwig EB: Chemistry of Bowen's disease. Relationship to arsenic. J Invest Dermatol 37:317–332, 1961.

302. Callen JP, Headington J: Bowen's and non-Bowen's squamous, intraepidermal neoplasia of the skin. Relationship to internal malignancy. Arch Dermatol 116:422–426, 1980.

303. Reymann F, Ravnborg L, Schau G, et al: Bowen's disease and internal malignant diseases. A study of 581 patients. Arch Dermatol 124:677–679, 1988.

304. Moller R, Nielsen A, Reymann F, et al: Squamous cell carcinoma of the skin and internal malignant neoplasms. Arch Dermatol 115:314–315, 1979.

305. Moller R, Nielsen A, Reymann F: Multiple basal cell carcinoma and internal malignant tumors. Arch Dermatol 111:584–585, 1975.

306. Andersen SLC, Nielsen A, Reymann F: Relationship between Bowen's disease and internal malignant tumors. Arch Dermatol 108:367–370, 1973.

307. Arbesman H, Ramshohoff DF: Is Bowen's disease a prediction for the development of internal malignancy? A methodological critique of the literature. JAMA 257:516–518, 1987.

308. Callen JP: Bowen's disease and internal malignant disease. Arch Dermatol 124:675–676, 1988.

309. King CM, Yates VM, Dare VK: Multicentric pigmented Bowen's disease of the genitalia associated with carcinoma in situ of the cervix. Br J Vener Dis 60:406–408, 1984.

310. Eliezri YD, Silverstein SJ, Nuevo GJ: Occurrence of human papilloma virus type 16 DNA in cutaneous squamous and basal cell neoplasms. J Am Acad Dermatol 23:836–842, 1990.

311. Ostrow RS, Shaver K, Turnquist S, et al: Human papillomavirus–16 DNA in a cutaneous invasive cancer. Arch Dermatol 125:666–669.

312. Cobb MW: Human papilloma virus infection. J Am Acad Dermatol 22:547–566, 1990.

313. Kawashima M, Jablonska S, Favre M, et al: Characterization of a new type of human papillomavirus found on a lesion of Bowen's disease of the skin. J Virol 57:688–692, 1986.

314. Abell MR, Gosling JRG: Intraepithelial and infiltrative carcinoma of vulva: Bowen's type. Cancer 14:318–329, 1961

315. Durst M, Gissmann L, Ikenberg H, et al: A papillomavirus DNA from a cervical carcinoma and its prevalence in cancer biopsy samples from different geographic regions. Proc Natl Acad Sci 80:3812–3815, 1983.

316. Ikenberg H, Gissmann L, Gross G, et al: Human papillomavirus type–16 related DNA in genital Bowen's disease and Bowenoid papulosis. Int J Cancer 32:563–565, 1983.

317. Crum CP, Mitao M, Levine RU, et al: Cervical papilloma viruses segregate within morphologically distinct precancerous lesions. J Virol 54:675–681, 1985.

318. Lorincz AT, Temple GF, Kukeman RT, et al: Oncogenic association of specific human papillomavirus types with cervical neoplasia. J Natl Cancer Inst 79:671–677, 1987.

319. DiLuca D, Pilotti S, Steffanon B, et al: Human papillomavirus type 16 DNA in genital tumors: a pathological and molecular analysis. J Gen Virol 67:583–589, 1986.

320. ZurHausen H: Papillomaviruses in human cancer. Cancer 59:1692–1696, 1987.

321. Noumoff JS, Farber M: Tumors of the vulva. Int J Dermatol 25:552–563, 1986.

322. Woodruff JD: Carcinoma in situ of the vulva. Clin Obstet Gynecol 28:230–239, 1985.

323. Obalek S, Jablonska S, Beaudenon S, et al: Bowenoid papulosis of the male and female genitalia. Risk of cervical neoplasia. J Am Acad Dermatol 14:433–444, 1986.

324. Macnab JCM, Walkenshaw SA, Cordiner JW, et al: Human papillomavirus in clinically and histologically normal tissue of patients with genital cancer. N Engl J Med 315:1052–1058, 1986.

325. Halpert R, Butt KMH, Sedles A, et al: Human papillomavirus infection and lower genital neoplasia in female renal allograft recipients. Transplant Proc 17:93–95, 1985.

326. Buscema J, Woodruff JD, Parmley TH, et al: Carcinoma in situ of the vulva. Obstet Gynecol 55:225–230, 1980.

327. Sutton GP, Stehman FB, Ehrlich CE, et al: Human papillomavirus deoxyribonucleic acid in lesions of the female genital tract. Evidence for type 6/11 in squamous carcinoma of the vulva. Obstet Gynecol 70:564–568, 1987.

328. Kawashima M, Farre M, Obalek S, et al: Premalignant lesions and cancers of the skin in the general population: evaluation of the role of human papillomavirus. J Invest Dermatol 95:537–549, 1990.

329. Baggish MS, Dorsey JH: CO_2 laser for the treatment of vulvar carcinoma in situ. Obstet Gynecol 57:371–375, 1981.

330. Kraus FT, Perez-Mesa C: Verrucous carcinoma. Clinical and pathologic study of 105 cases involving the oral cavity, larynx and genitalia. Cancer 19:26–38, 1966.

331. Demian SDE, Bushken FL, Echevarria RA: Perineural invasion and anaplastic transformation of verrucous carcinoma. Cancer 32:395–401, 1973.

332. Schwartz RA: Buschke-Lowenstein tumor. Verrucous carcinoma of the penis. J Am Acad Dermatol 23:723–727, 1990.

333. Okgagake T, Clark BA, Zachow KR, et al: Presence of human papillomavirus in verrucous carcinoma (Ackerman) of the vagina. Immunocytochemical ultrastructural, and DNA hybridization studies. Arch Pathol Lab Med 108:567–570, 1984.

334. Abramson AL, Brandsma J, Steinberg B, et al: Verrucous carcinoma of the larynx. Possible human papillomavirus etiology. Arch Otolaryngol 111:709–715, 1985.

335. Mikhail GR: Cancers, precancers, and pseudocancers on the male genitalia. A review of clinical appearances, histopathology, and management. J Dermatol Surg Oncol 6:1027–1035, 1980.

336. Mohs FE, Sahl WJ: Chemosurgery for verrucous carcinoma. J Dermatol Surg Oncol 5:302–306, 1979.

337. Kao GF, Graham JH, Helwig EB: Carcinoma cuniculatum (verrucous carcinoma of the skin). A clinicopathologic study of 46 cases with ultrastructural observations. Cancer 49:2395–2403, 1982.

338. Perez CA, Kraus FF, Evans JC, et al: Anaplastic transformation in verrucous carcinoma of the oral cavity after radiation therapy. Radiology 86:108–115, 1966.

339. Nguyen KQ, McMarlin SL: Verrucous carcinoma of the face. Arch Dermatol 120:383–385, 1984.

340. Coldiron BM, Brown FC, Freeman RG: Epithelioma cuniculatum (carcinoma cuniculatum) of the thumb. A case report and literature review. J Dermatol Surg Oncol 12:1150–1154, 1986.

341. Brownstein MH, Shapiro L: Verrucous carcinoma of the skin: epithelioma cuniculatum plantare. Cancer 38:1710–1716, 1976.

342. Balazs M: Busche-Lowenstein tumor. A histologic and ultrastructural study of six cases. Virchows Arch A 410:83–92, 1986.

343. Proffitt SD, Spooner TR, Kosek JC: Origin of undifferentiated neoplasm for verrucous epidermal carcinoma of oral cavity following irradiation. Cancer 26:389–393, 1970.

344. Duthie MB, Gupta NK, Pointon RCS: Head and neck. In: Easson EC, Pointon RCS (eds): The Radiotherapy of Malignant Disease. Springer-Verlag, New York, 1978, pp 153–214.

345. Wade TR, Kopf AW, Ackerman AB: Bowenoid papulosis of the penis. Cancer 42:1890–1903, 1978,

346. Wade TR, Kopf AW, Ackerman AB: Bowenoid papulosis of the genitalia. Arch Dermatol 115:306–308, 1979.

347. Emmerson RW: Multicentric pigmented Bowen's disease of the perineum. Proc R Soc Med 68:345–346, 1975.

348. Lloyd KM: Multicentric pigmented Bowen's disease of the groin. Arch Dermatol 101:48–51, 1970.

349. Berger BW, Hori Y: Multicentric Bowen's disease of the genitalia: spontaneous regression of lesions. Arch Dermatol 114:1698–1699, 1978.

350. Guillet GY, Barun L, Masse R, et al: Bowenoid papulosis: demonstration of human papillomavirus (HPV) with anti-HPV immune serum. Arch Dermatol 120:514–516, 1984.

351. Gross G, Hagedorn M, Ikenberg H, et al: Bowenoid papulosis. presence of human papillomavirus (HPV) structural antigens and of HPV 16 related DNA sequences. Arch Dermatol 121:858–863, 1985.

352. Stone MS, Noonan CA, Tschen J, et al: Bowen's disease of the feet: presence of human papillomavirus 16 DNA in tumor tissue. Arch Dermatol 123:1517–1520, 1987.

353. Abdennader S, Lessana-Leibowitch M, Pelisse M: An atypical case of penile carcinoma in situ associated with human papillomavirus DNA type 18. J Am Acad Dermatol 20:887–889, 1989.

354. Kimura S, Hirac A, Harada R, et al: So-called multicentric pigmented Bowen's disease: report of a case and a possible etiologic role of human papillomavirus. Dermatologica 157:229–237, 1978.

355. Patterson JW, Kao GF, Graham JH, et al: Bowenoid papulosis: a clinicopathologic study with ultrastructural observations. Cancer 57:832–836, 1986.

356. Skinner MS, Steinberg WH, Ichinose H, et al: Spontaneous regression of Bowenoid atypia of the vulva. Obstet Gynecol 42:40–46, 1973.

357. Halasz C, Silvers D, Crum CP: Bowenoid papulosis in a three year old girl. J Am Acad Dermatol 14:326–330, 1986.

358. Friedrich EG: Reversible vulvar atypia. A case report. Obstet Gynecol 39:173–181, 1972.

359. Obalalak S, Jablonska S, Orth G: HPV-associated intraepithelial neoplasia of the external genitalia. Clin Dermatol 3:104–113, 1985.

360. DeVillez RL, Stevens CS: Bowenoid papules of the genitalia: a case progressing to Bowen's disease. J Am Acad Dermatol 3:149–152, 1980.

361. Feldman SB, Sexton FM, Glenn JD, et al: Immunosuppression in men with bowenoid papulosis. Arch Dermatol 125:651–654, 1989.

362. Richart RM: Causes and management of cervical intraepithelial neoplasia. Cancer 60:1951–1959, 1987.

363. Brownstein MH, Rabinowitz AD: The precursors of cutaneous squamous cell carcinoma. Int J Dermatol 18:1–16, 1979.

364. Schwartz RA, Janniger CK: Bowenoid papulosis. J Am Acad Dermatol 24:261–264, 1991.

365. Gross G, Roussaki A, Papendick U: Efficacy of interferons on bowenoid papulosis and other precancerous lesions. J Invest Dermatol 95:1525–1575, 1990.

366. Queyrat L: Erythroplasie du gland. Bull Soc Fr Dermatol Syph 22:378–382, 1911.

367. Graham JH, Helwig EB: Erythroplasia of Queyrat: a clinico-pathologic and histochemical study. Cancer 32:1396–1414, 1973.

368. Bernstein G, Forgaard DM, Miller JE: Carcinoma in situ of the glans penis and distal urethra. J Dermatol Surg Oncol 12:450–455, 1986.

369. Blau S, Hyman AB: Erythroplasia of Queyrat. Acta Dermatol Venerol 35:341–378, 1955.

370. Williamson JJ: Erythroplasia of Queyrat of the buccal mucous membrane. Oral Surg Med Pathol 17:308–318, 1964.

371. Gorlin RJ: Bowen's disease of the mucous membrane of the mouth: a review of the literature and a presentation of six cases. Oral Surg Med Pathol 3:35–51, 1950.

372. Dixon RS, Mikhail GR: Erythroplasia (Queyrat) of conjunctiva. J Am Acad Dermatol 4:160–165, 1981.

373. Goette DK, Carson TE: Erythroplasia of Queyrat: treatment with topical 5-fluorouracil. Cancer 38:1498–1502, 1976.

374. Milstein HG: Erythroplasia of Queyrat in a partially circumcised man. J Am Acad Dermatol 6:398, 1982.

375. Sonnex TS, Ralfs IG, Plaza de Lanza M, et al: Treatment of erythroplasia of Queyrat with liquid nitrogen cryosurgery. Br J Dermatol 106:581–584, 1982.

376. Rosenberg SK, Fuller TA: Carbon dioxide rapid superpulsed laser treatment of erythroplasia of Queyrat. Urology 16:181–182, 1980.

377. Moy RL, Eliezri YD, Nuovo GJ, et al: Human papillomavirus type 16 DNA in periungual squamous cell carcinomas. JAMA 261:2669–2673, 1989.

378. Dietman DF: Bowen's disease of the nailbed. Arch Dermatol 108:577–578, 1973.

379. Mikhail GR: Bowen's disease and squamous cell carcinoma of the nail bed. Arch Dermatol 110:267–270, 1974.

380. Guitart J, Bergfeld WF, Tuthill RJ, et al: Squamous cell carcinoma of the nailbed: a clinicopathological study of 12 cases. Br J Dermatol 123:215–222, 1990.

381. Mikhail GR: Subungual epidermoid carcinoma J Am Acad Dermatol 11:291–298, 1984.

382. Baran RL, Gormley DE: Polydactylous Bowen's disease of the nail. J Am Acad Dermatol 17:201–204, 1987.

383. Attiyeh FF, Shah J, Booker RJ, et al: Subungual squamous cell carcinoma. JAMA 241:262–263, 1979.

384. Inlow PM: Cancer of the nailbed. JAMA 241:239, 1979.

385. Brown MD, Zachary CB, Grekin RC, et al: Penile tumors: their management by Mohs micrographic surgery. J Dermatol Surg Oncol 13:1163–1167, 1987.

386. Bissada NK, Morcos RR, El-Snorissi M: Postcircumcision carcinoma of the penis. I. Clinical aspects. J Urol 135:283–285, 1986

387. Onuigbo WIB: Carcinoma of skin of penis. Br J Urol 57:465–466, 1985.

388. Villa LL, Lopes A: Human papillomavirus DNA sequences in penile carcinoma in Brazil. Int J Cancer 37:853–855, 1986.

389. Barrasso R, DeBrux J, Croissant O, et al: High prevalence of papillomavirus-associated penile intraepithelial neoplasia in sexual partners of women with cervical intraepithelial neoplasia. N Engl J Med 307:916–923, 1987.

390. Boshart M, Gissmann L, Ikenberg H, et al: A new type of

papilloma-virus DNA: its presence in genital cancer biopsies and in cell lining derived from cervical cancer. EMBO J 3:1151–1157, 1984.

391. Rhatigan RM, Jimenez S, Chopskie EJ: Condyloma acuminata and carcinoma of the penis. South Med J 65:423–428, 1972.

392. McCance DJ, Kalache A, Ashdown K, et al: Human papillomavirus types 16 and 18 in carcinoma of the penis from Brazil. Int J Cancer 37:55–59, 1986.

393. Kovi J, Tillman L, Lee SM: Malignant transformation of condyloma acuminatum. A light microscopic and ultrastructural study. Am J Clin Pathol 61:702–710, 1974.

394. deKernion JB: The case for partial penectomy in the treatment of localized carcinoma of the penis. In: Carlton CE Jr (ed): Controversies in Urology. Year Book Medical, Chicago, 1989, pp 305–307.

395. Das S, Crawford ED: Carcinoma of the penis: management of the primary. In: Crawford ED, Das S (eds): Current Genitourinary Cancer Surgery. Lea & Febiger, Philadelphia, 1990, pp 367–372.

396. Nelson RP, Derrick FC, Allen WR: Epidermoid carcinoma of the penis. Br J Urol 54:172–175, 1982.

397. Fraley EE, Zhang G, Sazama R, et al: Cancer of the penis: prognosis and treatment plans. Cancer 55:1618–1624, 1985.

398. Wells AD, Pryor JP: Radiation induced carcinoma of the penis. Br J Urol 58:325–326, 1986.

399. Ash DV: The case for primary radiotherapy in the treatment of localized carcinoma of the penis. In: Carlton CE Jr (ed): Controversies in Urology. Year Book Medical, Chicago, 1989, pp 307–310.

400. Mohs FE, Snow SN, Mossing EM, et al: Microscopically controlled surgery in the treatment of carcinoma of the penis. J Urol 133:961–966, 1985.

401. Madej G, Meyza J: Cryosurgery of penile carcinoma. Oncology 39:350–352, 1982.

402. Cabanas RM: An approach to the treatment of penile carcinoma. Cancer 39:456–466, 1977.

403. Scappini P, Piscioli F, Pasio T, et al: Penile cancer: aspiration biopsy cytology for staging. Cancer 58:1526–1533, 1986.

404. Richie JP: Delayed inguinal lymphadenectomy in the management of carcinoma of the penis. In: Carlton CE Jr (ed): Controversies in Urology. Year Book Medical, Chicago, 1989, pp 314–316.

405. Das S, Crawford ED: Carcinoma of the penis: management of the regional lymphatic drainage. In: Crawford ED, Das S (eds): Current Genitourinary Cancer Surgery. Lea & Febiger, Philadelphia, 1990.

406. Catalano WJ: Lymphadectomy in the management of carcinoma of the penis. In: Carlton CE Jr (ed): Controversies in Urology. Year Book Medical, Chicago, 1989, pp 311–314.

407. Townsend DE, Levine RU, Richart RM, et al: Management of vulvar intraepithelial neoplasia by carbon dioxide laser. Obstet Gynecol 60:49–52, 1982.

408. Albright TM, Stehman FB, Roth LM, et al: Bowenoid dysplasia of the vulva. Cancer 50:2910–2919, 1982.

409. Lynch PJ: Condylomata acuminata (anogenital warts). Clin Obstet Gynecol 28:142–151, 1985.

410. Hart WR, Norris HJ, Helwig EB: Relation of lichen sclerosis et atrophicus of the vulva to development of carcinoma. Obstet Gynecol 45:369–377, 1975.

411. Crum CP, Liskow A, Petras P, et al: Vulva and intraepithelial neoplasm (severe atypia and carcinoma in situ): a clinicopathologic analysis of 41 cases. Cancer 54:1429–1434, 1984.

412. Reid R: Superficial laser vulvectomy: a new surgical technique for appendage-conserving ablation of refractory condylomas and vulvar intraepithelial neoplasia. Br J Obstet Gynecol 152:504–509, 1985.

413. Eliezri YD: The toluidine blue test: an aid in the diagnosis and treatment of early squamous cell carcinomas of mucous membranes. J Am Acad Dermatol 18:1339–1349, 1988.

414. Baker EJ, Hobbs ER: Enhancement of the clinical margins of Bowen's disease by acetowhitening. J Dermatol Surg Oncol 16:846–850, 1990.

415. Sillman FH, Boyce JG, Macasaet MA, et al: 5 Fluorouracil chemosurgery for intraepithelial neoplasia of the lower genital tract. Obstet Gynecol 58:356–360, 1981.

416. Kaufman RH, Friedrich EG: The carbon dioxide laser in the treatment of vulvar disease. Clin Obstet Gynecol 28:220–229, 1985.

417. DiSara P: Management of superficially invasive vulva carcinoma. Clin Obstet Gynecol 28:196–203, 1985.

418. Iversen T: New approaches to treatment of squamous cell carcinoma of the vulva. Clin Obstet Gynecol 28:204–210, 1985.

419. Wilkerson EJ: Superficial invasive carcinoma of the vulva. Clin Obstet Gynecol 28:188–195, 1985.

420. Barnes AE, Crissman JD, Schellhas HF, et al: Microinvasive carcinoma of the vulva: a clinicopathologic evaluation. Obstet Gynecol 56:234–238, 1980.

421. Dvoretsky PM, Bonfiglio TA, Helmkamp BF, et al: The pathology of superficially invasive thin vulvar squamous cell carcinoma. Int J Gynecol Pathol 3:331–342, 1984.

422. Hussein Zadeh N, Zaino R, Nahhas WA, et al: The significance of histologic findings in predicting nodal metastases in invasive squamous cell carcinoma of the vulva. Gynecol Oncol 16:105–111, 1983.

423. Andreasson B, Nyboe J: Predictive factors with reference to low-risk of metastases in squamous cell carcinoma in the vulvar region. Gynecol Oncol 21:196–206, 1985.

424. Mohs FE: Carcinoma of the vulva. In: Chemosurgery—Microscopically Controlled Surgery for Skin Cancer. Charles C Thomas, Springfield, IL, 1978, pp 215–222.

425. Batsakos JG: Squamous cell carcinomas of the oral cavity and the oropharynx. In: Tumors of the Head and Neck. Clinical and Pathological Considerations. Williams & Wilkins, Baltimore, 1979, pp 149–152.

426. Schwarz H II, Lesser JC: Cancer of the lip: Control of the primary lesion. Mo Med 51:355–359, 1954.

427. Mohs FE: Carcinoma of the lips. In: Chemosurgery—Microscopically Controlled Surgery for Skin Cancer. Charles C Thomas, Springfield, IL, 1978, pp 165–178.

428. Berktold RE: Carcinoma of the oral cavity. Selective management according to site and stage. Otolaryngol Clin North Am 18:445–450, 1985.

429. Baker SR, Krause CJ: Carcinoma of the lip. Laryngoscope 90:19–27, 1980.

430. Mehregan DA, Roenigk RK: Management of superficial squamous cell carcinoma of the lip with Mohs micrographic surgery. Cancer 66:463–468, 1990.

431. Stanley RJ, Roenigk RK: Actinic cheilitis. Treatment with the carbon dioxide laser. Mayo Clin Proc 63:23–25, 1988.

432. DuFresne RG Jr, Garrett AB, Bailin PL, et al: Carbon dioxide laser treatment of chronic actinic cheilitis. J Am Acad Dermatol 19:876–878, 1988.

433. Whitaker DC: Microscopically proven cure of actinic cheilitis by CO_2 laser. Lasers Surg Med 7:520–523, 1987.

CHAPTER 58

Use of Retinoids and Vitamin A in Cutaneous Oncology

JON C. STARR and RONALD G. WHEELAND

Even though the ancient Egyptians recognized the existence of a substance for the treatment of night blindness, it was not until the early 1900s that vitamin A, a fat-soluble extract, was isolated from egg yolk, butter fat, and fish oils.[1-3] Initially called fat-soluble A, the name was later changed to vitamin A.[3] The structure of vitamin A was first defined in 1931, and its synthesis was accomplished in 1937.[4]

The modern clinical significance of vitamin A and its role in cancer treatment began in 1926 when vitamin A deprivation was noted to be associated with gastric carcinoma.[5] During the ensuing years, many investigators reported the beneficial effects of vitamin A in the treatment of skin diseases secondary to abnormal keratinization[6-8] and chemically induced tumors.[9] Clinical applicability, however, was somewhat limited because of the severe toxicity produced when vitamin A was administered in therapeutic doses. Consequently, it was not until the development of vitamin A analogs, which demonstrated reduced toxicity while maintaining therapeutic effects, that the evolution of retinoid therapy truly began. Since the mid–1960s, more than 2000 retinoid compounds have been synthesized.[10] Clinically, the most important of these are all-*trans*-retinoic acid (tretinoin); 13-*cis*-retinoic acid (isotretinoin); the aromatic derivative etretinate and its metabolite, motretinid, and the third-generation arotinoids.

Chemical Interaction and Biologic Role

Physiologically, vitamin A (retinol) may act directly or indirectly to effect a cellular response. Indirectly, it can be oxidized to retinoic acid or, in a reversible oxidative process, converted into the aldehyde, retinal. These compounds are exceedingly important for vision and reproduction, as well as for the promotion of cell growth and differentiation.

Vitamin A is the prototype compound for retinoids, a term used to describe synthetic vitamin A analogs. The basic structure of retinol consists of a cyclic end group with a polyene side chain having a polar end group (Fig. 58–1). All retinoids represent basic modifications of this compound.

The first-generation retinoids, represented by tretinoin and isotretinoin, resulted from modification of the polar end group and polyene side chain. The second-generation aromatic retinoids, represented by etretinate, are derived from modification of the cyclic end group. The third-generation retinoids were created by cyclization of the polyene side chain and are represented by arotinoid, a potent derivative without significant additional toxicity.

Characterization of the biologic activity of the recently synthesized retinoids is based on several screening assays. For example, in the tumor-promotion assay, biologically active retinoids are noted to reverse or block the development of tumors on mouse skin that were induced by tumor promotors such as 7,12-dimethylbenz[a]-anthracene (DMBA), croton oil, or 12-O-tetradecanoylphorbol–13-acetate (TPA).[10, 11] Similarly, retinoids can also be assayed for their ability to induce differentiation in neoplastic tissue cultures.[12, 13] Another group of assays studies ornithine decarboxylase (ODC), an enzyme that increases its activity early in cellular hyperproliferation.[14] ODC activity can be experimentally increased either by chemical promotors, such as TPA, or by repetitive trauma, such as tape stripping. The ability of a retinoid to inhibit ODC induction has been shown to correlate with its biologic activity.[14, 15]

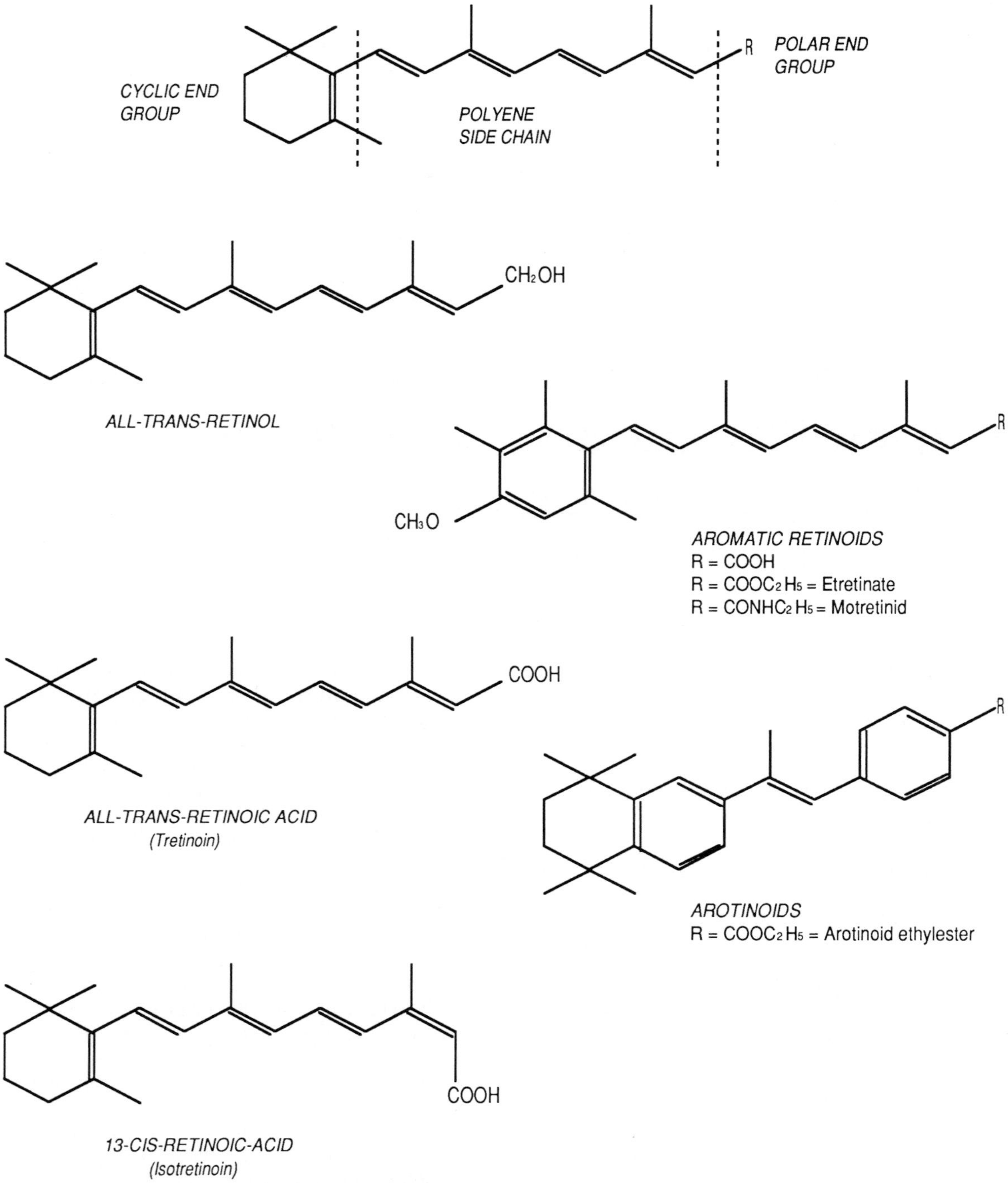

Figure 58–1. Chemical structures of the common retinoids.

While these screening tests are very effective, additional assays must be developed to identify other potentially effective retinoids.

Metabolism

It is necessary to discuss the metabolism of vitamin A and the retinoids to understand why these compounds demonstrate substantial differences in their efficacy. Two dietary sources contribute to vitamin A stores[16]: the carotenoids, found in plants and characterized primarily by the red and yellow pigments of β-carotene; and vitamin A, or retinol, found in milk, eggs, and meat. Absorption of both β-carotene and retinol is dependent on the presence of micelles in the intestinal lumen. At the gastrointestinal mucosa, β-carotene is cleaved and reduced to retinol (Fig. 58–2). Retinol is subsequently transported to the liver via chylomicrons after esterification to long-chain fatty acids. Hepatic Ito "fat cells" store retinol and regulate its release to maintain constant circulating serum levels. On release,

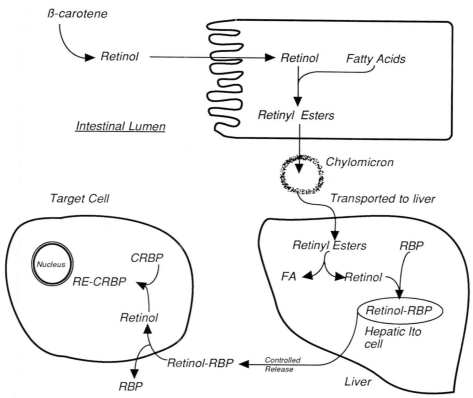

Figure 58–2. Absorption and transport of β-carotene and retinol. CRBP, Cellular retinol-binding protein; FA, fatty acid; RBP, retinol-binding protein; RE, retinoid.

retinol is bound to hepatic retinol-binding protein (RBP) for delivery to target tissues. Retinoids, on the other hand, are not stored in the liver and are not under the same physiologic control as their natural precursors. As a consequence, the tissue levels of retinoids are directly influenced by the dosing regimen.

Mechanisms of Retinoid Action in Malignancy

There are a number of hypotheses that attempt to explain the mechanism of action of retinoids in cancer, and the most promising theoretic mechanisms can be both supported and contradicted by published research. The following information should be considered only an introduction to these concepts. No attempt is made to support or discredit any of these theories, but instead they are discussed to demonstrate the array of possibilities that exist. Subjects for consideration include the effects of retinoids on (1) membrane structure regulation, (2) immune modulation, (3) enzyme system control, and (4) the steroid hormonal model.

MEMBRANE EFFECTS

One active area of research seeks to understand the effect of retinoids on gap junction density. Gap junctions, or nexi, are important structures for cell-to-cell communication. Current hypotheses relevant to cell

communication suggest that gap junctions can transmit growth-controlling signals.[17] Transformed cells have been shown to have reduced densities of gap junctions[18] and to communicate poorly with nontransformed cells.[19] Administration of retinoids has been shown to both significantly increase the number of gap junctions[20, 21] and enhance communication through these nexi.[19] This improvement in communication may in turn promote exchange of messages critical to the suppression of transformed cells.

Another possible mechanism of retinoids' influence on malignancy relates to retinoid-induced changes in membrane glycoconjugates.[22] It appears that once a retinoid is phosphorylated by phosphokinase, it may accept and transfer an oligosaccharide to a membrane glycoprotein.[23] Modifications of this type are known to affect those cell functions related to adhesion, contact inhibition, migration, differentiation, and growth.[10] Enhanced control of these functions through the action of the retinoids could limit the expression of malignant tissues.

Retinoids have also been hypothesized to have an effect on membrane surface fibronectin. Previous studies have shown that carcinogenesis induced by TPA is associated with a reduction in membrane fibronectin content.[24] Retinoic acid, however, inhibits the TPA-induced release of fibronectin.[25] Consequently, any tissue that requires fibronectin release for the expression of malignant change would be effectively suppressed by the administration of retinoids.

IMMUNE MODULATION

Retinoids may also influence the immunologic system in a variety of ways. For example, in physiologic doses, retinoids have been shown to stimulate killer T-cell induction.[26] This may be related to the retinoid-induced helper T-cell release of interleukin–2.[27] Additionally, retinoids are also known to inhibit prostaglandin synthesis,[28] which may improve macrophage function that is normally inhibited by prostaglandins. These immunopotentiating effects may be advantageous in the management of some cancer patients through enhanced immune responsiveness to tumors to which these patients are susceptible.

ENZYMATIC EFFECTS

Another hypothetical effect of retinoids in oncology relates to the inhibition of ODC. ODC is the rate-limiting enzyme in the production of polyamines, which control the synthesis of nucleic acids and proteins involved in cell proliferation and differentiation.[29] During carcinogenesis, it has been shown that ODC activity is increased,[30] but because retinoids inhibit ODC, this may be a key factor in retinoid-induced differentiation.[10] The site of retinoid action is not yet clear, but recent evidence demonstrates that retinoid-induced ODC inhibition is preceded by a reduction in ODC messenger RNA (mRNA) production.[31] Whether this inhibition is mediated at the genomic level or is dependent on a second messenger is not known.

Additionally, retinoids have been implicated in the control of many other enzyme systems, including cyclic adenosine monophosphate (cAMP), alkaline phosphatase, 2'-5'-oligoadenylate synthetase, cytochrome P-450 isoenzymes, and glutathione reductase. In each of these systems, retinoids appear to act in a manner consistent with their anticarcinogenic activity.[10]

Retinoids have recently been shown to inhibit protein kinase-C (PKC), a cell surface enzyme that acts in carcinogenesis via a transduction pathway.[32] PKC is known to activate ODC, increasing polyamine synthesis and enhancing malignant transformation. Retinoids, when bound to cellular retinoic acid–binding protein (CRABP), inhibit PKC activity[33] and thereby prevent the expression of ODC. Several enzyme systems that have a recognized role in carcinogenesis are associated with the PKC cascade and are also inhibited by the administration of retinoids,[32] which thus further inhibit malignant transformation. In fact, it has been suggested that PKC inhibition may be a unifying factor, possibly affecting all of the systems implicated in retinoid activity.[34]

ONCOGENE SUPPRESSION

DNA sequences that code for specific transforming polypeptides known to cause malignant changes are known as oncogenes.[35] Normally, these genes are suppressed by the repressor systems of the cell. However, repressor systems may be damaged by tumor initiators (e.g., ionizing radiation and alkylating agents), which results in the production of transforming polypeptides. These polypeptides have been shown to be inhibited by retinoids,[36] and in this way the retinoids may suppress malignant transformation of a cell, not by correcting the damage done by some carcinogenic factor, but by repressing malignant expression of the cell itself.

STEROID HORMONE MODEL

Numerous studies have demonstrated intracellular binding of retinoids to both cellular retinol-binding protein (CRBP) and CRABP.[37] While early hypotheses suggested that the retinoid–retinoid-binding protein complex binds directly to nuclear DNA and influences changes analogous to the steroid hormones, only nuclear membrane CRBP/CRABP receptors have been identified.[38] Recently, however, two novel retinoic acid receptors (RAR-α and RAR-β), which exhibit remarkable similarity to the steroid and thyroid hormone receptors, have been characterized.[39, 40] Although not yet proven, the hormone-receptor complex could regulate a specific set of genes that may induce a cascade of regulatory events.

Clinical Conditions and Retinoid Treatment

ACTINIC KERATOSES

Actinic keratoses (AKs), premalignant lesions typically found on sun-damaged skin, are normally treated with some form of destructive therapy. Retinoids offer a new treatment approach. The choice of topical or oral retinoid therapy is dependent on the region being treated and the long-term goal of therapy.

The most commonly used oral retinoid for the treatment of AKs is etretinate. Studies have shown that etretinate not only reduces AK density, but may also provide a protective effect as well. In an 8-month, double-blind, crossover study (4 months placebo/4 months etretinate at 1 mg/kg/day) of 15 patients with multiple AKs, 14 of the 15 patients improved while using etretinate.[41] Furthermore, the authors reported that during the first 4 months of the study, the AK density increased in five of the six patients who were receiving placebo.[41] In an uncontrolled trial using etretinate for AKs (1 mg/kg/day for 3 months with subsequent dose reduction to ≤0.5 mg/kg/day for another 4 to 5 months), complete clearing was reported in 75% of the 46 patients treated.[42] However, after completion of the study, 76% of those patients who responded relapsed within 12 months. To minimize recurrence, the authors suggest therapy consisting of an annual 2-month course of etretinate (1 mg/kg/day). The newer retinoids have also been used in the treatment of AKs, but clinical trials with arotinoid failed to demonstrate a significant advantage over etretinate in AK therapy.[43–45]

Topical retinoid treatment of AKs has also been shown to have beneficial results. In a study of 93 patients using topical retinoic acid cream for treatment of AKs, a complete response was noted in 49%, and a partial response was noted in the remainder.[46] Subsequent studies confirmed these results with similar response rates.[47] The poorest responses were reported with AKs on the hands and forearms. However, a 100% response for AKs in these areas occurred with the use of a combination of topical 5-fluorouracil (5-FU) and topical tretinoin.[48]

ARSENICAL KERATOSES

While only a few studies have focused on the treatment of arsenical keratoses with retinoids, many reports describe the use of retinoids for treatment of arsenic-related basal cell carcinomas (BCCs).[43, 49, 50] One report discussed the retinoid treatment of a patient with numerous arsenical keratoses, two bowenoid plaques, and seven intraepidermal squamous cell carcinomas.[51] After a 12-week course of etretinate (1 mg/kg/day), an 80% reduction in the number of keratoses was noted, although there was persistence of the bowenoid plaques. At a 15-month follow-up examination, no new keratoses were observed. By controlling the growth of the keratotic lesions, there is an expected reduction in the incidence of malignancy in addition to an improvement in appearance. Future studies in this area are clearly necessary.

SQUAMOUS CELL CARCINOMA

The use of retinoids for the treatment of squamous cell carcinoma (SCC) has also shown some success. Initially, only sporadic case reports of tumor regression were noted.[52–54] Subsequently, Lippman and colleagues reported on the results of a broad phase II trial of isotretinoin in the treatment of 38 patients with head and neck SCC.[55] Overall, 16% of the patients had a positive objective response, which is comparable to established single-agent responses to 5-FU (15%), bleomycin (18%), and cisplatin (24%). Clearly, not all patients experience objective responses, and in fact, variability of responses is common,[53, 56] which complicates interpretation. However, a certain percentage of patients can be expected to experience a reduction in tumor mass. Prognostic indicators to identify responders have yet to be elucidated. Because these data include all head and neck SCCs, the majority of which were aerodigestive in origin, it is unclear whether this information can be accurately extrapolated to the treatment of cutaneous SCC.

In addition to regression of an established tumor, chemoprevention of SCC with retinoid therapy holds considerable promise. This effect has been studied in patients with treated oropharyngeal SCC because of their known high rate of second primary SCCs (ranging from 10 to 40%).[57] In one prospective randomized study, 103 patients received placebo or isotretinoin for 12 months. After 32 months, the isotretinoin group had a 4% incidence of second primary tumors, while the control group experienced a 24% incidence of second primary tumors.[57] Interestingly, the incidence of primary tumor progression was not significantly different between the two groups. These data suggest that isotreti-

noin is especially effective in preventing the initiation and promotion of cells but has little or no effect on transformed cells.

In summary, isotretinoin has demonstrated some promise in the treatment of established SCC, but has the greatest potential significance in chemoprevention. More research in this area is necessary before final conclusions can be reached and appropriate treatment regimens established.

BASAL CELL CARCINOMA

A number of studies have reported on the treatment of BCC using retinoids.[46, 49, 50, 58–66] Two basic conclusions have been reached in retinoid therapy of BCC: (1) tumor regression is variable but predictable,[58] and (2) continuous maintenance therapy is necessary for maintaining a disease-free state. However, the optimal dosing regimen for the retinoids has not yet been defined. Because partial tumor regression usually occurs with retinoid therapy (with a remarkable reduction in tumor mass occurring on occasion[59]), it has been suggested that a course of retinoids be administered before treatment of BCCs in cosmetically sensitive regions.[59, 60] This may have a significant impact on the surgical care of specific patients, but no randomized prospective studies have examined this particular question. While an accurate prediction of the response is not possible, it appears that BCCs measuring less than 5 mm in diameter are most likely to regress during systemic retinoid therapy.[58, 64] The treatment of BCCs with topical retinoids, typically tretinoin, has demonstrated tumor responses that are similar to those results obtained with oral therapy.[62, 64]

Chemoprophylaxis with retinoids is one of the most exciting developments for treatment of patients with multiple BCCs (e.g., basal cell nevus syndrome and arsenic toxicity). Isotretinoin in doses of 0.25 to 3 mg/kg/day in one patient with multiple BCCs[49] prevented the development of new tumors during an 8-year treatment period, despite a pretreatment incidence of five new tumors per year. However, 17 months after discontinuing the isotretinoin, the patient developed his first BCC in 9 years. In another patient with basal cell nevus syndrome who had a pretreatment tumor incidence of 25 new cancers per year, only seven BCCs developed during a 7-year treatment period. Thirteen months after discontinuing retinoid treatment, the patient developed 29 new BCCs.[49] Other studies have shown similar reductions in tumor incidence followed by rapid recurrence soon after discontinuing therapy.[59, 65, 66] While the optimal dosing regimen for effective chemoprophylaxis is unknown, the most common recommendation is a dose of 0.25 to 1 mg/kg/day of either isotretinoin or etretinate. It is clear, however, that long-term therapy is necessary to maintain the tumor-free state. More rigorous and controlled trials on this subject are discussed in the section "Xeroderma Pigmentosum."

MALIGNANT MELANOMA

Clinical experience with the use of retinoids in the treatment of melanoma has been limited. In vitro studies on different human melanoma cell lines have shown mixed responses to retinoids ranging from strong inhibition to stimulation.[67] These data suggest that each patient with melanoma may respond differently to retinoid therapy, a fact supported by several clinical trials. In an early study of two melanoma patients with intracutaneous metastases, one patient demonstrated complete regression using once-daily topical application of 0.05% tretinoin solution under occlusive tape.[68] However, in the second patient a response was noted in only 3 of 22 metastases treated similarly. In a phase II trial of 15 melanoma patients treated with oral retinol (200,000 U/m²), only two patients experienced a partial response.[69] In a phase II trial with oral isotretinoin (3 mg/kg/day), only 1 of 13 melanoma patients exhibited a clinical response.[70] These results suggest that the currently available retinoids probably have little beneficial role in the therapeutic management of melanoma patients.

LEUKOPLAKIA

The treatment of leukoplakia, a presumed precancerous condition of the oral mucosa, has long been problematic for both physician and patients.[71] While surgical therapy remains the standard of care, it fails to correct the underlying impairment of cellular differentiation.[72] For this reason, treatment of leukoplakia with retinoids has some theoretical basis; clinical trials have supported this suggestion.

In a study of 48 leukoplakia patients treated with vitamin A or vitamin A analogs,[72] a 58% permanent complete or permanent partial response rate was seen even 24 months after completion of therapy. To limit relapse, repeat courses of oral etretinate (50 mg/day) and 0.1% aromatic retinoid paste applied topically once daily for 6 weeks were used as required for control. In a prospectively controlled trial, the efficacy of oral isotretinoin in treating oral leukoplakia was established.[73] However, systemic toxicity and a high relapse rate of 50% within 3 months complicated treatment. Preliminary data from a follow-up study found that 3 months of induction using isotretinoin (1.5 mg/kg/day) followed by 9 months of maintenance with isotretinoin (0.5 mg/kg/day) reduced toxicity and improved the response rate to approximately 50%.[74] Whether retinoids can reduce the incidence of malignant change better than can surgical therapy, however, remains unproved.

XERODERMA PIGMENTOSUM

Xeroderma pigmentosum (XP) is a rare, autosomal recessive disorder in which repair mechanisms for DNA damaged by ultraviolet light are defective. The frequency of skin cancers in these patients is approximately 1000 times higher than that in the general population. The chemopreventative properties of isotretinoin were conclusively demonstrated in a controlled prospective study.[75] Five XP patients were studied and found to have a combined tumor incidence of 121 skin cancers during a 2-year pretreatment interval. During the 2 years of treatment with isotretinoin (2 mg/kg/day), a combined total of only 25 new tumors occurred. After discontinuing retinoid treatment, however, tumor incidence increased 8.5-fold in the study group. Follow-up studies are currently in progress and should help identify dosage guidelines.

While these data seem to suggest that isotretinoin has a definite place in the management of XP patients, the risks and benefits must be considered in each patient. This is especially important since the chronic use of oral retinoids is associated with many potentially serious side effects that may not be reversible and can be of particular concern in children or adolescents.

Use of β-Carotene

Numerous reports have correlated low serum levels of the carotenoid β-carotene with an increased risk for developing cancer.[76] Whether the protective effect of β-carotene results from direct administration of β-carotene or dietary manipulation is not clear. A large 5-year study of 1805 patients with a history of nonmelanoma skin cancer failed to demonstrate that β-carotene supplementation prevented new skin cancers. The authors concluded that the data were insufficient to justify prescribing supplemental β-carotene for the prevention of nonmelanoma skin cancer.

Side Effects and Toxicity of Retinoids

Just as each type of retinoid demonstrates a fairly unique spectrum of clinical efficacy, the toxicity profiles of each derivative are also unique. This section deals with the common side effects (Table 58–1), chronic toxicity, and teratogenicity of the major retinoids.

COMMON SIDE EFFECTS

Etretinate. The acute and largely reversible side effects of orally administered etretinate include erythema and desquamation of the skin associated with dryness of mucous membranes (Table 58–2). A higher incidence of side effects can be expected with higher doses; these side effects lessen with dose reduction. Tolerance can be expected to develop over time (Table 58–2).[77] Most of these side effects resolve after cessation of treatment, which demonstrates the reversibility of etretinate toxicity.

Isotretinoin. The most common side effects of isotretinoin are strikingly similar to those seen with etretinate (Table 58–3). However, isotretinoin adversely affects the function of internal metabolism, causing abnormal laboratory parameters to be seen much more commonly than with etretinate. Once again, however, the laboratory and clinical side effects are similarly reversible on discontinuation of therapy.[78] As a generalization, isotretinoin causes much less thinning of the hair and palmoplantar desquamation than etretinate, but facial scaling is more common.[78]

TABLE 58–1. **RETINOID SIDE EFFECTS**

Acute mucocutaneous effects	Acute laboratory effects
Cheilitis	Hyperlipidemia
Dermatitis	Increased triglyceride levels
Xerosis	Increased cholesterol levels
Dry nasal mucosa	Decreased high-density
Pruritus	lipoprotein levels
Epistaxis	Eruptive xanthoma
Stratum corneum fragility	Elevated liver enzyme levels
Desquamation	(AST, ALT, GGT, LDH,
Paronychia	alkaline phosphatase)
Nail plate abnormalities	Hyperbilirubinemia
Pili torti	Hyperuricemia
Alopecia	Hypercalcemia
Excess granulation tissue	Elevated creatine kinase levels
Pyogenic granuloma	Leukopenia
Bruising	Anemia
Photosensitivity	Thrombocytosis
Pityriasis rosea	Thrombocytopenia
Nasal colonization by	Elevated amylase levels
Staphylococcus aureus	Acute systemic effects
Impetigo	Headache
Erythema multiforme	Pseudotumor cerebri
Acute ophthalmic effects	Teratogenicity (head, ear,
Blepharoconjunctivitis	thymic, cardiac, and skeletal
Contact lens intolerance (dry	abnormalities)
eyes)	Acute hemorrhagic pancreatitis
Corneal erosions and opacities	Spontaneous abortion
Myopia	Mental depression
Papilledema	Acute hepatotoxic reactions
Optic neuritis	Exercise-induced
Phototoxicity	bronchoconstriction
Cataracts	Irregular menses
Impaired night vision	Arthralgia
	Fatigue
	Myalgia
	Chronic systemic effects
	Diffuse idiopathic skeletal
	hyperostosis
	Osteophyte formation
	Spinal ligament calcification
	Tendon and ligament
	calcification
	Premature epiphyseal closure
	Long-bone osteoporosis

ATL, Alanine aminotransferase; AST, aspartate aminotransferase; GGT, gamma-glutamyl transferase; LDH, lactate dehydrogenase.

Tretinoin. Because of the high incidence of central nervous system (CNS) toxicity reported with oral tretinoin (i.e., headache, personality changes, pseudotumor cerebri, and coma), only topical tretinoin preparations are currently being used.[79] For this reason, local cutaneous reactions constitute most side effects reported. With recent reports describing reversal of chronic sun damage, especially fine wrinkles, with the use of topical tretinoin, there has been a significant increase in its use. As a consequence, the incidence of side effects from this topical agent may be anticipated to increase substantially.

Lipid Metabolism Effects

Hyperlipidemia is a common acute side effect associated with retinoid use (Table 58–4). The elevation in lipid levels is proportional to the retinoid dose and typically reverses within 8 weeks after discontinuing the drug.[80] Such elevation can be acutely dangerous on

TABLE 58–2. **CLINICAL SIDE EFFECTS OF ETRETINATE**

	Side Effect Present (%)	
	After First Month	After Third Month
Skin		
Erythema	65	17
Desquamation	50	0
Atrophy of the skin	4	0
Burning	2	0
Pruritus	23	6
Alopecia	4	3
Splitting of nails	0	0
Paronychia	8	
Mucous membranes		
Lip dryness	77	42
Nasal mucosa dryness	56	33
Oral mucosa dryness	48	14
Conjunctivitis	10	0
Mucosal erosions	10	0

rare occasions, causing acute pancreatitis. Predisposing factors for retinoid-induced hyperlipidemia include obesity, alcoholism, diabetes, and pre-existing serum hypertriglyceridemia.[81] Both etretinate and isotretinoin adversely affect serum lipid profiles. Triglyceride very low density lipoprotein and cholesterol low-density lipoprotein levels increase, while cholesterol high-density lipoprotein levels decrease.[82] These unfavorable shifts in lipid levels tend to be more severe with isotretinoin. Moderate elevations in triglyceride or cholesterol levels can frequently be managed with alterations in diet. However, dosage adjustment or lipid-lowering medications may be indicated in more recalcitrant cases. Elevations of more than 800 mg/dl are associated with pancreatitis and require immediate intervention.[83]

TABLE 58–3. **CLINICAL AND LABORATORY FINDINGS WITH ISOTRETINOIN THERAPY**

Findings	Incidence (%)
Clinical	
Cheilitis, dry lips	90
Dry mouth	30
Xerosis and desquamation	30
Pruritus	25
Palmoplantar desquamation	5
Alopecia	10
Epistaxis and petechiae	25
Conjunctivitis	50
Musculoskeletal symptoms	15
Lethargy and fatigue	10
Headache	10
Nausea, vomiting, other gastrointestinal	20
symptoms	
Laboratory	
Elevated sedimentation rate	50
Elevated triglyceride levels	25
Decreased red blood cell counts	10
Decreased white blood cell counts	10
Increased platelet counts	10
Pyuria	10
Elevated liver enzymes	10

TABLE 58–4. MONITORING GUIDELINES

Pretreatment laboratory screening
  Complete blood cell count with differential
  Chemistry panel, including liver enzyme and lipid levels
  Serum pregnancy test (if applicable)
Follow-up
  Repeat laboratory tests 2 wk after initiation of therapy; repeat
    every 2 to 3 wk until abnormalities stabilize
  Repeat pretreatment laboratory screening studies every month for
    ensuing 6 mo of therapy; thereafter, repeat laboratory tests
    every 2 to 3 mo
  Serum pregnancy test every month (if applicable)
  Annual radiologic examination
  Ophthalmologic examination if patient notes visual changes or
    persistent headache
  Review of patient complaints and physical examination every
    month

Central Nervous System Effects

While headaches are a common complaint of patients taking retinoids, the association with pseudotumor cerebri cannot be overemphasized. In a review of 237 patients who reported ocular complaints while taking isotretinoin, 18 were noted to have papilledema, and seven developed pseudotumor cerebri.[84] A complaint of headache associated with visual changes should prompt an immediate ophthalmologic evaluation. These symptoms usually develop early in the course of therapy.[81] The concomitant use of minocycline or tetracycline is believed to increase the risk of pseudotumor cerebri, and as a consequence, this combination of medications is not advised. Discontinuation of the retinoid typically eliminates the CNS side effects.

CHRONIC TOXICITY OF RETINOID THERAPY

The continuous long-term retinoid therapy that is required in treatment of some conditions raises important concerns of chronic toxicity. In addition to the well-documented acute effects, bony abnormalities may also occur.[81] These skeletal changes include hyperostosis, osteophyte formation, nasal osteophytosis, premature epiphyseal closure, and long-bone osteoporosis. Additionally, tendon and ligament calcification, especially of the anterior spinal ligament, feet, knees, hips, and pelvis, is common. Regular radiologic examinations may be indicated to limit these types of changes since symptoms are frequently absent in patients with radiographically proved changes.[81] Whether the bony changes are reversible and whether they also may develop from chronic intermittent therapy are unclear. Because premature epiphyseal closure is presumably not reversible, patients judged at risk should be carefully monitored for this side effect.

Wound Repair

Keloid and hypertrophic scar formation is an uncommon complication in patients who received isotretinoin prior to dermabrasion or argon laser therapy.[85, 86] For example, one report described several patients who received identical surgical treatment before and after receiving isotretinoin.[86] Those areas treated before isotretinoin therapy healed normally, while the areas treated after initiation of isotretinoin healed with keloids. The mechanism for this complication is unknown. Some studies have demonstrated that retinoids can inhibit fibroblasts and decrease collagen production,[87] while other studies suggest that retinoids inhibit collagenase.[88] This collagenase inhibition may primarily contribute to excess scar formation. Patients typically develop keloids between 1 and 3 months postoperatively, but even longer intervals have been seen. Some patients who developed keloids were concurrently receiving isotretinoin, but others had completed therapy from several months to up to 1 year before surgery. No guidelines for avoiding keloid formation exist, but it is advisable to postpone elective surgical procedures for a minimum of 6 months, and perhaps for as long as 2 years, after a patient has stopped retinoid use. Of course, in some cases the benefit to the patient, when compared with the risks, may favor shortening this delay interval.

TERATOGENICITY OF RETINOIDS

The teratogenic effects of retinoids are well documented and must be taken seriously. These effects include an increased incidence of spontaneous abortions, as well as malformations of bony craniofacial structures, the cardiovascular system, and the CNS.[89] For this reason, concomitant use of some form of contraception during retinoid therapy is mandatory for fertile women. The half-life of isotretinoin is 12 to 20 hours,[82] and pregnancy should also be avoided for a minimum of one full menstrual cycle after completing this form of therapy. The extended half-life of etretinate (80 to 100 days) suggests that subsequent pregnancy is probably never totally safe, but established guidelines do not exist. Through the development of new retinoids that have very short half-lives, it is hoped that this side effect can be greatly minimized.

SUMMARY

The development of synthetic vitamin A analogs, or retinoids, that exhibit improved clinical efficacy with reduced toxicity offers many novel therapeutic approaches for the cutaneous oncologist. While the mechanism of action is not completely understood, research points to a concert of genomic and enzymatic effects. The best established uses of retinoids focus on chemoprevention, especially of basal cell carcinomas, but effects are also favorable for chemoprevention of squamous cell carcinomas, leukoplakia, and actinic keratoses. It is clear that continued treatment is required to maintain the chemopreventive effects, but ideal dosage regimens are not yet defined. Established cutaneous malignancies have also shown some responsiveness to retinoids, but results are variable and not yet predictable.

REFERENCES

1. Stepp W: Versuche uber futterung mit lipoidfreier nahrung. Biochem Z 22:452–460, 1909.
2. McCollum EV, Davis M: The necessity of certain lipids in the diet during growth. J Biol Chem 15:167–175, 1913.
3. Drummond JC: The nomenclature of so-called accessory food factors (vitamins). Biochem J 14:660, 1920.
4. Kuhn R, Morris CJDR: Synthese von vitamin A. Chemische Berichte (Weinhein) 70:853–858, 1937.
5. Fujumaki Y: Formation of gastric carcinoma in albino rats fed on deficient diets. J Cancer Res 10:469–477, 1926.
6. Peck SM, Chargin L, Sobotka H: Keratosis follicularis (Darier's disease), a vitamin A deficiency disease. Arch Dermatol Syphilol 43:223–229, 1941.
7. Porter AD: Vitamin A in some congenital anomalies of the skin. Br J Dermatol 63:123–127, 1951.
8. Burgoon CF Jr, Graham JH, Urbach F, Musgnug R: Effect of vitamin A on epithelial cells of skin. Arch Dermatol 87:63–80, 1963.
9. Saffiotti V, Montesano R, Sellakumar AR, Borg SA: Experimental cancer of the lung. Inhibition by vitamin A of the induction of tracheobronchial squamous metaplasia and squamous cell tumors. Cancer 20:857–864, 1967.
10. Lippman SM, Kessler JF, and Meyskens FL Jr: Retinoids as preventive and therapeutic anticancer agents (part I). Cancer Treat Rep 71:391–405, 1987.
11. Bollag W: Therapeutic effects of an aromatic retinoic acid analog on chemically induced skin papillomas and carcinomas of mice. Eur J Cancer 10:731–737, 1974.
12. Clamon GH, Sporn MB, Smith JM, et al: Alpha- and beta-retinyl acetate reverse metaplasias of vitamin A deficiency in hamster trachea in organ culture. Nature 250:64–66, 1974.
13. Strickland S, Mahdavi V: The induction of differentiation in teratocarcinoma stem cells by retinoic acid. Cell 15:393–403, 1978.
14. Verma AK, Shapas BG, Rice HM, et al: Correlation of the inhibition by retinoids of tumor promotor-induced mouse epidermal ornithine decarboxylase activity and of skin tumor promotion. Cancer Res 39:419–425, 1979.
15. Bouclier M, Shroot B, Eustache J, Hensby CN: Rapid and simple test system for evaluation of the inhibitory activity of retinoids on induced ornithine decarboxylase activity in the hairless rat epidermis. J Pharmacol Methods 16:151–160, 1986.
16. Wolf G: Multiple functions of vitamin A. Physiol Rev 64:873–937, 1984.
17. Loewenstein WR: Junctional intercellular communication and the control of growth. Biochem Biophys Acta 560:1–65, 1979.
18. McNutt NS, Weinstein RS: Carcinoma of the cervix: deficiency of nexus intercellular junctions. Science 165:597–599, 1969.
19. Hossain MZ, Wilkens LR, Mehta PP, et al: Enhancement of gap junctional communication by retinoids correlates with their ability to inhibit neoplastic transformation. Carcinogenesis 10:1743–1748, 1989.
20. Prutkin L: Mucous metaplasia and gap junctions in the vitamin A acid-treated skin tumor, keratoacanthoma. Cancer Res 35:364–369, 1975.
21. Elias PM, Grayson S, Gross EG, Peck GL, McNutt NS: Influence of topical and systemic retinoids on basal cell carcinoma cell membranes. Cancer 48:932–938, 1981.
22. Nemanic MK, Fritsch PO, Elias PM: Perturbations of membrane glycosylation in retinoid-treated epidermis. J Am Acad Dermatol 6:801–808, 1982.
23. Lotan R: Effects of vitamin A and its analogs (retinoids) on normal and neoplastic cells. Biochim Biophys Acta 605:33–91, 1980.
24. Zerlauth G, Wolf G: Release of fibronectin is linked to tumor promotion: response of promotable and non-promotable clones of a mouse epidermal cell line. Carcinogenesis 6:73–78, l985.
25. Zerlauth G. Wolf G: Studies on the tumour promoter-induced release of fibronectin from human lung fibroblasts, and its counteraction by retinoic acid. Carcinogenesis 6:531–534, 1985.
26. Dennert G, Lotan R: Effects of retinoic acid on the immune system: stimulation of T killer cell induction. Eur J Immunol 8:23–29, 1978.
27. Dennert G: Immunostimulation by retinoic acid. In: Nugent J, Clark S (eds): Retinoids, Differentiation, and Disease. Pitman, London, 1985, pp 117–131.
28. Ziboh VA, Price B, Fulton J: Effects of retinoic acid on prostaglandin biosynthesis in guinea-pig skin. J Invest Dermatol 65:370–374, 1975.
29. Russell DH, Durie BGM: Polyamines as biochemical markers of normal and malignant growth. In: Progress in Cancer Research and Therapy. Raven Press, New York, 1978.
30. Russell DH: Ornithine decarboxylase: a key regulatory enzyme in normal and neoplastic growth. Drug Metab Rev 16:1–88, 1985.
31. Olsen DR, Hickok NJ, Uitto J: Suppression of ornithine decarboxylase gene expression by retinoids in cultured human keratinocytes. J Invest Dermatol 94:33–36, 1990.
32. Nishizuka Y: Studies and perspectives of protein kinase-C. Science 233:305–312, 1986.
33. Cope FO, Howard BO, Boutwell RK: The in vitro characterization of the inhibition of mouse brain kinase-C by retinoids and their receptors. Experientia 42:1023–1027, 1986.
34. Lippman SM, Meyskens FL Jr: Results of the use of vitamin A and retinoids in cutaneous malignancies. Pharmacol Ther 40:107–122, 1989.
35. Todaro GJ, Huebner RJ: The viral oncogene hypothesis: new evidence. Proc Natl Acad Sci USA 69:1009–1015, 1972.
36. Todaro GJ, De Larco JE, Sporn MB: Retinoids block phenotypic cell transformation produced by sarcoma growth factor. Nature 276:272–274, 1978.
37. Chytil F, Sherman DR: How do retinoids work? Dermatologica 175(suppl 1):8–12, 1987.
38. Sherman MI, Gubler ML, Barkai U, et al: Role of retinoids in differentiation and growth of embryonal carcinoma cells. In: Nugent J, Clark S (eds): Retinoids, Differentiation, and Disease. Pitman, London, 1985, pp 42–60.
39. Giguere V, Ong ES, Segui P, Evans RM: Identification of a receptor for the morphogen retinoic acid. Nature 330:624–628, 1987.
40. Brand N, Petkovich M, Krust A, et al: Identification of a second human retinoic acid receptor. Nature 332:850–853, 1988.
41. Watson AB: Preventive effect of etretinate therapy on multiple actinic keratoses. Cancer Detect Prev 9:161–165, 1986.
42. Grupper CH, Berretti B: Cutaneous neoplasia and etretinate. In: Spitzy KH, Karrer K (eds): Proceedings of the 143rd International Congress of Chemotherapy. VH Egermann, Vienna, 1983, pp 201/24–27.
43. Berretti B, Gruper C, Edelson Y, Bermejo D: Aromatic retinoid in the treatment of multiple superficial basal cell carcinoma, arsenic keratosis and karatoacanthoma. In: Orfanos CE, Braun-Falco O, Farber EM, et al (eds): Retinoids, Advances in Basic Research and Therapy. Springer-Verlag, Berlin, 1981, pp 397–399.
44. Kingston T, Gaskell S, Marks R: The effects of a novel potent oral retinoid (Ro13–6298) in the treatment of multiple solar keratoses and squamous cell epithelioma. Eur J Cancer Clin Oncol 19:1201–1205, 1983.
45. Merot Y, Canenzind M, Geiger J, Saurat J: Arotinoid ethyl ester (Ro 13–6298): a long term pilot study in various dermatoses. Acta Derm Venereol (Stockh) 67:237–242, 1987.
46. Belisario JC: Recent advances in topical cytotoxic therapy of skin cancer and pre-cancer. In: McCarthy WH (ed): Melanoma and Skin Cancer: Proceedings of the International Cancer Conference. Blight, Sydney, Australia, 1972, pp 349–365.
47. Thorne EG, Roach JB, McElroy J: Topical tretinoin in the treatment of actinic (solar) keratoses—results presented 1990 American Academy of Dermatology.
48. Robinson TA, Kligman AM: Treatment of solar keratoses of the extremities with retinoic acid and 5-fluorouracil. Br J Dermatol 92:703–706, 1975.
49. Peck GL: Long-term retinoid therapy is needed for maintenance of cancer chemopreventive effect. Dermatologica 175(suppl 1):138–144, 1987.
50. Peck GL, Gross EG, Butkus D, DiGiovanna JJ: Chemoprevention of basal cell carcinoma with isotretinoin. J Am Acad Dermatol 6:815–823, 1982.
51. Sharma SC, Simpson NB: Treatment of arsenical keratosis with etretinate. Acta Derm Venereol (Stockh) 63:449–452, 1983.
52. Levine N, Miller RC, Meyskens FL Jr: Oral isotretinoin therapy: use in a patient with multiple cutaneous squamous cell carcinomas and keratoacanthomas. Arch Dermatol 120:1215–1217, 1984.

53. Meyskens FL Jr, Gilmartin E, Alberts DS, et al: Activity of isotretinoin against squamous cell cancers and preneoplastic lesions. Cancer Treat Rep 66:1315–1319, 1982.

54. Lippman SM, Meyskens FL Jr: Treatment of advanced squamous cell carcinoma of the skin with isotretinoin. Ann Intern Med 107:499–501, 1987.

55. Lippman SM, Garewal HS, Meyskens FL Jr: Retinoids as potential chemopreventive agents in squamous cell carcinoma of the head and neck. Prevent Med 18:740–748, 1989.

56. Quintal D, Jackson R: Aggressive squamous cell carcinoma arising in familial acne conglobata. J Am Acad Dermatol 14:207–214, 1986.

57. Hong WK, Lippman SM, Itri LM, et al: Prevention of second primary tumors with isotretinoin in squamous-cell carcinoma of the head and neck. New Engl J Med 323:795–801, 1990.

58. Peck GL: Retinoids in the treatment of skin cancer. J Dermatol Surg Oncol 11:807, 1985.

59. Cristofolini M, Zumiani G, Scappini P, Piscioli F: Aromatic retinoid in the chemoprevention of the progression of nevoid basal-cell carcinoma syndrome. J Dermatol Surg Oncol 10:778–781, 1984.

60. Sanchez-Conejo-Mir J, Cammacho F: Nevoid basal cell carcinoma syndrome: combined etretinate and surgical treatment. J Dermatol Surg Oncol 15:868–871, 1989.

61. Peck GL, Yoder FW, Olsen TG, et al: Treatment of Darier's disease, lamellar ichthyosis, pityriasis rubra pilaris, cystic acne, and basal cell carcinoma with oral 13-cis-retinoic acid. Dermatologica 157(suppl):11–12, 1978.

62. Sankowski A, Janik P, Bogacka-Zatorska E: Treatment of basal cell carcinoma with 13-cis-retinoic acid. Neoplasma 31:615–618, 1984.

63. Bollag W, Ott F: Vitamin A acid in benign and malignant epithelial tumours of the skin. Acta Derm Venereol (Stockh) Suppl 74:163–166, 1975.

64. Peck GL: Topical tretinoin in actinic keratosis and basal cell carcinoma. J Am Acad Dermatol 15:829–835, 1986.

65. Hodak E, Ginzburg A, David M, Sandbank M: Etretinate treatment of the nevoid basal cell carcinoma syndrome: therapeutic and chemopreventive effect. Int J Dermatol 26:606–609, 1987.

66. Verret JL, Schnitzler L, Avenel M, Smulevici A: Etretinate and skin cancer prevention; a 6.5-year follow-up study. In: Saurat JH (ed): Retinoids: New Trends in Research and Therapy. Retinoid Symposium. Karger, Basel, Switzerland, 1984, pp 355–359.

67. Meyskens FL Jr, Edwards L, Levine NS: Role of topical tretinoin in melanoma and dysplastic nevi. J Am Acad Dermatol 15:822–825, 1986.

68. Levine N, Meyskens FL: Topical vitamin-A-acid therapy for cutaneous metastatic melanoma. Lancet 2:224–226, 1980.

69. Goodman GE: Phase II trial of retinol in patients with advanced cancer. Cancer Treat Rep 70:1023–1024, 1986.

70. Meyskens FL Jr: Studies of retinoids in the prevention and treatment of cancer. J Am Acad Dermatol 6:824–827, l982.

71. Dorey JL, Blasberg B, Conklin RJ, Carmichael RP: Oral leukoplakia, current concepts in diagnosis, management, and malignant potential. Int J Dermatol 23:638–642, 1984.

72. Koch HF: Effects of retinoids on precancerous lesions of oral mucosa. In: Orfanos CE, Braun-Falco O, Farber EM, et al (eds): Retinoids, Advances in Basic Research and Therapy. Springer-Verlag, Berlin, 1981, pp 307–312.

73. Hong WK, Endicott J, Itti LM, et al: 13-cis-retinoic acid in the treatment of oral leukoplakia. N Engl J Med 315:1501–1505, 1986.

74. Lippman SM, Toth BB, Batsakis JG, et al: Low-dose 13-cis-retinoic acid (13cRA) maintains remission in oral premalignancy: more effective than β-carotene in randomized trial. Proc Am Soc Clin Oncol 9:59, 1990.

75. Kramer KH, Digiovanna JJ, Moshell AN, et al: Prevention of skin cancer in xeroderma pigmentosum with the use of oral isotretinoin. N Engl J Med 318:1633–1637, 1988.

76. Greenberg ER, Brown JA, Stukel TA, et al: A clinical trial of beta carotene to prevent basal-cell and squamous-cell cancers of the skin. N Engl J Med 323:789–795, 1990.

77. Lassus A: Systemic treatment of psoriasis with an oral retinoic acid derivative (Ro 10–9359). Br J Dermatol 102:195–202, 1980.

78. Windhorst DB, Nigra T: General clinical toxicology of oral retinoids. J Am Acad Dermatol 6:675–682, 1982.

79. Elias PM, Williams JL: Retinoids, cancer, and the skin. Arch Dermatol 117:160–180, 1981.

80. David M, Hodak E, Lowe NJ: Adverse effects of retinoids. Med Toxicol 3:273–288, 1988.

81. Giovanna JJ, GL Peck: Retinoid toxicity. Progr Dermatol 21:1–8, 1987.

82. Vahlquist C, Michaelsson G, Vahlquist A, Vessby B: A sequential comparison of etretinate (Tigason) and isotretinoin (Roaccutane) with special regard to their effects on serum lipoproteins. Br J Dermatol 112:69–76, 1985.

83. Shalita AR, Cunningham WJ, Leyden JJ, et al: Isotretinoin treatment of acne and related disorders: an update. J Am Acad Dermatol 9:629–638, 1983.

84. Fraunfelder FT, Labraico JM, Meyer SM: Adverse ocular reactions possibly associated with isotretinoin. Am J Ophthalmol 100:534–537, 1985.

85. Rubenstein R, Roenigk HH Jr, Stegman SJ, Hanke CW: Atypical keloids after dermabrasion of patients taking isotretinoin. J Am Acad Dermatol 15:280–285, 1986.

86. Zachariae H: Delayed wound healing and keloid formation following argon laser treatment or dermabrasion during isotretinoin treatment. Br J Dermatol 110:703–706, 1988.

87. Oikarinen H, Oikarinen AI, Tan EM, et al: Modulation of procollagen gene expression by retinoids in human skin fibroblast cultures. Clin Res 32:142a, 1984.

88. Bauer EA, Seltzer JL, Eisen AZ: Inhibition of collagen degradative enzymes by retinoic acid in vitro. J Am Acad Dermatol 6:603–607, 1982.

89. Lippman SM, Kessler JF, Meyskens FL Jr: Retinoids as preventive and therapeutic anticancer agents (part II). Cancer Treat Rep 71:493–515, 1987.

CHAPTER 59

Management of Malignant Melanomas

DAVID M. AMRON and RONALD L. MOY

Although early descriptions of melanoma appear to date back to Hippocrates in the fifth century BC, it was not until 1787 that John Hunter provided the first published description of melanoma in one of his patients. In the century that followed, numerous case reports appeared both in Europe and America.[1-5] Initially the tumor was usually described as a fungal mass. In 1812 Rene Laennec coined the term melanosis, derived from the Greek word meaning "black,"[1] and the term "melanoma" was first used by Robert Carswell in 1838.[6]

The incidence of melanoma is increasing faster than that of any other cancer, except, perhaps, for lung carcinoma in women. Currently, about one in 120 Americans will develop malignant melanoma in his or her lifetime,[7] and it has been projected that more than 27,000 new cases and nearly 6000 deaths from the cancer will occur each year.[8]

However, in the midst of what has been termed an "epidemic of malignant melanoma," survival rates for the disease have never been better.[9-11] The increased survival rates may be attributed to earlier diagnosis of melanoma brought about by increased public awareness and education with regard to self-examination and increased physician awareness for the need to perform regular complete cutaneous examinations and biopsies of suspicious lesions. When malignant melanoma is detected at an early stage, the patient's prognosis is usually excellent. Improvements in the understanding of defined prognostic variables such as tumor thickness, level of invasion, histologic type, and presence of nodal involvement have enabled surgeons to better tailor the treatment to fit the individual patient.

Biopsy Techniques

In many instances, clinical inspection alone is not enough to exclude a diagnosis of melanoma. It has been shown that more than one third of biopsy-proven melanomas are misdiagnosed before biopsy.[12] Therefore, the importance of performing early biopsy of suspicious lesions cannot be overemphasized. Also, several studies have disproved previously held notions that biopsy performed before definitive surgery adversely affects the final outcome by promoting dissemination.[13-17]

There are several methods currently employed for biopsy of suspected melanoma lesions, including excisional, incisional, punch, and shave biopsy. Of these, excisional biopsy is by far the most common, since most melanomas are relatively small.[13] When feasible, the biopsy should be excisional with narrow margins and should include full-thickness skin along with subcutaneous fat. Punch or incisional biopsies are acceptable only when an excisional biopsy would be difficult to perform because of the size or location of the lesion. Shave biopsies or curettage are not recommended, as the pathologist is unable to provide information on tumor thickness. If a punch or incisional biopsy is used, the most raised site (or the darkest area if the lesion is flat) should undergo biopsy. However, determination of the final prognosis should be made only after the entire lesion has been removed and thoroughly examined histologically by performing multiple sections through the specimen.

Fear of performing incisional biopsies was based on the theory that transecting the lesion could cause dissemination of malignant cells. In 1980 one report showed a

TABLE 59–1.
CLARK'S LEVELS OF INVASION[35]

Level I	All tumor cells above basement membrane; also termed in situ melanoma
Level II	Tumor cells have broken through basement membrane and extend into papillary dermis but have not entered reticular dermis
Level III	Tumor cells have invaded ill-defined interface between papillary and reticular dermis
Level IV	Neoplastic cells are seen between collagen bundles of reticular dermis
Level V	Neoplastic cells have invaded subcutaneous tissue

TABLE 59–2. FIVE-YEAR SURVIVAL RATE FOR CLINICAL STAGE I MELANOMA ACCORDING TO BRESLOW THICKNESS

Tumor Thickness (mm)	% Survival		
	Balch et al[68]	Wanebo et al[69]	Breslow[36]
0–1	95	100	100
1–2	68	89	74
2–3	65	82	80
3–4	65	58	30
>4	20	55	25

16% decrease in the 5-year survival rate in patients with melanoma who had undergone incisional biopsy, compared with those who had undergone excisional biopsy.[18] However, in this study, patients were not stratified according to known prognostic variables, especially tumor thickness. It has since been shown that when prognostic variables, especially tumor thickness, are taken into consideration, no significant difference in survival exists for incisional versus excisional biopsy. These results are in agreement with many other published reports that studied the role of incisional biopsy in melanoma.[17, 19–22] Thus, incisional biopsy has not been proven to adversely affect the prognosis of melanoma patients.

It has also not been substantiated that biopsy performed before definitive surgery has an adverse effect on outcome.[16, 22–24] In a study of 954 patients with melanoma who had undergone either narrow excisional biopsy followed by delayed wide excision (319 patients) or primary wide excision alone (635 patients), no differences were found in either 5-year disease-free rates or 5-year survival rates.[23] Additionally, the time interval between excisional biopsy and delayed wide excision was found to have no influence on patient outcome. On this basis, it was concluded that excisional biopsy of melanoma followed by delayed wide excision was safe.[23] Thus, biopsy performed before definitive surgery also appears to have no effect on prognosis, although excisional biopsy is preferable.

Surgical Margins

HISTORICAL PERSPECTIVE

The width of the surgical margin for excision of primary melanoma of the skin has been the object of much debate among cutaneous surgeons for many years.[25–30] In 1907, W. Sampson Handley, in a lecture to the Royal College of Surgeons, recommended an excision margin of about 1 inch for melanoma.[31] His recommendation was based on observing the pattern of metastasis in a single patient who had died from malignant metastatic melanoma. For many years, the 5-cm surgical margin for melanomas was viewed as a requirement, regardless of the thickness of the tumor. However, Handley never mentioned a 5-cm margin, and he did not study primary melanoma. Nevertheless, apparent justification for employing the 5-cm rule began to

appear in the literature. The presence of atypical melanocytes were noted in normal skin 5 cm from the border of cutaneous melanoma lesions,[32] and an increased number of melanocytes were observed in the area surrounding a melanoma.[33] One study even recommended that the margin be widened to 15 cm.[34]

LEVELS AND THICKNESS OF MELANOMA

The work of Clark and Breslow provided the primary prognostic data that allowed for more conservative treatment of cutaneous melanoma. In 1969, Clark correlated the actual histologic level of invasion of melanoma with biologic behavior of the tumor.[35] Depth of invasion was defined according to five histologic levels (Table 59–1). These observations were supported by the fact that nodular melanoma, with the most prominent vertical growth phase of all melanomas, had a significantly higher mortality rate than either superficial spreading or lentigo maligna melanoma.

Breslow, using an ocular micrometer to measure depth of invasion, reviewed 98 patients in whom tumor thickness was no greater than 0.76 mm.[36] At 5 years after surgery, all of these patients were alive, and none had any evidence of melanoma. To date, tumor thickness remains the most reliable prognostic indicator in determining the 5-year survival rate in clinical stage I melanoma (Tables 59–2, 59–3).

CURRENT TRENDS

Since the 1970s, the trend has been toward more conservative approaches to the management and treatment of primary cutaneous melanoma. As our understanding of prognostic factors has become more clearly defined, surgical treatment has become less radical.

TABLE 59–3. FIVE-YEAR SURVIVAL RATE FOR CLINICAL STAGE I MELANOMA ACCORDING TO CLARK'S LEVEL OF INVASION

Clark's Level	% Survival		
	Balch et al[68]	Wanebo et al[69]	Breslow[36]
II	85	100	97
III	73	88	76
IV	57	66	43
V	28	15	33

TABLE 59–4. **STAGING OF CUTANEOUS MELANOMA**

Stage I	Localized disease (rarely including satellitosis or local recurrence within 5 cm of primary tumor or in-transit metastases)
Stage II	Regional lymph node involvement (documented by histology)
Stage III	Distant metastatic disease (documented by histology)

Many clinical studies have shown that the width of surgical margins is unrelated to the 5-year survival rate for clinical stage I disease.[9, 37–40]

The first study to challenge the conventional 5-cm excision rule was published in 1966.[41] This study of 456 patients showed that survival was unrelated to the width of the surgical margin. These results were confirmed in a subsequent study of 62 patients with cutaneous melanomas less than 0.76 mm thick in whom the width of resection margins varied from 0.10 to 5.15 cm. Of those patients who were followed for 5 years or more, none showed evidence of local recurrence. This suggested that the optimal width of the resection margins should be determined by tumor thickness.[26]

There have also been many reports showing that for thin melanomas, survival is not influenced by the extent of the surgical excision margin.[42–44] A World Health Organization (WHO) study of 593 patients found that tumor recurrence increased with increasing tumor thickness and decreased with increasing margins of resection.[42] However, the survival rate in patients with clinical stage I melanoma was not influenced by the width of the resection margin.[42] From this it was concluded that both thick and thin melanomas could be treated with a narrower resection margin.[37] It was cautiously and empirically recommended that 1.5-cm margins be used for all lesions less than 0.85 mm thick and for melanomas not on the back, neck, or scalp between 0.85 and 1.69 mm thick; other lesions should have a 3-cm margin.

TUMOR STAGING AND EXCISION MARGINS

Melanoma has traditionally been divided into stage I, stage II, and stage III disease (Table 59–4). In one retrospective review,[45] more than three fourths of 118 patients with clinical stage I melanoma had excision margins of 3 cm or less. The mortality rate was found to increase if margins less than 2 cm were used in tumors greater than 1 cm in diameter or more than 2 mm deep. With margins of 2.5 cm, the survival rate was increased, but the mortality rate did not change, even when the margins were greater than 3 cm. Recurrences were seen in patients with satellitosis, unrecognized subclinical stage II disease, or disseminated stage III disease. These authors suggested that thin lesions, especially those less than 0.76 mm thick, could probably be cured with a resection margin less than 2 cm. For lesions deeper than 2 mm, a 3-cm resection margin was recommended.[45, 46]

However, despite the growing evidence from retrospective reviews that narrower resection margins were safe for thin melanomas, the majority of surgeons still performed wide excision for most melanoma patients. A 1984 National Cancer Institute of Canada survey showed that nearly two thirds of surgeons still used a 3- to 5-cm excision margin for melanomas less than 1.5 mm in depth.[47] Another study found that only 5% of 800 patients had surgical excision margins of less than 2 cm.[42] Among these surgeons, 24% were found to perform routine, prophylactic lymph node dissection.

It was not until 1988 that an accurate, reliable WHO study for clinical stage I melanoma less than 2 mm thick was performed.[40] This well-designed, randomized prospective study compared survival rates with excision margins of 1 cm (narrow excision) and 3 cm (wide excision) for primary melanomas less than or equal to 2 mm in thickness. A total of 305 narrow-excision patients and 307 wide-excision patients were followed for a mean duration of 55 months. Mean thickness of the lesions was 0.99 mm in the narrow-excision group and 1.02 mm in the wide-excision group. Both disease-free survival and overall survival rates were similar in the two groups. The rate of subsequent development of metastatic disease involving regional lymph node and distant organs was also similar in the two groups. In patients with melanoma less than 1 mm thick, no local recurrences were observed. It was concluded that a 1-cm excision margin down to the muscular fascia is as effective as wide excision for stage I cutaneous melanomas no thicker than 2 mm.[40] However, it should be remembered that these are only preliminary results, and for some patients, a 5-year follow-up period may not be sufficient to accurately evaluate treatment.

To further determine the effectiveness of narrower excision margins for thin melanomas, the presence of "microscopic satellites" in the reticular dermis and subcutaneous tissue of patients with clinical stage I cutaneous melanoma was studied.[48] In 596 patients, no satellites were found by microscopy when the lesion was less than 0.75 mm thick. The presence of these satellites was noted to increase dramatically as the thickness of the primary lesion increased. Results of other studies also suggested that a minimum 1-cm margin be used for thin primary melanomas less than 1 mm thick. Nearly a tenfold increase in the in situ melanoma recurrence rate was found with resection margins of 0.1 to 0.9 cm when compared with margins between 1.0 and 1.9 cm.[49] It was further shown that if the recurrence is re-excised early, survival may not be affected.

These studies on surgical margins suggest that the biologic behavior of melanoma is one of continuous growth until the tumor metastasizes. The older idea that melanoma can spread locally with noncutaneous microscopic satellites and without metastasizing is incorrect. For this reason, once the tumor has been excised, wider surgical margins to theoretically include nearby satellites cannot improve survival.

THICK MELANOMAS

For melanomas more than 2 mm thick, the evidence defining guidelines for resection margins remains unclear. Margins of more than 3 cm offer no additional protection for lesions more than 2 mm deep.[45] A higher incidence of local recurrence was noted when margins were less than 3 cm in patients with high-risk melanoma.[50] However, survival rates remained unchanged. At the Massachusetts General Hospital, the empirical guidelines for clinical stage I melanomas have been an excision margin of 1.5 cm with primary closure for lesions 1 to 1.5 mm thick and a 3-cm margin for melanomas more than 1.5 mm thick.[51]

Well-conducted prospective randomized clinical studies are clearly needed, and a number of such studies are currently in progress. Until the results are published and standards are established, decisions regarding margin depth and width may be arbitrary and empirical. One randomized prospective study currently under way to assess margins for thicker melanomas is the Intergroup Melanoma Trial, in which more than 300 patients with melanomas 1 to 4 mm deep are being studied using either 2- or 4-cm surgical margins.[52]

Surgical excision for melanoma is carried down to the deep subcutaneous tissue by many cutaneous surgeons. In the past it had been customary to resect the muscle fascia along with wide excision of the melanoma. However, no evidence exists to support the need for removal of the fascia. A retrospective study of 212 patients demonstrated no statistically significant difference in recurrence or survival rates at 5-year follow-up for patients who had their fascia excised as opposed to those who did not.[53] Only when the fascia is infiltrated by melanoma is there need for its resection.[54] Excisions extending through the underlying fascia in stage I melanoma were associated with a higher rate of subsequent lymph node metastases than those in which the fascia was left intact.[41] However, it is possible that in this study the fascia was resected more frequently for thicker melanomas, as the study was done before knowledge of the prognostic significance of Breslow thickness. Until more definitive studies are produced, it appears safe to leave the fascia intact when treating most melanomas. Fascial resection appears to only lengthen postoperative morbidity and delay healing.

On the basis of currently available evidence, the following recommendations are valid for the surgical treatment of melanoma:

1. A surgical margin of 1 to 1.5 cm is indicated for melanomas less than 2 mm thick.

2. A surgical margin of 3 cm is appropriate for melanomas more than 2 mm thick.

Mohs Micrographic Surgery

Mohs micrographic surgery is a controversial surgical technique when used in the treatment of melanoma because of the possibility of narrower margins and the difficulty encountered in microscopically identifying melanoma cells on frozen sections. When used for the treatment of basal cell carcinomas and squamous cell carcinomas, Mohs micrographic surgery has proved to have better cure rates with less sacrifice of normal tissue than any other type of surgery, because it traces out the tumor extensions microscopically. It is possible that

Mohs micrographic surgery, when used to treat melanomas, will provide cure rates similar to those provided by conventional surgery while sparing normal tissue. For this reason, Mohs micrographic surgery may be especially valuable in specific anatomic areas where conventional surgery for melanoma can cause significant cosmetic deformity.

TECHNICAL ASPECTS

Mohs micrographic surgery is different from conventional surgery in that frozen sections are used to assess whether all surgical margins are clear of atypical melanocytes. This method differs from standard operating room frozen sections in that 100% of the surgical margin—the entire periphery and undersurface of the specimen—is examined, compared with the 0.1% of the surgical margin examined with conventional frozen sections.[55] The visible tumor is excised with a 6-mm surgical margin, extending down to subcutaneous fat. A 2-mm surgical margin is then taken around this wound so that all of the periphery and bottom surface of the specimen will be examined by the horizontal frozen sections.[56]

ACCURACY OF FROZEN SECTION

The reliability of interpretation of frozen sections compared with that of paraffin sections has been clearly demonstrated in an evaluation of surgical margins in melanoma.[57] In one study of 221 specimens in 59 patients, the interpretations of frozen and paraffin sections from the same block were compared. Frozen sections were 100% sensitive and 90% specific in detecting melanoma, when present. In no specimen was melanoma missed on frozen section when also present on paraffin sections. However, 16 specimens were incorrectly interpreted as being melanoma on frozen sections but showed only actinic keratosis on paraffin sections. Frozen sections for diagnosis have been demonstrated in other melanoma studies[58–60] to be 95 to 99% accurate when interpreted by experienced pathologists.[61–64] In another study of 482 frozen sections with paraffin sections of various tumors, frozen sections were 100% accurate in the evaluation of resection margins and 97% accurate in identification of benign or malignant processes.[65] These and other studies of melanoma excised by Mohs micrographic surgery document the accuracy of frozen sections for evaluating surgical margins.[56–60]

CURE RATES

Mohs micrographic surgery has provided cure rates comparable to those of conventional wide excision when used to treat melanoma. In one study, 103 patients were stratified according to Clark's levels, and the survival rate of patients treated by fixed tissue Mohs surgery compared favorably with that of patients who had wide excisions by standard surgery. The value of Mohs micrographic surgery in the treatment of melanoma of the periauricular area and of familial melanoma was also described. Data on 200 patients treated between 1980 and 1988 with fresh tissue Mohs micrographic surgery

TABLE 59–5. EFFECT OF TUMOR THICKNESS ON SURVIVAL OF PATIENTS WITH MELANOMA TREATED BY THE FRESH TISSUE MOHS SURGICAL TECHNIQUE

Tumor Thickness	Determinate Patients Followed 2.5 Yr (N = 77)			Determinate Patients Followed 5 Yr (N = 26)		
	No. of Patients	Expected Deaths	Actual Deaths	No. of Patients	Expected Deaths	Actual Deaths
In situ	12	—	0	6	—	0
≤0.85 mm	38	0.38	0	10	0.10	0
0.86–1.69 mm	11	0.33	1	4	0.24	1
1.70–3.64 mm	12	1.44	0	4	0.96	0
>3.64 mm	4	1.72	0	2	1.08	0
Total	77	3.87	1	26	2.38	1

show that survival and local recurrence rates compared favorably with those of historical controls from the same period (Table 59–5).[56] These studies from different investigators support the use of Mohs micrographic surgery for melanoma.

The use of Mohs microscopic surgery has demonstrated that the visible melanoma tumor has contiguous microscopic extensions. The width of these microscopic extensions is unrelated to the depth of the melanoma and is unpredictable. In one study of 200 patients, the subclinical extensions of melanoma measured as far as 1.5 cm from the visual clinical margin. Most tumors (80%) had extensions of less than 6 mm. These data suggest that narrowing the surgical margins to less than 1.5 cm in thin melanomas may result in an increased risk of local recurrence.

ADVANTAGES

The main advantage of Mohs micrographic surgery is the removal of subclinical extensions while sparing normal tissue. Results show that in 80% of the patients treated with Mohs micrographic surgery, the tumor can be excised with a 6-mm margin instead of a wider surgical margin. This sparing of normal tissue may be very important cosmetically and functionally for melanomas on the face, digits, ears, or genitalia, although it may not be important on the trunk or extremities. Mohs micrographic surgery with frozen section control may also be useful during excisions of melanomas with poorly defined margins (e.g., lentigo maligna melanoma, lentigo maligna, amelanotic melanoma, desmoplastic melanoma, and subungual melanoma).

Elective Regional Lymph Node Dissection

Elective lymphadenectomy for malignant melanoma has been and continues to be extremely controversial.[66–74] The rationale for elective regional lymph node dissection for melanoma almost certainly stems from Handley's original description of lymphatic permeation in 1907.[31] It has been hypothesized that melanoma metastasizes sequentially from primary site to regional lymph nodes to distant sites.[75] However, almost one fourth of melanomas were found to recur at distant sites without previous lymph node involvement.[76]

GOAL

The aim of elective lymphadenectomy is to improve the survival of those patients who have had a metastasis to a regional lymph node but have not yet suffered systemic dissemination of melanoma. The biologic concept accepted by proponents of prophylactic lymph node dissection is that regional lymph nodes act as a biologic filter, stopping melanoma from metastasizing. The problem with this theory is that it does not apply to any other types of cancer or to any analogous model. Prophylactic lymph node dissection does not improve the survival rate in head and neck cancers, breast cancer, or thin or thick melanomas. It follows that patients with thin melanomas (less than 1 mm thick) who have a very low likelihood of metastasis and patients with lesions more than 4 mm thick and who have a poor prognosis will clearly not benefit from elective lymphadenectomy.[77] However, patients with melanomas of intermediate thickness (1 to 4 mm) might possibly benefit from elective node dissection. Several large, prospective but nonrandomized clinical studies describe the benefit of elective lymphadenectomy for intermediate-thickness melanoma.[71–73] However, selection biases or some other unidentified prognostic factors could have affected the results.

Since the 1960s there has been a decline in the number of elective node dissections performed for malignant melanoma in the United States. In Canada, 24% of surgeons perform prophylactic node dissections on patients with melanomas 1.5 mm or more in depth. However, 66% still wait until clinically palpable nodes are evident before proceeding with nodal dissection.[47] Most surgeons in the United States and Europe also now choose to wait and maintain close follow-up until there is clinical suspicion of nodal metastasis.

CURRENT STATUS

Currently there is no clear answer regarding the benefit of elective regional lymph node dissection. Even for the subgroup of patients with intermediate-thickness melanoma, a consensus does not yet exist. The issue becomes even more confusing when lymph nodes appear clinically negative or when drainage to nodes from certain areas, such as the trunk, is multidirectional.[14]

Most proponents of elective lymphadenectomy base their views on the results of several large but nonrandomized retrospective studies.[67, 69, 70] A 1979 study examined the benefit gained from prophylactic node dissection in 151 patients with malignant melanoma of the lower extremity.[67, 78] For lesions 1.5 to 3.99 mm thick, a nodal dissection was associated with only about a two-fold increase in survival rate at 5 years. For melanomas between 1.6 and 3 mm thick, there was only a 50% survival advantage, and this only for men with extremity lesions.[70] A retrospective bicenter European study of more than 800 patients with clinical stage I melanoma treated with either wide excision alone or wide excision with elective lymph node dissection and followed for 4 to 18 years reported an improved survival rate only in men with primary tumors 1.51 to 3 mm thick.[79]

Prospective randomized studies published to date show no therapeutic benefit associated with elective lymph node dissection.[80–83] However, possible inherent weaknesses exist within the two major prospective studies most often referred to by opponents of elective lymphadenectomy. In the Mayo Clinic study, almost two thirds of the patients had lesions less than 1.5 mm thick.[82] Only a small number of patients had lesions of intermediate thickness. The later WHO study has been criticized, because it contained a disproportionately large number of patients with favorable prognostic factors[83] (i.e., women and patients with melanomas of the limbs). The patients in these two studies also were not stratified according to Breslow thickness, since the studies were begun before general acceptance of this technique. However, a fairly comparable patient distribution with regard to lesion thickness has been found by subsequent retrospective analysis.

PREDICTING LYMPH NODE METASTASIS

Tumor thickness is the most important factor in predicting nodal metastasis. The incidence of nodal involvement was studied in 151 patients with melanoma of the extremity[69]; 22% of patients with lesions 2.1 to 3 mm thick and 39% of patients with lesions more than 3 mm thick had evidence of nodal involvement. The incidence of nodal involvement relative to Clark's levels was determined to be 4% for level II, 7% for level III, 25% for level IV, and 70% for level V.[69] Other subsequent studies have confirmed the finding of more frequent nodal metastasis with increasing depth of melanoma invasion and tumor thickness.[84, 85] In a prospective study of patients with stage I malignant melanoma, no evidence of nodal micrometastases was found in patients with lesions less than 1 mm thick.[74] Nodal involvement was assessed by serial sections of lymph nodes prophylactically removed at the time of surgery. In this study, the incidence of positive nodal involvement was 27% for intermediate-thickness melanomas (i.e., between 1 and 4 mm thick).

Anatomic location of the primary tumor is also a factor that affects regional lymph node involvement and subsequent prognosis in melanoma patients. An almost 50% 5-year mortality rate was demonstrated in patients who had one or two positive lymph nodes with the primary tumor in the head and neck region.[86] Others have corroborated the poor prognosis of patients with head or neck melanoma and regional nodal involvement.[87, 88]

Head and Neck Melanoma

The pattern of metastasis to lymph nodes was examined in patients with head and neck melanomas. It was found that metastasis did not "skip" nodal groups but could usually be identified in the nodes immediately adjacent to the site of surgery.[88] On the basis of these and similar findings,[89] it was suggested that elective lymphadenectomy be performed, using a modified version of the standard neck dissection, for head and neck melanomas more than 1 mm thick when there was no evidence of clinically palpable nodes.[90] A conventional radical neck dissection was thought to be virtually unnecessary. However, because of the ambiguous lymphatic drainage patterns seen with midline head and neck lesions, elective nodal dissection significantly increases morbidity without clearly improving survival in patients with such lesions.

Trunk Melanoma

The route of lymphatic drainage in the trunk is even less predictable than that in midline head and neck lesions. Close to one half of patients have a multidirectional lymphatic flow from cutaneous lesion sites as demonstrated by preoperative lymphoscintigraphy performed with technetium 99m.[91] Surgical oncologists have used a dye to help determine lymph node drainage, only performing a biopsy on nodes that take up the dye; in this way, fewer radical surgeries are performed. However, the value of this technique is still unclear. Thus, for most patients, elective lymph node dissection for cutaneous melanoma of the trunk may offer no therapeutic benefit because of unpredictable drainage patterns.[92]

Melanoma of the Extremities

With regard to other anatomic locations, the extremities usually have a fairly consistent and predictable pattern of lymphatic drainage. However, the data regarding the benefit of elective lymphadenectomy remain inconclusive, even in these areas.[93–96] In a study of 490 patients with clinical stage I or II melanoma of the upper or lower extremity, 107 patients (22%) were found to have regional nodal involvement on histologic examination.[93] A total of 13% of patients who had undergone nodal dissection and 60% of patients who had positive nodal metastases had no clinical evidence of regional nodal involvement on physical examination. At the present time, more studies and data should be generated before prophylactic lymph node dissection is recommended to patients. It is possible that if there is any survival advantage to elective lymphadenectomy, the benefits may be small and may not become apparent for many years after surgery.[75] Until the value of prophylactic lymph node dissection is proved in a well-designed, large prospective study, the surgical technique may only add significant morbidity to patients without improving the survival rate.

THERAPEUTIC LYMPHADENECTOMY

The general consensus among most surgeons is that without demonstrable evidence of disseminated systemic metastasis, melanoma patients with clinically palpable lymph node metastasis should undergo regional nodal dissection. However, for many patients the presence of clinically evident nodal involvement is probably an indication of more distant metastases. It is possible that lymphadenectomy will do little to alter the clinical course of such patients. With the possibility of lymphatic obstruction or ulceration, resection of involved lymph nodes should be pursued for confirmatory prognostic reasons. The extent of surgery needed for nodal metastasis (i.e., deep versus superficial inguinal dissection or modified versus radical neck dissection) still remains controversial with regard to therapeutic benefit.[94–96]

Nonsurgical Treatment Modalities

REGIONAL PERFUSION

The technique of isolated limb perfusion was developed in the late 1950s.[97] The initial goal of this method was to increase the dose of the chemotherapeutic agent to an isolated area while decreasing the agent's systemic toxicity. Predictably, the technique is only appropriate for melanomas of an extremity. The drug most widely employed for regional perfusion is melphalan (L-phenylalanine mustard) used either alone or in combination with other alkylating agents.

Much controversy centers around the use of isolated perfusion therapy for melanoma.[98–106] Perfusion has been used either in combination with surgery or alone, the latter mostly for cases of in-transit metastasis. A combination of chemotherapy and perfusion has been shown to yield better results than perfusion alone.[99, 107] In a 1988 study, excision alone was compared with excision plus limb perfusion with melphalan in patients with stage I, II, or III melanoma of the extremity.[108] In this randomized prospective study, a survival benefit was demonstrated when perfusion was used as adjunctive therapy to surgery. A more than threefold increase in survival rate in patients with in-transit metastases was found when hyperthermic perfusion was employed.[99] One study showed an improved disease-free survival rate for patients with stage I melanoma more than 1.5 mm thick who received adjuvant regional perfusion.[109] However, another study failed to demonstrate a benefit from adjuvant perfusion. In this study of more than 450 patients with stage I melanoma of the extremity thicker than 1.5 mm,[104] no differences were noted in terms of the disease-free interval, time to distant metastases, or survival rate when patients received regional limb perfusion in addition to wide excision of their melanoma.

Presently, regional perfusion is not widely accepted for melanoma treatment. Additional studies with accurate patient stratification, performed according to known prognostic variables, are needed to properly evaluate the benefit from isolated limb perfusion, especially for patients with higher risk primary melanomas. Patients with thicker melanomas may have in-transit metastases or occult micrometastases, which have been shown to respond to regional perfusion.[107, 110] In these individuals, progression to systemic spread of their melanoma may be halted by perfusion therapy. A prospective, randomized WHO study is currently in progress.

CHEMOTHERAPY

Adjuvant Chemotherapy

The rationale behind combining chemotherapy with surgery for melanoma is to attack micrometastases that may have been missed by primary resection of the tumor but whose cells are vulnerable to the effects of chemotherapeutic agents. Patients with lymph node metastases are especially prone to recurrent disease and may benefit from systemic adjuvant therapy. At present, the most commonly used and most effective chemotherapeutic agent is 5(or 4)-(dimethyltriazeno)imidazole-4(or 5)-carboxamide (DTIC).

No beneficial effect has been adequately demonstrated for the use of adjuvant chemotherapy in malignant melanoma.[111–113] A study by the Central Oncology Group (COG) found that patients with high-risk melanomas who received DTIC as adjuvant therapy actually had a worse survival rate than those who had surgery alone.[104] A WHO study also failed to show a survival advantage for patients receiving DTIC in addition to surgery.[113]

Chemotherapy as Sole Treatment for Metastatic Melanoma

Systemic chemotherapy for malignant melanoma that has metastasized, although beneficial in a minority of patients, usually provides only a temporary and incomplete response. Most current chemotherapeutic agents do not have a significant antitumor effect on metastatic melanoma. Combination drug therapy is becoming increasingly popular, but its advantage over traditional single-agent treatment is still questionable. The benefit to the patient must always be weighed against side effects before beginning systemic chemotherapy.

The most commonly used and probably the most effective single agent for metastatic melanoma is DTIC. It is usually given daily[114] for 5 days every 4 weeks at a dose of 150 to 400 mg/m². Response rates have usually averaged from 15 to 25%.[115, 116] The complete response rate is significantly lower. Success is usually much greater for soft tissue and lymph node metastases as opposed to visceral metastases, which show a less than 10% response rate with single-agent therapy. The most common side effects of DTIC are gastrointestinal (e.g., nausea and vomiting), but it is also toxic to the bone marrow.

Other chemotherapeutic agents that have been used with varying success against metastatic melanoma include actinomycin D, cisplatin, the nitrosoureas, dibromodulcitol, taxol, and detorubicin.[117–120] While some of these newer agents show promise, response rates have been no greater than with DTIC.

Many of the more effective single agents have been used in combination regimens against advanced metastatic melanoma. In many instances, toxicity is increased without a concomitant increase in tumor regression. While some of these regimens report response rates as high as 40 to 50%, results have not been reproducible, and responses are only temporary.[121, 122] A three-drug regimen of cisplatin, vinblastine, and DTIC was evaluated,[123] and the most notable finding was that the response rate for visceral metastases was significantly higher for the combination chemotherapy than for DTIC alone. Increased response was also noted for metastases to bone, for which therapy with DTIC alone has been fairly ineffective. These results are encouraging, especially since the regimen was quite well tolerated.

IMMUNOTHERAPY

One of the most exciting areas to develop in the treatment of melanoma is immunotherapy. Several types of immunologically based treatments are currently being evaluated or employed.

Adoptive Immunotherapy

Adoptive immunotherapy is a pioneering biologic approach to melanoma treatment. Interest in the development of this technique stemmed from observations, although rare, of spontaneous regression and disappearance of cancer, in which the immune system is thought to be obviously playing a central role.[124] Disseminated melanoma has shown one of the most promising responses to adoptive immunotherapy.

Two basic forms of treatment constitute adoptive immunotherapy: lymphokine-activated killer cell (LAK) and tumor-infiltrating lymphocyte (TIL) therapy. LAK therapy involves isolating a patient's lymphocytes and growing them in culture in the presence of interleukin–2.[125] These stimulated lymphocytes are then infused back into the patient, where they cause regression of the tumors. Interleukin–2, which is produced naturally by helper T cells but can also be generated in great quantity by recombinant DNA technology, may also cause regression of the tumor when administered alone in high doses. For advanced metastatic melanoma, a 10% complete regression rate has been reported, and in another 10% of patients, at least a 50% tumor regression has been seen.[124]

In TIL therapy, a melanoma nodule is surgically removed, and its cells are cultured in the presence of interleukin–2. After about a month, the tumor cells are completely replaced by the proliferating lymphocytes. These lymphocytes, which are more specific and tumoricidal than those derived from LAK therapy, are then infused into the patient with interleukin–2.[125] Preliminary reports suggest that TIL therapy may be more effective with fewer side effects than LAK therapy.[126] Research is currently being done to try to insert the genes for cytokines with antitumor activity, such as alpha-interferon or tumor necrosis factor, into the TILs.[124] Melanoma appears to be one of the most responsive tumors to adoptive immunotherapy. Dosages and treatment schedules must be fine tuned, but the results of the work in immunotherapy are extremely promising for metastatic melanoma patients.

Tumor Vaccines

The use of tumor vaccines to increase patients' immune response to melanoma-associated antigens has also been employed. In initial trials, bacille Calmette-Guérin (BCG) and *Corynebacterium parvum* were the agents most commonly studied. Both of these agents stimulate the immune system nonspecifically. While initial studies showed some promise in terms of prolonging recurrence-free intervals,[127–129] subsequent trials have failed to show a statistically significant benefit in melanoma patients treated with either BCG or *C. parvum*.[130–132]

Other tumor vaccines have also been evaluated and appear to show some promise, although these studies have not been confirmed by randomized clinical trials.[133, 134] A purified melanoma tumor-associated antigen has been used in patients with stage III melanoma, and a response was seen in almost one third of patients who received the antigen alone.[133] A novel approach to immunization has also been developed using a polyvalent vaccine for melanoma.[134] This is significant, since the various melanoma subtypes have differing surface antigens. Immune stimulation was seen in approximately one half of the patients studied.

RADIOTHERAPY

Melanoma is far more radioresistant than most other tumors.[135, 136] For many years it was thought that there was no place for the use of radiation in the treatment of malignant melanoma. However, with improved understanding of the biology of melanoma and the use of refined dosing schedules, radiation therapy has been used with much greater success.

Response rates have been significantly improved by using fewer fractions in conjunction with high-dose radiation, usually in the range of 400 to 800 rad.[137–139] In a retrospective review of patients with melanoma metastatic to soft tissue, brain, spinal cord, and bone who had undergone radiation therapy,[140] response rates were significantly greater in those patients who had received high-dose radiation fractions. It was concluded that fraction size was the most important factor determining the response to treatment. However, increasing tumor volume also appears to adversely affect the response rate.[141]

At present, the use of radiotherapy in melanoma is primarily for palliation in selected patients with symptomatic metastases and as adjuvant treatment after excision of cutaneous melanomas of the head and neck. For head and neck melanomas, when wide excision would be either dangerous or grossly mutilating, local excision followed by high-dose radiotherapy may be considered.[142] When nodal metastases are unresectable or when there are multiple skin lesions that cannot be surgically excised, radiotherapy may also be used for palliation.

Radiation therapy has also been used for the treatment of lentigo maligna (LM) and lentigo maligna melanoma (LMM). As these lesions are commonly quite large, radiotherapy offers the advantage of significantly improved cosmesis. In some centers, radiotherapy remains the treatment of choice for LM and LMM, with response rates of more than 90% being reported.[142] Only one of eight cases of LM and 1 of 15 cases of LMM were found to recur after irradiation.[143] No cure rates for LMM treated by radiation therapy could be found. However, some cutaneous surgeons support the recommendation that surgical excision is the treatment of choice for these lesions.[144]

Lentigo Maligna and Lentigo Maligna Melanoma

Nearly 100 years ago, Hutchinson described the lesion of LM.[145] LM is a slowly enlarging macular lesion that occurs primarily on sun-exposed skin in elderly, light-skinned individuals. It often reaches a rather large size before the diagnosis is established and treatment is instituted. It still remains unclear what proportion of these precancerous LM lesions eventually progress to invasive LMM; most sources place the incidence between 33 and 50%.[146, 147] However, one study suggests a less than 1% progression rate per year for patients older than 45 years.[148] More than 90% of LMM lesions occur in the head and neck region.[149] In contrast to the widely held belief that LMM carries a better patient prognosis than other melanomas, it was found that after accounting for primary tumor thickness and site, LMM and non-LMM lesions have the same patient prognosis.[150]

Various approaches to the management and treatment of LM exist. Because the progression rate of LM to LMM was as high as 50% in early studies, combined with a 10% eventual rate of metastatic spread of the LMM, complete surgical excision of LM has been the customary treatment.[144, 146, 151, 152] A high percentage of lesions diagnosed as LM by clinical inspection were actually found to be LMM by subsequent thorough histologic examination.[146] Many researchers believe it is possible to adequately assess the biologic potential of the lesion only when the entire lesion is evaluated histopathologically.[153] In a retrospective review of 38 cases of LM and 22 cases of LMM, it was found that surgical excision provided a cure rate of 90% versus an overall 45% cure rate for all other treatment modalities.[153] Patients who had undergone radiotherapy were not included in this study.

Another study also found the lowest recurrence rate with surgical excision of LM lesions.[144] After a biopsy of at least a portion of the lesion confirms LM, excision with a 5- to 10-mm margin of normal skin is recom-

TABLE 59–6. CHANCE OF INITIAL RECURRENCE OF MELANOMA IN FIRST AND FIFTH YEARS AFTER DIAGNOSIS BASED ON BRESLOW THICKNESS[159]

Melanoma Thickness (mm)	Recurrence Rate in First Yr (%)	Recurrence Rate at Fifth Yr (%)
<0.76	1	0.7
0.76–1.50	5.7	3.1
1.51–4.0	18.8	4.7
>4.0	33.6	5.0

mended.[144] For lesions suspected to be LMM by clinical examination, a full-thickness biopsy was recommended. If histologically proved LMM is found, a 2- to 5-cm margin is used.[144]

To achieve the best cosmetic results, many alternative forms of treatment have been used for LM. These include topical 5-fluorouracil (5-FU), cryosurgery, topical azelaic acid, radiotherapy, electrodesiccation and curettage, and dermabrasion.[143, 152, 154–158] In a study of 42 patients with LM, a 9% recurrence rate was found in those patients who had undergone surgical excision.[144] In LM patients who underwent a destructive form of primary treatment such as radiotherapy, curettage, electrodesiccation, or cryosurgery, the overall recurrence rate was 35%.[144] While encouraging results have been reported for topical 5% 5-FU in the treatment of LM,[154] another study found that all patients with LM treated with topical 5-FU suffered recurrence.[153]

Follow-up and Risk of Recurrence

The risk of recurrence should be considered when formulating a follow-up regimen. At present, Breslow thickness is the factor most strongly correlated with risk of recurrence for clinical stage I melanomas.[159–161] Of 295 patients who initially presented with clinical stage I melanoma but subsequently developed metastatic disease,[159] the risk of recurrence was directly related to tumor thickness. The data from this study can be summarized as follows: melanomas less than 0.76 mm thick carried an annual risk of recurrence of approximately 1%; for tumors between 0.76 and 1.5 mm thick, the recurrence rate was found to be relatively constant at about 5% per year; tumors between 1.5 and 4 mm thick have a significantly higher recurrence risk in the first few years after diagnosis, but this gradually decreases to 5% annually by the fifth year; for melanomas more than 4 mm thick, the recurrence rate jumps to greater than 30% in the first year and gradually declines to 5% by the fifth year[159] (Table 59–6).

Based on these data, the following guidelines have been suggested: patients with thin melanomas (less than 0.76 mm thick) should be seen twice for follow-up in the first year and annually thereafter; patients with lesions between 0.76 and 1.5 mm thick should be seen

TABLE 59–7. FOLLOW-UP RECOMMENDATIONS ACCORDING TO TUMOR THICKNESS FOR PATIENTS WITH STAGE I MALIGNANT MELANOMA[168]

Lesions <0.76 mm in thickness
  Screening: No studies
  Follow-up: Yearly for life (history and physical)
  Laboratory evaluation: Only to confirm clinical suspicion
Lesions 0.76–1.50 mm in thickness
  Screening: Chest radiograph
  Follow-up: Chest radiograph yearly for 5 yr
       History and physical: Every 6 mo for 3 yr; every yr thereafter
Lesions >1.50 mm in thickness
  Screening: Chest CT scan + serum LDH; if LDH elevated, then abdominal CT scan
  Follow-up, first and second years:

1.51–3 mm thick:	Chest radiograph every yr
	Physician visit every 3 mo
>3 mm thick:	Chest radiograph every 6 mo first yr; every yr thereafter
	Physician visit every 3 mo
	LDH at end of second yr
Follow-up, third and fourth yr:	Chest radiograph every yr
	Physician visit every 6 mo
Follow-up, fifth yr and beyond:	Physician visit every yr
	Laboratory evaluation only to confirm clinical suspicion

at 6-month intervals indefinitely; patients with tumors 1.5 to 4 mm thick carry an elevated risk of recurrence and should be followed at 3-month intervals for the first year, 4-month intervals for the next 3 years, and every 6 months thereafter; patients with melanomas thicker than 4 mm should be seen even more frequently in the first year, when the risk of recurrence is highest.[159]

LATE RECURRENCES

There have been several reports of sporadic "late" recurrences after a disease-free interval of more than 10 years, even for thin melanomas.[162] The rate at which "late" recurrence occurs, however, is under speculation but has been variously reported to be 0.93% (51/586),[163] 2.7% (34/1283),[164] and 6.7% (7/105).[165]

However, these studies may be criticized for two reasons. First, the follow-up period for some of the patients was as short as 11 years, and recurrences as late as 33 years after diagnosis have been reported.[161] Therefore, it is possible that some of these patients may present with a relapse of their disease in the future. Second, patients who died of other causes without suffering a recurrence in the first 10 years after initial treatment were not taken into account.[166] For these reasons, true late recurrence rates may actually be higher than those reported.

Because most patients currently present with early disease, it is difficult to predict the benefit of life-long follow-up for melanoma patients. However, it is prudent to have at least yearly total body skin examinations when there is a history of melanoma. This provides the advantage of not only detecting recurrences but also identifying new melanomas. Since 69% of patients initially identify their own recurrences, the value of proper patient education with regard to self-examination cannot be overlooked.[167] General guidelines for recommended follow-up have been developed and are based on primary tumor thickness (Table 59–7).

SUMMARY

Recent increases in the incidence of melanoma, presumably because of excessive ultraviolet light exposure, have resulted in dramatic changes in our understanding of the biology of this serious cutaneous malignancy. As our basic knowledge has grown, so has our ability to provide the most appropriate care for each affected individual. Treatment recommendations and patient evaluation techniques are constantly being refined, and it is exceedingly important for the cutaneous surgeon to be aware of these important advances.

REFERENCES

1. Laennec RTH: Sur les melanoses. Bull Faculte Med Paris 1:2, 1812.
2. Halliday A: Case of melanosis. London Medical Repository 19:442, 1823.
3. Norris W: Case of fungoid disease. Edinb Med Surg J 16:562, 1820.
4. Parrish I: Case of melanosis. Am J Med Sci 20:266, 1837.
5. Coats J: On a case of multiple melanotic sarcoma. Glasgow Med J 24:92, 1885.
6. Carswell R: Illustrations of the elementary forms of disease. Longman, Orme, Brown, Green, & Longman, London, 1838.
7. Rigel DS, Kopf AW, Friedman RJ: The role of malignant melanoma in the United States: are we making an impact? J A Acad Dermatol 17:1050–1053, 1987.
8. Silverberg E: Cancer statistics. CA 39:13, 1989.
9. Day CL, Mihm MC, Sober AJ, et al: Narrower margins of clinical stage I malignant melanoma. N Engl J Med 306:479–481, 1982.
10. Landthaler M, Braun-Falco O, Leitl A, et al: Excisional biopsy as the first therapeutic procedure version primary wide excision of malignant melanoma. Cancer 64:1612–1616, 1989.
11. Davis NC: Cutaneous melanoma: the Queensland experience. Curr Probl Surg 13:1–63, 1976.
12. Kopf AW, Mintzis M, Bart RS: Diagnostic accuracy in malignant melanoma. Arch Dermatol 111:1291–1292, 1975.
13. Bharwani N: Initial management of cutaneous malignant melanoma. Can Med Assoc J 135:128, 1986.
14. White MJ, Polk AC: Therapy of primary cutaneous melanomas. Med Clin North Am 70:71, 1986.

15. Lederman JS, Sober AJ: Does biopsy type influence survival in clinical stage I cutaneous melanoma? J Am Acad Dermatol 13:983–987, 1985.

16. Verones U, Cascinelli N: Surgical treatment of malignant melanoma of the skin. World J Surg 3:279, 1979.

17. Drzewiecki KT, Ladefoged LC, Christensen HE: Biopsy and prognosis for cutaneous melanomas in clinical stage I. Scand J Plast Reconstr Surg 14:141, 1980.

18. Rampen FH, Van Horton WA: Incisional procedures and prognosis in malignant melanoma. Clin Exp Dermatol 5:313, 1980.

19. Jones WM, Williams WJ, Roberts MM, et al: Malignant melanoma of the skin: prognostic value of clinical features and the role of treatment in 111 cases. Br J Cancer 22:437, 1968.

20. Bagley FH, Cady B, Lee A: Changes in clinical presentation and managment of malignant melanoma. Cancer 47:2126, 1981.

21. Chanda JJ, Callen JP: Adverse effect of melanoma incision. J Am Acad Dermatol 13:519–521, 1985.

22. Epstein E, Bragg K, Linden G: Biopsy and prognosis of malignant melanoma. JAMA 208:1369, 1969.

23. Landthaler M, Braun-Falco O, Leitl A, et al: Excisional biopsy as the first therapeutic procedure versus primary wide excision of malignant melanoma. Cancer 64:1612, 1989.

24. Knutson CO, Hori JM, Spratt JS Jr: Melanoma. Curr Probl Surg December:3–55, 1971.

25. Davis NC: Cutaneous melanoma: the Queensland experience. Curr Probl Surg 13:30, 1976.

26. Breslow A, Macht SD: Optimal size of resection margin for thin cutaneous melanoma. Surg Gynecol Obstet 145:691–692, 1977.

27. Aitkin DR, Clausen K, Klein JP, James AG: The extent of primary melanoma excision. A re-evaluation—how wide is wide? Ann Surg 198:634–641, 1983.

28. Cosimi AB, Sober AJ, Mihm MC, Fitzpatrick TB: Conservative surgical management of superficially invasive cutaneous melanoma. Cancer 53:1256–1259, 1984.

29. Fisher JC: Safe margins for melanoma excision. Ann Plast Surg 14:158, 1985.

30. Olsen G: The malignant melanoma of the skin: new theories, based on a study of 500 cases. Acta Chir Scand (Suppl) 365:1, 1966.

31. Handley WS: The pathology of melanotic growths in relation to their operative treatment. Lancet 1:927, 1907.

32. Wong CK: A study of melanocytes in the normal skin surrounding malignant melanomata. Dermatologica 141:215, 1970.

33. Cochran AJ: Studies of the melanocytes of the epidermis adjacent to tumors. J Invest Dermatol 57:35, 1971.

34. Peterson NC: Malignant melanomas of the skin: a study of the origin, development, aetiology, spread, treatment and prognosis. Br J Plast Surg 15:49, 1962.

35. Clark WH Jr: The histogenesis and biologic behavior of primary human malignant melanoma of the skin. Cancer Res 29:705, 1969.

36. Breslow A: Thickness cross-sectional areas and depth of invasion in the prognosis of cutaneous melanoma. Ann Surg 172:902, 1970.

37. Day CL Jr, Mihm MC Jr, Sober AJ, et al: Narrower margins for clinical stage I melanoma patients. N Engl J Med 306:479–481, 1982.

38. Elder DE, Guessy D IV, Heiberger RM, et al: Optimal resection margin for cutaneous malignant melanoma. Plast Reconstr Surg 71:66, 1983.

39. Goldman LI, Byrd R: Narrowing resection margins for patients with low risk melanoma. Am J Surg 155:242, 1988.

40. Veronesi U, Cascinelli N, Adamus J, et al: Thin stage I primary cutaneous malignant melanoma. N Engl J Med 318:1159, 1988.

41. Olsen G: The malignant melanoma of the skin: new theories based on a study of 500 cases. Acta Chir Scand (Suppl) 365:1–220, 1966.

42. Cascinelli N, Van der Esch EP, Breslow A, et al: Stage I melanoma of the skin: the problem of resection margins. Eur J Cancer 16:1079, 1980.

43. Bagley FH, Cady B, Lee A, Legg MA: Changes in clinical presentation and management of malignant melanoma. Cancer 47:2126, 1981.

44. Hansen MG, McCarten AB: Tumor thickness and lymphocytic infiltration malignant melanoma of the head and neck. Am J Surg 128:557, 1974.

45. Aitken DR, Clausen K, Klein JP, James AG: The extent of primary melanoma excision: a re-evaluation—how wide is wide? Ann Surg 198:634–641, 1983.

46. Aitken DR, James AG, Carey LC: Local cutaneous recurrence after conservative excision of malignant melanoma. Arch Surg 119:643, 1984.

47. Shelley W, Kersey P, Quirt I, Pater J: Survey of surgical management of malignant melanoma in Canada: optimal margins of excision and lymph node dissection. Can J Surg 27:190, 1984.

48. Day CL, Harrist TJ, Gorstein F, et al: Malignant melanoma: parogrostic significance of "microscopic satellites" in the reticular dermis and subcutaneous fat. Ann Surg 194:108–112, 1981.

49. Kelly JW, Sagebiel RW, Calderon W, et al: The frequency of local recurrence and microsatellites as a guide to re-excision margins for cutaneous melanoma. Ann Surg 200:759, 1984.

50. Bockelbrink A, Bockelbrink H, Ristler H, Braunfalco O: Is wide excision necessary in malignant melanom? Abstract. Int J Dermatol 76:424, 1981.

51. Ho VC, Sober AJ: Therapy for cutaneous melanoma: an update. J Am Acad Dermatol 22:159–176, 1990.

52. Boddie AW, Balch CM: Three unresolved issues in the surgical treatment of melanoma. Oncology 2:39, 1988.

53. Kenady DE, Brown BW, McBridge CM: Excision of underlying fascia with a primary malignant melanom: effect on recurrence and survival rates. Surgery 92:615, 1982.

54. Cascinelli N, Santinami M, Urist MM, et al: Indications for managment of primary melanoma. In: Veronesi U, Cascinelli N, Santinomi M (eds): Cutaneous Melanoma. Status of Knowledge and Future Perspective. Karger, Basel, 1987, pp 545–553.

55. Abide JM, Nahai F, Bennett RG: The meaning of surgical margins. Plast Reconstr Surg 73:492, 1984.

56. Zitelli JA, Mohs FE, Larson P, Snow S: Mohs micrographic surgery for melanoma. Dermatol Clin 7:833, 1989.

57. Zitelli JA, Moy RL, Abell E: The reliability of frozen sections in the evaluation of surgical margins for melanoma. J Am Acad Dermatol 24:102–106, 1991.

58. Mohs FE: Chemosurgery for melanoma. Arch Dermatol 113:285–291, 1977.

59. Mohs FE, Bloom RF, Sahl WL: Chemosurgery for familial malignant melanomas. J Dermatol Surg Oncol 5:127–131, 1979.

60. Mohs FE: Microscopically controlled surgery for periorbital melanoma: fixed-tissue and fresh-tissue techniques. J Dermatol Surg Oncol 11:284–291, 1985.

61. Sawady J, Berner JJ, Siegler EE: Accuracy of and reasons for frozen section: a correlative, retrospective study. Hum Pathol 19:1019, 1988.

62. Little JH, David NC: Frozen section diagnosis of suspected malignant melanomas of the skin. Cancer 34:1163, 1974.

63. Milton GW, Jelihovsky T: Frozen section examination in the diagnosis of cutaneous malignant melanoma (melanoblastoma). Med J Aust 37:503, 1962.

64. Shafir R, Hiss J, Tsur H, Bubis JJ: Pitfalls in frozen section diagnosis of malignant melanoma. Cancer 51:1168, 1983.

65. Hirst E, Cains GD, Bale PM, et al: Diagnosis by frozen section examination, II: results in skin lesions. Aust NZ J Surg 38:216, 1969.

66. Guiss LW, MacDonald I: The role of radical regional lymphoadenectomy in treatment of melanoma. Am J Surg 104:135, 1962.

67. Balch CM, Murad TM, Soong SJ, et al: Tumor-thickness as a guide to surgical management of clinical stage I melanoma patients. Cancer 43:883, 1979.

68. Balch CM, Murad TM, Soong SJ, et al: A multifactorial analysis of melanoma: prognostic histopathological features comparing Clark's and Breslow's staging methods. Ann Surg 188:732, 1978.

69. Wanebo HJ, Fortner JG, Woodruff J, et al: Selection of the optimum surgical treatment of stage I melanoma by depth of microinvasion: use of combined microstage technique (Clark-Breslow). Ann Surg 182:302, 1975.

70. Milton GW, Shaw HM, McCarty WH, et al: Prophylactic lymph node dissection in clinical stage I cutaneous malignant melanoma: results of surgical treatment in 1319 patients. Br J Surg 69:108, 1982.

71. Reintgen DS, Cox EB, McCarthy RS Jr, et al: Efficacy of elective lymph node dissection in patients with intermediate thickness primary melanoma. Ann Surg 196:379–385, 1983

72. McCarthy WH, Shaw HM, Milton GW: Efficacy of elective

lymph node dissection in 2347 patients with clinical stage I malignant melanoma. Surg Gynecol Obstet 161:575, 1985.

73. Koh HR, Sober AJ, Day CL, et al: Prognosis of clinical stage I melanoma patients with positive elective regional node dissection. J Clin Oncol 4:1238–1244, 1986.

74. Roses DF, Harris MV, Hidalgo D, et al: Correlation of the thickness of melanoma and regional lymph node metastases. Arch Surg 117:921, 1982.

75. Balch CM: The role of elective lymph node dissection in melanoma: rationale, results, and controversies. J Clin Oncol 6:163, 1988.

76. Cascinelli N, Preda F, Vaglini M, et al: Metastatic spread of stage I melanoma of the skin. Tumori 69:449, 1983.

77. Rhodes AR, Weinstock MA, Fitzpatrick TB, et al: Risk factors for cutaneous melanoma: a practical method of recognizing predisposed individuals. JAMA 258:3146–3154, 1987.

78. Balch CM, Soong SJ, Murad TM, et al: A multifactorial analysis of melanoma. Prognostic factors in patients with stage I (localized) melanoma. Surgery 86:343, 1979.

79. Bieb B, Brcker EB, Drepper H, et al: Should elective lymph node dissection be used for treatment of primary melanoma? J Cancer Res Clin Oncol 115:470, 1989.

80. Veronesi U, Adamus J, Bandiera DC, et al: Inefficacy of immediate node dissection in stage I melanoma of the limbs. N Engl J Med 297:627, 1977.

81. Sim FH, Taylor WT, Ivins TC, et al: A prospective randomized study of the efficacy of routine lymphadenectomy in management of malignant melanoma. Cancer 41:948, 1978.

82. Sim FH, Taylor WT, Pritchard DJ, Soule EH: Lymphadenectomy in the management of stage I malignant melanoma: a prospective randomized study. Mayo Clin Proc 61:697, 1986.

83. Veronesi U, Butalino R, Cascinelli N, et al: Long term results of randomized trial comparing immediate versus delayed node dissection in stage I melanoma of the limbs. Dev Oncol 25:165, 1984.

84. Holmes EC, Mosely HS, Morton DL, et al: A rational approach to the surgical management of melanoma. Ann Surg 186:481, 1977.

85. Das Gupta TK: Results of treatment of 269 patients with primary cutaneous melanoma: a five-year prospective study. Ann Surg 186:201, 1977.

86. Olson RM, Woods JC, Soule EH: Regional lymph node management and outcome in 100 patients with head and neck melanoma. Am J Surg 142:470, 1983.

87. Southwick HW, Slaughter DP, Hinkamp JS: Malignant melanoma of the skin of the head and neck. Am J Surg 106:852, 1963.

88. Roses DF, Harris MN, Grunberger I, et al: Selective surgical managment of cutaneous melanoma of the head and neck. Ann Surg 192:629, 1980.

89. Byers RM, Medina JE, Wolf PF: Regional node dissection of the head and neck. In: Balch CM (ed): Surgical Approaches to Cutaneous Melanoma. Karger, New York, 1985, p 83.

90. Harris MN, Roses DF: Managment of head and neck melanoma. In: Nussbaum M (ed). Modern Techniques of Surgery. Futura Publishing, Mt Kisko, NY, 1981.

91. Lock-Anderson J, Rossing N, Drzewieck KT: Preoperative cutaneous lymphoscintigraphy in malignant melanoma. Cancer 63:77, 1989.

92. Byers RM: The role of modified neck dissection in the treatment of cutaneous melanoma of the head and neck. Arch Surg 121:1338–1341, 1986.

93. Roses DF, Harris MN, Gumpert SL, et al: Regional lymph node dissection in malignant melanoma of the extremities. Surgery 89:654, 1981.

94. Korakousis CP, Emrich LJ, Rao U: Groin dissection in malignant melanoma. Am J Surg 152:491–495, 1986.

95. Finck SJ, Giuliano AE, Mann BD, et al: Results of ilioinguinal dissection for stage II melanoma. Ann Surg 196:180–186, 1982.

96. Coit DG, Brennan MF: Extent of lymph node dissection in melanoma of the trunk or lower extremity. Arch Surg 124:162–166, 1989.

97. Creech O Jr, Krementz ET, Ryan RF, et al: Chemotherapy of cancer. Regional perfusion utilizing an extracorporeal circuit. Ann Surg 145:616, 1958.

98. Cavaliere R, Ciocatto EL, Gionavella BL, et al: Selective heat

99. Stehlin JS, Giovanella BC, de Ipolyi PD, et al: Results of hyperthermic perfusion for melanoma of the extremities. Surg Gynecol Obstet 140:339, 1975.

100. Janoff KA, Moseson D, Nohigren J, et al: The treatment of stage I melanoma of the extremities with regional hyperthermic isolation perfusion. Ann Surg 196:316, 1982.

101. McBride CM, Sugarbaker EV, Hickey RC: Prophylactic isolation-perfusion as the primary therapy for invasive malignant melanoma of the limbs. Ann Surg 182:316, 1972.

102. Wagner DE: A retrospective study of regional perfusion for melanoma. Arch Surg 111:410, 1976.

103. Stehlin JS Jr: Hyperthermic perfusion for melanoma of the extremities: experience with 165 patients, 1967 to 1979. Ann NY Acad Sci 335:352, 1980.

104. Franklin HR, Koopf HS, Oldoff J, et al: To perfuse or not to perfuse? A retrospective study to evaluate the effect of adjuvant isolated regional perfusion in patients with stage I extremity melanoma with a thickness of 1.5 mm or greater. J Clin Oncol 6:701–708, 1988.

105. Martjin H, Schraffordt-Koops H, Milton GW, et al: Comparison of two methods of treating primary malignant melanomas Clark IV and V, and thickness 1.5 mm and greter, localized on the extremities: wide surgical excision with and without adjuvant regional perfusion. Cancer 57:1923–1930, 1986.

106. Ghussen F, Nagel K, Groth W, et al: A prospective randomized study of regional extremity perfusion in patients with malignant melanoma. Ann Surg 200:764–768, 1984.

107. Krementz ET, Ryan RF, Carter RD, et al: Hyperthermic regional perfusion for melanoma of the limbs. In: Balch CM, Milton GW (eds): Cutaneous Melanoma: Clinical Management and Treatment Results Worldwide. JB Lippincott, Philadelphia, 1985.

108. Ghussen F, Kruger I, Groth W, et al: The role of regional hyperthermic cytostatic perfusion in the treatment of extremity melanoma. Cancer 61:654, 1988.

109. Rege VB, Leone LA, Soderberg CH, et al: Hyperthermic adjuvant perfusion chemotherapy for stage I malignant melanoma of the extremity with literature review. Cancer 52:2033, 1983.

110. Storm FK, Morton DL: Value of therapeutic hyperthermic limb perfusion in advanced recurrent melanoma of the lower extremity. Am J Surg 150:32, 1985.

111. Hill JG, Moss SE, Golomb FM, et al: DTIC and combination therapy for melanoma III. DTIC (NSC 45388) surgical adjuvant study COG protocol 7040. Cancer 47:2556–2562, 1981.

112. Tranum BL, Dixon D, Quagliana J, et al: Lack of benefit of adjunctive chemotherapy in stage I malignant melanoma: a Southwest Oncology Group study. Cancer Treat Rep 71:643, 1987.

113. Veronesi U, Adamus J, Aubert C, et al: A randomized trial of adjuvant chemotherapy and immunotherapy in cutaneous melanoma. N Engl J Med 307:913–916, 1982.

114. Comis RL: Systemic therapay of malignant melanoma. Curr Concept Oncol 4:18, 1982.

115. McClay EF, Mastrangelo MJ: Systemic chemotherapy for metastatic melanoma. Semin Oncol 15:169, 1988.

116. Luce JK: Chemotherapy of melanoma. Semin Oncol 2:179, 1975.

117. Young RC, Canellos GP, Chabner BA, et al: Treatment of malignant melanoma with methyl CCNU. Clin Pharmacol Ther 15:617, 1974.

118. Wiernik PH, Schwartz KEL, Einzig A, et al: Phase I trial of taxol given as a 24 hour infusion every 21 days: responses observed in metastatic melanoma. J Clin Oncol 8:1232, 1987.

119. Chawla SP, Legha SS, Benjamion RS: Detrorubicin—an active anthrocycline in untreated metastatic melanoma. J Clin Oncol 3:1529, 1985.

120. Bellet RE, Catalano RB, Mastrangelo MJ, et al: Positive phase II trial of dibromodulcitol in patients with metastatic melanoma refractory of DTIC and a nitrosourea. Cancer Treat Rep 69:65, 1985.

121. Nathanson L, Kaufman SD, Carey RW: Vinblastine, infusion, bleomycin, and cis-dichlorodiammine-platinum chemotherapy in metastatic melanoma. Cancer 48:1290, 1981.

122. Seigler HF, Lucas VS, Pickett NJ, et al: DTIC, CCNU, bleo-

mycin and vincristine in metastatic melanoma. Cancer 46:2346, 1980.

123. Legha SS: Cisplatin, vinblastine and DTIC chemotherapy for advanced melanoma. Melanoma Lett 8:1–4, 1990.

124. Rosenberg SA: Adoptive immunotherapy for cancer. Sci Am 262:62, 1990.

125. Rosenberg SA, Lotze MT, Muul LM, et al: A progress report on the treatment of 157 patients with advanced cancer using lymphokine activated killer cells and interleukin-2 or high-dose interleukin-2 alone. N Engl J Med 316:889–897, 1987.

126. Rosenberg SA, Packard BC, Abersold PM, et al: Use of tumor infiltrating lymphocytes and interleukin–2 in the immunotherapy of patients with metastatic melanoma: A preliminary report. N Engl J Med 319:1676–1680, 1988.

127. Eilber FR, Townsend CM Jr, Morton DL: Results of BCG adjuvant immunotherapy for melanoma of the head and neck. Am J Surg 132:476, 1976.

128. Eilber FR, Morton DL, Holmes EL: Adjuvant immunotherapy with BCG in treatment of regional lymph node metastases from malignant melanoma. N Engl J Med 294:237, 1976.

129. Lipton A, Harvey HA, Lawrence B, et al: *Corynebacterium parvum* versus BCG adjuvant immunotherapy in human malignant melanoma. Cancer 51:57, 1983.

130. Silver HKB, Ibrahim EMA, Evers JW, et al: Adjuvant BCG immunotherapy for stage I and II malignant melanoma. Can Med Assoc J 128:1291, 1983.

131. Fisher RI, Terry WD, Hodes RJ, et al: Adjuvant immunotherapy of chemotherapy for malignant melanoma. Surg Clin North Am 61:1267–1277, 1981.

132. Hilal EY, Pinsky CM, Hirshaut Y, et al: Surgical adjuvant therapy of malignant melanoma with *Corynebacterium parvum*. Cancer 48:245, 1981.

133. Hollinshead A, Arlen M, Yonemoto R: Pilot studies using melanoma tumor-associated antigens (TAA) in specific-active immunochemotherapy of malignant melanoma. Cancer 49:1387, 1982.

134. Bystryn JC, Oratz R, Harris MN, et al: Immunogenicity of a polyvalent melanoma antigen vaccine in humans. Cancer 61:1065, 1988.

135. Adair FE: Treatment of melanoma: report of four hundred cases. Surg Gynecol Obstet 62:406, 1936.

136. Barranco SC, Romsdahl MM, Humphrey RM: The radiation response of human malignant melanoma cells grown in vitro. Cancer Res 31:830, 1971.

137. Hornsey S: The relationship between total dose, number of fractions and fraction size in the response of malignant melanoma in patients. Br J Radiol 51:905, 1978.

138. Habermaiz HJ, Fischer TJ: Radiation therapy of malignant melanoma: experience with high individual treatment doses. Cancer 38:2258, 1976.

139. Hellriegel W: Radiation therapy of primary and metastatic melanoma. Ann NY Acad Sci 100:131, 1963.

140. Strauss A, Dritschilo A, Nathanson L, et al: An evaluation of clinically used fractionation schemes. Cancer 47:1262, 1981.

141. Harwood AR, Cummings BJ: Radiotherapy for malignant melanoma: a re-appraisal. Cancer Treat Rev 8:271, 1981.

142. Harwood AR, Dancuart F, Fitzpatrick PJ: Radiotherapy in nonlentiginous melanoma of the head and neck. Cancer 48:2599, 1981.

143. Duancuart F, Harwood AR, Fitzpatrick PJ: The radiotherapy of lentigo maligna and lentigo maligna melanoma of the head and neck. Cancer 45:2279, 1980.

144. Pitman GH, Kopf AW, Bart RS, Casson PR: Treatment of lentigo maligna and lentigo maligna melanoma. J Dermatol Surg Oncol 9:727–737, 1979.

145. Hutchinson J: Senile freckles (cases III, IV, V, VI). Arch Surg 3:319, 1892.

146. Wayte DM, Helwig EB: Melanotic freckle of Hutchinson. Cancer 21:893, 1968.

147. Sober AJ, Mihm MC Jr, Fitzpatrick TB, et al: Malignant melanoma of the skin, and benign neoplasms and hyperplasias of melanocytes in the skin. In: Fitzpatrick TB, Eizen AZ, Wolff K, et al (eds): Dermatology in General Medicine. McGraw-Hill, New York, 1979, p 629.

148. Weinstock MA, Sober AJ: The risk of progression of lentigo maligna to lentigo maligna melanoma. Br J Dermatol 116:303, 1987.

149. Sober AJ, Day CL, Koh HK, et al: Melanoma in the northeastern United States: experience of the melanoma clinical cooperative group. In: Balch CM, Milton GW (eds): Cutaneous Melanoma. JB Lippincott, Philadelphia, 1985.

150. Koh HK, Michalik E, Sober AJ, et al: Lentigo maligna melanoma has no better prognosis than other types of melanoma. J Clin Oncol 2:994, 1984.

151. Davis J, Pack GT, Higgins GK: Melanotic freckle of Hutchinson. Am J Surg 113:457, 1967.

152. Becker F: Lentigo maligna: cut out or freeze? J Dermatol Surg Oncol 6:691–700, 1980.

153. Coleman WP III, David RS, Reed RJ, et al: Treatment of lentigo maligna and lentigo maligna melanoma. J Dermatol Surg Oncol 6:476–479, 1980.

154. Litwin MS, Krementz ET, Mansell PW: Topical chemotherapy of lentigo maligna melanoma with 5-fluorouracil. Cancer 35:721, 1975.

155. Ryan RF, Krementz ET, Litwin MS: A role for topical 5-fluorouracil therapy in melanoma. J Surg Oncol 38:250, 1988.

156. Graham GF, Stewart R: Cryosurgery for unusual cutaneous neoplasms. J Dermatol Surg Oncol 3:437–444, 1977.

157. Nazzaro-Porro M, Passi S, Zina G, et al: Ten years experience of treating lentigo maligna melanoma with topical azelic acid. Acta Derm Venereol (Suppl) (Stockh) 143:49, 1989.

158. Harwood AR, Cummings BJ: Radiotherapy for malignant melanoma: a re-appraisal. Cancer Treat Rev 8:271, 1981.

159. Kelly JW, Blois MS, Sagebiel RW: Frequency and duration of patient follow-up after treatment of a primary malignant melanoma. J Am Acad Dermatol 13:756–760, 1985.

160. Milton GW, Shaw HW, Farrago GA, et al: Tumour thickness and the site and time of first recurrence in cutaneous malignant melanoma (stage I). Br J Surg 67:543, 1980.

161. McCarthy WH, Shaw HM, Thompson JF, et al: Time and frequency of recurrence of cutaneous stage I malignant melanoma with guidelines for follow-up study. Surg Gynecol Obstet 166:497–502, 1988.

162. Naruns PL, Nizze JA, Cochran AJ, et al: Recurrence potential of thin primary melanomas. Cancer 57:545–548, 1986.

163. Calloway MP, Briggs JC: The incidence of late recurrence (greater than 10 year): an analysis of 536 consecutive cases of cutaneous melanoma. Br J Plast Surg 42:46, 1989.

164. Shaw HM, Beattie CW, McCarthy WH, et al: Late relapse from cutaneous stage I malignant melanoma. Arch Surg 120:1155, 1985.

165. Briele HA, Beattie CW, Ronana SG, et al: Late recurrence of cutaneous melanoma. Arch Surg 118:800, 1983.

166. McEwan L, Smith JG, Matthews JP: Late recurrence of localized cutaneous melaneous melanoma: its influence on follow-up policy. Plast Reconstr Surg 86:527, 1980.

167. Regan MW, Reid CD, Griffiths RW, et al: Malignant melanoma: evaluation of clinical follow-up by questionnaire survey. Br J Plast Surg 38:11, 1985.

168. Rogers GS: Advances in diagnostic technique. J Dermatol Surg Oncol 15:605–607, 1989.

CHAPTER 60

Management of Uncommon Malignant Tumors

DAVID P. CLARK

The association of ultraviolet light exposure with the subsequent development of the three most common forms of skin cancer—basal cell carcinoma, squamous cell carcinoma, and melanoma—has been the subject of many publications in both professional journals as in the lay press. With 600,000 new cases of these types of skin cancer being reported in the United States each year, the importance of disseminating this information is readily obvious. However, other important but less common types of cutaneous tumors may also be encountered by the cutaneous surgeon. For this reason, an awareness of these other tumors is necessary because of their potential for locally aggressive behavior, occasional association with previously unrecognized internal malignancies, and grave prognosis for some types if an accurate diagnosis is not established early in the course of the disease.

Dermatofibrosarcoma Protuberans

Dermatofibrosarcoma protuberans (DFSP) is a low-grade malignant tumor arising in the dermis. First described in 1924,[1] the neoplasm can be characterized as a fibrohistiocytic sarcoma with little propensity for distant metastasis but with a strong tendency for extensive infiltration and frequent local recurrences after excision.[2–7]

Patients having DFSPs report a slow-growing, firm plaque (Fig. 60–1) with multiple irregular projections above the skin surface. Although they are most common on the trunk, they have also been reported in virtually all locations, including the vulva, eyelids, and toes.[2–12] Most patients are between 20 and 50 years of age, but the tumor may be found in all age groups. DFSP tumors may attain a large size, often 20 cm in diameter,[4, 5] before therapy is sought. One elderly patient had a DFSP removed that had reportedly been present since early childhood, an indication of the indolent pattern of growth.[13] Only 25% of 115 patients with DFSPs reported local pain associated with their tumor.[7] This tumor has frequently been reported in association with traumatic and surgical scars and burns,[4, 7, 14] and many patients relate a single memorable traumatic event seemingly linked to the development of their DFSP. Some uncommon associations with DFSPs have also been described, including pregnancy, chronic arsenic ingestion, and vaccination scars.[14, 15]

METASTASIS

In a review of 600 cases, only 34 cases of proven metastasis were found.[2] For most patients with metastatic DFSP, the spread of the disease is hematogenous.[16–20] However, seven well-documented examples of lymphatic spread have also been reported.[16] One patient had long-term survival after resection of a lung metastasis.[18] Some DFSPs on the scalp directly invade the brain. Metastases are most commonly found in patients who had developed local recurrences of the tumor.[6]

HISTOLOGY

Histologically, DFSPs are composed of spindle-shaped cells arranged in cartwheel-like configurations, referred to as a storiform pattern (Fig. 60–2). These bands and whorls of fibroblasts surround collagenous centers, extend to the borders of the reticular dermis, and may infiltrate the subcutaneous fat.[21] The storiform

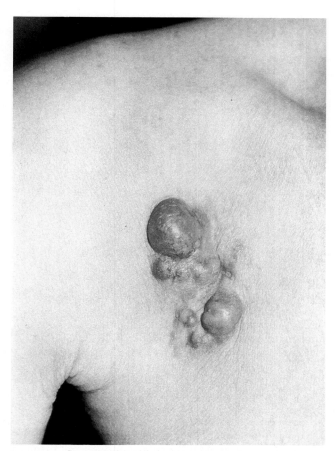

Figure 60–1. Dermatofibrosarcoma protuberans on the anterior chest of a 62-year-old man.

pattern is not unique to DFSPs and can be seen also in dermatofibromas (DFs), malignant fibrohistiocytomas, and atypical fibroxanthomas. In a study of 40 cases of DFSPs and 185 examples of DFs involving the dermis,[22] DFSPs were found to have two patterns of extension: slender, spindle cells that extended along fibrous septa and fat cells in a lacelike pattern, and bundles of spindle cells oriented in a multilayered arc parallel to the skin surface. These infiltrating types of growth contrast with that of DFs, which extend into the dermis in a vertical or radial fashion and have a smooth and well-demarcated margin that pushes into the subcutaneous fat. Simple stains are not generally helpful in distinguishing DF from DFSP, and immunohistochemistry has also not been of practical benefit.[21] However, simple polarization under light microscopy often assists the diagnosis. The collagen found in DFs demonstrates distinctive polarization, while that found in DFSPs does not.[23] DFSPs are not encapsulated and have many irregular downward projections that infiltrate between normal collagen fibers, subcutaneous fat, muscle, and underlying fascia. Individual tumor cells have nuclei with mild to moderate pleomorphism but little mitotic activity. Giant cells, hemosiderin-laden macrophages, and xanthoma cells are rare and, if present, are not cytologically atypical. Frequently, a zone of the upper dermis is spared. Pilosebaceous units are often surrounded, but not damaged,

by the tumor. Small focal areas of hemorrhage may be present, and small, thin-walled capillaries are frequently seen.[24] Unlike in DFs, overlying epidermal hyperplasia is uncommon in DFSPs.[21]

VARIANTS OF DFSP

A myxoid variant of DFSP is known.[25–27] While many DFSPs demonstrate small focal myxoid areas in the stroma because of hyaluronic acid deposition, large deposits are uncommon. Only 15% of all DFSPs[27] have widespread myxoid features. A darkly pigmented variant of DFSP containing melanin granules that proved to be mature membrane-bound melanosomes has been reported.[28] The number of pigmented cells in DFSP varies with each tumor, and pigment can only occasionally be seen grossly.[29] It has been suggested that this tumor is of neural origin.[28–31]

Another rare tumor, the giant cell fibroblastoma, has immunohistologic findings consistent with DFSPs.[32, 33] DFSPs may contain focal areas that are identical to those seen in a fibrosarcoma.[34, 35] Nine cases of DFSP[35] with focal areas of fibrosarcoma-like changes have been reported. These tumors occurred primarily on the trunk and demonstrated aggressive biologic activity. Eight of these patients had local recurrences, and one patient had distant metastasis. A rare case of an elderly woman who developed a malignant fibrous histiocytoma at the site of a recurrent DFSP has also been reported.[36]

HISTOGENESIS

The histogenesis of DFSP remains somewhat controversial, with some authors considering this tumor to be of perineural derivation[27–30] and other authors arguing for a fibroblastic-histiocytic derivation.[21, 37–40] Immunohistochemical studies of DFSPs demonstrate a positive reaction to vimentin, an antigen found in cells of mesenchymal origin, but negative staining with antibodies to S-100 protein or other antigens found in neural and melanocytic-derived tumors.[41–43] However, markers for

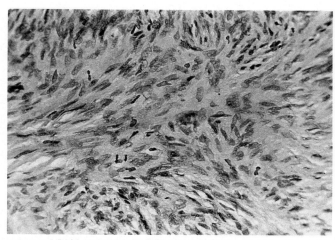

Figure 60–2. Photomicrograph of a dermatofibrosarcoma protuberans showing fasicles of tumor with a cartwheel or storiform configuration (original magnification, × 100).

histiocytic cell lines have been variably present on the cells of DFSP. There are conflicting studies on stains of DFSP to lysozyme or anti-chymotrypsin.[21, 42, 43] Cell culture lines developed from DFSPs produce cells with features of both fibroblasts and histiocytes.[6, 44] Two distinctly abnormal clones were found in one DFSP when cytogenetic analysis was performed.[45] DNA analysis of DFSPs demonstrated a high rate of aneuploidy,[6, 46] which correlated with a high degree of cellular atypia and may be of some use in predicting the biologic behavior of the tumor.[6, 46, 47] Ultrastructural analysis with electron microscopy has shown that DFSPs are of fibroblast origin.[38] Despite the suggestion of perineural differentiation,[30] DFSP is best considered a fibrohistiocytic tumor derived from an undifferentiated mesenchymal cell.

MANAGEMENT

Therapy for DFSPs should be based on a thorough understanding of this tumor's unique biologic activity. Because DFSPs are locally aggressive tumors with a low metastatic potential, the standard surgical approach has been wide excision with at least a 3-cm margin.[2–5, 48] Despite these aggressive procedures, however, several authors have demonstrated significant recurrence rates.[7, 48, 49] These reports are difficult to evaluate, because the precise surgical procedure was not clearly stated and the extent of the surgical margins in all cases is unknown. A 41% recurrence rate[48] has been noted when surgical margins of less than 2 cm were used. Recurrences often develop within 3 years but may be delayed for up to 19 or 20 years.[2–5, 7] In one study,[7] a 49% overall recurrence rate was noted, with 75% of these occurring within 3 years. In another study of 27 patients treated surgically with at least a 3-cm surgical margin and including the fascia, a 2% recurrence rate was seen.[4]

Experience with Mohs micrographic surgery (MMS) suggests that this offers a significant improvement in treatment.[25, 50–56] Use of MMS[57] requires experience to identify the subtle infiltrating tumor cells at the margins, but the current literature supports MMS as an effective tool that provides high cure rates with maximal preservation of normal tissue.[25, 50–56] A group of 18 patients treated with MMS remained disease free after 4 years.[50] More than 40 patients have been studied with 4 to 10 years of follow-up, and no recurrences have been reported.[25, 50–56]

Soft tissue sarcomas have proved relatively resistant to radiation therapy. In a study of 10 patients with DFSPs who received radiation either as primary or adjunctive therapy,[58] two of the three patients who received radiation therapy only were disease free after 2 years of follow-up. Six of the seven patients who received postoperative radiation for microscopic residual disease had no recurrence during a follow-up period of 16 to 105 months.

DFSP is an indolent tumor with low metastatic potential and a high local recurrence rate. Adequate surgical excision remains the treatment of choice. MMS (Table 60–1) is an important improvement in the treatment of patients with DFSPs (Table 60–2).

TABLE 60–1. MOHS MICROGRAPHIC SURGERY IN TREATMENT OF DERMATOSARCOMA PROTUBERANS

Reference	No. of Patients	Recurrence Rate (%)
Hobbs et al[54]	10	0
Robinson[55]	5	0
Mohs[52]	5	0
Peters et al[53]	1	0
Hess et al[25]	1	0
Mikhail and Lynn[56]	2	0
Brown and Swanson[50]	18	0
Goldberg and Maso[51]	1	0

Merkel Cell (Primary Neuroendocrine) Carcinoma

Primary neuroendocrine carcinoma (PNEC) of the skin is a rare and comparatively undifferentiated skin malignancy that was first described in 1972 as a trabecular carcinoma.[59] Other equivalent terms include extrapulmonary small cell carcinoma of the skin, primary undifferentiated carcinoma of the skin, and Merkel cell carcinoma. In 1875, Merkel[60] described a peculiar epithelial clear cell in normal human skin that now bears his name. Often associated with epithelial nerve endings, Merkel cells are found singly in both the epidermis and the dermis.[61, 62] This nondendritic, nonkeratinocytic cell is believed to be derived from the foregut.[61–63] Ultrastructural studies of Merkel cells demonstrate distinctive neurosecretory granules.[64–66] Because of these intracytoplasmic granules and a close association with nerve fibers, a neuroendocrine function for Merkel cells has been postulated.[67, 68] Both normal neuroendocrine cells and neoplastic neuroendocrine cells share the ability to take up amino acid precursors and decarboxylate them.[69] The term amine precursor uptake and decarboxylation (APUD) has been used to describe a diverse biochemical system involving several tissues and cells. Integral to any description of these anatomic constituents of the body's APUD system is the fact that the cells must synthesize peptide hormones, possess numerous cytoplasmic esterases, and contain distinctive dense-core neurosecretory cytoplasmic granules.[69, 70] Because Merkel cells have these special intracytoplasmic granules[71–74] and are often found in close association with nerve fibers,[75] it has been suggested that these cells should be

TABLE 60–2. STANDARD SURGERY IN THE TREATMENT OF DERMATOSARCOMA PROTUBERANS

Reference	No. of Patients	Surgical Margins (cm)	Recurrence Rate (%)
McPeak et al[4]	27	3	11
Hajdu[49]	119	"Wide"	54
Roses et al[48]	10	3	20
Bendix-Hansen et al[2]	7	3	0
Taylor and Helwig[7]	98	"Wide"	49

included as special APUD cells found in the skin.[66] However, attempts to demonstrate monoamine metabolism or cholinesterase or catecholamine secretion in Merkel cells have been unsuccessful.[76, 77] While the neuropeptide met-enkephalin[78] and the enzyme neuron-specific enolase[79–82] have been found in Merkel cells, apparently giving these cells some neuroendocrine function,[83, 84] they cannot be considered members of the APUD group. It also remains uncertain whether Merkel cell tumors are actually malignant tumors of the classic Merkel cells observed in the normal skin. Benign tumors of the Merkel cell have not been described.[85]

CLINICAL FEATURES

The original clinical description of Merkel cell carcinomas concerned five patients, all 65 years of age or older, who had poorly differentiated dermal tumors. Three of the five had nodal metastasis, two had local recurrences, and one patient died of disseminated tumor within 3 years.[59] Since this original description, more than 400 cases of PNEC have been reported.[86] The average age of patients with PNEC (Table 60–3) has been found to be 68 years, with a range of 24 to 92 years.[87] PNEC usually presents as an asymptomatic, pink or violaceous, slowly growing, firm nodule or plaque (Fig. 60–3). Manipulation of the lesion often produces bleeding, and ulceration is common.[88, 89] Approximately 50% of all PNEC tumors occur on the head and neck,[90–97] 25% on the upper extremities, 18% on the lower extremities, and the remainder on the trunk.[90] Occasionally, tumors also occur on the vulva,[98] eyelid,[99] lip,[100, 101] thigh,[102] and pinna.[103] Although PNEC often occurs as a single tumor, multiple tumors have also been reported.[90–105] At the time of initial diagnosis, 12% of patients with PNEC[88] have metastasis to regional lymph nodes, and 40 to 60% of patients can be expected to develop local lymph node metastases at some time during the course of the disease.[86, 88–92] Distant metastasis can be found in up to 49% of patients within 2 years of diagnosis.[86, 88–92, 106–109] The most common sites of metastasis include liver, brain, lung, and bone. Although therapy seem to be effective, 40% of all tumors recur with a mean time of only 10 months.[86, 88, 89]

TABLE 60–3. CLINICAL FEATURES OF PRIMARY NEUROENDOCRINE (MERKEL CELL) CARCINOMA AT PRESENTATION

Age (years)	
Range (N = 332)	15–97
Mean (N = 269)	68.2
Sex (N = 316)	
Male	48.1%
Female	51.9%
Primary lesion site (N = 315)	
Head and neck	48.9%
Upper extremities	15.6%
Lower extremities	20.3%
Trunk	3.8%
Multiple	1.5%

From Hitchcock CL, Bland KI, Laney RG, et al: Neuroendocrine (Merkel cell) carcinoma of the skin: its natural history, diagnosis, and treatment. Ann Surg 207:201–207, 1988.

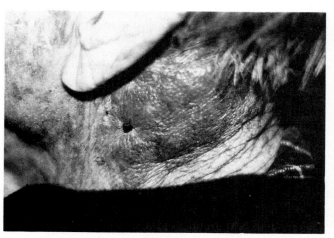

Figure 60–3. Primary neuroendocrine (Merkel cell) carcinoma on the posterior neck of a 78-year-old man.

An association between PNEC and other skin neoplasms has been noted.[65, 90, 110–113] Of 32 patients with PNEC, 11 had a previous or concomitant squamous cell carcinoma (SCC) in the same anatomic area.[110] In two instances, the SCC and PNEC tumors were admixed. Bowen's disease has also been described overlying a PNEC tumor.[65, 90, 112] In another study,[112] 20% of patients with PNEC reported removal of an SCC in the same area. There is also a report of a young woman who developed a PNEC tumor during pregnancy and died of extensive metastatic disease 23 months later, despite aggressive therapy.[114] Previous radiation therapy may also predispose patients to the development of PNEC.[115]

HISTOLOGY

The classic histologic description of PNEC by routine light microscopy[59, 66, 73–78] is that of an organoid tumor with a fibrovascular stroma and nests of cells found in the dermal lymphatics. The ill-defined tumor is found predominantly in the dermis with extensions into subcutaneous fat or muscle. Involvement of the epidermis is rare, and pilosebaceous units often are surrounded but only occasionally destroyed by tumor. Tumor cords or single cells extend between collagen fibers at the borders, and bizarre mitotic figures are common. Tumors usually consist of small cells of uniform size and shape, with oval to round nuclei that contain hyperchromatic, stippled chromatin and scanty acidophilic granular cytoplasm. Although tumors with the classic microscopic pattern of trabecular growth are seen, great variability is common.[85, 86, 116–118] Often a sheetlike or medullary growth pattern is seen with central necrosis of tumor aggregates and individual cell necrosis. The individual cells can be oval, with evenly distributed hyperchromatic chromatin and scanty cytoplasm[85]; small with marked pleomorphism; or a combination of the classic, small cells and an intermediate cell.

PNEC tumors can be categorized as the trabecular type, with its distinctive organoid growth pattern; the intermediate type, with a diffuse growth pattern, ne-

TABLE 60–4. HISTOLOGIC DIFFERENTIAL DIAGNOSIS OF PRIMARY CUTANEOUS NEUROENDOCRINE (MERKEL CELL) CARCINOMA

Lymphoma
Small cell melanoma
Sweat gland carcinoma
Metastatic small cell lung carcinoma
Metastatic neuroblastoma
Extraosseous Ewing's sarcoma
Squamous cell carcinoma
Cutaneous carcinoid tumor
Embryonal rhabdomyosarcoma
Cloacagenic carcinoma

crotic areas, numerous mitoses, and lymphocytic infiltrates; and the small cell type, composed of solid sheets of cells separated by stroma. These descriptions point out the morphologic heterogeneity of PNEC. However, light microscopy is often inadequate to distinguish PNEC from other small cell tumors of the dermis (Table 60–4).

Electron microscopy (EM) and immunohistochemical (IHC) studies may be essential in making the correct diagnosis of PNEC.[66, 69, 71, 73, 117–122] Ultrastructural analysis of PNEC by EM demonstrates abundant Golgi bodies with neurosecretory granules 100 to 150 nm in diameter. These electron-dense granules may also be located at the cell periphery, enmeshed in microfilaments, or found within the cell membrane bound to cytoplasmic processes. These EM findings are also consistent with other small cell neuroendocrine carcinomas.[72, 118, 123, 124] A second distinctive EM finding is a collection of whorls and bundles of low-electron-density, intermediate microfilaments around the nucleus. These microfilaments have been reported in other neuroendocrine tumors such as bronchogenic, thymic, and islet cell carcinomas.[72, 123]

IHC techniques have aided greatly in making a definitive diagnosis of PNEC.[74, 78–83, 118, 124] Merkel cell carcinomas routinely stain positively for neuron-specific enolase (NSE) and neurofilaments (NFs), but some tumors have also been reported to react positively with antibodies to vasoactive intestinal polypeptides (VIPs).[83] Antibodies to S-100 protein, met-enkephalin, cytokeratin, and serotonin stains in PNEC are routinely negative.[66, 74, 86, 118] Differences in IHC staining for PNEC and non-PNEC tumors are relative and cannot provide a definitive differentiation between these tumors.[78, 124, 125] However, because both therapy and prognosis vary greatly among the various tumors easily confused with PNEC, it is essential to obtain an accurate histopathologic diagnosis.[126]

PROGNOSIS

PNEC is an aggressive tumor, and the small cell variety has proved the most difficult to treat (Table 60–5). In one study,[85] all patients with the small cell type developed regional or generalized metastases within 2 years. The trabecular form of PNEC appears to have the best patient prognosis. In one group,[86] no deaths occurred, but two of four patients had regional lymph node involvement. Spontaneous regression of PNEC has been noted[127, 128] but is rare. The overall survival rate for PNEC is 72% at 2 years and 55% at 3 years.[86]

MANAGEMENT

A variety of methods have been used to treat PNEC. Surgical excision for PNEC with 2- to 4-cm margins has been recommended.[88–93] MMS has been used to achieve complete tumor extirpation,[92, 129] but MMS alone was unable to control PNEC.[92] The best management of regional lymph nodes also remains unclear. There is a 75% failure rate in patients with head and neck PNEC and untreated neck lymph nodes[91] and thus elective lymph node dissection for all patients with head and neck PNEC has been proposed. Elective lymph node dissections for all patients with palpable lymph nodes and for those patients at high risk (i.e., those with tumors larger than 2 cm, showing high mitotic rates, or with histologic evidence of vascular invasion) has been suggested.[112]

Because it is a radiosensitive tumor,[87] PNEC is amenable to radiation therapy.[87, 130–133] Doses in excess of 4500 rads have produced no treatment failures.[112] Radiation therapy should be considered when the tumor is close to or in the surgical margins, there is histologic evidence of vascular invasion, or nodal metastasis is present.[88] Uniform postoperative radiation to the local site and regional lymphatic vessels has also been recommended.[130]

Experience is sparse using chemotherapy in the treatment of PNEC, but a favorable response of PNEC to some cytotoxic regimens has been noted.[134–137] Chemotherapy regimens that include cisplatin, lomustine, vin-

TABLE 60–5. CLINICAL BEHAVIOR OF NEUROENDOCRINE CARCINOMA

	No. of Patients	(%)
Local recurrence		
Patients with ≥ 6 mo follow-up	80/220	(40.0)
Number of recurrences (range, 2–9)	30/88	(34.1)
Time from initial diagnosis to first local recurrence: 1–54 mo (mean, 10.1 mo)		
Regional lymph node metastasis		
All patients		
At presentation	31/254	(12.2)
After initial diagnosis	86/187	(46.0)
Patients with 12 mo follow-up	107/193	(55.4)
Time from initial diagnosis to nodal metastasis: 1–202 mo (mean, 13.4 mo)		
Distant metastasis		
All patients	82/226	(36.3)
Multiple sites	10/82	(12.2)
Patients with ≥24 mo follow-up	73/148	(49.3)
Time from initial diagnosis to distant metastasis: 11 days to 96 mo (mean follow-up of 18.3 mo)		

From Hitchcock CL, Bland KI, Laney RG, et al: Neuroendocrine (Merkel cell) carcinoma of the skin: its natural history, diagnosis, and treatment. Ann Surg 207:201–207, 1988.

cristine, doxorubicin, cyclophosphamide, and etoposide have been used with moderate success. Although tumor response is often swift, rapid tumor recurrence is the rule.

Other experimental methods used to treat PNEC have resulted in some favorable responses. One patient treated with intralesional injection of tumor necrosis factor (TNF) demonstrated a complete response and remained disease free after 1 year.[138] A trial of local hyperthermia in conjunction with low dose radiation therapy was also reported to be successful in two patients.[139] Finally, two reports note spontaneous regression of PNEC in three patients.[127, 128]

CONCLUSION

Because PNEC is an aggressive tumor, excision with wide surgical margins followed by postoperative radiation therapy seems to be a prudent form of treatment. Local recurrences and regional metastases often require multiple modalities, including surgery, radiation, and chemotherapy, to control tumor growth.

Paget's Disease

In 1874, the English surgeon Sir James Paget[140] reported a patient with a distinctive chronic scaling disorder of the nipple and areola associated with an underlying intraductal mammary gland carcinoma. A male patient with a similar scaly eruption on the penis and scrotum that showed the same histologic features was described 15 years later.[141] Since these late nineteenth century descriptions, many authors have confirmed the accuracy of these first reports concerning mammary Paget's disease (PD) and extramammary Paget's disease (EMPD).[142–146] While many similarities exist between the two conditions, there are also several important differences.[147–150]

Mammary PD, with few exceptions, is always associated with an intraductal mammary gland adenocarcinoma.[140, 144–146, 149, 151–160] The Paget cells are assumed to be epidermotropic, migrating through the intact lactiferous ductal epithelium into the skin.[150, 155, 156, 161] The nature of EMPD remains more controversial.[162–166] In most cases EMPD appears to begin in the epidermis as a sweat gland with subsequent extension into the dermis and beyond.[167–174] Occasionally, as in PD, the epidermal tumor results from direct contiguous extension of an adenocarcinoma located in the deeper tissues.[175–177] Patients affected with EMPD have a high incidence of concomitant underlying malignancy.[178]

MAMMARY PAGET'S DISEASE

Clinical Presentations

Mammary PD typically affects older women, with an average age at presentation of 54 years (range, 28 to 82 years).[144] Most patients seek medical attention (Table VI) for a scaling or ulcerating nipple lesion (Table 60–6),[144–146] which begins as an eczematous disorder with

TABLE 60–6. PRESENTING SIGNS AND SYMPTOMS IN 50 PATIENTS WITH PAGET'S DISEASE OF THE BREAST

Primary Presenting Signs and Symptoms	No. of Patients (%)	
Localized to nipple		
Eczema or ulceration	17	(34)
Discharge or bleeding	13	(26)
Abnormal sensation	7	(14)
Dermatitis	5	(10)
Inversion	3	(6)
Breast mass only	5	(10)

From Paone J, Baker RR: Pathogenesis and treatment of Paget's disease of the breast. Cancer 48:825–829, 1981.

erythema, thickening, and scaling (Fig. 60–4). With time, a well-demarcated plaque forms with erosions, ulcers, and crusts (Fig. 60–5). Often PD is asymptomatic, but the secondary skin changes frequently produce pain or pruritus.[144–146, 179] Because clinical presentations are often subtle, early diagnosis of PD may be difficult. The time between onset of the symptoms and confirmation of the diagnosis is often greater than 10 months.[180] Any eczema of the areola and nipple that is unresponsive to standard treatment should be considered suspect, and a definitive histologic diagnosis should be made (Table 60–7).

On physical examination, 25 to 50% of patients with PD will have a palpable breast mass.[144, 145, 152–154, 180] Although most masses are adjacent to the affected nipple, deep masses in the breast are also occasionally noted. Approximately two thirds of patients with a palpable neoplastic mass associated with PD have metastasis to axillary lymph nodes.[180] A breast mass concomitant with PD is associated with a worse prognosis. In the patient group without a breast mass, the 5-year survival rate was 94%,[152] compared with only 40% in those with a mass.[146] Metastasis to the lymph nodes was reported in 58% of patients with PD,[158] and only 29% of them survived 5 years. The cumulative 5-year survival rate was only 22% and the 10-year rate only 10%.[180]

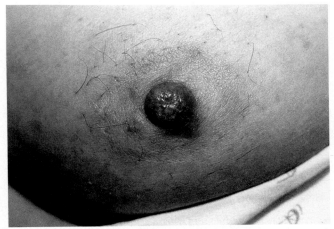

Figure 60–4. Early Paget's disease of the breast in a 59-year-old woman with an underlying ductal carcinoma found on mammography.

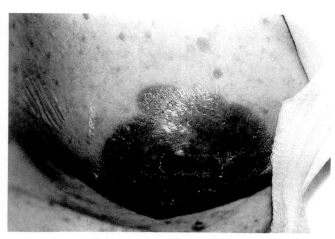

Figure 60–5. Advanced Paget's disease of the breast in an 80-year-old woman with an underlying ductal carcinoma and regional lymph node metastasis.

Mammary PD is typically thought of as a unilateral disease, but bilateral disease has also been reported.[181] PD in association with underlying intraductal carcinoma has also been found in ectopic breast tissue,[182] in residual breast tissue after subcutaneous mastectomy,[159] and in a preserved nipple after mastectomy.[183] It has been estimated that PD comprises 3% of all female breast cancers. PD of the male breast is much less common and may be associated with a worse prognosis.[151, 154, 157]

Histology

Paget cells are large, round, clear cells and are found scattered throughout an otherwise normal epidermis.[140, 145, 146] These cells have abundant pale cytoplasm that compresses the hyperchromatic nucleus into the periphery of the cell. Although most Paget cells appear quite banal, they can also have grossly abnormal nuclei and mitotic figures. The resident epidermal cells get compressed as the number of Paget cells increases. The Paget cells may invade the epithelium of hair follicles, which is accompanied by a brisk dermal inflammatory reaction, but they rarely traverse into the dermis.[144–147, 149] Examination of mammary glands and ducts demonstrates malignant transformation in almost all cases.[180] With progression of an underlying ductal breast

TABLE 60–7. CLINICAL CONDITIONS CONFUSED WITH PAGET'S DISEASE

Eczematous dermatitis
Benign intraductal papilloma
Erosive adenomatosis
Tinea
Impetigo
Bowen's disease
Malignant melanoma
Hailey-Hailey disease
Papulosquamous disease
Basal cell carcinoma
Metastatic carcinoma

cancer, tumor cells can be found in both the underlying connective tissue and lymphatics.[153, 156, 158] Although the usual malignant pattern starts with transformation in the mammary duct followed by extension into the epidermis, rare cases of malignant changes confined entirely to the epidermis have been reported.[155]

Immunochemistry

IHC techniques IHC have helped to improve our understanding of the origin and histogenesis of Paget cells. These studies support the theory that Paget cells are derived from sweat gland precursors.[184, 185] IHC staining with antibodies to carcinoembryonic antigen (CEA), originally found in fetal tissues and in some gastrointestinal malignancies, is frequently demonstrated in Paget cells.[186–189] CEA staining has been demonstrated to be positive in eccrine and apocrine sweat glands, as well as in sweat gland tumors.[190] The positive CEA reaction combined with negative staining for antibodies to epidermal keratin suggests a glandular origin for Paget cells and allows discrimination of Paget cells from melanocytes and keratinocytes.[189, 191, 192] Epidermal Paget cells and the underlying breast tumor cells show staining similar to that demonstrated by apocrine epithelial antigens.[188] In addition, the KA4 monoclonal antibody, found in the living cells of normal eccrine and apocrine ducts,[162] also reacts strongly with Paget cells. Monoclonal antibodies to the membrane of human milk fat globules also react strongly with Paget cells and breast carcinoma cells.[193] Finally, two lectins, peanut agglutinin and wheat germ agglutinin, are found in both normal apocrine glands and breast carcinoma.[194] Paget cells stain readily for these lectins, but no staining is seen in keratinocytes, normal breast tissue, or eccrine gland cells. Enzyme histochemical studies demonstrate strong staining of Paget cells to the enzymes found in apocrine glands.[149, 195, 196] EM studies of Paget cells show glandular structures such as microvilli, lumina, and secretory vacuoles.[197] However, tonofilaments and desmosomes found between cells on EM studies have suggested an epithelial origin for Paget cells.[179, 197]

Histogenesis

In mammary PD an underlying breast malignancy[144–146] is found in almost all cases, providing strong support for the view that intraepidermal Paget cells migrate from an underlying intraductal neoplasm through the lactiferous ducts. A primary breast carcinoma rarely can invade the epidermis directly and produce a lesion histologically similar to mammary PD. Documented cases of mammary PD without an underlying malignancy have led some investigators to suggest an epidermal origin for Paget cells.[144, 147, 156] However, most evidence strongly favors derivation of mammary PD cells from an underlying intraductal breast malignancy.

Treatment

The primary treatment of mammary PD is surgical,[144–146, 152, 153, 156, 180] but as always, the operative approach varies with the clinical presentation. Sixty per cent of patients with PD and a palpable mass have lymph node metastasis.[144] The 10-year survival rate in this group varies from 20 to 33%, and as a result, these patients are generally treated with modified radical mastectomy. Patients who have no palpable breast mass are generally treated with at least a total simple mastectomy.[152, 156, 180] Consideration should also be given to axillary lymph node resection, as up to 30% of patients without a mass have axillary lymph node metastasis.[144, 153, 180] The 10-year survival rates for patients with mammary PD and no palpable breast mass may be as high as 90%.[146, 152]

EXTRAMAMMARY PAGET'S DISEASE

EMPD[164-177] is most commonly found on the vulva and perineum but has been described in the external ear canal, tongue, eyelid, and esophagus[198-202] (Table 60–8). Although EMPD most commonly presents as a single lesion,[142, 143] multiple or multifocal lesions have been reported. The average age of EMPD patients is 62 years (range, 44 to 80 years), and there is a female-to-male ratio of 4.5:1, which reflects the predominance of vulvar EMPD relative to EMPD in other locations.

Clinical Features

In the usual clinical presentation of EMPD, patients show a chronic, red, scaly patch or plaque[142, 143, 164-177, 203-207] of variable size, with crusting and ulceration (Fig. 60–6). These lesions can be confused with superficial fungal infection or Bowen's disease. Pruritus or burning can occur but may be a result of secondary skin changes. Patients often ignore EMPD for many decades, which results in an average delay in seeking medical attention of 20.4 months.[167] The duration of symptoms correlates with the histologic evidence of tumor extension into the dermis. In a review of 98 patients,[207] invasion of sweat glands by EMPD was associated with 3 to 4 years of symptoms, while direct dermal invasion had an average symptom duration of 6.9 years.

EMPD most commonly behaves as an in situ adenocarcinoma of the skin.[147-149] In contrast, PD appears to be a skin extension of an underlying intraductal adenocarcinoma. However, numerous series have documented patients with a primary adnexal adenocarcinoma and

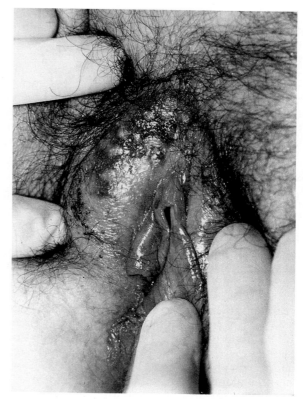

Figure 60–6. Preoperative photograph of a 57-year-old woman with extramammary Paget's disease without evidence of an underlying malignancy.

direct extension to the skin.[165, 175-177] Although most patients with EMPD do not have an underlying adenocarcinoma, a definite association exists between EMPD and other cancers.[173-178, 205] In a review of 196 cases of EMPD,[178] 25% of patients had an associated underlying cutaneous adnexal carcinoma, 12% had an underlying visceral malignancy, and an additional 17% had a non-concurrent internal malignancy. There is a strong association of perirectal EMPD with underlying rectal cancer (86%).[205] In contrast, in a series of 200 patients with vulvar EMPD,[143] only 15 patients were found to have associated underlying visceral malignancy. The underlying malignancy correlates with the cutaneous site affected by EMPD, so vulvar and scrotal EMPD are highly associated with genitourinary neoplasms, while perianal lesions are more commonly seen in association with gastrointestinal malignancy.[178]

Patients with in situ EMPD who do not have underlying malignancy rarely die of EMPD.[164-174] However, the overall mortality rate for patients with EMPD and an underlying adenocarcinoma is as high as 80%[169]; for patients with underlying adnexal carcinoma, 46%[178]; and for patients with rectal carcinoma, 75%. The mortality rate of patients without underlying malignancy is reported to be 18%.[169, 207] The internal malignancy and EMPD need not occur simultaneously. If both the concurrent incidence and the nonconcurrent incidence of EMPD with internal malignancy are recorded, about 30% of patients with EMPD will be affected.[178] Certain

TABLE 60–8. SITES OF EXTRAMAMMARY PAGET'S DISEASE

Site	No.
Vulva	39
Scrotum	5
Axillae	4
Perianal	3
Groin	2
Buttock	1
Pubis	1
Total	55

Adapted from Jones R: Extramammary Paget's disease. A critical reexamination. Am J Dermatopathol 1:101–132, 1979.

anatomic areas appear to have a higher correlation with internal tumors. In one study, 86% of 14 patients with perianal EMPD had rectal cancer, and 75% of these patients died of invasive disease.[205] Two other series have confirmed the high incidence of underlying regional internal cancer with perianal EMPD.[163, 205] Patients without an underlying malignancy, either adnexal or internal, rarely die of EMPD. However, 46% of patients with EMPD associated with an adnexal carcinoma died of metastatic disease.[178]

Histology

Mammary PD and EMPD have many histologic features in common.[147, 149] Paget cells are found singly and in groups in both diseases and often are cytologically indistinguishable.[147] Paget cells in EMPD stain more commonly for mucin than do Paget cells found in PD.[149] One difference is that Paget cells of EMPD can be found throughout the pilosebaceous unit, a rare feature in PD.[149] EMPD confined to the epidermis remains an in situ carcinoma. However, with progression, the expanding cell mass can extend into the dermis, the fascia, or even the underlying structures.[203] Direct extension to the epidermis from an underlying malignancy to the epidermis will produce EMPD of the skin,[150, 163, 165] which is most commonly seen with adenocarcinoma of the rectum[205] but has also been reported with bladder and uterine cancers.[150, 163, 165, 172] Many IHC and ultrastructural studies have been unable to establish reproducible differences between the Paget cells found in EMPD and those found in PD. IHC studies suggest that the extramammary Paget cells have a glandular origin. Positive staining to the CEA antigen and to the secretory portion of sweat glands has strengthened the argument that extramammary Paget cells have a sweat gland origin.[184–192]

Pathogenesis

The pathogenesis of EMPD remains controversial, and three theories currently exist.[149, 166] The first is that the Paget cells in the epidermis originate from an in situ adenocarcinoma of underlying sweat glands (Table 60–9), and malignant cells migrate along apocrine or eccrine ducts to the epidermis. The second theory is that Paget cells are derived from an adenocarcinoma originating in pluripotential cells that are distributed multifocally in the epidermis. Paget cells may remain confined to the epidermis, extend downward into the underlying adnexal structures, or invade the dermis directly. The third

TABLE 60–9. ADNEXAL CARCINOMA ASSOCIATED WITH EXTRAMAMMARY PAGET'S DISEASE

Reference	No. of Patients	Underlying Adnexal Carcinoma (%)
Helwig and Graham[205]	40	33
Chanda[178]	194	24

TABLE 60–10. RECURRENCE RATES FOR EXTRAMAMMARY PAGET'S DISEASE AFTER SURGICAL EXCISION

Reference	No. of Patients	Recurrence Rate (%)
Jones et al[147]	55	35
Breen et al[207]	13	12
Creasman et al[174]	11	36
Koss et al[172]	10	20
Mohs and Blanchard[215]	5	0

and final theory is that Paget cells result from the multicentric effect of an unknown carcinogenic stimulus exerted on the epidermis as well as on underlying adnexal structures and adjacent organs of the gastrointestinal and genitourinary tracts. Support for the first theory derives from isolated cases that clearly demonstrate extension of an underlying sweat gland adenocarcinoma into the skin.[66, 61, 102, 171, 172, 208] The large number of EMPD patients that lack histologic proof of a sweat gland malignancy may represent a sectioning error when the vast number of sweat glands present beneath are considered.[171] IHC studies strongly suggest that the Paget cell may be of a sweat gland origin. However, neither ultrastructural nor current IHC techniques can separate a pluripotential epidermal cell with glandular differentiation from a glandular cell that has migrated to the epidermis. An exhaustive study of four patients with EMPD showed that the area involved was more extensive histologically than was clinically evident.[166] Furthermore, despite finding multiple foci of cancer, only an occasional Paget cell was seen in the underlying sweat glands or ducts. The multiple cancers associated with EMPD support the idea of a carcinogenic stimulus acting on multiple organs. It can be concluded that Paget cells in EMPD appear to arise from a pluripotential epidermal precursor cell, are of glandular origin, and usually manifest some apocrine differentiation.

Treatment

Before treatment can be planned, a complete workup must be performed in patients with EMPD to exclude an underlying adnexal or internal malignancy. Surgery remains the mainstay of therapy for EMPD,[164–175, 209] but local recurrence after excision is common (Table 60–10). Recurrence rates of 12 to 60% have been reported after modified and radical vulvectomies for vulvar EMPD.[142, 143, 164–168, 174, 210, 211] The extensive subclinical involvement of skin by tumor and difficulties in accurately accessing tumor margins probably contribute to the number of inadequate excisions. Because of the indolent nature of EMPD, other treatment modalities have also been used, including radiation therapy. However, in one study,[178] 9 of 11 patients treated with radiation had recurrent disease and died of distant disease. Metastatic lesions have shown a variable response to radiation therapy,[174] but one patient treated with local irradiation for EMPD remained disease free at 10 years.[212]

Although 5-fluorouracil (5-FU) has some tumoricidal effect when applied topically to EMPD,[164] clinical benefit has been disappointing.[211] Topical 1% 5-FU applied to scrotal and perianal EMPD produced only partial clearing at 12 weeks, and subsequent biopsies demonstrated persistent tumor.[211] A 5% 5-FU ointment applied extensively was reported to produce complete clinical clearing, but unfortunately, biopsies continued to show histologic evidence of tumor.[202] Topical 5-FU has been shown to poorly penetrate the epithelium of the pilosebaceous unit, which may explain the 5-FU treatment failures. Involvement of the hair shaft by EMPD may also partly explain the failure of cryosurgery and electrodesiccation and curettage to effect a cure.[178, 213]

Treatment failures may also be a result of the extensive subclinical and widely multifocal nature of EMPD.[166] Complete removal of the in situ epidermal malignancy should be the goal of therapy.[214] Every effort should be made to cure EMPD in the in situ stage, as invasive disease is associated with a poor patient prognosis, regardless of the therapy used. Methods used to improve cure rates include increased histologic control, multiple satellite biopsy specimens,[213] MMS (Figs. 60–7, 60–8),[213, 215, 216] or multiple frozen sections.[169, 171, 217] MMS seems to offer conservative excision with histologic control to obtain a tumor-free margin. Combination therapy using preoperative topical 5-FU was reported to help delineate the extent of disease before performing Mohs MMS.[213] Rarely, despite apparently adequate treatment, EMPD still progresses to invasive carcinoma.

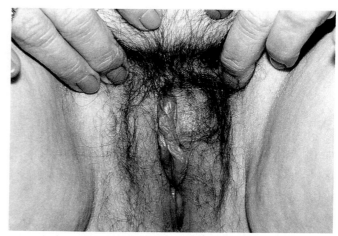

Figure 60–8. Clinical appearance at 3 months postoperatively showing a completely healed wound.

In contrast, remission of metastatic EMPD in a patient treated with radiation therapy, chemotherapy, and surgery has also been seen.[218] However, the bulk of patients with EMPD can be managed with conservative surgical excision and careful follow-up.[167–170, 219]

Atypical Fibroxanthoma

Atypical fibroxanthoma (AFX) of the skin is a benign neoplasm that morphologically mimics a more malignant soft tissue sarcoma or squamous cell carcinoma.[220–223] AFX typically occurs in elderly patients as a solitary, often ulcerative nodule on sun-exposed skin.[224–235] While the histologic characteristics of an AFX often appear ominous, long-term studies suggest that this tumor's biologic behavior is benign.[236] AFX is thought to be a reparative or reactive process that only rarely metastasizes.

CLINICAL DESCRIPTION

The vast majority of AFX tumors occur in the areas of actinically damaged skin of elderly individuals[224–235] but may also occur in previously irradiated sites (Fig. 60–9). Although tumors have been reported at all sites on the head and neck,[237–240] the nose and ears are most commonly affected.[224–235, 241] The average age of patients is 69 years.[220] A second, smaller subset of histologically similar tumors occur on the trunk and extremities of a younger patient population[231] (average age, 39 years). These tumors have a slightly different clinical presentation but similar histology, biology, and long-term patient prognosis.[231] AFX tumors are typically asymptomatic, small (less than 2 cm), and often present for less than 1 year. They are frequently misdiagnosed as pyogenic granulomas (Fig. 60–10),[242] basal cell carcinomas,[233] or sebaceous cysts.[233] In the older literature, these tumors were called paradoxical fibrosarcomas, pseudosarcomatous dermatofibromas, and pseudosarcomatous reticulohistiocytomas.[220, 231, 243]

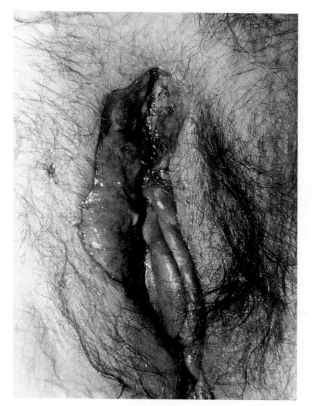

Figure 60–7. Clinical appearance 3 weeks after Mohs micrographic surgery. The wound was allowed to heal by second intention.

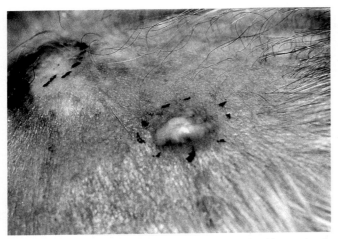

Figure 60–9. Two atypical fibroxanthomas arising in skin previously treated with radiation therapy.

HISTOLOGY

AFX lesions are located in the superficial dermis without extension into deep fascia.[220, 230, 233] The surrounding skin shows actinic damage, while the overlying epidermis is thinned or ulcerated. The tumor is highly cellular and composed of multiple spindle cells; large, pleomorphic, polyhedral histiocytic cells[227, 230]; and bizarre multinucleated giant cells.[244] These hyperchromatic cells often have multiple fused nuclei and a foamy cytoplasm. Cells with both normal and abnormal mitotic figures are identified.[220, 227–229, 244–246] Although lesions are commonly confined to the dermis and dilated capillaries are seen at the periphery of the lesion,[230, 232] the lesions do not have capsules. Hemorrhage, hemosiderin deposition, and myxomatous changes are found in the adjacent tissue.[232]

IHC studies have proved valuable in confirming the diagnosis of AFX,[230, 232, 247–249] since they demonstrate negative staining for epidermal cytokeratins and S-100 protein. Some S-100 antibody staining of certain AFX lesions has been reported, but these cells were at the periphery of the central tumor.[250] The spindle cell population, as well as the polygonal and giant cell population, stained with recognized tissue histiocyte markers alpha$_1$-antichymotrypsin and alpha$_1$-antitrypsin.[232] Vimentin, a marker of mesenchymal cell origin, was also uniformly positive. IHC methods are exceedingly helpful when attempting to differentiate spindle cell tumors that have similar histologic appearances. Historically, spindle cell variants of squamous cell carcinoma have been confused with AFX.[230, 233, 236] In some cases, careful routine histologic techniques often demonstrate a connection of the dermal tumor to the epidermis. A reaction to antikeratin antibodies is confirmation of the epidermal origin[230, 232, 247, 248] of squamous cell carcinomas.

A more difficult problem is to differentiate AFX from a malignant fibrous histiocytoma (MFH),[230, 231, 233] since some authors feel these lesions are closely related.[224, 233, 247, 248] However, MFH usually occurs in younger patients, originates in the deep fascia, and involves the superficial dermis only as a secondary event.[231] The biologic behavior of MFH is decidedly more malignant than that of AFX. As determined by ultrastructural (Table 60–11) and IHC (Table 60–12) methods, MFH tumors arise out of histiocytic cell lines and may be indistinguishable from an AFX.[247] No diagnosis of AFX is certain until these confirming tests are complete. On the basis of these studies, most authors have concluded that the cells of a true AFX have a fibrohistiocytic origin.[220, 230–232, 239, 247, 251]

PROGNOSIS

AFXs recur in 7% of cases,[231, 233] usually within 3 months. Metastasis, although rare, has been documented.[238, 252–254] In an analysis of metastatic AFX, the factors that identify a high-risk patient are histologic evidence of vascular invasion, recurrent or inadequately excised lesions, previous irradiation, or an immunocompromised host.[231]

TREATMENT

For most patients with AFX, surgical treatment is standard. Simple excision with conservative margins is curative in most patients.[220, 224–235] Histologic evidence of complete tumor extirpation is advisable, and re-excision of inadequately removed tumors is prudent. MMS may

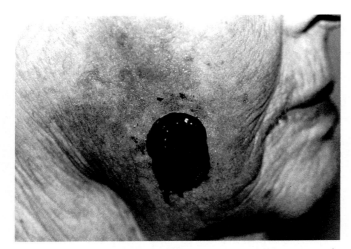

Figure 60–10. An atypical fibroxanthoma that mimics a pyogenic granuloma in its rapid growth over a 6- to 8-week period.

TABLE 60–11. HISTOLOGIC DIFFERENTIAL DIAGNOSIS OF SPINDLE CELL LESIONS OF SKIN

Atypical fibroxanthoma
Squamous cell carcinoma
Malignant melanoma
Kaposi's sarcoma
Soft tissue sarcoma
Spitz nevus
Malignant fibrous histiocytoma
Dermatofibrosarcoma protuberans
Schwann's cell tumors

TABLE 60–12. IMMUNOHISTOCHEMICAL STUDIES OF SPINDLE CELL TUMORS OF SKIN

	S-100 Protein	Cytokeratins	Vimentin	AAT	AACT	Desmin
Squamous cell carcinoma	−	+	−	−	−	−
Malignant melanoma	+	−	+	−	−	−
Spitz nevus	+	−	−	−	−	−
Leiomyosarcoma	−	−	±	−	−	+
Malignant fibrous histiocytoma	−	−	−	+	+	−
Sarcomas	−	−	+	−	−	±
Atypical fibroxanthoma	−	−	n/a	+	+	n/a

AACT, Alpha$_1$-antichymotrypsin; AAT, alpha$_1$-antitrypsin.

have a role in the treatment of AFX, as this method conserves tissue and ensures histologic control of the tumor margins.[255] AFX tumors arising in irradiated skin[256] or in immunocompromised patients[254] must be treated aggressively. In addition, AFX tumors arising in periocular locations commonly behave very aggressively. However, most patients with AFX require diagnostic expertise and therapeutic restraint for proper management.

Microcystic Adnexal Carcinoma

Microcystic adnexal carcinoma (MAC) is a neoplasm with features of pilar and eccrine differentiation. First described in 1982,[257] MAC is currently a well-recognized entity.[258–260] This tumor is typically a slow-growing, firm, dermal nodule located on the upper lip of middle-aged women. One patient with MAC present on the cheek for 16 years before treatment has been reported.[261] MAC has also occurred in the axilla.[259] These tumors have a characteristic histologic appearance consisting of keratinous cysts, dense desmoplastic stroma, abortive follicular structures, ducts, and occasional glandlike structures.[257–259, 262] MAC frequently invades deeply and often demonstrates perineural tissue involvement in addition to involvement of skeletal muscle.[259] Although it is locally quite invasive, cytologic atypia and mitoses are rare. One or more local recurrences have been reported in up to 40% of patients.[259] One tumor recurred 30 years after the initial surgical treatment.[260] There have been no reports of distant metastasis, and only one patient with lymph node involvement resulting from the direct extension of tumor has been noted.[259]

Treatment of MAC typically consists of surgical excision. However, because of the ill-defined nature of this neoplasm, MMS is also an excellent form of treatment.[261] Regardless of the type of treatment, the incidence of local recurrences suggests a continued need for frequent and meticulous re-examination by the cutaneous surgeon.[258, 259]

Sebaceous Carcinoma

Sebaceous carcinoma (SC) is a rare neoplasm, most commonly found on periocular skin but occasionally present at other cutaneous sites.[263–275] Although this malignant neoplasm frequently has a banal clinical appearance, SC can be an aggressive tumor and is commonly associated with frequent local recurrence and distant metastasis.

PERIOCULAR TUMORS

SC accounts for only a small proportion (3%) of all malignant tumors of the eyelid.[263, 265, 268, 272] Most SCs originate in meibomian glands or the glands of Zeis.[271, 273] Rarely, the sebaceous glands associated with fine lanugo hairs, the sebaceous glands of the lacrimal apparatus, or the sebaceous glands in the eyebrows can also be the site of SC.[264, 271, 273] The upper eyelids are involved far more often than the lower eyelids, and multicentric involvement occurs[268, 275] in approximately 6% of patients.[271]

CLINICAL FEATURES

The typical patient with SC is a woman in her late fifties with a painless nodule or a recurrent sty.[263–276] SC may often masquerade as blepharoconjunctivitis, a chalazion, or a cutaneous horn.[276] Clinical features[272] that should alert the clinician to suspect SC include recurrent chalazia (Fig. 60–11), a nodular tumor of the eyelids associated with loss of cilia (Fig. 60–12) or yellow discharge, persistent unilateral blepharoconjunctivitis unresponsive to therapy, an orbital or eyelid mass that develops after removal of an eyelid tumor, and a tumor

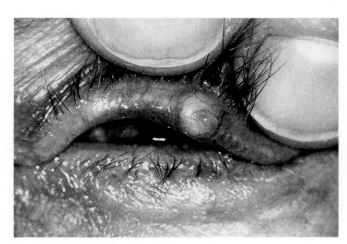

Figure 60–11. Clinical appearance of a sebaceous carcinoma on the upper lid of a 65-year-old woman.

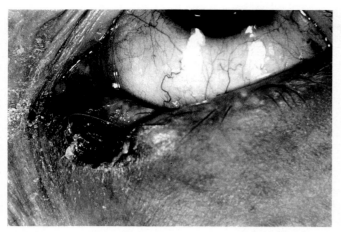

Figure 60–12. A sebaceous carcinoma on the lower lid that appears as a chronic ulcerative nodule and is associated with a loss of cilia.

arising in a previously irradiated site. The average age of patients with SC is 57 years, and women outnumber men 2:1.[269] SC also appears to be more common in the Asian population[268, 270] and in those with a history of previous radiation therapy.[265, 267, 268, 271, 277–279]

HISTOLOGY

SC is characterized by lobules of cells having variable differentiation and a high mitotic index.[265, 268, 271, 273, 280] In well-differentiated tumors, the cells have foamy, vacuolated cytoplasm and round nuclei. Areas of lesser differentiation have cells with basophilic cytoplasm, hyperchromatic nuclei,[273, 274] atypical and bizarre mitotic figures (Fig. 60–13), and areas of necrosis. Often SCs differ greatly in their degree of cytologic atypia and tissue infiltration.[273, 280] Those SCs that show sheetlike medullary growth and marked infiltration of connective tissue, vessels, and nerves have a high risk of associated metastatic disease.[265, 271] Tumor cells from SC are frequently found in the surrounding epidermis,[268, 271–273]

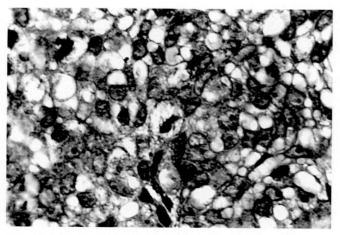

Figure 60–13. Light microscopic findings of a sebaceous carcinoma showing pleomorphic cells with bizarre nuclei and a high mitotic index.

which is characterized by a pagetoid type of growth. When collections of tumor cells are found within the overlying or surrounding epidermis, there is an associated increased risk of mortality.[281–285] Intraepithelial involvement with cells from an underlying SC is often not apparent clinically and may contribute to the high local recurrence rate.[285]

PROGNOSIS

SCs of the periocular tissue frequently recur after treatment,[263–275] with approximately one third of all patients developing a local recurrence and 30% of these having a distant metastasis.[265, 271] Lower lid lesions have a better patient prognosis, but the outlook is poor if both lids are involved. An overall 4-year survival rate of 29% has been reported in patients with SC.[268]

SC OF NONOCULAR TISSUE

While SC of nonocular tissue is unusual,[286–288] 70% of nonocular SC lesions occur on the head and neck.[267, 287] The biologic behavior of SCs found in these sites is about the same as that of ocular SC.[289] Initially, a more benign behavior was suggested,[286] but a summary[289] of the reported cases of SCs arising at nonocular sites found a local recurrence rate of 34% and a distant metastasis rate of 32%. Sebaceous neoplasms, including SC, have been associated with internal malignancies, especially colonic cancer.[290] Sebaceous tumors are distinctly unusual, and the presence of an SC should prompt an examination of the gastrointestinal tract for cancer.[291–297]

TREATMENT

Treatment of SC requires careful diagnosis and workup. Accurate pathologic diagnosis typically requires a full-thickness biopsy. An evaluation to exclude the possibility of tumor spread requires careful radiologic examination of the orbits and a search for distant metastasis.

The mainstay of treatment for SC is surgical excision.[263–275, 298, 299] Because of the tendency for this tumor to recur, excision with wide surgical margins and including orbital exenteration and multiple frozen section biopsies taken at the time of tumor removal has been suggested.[265, 271, 289, 285] The pagetoid spread of tumor cells within the epidermis is often difficult to appreciate histologically on small samples of frozen tissue. Furthermore, the tendency for multicentric growth makes random frozen sections of little value.

MMS has been successfully used to improve margin control and conserve tissue.[281, 288, 298–302] A zero recurrence rate has been reported (Table 60–13) from a small study of patients with periocular SC treated with MMS.[301] Because of difficulties in evaluating the surgical margins, exclusion of intraepidermal tumor requires great experience and care, and recurrences have been reported after adequate MMS.[281, 302] In an attempt to improve cure rates, cryotherapy for tissue surrounding the tumor excision site has been suggested to eradicate occult intraepithelial foci of SC.[282] Radiation therapy,

TABLE 60–13. EXPERIENCE WITH SEBACEOUS CARCINOMA TREATED WITH MOHS MICROGRAPHIC SURGERY

Reference	No. of Patients	Residual Tumor or Tumor Recurrence (%)	Length of Follow-up
Harvey and Anderson[298]	3	0	2 yr
Dixon et al[299]	1	0	30 mo
Ratz et al[301]	3	0	35 mo
Folberg et al[281]	3	2	Short
Dzubow[302]	2	1	Short

both as a primary modality and after surgery, has also been used to treat SCs.[281, 303–305] Primary treatment of ten patients with SC using radiation therapy resulted in a 96% 5-year survival rate.[305] Extension of an SC into the orbit significantly worsens the prognosis. For that reason, orbital exenteration has been suggested as the best therapy for orbital invasion.[265, 281] Metastasis usually involves the preauricular lymph nodes, parotid gland, and the ipsilateral cervical lymphatic chain.[265, 271, 281, 305] Aggressive surgical management with lymph node dissection is indicated in these cases, since a 50% 5-year survival rate has been noted in patients with regional lymph node metastasis who were treated aggressively. The number of patients treated with radiation therapy and radical neck dissection is too small at present to reach a firm conclusion about the efficacy of this form of treatment.[306]

SUMMARY

Despite the prevalence of basal cell and squamous cell carcinomas, it is extremely important that the cutaneous surgeon also have a thorough knowledge of less common types of cutaneous tumors. The establishment of an accurate and early diagnosis of these various tumors remains the most important factor in determining prognosis, reducing morbidity, limiting scarring, and minimizing functional impairment. For all these reasons, an awareness of the clinical appearance and biologic activity of each of these uncommon tumors is vital for every cutaneous surgeon.

REFERENCES

1. Darier J, Ferrand M: Dermatofibromas progressits et recidwants ou fibrosarcomes de le peau. Ann Dermatol Syphil 5:545, 1924.
2. Bendix-Hansen K, Myhre-Jensen O, Kaae S: Dermatofibrosarcoma protuberans. a clinicopathological study of nineteen cases and review of world literature. Scand J Plast Reconstr Surg 17:247–252, 1983.
3. Burkhardt BR, Soule EH, Winkelmann RK, Ivins JC: Dermatofibrosarcoma protuberans: study of fifty-six cases. Am J Surg 111:638–644, 1966.
4. McPeak CJ, Cruz T, Nicastri AD: Dermatofibrosarcoma protuberans: an analysis of 86 cases-five with metastasis. Ann Surg 166:803–816, 1967.
5. Pack GT, Tabah EJ: Dermatofibrosarcoma protuberans: thirty-nine cases. Arch Surg 62:391–402, 1951.
6. Rockley PF, Robinson JK, Magid M, Goldblatt D: Dermatofibrosarcoma protuberans of the scalp: a series of cases. J Am Acad Dermatol 21:278–283, 1989.
7. Taylor HB, Helwig EB: Dermatofibrosarcoma protuberans: a study of 115 cases. Cancer 15:717–725, 1962.
8. Barnhill DR, Boling R, Nobles W, et al: Vulvar dermatofibrosarcoma protuberans. Gynecol Oncol 30:149–152, 1988.
9. Barnes L, Coleman JA, Johnson JT: Dermatofibrosarcoma protuberans of the head and neck. Arch Otolaryngol 110:398–404, 1984.
10. Coles M, Smith M, Rankin EA: An unusual case of dermatofibrosarcoma protuberans. J Hand Surg 14:135–138, 1989.
11. Kraemer BA, Fremling M: Dermatofibrosarcoma protuberans of the toe. Ann Plast Surg 25:295–298, 1990.
12. Sagi A, Ben-Yaher Y, Mahler D: A ten-year old boy with dermatofibrosarcoma protuberans of the face. J Dermatol Surg Oncol 13:82–83, 1987.
13. Weber PJ, Gretzula JC, Hevia O, et al: Dermatofibrosarcoma protuberans. J Dermatol Surg Oncol 14:555–558, 1988.
14. McLelland J, Chn T: Dermatofibrosarcoma protuberans arising in a BCG vaccination scar. Arch Dermatol 124:496–497, 1988.
15. Schneidman D, Belizaire R: Arsenic exposure followed by the development of dermatofibrosarcoma protuberans. Cancer 58:1586–1587, 1986.
16. Brenner W, Schaefler K, Chabra H, Postel A: Dermatofibrosarcoma protuberans metastatic to a regional lymph node. Cancer 36:1897–1902, 1975.
17. Hirabayashi S, Kajikawa A, Kanazawa K, Mimoto K: Dermatofibrosarcoma protuberans with regional lumph node metastasis: a case report. Head Neck 11:562–564, 1989.
18. Kahn LB, Saxe N, Gordon W: Dermatofibrosarcoma protuberans with lymph node and pulmonary metastases. Arch Dermatol 114:559–601, 1978.
19. Hausner RJ, Vargas-Cortes F, Alexander RW: Dermatofibrosarcoma protuberans with lymph node involvement. A case report of simultaneous occurrence with atypical fibroxanthoma of the skin. Arch Dermatol 114:88–93, 1978.
20. Fisher ER, Hellstrom HR: Dermatofibrosarcoma with metastases simulation Hodgkin's disease and reticulum cell sarcoma. Cancer 19:1165–1171, 1966.
21. Fletcher CDM, Evans BJ, Macartney JC, et al: Dermatofibrosarcoma protuberans: a clinicopathological and immunohistochemical study with a review of the literature. Histopathology 9:921–938, 1985.
22. Kamino H, Jacobson M: Dermatofibroma extending into the subcutaneous tissue. Differential diagnosis from dermatofibrosarcoma protuberans. Am J Surg Pathol 14:1145–1164, 1990.
23. Barr RJ, Young EM, King DF: Nonpolarizable collagen in dermatofibrosarcoma protuberans: a useful diagnostic aid. J Cutan Pathol 13:339–342, 1986.
24. Manivel JC, Dehner LP, Wich MR: Nonvascular sarcomas of the skin. In: Wick MR (ed): Pathology of Unusual Malignant Cutaneous Tumors. Marcel Dekker, New York, 1985.
25. Hess KA, Hanke CW, Estes NC, Shideler SJ: Chemosurgical reports: myxoid dermatofibrosaroma protuberans. J Dermatol Surg Oncol 11:268–271, 1985.
26. Frierson HF, Cooper PH: Myxoid variant of dermatofibrosarcoma protuberans. Am J Surg Pathol 7:445–450, 1983.
27. Allen PW: Myxoid tumors of soft tissues. Pathol Annu 15:133–192, 1980.
28. Bednar B: Storiform neurofibromas of the skin, pigmented and nonpigmented. Cancer 10:368–376, 1957.
29. Dupree WB, Langloss JM, Weiss SW: Pigmented dermatofibrosarcoma (Bednar tumor): a pathologic ultrastructural and immunohistochemical study. Am J Surg Pathol 9:630–639, 1985.
30. Hashimoto K, Brownstein MH, Jakobiec FA: Dermatofibrosar-

coma protuberans: a tumor with perineural and endoneural cell features. Arch Dermatol 110:874–875, 1974.

31. Nakamura T, Ogata H, Katsuyama T: Pigmented dermatofibrosarcoma protuberans: report of two cases as a variant of dermatofibrosarcoma protuberans with partial neural differentiation. Am J Dermatopathol 9:18–25, 1987.

32. Shmookler BM, Enzinger FM, Weiss SW: Giant cell fibroblastoma: a juvenile form of dermatofibrosarcoma protuberans. Cancer 64:2154–2161, 1989.

33. Beham A, Fletcher CD: Dermatofibrosarcoma protuberans with areas resembling giant cell fibroblastoma: report of two cases. Histopathology 17:165–167, 1990.

34. Wrotnowski V, Cooper PH, Shmookler BM: Fibrosarcomatous change in dermatofibrosarcoma protuberans. Am J Surg Pathol 12:287–293, 1988.

35. Ding J, Hashimoto H, Enjoji M: Dermatofibrosarcoma protuberans with fibrosarcomatous areas. A clinicopathologic study of nine cases and a comparison with allied tumors. Cancer 64:721–729, 1989.

36. O'Dowd J, Lardler P: Progression of dermatofibrosarcoma protuberans to malignant fibrous histiocytoma: report of a case with implications for tumor histogenesis. Hum Pathol 19:368–370, 1988.

37. Lautier R, Wolff HH, Jones RE: An immunohistochemical study of dermatofibrosarcoma protuberans supports its fibroblastic character and contradicts neuroectodermal or histiocytic components. Am J Dermatopathol 12:25–30, 1990.

38. Alguacil-Garcia A, Unni KH, Goellner JR: Histogenesis of dermatofibrosarcoma protuberans. An ultrastructural study. Am J Clin Pathol 69:427–434, 1978.

39. Volpe R, Carbone A: Dermatofibrosarcoma protuberans metastatic to lymph nodes and showing a dominant histiocytic component. Am J Dermatopathol 5:327–334, 1983.

40. Fisher ER, Vuzevski VD: Cytogenesis of schwannoma (neurilemoma), neurofibroma, dermatofibroma and dermatofibrosarcoma as revealed by electron microscopy. Am J Clin Pathol 9:141–154, 1968.

41. Kuhn LB, Martes A, Thom H, Bunmu R: Role of antibody to S-100 protein in diagnostic pathology. Am J Clin Pathol 79:341–347, 1983.

42. DuBonlay CEH: Demonstration of alpha-1-antitrypsin and alpha-1-antichymotrypsin in the fibrous histiocytomas using the immunoperoxidase technique. Am J Surg Pathol 6:559–564, 1982.

43. Kindblom LG, Jacobsen GK, Jacobsen M: Immunohistochemical investigations of tumors of supposed fibroblastic-histiocytic origin. Hum Pathol 13:834–840, 1982.

44. Ozzello L, Hamels J: The histiocytic nature of dermatofibrosarcoma protuberans: tissue culture and electron microscopic study. Am J Clin Pathol 65:136–148, 1976.

45. Bridge JA, Neft JR, Sandberg AA: Cytogenetic analysis of dermatofibrosarcoma protuberans. Cancer Genet Cytogenet 42:199–202, 1990.

46. Ericksen BL, Bauer KD, Caw WA, Roth SI: DNA analysis with cytologic and clinical correlation of dermatofibrosarcoma protuberans. Lab Invest 58:28A, 1988.

47. Perry MD, Furlong JW, Johnston WW: Fine needle aspiration cytology of metastatic dermatofibrosarcoma protuberan—a case report. Acta Cytol 30:507–512, 1986.

48. Roses DF, Valensi Q, LaTrenta G, Harris MN: Surgical treatment of dermatofibrosarcoma protuberans. Surg Gynecol Obstet 162:449–452, 1986.

49. Hajdu SI: Pathology of Soft Tissue Tumors. Lea & Febiger, Philadelphia, 1979, pp 60–83.

50. Brown M, Swanson N: Dermatofibrosarcoma protuberans treated with Mohs micrographic surgery. Presented at the American Academy of Dermatology, Atlanta, December, 1990.

51. Goldberg DJ, Maso M: Dermatofibrosarcoma protuberans in a 9 year old child: treatment by Mohs micrographic surgery. Pediatr Dermatol 7:57–59, 1990.

52. Mohs FE: Chemosurgery: Microscopically Controlled Surgery for Skin Cancer. Charles C Thomas, Springfield, IL, 1978.

53. Peters W, Hanke CW, Pasarell HA, Bennett JE: Dermatofibrosarcoma protuberans of the face. J Dermatol Surg Oncol 8:823–826, 1982.

54. Hobbs ER, Wheeland RG, Bailin PL, et al: Treatment of dermatofibrosarcoma protuberans with Mohs micrographic surgery. Ann Surg 207:102–107, 1988.

55. Robinson JK: Dermatofibrosarcoma protuberans resected by Mohs surgery (chemosurgery). J Am Acad Dermatol 12:1093–1098, 1985.

56. Mikhail GR, Lynn BH: Dermatofibrosarcoma protuberans. J Dermatol Surg Oncol 4:81–84, 1978.

57. Andrew JE, Silvers DN, Lattes R: Sarcomas involving the skin and superficial tissues. In: Friedman RJ, Rigel DS, Kopf AW, et al (eds): Cancer of the Skin. WB Saunders, Philadelphia, 1991, pp 263–287.

58. Marks LB, Suit HD, Rosenberg AE, Wood WC: Dermatofibrosarcoma protuberans treated with radiation therapy. Int J Radiat Oncol Biol Phys 17:379–384, 1989.

59. Toker C: Trabecular carcinoma of the skin. Arch Dermatol 105:107–123, 1972.

60. Merkel F: Tastzellen and Tastkorperchen bei den Haustieran und beim Menshen. Arch Microsk Anat 11:636, 1875.

61. English KB: Morphogenesis of Haarscheiben in rats. J Invest Dermatol 69:58–67, 1977.

62. English KB: The ultrastructure of cutaneous type 1 mechanoreceptors (Haarscheiben) in cats following denervation. J Comp Neurol 172:137–164, 1977.

63. Smith KR: The Haarscheibe. J Invest Dermatol 69:68–74, 1977.

64. Gohscaldt R-M, Vahle-Hinz C: Merkel cell receptors: structure and transducer function. Science 214:183–186, 1981.

65. Frigerio B, Capella C, Euscabi V, et al: Merkel cell carcinoma of the skin: the structure and origin of normal Merkel cells. Histopathology 7:229–249, 1983.

66. Warner T, Uno H, Hafez GR, et al: Merkel cells and merkel cell tumors: ultrastructure, immunocytochemistry and review of the literature. Cancer 52:238–245, 1983.

67. Winklemann RK: The Merkel cell system and a comparison between it and the neurosecretory of APUD cell system. J Invest Dermatol 69:41–46, 1977.

68. Pearse AGE: The neuroendocrine (APUD) cells of the skin. Am J Dermatopathol 2:121–123, 1980.

69. Pearse AGE: Common cytochemical and ultrastructural characteristics of cells producing polypeptide hormones (the APUD series) and their relevance to thyroid and ultimobranchial C-cells and calcitonics. Proc R Soc Lond Biol 170:71–80, 1968.

70. Pearse AGE: The cytochemistry and ultrastructure of polypeptide hormone-producing cells (the APUD series) and the embryologic, physiologic, and pathologic implications of the concept. J Histochem Cytochem 17:303–313, 1969.

71. Sibley RK, Dehner LP, Rosai J: Primary neuro-endocrine (Merkel cell?) carcinoma of the skin: a clinicopathological and ultrastructural study of 43 cases. Am J Surg Pathol 9:95–108, 1985.

72. Sidhu GS: The endodermal origin of digestive and respiratory tract APUD cells: histopathologic evidence and a review of the literature. Am J Pathol 96:5–20, 1979.

73. Sidhu GS, Feiner H, Flotte TJ, et al: Merkel cell neoplasms: histology, electron microscopy, biology, and histogenesis. Am J Dermatopathol 2:101–119, 1980.

74. Gould VE, Dardi LE, Memoli VA: Neuroendocrine carcinoma of the skin: light microscopic, ultrastructural and immunohistochemical analysis. Ultrastruct Pathol 1:499–509, 1980.

75. Hashimoto K: The ultrastructure of the skin of human embryos. X. Merkel tactile cells in the finger and nail. J Anat 111:99–120, 1972.

76. Munger BL: Neural-epithelial interactions in sensory receptors. J Invest Dermatol 69:27–40, 1977.

77. Hartschuh W, Weihe E, Buchler M, Kalmbach P: Experimental investigation of the Merkel cell. J Invest Dermatol 72:276–277, 1979.

78. Hartschuh W, Weihe E, Buchler PR, et al: Metenkephalin-like immunoreactivity in Merkel cells. Cell Tissue Res 201:343–348, 1979.

79. Gu J, Polah JM, Tapia FJ, et al: Neuron-specific enolase in the Merkel cells of mammalian skin: the use of specific antibody as a simple and reliable histologic marker. Am J Pathol 104:63–68, 1981.

80. Wich MR, Scheithauer BW, Kovacs K: Neuron-specific enolase in neuroendocrine tumors of the thymus, bronchus, and skin. Am J Clin Pathol 79:703–707, 1983.

81. Kirkham N, Isaacson P: Merkel cell carcinoma: a report of three cases with neurone-specific enolase activity. Histopathology 7:251–259, 1983.

82. Johansson L, Tennvall J, Akerman M: Immunohistochemical examination of 25 cases of Merkel cell carcinoma: a comparison with small cell carcinoma of the lung and oesophagus, and a review of the literature. APMIS 98:741–752, 1990.

83. Sibley RK, Dahl D: Primary neuroendocrine (Merkel cell?) carcinoma of the skin. An immunocytochemical study of 21 cases. Am J Surg Pathol 9:109–116, 1985.

84. Visscher D, Cooper PH, Zarbo RJ, Crissman JD: Cutaneous neuroendocrine (Merkel cell) carcinoma: an immunophenotypic, clinicopathologic and flow cytometric study. Mod Pathol 4:331–338, 1989.

85. Gould E, Moll R, Moll I, et al: Endocrine (Merkel) cells of the skin: hyperplasias, dysplasias, and neoplasms. Lab Invest 52:334–476, 1985.

86. Bayrou O, Avril F, Charpentie P, et al: Primary neuroendocrine carcinoma of the skin. J Am Acad Dermatol 24:198–207, 1991.

87. Raaf JH, Urmacher C, Knappa EK, et al: Trabecular (Merkel cell) carcinoma of the skin. Cancer 57:178–182, 1986.

88. Hitchcock CL, Bland KI, Laney RG, et al: Neuroendocrine (Merkel cell) carcinoma of the skin: its natural history, diagnosis, and treatment. Ann Surg 207:201–207, 1988.

89. Mercer D, Brandler P, Liddell K: Merkel cell carcinoma: the clinical course. Ann Plast Surg 25:136–141, 1990.

90. Kroll MH, Toker C: Trabecular carcinoma of the skin. Arch Pathol Lab Med 106:404–408, 1982.

91. Goeptert H, Remmler D, Silva E, Wheeler B: Merkel cell carcinoma (endocrine carcinoma of the skin) of the head and neck. Arch Otolaryngol 110:707–712, 1984.

92. Hanke CW, Conner C, Temofeew RK, Lingeman E: Merkel cell carcinoma. Arch Dermatol 125:1096–1100, 1989.

93. Meland NB, Jackson IT: Merkel cell tumor: diagnosis, prognosis, and management. Plast Reconstr Surg 77:632–638, 1986.

94. Murphy RX, Li JK, Mincer FK, Strauch B: Trabecular (neuroendocrine) carcinoma of the skin. Report of four cases and review of the literature. NY State J Med 90:35–38, 1990.

95. Pilotti S, Rilke F, Bartoli A, Grisotti A: Clinicopathologic correlations of cutaneous neuroendocrine Merkel cell carcinoma. J Clin Oncol 6:1863–1873, 1988.

96. Szadowska A, Wozniak L, Lasota J, et al: Neuroendocrine (Merkel cell) carcinoma of the skin: a clinicomorphological study of 13 cases. Histopathology 15:483–493, 1989.

97. Domarus H, Johanisson R, Schmauz R: Merkel cell carcinoma of the face. J Maxillofac Surg 13:39–43, 1985.

98. Bottles K, Lacey CG, Goldberg J, et al: Merkel cell carcinoma of the vulva. Obstet Gynecol 63:615–655, 1984.

99. Beyer CK, Goodman M, Dickersin GR, Dougherty M: Merkel cell tumor of the eyelid. Arch Opthalmol 101:1093–1101, 1983.

100. Dolezal RF, Cohen M, Taxyl JB: Merkel tumor of the lower lip. J Surg Oncol 37:123–127, 1988.

101. Boysen M, Wetteland P, Hovig T, Brandtzaeg P: Neuroendocrine carcinoma of the lip (Merkel cell tumor) examined by electron microscopy and immunohistochemistry. J Laryngol Otol 103:519–523, 1989.

102. Lindae ML, Nickoloff BJ, Greene I: Merkel cell tumor of the thigh. J Dermatol Surg Oncol 14:413–417, 1988.

103. Hanna GS, Ali MH, Akosa AB, Maher EJ: Merkel-cell carcinoma of the pinna. J Laryngol Otol 102:608–611, 1988.

104. Bourne RG, O'Rourke MG: Merkel cell tumour. Aust NZ J Surg 58:971–974, 1988.

105. Karam F, Nussey J, Nawab R: Trabecular or Merkel's cell carcinoma. South Med J 83:1354–1356, 1990.

106. Grosh WW, Giannone L, Handi KR, Johnson DH: Disseminated Merkel cell tumor. Treatment with systemic chemotherapy. Am J Clin Oncol 10:227–230, 1987.

107. Tennvale J, Biorklund A, Johansson L, Akerman M: Merkel cell carcinoma: management of primary, recurrent and metastatic disease. Eur J Surg Oncol 15:1–9, 1989.

108. Small KW, Rosenwasser GO, Alexander E, et al: Presumed choroidal metastasis of Merkel cell carcinoma. Ann Ophthalmol 22:187–190, 1990.

109. Ro JY, Ayala AG, Tetu B, et al: Merkel cell carcinoma metastatic to the testis. Am J Clin Pathol 94:384–389, 1990.

110. Gomez LG, DiMaw S, Silva EG, Machay B: Association between neuroendocrine (Merkel cell) carcinoma and squamous carcinoma of the skin. Am J Surg Pathol 7:171–177, 1983.

111. Nelson EL, Houghton DC: Concurrent spindle cell peripheral pulmonary carcinoid tumor and Merkel cell tumor of the skin. Arch Pathol Lab Med 114:420–423, 1990.

112. Silva EG, Mackay B, Goepfert H, et al: Endocrine carcinoma of the skin (Merkel cell carcinoma). Pathol Annu 19:1–30, 1984.

113. Jones CS, Tyring SK, Lee PC, Fine JD: Development of neuroendocrine (Merkel cell) carcinoma mixed with squamous cell carcinoma in erythema ab igne. Arch Dermatol 124:110–113, 1988.

114. Chao TC, Park JM, Rhee H, Greager JA: Merkel cell tumor of the back detected during pregnancy. Plast Reconstr Surg 86:347–351, 1990.

115. Tuneu A, Pujol RM, Moreno A, et al: Postirradiation Merkel cell carcinoma. J Am Acad Dermatol 20:505–507, 1989.

116. Heenan PJ, Cole JM, Spagnolo DV: Primary cutaneous neuroendocrine carcinoma (Merkel cell tumor). An adnexal epithelial neoplasm. Am J Dermatopathol 12:7–16, 1990.

117. Sibley RK, Rosai J, Foucar E, et al: Neuroendocrine (Merkel cell) carcinoma of the skin: a histologic and ultrastructural study of two cases. Am J Surg Pathol 4:211–221, 1980.

118. Wich MR, Goellner JR, Scheithauer BW, et al: Primary neuroendocrine carcinoma of the skin (Merkel cell tumors). A clinical, histologic and ultrastructural study of thirteen cases. Am J Clin Pathol 79:6–13, 1983.

119. Tang CK, Toker C: Trabecular carcinoma of the skin. An ultrastructural study. Cancer 42:2311–2321, 1978.

120. Haneke E: Electron microscopy of Merkel cell carcinoma from formalin-fixed tissue. J Am Acad Dermatol 12:487–492, 1985.

121. Abucj IF, Zak FG: Multicentric amyloid-containing cutaneous trabecular carcinoma. Case report with ultrastructural study. J Cutan Pathol 6:292–303, 1979.

122. Wich MR, Thomas JR III, Scherthauer BW, Jackson I: Multifocal Merkel's cell tumors associated with cutaneous dysplasia syndrome. Arch Dermatol 119:409–414, 1983.

123. Wich MR, Scheithauer BW: Oat-cell carcinoma of the thymus. Cancer 49:1652–1657, 1982.

124. Wich MR, Millns JL, Sibley RK, et al: Secondary neuroendocrine carcinomas of the skin. An immunohistochemical comparison with primary neuroendocrine carcinoma of the skin. J Am Acad Dermatol 13:134–142, 1985.

125. Battifora H, Silva EG: The use of antikeratin antibodies in immunohistochemical distinction between neuroendocrine (Merkel cell) carcinoma of the skin, lymphoma, and oat cell carcinoma. Cancer 58:1040–1047, 1986.

126. Dudley TH, Moinuddin S: Cytologic and immunohistochemical diagnosis of neuroendocrine (Merkel cell) carcinoma in cerebrospinal fluid. Am J Clin Pathol 91:714–717, 1989.

127. O'Rourke MGE, Bell JR: Merkel cell tumor with spontaneous regression. J Dermatol Surg Oncol 12:994–1000, 1986.

128. Kayashima K, Ono T, Johno M, et al: Spontaneous regression in Merkel cell (neuroendocrine) carcinoma of the skin. Arch Dermatol 27:550–553, 1991.

129. Roenigk RK, Goltz RW: Merkel cell carcinoma—a problem with microscopically controlled surgery. J Dermatol Surg Oncol 12:332–336, 1986.

130. Cotter AM, Gate JO, Gibbs FA: Merkel cell carcinoma: combined surgery and radiation therapy. Am Surg 52:159–164, 1986.

131. Ashby MA, Jones DH, Tasker AD, Blackshaw AJ: Primary cutaneous neuroendocrine (Merkel cell or trabecular carcinoma) tumor of the skin: a radioresponsive tumor. Clin Radiol 40:85–87, 1989.

132. Marks ME, Kim RY, Sulter MM: Radiotherapy as an adjunct in the management of Merkel cell carcinoma. Cancer 65:60–64, 1990.

133. Morrison WH, Peters LJ, Silva EG, et al: The essential role of radiation therapy in securing locoregional control of Merkel cell carcinoma. Int J Radiat Oncol Biol Phys 19:583–591, 1990.

134. George TK, Santangese AD, Bennell JM: Chemotherapy for metastatic Merkel cell carcinoma. Cancer 56:1034–1038, 1985.

135. Wynne CJ, Kearsley JH: Merkel cell tumor: a chemosensitive skin cancer. Cancer 62:28–31, 1988.

136. David MP, Miller EM, Rau RC, et al: The use of VP 16 and

cisplatin in the treatment of Merkel cell carcinoma. J Dermatol Surg Oncol 16:276–278, 1990.

137. Feun LG, Savaraj N, Legha S, et al: Chemotherapy for metastatic Merkel cell carcinoma. Cancer 62:683–685, 1988.

138. Ito Y, Kawamura K, Miura T, et al: Merkel cell carcinoma: a successful treatment with tumor necrosis factor. Arch Dermatol 125:1093–1095, 1989.

139. Knox SJ, Kapp DS: Hyperthermia and radiation therapy in the treatment of recurrent Merkel cell tumors. Cancer 62:1479–1486, 1988.

140. Paget J: On disease of the mammary areola preceding cancer of the mammary gland. St Barth Hosp Rep 10:87, 1874.

141. Cocker HR: Paget's disease affecting the scrotum and penis. Trans Pathol Soc Lond 40:187–189, 1889.

142. Dubreuilh W: Paget's disease of the vulva. Br J Dermatol 13:407, 1901.

143. Degetu S, O'Quinn AG, Dhurandhar HN: Paget's disease of the vulva and urogenital malignancies: a case report and review of the literature. Gynecol Oncol 25:347–356, 1986.

144. Ashikari R, Park K, Juvos A, Urbun J: Paget's disease of the breast. Cancer 26:680–685, 1970.

145. Kister SJ, Haagensen CD: Paget's disease of the breast. Am J Surg 119:606–611, 1970.

146. Salvadori B, Fariselli G, Saccozzi R: Analysis of 100 cases of Paget's disease of the breast. Tumor 62:529–536, 1976.

147. Jones RE, Austin C, Ackerman AB: Extramammary Paget's disease. A critical reexamination. Am J Dermatopathol 1:101–132, 1979.

148. Balducci L, Crawford ED, Smith GF, et al: Extramammary Paget's disease: an annotated review. Cancer Invest 6:293–303, 1988.

149. Sitakalin C, Ackerman AB: Mammary and extramammary Paget's disease. Am J Dermatopathol 7:335–340, 1985.

150. Wich MR, Goellner JR, Wolfe T, Su WPD: Vulvar sweat gland carcinomas. Arch Pathol Lab Med 109:43–47, 1985.

151. Crichlow RW, Czernobilsky B: Paget's disease of the male breast. Cancer 24:1033–1040, 1969.

152. Freund H, Maydovik M, Lauter N: Paget's disease of the breast. J Surg Oncol 9:93–100, 1977.

153. Greenwood SM, Minkowitz S: Paget's disease in metastatic breast carcinoma. Arch Dermatol 104:312–319, 1971.

154. Gupta S, Khanna NN, Khanna S, Cupta S: Paget's disease of the male breast: a clinicopathologic study and a collective review. J Surg Oncol 22:151–157, 1983.

155. Jones RE: Mammary Paget's disease without underlying carcinoma. Am J Dermatopathol 7:361–365, 1985.

156. Lagios MD, Westdahl PR, Rose MR, Concannon S: Paget's disease of the nipple: alternative management in cases without or minimal extent of underlying breast carcinoma. Cancer 54:545–555, 1984.

157. Lancer HA, Moschella SL: Paget's disease of the male breast. J Am Acad Dermatol 7:393–396, 1982.

158. Nance FC, DeLoach DH, Welsh RA, Becher WF: Paget's disease of the breast. Ann Surg 171:864–874, 1970.

159. Plowman PN, Bilmore OJA, Curling M, Janvrin SB: Paget's disease of the nipple occuring after conservation management of early infiltrating breast cancer. Br J Surg 73:45–50, 1986.

160. Satiani R, Powell RW, Mathews WH: Paget's disease of the male breast. Arch Surg 112:587–592, 1977.

161. Jones RR, Spaull J, Fusterson B: The histogenesis of mammary and extramammary Paget's disease. Histopathology 14:409–416, 1989.

162. Nagle RB, Lucas DO, McDoniel KM, et al: New evidence linking mammary and extramammary Paget cells to a common cell phenotype. Am J Clin Pathol 83:431–436, 1985.

163. Merot Y, Mazoujian G, Pinkus G, et al: Extramammary Paget's disease of perianal and perineal regions. Evidence of apocrine derivation. Arch Dermatol 121:750–752, 1985.

164. Fetherston W, Friedrich EG: The origin and significance of vulvar Paget's disease. Obstet Gynecol 39:735–744, 1972.

165. Feuer GA, Shevchuh M, Calanog A: Vulvar paget's disease: the need to exclude an invasive lesion. Gynecol Oncol 38:81–89, 1990.

166. Gunn RA, Gallager HS: Vulvar Paget's disease: a topographic study. Cancer 46:590–594, 1980.

167. Taylor PT, Stenwig JT, Klausen H: Paget's disease of the vulva. Report of 18 cases. Gynecol Oncol 3:36–60, 1975.

168. Pliskow S: Vulvar Paget's disease. Clinicopathological review of 14 cases. J Fla Med Assoc 77:667–671, 1990.

169. Pitman GH, McCarthy JF, Perzin KH, Herter FP: Extramammary Paget's disease. Plast Reconstr Surg 69:238–244, 1982.

170. Perez MA, LaRossa DD, Tomaszewski JE: Paget's disease primarily involving the scrotum. Cancer 63:970–975, 1989.

171. Lee SC, Roth L, Ehrlich C, Hall J: Extramammary Paget's disease of the vulva. Cancer 39:2540–2549, 1977.

172. Koss LG, Ladinsky S, Brockunier A: Paget's disease of the vulva. Report of 10 cases. Obstet Gynecol 31:513–525, 1968.

173. Fann ME, Morley GW, Abell MR: Paget's disease of the vulva. Obstet Gynecol 38:660–670, 1971.

174. Creasman WT, Gallager HS, Rutledge F: Paget's disease of the vulva. Gynecol Oncol 3:133–148, 1975.

175. Sasaki M, Terada T, Nakanuma Y, et al: Anorectal mucinous adenocarcinoma associated with latent perianal Paget's disease. Am J Gastoenterol 85:199–202, 1990.

176. deBlois GG, Patterson JW, Hunter SB: Extramammary Paget's disease. Arising in knee region in association with sweat gland carcinoma. Arch Pathol Lab Med 108:713–719, 1984.

177. Armitage NC, Kass JR, Richman PI, et al: Paget disease of the anus: a clinicopathologic study. Br J Surg 76:60–63, 1989.

178. Chanda JS: Extramammary Paget's disease: prognosis and relationship to internal malignancy. J Am Acad Dermatol 13:1009–1014, 1985.

179. Orr JW, Parish DJ: The nature of the nipple changes in Paget's disease. J Pathol Bacteriol 84:201–208, 1962.

180. Paone JF, Baker RR: Pathogenesis and treatment of Paget's disease of the breast. Cancer 48:825–832, 1981.

181. Anderson WR: Bilateral Paget's disease of the nipple: case report. Am J Obstet Gynecol 134:877–880, 1979.

182. Kao GF, Graham JH, Helwig EB: Paget's disease of the ectopic breast with an underlying intraductal carcinoma: report of a case. J Cutan Pathol 13:59–63, 1986.

183. Mendez-Fernandez MA, Henly WS, Geis RC, et al: Paget's disease of the breast after sub-cutaneous mastectomy and reconstruction with a silicone prosthesis. Plast Reconstr Surg 65:683–687, 1980.

184. Kashimura Y, Kashimura M, Horle A: Cytologic, histologic, DNA ploidy and electron microscopic analysis of a case of vulvar Paget's disease. Anal Quant Cytol Histol 11:413–418, 1989.

185. Kariniemi AL, Ramaeker F, Lehto P, Virtanen I: Paget cells express cytokeratins typical of glandular epithelia. Br J Dermatol 112:179–183, 1985.

186. Mori O, Hachisuka H, Sasai Y: Immunohistochemical demonstration of epithelial membrane antigen (EMA), carcinoembryonic antigen (CEA), and keratin on mammary and extramammary Paget's disease. Acta Histochem 85:93–100, 1989.

187. Reed W, Oppedal BR, Eeg Larsen T: Immunohistology is valuable in distinguishing between Paget's disease, Bowen's disease and superficial spreading malignant melanoma. Histopathology 16:583–588, 1990.

188. Guarner J, Cohen C, DeRose PB: Histogenesis of extramammary and mammary Paget cells. An immunohistochemical study. Am J Dermatopathol 11:313–318, 1989.

189. Nadji M, Morales AR, Girtanner RE, et al: Paget's disease of the skin: a uniting concept of histogenesis. Cancer 50:2203–2206, 1982.

190. Penneys NS, Nadji M, Morales A: Carcinoembryonic antigen in benign sweat gland tumors. Arch Dermatol 118:225–227, 1982.

191. Yoneda K: Immunohistochemical staining properties of keratin type intermediate filaments in mammary and extramammary Paget's disease. J Dermatol 16:47–53, 1989.

192. Glasgow BJ, Wen D-R, Al-Jitawi S, Cochran AJ: Antibody to S-100 protein aids the separation of pagetoid melanoma from mammary and extramammary Paget's disease. J Cutan Pathol 14:223–229, 1987.

193. Kirkham N, Berry N, Jones DB, Taylor-Papadimitriow J: Paget's disease of the nipple. Cancer 55:1510–1512, 1985.

194. Tamaki K, Hino H, Ottara K, Furul M: Lectin-binding sites in Paget's disease. Br J Dermatol 113:17–24, 1985.

195. Belcher RW: Extramammary Paget's disease. Enzyme histochemical and electron microscopic study. Arch Pathol 94:59–64, 1972.

196. Urano Y, Watanabe K, Sukaki A, et al: Immunohistochemical demonstration of peptidylarginine deiminase in human sweat glands. Am J Dermatopathol 12:249–255, 1990.
197. Sagebiel RW: Ultrastructural observations on epidermal cells in Paget's disease of the breast. Am J Pathol 57:49–60, 1969.
198. Fliegel Z, Kenako M: Extra-mammary Paget's disease of the external ear canal in association with ceruminous gland carcinoma. Cancer 36:1072–1076, 1975.
199. Changus GW, Yonan TN, Barolome JS: Extramammary Paget's disease of the tonque. Laryngoscope 81:1621–1623, 1971.
200. Knauer WJ, Whorton CM: Extramammary Paget's disease originating in Moll's gland of the lids. Trans Am Acad Ophthalmol Otolaryngol 67:829–833, 1963.
201. Kates DR, Koss LG: Paget's disease of the esophageal epithelium: report of first case. Arch Pathol Lab Med 86:447–450, 1968.
202. Kawatsu T, Miki Y: Triple extramammary Paget's disease. Arch Dermatol 104:316–319, 1971.
203. Hart WR, Millman J: Progression of intra epithelial Paget's disease of the vulva to invasive carcinoma. Cancer 40:2333–2337, 1977.
204. Shutze WP, Gleysteen JJ: Perianal Paget's disease. Classification and review of management: report of 2 cases. Dis Colon Rectum 33:502–507, 1990.
205. Helwig EG, Graham AH: Anogenital Paget's disease. A clinicopathologic study. Cancer 16:387–403, 1963.
206. Grow JR, Kshirsagar V, Tolentino M, et al: Extramammary perianal Paget's disease. Dis Colon Rectum 20:436–442, 1977.
207. Breen J, Smith C, Gregori CA: Extramammary Paget's disease. Clin Obstet Gynecol 2:1107–1115, 1978.
208. Roth LM, Lee SC, Ehrlich CE: Paget's disease of the vulva: a histogenetic study of 5 cases including ultrastructural observations and review of the literature. Am J Surg Pathol 1:193–201, 1977.
209. Lai CS, Lin SD, Yang CC, Chou CK: Surgical treatment of the penoscrotal Paget's disease. Ann Plast Surg 23:141–146, 1989.
210. Misas JE, Larson JE, Podezaski E, et al: Recurrent Paget disease of the vulva in a split-thickness graft. Obstet Gynecol 76:543–544, 1990.
211. Haberman HF, Goodall J, Llewellyn M: Extramammary Paget's disease. Can Med Assoc J 118:161–162, 1978.
212. Thirlby RC, Hammer CJ Jr, Balagan KA, et al: Perianal Paget's disease: successful treatment with combined chemoradiotherapy. Report of a case. Dis Colon Rectum 33:150–152, 1990.
213. Eliezri YD, Silvers DN, Horan DB: Role of preoperative topical 5-fluorouracil in preparation for Mohs micrographic surgery of extramammary Paget's disease. J Am Acad Dermatol 17:497–505, 1987.
214. Bergen S, DiSaia PJ, Liao SY, Berman ML: Conservative management of extramammary Paget's disease of the vulva. Gynecol Oncol 33:151–156, 1989.
215. Mohs FE, Blanchard L: Microscopically controlled surgery for extramammary Paget's disease. Arch Dermatol 115:706–709, 1979.
216. Wagner RF, Cottel WI: Treatment of extensive extramammary Paget disease of male genitalia with Mohs micrographic surgery. Urology 31:415–418, 1988.
217. Misas JE, Cold CJ, Hall FU: Vulvar Paget disease: Fluorescein-aided visualization of margins. Obstet Gynecol 77:156–159, 1991.
218. Balducci L, Athar M, Smith GF, et al: Metastatic extramammary Paget's disease in dramatic response to combined modality treatment. J Surg Oncol 38:38–44, 1988.
219. Archer CB, Loubach JB, MacDonald DM: Spontaneous regression of perianal extramammary Paget's disease after partial surgical excision. Arch Dermatol 123:379–382, 1987.
220. Fretzin DF, Helwig EB: Atypical fibroxanthoma of the skin. Cancer 31:1541–1552, 1973.
221. Helwig EB: Atypical fibroxanthoma tumor seminar. Proceedings of 18th annual tumor seminar of San Antonio Society of Pathologists. Tex J Med 59:664–667, 1963.
222. Halpert B, Hachney VC: Fibrosarcoma of the helix of the ear. Arch Pathol 48:218–220, 1949.
223. Gentele H: Malignant fibroblastic tumors of the skin. Acta Derm Venereol 31:1–180, 1951.
224. Alguacil-Garcia A, Unni K, Goellner JR, Winkelmann RK: Atypical fibroxanthoma of the skin. Cancer 40:1471–1480, 1977.
225. Fukamizu H, Oku T, Inoul K, et al: Atypical ("pseudosarcomatous") cutaneous histiocytoma. J Cutan Pathol 10:327–333, 1983.
226. Soares HL, Silveira JG, Fantini A, Soares ME: Atypical fibroxanthoma. J Dermatol Surg Oncol 7:915–916, 1981.
227. Hudson AW, Winkelmann RK: Atypical fibroxanthoma of the skin: a reappraisal of 19 cases in which the original diagnosis was spindle-cell squamous carcinoma. Cancer 29:413–422, 1972.
228. Kempson RL, McGavran M: Atypical fibroxanthomas of the skin. Cancer 17:1463–1471, 1964.
229. Lanigan S, Gilkes J: Spectrum of atypical fibroxanthoma of the skin. J R Soc Med 77:27–30, 1984.
230. Silvis NG, Swanson PE, Manivel JC, et al: Spindle-cell and pleomorphic neoplasms of the skin. A clinicopathologic and immunohistochemical study of 30 cases, with emphasis on "atypical fibroxanthomas." Am J Dermatopathol 10:9–19, 1988.
231. Helwig EB, May D: Atypical fibroxanthoma of the skin with metastasis. Cancer 57:368–376, 1986.
232. Leong ASY, Milios J: Atypical fibroxanthoma of the skin: a clinicopathological and immunohistochemical study and a discussion of its histogenesis. Histopathology 11:463–475, 1987.
233. Starink TM, Hausmam R, Van Delden L, Neering H: Atypical fibroxanthoma of the skin: presentation of 4 cases and review of the literature. Br J Dermatol 97:167–177, 1977.
234. Vargar-Cortex R, Winkelmann RK, Soule EH: Atypical fibroxanthomas of the skin. Further observations with 19 additional cases. Mayo Clin Proc 48:211–218, 1973.
235. Kempson RL, Kyriakos M: Fibroxanthoma of the soft tissues. Cancer 29:961–976, 1972.
236. Connors RC, Ackerman AB: Histologic pseudomalignancies of the skin. Arch Dermatol 112:1767–1780, 1976.
237. Berschadsky M, Gianetti C, David A, LoVerne S: Atypical fibroxanthoma in the pharynx. Plast Reconstr Surg 52:443–445, 1973.
238. Boynton JR, Markowitch W, Searl SS: Atypical fibroxanthoma of the eyelid. Ophthalmology 96:1480–1484, 1989.
239. High AS, Hume WJ, Dyson D: Atypical fibroxanthoma of oral mucosa: a variant of malignant fibrous histiocytoma. Br J Oral Maxillofac Surg 28:268–271, 1990.
240. Kemmett D, Gawkrodger DJ, Mclaren KM, Hunter JA: Two atypical fibroxanthomas arising separately in x-irradiated skin. Clin Exp Dermatol 13:382–384, 1988.
241. Dahl I: Atypical fibroxanthoma of the skin. Acta Pathol Microbiol Scand 84:183–197, 1976.
242. Goette DK, Odom RB: Atypical fibroxanthoma masquerading as a pyogenic granuloma. Arch Dermatol 112:1155–1157, 1976.
243. Bourne RG: Paradoxical fibrosarcoma of skin (pseudosarcoma). Med J Aust 15:504–509, 1963.
244. Barr RJ, Wuerker RB, Graham JH: Ultrastructure of atypical fibroxanthoma. Cancer 40:736–743, 1977.
245. Markow LP, Frich JC, Sliflan M, et al: Ultrastructure of a fibroxanthosarcoma (malignant fibroxanthoma). Cancer 28:372–383, 1971.
246. Weedon D, Ken JFR: Atypical fibroxanthoma of skin: an electron microscope study. Pathology 7:173–177, 1975.
247. Eckert F, Burg G, Braun-Talco O, et al: Immunostaining in atypical fibroxanthoma of the skin. Pathol Res Pract 184:27–34, 1988.
248. Kuwano H, Hashimoto H, Enjoji M: Atypical fibroxanthoma distinguishable from spindle cell carcinoma in sarcoma-like skin lesions. Cancer 55:172–180, 1985.
249. Pennys NS, Nadji M, Ziegels-Weissman J, et al: Prekeratin in spindle cell tumors of the skin. Arch Dermatol 119:476–479, 1983.
250. Winkelmann RK, Peters MS: Atypical fibroxanthoma: a study with antibody to S-100 protein. Arch Dermatol 121:753–785, 1985.
251. Wilson R, Strutton GM, Stewart MR: Atypical fibroxanthoma: two unusual variants. J Cutan Pathol 16:93–98, 1989.
252. Glavin FL, Cornwell ML: Atypical fibroxanthoma of the skin metastatic to a lung. Am J Dermatopathol 7:57–63, 1985.
253. Jacobs DS, Edwards WD, Ye R: Metastatic atypical fibroxanthoma of skin. Cancer 35:457–463, 1975.
254. Kemp JD, Stenn KS, Arons M, Fischer J: Metastasizing atypical fibroxanthoma. Arch Dermatol 114:1533–1535, 1978.
255. Brown MD, Swanson NA: Treatment of malignant fibrous his-

tiocytoma and atypical fibrous xanthomas with micrographic surgery. J Dermatol Surg Oncol 15:1287–1292, 1989.

256. Rachmaninoff N, McDonald JR, Cook JC: Sarcoma-like tumors of skin following irradiation. Am J Clin Pathol 36:427–437, 1961.

257. Goldstein DJ, Barr RJ, Santa Cruz DJ: Microcystic adnexal carcinoma: a distinct clinicopathologic entity. Cancer 50:566–572, 1982.

258. Cooper PH, Mills SE, Leonard DD, et al: Sclerosing sweat duct (syringomatous) carcinoma. Am J Surg Pathol 9:422–433, 1985.

259. Cooper PH, Mills SE: Microcystic adnexal carcinoma. J Am Acad Dermatol 10:908–914, 1984.

260. Lupton GP, McMarlin SL: Microcystic adnexal carcinoma: report of a case with 30-year follow-up. Arch Dermatol 122:286–289, 1986.

261. Fleischmann HE, Roth FJ, Wood C, et al: Microcystic adnexal carcinoma treated by microscopically controlled excision. J Dermatol Surg Oncol 10:873–875, 1984.

262. Nickoloff BJ, Fleischmann HE, Carmel J, et al: Microcystic adnexal carcinoma. Immunohistologic observations suggesting dual (pilar and eccrine) differentiation. Arch Dermatol 122:290–294, 1986.

263. Abe M, Ohnishi Y, Hara Y, et al: Malignant tumors of the eyelid: clinical survey during 22-year period. Jpn J Ophthalmol 27:175–186, 1983.

264. Boniuk M, Zimmerman LE: Sebaceous carcinoma of the eyelid, eyebrow, caruncle, and orbit. Trans Am Acad Ophthalmol Otolaryngol 72:619–642, 1968.

265. Doxanas MT, Green WR: Sebaceous gland carcinoma: review of 40 cases. Arch Ophthalmol 102:245–249, 1984.

266. Ginsberg J: Present status of Meibomian gland carcinoma. Arch Ophthalmol 73:271–276, 1965.

267. Miller RE, White JJ: Sebaceous gland carcinoma. Am J Surg 114:958–964, 1981.

268. Ni C, Kuo PK: Meibomian gland carcinoma: a clinico-pathological study of 156 cases with long-period follow-up of 100 cases. Jpn J Ophthalmol 23:388–397, 1979.

269. Ni C, Searl SS, Kuo PK, et al: Sebaceous cell carcinoma of the ocular adnexa. Int Ophthalmol Clin 22:23–41, 1982.

270. Parsa FD: Sebaceous gland carcinoma of the eyelids in Hawaii. Hawaii Med J 48:165–166, 1989.

271. Rao NA, Hidayat AA, McLean IW, Zimmerman LE: Sebaceous carcinomas of the ocular adnexa: a clinicopathologic study of 104 cases with five year follow-up data. Hum Pathol 13:113–134, 1982.

272. Rodriguez-Sains RS: The role of the ophthalmologist in management of skin cancers. In: Friedman RJ, Rigel DS, Kopf AW, et al (eds): Cancer of the Skin. WB Saunders, Philadelphia, 1991, pp 589–602.

273. Urban FH, Winkelmann RK: Sebaceous malignancy. Arch Dermatol 84:63–67, 1961.

274. Wright JD, Font RL: Mucinous sweat gland adenocarcinoma of eyelid. Cancer 44:1757–1768, 1979.

275. Cavanagh HD, Green WR, Goldberg HK: Multicentric sebaceous adenocarcinoma of meibomian gland. Am J Ophthalmol 77:326–332, 1974.

276. Wagoner MD, Beyer CK, Gonder JR, Albert DM: Common presentations of sebaceous gland carcinoma of the eyelid. Ophthalmology 14:159–163, 1982.

277. Hood IC, Qizilbash AH, Salama SS, et al: Sebaceous carcinoma of the face following irradiation. Am J Dermatopathol 8:505–508, 1986.

278. Schlernitzauer DA, Font RL: Sebaceous gland carcinoma of the eyelid. Arch Ophthalmol 94:1523–1525, 1976.

279. Justi RA: Sebaceous carcinoma: report of case developing in area of radiodermatitis. Arch Dermatol 77:195–198, 1958.

280. Wolfe JT, Yeatts RP, Wich MR, et al: Sebaceous carcinomas of the eyelid: errors in clinical and pathologic diagnosis. Am J Surg Pathol 8:597–601, 1984.

281. Folberg R, Whitaker DC, Tse DT, Nerad JA: Recurrent and residual sebaceous carcinoma after Mohs excision of the primary lesion. Am J Ophthalmol 103:817–823, 1987.

282. Lisman RD, Jukobiec FA, Small P: Sebaceous carcinoma of the eyelids. The role of adjunctive cryotherapy in the management of conjunctival pagetoid spread. Ophthalmology 96:1021–1026, 1989.

283. Lee SC, Roth LM: Sebaceous carcinoma of the eyelid with pagetoid involvement of the bulbar and palpebral conjunctiva. J Cutan Pathol 4:134–137, 1977.

284. Russell WG, Page DL, Hough AJ, Rogers LW: Sebaceous carcinoma of meibomian gland origin. The diagnostic importance of pagetoid spread of neoplastic cells. Am J Clin Pathol 73:504–508, 1980.

285. Putterman AM: Conjunctival map biopsy to determine pagetoid spread. Am J Ophthalmol 102:87–90, 1986.

286. Rulon DB, Helwig EB: Cutaneous sebaceous neoplasms. Cancer 33:82–102, 1974.

287. Oppenheim AR: Sebaceous carcinoma of the penis. Arch Dermatol 117:306–309, 1981.

288. Mellette JR, Amonette RA, Gardner JH, Chesney T: Carcinoma of sebaceous glands on the head and neck: a report of 4 cases. J Dermatol Surg Oncol 7:404–409, 1981.

289. Wolfe JT, Wich MR, Campbell RJ: Sebaceous carcinoma of the oculocutaneous adnexa and extraocular skin. In: Wich MR (ed): Pathology of Unusual Malignant Cutaneous Tumors. Marcel Dekker, New York, 1985.

290. Torre D: Multiple sebaceous tumors. Arch Dermatol 98:549–554, 1968.

291. Burgdorf WHC, Pitha J, Fahmy A: Muir-Torre syndrome: histologic spectrum of sebaceous proliferations. Am J Dermatopathol 8:202–208, 1986.

292. Graham R, McKee P, McGibbon D, Heyderman E: Torre-Muir syndrome: an association with isolated sebaceous carcinoma. Cancer 55:2868–2873, 1985.

293. Householder MS, Zeligman I: Sebaceous neoplasms associated with visceral carcinomas. Arch Dermatol 115:862–868, 1980.

294. Leonard DD, Deaton WR: Multiple sebaceous gland tumors and visceral carcinomas. Arch Dermatol 110:917–920, 1974.

295. Muir EG, Yates Bell AJ, Burlow KA: Multiple primary carcinomata of the colon, duodenum and larynx associated with keratoacanthoma of the face. Br J Surg 54:191–195, 1967.

296. Rothenberg J, Lambert WC, Vail JT, et al: The Muir-Torre (Torre's) syndrome: the significance of a solitary sebaceous tumor. J Am Acad Dermatol 23:638–640, 1990.

297. Schwartz RA, Goldberg DJ, Mahmood F, et al: The Muir-Torre syndrome: a disease of sebaceous and colonic neoplasm. Dermatologica 178:23–28, 1989.

298. Harvey JT, Anderson RL: The management of meibomian gland carcinoma. Ophthalmic Surg 13:56–61, 1982.

299. Dixon RS, Mikhail GR, Slater HC: Sebaceous carcinoma of the eyelid. J Am Acad Dermatol 3:241–243, 1980.

300. Callahan A, Monheit GD, Callahan MA: Cancer excision from eyelids and ocular adnexa: the Mohs fresh tissue technique and reconstruction. CA 32:322–330, 1982.

301. Ratz JL, Lun-Duong S, Kulwin DR: Sebaceous carcinoma of the eyelid treated with Mohs surgery. J Am Acad Dermatol 14:668–673, 1986.

302. Dzubow LM: Sebaceous carcinoma of the eyelid. Treatment with Mohs surgery. J Dermatol Surg Oncol 11:40–44, 1985.

303. Hendley RL, Reiser JC, Cavanagh HD, et al: Primary radiation therapy for meibomian gland carcinoma. Am J Ophthalmol 87:206–210, 1979.

304. Ide CH, Ridingr GR, Yamashota T, Buesseler JA: Radiotherapy of current adenocarcinoma of the meibomian gland. Arch Ophthalmol 79:540–545, 1968.

305. Pardo FS, Wang CC, Albert D, Stracher MA: Sebaceous carcinoma of the ocular adnexa: radiotherapeutic management. Int J Radiat Oncol Biol Phys 17:643–647, 1989.

306. Nunery WP, Welsh MG, McCord CD: Recurrence of sebaceous carcinoma of the eyelid after radiation therapy. Am J Ophthalmol 96:1015, 1983.

CHAPTER 61

Cryosurgery for Benign, Premalignant, and Malignant Lesions

GLORIA F. GRAHAM

The first known medical use of cryotherapy was by the Egyptians,[1] who, as early as 2500 BC, employed cold to soothe injuries. In the fifth century, Hippocrates[2, 3] used hypothermia for treating edema, bleeding, and pain. Baron Dominique Jean Lorrey,[4] a surgeon serving with Napoleon during his historic retreat from Moscow, noted the anesthetic and sedative effects of cold. In the mid-nineteenth century, London physician James Arnott[5] used cold for the treatment of neuralgias and as palliative therapy for cancerous tumors in terminally ill patients; the latter was accomplished by lowering the temperature of the tumors to $-24°C$ with a brine solution. Contributions in the liquefaction of gases were made in 1877 by the French scientist Cailletet,[6] who liquified small quantities of oxygen and carbon monoxide, and the Swiss engineer Pictet,[7] who liquified oxygen. In 1883, two Polish scientists, Wroblewski and Olszewski,[8] were able to convert oxygen and nitrogen into a liquid state.

Modern cryosurgery was made possible in 1895 when Linde commercially produced large quantities of liquid air and nitrogen. The development of the vacuum flask by Dewar in 1898 was another significant contribution.[9] In 1899, White,[10] a New York dermatologist, became the first cryosurgeon when he dipped a cotton-tipped applicator into liquefied air and successfully treated warts, nevi, precancerous lesions, and some skin cancers.[11] His statement that "epithelioma treated early will always be cured"[12] shows that he recognized, even before the twentieth century, the value of cryosurgery in the management of skin cancer. In 1907 Whitehouse,[13] another New York dermatologist, developed a spray method using a laboratory wash bottle that gave excellent results in treating multiple skin cancers and led to the pioneering work of Zacarian, who conceived the idea of a hand-held cryosurgical unit, the Kryospray, for treating malignant tumors.[14]

In 1907, Pusey[15] was the first dermatologist in the United States to use liquid carbon dioxide for treating nevi and acne, and in the 1940s, Allington[16] introduced liquid nitrogen. Torre,[17] in 1967, pioneered a spray of liquid nitrogen for the treatment of malignant lesions of the skin based on instrumentation developed by Cooper, a neurosurgeon. Torre is currently working to develop liquid helium instrumentation for performing cryosurgery.[18] The ease of operation, efficiency in terms of time and cost, cosmetic results, and cure rates all make cryosurgery among the most widely used modalities in cutaneous surgery. Virtually every office can be inexpensively equipped to perform cryosurgery efficiently. It is particularly recommended for patients considered to be poor surgical candidates (e.g., children, the elderly, or those who have a variety of bleeding disorders). Cryosurgery can also be used in patients who have radiation damage and is particularly advantageous in the treatment of multiple lesions in a single visit.

Equipment

A number of cryogens (Table 61–1) and delivery systems have been used over the years, including dry ice slush, the Kidde apparatus, liquid nitrogen applied with a cotton swab (Fig. 61–1A), and various types of nitrous oxide and liquid nitrogen instruments. The original cryosurgical device was a small hand-held unit, the

TABLE 61–1. COMMON CRYOGENS USED IN CUTANEOUS SURGERY

Agent	Temperature
Freon 12	−29.8°C
Freon 22	−40.8°C
Solid CO_2	−79.0°C
Liquid N_2O	−88.5°C
Liquid nitrogen	−195.8°C
Helium	−185°C

Kryospray, developed by Brymill Corporation and based on the work of Zacarian.[19] Subsequently, the Frigitronics CE8 mobile unit, utilizing a 32-liter Dewar flask containing liquid nitrogen, became available with both spray and probe capabilities. Frigitronics developed a tabletop unit, the CS76, that held liquid nitrogen in two sections, one for priming the unit and the other for spraying. This unit had both probe and spray capabilities, as well as open cones that could be attached to the unit. Frigitronics' smaller thermos-type unit, the Cryo-Surg (Fig. 61–1*B*), holds 500 ml of liquid nitrogen and can be used with various sizes of spray and probe tips. The Brymill Corporation has developed several new small Cry-Ac units (Fig. 61–1*C*) that are lightweight (only about 1.5 to 2 pounds) and capable of holding liquid nitrogen for 12 to 24 hours. A variety of probes and spray attachments are also available (Fig. 61–2*A*). In addition, a number of devices are available for eye protection (Fig. 61–2*B*). Another cryosurgical device is the Fern Cryoprobe (Fig. 61–3), a convenient self-contained unit with a flexible hose that can be sterilized.[13, 20, 21] Various types of thermocouples are also available to accurately measure the tissue temperature (Fig. 61–4).

CRYOGENS

One group of cryogens, the Freons, have been primarily used as sprays to provide temporary anesthesia

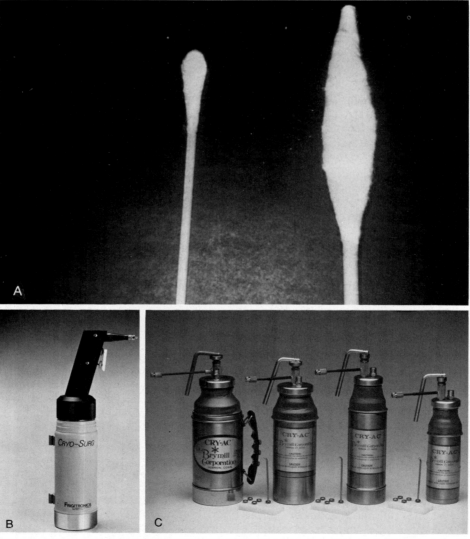

Figure 61–1. *A,* The first and simplest cryosurgical delivery system using cotton-tipped applicators of different sizes. *B,* Frigitronics' thermos-type unit called the Cryo-Surg. *C,* Brymill Corporation has developed several Cry-Ac units with a static holding time for liquid nitrogen of 12 to 24 hours and a full weight of 2.15 to 4.22 pounds.

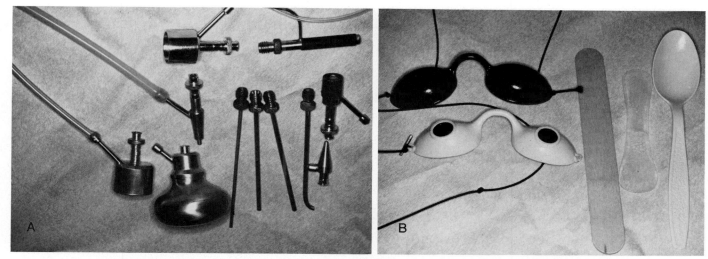

Figure 61–2. *A,* Stainless steel probes and spray attachments. *B,* Various equipment used for eye protection.

before the removal of small skin lesions and to prepare the skin for dermabrasion. Carbon dioxide has been used, especially as a "snow," for the treatment of acne and acne scarring. Nitrous oxide has been most commonly used in gynecology for treating disorders of the cervix and in ophthalmology for the treatment of cataracts.

Currently the cryogen most commonly used in cutaneous surgery is liquid nitrogen. It has the lowest temperature of all the common cryogens ($-195.8°C$) and a proven uniform effectiveness in the treatment of cutaneous malignancies. It is possible that future cryosurgical instruments using liquid helium as the cryogen will eventually replace liquid nitrogen in the clinical setting.

Storage of Liquid Nitrogen

Liquid nitrogen is available in most parts of the country from welding supply companies, which routinely

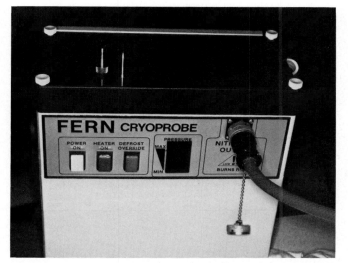

Figure 61–3. The Fern Cryoprobe unit with spray and probe capabilities.

service physicians' offices. It is typically stored in the office in 20- to 30-liter insulated Dewar flasks (Fig. 61–5).

Evidence[22] has shown that viral contamination of liquid nitrogen (LN_2) may occur when treating warts or other infectious lesions if a "dipstick" method (i.e., repeated dipping of cotton swabs or solid probes into the main liquid nitrogen storage container) is used. For this reason, it is usually preferable to dispense a small amount of LN_2 into a Styrofoam cup and discard any remaining LN_2 after treatment with the dipstick technique. The small, hand-held units are most convenient for treatment of infectious lesions because of the ease of carrying them from room to room.

Cryotherapy for Benign and Precancerous Lesions

For treatment of benign and most precancerous lesions, the depth and duration of liquid nitrogen spray (LNSP) or liquid nitrogen probe (LNPR) need not be as long as those used in the treatment of malignant lesions. Cosmetic results are of prime importance but are usually satisfactory regardless of the anatomic location. Placement of thermocouples (Fig. 61–4) is rarely required for treating benign lesions but may be used for certain precancerous lesions, especially lentigo maligna.

PATIENT SELECTION

Because of the wide variety of treatment methods available for many different skin conditions, the method selected often depends on the skin type, the general health of the patient, and individual preference.

INDICATIONS

Patients taking anticoagulants, those with a previous history of poor wound healing after standard surgical

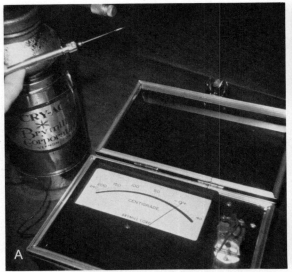

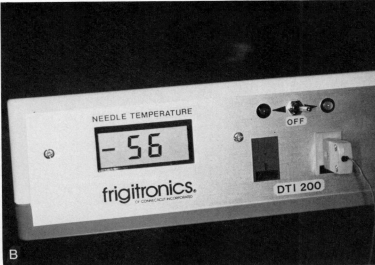

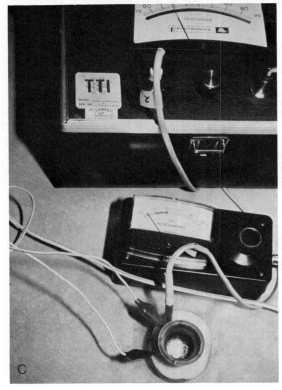

Figure 61–4. Various types of thermocouples. *A,* Brymill device with solid needle and pyrometer. *B,* Frigitronics digital readout pyrometer. *C,* Ezee cryometer, thermocouple, and ampmeter (Courtesy of D. Torre, M.D., New York, NY.)

Figure 61–5. Liquid nitrogen is commonly stored in a 32-L Dewar flask, although smaller sizes are also available.

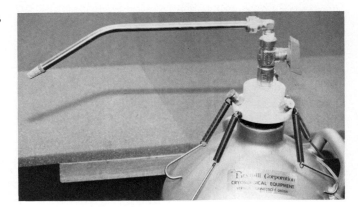

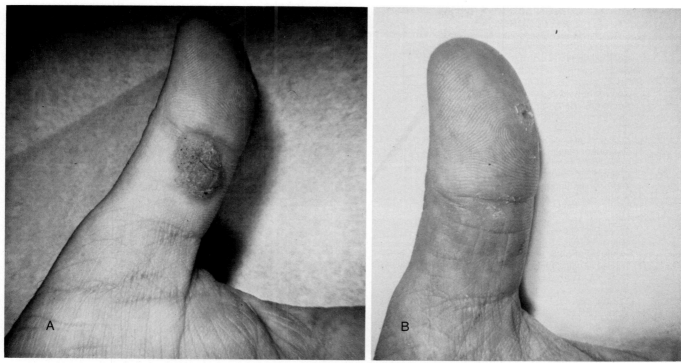

Figure 61–6. *A,* Preoperative appearance of a typical verruca. *B,* Complete resolution after one cryosurgical treatment.

procedures, and those with fair skin are often the best candidates for cryosurgery. Patients with multiple large lesions are also excellent candidates, while those with many small (1- to 2-mm) lesions are often best treated with other techniques.

Cryotherapy is the preferred modality in the treatment of warts (Fig. 61–6) and molluscum contagiosum in persons infected with the human immunodeficiency virus (HIV). However, treatment with podophyllin, topical keratolytics, intralesional chemotherapeutic agents, electrosurgery, or laser may also be considered appropriate. In these patients, cutaneous infections are often very extensive, may have atypical patterns, and tend to be recalcitrant to therapy. For these reasons, topical and systemic antifungal, antibacterial, and antiviral agents are often used in addition to cryosurgery to manage many cutaneous infections in persons infected with HIV.

There are also many advantages to performing cryosurgery in nursing home patients: it is easily performed, has few associated complications, and requires only minimal postoperative wound care. In addition, most patients do not require injection of a local anesthetic when treating benign and premalignant lesions of the skin.

CONTRAINDICATIONS

Cryosurgery is contraindicated in patients with cryoglobulinemia or cryofibrinogenemia, especially if large areas are to be treated. Delayed healing has been reported when treating acne scarring in a patient later found to have cryofibrinogenemia.[23]

The choice of surgical method may also depend on the location of the lesion and the patient's natural skin color. If an area of alopecia resulting from cryosurgical treatment of the scalp would be cosmetically unacceptable, surgical excision might be a preferable form of therapy. However, large areas of actinic damage on a bald head are often best treated by cryosurgery. An actinic keratosis that curves over the pinna of the ear is probably better treated by cryosurgery than by electrodesiccation and curettage, as the former will avoid a notched scar. A lesion on the tip of the nose of a dark-skinned patient is probably best treated with some technique other than cryosurgery because of the anticipated hypopigmentation that is likely to follow.

A history of previous radiation therapy with secondary radiation dermatitis may make surgical excision a poor choice, as healing may be impaired. However, cryosurgery in this situation rarely causes any significant problem with healing, except that it may be slightly slower than normal. If there is evidence of significant arteriosclerosis in the lower leg, cryosurgery should be avoided. However, if the circulation is good in the lower leg, healing may be somewhat slower than elsewhere on the body but will usually take place in a reasonable period of time. It is always appropriate to evaluate the patient's general health, psychological makeup, and expectations and the cost of the procedure when considering cryosurgery.[24]

LESION SELECTION

Because a large number of benign, premalignant, and malignant lesions can be effectively treated by cryosur-

TABLE 61–2. BENIGN LESIONS TREATED WITH CRYOSURGERY

Acne rosacea
Acne vulgaris
Angiokeratoma of Fordyce
Angiokeratoma, solitary type
Angiolymphoid hyperplasia
Angioma, cherry and spider
Chondrodermatitis chronicus helicus
Dermatofibroma
Disseminated superficial actinic porokeratosis
Epidermal nevus
Granuloma faciale
Granuloma fissuratum
Hidradenitis suppurativa
Keloid
Keratoacanthoma
Leishmaniasis
Lentigines (simplex or solar types)
Lichen planus
Lichen sclerosus et atrophicus
Lichen simplex chronicus
Molluscum contagiosum
Mucocele
Myxoid cyst
Porokeratosis of Mibelli
Porokeratosis plantaris discreta
Prurigo nodularis
Psoriatic plaques
Pyogenic granuloma
Sebaceous hyperplasia
Seborrheic keratosis
Steatocystoma multiplex
Syringoma
Trichiasis
Venous lake
Verrucae
   Condyloma acuminatum
   Periungual verrucae
   Verruca plana
   Verruca palmaris and plantaris
   Verruca vulgaris

gery (Tables 61–2, 61–3, 61–4), a number of factors must be considered in determining whether cryosurgery is the treatment of choice. These factors include a determination of the desired freezing time, the required depth of freeze, the need for use of thermocouples, the proper tip size, and the desired final result.

TREATMENT TECHNIQUE

The technique used for the treatment of benign lesions involves freezing the lesion until a 1- to 2-mm rim of normal tissue has been frozen (Table 61–5). Although freezing can be performed with a continuous spray,

TABLE 61–3. PRECANCEROUS LESIONS OR TUMORS OF UNCERTAIN BEHAVIOR

Actinic cheilitis
Actinic keratosis
Bowenoid papulosis
Keratoacanthoma
Lentigo maligna
Leukoplakia

TABLE 61–4. MALIGNANT LESIONS TREATED WITH CRYOSURGERY

Basal cell carcinoma
Bowen's disease (carcinoma in situ)
Kaposi's sarcoma
Metastatic melanoma (palliative treatment)
Squamous cell carcinoma
   Actinic keratosis with squamous cell carcinoma
   Adenoid type
   De novo type

better control is often obtained with the use of an intermittent spray technique or contact probes. Probe tips are selected so that they approximate the size of the lesion or are slightly smaller.

SIDE EFFECTS AND COMPLICATIONS

Cryosurgery is a safe procedure with a low incidence of complications. Certain common side effects such as edema, vesicles, bullae, weeping, and eschar formation can be expected as a normal result of the inflammatory reaction. However, these are transient and usually subside within 1 to 2 weeks after treatment of benign lesions and within 4 to 6 weeks after treatment of malignant lesions.

Pain

Some patients will experience mild pain during freezing and thawing, particularly when the fingers, toes, or plantar surfaces of the feet are treated. Because local anesthesia is used before the treatment of most malignancies, little pain will be experienced. Although patients only rarely experience significant pain after cryosurgery, treatment of warts on the fingers or feet may

TABLE 61–5. APPROXIMATE FREEZE TIMES FOR COMMON BENIGN LESIONS*

Lesions	Freeze Times (seconds)
Verruca plana	5
Lentigo	7
Sebaceous adenoma	5–10
Actinic keratosis	5–10
Seborrheic keratosis	10–15
Verruca vulgaris	15–20
Prurigo nodularis	30
Keloid	30
Hemangioma	60+
Keratoacanthoma	30
Dermatofibroma	60+
Granuloma faciale	30
Granuloma annulare	20
Chondrodermatitis	30
Psoriasis plaque	15–30
Cherry angioma	10
Nevus	10
Leukoplakia	15
Mucocele	30
Molluscum contagiosum	5–10

*Using Brymill Cry-AC with a B tip.

require use of pain medications for 24 to 48 hours. Transient headaches often develop during treatment of tumors of the scalp, forehead, or temple. Because fainting may also occur after some cryosurgical procedures, especially on the fingers, patients should be carefully watched during thawing, and if pallor develops, they should lie down immediately.

Bleeding

Tissue necrosis resulting from cryosurgery for cancers or other deep tumors can be associated with bleeding. Capillary bleeding may occur once the necrotic tissue begins to separate. After debulking procedures, bleeding may result, but aluminum chloride or Monsel's solution is usually effective in controlling this problem, even in patients on anticoagulants or aspirin.

Infection

Rarely does infection occur, even when extensive areas are treated. This low rate of infection after cryosurgery is probably a result of maintenance of an intact basement membrane and the rapid reepithelialization that occurs after treatment of benign and premalignant lesions. Destruction of bacteria on the surface of the skin during freezing may also partially account for the low incidence of infection. Patients should be cautioned that if increased warmth, redness, or any other evidence of infection occurs, they should return to see the physician promptly.

Abnormal Scarring

Because the normal dermal fibrous network is maintained after freezing and aids in the rapid regeneration of the epidermis, many lesions can be frozen with little or no resultant scarring. Because of this, hypertrophic or atrophic scarring is rarely seen after treatment of benign and premalignant lesions. The most common scar seen after cryosurgery is a soft, slightly lighter-colored, minimally atrophic area with a shiny surface. Even with aggressive treatment, the hair follicles are often maintained, but loss of pore structure can occur after cryosurgery. Linear hypertrophic scarring occurs with some frequency on the nose and upper lip but usually disappears with time. When the eyelid is treated cryosurgically, an ectropion only rarely results, but loss of eyelashes may occur.

Nerve Damage

Damage to underlying nerves after cryosurgery has been reported only rarely when treating benign and premalignant lesions. However, digital neuropathy after cryosurgery for a wart on the finger using a cotton-tipped applicator has been reported.[25] The sensory loss that occurs after cryosurgery usually fully resolves, although this may take 6 to 12 months.[26] This recovery occurs more rapidly in younger patients, and the sense of touch recovers more quickly than the sensations of pain and cold.

Insufflation of Soft Tissue

If a biopsy has been performed and liquid nitrogen spray is delivered directly to the biopsy site, the gas may spread under the skin, causing crepitation and a very dramatic inflation of the tissue. Pressure on the area will result in expulsion of the liquid nitrogen. Use of a cone placed around the biopsy site will help prevent this complication from occurring, as will spraying tangentially to seal the tissue defect with the cryogen.

Traumatic Exfoliation

If the probe is not pre-chilled, adherence can result in stripping off of the mucous membrane when the probe is removed. The probe should be allowed to thaw completely before pulling it off the skin surface. In this way, it will come off the skin without traumatizing the tissue through forceful exfoliation.

Cartilage Necrosis

Necrosis of cartilage is rare but can occur after cryosurgery. It is particularly common on the helix of the ear, especially if a through-and-through freezing technique has been employed.

Abnormal Pigmentation

One side effect that can be anticipated in many patients is hypopigmentation. For this reason, cryosurgery should not be performed on dark-skinned or tanned individuals without first explaining that hypopigmentation may result. In treating keloids on the ear, for instance, hypopigmentation of the posterior earlobe may not be a significant problem for the patient, but the same discoloration occurring on the anterior surface may be. The pigment cell is extremely sensitive to cold and will be destroyed at a temperature of only $-4°C$.[27] Consideration of this point will often help in the proper selection of patients to prevent the use of cryosurgery where pigment loss would be a source of significant cosmetic disability. Hyperpigmentation also can occur after cryosurgery, most often on the lower leg and at the outer edge of treated lentigines on the face and hands, even after only short exposures.

Miscellaneous Complications

Other permanent complications of cryosurgery include alopecia, notching of the eyelid margin if freezing is done near this anatomic structure, and notching and atrophy of the nose tip, margin of the ear, or the border of the upper lip.

Cryosurgery of Specific Lesions

Actinic Keratosis. Because actinic keratosis (AK) is a very common cutaneous lesion treated by cryosurgery, it will be used as a focal point for the discussion of the proper treatment techniques, postoperative care, and

TABLE 61–6. **TREATMENT PARAMETERS FOR CRYOSURGERY***

Lesion Type	Treatment	Tip	Time (sec)	Target (mm)	Technique	Thermocouple Required	Result
Hypertrophic actinic keratosis	√Choice Alternate Adjunct	B	F = 20–30 T = 30–40	2	√Cryospray Cryoprobe 1 Cryocycle	No	Excellent to good
Seborrheic keratosis	Choice √Alternate √Adjunct	B	F = 10–20 T = 20–30	2.5	√Cryospray Cryoprobe 1 Cryocycle	No	Good to fair
Dermatofibroma	√Choice √Alternate Adjunct	Probe	F = 20–30 T = 30–40	3–4	√Cryospray √Cryoprobe 1 Cryocycle	No	Good to fair
Basal cell carcinoma	√Choice √Alternate Adjunct	A (>1 cm) B (<1 cm)	F = 60–120 T = 60–180	3–4	√Cryospray √Cryoprobe 2–3 Cryocycles	Yes	Good to fair
Lentigo maligna	√Choice Alternate Adjunct	A or B	F = 60–120	3–4	√Cryospray √Cryoprobe 2–3 Cryocycles	Yes	Excellent to good

*Using Brymill Cry-Ac.
F, freeze time; T, thaw time.
√, preferred technique or treatment.

methods to avoid side effects. Cryosurgery is an excellent method for the treatment of AKs, because it is rapid and relatively free of complications. The spray technique is especially well suited to treat many lesions quickly in a single session, especially those with irregular shapes, but the dipstick method can also work well (Table 61–6).

Treatment Technique. Outlining the margins of the AK before treating with LNSP ensures uniform freezing of the entire lesion. During spraying, a distinctive appearance often helps to more clearly show the full extent of the lesion. An intermittent spray of 8 to 10 seconds is normally used for small, flat AKs, while a 10- to 20-second exposure is required for hypertrophic AKs. For larger lesions, a back-and-forth "paintbrush" method is used, while smaller lesions are treated using a direct intermittent spray. The intermittent technique helps to avoid excess lateral spreading of the freeze.

When treating around the eye, ear, and nose, extra precautions must be used. The eye may be protected with a tongue blade (Fig. 61–7), Styrofoam, or Jaeger retractor, but a metal shield should never be used during freezing. When treating around the nose, a wooden tongue blade is especially useful in preventing vapor from entering the nostril (Fig. 61–8). The cryoprobe may be advantageous to use in difficult locations such as around the eye or in the ear canal. When treating the ear, angling the spray can reduce the potential for liquid nitrogen to enter the external ear canal and damage the tympanic membrane. When freezing the pinna, it is also helpful to watch the opposite side of the ear for ice formation, as cartilage is very cryosensitive. The potential for causing cartilage damage can be reduced by not excessively freezing normal skin.

The cryoprobe is useful on the scalp and nose when a greater depth of freeze is needed with less lateral spread. Thaw times for common AKs range from 10 to 15 seconds, while hypertrophic AKs may require 30 to 40 seconds (Fig. 61–9). Freezing is continued until a 1- to 2-mm halo of freeze is obtained around the lesion (Fig. 61–10).

The three basic spray patterns are solid central, spiral circular, and paintbrush (Fig. 61–11). The art of freezing AKs may be enhanced by varying the spray patterns. A solid central spray may be used on lesions smaller than 0.5 cm; a circular intermittent pattern can be used for slightly larger, 1- to 2-cm lesions; and a paintbrush

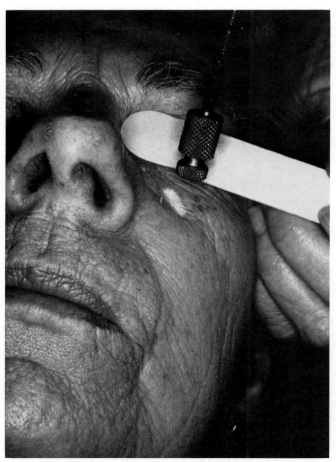

Figure 61–7. The eye is protected with a tongue blade during freezing.

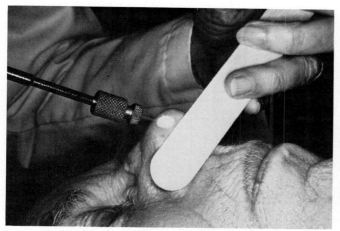

Figure 61–8. The nares are protected during freezing with a wooden tongue blade.

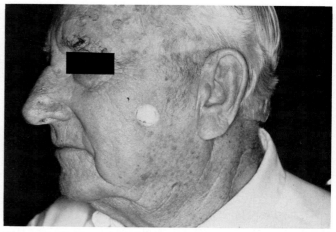

Figure 61–10. Freezing is continued until a 1- to 2-mm rim of normal tissue is included.

pattern is used for lesions greater than 2 cm. In addition, each surgeon will develop an individual style and technique for performing cryosurgery that may alter freeze times by 5 to 10 seconds or more. If a lesion thaws more quickly than anticipated, a second freeze-thaw cycle may be performed, but this is not often necessary in the treatment of benign and precancerous lesions (Figs. 61–12, 61–13). Alternately, a cryoprobe can be used to treat large, deep, or thick lesions (Fig. 61–14).

Postoperative Course and Wound Care. Initially, erythema and edema develop, usually within 5 to 15 minutes after freezing. Absorbent pads may be useful during the early healing process, as vesicles or bullae typically appear within several hours. After drying of the bulla, a small eschar forms. During the later stages of healing, simple cleansing with soap and water is all that is needed. Although secondary infection is rare, should this develop, topical cleansing with 3% hydrogen peroxide followed by application of a topical antibiotic ointment is usually sufficient, as systemic antibiotics are seldom required. Normally, healing occurs within 10 to 14 days, but thicker lesions may require 3 weeks.

Healing may be somewhat slower on the helix of the ear, the scalp, the dorsum of the hand, and the lower leg. Hydrocolloid dressings have proved useful in speeding healing after cryosurgery on the legs. The final cosmetic appearance is a soft, hypopigmented macular area with slight textural change. The overall cure rate for AKs followed for at least 1 year[28] has been reported to be 98%. However, hyperkeratotic lesions sometimes require retreatment.

Leukoplakia. Leukoplakia of the lip and buccal mucosa is particularly well suited to cryosurgery using the LNSP technique.[29] Cryoprobes may be used for small lesions in the mouth, but LNSP is preferable for both lip lesions and larger lesions in the mouth. Usually one half of a large lip lesion is treated at each session using a freeze time of about 15 seconds, which yields a thaw time of 30 to 60 seconds (Figs. 61–15, 61–16). Large areas on the tongue can also be eradicated by cryosurgery. Some simple devices can be made to help localize the spray. One design uses the plastic part of a syringe cylinder to which the spray nozzle can be attached. When LNSP is used intraorally, a dental suction is helpful for removing the resulting fog. In addition, having the patient take a deep breath and exhale slowly while the spraying progresses dissipates the fog more readily.

One technique[30] for treating leukoplakia on the lip uses LNSP, starting near the lateral commissure and working toward the center, resulting in a solid freeze. The total thaw time may be 1 minute or more. Ballottement is a valuable guide in determining the adequacy

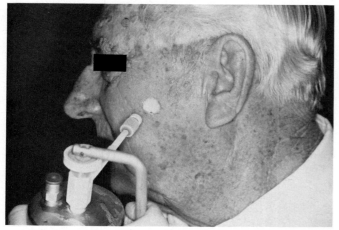

Figure 61–9. The Cry-Ac by Brymill is used to freeze an actinic keratosis on the cheek.

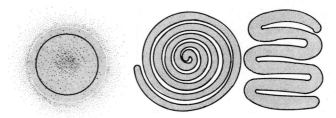

Figure 61–11. Basic spray patterns: solid central *(left)*, circular *(center)*, and paintbrush *(right)*.

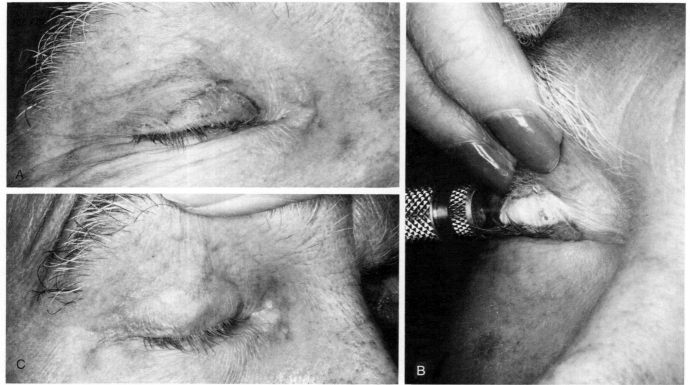

Figure 61–12. *A,* Actinic keratosis of the eyelid. *B,* Appearance during freezing. *C,* An excellent cosmetic result is seen after cryosurgery.

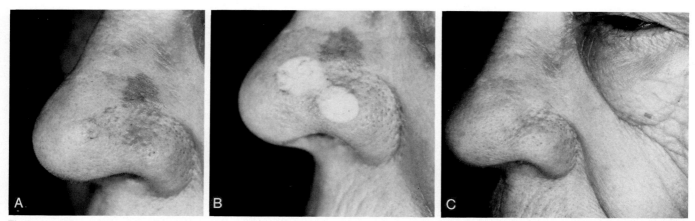

Figure 61–13. *A,* Preoperative appearance of a pigmented actinic keratosis on the nose. *B,* The inferior portion is treated with liquid nitrogen spray for 15 seconds. *C,* Seven months after two treatments, there is a very satisfactory clearing.

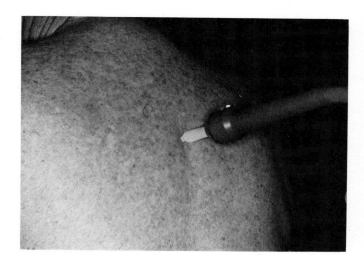

Figure 61–14. The Fern Cryoprobe is used to treat an actinic keratosis on the back to permit greater depth of freeze with less lateral spread.

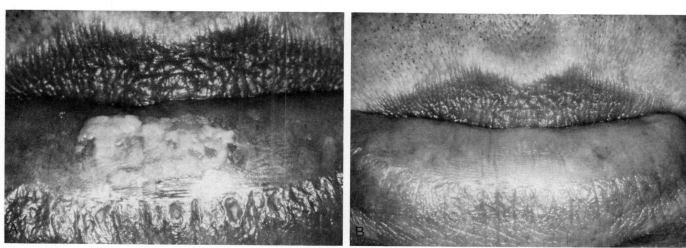

Figure 61–15. *A,* Preoperative appearance of leukoplakia of the lip. *B,* Appearance after cryosurgery. (Courtesy of J. Zakrzewska, M.D., London, England.)

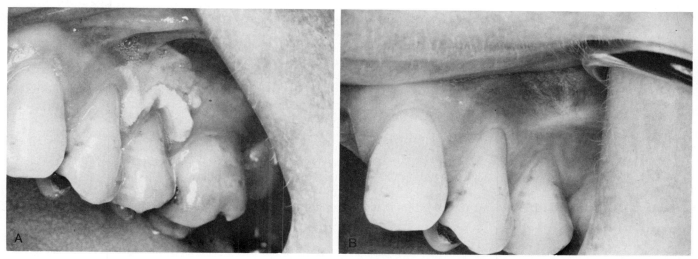

Figure 61–16. *A,* Preoperative appearance of leukoplakia of the alveolar ridge. *B,* Clearing after cryosurgery. (Courtesy of J. Zakrzewska, M.D., London, England.)

of the freeze. The entire lip may be treated in one session, although it is often preferable to do one half at a time. A 96% cure rate using LNSP for premalignant leukoplakia of the lip has been reported.[31] Lesions on the tongue may be treated with LNSP for 10 to 15 seconds, but scarring has resulted, especially on the lateral aspect.[29] Squamous cell carcinoma should be treated aggressively, as leukoplakia may develop.[32]

Adenoma Sebaceum. These facial tumors are commonly found in patients with tuberous sclerosis, and treatment is often desirable because of the extreme cosmetic disfigurement that they may produce. One technique that provides a satisfactory cosmetic result without significant scarring[33] divides the face into sections that are individually treated at 3-week intervals. Several sessions are typically required to obtain complete flattening of the lesions.

Spider Angioma. Electrodesiccation and laser photocoagulation may provide effective treatment for spider angiomas, but these lesions are also amenable to freezing. A small, pointed cryoprobe is applied to the elevated central arteriole, and moderate pressure is applied until a 1- to 2-mm halo around the lesion is obtained. The patient should be forewarned that several treatments may be necessary to avoid excessive freezing, which may result in atrophy and hypopigmentation.

Dermatofibroma. Although many patients are reassured to know that dermatofibromas are benign and do not require removal, a significant number of patients will request treatment. In a retrospective study of 393 dermatofibromas treated with liquid nitrogen (Fig. 61–17), 64.8% were free of the visible and palpable lesion, although pigmentation remained in 9.4%.[34] Of the remaining group, 9.4% had residual palpable fibrosis, 6.4% were classified as partial failures (25 to 75% of the fibrosis remaining), and 9.7% were classified as complete failures (little or no response). Of the 277 lesions in which the fibrosis cleared completely, only 15 required more than two treatments, and a third treatment cured only another 6%. Of the lesions that cleared, 71% did so with only a single treatment.[34–36]

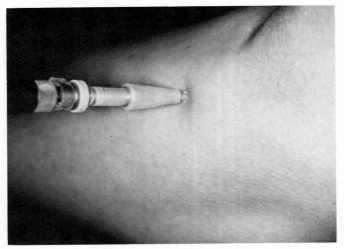

Figure 61–17. Dermatofibroma on the leg during liquid nitrogen cryosurgery.

One effective technique modification is to tangentially excise the elevated portion of the fibroma and then spray the base until a 1- to 2-mm frozen rim develops (Table 61–6). Spraying into a neoprene cone can increase the depth of freeze while limiting the lateral spread. A frequent side effect of treatment is central hypopigmentation and peripheral hyperpigmentation, especially in dark-skinned individuals. The hyperpigmentation may take months to clear completely, but occasionally persistent hypopigmentation is seen. Several treatments with shorter thaw times may provide better cosmetic results.[37]

Granuloma Faciale. Many different types of treatment have been used for granuloma faciale, but some cases prove to be resistant. Cryosurgery has proved successful in managing some of these lesions[38] using the spray technique with a relatively long single freeze cycle of 1 minute.

Capillary Hemangiomas. Although many capillary hemangiomas spontaneously regress, some located around the eye or mouth can compromise function and may require treatment. A technique using cryosurgery to treat angiomas and other vascular birthmarks—not only for those lesions of enormous size and in locations that impair function, but also those that proliferate rapidly—has been developed. It appears that the earlier treatment is initiated, the simpler the procedure and the better the results. The technique used to treat hemangiomas uses a flat, round, or doorknob-type cryoprobe with a diameter that approximates the size of the lesion. The cryoprobe is first chilled to prevent adherence to the lesion, which can make the probe more difficult to remove and unnecessarily traumatizes the patient. The probe is then applied to the center of the tumor to force out the blood. Freezing is continued until a 1- to 1½-mm halo of ice extends beyond the visible margin of the lesion (Fig. 61–18).

Cavernous Hemangioma. The technique for managing cavernous hemangiomas is similar to that used for capillary hemangiomas. However, because they are deeper lesions, a double freeze-thaw cycle is often required. A cryoprobe has been designed for intralesional use in treating deep cavernous hemangiomas, even large lesions under the eye (Fig. 61–19).

Port-wine Stains. Although the macular component of port-wine stains is resistant to cryotherapy, the exophytic areas may be flattened and the more darkly colored areas may be lightened by freezing for 30 to 60 seconds. Because cryosurgery can result in atrophy and scarring, laser surgery is usually preferable.[39]

Angiolymphoid Hyperplasia with Eosinophilia. Although this tumor is often difficult to eradicate, a good response can be obtained with cryosurgery. Several treatments may be required for extensive lesions involving the pinna and the external auditory canal, and monitoring is often necessary to ensure a sufficient depth of freeze.[40]

Keloids. Excellent results can be obtained when treating some keloids if cryosurgery is done in conjunction with either intralesional steroid injection or preliminary excision of the bulk of the keloid.[41] In this treatment,

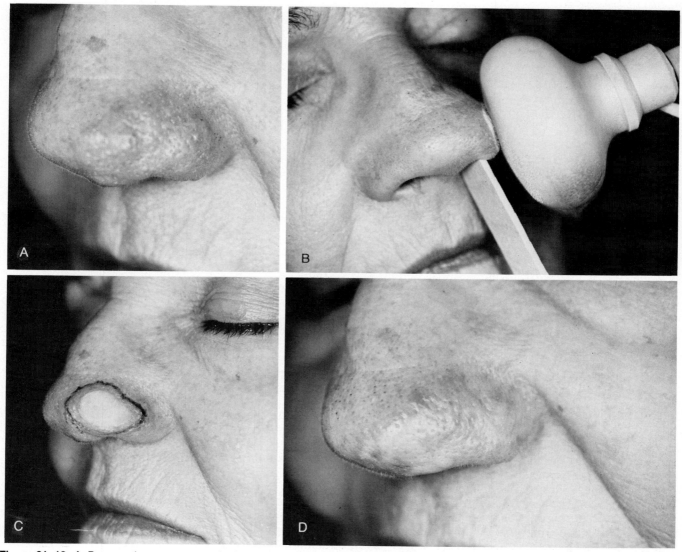

Figure 61–18. *A,* Preoperative appearance of a hemangioma on the nose. *B,* Application of liquid nitrogen using a doorknob-type probe. *C,* Appearance immediately after completion of cryosurgery. *D,* Appearance 2 months after cryosurgery.

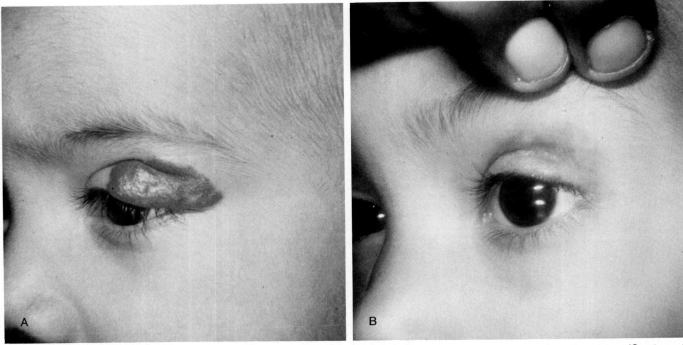

Figure 61–19. *A,* Preoperative appearance of a hemangioma on the eyelid. *B,* Appearance of the hemangioma after cryosurgery. (Courtesy of Gilberto Castro-Ron, M.D., Caracas, Venezuela.)

first the base is injected with intralesional steroids and then the keloid is frozen for 1 minute (Fig. 61–20). Monthly retreatments of persistent areas can usually provide a very satisfactory final cosmetic result.[33]

Keratoacanthoma. Keratoacanthomas are best treated by first performing shave excision and then freezing the base for 30 to 60 seconds (Fig. 61–21).

Solar Lentigines. These very common lesions, especially larger lesions on the face and darker lesions on the chest or hands, can also be successfully treated with cryosurgery. Pretreating the skin with topical tretinoin and hydroquinone will often provide better cosmetic results after freezing. In addition, patients should use sunscreen lotions for at least 3 to 6 months before cryosurgery is performed. If the lesions do not clear completely, they will often be lighter in color. A total of 7 to 8 seconds of intermittent freezing is usually sufficient to treat these lesions, and either the spray or the probe technique may be used. Sunscreen lotions that provide ultraviolet A and B (UVA and UVB) protection are essential postoperatively to prevent recurrences. Smoker's melanosis of the lips will also respond quite satisfactorily to cryosurgery (Fig. 61–22).

Molluscum Contagiosum. The multitude of lesions that are frequently present with this infection make freezing an uncomfortable and rather time-consuming method of treatment. Cryosurgeons sometimes spray with fluoroethyl and then curette the lesions or use a comedo extractor to press the central core of the lesion. Freezing lightly with a liquid nitrogen spray for 5 to 10 seconds is also usually effective. In the pediatric age group, multiple lesions of the eyelids can be treated with a tiny probe while protecting the eye with a Jaeger

retractor.[42] However, considerable postoperative edema can be expected.

Mucocele. Although mucoceles may respond well to cryosurgery, only 50 to 60% can be expected to resolve after the first treatment. With the second treatment, however, 80 to 90% of lesions are usually eradicated. It is not necessary to drain the lesions first, but this may be helpful at times for the larger lesions. When the probe is used, it should first be pre-chilled and then moved around for a few seconds so that it does not adhere to the lesion. This prevents tearing the mucous membrane on removal. Retreatment may be performed after 1 to 2 months.

Porokeratosis Plantaris Discreta (Conical Callus). Cryosurgery has been successfully used to treat conical calluses by combining freezing with surgical paring at 2-week intervals until lesions have completely healed.[43, 44] This combination appears to be the treatment of choice for this problem, but surgery to correct underlying bony abnormalities still may be required.

Epidermal Nevi. Inconsistent results have been achieved when treating epidermal nevi with cryosurgery.[45] Total regression occurs more frequently in young children,[33] but significant hypopigmentation may result before complete eradication of the nevus occurs.

Junctional Nevi. While nevi may respond erratically to freezing,[46] promising results have been reported.[36] The response of junctional nevi has been studied in carefully selected patients with large numbers of small (2- to 4-mm) benign-appearing lesions.[47] To determine the correct freeze times, many lesions have been surgically removed and examined histologically 1 month after freezing. For most junctional lesions, 10 to 15

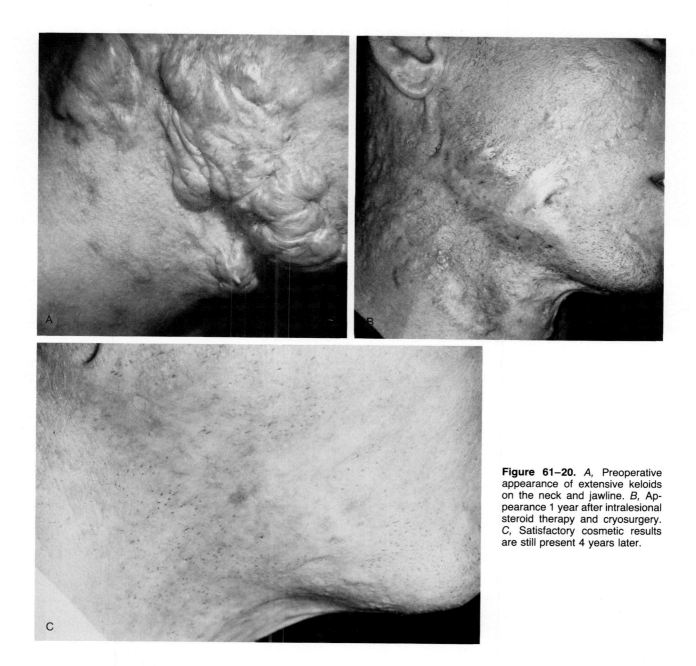

Figure 61–20. *A,* Preoperative appearance of extensive keloids on the neck and jawline. *B,* Appearance 1 year after intralesional steroid therapy and cryosurgery. *C,* Satisfactory cosmetic results are still present 4 years later.

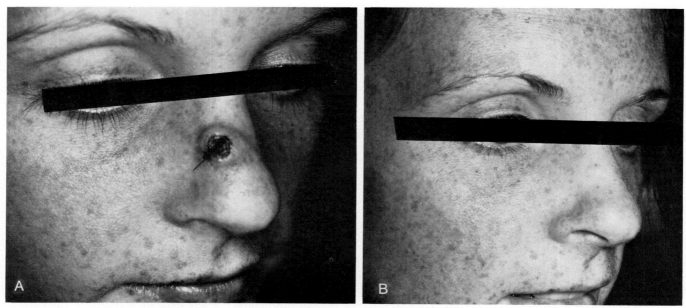

Figure 61–21. *A,* Preoperative appearance of a biopsy-proven keratoacanthoma of the nose. *B,* Complete resolution after cryosurgery.

seconds of freezing has been found to be sufficient to destroy the entire lesion. Despite this fact, if pigment persists after cryosurgery, the lesion should be surgically removed. Although cryosurgery is not advocated as a form of therapy for all nevi, there are situations in which the cosmetic results from such treatment can be outstanding. In this technique, after shave excision of the nevus, any persistent pigment is treated with 10 to 15 seconds of freezing with LNSP or cryoprobe.

Prurigo Nodularis. Despite the fact that lesions of prurigo nodularis are difficult to eradicate with most forms of therapy, cryosurgery is often considered to be the treatment of choice for recalcitrant lesions.[48] The C nerve fibers may be altered by freezing, decreasing

pruritus and reducing the trauma caused by scratching. Freeze times vary from 20 to 30 seconds because of differences in lesion thickness.[49] While the spray technique is effective, the contact probe with pressure may also be used.

Sebaceous Hyperplasia. These lesions rarely require treatment, but those large enough to cause a cosmetic problem may be effectively eradicated, with minimal scarring, using a cryoprobe placed into the central pore of the lesion. Many lesions may be treated quickly in a single session, with results comparable to those produced by platinum needle electrodesiccation. With the cryoprobe, 5 to 10 seconds of freezing is usually sufficient.[37] Retreatments are frequently necessary, but

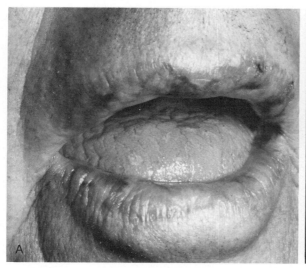
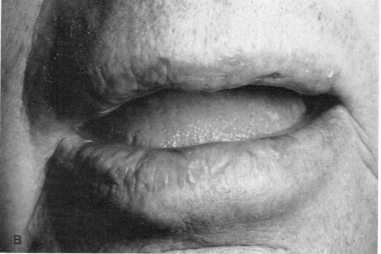

Figure 61–22. *A,* Preoperative appearance of a patient with diffuse macular pigmentation (smoker's melanosis) of the lip. *B,* Complete resolution has occurred 2 months after spray cryosurgery (3 to 10 seconds per lesion) was performed.

about two thirds of patients are satisfied with the results obtained from a single treatment.

Seborrheic Keratoses. Cryosurgery alone may eradicate many seborrheic keratoses (SKs), but freezing of the lesion followed by curettage is often preferable for thicker lesions. Many patients request removal of these lesions because they are pruritic, unsightly, or irritated by clothing. Sometimes topical application of castor oil or alpha-hydroxy acid lotions before cryosurgery provides substantially improved results.

The preferred treatment for scalp SKs is liquid LNSP plus curettage.[35] For macular SKs on the cheek, LNSP alone is often successful.[50] For multiple SKs on the trunk, removal is accomplished by light freezing followed by curettage (Table 61–6). Covering the wound with Second Skin for 24 hours decreases the postoperative discomfort.[37] After that period, soap and water cleansing is done twice daily until healing is complete.

For flat SKs, LNSP for 10 to 15 seconds with a frost halo of 2 to 3 mm gives excellent results. The proper duration of LNSP for thick SKs is unpredictable, and thus light freezing for 5 seconds followed by curettage is often used initially. Aluminum chloride solution is used topically to provide hemostasis. Mild hypopigmentation may develop in the treated sites, but the intense pruritus usually resolves. SKs should not be frozen excessively, as they become more difficult to remove

with the curette, and this technique also causes more hypopigmentation. Clinical experience is required to achieve the best results. The end result is often a central hypopigmented area with slight peripheral hyperpigmentation that fades with time. Often there is significant pigmentary loss after treating lesions on the back with LNSP.

Pyogenic Granulomas. The vascular lesions of pyogenic granuloma may be quite recalcitrant to freezing, but the cosmetic results are good. Small lesions are best treated using a cryoprobe with a freeze time of 30 to 45 seconds, while larger lesions may require 1 to 2 minutes of freezing.

Pseudopyogenic Granuloma of Wilson-Jones. These tumors may mimic pyogenic granulomas but are very resistant to treatment and may be difficult to eradicate. For extensive lesions involving the pinna and the external auditory canal,[38] it is best to monitor the temperature with thermocouples to ensure a sufficient depth of freeze. Freeze times range from 1 to 4 minutes, and the thaw time may be up to 6 minutes.

Venous Lake. A contact cryoprobe is employed to treat venous lakes, using external pressure to compress the lesions before and during cryosurgery. Good cosmetic results can often be obtained with this technique (Fig. 61–23).

Trichiasis. Cryosurgery is often the treatment of

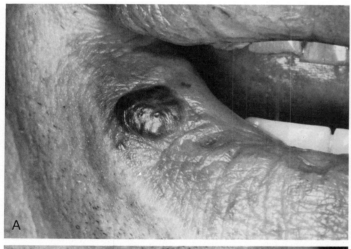
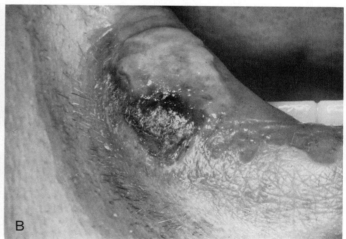
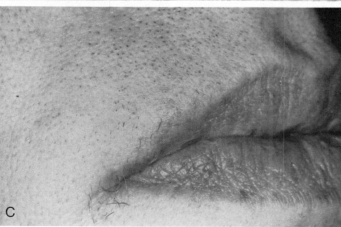

Figure 61–23. *A,* Preoperative appearance of a venous lake of the lip. *B,* Eschar has formed after cryosurgery. *C,* Complete resolution is seen without scarring.

choice for this uncomfortable condition of the eyelids in which eyelashes become inverted and irritate the eyes. This commonly results in entropion and nearly inevitably in ocular pemphigus, or essential shrinkage of the eye.[51] Thermocouple monitoring at the base of the follicles is necessary to ensure that the lid is frozen to about −15°C. Retreatment at 8-week intervals may be necessary to completely destroy the hair follicles.

Verrucae. Verrucae are commonly treated cryosurgically (Fig. 61–6), but with extremely variable cure rates.[52, 53] Digital warts respond well to the spray technique by freezing a small surrounding rim of normal tissue. Periungual warts are sometimes very refractory to treatment, but often the spray technique is required to extend the zone of freeze under the nail plate. However, for smaller lesions, the cryoprobe gives a better depth of freeze with less lateral spread. Some cryosurgeons prefer to use a cotton-tipped applicator (dipstick method) on periungual warts. Pain can be a problem but may be reduced by pretreatment with acetaminophen or aspirin, which is continued after completion of treatment.[52] Syncopal episodes are common after freezing of periungual warts. Ridging of the nail plate may occur after cryosurgery, but permanent damage to the nail plate is extremely rare.

Both the dipstick and the spray techniques are excellent for the treatment of warts, but cryoprobes are especially helpful for the treatment of small warts, even though the procedure can take longer to perform. If spray freezing is used, a cone placed around the wart will allow greater depth of freeze with less lateral spread. Cure rates for warts after one cryosurgical procedure range from 65 to 75%. Multiple short treatments performed every 3 weeks can yield higher cure rates. Pretreatment with topical application of salicylic acid, especially TransVerSal pads, may allow deeper penetration and better destruction of the wart.[54] Fortunately, these modifications of the traditional therapeutic technique have provided for the successful management of a larger number of patients.[54]

Freezing of verrucae on children may be an unpleasant experience. It may help to tell children that a "snowman" will form on their hand. They are often fascinated while watching this develop, sometimes for the entire 8- to 10-second period that is necessary to accomplish the procedure. There are different opinions about whether the bullae that form after cryosurgery should be drained. Leaving the bullae intact is probably best unless there is excessive pain from the pressure. It appears that treated warts that develop hemorrhagic bullae often resolve, but despite this fact, every patient should recognize that multiple treatments may still be required for effective management of periungual verrucae and verruca vulgaris. Verrucae can often be made more responsive to cryosurgery by pretreatment with topical retinoic acid, castor oil, or salicylic or lactic acid.[55]

Verruca Plana. Either spray or a cryoprobe can be used to treat the individual lesions of verruca plana. If a significant area is involved, a superficial spray technique of only a few seconds is often preferable. Treatment with topical tretinoin before freezing is also useful

and may enhance the development of an immune response in these very recalcitrant and recurrent lesions.[55]

Plantar and Palmar Verrucae. Cryosurgery alone is not always effective in the management of plantar and palmar verrucae. For that reason, it is commonly used in conjunction with other techniques to reduce the number of recurrences. The dipstick, spray, or cryoprobe technique may be used, but many cutaneous surgeons prefer the spray. Pretreatment with Transplantar pads or salicylic acid is often useful. For very hyperkeratotic lesions, soaking in water and paring the warts before treatment also yields a higher cure rate than trying to freeze through the lesions.[56, 57] Local anesthesia makes it possible to obtain a more adequate freeze and reduces the pain of the procedure, but many children will not tolerate the injection of the anesthetic. Bleomycin injections may also be useful in treating select cases.[58]

Condylomata Acuminata. Multiple treatments exist for these often recalcitrant lesions, including podophyllin therapy,[59, 60] trichloroacetic acid, cryotherapy,[60, 61] electrodesiccation,[60] surgical excision,[62, 63] laser surgery,[64] and interferon therapy.[65, 66] Experience has shown that several courses of podophyllin therapy followed by cryosurgery can often give the best results. These treatments may be done simultaneously or performed separately several weeks apart. Reliable patients can use podophyllin[59] at home, returning to the office only for the cryosurgical procedure.

Cryosurgical treatment of condylomata of the anogenital area generally produces no scars when the technique consists of freezing only a 5-mm margin of healthy skin around each lesion.[33] Freezing times range from a few seconds to more than 30 seconds. For extensive areas, the freezing must extend 10 to 20 mm beyond visible lesions,[33] as the virus may be present in normal-appearing skin.[67] In anogenital condylomata, a 90% cure rate can be obtained with cryosurgery,[61, 68] while the cure rate reported with interferon[65, 66] has not been as high; carbon dioxide laser vaporization yields an approximate 80% cure rate.[64]

Complications Associated With Verruca Vulgaris. An unusual case of pyogenic granuloma has been reported after dual cryosurgery and 27% salicylic acid treatment for a verruca vulgaris.[69] There have been two other reported cases of pyogenic granuloma occurring after freezing alone.[70, 71]

Lentigo Maligna. Lentigo maligna (LM) is a premalignant, slowly growing lesion that occurs most commonly on the face in elderly patients. LM may be present for decades before progressing into lentigo maligna melanoma (LMM). If LM is left untreated, approximately 30 to 50% of lesions will progress to LMM.[72] Cryosurgery is the preferred treatment modality,[72] because it selectively destroys pigment-producing cells,[27] has minimal morbidity, can be performed in an outpatient setting with easily learned techniques using portable equipment, and has a high rate of cure (Fig. 61–24). Among 206 cases of LM treated by cryosurgeons, a cure rate of 96.1% was reported, with only eight recurrences.[73–77] However, multiple pretreatment biopsies

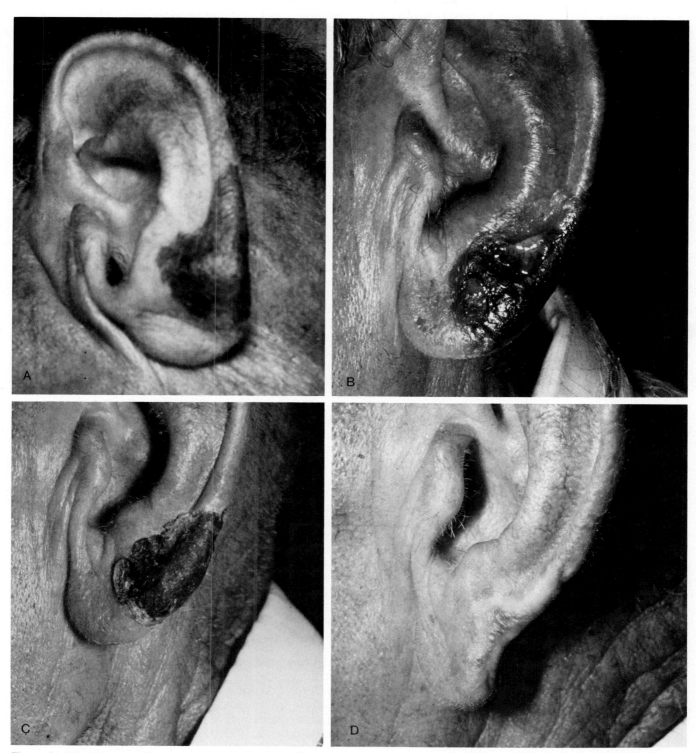

Figure 61–24. *A,* Preoperative appearance of a lentigo maligna on the left ear. *B,* Appearance 1 week after cryosurgery. *C,* Appearance 2 weeks after cryosurgery. *D,* Appearance 2 months after cryosurgery.

performed at various sites within the LM are extremely important to verify the diagnosis, determine the depth of invasion, and rule out possible transformation to LMM. Tumors more than 2 cm in diameter may require two or more biopsies.[72]

The technique used in the treatment of LM is relatively simple and straightforward. First, a margin 5 mm beyond the visible margins of the tumor is outlined. The thermocouple needle is then implanted at least 3 mm below the surface of the skin. This is important so that the lesion is frozen sufficiently to destroy all abnormal melanocytes that may have invaded the follicular epithelium. An intermittent spray technique is used to deliver LN_2 to the center of the tumor. Freezing is continued until the monitor registers $-50°C$ and the icefront extends 3 mm beyond the tumor margins (Table 61-6). The treated area is allowed to thaw completely before freezing a second time to $-50°C$.[76] When the Freeze-Depth Indicator is used, the electrode needles are inserted perpendicularly and equidistant from each other across the tumor at a depth of 5 mm below the surface. The LN_2 is delivered until 2 mΩ of resistance is registered.[72]

Cryosurgery for LM only rarely results in complications such as secondary infection and hypertrophic scarring, but depigmentation can be anticipated. Because of the large size of some of the lesions being treated, there will be significant formation of eschar, which is routinely treated with soap and water. Should the eschar require removal, however, a hydrocolloid surgical dressing or topical antibiotic may be applied.

INFREQUENT USES OF CRYOSURGERY

Acne and Acne Rosacea. Cryosurgical treatment of acne, acne rosacea, and acne scarring was once very common,[41, 78] but with the advent of newer therapies, cryosurgical techniques currently are used only infrequently for these conditions.

Alopecia. For managing androgenetic alopecia, weekly treatment with cryosurgery using liquid nitrogen and an open spray technique has been effective.[79] The duration of each treatment is 60 to 90 seconds, or until erythema is produced. After four to six treatments, hair loss is reduced (presumably because of a prolonged anagen phase), a decrease occurs in the number of vellus hair follicles, and an increase in terminal hair follicles is seen. The improvement is thought to be secondary to vasodilation, improved circulation, stimulation of hair follicle epithelium, or interference with the effect of androgen on the follicle.

Lichen Sclerosus et Atrophicus (LS&A). These atrophic lesions are often present on the genitalia but may also be seen on the shoulders, breasts, thighs, and abdomen. Lesions up to 2 cm in size may be satisfactorily treated by LNSP for 10 to 15 seconds.

Chromomycosis. Localized chromomycosis, which rarely occurs in the United States, has been successfully treated with cryosurgery.[30, 80, 81] Freezing with liquid nitrogen is performed in two cycles and repeated weekly until complete healing with scar formation occurs, usually in 6 to 8 weeks.

Idiopathic Guttate Hypomelanosis. Fewer dopa-positive melanocytes are found in these white macular areas than in normal skin. Light freezing can result in repigmentation in 6 to 8 weeks, apparently by removing the defective epidermal melanin unit.[82]

Cryosurgery for Malignant Lesions: General Considerations

Comparative Review. Cryosurgery for the treatment of cutaneous malignancies has become a standard form of therapy since the 1960s. The very acceptable cosmetic results, high cure rates, and cost effectiveness associated with this procedure often make it the treatment of choice for a wide variety of skin cancers, especially those overlying cartilage.[83–88]

There are specific instances, however, when cryosurgery should not be the treatment of choice. Some tumors, such as morpheaform and metatypical basal cell carcinomas and some de novo squamous cell carcinomas, are best managed by Mohs micrographic surgery or excisional surgery. Recurrent carcinomas are typically referred for Mohs micrographic surgery, especially when the recurrence is deep to the center of the tumor. Marginal recurrences can often be satisfactorily treated with cryosurgery.

Scalp Tumors. Although a lower cure rate has been described for tumors treated cryosurgically on the scalp, aggressive cryosurgery with fixation of the iceball to the underlying calvarium has yielded very acceptable cure rates.[84–87] Considering the difficulty of managing many scalp tumors, cryosurgery has proved to be an excellent method for treating selected tumors in this anatomic location.

Tissue Sparing. Patients with multiple skin cancers (e.g., in the nevoid basal cell carcinoma syndrome or after arsenic exposure or radiation therapy) appreciate the speed, efficiency, and effectiveness of cryosurgery. In addition, the tissue sparing that results from cryosurgery in these patients is very important. The back and temple are especially good sites for cryosurgery.

Curettage and Freeze Cycles. Curettage followed by cryosurgery is the preferred method for an increasing number of cryosurgeons.[84, 85, 88] This method consists of first thoroughly curetting the cancer to detect any deeper extensions and then performing a single or double freeze. This technique has yielded excellent cosmetic results and high cure rates.[84, 85]

Dermatopathology, Ultrasound, and Depth of Freeze. Dermatopathologists can obtain valuable information concerning tumor thickness from ultrasound studies and thereby can more accurately determine the appropriate depth of freeze before performing the procedure. Ultrasound may also help to determine when a tumor may be too deep to manage with cryosurgery alone. Ultrasound control also provides information that allows for more accurate placement of thermocouple needles.[89, 90]

Lateral Spread of Freeze. The lateral spread of freeze correlates well with depth of freeze,[21, 91] and this correlation is so accurate that, with sufficient clinical experience, thermocouple monitoring is no longer required in many cases. Thermocouple monitoring may be reserved for treating deeper tumors or tumors found in critical locations, such as the eyelid. Monitoring techniques remain very useful in helping to learn the proper surgical technique for performing cryosurgery.

Treatment of Malignant Lesions

Cryosurgery using a single or double freeze-thaw cycle is employed to bring about tumor destruction. Although a single cycle of freezing is sufficient for most superficial tumors, a double cycle of freezing is used for tumors that are 3 mm or more in depth. After treatment, an edematous, weeping reaction develops, followed by eschar formation. In about 1 month, the area heals by second intention, leaving a hypopigmented soft scar.

EQUIPMENT

The equipment needed may be a thermos-type container with a spray attachment or a more complex unit, such as the Frigitronics portable tabletop cryosurgical instrument. A thermocouple monitoring unit is used for treating deeper tumors (Figs. 61–4, 61–25). The use of thermocouples can provide greater accuracy in determining the depth of freeze, although effective use requires proper placement of the needles. The use of thermocouples may lead to a longer freeze time than would have been suggested by clinical judgment alone.[92]

The skin is frozen for at least 1 minute so that the lateral spread of freeze is 5 mm beyond the margin of the tumor or until the pyrometer registers $-50°C$. A halo thaw time of at least 1 minute correlates closely with this degree of tissue damage. The lethal temperature for cells has been reported as $-25°C$, $-35°C$, $-50°C$, or $-55°C$, but temperatures of about $-40°C$ have been confirmed by electrical resistance monitoring systems to cause tissue destruction.[93] A battery-powered device, the Ezee Cryometer, has been shown to correlate well with thermocouple readings and lateral spread of freeze.[21]

PROTECTIVE DEVICES

Goggles may be used for covering the eyes, but a simple tongue blade manually held at the medial canthal region also provides satisfactory protection. For treating tumors on the lid margins, a plastic Jaeger retractor is probably best for protecting the eye, but a plastic spoon may also be used. Cotton balls or dental rolls may be placed in the ear canals or the nares to protect these structures.

BIOPSY

A preoperative biopsy is generally recommended when treating malignant lesions cryosurgically. However, when little doubt exists as to the diagnosis, biopsy and treatment may be carried out during the same visit. If the clinical diagnosis is uncertain, treatment should be delayed until the pathology results of the biopsy return.

TECHNIQUE

A local anesthetic with epinephrine is injected before initiating cryosurgery. The epinephrine provides sufficient vasoconstriction to lengthen the thaw time. A marked outline around the lesion helps to ensure treatment of the full extent of the tumor, because once freezing begins, the margins often become blurred.

The traditional technique involves first taking a deep shave biopsy, curetting the base, and then carrying out the cryosurgical procedure. Cure rates may be higher and cosmetic results better using this technique, since the freezing is performed directly on the remaining deepest part of the tumor. Longer freeze times will be required if reepithelialization occurs after biopsy. Liquid nitrogen is most often applied with an intermittent spray technique using a paintbrush, circular, or central spray pattern. Spraying is continued until the thermocouple needle registers $-50°C$ or $-55°C$ or until the lateral spread of freeze extends 5 mm beyond the tumor margins, usually about 1 minute. The halo thaw time (HTT),

Figure 61–25. A diagrammatic representation of a 1-cm iceball extending to a 5-mm depth with a lateral extension of 5 mm beyond the tumor. Halo TT, Halo thaw time; Complete TT, complete thaw time; FT, Freeze time 1.0′.

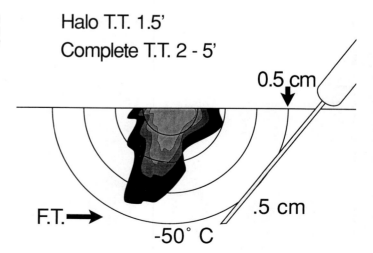

Halo T.T. 1.5′
Complete T.T. 2 - 5′
0.5 cm
.5 cm
F.T. →
-50° C

or the time necessary for the freeze to thaw to the inked margins, is recorded and should be between 1 and 1½ minutes. If it is less than this period of time, a repeat cycle of freezing is performed and the first freeze is not counted. This is especially important if thermocouple monitoring is not being used. The total thaw time of the lesion, which often takes 1½ to 5 minutes, should also be recorded. The second or third cycle of freezing is not performed until after complete thawing has occurred. Some cryosurgeons wait 5 minutes before beginning the second freeze.[87]

Use of Cones

Cones (Fig. 61–26) may be used to obtain a deeper freeze without causing the lateral damage that sometimes results from use of a spray technique. Cones will also prevent the spray from getting in the eyes, nose, or ears.[21]

POSTOPERATIVE CARE

The care of cryosurgical sites involves washing the wound with soap and water daily while leaving the treated areas open. The cryosurgical site acts as its own biologic dressing once the bullous reaction subsides in 5 to 7 days, forming a dry eschar. Some cryosurgeons prefer to remove the eschar and apply topical antibiotic ointment until healing is complete, while others allow the eschar to remain in place until it separates naturally in 3 to 6 weeks.

PATIENT SELECTION

Certain patients and particular tumor types (see Table 61–4) lend themselves well to cryosurgery. The versatility of the procedure and the cosmetic acceptability permits patients having even large numbers of skin cancers to be effectively treated (Figs. 61–27 through 61–31).

Side Effects and Complications of Cryosurgery

There are relatively mild and transient side effects as well as normal reactions that follow cryosurgery. The resulting inflammatory reaction produces vesicles, bullae (Figs. 61–32, 61–33), edema (Fig. 61–34), weeping, and eschar formation (Figs. 61–35, 61–36). After treatment of benign lesions, these effects typically disappear in 1 to 2 weeks, but after treatment of malignant lesions, 4 to 6 weeks may be required for these effects to resolve. In some locations, such as the lower leg, back, neck, and scalp, the effects of cryosurgery may remain apparent for several months.

Pain. Pain is common after cryosurgery of the fingers and soles. Cryosurgery of a malignancy on the temple may result in a migraine-type headache that lasts a few minutes or several hours. Throbbing pain can persist for several hours after cryosurgery for a tumor on the scalp. Because local anesthesia is used before the treatment of most cutaneous malignancies, little pain is felt immediately. However, patients will occasionally require pain medication for 24 to 48 hours postoperatively.

Edema. Edema is a problem when freezing tumors on the forehead or around the eye. Periorbital edema may persist for 3 to 5 days and occasionally longer (Fig. 61–34). Systemic steroids[94] given at the time of the procedure can help reduce the postoperative edema but may also delay wound healing.

Hemorrhage. Capillary bleeding may occur as a result of tissue necrosis when cryosurgery is used to treat skin cancers or other deep lesions. After debulking procedures, bleeding may also occur, but aluminum chloride solution or Monsel's solution can effectively control this problem, even in patients taking anticoagulants or aspirin. On rare occasions, patients may experience bleeding 2 or 3 weeks after cryosurgery for lesions of the temple, nasal tip, or lip. Pressure and, rarely, suturing may be required to control bleeding in these cases.

Gas Insufflation. If freezing is performed on an area of lax skin after a biopsy, the tissue may separate as the

Text continued on page 863

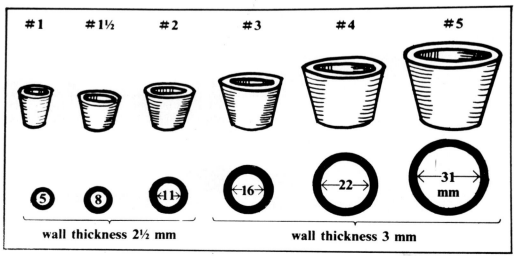

Figure 61–26. Neoprene cones in a variety of sizes.

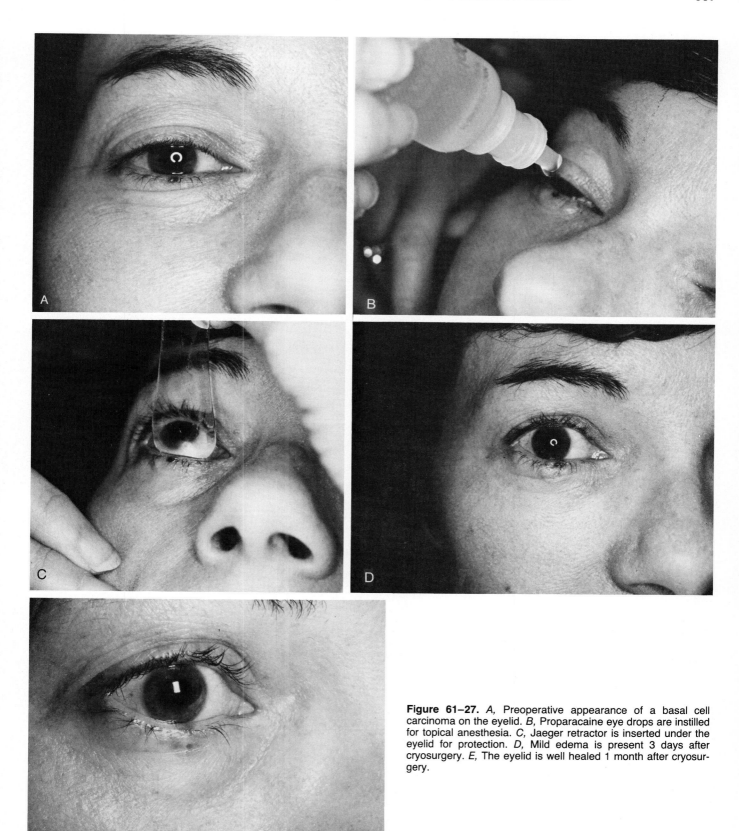

Figure 61–27. *A,* Preoperative appearance of a basal cell carcinoma on the eyelid. *B,* Proparacaine eye drops are instilled for topical anesthesia. *C,* Jaeger retractor is inserted under the eyelid for protection. *D,* Mild edema is present 3 days after cryosurgery. *E,* The eyelid is well healed 1 month after cryosurgery.

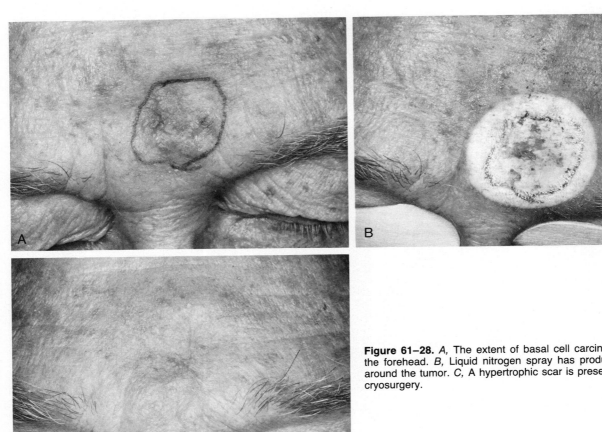

Figure 61–28. *A,* The extent of basal cell carcinoma is marked on the forehead. *B,* Liquid nitrogen spray has produced a 5-mm halo around the tumor. *C,* A hypertrophic scar is present 10 months after cryosurgery.

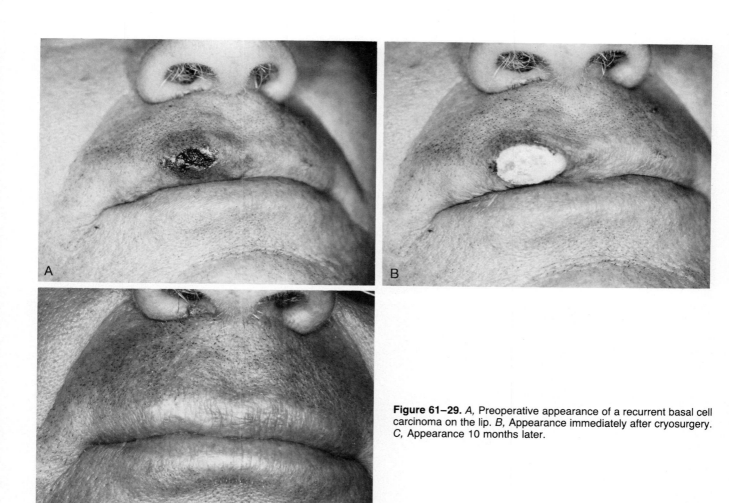

Figure 61–29. *A,* Preoperative appearance of a recurrent basal cell carcinoma on the lip. *B,* Appearance immediately after cryosurgery. *C,* Appearance 10 months later.

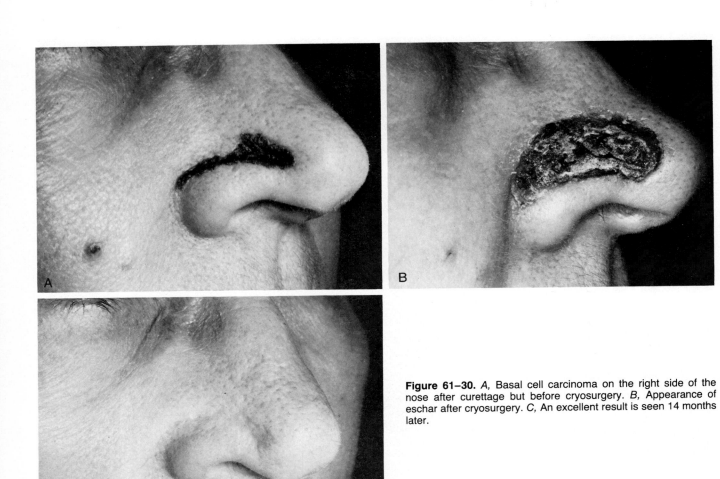

Figure 61–30. *A*, Basal cell carcinoma on the right side of the nose after curettage but before cryosurgery. *B*, Appearance of eschar after cryosurgery. *C*, An excellent result is seen 14 months later.

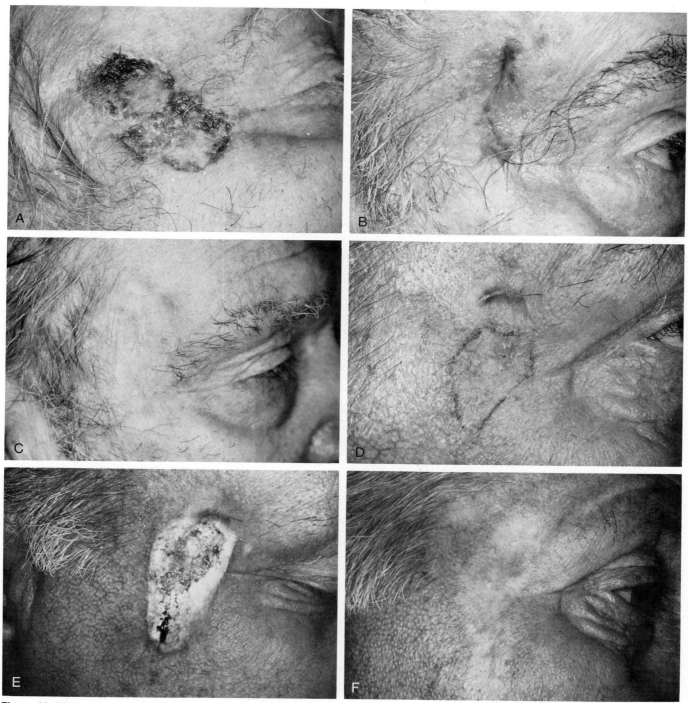

Figure 61–31. *A,* Large basal cell carcinoma on the temple was treated with curettage and electrodesiccation. *B,* A linear hypertrophic scar is seen early after healing. *C,* The scar has become soft and flat several months later. *D,* Another patient who has developed a new lesion adjacent to a previous treatment site. *E,* The recurrence is treated with cryosurgery. *F,* Final appearance 8 months later.

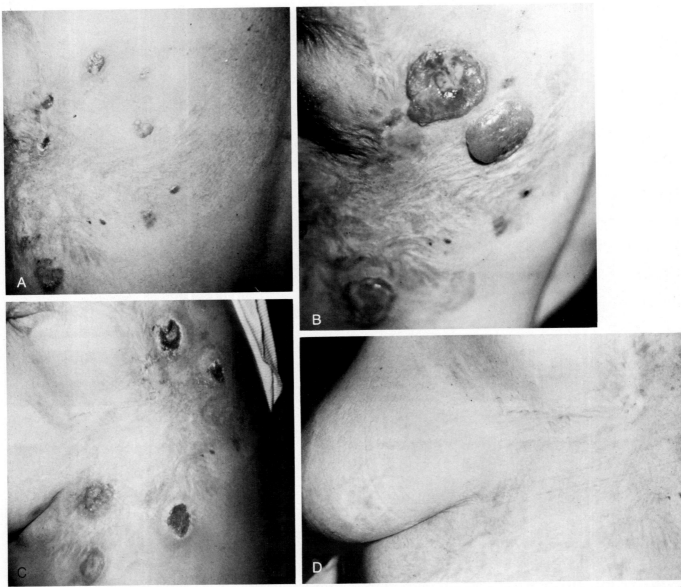

Figure 61–32. *A,* Multiple basal cell carcinomas have developed in an old irradiation scar. *B,* Bullae have formed 1 week after cryosurgery. *C,* Eschar has developed 2 months later. *D,* Appearance 4 years after cryosurgery.

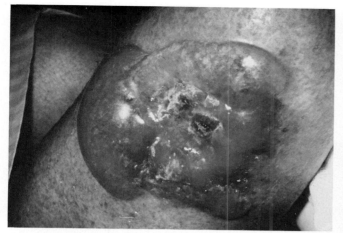

Figure 61–33. Large bulla of the leg after cryosurgery.

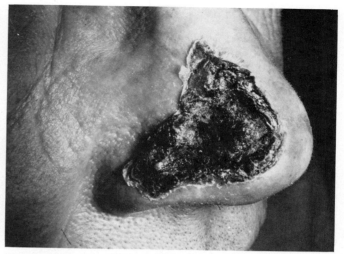

Figure 61–35. Large eschar has developed 2 weeks after cryosurgery for a basal cell carcinoma.

liquid nitrogen gas accumulates directly under the skin. Pressure on the treated area will allow the trapped gas to dissipate. Spraying into a cone or onto the normal skin before spraying the curetted area will help prevent this complication.

Syncope. Syncopal episodes are very rare but occur most commonly with treatment of skin cancers. For this reason, each patient should be monitored carefully for this reaction after completion of the procedure.

Nerve Injury. Damage to underlying nerves has been reported after cryosurgery.[25] Paresthesias may persist for 1 to 3 months after treatment of some deeper lesions, but permanent nerve damage is rare. Full recovery of nerve transmission, including sensory motor nerve func-

tion, has been reported after cryosurgery.[26] A slight decrease in sensation may be useful palliative therapy in managing some extensive cancers and in the treatment of lichen simplex chronicus and prurigo nodularis.

Scar Formation. Because the preserved dermal fibrous network aids in the rapid regeneration of the epidermis, many lesions may be treated with cryosurgery with little or no resultant scarring. Hypertrophic scarring after cryosurgery is uncommon, but when it occurs (Figs. 61–37 through 61–39), the scar can be expected to soften and flatten over time or with the use of potent topical or intralesional steroids. Loss of pore structure and mild

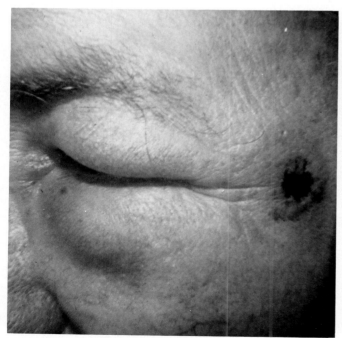

Figure 61–34. Periorbital edema seen 2 days after cryosurgery for a basal cell carcinoma on the temple.

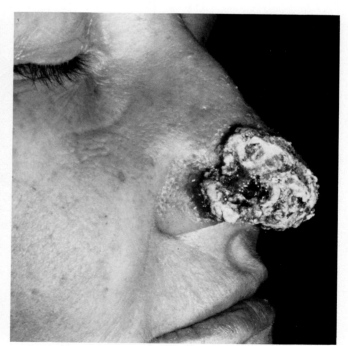

Figure 61–36. Large eschar is seen 2 weeks after cryosurgery for basal cell carcinoma of the nose.

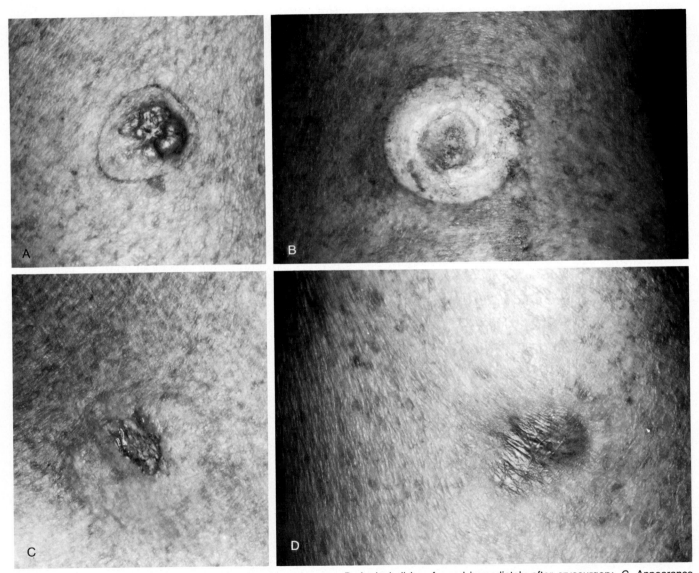

Figure 61–37. *A,* Patient with a basal cell carcinoma on the arm. *B,* An iceball has formed immediately after cryosurgery. *C,* Appearance immediately after total thawing. *D,* Hypertrophic scar has developed 4 months after cryosurgery.

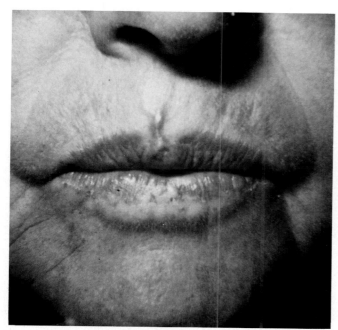

Figure 61–38. Hypertrophic scar on the lip after cryosurgery.

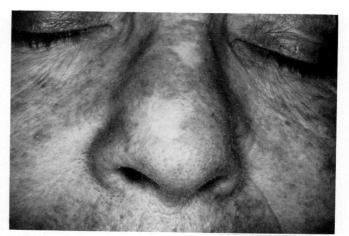

Figure 61–40. Hypopigmented scar on the nose 3 years after cryosurgery.

atrophy may also occur after cryosurgery. Freezing for more than 15 to 20 seconds may cause hair follicle loss. Hypertrophic scarring may occur in a linear fashion on the nose and upper lip. Fortunately, ectropion is rare after freezing of eyelid tumors.

Cartilage Necrosis. Although necrosis of cartilage is rare, it can and does occur, especially on the helix of the ear. This is most common when through-and-through cryosurgery is used to treat a malignancy.

Pigment Alteration. The most disconcerting change after cryosurgery is hypopigmentation (Fig. 61–40). Pigment loss occurs because the pigment cell is extremely sensitive to cold, and destruction may result from freez-

ing to a temperature of only −4° to −7°C. Prolonged freezing of 30 to 60 seconds or more may cause permanent pigmentary loss. The association of freezing with pigmentation loss must always be considered when treating a patient with dark skin, as such treatment could result in a potentially unacceptable cosmetic result. Patients with freckles or prominent facial blood vessels may also experience sufficient changes in the treated areas to cause a cosmetic deficit, even though the treated skin may actually be more "normal" than the untreated skin.

Infection. Although postoperative infection is quite uncommon after cryosurgery, it does occur occasionally and may require traditional treatment with antibiotics.

Reactive Changes. Milia formation and pseudoepitheliomatous hyperplasia may occur after cryosurgery but usually resolve with treatment. Pseudotumor recidive, a form of pseudoepitheliomatous hyperplasia, occasionally develops on the nose 1 to 3 months after cryosurgery (Fig. 61–41). This reaction may mimic a recurrent tumor

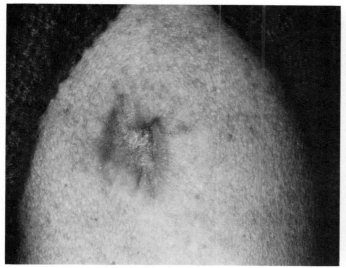

Figure 61–39. Hypertrophic scar on the arm 4 months after cryosurgery.

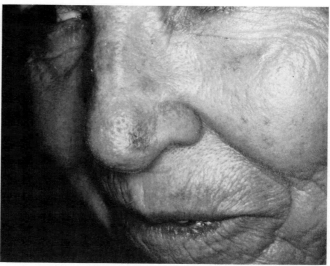

Figure 61–41. A pseudotumor recidive has formed on the nose after cryosurgery.

but usually regresses spontaneously within a few months. Excess formation of granulation tissue (Fig. 61–42) also occurs rarely during the healing of some cryosurgical wounds. This usually resolves spontaneously or with topical treatment using silver nitrate.

Cure Rates

Cryosurgery is a safe, effective, and time-efficient method for treating skin cancers, yielding good cosmetic results and overall cure rates of 97 to 99%.[83–86, 88] The most recent statistics (Tables 61–7 through 61–10) regarding cure rate by size, method, and site of lesion show that the most effective methods of treatment are curettage with double-freeze cryosurgery and deep shave excision with cryosurgery. The dermatopathologist can provide information about tumor depth, which will help in selecting the best method of treatment. Improvements in skin cancer cure rates result from better patient selection, increased skill in the cryosurgical techniques, use of single- or double-freeze techniques, development of monitoring devices, and assistance rendered by the dermatopathologist in defining tumor depth and histologic subtypes. Classification of basal cell carcinoma and squamous cell carcinoma is also important in determining tumor biology and prognosis. The determination of tumor depth before freezing may aid in the proper selection of treatment times for managing a particular lesion.

Cure rates can also be evaluated according to tumor size. Larger basal and squamous cell carcinomas (more than 2.4 cm in diameter) show the highest cure rates after cryosurgery, presumably because they are more superficial. Basal cell carcinomas that measure 1.3 to 2.4 cm in diameter have a lower cure rate (94.1%) and should be treated more aggressively. The 97% cure rate for squamous cell carcinomas of all sizes is due in part to the fact that many of these tumors are actinic kera-

TABLE 61–7. CURE RATES OF PRIMARY TUMORS ACCORDING TO SIZE (IN CENTIMETERS)

	0–0.5	0.6–1.2	1.3–2.4	2.4+
Basal cell carcinoma	97.6%	97.1%	94.1%	97.8%
Number of cases treated	834	1218	373	92
Squamous cell carcinoma	96.4%	97.8%	96.5%	100%
Number of cases treated	139	313	86	17

tosis–squamous cell carcinomas (AK-SCC). The term AK-SCC is used only for those lesions with definite dermal invasion by atypical squamous keratinocytes.

SUMMARY

The role modern cryosurgery plays in the treatment of a host of benign, premalignant, and malignant lesions makes it an extremely important modality for many cutaneous surgeons. When the patient and lesion are properly selected and good surgical technique is used, cryosurgery can provide a superb cosmetic result in the removal of many benign lesions, without producing a discernible scar. The development of thermocouple monitors and liquid nitrogen spray devices has allowed cryosurgery to be successful even in patients with multiple medical conditions for whom conventional surgery would be contraindicated. Cryosurgery has high cure rates in the treatment of many cutaneous malignancies while requiring only minimal postoperative care and causing few complications. As standardized treatment parameters have become established, the effective use of cryosurgery has expanded to include the successful management of many uncommon and therapeutically problematic conditions. As other cryogens are discovered and new devices are developed to use them, cryosurgery will remain a useful modality in the future.

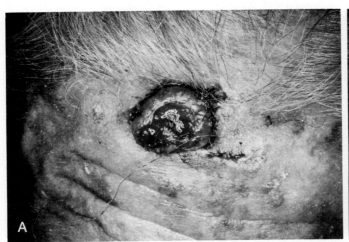 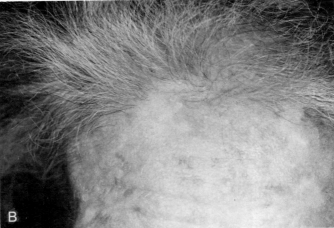

Figure 61–42. *A,* Granulation tissue has formed after cryosurgery for a basal cell carcinoma of the forehead. *B,* Resolution after treatment with topical silver nitrate.

TABLE 61–8. **CURE RATES FOR TREATMENT OF PRIMARY TUMORS ACCORDING TO CRYOSURGICAL TECHNIQUE**

	Shave and Freeze	Curettage and Freeze	Single Freeze	Double Freeze	Curettage and Double Freeze	Shave and Double Freeze
Basal cell carcinoma	100%	97.7%	95.8%	96.3%	98.4%	100%
Number of cases treated	56	731	566	711	788	83
Number recurrent	0	17	24	26	13	0
Percent recurrent	0	2.3	4.2	3.7	1.6	0
Squamous cell carcinoma	100%	97.6%	97.9%	95.1%	100%	100%
Number of cases treated	32	211	144	143	105	23
Number recurrent	0	5	3	7	0	0
Percent recurrent	0	2.4	2.1	4.9	0	0

TABLE 61–9. **CURE RATE ACCORDING TO TUMOR SITE**

Location	Basal Cell Carcinoma				Squamous Cell Carcinoma			
	No. Recurrent	No. Treated	% Recurrent	Cure Rate (%)	No. Recurrent	No. Treated	% Recurrent	Cure Rate (%)
Ear	4	198	2.0	98.0	1	85	1.2	98.8
Nose	29	728	4.0	96.0	5	53	9.4	90.6
Eyelids	1	24	4.2	95.8	1	4	2.5	75.0
Nasolabial fold	3	51	5.9	94.1	0	2	0	100.0
Other face	28	984	2.8	97.2	5	234	2.1	97.9
Trunk	2	354	0.6	99.4	1	17	5.9	94.1
Arm	2	133	1.5	98.5	1	156	0.6	99.4
Legs	0	33	0	100.0	0	11	0	100.0
Lips	3	44	6.8	93.2	0	21	0	100.0
Scalp	2	42	4.8	95.2	1	11	9.1	90.9
Neck	2	158	1.3	98.7	0	44	0	100.0
Other areas	5	295	1.7	98.3	0	39	0	100.0
Total	81	3944	2.7*	97.3†	15	677	2.2*	97.8†

*Average recurrence rate.
†Average cure rate.

TABLE 61–10. **CURE RATES OF PRIMARY TUMORS BY DATE OF TREATMENT**

	1968–1970	1971–1975	1976–1980	1981–1985	1985 +	Total
Basal cell carcinoma	95.3%	94.5%	96.3%	98.0%	99.4%	96.9%
No. treated	236	438	779	712	469	2634
Squamous cell carcinoma	91.2%	98.3%	98.3%	97.5%	98.5%	97.3%
No. treated	68	117	230	80	68	563

REFERENCES

1. Squazzi A, Bracco D: A historical account of the technical means used in cryotherapy. Minerva Med 65:3718–3722, 1974.
2. Bracco D: Historical development. In: Ablin RK (ed): Handbook of Cryosurgery. Marcel Dekker, New York, 1980.
3. Hippocrates: Greek Medicine. Translated by AJ Brock. Dent, London, 1929.
4. Lorrey DJ: Memoires de Chirurgie Militaire et Campagnes, 1812–1817. Philadelphia, Carey & Lea, 1832.
5. Arnott J: On the Treatment of Cancers by Regulated Application of an Anaesthetic Temperature. Churchill Livingstone, London, 1855.
6. Cailletet L: Annales de Chemie et de Physique 15:113, 1878.
7. Pictet R: Annales de Chemie et de Physique 13:145, 1878.
8. Wroblewski SU, Olszewski KS: Wiedemann's Annalen de Physik 20:256, 1883.
9. Dewar L: Collected Papers of Sir James Dewar. Cambridge University Press, Cambridge, England, 1927.
10. White AC: Liquid air in medicine and surgery. Med Rec 56:109–112, 1899.
11. White AC: Possibilities of liquid air to the physician. JAMA 36:426–428, 1901.
12. White AC: Liquified oxygen and x-ray treatment of malignant growths. Interstate Med J 9:657, 1902.
13. Whitehouse HH: Liquid air in dermatology: its indications and limitations. JAMA 49:371–377, 1907.
14. Zacarian SA: Cryogenics: the cryolesion and the pathogenesis of cryonecrosis. In: Zacarian SA (ed): Cryosurgery for Skin Cancer and Cutaneous Disorders. CV Mosby, St. Louis, 1985, pp 2–3.
15. Pusey WA: The use of carbon dioxide snow in the treatment of nevi and other lesions of the skin. JAMA 49:1354–1356, 1907.
16. Allington HD: Cryosurgery. Calif Med 72:153–155, 1950.
17. Torre D: Cradle of cryosurgery. NY State J Med 67:465–467, 1967.
18. Torre D: Cryosurgical instrumentation and depth dose monitoring. In: Breitbart E, Dachow-Siwiec E (eds): Clinics in Dermatology: Advances in Cryosurgery. Elsevier, New York, 1990, p 59.
19. Zacarian SA, Adham MI: Cryotherapy of cutaneous malignancy. Cryobiology 2:212–218, 1966.
20. Gage AA, Kuflik EG: Cryosurgical Treatment for Skin Cancer. Igaku-Shoin, New York, 1990, pp 65–82.
21. Torre D: Cryosurgical instrumentation and depth dose monitoring. In: Breitbart E, Dachow-Siwiec E (eds): Clinics in Dermatology: Advances in Cryosurgery. Elsevier, New York, 1990, p 48.
22. Jones SK, Darville JM: Transmission of virus by cryotherapy and multi-use caustic pencils: a problem for dermatologists? Br J Dermatol 12:481–486, 1989.
23. Stewart RH, Graham GF: A complication of cryosurgery in a patient with cryofibrinogenemia. J Dermatol Surg Oncol 4:743–744, 1978.
24. Spiller WF, Spiller RF: Cryosurgery in dermatology office practice. South Med J 69:157, 1975.
25. Nix TW Jr: Liquid nitrogen neuropathy. Arch Dermatol 92:185, 1965.
26. Burge SM, Dawber RPD: Hair follicle destruction and regeneration in guinea pig skin after cutaneous freeze injury. Cryobiology 27:153–163, 1990.
27. Gage AA, Meenaghan M: Sensitivity of pigmented mucosa and pigmented cells in skin due to freezing injury. Cryobiology 16:348–361, 1979.
28. Lubritz RR, Smolewski SA: Cryosurgery cure rate of actinic keratoses. J Am Acad Dermatol 7:631–632, 1982.
29. Zakrzewska J: Cryosurgery and comparisons. Report from 10th Annual American College of Cryosurgery Meeting, Margarita Island, Venezuela. Dermatol News 11:3, 1989.
30. Lubritz RR: Cryosurgical approach to benign and precancerous tumors of the skin. In: Zacarian SA (ed): Cryosurgery for Skin Cancer and Cutaneous Disorders. CV Mosby, St. Louis, 1985, pp 45–50.
31. Lubritz RR, Smolewski SA: Cryosurgery cure rate of premalignant leukoplakia of the lower lip. J Dermatol Surg Oncol 9:235–237, 1983.
32. Banoczy J: Follow up studies in oral leukoplakia. J Oral Maxillofac Surg 5:69–75, 1977.
33. Dachow-Siwiec E: Treatment of cryosurgery in premalignant and benign lesions of skin. In: Breitbart E, Dachow-Siwiec E (eds): Clinics in Dermatology: Advances in Cryosurgery. Elsevier, New York, 1990, pp 75–79.
34. Vesper LJ: Cryosurgery is called effective option for treating dermatofibromas. Dermatol News 23:1, 1990.
35. Spiller WF, Spiller RF: Cryosurgery in dermatologic office practice. South Med J 68:175–177, 1975.
36. Torre D: Cryosurgery of premalignant and malignant skin lesions. Cutis 11:123–129, 1971.
37. Lubritz RR: Cryosurgical approach to benign and precancerous tumors of the skin. In: Zacarian SA (ed): Cryosurgery for Skin Cancer and Cutaneous Disorders. CV Mosby, St. Louis, 1985, pp 44–48.
38. Graham G, Stewart R: Cryosurgery for unusual cutaneous neoplasms. Dermatol Surg Oncol 3:437–442, 1977.
39. Castro-Ron G: Cryosurgery of angiomas and birth defects. In: Zacarian SA (ed): Cryosurgery for Skin Cancer and Cutaneous Disorders. CV Mosby, St. Louis, 1985, pp 77–90.
40. Castro-Ron G: Personal communication, December, 1991.
41. Graham G: Cryosurgery for acne. In: Zacarian SA (ed): Cryosurgery for Skin Cancer and Cutaneous Disorders. CV Mosby, St. Louis, 1985, pp 67–71.
42. Biro L: Pediatric cryosurgery. Syllabus for basic cryosurgery course. American Academy of Dermatology, Evanston, IL, 1990, p 21.
43. Limmer BL: Cryosurgery of porokeratosis plantaris discreta. Arch Dermatol 115:582–584, 1979.
44. Waller J: Porokeratosis plantaris discreta (conical callus): cone spray freeze method. Presented at the First Annual Meeting of the American College of Cryosurgery, New Orleans, LA, March 13, 1978.
45. Lubitz RR: Cryosurgery of benign and premalignant cutaneous lesions. In: Zacarian SA (ed): Cryosurgical Advances in Dermatology and Tumors of the Head and Neck. Charles C Thomas, Springfield, IL, 1977.
46. Lindo SD, Daniels F Jr: Cryosurgery of junction nevi. Cutis 16:426–427, 1975.
47. Graham G, Graham J: Cryosurgery: combination and comparison report from American College of Cryosurgery Meeting in Margarita Island, Venezuela. Dermatol News 11:3, 1989.
48. Stoll DM, Fields JP, King LE Jr: Treatment of prurigo nodularis: use of cryosurgery and intralesional steroids plus lidocaine. J Dermatol Surg Oncol 9:922–924, 1983.
49. Waldinger TP, Wong RC, Taylor WB, et al: Cryotherapy improves prurigo nodularis. Arch Dermatol 120:1598–1600, 1984.
50. Torre D: Cryosurgery. In: Newcomer VD, Young EM (eds): Geriatric Dermatology. Igaku-Shoin, New York, 1988, pp 55–59.
51. Fraunfelder FT: The role of cryosurgery in external ocular and periocular disease. Trans Am Acad Ophthalmol Otolaryngol 83:713–714, 1977.
52. Keefe M, Dich DC: Cryotherapy of hand warts—a questionnaire survey of "consumers." Clin Exp Dermatol 15:260–263, 1990.
53. Hopkins P: Treatment of warts with liquid nitrogen. J R Coll Gen Pract 59:173–174, 1989.
54. Mottaz JH, McKeever PJ, Zelickson AS, et al: Transdermal delivery of salicylic acid in the treatment of viral papillomas. Int J Dermatol 27:596–600, 1988.
55. Arnold HL, Odom RB, James WD: Andrews' Diseases of the Skin. 8th ed. WB Saunders, Philadelphia, 1990, pp 468–475.
56. Limmer BL, Bogy LT: Cryosurgery of plantar warts. J Am Podiatr Assoc 69:713–715, 1979.
57. Prieto A: Cryosurgery for plantar and palmar verrucae. Presented at the Third International Symposium on Plastic Surgery, New Orleans, May, 1979.
58. Shumer SM, O'Keefe EJ: Bleomycin in the treatment of recalcitrant warts. J Am Acad Dermatol 9:91–96, 1983.
59. Greenberg MD, Rutledge LH: A double-blind, randomized trial of 0.5% Podofilox and placebo for the treatment of genital warts in women. Obstet Gynecol 75:737–739, 1991.
60. Stone KM, Becker TM, Hadga A, et al: Treatment of external genital warts: a randomized clinical trial comparing podophyllin, cryotherapy and electrodesiccation. Gentourin Med 66:16–19, 1990.

61. Ghosh AK: Cryosurgery of genital warts in cases which podophyllin treatment failed or was contraindicated. Br J Vener Dis 53:49–53, 1977.

62. Thompson PS, Grace RH: The treatment of perianal and anal condylomata acuminata: a new operative technique. J R Soc Med 71:180–185, 1978.

63. Gollock SM, Slatford K, Hunter JM: Scissor excision of anogenital warts. Br J Vener Dis 58:400–401, 1982.

64. Badieramonte G, Chiesa F, Lupi M, et al: Laser microsurgery in oncology: indications, techniques, and results of a 5 year experience. Lasers Surg Med 7:478–486, 1987.

65. Gall SA, Hughes CE, Trofatter K: Interferon for the therapy of condylomata acuminata: a new operative technique. J R Soc Med 7:180–185, 1978.

66. Eron LJ, Judson F, Tucker S, et al: Interferon therapy for condylomata acuminata. N Engl J Med 315:1059–1064, 1986.

67. Ferenczy A, Masaru M, Nagai N, et al: Latent papillomavirus and recurring genital warts. N Engl J Med 313:784–788, 1985.

68. Dodi G, Infantino A, Moretti R, et al: Cryotherapy of anorectal warts and condylomata. Cryobiology 19:287–288, 1982.

69. Kolbusz RB, O'Donoghue MA: Pyogenic granuloma following treatment of verruca vulgaris with cryotherapy and Duoplant. Cutis 47:204, 1991.

70. Greer KE, Bishop GE: Pyogenic granuloma as a complication of cutaneous cryosurgery. Arch Dermatol 111:1536–1537, 1975.

71. Elton RF: Complications of cutaneous cryosurgery. J Am Acad Dermatol 8:513–519, 1983.

72. Zacarian SA: Cryosurgery of lentigo maligna. In: Zacarian SA (ed): Cryosurgery for Skin Cancer and Cutaneous Disorders. CV Mosby, St. Louis, 1985, pp 199–214.

73. Coleman WP III, Davis RS, Reed RJ, Krementz ET: Treatment of lentigo maligna and lentigo maligna melanoma. J Dermatol Surg Oncol 6:476–479, 1980.

74. Dawber RPR, Wilkinson SD: Pelantic freezing Hutchinson treatment macular and nodular phases with cryotherapy. Br J Dermatol 101:47, 1979.

75. Graham GF, Stewart R: Cryosurgery for unusual cutaneous neoplasms. J Dermatol Surg Oncol 3:437–444, 1977.

76. Kuflik EG: Cryosurgery for lentigo maligna: a report of four cases. J Dermatol Surg Oncol 6:432, 1982.

77. Lorenc E: Cryosurgery for melanotic freckle. Dermatol Times 4:29, 1983.

78. Graham GF: Cryotherapy in the treatment of acne. In: Epstein E, Epstein E Jr (eds): Skin Surgery. Charles C Thomas, Springfield, IL, 1982, pp 680–697.

79. Martins O: Alopecia may respond to weekly cryotherapy. Dermatol Times 11:1–36, 1990.

80. Lubritz RR, Spence JE: Chromoblastomycosis: cure by cryosurgery. Int J Dermatol 17:380–381, 1978.

81. Pimentel ER, Castro LG, Cude LC, et al: Treatment of chromomycosis by cryosurgery with liquid nitrogen: a report on 11 cases. J Dermatol Surg Oncol 15:72–77, 1989.

82. Plogsangam T, Dee-Ananlap S, Suvanprakorn P: Treatment of idiopathic guttate hypomelanosis with liquid nitrogen: liquid and section microscopic studies. J Am Acad Dermatol 23:681–684, 1990.

83. Zacarian SA: Cryosurgery for cancer of the skin. In: Zacarian SA (ed): Cryosurgery for Skin Cancer and Cutaneous Disorders. CV Mosby, St. Louis, 1985, pp 96–162.

84. Graham GF, Clark LC: Statistical update in cryosurgery for cancers of the skin. In: Zacarian SA (ed): Cryosurgery for Skin Cancer and Cutaneous Disorders. CV Mosby, St. Louis, 1985, pp 298–305.

85. Graham GF, Clark LC: Statistical analysis in cryosurgery of skin cancer. In: Breitbart E, Dachow-Siwiec E (ed): Clinics in Dermatology. Advances in Cryosurgery. Elsevier, New York, 1990, pp 101–107.

86. Kuflik EG, Gage AA: The five-year cure rate achieved by cryosurgery for skin cancer. J Am Acad Dermatol 24:1002–1004, 1991.

87. Holt PSA: Cryotherapy for skin cancer: results over a 5-year period using liquid nitrogen spray. Cryosurgery 119:231–240, 1988.

88. Spiller WF: Combination curettage and cryosurgery for basal cell carcinoma. Syllabus for basic cryosurgery course. American Academy of Dermatology Annual Meeting, 1990, pp 26–27.

89. Graham GF: Ultrasound as an aid in cryosurgery. Syllabus for basic cryosurgery course. American Academy of Dermatology Annual Meeting, 1990, pp 38–40.

90. Clark LC, Graham GF: Plasma selenium and skin neoplasm: a case control study. Nutr Cancer 6:13–31, 1984.

91. Torre D, Torre S: Gadgets and gimmicks. Cutis 12:93–94, 1973.

92. Brodthagen H: Local freezing of the skin by carbon dioxide snow. Acta Dermatovener (Stockh) 41(Suppl 44):1–150, 1961.

93. LePivert P: Predictability of cryonecrosis by tissue impedancemetry. Low Temp Med 4:129–138, 1977.

94. Kuflik EG, Webb W: Effects of systemic corticosteroids on postcryosurgical edema and other manifestations of the inflammatory response. J Dermatol Surg Oncol 11:464–468, 1985.

CHAPTER 62

Mohs Surgery: Fixed Tissue Technique

PAUL O. LARSON

Mohs micrographic surgery using the fixed tissue technique for treatment of skin cancer was first performed by Dr. Frederic E. Mohs in 1936.[1] This technique involves in situ fixation of cancer tissue, followed by layered excision and microscopic examination of the under surface of each layer. This process, termed chemosurgery,[2] is repeated until a tumor-free plane is reached. The name was changed in 1986 to Mohs micrographic surgery—fixed tissue technique to more clearly describe the procedure and to honor the man who developed it.

Mohs surgery using the fixed tissue technique is a direct extension of the cancer research that was initiated by Mohs at the University of Wisconsin in the early 1930s as a medical student.[1, 2] Mohs was investigating agents that kill cancers when injected into a tumor. It was noted that zinc chloride solution caused fixation with little microscopic distortion of the tissues.[3] He reasoned he could microscopically examine the perimeter of fixed tissue, tracing silent outgrowths of cancer until he reached a tumor-free plane. Fixation decreased the risk of intraoperative seeding of cancer cells and yet permitted preservation of the maximum amount of normal tissue. In this way, Mohs surgery using the fixed tissue technique was developed.

Mohs subsequently applied the fixed tissue technique to a variety of diseases, including skin cancers, breast cancers, laryngeal cancers, and gangrene, but it has found its greatest acceptance in the treatment of skin cancers.[1] The fixed tissue technique was used almost exclusively until 1974, when Dr. Theodore A. Tromovitch[4] reported high cure rates for skin cancer in 75 patients using the fresh tissue technique.[1] Mohs had first used the fresh tissue technique in 1953 for treatment of an eyelid cancer[1] and in 1969 reported on a series of 70 patients with eyelid cancers in whom the fresh tissue technique was used. Despite this, before Tromovitch's reported results, Mohs doubted that the fresh tissue technique would be accepted, because "it was a rather bloody, untidy procedure."[1] Since 1974, the fresh tissue technique has almost completely replaced the fixed tissue technique.[5–7] Fixed tissue excision currently has only limited clinical application, and very few Mohs surgeons have had much experience using it. However, it remains useful in the treatment of melanomas, gangrene, chronic ulcers, and penile cancers.

Procedure

ZINC CHLORIDE FIXATIVE

The zinc chloride fixative paste (Fig. 62–1) is a concentrated solution of zinc chloride held in suspension in an 80-sieve-mesh stibnite, a coarse antimony ore.[2] Sanguinaria is used as a binder to maintain proper consistency and prevent separation of the paste (Table 62–1). Because the zinc chloride paste is highly hygroscopic,[2] it can rapidly turn into an unusable slurry during the humid summer months. With low humidity, the paste becomes hard and unmanageable. Thus, to maintain the proper consistency, the fixative paste should be stored in a desiccator. Zinc chloride paste–impregnated gauze[8] that has been cut into small, variably sized pieces called Z-squares (Fig. 62–2) can be used to apply thin layers of zinc chloride or to hold the paste in place.* Consid-

---

*The zinc chloride paste can be purchased by qualified individuals from the School of Pharmacy, University of Wisconsin, Madison, WI 53706.

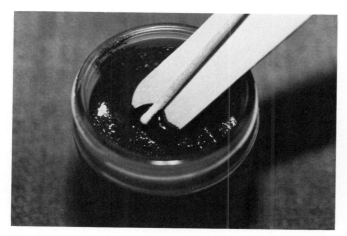

Figure 62–1. Zinc chloride is held in suspension in a coarse stibnite ore, forming a thick, black paste.

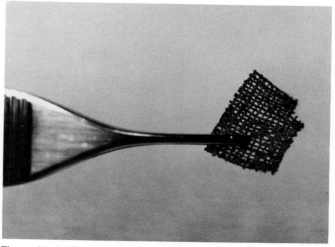

Figure 62–2. "Z-squares" are made by impregnating gauze with zinc chloride paste.

erable experience is necessary to know how to correctly apply the zinc chloride fixative.[2, 8–12]

BIOPSY USING THE FIXED TISSUE TECHNIQUE

The fixed tissue technique can be used to biopsy suspicious skin lesions. Using this technique, the zinc chloride paste is applied to the suspicious lesion (Fig. 62‑3). The fixed tissue is excised, usually after 24 hours, and processed for routine microscopic examination.

Biopsies using standard fresh tissue methods can also be done prior to fixed tissue excision of the cancer. The clear advantage of biopsy by fresh tissue excision is that it permits standard histologic examination. This is very helpful in the staging of melanoma, as fixation artifact can make interpretation of zinc chloride–fixed tissue difficult. Theoretically, there is a risk of intraoperative spread of melanoma or squamous cell carcinoma if tumor cells are dislodged during fresh tissue biopsy.[2] Previous studies, however, show no increase in mortality in patients with melanomas that underwent biopsy before definitive surgery.[13–15] In spite of these findings, it seems prudent in highly suspicious lesions to use excisional rather than incisional biopsy. The base of the biopsy site in lesions highly suspicious for melanoma or squamous cell carcinoma should be chemically cauterized immediately with dichloroacetic acid (DCA) or trichloroacetic acid (TCA) to reduce the risk of seeding by tumor cells.

SITE PREPARATION

Before applying fixative paste to the skin, the stratum corneum must be rendered permeable. To do this, the

skin is first anesthetized by local infiltration, making sure that the needle is well outside of the zone of implantable tumor.[2] A concentrated solution of DCA or 50% TCA[12] is then applied to the desired area of skin (Figs. 62–4, 62–5) until the skin whitens.[2, 10] Once whitening appears, the zinc chloride fixative paste is applied. If the tumor site has recently undergone biopsy and suturing, the sutures can be removed and the wound allowed to dehisce before application of the fixative. Debulking the cancer before application of the fixative may expedite complete excision.[16]

APPLICATION OF ZINC CHLORIDE FIXATIVE

Zinc chloride paste is applied to the acid-prepared skin with a small stick applicator.[2] Clumps of paste 2 to 3 mm in size are twisted onto the surface to be treated and then smoothed to the desired thickness (Fig. 62–6). A relatively thick layer of fixative (2 to 3 mm) is initially

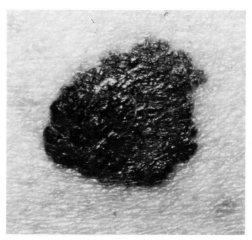

Figure 62–3. Malignant melanoma may theoretically spread by intraoperative seeding, but in situ fixation of melanoma may prevent this complication.

TABLE 62–1. **FORMULA FOR ZINC CHLORIDE FIXATIVE PASTE**

Zinc chloride (saturated solution)	34.5 ml
Stibnite (80 mesh sieve)	40.0 gm
Sanguinaria canadensis	10.0 gm

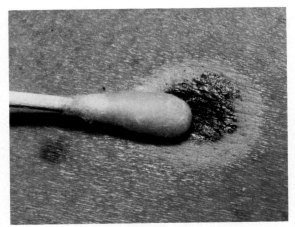

Figure 62–4. Dichloroacetic acid is applied to the treatment site to render the skin permeable to zinc chloride paste.

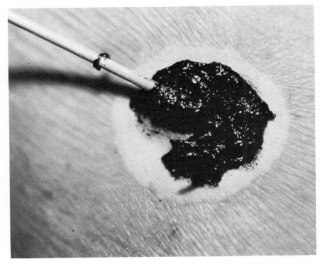

Figure 62–6. Zinc chloride paste is applied with small applicator sticks to the denatured skin.

applied to penetrate the epidermis and dermis.[8, 17] Thin skin and subsequent layers of fixation require much less fixative, typically only 0.1 to 0.5 mm in thickness.

Experience with the fixative is most helpful in determining the thickness of each application. Excised tissue should always have been recently fixed. If the skin is fixed for longer than 24 hours, the tissue becomes friable, and the histologic specimens will be of poor quality. Zinc chloride–impregnated gauze (Z-squares) can be laid over the top of the paste to hold the fixative in place (Fig. 62–7). Z-squares can also be used alone for fixation on thin skin such as on the eyelid or penis.

DRESSINGS

A surface dressing must be applied over the zinc chloride paste to hold it in place.[2, 10] If the air is humid, the paste may become moist and spread onto adjacent skin, resulting in unintended and unneeded fixation. A thin layer of dry cotton is applied to hold the paste in place (Fig. 62–8). This is covered with a petrolatum gauze or Adaptic gauze to help prevent ambient humid-

ity from affecting the consistency of the paste.[8] A barrier to protect the surrounding skin can be made by cutting a hole in the center of a hydrocolloid dressing and applying it around the treatment site. Fixation of the skin may take as little as several hours in thin skin, but the dressing is usually is left in place for 24 hours before proceeding with excision.

EXCISION AND MAPPING

When the patient returns in 24 hours, the dressings and all residual zinc chloride paste are removed (Fig. 62–9). The excision and mapping of fixed tissue are very similar to those used in fresh tissue excision.[2] Fixed tissue, however, has a hard, cardboard-like consistency.

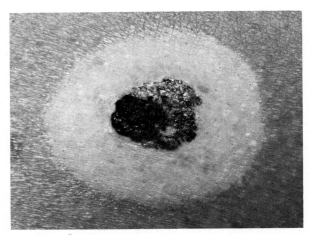

Figure 62–5. Completed zone of denaturation after dichloroacetic acid application.

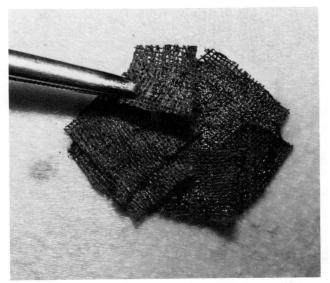

Figure 62–7. "Z-squares" are applied over the paste to hold the paste in place.

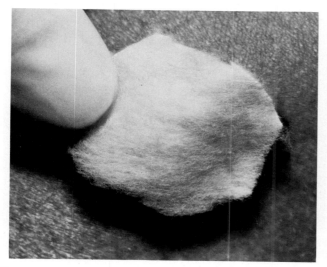

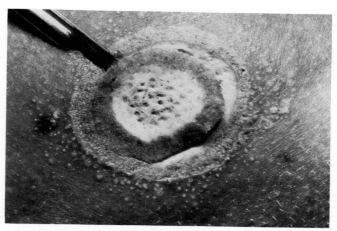

Figure 62–10. Excision site after debulking a melanoma. A second layer of fixed tissue is removed with smooth sweeps of the scalpel.

Figure 62–8. Dry cotton wadding is applied over the zinc chloride paste to further stabilize the placement of the paste.

Thin layers are excised as saucer-like disks using smooth sweeps of the scalpel (Fig. 62–10). Because the tissue is already fixed, no pain or bleeding occurs during the excision, unless the surgeon inadvertently cuts through an unfixed margin.[16] If bleeding is encountered, zinc chloride paste or a Z-square is applied over the bleeding point[8] and pressure held with an applicator for several minutes.

Excised tissue is marked in a standard fashion (Figs. 62–11, 62–12) using red, blue, or black dyes, and a map is made of the excision site.[2, 10] With the fixed tissue technique, an outline of each excised specimen can be drawn directly onto the excision site with tissue dyes. Fixed tissue specimens can be friable and require careful handling; microtome sections may have to be cut thicker than standard fresh tissue sections because of this friability. Stained sections are examined microscopically to locate the exact position of any remaining cancer,[2] and fixative paste is reapplied to the areas of residual tumor

(Fig. 62–13). The additional tissue is re-excised in serial fashion until a tumor-free plane is reached.[17]

Bone can be fixed with zinc chloride paste in a fashion similar to that used for soft tissue. After fixation, bone is chiseled or rongeured, and specimens are numbered, mapped, decalcified, stained, and then examined microscopically as in the traditional method.[2] A layer of fixed bone will spontaneously demarcate and slough off several weeks after fixation.

INTRAOPERATIVE AND POSTOPERATIVE CARE

In situ fixation causes a moderate degree of pain during the fixation process. The pain is usually well controlled with either nonprescription or narcotic oral pain medications.[2] The fixed tissue technique causes an intense inflammatory reaction 2 to 5 days after application (Fig. 62–14). The patient may be quite uncomfortable at this stage and very anxious if not well prepared in advance for the inflammatory reaction. Fever, myalgia, and general malaise are not uncommon symptoms

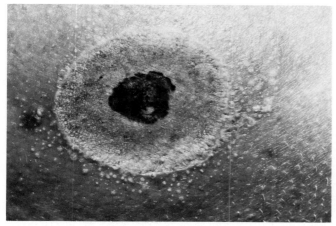

Figure 62–9. Appearance of the fixed melanoma and surrounding skin 24 hours after application of zinc chloride paste.

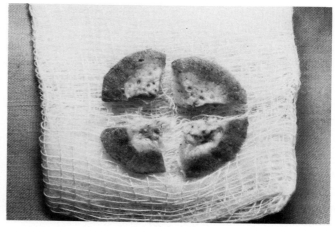

Figure 62–11. The fixed tissue is oriented and cut into specimens of a size that can be processed in the cryostat.

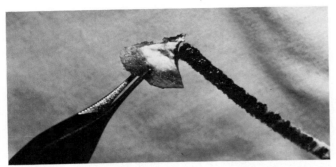

Figure 62–12. Specimens are marked with tissue dyes using the standard Mohs surgical technique.

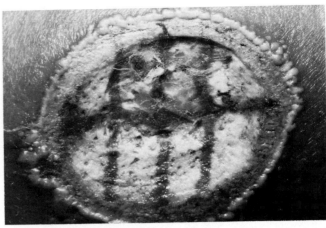

Figure 62–14. Intense inflammation surrounds the fixative site 2 to 5 days after completion of fixation.

at this stage, and supportive care is invaluable.[18] The wound resulting from the fixed tissue excision must be kept clean and moist. Topical antibiotic ointment and sterile absorbent dressings are applied to the wound. Five to 10 days after the excision is completed, the necrotic devitalized soft tissue will separate sharply from the viable tissue (Fig. 62–15),[2, 7] but tendon or bone may require 1 to 2 months for final separation to occur.[19] The line of demarcation is remarkably sharp with the fixed tissue technique, and the underlying granulating defect is very clean (Fig. 62–16). The defect will heal by second intention, usually within 1 month.[20] The resultant mature scar ordinarily heals flush with the surrounding skin and is supple and strong (Fig. 62–17).

Indications for Fixed Tissue Mohs Surgery

MELANOMA

The strongest indication for Mohs surgery using the fixed tissue technique is in the treatment of malignant melanoma.[2, 21–24] The rationale for using the fixed tissue technique is twofold. First, the application of zinc chloride paste causes in situ fixation of tumor, which de-

creases the risk of intraoperative metastasis, since excision of the tumor is made through completely fixed and devitalized tissue. This seems to be confirmed by the very low rate of satellite metastasis and in-transit metastasis using the fixed tissue technique. Second, the use of microscopically controlled excision permits excision of a minimum amount of normal tissue with maximum assurance of complete removal of the melanoma. The question of the width of excision frequently arises with regard to fixed tissue excision. The conventional width of excision is predetermined based on the lesion's Clark level or Breslow thickness. Mohs surgery using the fixed tissue technique is based purely on reaching a tumor-free border as determined microscopically. An additional fixed tissue layer is routinely taken as an extra measure of assurance once that level has been reached.

The results of melanoma excision using the fixed tissue technique have been very promising (Table 62–2). In a series of 200 melanoma patients treated with the fixed tissue technique, an overall 5-year cure rate of 65.2% was achieved.[25] The 5-year cure rate ranged from 89%

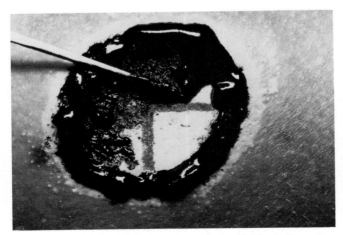

Figure 62–13. Zinc chloride paste is reapplied to histologically positive areas or to provide an extra margin of safety.

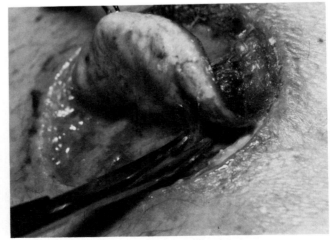

Figure 62–15. The final layer of fixed tissue will spontaneously separate but can usually be removed with gentle excision along the line of demarcation.

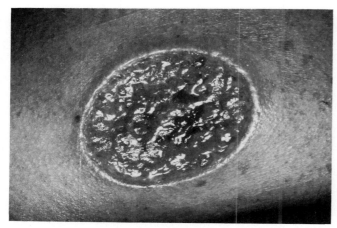

Figure 62–16. The underlying defect has a clean granulating surface that is generally left to heal by second intention.

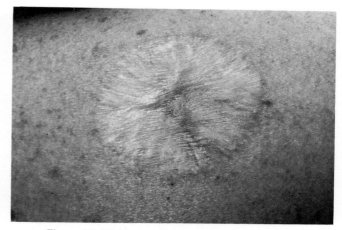

Figure 62–17. The resultant scar is soft and supple.

in Clark's level I disease to 38% in Clark's level V disease. These data take into account the fact that if there was a recurrence any time after surgery, the patient was considered to be a treatment failure.[2, 26] Most current statistics are evaluated by determining the 5-year survival rate, which means that a patient who has survived for 5 years is a treatment success, even though he or she may have had a recurrence.

OTHER TUMORS

Aggressive skin cancers that invade bone,[27] extend deeply into the ear canal, or are exceedingly vascular are also amenable to treatment with the fixed tissue technique.[7, 28] Because squamous cell carcinomas are highly transplantable, the in situ fixation of these cancers by the fixed tissue technique may prevent transplantation or metastasis. A total of 2249 reported cases of squamous cell carcinomas treated by fixed tissue technique between 1936 and 1968[2] yielded an overall 5-year cure rate of 94%. The fixed tissue technique has also been used to debulk large, unresectable, malodorous cancers.[7]

PENILE CANCERS

Cancer of the penis is difficult to treat, and the use of conventional surgery may necessitate amputation.

Mohs surgery using the fresh tissue technique for treatment of penile cancer is often difficult, because obtaining hemostasis is very laborious. However, the fixed tissue Mohs surgical technique[2, 7, 29] permits excision of the cancer in a bloodless field (Figs. 62–18 through 62–20) and also permits maximum preservation of normal tissue. A series of 29 patients with squamous cell carcinoma of the penis treated with the fixed tissue technique[29] showed an overall 5-year cure rate of 68%. The primary carcinoma was eradicated in 92% of the patients, a rate that compares very favorably with that produced by conventional surgery. Treatment may require the placement of a urethral or suprapubic catheter to prevent intraoperative urinary obstruction.

PATIENTS WITH AIDS

Patients who are HIV positive present a significant risk to Mohs surgeons, nursing staff, and laboratory personnel. However, in situ fixation may help reduce the risk of transmitting the HIV organism. One patient with AIDS was treated with the fixed tissue technique and later had delayed reconstruction.[30]

GANGRENE

Fixed tissue excision for treatment of gangrene has been used for many years.[2, 31, 32] Gangrenous skin is first

TABLE 62–2. **CORRELATION OF CLARK'S LEVEL WITH 5-YEAR SURVIVAL RATE**

Reference	Survival Based on Clark's Level			
	II	*III*	*IV*	*V*
McGovern[55]	84	65	49	29
Balch et al[56]	85	73	57	28
Eldh et al[57]	100	87	72	35
Breslow[58]*	97	76	43	33
Blois et al[59]	98	80	70	45
Wanebo et al[60]	100	88	66	15
DeVita and Fisher[61]	83	62	51	37
Zitelli et al[25]†	89	88	63	38

*Based on 5-year disease free interval.
†Recurrence after 5 years is considered a treatment failure.

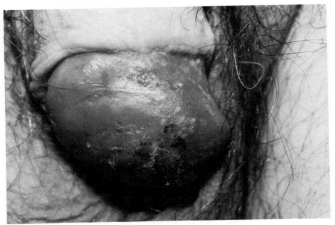

Figure 62–18. A biopsy-proven squamous cell carcinoma of the penis.

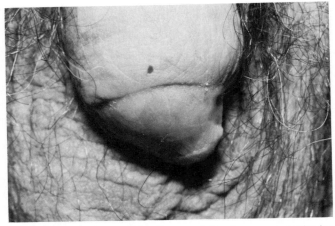

Figure 62–20. A portion of the glans penis has been preserved using the Mohs fixed tissue technique.

rendered permeable by application of DCA. Zinc chloride is applied to the gangrenous tissue. Standard dressings are then applied over the fixative, and the patient is instructed to return 24 hours later. The fixed gangrenous tissue is excised until viable tissue is reached (Figs. 62–21 through 62–23). Cartilage exposed by disarticulation must be removed to support granulation tissue formation. Wound care must be meticulous in areas where circulation is compromised to prevent infection and promote wound healing. If the fixed tissue excision is not successful, the area must be amputated proximal to the gangrenous tissue by conventional surgery. A success rate of 72% has been reported in 521 patients with gangrenous lesions treated with conservative fixed tissue amputation.[2]

OSTEOMYELITIS

Infections, including osteomyelitis, have been treated with the fixed tissue technique. Successful treatment of osteomyelitis of 67 year's duration with the fixed tissue

technique has been described.[33] Fixation sterilizes the tissue, allows clean separation of fixed bone, and stimulates formation of new granulation tissue.

CHRONIC ULCERS

Chronic ulcers have also been successfully treated with fixed tissue technique.[34] Zinc chloride paste is applied to the ulcer, and the fixed tissue is subsequently removed. After final separation of the fixed tissue, granulation tissue fills the defect, providing a wound suitable for grafting. The healed defect is generally very supple and pliable.

Advantages of the Fixed Tissue Technique

IN SITU FIXATION OF CANCER CELLS

The fixation of cancer cells in situ is one of the most important advantages offered by the fixed tissue technique. To test this theory, the incidence of metastasis

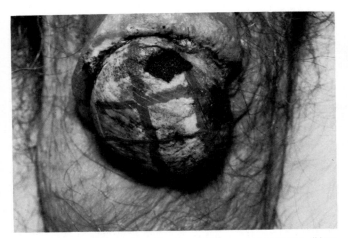

Figure 62–19. Glans penis after the first layers of excision. (Note mercurochrome markings for orientation and "Z-squares" for additional fixation.)

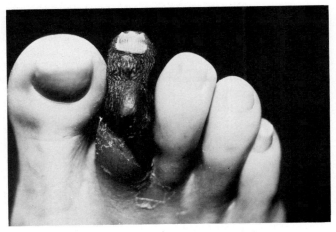

Figure 62–21. Gangrenous toe in a diabetic man.

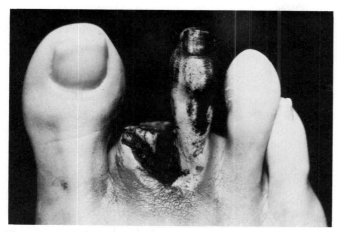

Figure 62–22. The gangrenous toe has been excised using the fixed tissue technique. (Note that the middle toe has also been fixed but has not yet been excised.)

was examined in incompletely treated rats with Flexner-Jobling carcinoma. Repeated subcurative zinc chloride fixation was used to see whether metastases would be induced. The rate of metastasis in the zinc chloride–treated group was 28%, compared with a metastasis rate of 41.5% in the control group.[35] The decreased rate of metastasis in the zinc chloride–treated group was attributed to the in situ fixation of cancer cells with the zinc chloride. This is the rationale for using the fixed tissue technique in highly transplantable cancers such as malignant melanoma, aggressive squamous cell carcinomas, and perhaps Merkel cell carcinoma. The fixed tissue technique is not generally needed in routine basal cell carcinomas, where the risk of implantation or metastasis is small. However, in situ fixation is useful in treating multiply recurrent dedifferentiated basal cell carcinomas.

MICROSCOPIC MARGIN CONTROL

The rationale for using zinc chloride for fixation is that it permits microscopic examination of the fixed

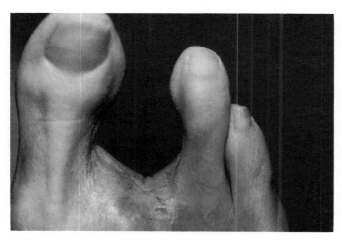

Figure 62–23. Excision site after healing by second intention.

tissue.[16] A variety of fixatives were tested before zinc chloride was finally selected for use in the fixed tissue surgical procedure. Zinc chloride was chosen largely because it caused the least amount of tissue distortion. Actively fixed tissue (fixed within 24 hours) generally has good microscopic detail. Tissue fixed longer than 24 hours, however, is friable and difficult to interpret microscopically. Excellent tissue detail using the fixed tissue technique requires excision through tissue that has been recently fixed.

HIGH CURE RATES

As with the fresh tissue technique, the fixed tissue technique provides a high assurance of cure of skin cancers, as all margins are checked microscopically.[9] In conventional excision with a representative margin check, less than 1% of the peripheral border may be examined, thus increasing the risk of missing outgrowths of cancer.[36] In a series of 72 patients, it has been shown that subclinical extension of tumor ranged from 4.6 mm to more than 10 mm beyond the apparent margin of the tumor.[37] In a series of 13,015 patients treated by the fixed tissue technique, the overall cure rate for basal cell carcinoma was 99.3% and for squamous cell carcinoma, 94%.[2] In another series of 100 recurrent basal cell carcinomas treated between 1966 and 1971 with the fixed tissue technique,[17] the reported recurrence rate was 4%. A different group of Mohs surgeons reported a 5-year cure rate of 93.1% in 102 patients with recurrent cutaneous cancers.[38] The 5-year cure rate using the fixed tissue technique compiled from 13 different authors, for treatment of basal cell carcinomas, is 99%.[39, 40]

TISSUE SPARING

The fixed tissue technique has the same advantage as the fresh tissue technique in preserving normal tissues.[2, 9, 16] Mohs surgery with the fresh tissue technique used to treat cancer of the ear, has been shown to conserve tissue in 100% of 17 cases when compared with conventional surgery.[41] Conventional surgery removed an excess amount of skin totaling 180% in primary excisions and 347% in recurrent lesions when compared with actual tumor size as determined by Mohs surgery.

BLOODLESS FIELDS

In situ fixation with zinc chloride paste results in the creation of bloodless, nonviable tissue,[42] and excision through the fixed tissue causes no bleeding. This is of particular value when treating penile cancers and large complicated cancers in which hemostasis is difficult.[1, 7] Although zinc chloride provides a completely bloodless field for excision, late perforation through larger blood vessels may result in delayed bleeding.[43, 44] Patients should be made aware of this possibility and given instructions as to what to do if this does happen.

STERILIZATION

Zinc chloride fixation will sterilize the operative field to which it is applied. Although marked inflammation results from fixation, fixed tissue excisions rarely become infected. Zinc chloride paste can be used to sterilize osteomyelitis[33] and chronic ulcers[34] and has also been used to treat the local occurrence of tetanus.[45]

WOUND HEALING

Fixed tissue excisions tend to heal with surprisingly smooth scars.[46, 47] This is especially remarkable, since the wound after final excision appears crater-like. The underlying tissue first granulates to the level of the skin, and then the wound reepithelializes from the margins of the defect. The scar may at first be erythematous and firm but naturally matures to a soft, flat, supple scar.

Disadvantages of the Fixed Tissue Technique

HISTOPATHOLOGIC INTERPRETATION

Perhaps the most criticized aspect of using the fixed tissue technique relates to the difficulty experienced in interpreting the histologic slides. This difficulty occurs as a result of inflammation,[16] tissue distortion, and other artifacts and may be due in part to differences in technique and operator experience. There is no doubt, however, that fixed tissue slides do not have the same tissue detail as seen in fresh tissue paraffin-embedded specimens. In spite of this loss of tissue detail, Mohs surgery using either the fixed or fresh tissue technique is the most reliable method for treating skin cancers.[48, 49]

PAIN

The application of zinc chloride fixative and DCA used to render the skin permeable is quite painful.[8, 16, 19, 42, 43, 50] The intense inflammation that develops at the treatment site after about 3 to 5 days is also painful. The pain of applying DCA can be controlled with previous infiltration of local anesthesia. The discomfort of slow fixation and the secondary inflammation is generally well controlled with analgesics such as acetaminophen or acetaminophen with codeine. If patients know what to expect in advance, the fixation process can generally be tolerated very well.

EFFICIENCY

Fixed tissue excision can be time consuming for the patient.[8, 9, 16, 19, 42, 50, 51] The patient must return to the Mohs surgery unit for layered excisions, usually at 24-hour intervals, until the cancer is completely removed. In addition, the patient must usually return 1 to 2 weeks after completion of Mohs surgery to have the fixed tissue eschar removed from the treatment site. This can be inconvenient for actively working, productive individuals.

DELAYED RECONSTRUCTION

Treatment with the fixed tissue technique generally precludes primary closure.[6, 42] Although healing by second intention is often satisfactory,[6] it can at times be unpredictable.[52] Scar revision is usually delayed for 6 to 12 months to ensure that there is no recurrence.[40] Again, this may not be acceptable for individuals who are actively working or "in the public eye." Defects resulting from fixed tissue excision can be closed by either excising the fixed tissue eschar or waiting until it sloughs spontaneously[2, 51] before proceeding with a delayed primary closure. However, this is usually inefficient, as it requires at least one additional surgical procedure.

NONSTANDARD SURGICAL TECHNIQUE

A final disadvantage of Mohs surgery using the fixed tissue process is that the techniques used are not well understood by most cutaneous surgeons.[50] In addition, any follow-up or emergency care provided by another physician is often difficult, because the examining physician may not know how to interpret the clinical appearance of the wound. Thus, patients should be given as much information as possible about their treatment; preprinted information sheets can be invaluable for both the patient and the attending physicians.

Role of the Fixed Tissue Technique

The role of Mohs surgery using the fixed tissue technique has changed dramatically since the widespread acceptance of the fresh tissue technique.[53] Fresh tissue excision is usually more efficient, better tolerated by the patient, and lends itself to primary closure.[54] However, Mohs surgery using the fixed tissue technique is not obsolete because of the potential benefit of the intense inflammatory response,[16] which may act in a specific or nonspecific way to prevent metastasis of melanomas.[55–61] The lymphocytic infiltrate may act as a specific or nonspecific "scavenger" system to kill single-cell metastases in the lymphatic drainage system or in the regional nodes. While many questions remain to be answered, it seems unwise to consider the fixed tissue technique outdated.

SUMMARY

Mohs surgery using the fixed tissue technique is a viable option for treating certain skin cancers, especially melanoma, aggressive squamous cell carcinomas, and cancers of very vascular areas such as the penis. The fixed tissue technique may also be helpful for the treatment of unresponsive ulcers, gangrene, and osteomyelitis. Additional critical studies are needed to evaluate properly the potential role of the fixed tissue technique in each of these areas.

REFERENCES

1. Mohs FE: Frederic E. Mohs, M.D. J Am Acad Dermatol 9:806–814, 1983.
2. Mohs FE: Chemosurgery: Microscopically Controlled Surgery for Skin Cancer. Charles C Thomas, Springfield, IL, 1978.

3. Mohs FE, Guyer MF: Pre-excisional fixation of tissues in the treatment of cancer in rats. Cancer Res 1:49–51, 1941.
4. Tromovitch TA, Stegman SJ: Microscopically controlled excision of skin tumors. Arch Dermatol 110:231–232, 1974.
5. Swanson NA: Mohs surgery: technique, indications, applications, and the future. Arch Dermatol 119:761–773, 1983.
6. Robins P: Chemosurgery: my 15 years of experience. J Dermatol Surg Oncol 7:779–789, 1981.
7. Braun M: The case for Mohs' surgery by the fixed-tissue technique. J Dermatol Surg Oncol 7:634–640, 1981.
8. Tolman EL: Chemosurgery (Mohs' technique) in the treatment of epitheliomas. Med Clin North Am 56:739–745, 1972.
9. Szujewski HA: Microscopic guidance in the treatment of skin cancer. Plast Reconstr Surg 5:524–531, 1950.
10. Robins P: Chemosurgery of the treatment of skin cancer. Hosp Pract 5:40–50, 1970.
11. Mikhail GR: The application of "chemosurgery" in cancer. Henry Ford Hosp Med J 17:217–224, 1969.
12. Loney WRR: Chemosurgical treatment of skin cancer. J Okla State Med Assoc 60:165–168, 1967.
13. Landthaler M, Braun Falco O, Leitl A, et al: Excisional biopsy as the first therapeutic procedure versus primary wide excision of malignant melanoma. Cancer 64:1612–1616, 1989.
14. Lederman JS, Sober AJ: Does wide excision as the initial diagnostic procedure improve prognosis in patients with cutaneous melanoma. J Dermatol Surg Oncol 12:697–699, 1986.
15. Lederman JS, Sober AJ: Does biopsy type influence survival in clinical stage I cutaneous melanoma? J Am Acad Dermatol 13:983–987, 1985.
16. Lunsford CJ, Templeton HJ, Allington HV, Allington RR: Use of chemosurgery in dermatologic practice. Arch Dermatol Syph 68:148–156, 1953.
17. Robins P, Amonette R: Basal cell carcinoma: treatment by the Mohs technique. Laryngoscope 82:965–972, 1972.
18. Stanewick B: Chemosurgery in skin cancer. AORN J 22:351–359, 1975.
19. Mikhail GR: Subungual epidermoid carcinoma. J Am Acad Dermatol 11:291–298, 1984.
20. Phelan JT, Milgrom H, Stoll H, Traenkle H: The use of Mohs' chemosurgery technique in the management of superficial cancers. Surg Gynecol Obstet 114:25–30, 1962.
21. Mohs FE: Chemosurgery for melanoma. Arch Dermatol 113:285–291, 1977.
22. Mohs FE: Micrographic surgery for satellites and in-transit metastases of malignant melanoma. J Dermatol Surg Oncol 12:471–476, 1986.
23. Mohs FE: Chemosurgical treatment of melanoma: a microscopically controlled method of excision. Arch Dermatol Syph 62:269–279, 1950.
24. Mohs FE: Microscopically controlled surgery for periorbital melanoma: fixed-tissue and fresh-tissue techniques. J Dermatol Surg Oncol 11:284–291, 1985.
25. Zitelli JA, Mohs FE, Larson P, Snow S: Mohs micrographic surgery for melanoma. Dermatol Clin 7:833–843, 1989.
26. Mohs F, Larson P, Iriondo M: Micrographic surgery for the microscopically controlled excision of carcinoma of the external ear. J Am Acad Dermatol 19:729–737, 1988.
27. Mohs FE, Zitelli JA: Microscopically controlled surgery in the treatment of carcinoma of the scalp. Arch Dermatol 117:764–769, 1981.
28. Phelan JT: The use of the Mohs' chemosurgery technic in the treatment of basal cell carcinoma. Ann Surg 168:1023–1029, 1968.
29. Mohs FE, Snow SN, Messing EM, Kuglitsch ME: Microscopically controlled surgery in the treatment of carcinoma of the penis. J Urol 133:961–966, 1985.
30. Hruza GJ, Snow SN: Basal cell carcinoma in a patient with acquired immunodeficiency syndrome: treatment with Mohs micrographic surgery fixed-tissue technique. J Dermatol Surg Oncol 15:545–551, 1989.
31. Mohs FE, Severinghaus EL, Schmidt ER: Conservative amputation of gangrenous parts by chemosurgery. Ann Surg 114:274–282, 1941.
32. Mohs FE: Chemosurgical amputation for gangrene. Surgery 57:247–253, 1965.
33. Bennett RG, Goldman MP: Chemosurgical debridement of osteomyelitic bone by zinc chloride fixative. J Dermatol Surg Oncol 13:771–775, 1987.
34. Falanga V, Iriondo M: Zinc chloride paste for the debridement of chronic leg ulcers. J Dermatol Surg Oncol 16:658–661, 1990.
35. Mohs FE: Chemosurgical treatment of cancer of the facial orifices. Minn Med 42:381–387, 1959.
36. Davidson TM, Haghighi P, Astarita R, et al: Mohs for head and neck mucosal cancer: report on 111 patients. Laryngoscope 98:1078–1083, 1988.
37. Burg G, Hirsch RD, Konz B, Braun-Falco O: Histographic surgery: accuracy of visual assessment of the margins of basal-cell epithelioma. J Dermatol Surg 1:21–24, 1975.
38. Tromovitch TA, Beirne G, Beirne C: Mohs' technique (cancer chemosurgery). Treatment of recurrent cutaneous carcinomas. Cancer 19:867–868, 1966.
39. Crissey JT: Curettage and electrodesiccation as a method of treatment for epitheliomas of the skin. J Surg Oncol 3:387, 1969.
40. Mikhail GR: Chemosurgery in the treatment of cancer. Int J Dermatol 14:33–38, 1975.
41. Bumsted RM, Ceilley RI: Auricular malignant neoplasms. Identification of high-risk lesions and selection of method of reconstruction. Arch Otolaryngol 108:225–231, 1982.
42. Stegman SJ, Tromovitch TA: Modern chemosurgery: microscopically controlled excision. West J Med 132:7–12, 1980.
43. Phelan JT, Juardo J: Chemosurgical management of carcinoma of the nose. Surgery 53:310–314, 1963.
44. Szujewski HA: Treatment of facial cancer in the geriatric patient: chemosurgery. J Am Geriatr Soc 12:90–94, 1964.
45. Davila de Pedro RL, Mohs FE: Extirpation of a nidus of infection with tetanus bacilli by chemosurgery. J Dermatol Surg Oncol 7:629–631, 1981.
46. Phelan JT, Juardo J: Mohs' chemosurgery technique in basal cell carcinoma of the chin and cheek areas of the face. Arch Surg 87:212–214, 1963.
47. Robins P: Basal cell epitheliomata, case reports. Arch Dermatol 97:481, 1968.
48. Larson PO: Topical hemostatic agents for dermatologic surgery. J Dermatol Surg Oncol 14:623–632, 1988.
49. Dzubow LM: False-negative tumor-free margins following Mohs surgery. J Dermatol Surg Oncol 14:600–602, 1988.
50. Swanson NA, Taylor WB, Tromovitch TA: The evolution of Mohs' surgery. J Dermatol Surg Oncol 8:650–654, 1982.
51. Moraites RS: Chemosurgery in Cincinnati. Cutis 5:559–562, 1969.
52. Baylis HI, Cies WA: Complications of Mohs' chemosurgical excision of eyelid and canthal tumors. Am J Ophthalmol 80:116–122, 1975.
53. Mohs FE: Mohs micrographic surgery. A historical perspective. Dermatol Clin 7:609–611, 1989.
54. Mohs FE: Cancer of the eyelid. Bull Am Coll Chemosurg 3:10–11, 1970.
55. McGovern VJ: The classification of melanoma and its relationship with prognosis. Pathology 2:85–98, 1970.
56. Balch CM, Murad TM, Soong SJ, et al: A multifactorial analysis of melanoma: prognostic histopathological features comparing Clark's and Breslow's staging methods. Ann Surg 188:732–742, 1978.
57. Eldh J, Boeryd B, Peterson LE: Prognostic factors in cutaneous malignant melanoma in stage I. A clinical, morphological and multivariate analysis. Scand J Plast Reconstr Surg 12:243–255, 1978.
58. Breslow A: Thickness, cross-sectional areas and depth of invasion in the prognosis of cutaneous melanoma. Ann Surg 172:902–908, 1970.
59. Blois MS, Sagebiel RW, Abarbanel RM, et al: Malignant melanoma of the skin. I. The association of tumor depth and type, and patient sex, age, and site with survival. Cancer 52:1330–1341, 1983.
60. Wanebo HJ, Fortner JG, Woodruff J, et al: Selection of the optimum surgical treatment of stage I melanoma by depth of microinvasion: use of the combined microstage technique (Clark-Breslow). Ann Surg 182:302–315, 1975.
61. DeVita VT Jr, Fisher RI: Natural history of malignant melanoma as related to therapy. Cancer Treat Rep 60:153–157, 1976.

CHAPTER 63

Mohs Surgery: Fresh Tissue Technique

RAYMOND G. DUFRESNE, JR.

Mohs micrographic surgery has represented a major advance in the treatment of cutaneous carcinoma since its development in the 1930's by Dr. Frederick Mohs.[1-3] This technique, now commonly referred to as Mohs surgery, included application of the zinc chloride fixative, sequential excision of tumor, detailed marking and mapping of the removed tissues, and horizontal sectioning of the excised material with complete margin control. Dr. Mohs initially used the "fresh technique" in 1953 when he excluded the fixative in the treatment of an eyelid tumor but continued the other essential elements of Mohs surgery (Table 63–1).[4] The fresh tissue variant, popularized by Dr. Theodore Tromovitch, proved to have the same high cure rates as the original fixed tissue technique.[5-9]

The fresh technique afforded several advantages over the original chemosurgical technique (Table 63–2).[6, 10] The time delay required for tissue fixation with the zinc chloride paste was avoided; the use of local anesthesia resulted in a relatively painless procedure; and the elimination of the fixative avoided the local tissue irritation and the possibility of overpenetration by the zinc chloride fixative. Also, immediate reconstruction of the defect became technically possible and interdisciplinary approaches more feasible. Because of these factors, the fresh technique has enjoyed great popularity, although the fixed technique is still useful to treat certain vascular tumors or tumors in vascular sites, very large or deeply invasive tumors and tumors invading bone.[11]

Operative Technique

PREOPERATIVE EVALUATION

A general history taking and physical examination are performed to ascertain the medical status of the patient. Allergies, medications, bleeding tendencies, healing abnormalities, and cardiovascular and neurologic status should be noted. Pertinent information such as the duration of the lesion, previous treatment, and risk factors of petrochemical, arsenic, radiation, and ultraviolet exposure should be obtained. The site and size of the lesion, regional nerve function, and the presence or absence of adenopathy should also be noted. This evaluation may also suggest the need for additional laboratory tests, electrocardiography, magnetic resonance imaging (MRI) or x-ray studies, and possible consultation with other specialists. During the preoperative evaluation, the etiology, natural history, and prognosis of the skin cancer, details of Mohs surgery;[12, 13] possible plans for reconstruction, the risks and complications of the procedure, and alternative forms of treatment are always discussed.

PROCEDURE

The surgery is usually performed in an outpatient suite or office setting. General anesthesia and a full operating suite are typically required only for exceptional cases. This outpatient approach involves minimal alteration of patients' daily routine, including use of medications, and results in a very safe procedure that

TABLE 63–1. **ESSENTIALS OF MOHS SURGERY**

Thin layers are excised
Color coding of tissues is performed
Tissue mapping is created
Horizontal frozen sections are processed in the Mohs unit as integral part of technique
Tissue sections are evaluated by Mohs surgeon

TABLE 63–2. **ADVANTAGES OF FRESH VERSUS FIXED TECHNIQUE**

Speed
Reduced pain
Improved tissue conservation
Immediate reconstruction is possible
Interdisciplinary approach can be used

can be performed with low morbidity and very low mortality risks. Although patient restrictions are minimal, aspirin should be avoided for 2 to 4 weeks and alcohol for a few days preoperatively to reduce the risk of bleeding. In most instances, patients can continue normal use of routine medicines, and preoperative fasting is not a requirement. Family members are encouraged to accompany patients and bring whatever may help them to relax and be comfortable. Properly prepared patients in a relaxed environment usually tolerate the procedure quite well.

The Mohs excision is performed in a clean manner using standard surgical preparation of the skin along with sterile instruments and drapes. Local anesthesia is generally performed by infiltration with lidocaine 1% with epinephrine (1:100,000 to 200,000). The addition of bicarbonate buffers to the anesthetic solution decreases the pain of injection and increases the tolerance.[14] A long acting local anesthetic such as bupivacaine (Marcaine) can help to provide prolonged anesthesia. A peripheral field block around the tumor, rather than direct infiltration with the anesthetic, should be performed in tumors that have the potential of implantation. Regional blocks may be used in certain circumstances to increase patient tolerance and minimize the total dosage of anesthetic.[15]

The first stage of Mohs surgery consists of debulking the tumor (Figs. 63–1, 63–2). Gross surgical debulking is especially helpful for treating larger tumors, but simple curettage of even small tumors can help to further grossly define tumor margins. In delicate areas or treatment of small tumors, debulking is often omitted to avoid the risk of unnecessary adjacent epidermal injury

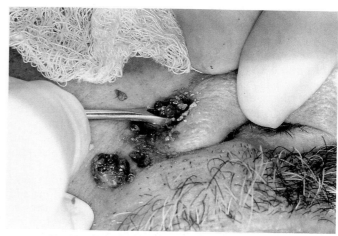

Figure 63–2. Curettage is performed for debulking.

which may reduce the normal tissue conservation that is possible with this surgical technique. The risk of implantation of tumor should be considered during debulking. The resultant debulked defect, any areas suspicious for tumor, and any scar tissue from previous treatment are then excised (Fig. 63–3).

The initial surgical margins vary with the clinical situation.[16–19] A small primary nodular basal cell may require only a 2-mm margin, while larger margins such as 5 mm are appropriate for morpheaform tumors, large tumors, recurrent tumors, and tumors that have been present for many years. Larger initial margins are also prudent for tumors of great infiltrating potential such as dermatofibrosarcoma protuberans. Despite the increased size of the initial stage of Mohs surgery, these surgical margins are still generally less than what would be necessary without complete microscopic control.

A No. 15, or in larger excisions a No. 10 blade, on a No. 3 Bard-Parker handle can be used to remove the tissue in a horizontal fashion. Many Mohs surgeons prefer to use a round scalpel handle such as the Siegle or the Beaver system handles and blades to harvest the

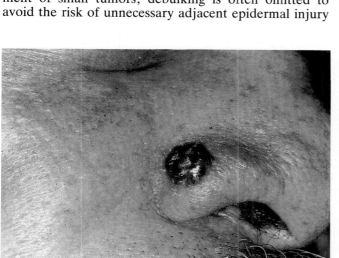

Figure 63–1. Preoperative appearance of a tumor on the right ala.

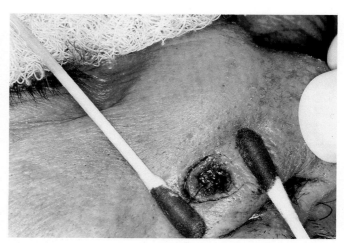

Figure 63–3. The excision is outlined with conservative margins and skin nicks for proper orientation.

tissue horizontally. The angle of the excision is usually tapered to allow easier processing of the lateral margins. The tumor is marked to identify the sites of origin of the separate pieces of tissue. The specimens are generally limited to 1 to 2 cm by the size of the microtome chuck and technical limits on the quality of the slides. Identifying marks such as skin nicks, scored lines, or hash marks are made on the patient to identify the origins of each specimen (Fig. 63–3). Staples may also be helpful to mark extensive or complex excisions,[20] and instant photography may also be used to assist this process.[21]

The tissue may then be removed in sections and marked (Fig. 63–4), or removed in en bloc fashion, and later divided as marked on the patient. The latter is preferable in tumors that are implantable, to minimize manipulation of the tumor. Once excised and divided, each tissue specimen is mapped according to its origin and marked with a system of different colored inks to maintain proper orientation and verification of complete tissue sectioning. The inks normally used include Mercurochrome, laundry blueing, and Indian ink. Commercial inking kits are now readily available in additional colors (Fig. 63–5). After marking, the specimens are placed on a moist filter paper in a Petri dish and transported to the laboratory (Fig. 63–6).

PROCESSING

The processing should be performed in the Mohs unit under the supervision of the Mohs surgeon by a specially trained technician to ensure proper handling and processing.[22] The tissue blocks are imbedded on a chuck in a medium such as OCT and quick frozen in liquid

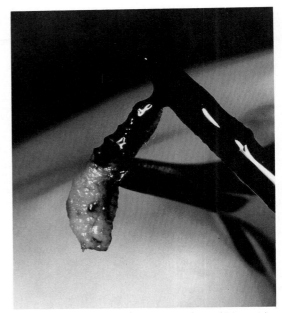

Figure 63–5. Inks are used to color-code each specimen.

nitrogen (Fig. 63–7). The outer edge of the tissue may be molded with a warmed handle blade to ensure sectioning of the entire lateral margin (Fig. 63–8). Alternatives to achieve this lateral processing include the Miami special and cromold or tissue processors such as those made by American Optics or of special design.[23]

The block on the chuck is then sectioned at 4 to 10 microns in the cryostat (Figs. 63–9, 63–10). Several representative cuts are placed on the microscopic slide (Fig. 63–11) and then stained with standard hematoxylin and eosin.[24] Toluidine blue is an excellent alternative stain for basal cell carcinoma.[25] These slides are then interpreted by the Mohs surgeon, an essential part of the procedure.[4, 26–28] If residual tumor is demonstrated, the location of the tumor in the block can be identified and noted on the map, and re-excision performed in the

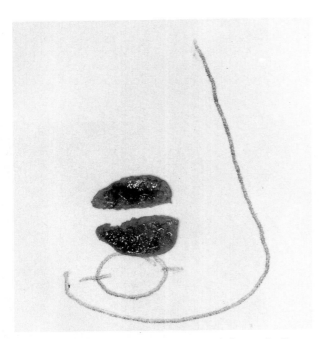

Figure 63–4. The specimen is placed on an index card with appropriate anatomic features to delineate precisely the treatment site and maintain orientation during processing.

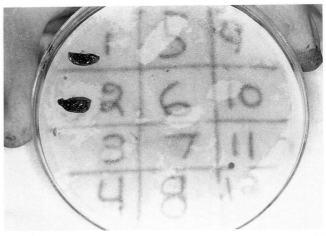

Figure 63–6. Specimens are placed on a moistened filter paper with numbers visible on the back of the dish.

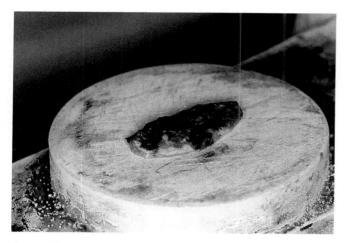

Figure 63–7. Each piece of tissue is placed upside down on a microtome chuck in the medium OTC for processing.

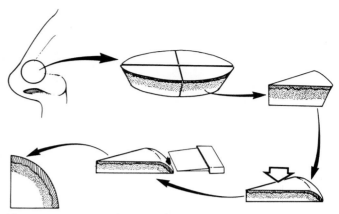

Figure 63–9. Schematic representation of the horizontal sectioning technique used in processing tissue with the Mohs technique.

corresponding area on the patient (Fig. 63–12). This cycle is repeated until the entire tumor is removed. An additional margin of normal tissue is sometimes removed in aggressive tumors.

SPECIAL CONSIDERATIONS

The clinical circumstances may occasionally require modification of the normal excisional procedure. The carbon dioxide laser can be used to provide hemostasis without causing significant histologic tissue artifact.[29] This may prove helpful in highly vascular areas, in patients with coagulation complications, and for accurately marking the excisional bed. Exposed bone requires bur,[30] chisel,[31] or laser perforations[32] to allow granulation tissue to form. More extensive resections require a multispecialty approach.

Modifications to the processing may also be required. The removal of bone requires special tissue processing for decalcification. Paraffin-fixed sections rather than standard fresh frozen sections can be used to delineate margins in difficult cases. Oil red O staining may be

helpful in the final delineation of sebaceous carcinoma and a diastase periodic acid Schiff (DPAS) stain may assist the treatment of extramammary Paget's disease. New advances using special stains, immunoperoxidase, or immunofluorescence may find a role in the delineation of tumors.[33, 34]

POSTOPERATIVE CONSIDERATIONS

One of the benefits of the fresh technique is the ability to proceed with reconstruction of the defect immediately after tumor extirpation.[35–42] This approach offers increased convenience for the patient, protection of critical structures, and sometimes a superior cosmetic outcome. Reconstruction may help to avoid complications such as osteomyelitis[43] and tendon rupture[44] that rarely may occur with second-intention healing.

Alternatively, second-intention healing should be considered as a simple, cost-effective, and safe approach offering equal or superior cosmetic results[45–47] in some cases compared with reconstructed wounds. This is especially true for concave or flat areas such as the temple, for small or superficial lesions, and for defects

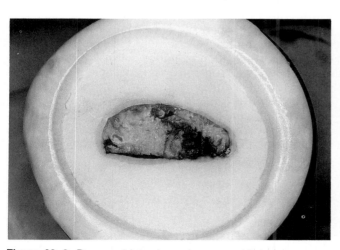

Figure 63–8. Deep and lateral margins are molded on a custom-made tissue processor.

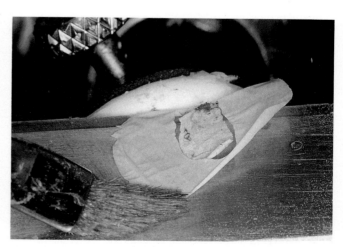

Figure 63–10. Thin sections of tissue are cut using the cryostat.

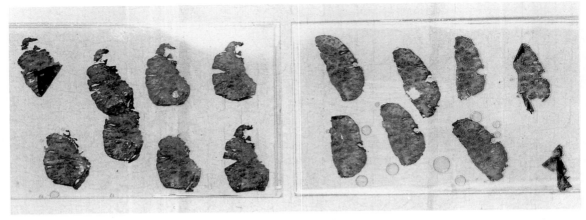

Figure 63–11. Representative sections are mounted on slides for subsequent microscopic examination.

at sites of lax skin. However, convex areas heal poorly with prominent scars.[48] For high-risk tumors treated with Mohs surgery, second-intention healing may be chosen because it permits observation of the wound bed for possible early detection of recurrence and avoids further alteration of tissue planes that may provide avenues for tumor growth.[49]

If a wound is allowed to heal by second intention, hemostatic agents such as Monsel's solution may be applied to the wound. Topical antibiotic ointment and a nonstick dressing is all that is generally needed.[6] Semipermeable dressings offer faster healing, decrease the frequency of dressing changes, possibly reduce pain, and provide more cosmetically acceptable scars.[50, 51] Multiple synthetic surgical dressings are now available to help meet the many different needs of patients' wounds.

Postoperative narcotics are not generally needed, since an ice pack and acetaminophen are usually sufficient to provide pain relief. Patients with deeper wounds involving cartilage or muscle or requiring tight surgical closures may occasionally need a narcotic analgesic. Perioperative antibiotics also are not routinely required

when second-intention healing is chosen. However, the standard indications for the use of antibiotics in cutaneous surgery may be followed if the wound is closed primarily.[52, 53]

BENEFITS

The fresh tissue Mohs surgical technique offers several benefits to patients with a cutaneous carcinoma, including cost effectiveness, tissue conservation, and the highest possible cure rate of any technique available for the treatment of cutaneous carcinomas. It is a very cost-effective procedure because it is often used for outpatient ambulatory management of complex tumors that otherwise would frequently require hospitalization, general anesthesia, and significant facility fees. The cost effectiveness is further multiplied since recurrent tumors are minimized by the higher cure rates achieved with the Mohs technique. The technique also gives the surgeon confidence in the adequacy of the surgical margins. This allows conservative excisions to be performed without compromising the cure rates, which may make a crucial difference in areas such as the midface or ears,[54] digits, or penis.

Since the margins of a Mohs excision are more conservative than generally used in excision of cutaneous malignancies, this may allow for simpler reconstructive surgery. If multiple layers of excision are required, tissue conservation is further magnified because the extensions of the tumor are generally asymmetric. Even in small primary tumors of the nose, tissue conservation can be in excess of 30%.[55] In auricular neoplasms, an adequate standard excision would result in 180% more tissue removal for primary tumors and 347% more for recurrent tumors than was necessary with the Mohs approach.[56]

Basal Cell and Squamous Cell Carcinomas

Although the fresh technique was first applied to eyelid tumors in 1953, the effectiveness of the fresh

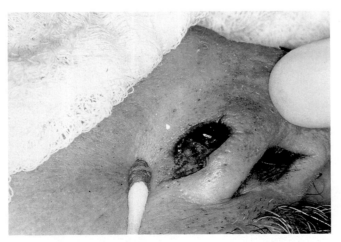

Figure 63–12. Limited re-excision of areas with persistent tumor is performed.

technique was not fully appreciated until the 1970s. A total of 532 tumors were reported in the classic 1978 article,[6] with an overall cure rate of 97.2%. With follow-up periods of more than 1 year, successful treatment was reported in 99.8% of all basal cell carcinomas (3466 cases) and 98.8% of 822 cases of squamous cell carcinoma (SCC) followed for at least 1 year.[3] Similar high cure rates for both basal cell and squamous cell carcinomas[7, 8] have been demonstrated by other authors. The fresh technique is now firmly established as a highly successful treatment of cutaneous carcinoma that is as effective as the fixed technique. This unparalleled effectiveness demanded its implementation in the management of difficult recurrent tumors and high risk primary tumors (Table 63–3).[57]

Recurrent tumors are a prime indication for Mohs surgery. These tumors appear to be more aggressive from the onset[18] and are complicated by the scar tissue and anatomic alterations resulting from the previous surgery. This creates further problems in accurately assessing the extent of a tumor. Traditional treatment of recurrent basal cell carcinomas[57] is associated with an even higher recurrence rate, generally 20 to 50%.[58, 59] These tumors can be successfully treated by Mohs surgery with only slightly less effectiveness than for primary tumors, consistently in the 94 to 97% success range.[3, 7, 8] Mohs surgery appears to be almost equally effective in the treatment of recurrent SCC.[60] However, other factors such as tumor size and site significantly affect the outcome and must be taken into consideration when discussing prognosis.

HIGH-RISK BASAL CELL CARCINOMAS

Because of the exceptionally high cure rates, despite the referral bias that tends to select high-risk tumors, Mohs surgery is clearly indicated in the treatment of primary basal cell carcinomas at high risk for recurrence. These tumors can be identified from clinical and histologic data[61–64] as tumors larger than 2 cm and those that have poorly defined margins, arise in a scar,[65] or have aggressive histologic subtypes,[58, 66] including infiltrating,[67] morpheaform, adenoid, basosquamous, and multifocal patterns. Tumors that have small spike-shaped cells, strands of microfoci, and other poorly organized histologic patterns are commonly very aggressive. Recurrences of basal cell carcinomas can also be predicted by the anatomic location. These sites include the midface and periauricular areas, probably because tumors in these locations can invade deeply in anatomic folds, spread along tissue planes, perichondrium, or bone; and skip along nerves.[68–73] These are all areas highly recommended for Mohs surgery because of the higher risk of recurrence and need for maximal tissue conservation.

Eyelid Tumors

Periorbital tumors often represent a management problem since they can invade early and deeply in the medial canthal area and on the eyelids, spread along nerves[68] and into the lacrimal system, or erode through

TABLE 63–3. INDICATIONS FOR MOHS SURGERY

Tissue conservation
  Penis, digits, nose, lips, ears, eyes
  Basal cell nevus syndrome
Lesions at risk for recurrence
  Recurrent lesions
  Tumors arising in scars
  Large tumors (>2 cm)
  Tumors with ill-defined or vague borders
Anatomic locations with high risk of recurrence
  Mid-face
    Ear, lip, nose
  Temple
  Lower limb, trunk
  Penis, mucosa
Lesions with aggressive histology
  Basal cell carcinoma
    Morpheaform
    Infiltrating
    Adenoid
    Basosquamous
    Multifocal
    Perineural involvement
  Squamous cell carcinoma
    Poorly differentiated
    Deeply invasive
    Perineural involvement
Immunosuppressed patients

the thin bones of the periorbital area. Tissue conservation is also of critical importance in this area for a good functional result. A 99% cure of basal cell carcinomas on the lids and canthal areas has been reported with Mohs surgery, and yet tissue conservation is maximized.[69] Critical lid tissue and elements of the lacrimal system may be salvaged with this technique, and even deep orbital tumors can be successfully removed without exenterations.[70] The complete sectioning of the tissue may allow for better recognition and subsequent treatment of any spread of tumor cells in the perineural or perilacrimal system. At times a combined multispecialty approach may be best for complete resection of very aggressive tumors of the orbit in order to obtain optimal function and cosmesis. In many cases, immediate reconstruction may be performed without compromising the eventual outcome.[71, 72] However, reconstruction should still be postponed, if possible, for tumors at higher risk for recurrence, such as after radiation. In this situation, even Mohs surgery has a failure rate of over 16%.[73]

Periauricular Tumors

Periauricular tumors are often treated with Mohs surgery because of the high cure rates achievable even in an area at risk for recurrence, as well as the need for tissue conservation.[74–79] In this area, tumor spread can be extensive, along the cartilage or into the external ear canal.[79] Even small primary tumors of the ear would be incompletely resected in 13% of patients if conventional excision were performed.[78] Although periauricular tumors are highly amenable to Mohs surgery, special attention is required in the posterior auricular fold, the site of highest recurrence (over 16%), after Mohs surgery.[7] An additional margin of tissue beyond the established clear margins and second intention healing should be used in this site. When the tumor is extensive or involves the ear canal,[79] parotid gland,[80] or facial nerve, a multispecialty approach with the fresh tissue technique can be satisfactory.

Nasal Tumors

The nose is the most common site for basal cell carcinoma and unfortunately is the highest site of recurrence, with a relative risk of 2.38-fold[8] from conventional surgical procedures. Tumors may invade into muscle or spread along nasal cartilage or bone.[81, 82] Despite these potential problems, Mohs surgery offers a 97 to 99% cure rate for basal cell carcinomas in this location.[3, 7] Thus, Mohs surgery is recommended, even for small primary tumors of the nose, since asymmetric extension beyond a standard 2 mm margin is common.[55] Tissue conservation made possible with Mohs surgery may result in more superficial[83] or smaller defects and may well permit salvaging the alar rim, which helps to avoid full-thickness defects. When large tumors, especially morpheaform and recurrent types, deeply involve folds or the nasal septa, a multispecialty approach may be best.[81, 82]

Squamous Cell Carcinomas

SCCs are common management problems because of the risk of recurrence and metastasis coupled with the desire for maximal tissue conservation.

Lip Tumors

SCC of the lip is very amenable to treatment with Mohs surgery, with a reported 94.2% cure rate in 1448 patients.[84] A 1990 report of 41 thin SCCs of the lower lip with a 100% success rate attests to the efficacy of the Mohs surgical technique[85] in early lesions. The tissue conservation made possible with this technique helps to avoid the standard deforming wedge resection.

Genital Tumors

SCC of the genitalia may be a serious problem commonly associated with regional metastasis. The fixed tissue Mohs surgical technique is often effective in treatment of these locations, especially in distal or primary tumors.[86] Although the hemostatic nature of the fixed technique is good for this site, the fresh technique can also be used effectively, especially for smaller lesions, while producing less pain and providing more rapid treatment. SCCs of the penis were treated with Mohs surgery in 11 patients.[87] Although local control was achieved in all but one of these patients, four developed regional lymph node involvement. Evaluation by a urologist is recommended in caring for these types of patients.

Digital Tumors

Mohs surgery is also effective for tumors of the digit.[88–92] In a report of 24 lesions, only two recurrences were noted.[88] The fresh tissue technique can be used in most instances, although the fixed technique is preferable for tumors invading bone. The main benefit of the Mohs approach to digital tumors is that it avoids amputation of the digit without compromising the cure rate.

Oral Cavity Tumors

SCCs of the oral cavity are often difficult to manage. The fresh technique is most appropriate for smaller tumors.[3] In a report of 43 cases of oral carcinoma treated with the Mohs technique, 24 of 34 evaluable patients were alive and tumor-free.[93] Larger margins than recommended for cutaneous carcinomas have been recommended: 1 to 2 cm.[93, 94] The use of Mohs surgery in a multidisciplinary team has also been advocated[94] for oral tumors.

Risk Factors for Recurrences

Despite the high overall success rate of Mohs surgery in the treatment of SCCs, there remain several problems that must be considered, including local recurrences and metastasis. Several risks for recurrence of cutaneous SCC after Mohs surgery have been identified: tumors found on the lower extremity in patients under 39 years of age, lesions greater than 5 cm in diameter, and those requiring more than four layers of excision had high recurrence rates.[60, 95] Removal of an additional tissue margin after achieving a tumor-free plane has been recommended to improve local control of large recurrent tumors.[60, 95] High-risk tumors arising in scars, ulcers, or radiation sites can likewise be considered for Mohs surgery for improved local control of disease despite the recognized high metastatic potential.

Perineural involvement by SCC is another high-risk situation. Perineural spread tumor of SCC,[96–98] and less commonly basal cell carcinoma,[99–102] may occur, usually along terminal branches of the trigeminal and facial nerves. Pain, dysesthesia, and motor dysfunction may be noted, but perineural involvement may also present as a histologic finding on tissue processing. The complete margin processing with the Mohs surgical technique allows the recognition of perineural tumor and enables tumor to be traced out to its full extent. Skipping tumor has been described with SCC, and an additional surgical margin beyond identifiable tumor or perineural inflammation, suggestive of adjacent tumor, should be considered.[97] The patient who is thought to be at higher risk for nodal spread and metastasis should be considered for adjunctive therapy such as radiation or prophylactic lymph node dissection. Unfortunately, clear treatment guidelines do not yet exist. Interspecialty consultation may be helpful in ensuring delivery of the best care of these high-risk patients.

Other forms of SCC can also be effectively managed with the Mohs fresh tissue technique. These include tumors of the scalp, which can be quite extensive, can invade deeply down to or into bone, and have striking peripheral silent extensions. The largest series of 131 SCCs of the scalp reported almost a 99% cure.[102] This compares most favorably with earlier reports of 5-year cures in the 80% range with traditional therapy.[103] Mohs surgery has also been reportedly used with success to treat several exceptionally large tumors.[102–108]

Special Indications

There are a few other situations and tumors in which Mohs surgery also represents a superb form of treatment (Table 63–4). The types of tumors treated by Mohs surgery continue to expand as the technique is applied to less common malignancies.

MOHS CHECK

If a patient has a subtotally resected tumor, the overall recurrence rate for basal cell carcinomas is approximately 35%. However, this rate is much higher (82%) around the eyes, ears, and nose.[109] A conservative re-excision with a Mohs check[110] is sometimes indicated for these locations. This is performed by excising the scar with conservative margins, bisecting the tissue along the long axis, and then processing the outer margins using the standard Mohs processing technique.

BASAL CELL NEVUS SYNDROME AND IMMUNOSUPPRESSED PATIENTS

Patients with the basal cell nevus syndrome have multiple lesions that demand the maximal tissue conservation and effectiveness offered by the Mohs surgical technique.[111] Patients who are immunosuppressed as a result of organ transplantation, leukemia, lymphoma, or chronic use of oral corticosteroids develop a high number of tumors, predominantly SCCs, that may behave very aggressively and result in metastasis.[112] These patients also would obviously benefit from Mohs surgery.

TABLE 63–4. TUMORS TREATED WITH MOHS FRESH TECHNIQUE

Basal cell carcinoma
Squamous cell carcinoma (SCC)
  SCC in situ
  Bowen's disease
  Erythroplasia of Queyrat
  Verrucous carcinoma
Keratoacanthoma
Dermatofibrosarcoma protuberans
Atypical fibroxanthoma
Malignant fibrous histiocytoma
Sebaceous carcinoma
Extramammary Paget's disease
Melanoma
Lentigo maligna
Eccrine adenocarcinoma
Merkel's cell tumor
Adenocystic carcinoma
Leiomyosarcoma
Angiosarcoma
Granular cell tumor
Apocrine adenocarcinoma

VERRUCOUS CARCINOMA

This tumor, considered a variant of SCC, may occur on the foot, scalp, and genitalia or in the mouth. Recurrences with other forms of treatment are common, and more aggressive behavior after radiation has also been described. There are several reports of successful treatment of this tumor by the Mohs fresh tissue technique,[87, 113–119] documenting its effectiveness and tissue conservation. In this way, amputation of the penis or foot may be avoided.

BOWEN'S DISEASE

This tumor typically can be easily treated by many different modalities, and Mohs surgery is usually unnecessary. However, for some critical sites such as a digit, the need for tissue conservation may warrant use of Mohs surgery.[119] The potentially more aggressive erythroplasia of the penis can be treated with several destructive modalities as well as the classic fixed tissue Mohs surgical technique. This SCC in situ can also be treated via the fresh tissue Mohs surgical approach with a high level of confidence.[87]

KERATOACANTHOMAS

The Mohs technique can be very effective for these tumors. In one report of 115 keratoacanthomas treated by the fresh tissue technique, almost complete success was achieved, although one tumor was subtotally resected and its eradication was completed with topical 5-fluorouracil.[3] The effectiveness was demonstrated again in another reported series of 42 keratoacanthomas with only a single recurrence.[120] Clearly, Mohs surgery is a tissue-sparing excisional technique of exceptional value that should be considered in several situations: large or recurrent lesions, lesions that threaten an important structure, and patients who are immunosuppressed.[121]

DERMATOFIBROSARCOMA PROTUBERANS

These tumors tend to invade widely, far beyond the clinically eivdent margins. Recurrences, even when using margins of 3 cm width, are not uncommon. There are several case reports of successful treatment of this tumor and malignant fibrous histiocytoma by the fresh tissue Mohs technique.[122–126] Two series have established this treatment as the one of choice for dermatofibrosarcoma protuberans. One report of four cases showed no recurrences for at least 5 years.[127] In three of these cases, subtotal excision would have resulted if traditional 3 cm margins were used. Another report of ten patients followed for an average of 3.5 years confirmed the value of this technique.[128] Finally, another 13 cases without recurrence have been reported,[129] further substantiating the fact that Mohs surgery is indicated in the treatment of this tumor.

Other fibrous tumors, including malignant histiocytomas,[3, 126, 129] can also be effectively managed with fresh tissue Mohs surgical technique. In a series of 17 malignant fibrous histiocytomas treated with the fresh technique, two recurrences were reported. Although one patient died of metastatic disease, the other was successfully treated with a second Mohs procedure.[129] Atypical fibroxanthomas, a low-grade histiocytic tumor that rarely metastasizes, have also been treated with the fresh tissue Mohs technique with no reported recurrences.[129]

EXTRAMAMMARY PAGET'S DISEASE

This condition is associated with wide, clinically unapparent tumor spread, an obvious indication for Mohs surgery. Recurrent extramammary Paget's disease has been treated by the fresh technique.[3, 130] Tumor extension was detected far beyond the clinical margins. No recurrences were reported during a follow-up period ranging from 4 months to 9 years. Additional instances of successful treatment of Paget's disease have also now been described.[131, 132] One useful modification in the approach to this tumor is a 10-day preoperative course of topical 5-fluorouracil to help highlight the tumor.[132] Periodic acid–Schiff (PAS) staining with diastase digestion may also assist identification of the Paget cells.[131]

MICROCYSTIC ADENOCARCINOMA

This slow-growing, relatively benign tumor is not typically associated with metastasis, and local nodal spread is also rare. Two patients with extensive disease treated with Mohs surgery have been reported. Each required multiple layers of excision despite having primary tumors less than 2 cm in size.[135] The nature of this tumor make it ideal for treatment by Mohs surgery.

SEBACEOUS CARCINOMA OF EYELID

This tumor is a rare and aggressive carcinoma associated with local recurrence and metastatic spread. A few reported cases have been successfully approached with the fresh tissue Mohs technique,[136–138] but recurrences after apparent successful excisions have also been reported.[139] The potential for skip areas and irregular pagetoid spread suggests that a guarded confidence in a conservative Mohs excision is appropriate.[139, 140] The sebaceous cell carcinoma cells stain positively with oil red O stain, which may help histologic recognition of the tumor cells.[140]

ECCRINE-ASSOCIATED TUMORS

These tumors can also be effectively treated with Mohs surgery. Three cases of eccrine epithelioma, an invasive tumor of the scalp, have been reported.[141] More serious eccrine adenocarcinomas have also been treated using the fresh Mohs surgical approach, as have three cases of syringoid adenocarcinoma.[142] Mohs surgery may improve the ability to trace out these eccrine tumors, but if discontinuous tumor growth occurs, there is limited benefit from the Mohs surgical technique.[143] Eccrine-associated tumors are a varied group of tumors with great differences in behavior[144] that must be individually evaluated.

MELANOMA

The use of the fixed technique for melanoma has been advocated for decades, because of the lack of tumor manipulation. However, use of the fresh tissue technique for periorbital tumors of the eyelid margin and bulbar conjunctiva was reported in 1985,[145] and for a single small ear lesion in 1988.[146] The experience was substantially broadened by a report of 200 patients treated with the fresh technique.[147] Despite this, the use of fresh or fixed tissue Mohs surgery for melanoma is still a matter of considerable debate. However, it may be considered as an alternative to traditional resection of amelanotic tumors, tumors of poor definition, or tumors in areas where maximal tissue conservation is an important consideration. Lentigo maligna can also be treated with the fresh tissue technique.[147] Since this tumor is less aggressive, the use of Mohs surgery is less controversial.

MISCELLANEOUS TUMORS

Other tumors treated with the fresh tissue technique include Merkel's cell carcinoma,[148] giant granular cell tumor, adenoid cystic carcinoma,[149] angiosarcoma,[150] leiomyosarcoma,[87] and apocrine adenocarcinoma.[151] The fresh tissue approach has also been reported to have encouraging success in extracutaneous head and neck tumors.[93, 94, 152]

SUMMARY

The fresh tissue Mohs surgical technique has greatly improved the treatment of cutaneous carcinomas. Any tumor with relatively low metastatic potential that grows in a contiguous manner can be considered appropriate for Mohs fresh tissue excision. This is especially true if recurrences are frequent owing to subtotal resection with conventional surgical techniques, or if there is a need for maximal tissue conservation. This technique is now firmly established in the surgical armamentarium for the effective management of many different types of skin cancer. As experience with the technique continues to grow, it is certain that further indications will be recognized in the future.

The author wishes to thank Mr. David Gresh for his assistance with the photographic illustrations in this chapter.

REFERENCES

1. Mohs FE: Mohs micrographic surgery: a historical perspective. Dermatol Clin 7:609–612, 1989.
2. Mohs FE: Microscopically controlled surgery for skin cancer—past, present and future. J Dermatol Surg Oncol 4:41–53, 1978.
3. Mohs FE: Chemosurgery: Microscopically Controlled Surgery for Skin Cancer. Charles C Thomas, Springfield, IL, 1978.
4. Cottel WI, Bailin PL, Albom MJ, et al: Essentials of Mohs micrographic surgery. J Dermatol Surg Oncol 14:11–13, 1988.
5. Tromovitch TA, Stegman SJ: Microscopically controlled excision of skin tumors: chemosurgery (Mohs) fresh technique. Arch Dermatol 110:231–232, 1974.
6. Tromovitch TA, Stegman SJ: Microscopic-controlled excision of

cutaneous tumors: chemosurgery, fresh tissue technique. Cancer 41:653–658, 1978.

7. Robins P: Chemosurgery: my 15 years of experience. J Dermatol Surg Oncol 7:779–789, 1981.

8. Roenigk, RK, Ratz JL, Bailin PL, Wheeland RG: Trends in the presentation and treatment of basal cell carcinomas. J Dermatol Surg Oncol 12:860–865, 1986.

9. Swanson NA, Taylor WB, Tromovitch TA: Commentary: the evolution of Mohs surgery. J Dermatol Surg Oncol 8:650–654, 1982.

10. Swanson NA: Mohs surgery: the technique, indications, applications, and the future. Arch Dermatol 119:761–773, 1983.

11. Braun M: The case for Mohs surgery by the fixed tissue technique. J Dermatol Surg Oncol 7:634–640, 1981.

12. Cottel WI, Proper S: Mohs surgery, fresh tissue technique: our technique with a review. J Dermatol Surg Oncol 8:576–587, 1982.

13. Lang PG: Mohs micrographic surgery. Fresh tissue technique. Dermatol Clin 7:613–626, 1989.

14. Stewart JH, Chinn SE, Cole GW, Klein JA: Neutralized lidocaine with epinephrine for local anesthesia—II. J Dermatol Surg Oncol 16:842–845, 1989.

15. Panje WR: Local anesthesia of the face. J Dermatol Surg Oncol 5:311–315, 1979.

16. Burg G, Hirsch RD, Konz B, et al: Histographic surgery: accuracy of visual assessment of the margins of basal cell carcinoma. J Dermatol Surg 1:21–24, 1975.

17. Wolf DJ, Zitelli JA: Surgical margins for basal cell carcinoma. Arch Dermatol 123:340–344, 1987.

18. Lange PG, Maize JC: Histologic evolution of recurrent basal cell carcinoma and treatment implications. J Am Acad Dermatol 14:186–196, 1986.

19. Salasche SJ, Amonette RA: Morpheaform basal cell epitheliomas. A study of subclinical extensions in a series of 51 cases. J Dermatol Surg Oncol 7:387–394, 1981.

20. Larson PO: Staple and double staple method of tissue orientation in Mohs micrographic surgery. J Dermatol Surg Oncol 13:732–734, 1987.

21. Koranda FC, Heffron ET, Modert CW, Perkins LL: Photomapping for microscopically controlled surgery. J Dermatol Surg Oncol 8:463–465, 1982.

22. Picoto AM, Picoto A: Technical procedures for Mohs fresh tissue surgery. J Dermatol Surg Oncol 12:134–138, 1986.

23. Hanke CW, Lee MW: Cryostat use and tissue processing in Mohs micrographic surgery. J Dermatol Surg Oncol 15:29–32, 1989.

24. Bentley TJ, Koranda FC, Miller LM: Histologic evaluation of horizontal frozen sections. Improved staining and special staining techniques. J Dermatol Surg Oncol 8:466–470, 1982.

25. Rustad OJ, Kaye V, Cerio R, Zachary CB: Postfixation of cryostat sections improves tumor definition in Mohs surgery. J Dermatol Surg Oncol 15:1262–1267, 1989.

26. Grabski WJ, Salasche SJ, McCollough ML, et al: Interpretation of Mohs micrographic frozen sections: a peer review comparison study. J Am Acad Dermatol 20:670–674, 1989.

27. Dzubow LM: Recurrence (persistence) of tumor following excision by Mohs surgery. J Dermatol Surg Oncol 13:27–30, 1987.

28. Rapini RP: Pitfalls of Mohs micrographic surgery. J Am Acad Dermatol 22:681–686, 1990.

29. Bailin PL, Ratz JL, Lutz-Nagey L: CO_2 laser modification of Mohs surgery. J Dermatol Surg Oncol 7:621–623, 1981.

30. Ceilley RI, Bumsted RM, Panje WR: Delayed skin grafting. J Dermatol Surg Oncol 9:288–293, 1983.

31. Vanderveen EE, Stoner JG, Swanson NA: Chiseling of exposed bone to stimulate granulation tissue after Mohs surgery. J Dermatol Surg Oncol 9:925–928, 1983.

32. Bailin PL, Wheeland RG: Carbon dioxide (CO_2) laser perforation of exposed bone to stimulate granulation tissue. Plast Reconstr Surg 75:898–902, 1985.

33. Silvis NG, Swanson PE, Manivel JC, et al: Spindle cell and pleomorphic neoplasms of the skin—a clinicopathologic and immunohistochemical study of 30 cases with emphasis on "atypical" fibroxanthoma. Am J Dermatopathol 10:9–19, 1988.

34. Oseroff AR, Roth R: Use of a murine monoclonal antibody which binds to malignant keratinocytes to detect tumor cells in microscopically controlled surgery. J Am Acad Dermatol 8: 616–619, 1983.

35. Larrabee WF: Immediate repair of facial defects. Dermatol Clin 7:661–676, 1989.

36. Robins P, Pollack SV, Robinson JK: Immediate repair of wounds following operations by Mohs' fresh technique. J Dermatol Surg Oncol 5:329–336, 1979.

37. Casson PR, Baker DC: Reconstruction of defects following Mohs surgery. J Dermatol Surg Oncol 7:811–813, 1981.

38. Smith JD: Surgical repair of defects resulting from the serial fresh tissue technique of Mohs. J Dermatol Surg Oncol 3:184–187, 1977.

39. Bennett RG, Robins P: Repair of tissue defects resulting from removal of cutaneous neoplasms. J Dermatol Surg Oncol 3:512–517, 1977.

40. Becker FF: Reconstruction of facial defects resulting from Mohs chemosurgical procedures. J Dermatol Surg Oncol 4:69–76, 1978.

41. Whitaker DC, Birkby CS: An approach to cutaneous surgical defects of forehead and eyebrow following Mohs micrographic surgery. J Dermatol Surg Oncol 13:1312–1317, 1987.

42. Whitaker DC, Goldstein GD: Lateral nose and perinasal defects: options in management following Mohs micrographic surgery for cutaneous carcinoma. J Dermatol Surg Oncol 14:177–183, 1988.

43. Snyder PA, Alper JC, Albom MJ: Osteomyelitis complicating Mohs chemosurgery. J Am Acad Dermatol 11:513–516, 1984.

44. Gaspari AA, Surge d'Aubermont PC, Bennett RC: Delayed extensor tendon rupture: a complication of Mohs surgery. J Dermatol Surg Oncol 10:721–723, 1984.

45. Barton FE, Cottel WI, Walker B: The principles of chemosurgery and delayed primary reconstruction in management of difficult basal cell carcinomas. Plast Reconstr Surg 68:746–752, 1981.

46. Goldwyn RM, Rueckert F: The value of healing by second intention for sizable defects of the face. Arch Surg 112:285–292, 1977.

47. Panje WR, Bumsted RM, Ceilley RI: Secondary intention healing as an adjunct to the reconstruction of mid facial defects. Laryngoscope 90:1149–1154, 1980.

48. Zitelli JA: Wound healing by second intention: a cosmetic appraisal. J Am Acad Dermatol 9:407–415, 1983.

49. Albom MJ: Surgical gems: the management of recurrent basal-cell carcinomas. Please, no grafts or flaps at once. J Dermatol Surg Oncol 3:382–384, 1977.

50. Roth RR, Winton GB: A synthetic skin substitute as a temporary dressing in Mohs surgery. J Dermatol Surg Oncol 15:670–672, 1989.

51. Hien NT, Prawer SE, Katz HI: Facilitated wound healing using transparent film dressing following Mohs micrographic surgery. Arch Dermatol 124:903–906, 1988.

52. Sebben JE: Sterile technique and the prevention of wound infection in office surgery—Part I. J Dermatol Surg Oncol 14:1364–1371, 1988.

53. Sebben JE: Sterile technique and the prevention of wound infection in office surgery—Part II. J Dermatol Surg Oncol 15:38–48, 1989.

54. Bailin PL, Levine HL, Wood HL, Tucker H: Tissue conservation in treatment of cutaneous neoplasms of the head and neck. Arch Otolaryngol 105:140–144, 1979.

55. Dufresne RG, Garrett AG, Bailin PL, Ratz JL: Mohs surgery of 500 small primary tumors of the nose: patterns of spread. Presented at the American College of Mohs Micrographic Surgery and Oncology, Fort Lauderdale, FL, March, 1988.

56. Bumsted RM, Ceilley RI: Auricular malignant neoplasms. Arch Otolaryngol 108:225–231, 1982.

57. Albright SD: Treatment of skin cancers using multiple modalities. J Am Acad Dermatol 7:143–171, 1982.

58. Menn H, Robins P, Kopf AW, et al: The recurrent basal cell epithelioma. A study of 100 cases of recurrent retreated basal cell epithelioma. Arch Dermatol 103:628–631, 1971.

59. Rowe DE, Carroll RJ, Day CL: Mohs surgery is the treatment of choice for recurrent (previously treated) basal cell carcinoma. J Dermatol Surg Oncol 15:424–431, 1989.

60. Dzubow LM, Rigel DS, Robins P: Risk factors for local recurrence of primary cutaneous squamous cell carcinoma. Arch Dermatol 118:900–902, 1982.

61. Levine HL, Bailin PL: Basal cell carcinoma of the head and

neck. Identification of the high risk patient. Laryngoscope 90:955–961, 1980.

62. Sloan JP: The value of typing basal cell carcinoma and predicting recurrence after surgical excision. Br J Dermatol 96:127–132, 1977.

63. Taylor GA, Barison D: Ten years experience in the surgical treatment of basal cell carcinoma: a study of factors associated with recurrence. Br J Surg 60:522–525, 1973.

64. Koplin L, Rarem HA: Recurrent basal cell carcinoma. A review concerning the incidence, behavior and management of recurrent basal cell carcinoma with emphasis on the incompletely excised lesion. Plast Reconstr Surg 65:656–663, 1980.

65. Noodleman R, Pollack SV: Trauma as a possible etiologic factor in basal cell carcinoma. J Dermatol Surg Oncol 12:841–846, 1986.

66. Jacobs GH, Rippey JJ, Altini M: Prediction of aggressive behavior in basal cell carcinoma. Cancer 49:533–557, 1982.

67. Siegle RJ, MacMillan J, Pollack SV: Infiltrating basal cell carcinoma: a nonsclerosing type. J Dermatol Surg Oncol 12:830–836, 1986.

68. Weimar MW, Ceilley RI: Basal cell carcinoma of a medial canthus with invasion of supraorbital and supratrochlear nerves: report of a case treated by Mohs technique. J Dermatol Surg Oncol 5:279–282, 1979.

69. Mohs FE: Micrographic surgery for the microscopically controlled excision of eyelid tumors. Arch Ophthalmol 104:901–909, 1986.

70. Monheit GD, Callahan MA, Callahan A: Mohs micrographic surgery for periorbital skin cancer. Dermatol Clin 7:677–697, 1989.

71. Ceilly RI, Anderson RL: Microscopically controlled excision of neoplasms on and around eyelids followed by immediate surgical reconstruction. J Dermatol Surg Oncol 4:55–62, 1978.

72. Anderson RL: Mohs micrographic technique. Arch Ophthalmol 104:818–819, 1986.

73. Robins P, Rodriguez-Sains R, Rabinovitz H, Rigel D: Mohs surgery for periocular basal cell carcinoma. J Dermatol Surg Oncol 11:1203–1207, 1985.

74. Ceilley RI, Bumsted RM, Smith WH: Malignancies on the external ear: methods of ablation and reconstruction of defects. J Dermatol Surg Oncol 5:762–767, 1979.

75. Bailin PL, Levine HL, Wood HL, Tucker HM: Cutaneous carcinoma of the auricular and preauricular region. Arch Otolaryngol 106:692–696, 1980.

76. Levine HL, Kinney SE, Bailin PL, Roberts JK: Cancer of the periauricular region. Dermatol Clin 7:781–795, 1989.

77. Clarke DP, Hanke CW: Neoplasms of the conchal bowl: treatment with Mohs micrographic surgery. J Dermatol Surg Oncol 14:1223–1228, 1988.

78. Bumsted RM, Ceilley RI, Panje WR, Crumley RL: Auricular malignant neoplasms: when is chemotherapy (Mohs' technique) necessary? Arch Otolaryngol 107:721–724, 1981.

79. Hanke CW, Temofeew RK, Miyamoto RT, Lingeman RE: Basal cell carcinoma involving the external auditory canal: treatment with Mohs micrographic surgery. J Dermatol Surg Oncol 11:1189–1194, 1985.

80. Hanke CW, Weisberg EC: Invasion of parotid gland by basal cell carcinoma: implications for therapy. J Dermatol Surg Oncol 12:849–852, 1986.

81. Siegle RJ, Schuller DE: Multidiscplinary surgical approach to the treatment of perinasal nonmelanoma skin cancer. Dermatol Clin 7:711–731, 1989.

82. Baker SR, Swanson NA: Management of nasal cutaneous malignant neoplasms. An interdisciplinary approach. Arch Otolaryngol 109:473–479, 1983.

83. Grabski WJ, Salasche SJ: Razor blade excision of Mohs surgery for superficial basal cell carcinoma of the distal nose. J Dermatol Surg Oncol 14:1290–1292, 1988.

84. Mohs FE, Snow SN: Microscopically controlled surgical treatment for squamous cell carcinoma of the lower lip. Surg Gynecol Obstet 160:37–41, 1985.

85. Mehregan DA, Roenigk RK: Management of superficial squamous cell carcinoma of the lip with Mohs micrographic surgery. Cancer 66:463–468, 1990.

86. Mohs FE, Snow SN, Messing EM, Kuglitsch ME: Microscopi-

cally controlled surgery in the treatment of carcinoma of the penis. J Urol 133:961–966, 1985.

87. Brown MC, Zachary CB, Grekin RC, Swanson NA: Penile tumors: their management by Mohs micrographic surgery. J Dermatol Surg Oncol 13:1163–1167, 1987.

88. Mikhail GK: Subungual epidermoid carcinoma. J Am Acad Dermatol 1:291–298, 1984.

89. Tomsick RS, Menn H: Squamous cell carcinoma of the fingers treated with chemosurgery. South Med J 77:1124–1126, 1984.

90. Albom MJ: Squamous cell carcinoma of the finger and nail bed. A review of the literature and treatment by the Mohs surgical technique. J Dermatol Surg 1:473–477, 1975.

91. Goldberg DJ, Robins P: Subungual squamous cell carcinoma treated by Mohs surgery in a patient with sarcoidosis. J Dermatol Surg Oncol 12:972–974, 1986.

92. Mikhail GR: Subungual basal cell carcinoma. J Dermatol Surg Oncol 11:1222–1223, 1985.

93. Davidson TM, Haghigi P, Artarita R, et al: Mohs for head and neck mucosal cancer: report on 111 patients. Laryngoscope 98:1078–1083, 1988.

94. Baker SR, Swanson NA: Cancer of the oral cavity and Mohs surgery. Dermatol Clin 7:815–824, 1989.

95. Robins P, Dzubow LM, Rigel DS: Squamous cell carcinoma treated by Mohs surgery. An experience with 414 cases in a period of 15 years. J Dermatol Surg Oncol 7:800–801, 1981.

96. Weimar VM, Ceilley RI, Babin RW: Squamous cell carcinoma with invasion of the facial nerve and underlying bone and muscle: report of a case. J Dermatol Surg Oncol 5:526–530, 1979.

97. Cottel WI: Perineural invasion by squamous cell carcinoma. J Dermatol Surg Oncol 8:589–600, 1982.

98. Birkby CS, Whitaker DC: Management considerations for cutaneous neurophilic tumors. J Dermatol Surg Oncol 14:731–737, 1988.

99. Morris JGL, Joffe R: Perineural spread of cutaneous basal cell and squamous cell carcinoma. Arch Neurol 40:424–429, 1983.

100. Mark GJ: Basal cell carcinoma with intraneural invasion. Cancer 40:2181–2187, 1977.

101. Hanke CW, Wolf RL, Hichman SA, O'Brian JJ: Perineural spread of basal cell carcinoma. J Dermatol Surg Oncol 9:742–747, 1983.

102. Mohs FE, Zitelli JA: Microscopically controlled surgery in the treatment of carcinoma of the scalp. Arch Dermatol 117:764–769, 1981.

103. Conley JJ: Malignant tumors of the scalp: analysis of 92 cases of malignant epithelial and somatic tumors of the scalp. Plast Reconstr Surg 33:1–15, 1964.

104. Binstock JH, Stegman SJ, Tromovitch TA: Large aggressive basal cell carcinoma of the scalp. J Dermatol Surg Oncol 7:565–568, 1981.

105. Peters CR, Dinner MI, Dolsky RL, et al: The combined multispecialty approach to invasive basal cell carcinoma of the scalp. Ann Plast Surg 4:199–204, 1980.

106. Hanke CW, Weisberger EC, Lingeman RE: Cancer of the scalp. Dermatol Clin 7:797–814, 1989.

107. Bekamjian VY, Morain WD, Phelan JT: Massive basal cell carcinoma of the scalp: successful management by cooperation of the chemosurgeon and reconstructive surgeon. Ann Plast Surg 1:421–428, 1978.

108. Bloom RF, Mohs FE, Way BH: Chemosurgical excision of recurrent basal cell carcinoma of the scalp. Cutis 22:602–603, 1978.

109. Thomas P: Treatment of basal cell carcinomas of the head and neck. Rev Surg 27:293–294, 1970.

110. Swanson NA, Tromovitch TA, Stegman SJ, Glogau RG: A novel method of re-excising incompletely excised basal cell carcinomas. J Dermatol Surg Oncol 6:438–439, 1980.

111. Mohs FE, Jones DC, Koranda FD: Microscopically controlled surgery for carcinomas in patients with nevoid basal cell syndrome. Arch Dermatol 116:777–779, 1980.

112. Dinehart SM, Chu DZJ, Maners AW, Pollack SV: Immunosuppression in patients with metastatic squamous cell carcinoma from the skin. J Dermatol Surg Oncol 16:271–274, 1990.

113. Mohs FE, Sahl WJ: Chemosurgery for verrucous carcinoma. J Dermatol Surg Oncol 5:302–306, 1979.

114. Mallatt BD, Ceilley RI, Dryer RF: Management of verrucous

carcinoma on a foot by a combination of chemosurgery and plastic repair: Report of a case. J Dermatol Surg Oncol 6:532–534, 1980.

115. Swanson NA, Taylor WB: Plantar verrucous carcinoma. Literature and treatment by the Mohs chemosurgical technique. Arch Dermatol 116:794–797, 1980.

116. Mora RG: Microscopically controlled surgery (Mohs chemosurgery) for treatment of verrucous squamous cell carcinoma of the foot (epithelioma cuniculatum). J Am Acad Dermatol 8:354–362, 1983.

117. Padilla RS, Bailin PL, Howard WR, Dinner MI: Verrucous carcinoma of the skin and its management by Mohs surgery. Plast Reconstr Surg 73:442–447, 1984.

118. Hanke CW, Bailin PL, O'Brian JJ: Plantar verrucous carcinoma in black women. J Dermatol Surg Oncol 10:90–93, 1984.

119. Baran RL, Gormley DE: Polydactylous Bowen's disease of the nail. J Am Acad Dermatol 17:201–204, 1987.

120. Larson PO: Keratoacanthomas treated with Mohs' micrographic surgery (chemosurgery). J Am Acad Dermatol 16:1040–1044, 1987.

121. Piscioli F, Zumian G, Boi S, et al: A giant metastasizing keratoacanthoma. Am J Dermatopathol 6:123–129, 1984.

122. Mikhail GR, Lynn BH: Dermatofibrosarcoma protuberans. J Dermatol Surg Oncol 4:81–84, 1978.

123. Dzubow LM: Spindle cell fibrohistiocytic tumors: classification and pathophysiology. J Dermatol Surg Oncol 14:490–485, 1988.

124. Hess KA, Hanke CW, Estes NC, Shideler SJ: Myxoid dermatofibrosarcoma protuberans. J Dermatol Surg Oncol 11:268–271, 1985.

125. Goldberg DJ, Maso M: Dermatofibrosarcoma protuberans in a 9 year old child: treatment by Mohs micrographic surgery. Pediatr Dermatol 7:57–59, 1990.

126. Weimar VM, Ceilley RI: A myxoid variant of malignant fibrous histiocytoma: report of a case treated by Mohs technique with a slight modification. J Dermatol Surg Oncol 5:16–18, 1979.

127. Robinson JK: Dermatofibrosarcoma protuberans resected by Mohs surgery (chemosurgery). J Am Acad Dermatol 12:1093–1098, 1985.

128. Hobbs ER, Wheeland RG, Bailin PL, et al: Treatment of dermatofibrosarcoma protuberans with Mohs micrographic surgery. Ann Surg 207:102–107, 1988.

129. Brown MD, Swanson NA: Treatment of malignant fibrous histiocytoma and atypical fibrous xanthomas with micrographic surgery. J Dermatol Surg Oncol 15:1287–1292, 1989.

130. Mohs FE, Blanchard L: Microscopically controlled surgery for extramammary Paget's disease. Arch Dermatol 115:706–708, 1979.

131. Wagner RF, Cotell WI: Treatment of extensive extramammary Paget disease of male genitalia with Mohs micrographic surgery. Urology 16:415–418, 1988.

132. Eliezri YD, Silvers DN, Horan DB: Role of preoperative topical 5-fluoruracil in preparation for Mohs micrographic surgery of extramammary Paget's disease. J Am Acad Dermatol 17:497–505, 1987.

133. Cooper PH: Sclerosing carcinomas of sweat ducts (microscopic adnexal carcinoma). Arch Dermatol 122:261–264, 1986.

134. Fleischmann HE, Roth RJ, Wood CC, Nickoloff BJ: Microcystic adnexal carcinoma treated by microscopically controlled excision. J Dermatol Surg Oncol 10:873–875, 1984.

135. Nickoloff BJ, Fleischmann HE, Carmel J, et al: Microcystic adnexal carcinoma. Immunohistologic observations suggesting dual (pilar and eccrine) differentiation. Arch Dermatol 122:290–294, 1986.

136. Dixon RS, Mikhail GR, Slater HC: Sebaceous carcinoma of the eyelid. J Am Acad Dermatol 3:241–243, 1980.

137. Harvey JT, Anderson RL: The management of meibomian gland carcinoma. Ophthalmic Surg 13:56–61, 1982.

138. Ratz JL, Luu-Duong S, Kulwin DR: Sebaceous carcinoma of the eyelid treated with Mohs' surgery. J Am Acad Dermatol 14:668–673, 1986.

139. Folberg R, Whitaker DC, Tse DT, Nerad JA: Recurrent and residual sebaceous carcinoma after Mohs excision of the primary lesion. Am J Ophthalmol 103:817–823, 1987.

140. Dzubow LM: Sebaceous carcinoma of the eyelid: treatment with Mohs surgery. J Dermatol Surg Oncol 11:40–44, 1985.

141. Hanke CW, Temofeew RK: Basal cell carcinoma with eccrine differentiation (eccrine epithelioma). J Dermatol Surg Oncol 12:820–824, 1986.

142. Mehregan AH, Hashimoto K, Rahbari H: Eccrine adenocarcinoma: a clinicopathologic study of 35 cases. Arch Dermatol 119:104–114, 1983.

143. Weber PJ, Gretzula JC, Garland LD, et al: Syringoid eccrine carcinoma. J Dermatol Surg Oncol 13:64–67, 1987.

144. Dzubow LM, Grossman DJ, Johnson B: Eccrine adenocarcinoma—report of a case, treatment with Mohs surgery. J Dermatol Surg Oncol 12:1049–1053, 1986.

145. Mohs FE: Microscopically controlled surgery for periorbital melanoma: fixed-tissue and fresh-tissue techniques. J Dermatol Surg Oncol 11:284–291, 1985.

146. Mohs FE: Fixed tissue micrographic surgery for melanoma of the ear. Arch Otolaryngol 114:625–631, 1988.

147. Zitelli JA, Mohs FE, Larson P, Snow S: Mohs micrographic surgery for melanoma. Dermatol Clin 7:833–843, 1989.

148. Roenigk RK, Goltz RW: Merkel cell carcinoma—a problem with microscopically controlled surgery. J Dermatol Surg Oncol 12:332–336, 1986.

149. Dzubow LM, Kramer EM: Treatment of a large, ulcerating, granular cell tumor by microscopically controlled excision. J Dermatol Surg Oncol 11:392–395, 1985.

150. Lang PG, Metcalf JS, Maize JC: Recurrent adenoid cystic carcinoma of the skin managed by microscopically controlled surgery (Mohs surgery). J Dermatol Surg Oncol 12:395–398, 1986.

151. Dhawan RS, Nanda VS, Grekin S, Rabinovitz HS: Apocrine adenocarcinoma: case report and review of the literature. J Dermatol Surg Oncol 16:468–470, 1990.

152. Davidson TM, Haghighi P, Astarita R, et al: Microscopically oriented histologic surgery for head and neck mucosal cancer. Cancer 60:1856–1861, 1987.

CHAPTER 64

Healing by Second Intention

MANUEL IRIONDO

Probably the earliest discovered tumor is a hemangioma found in a fossilized bone of a Mesozoic dinosaur. With other fossils providing numerous examples of fractures, dental caries, and parasitic diseases,[1] there is abundant evidence that both disease and injury have plagued even the earliest forms of life on earth. The biologic adaptation of wound repair therefore represents a process linked to the survival of complex, multicellular organisms.[2]

Another biologic adaptation, instinct, is defined as the innate aspect of behavior that is unlearned, complex, and normally adaptive.[3] One example of this behavior can be seen in animals who instinctively lick their wounds to lessen pain. Also, monkeys are known to be capable of instinctively removing foreign bodies from their own skin. The earliest form of medicine practiced by our distant ancestors was most likely instinctive in nature. Perhaps the most ancient form of medical assistance was the help given to a pregnant or parturient woman!

Instinctive medicine subsequently led to the development of empirical medicine, which is guided by practical experience and not theory. An example of empirical medicine pertaining to wound healing can be found in the writings of Ambroise Paré, considered the greatest surgeon of the Renaissance. While serving as a surgeon in the French Army, he abolished the practice of applying cautery and boiling oil to gunshot wounds. In 1536, during a battle in which the supply of oil ran out, Paré was forced to use simple bandages! He writes:

I feared that the next day I should find them dead, or at the point of death by the poyson of the wound, whom I had not dressed with the scalding oyle. Therefore, I rose early in the morning, I visited my patients, and beyond expectation, I found such as I had dressed with a digestive [made of the yolke of an egg, oyle of roses, and turpentine] only, free from

vehemencie of paine, to have had good rest, and that their wounds were not inflamed nor tumifyed; but on the contrary, the others that were burnt with the scalding oyle were feverish, tormented with much paine, and the parts about their wounds were swolne.[4]

Paré's observation revolutionized the treatment of wounds and demonstrated the great healing force of nature.

Classification of Skin Wounds

Skin wounds are classified as either partial or full thickness depending on the depth of injury. A partial-thickness wound involves either just the epidermis or both the epidermis and a portion of the dermis. A full-thickness wound extends through the entire dermis. The term open wound refers to either a full-thickness or partial-thickness wound that has not been closed.

There are three mechanisms by which full-thickness open wounds heal: (1) primary intention, (2) delayed primary closure, and (3) second intention. Primary-intention healing occurs when the edges of a wound are brought together (coapted) shortly after an incision or laceration has occurred. Prerequisites for this type of healing include an adequate blood supply to the wound margins, removal of foreign bodies and nonviable tissue (debridement), and a wound bacterial colony count that is less than 1×10^5 organisms per gram of tissue.

In primary-intention healing, epithelialization and contraction are not important factors in the wound healing process. The major factor that contributes to wound strength is collagen cross-linking, which in turn is dependent on the orderly synthesis, deposition, and degradation of collagen.

A second mechanism by which full-thickness open

wounds can heal (or close) is delayed primary closure. This method is advantageous in grossly contaminated skin wounds because the delay in closure allows time for the patient's immune response to control bacterial contamination. In addition, delayed primary closure does not delay the development of wound strength, so that a contaminated wound that is not closed until the third day after injury has the same tensile strength on the seventh day as a clean wound closed by primary intention closure.

A third mechanism by which full-thickness open wounds can heal is second-intention healing. Well known to Mohs micrographic surgeons, this type of healing involves all three elements of wound healing: collagen deposition, epithelialization, and contraction (Fig. 64–1). The most important of these three elements in the spontaneous closure of wounds is contraction.[5] To better understand second-intention healing, it is important first to briefly review some of the basic biology of wound healing. This is covered in greater detail in Chapter 10.

Biology of Wound Healing

Wound healing begins immediately after injury as a clot forms in the wound. Fibrinogen molecules from the blood rapidly form interconnected strands of fibrin, providing a network that weakly joins the edges of the wound. After clot formation the injured tissue induces the release of substances that make blood vessels permeable to serum and proteins such as globulin, albumin, and antibodies. The main function of this fluid appears to be the sustenance of white blood cells that begin to migrate into the wound about 6 hours after injury.

The first cells to arrive are the neutrophils (polymorphonuclear leukocytes). These cells are able to slip through the blood vessel walls from the bloodstream into the wound by forcing apart the endothelial cells. The neutrophils contain few cytoplasmic organelles and do not divide. In addition, since they cannot synthesize protein, these cells characteristically have a life span of only several days. Once in the wound, neutrophils ingest foreign debris and infectious organisms by phagocytosis. Neutrophils kill bacteria and digest most of their remains. When a neutrophil dies, its outer membrane ruptures, releasing enzyme granules into the wound. These enzymes attack extracellular debris in the wound, which facilitates the removal of such material by monocytes that subsequently appear.

Within the first 12 hours after injury, monocytes migrate into the wound from the bloodstream and become macrophages. A macrophage is a phagocytic cell that ingests and partially digests most of the debris in the wound. Unlike neutrophils, monocytes have a fairly long life span, can synthesize proteins (like en-

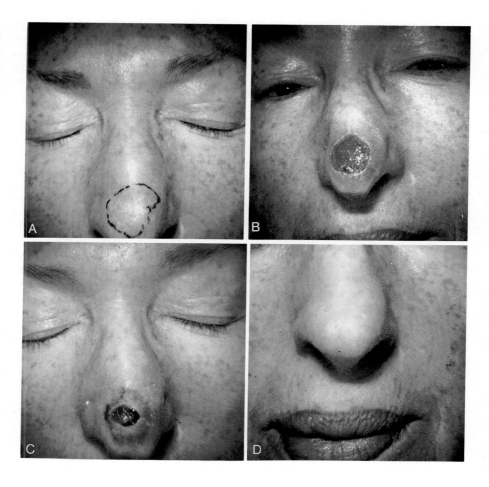

Figure 64–1. Second-intention healing associated with Mohs surgery. *A*, Preoperative appearance of a basal cell carcinoma of the nasal tip. *B*, Clinical appearance following completion of Mohs surgery. *C*, Partial wound contraction has occurred by 2 weeks. *D*, Final appearance of the healed scar after 3 years.

zymes used in phagocytosis), and remain active to the end of the inflammatory phase of wound repair. Current evidence suggests that monocytes do not divide.

Toward the end of the inflammatory phase of wound repair, fibroblasts[6, 7] appear in the wound from the nearby connective tissue and begin to produce collagen and protein polysaccharides that form scar tissue. As the fibroblasts are synthesizing collagen and protein polysaccharides, large numbers of small blood vessels begin to form in the wound. These capillaries originate from nearby vessels and appear as budlike structures that grow into loops, which then branch throughout the wound. This network of capillaries supplies the oxygen, creating a gradient that stimulates new blood vessel formation.[8] After wound repair is complete, regression of these new blood vessels occurs.

As the dermal scar tissue develops, the epidermal cells begin to close the wound surface. The fibrin network derived from the clotted blood acts as a guide for the migrating epidermal cells. An unusual feature of these mobile epidermal cells is that they ingest and digest the strands of fibrin in their path. This process is similar to the neutrophil and monocyte phagocytosis[9, 10] that occurs deeper in the wound and serves to remove debris. After the epidermal cells meet in the center of the wound and form a continuous layer, they regain their normal shape and growth rate. It has been observed in tissue culture that keratinocytes stop dividing once they make contact with one another, a process known as contact inhibition. This same effect may also occur in healing wounds.

Collagen Types

There are at least five types of collagen molecules in humans.[11] Each molecule is composed of three individual polypeptide chains known as alpha chains, which wrap around each other in a triple helix. Type I collagen constitutes 80 to 85% of dermal collagen and provides structural support for almost all body tissues. The other 15 to 20% of dermal collagen is composed of type III collagen, which is also prominently found in distensible structures such as blood vessels and visceral organs. Type IV collagen, which resists cleavage by human skin collagenase,[12] is present in the skin basement membrane. Type V collagen is found in fetal membranes, cornea, and heart valves but is only a minor component of skin. Lastly, type II collagen is found only in cartilage and vitreous humor[11–13] and does not occur in skin.

Collagen Metabolism

Injured tissue can stimulate messenger RNA specific for collagen synthesis, and inflammation appears to be an important factor in this process. A decrease in the amount of collagen deposition occurs in wounds depleted of macrophages,[9] while increased collagen synthesis occurs in wounds injected with macrophage-conditioned media.[10]

Within the fibroblast, hydroxylation of proline and lysine is required for the synthesis of the collagen protein. This hydroxylation reaction is catalyzed by the enzymes lysyl and prolyl hydroxylase with alpha-ketoglutarate, ascorbate, iron, and oxygen as cofactors. The synthesized collagen is then secreted in a triple-helical form and cross-linked in the extracellular space. It is this cross-linking of collagen that gives the wound its strength.

Vitamin C deficiency results in the production of underhydroxylated collagen, which cannot cross-link properly and thus compromises both wound strength and integrity, as in scurvy. Corticosteroids also interfere with prolyl and lysyl hydroxylase activity, resulting in poor wound healing. Equally important to collagen synthesis is collagen degradation, which is mediated by the enzyme collagenase. In the normal dermis there is an equilibrium between collagen synthesis and degradation, but in a wound the rates of collagen synthesis and degradation are altered to produce enough collagen for healing. Exactly how this balance is regulated remains unknown at present. It is known, however, that during the remodeling phase the randomly oriented collagen fibers formed early in the wound healing process are degraded and reorganized into large bundles. The collagen bundles then become aligned in the direction of stresses in the wound. These structural changes, along with increased collagen cross-linking, give scar tissue its great strength.[2, 5]

Contraction

The term wound contraction refers to the gradual shrinkage of a wound that occurs during healing.[14] Wounds contract by the centripetal movement of the surrounding skin, which is similar to closing the aperture of a camera (Fig. 64–2). Contraction coincides with the formation of granulation tissue in the wound (Fig. 64–3). Granulation tissue is composed of new capillaries, fibroblasts, collagen, and protein polysaccharides. The fibroblasts appear to be primarily responsible for the contractile property of granulation tissue.[15] On electron microscopy the fibroblasts in granulation tissue develop characteristics similar to those of smooth muscle cells. The name myofibroblast has been given to these contractile cells.[14, 15]

Wound contraction begins about 1 week after the wound is created and continues even after the wound is covered with epithelium. Contraction occurs at a rate of approximately 0.6 to 0.15 mm per day from the fifth to about the twelfth day. After this period the rate of contraction diminishes while collagen deposition increases. This supports the hypothesis that the myofibroblasts contract the wound and collagen holds the contracted tissues in place.

Contraction of surface wounds may lead to limited joint mobility or an aesthetic deformity known as a contracture. This may also occur internally and is a serious complication with high morbidity and mortality. One example of internal contracture is an esophageal stricture.[5, 16]

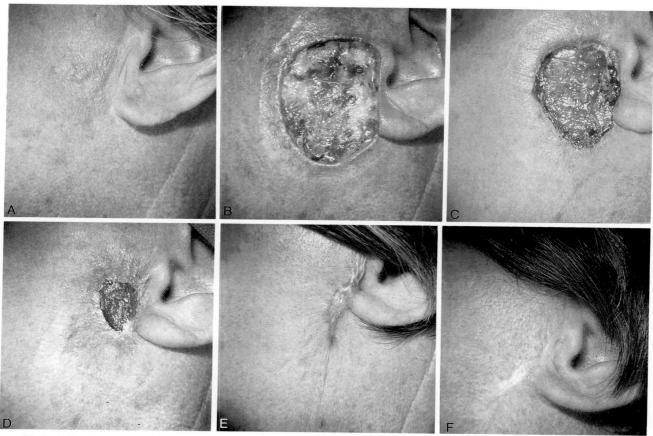

Figure 64–2. *A,* Preoperative appearance of an ill-defined basal cell carcinoma of the left preauricular area. *B,* Clinical appearance of the wound after Mohs surgery. *C, D,* Approximately 30% and 70% wound contraction has occurred by 2 and 4 weeks postoperatively, respectively. *E,* Healed, hypertrophic scar is evident after 3 months. *F,* Final appearance of the remodeled scar 18 months after completion of the surgical procedure.

Epithelialization

Successful healing of a full-thickness wound by second intention requires wound contraction to bring the dermal edges of the wound together. Even if epidermal cells cover the entire wound surface, the wound will break down until contraction causes coaptation of the dermis. It is, therefore, important to recognize that epithelialization contributes little to the strength of a wound. It has been proposed that because both the epidermis and dermis heal simultaneously, there is interdependency between these two components of the skin during wound healing. One example of this is the epidermal production of collagenase that is necessary for the remodeling of collagen.

Both mitosis and migration of keratinocytes are necessary for the restoration of epidermal continuity.[17] However, increased mitotic activity does not occur at the leading edge of the epidermal cells. It appears that cellular migration is the major factor in the epithelialization of wounds. In two models the epidermal cells appear to migrate by rolling or sliding over each other.[17] It has been observed that the leading epidermal cell extends a pseudopod that attaches to the basal lamina

by the formation of new hemidesmosomes. With part of the cell now attached to a substratum, the trailing portion of the cell moves forward along with other epidermal cells joined to it via the intercellular junctions or desmosomes. The epidermal cell connected superiorly to an advancing cell moves forward by rolling or sliding over the inferiorly positioned cell. This pattern of movement has been called "leap-frog" migration.

When the pattern of epidermal cell migration is studied in models consisting of both intact and open blisters, a striking difference in the rate of epidermal repair is seen. Epithelialization occurs faster in the intact blister model, possibly for several reasons. First, the intact blister has a continuous substratum, the basal lamina, which is not found in the open blister. Second, there is little debris in the intact blister, while the open blister is congested with fibrin and cellular fragments, which probably slow down the rate of the migrating epidermal cells. Third, greater amounts of phagocytosis occur in the open system, which requires energy that could be used for migration. Fourth, dehydration occurs in the open blister, whereas the intact blister fluid provides a constant physiologic environment for migrating cells.[5, 17] Studies have led to the conclusion that epithelialization occurs at a faster rate in moist, covered wounds.[17, 18] In

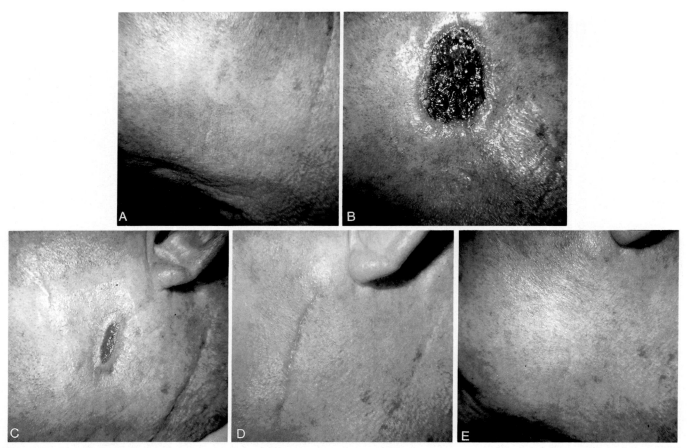

Figure 64–3. *A,* Preoperative appearance of a basal cell carcinoma of the left side of the neck. *B,* Granulation tissue has developed in the base of the wound by 2 weeks. *C,* Approximately 80% wound contraction has occurred by 4 weeks postoperatively. *D,* A healed linear scar is evident after 3 months. *E,* The scar is almost invisible after 10 months.

fact, it has been calculated that the epidermal migration rate in moist, covered wounds is double that in dehydrated or crust-covered wounds.[19]

Clinical Aspects

With this brief review of the specific cellular events that contribute to wound healing, it becomes easier to understand the clinical aspects that occur during second-intention healing. Once a defect has been created, perhaps after a skin cancer has been removed by Mohs micrographic surgery, a decision is made whether to repair the defect or to allow it to heal by second intention. Certain anatomic locations may require immediate repair: for example, when supporting eyelid ligaments are severed. However, there are many situations in which second-intention healing can be either the preferred choice or an effective alternative method of healing.

Dr. Frederic E. Mohs, the developer of the micrographic surgical technique for the treatment of skin cancers, has championed second intention wound healing for many years. He clearly has the largest and the most impressive series of wounds allowed to heal by this method. In addition to providing excellent cosmetic results in many locations, second intention healing allows the physician to better observe a skin cancer treatment site for signs of possible recurrence. When residual tumor is covered by a flap or a graft, a long time may elapse before it can be detected.[20] Other advantages of second-intention healing include the requirement for only simple postoperative wound care, minimal pain, rare bleeding and infection, a lack of need for hospitalization in most cases, and avoidance of possible complications associated with reconstructive surgery.

Patients are often concerned about the final cosmetic results obtained in wounds allowed to heal by second intention. Location seems to be the most important factor in predicting the final appearance of a healed wound. Wounds found on concave surfaces tend to heal by second intention with better cosmetic results than those on convex surfaces.[21] The concave areas of the *n*ose, *e*ye, *e*ar, and *t*emple (termed the NEET areas) heal by second intention with the best cosmetic results (Fig. 64–4). However, wounds on convex surfaces such as the *n*ose, *o*ral lips, *c*heeks or *c*hin, and *h*elix of the ear (termed the NOCH areas) heal by second intention with poor cosmetic results and very noticeable scars (Figs. 64–5, 64–6). Less predictable intermediate results occur in wounds found on flat areas of the *f*orehead,

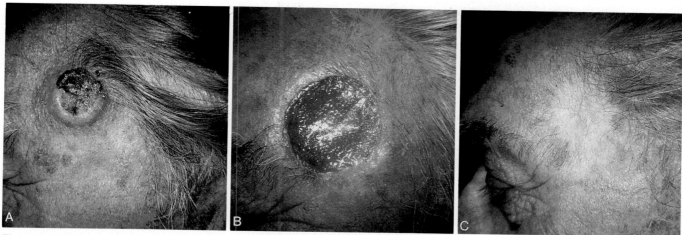

Figure 64–4. Good cosmetic result at a nose, eye, ear, and temple (NEET) location. *A*, Preoperative appearance of a large squamous cell carcinoma of the temple. *B*, Granulation tissue has formed by 10 days after Mohs surgery. *C*, Final appearance showing a soft, flat, round scar.

Figure 64–5. Poor cosmetic result from second-intention healing. *A*, Preoperative appearance of a basal cell carcinoma of the eyebrow. *B*, Tumor-free plane after Mohs surgery. *C*, Wound contraction after 1 month. *D*, Distorted brow with depressed scar seen after 3 months.

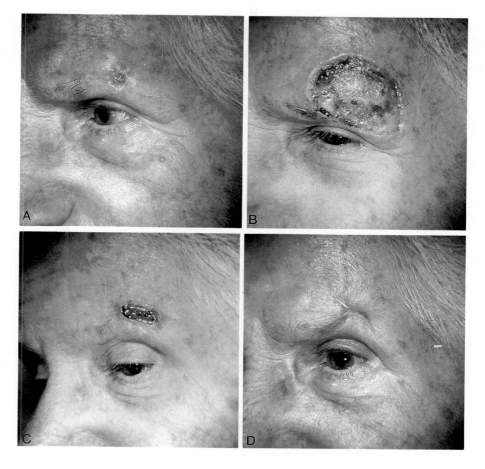

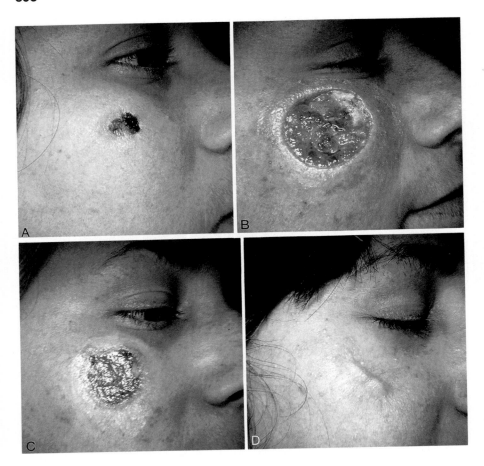

Figure 64–6. Poor cosmetic result after second-intention healing. *A*, Preoperative view of a basal cell carcinoma of the right cheek. *B*, Appearance of the wound after Mohs surgery. *C*, Early contraction and granulation tissue formation after 12 days. *D*, A raised, linear, hypertrophic scar is seen 7 months postoperatively.

*a*nthelix, *e*yelids (*I*), and the *r*emainder (termed the FAIR areas) of the cheeks, lips, and nose (Fig. 64–7).

Aside from location, factors such as wound depth, wound size, and skin color also contribute to the final cosmetic result obtained for wounds allowed to heal by second intention. Small, superficial wounds tend to heal by second intention with less noticeable scars than large, deep wounds. Because these scars typically are somewhat hypopigmented, they tend to be less noticeable in fair-skinned individuals[21, 22] than similar wounds occurring in patients with dark complexions.

Wound Management

Using the example of Mohs surgery to treat malignant skin tumors, similar full-thickness defects may result from either the fixed tissue or fresh tissue technique. In addition, postoperative wound care is similar for both techniques. After completion of the Mohs micrographic surgery using zinc chloride fixative, the final layer of fixed tissue sloughs off over several days (Fig. 64–8). As the final layer of fixed tissue loosens and separates,

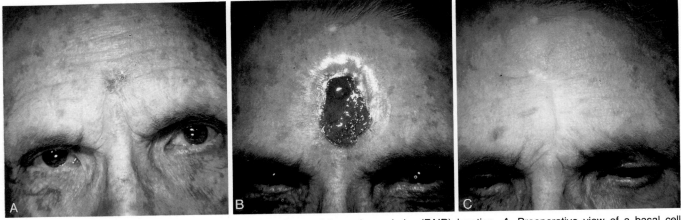

Figure 64–7. Good cosmetic result at a forehead, anthelix, eyelids, and remainder (FAIR) location. *A*, Preoperative view of a basal cell carcinoma of the midforehead. *B*, Appearance of the wound 3 weeks after Mohs surgery. *C*, Final appearance of the scar after 18 months.

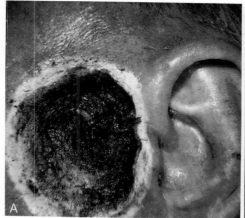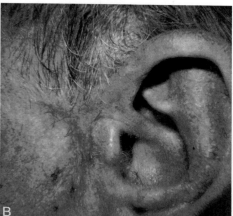

Figure 64–8. Fixed tissue Mohs surgery. *A,* Clinical appearance of the treatment site as the final layer of fixed tissue sloughs off over a period of several days. *B,* Postoperative view of the completely healed scar after 8 months.

bright red granulation tissue appears. The chemical fixation is omitted in the fresh tissue technique, and formation of granulation tissue begins about 1 week postoperatively.

Whether the technique used is fixed tissue or fresh tissue, patients should be given verbal and written instructions to clean the wound with 3% hydrogen peroxide solution daily. After the wound is clean and dry, a small amount of either polymyxin B–bacitracin ointment or mupirocin ointment 2% is applied to the wound surface with a clean cotton-tipped applicator. A nonadherent dressing is cut to fit the size of the wound and placed over the surface of the wound. A layer of gauze is added over the nonadherent pad for pressure and to absorb any exudate or serum drainage. Flesh-colored tape is used to seal the dressing completely.

For wounds allowed to heal by second intention when bone or cartilage is exposed, wound care is similar except that a more liberal application of ointment is recommended to prevent desiccation. Areas of exposed bone or cartilage that measure less than 1 cm in diameter usually heal without complications. When treating larger wounds that are greater than 1 cm in diameter, there may not be prompt coverage with granulation tissue. In these patients it may be necessary to remove small areas of the exposed bone or cartilage to allow granulation tissue to form. With cranial bone, a chisel and small mallet are employed to remove a thin portion of the outer table of the skull until small bleeding points are visualized. Alternatively, a drill or carbon dioxide laser can be used to make small perforations in the outer table of the skull through which granulation tissue can grow.[23] Since cartilage is softer than bone, a 3-mm punch can be used to cut a small window to the perichondrium on the opposite side. These procedures can be carried out quickly and painlessly in an outpatient setting.[20, 21, 24]

In cases of wound hemorrhage, patients are instructed to apply continuous pressure with a gauze pad directly on the wound for 30 minutes. If the bleeding has not stopped after 30 minutes of continuous pressure, patients are advised to proceed to the nearest emergency room.

Complications

Apart from bleeding, complications from second-intention healing are rare. Since granulation tissue is very vascular, it is resistant to infection. The time required for healing by second intention in most common wounds varies from 2 to 8 weeks, although longer periods may be required for leg wounds. This is not a true complication, since even these wounds eventually heal. The slower rate of healing for leg wounds is attributed to poor circulation. Drainage of clear lymphatic fluid from leg wounds is sometimes reported by patients.[25]

SUMMARY

All three mechanisms by which full-thickness open wounds heal have certain advantages and disadvantages. Despite some distinct drawbacks, second-intention wound healing is a superb method of healing for selected wounds and should be used to the fullest advantage to help patients obtain the most desirable result.

REFERENCES

1. Castiglioni A. In: Krumbhaar EB (ed): A History of Medicine. Jason Aronson, New York, 1975, pp 13–14.
2. Ross R: Wound healing. Sci Am 220:40–50, 1969.
3. Morris W (ed): The American Heritage Dictionary of the English Language. Houghton Mifflin, New York, 1973.
4. Singer DW: Selections from the works of Ambroise Paré. Bale, London, 1924.
5. Goldsmith LA (ed): Biochemistry and Physiology of the Skin. Oxford University Press, New York, 1983, pp 462–463.
6. Grillo HC: Derivation of fibroblasts in the healing wound. Arch Surg 88:218–224, 1964.
7. Van Winkle W Jr: The fibroblast in wound healing. Surg Gynecol Obstet 124:369–386, 1967.
8. Knighton DR, Hunt TK, Schevenstuhl H, Halliday BJ: Oxygen tension regulates the expression of angiogenesis factor by macrophages. Science 221:1283-1285, 1983.
9. Leibovich SV, Ross R: The role of the macrophage in wound repair. Am J Pathol 78:71–100, 1975.
10. Diegelmann RF, Kaplan AM, McCoy BJ, Cohen IK: Macrophage

stimulation of fibroblast proliferation and collagen synthesis in vivo and in vitro. XI Int Cong Biochem 7:502–503, 1979.

11. Goldsmith LA (ed): Biochemistry and Physiology of the Skin. Oxford University Press, New York, 1983, pp 385–388.

12. Liotta LA, Abe S, Robey PG, Martin GR: Preferential digestion of basement membrane collagen by an enzyme derived from a metastatic murine tumor. Proc Natl Acad Sci USA 76:2268–2272, 1979.

13. Uitto J, Booth BA, Polak KL: Collagen biosynthesis by human skin fibroblasts. II. Isolation and further characterization of type I and type III procollagens synthesized in culture. Biochem Biophys Acta 624:545–561, 1980.

14. Majno G, Gaddiani G, Hirschel BJ, et al: Contraction of granulation tissue in vitro: similarity to smooth muscle. Science 173:548–550, 1971.

15. Montandon D, Gabbiani G, Ryan GB, Majno G: The contractile fibroblast. Its relevance in plastic surgery. Plast Reconstr Surg 52:286–290, 1973.

16. Harris DR: Healing of the surgical wound. J Am Acad Dermatol 1:197–207, 1979.

17. Krawczyk WS: A pattern of epidermal cell migration during wound healing. J Cell Biol 49:247–263, 1971.

18. Mertz PM, Eaglstein WH: The effect of a semi-occlusive dressing on the microbial population in superficial wounds. Arch Surg 119:287–289, 1984.

19. Winter GD: Formation of the scab and the rate of epithelialization of superficial wounds in the skin of the young domestic pig. Nature 193:293–294, 1962.

20. Mohs FE: Chemosurgery: Microscopically Controlled Surgery for Skin Cancer. Charles C Thomas, Springfield, IL, 1978, pp 7–29.

21. Zitelli JA: Wound healing by secondary intention. J Am Acad Dermatol 9:407–415, 1983.

22. Ellner KM, Goldberg LH, Sperber MA: Comparison of cosmesis following healing by surgical closure and second intention. J Dermatol Surg Oncol 13:1016–1020, 1987.

23. Bailin PL, Wheeland RG: Carbon dioxide (CO_2) laser perforation of exposed cranial bone to stimulate granulation tissue. Plast Reconstr Surg 75:898–902, 1985.

24. Mohs FE, Larbon PO, Iriondo M: Micrographic surgery for the microscopically controlled excision of carcinoma of the external ear. J Am Acad Dermatol 19:729–737, 1988.

25. Moranz JF, Siegle RF, Barrett JL: Lymphatic bullae arising as a complication of second-intention healing. J Dermatol Surg Oncol 15:874–877, 1989.

CHAPTER 65

Facial Prosthetics in Cutaneous Surgery

THOMAS R. COWPER and SALVATORE J. ESPOSITO

In this age of television filled with almost perfect-looking individuals presenting solutions and prescriptions for retaining looks and youth, we are constantly reminded of how significant appearance is to careers and personal success. We do, in fact, greet the world with our faces! Films and literature reinforce the concept that a disfigured face denotes anger, evil, and usually self-destruction. In this context, what can be said to those individuals who have been subjected to disfiguring facial surgical procedures? Sadly, more than ever, in this era of technical and medical marvels, it is simply not enough to cure a patient. Rather, patients demand not only to be able to resume their daily routines, but also to do so totally unimpaired and without a hint of significant disability. This is not to imply that rehabilitation has been neglected in the past. "Almost three quarters of a century ago, the distinguished physician, Dr. William J. Mayo, boldly predicted that 'Rehabilitation will be a master word in medicine.' Bold words, indeed, for the 1920s."[1]

Never before has disfigurement and rehabilitation, particularly facial rehabilitation, loomed so significant in our society. Never has the public demanded so much of its health care professionals or been so ready to reprimand them for their failure to meet expectations. As the sphere of technology and knowledge enlarges and training becomes more complex, the traditional boundaries of medical and surgical specialties often overlap and become blurred. Cutaneous surgeons have pioneered and developed many new technical procedures that are currently being used by many different specialties to better manage a host of medical problems. Increased awareness and knowledge are needed regarding the principles of prosthetic rehabilitation and what this technical procedure can offer to patients and their physicians in the management of otherwise psychologically catastrophic disease.

History

Currently, the dental subspecialty of maxillofacial prosthetics dominates the prosthetic rehabilitation of facial defects.[2–5] Historically, it is difficult to determine accurately when prostheses were first used to restore facial deformities. It has been recognized that prosthetic devices, presumably made by craftsmen and artisans, were employed long before dentistry was practiced. Examination of Egyptian mummies reveals that artificial noses, ears, and eyes were used to restore missing anatomy, at least in death.[6] Therefore, it seems logical to conclude that prosthetic restorations have probably been attempted since man first suffered facial disfigurement.

Historically, the use of prostheses is entwined with the discovery and development of materials that could serve as substitutes for human tissues. Materials that could be easily shaped or carved (e.g., wood, ivory, glass, and certain malleable metals) were all known to serve in this regard. Later, with the discovery of the lost-wax technique, which is still used, it became possible to cast custom shapes in low-fusing metals. Although such techniques were most often employed in more common endeavors such as jewelry making, they were also used to fabricate facial prostheses as well. One famous example of this is Tycho Brahe, the famous sixteenth century Danish astronomer, who fashioned a prosthetic nose for himself after a dueling injury. Using wax, he reshaped the missing structure, made a mold and, employing the lost-wax technique, cast it in gold or copper. The prosthesis was said to be colored with oil paint to match his skin color and attached to his face with a glutinous adhesive. Brahe successfully wore this prosthesis for 35 years until his death, and it was said that it actually looked better than his real nose.[7]

Another celebrated case reported in the *London Medical Gazette* of 1832 described the "gunner with the silver mask," a French soldier named Alponse Louis, who sustained a disfiguring facial injury in battle. A silver prosthesis, which would be considered a combination prosthesis today, was designed for Louis. The prosthesis reportedly replaced his left mandible, lower lip, and part of his left maxilla and was colored with oil paints to match his skin tones. It was retained by straps hidden by his hair, a tactic still employed to cover defects of this size. Ambroise Paré, a sixteenth century French surgeon and one of the earliest pioneers of maxillofacial prosthetics, was the first to extensively describe the use of extraoral prostheses in repairing facial defects. Gold and silver ocular prostheses, ingeniously colored with enamel to match the eye color, were reportedly fabricated by Paré.[8] Other early pioneers of maxillofacial prosthetics were Pierre Fauchard (1678–1761), the proclaimed "father of dentistry," who improved the design for maxillary obturators, and Tetamore, who in 1894[9] described nine cases of nasal deformities in which prosthetic restorations were made from a light plastic-like material.[9] Tetamore also first described the use of impression techniques, which are still employed.[9, 10]

In the latter half of the nineteenth century, it was recognized that dentistry was most familiar and equipped to deal with facial defects. Kingsley pointed out that their knowledge of anatomy and understanding of materials allowed dentists to lead the way in treating such patients.[11] As would be expected, the materials utilized were those familiar to dentistry (e.g., plastic compounds such as cellulose nitrates and vulcanite, a rubber-like compound used in denture construction). In the early twentieth century, the first flexible materials were developed, including gelatin glycerin compounds and, later, a prevulcanized liquid latex developed by Clarke and Bulbulian.[10, 12]

During this period, dentists and surgeons began to collaborate on prosthetic restorations. Unfortunately, it required the misfortunes of World War I to stimulate efforts in prosthetic rehabilitation when soldiers on both sides returned with large facial deformities, and many dentists took control of the surgical and prosthetic rehabilitation of numerous British soldiers. Although many innovative surgical reconstructive techniques were pioneered simultaneously, facial prosthetics were continuously employed, and their great value was recognized.[13]

With the introduction of polymethyl methacrylate (acrylic) to dentistry in the 1930s and its subsequent improvement by cross-linking during World War II, dramatic improvements were possible for facial restorations.[4] This was particularly true for the ocular prosthesis, which had previously been fashioned only from glass. However, aside from the efforts of a few innovative individuals, prosthetic restoration of head and neck deformities was still largely ignored by the medical and dental professions until 1953, when a group of dentists founded the American Academy of Maxillofacial Prosthetics. Through the efforts of this group, the American Dental Association was convinced to recognize the subspecialty of maxillofacial prosthetics within the specialty of prosthodontics, and currently almost all patients with head and neck defects are referred to prosthodontists for rehabilitation. Most of these practitioners are members of surgical teams and can be found in major cancer treatment centers throughout America, where formal training programs have been established, usually in association with head and neck oncology teams.

Causes of Facial Disfigurement

Although treatment of tumors by radiation or chemotherapy can result in significant loss of tissue, surgical resection of neoplasms is probably the most frequent cause of facial deformities requiring prosthetic restoration[14]; other causes include congenital malformations and iatrogenic mishaps. However, epithelial tumors of the face and neck account for most of the destruction observed. Of these neoplasms, basal cell carcinoma, squamous cell carcinoma, and malignant melanoma are the most common. Although squamous cell carcinoma and malignant melanoma are well known for their destructive potential, basal cell carcinoma, due to its frequently insidious nature, is often the cause of the most extensive tissue defects encountered (Fig. 65–1). Actinic radiation is thought to be a significant factor[15, 16] in the formation of such tumors, although low-level radiation therapy for acne, practiced in the 1940s and 1950s,[17] is a common finding in the medical histories of many patients with large facial deformities.

Surgical correction of these deformities is often difficult and limited by the amount of tissue available for reconstruction, a compromised vascular bed (as a result of radiation therapy), and the overall poor physical condition of the patient. When these conditions exist, a prosthesis may be the treatment of choice. Of the facial structures involved, the orbit, nose, and pinnae are most often candidates for prosthetic rehabilitation, although occasionally these and regional extensions beyond may require more complex restorations known as composite or combination prostheses. Again, basal cell carcinoma most frequently requires such large composite resections and prostheses. Relatively small initial resections of apparently small skin cancers of the nose occasionally result in the creation of devastating defects involving the entire midface (Fig. 65–1), maxillae, and orbital contents. Similarly, seemingly small basal cell cancers of the infraorbital region have been observed to ultimately destroy the orbit and frontal processes of the cranium. In such cases, surgical rehabilitation is either impossible or imprudent, and prosthetic reconstruction is often the best choice.

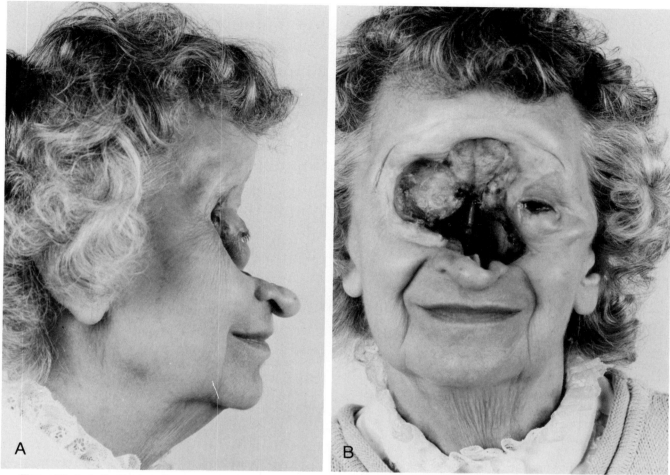

Figure 65–1. *A,* Profile view of an extensive facial defect after treatment of multiple recurrent basal cell carcinomas. *B,* Frontal view.

Preoperative Considerations

It would seem at first glance that the primary indication for prosthetic reconstruction of a missing structure is the inability to surgically reconstruct the affected structure. Although this is often true, many other factors must be considered. Chief among these is the patient's desires, which requires that the patient has been completely advised of the range of treatment alternatives, both surgical and prosthetic, before definitive therapy is performed. Only after patients have been made thoroughly aware of the advantages, disadvantages, and limitations of all possible approaches can they make an intelligent decision on the course of treatment.

It is equally inappropriate for the prosthodontist to render an opinion regarding the surgical considerations in treating a patient, as for the surgeon to provide the sole description of the prosthetic possibilities. Instead, both the cutaneous surgeon and the prosthodontist should collaborate to provide the patient and each other with a complete range of alternatives so that the best course of action can be followed. Lack of familiarity with prosthetic rehabilitative techniques is often a result of the unavailability of such specialists in many training

programs and medical centers. Therefore, it is important for surgeons who treat such patients to work with a prosthodontist so as to permit appropriate patient referral. Patients should not be denied information on the prosthetic possibilities out of ignorance.

Another pitfall in contemplating the treatment of such patients is to assume an "either/or" mentality with regard to surgical or prosthetic rehabilitation. Often, prosthetic rehabilitation can serve as an extremely successful interim form of treatment before final surgical reconstruction is performed. An example of this is reconstruction of the nasal tip or ala, in which an interim prosthesis can serve admirably before the definitive surgical reconstruction (Fig. 65–2). In such instances, interim prostheses can aid the patient and surgeon in evaluating this type of rehabilitation and help determine whether additional surgical rehabilitation is indicated or even desired by the patient.

Another important consideration that is frequently overlooked is the need to refer the patient for a preoperative dental evaluation. The dentition serves as the foundation for the functional and aesthetic integrity of the lower third of the face. Loss of teeth at birth or through trauma or surgery can have dire consequences

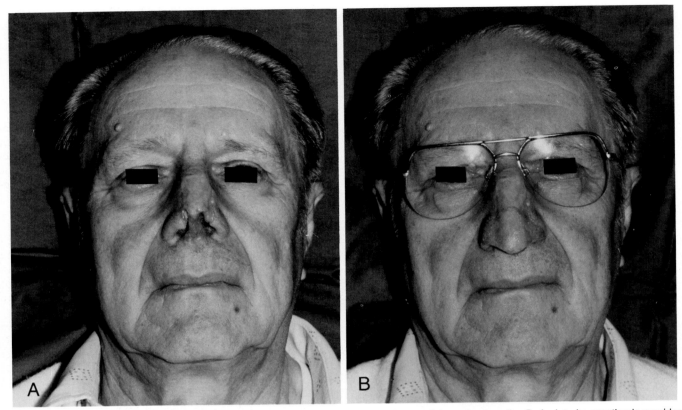

Figure 65–2. *A*, Mohs surgical defect after removal of a basal cell carcinoma of the nasal tip and columella. *B*, An interim prosthesis provides a superb result until the delayed definitive procedure can be performed.

for the subsequent surgical or prosthetic rehabilitation of the affected patient. In oncologic cases, in which radiation and chemotherapy are often employed, the dentition and supporting alveolar structures can be detrimentally affected both directly and indirectly. Although both radiation and chemotherapy usually produce reversible acute effects, radiation therapy can also result in permanent xerostomia, trismus, and compromised resistance.[18] Such side effects, if left untreated, can lead to "radiation caries," loss of teeth, and, in the most serious instance, osteoradionecrosis.[19] Worst of all, in situations where the dentition may serve to support an intraoral, extraoral, or combination prosthesis, its compromise may severely jeopardize the restorative prognosis. However, if the patient is referred preoperatively, both potential and actual abnormalities can be readily identified and treated. The teeth that are most important to the ultimate prosthetic or surgical rehabilitation can be identified and strict protocols, in the case of the irradiated patient, instituted to prevent complications.[20–22] There is potentially much to be gained and little to be lost in referring patients for preoperative prosthetic consultation. Such referrals may spell the difference between rehabilitative success and failure and even between excellence and malpractice.

Indications

A number of factors can help determine which patients are best suited for surgical rehabilitation and reconstruction (Table 65–1).[23] In most instances, if the patient can be surgically reconstructed, this is the preferred treatment of choice. The strictest indication for prosthetic rehabilitation is the inability to surgically reconstruct the affected part, although it is important to add that the patient must be psychologically capable of accepting this alternative. Indeed, a small number of patients would prefer a dressing to cover a defect rather than what seems to them to be a glaringly artificial prosthetic device.[24, 25] In these cases, it may be advisable simply to fabricate a prosthetic dressing that gives the illusion of a normal anatomic structure under the dressing. This is often much easier for the patient to utilize on a day-to-day basis than a more complex or extensive prosthesis. However, it can be difficult to recognize these patients until after treatment; and it is generally agreed that most patients desire and succeed with prosthetic rehabilitation.[26–29]

TABLE 65–1. **CHARACTERISTICS REQUIRED FOR A SUCCESSFUL POSTOPERATIVE AND REHABILITATION PERIOD**

Good past medical and surgical experience
Good relationships with family members
Good social relationships in general
Good relationships with previous physicians
Ability to verbalize fears openly
Good adaptation to previous stressful situations
Good work record

TABLE 65–2. INDICATIONS FOR PROSTHETIC REHABILITATION

Patient desires
Poor prognosis
Poor surgical risk
Inability to surgically reconstruct
Unavailability of surgical expertise
High possibility of regional recurrence
Delayed surgical reconstruction
Large resection defect

Even though a defect can be surgically reconstructed, a number of factors may influence that decision. For example, the patient's age, prognosis, desires, and overall health may weigh against surgical reconstruction and suggest the value of prosthetic rehabilitation (Table 65–2). In addition, the number of stages, financial considerations, and the concern of masking regional recurrence can preclude immediate or long-term surgical rehabilitation.[30] Most importantly, the ability to surgically reconstruct a defect does not implicitly demand that this action be taken immediately; instead, it can be delayed for a variable period of time. Finally, the inaccessibility of adequate prosthetic expertise can sometimes modify the appropriate course of rehabilitation, although in such a case it is preferable to refer the patient to a center where this service is available.

AGE

Prosthetic rehabilitation, with the exception of ocular rehabilitation, is generally contraindicated in infants and young children.[4, 12] Potential dislodgement of the prosthesis, which can cause significant psychological trauma to the child, is of principal concern in this age group. In adolescents, surgical rehabilitation of deformed facial structures is preferable whenever possible. However, there are occasional instances when prosthetic restoration may be the only alternative (e.g., complete loss of the nose or eye). Most surgeons believe that deformities of the ear can be adequately reconstructed surgically. Although extensive defects can be surgically reconstructed in multiple stages, the patient may be best served aesthetically and practically by a prosthesis. In such circumstances, the psychological trauma of multiple surgical procedures and less-than-ideal aesthetic outcome must be weighed against the potential for dislodging the prosthesis during the formative years. It has become increasingly clear that untreated congenital deformities can lead to permanent psychosocial trauma, especially in adolescents. The responses on the Cornell Medical Index (CMI) of 102 adolescents with varying facial deformities showed high scores in inadequacy, low self-esteem, and perceptions of unsuccessful coping.[31]

In some cases the noninvasive nature of prosthetic treatment argues for this approach, since surgical reconstruction can always be instituted if the patient or parents desire. In addition, prosthetic rehabilitation is reversible, whereas a poor surgical result may be extremely difficult, if not impossible, to revise.

In the young and middle-aged adult, surgical rehabilitation is preferred when possible. Nevertheless, treatment strategies must be balanced by other factors such as prognosis and patient desires. In the older adult, however, prosthetic intervention may be the therapy of choice because of frail health or the desire of the patient or surgeon to avoid additional surgical procedures.

PROGNOSIS

Other than the inability to adequately surgically reconstruct the defect, the overall prognosis of the patient is probably the most influential determinant in convincing both patient and surgeon of the need for prosthetic rehabilitation. Obviously, a patient with a poor prognosis is not an ideal candidate for extensive surgical reconstruction, and a prosthesis may be the only alternative. Likewise, the fear of masking local or regional recurrence may also influence the reconstructive decision. A removable prosthesis can readily provide the patient, surgeon, and prosthodontist with the opportunity to inspect the region on a regular basis. Additionally, if the prognosis requires an extensive delay before surgical reconstruction, a prosthesis can provide an interim solution that enables the patient to return to normal activities rather than becoming unemployed or, worse yet, a recluse. Finally, in considering the patient's prognosis, the tremendously important psychological benefits of "feeling whole" in some individuals cannot be overstated. Prosthetic restoration of a missing facial structure can provide some solace to a patient who otherwise has a rather dismal future. In fact, a number of terminally ill patients seek a prosthesis solely for the purpose of preparing for a presentable funeral.

PATIENT DESIRES

The patient must make the final decision as to the course of treatment that will be pursued. However, for a decision to be intelligent, it must be an informed one. This means all reconstructive alternatives must be considered before therapy begins, as the decision to pursue one path may influence the technical treatment considerations throughout. The extent of the resection may be different if the patient has decided that further surgical reconstruction is undesirable. Conversely, a different approach may be indicated if the patient decides to proceed with surgical reconstruction. More specifically, on occasion a particular anatomic structure may prove useful in surgical reconstruction but will interfere with successful prosthetic rehabilitation. The bony and cartilaginous septa of the nose illustrate this point. Although they are possibly useful in surgical reconstruction, these two structures are most often obstacles to providing an aesthetic nasal prosthesis (see Fig. 65–2). Clearly, it is not the surgeon's responsibility to decide which structures are prosthetically important or what the advantages and limitations of prosthetic reconstruction are. However, to best serve the patient, the surgeon is obligated to make the patient aware of these considerations through communication and consultation with the prosthodontist. Only then will the patient be fully informed and have a sufficient understanding of all treatment options and their limitations to make a realistic and intelligent decision.

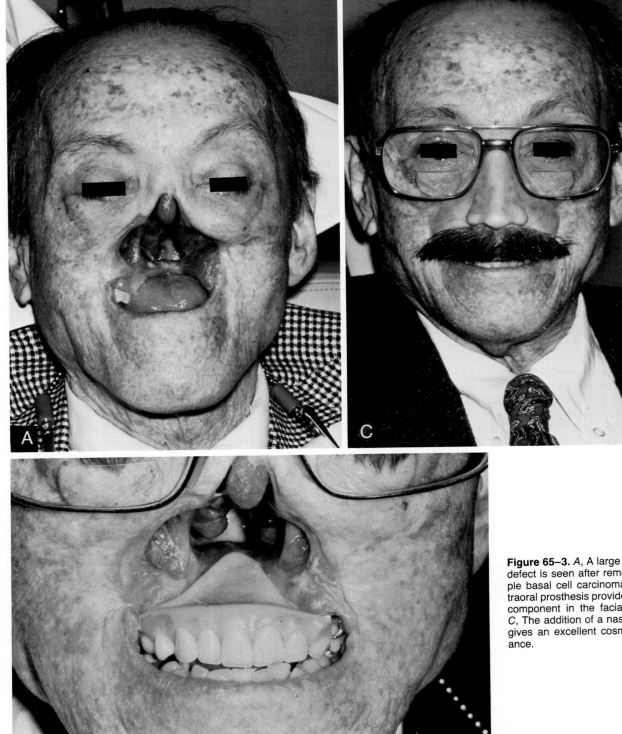

Figure 65–3. *A*, A large central facial defect is seen after removal of multiple basal cell carcinomas. *B*, An intraoral prosthesis provides an integral component in the facial restoration. *C*, The addition of a nasal prosthesis gives an excellent cosmetic appearance.

DELAYED SURGICAL RECONSTRUCTION

Patients who are not considered to be good candidates for immediate facial reconstruction can often benefit most from interim prosthetic rehabilitation. Frequently, such patients present with limited defects that are quite disfiguring (Fig. 65–2). A patient who is at high risk for local recurrence (e.g., from radiation-induced basal cell cancer) is a good example. In these patients, temporary prosthetic rehabilitation can provide the surgeon with the opportunity to clearly evaluate the postoperative site while allowing the patient to avoid obvious disfigurement. Additionally, an interim prosthesis can be employed extremely successfully during staged reconstruction when the final cosmetic or functional result has not yet been achieved and the defect is still quite aesthetically unappealing in appearance. In many instances, this can make the difference between normal physical and psychological re-entry to society or long-term disability.

SIZE OF THE RESECTION

As the size of the contemplated defect increases, the likelihood of prosthetic reconstruction also increases. Large defects, which are difficult or impossible to reconstruct surgically, can frequently be successfully restored prosthetically. This can help avoid multiple or complex surgical reconstructive procedures with a low probability of good aesthetic or functional results. As an example, extensive defects involving multiple structures such as the eye, nose, and cranium have been successfully restored prosthetically (Fig. 65–3). As the anticipated extent of the defect increases in size, the need for prosthetic consultation before surgery increases correspondingly to allow for provision of a defect that can be adequately restored prosthetically.

Types of Facial Prostheses

AURICULAR PROSTHESIS

The auricular prosthesis is probably one of the most successful of all prosthetic devices, primarily because of the ability to disguise much of the marginal interface with hair and the natural skin folds of the temporal region (Fig. 65–4). In addition, the ear is not a prominent facial structure like the eyes or nose. Both total and partial amputation of the ear can be admirably prosthetically restored, and in most instances such restoration is aesthetically superior to surgical reconstruction. Although retention of the auricular prosthesis might seem to be problematic, this is usually not the case because of the broad surface area available for adhesion. With the advent of successful craniofacial implants, retention is of even less concern, as the temporal bone can readily and successfully accommodate implant fixtures that can be used to retain the prosthesis either mechanically or magnetically.[32] Even without the use of implant fixtures, auricular prostheses can be worn during swimming or other strenuous activities without fear of loosening.

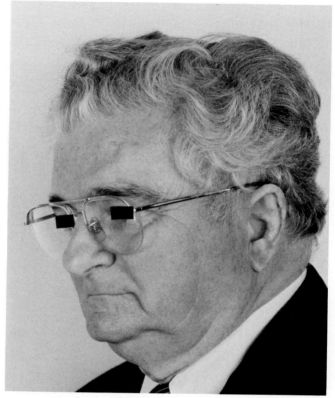

Figure 65–4. The auricular prosthesis is very successful because it is easily disguised by the surrounding hair and natural skin folds.

Surgical Considerations

Prosthetic rehabilitative treatment usually commences between 8 and 10 weeks postoperatively, unless radiotherapy is anticipated, in which case treatment is not begun until several weeks after this therapy is completed. To optimize the site for receiving an auricular prosthesis, it is often necessary to remove redundant, loose tissue that interferes with both retention and the overall appearance of the prosthesis. Unfortunately, this frequently makes it necessary to alter the sites of previous surgical reconstructive attempts, which may compromise prosthetic rehabilitation. This is especially true for patients with congenitally microtic ears, regardless of whether surgical reconstruction has been attempted, as often the residual soft tissue serves only to obstruct an aesthetically pleasing prosthetic reconstruction (Fig. 65–5). Most of the redundant structures, including the lobule, should be removed, although some residual cartilage may be retained to aid the patient in properly orienting the prosthesis.[33]

In addition, the tragus, which serves as both a landmark for orientation and a disguise for a portion of the anterior margin of the prosthesis, should be preserved if possible (Fig. 65–6). The surgical site should be comprised of firm, immobile tissue with some surface irregularities, which aid in positioning the prosthesis.[34]

Ideally, the area to receive the "base" of the prosthesis should be inset with a split-thickness skin graft to create a "step" defect along the anticipated superoan-

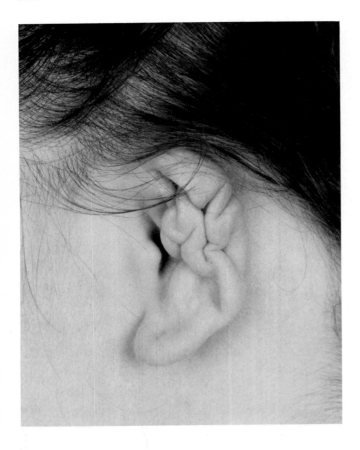

Figure 65–5. A congenital microtic left ear.

terior margin of the prosthesis. This allows for adequate thickness of the prosthetic margin without giving the prosthesis an aesthetically unpleasing, bulky appearance.

OCULAR PROSTHESIS

By necessity, loss of the orbital contents requires prosthetic rehabilitation. If simple enucleation or evisceration of the globe can be accomplished as definitive treatment, an ocular prosthesis can successfully replace the missing structures. Before 1940, such prostheses were fashioned of glass. However, the quality was dramatically improved with the introduction of polymethyl methacrylate by prosthodontists during World War II.[35] Indeed, the ocular prosthesis is probably the most successful of all prosthetic devices. It is extraordinarily realistic and can be worn for long periods of time, even months, without removal (Fig. 65–7). Additionally, it is the only extraoral prosthesis that should be used in infancy and maintained through adolescence and maturity, as its volume promotes normal growth and development of the remaining structures.[36] Furthermore, its presence maintains proper lid and tear function by providing contours in close proximity to what would have been the native scleral and corneal surfaces. As in the case of the auricular prosthesis, prosthetic rehabilitative treatment usually begins 8 to 10 weeks postoperatively, unless radiotherapy is anticipated, in which case treatment is delayed until several weeks after therapy.

Surgical Considerations

Although some controversy still exists regarding evisceration[37] versus enucleation of the globe, evisceration is preferred, if possible. This is because much of the orbital volume, muscular relationships, and muscle attachments can be maintained, resulting in an overlying prosthesis with exceptional motility. If enucleation is indicated, then placement of an appropriately sized motility implant is desirable to prosthetically maintain some of the orbital volume. This also reduces the otherwise bulky size of the overlying prosthesis and improves the ultimate mobility, although overall mobility will still be less than with evisceration. The reduced mobility seen in enucleation is probably a result of failure of the ocular muscles to truly attach to the underlying polymethyl methacrylate implant. Motility implants fabricated from coralline hydroxyapatite, which was originally used as a dental implant material, may provide a superior method of maintaining orbital volume and muscle function.[38]

Although restoring orbital volume is an important surgical consideration, care must be taken not to overfill the orbit, not to in any way obliterate or foreshorten the natural fornices that retain the prosthesis, and to allow for adequate lid drape and support. An acrylic conformer placed immediately postoperatively and allowed to remain for an additional 6 weeks is necessary to maintain these fornices. Consultation with an ophthalmologist and prosthodontist before such surgery is imperative to obtaining a successful outcome.

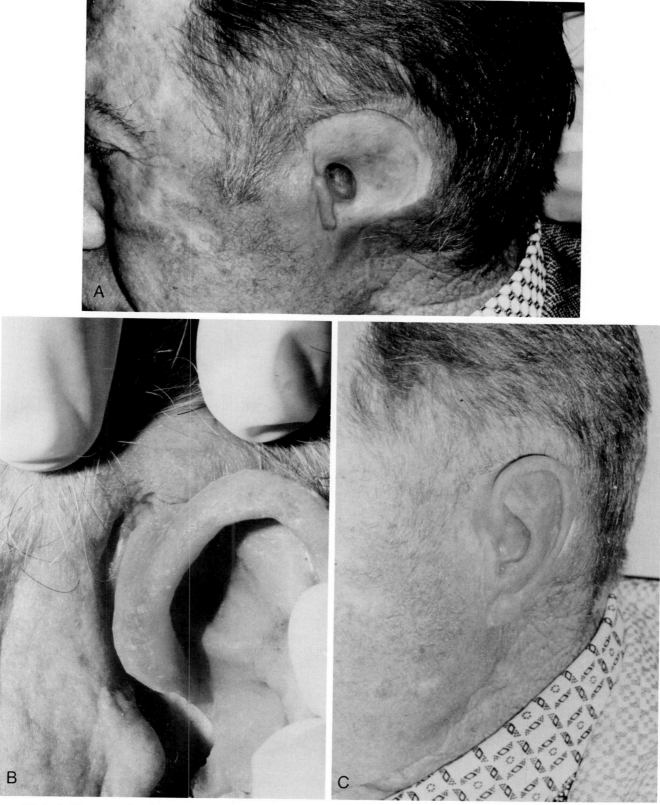

Figure 65–6. *A,* The tragus has been retained for proper orientation. *B,* This also helps disguise a portion of the anterior margin of the prosthesis. *C,* A broad surgical bed has been lined with a split-thickness skin graft and a step defect to allow a thick strong margin flush with the skin surface.

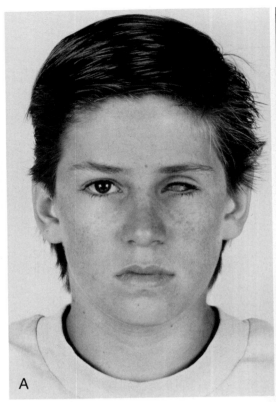

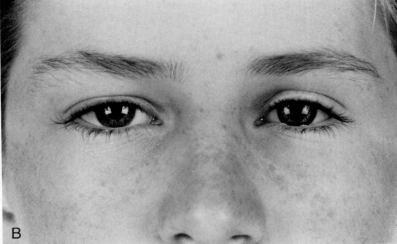

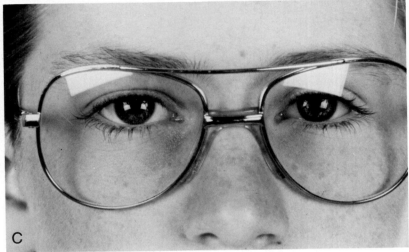

Figure 65–7. *A*, Preliminary appearance of a young man with simple enucleation. *B*, An excellent aesthetic appearance is possible with an ocular prosthesis. *C*, An even greater improvement in the appearance is possible with glasses to help disguise the prosthesis.

ORBITAL PROSTHESIS

If simple enucleation cannot satisfy the surgical treatment plan, then exenteration of the orbital contents and placement of an orbital prosthesis supplying both the globe and adjacent eyelid structures may be necessary. Unlike the ocular prosthesis, the orbital prosthesis is aesthetically far less successful, since it is currently impossible to artificially provide movement of the globe or lids. However, such a prosthesis still attracts less attention than a patch or bandage, attention that is undoubtedly of great psychological impairment to most patients. The orbital prosthesis is not intended to pass unnoticed under close scrutiny, but rather to provide an illusion of normalcy at a distance. Glasses are always useful in distracting attention from the prosthesis, which has some relevance to the surgeon when planning the surgical margins. Clearly, the aesthetic and functional success of the orbital prosthesis depends heavily on the preoperative surgical skills used to prepare the site. Care must be taken to provide adequate volume and retentive contours for the anticipated prosthesis. Treatment usually does not begin until 6 to 8 weeks postop-

eratively, unless radiation therapy is contemplated, in which case a delay of 2 to 3 weeks should be given after completion of radiotherapy.

Surgical Considerations

If the patient's condition allows, preservation of the bony orbital structures, especially the bony orbital rims, greatly enhances the success of the subsequent prosthesis. In addition, it is useful to maintain the naturally overlying soft tissue at the edge of the defect margin. The resulting defect will then provide a well-circumscribed, firm and yet flexible periphery that permits the slightly oversized posterior aspect of the prosthesis to slide by and thus engage the defect for added retention. In most instances, preservation of the eyelids is undesirable, as they are easily irritated, and the residual lashes are difficult to keep clean (Fig. 65–8). Instead, the defect is best lined with a split-thickness skin graft (Fig. 65–9).

Loss of the inferior bony rim is undesirable, as it results in a less stable "bed" for the prosthesis. In this instance, the inferior soft tissue will quickly stretch, and

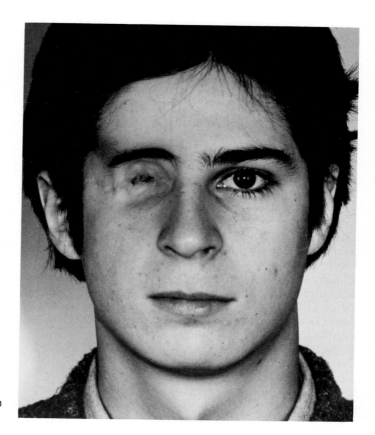

Figure 65–8. Preserved eyelids and lashes serve as a common source of irritation and a nidus for infection after enucleation.

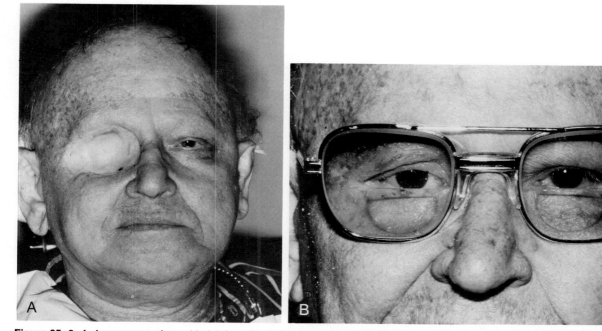

Figure 65–9. *A*, Appearance of an orbital defect after being lined with a split-thickness skin graft. The margins closely approximate the eyeglass frames. *B*, Preservation of the orbital rim provides a well-circumscribed and stable bony defect.

the prosthesis will take on a proptotic appearance. If the bony floor of the orbit must be sacrificed, it is preferable to maintain as much of the inferior orbital rim as possible. If the inferior orbital rim and other associated inferior structures must be sacrificed, the more conservative the resection is inferiorly, the better the chances of a stable prosthesis.

Conversely, the greater the resection inferiorly, the more difficult it will be to obtain a stable prosthesis. Wherever possible, care should be taken not to extend the resection onto movable facial tissues, which could break the adhesive bond during expressive facial activity. Similarly, if the superior orbital rim, including the overlying eyebrow, can be maintained, this will result in a superior prosthetic restoration. Despite these precautions, overly conservative surgery in a seemingly laudable attempt to aid in rehabilitation can actually be detrimental to overall prosthetic success. Particular care must be taken to provide enough volume anteroposteriorly for an adequately sized prosthesis, or an exophthalmic or similarly aesthetically unpleasing appearance can ensue. Ideally, if the margins of the resection can be made to fall at the approximate periphery of spectacle frames, the prosthetic cutaneous margins can then be readily camouflaged by appropriate selection of glasses at the time of prosthetic restoration (Fig. 65–9*B*).

Placement of a thin split-thickness skin graft in the surgical site provides for accelerated healing and a cleaner, drier defect that is more conducive to prosthetic rehabilitation than one that is allowed to "granulate in."

The latter approach should be avoided, because it often produces a shallow, conical defect with unfavorable architecture for retaining a prosthesis in an aesthetically pleasing manner.[34] Again, preoperative consultation with the prosthodontist can be extremely helpful.

NASAL PROSTHESIS

Even small nasal defects, because of their location, can produce glaring cosmetic deformities that are difficult to disguise. Although such defects are amenable to surgical reconstruction, a significant waiting period is often required before such surgery can be performed. Although small nasal defects are best reconstructed surgically, interim prosthetic rehabilitation is often an effective way to "bridge" the time between resection and reconstruction. Occasionally, a patient will either defer or cancel further surgical rehabilitation because of the success of such a prosthesis. Larger defects are notoriously difficult to reconstruct surgically and, because of the underlying condition or the patient's age, may require a period of years before a multiple-staged reconstruction is considered, if at all. Again, in these instances, prosthetic reconstruction may serve as an excellent interim or permanent solution (Fig. 65–10).

As in other defects, prosthetic rehabilitative treatment usually begins approximately 8 to 12 weeks postoperatively, unless radiotherapy is anticipated, in which case treatment is postponed until several weeks after completion of such therapy.

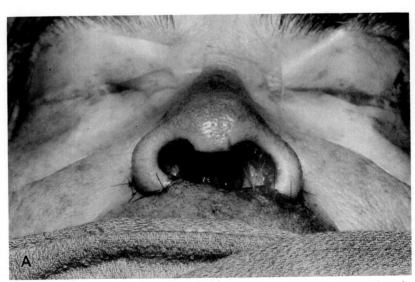
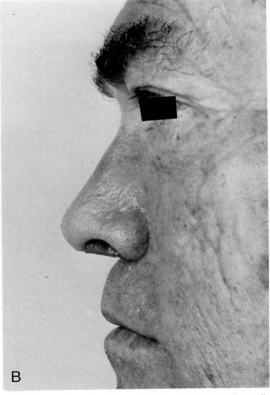

Figure 65–10. *A,* Columellar septal defect and interim prosthetic reconstruction after resection for basal cell carcinoma. *B,* The small acrylic prosthesis served as a postsurgical stent to minimize contracture of the nasal tip while the reconstruction was delayed 1 year.

Surgical Considerations

When planning a partial or complete nasal resection, a presurgical facial moulage is invaluable to subsequent prosthetic reconstruction, since the nose is a midline structure with no mirror image counterpart to copy. The cast obtained from such an impression can also be used for presurgical planning of "ideal" surgical margins, providing, of course, that the underlying condition will allow this maneuver.

When anticipating complete or partial resection of the nose, the primary prosthetic consideration is the failure to remove adequate tissue to allow for an aesthetically pleasing prosthesis (see Fig. 65–2). In large resections in which prosthetic reconstruction is anticipated, removal of the bulk of the nose, including the nasal cartilagineous and bony septa, is preferable, as these structures serve only to obstruct the prosthetic reconstruction. The exception to this is the bridge of the nose, which should be retained for support of the prosthesis. The lateral margins of the resection, whether unilateral or bilateral, should extend to or near the natural folds of soft tissue in the nasolabial area to help disguise the margins of the prosthesis. Wherever possible, care should be taken not to extend the resection onto mobile facial tissues, which may invite loosening of the adhesive bond during expressive facial activity. However, this is not always possible because of the location of the disease (Fig. 65–11).

COMBINATION PROSTHESES

Unfortunately, extensive resections can result in defects of multiple facial structures that require a combination of one or more different prostheses to restore. Such resections may involve the oral cavity, maxilla, nose, orbit, and cranium in any combination (Fig. 65–12). In instances in which the oral cavity and overlying maxillary structures are affected, it is best to restore the intraoral defect initially, as such a defect can alter the soft tissue contours of the adjacent facial defect. Infrequently, the intraoral prosthesis may serve as a supporting foundation for a facial prosthesis; in such cases the prosthodontist should evaluate the remaining teeth and associated oral structures preoperatively (Fig. 65–13). Similarly, other seemingly unlikely structures, such as the floor of the orbit or residual nasal septum, may have significance in terms of prosthetic retention and support. Special attention to preserving strategic soft tissue undercuts may be of tremendous help in the ultimate successful retention of these large prostheses.

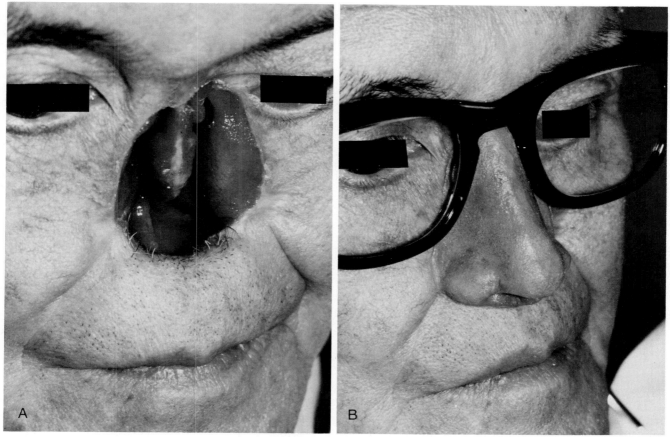

Figure 65–11. *A*, Nasal defect, with retention of part of the bridge of the nose, after resection for recurrent basal cell carcinoma. *B*, The prosthesis fits well, since all aesthetically obstructive structures have been removed.

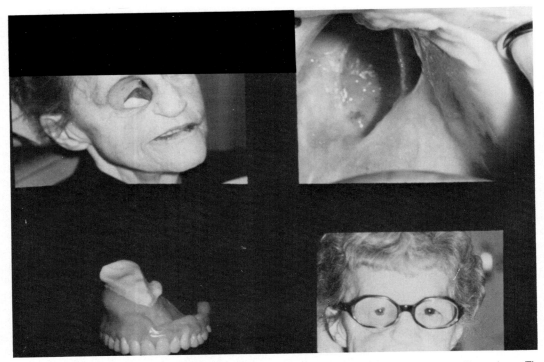

Figure 65–12. Maxillectomy and orbital exenteration for squamous cell carcinoma of the maxilla and maxillary sinus. The patient has a combination prosthesis with extra- and intraoral components.

Surgical Considerations

Traditionally, prosthodontists have relied on opposing soft tissue undercuts of defects to aid in the retention of large combination prostheses. For this reason, care must be taken during surgical planning to provide sufficient access to areas of the defect that may aid in support and retention (Fig. 65–14). Occasionally, bulky flaps used to reduce the volume of a large defect have, despite the surgeon's good intentions, served to interfere with the retention and aesthetics of the prosthesis. Attempts to transfer large volumes of tissue into a combination defect have actually prevented an extra- or intraoral prosthesis from being effective. In defects involving the oral structures, particular care must be paid to the status and significance of the remaining dentition, as often the teeth can help to retain and stabilize large combination prostheses (Fig. 65–12). Again, preoperative or intraoperative consultation with a prosthodontist can help to avoid many later difficulties.

Implant Prostheses

Implant prostheses can be divided into percutaneous and subcutaneous types. Custom subcutaneous implants made of various materials (i.e., metal, acrylic, and silicone rubber) have been used successfully for many years in the repair of craniofacial defects.[39] Coralline hydroxyapatite, first used in dental implants, has gained popularity as an alloplastic material for implants in extraoral sites. Unlike its relatively mobile silicone predecessors whose surface alone is encapsulated by fibrous

tissue soon after implantation,[40] hydroxyapatite has been shown to completely incorporate the surrounding fibrous tissue, thereby becoming relatively immobile soon after its placement.[41] This property has made it increasingly popular for ocular motility implants, since the remaining muscles appear to attach more effectively, producing greater movement of the overlying ocular prosthesis. Previously, only well-circumscribed bony defects of the cranium into which the alloplastic implant could be set without fear of migration over time were considered appropriate for such treatment. Facial soft tissue deficits restored by such implants eventually demonstrated migration of the implant secondary to gravity or muscular influence.[42, 43] Whether coralline hydroxyapatite will prove to be advantageous in these areas in the future remains to be seen.

Percutaneous implants, which have successfully revolutionized prosthetic dentistry,[44] also hold great promise as an adjunct for facial prosthetic restoration. Commercially pure titanium fixtures have been successfully placed in various locations of the cranium and face to provide support for and aid in retaining an overlying prosthesis.[32] Adhesives are replaced by magnets or other underlying retainers attached to these fixtures, which increases the ease of use, as well as the longevity, of the prosthesis. Prostheses that in the past may have been considered difficult to retain because of the configuration or extent of the surgical defect can now be successfully placed using such percutaneous implants as retentive abutments. Although such implants are still considered experimental in the United States, they have been effectively employed in Europe for a number of years, with few complications.[16, 45]

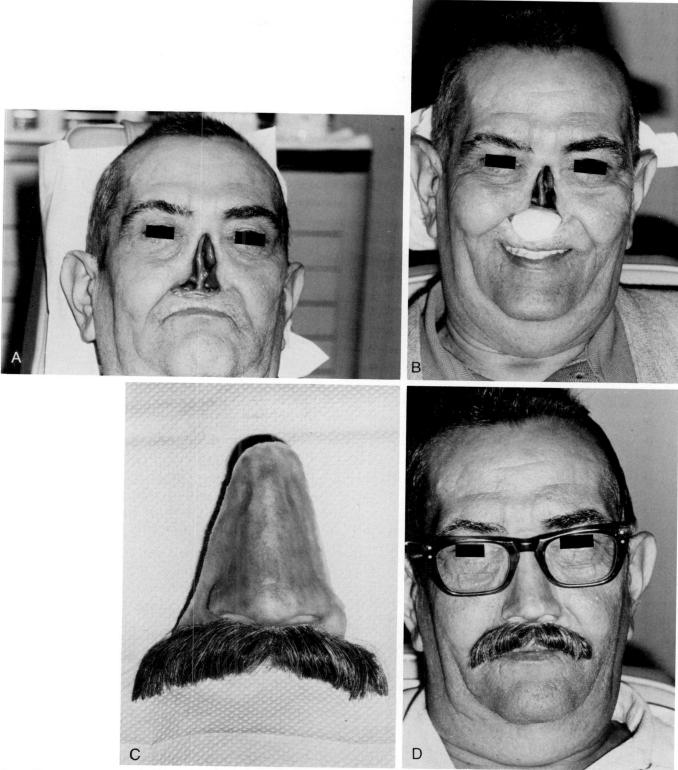

Figure 65–13. *A*, Defect after extensive surgery for cutaneous malignancy. *B*, A combination prosthesis is partially fabricated from an intraoral (silicone) obturator. *C*, A hair-bearing nasal component is also used to further improve the appearance. *D*, Final appearance with glasses to help disguise the prosthesis.

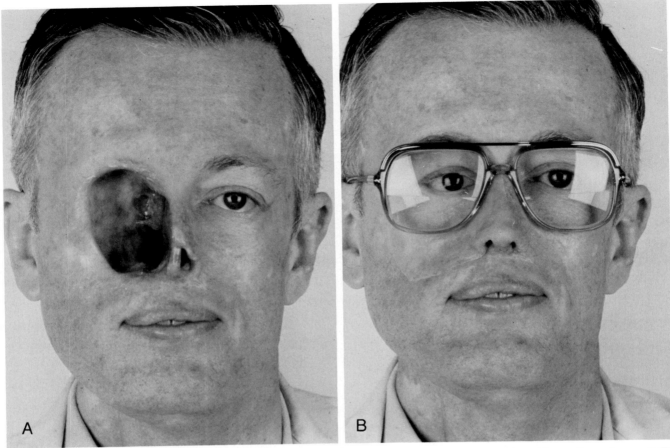

Figure 65–14. *A,* Large resection and prosthetic rehabilitation for recurrent basal cell carcinoma involving the orbit, maxilla, and nose. *B,* The opposing tissue undercuts are engaged by the flexible aspects of the prosthesis and aid in traditional retention. In addition, the defect is well circumscribed, with bone underlying the margins lending stability to the prosthesis.

SUBCUTANEOUS IMPLANTS

Surgical Considerations

Preoperative prosthetic consultation and coordination are of critical concern when contemplating the use of subcutaneous or percutaneous implants. Conventional custom subcutaneous implants are best employed in well-circumscribed bony defects of the cranium where there is little chance of subsequent migration of the implant (Fig. 65–15). Such implants, usually fashioned of metal or acrylic, have been best utilized in delayed reconstruction of these defects when a preoperative moulage impression could be obtained before the secondary reconstructive operation for evaluation and fabrication of the implant. This minimizes alterations and operative time during the actual reconstructive procedure. Reformatted three-dimensional computed tomographic (CT) imaging of bony defects can be used to obtain a more accurate master model from which a customized implant can be fabricated.[46] It is best to delay 3 to 8 months to allow adequate bony recontouring to occur before reconstructing these defects.

Because of its flexibility, silicone rubber (Silastic) has traditionally been employed in facial implants when mobility of the surrounding tissues is an anticipated problem. Preoperative coordination with the prostho-dontist again is of vital importance, as is obtaining a presurgical impression and master model for fabrication of the appropriately contoured implant. However, with few exceptions, facial implants, because of their increased propensity for migration with time, enjoy limited long-term success and should probably be avoided if possible.

PERCUTANEOUS IMPLANTS

Surgical Considerations

Prosthodontic and radiologic presurgical planning is imperative in anticipating the use of percutaneous implants. It is essential not only that bone be of adequate thickness to place the fixtures, but also that the location of the fixtures be correct with respect to the overlying prosthesis.

An implant fixture successfully integrated into bone is of no use to the prosthodontist if its position obstructs the aesthetic contours of the superimposed prosthesis. In such instances, the first presurgical step is to fabricate a conventional prosthesis to establish the limits and contours necessary for an aesthetically pleasing result. Three-dimensional CT imaging of the underlying bone is then performed to locate areas of adequate thickness

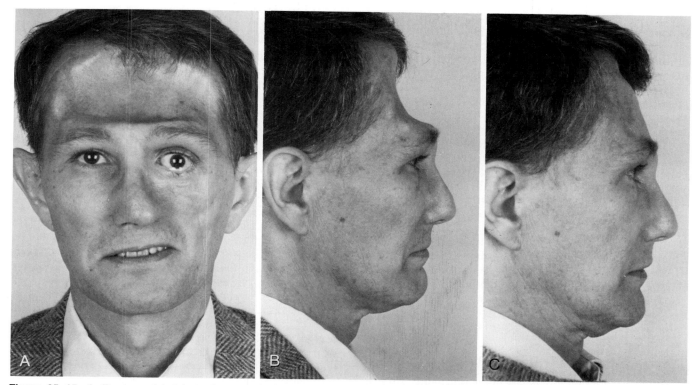

Figure 65–15. *A,* Frontocranial defect after resection for rare Ewing's sarcoma, illustrating ideal conditions for a subcutaneous implant prosthesis. *B,* The defect is circumscribed with bony margins and immobile tissue, which prevent migration of the implant. *C,* Defects of the vertical face rarely exhibit these favorable conditions, and traditional subcutaneous implants often migrate or extrude with time.

and density for the required two to three fixtures. Finally, a surgical template, which will help the surgeon to correctly place the fixtures, is constructed. Percutaneous implants are then placed and buried for 3 to 5 months until appropriate healing has occurred, after which they are re-exposed; a transcutaneous post is then connected before prosthetic rehabilitation. Secondary soft tissue recontouring may be necessary during this last procedure. Placing percutaneous fixtures without using these steps techniques invites almost certain failure.

Materials

Since the 1970s, much effort has been expended to develop a material that would meet all of the requirements of an ideal facial restoration.[47] Although much progress has been made, a material that would satisfy all the desirable physical, biologic, and chemical properties necessary to achieve clinical success and patient acceptance has not yet been developed. In short, no artificial material has been found that can duplicate the remarkable flexibility, elasticity, and toughness of human skin.

CHARACTERISTICS OF IDEAL PROSTHETIC MATERIALS

A consensus report resulting from a workshop on materials held at the thirteenth annual meeting of the

American Academy of Maxillofacial Prosthetics stated that the ideal material should possess some general characteristics (Table 65–3). First, the material should reproduce the missing or defective facial anatomy with accurate color, texture, and form to provide optimal aesthetic results. Of vital importance is the reproduction of the actual pigmentation of skin, re-creating the coloration caused by the combined presence of melanin, hemoglobin, and carotene. The completed prosthesis should be virtually undetectable in public and should allow the patient to function normally in society. A conspicuous prosthesis will increase, not decrease, the

TABLE 65–3. REQUIREMENTS FOR AN IDEAL PROSTHETIC MATERIAL

Nontoxic, nonallergenic
Resistant to microorganisms
Chemically inert
Dimensionally stable
Strong and elastic with high tear strength
Flexible under all conditions
Poor thermal conductor
Resistant to wear, weathering
Lightweight
Color stable
Compatible with adhesives or other retention means
Easily processed and colored
Readily repaired and modified
Easily cleaned
Readily available commercially
Inexpensive

anxiety of the patient and will often result in failure. Second, the material should be lightweight and dimensionally very stable, yet remain flexible under all conditions. It must possess adequate tensile strength to resist tearing and allow for thinning of the edges of the prosthesis to permit blending them with the soft tissue bed. This tensile quality should be close to that of living tissue for comfortable use on the movable skin that supports the prosthesis.

Third, an optimal prosthetic material must be chemically inert, odorless, nonflammable, and a poor thermal conductor. In addition, the material should also be color stable when exposed to sunlight, thermal changes, and adhesives and their solvents. Fourth, the ideal facial prosthetic material should have excellent tissue biocompatibility or receptivity. It must be nontoxic, noncarcinogenic, and nonallergenic, as well as resistant to microorganisms. The material should also be hygienic, capable of being washed and disinfected in appropriate solutions. Finally, the material should be relatively inexpensive to purchase and readily available commercially. It should be easy to work with, requiring no complicated or extensive equipment for fabrication of the prosthesis.

TYPES OF PROSTHETIC MATERIALS

The most popular materials currently being used for the fabrication of facial prostheses are acrylic resins, polyurethane elastomers, and silicone elastomers.

Acrylic Resins

Many maxillofacial prosthodontists consider heat-polymerizing polymethyl methacrylate (acrylic resin) to be the facial restorative material of choice. Heat-polymerizing acrylic is preferable to the autopolymerizing type because of the presence of the toxic tertiary amine, dimethyl-*p*-toluidine, in the latter. Acrylic resin has many excellent properties that make it suitable as a facial restorative material. It is a transparent material that can be colored or tinted to almost any shade or degree of translucence. It can be used very effectively in interim prostheses in recently healed surgical patients, since its ease of modification makes it particularly suitable during the initial stages of rehabilitation. Its physical and chemical properties are extremely stable, changing very little under most environmental conditions. Because of its rigidity, polymethyl methacrylate is particularly effective in areas where there is little or no movement of the surrounding tissue (Fig. 65–16). This quality also allows the edges of the prosthesis to be tapered into the soft tissue bed, rendering them virtually undetectable. In addition, any of the available adhesive systems can be used effectively with acrylic resin prostheses. The rigidity of the acrylic resin remains its primary disadvantage, as it often causes discomfort in beds of mobile tissue. Patients also find the rigid material less acceptable because the prostheses do not feel like skin. In addition, duplicate prostheses are not possible when acrylic is used, because the molds are lost during fabrication.

Polyurethane Elastomers

The polyurethane elastomers are long-chain polyesters or polyethers reacted with isocyanates. By varying the amount of isocyanates, the physical properties of the material change significantly. Although used infre-

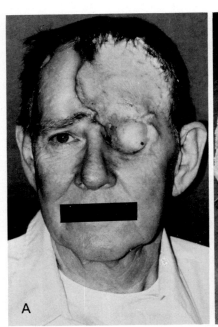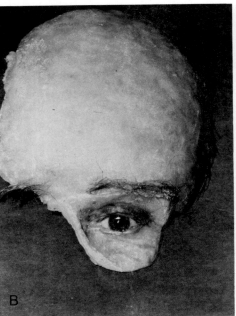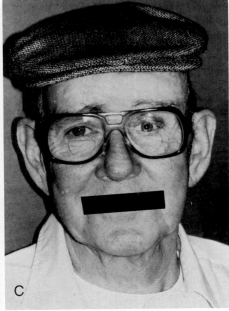

Figure 65–16. *A,* Large composite resection for recurrent basal cell carcinoma. *B,* Restoration was accomplished with an acrylic prosthesis that is strong, long-lasting, and color stable and has margins that can be "feathered" aesthetically. *C,* The inflexibility of the prosthesis requires immobile margins and feels more "foreign" to patients.

quently by practitioners, this restorative material possesses excellent properties, including softness, inertness, flexibility, resistance to solvents, and high tensile and tear strength.[48] It is especially ideal for movable tissues. The material can be colored both intrinsically and extrinsically, with excellent cosmetic results. One problem that makes the isocyanates unpopular among clinicians is that they are so moisture sensitive that consistent processing is difficult. The color stability of the urethanes on exposure to ultraviolet light is poor. Tinnivian has been used in an attempt to make the material more colorfast; however, there has been much concern regarding the carcinogenicity of this material. In addition, the external coloration seems to deteriorate quickly, and although there is an initial excellent aesthetic result, optimum long-term results are the exception rather than the rule.

Silicone Elastomers

Silicones are the most popular facial material used by prostheticians. First developed during World War II for use in military aircraft, silicones were introduced as a medical material several years later when employed as an implant material for shunts in patients suffering from cerebrovascular accidents. In 1960, silicone elastomer was first utilized for facial prostheses; since then, various formulations of silicone have made it the most popular facial restorative material. Medical-grade silicone, or polydimethylsiloxane, contains none of the toxic additives found in industrial silicones. Vulcanization to the clinically useful formulation takes place when chains of silicone polymers become cross-linked. This process occurs either with or without heat, depending on the cross-linking agent and the catalyst used. Although heat-catalyzed silicone polymers are occasionally used, the elastomers most commonly employed for facial

prostheses are either room-temperature vulcanizing (RTV) or single-component adhesive systems. The original RTV silicones, such as Silastic 399, had many excellent properties that made them very popular when first introduced. They were biocompatible, inert, color stable,[49] and easy to fabricate using simple dental gypsum molds, which were readily available. However, they were difficult to colorize and had poor edge strength.

In the late 1970s, MDX 4-4210 was developed by Dow Corning. This silicone elastomer had all the desirable properties of earlier RTV materials but was more easily colored and had improved tensile strength. Because of these advantages, particularly its increased edge strength, MDX 4-4210 currently is the most popular silicone material used. It is strong yet flexible, and its resilience even allows characterization with eyelashes and eyebrows, which can literally be sewn into the material (Fig. 65–17). Like earlier silicones, however, its color stability is short-lived when it is subjected to ultraviolet light. A new silicone polymer, A-2186, has been introduced that is softer than MDX 4-4210 but has better tear resistance and edge strength.[50]

Silicone adhesive, or Silastic 382, although currently used primarily for repairs and surface color characterization, was previously employed as a definitive restorative material. Stored in tubes, this silicone vulcanizes rapidly on exposure to atmospheric moisture. However, its usefulness as a primary facial restorative material is minimal, because it is difficult to color and has poor edge strength. Nonetheless, it is still occasionally used as an additive to create a composite material with intermediate properties. Significantly, composite formulations hold great promise for achieving the goal of an ideal skinlike material. However, because of the small number of patients needing these types of prostheses, such materials will likely be slow to develop.

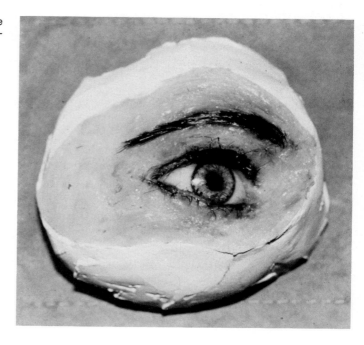

Figure 65–17. The silicone orbital prosthesis is flexible and more skinlike, and because of its resilience, hair can be sewn into appropriate places for increased realism.

SUMMARY

Patients who have had disfiguring facial trauma or surgery should be provided with the best form of rehabilitation until definitive reconstructive surgery can be performed. To do this, every cutaneous surgeon must be aware of the indications and benefits of maxillofacial prostheses. By using a team approach, many patients can be returned to full productivity and function in a relatively short period of time. Prosthetic restoration also allows patients who must be evaluated for prolonged periods of time postoperatively to exclude possible recurrences of head and neck cancers and function more normally both psychologically and socially.

REFERENCES

1. Argerakis GP: Psychosocial considerations of the posttreatment of head and neck cancer patients. Dent Clin North Am 34:285–305, 1990.
2. Ackerman AJ: Maxillofacial prosthetics. Oral Surg 6:176–200, 1953.
3. Chalian VA, Drane JB, Standish MS: Maxillofacial Prosthetics. Williams & Wilkins, Baltimore, 1971.
4. Reisburg DJ, Habakuk SW: A history of facial and ocular prosthetics. Adv Opthalmol Plast Reconstr Surg 8:11–24, 1990.
5. Ring ME: The history of maxillofacial prosthetics. Plast Reconstr Surg 87:174–184, 1991.
6. Bulbulian AH: Facial Prosthesis. Charles C Thomas, Springfield, IL, 1973.
7. Lee DC: Tycho Brahe and his sixteenth century nasal prosthesis. Plast Reconstr Surg 50:332, 1972.
8. The Works of that Famous Chirurgion, Ambroise Paré, Translated from Latin and compared with the French by Thomas Johnson. Richard Cotes & William DuGard, London, 1649, pp 578–579.
9. Tetamore FLR: Deformities of the Face and Orthopedics, Treatment of Spinal Curvatures with New Aluminum Shell Jackets, Artificial Devices for Deformities of the Face, Also Report of Operations on Children Under Three Years of Age for Angular Deformities of the Legs. Brooklyn, 1894.
10. Bulbulian AH: Facial Prosthetics. Charles C Thomas, Springfield, IL, 1973, 40–67.
11. Kingsley NA: A Treatise on Oral Deformities. Appleton-Century-Crofts, New York, 1880, pp 215–312.
12. Gonzalez JB: Recently developed elastomers for facial prostheses. Mayo Clin Proc 53:423–431, 1978.
13. Deranian HM: The miracle man of the western front: The story of Dr. Varaazstad Kazanjian. Bull Hist Dent 32:92, 1984.
14. Beumer J, Curtis TA, Firtell DN: Maxillofacial Rehabilitation. CV Mosby, St. Louis, 1979.
15. Montgomery H: Precancerous dermatosis and epithelioma in situ. Arch Dermatol 39:387, 1939.
16. Anderson NP, Anderson HE: Development of basal cell epithelioma as a consequence of radiodermatitis. Acta Dermatol Syphilol 63:586–596, 1951.
17. Goldschmidt H: Dermatologic radiotherapy and thyroid cancer: dose measurements and risk quantification. Arch Dermatol 119:383, 1983.
18. Beumer J III, Curtis T, Harrison R: Radiation therapy of the oral cavity: sequelae and management. Head Neck Surg 1:392–408, 1979.
19. Friedman RB: Osteoradionecrosis: causes and prevention. NCI Monogr 9:145–149, 1990.
20. Myers RA, Marx RE: Use of hyperbaric oxygen in postradiation head and neck surgery. NCI Monogr 9:151–157, 1990.
21. Carl W: Managing the oral manifestations of cancer therapy: head-and-neck radiation therapy. Compendium 9:306–312, 1988.
22. Carl W: Managing the oral manifestations of cancer therapy: chemotherapy. Compendium 9:376–378, 1988.
23. Miller RN: Psychological problems of patients with head and neck cancer. In: Miller RN (ed): Rehabilitation of the Cancer Patient. Year Book Medical, Chicago, 1972, pp 1946–1957.
24. Jani RM, Schaaf NG: An evaluation of facial prostheses. J Prosthet Dent 39:546–550, 1978.
25. Roefs AJ, van Oort RP, Schaub RM: Factors related to the acceptance of facial prostheses. J Prosthet Dent 52:849–852, 1984.
26. Chen MS, Udagama A, Drane JB: Evaluation of facial prostheses for head and neck cancer patients. J Prosthet Dent 46:538–544, 1981.
27. Gillis RE Jr, Swenson WM, Laney WR: Psychological factors involved in maxillofacial prosthetics. J Prosthet Dent 41:183–188, 1979.
28. Marunick MT, Harrison R, Beumer J: Prosthodontic rehabilitation of midfacial defects. J Prosthet Dent 54:553–560, 1985.
29. Sela M, Lowental U: Theraputic effects of maxillofacial prostheses. Oral Surg Oral Med Oral Pathol 50:13–16, 1980.
30. Woods JE: Facial prostheses or surgical reconstruction? Mayo Clin Proc 53:473, 1978.
31. Beder OE, Weinstein P: Explorations of the coping of adolescents with orofacial anomalies using the Cornell Medical Index. J Prosthet Dent 43:565–567, 1980.
32. Albrektsson T, Brönemark P-I, Jacobsson M, Tjellström A: Present clinical applications of osseointegrated percutaneous implants. Plast Reconstr Surg 79:721–730, 1987.
33. Suen JY, Myers MN: Maxillofacial prosthetic rehabilitation. In: Aramany MA, Myers MN (eds): Cancer of the Head and Neck. Churchill Livingstone, New York, 1981, pp 165–184.
34. Parr GR, Goldman BM, Rahn AO: Maxillofacial prosthetic principles in the surgical planning for facial defects. J Prosthet Dent 46:323–324, 1981.
35. Pitton RD, Murphy PJ, Schlossberg L, Harris LW: The development of acrylic eye prosthesis at the National Naval Medical Center. J Am Dent Assoc 32:1227–1244, 1945.
36. Bartlett SO, Moore DJ: Ocular prosthesis: a physiologic system. J Prosthet Dent 29:450–459, 1973.
37. Green WR, Maumenee AE, Sanders TE, et al: Sympathetic uveitis following evisceration. Trans Am Acad Opthalmol Otol 76:625, 1972.
38. Arthur Perry, M.D.: Personal communication, January, 1991.
39. Beumer J, Firtell DW, Curtis TA: Current concepts in cranioplasty. J Prosthet Dent 42:67, 1979.
40. Lilla JA, Vistnes LM: Long term study of reactions to various silicone implants in rabbits. Plast Reconstr Surg 57:637, 1976.
41. Jarcho M, Kay JF, Gumaer KI, et al: Tissue, cellular and subcellular events at a bone-ceramic hydroxyapatite interface. J Bioeng 1: 79–92, 1977.
42. Davis PK: The complications of silastic implants. Experience with 137 consecutive cases. Br J Plast Surg 24:405, 1971.
43. Milward TM: The fate of Silastic and vitrathene nasal implants. Br J Plast Surg 25:276, 1972.
44. Zarb GA, Schmitt A: The longitudinal clinical effectiveness of osseointegrated dental implants: the Toronto study. Part I: surgical results. J Prosthet Dent 63:451–457, 1990.
45. Parel SM, Tjellstrom A: The United States and Swedish experience with osseointegration and facial prostheses. Int J Oral Maxillofac Implants 6:75–79, 1991.
46. Marsh JL, Vannier MV, Stevens WG, et al: Computerized imaging for soft-tissue and osseous reconstruction in the head and neck. Clin Plast Surg 12:279, 1985.
47. Moore DJ, Glasser ZR, Tabacco MJ, Linebaugh MG: Evaluation of polymeric materials for maxillofacial prosthetics. J Prosthet Dent 38:319, 1977.
48. Gonzalez JB, Chao EYS, An KN: Physical and mechanical behavior of polyurethane elastomers formulations used for facial prosthesis. J Prosthet Dent 39:307, 1978.
49. Bell WT, Chalian BA, Moore BK: Polymethyl siloxane materials in maxillofacial prosthodontics: evaluation and comparison of physical properties. J Prosthet Dent 54:404, 1985.
50. Sanchez RA, Moore DJ, Cruz DL, Chappell R: Comparison of the physical properties of two types of polydimethyl siloxane for fabrication of facial prostheses. J Prosthet Dent 67:679, 1992.

CHAPTER 66

Management of Surgical Complications and Suboptimal Results

MARY E. MALONEY

Complications during cutaneous surgery range from minimal problems such as slightly increased bleeding intraoperatively to cardiac arrhythmia or arrest. Anything that increases the difficulty of the procedure or the length of the postoperative recovery is considered a complication. It is often unexpected and changes the surgical approach or the long-term outcome. Complications may occur intraoperatively, in the immediate postoperative period, or even after what is considered the normal postoperative period. Within each of these time frames there are certain complications that are more likely to occur and that the surgeon should be ready to handle.

Complications are often interrelated. For example,

hematoma formation may result in tissue swelling, which places tension on the wound, which in turn increases the risks of infection, dehiscence, and wound necrosis. This cascade of complications (Fig. 66–1) is important to recognize so that the chain of events can be interrupted as soon as possible.

Bleeding

Bleeding is both an expected part of every surgery and the most common of all surgical complications. It may lead to other complications such as infection or dehiscence or may be a continuing complication by itself.

Figure 66–1. Interrelationships of common surgical complications.

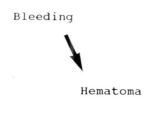

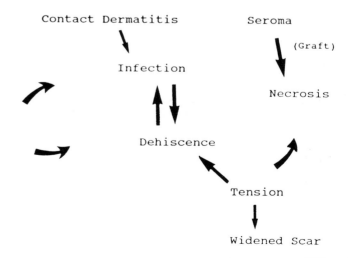

Obtaining meticulous hemostasis during a surgical procedure is as important as identifying the risk factors associated with postoperative bleeding.

HEMOSTATIC PATHWAYS

Understanding the hemostatic pathway is important in the management of bleeding. Primary hemostasis occurs when a platelet plug rapidly forms after vascular injury. This stops additional blood loss from capillaries, small arterioles, and venules. Any platelet dysfunction, either intrinsic or secondary to the use of medications, will cause difficulty in obtaining hemostasis. Continued oozing will require great attention to bring this under control. Secondary hemostasis, also known as fibrin formation, results from the reactions of the plasma coagulation system and requires a longer time to complete its portion of final clot formation. In essence, fibrin strands strengthen a primary hemostatic or platelet plug. This portion of the hemostatic pathway is particularly important for larger vessels and also prevents secondary bleeding from occurring within several hours or days after the initial injury or surgery. Many genetic disorders and medications (e.g., warfarin) interfere with this particular pathway. These two aspects of hemostasis will be reviewed in more detail.

Vascular injury allows exposure of the collagenous components of the subendothelial connective tissue. It is this subendothelial connective tissue to which platelets adhere. This adherence is facilitated by von Willebrand's factor with the formation of a cross-link between the platelet receptor sites and the exposed collagen fibrils. This binding of collagen to the platelet cell receptors activates the platelets to secrete a number of mediators and activates phospholipase C and phospholipase A_2. The end result of this pathway (Fig. 66–2) is the release of thromboxane A_2 and prostacyclin. Thromboxane A_2 leads to further platelet aggregation, causing platelets to adhere to each other rather than the collagenous endothelial substrate. Thromboxane A_2 also stimulates phospholipase C, amplifying the process. Prostacyclin is part of the internal control and inhibits platelet activation by inhibiting phospholipase C.

As platelets adhere to one another and become part of the primary platelet aggregation, they are activated to secrete substances into both the surrounding tissue and the circulation. Of the many substances secreted, adenosine diphosphate modifies the surface of the platelets so that fibrinogen can link platelets and cause clot maturation. The platelet plug initiates the clotting process and is probably most important for providing the hemostasis that occurs intraoperatively.

At essentially the same time that the platelet plug is forming, the secondary phase of clot formation is occurring. Plasma proteins, Hageman's factor (Factor XII), high-molecular-weight kininogen (HMWK) and prekallikrein (PK) complex with exposed endothelial collagen. This means that exposed collagen is important in both phases of clot formation. The clotting cascade moves through the extrinsic and intrinsic pathways (Fig. 66–3) and converts prothrombin (Factor II) to thrombin. Thrombin then converts fibrinogen to fibrin, which po-

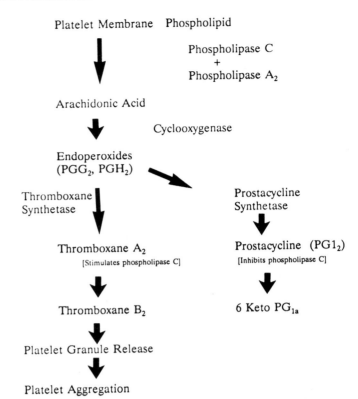

Figure 66–2. The cascade leading to platelet aggregation.

lymerizes with the platelet aggregate to an insoluble gel. The final step is stabilization by cross-linking, which leads to the development of the final mature clot. By understanding these pathways, the cutaneous surgeon will be better prepared to deal with complications related to hemostasis.

INTERFERENCE WITH NORMAL CLOT FORMATION

A number of factors interfere with normal hemostasis at various points in the clotting pathway. These include mechanical factors, thrombocytopenia, platelet dysfunction, pharmacologic interference, and acquired or genetic defects in the clotting cascade.

Vasoconstriction

Vasoconstriction itself plays a major role in clotting. When a vessel is cut, it immediately constricts, reducing the diameter that has to be filled by platelet aggregation. This vasoconstriction also decreases the volume of blood lost before platelet aggregation can occur. Surgeons have used epinephrine in local anesthetics to preconstrict the vessels and provide a clean or bloodless field during surgery. The duration of this epinephrine effect is variable, but the risk in using epinephrine is that a small vessel may be so vasoconstricted that it may not actually bleed during the procedure. However, as the epinephrine effect resolves and the vessel returns to its normal diameter, bleeding may occur suddenly. This bleeding usually begins within 30 minutes after completion of the

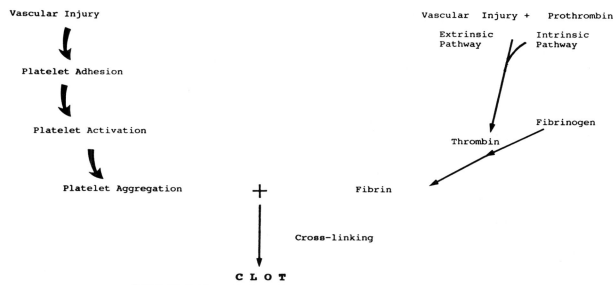

Figure 66–3. The extrinsic and intrinsic pathways of the clotting cascade.

surgical procedure, although it may be delayed as long as 2 to 3 hours. If the vessel is small, 10 to 15 minutes of direct pressure may resolve the bleeding. However, in some instances the incision may need to be reopened, the bleeding vessel identified and cauterized, and the wound reclosed, all by means of sterile technique. Although epinephrine is a convenient surgical aid, this unpredictable complication has led some cutaneous surgeons to use epinephrine only for longer procedures in which the benefit of prolonged anesthesia will not be outweighed by the risk of a missed cut blood vessel.

Alcohol is a potent vasodilator and, when consumed postoperatively, may restart bleeding, because as the vessel dilates, the maturing clot may be dislodged. Pressure may be sufficient to control this bleeding, but occasionally the wound may need to be reopened. For this reason, alcohol should be avoided for several days postoperatively.

Platelets

Platelets may be either absent or nonfunctional (Table 66–1). Thrombocytopenia may be the result of impaired production, as in patients with nonfunctioning bone marrow or bone marrow that is involved with leukemia or metastatic cancer. There may also be excessive destruction through immune mechanisms (e.g., idiopathic thrombocytopenic purpura, or ITP) or a drug reaction or as a result of disseminated intravascular coagulation (DIC), vasculitis, or even abnormal sequestration in the spleen or a hemangioma. Cutaneous surgery, when indicated, can be performed in patients with platelet counts of more than 50,000. Surgery can be performed when absolutely necessary, even in those with lower platelet levels, but great care should be taken to have meticulous hemostasis. Extensive undermining that could produce hidden bleeding sites at a distance from the actual incision should be avoided if possible.

Nonfunctioning platelets are far more commonly en-

countered in the surgical setting. The most common cause of this platelet dysfunction is aspirin use. Aspirin irreversibly inactivates phospholipase, which inhibits platelet aggregation. This irreversible inactivation will affect the platelet for its entire life cycle. Bleeding caused by aspirin consumption and the resulting platelet inhibition is immediate and can be recognized at the time the incision is made. Fortunately, the use of aspirin several days postoperatively does not affect the stability of a previously formed clot.

TABLE 66–1. CAUSES OF THROMBOCYTOPENIA

Impaired production
  Aplastic marrow
  Preleukemia/leukemia
  Metastatic cancer
  Drugs
    Chemotherapeutic agents
    Parenterally administered gold
Excess platelet destruction
  Immune causes
    Acute idiopathic thrombocytopenic purpura
    Chronic idiopathic thrombocytopenic purpura
  Medications
    Antibiotics
    Quinidine
    Quinine
    Sedatives
    Anticonvulsants
    Digoxin
    Methyldopa
  Idiopathic causes
  Disseminated intravascular coagulation (DIC)
  Vasculitis
  Vascular prosthesis
  Abnormal sequestration
    Malignancy
    Liver disease
    Storage disorders
      Splenomegaly
      Proliferating capillary hemangiomas

Aspirin is contained in many over-the-counter allergy, headache, and cold remedies. Patients are frequently unaware that they are consuming aspirin or are under the mistaken impression that the effect is only short-lived and that there will not be any effect 2 to 3 days after consumption. Aspirin currently is commonly used as prophylaxis for myocardial infarction and strokes. Therefore, a large number of elderly patients are taking a single aspirin daily, which adversely affects hemostasis during skin surgery.

Although cutaneous surgery can be done safely when a patient has been taking aspirin, it is imperative to know about this before the procedure begins. Many patients do not consider aspirin a medication and neglect to inform the surgeon when they are asked about current medication use. It is therefore important to ask about all prescription and nonprescription medications the patient may be taking. If the surgeon is anticipating a particularly bloody procedure, it may be prudent to have the patient discontinue aspirin 10 to 14 days beforehand. Again, it is important to instruct the patient not to take any over-the-counter medication without first checking very carefully for the presence of aspirin.

Nonsteroidal anti-inflammatory drugs (NSAIDs) reversibly bind at the same point as aspirin in the cyclo-oxygenase pathway. All NSAIDs inhibit platelet function.[1, 2] The duration of platelet dysfunction is directly related to the half-life of NSAIDs. Longer-acting drugs have a longer effect on the platelet. The pharmacologic effect should be undetectable after four half-lives. However, no study has documented increased intraoperative or postoperative bleeding associated with the use of NSAIDs.[3]

INHERITED CLOTTING DEFECTS

There are a large number of inherited clotting defects that may adversely affect a surgical procedure.[4, 5] The more important of these will be discussed individually.

Von Willebrand's Disease

Von Willebrand's disease is the most common of the inherited bleeding disorders and is inherited as an autosomal dominant trait. Because of this inheritance pattern, some von Willebrand's factor is produced by the normal allele. For this reason, laboratory measurements of von Willebrand's factor may fluctuate. The factor facilitates platelet adhesion, especially in high-flow situations, and also serves as the plasma carrier for Factor VIII. Consequently, decreased levels of von Willebrand's factor may also decrease circulating levels of Factor VIII. In mild cases of von Willebrand's disease, extensive bleeding may occur only with surgery or trauma, making this disorder unrecognizable preoperatively. It is common for this disease to first be suspected when bleeding occurs after a surgical procedure has been performed, and it may be diagnosed only after full postoperative investigation.

On evaluation, a prolonged bleeding time and a decrease in the quantitative von Willebrand's factor in plasma are found. With the decreased von Willebrand's factor, plasma Factor VIII may also be decreased on evaluation. There is also an acquired form of the disease in which antibodies block function. In this variant, von Willebrand's factor levels will be normal.

Hemophilia A (Factor VIII Deficiency)

Factor VIII regulates the activation of Factor X and circulates complexed to the von Willebrand factor. Bleeding may occur hours or days after injury, and thus immediately after surgery there may be no suspicion of continued bleeding. The disorder may be quantitated as severe (with less than 1% of Factor VIII activity), moderate (with 1 to 5% Factor VIII activity), or mild (patients with greater than 5% of Factor VIII activity). If surgery is required in these patients, Factor VIII levels should be maintained at greater than 50% for 10 to 14 days after surgery to prevent late postoperative bleeding.

Hemophilia B (Factor IX Deficiency, Christmas Disease)

Hemophilia B is a deficiency of Factor IX and occurs only in males. Clinically, this disorder cannot be distinguished from hemophilia A, but cryoprecipitate (Factor VIII) will not correct the bleeding defect. Fresh frozen plasma is required for correction.

Factor XI Deficiency

Factor XI deficiency is inherited as an autosomal recessive trait; the factor itself is part of the intrinsic pathway. Spontaneous bleeding is usually minimal, and patients with this problem may not be diagnosed until the perioperative period. Daily infusion of fresh frozen plasma will correct this defect; such correction is important to prevent late postoperative bleeding.

Fibrinogen

Fibrinogen may be either absent or dysfunctional. When the fibrinogen is only dysfunctional, circulating levels will be normal, and the cause of a bleeding disorder may be difficult to diagnose. Spontaneous bleeding will vary from minimal to moderate.

Factor XIII

Factor XIII is a transglutaminase that cross-links by fibrinogen and is therefore essential in clot stabilization. Bleeding occurs in the late postoperative period as clot retraction and stabilization become important. Fresh frozen plasma can be used to correct this defect. Assaying for the level of Factor XIII is the only laboratory technique that will detect this disorder.

Activation Pathway Deficiencies (Factor XII, HMWK, and PK)

Deficiencies of these factors are rare and do not produce clinical bleeding. However, there will be an

TABLE 66–2. EVALUATION OF THE HEMOSTATIC HISTORY

1. History of excessive or prolonged bleeding with previous surgery, including dental procedures
2. Previous need for a transfusion to replace blood loss or to stop bleeding
3. History of spontaneous bleeding or excess bleeding with minor trauma
4. A bleeding problem present as child
5. Concurrent medical problems
6. Medications including the date of last use of aspirin or a nonsteroidal anti-inflammatory drug (NSAID)

increase in the partial thromboplastin time (PTT), and preoperative screening may trigger a full evaluation. Identification of this problem is important in explaining the increased PTT.

PREOPERATIVE EVALUATION FOR BLEEDING

The most important part of the preoperative evaluation is the history (Table 66–2). The medical history will identify patients who may be at risk for bleeding, and testing can then be used to identify the specific defect. Routine laboratory evaluation should *not* be used to replace the history; rather, it should supplement it. If there is no history of bleeding complications and the patient is otherwise well, laboratory testing is usually unnecessary. However, when testing is indicated, it is important to know which tests are appropriate (Table 66–3). A platelet count will identify only a quantitative problem. A low count may be the result of marrow failure (aplastic anemia, hematologic malignancy, metastatic disease, or drugs such as gold or chemotherapeutic medications), sequestration of platelets in the spleen, a hemangioma, or immunologic destruction.

Platelet function is measured by the bleeding time. A decrease in platelets produces a prolonged bleeding time. Dysfunctional platelets may be the result of med-

TABLE 66–3. LABORATORY TESTS TO DETECT BLEEDING DISORDERS

Platelet count
  Qualitative numbers only
  Does not reflect platelet dysfunction
Bleeding time (BT)
  Indicator of platelet function
  Indirectly reflects a decreased number of platelets
  Aspirin and NSAIDs both cause prolongation
Prothrombin time (PT)
  Reflects defects in both extrinsic and common coagulation pathways
  Warfarin affects this test early in its administration
Partial thromboplastin time (PTT)
  Reflects defects in both intrinsic and common coagulation pathways
  Abnormal with heparin administration
  Also reflects warfarin activity
Thrombin time (TT)
  Measures conversion of fibrinogen to fibrin

NSAID, Nonsteroidal anti-inflammatory drug.

ications, congenital platelet defects, or von Willebrand's disease. The bleeding time may be prolonged by interference with platelet adhesion.

The prothrombin time (PT) can be used to determine a defect in the extrinsic clotting pathway, while the activated partial thromboplastin time (aPTT) can detect a defect in the intrinsic pathway. When results of both tests are abnormal, there is a defect in the portion of the pathway shared by the two. When the PT or aPTT is abnormal, further testing may be needed to definitively identify the specific defect (Table 66–4). It should be remembered that Factor XII, PK, and HMWK may cause an abnormal aPTT level but are not associated with clinical bleeding.

SURGICAL COMPLICATIONS FROM BLEEDING

A bleeding complication may occur in one of several forms: acute bleeding (during surgery), immediate postoperative bleeding (first few hours postoperatively), or late postoperative bleeding (several days after surgery), which correlates with impaired clot retraction.

TABLE 66–4. CAUSES OF ABNORMAL LABORATORY TEST RESULTS

Abnormal platelet count
  Marrow failure
  Consumption
    ITP
    DIC
  Sequestration
Abnormal bleeding time
  Drugs
    Aspirin
    NSAIDs
  von Willebrand's disease
  Nonfunctional platelets
  Renal or liver disease
Abnormal prothrombin time (PT)
  Factor VII deficiency
  Vitamin K deficiency (mild) affecting Factors II, VII, IX, and X
  Warfarin (early effect)
  Liver disease
Abnormal activated partial thromboplastin time (aPTT)
  Hemophilia A (Factor VIII deficiency)
  Hemophilia B (Factor IX deficiency)
  Factor XI deficiency
  Warfarin
  Liver disease
  Heparin
  Lupus anticoagulant
  Vitamin K deficiency (severe)
  von Willebrand's disease
  Factor XII deficiency
  Prekallikrein
  High-molecular-weight kininogen (HMWK)
Abnormal prothrombin and activated partial thromboplastin time
  Vitamin K deficiency (late) affecting Factors II, VII, IX, and X
  Warfarin (late)
Abnormal thrombin time
  Heparin
  Dysfibrinogenemia
  Paraproteinemia

DIC, Disseminated intravascular coagulation; ITP, idiopathic thrombocytopenic purpura; NSAID, nonsteroidal anti-inflammatory drug.

Acute Intraoperative Bleeding

Acute intraoperative bleeding is most frequently related to transecting or unroofing an arterial bleeder. The unroofing process occurs when the vessel is not fully transected. A vessel damaged in this way is usually more easily located but may bleed more profusely than the fully transected arterial bleeder. The transected vessel tends to retract and constrict, thereby decreasing the volume of blood flowing into the wound. The unroofed or partially transected vessel does not have the ability to retract and constrict and therefore may cause more copious bleeding. Such arteriolar bleeding is stopped by clamping the vessel immediately and treating it either with electrocautery or by tying it off with an appropriate suture ligature. The figure-of-eight suture is most commonly used for ligating an interrupted artery. It is usually important to treat both ends of a bleeding artery identically, as many arteries have sufficient backflow from the upstream end of the artery to cause significant bleeding or hematoma formation.

The other acute bleeding problem is the vigorous oozing related to aspirin use. Virtually all vessels in the wound contribute to this ooze, and it is impossible to identify a single blood vessel source or to rapidly stop the oozing process. In such patients, several steps are absolutely imperative. Meticulous hemostasis should be obtained with electrocautery before initiating wound closure. If possible, a dry field should be obtained, waiting 10 to 15 minutes, if possible, to be certain that there is complete hemostasis before closing the wound.

In those instances when aspirin use is known preoperatively, some surgeons may choose to avoid using epinephrine in lidocaine. This will prevent immediate small arteriolar vasoconstriction and increase intraoperative bleeding but will avoid dilation of an uncauterized vessel once the epinephrine effect wears off, resulting in bleeding 1 to 3 hours later. A hemostatic scalpel (Shaw scalpel) or carbon dioxide laser, if available, may be used in these instances. Each of these instruments seals blood vessels as the incision is being made and may make the procedure somewhat less difficult to perform.

Early Postoperative Bleeding

Early postoperative bleeding is usually sudden in onset and moderate in amount. Most of these bleeding vessels will be found at the most distal extent of undermining or in a muscle that has been cut or exposed. If this bleeding occurs while the patient is still in the operating room, the wound should be reopened and explored in sterile fashion. The use of epinephrine in the local anesthetic should be avoided so as not to mask the bleeding site by vasoconstriction. Skin hooks are an important aid in adequately visualizing the entire wound. Immediate wound exploration is more expeditious than a late-night return to the emergency department. If wound takedown is done using sterile technique and the wound is immediately resutured in a sterile fashion, there is no need to use prophylactic antibiotics.

If bleeding occurs after the patient has gone home, 10 to 15 minutes of direct pressure on the wound may control it. This requires the patient to remove the saturated dressing, apply a clean dressing, and put direct pressure on the wound. This possible complication should be included in the postoperative wound care sheet and should be part of the postoperative wound care instructions given to all patients so that they will be able to deal satisfactorily with the problem. This will also reduce much of the anxiety that patients typically have when their bandage becomes saturated with blood. However, if bleeding is not controlled with pressure, the surgeon should meet the patient in the office or emergency department.

Late Postoperative Bleeding

The cause of late postoperative bleeding may be interference with clot retraction or trauma to the wound during the postoperative period. It is not uncommon for a hematoma to form late in the course of wound healing after complete reepithelialization and partial collagen deposition have occurred. If the hematoma produces sufficient pressure to result in necrosis of the surrounding tissue or to cause partial wound dehiscence, the wound must be opened and the hematoma evacuated. At this point, it is most prudent to allow this wound to heal by second intention. This should be fully explained to the patient so that it is understood that if a cosmetically acceptable scar does not result, scar revision can be performed at a later time. Occasionally, a hematoma can be evacuated with the use of a large-bore needle and syringe or extracted with the removal of a single suture. In these instances, the expected cosmetic result of the procedure is not significantly altered, and an excellent outcome can be predicted.

Many patients may not detect or report hematoma formation and may return for suture removal with a firm, deeply fibrotic, resolving hematoma. In these instances, no intervention should be performed, as such swelling will resolve spontaneously over several months. Often gentle massage or a single injection of intralesional steroids may be useful in speeding resolution of this process.

Occasionally, ecchymoses develop at sites distant to the surgical site. These are the result of blood diffusing along the natural tissue planes and collecting at distant dependent sites. This complication requires patient reassurance only; resorption of the blood may be hastened by heat applied with hot towels or a heating pad.

Seroma

Seromas are the result of transudating serum into a closed space. This frequently occurs if dead space is not obliterated at the depth of the wound and is a common complication of skin grafting (Table 66–5). A seroma in a sutured wound may be easily extracted with a large-bore needle and syringe at any time after it has been identified. A seroma that forms under a skin graft can

TABLE 66–5. **SPECIFIC COMPLICATIONS OF VARIOUS SURGICAL PROCEDURES**

Random-pattern flaps
   Trapdoor defect
   Necrosis
Full-thickness grafts
   Seroma
   Hematoma
   Necrosis
Dermabrasion and chemical peels
   Keloids
   Hypertrophic scars
   Irregular pigmentation
     Hypopigmentation
     Hyperpigmentation

"float" the graft off the recipient bed and interfere significantly with graft survival. Therefore, it is important to identify a seroma beneath a skin graft as soon as it occurs. Seromas can be evacuated through a small nick made in the skin graft with a 22-gauge needle (a technique known as "pie-crusting"). If they are near the margin of the skin graft, they can be rolled to the graft margin with cotton swabs.

Allergic Reactions

Allergic reactions may consist of the type I anaphylaxis or type IV contact sensitivity. These reactions may occur to virtually any substance or medication used during the surgical procedure. Therefore, it is absolutely vital to obtain an accurate history, recording all known allergies in the patient's chart preoperatively. Many patients report tachycardia as an allergic reaction to epinephrine when it is simply a direct adrenergic effect. It is vital to differentiate these types of reactions from a true allergy.

INTRADERMAL LOCAL ANESTHETICS

Local anesthetics fall into one of two major groups: ester or amide type anesthetics. The ester type, represented by procaine (Novocain), cross-reacts with para-aminobenzoic acid (PABA) esters and other related compounds. The ester group has been associated with a higher incidence of allergic reactions and for this reason are not commonly used in medicine or dentistry at this time.

Amide anesthetics include lidocaine, bupivacaine, etidocaine, and prilocaine. Of these, lidocaine is the most commonly used, although the others have their proponents and their indications for particular uses. A few allergic reactions with this class of anesthetic have been reported. Because these agents are injected, the reaction may begin immediately with local edema, generalized urticaria, or anaphylaxis. Immediate treatment with epinephrine, antihistamines, and circulatory support is often required, and therefore these agents must be immediately available in the surgical suite for the rare but life-threatening reaction (see Chap. 13).

There have been rare reports of contact sensitivity to the amide anesthetics. The method of sensitization is usually through over-the-counter application to mucosal surfaces (e.g., with hemorrhoidal preparations) or to otherwise damaged skin with products such as sunburn creams or sprays. Cross-sensitivity between compounds of the same ester or amide group does occur.

SKIN PREPARATION AGENTS

Povidone-iodine is an iodophor that slowly releases a low concentration of iodine. Iodophor compounds have been shown to cause an acute contact dermatitis in the sensitized patient. This contact dermatitis, consisting of vesiculation and weeping, may develop in the area of application and predispose the patient to secondary infection. Treatment should include application of wet dressings and topical steroids. Occasionally, systemic steroids may be required if the reaction is extensive and severe. However, the best advice is to avoid the use of these compounds in the known sensitized patient.

Chlorhexidine gluconate has become very popular as a surgical skin preparation agent and surgical scrub. It causes very little skin irritation, has a very weak sensitizing potential,[6] and provides a prolonged bactericidal effect. Application has been reported to cause contact allergy[7] in a few patients, and there has been one report of anaphylaxis associated with mucosal application.[8]

TOPICAL ANTIBIOTICS

Topical antibiotics are known to produce contact sensitivity and may be a problem for many patients, as they are available over the counter and are frequently used by patients for a variety of problems. The most common sensitizer is neomycin, which causes sensitization in as many as 6 to 8% of patients.[9, 10] Neomycin sensitivity and bacitracin sensitivity frequently occur in the same patient.[11, 12] This is probably an independent but simultaneous sensitivity, as both medications are frequently found in the same over-the-counter preparations. Bacitracin, when used as a single agent, does not appear to be a potent sensitizer. Any topical antibiotic can be a sensitizer, and the cutaneous surgeon using such products should be aware of that possibility. The use of single agents in a petrolatum base will decrease the risk of dual sensitization and may help to identify the causes of a contact sensitivity.

A mild contact dermatitis may be mistaken for a wound infection. It is important to look carefully for early vesiculation and to determine whether the configuration corresponds to the site of application of the topical antibiotic ointment. Many patients apply the ointment over an increasingly wider area as the contact dermatitis increases in severity or extent of involvement. The physician should look carefully for involvement up to the incision line, which is an indication of contact sensitivity to a topical product used in wound care, as opposed to tape or dressing irritation, which usually does not involve the incision itself.

TAPE ALLERGY

Many patients react severely to adhesive tape application. Some react with a rapid severe blistering, while others have a more chronic erythema with skin irritation. A change to hypoallergenic tape is helpful, but a few patients also react to these tapes. In some locations, dressings may be held in place with circumferential gauze wraps or elastic bandages without adhesives to avoid tape application in the severely allergic or reactive patient. For other wounds, dressings should be discontinued as soon as possible, usually after 24 hours.

Infection

Infection rates vary by institution and by procedure. An infection in a closed wound is a much greater problem than a superficial infection in an open wound. Infections may range in severity from those with mild erythema to those with severe abscess formation. The two different complications that may be seen with infection are local infection and systemic infection resulting from bacteremia.

WOUND INFECTION

A mild wound infection may be difficult to distinguish from a normally healing wound or a mild irritative or allergic dermatitis around a wound. Often the normal wound demonstrates mild erythema and mild tenderness as the result of the surgical trauma. In many patients there is an inflammatory response to the suture material itself, causing erythema around each individual suture. This should not be confused with a wound infection. Wound infections usually develop 4 to 10 days postoperatively, rather than immediately postoperatively, when pain would be expected to be greatest. One point that may be helpful in determining the presence of a wound infection is that with an infection, pain continues to increase rather than diminish postoperatively; true postincisional pain decreases postoperatively. Still, differentiating the normal healing process from a mild wound infection can be difficult. Most surgeons prefer to treat the patient with an antibiotic that provides *Staphylococcus aureus* coverage. If purulent drainage is present, it is prudent to perform Gram stains and cultures of the drainage before starting antibiotics. However, in very mild wound infections, drainage is not usually present.

As the severity of the wound infection increases, there is increasing erythema, swelling, and tenderness. This host inflammatory response has a negative effect on wound healing. Proteolytic enzymes are released from the inflammatory cells into the surrounding tissue. These enzymes will speed the resorption of buried sutures, thereby decreasing wound support and increasing the risk of wound dehiscence.

The most common organism identified in cutaneous surgical wound infections is *S. aureus*. Many organisms may be responsible for infections in other locations. For example, the ear and perineal area are particularly susceptible to gram-negative infections. In all cases of infection, specimens should be obtained for culture and a Gram stain done to help direct therapy. If a Gram stain is not helpful, initial therapy should be broad and directed toward the most likely organisms for the location of the wound infection. Wounds should be opened and drained completely. In some instances, this does not mean removing all sutures, but a significant proportion of the sutures will certainly need to be removed, which will unquestionably affect the final cosmetic outcome. Deep wounds may require packing with sterile or iodoform gauze, which will need to be changed daily.

Rarely is a wound infection from cutaneous surgery serious enough to necessitate hospitalization, unless the patient has a contraindication to the available recommended oral antibiotic or an underlying condition that impairs tissue penetration of antibiotics (e.g., diabetes) (Table 66–6). The one exception is malignant external otitis, which represents a severe infection of the external auditory canal with *Pseudomonas* organisms. If this infection is not recognized early, there may be loss of the ear, or *Pseudomonas* sepsis, with its associated high mortality rate, may occur.[13] Hospitalization and use of intravenous antibiotics, at least until the organism's sensitivity to oral antibiotics becomes known, are prudent in this condition. When a severe wound infection compromises a surgical procedure, it is important to explain to the patient that future scar revision is available if the cosmetic outcome is either unacceptable or suboptimal. This frequently reduces the patient's fears about the final outcome and allows the physician to deal appropriately with the wound infection.

BACTEREMIA

Systemic infection resulting from cutaneous surgery is rare. A transient bacteremia may occur, especially in

TABLE 66–6. DISEASES THAT MAY AFFECT THE COMPLICATION RATE OR DELAY HEALING

Metabolic disorders
  Diabetes mellitus
  Renal failure
  Adrenal disease (Cushing's syndrome)
  Thyroid disease (hyper- or hypothyroidism)
  Malnutrition or starvation
  Chronic liver disease
Immunosuppression
  Organ transplantation
  Malignancy
    Lymphoma
    Leukemia
Autoimmune disorders
  Systemic lupus erythematosus
Pulmonary insufficiency
Vascular disorders
  Coronary insufficiency
  Chronic congestive heart failure
  Hypertension (uncontrolled)
  Valve replacement
Coagulation disorders
  Hereditary
  Medication-related
  Acquired

cases where there is an eroded but not clinically infected skin lesion.[14] Care must be taken in patients with underlying conditions that could lead to seeding of infection, such as an artificial heart valve, mitral valve prolapse, or joint prostheses.

Dehiscence

Dehiscence is almost always related to another complicating event, the most common being hematoma, wound infection, or premature suture removal. A severe wound infection will require premature suture removal so that the wound can be opened and drained. In some instances, hematomas require evacuation, which also necessitates opening the wound. On occasion, a hematoma that is not evacuated surgically will significantly interfere with the tensile strength of the wound, causing dehiscence when the sutures are removed at the normal time.

Although the normal events and time course of wound healing are understood, not all patients heal at the same rate. Healing may be affected by wound tension, external trauma, underlying medical conditions, and smoking. Any or all of these factors may cause a wound to dehisce when sutures are removed at what would otherwise be deemed the appropriate time. Adhesive strips add a little security to a wound once the sutures are removed. However, wound tension, trauma, or patient activity can still cause a wound to open.

Management of the dehisced wound depends directly on the cause. Wounds that have been surgically opened for hematoma evacuation or wound infection need to heal by second intention, and a second surgical repair may be required to improve cosmesis. A wound that opens because of nonspecific factors may be resutured if it is brought to the attention of the physician within 24 hours. Unless there is nonviable material at the base or margins of the incision, "freshening" of the edges is not absolutely required. The wound should be cleaned and prepared for closure, which is done using sterile technique. In these instances, selection of the least traumatic suture material (e.g., monofilament nylon) is indicated. The use of prophylactic antibiotics is controversial, and many physicians believe that they are not required in this situation. Others use prophylactic antibiotics to cover *S. aureus*.

Necrosis

Necrosis of a wound is almost always the result of some other complication. In an excisional wound, necrosis may result from hematoma, a very large seroma, undue tension, infection, or an inadequate blood supply. Any of these can cause full-thickness tissue loss and require healing by second intention or a second-stage repair.

Flap survival is dependent on the circulation from the base to the distal tip, and a number of factors may compromise that circulation. The first is poor flap design in which the base is too narrow for the length of the flap. Flaps require a minimal 3:1 length-to-base ratio (i.e., the length of the flap should be no more than three times the width of its base).[15] When that ratio is changed, the distal circulation may be compromised. A common mistake in flap movement is the correction of a dogear at the base of the pedicle so as to narrow the base beyond its initial design.[15] Dogears that form with flap surgery must be corrected away from the base or corrected as a later second procedure after full healing and establishment of a secondary blood supply to the flap (Table 66–5).

A second cause for flap necrosis is inadvertent cutting, cauterization, or ligation of a single arterial feeder to the flap. This may decrease blood flow, which compromises the viability of the flap. Wound tension, especially of the flap tip, may result in ischemia sufficient to cause flap necrosis. The surgeon must ensure that the tension of the flap not involve the flap tip. Occasionally, this cannot be avoided, and if tension is excessive, the tip may be compromised.

Necrosis of a graft is a recognized complication and constitutes a lack of a graft "take." Again, this is usually the result of another complication. Anything that keeps the graft from contacting the recipient bed will compromise the graft. A seroma or hematoma will float the graft off the underlying base and prevent nutrient exchange with the graft. The graft can survive for 24 to 48 hours in this setting, but to maximally preserve the graft, hematomas and seromas must be evacuated as soon as they are detected. Tension on the graft itself will also result in tissue ischemia and may cause graft failure. Tension is usually the result of having a graft that is too small for the recipient site. Care must be taken to design and harvest a graft of adequate size to allow it to lie gently in the recipient site, with sutures acting only to hold it in place; it should not be stretched to fit the recipient site. Patient hypoxemia also decreases oxygen tension and occasionally compromises a graft. A general rule is that patients who smoke one to two packs of cigarettes per day may have sufficient hypoxemia to cause graft failure.

When necrosis occurs, early debridement should be performed only if there is evidence of infection; otherwise the necrosis should be allowed to fully demarcate so that healthy tissue is not removed with the necrotic tissue. Patients with full or partial necrosis need support throughout their course and should be followed up closely.

Tension

Tension has been cited as a cause of both wound dehiscence and tissue necrosis. It may lead to immediate postoperative pain or discomfort and to scar widening as a long-term complication. Sutures are often made very tight when there is excessive wound tension at the time of closure; this frequently leads to "railroad track" scars.

Wound tension should be evaluated thoroughly at the time of surgery to avoid these complications. Occasionally, tension, if not excessive, may be acceptable. There are three surgical techniques that can be used if undue tension is present at the time of wound closure. First, a relaxing incision may be performed 2 to 3 cm from the wound edge and in a direction parallel to it. The initial wound is closed, and the secondary wound is then fully undermined and closed. This method shares tension over a larger area and is especially useful on the scalp, where a second scar will not be a cosmetic problem.

The second method for dealing with tension is to perform immediate tissue expansion. This may be done with formal tissue expanders, Foley catheters,[16] or even intraoperative sutures (see Chap. 28).

Partial closure is a third acceptable method of avoiding tension that would otherwise cause tissue necrosis. In this technique, the wound is closed to the point of tension, and the remainder of the defect is allowed to heal by second intention. Sutures may be taken out after a normal interval, since it is not necessary to wait for full healing of the granulating wound. This type of closure can yield an excellent cosmetic result in some cases.

Excess Granulation Tissue

Hypergranulation is also known as simple granulation tissue formation (Fig. 66–4) or "proud flesh." It consists of an overgrowth of fibroblasts and endothelial cells, and such tissue may be both friable and secondarily infected. It occurs almost exclusively in wounds allowed to heal by second intention, including wounds created by electrodesiccation and curettage, wounds in which complications have arisen and the opened wound has been allowed to heal by second intention, and wounds that have been partially closed (Fig. 66–5). Rarely, hypergranulation may occur even in a sutured wound. In this setting, granulation tissue extends well above the skin surface and prevents reepithelialization. Without removal of this granulation tissue, the wound will not heal.

Granulation tissue may be removed in one of several ways. Most easily, the wound is reanesthetized after being prepared in a sterile fashion, the granulation tissue

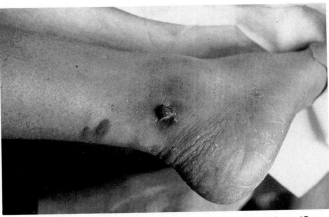

Figure 66–4. Granulation tissue at the site of vascular injury. (Courtesy of John Scully, M.D.)

is curetted, and hemostasis is obtained with either a cautery or aluminum chloride. An alternative method is to treat the tissue with silver nitrate. This is an effective method and does not require anesthesia. However, the silver nitrate may cause pigment deposition or "tattooing" of the resulting scar. Various visible light lasers have also been used to photocoagulate the excess capillaries without anesthesia.

Suturing Complications

There are a wide variety of complications from suture materials and the techniques with which they are used. Sutures may be tied too tightly, causing ischemia and even necrosis of the underlying tissue. During suturing, the tendency is to lightly coapt the wound margins and then cinch the suture knots tightly. Almost all wounds have some degree of swelling postoperatively, and if no allowance is made for this swelling, a knot that is initially tight may cause local tissue strangulation. The loop stitch prevents sutures from being tied too tightly and allows for tissue swelling to prevent ischemia.[17] The square knot is cinched on the second throw, with a loop being left between the first and second throw.

Conversely, if the last throws of knot placement are not cinched down tightly or extra throws are not used with monofilament nonabsorbable sutures, especially polypropylene, the sutures may slowly unravel because of their high "memory" and may come completely untied by the time of suture removal. Similarly, men may inadvertently shave off sutures in the beard area. It is very important to warn them of this possibility and ask them to avoid shaving the sutured area to prevent this complication.

Many wounds require sutures to be left in place for more than 1 week. As the wound reepithelializes, the tracts of the sutures also reepithelialize. After the sutures have been removed, the epithelialized tracts remain. This may set up an inflammatory response and lead to a "stitch abscess," which is a sterile pustule secondary to the inflammatory response in this tract. Similarly, milia may develop at these points; these will need to be expressed. Although these complications are annoying, they should not lead to premature suture removal, as wound dehiscence will leave a much more noticeable scar.

Extrusion of buried sutures is another common postoperative complication. The factors leading to extrusion or "spitting" of buried sutures are poorly defined. There is some suggestion that buried sutures that are placed too close to the skin surface work themselves more easily to the surface and extrude. When the surgical knot is tied at the surface rather than at the depth of a buried suture, it may cause a lump to form in the wound margin and may allow the suture to work to the surface. However, even a properly placed buried suture may work to the surface. In these instances, often a small crust first appears, followed by a small erosion; then a tuft of suture material will extrude or poke through the surface. Patients are usually very worried about this complication, which can occur as early as 2 weeks and

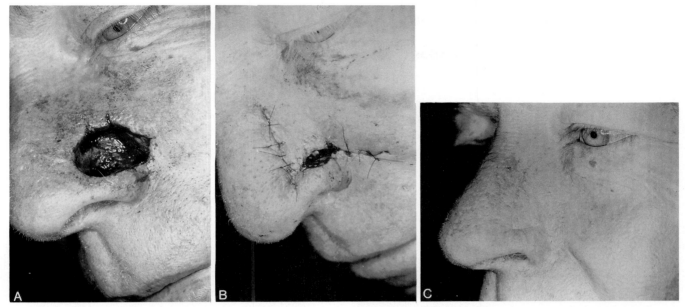

Figure 66–5. *A,* Postoperative defect after Mohs surgery. *B,* Partial closure of the defect (note the infraorbital ecchymosis). *C,* Excellent result without ala deformity.

as late as 6 weeks postoperatively, and they frequently contact the physician about it. It is important to see patients as soon as possible in these situations to allay their fears and remove this focus of inflammation. This complication usually does not adversely affect the long-term outcome of the wound in regard to strength or final cosmetic appearance.

Long-term Postoperative Complications of Wound Appearance

HYPERTROPHIC SCARRING

Hypertrophic scars are thickened, raised, and frequently symptomatic (Figs. 66–6, 66–7). They differ from keloids in that they do not extend beyond the margins of the wound. Hypertrophic scarring occurs most commonly on the chest, shoulders, upper back, and breasts. It may occur in response to acne, dermabrasion (see Table 66–5), or electrodesiccation and curettage or in sutured wounds. Patients with a history of hypertrophic scarring are at greater risk of developing similar scars with other surgical procedures.

It is important to recognize this complication early and to initiate treatment with either high potency topical steroids or intralesional steroid injections. This will decrease the erythema, itching, or pain and should also flatten the scar. However, these methods will not return a scar to normal in that the scar will always be wide and have an irregular texture. The possibility of hypertrophic scar formation should be discussed preoperatively with any patient having a procedure in a known high-risk area or with a history of hypertrophic scarring.

KELOIDS

Keloids are excessive and extensive scars that have formed well beyond the original site of trauma or surgery. These scars are often painful and may be massive in size and may complicate ear piercing or any traumatic or surgical injury. The populations at greatest risk for keloid development include blacks and people of Mediterranean descent. However, keloids may develop in any patient at any time. Sites of predilection include the earlobes (Fig. 66–8), neck, and upper trunk (Fig. 66–9). However, they may occur at any body location and may be disfiguring almost anywhere.

Treatment of keloids is very difficult. In some cases, injected steroids produce a favorable response to the point that the keloidal scar is acceptable to the patient. However, in many patients regression is insignificant

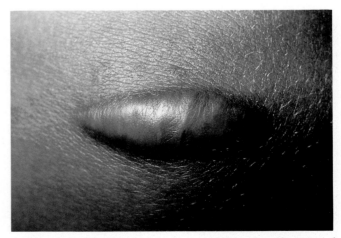

Figure 66–6. Hypertrophic scar at an excision site. (Courtesy of James Marks, Jr., M.D.)

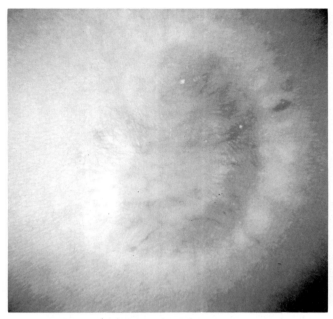

Figure 66–7. Hypertrophic scar at the site of the shave removal of a nevus. (Courtesy of John Scully, M.D.)

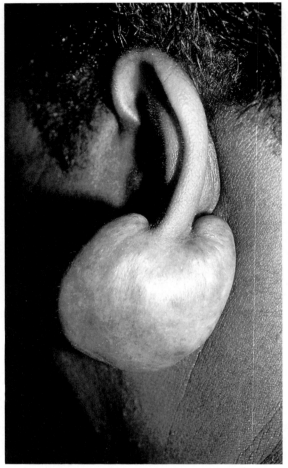

Figure 66–8. Keloid that has developed at the site of ear piercing.

with this approach. Conventional surgery puts the patient at high risk for development of another keloid in the surgical scar and may be self-defeating in that each surgical scar is a little larger than the original keloid and the original keloids themselves are larger than the scar from the original surgical procedure. Sutures themselves may act as a nidus for additional keloid formation. Surgery using the carbon dioxide laser has produced dramatic results in many patients in particular locations. However, the laser appears to be best suited for keloids of the head and neck, particularly of the earlobes. It has not been as successful in treating keloids of the trunk.

WIDENED SCARS

Scars widen over time as the result of forces of tension (Fig. 66–10). More than 80% of the widening occurs in the first 6 months postoperatively.[18] These forces may be the result of a large excision in which tension was unavoidable or inadequate undermining of a wound. In many wounds, buried sutures may reduce some of the tension, which in turn decreases the tendency for a scar to widen. In these instances it is important to use a buried suture that will retain its tensile strength as long as possible. Scar widening also occurs in some locations (e.g., chest, shoulders, and upper back) irrespective of wound management. This should be discussed preoperatively with the patient when any procedure is being performed in these areas.

Prevention of this complication is more important than treatment. When possible, the avoidance of cosmetic procedures in these high-risk areas is always prudent. If a surgical procedure is unavoidable, support of the wound with a nonabsorbable buried suture may be helpful in decreasing scar widening,[19] as may the

newer slowly absorbing sutures. Postoperative external support with adhesive strips will not usually affect the long-term scar outcome.

A patient who is relatively sedentary and does not perform heavy physical activities is at less risk of developing scar widening, as long-term stresses and collagen remodeling occur with greater levels of physical activity. This means that very active people are more prone to

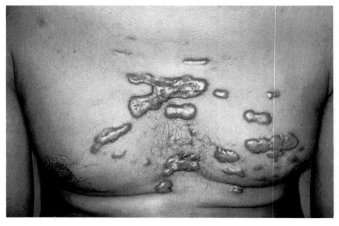

Figure 66–9. Keloids of the chest complicating acne.

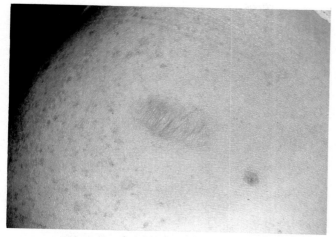

Figure 66–10. Widened scar of the shoulder.

scar spreading over time. It is important to remember that scars may spread for a full year after surgical wounding.

PIGMENTARY CHANGES

Pigmentary changes are the result of many factors. Postinflammatory hyperpigmentation may occur in inflammatory dermatoses as well as in surgical wounds. This may be the result of hemoglobin pigments as well as increased melanin, possibly as the result of various inflammatory and growth factors. "Tattooing" may also occur if ferrous subsulfate or silver nitrate is used in the hemostatic process. Postinflammatory changes that occur as a response to ultraviolet light may either accentuate or inhibit tanning and will leave a mottled appearance. Although most Asians experience hyperpigmentation after surgery and some blacks have hypopigmentation at the wound site, most pigmentary changes are unpredictable in a given patient.

Some procedures have a higher incidence of postoperative pigmentary changes. Dermabrasion and chemical peeling may leave a mottled appearance, most commonly hyperpigmentation, but this may be related to focal areas of hypopigmentation. Sclerotherapy may be associated with linear hyperpigmentation, and laser surgery is likely to cause hypopigmentation. Electrodesiccation and curettage are commonly associated with hypopigmented scars.

It is important to select patients carefully for cosmetic procedures in which pigmentary changes may overshadow the cosmetic benefits. When a procedure such as dermabrasion is being considered, especially in a high-risk patient, a 1- to 2-cm area should first be tested in a cosmetically hidden location. The possibility of postinflammatory hyperpigmentation should be discussed with the patient whenever indicated.

TRAPDOOR DEFORMITY

The trapdoor, or "pin-cushion," deformity is most commonly seen as a complication of the transposition flap but can also be seen in rhomboid flaps. The margins

of the flap lie at the normal skin level, but elevation is seen centrally. This may be the result of excess subcutaneous tissue on the undersurface of the flap or of fibrous bands that develop at the flap margins. To minimize this effect, the flap should be thinned so as not to move subcutaneous tissue into the recipient site. By widely undermining the edges of the recipient site, the tendency to develop a buckled scar may be reduced.[20]

If this complication arises, the initial treatment should include steroid injections of the margin with massage to the entire flap. If this is ineffective, a corrective defatting of the flap with undermining of the scarred bands at the incision margins will help to improve the flap's final appearance.

Medical Conditions Affecting Wound Healing and Complications

A multitude of underlying medical conditions (Table 66–6) and medications (Table 66–7) may dramatically affect wound healing and the final cosmetic outcome. It is important to be fully aware of each patient's medical conditions and medications so as to make appropriate decisions in wound management. Medical conditions that may affect circulation include diabetes, coronary insufficiency, congestive heart failure, and hypertension. Pulmonary diseases may decrease oxygen saturation of the blood, causing a delay in wound healing. Immunosuppression and any debilitating chronic disease can predispose the patient to a secondary infection. Coagulation disorders predispose the patient to hematoma formation, which can lead to a multitude of other complications.

Medications may also reproduce the effects of some medical disorders. Glucocorticoid therapy not only may cause immunosuppression but also may delay healing, resulting in many of the complications seen in patients with diabetes. Chemotherapeutic agents and cyclosporine cause immunosuppression, while penicillamine and β-aminopropionitrile can interfere with the development of wound tensile strength. Underlying medical conditions or medications should not preempt performance of an indicated surgical procedure. However, it is imperative for the surgeon to know the patient's medications and coexistent medical problems so as to manage surgical wounds appropriately.

TABLE 66–7. **MEDICATIONS THAT AFFECT WOUND HEALING**

Glucocorticoids
Chemotherapeutic agents
Cyclosporine
Penicillamine
Metronidazole
β-Aminopropionitrile

Life-threatening Complications

Seizures, anaphylaxis, and arrhythmias are rare but are the most common life-threatening complications seen in cutaneous surgery. To manage these complications, emergency equipment and medications should be immediately available, and the staff, as well as the surgeon, should be fully trained in cardiopulmonary resuscitation. It is recommended that office staff members be trained so that someone will always be available to assist with resuscitation in the event that a situation occurs when not all staff members are available.

The most common cause of seizures in the surgical suite is a vasovagal event. In many instances, patients can identify themselves as "fainters," and when this is the case, even the most minor procedure should done in a setting where the surgical table can be placed in the Trendelenburg position and emergency equipment is immediately available. This emergency equipment should include a bite stick to aid patients with seizures.

In many instances, a seizure complicates fainting simply because of decreased blood flow to the brain. Except in patients with a known seizure disorder from another cause, such a seizure usually does not indicate an underlying seizure disorder. However, the patient is at risk for aspiration, and the airway must be appropriately managed to prevent anoxic brain damage. These patients should be referred to their primary physician for further evaluation. Fainting with resultant seizure activity should be clearly noted in the chart and appropriately indicated so that future minor surgical procedures can be undertaken in the most advantageous of circumstances.

Anaphylaxis requires immediate recognition and treatment. Circulatory collapse can occur unless epinephrine and fluids are immediately administered. Thus these items should be immediately available, and all staff members should know the location of these items and be able to respond immediately to an emergency. Many commercially available kits provide all of these items in a portable case. A "crash cart" may be available at large institutions and should be readily accessible. Epinephrine must be administered emergently, an intravenous line started, and fluids begun. Transfer to a hospital setting should be accomplished as soon as the patient is sufficiently stable.

Cardiac complications, including a myocardial infarction or arrhythmia, may occur as a result of preoperative anxiety or medications administered during the procedure. In either instance, a careful preoperative history will alert the surgeon to patients at highest risk and allow for careful intraoperative monitoring when appropriate. Monitoring equipment is reasonably priced, and virtually every office performing large, complex, or extensive cosmetic procedures should be so equipped. Patients who develop chest pain or arrhythmias should have an intravenous line established and should be immediately transferred to an emergency department when stable. Additional medications should be administered only if the attending physician is qualified to select them. In offices where extensive cutaneous surgery is performed, the physicians should be certified in Advanced Cardiac Life Support, and the entire staff should be certified in Basic Life Support.

SUMMARY

A multitude of surgical and medical complications can occur during cutaneous surgery. With a careful physical examination and a detailed medical history, many potential complications can be reduced in severity or eliminated entirely. Proper management of surgical complications can provide the patient with a successful outcome in most situations.

REFERENCES

1. Simon LS, Mills JA: Nonsteroidal antiinflammatory drugs. I. N Engl J Med 302:1179–1185, 1980.
2. Simon LS, Mills JA: Nonsteroidal antiinflammatory drugs. II. N Engl J Med 302:1237–1242, 1980.
3. Gardner GC, Simkin PA: Adverse effects of NSAID's. Drug Ther 20:50–60, 1990.
4. Gordon RA, Ballard JO, Kammerer WS, Gros RJ: Hematology. In: Kammerer WS (ed): Medical Consultation. Williams & Wilkins, Baltimore, 1990, pp 325–330.
5. Handin RI: Bleeding and thrombosis. In: Braunwald E, Isselbacher KI, Petersdorf RG, et al (eds): Harrison's Principles of Internal Medicine. McGraw-Hill, New York, 1987, pp 266–272.
6. Goh CL: Contact senstivity to topical medicaments. Int J Dermatol 28:25–28, 1989.
7. Ljunggren B, Moller H: Eczematous contact allergy to chlorhexidine. Acta Dermatol 52:308–310, 1972.
8. Okano M, Nomura M, Hata S, et al: Anaphylactic symptoms due to chlorhexidine gluconate. Arch Dermatol 125:50–52, 1989.
9. Prystowsky SD, Allen AM, Smith RW, et al: Allergic contact hypersensitivity to nickel, neomycin, ethylenediamine, and benzocaine. Arch Dermatol 115:959–962, 1979.
10. Goh CL: Contact sensitivity to topical antimicrobials. Contact Dermatitis 21:166–171, 1989.
11. Pirila V, Forstrom L, Rouhunkoski S: Twelve years of sensitization to neomycin in Finland. Acta Dermatol Venereol 47:419–425, 1967.
12. Gette MT, Marks JG, Maloney ME: The frequency of postoperative allergic contact dermatitis to topical antibiotic. 128:365–367, 1992.
13. Scherbenske JM, Winton GB, James WD: Acute pseudomonas infection of the external ear (malignant external otitis). J Dermatol Surg Oncol 14:165–169, 1988.
14. Sabetta JB, Zitelli JA: The incidence of bacteremia during skin surgery. Arch Dermatol 123:213–215, 1987.
15. Stegman SJ, Tromovitch TA, Glogan RG: Basics of Dermatologic Surgery. Year Book Medical, Chicago, 1982.
16. Greenbaum SS, Greenbaum CH: Intraoperative tissue expansion using a Foley catheter following excision of a basal cell carcinoma. J Dermatol Surg Oncol 16:45–48, 1990.
17. Bernstein G: The loop stitch. J Dermatol Surg Oncol 10:587, 1984.
18. Sommerlad BC, Creasey JM: The stretched scar: a clinical and histological study. Br J Plast Surg 31:34–45, 1978.
19. Elliott D, Mahaffey PJ: The stretched scar: the benefit of prolonged dermal support. Br J Plast Surg 42:74–78, 1989.
20. Salasche SJ, Grabski WJ: Complications of flaps. J Dermatol Surg Oncol 17:132–140, 1991.

CHAPTER 67

Psychiatric Aspects of Cutaneous Surgery

JOHN Y. M. KOO

There are two situations in which the understanding of psychiatric issues becomes critical in the management of cutaneous surgery patients. The first involves the patient who demands a cosmetic surgical procedure for an alleged cosmetic defect that is minimal or nonexistent. The second arises when a patient who has undergone an extensive cutaneous surgical procedure, such as removal of a large neoplasm, experiences significant psychological problems because of the disfigurement that resulted from the surgery. These two different situations will be discussed in detail with an emphasis on understanding the psychiatric differential diagnoses and their management, along with advice as to how best to interact with these patients.

Patients Who Exaggerate Their Cosmetic Defects

When encountering a patient who demands a surgical procedure for the correction of a "cosmetic defect" that is minimal or nonexistent, the first step required in managing such a case involves making an attempt to understand the nature of the underlying psychopathology. Although many psychiatric conditions can create an exaggerated perception of an alleged cosmetic defect (Table 67–1), four disorders are most commonly seen among this group of patients. These disorders are monosymptomatic hypochondriacal psychosis (MHP), somatization of depression, chronic anxiety disorder, and borderline personality disorder.

MONOSYMPTOMATIC HYPOCHONDRIACAL PSYCHOSIS

MHP refers to a group of disorders characterized by an encapsulated delusional belief system that is hypo-chondriacal in nature (Table 67–2).[1] A delusional disorder is typified by a false idea that is rigidly held by the patient and is not shared by other people in the same social or cultural group. MHP is frequently a chronic condition but is easily distinguished from other forms of chronic psychosis, such as schizophrenia, by its encapsulated nature. Patients with MHP may appear quite normal except when expressing concern about the hypochondriacal delusional idea. This is in contrast to schizophrenic patients who, in addition to a delusional belief system, may develop many other psychiatric symptoms such as auditory hallucinations, flat or inappropriate affect, and deterioration in interpersonal relationships.[2]

Dysmorphophobia, one type of MHP, is a condition in which the patient is preoccupied by an exaggerated or imaginary cosmetic defect.[3] However, concern has been raised that this term is actually a misnomer for a large proportion of the patients who present with such a complaint but are delusional,[4] not phobic. In phobias,

TABLE 67–1. **COMMON PSYCHIATRIC CONDITIONS CHARACTERIZED BY AN EXAGGERATED PERCEPTION OF COSMETIC DEFICIENCIES**

Monosymptomatic hypochondriacal psychosis
Major depression with somatization
Chronic anxiety disorder
Borderline personality disorder
Dysmorphophobia
Body dysmorphic disorder
Schizophrenia
Schizoaffective disorder
Bipolar disorder
Gender identity disorder

TABLE 67–2. FEATURES OF MONOSYMPTOMATIC HYPOCHONDRIACAL PSYCHOSIS

Hypochondriacal complaints
Chronic in nature
Encapsulated delusional belief system
Patient is normal in other respects

patients usually recognize that their fear is exaggerated or irrational. However, in delusions, patients truly believe in the distorted perception and exhibit very little psychological insight. Therefore, the preferred term to describe this subset of delusional patients is "delusions of dysmorphosis."

The term MHP is most often used in Europe. In American psychiatric nosology, this group of disorders can be classified under delusional disorder, somatic subtype, or atypical psychosis.[5] In general dermatology practices, many other subsets of MHP can be seen, such as delusions of parasitosis and delusions of bromosis. In delusions of bromosis, patients believe they are emitting a bad odor that offends people and drives them away. In a cutaneous surgical practice, however, delusional concerns regarding the cosmetic appearance typically predominate.[6]

SOMATIZATION OF DEPRESSION

Patients may develop exaggerated physical complaints when suffering from major depressive episodes. This phenomenon, in which the depressed patient presents to the physician with an exaggerated physical complaint without recognizing its relationship to the underlying depression, is called somatization of depression.[7] To make this diagnosis, it must be ascertained that the patient has sufficient depressive symptoms (Table 67–3) to meet the diagnostic criteria of a major depressive episode[5, 8] (i.e., the patient must exhibit symptoms and signs such as a prevailing depressed mood, markedly diminished interests or pleasure in daily activities, significant weight loss or weight gain, insomnia or hypersomnia, psychomotor agitation or retardation, fatigue, feeling of worthlessness, excessive guilt, diminished ability to concentrate, and possibly suicidal ideation or plans). Not every patient will exhibit all of these psychological symptoms and physiologic signs of major depression. Moreover, some patients may consciously or unconsciously deny some of the subjective symptoms,

TABLE 67–3. MAJOR DEPRESSIVE SYMPTOMS

Prevailing depressed mood
Significant weight loss (or gain)
Diminished interests
Reduced pleasure in daily activities
Insomnia (or hypersomnia)
Psychomotor agitation (or retardation)
Fatigue
Feeling of worthlessness
Excess guilt
Diminished ability to concentrate
Suicidal ideation (or plans)

TABLE 67–4. PHYSIOLOGIC MANIFESTATIONS OF ANXIETY DISORDERS

Trembling
Twitching
Restlessness
Shortness of breath
Palpitations
Tachycardia
Sweating
Dizziness
Nausea
Diarrhea
Difficulty swallowing
Hyperreactivity

such as a depressed mood. However, even in these cases, the diagnosis of major depression can be postulated if enough symptoms and signs of depression can be detected during the evaluation.

ANXIETY DISORDER

It is well known that patients with chronic anxiety disorder frequently experience many physical complaints (Table 67–4).[9] These complaints can be either psychophysiologic or purely psychiatric in nature. Psychophysiologic disturbances are exemplified by conditions such as stress-induced gastric ulceration or migraine headache, in which a real physiologic abnormality that is exacerbated by anxiety can be demonstrated. In contrast, there is no demonstrable physiologic abnormality when the physical complaint merely represents a psychological fixation on the part of the anxious patient. It has been speculated that a patient experiencing chronic recurrent anxiety finds the anxiety most unbearable when it is undefined and "free floating" in character. One way to make this amorphous anxiety more psychologically manageable is to "fixate" the anxiety onto some visible, concrete physical complaint.

To confirm the diagnosis of underlying anxiety, the physician should question these patients regarding any symptoms of generalized anxiety disorder. Just as in the case of depression, the manifestations of underlying anxiety disorder can be either subjective or physiologic.[10] Frequently, there are both subjective and physiologic symptoms and signs of anxiety disorders. Subjective symptoms of anxiety are manifested by an unrealistic or excessive anxiety that is often chronic and recurrent in nature. The physiologic manifestations of anxiety may include motor tension such as trembling, twitching, muscle tension, restlessness, and a feeling of "shakiness." Alternatively, hyperactivity of the autonomic nervous system, usually consisting of shortness of breath, palpitations, tachycardia, sweating, clammy hands, dry mouth, dizziness, nausea, diarrhea, hot flashes, frequent urination, and trouble in swallowing, may also be observed. At times, the patient may also exhibit hyperreactivity (e.g., an exaggerated startle response or irritability). If enough symptoms and signs are present, the physician can be certain that an underlying anxiety disorder is present.

TABLE 67–5. **FEATURES OF BORDERLINE PERSONALITY DISORDER**

Affects young women most frequently
Poorly defined sense of identity
Boredom
Chronic feelings of emptiness
Inappropriate anger
Impulsiveness
Unstable affect
Wide mood swings
Unstable interpersonal relationships
Distorted body image
Ill-defined long-term goals
Self-destructive behavior

BORDERLINE PERSONALITY DISORDER

Borderline personality disorder is a commonly encountered chronic personality disturbance that most frequently affects young women (Table 67–5).[11] One of the central deficits in this disorder consists of a sense of identity that is poorly defined, precarious, and unstable in nature. This instability of the sense of self may be manifested by chronic feelings of emptiness and boredom, inappropriate or intense feelings of anger, impulsiveness, and instability of affect whereby the patient may shift quickly from baseline mood to depression, irritability, or anxiety. This vague sense of self can also lead to a pattern of unstable and intense interpersonal relationships characterized by alternating extremes of overidealization and devaluation of the people with whom emotional attachments have been formed.

In addition to the characteristic problems with personal identity and interpersonal relationships, these patients frequently experience difficulties in regard to their body image. In this context, body image refers to patients' mental or psychological representation of their body. There are several well-known psychiatric disturbances (e.g., anorexia nervosa or bulimia) in which patients' body image diverges from their actual physical appearance. For example, anorectic patients typically engage in extreme forms of diet and exercise to lose weight, even though they are already emaciated.[12–14] This is because, in their body image, they see themselves as obese. Distortions in body image can also be seen with borderline personality disorder. Borderline patients may externalize their core problem and try to define their amorphous sense of self by altering their physical appearance.

Patients with borderline personality disorder can be classified into those with a high psychosocial functional level and those with a low psychosocial functional level. High-functioning borderline patients may appear fairly normal, except for a pattern of unstable and intense interpersonal relationships, uncertainty regarding self-image, ill-defined long-term goals, unknown preferred personal values, and a chronic feeling of emptiness. Low-functioning borderline patients may chronically engage in self-destructive behavior such as promiscuous sex, binge eating, reckless spending, repeated suicidal gestures, or other self-mutilating behaviors. With experience, it is not difficult to identify patients with borderline personality disorder merely by observing the way they look or talk to the physician. Their look is typically intense, with a touch of adoration, and the content of their verbal expression idealizes the physician. Borderline personality disorder is most frequently seen in young women, and consequently male physicians are more susceptible to becoming the focus of attention of these patients. Needless to say, the chronic sense of defective identity cannot be repaired by surgical correction of the exaggerated or imaginary cosmetic defects.

ALTERNATIVE PSYCHIATRIC DIAGNOSES

Even though most patients with exaggerated complaints regarding real or imaginary cosmetic defects fall into one of the four psychiatric diagnoses previously described, a minority of patients may fall into some other psychiatric diagnostic category, such as body dysmorphic disorder, schizophrenia, schizoaffective disorder, bipolar disorder, and gender identity disorder.

Body Dysmorphic Disorder

In body dysmorphic disorder, normal-appearing persons develop a preoccupation with some imagined defect in their appearance. Sometimes a slight physical anomaly may be present, but the patient's concern is grossly excessive. This condition can be distinguished from MHP because the patient's belief system is not of delusional intensity. In other words, the patient can acknowledge the possibility that the complaint may be exaggerated or that there may be no defect at all. Because their insight is relatively retained, these patients can be reassured that their concerns are exaggerated and that surgical correction is neither necessary nor advisable.[15]

Schizophrenia

In schizophrenia, patients may develop delusions concerning their physical appearance that are often bizarre in nature. However, it is relatively easy to diagnose schizophrenic patients because of their multiple psychological impairments, which include auditory hallucinations, flat or inappropriate affect, bizarre delusional belief system, and failure to establish any interpersonal rapport with the physician.[16]

Schizoaffective Disorder

Schizoaffective disorders are characterized by both schizophrenic and depressive symptoms.[17]

Bipolar Disorder

Patients with a bipolar disorder, such as manic-depressive illness, may also develop somatization during their depressive episodes. However, the diagnosis can usually be determined by asking about previous episodes of mania during which patients experienced symptoms that are the opposite of depression. During an episode of mania, patients may experience grandiosity with inflated self-esteem and exaggerated self-confidence, flights of ideas, racing thoughts, psychomotor agitation, pressured speech, distractibility, and recklessness manifested by spending sprees, sexual indiscretion, or involvement in unrealistic business ventures.[18]

Gender Identity Disorder

Patients who suffer from gender identity disorder are unsure whether they are psychologically male or female and may request a variety of cosmetic surgical procedures. However, the underlying diagnosis usually becomes apparent when the nature of gender confusion is generalized, and the patient's complaint represents only one small manifestation of this underlying confusion.[19]

Management

GENERAL CONCEPTS

In the ideal situation, management of patients with some form of psychopathology would simply involve making a referral to a mental health professional. However, in reality many of these patients may refuse to recognize the psychological nature of their condition or refuse a referral to a mental health professional, even if they do recognize the existence of their psychiatric disturbance. Therefore, it is useful for the cutaneous surgeon to have a general knowledge of how to manage these patients and of the forms of treatment available. This does not imply that the cutaneous surgeon must take the responsibility for treating the psychiatric disorder. However, even partial treatment administered by the surgeon may benefit the patient more than no treatment at all. Ultimately, each cutaneous surgeon must decide whether to treat those patients who refuse a referral to a mental health professional. Regardless, it is important to recognize that ways to manage these conditions differ greatly, depending on the psychiatric diagnosis.

MONOSYMPTOMATIC HYPOCHONDRIACAL PSYCHOSIS

By definition, patients with delusional beliefs cannot be persuaded to give up their delusion. Therefore, explanations and reassurances are unlikely to be helpful. Delusions of dysmorphosis and other forms of MHP were thought to be almost untreatable until an antipsychotic medication, pimozide (Orap), was discovered to be efficacious in the treatment of these conditions.[20] Pimozide is the most potent oral antipsychotic medication available in the United States. Because of its potency, treatment with pimozide should be started at a lower dosage level than that of other antipsychotic medications such as haloperidol (Haldol) and fluphenazine hydrochloride (Prolixin). Pimozide is available only as a 2-mg white tablet. The most conservative starting oral dosage is 1 mg daily. If the patient experiences sedation, pimozide should be given at bedtime. On the other hand, if the patient experiences increased energy levels, the medication should be taken in the morning. The dosage of pimozide can be increased by 1 mg every 3 to 4 days as tolerated until its clinical efficacy becomes evident. In the literature, dosages up to 10 mg per day have been used for psychocutaneous conditions. However, 4 mg or less per day is effective in most cases in decreasing the intensity of the somatic delusions.

The main side effects of pimozide are identical to those of other antipsychotic medications such as haloperidol. The most frequently encountered complaint involves an inner feeling of restlessness or akathisia. Stiffness in the joints and muscles is one of the manifestations of pseudoparkinsonism, an extrapyramidal side effect of pimozide. These side effects are easily controlled by concurrent use of a medication with anticholinergic effect (e.g., benztropine mesylate [Cogentin], 1 to 2 mg orally four times daily, or diphenhydramine hydrochloride [Benadryl], 25 mg orally four times daily) as needed. Benztropine mesylate has an advantage over diphenhydramine hydrochloride in that it has no sedative side effects. It is often difficult to convince this group of patients to take pimozide. Even if they do agree to take it, they may still have considerable ambivalence about doing so. As a consequence, if they experience these side effects and have no means to control them, they may refuse to take pimozide again. Therefore, even though many patients with MHP tolerate pimozide without experiencing akathisia or any extrapyramidal side effects, it may be advisable to prescribe a small supply of either benztropine mesylate or diphenhydramine hydrochloride so that they can control these side effects if they arise.

Other rare side effects of pimozide include acute dystonic reaction and tardive dyskinesia. In acute dystonic reaction, the patient experiences the onset of muscle spasms, especially of the neck and around the mouth. These spasms usually respond promptly to the administration of either benztropine mesylate or diphenhydramine hydrochloride. Cases of acute dystonic reaction involving the oral pharynx are very rare. However, this condition constitutes an emergency, because the patient's breathing may become compromised. For this reason, the patient should be instructed to go to an emergency department if a dystonic reaction is accompanied by any respiratory difficulties. Tardive dyskinesia is extremely rare with short-term use of pimozide. However, this condition may develop with long-term use, especially at high dosages. Tardive dyskinesia is manifested by involuntary movements, especially involving the oral musculature. Withdrawal dyskinesia is identical to tardive dyskinesia, except that the involuntary movements are of very mild intensity and typically appear as the medication is being tapered in dosage or discontinued. This reaction is extremely rare and is usually self-limiting. The only reason the physician should know of its existence is to be spared the anxiety resulting from mistaking the self-limited withdrawal dyskinesia for tardive dyskinesia.

SOMATIZATION OF DEPRESSION

Somatization of depression can be suspected both from the depressive symptoms and from the fact that patients who somatize may not hold their belief system as rigidly as patients with true delusion. Therapy for somatization of depression is directed at treatment of the underlying depression. There are many ways to treat depression, including individual psychotherapy, group therapy, and psychopharmacotherapy. If patients recognize the presence of depression but refuse to see a psychiatrist or other mental health professional, they may still be helped by antidepressant medications. However, before embarking on pharmacotherapy for depression, it is useful to determine to what extent the depression results from some difficulties in the patient's life and to what extent it might be endogenous in origin. If some real life issues such as stress at work or financial difficulty precipitated the episode of depression, an extra effort should be made to try to refer the patient to a psychotherapeutic setting where counseling can be provided.

Pharmacologic treatment of depression consists of both tricyclic and nontricyclic medications. Among the tricyclic antidepressants, newer agents such as desipramine hydrochloride (Norpramin, Pertofrane) have considerably fewer anticholinergic, sedative, and cardiac side effects than the older agents[21] such as amitriptyline hydrochloride (Elavil, Endep). This advantage is especially important for the management of older patients who may have conditions that may be exacerbated by the anticholinergic properties of tricyclic antidepressants (e.g., chronic constipation, acute-angle glaucoma, and urinary hesitation). Moreover, older patients are more susceptible to sedative side effects and also more likely to have coexisting cardiac disorders. The dosage of desipramine hydrochloride should be titrated, beginning with 25 mg orally per day and increasing by 25 mg every 4 to 7 days as tolerated up to the usual adult dosage of 150 to 300 mg per day. The optimal dosage for psychocutaneous patients may be in the lower end of this dosage range, since patients who have never taken psychotropic medications tend to require less medication than chronic psychiatric patients. After the therapeutic range for the medication has been reached, 2 weeks or more may be required for the antidepressant effect to become evident. Once the depressive symptoms are under control, the therapeutic dosage should be maintained for several months before the medication is gradually tapered. Side effects of desipramine hydrochloride, except for weight gain, are relatively rare in young, healthy patients. However, side effects such as orthostatic hypotension, constipation, urinary hesitation, and sedation are much more frequently seen in older patients. If the dosage is adequate and the patient shows no clinical response, the serum desipramine level should be determined to evaluate the adequacy of absorption and patient compliance.[22]

One nontricyclic antidepressant that is gaining widespread use is fluoxetine (Prozac), which offers the advantage of having little or no anticholinergic activity and is also not associated with weight gain.[23] The recommended oral dosage of 20 to 40 mg per day is generally well tolerated. However, side effects include anxiety, agitation, insomnia, nausea, diarrhea, and rash. There has been some concern that in depressed patients who become agitated on fluoxetine there may be an increased risk of suicide,[24, 25] and for this reason the physician should be alert for changes in patients' excitement level, especially if agitation is part of the clinical presentation. Fluoxetine should not be given simultaneously with monoamine oxidase inhibitors or tryptophan, as serotonin excess may result, leading to confusion, gastrointestinal distress, and tremor.[26] The patient taking monamine oxidase inhibitors should discontinue those drugs at least 3 weeks before starting fluoxetine treatment.

CHRONIC ANXIETY DISORDER

When the exaggerated cosmetic complaint is a manifestation of an underlying chronic anxiety disorder, the intensity of the mental fixation usually diminishes when the anxiety level is brought under control. It is again important to ascertain whether some outside psychosocial stress is causing the increased anxiety level. If an identifiable psychosocial stress is present, the patient might be directed to seek professional counseling to help solve those problems. Two types of antianxiety medications are used to lower anxiety levels. One type is quick acting but sedating and potentially addicting; the other is slow in onset but nonsedating and nonaddictive. The most frequently used rapid-action medication in the United States is alprazolam (Xanax), which differs from the older benzodiazepines such as diazepam (Valium) in three respects. First, alprazolam has both antidepressant and antianxiety effects.[27, 28] This is in contrast to other benzodiazepines, which, like alcohol, tend to have depressant rather than antidepressant effects. Second, the half-life of alprazolam is shorter and more predictable than that of diazepam, and therefore there is less risk of accumulation in the body when the medication is used for long periods. Third, alprazolam is the first medication in the United States to be approved for treatment of panic attacks.[29] A panic attack is distinguished from other forms of anxiety disorders by a sudden onset of anxiety of tremendous intensity.[30] In short-term use (2 weeks or less), the side effects of alprazolam are generally limited to sedation. However, sedation can be avoided by carefully titrating the dose. The safest approach is to start with a low dose and gradually increase it until the dose is sufficient to control the anxiety but not result in sedation. Alprazolam may be started at an oral dosage of 0.25 mg four times a day and gradually increased by 0.25 mg per day, if necessary, until effective control of the anxiety is obtained on a dosing schedule of three or four times per day. Once the anxiety is under control, the dosage can be gradually tapered. It is not recommended that alprazolam or any other benzodiazepine be abruptly discontinued, since this may result in a recurrence or exacerbation of the anxiety disorder. In addition, with long-term use, as with other benzodiazepines, there is a risk of addiction. Therefore, a psychiatrist should be consulted if usage beyond a 2- to 4-week period is required.

Buspirone hydrochloride (Buspar) represents the second type of antianxiety medication, which is not addictive or sedating. However, this medication must be taken on a regular (three or four times per day) basis, since it does not work well when taken "as needed." Two weeks or more may be required for the clinical effect of buspirone hydrochloride to become evident, and therefore it is used ideally for patients with a chronic anxiety disorder that is expected to last longer than 2 to 3 weeks per episode. The oral dosage of buspirone hydrochloride ranges from 5 to 10 mg three or four times daily. However, this must be individualized for each patient, beginning with the lowest dosage and titrating upward until the optimal dosage is reached. The side effects of buspirone hydrochloride include dizziness, nausea, headache, nervousness, lightheadedness, and excitement.

BORDERLINE PERSONALITY DISORDER

Borderline personality disorder represents a chronic psychological deficit that is not expected to change over a short period. For this reason, medications are of only limited usefulness in this condition and are generally used to treat anxiety or depression symptoms if they are present. The cutaneous surgeon cannot be expected to conduct long-term psychotherapy, which is the mainstay of treatment for these patients.[31] Therefore, this discussion will be limited to those aspects of the doctor-patient relationship that are important to recognize so that interpersonal problems can be minimized when dealing with borderline personality disorder patients. There are three issues that the clinician should watch for when dealing with a patient with this disorder: idealization, devaluation, and splitting.[32]

Patients with borderline personality disorder have a characteristic deficit: they can perceive people only in an idealized or devalued mode. Their perception is "black and white," with no gray zone. In idealization these patients, who are usually young women, idealize the physician. There is a seductive and flattering quality to this idealization that can sometimes result in the physician making an error in judgment by consenting to perform a surgical procedure that has no medical justification.

Devaluation is the opposite of idealization. If there is the slightest deviance from expectations, the patient with borderline personality disorder may suddenly shift behavior and treat the physician as if he or she is the worst physician ever encountered. This intense expression of devaluation and anger by the patient can also catch the physician off guard. In turn, the physician may respond with personal rage against the patient and not exercise proper medical or legal judgment.

The third characteristic of the patient with borderline personality disorder is a mental process called splitting. Splitting refers to the way the patient creates confusion and antagonism among different physicians or between the physician and the medical staff. This is partly accomplished by the process of idealization and devaluation and also partly by lying. By flattering the physician and the office staff, the patient idealizes while simultaneously bitterly criticizing those who have been devalued. Different stories are told to different staff members with the intention of splitting the caretakers and creating intense conflicts among them. One way to counter this devisive effect is for the staff to meet periodically and exchange information to make sure that everyone is in agreement on how to deal with these patients. Once the physician learns the characteristics of borderline personality disorder and the way havoc can be created in the office, interactions with the patient become easier and the physician is less vulnerable to these types of manipulation.

OTHER PSYCHIATRIC DISORDERS

Detailed discussion regarding the management of other, less frequently encountered psychiatric disturbances such as schizophrenia, schizoaffective illness, and bipolar disorder is beyond the scope of this chapter but can likely be found in any standard psychiatric textbook.

PSYCHIATRIC DISORDERS RESULTING FROM DISFIGUREMENT

Most patients who undergo significant cutaneous surgical procedures for the treatment of skin cancer or other diseases make a reasonable psychological adjustment to their cosmetic defects. However, a few patients develop significant psychiatric problems because of their disfigurement. This is understandable in light of the fact that society has been oriented to a very narrow standard of beauty.[33] Many psychological studies indicate that appearance correlates with the personality traits that people attribute to strangers. Attractive persons of both sexes are presumed to have more socially desirable traits, to be kinder and more intelligent, to have greater internal control and competence, and to have made greater achievements.[34-40] Many studies show that people respond differently to those who are physically handicapped, such as an amputee, compared with those who are visibly disfigured. Traits attributed to those who are visibly disfigured are more frequently negative in character.[41, 42] For example, studies have demonstrated that people are less likely to help a facially disfigured person than a nondisfigured person.[43] Therefore, it is understandable that patients who have extensive disfigurement from skin cancer surgery or trauma may encounter many difficulties, not only in terms of their personal emotional equilibrium, but also as a victim of negative perceptions from others.

Patients who develop significant psychiatric morbidity secondary to disfigurement may manifest their problem in terms of clinical depression, anxiety, and social phobia. Secondary psychiatric complications include social withdrawal and occupational difficulties. It is important to recognize the psychiatric consequences of surgical disfigurement, since many of these patients can be encouraged to seek professional help for their psychological difficulties. Moreover, unlike some chronic psychiatric patients, many of these patients have had reasonable premorbid psychological adaptation levels, and if they can be helped through the current crisis, they can become quite functional in society again.

Social Phobia

Social phobia refers to a condition in which the patient develops a persistent fear of social situations where he or she is likely to be scrutinized by others.[44] Sometimes even something as minor as receiving an invitation to attend a party may trigger phobic avoidance. Once social phobia has begun, it gradually becomes worse because of two factors. First, anticipatory anxiety gradually develops whenever the person is confronted with the necessity to enter a social gathering. Second, the patient's social performance can be impaired by this underlying anxiety, resulting in the development of a vicious cycle. At times, some patients with social phobias try to force themselves to endure the social situation despite their intense anxiety. Through this process, some may actually overcome their fears. However, many others with this condition will require professional counseling to cure their phobia. Otherwise, they may become progressively socially isolated to the point where they suffer serious social or occupational impairment. These patients usually retain their insight and recognize that their fears are excessive or unreasonable, even in view of their cosmetic disfigurement. Therefore, these patients tend to be receptive to the suggestion that they should obtain professional help from a psychiatrist or other mental health professionals.

Generally speaking, there are three types of therapies available for the treatment of social phobia. One is a behavioral therapy technique involving "exposure" or "flooding." In exposure, patients are presented with increasingly anxiety-provoking social situations, first in imagery and later in real life. At each stage of exposure, care is taken to make sure that the patient's anxiety level does not go out of control. In this process, known as systematic desensitization, the patient gradually learns not to fear the social situation.[45] In flooding, also known as implosion, the patient is rapidly exposed to an enormous volume of phobic material to try to overwhelm the phobic response. This technique can also be used either in imagery or in real life situations.

The second approach involves psychotherapy, in which the patient explores different psychological issues with the therapist. This approach can take many different forms, depending on the particular orientation of the therapist. Some therapists may be psychodynamic (i.e., emphasizing the use of Freudian principles), while others may be cognitive (i.e., actively trying to change the patient's thinking habits by challenging existing semiautomatic or automatic thought patterns).

The third approach is the use of medications, including antianxiety drugs to treat anxiety symptoms and antidepressants to treat phobic symptoms. However, the efficacy of medications such as tricyclic antidepressants and monoamine oxidase inhibitors in the treatment of social phobia has not been studied systematically.

SUMMARY

Many different psychiatric issues may arise in the practice of cutaneous surgery. Two such conditions include psychiatric disorders manifesting as a cutaneous surgical problem and the psychiatric consequences of traumatically or surgically induced disfigurement. Some treatment modalities have been described in detail, but cutaneous surgeons should not be expected to treat psychiatric problems on a regular basis. For these types of patients, referral to a psychiatrist should be made whenever feasible. If the patient refuses such a referral, as is frequently the case, it may still be possible to obtain a consultation from a psychiatrist or other mental health professional. This information should help the cutaneous surgeon more effectively handle psychological problems that may arise in the clinical setting.

REFERENCES

1. Bishop ER: Monosymptomatic hypochondriacal syndromes in dermatology. J Am Acad Dermatol 9:152–158, 1983.
2. American Psychiatric Association. DSM-III-R: Diagnostic and Statistical Manual of Mental Disorders. Washington, DC, 1987, pp 194–195.
3. Birtchnell SA: Dysmorphophobia—a centenary discussion. Br J Psychiatry 2:41–43, 1988.
4. Thomas CS: Dysmorphophobia: a question of definition. Br J Psychiatry 144:513–516, 1984.
5. American Psychiatric Association. DSM-III-R: Diagnostic and Statistical Manual of Mental Disorders. Washington, DC, 1987, pp 200, 211.
6. Woods LW: Psychiatry, body image, and cosmetic surgery. Appl Therapeut 10:451–454, 1968.
7. Kaplan HI, Freedman AM, Sadock J: Comprehensive Textbook of Psychiatry. Williams & Wilkins, Baltimore, 1980, p 691.
8. American Psychiatric Association. DSM-III-R: Diagnostic and Statistical Manual of Mental Disorders. Washington, DC, 1987, pp 222–224.
9. Glass RM, Allan AT, Uhlenhuth EH, et al: Psychiatric screening in a medical clinic. Arch Gen Psychol 35:1189–1195, 1978.
10. American Psychiatric Association. DSM-III-R: Diagnostic and Statistical Manual of Mental Disorders. Washington, DC, 1987, pp 252–253.
11. American Psychiatric Association. DSM-III-R: Diagnostic and Statistical Manual of Mental Disorders. Washington, DC, 1987, pp 346–347.
12. Heilbrun AB, Friedberg L: Distorted body image in normal college women: possible implication for the development of anorexia nervosa. J Clin Psychol 46:398–401, 1990.
13. Heilbrun AB, Witt N: Distorted body image as a risk factor in anorexia nervosa: replication and clarification. Psychol Rep 66:407–416, 1990.
14. Franzen U, Florin I, Schneider S, Meier M: Distorted body image in bulimic women. J Psychosom Res 32:445–450, 1988.
15. American Psychiatric Association. DSM-III-R: Diagnostic and Statistical Manual of Mental Disorders. Washington, DC, 1987, pp 255–256.
16. American Psychiatric Association. DSM-III-R: Diagnostic and Statistical Manual of Mental Disorders. Washington, DC, 1987, pp 187–198.
17. American Psychiatric Association. DSM-III-R: Diagnostic and Statistical Manual of Mental Disorders. Washington, DC, 1987, pp 208–210.
18. American Psychiatric Association. DSM-III-R: Diagnostic and Statistical Manual of Mental Disorders. Washington, DC, 1987, pp 225–226.
19. American Psychiatric Association. DSM-III-R: Diagnostic and Statistical Manual of Mental Disorders. Washington, DC, 1987, p 71.
20. Riding J, Munro A: Pimozide in the treatment of monosymptomatic hypochondriacal psychosis. Acta Psychol Scand 52:223–230, 1975.
21. Schatzberg AF, Cole JO: Handbook of Clinical Psychopharmacology. American Psychiatric Press, Washington, DC, 1986.

22. Cole JO: The drug treatment of anxiety and depression. Med Clin North Am 72:820, 1988.

23. Physicians' Desk Reference. 45th ed. Medical Economics, Oradell, NJ, 1991, pp 902–904.

24. Papp LA, Gorman JM: Suicidal preoccupation during fluoxetine treatment. Am J Psychol 147:1380, 1990.

25. Teicher MH, Glod C, Cole JO: Emergence of intense suicidal preoccupation during fluoxetine treatment. Am J Psychol 147:207–210, 1990.

26. Feighner JP, Boyer WF, Tyler DC, Neborsky RJ: Adverse consequences of fluoxetine-MAOI combination therapy. J Clin Psychol 51:222–225, 1990.

27. Robinson DS, Kayser A, Bennett B: Alprazolam: an antidepressant? Alprazolam, desipramine, and an alprazolam-desipramine combination in the treatment of adult depressed outpatients. J Clin Psychopharmacol 7:295–310, 1987.

28. Feighner JP, Aden GC, Fabre LF, et al: Comparison of alprazolam, imipramine, and placebo in the treatment of depression. JAMA 249:3057–3064, 1983.

29. Ballenger JC, Burrows GD, Dupont RL, et al: Alprazolam in panic disorder and agoraphobia: results from a multicenter trial. Arch Gen Psychol 45:413–422, 1988.

30. American Psychiatric Association. DSM-III-R: Diagnostic and Statistical Manual of Mental Disorders. Washington, DC, 1987, pp 235–239.

31. Chessick RD: Intensive psychotherapy of a borderline patient. Arch Gen Psychol 39:413–419, 1982.

32. Gunderson JG, Singer MT: Defining borderline patients: an overview. Am J Psychol 132:1–9, 1975.

33. Hill-Beuf A, Porter JDR: Children coping with impaired appearance: social and psychologic influences. Gen Hosp Psychol 6:294–301, 1984.

34. Dwyer J, Mcquiro J: Psychological effects of variations in physical appearance during adolescence. Adolescence 1:353–358, 1968.

35. Miller A: Role of physical attractiveness in impression formation. Psychosom Sci 19:103–109, 1970.

36. Dion K, Berscheid E, Walster E: What is beautiful is good. J Pers Soc Psychol 24:215–220, 1972.

37. Cash T, Begley PJ: Internal-external control, achievement orientation and physical attractiveness of college students. Psychol Rep 38:1205–1206, 1976.

38. McKelvie SJ, Mattews SJ: Effect of physical attractiveness and favorableness of character on liking. Psychol Rep 38:1223–1230, 1976.

39. Landy D, Sigall H: Beauty is talent. Task evaluation as a function of the performer's physical attractiveness. J Pers Soc Psychol 39:861–873, 1974.

40. Cash T, Kehr J, Polyson J, Freman V: Role of physical attractiveness in peer attribution of psychological disturbance. J Consult Clin Psychol 23:33–39, 1963.

41. Centers L, Centers R: Peer group attitudes toward the amputic child. J Soc Psychol 23:33–39, 1977.

42. Siller J, Ferguson L, Vann D, Holland B: Structure of attitudes toward the physically disabled: the disability factor scale: amputation, blindness, cosmetic conditions. Proceeds 76th Annual Convention Am Psychol Assoc 65:652, 1968.

43. Piliavin IM, Piliavin JA, Rodin J: Costs, diffusion and the stigmatized victim. J Pers Soc Psychol 32:429–438, 1975.

44. American Psychiatric Association. DSM-III-R: Diagnostic and Statistical Manual of Mental Disorders. Washington, DC, 1987, pp 241–243.

45. Cassell WA: Desensitization therapy for body image anxiety. Can Psychiatr Assoc J 22:239–242, 1977.

CHAPTER 68

Considerations for Performing Cutaneous Surgery in Black Patients

A. PAUL KELLY

Cutaneous surgery can be divided into two general categories: basic surgical procedures used in the removal of benign and malignant lesions and cosmetic surgical procedures that are performed at patients' request to enhance their appearance. Although most cosmetic procedures are not considered medical necessities, sometimes there is overlap. One example is when patients request removal of a painful keloid. Patients primarily want the keloid removed to eliminate the pain, but the procedure will also improve their appearance.

In the past, cosmetic surgical procedures were often withheld from black patients because of the surgeon's fear that they would develop keloids or dyspigmentation at the operative site. Black patients were frequently told that nothing could be done surgically to help them and that they would just have to learn to live with their problem. Some physicians even felt that blacks did not want or need any type of cosmetic procedure. Although such misconceptions are now rare, concerns about scarring and dyspigmentation may still be valid for some patients. However, most adverse cosmetic results secondary to cutaneous surgery can be avoided by obtaining a good history of the patient's previous response to surgery or cutaneous trauma and then using this information to make appropriate operative and postoperative decisions. The physician should also be aware of the possible psychological and vocational ramifications for the patient if the procedure is performed.

Basic Considerations

Several basic concepts should be recognized by the surgeon before performing cutaneous surgery on blacks.

Each cutaneous surgeon should be aware of these principles and, when appropriate, should explain them to the patient in detail preoperatively.

PIGMENTARY ABNORMALITIES

Changes in skin pigmentation may occur after cryosurgery. This is true even for procedures that require a freezing time of less than 20 seconds, which often results in hyperpigmentation that may last 6 to 12 months. Longer freezing times may produce hypopigmentation, which usually lasts 12 to 18 months or longer. Liquid nitrogen, when used as a topical freezing agent before dermabrasion, also often produces long-lasting dyschromia. Intralesional triamcinolone acetonide injections in concentrations of more than 3 mg/ml may produce hypopigmentation that usually persists for 6 to 12 months. Scars in blacks, whether flat or raised, are more often irregularly pigmented than similar scars in whites. The hyperpigmentation that occurs after injection sclerotherapy is more common in black patients than in whites.

PSYCHOLOGICAL CONSIDERATIONS

When black patients seek a particular cutaneous cosmetic procedure, they should be given the same psychiatric screening used for white patients. If they want to "look white," it is usually best to try to talk them out of the procedure. Black patients with skin cancerphobia should be told that skin cancer is rare in blacks, but malignant melanoma, if it develops, is usually found in acral and mucosal areas. As a consequence, it is especially important for patients to monitor these areas carefully for possible changes.

Special Surgical Procedures

Most of the basic cutaneous surgical techniques used in blacks are the same as those used in whites. However, certain disorders occur more frequently in blacks or require special surgical adaptations to be successfully performed in black patients. Some of these are punch grafts for vitiligo repigmentation, hair transplantation, dermatosis papulosa nigra, hidradenitis suppurativa, keloids, acne keloidalis, and dermabrasion. Each of these entities will be discussed individually.

PUNCH GRAFTS FOR VITILIGO REPIGMENTATION

Vitiligo is characterized by the loss of melanin pigment. Even though its incidence is approximately the same in blacks and whites, the lesions are considerably more noticeable in patients with darker complexions. For some black patients, vitiligo may even be psychologically malignant.

When patients no longer show improvement with psoralen plus ultraviolet A (PUVA) therapy, autologous punch grafts can be an excellent alternative for pigment restoration. This technique is performed in sterile fashion using local anesthesia (1% lidocaine with epinephrine). Multiple adjacent 2-mm superficial punch grafts, equivalent to a thin split-thickness graft, are harvested in rows. Longer grafts are trimmed to a thickness of 1 mm. The donor sites are either closed with 6–0 nylon sutures or allowed to heal by second intention. Next, superficial 2-mm plugs are taken from the areas of therapeutically resistant vitiligo. The recipient defects are spaced approximately 8 to 10 mm apart, since the pigmentation can be expected to migrate 3 to 6 mm from the borders of the graft. Harvested grafts from the donor sites are then placed in recipient areas, followed by the application of a thin layer of antibiotic ointment and a nonadherent dressing. The dressing is left in place for 5 to 7 days and then changed daily until healing is complete. Up to 50 autologous grafts can be inserted at each session. Postoperatively, PUVA therapy is continued to stimulate pigment dispersion, which usually begins approximately 2 months after grafting but may be seen as early as 6 weeks (Fig. 68–1). Superficial harvesting and meticulous placement of grafts usually eliminate scar formation or cobblestoning at the recipient sites. The success rate is much higher if autologous grafting is done after the patient has demonstrated maximal repigmentation response from PUVA therapy. Grafting without previous or ongoing PUVA therapy seldom produces adequate pigment dispersion.

DERMABRASION

Dermabrasion may be performed in black patients using the same technique and equipment employed in whites. However, before surgery is initiated, the patient

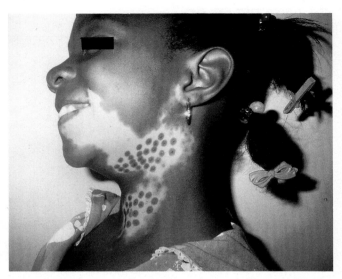

Figure 68–1. Pigment dispersion from the the tiny central transplanted grafts can be seen on the neck of this young vitiligo patient. (Courtesy of Pearl E. Grimes, M.D.)

should be informed about possible postoperative pigmentary changes. Preoperative photographs are of particular importance when dealing with cosmetic procedures such as dermabrasion. When obtaining preoperative photographs of black patients, the physician should normally open the lens one-half to one full stop to get high-quality photographs. Also, black patients who are prone to keloid or scar formation should not undergo dermabrasion. Dermabrasion is most commonly performed in blacks for correction of acne scarring and the removal of tattoos.

After dermabrasion, the patient should avoid direct sunlight exposure for at least 4 months to prevent development of hyperpigmentation. Twice-daily application of a sunscreen lotion after applying a hydroquinone preparation is often successful in attenuating the hyperpigmentation. The postoperative development of hypopigmentation can usually be avoided by not dermabrading too deeply. If elevated scars start to form postoperatively, daily application of a class 1 or 2 topical steroid, followed by application of a hydrocolloid surgical dressing, will usually prevent further development. However, long-term use of these products should be avoided to prevent temporary perilesional hypopigmentation. Silicone gel sheeting may also be used to help soften and flatten elevated scars.

Dermatosis Papulosa Nigra

Dermatosis papulosa nigra (DPN) consists of benign epidermal tumors of the face, neck, trunk, and upper arms that are found in 35 to 50% of all black Americans. They have also been reported in Mexican, Japanese, Vietnamese, and (rarely) European populations. The lesions usually appear during the second or third decade of life. Initially they are 1 to 2 mm in diameter, almost flat, annular, and hyperpigmented and may resemble

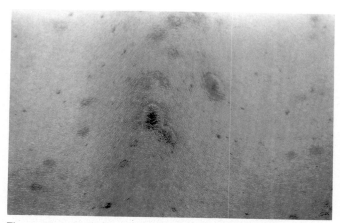

Figure 68–2. Small hypertrophic scars with dyspigmentation can be seen on the back after treatment with topical application of bichloracetic acid.

ephelides. They typically increase slowly in size and number until the fifth or sixth decade of life, after which new lesions seldom appear. While they do not undergo spontaneous involution or malignant transformation, they may continue to enlarge. Therapy is not usually indicated except when the patient requests removal for cosmetic reasons or when the lesions become symptomatic secondary to trauma.

Cryotherapy is often successful but usually causes 6 to 18 months of dyspigmentation. The same is true for treatment with bichloracetic acid, which may result in the development of small hypertrophic scars, especially on the back and shoulders (Fig. 68–2). Even when dermabrasion of DPN is performed with great caution, dyspigmentation secondary to inflammation is a common complication.

The usual treatment of choice is light electrodesiccation, which is done until the lesions turn gray. With minimal postoperative care, the lesions typically disappear in 7 to 14 days. Patients should be told that they may experience burning or itching at the treated sites for the first 48 hours postoperatively. Topical steroids usually prevent or attenuate this problem. However, if steroids are used within the first 24 hours, the inflammatory reaction necessary for the treated DPN to resolve may not occur, and the treatment will fail. Other excellent treatment options include direct cautery, laser vaporization, shaving with a razor blade, and removal with a sharp curette or scissors. Some patients can tolerate these procedures without anesthesia, but for removing or destroying lesions greater than 1 cm in diameter or for treating more than five or six lesions, local anesthesia is usually necessary. Newly developed topical anesthetic creams may prove to be ideal for eliminating the pain and discomfort of DPN removal, but this has not yet been determined. Postinflammatory hyperpigmentation, usually lasting a minimum of 4 to 6 months, is the most common complication with all of these procedures. It can often be prevented if a topical hydroquinone preparation is used immediately after the treated sites have healed. Cosmetics can be used to hide the dyspigmentation until it resolves spontaneously over time.

Hidradenitis Suppurativa

Hidradenitis suppurativa (HS) is a chronic, recurrent, suppurative disease of the apocrine gland–bearing areas of the body that occurs more often in blacks than in whites. Women are more likely to have axillary involvement, while men are more commonly affected by perianal HS. The exact etiology remains unknown, but poral occlusion along with secondary bacterial infection is considered to be the most likely cause. Tender erythematous abscesses that drain spontaneously are the hallmark of the initial lesions. Old lesions may reform, and new ones may develop. Long-term complications include marked fibrosis, sinus tracts extending into the subcutaneous tissue, anemia, interstitial keratitis, hypoproteinemia, secondary amyloidosis, and squamous cell carcinoma.

Although mild to moderate HS is sometimes managed medically, surgery is the most effective and successful form of therapy. However, before performing surgery, areas of drainage should be cultured for anaerobic and aerobic bacteria, and appropriate antibiotics should be started if indicated. The surgical technique for acute lesions involves first anesthetizing the involved area with 1% lidocaine with epinephrine. A probe is then inserted into the abscesses or sinus tracts, and the skin is cut over the probe to expose the involved area. The overhanging skin is removed using scissors, a process known as exteriorization. Next, the base of the abscess or sinus tract is scraped with a dermal curette and then electrocoagulated. If exteriorization is unsuccessful because of excess fibrous tissue or extensive involvement, the affected tissue must be completely removed; healing is accomplished by second intention or grafting. In one report of ten patients with bilateral axillary HS, better cosmetic results were obtained when full-thickness excision was followed by second-intention healing rather than by grafting.[1]

If grafting is performed, staples can tack down the grafts faster than can sutures (Fig. 68–3) and seldom cause increased morbidity. After surgery, the gauze dressing is placed on the lateral chest wall rather than the axilla, since this position allows a greater range of

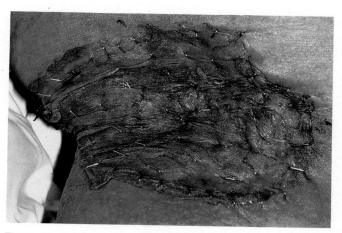

Figure 68–3. A large skin graft in the axilla has been rapidly tacked down using staples.

motion and at the same time holds the dressing in perfect apposition with the axilla whenever the arm is in its normal position (i.e., closely approximated with the lateral chest wall).

Keloids

Keloids result from the production of excess dermal connective tissue that forms in response to trauma in predisposed individuals. Blacks have a higher incidence than whites, but once keloids develop the recurrence rate after surgical removal is the same in both races. Keloids are found most often at the sites of ear piercing, surgical scars, burns, vaccinations, severe nodulocystic acne lesions, tattoos, and trauma. In addition, spontaneous keloids, usually on the middle chest, can arise without a history of antecedent trauma in patients with a strong family history of keloid formation.

Although earlobe keloids are common after ear piercing (Figs. 68–4, 68–5), they do not accurately predict the likelihood of keloids forming elsewhere. Other common areas of keloid formation include the anterior neck (Fig. 68–6), abdomen (Fig. 68–7), chest, shoulders, and upper back. Keloids rarely develop on the eyelids, hands, feet, genitalia, and mucous membranes.

Differentiation of keloids from hypertrophic scars may be difficult at times. Clinically, keloids extend onto normal skin beyond the area of the precipitating trauma and may increase or remain stable in size. Hypertrophic scars, on the other hand, usually remain limited to the

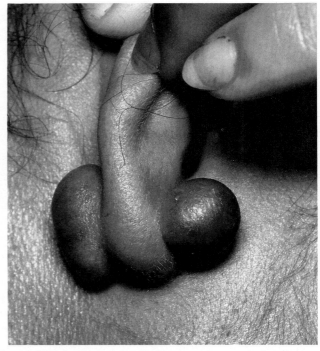

Figure 68–5. Dumbbell-shaped keloids commonly develop with components on both the anterior and posterior aspects of the earlobe.

traumatized area and regress spontaneously over 12 to 18 months. Both are usually asymptomatic, but keloids may be tender, painful, or pruritic. However, some patients may seek therapy for cosmetic rather than functional reasons.

Histologically, keloids are characterized by thick, glassy collagen bundles; an abundance of mucinous ground substance; a minimal number of inflammatory cells; and few fibroblasts.[2] Hypertrophic scars, on the other hand, have numerous foreign body giant cells and fibroblasts, but few glossy collagen bundles and scanty mucinous ground substance.[2]

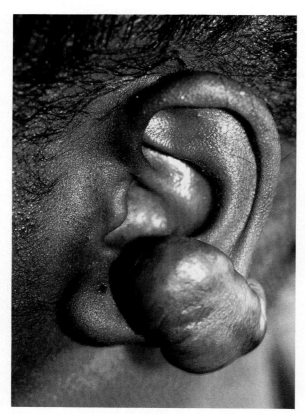

Figure 68–4. A large keloid wrapped around the inferior auricular rim after ear piercing.

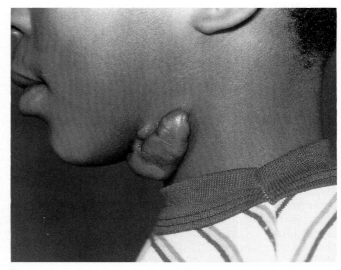

Figure 68–6. A common site for keloid formation is the anterior neck.

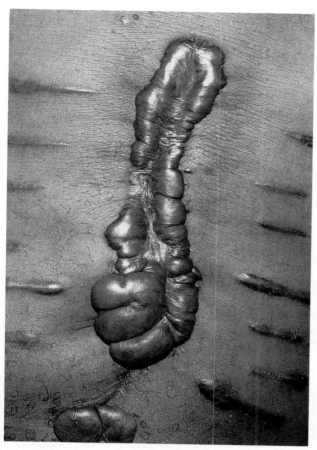

Figure 68–7. Another common site for keloid formation is the abdomen.

The cardinal rule of keloid therapy is prevention. Nonessential cosmetic surgery should be withheld from patients prone to keloid formation. However, those with only earlobe keloids and a negative family history should not be considered at increased risk. All surgical wounds should be closed with minimal tension, following skin creases whenever possible. Incisions should not cross joint spaces, and middle chest incisions should be avoided. A pressure gradient elastic garment (Fig. 68–8) should be worn at least 12 hours a day for 4 to 6 months after cutaneous trauma in patients at high risk for the development of keloids. There is no single therapeutic modality that is best for all keloids. The location, size, and depth of the lesion, as well as the age of the patient and history of past response to treatment, should all be considered when choosing the type of therapy.

Surgical removal of keloids is best accomplished when combined with liquid nitrogen, intralesional steroids, and pressure. To decrease the incidence of recurrence, corticosteroids should be injected into the keloid at 2-week intervals several times before surgery and at least four times after surgery. For keloids small enough to be excised and closed primarily with minimal wound tension, a simple excision, followed by undermining and closing with sutures, is usually sufficient. The base and edges of the wound are injected with 10 mg triamcino-

lone acetonide before wound closure. If a layered closure is necessary, buried polyglycolic acid sutures should be used because of their low tissue reactivity. Monofilament nylon may be used to close the superficial layers, although monofilament polybutester sutures are sometimes preferred because of their elasticity and low tissue reactivity. The sutures are left in place for 10 to 14 days, since premature removal may cause wound dehiscence. This reduced rate of healing is a result of the corticosteroids that were injected at the time of surgical removal.

For pedunculated keloids on the posterior earlobe, where the cosmetic result is not of paramount importance, shaving with a razor blade followed by pressure hemostasis may be a simple and efficient method of removal (Fig. 68–9). For pedunculated keloids with a wide base (Fig. 68–10), large nonpedunculated keloids, or wide-based keloids on other anatomic areas, surgical removal is more complex.[3] A half-moon or tonguelike incision approximately one fifth to one fourth the size of the lesion is made into the part of the keloid with the smoothest and flattest skin surface border. The attached keloid tissue is removed, creating a lip of skin like a thin split-thickness graft. The rest of the keloid is excised with a surgical blade held at a 30- to 45-degree angle

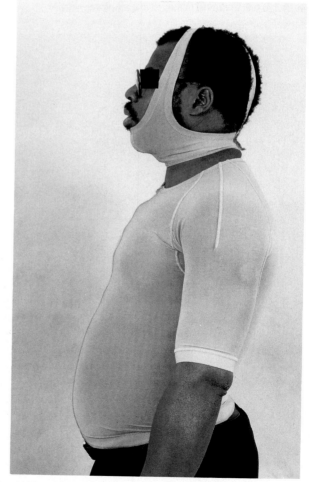

Figure 68–8. Clinical appearance of an elasticized pressure garment worn to reduce the risk of keloid formation in high-risk patients.

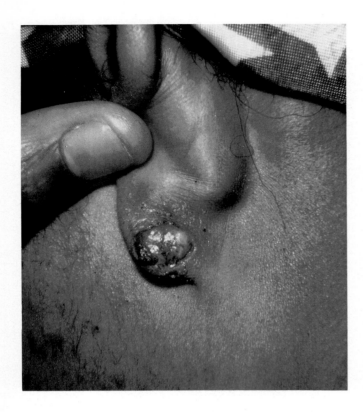

Figure 68–10. Preoperative appearance of a large, wide-based, pedunculated keloid on the posterior aspect of the earlobe.

Figure 68–9. A shallow wound has been created by shave removal of a pedunculated keloid on the posterior aspect of the earlobe.

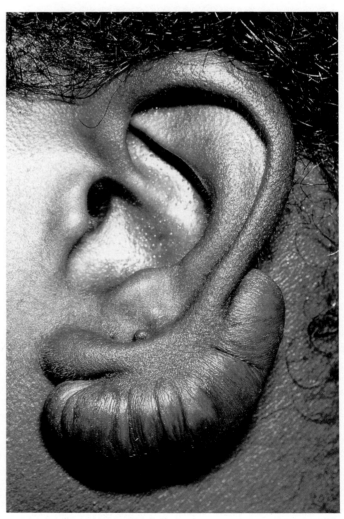

with the skin rather than the standard 90-degree angle. This angulation allows for removal and undermining at the same time. The overlying lip of skin is approximated with the excision borders using 5–0 or 6–0 monofilament nylon or monofilament polybutester (Fig. 68–11). If the lip of skin is large, absorbable subcuticular sutures are sometimes used to tack it down. Before the wound is closed, the base is injected with 10 mg triamcinolone.

Excision with second-intention healing or shaving of the keloid flush with or slightly below the level of the surrounding skin is rarely successful. However, keloid regrowth may possibly be prevented when these procedures are combined with postoperative intralesional steroid injections, class 1 topical steroids, occlusive hydrocolloid surgical dressings, and silicone gel sheeting.

Although laser therapy has been reported to be a successful and rapid way to treat keloids,[4, 5] it does not in itself always prevent recurrences. Postoperative use of intralesional steroids, pressure, and colloid dressings combined with topical steroids is usually necessary to prevent keloids from recurring.

Acne Keloidalis

Acne keloidalis (AK), also known as dermatitis papillaris capillitii or sycosis nuchae, occurs almost exclusively in black males. It typically begins after puberty as groups of firm, dome-shaped, follicular papules 2 to 4 mm in diameter that develop on the nape of the neck and on the posterior scalp (Fig. 68–12). As the disease progresses, the papules enlarge, and some coalesce to form plaques. These plaques are usually only 1 to 2 cm in diameter but may sometimes reach more than 10 cm in diameter (Fig. 68–13). The usual clinical appearance is that of a large area of scar tissue on the posterior scalp or neck composed of hard papules or plaques. The hair is usually lost in the large lesions, and the upper borders are often fringed with polytrichia hairs that resemble doll's hair (Fig. 68–14). Areas of chronic involvement typically have subcutaneous abscesses with draining sinuses and scarring alopecia.

Medical treatment is usually ineffective or only palliative at best. Before surgery is initiated, the inflammatory lesions should be cultured and the patient treated with appropriate antibiotics. Small papular lesions can be excised in full-thickness fashion with a dermal punch to a depth below the fibrous tissue; the wound is either closed primarily or allowed to heal by second intention. A more superficial excision is usually associated with a high incidence of recurrence.

For lesions with a width of less than 2 cm, a deep excision below the fibrous tissue to the fascia and primary closure after adequate undermining are usually recommended. After 4 to 6 months, the postoperative scar usually spreads to about one half the width of the initial excision. For larger lesions, deep excision to the fascia or deep subcutaneous tissue with second-intention healing is the method of choice.[6, 7] Even though the excised area is deep, skin grafting is not recommended, as it leaves a large, hairless, cosmetically unacceptable concavity and also prevents the wound from contracting. Primary closure of a large, deep, posterior nuchal wound

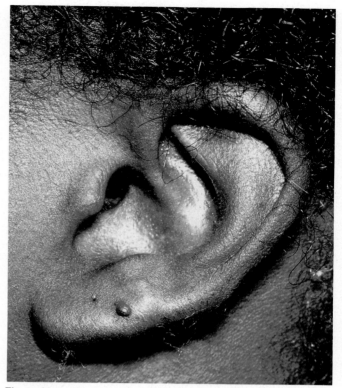

Figure 68–11. Postoperative appearance of the patient in Figure 68–10 after removal of the keloid using a "half-moon" excisional surgery technique.

often requires the patient to extend the neck to permit proper wound closure. This means that the patient will be unable to look straight ahead or down during the first week or two postoperatively.

The defect caused by excision with second-intention healing closes better if the resultant postoperative site is horizontally oriented and involves the posterior hairline. These wounds typically heal in approximately 8 weeks with a linear scar less than 1 cm wide that can usually be covered by the posterior hairline. After 4 to 6 months, the scar has a tendency to spread, often

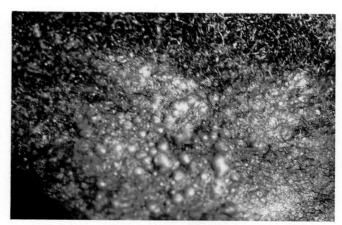

Figure 68–12. Typical clinical appearance of acne keloidalis nuchae, which consists of groups of small, firm, dome-shaped follicular papules.

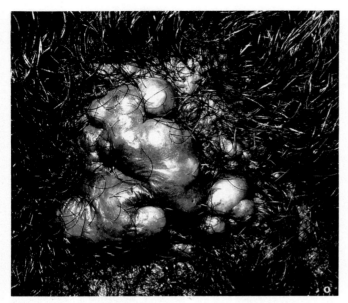

Figure 68–13. Larger plaques form in acne keloidalis nuchae as the disease progresses.

doubling or even tripling its initial width but seldom reaching the size of the scar from primary closure. Lesions removed with vertical ellipses or rectangular excisions take longer to heal and contract less than horizontal ellipses. When the excision involves the posterior hairline, there is better contraction and the postoperative scar can be hidden by the hair.

After surgery, oral antibiotic therapy is begun, and the patient is instructed to remove the surgical dressing after 36 hours. The wound is cleansed with hydrogen peroxide, a topical antibiotic ointment is applied to the base of the wound, and then a nonadherent dressing is placed on the surface of the wound. The dressing is changed daily until the wound has completely healed.

Sometimes, satellite fibrotic follicular papules can be identified peripheral to the excised area. These should be either removed with dermal punches and left to heal by second intention or closed primarily at the time of the major excision. Carbon dioxide laser vaporization

offers little therapeutic benefit, but laser excision carried down to a subfollicular depth with the wound allowed to heal by second intention has been successful.[8] Postoperative care after laser excision is the same as that after surgery.

Hair Transplantation

The standard technique of hair transplantation requires only a few minor modifications to be performed in black patients. The donor plugs, instead of being 0.5 mm larger, should be either the same size or only 0.25 mm larger than the recipient site. This is done to help prevent cobblestoning, which is more common in blacks than in whites. When the donor plugs and the recipient sites are the same size, there is a tendency in black patients for a ring of peripheral hyperpigmentation to form around each plug; this usually clears in 6 to 12 months.

Because of the curved nature of the hair follicles in blacks, better results are obtained with a very sharp manual punch that cuts the plug with minimal rotation. In addition, the scalp hair of blacks is not as dense as that of whites, and most plugs contain only eight to ten hairs. However, because of the curliness of the hair, the coverage provided will be at least as good as, if not better than, that in patients with straight hair.

SUMMARY

Cutaneous surgical procedures can be safely and effectively performed in most black patients. With careful preoperative evaluation (including a detailed personal history of wound healing), meticulous surgical technique, and diligent postoperative wound care, cosmetic surgery can be performed with good results. Knowledge of the technical modifications required to manage satisfactorily the more common types of surgical problems seen in black patients is an absolute prerequisite for a successful outcome.

REFERENCES

1. Morgan WP, Harding KG, Hughes LE: A comparison of skin grafting and healing by granulation, following axillary excision for hidradenitis suppurativa. Ann R Coll Surg (Engl) 65:235, 1983.
2. Blackburn WR, Cosman B: Histologic basis of keloid hypertrophic scar differentiation. Arch Pathol 82:65–71, 1966.
3. Kelly AP: Keloids. Dermatol Clin 6:413–424, 1988.
4. Kantor GR, Wheeland RG, Bailin PL, et al: Treatment of ear lobe keloids with carbon dioxide laser excision: a report of 16 cases. J Dermatol Surg Oncol 11:1063–1067, 1985.
5. Abergel PR, Dwyer RM, Meeker CA, et al: Laser treatment of keloids: a clinical trial in an in-vitro study with Nd:YAG laser. Lasers Surg Med 4:291–295, 1984.
6. Dinehart SM, Herzberg AJ, Kerns BJ: Acne keloidalis: a review. J Dermatol Surg Oncol 15:642–647, 1989.
7. Bennett RE, Davis LT, Kelly AP: Acne keloidalis. J Dermatol Surg Oncol 16:293–294, 1990.
8. Kantor GR, Ratz JL, Wheeland RG: Treatment of acne keloidalis nuchae with carbon dioxide laser. J Am Acad Dermatol 14:263–267, 1986.

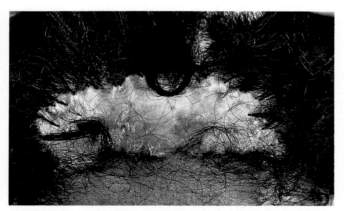

Figure 68–14. At the end stage of this disease, large scarred areas with central alopecia and fringes of polytrichia form on the posterior neck.

CHAPTER 69

Sclerotherapy

ROBERT A. WEISS and MARGARET A. WEISS

Protuberant and uncomfortable veins are a representation of mankind's losing struggle with the force of gravity. Until weightless environments are available, people will seek treatment for varicosities and telangiectases. In the United States, physician interest in sclerotherapy has blossomed since the 1980s, although the American medical community disparaged sclerotherapy for decades. Cutaneous surgeons have played a major role in advancing knowledge of the treatment of leg telangiectases by sclerotherapy, while European phlebologists, angiologists, and vascular surgeons have advanced knowledge of sclerotherapy treatment of varicose veins.[1] As a result of these efforts, sclerotherapy has become accepted as an important tool for the treatment of varicose veins of all sizes. Because telangiectases may often arise from larger vessels, effective use of sclerotherapy for leg veins requires a complete understanding of the anatomy of the venous system. In addition, it is important to be able to evaluate disorders of the venous system of the leg with appropriate diagnostic tools and to recognize patterns of disease.

Patient Interest

Of the many causes for the resurgence of interest in sclerotherapy, the primary one has been patient interest. One survey has shown that American women are more concerned with lower extremity telangiectases than with almost any other cosmetic problem[2] and refer to these vessels as "spider veins" or "broken vessels." Until relatively recently, these vessels have been thought to be entirely of cosmetic concern. However, superficial telangiectases and venulectases actually result in symptoms in approximately 50% of women who present for treatment.[3] It is important to realize that the term varicose veins may include anything from minor cosmetic blemishes to important venous hypertension with ulcers.[4] Therefore, physicians performing sclerotherapy should be familiar with symptoms caused by varicose veins of all sizes.

Prevalence

The demand for sclerotherapy should increase, as predicted by the high prevalence of varicose and telangiectatic veins in the adult population (estimated at between 10 and 20%).[5] It has been estimated that 24 million people in the United States have varicose veins.[6] Others have reported that 28.9 to 40.9% of American women have telangiectatic leg veins,[7] with some estimates as high as 50%.[2] In Great Britain, many hospitals have long waiting lists for operations on veins. Some surgeons will not see new patients with this complaint, primarily because of a lack of interest in treating venous disorders.[4] Proper treatment is often difficult to find in the United States, since modern surgical technique and sclerotherapy remain largely untaught in medical schools and residency training programs. Often, patients are simply told that they must live with the consequences of varicose and telangiectatic leg veins and that symptomatic relief can be obtained with the use of support hose. Sclerotherapy is frequently mentioned in negative terms, if at all, and is considered capable of offering little hope for success. Vascular surgeons trained in traditional ligation and stripping procedures typically advise patients to undergo such surgery.

Although heaviness and aching of the legs are often relieved by wearing compression hose,[8] patients usually want to be rid of the veins, whether large or small, rather than burdened with the required daily use of external support. Sclerotherapy, when performed properly, can be not only a markedly effective treatment for telangiectasia, but also a highly effective alternative or adjunct to surgery for varicose veins. Techniques for treating different types and sizes of varicose and telangiectatic leg veins vary greatly. One common mistake made by cutaneous surgeons is assuming that knowledge of venipuncture confers expertise in sclerotherapy. Expertise in sclerotherapy is gained only after observing trained cutaneous surgeons using meticulous technique, along with hours of subsequent practice. Proper technique is crucial to the success of the procedure and is of paramount importance. Understanding the history of sclerotherapy is the first step toward success.

History

Compression therapy for treatment of venous disease was actually first mentioned in the Old Testament. Hippocrates further documented this treatment in the fourth century BC,[9] and his blood-letting technique remained the treatment of choice for varicose veins until the Middle Ages. He also described the first surgical treatment with the use of "a slender instrument of iron" to cause thrombosis. Primitive stripping and cauterization were practiced by Celsus, while ligation was mentioned by Antillus in 30 AD. In the second century AD, Galen proposed tearing out the veins with hooks. Aeginata, in the seventh century AD, practiced ligation of the vein.

Fabricius of Aquapendete discovered valves and directional blood flow in the venous system in the 1580s. Paré[10] first associated leg ulcers with varicose veins and recommended support. This was not widely used until the introduction of the laced leather stocking in the late 1600s.[11]

In 1682, Zollikofer described the injection of acid into a vein to create a thrombus, thus introducing a crude type of sclerotherapy. By the late 1700s, the critical role of saphenofemoral reflux in the pathogenesis of varicose veins had been recognized by the Swiss surgeon, Rima. Because of excessive mortality, however, ligation of the saphenous vein could not be attempted. Reports of use of absolute alcohol as a sclerosing agent appeared between 1835 and 1840.[12] In 1851, in France, Pravaz attempted sclerotherapy, first on an arterial aneurysm and later on varicose veins, by injecting ferric chloride with his new device, the hypodermic syringe.[13] Despite this great technical advance, results were poor and fraught with complications, including mortality from sepsis, emboli, and other toxic phenomena.

With the advent of the sterile technique, surgery emerged as the treatment of choice for venous disease. After Trendelenburg's pioneering work in the 1890s, high ligation of the saphenous vein was widely practiced.[14] In 1905, Keller and Mayo combined ligation with stripping, setting a new standard of care.[15] Technical improvements in stripping devices allowed the surgical management of varicose vein disease to predominate for many years.

The foundation of modern sclerotherapy was laid during World War I when Linser and Sicard both noticed the sclerosing effect of intravenous injections used to treat syphilis.[14] They employed this technique in the treatment of varicose veins, injecting various hypertonic agents with some success. Tournay greatly refined the technique, being the first to drain intravaricose clots. Sclerotherapy became increasingly popular in Europe, but it was not until 1946, when a safe sclerosant, sodium tetradecyl sulfate (Sotradecol), was developed that sclerotherapy began to be seriously studied in the United States.[16]

Probably the single most important advance in the success and ultimate acceptance of the treatment of varicose veins by sclerotherapy has been the use of compression. Although the use of compression to treat the symptoms of venous insufficiency had long been described, it was not until the reports by Sigg[17] and Orbach[18] in the 1950s and Fegan[19] in the 1960s that the importance of combining compression bandaging with injections was discovered. With the compression technique, the results of sclerotherapy compared favorably with those of surgery. The successful use of the sclerosing agent sodium tetradecyl sulfate in an outpatient setting, with its relatively good safety profile, allowed sclerotherapy to become a medically accepted technique. However, it remained largely ignored by practitioners in mainstream American medicine.

The earliest report in the United States of the use of sclerotherapy for telangiectasia in the presence of occlusion of the deep venous circulation appeared in 1934.[20] However, it was not until the early 1970s that use of sclerotherapy was reported for the treatment of telangiectatic leg veins in a large group of patients.[21] As late as 1970, cutaneous surgeons were recommending cosmetic camouflage for telangiectases.[22] A renewed interest in sclerotherapy was sparked by reports of successful treatment of telangiectasias in more than 250 patients.[23, 24] A subsequent report promoted the technique among cutaneous surgeons by advocating the use of polidocanol (Aethoxysklerol) and hypertonic saline as safe and effective sclerosing solutions.[25]

In Europe, sclerotherapy has been accepted by the medical community since the 1960s and currently exists as the separate subspecialty of phlebology. American physicians have only relatively recently discovered the tremendous European experience in the treatment of varicose veins. Unfortunately, many cutaneous surgeons in the United States only use sclerotherapy routinely to treat telangiectases. The 1980s and 1990s have witnessed a new era of cooperation and interchange of knowledge between the European and American medical communities, which bodes well for future progress in the field of sclerotherapy.

Sclerotherapy Versus Surgery

In 1983, one study reported that of 66 patients who underwent sclerotherapy after traditional surgery, all preferred sclerotherapy.[26] According to the prevailing philosophy for surgery of varicose veins in the 1970s, the more extensive the surgery, the better.[27] However, the literature substantiated the need for postoperative sclerotherapy in up to 49% of patients.[28, 29] Because factors that cause varicose veins continue to promote further disease after any form of treatment, patients undergoing surgery are at high risk for recurrence and often require additional treatment. As a consequence, complete cure in all cases cannot be expected, no matter what method of treatment is used.[30] Claims of 85% good to excellent outcomes[31] for the results of surgery in the United States have been reported. Complications after surgery include a mortality rate of 0.02%,[30] as well as nerve injury, deep vein thrombosis, pulmonary embolism, delayed wound healing, ligation of the femoral vein, and inadvertent arterial stripping.[32]

Several randomized studies comparing surgery with compression sclerotherapy have demonstrated comparable results. For varicose veins below the knee, injection plus compression was the most effective, with 59% total resolution and 40% improvement.[32] In this study, incompetence of the saphenofemoral junction treated by compression sclerotherapy required subsequent ligation in only 9% of cases. In a follow-up study involving 404 legs treated by compression sclerotherapy versus 275 treated by surgery, it was found that superficial varicosities and incompetent lower leg perforator veins are best treated by compression sclerotherapy.[33] Other investigators have concluded that there is no statistical difference in results between surgery and sclerotherapy.[29, 34]

Interestingly, a study of cadaver legs with significant varicosities revealed an entirely normal saphenous system in more than half of the legs. It was concluded from these data that the procedure of vein stripping was therefore inappropriate in more than half of patients.[35] These data also suggest that sclerotherapy is a more physiologic approach to the treatment of varicosities.

In a 4- to 8-year follow-up of 1172 patients treated by compression sclerotherapy, good to excellent results were reported in 81 to 86% of patients. In addition, 15,000 patients were treated without any incidence.[36] Other authors have reported giving 42,000 injections without complications, with a relapse rate of only 15 to 25%.[37] Of 264 patients treated in one study,[38] good results were experienced by 91%. Serious complications, such as pulmonary emboli, were not reported by any of these authors and appear to be equal to, if not less frequent than, those in patients undergoing surgery. An additional benefit of sclerotherapy was a cure rate of 89% in nonobese patients with venous leg ulcers.[39]

These data strongly support compression sclerotherapy as an effective treatment for varicose veins. Sclerotherapy is preferred by patients, as it has less morbidity and is comparable in efficacy and recurrence rate to surgery. Additional advantages are lower cost and minimal patient inconvenience. It has been reported that surgery is five times as expensive as compression sclerotherapy[40] and that four times as many work days are lost with surgical treatment.[41] While newer microphlebectomy techniques may reduce the relative disadvantages of surgery somewhat, relatively few vascular surgeons in the United States currently offer this procedure. In most cases there is no time lost from work after sclerotherapy, and the actual cost is typically only one tenth that of surgery.

Evolving concepts among vascular surgeons, however, have led to the recommendation of more limited surgery in combination with sclerotherapy. After careful determination that saphenofemoral incompetence exists, a single groin incision is made, through which only the upper thigh portion of the saphenous vein is removed by an intraluminal stripper.[42] This stripping is accompanied by juxtafemoral saphenous vein ligation and subsequent sclerotherapy for remaining varicosities below the knee. Simple ligation of the saphenofemoral junction without limited stripping appears to yield poor long-term results.[42] Only long-term follow-up of thousands of patients will ultimately lead to a consensus as to the best treatment of larger varicosities. Patient preference, however, appears to be clearly in favor of sclerotherapy.

Anatomy and Physiology

Although the venous anatomy of the leg can be variable and complex, an understanding of the essentials of blood flow through the superficial venous system is crucial to perform sclerotherapy properly. The venous system of the leg is composed of a deep component—the "muscle pump," which normally carries 85 to 90% of venous return from the leg—and a superficial component, which carries 10 to 15%. Calf muscle contraction generates propulsive forces to move venous blood, somewhat like squeezing a tube of toothpaste (Fig. 69–1). During contraction of the calf, the valves of the perforating veins and superficial veins close, allowing blood to flow only proximally through the deep system. During relaxation the deep veins dilate, causing negative pressure, which draws blood from the superficial system through the perforating veins and main junctions into the deep system.

The superficial system consists primarily of the greater and lesser saphenous veins, multiple collateral accessory veins, and multiple perforator veins, which allow blood flow from the superficial to the deep system (Fig. 69–2). In phlebology, the points of connection between the superficial and the deep system are crucial, because these are the sites of leakage or reverse flow that leads to reflux. These sites include the greater saphenous-femoral vein junction, the lesser saphenous-popliteal vein junction, and multiple (50 to 100) perforating veins. Major perforating veins are more common below the knee than above the knee, where there are only 10 to 20. The perforating veins most commonly connect major tributaries of the saphenous system to the deep venous system but may also connect either of the saphenous veins directly to it.

The term primary varicose veins describes varicosities of the lower limb that develop spontaneously in the absence of deep venous thrombosis. Most patients seeking treatment for leg varicosities present with primary varicose veins. Most frequently the greater saphenous vein or its tributaries and perforators are involved, with only approximately 12% involving the lesser saphenous system.[43]

The long or greater saphenous vein originates on the foot at the confluence of the venous arch. It receives tributaries from the deep foot veins as it courses upward,

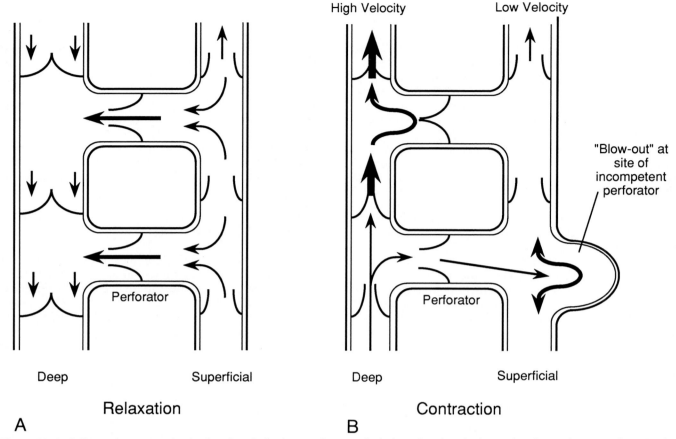

Figure 69–1. Calf muscle pump-and-valve function. *A,* As the muscle expands during relaxation, the internal or deep veins expand, generating negative pressure and "sucking" blood through the open valves of the perforating veins from the superficial veins. Retrograde flow is blocked in the internal system by the internal valves. *B,* The internal or deep venous system is compressed by surrounding muscles, generating high-velocity flow in a proximal direction. Perforating valves must close for proper pump function. The external valves may be closed, or open for low-velocity proximal flow with inspiration. A schematic of blood flow through an incompetent perforator valve during contraction is shown. Note that when the calf muscle is in the resting state without the contraction and relaxation cycle, venous blood flow is regulated by respiratory pressure changes and gravity. The respiratory cycle is responsible for the spontaneous sounds heard during Doppler examination.

just anterior to the medial malleolus. Below the ankle the valves of the tributary veins point outward, allowing flow from the deep to the superficial system. Above the medial malleolus, the valves of the perforating veins point inward, allowing emptying only. The greater saphenous vein continues up the anteromedial aspect of the thigh, receiving tributaries from the medial and lateral aspects. Just before the greater saphenous vein joins the femoral vein, it receives important tributary veins such as the lateral and medial femoral cutaneous branches, the external circumflex iliac vein, the superficial epigastric vein, and the internal pudendal vein. Under certain circumstances, these tributaries may also develop into varicose veins.

The lesser saphenous vein receives deep tributary veins from the lateral aspect of the dorsal venous arch of the foot. Other tributaries arise from the medial and lateral aspects of the calf. Multiple perforators communicate with the deep system. The lesser saphenous vein most commonly terminates in the popliteal vein at or slightly above the popliteal fossa. Occasionally, branches may continue up the posterior aspect of the thigh to join one of the final tributaries to the greater saphenous

vein. Important veins in the popliteal fossa that may exhibit reflux include the gastrocnemius veins, which terminate in the popliteal vein, and a popliteal-saphenous connection called the vein of Giacomini.

Although many names have been given to individual perforating veins, there is great variation in the number and exact position of the perforators serving both the greater and lesser saphenous veins and their tributaries. The greatest number of perforating veins demonstrating abnormal function without associated saphenofemoral or saphenopopliteal incompetence can be found on the lateral and medial aspects of the calf just below the knee. Doppler examination serves the cutaneous surgeon better than anatomic landmarks in the location of incompetent perforators.

Superficial vein walls are inherently weak, because they are supported only by subcutaneous tissue and skin, rather than by fascia and muscle. Primary varicosities are thought to develop when these veins are subject to pressure and turbulence caused by retrograde flow or reflux from a point of connection with the deep system. Reflux is the result of weak or defective valves. The valve is a bicuspid structure whose base expands into a

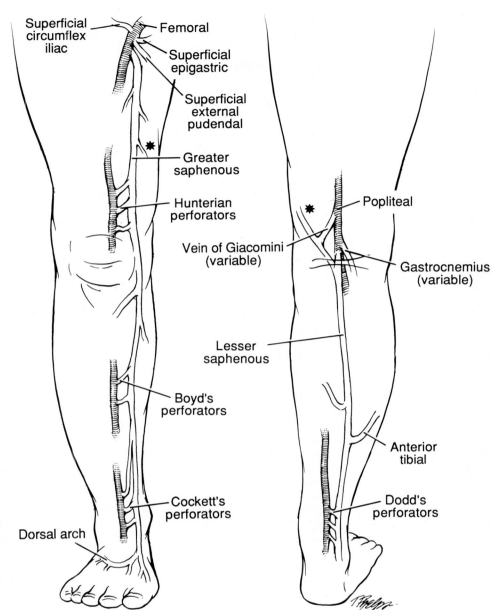

Figure 69–2. Simplified anatomy of the superficial venous system of the leg. This diagram is highly schematic and should serve only to illustrate important landmarks for treating varicose veins. The locations of the perforators are highly variable. Perforators connect directly with the saphenous system but also with tributaries of the saphenous system. The asterisks indicate a variable direct communication between the greater saphenous and the lesser saphenous veins.

sinus. When venous distention expands the sinus, the leaflets may not oppose, and a leak may ensue. After 5 or more hours of standing, venous distention leads to slight evidence of venous reflux in about one fifth of normal individuals.[44]

Sequential retrograde breakdown of the venous valves often follows a leak at one point, leading to propagation of a varicosity. With the reversal of blood flow through incompetent valves, the superficial veins dilate to accommodate the increased blood flow. Calf pump pressure can then be transmitted directly to the superficial veins in the area drained by the incompetent perforating vein. The increased pressure may be as great as 100 mm Hg in the cutaneous venules with the patient erect.[45] This may result in venular dilatation over a wide area of skin and may cause capillary dilatation as well.

Whether this process accounts for all telangiectases on the leg is open to question, but most cutaneous surgeons currently believe that transmission of abnormal venous pressure plays an important role. Therefore, the goal in treatment of a varicose vein is to stop the leak or reflux at its origin. Many of the specialized diagnostic procedures used in sclerotherapy are necessary to identify the reflux points and properly treat the correct site.

Causes of Varicose Veins

Although the specific cause of varicosities and incompetent valves is not known, hereditary factors are important. The incidence of reflux at the saphenofemoral junction was found to be twice as likely in children when a parent had a similar condition.[46] Patients seeking treatment frequently relate a positive family history of varicose veins. Susceptibility to valvular reflux also appears to be hereditary.

Pregnancy is another predisposing factor for the development of varicosities. The enlarged uterus compresses the inferior vena cava, causing venous hypertension with secondary distention in the legs.[47] To accommodate the higher volumes of blood required during pregnancy, venous capacity must expand. Multiple circulating hormonal and other factors contribute to the distensibility of the vein walls, which in turn predisposes the patient to valvular incompetence.[48] Because some spontaneous regression may occur after pregnancy, sclerotherapy is often postponed until several months after delivery.

Occupations requiring long hours of standing, or possibly those requiring prolonged sitting, may lead to valvular incompetence secondary to venous distention. Women are more susceptible than men because of the increased distensibility of the venous system that occurs with each menstrual cycle, presumably as a result of progesterone.[49] Advancing age itself will also cause vein walls to weaken as the elastic lamina becomes thinner, fragmented, and atrophic in combination with smooth muscle degeneration.[50] This weakened vein is more susceptible to pressure-induced distention. Population studies have shown an association between increasing age and onset of varicosities.[51]

Traumatic superficial thrombophlebitis or trauma without phlebitis can cause scarring of the vein walls and may compromise valve function. In the presence of occlusion of the deep venous circulation due to thrombosis or other factors, superficial varicosities must function as an accessory venous return system. As a consequence, the superficial system may dilate and become tortuous when the deep muscle pump no longer functions. This condition must be recognized, and sclerotherapy or surgery to treat varicosities avoided, as such treatment would eliminate the functioning venous return of the affected leg, with resultant dire consequences.

Signs and Symptoms of Venous Disease: Rationale for Treatment

Hypertension of the venous system from any cause with resulting dilation of the superficial veins leads to a predictable, progressive set of symptoms and complications. Galen aptly described one symptom of varicose veins as "a heavy and depressing pain."[52] Treatment of varicose and telangiectatic leg veins is undertaken to relieve pain, improve venous function, prevent complications, and achieve cosmetic improvement. When valvular insufficiency disrupts venous physiology, thereby interfering with normal venous circulation, venous pressure remains high, even during walking or exercise. This leads to "chronic venous insufficiency" manifested in the skin of the lower leg and ankle. The most common symptom is aching of the legs.[53] In a survey of 215 patients, the most common symptom reported with telangiectases was a sensation of muscle fatigue in the

TABLE 69–1. SYMPTOMS CAUSED BY TELANGIECTATIC OR VARICOSE LEG VEINS

Symptom	Incidence (%)
Aching pain in leg (may be associated with fatigue)	53
Muscle fatigue or tired legs (may be associated with ache)	27
Burning or pruritus (regional or focal)	26
Throbbing of varicosities or telangiectases	17
Night cramps	21
Edema or swelling	20

Reprinted by permission of the publisher from Weiss RA, Weiss MA. Resolution of pain associated with varicose and telangiectatic leg veins after compression sclerotherapy. J Dermatol Surg Oncol 16:333–336, 1990. Copyright 1990 by Elsevier Science Publishing Co., Inc.

affected legs with localized pain over groups of blood vessels or small varicosities.[3] Symptoms worsen with prolonged standing but can be partially relieved by wearing support hose while standing or by elevating and resting the legs. Surprisingly, the vessels causing symptoms may be only 1 to 2 mm or less in diameter. Larger varicosities may cause no complaints, while small-caliber veins may produce surprising discomfort.[53]

A closely related symptom of venous disease is fatigue or the sensation of aching or tired legs (Table 69–1). Swelling of the ankles is a symptom of mild venous physiologic disturbance, while pitting edema is a symptom of more progressive disease. Cramping of the calf muscles can occur and may occasionally awaken the patient at night. Some patients experience itching or burning, while others describe a throbbing sensation localized to an area of varicosities or telangiectases.[3]

The complications of varicose veins (Table 69–2) include pigmentation, stasis dermatitis, subacute cellulitis, ulceration, bleeding, and thrombophlebitis. It is important not to confuse the complications of altered venous hemodynamics with those that may occur from sclerotherapy. With persistent venous hypertension, capillaries become hyperpermeable, permitting proteinaceous fluid and red blood cells to escape into the subcutaneous tissue. An early sign of this process is pigmentation from the hemosiderin deposited in the subcutaneous tissue by pressure-forced extravasation of erythrocytes. This typically occurs in the medial distal third of the leg extending onto the ankle.[54] Treatment of varicosities may cause this pigmentation to slowly resolve.

TABLE 69–2. COMPLICATIONS OF VARICOSE VEINS

Pigmentation
Stasis dermatitis
Fibrosis
    Lipodermatosclerosis
    Atrophie blanche
Cellulitis
Ulceration
Bleeding or hemorrhage
Superficial thrombophlebitis

As the extravasated proteins and red blood cells organize, the subcutaneous tissue begins to undergo fibrosis, leading eventually to lipodermatosclerosis,[55] a condition characterized by fibrotic hypopigmented plaques on the ankle. The initial step is a dermatitis that begins as dry, scaly plaques but may progress to eroded, weeping erythematous areas. Itching often accompanies these changes, and the resulting excoriation worsens skin breakdown and may lead to subacute or acute cellulitis. Redness, tenderness, and induration then envelop the lower one half to one third of the leg, requiring treatment consisting of leg elevation, external compression, moist dressings of aluminum acetate solution, and systemic antibiotics.

It has long been believed that after pericapillary fibrinogen accumulation under conditions of chronic fluid extravasation, diffusion of oxygen into tissue is restricted, causing hypoxia of the skin.[56] Ulcers may then easily occur, either spontaneously or from superficial abrasion or minor trauma. However, this concept of tissue hypoxia leading to ulceration has been challenged, and an alternative mechanism has been proposed. This theory suggests that capillary occlusion by polymorphonuclear leukocytes with release of proteolytic enzymes results in tissue destruction.[57] Local treatment of venous ulcers by sclerotherapy of a varicosity in proximity to the ulcer may lead to rapid resolution of the ulcer.[39, 58]

A rare but serious complication of varicose veins is bleeding from an erosion through the wall of the varicosity. Spontaneous hemorrhage can be a medical emergency, but blood loss is not usually severe. After the acute bleeding is stopped using pressure and leg elevation, the offending vein should be treated, preferably by injection and compression sclerotherapy.[53]

Often occurring after a trivial injury to a prominent varicose vein, superficial thrombophlebitis presents as redness, tenderness, and induration of a varicosity. Early surgical removal of the thrombosed varicosity seems to shorten the disability time.[59] However, conservative treatment with compression and nonsteroidal anti-inflammatory drugs has also been recommended.[60] Occasionally, extension upward into the saphenous vein may occur; this may require more aggressive anticoagulant therapy.

It is important to realize that even when pain or other complications of varicosities are not present, the appearance of the veins may be so psychologically disturbing to female patients that they will not wear shorts or bathing suits at all. Thus these women are deprived of major sources of exercise, and their lifestyle is severely limited. Sclerotherapy offers these patients outstanding cosmetic results. For patients with symptomatic small varicosities, pain relief can also be expected from sclerotherapy (85% success rate).[3]

Evaluation of the Patient With Varicosities and Telangiectases

Each patient evaluation should begin with a complete history (Fig. 69–3). Relevant information includes pa-

tient symptoms, a history of worsening with pregnancy, previous trauma, and previous use of exogenous hormones. Hormone therapy may hinder the progress of sclerotherapy, and patients should be so informed.[61] A positive family history of varicosities indicates a greater likelihood of primary varicose veins owing to valvular reflux without complicating factors. Patients with a history of deep venous thrombosis, arterial occlusive disease, or diabetes are poor candidates for sclerotherapy. When a patient gives a history of poor tolerance of support hose or worsening of symptoms with use of support hose having a pressure gradient of at least 20 to 30 mm Hg, treatment by sclerotherapy should be reconsidered for two reasons. First, the possibility that the superficial venous system serves a vital role in venous outflow secondary to deep venous obstruction should be considered. Second, the use of support hose for compression is necessary after sclerotherapy of varicosities.

Complete physical examination of the lower extremities allows recognition of signs and complications of venous insufficiency. Although judgment varies from physician to physician, selection for noninvasive office testing should be based on the presence of symptoms and the size of grouped telangiectases or varicosities. Patients with scattered, isolated, asymptomatic telangiectases approximately 1 mm in diameter or less with no obvious associated reticular or blue venulectases or varicose veins and a negative history need no further testing.

If physical examination reveals varicosities, usually greater than 3 mm in diameter, some simple maneuvers without instrumentation may help to define the etiology. These include the Perthes test, in which a thigh tourniquet is applied while the patient stands. After ten steps in place, the varicosities should decrease if the deep muscle pump is effective. If the varicosities remain large, the patient then lies down with the tourniquet in place, and the leg is elevated (Linton test) to test for deep venous outflow obstruction. If varices distal to the tourniquet fail to drain after a few seconds, obstruction is suspected.

To analyze the competency of the saphenofemoral junction, a tourniquet is applied just below the groin of an elevated leg in a recumbent patient (Trendelenburg II test). The patient then stands, and the tourniquet is removed; if proximal valves are incompetent, the varices fill immediately. Much of the value of these tests is diminished by the availability of the hand-held Doppler instrument.[62] In most cases, a Doppler examination to locate the source of reflux and to guide selection of entry points for treatment with sclerotherapy is the preferred technique.

When varicosities extend into the groin or are located on the calf or popliteal fossa or if large groups of symptomatic telangiectases in association with a venulectasia or reticular vein are seen, further noninvasive examination is indicated. Using a simple hand-held Doppler instrument, the cutaneous surgeon can rapidly assess the lower extremity venous system (Fig. 69–4). The purpose of this assessment is to identify the competence of the saphenofemoral and lesser saphenous-popliteal vein junctions bilaterally and to listen for

VASCULAR PATIENT HISTORY

Name_____   Date_____

Diagnosed Conditions
    Diabetes   [   ]
    Hypertension   [   ]
    Hyperlipidemia   [   ]
    Stroke   [   ]
    Heart Disease   [   ]
    Varicose Veins   [   ]
    Previous Vascular Surgery   [   ]
    History of Phlebitis   [   ]
    History of Blood Clots   [   ]
    Other _____   [[

Risk Factors (Past and Present)
    Oral Contraceptives   [   ]_____
    Hormone Supplements   [   ]_____
    Family History of Veins   [   ]
    Past Pregnancies   [   ] #____

Current Symptoms in Legs
    Weakness   [   ]
    Heaviness/Fatigue/Pressure   [   ]
    Skin Discoloration   [   ]
    Stasis Dermatitis   [   ]
    Ulcerations   [   ]
    Swelling with Menstruation   [   ]
    Dull Aches   [   ]
    Nighttime Cramps   [   ]
    Burning Sensation   [   ]
    Throbbing   [   ]
    Other _____   [   ]

What seems to bring on discomfort?

    Prolonged sitting   [   ]
    Prolonged standing   [   ]
    Other _____   [   ]

Does the pain/discomfort increase in the evening?   [   ]

Is the pain/discomfort worse in warm weather?   [   ]

Is the pain/discomfort worse during menstruation?   [   ]

What seems to relieve the pain/discomfort?

    After a good night's sleep   [   ]
    Elevating the legs   [   ]
    Exercise   [   ]
    Support hose   [   ]

Figure 69–3. History form, allowing the nurse or the patient to rapidly check off those items that apply.

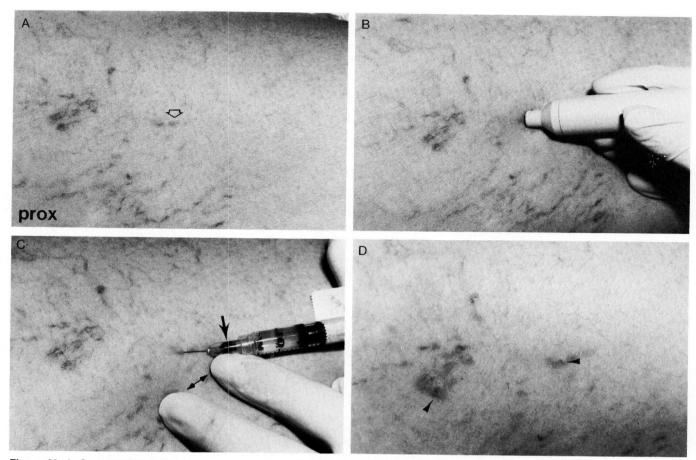

Figure 69–4. Grouped telangiectases associated with a reticular vein. *A,* The lateral thigh is shown with a central blue reticular varicosity *(arrowhead),* which is actually much more prominent than it appears in this black-and-white reproduction. The telangiectases are located proximal (prox) to this reticular vein, paradoxically against the force of gravity. *B,* The Doppler probe is placed gently over the reticular vein at a 45- to 60-degree angle after application of ultrasound gel. Three fingers of the dominant hand create a platform to keep the probe steady as it is held between the thumb and index finger (similar to holding the syringe for injecting sclerosing solution). The nondominant hand is used to compress the thigh or upper calf distal to the Doppler probe. When compression is released, a whooshing sound of free reflux is heard for several seconds. A normal vein would yield a very brief sound until competent valves snap shut. *C,* The initial site of treatment is in the reticular vein. Blood is drawn back through the 30-gauge needle *(large arrow)* to ensure intraluminal placement of the needle. A transparent hub needle is therefore recommended. Note the use of the nondominant hand to stretch the skin tightly and also allow further support of the needle hub; this allows extremely fine movement back and forth for minor adjustments of needle position. 0.5 ml of solution is injected. *D,* Several minutes later, all the vessels in the region exhibit urtication. This phenomenon allows easy identification of all treated telangiectases, including those not directly treated but receiving sclerosing solution through the injected incompetent reticular vein. The two injection points indicated by the arrowheads show greater swelling. Urtication resolves spontaneously within 1 to 2 hours.

points of reflux through suspected incompetent perforating veins in the calf, thigh, and ankle. In addition, an estimate of venous outflow from the femoral vein can be made.

For superficial veins, an 8-MHz transducer is used with the patient relaxed and sitting or the leg slightly dependent in a warm room. With very light or no pressure, the transducer is placed on the area of interest after liberal application of ultrasonic gel. The physician usually begins at the medial groin, locates the femoral arterial signal, and then proceeds to listen for the normal changes with respiratory excursions in the adjacent medial femoral vein (Fig. 69–5). Manual distal thigh compression produced by the hand that is not holding the transducer should rapidly and briefly enhance the signal.

Once normal venous outflow is established, the probe is moved distally approximately 4 cm. While a short series of thigh compressions are performed with the other hand to generate a venous flow signal, the transducer is moved side to side to locate the greater saphenous vein. If the physician can see a varix in this region, the probe can be placed directly over it. Gentle external compression and release of the thigh distal to the transducer should lead to a transient increase in signal frequency or amplitude, followed by rapid decrease in the signal as competent valves snap shut. With valvular insufficiency at the saphenofemoral junction, the initial increase is followed by a prolonged backflow signal. If the result is equivocal, manual external compression and release can be performed proximal to the Doppler transducer, causing a very brief sound if normal valve

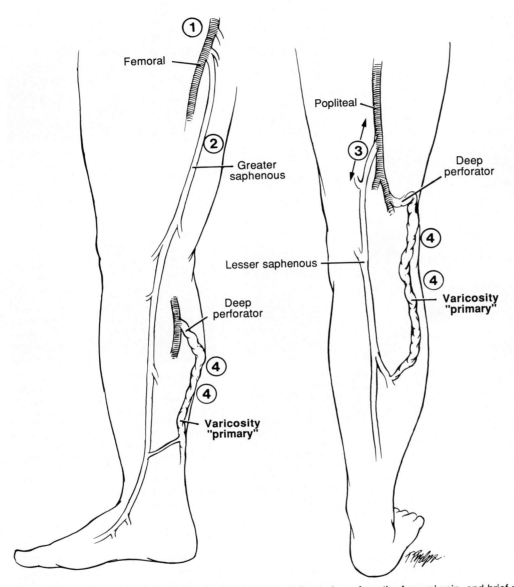

Figure 69–5. Anatomic locations for Doppler examination. 1, Femoral vein. The patient is placed supine, and a transducer is placed below the inguinal ligament. Listen for the normal spontaneous sound ("windstorm"-type sound) of the femoral vein just medial to the pulsatile arterial sound. Brief manual compression of the distal thigh with the hand not holding the Doppler probe should cause rapid augmentation of the femoral vein sound. Sounds should be equal bilaterally. Absence of any of these sounds may indicate deep venous obstruction. Further evaluation with duplex ultrasound may be of value if these sounds are absent. 2, Greater saphenous–femoral vein junction (saphenofemoral junction [SFJ]). The patient remains supine or sitting. The transducer is moved 1 to 4 cm below the inguinal ligament, following the course of the greater saphenous vein. Normal sounds include a brief flow upward with manual distal compression, but immediate cessation of sound on release of compression as the competent SFJ valve snaps shut. Reflux across the SFJ is revealed by a long sound on release of distal compression. More important, a Valsalva maneuver in the presence of SFJ incompetence yields a long "windstorm" sound toward the Doppler probe (a Valsalva maneuver should yield no sound normally). 3. Lesser saphenous–popliteal vein junction (saphenopopliteal junction [SPJ]). The site of this junction is variable and may appear in the lower posterior thigh rather than the popliteal fossa. The patient is usually standing for this portion of the examination. The popliteal vein is adjacent to the pulsatile sound of the popliteal artery. Spontaneous sounds may be heard similar to those from the femoral vein, and brief manual compression should lead to a brief augmentation. If reflux across this junction exists, compression and release distal to the Doppler probe should lead to a long reflux sound upon compression release. Alternatively, if reflux exists, compression *proximal* to the Doppler probe should lead to a sound of retrograde flow on active compression and the normal forward flow on release. Distal manual compression is a more reliable method to detect valve incompetence with reflux. Abnormal flow during a Valsalva maneuver may not occur often enough to be a reliable indicator of reflux in this location. 4, Perforators. If additional varicose veins are present with a totally normal examination up to this point, or if the varicose veins appear not to be associated with the main saphenous system, the Doppler probe is held over the bulges of the veins. Distal and proximal (to the Doppler probe), augmentation of sounds by manual compression is performed as above. Incompetent perforators demonstrate a long sound upon *distal compression release.* To confirm the reflux, a compression proximal to the vein should cause augmentation of sound *during compression.* A Valsalva maneuver may cause augmentation of sounds if reflux exists.

function exists or, alternatively, a prolonged sound with compression, indicating reflux with valve leakage. If the patient then performs a Valsalva maneuver and a continuous and pronounced reflux signal is produced, this is a reliable sign of valvular insufficiency. However, a mild and brief reflux can be found in 15% of normal individuals.[63]

A similar sequence of external compression and release can be performed for the lesser saphenopopliteal vein junction in the lateral third of the popliteal fossa. Usually the patient is standing for this examination. The location of the saphenopopliteal junction lies adjacent to the popliteal artery and can be located rapidly by listening for the arterial signal and moving laterally. Light compression of the calf distal to the Doppler probe is the best method to demonstrate reflux occurring with decompression.[64] The Valsalva maneuver is less likely to reveal reflux in this area, since connection to the abdominal cavity is not direct.[65]

If reflux is not detected at the saphenofemoral or saphenopopliteal junctions but varicose veins are present, the physician must next look for incompetent perforating veins. Location of insufficient perforating veins, usually below the knee, is performed clinically by palpation of fascial gaps along varicosities through which the perforating veins travel. Bulges along the course of a varix may correlate with the sites of perforators. Doppler ultrasound can help localize reflux from perforating veins; this is done by manual distal compression

and release and then detecting the point of loudest amplitude of the signal by moving the Doppler probe slowly around the suspected area of the blowout bulge. Blocking of the varices a few centimeters distally to the blowout bulge with a tourniquet is recommended.[65] Compression of the calf then forces blood through the deep system, not through the varicosity, and reflux is heard only across an incompetent perforating valve. Identification of the leaky perforator site is necessary to guide injection of the sclerosing solution.

It is clear that experience with the Doppler increases accuracy of the examination. A wide range of accuracy for Doppler diagnosis (49 to 96%) has been reported and probably reflects the wide range of experience of the examiners.[66, 67] Instruction in the technique is given regularly at symposia and meetings of the North American Society of Phlebology (NASP, 523 Encinitas Blvd., Suite 108, Encinitas, CA 92024). There are many possible abnormal findings in a Doppler examination (Table 69–3), and proper interpretation of the results by the novice may be difficult.

Although Doppler detects valvular incompetence, photoplethysmography (PPG) offers a simple, reproducible technique for the evaluation of the effectiveness of the calf muscle pump and quantification of the degree of venous insufficiency. It is not as dependent as the hand-held Doppler examination on examiner experience for accuracy. Excellent correlation of PPG results with direct invasive venous pressure measurements has been

TABLE 69–3. KEY ABNORMAL FINDINGS ON DOPPLER EXAMINATION

Figure Location*	Anatomic Site	Spontaneous Sound	Augmented Sound by Manual Compression and Release	Valsalva Maneuver	Conclusion
1	Femoral vein	Absent	No sound or sudden, sharp, high-pitched sound on distal compression	No sound	Deep venous obstruction below level of femoral vein
2	Saphenofemoral junction (SFJ)	May be present	Loud, long sound with release of distal compression	Loud sound	Reflux at SFJ
3	Saphenopopliteal junction (SPJ)	May be present	Loud, long sound with release of distal compression	Sound may be present	Reflux at SPJ
4	Perforators (various locations) Anteromedial Anterolateral Posterlateral	Not present	Loud, long sound with release of distal compression or continuous sound during proximal compression	If sound is present, recheck SFJ	Reflux at perforator; sound usually loudest at reflux point; may confirm with tourniquet and distal compression (see text)

Therapeutic Decisions Based on Interpretation of Doppler Examination

1. If spontaneous sound is absent at femoral vein, suspect outflow obstruction with deep venous disease. Duplex ultrasound is advisable.
2. If saphenofemoral or saphenopopliteal reflux exists by abnormal augmented sounds, these must first be treated surgically (or with sclerotherapy by a phlebologist experienced at sclerosing SFJ or SPJ).
3. If incompetent perforators exist in presence of junctional (SFJ or SPJ) reflux, junctional reflux must be treated first.
4. Incompetent perforators in absence of junctional reflux (SFJ or SPJ) may be treated by sclerotherapy alone.
5. Treatment progress may be monitored by repeat Doppler examination. If patient returns with a sudden increase in symptoms, an untreated or recurrent area of venous reflux can be rapidly identified by Doppler ultrasonography.
6. If results of Doppler examination are equivocal or if deep venous reflux is suspected, a photoplethysmographic (PPG) examination is advised to measure deep venous system function. PPG examination reveals a good candidate for sclerotherapy when muscle pump function is normal (competent deep venous system) or is easily corrected by external compression of superficial varicosities.

*Corresponds to numbers on diagram in Figure 69–5.

shown.[68] The cost of the apparatus is around $10,000, making it feasible for the office-based cutaneous surgeon to own.

In PPG, a light source illuminates a small area of skin, and an adjacent photoelectric sensor measures the reflectance of light. The amount of reflectance is then related to the blood volume in the area of the probe. By convention, the patient sits with the knees bent at a 90-degree angle. A small PPG probe is taped to the medial aspect of the lower leg about 10 cm above the medial malleolus (Fig. 69–6). The patient then pumps the foot ten times, which empties the deep venous system. After the calf muscle pumping ceases, the tracing slowly returns to its initial resting value[63] as the deep veins refill. A refilling time of less than 20 seconds indicates venous valvular insufficiency,[68, 69] while normal longer refilling times indicate a normal muscle pump function. If the initial test indicates a short refill time, the test is repeated using a thigh tourniquet inflated to a pressure of approximately 60 mm Hg. The tracing should return to normal if the source of reflux is at the saphenofemoral junction or the Hunterian mid-thigh perforators. If the PPG refilling time remain less than 20 seconds with the thigh tourniquet, the test is repeated with a calf tourniquet. Repeating the PPG with the calf tourniquet is indicated only if varicosities are noted below the knee. The refill time should return to more than 20 seconds if reflux in calf perforators or at the saphenopopliteal junction exists. A PPG refilling time that remains less than 20 seconds with the calf tourniquet indicates that the muscle pump is functioning poorly as a result of deep venous system disease or some other problem, and sclerotherapy should not be performed without further evaluation. However, a patient with a normal PPG refill time or a PPG refill time correctable by a tourniquet is a candidate for sclerotherapy. In fact, the success of treatment can be measured by normalization of a PPG refill time that required external compression for correction before sclerotherapy.

The ultimate in noninvasive examination of the venous system is real-time B-mode ultrasonography, or duplex ultrasound, which allows direct visualization of the normal veins as easily compressible structures (as opposed to arteries, which do not compress) and easy identification of valves within veins. Valve movement can be studied in real time as well. A complete mapping of the venous system can be performed with precise identification of venous reflux.[70] In one study, most of the 250 patients presenting for treatment of cosmetic leg veins were demonstrated to have superficial venous valvular incompetence by duplex ultrasound.[71] Duplex ultrasound allows direct visualization of the saphenofemoral junction when performing sclerotherapy of this site and probably leads to lower complication rates.[72] Presently this instrumentation is too costly for routine office use but is commonly available in hospitals and vascular surgery centers.

Once the evaluation of the patient is complete, the presence and source of significant venous reflux should be identified. If the patient has significant saphenofemoral reflux, the cutaneous surgeon should consider referring the patient to a vascular surgeon for simple ligation of the junction and its tributaries without extensive stripping. Experienced European or Canadian phlebologists may first attempt to sclerose the saphenofemoral junction, as there is a 93% reported success rate with strong sclerosing solutions not available in the United States.[73] Most patients with varicosities and telangiectases are good candidates for sclerotherapy and have no evidence of deep system disease or significant reflux of the saphenofemoral or saphenopopliteal junction. A combination of Doppler ultrasound and PPG studies readily identifies those patients who need surgical ligation of incompetent junctions.

The final step in the evaluation process is to show photographs of complications of sclerotherapy to the patient and obtain informed consent (Fig. 69–7). The risks and complications, explained in detail, include no improvement, recurrence, ulceration, persistent hyperpigmentation, telangiectatic matting, allergic reactions, thrombophlebitis, and lumpiness of the treated vessel. Once the consent form is signed, 35-mm color slides are taken of each affected area. It is important during the early stages of sclerotherapy to show patients their "before" photographs, as they may become discouraged by their apparently slow rate of improvement. Surprisingly, even after as much as 75% improvement, patients may still find it difficult to recognize improvement, focusing instead on the remaining vessels or pigmentation. Frequently patients believe that the remaining vessels adjacent to treated areas are new unless they are shown their preexistence on the initial photos. Investment in a high-quality rear-projection system, such as the Telex Caramate 4000, helps to clearly show the results of treatment to patients. Patient satisfaction increases dramatically when progress can be clearly demonstrated. After consent, a small area of vessels is treated as a "test," particularly when telangiectases are involved. Occasionally the test injections are performed in two or more areas using different sclerosing solutions to help evaluate the patient's response to each agent. This can be helpful when patients are concerned about the discomfort caused by hypertonic saline. Four to 6 weeks later the test sites are evaluated, and treatment is begun with the chosen solution. When treating varicosities, patients are encouraged to call as soon as possible if any tender lumpiness or swelling occurs. At the follow-up visit the patient may express concern about reactions to compression tape, hyperpigmentation, or other side effects of sclerotherapy. Typically, the more detailed the consent process, the less likely patients are to worry about these reactions.

Comparison of Sclerosing Solutions

Whether varicose or telangiectatic veins are treated, production of endothelial damage with subsequent fibrosis of the entire vein wall without recanalization is the goal of sclerotherapy. The ideal sclerosing solution produces local endothelial destruction extending to the

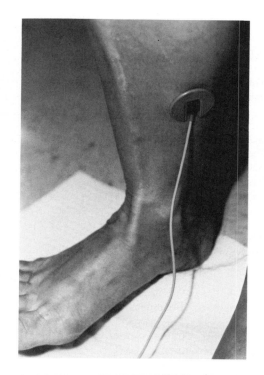

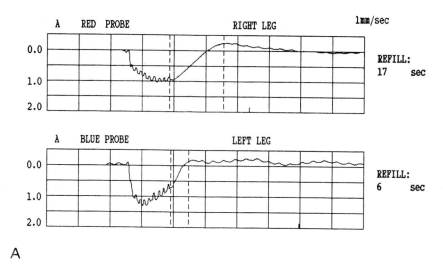

A

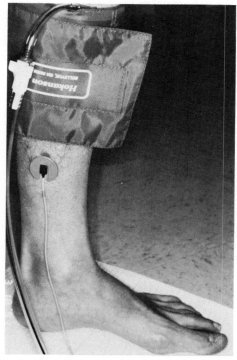

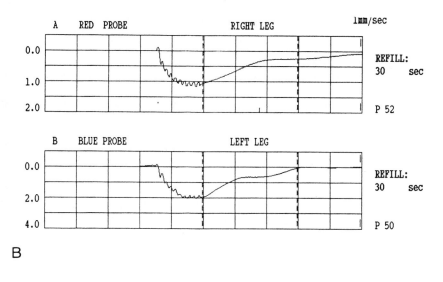

B

Figure 69–6. Photoplethysmography (PPG). A small PPG probe is taped to the medial aspect of the lower leg about 10 cm above the medial malleolus. *A,* These tracings show simultaneous recording of the refill time of both legs. The initial portion of the tracings reflects pumping of the calf ten times. The first dashed line marks the completion of pumping; the second indicates the return to baseline. The distance between these dashed lines reflects the refill time. A normal tracing would show a refill time of more than 20 seconds. In this patient, the right leg's venous system just fails with a refill time of 17 seconds. The varicosities in the left leg appear to be more hemodynamically significant, with a refill time of only 6 seconds. Repeating the test with a thigh tourniquet did not lead to correction of the refill time. *B,* Since this patient had obvious varicosities only in the calf, the test was repeated with a calf tourniquet at 50 mm Hg as shown. The right leg corrects to a refill time of 30 seconds (normal >20) and the left leg also corrects to 30 seconds. The proper interpretation of this test is that both legs have incompetent valves in the superficial veins, since elimination of the varicosity by external compression leads to normalization of the refill time. The site of the incompetence is probably the calf perforators or saphenopopliteal junction, and not the saphenofemoral junction or hunterian perforators, since a thigh tourniquet did not correct the PPG refill time. The Doppler examination will help to elucidate further.

CONSENT FOR TREATMENT OF LEG VEINS

There have been many methods tried to remove unsightly "broken" or enlarged veins on the legs. Most do not work, and have been abandoned. The doctor uses a technique called sclerotherapy, which involves the following:

A tiny needle is threaded into the blood vessel and a small amount of a sclerosing agent is gently injected. This may sting for 20-30 seconds or cause a slight cramp. The injection "flushes" out the red blood cells temporarily, leading to an inflammatory reaction. This reaction causes "sclerosis", or the formation of fibrous tissue within the vessel, leading to the gradual disappearance of the vessel. This fading can take from a few weeks to a few months. Most areas will require between three to five treatments to fade.

A test area is injected first and observed for 4-6 weeks to see how well the procedure and particular solution achieves the desired result in that particular patient.

Some of the possible risks include:

1. The appearance of the veins may not improve. However, over 90% of patients see improvement.

2. Brown spots may appear that look like bruises or follow the path of the vein. These brown areas take several weeks to months to go away. It is rare for any discoloration to be permanent.

3. Blistering, redness, itching and irritation may develop as reaction to the adhesive tape used for compression.

4. Blistering, infection, ulceration, and scarring may develop if someone is exceptionally sensitive to the tiny amount of solution that may leak out during the injection. This occurs in less than 1% of patients. An allergic reaction to some of the solutions is also a rare possibility.

5. Tenderness, bruising, or a firmness (especially along the larger vessels) in the treated area may last for varying periods of time. This can be minimized by the use of support hose after the treatment.

6. Some people (less than 10%) may develop a "matt", or pink blush of the skin, which comes from a temporary enlargement of the tiny capillaries. This is rarely permanent, and can be treated.

7. Sometimes blood may accumulate in the larger veins treated by sclerotherapy. These accumulations may be treated by the physician to decrease any discomfort. Strict use of support hose minimizes this possibility.

8. Rarely, this accumulation of blood may form a clot. Although this is usually trapped in the treated vein, an extremely rare possibility is the extension of this clot into a deeper vessel causing phlebitis. The risk of this occurring is much less than 1%.

9. People with significant circulatory problems or diabetes should not undergo this procedure.

CONSENT

By signing this form, I attest that I have read and understand the procedure and its risks, and that it has been explained to my satisfaction.

PATIENT_____

WITNESS_____

Figure 69–7. Sclerotherapy consent form.

adventitia of the vessel wall, with a minimum of thrombus formation, and is rapidly inactivated to prevent damage beyond the injection site. The degree of endothelial cell destruction can be modulated by the concentration of the sclerosing solution employed.[74, 75] Depending on the mechanism of endothelial cell injury, sclerosing solutions can be classified into three categories: hypertonic, detergent, and chemical irritants (toxins) (Table 69–4). The hypertonic, or hyperosmotic, solutions include hypertonic saline (HS) and the combination of hypertonic glucose and saline (Sclerodex). The detergent solutions include polidocanol (POL) (Aethoxysklerol), sodium tetradecyl sulfate (STS) (Sotradecol), ethanolamine oleate, and sodium morrhuate. The only sclerosing solutions approved by the U.S. Food and Drug Administration (FDA) are these in the detergent category, with the exception of polidocanol, which may receive FDA approval soon.[76] The chemical irritants, infrequently used in the United States, include chromated glycerin and polyiodine iodide. Other agents utilized for sclerosing esophageal varices, but not commonly employed in leg veins, are ethanol concentrations of 50 to 90% and phenol in almond oil.[77]

HYPERTONIC SOLUTIONS

Hypertonic solutions are thought to crenate the endothelial cell, probably disrupting the tight junctions between cells. This damages the intima and allows subsequent layers to be injured by the hyperosmotic gradient and resultant edema. The osmotic gradient must be of sufficient intensity to diffuse through the entire vessel wall to cause complete destruction.[78] Hypertonic agents are the slowest acting of all classes of sclerosing agents, requiring minutes rather than seconds for endothelial destruction.[79] Therefore, the greatest success using these agents is obtained in a low-flow-rate vessel such as a leg telangiectasia.

Hypertonic Saline

Although approved by the FDA only for use as an abortifacient, HS in a concentration of 23.4% is currently the most commonly employed solution by cutaneous surgeons in the United States. The advantage of HS is its theoretical total lack of allergenicity when there have been no additives. Using a rabbit ear vein model,

TABLE 69–4. CHARACTERISTICS OF COMMON SCLEROSING SOLUTIONS

Sclerosing Solution	Category	Use and Concentration	Advantages	Disadvantages	Session Dose
Hypertonic saline 23.4% (HS)	Hypertonic	Telangiectasia (11.7–23.4%) Reticular veins (20–23.4%) Varicose veins up to 4 mm (23.4%)	No allergenicity Easy to obtain	Painful to inject* Skin necrosis	Rarely more than 6 ml due to pain
Combination dextrose (250 mg/ml) and NaCl (100 mg/ml) (Sclerodex)	Hypertonic	Telangiectasia (undiluted) Reticular veins (undiluted)	Less pain than with HS Low allergic potential	Skin necrosis No FDA approval	10 ml
Polidocanol (POL) (Aethoxysklerol)— 0.5%, 1%, 2%, 3%	Detergent	Telangiectasia (0.25–0.75%) Reticular veins (0.5%–1%) Varicose veins (1–3%)	No pain Low risk of skin necrosis	No FDA approval	10 ml of 1%
Sotradecol (STS)—1.0% or 3.0%	Detergent	Telangiectasia (0.1–0.3%) Reticular veins (0.1–0.5%) Varicose veins, all sizes (0.5–3%)	FDA approved Far less pain than with HS	Skin necrosis* Pigmentation* Rare anaphylaxis potential	10 ml of 1%
Sodium morrhuate	Detergent	Varicose veins (undiluted)	FDA approved	Frequent skin necrosis High allergenicity	10 ml
Polyiodinated iodine (Varigloban)— 2%–12%	Chemical irritant	Largest varicose veins (2–8%)	Strong enough to treat largest varicosities	No FDA approval Skin necrosis Sensitivity/allergy (rare)	3 ml
72% glycerin with chromium salt (Scleremo)	Chemical irritant	Telangiectasia (undiluted or diluted [50% or 25%])	Rare allergy Rare necrosis Rare pigmentation	No FDA approval Viscous to inject	3–5 ml

*Concentration dependent

HS has demonstrated complete endothelial cell destruction 1 hour after exposure.[74] HS has been used in concentrations ranging from 10 to 30% and with the addition of heparin, procaine, or lidocaine. Heparsal, a patented solution that contains 20% hypertonic saline, 100 units/ml of heparin, and 1% procaine, was developed to reduce pain and prevent thrombus formation in deep vessels.[23] However, a study of 800 patients demonstrated that the addition of heparin to HS provided no real benefit.[80] HS is currently used primarily in its pure form, as the claims of pain reduction from the addition of procaine or lidocaine seem to be exaggerated. Informed patients appear to choose HS primarily because of its low allergenicity in its pure form. In our experience, no allergic reactions have been seen after treatment of 1200 patients with more than 50,000 injections of 23.4% HS. HS proved highly successful in the treatment of telangiectases in nearly 300 patients, with few complications reported.[3]

Some patients abandon HS in spite of the low risk of allergic reactions after experiencing burning pain or muscle cramping immediately after injection. Because hypertonic solutions affect all cells in the path of the osmotic gradient, nerve endings in the vessel adventitia or the underlying muscle may be stimulated, causing a burning pain or cramping sensation lasting from seconds to minutes. The duration is rarely longer than 5 minutes.[3] Many modifications in the sclerotherapy technique have been attempted to minimize the pain of HS injection, including limitation of sclerosant volume, air bolus, massage, and dilution of the sclerosing solution.

With hypertonic solutions, damage of tissue adjacent to injection sites can occur. Large ulcers may be produced by extravasation at the injection site, particularly when injecting very close to the skin surface. Intradermal injection of 0.1 ml HS in rabbit skin produces necrosis.[81] Immediate intense pain on extravasation warns against further injection at the site. Meticulous technique with absolutely minimal extravasation is necessary for safe use of HS.

Use of diluted HS in small volumes to limit destruction was originally advocated[24] for treatment of telangiectases. More recently, the use of HS diluted to 11.7% has been advocated to reduce the pain of injection and other side effects, particularly in smaller varicosities.[82] In this study, no difference in effectiveness was seen when 23.4% HS and 11.7% HS were compared in varicosities smaller than 4 mm, although the volumes of sclerosing solution were limited to only 2 ml per treatment session. Limitation of volume, typically 2 to 8 ml per session, is necessary to reduce cramping and burning. Use of larger volumes of HS theoretically may exacerbate hypertension. There is great variability from patient to patient in the perception of discomfort and pain with HS injection, with approximately 20% of patients able to tolerate small volumes of HS with minimal pain. Another 30 to 50% can tolerate what they describe as moderate pain. In patients who tolerate HS, one benefit may be faster clearing of telangiectasia than with other sclerosing agents.[83]

Hypertonic Dextrose–Hypertonic Saline

Hypertonic dextrose–hypertonic saline (Sclerodex, Omega Laboratories, Ltd., Montreal, Canada) is a mixture of dextrose (250 mg/ml), sodium chloride (100 mg/ml), propylene glycol (100 mg/ml), and phenethyl alcohol (8 mg/ml). It is advertised as a relatively weak sclerosant recommended for the treatment of small vessels; the total injection volume should not exceed 10 ml per visit, with 0.1 to 1 ml per injection site.[84] Sclerodex has been used predominantly in Canada and, although it causes slight pain on injection,[85] is reported to result in less discomfort than hypertonic saline. The lower concentration of saline combined with the nonionic dextrose causes a hypertonic injury without the intense nerve ending stimulation produced by pure HS. Sclerodex has fewer complications but a similar incidence of pigmentation when compared with polidocanol and sotradecol.[86] The advantage of decreased pain on injection is slightly offset by the potential increased allergenicity of the phenethyl alcohol component of Sclerodex, with a reported incidence of allergic reactions of 1/500.[85] Limited side-by-side comparison of HS and Sclerodex confirms that Sclerodex is far less painful than HS, while achieving similar results. Whether Sclerodex will gain widespread acceptance in the United States remains to be seen.

DETERGENT SOLUTIONS

A detergent molecule has a hydrophobic and a hydrophilic portion. Presumably, cell membranes of the endothelium are immediately disrupted or dissolved as the hydrophobic portion aligns with the lipid cell membrane and reduces surface tension with the surrounding aqueous environment. In theory the solution must make good contact with the vessel wall to cause destruction. Compression of the varicosity after the instillation of a detergent sclerosant may increase contact and possibly enhance efficacy. Maceration of the endothelium has been shown to occur within seconds,[79] and intimal damage follows shortly when strong detergent agents are used.

The dorsal rabbit ear vein model has shown that when 0.25 ml of 0.5% STS is injected and compression is used for 20 seconds, reproducible endothelial damage occurs within 1 hour.[74] This process is followed by the formation of a thrombus. The extent of damage and relative efficacy can be modified by varying the concentrations of the detergent solutions.

Polidocanol

POL (Aethoxysklerol, Chemische Fabrik Kreussler & Co., Wiesbaden-Biebrich, Germany; Aetoxisclerol, Laboratories Pharmaceutiques Dexo, Nanterre, France; Sclerovein, Resinag AG, Zurich, Switzerland) is a urethane compound originally developed as an anesthetic. It was subsequently found to sclerose small-diameter blood vessels after intradermal injection. POL contains hydroxypolyethoxydodecane dissolved in distilled water with 5% ethanol as a stabilizer. POL is used as a dough emulsifier in certain baked goods[76] and appears to be safe for human consumption. Although first used in the late 1960s in Germany as a sclerosing agent,[87] POL has only relatively recently been introduced to U.S. cutaneous surgeons.[25, 88] It is presently the second most popular sclerosing solution among cutaneous surgeons in the United States, although it can be difficult to obtain. Its advantages include painless injection and an extremely rare incidence (less than 1%) of cutaneous necrosis with intradermal injection.[81] To be totally painless, POL must be diluted to reduce the 5% ethanol content. POL is a safe solution with a high degree of efficacy and low incidence of side effects. Allergic reactions have been reported in only four patients in a review of the literature.[89]

The risk of cutaneous necrosis is so low with POL 0.5% that its use has been advocated for intradermal injection in telangiectasia too small to inject intravascularly.[90] This practice is not generally recommended, as a small area of cutaneous necrosis has been observed with 1% POL. Equally rare is mild prolonged bronchospasm suspected to have resulted from injection of 4 ml of 1% POL. To minimize risks, the concentration of POL should be adjusted according to vessel size. Superficial telangiectases smaller than 1 mm are treated with a 0.25% to 0.75% solution,[83] with the ideal concentration probably being about 0.5%.[91] The manufacturer of POL (Kreussler) recommends 3% POL for varicose veins that measure 4 to 8 mm in diameter, 2% POL for veins 2 to 4 mm in diameter, and 1% POL for veins 1 to 2 mm in diameter. The maximum dosage for POL per session is approximately 6 ml of 3% POL or the equivalent.

In the rabbit ear dorsal vein model, 1% POL is equivalent to 0.5% STS and HS.[74] As determined by extrapolating from several clinical studies, 0.5% POL, when used on human telangiectasia, appears to be equivalent to HS and 0.1 to 0.2% STS. A higher incidence of hyperpigmentation with 1% POL compared with HS in one study may indicate that 1% POL is a stronger sclerosant than HS.[92] Lower concentrations of POL have demonstrated a lower incidence of hyperpigmentation than seen with HS or STS.[83]

Sodium Tetradecyl Sulfate

STS (Sotradecol, Wyeth-Ayerst Laboratories, Philadelphia, PA; S.T.D. Injection, S.T.D. Pharmaceuticals, United Kingdom; Thromboject, Omega Labs, Montreal, Canada) is a long-chain fatty acid salt with strong detergent properties. It is a very effective sclerosing agent approved for use in the United States. Although popular with vascular surgeons since the 1960s[19, 32, 33] and first described for use in telangiectases in the 1970s,[21] STS has proved unpopular with cutaneous surgeons. This is a result of the relatively high incidence of postsclerosis pigmentation and the possibility of cutaneous necrosis even in the absence of extravasation[93] reported with 1% STS. The incidence of cutaneous

necrosis, reported to be as high as 60 to 70% with 1% STS, can be reduced to 3% by using 0.33% STS.[93] Intradermal injection of 0.1 ml of 0.5% STS into rabbit skin leads to dermal and epidermal necrosis.[81] Because of the usual lack of pain that occurs with extravasation (compared with HS, which is extremely painful), the potential to unknowingly extravasate larger volumes, with the subsequent consequence of severe necrosis, is potentially greatest with STS.

Although allergic reactions such as generalized urticaria, bronchospasm, anaphylactic shock, and even death have been reported,[94, 95] the actual incidence of allergic reactions to STS has been estimated at approximately 0.3%.[89] In a study of 16,000 patients, only 15 cases of a stinging pain in the skin accompanied by erythema 30 to 90 minutes after STS injection were reported.[96] Premedication with antihistamines prevents this reaction. Although all patients treated with STS do need not to be given prophylactic antihistamines, physicians should be aware that delayed reactions can occur even several hours after treatment.[97] Despite the slightly higher risks of allergic reactions with STS when compared with HS and POL, STS remains very popular among vascular surgeons because of its potency and relative painlessness in treating large varicosities.

One study in which STS 0.1% was used on telangiectases in 38 patients indicates safety and effectiveness comparable to those of POL and HS.[98] Scattered punctate erosions at the site of STS 0.1% injection into telangiectases smaller than 0.5 mm were noted in two patients and were not seen when POL or HS was used in these same patients. Studies in the dorsal rabbit ear vein model indicate that although endothelial damage occurs with STS 0.1%, histologic recanalization is evident after 30 days; similar changes occur even with STS at a concentration of 0.5%.[75] Interpretation of available data has led to recommended concentrations of 0.1 to 0.3% for telangiectases up to 1 mm, 0.3 to 0.5% for reticular veins or small varicosities 1 to 3 mm in diameter, and 1% for larger varicosities related to major sites of valvular reflux. The maximum recommended dose per treatment session is 10 ml of 3% solution.

Sodium Morrhuate

Sodium morrhuate (Scleromate, Palisades Pharmaceuticals, Inc., Tenafly, NJ) is a mixture of the salts of saturated and unsaturated fatty acids in cod liver oil. It is available as a 5% solution. Surprisingly, 20.8% of its fatty acid composition is unknown.[99] Although promoted as an effective sclerosing agent,[100] its use is limited by reports of fatalities secondary to anaphylaxis.[101] This agent is most popular in the United States for sclerosis of esophageal varices, but the incidence of complications, including allergic reactions, is reported to be as high as 17 to 48%.[77]

Sodium morrhuate is approved for the sclerosis of varicose veins. Because of the relatively high incidence of allergic reactions, however, most cutaneous surgeons do not use this agent. It is a caustic solution that has a great potential for causing cutaneous necrosis with extravascular injection and is not recommended for the treatment of telangiectases.

Ethanolamine Oleate

Ethanolamine oleate (Ethamolin, Block Drug Co., Piscataway, NJ) is a synthetic agent containing an organic base combined with oleic acid and is used as a 5% solution. It has been approved for the treatment of esophageal varices. Ethanolamine oleate is an oily, viscous solution that is difficult to inject. It has been used extensively in the United Kingdom for control of acute esophageal variceal bleeding and is reported to have a complication rate similar to that of sodium morrhuate but far greater than that of STS.[102] Also, allergic reactions have been reported with its use in leg varicosities.[103] It is a caustic agent similar to sodium morrhuate and thus is also not recommended for telangiectases.

CHEMICAL IRRITANTS

The chemical irritants are thought to have a direct toxic effect on the endothelium. After injection of polyiodinated iodine (Varigloban), the endothelium is destroyed within seconds but only near the site of injection because of rapid inactivation. The exposed subendothelial layers are rapidly covered by deposited fibrin.[104] At the sites of endothelial destruction, the chemical can penetrate further and diffuse into deeper layers of the vessel wall, causing additional damage. One preliminary study indicates that no activation of blood coagulation occurs with sodium iodide, indicating little risk of propagation of a thrombus.[105]

The chemical irritants may be the most specific sclerosing agents as a result of their ability to target injury to the site of injection and quickly become inactivated by blood proteins. This is accompanied by minimal thrombus formation and deep diffusion into the vessel wall. The chemical irritants are presently underutilized in the United States because of a paucity of published data in major American journals and a lack of FDA approval.

Polyiodide Iodine

Polyiodide iodine (Varigloban, Kreussler & Co., Wiesbaden-Biebrich, Germany) is a stabilized water solution of iodide ions, sodium iodine, and benzyl alcohol. The active ingredient is sodium iodine. Varigloban is dark brown in color and available in concentrations ranging from 2 to 12%. Its color makes confirmation of the intravascular position of the needle more difficult during sclerotherapy, because blood withdrawal into the syringe is not easily seen.

Varigloban is slightly painful when injected extravascularly and produces tissue necrosis by its caustic effect. Injection should proceed carefully when pain is reported by the patient. Varigloban is used primarily by French, Swiss, German, and French Canadian phlebologists for injection of incompetent saphenofemoral junctions and

other very large varicosities. Concentrations of 4 to 8% are used, with no more than 3 ml injected per session. When used by skilled practitioners, complications and side effects are comparable to those of other sclerosing agents. One study reported a 1.3% incidence of self-limited hypersensitivity reactions consisting of fever, flulike symptoms, and shortness of breath in more than 2000 patients treated for incompetence of the saphenofemoral junction with Varigloban.[106] No more than 2 ml of 3% solution was used per treatment session. Although this required three to five treatment sessions, Varigloban was 90% successful at occluding the saphenofemoral junction, and only one patient developed deep venous thrombosis.

Chromated Glycerin

Chromated glycerin (Scleremo, Laboratories E. Boutielle, Limoges, France; Chromex, Omega Laboratories, Montreal, Canada) is the most widely used sclerosing agent in the world, but is used only rarely in the United States.[99] It is composed of glycerin (720 mg/ml) and chrome potassium alum, (8 mg/ml), which is a chrome salt, in an aqueous base. The Europeans advocate its use as a mild sclerosant to treat the smallest telangiectases with minimal side effects. Chromated glycerin may be used full strength or diluted by 25 to 50%. In its undiluted form, chromated glycerin is quite viscous and may cause pain on injection, particularly if injected extravascularly. When diluted by 50%, chromated glycerin injection is easily performed through the smallest gauge needle, and patients typically experience no discomfort.

The incidence of adverse sequelae such as allergic or hypersensitivity reactions to chromated glycerin is very low, and a small amount can be injected extravascularly without causing necrosis or sloughing.[107] Pigmentation and bruising are relatively rare as well.[108] The relatively "weak" nature of chromated glycerin is confirmed in rabbit dorsal ear vein studies with endothelial damage equivalent to that produced by 0.25% polidocanol.[75]

Glycerin is rapidly absorbed and transformed into glycogen or used for the synthesis of fatty acids and theoretically must be used with caution in diabetics. Additionally, glycerin will lyse red blood cells, and excessive quantities may induce hematuria.[107] The maximum recommended volume per injection session is 10 ml of undiluted solution. As more reports appear in the English literature, glycerin use, primarily for the treatment of small telangiectases, may increase in the United States, pending FDA approval.

Sclerotherapy Techniques

TREATMENT OF TELANGIECTASIA: MICROSCLEROTHERAPY

Once patients have been properly evaluated, informed consent has been obtained, and photographs have been taken, the abnormal vessels may be treated. Patients are told to wear shorts and not to use moisturizers or shave their legs on the day of treatment. They are encouraged to eat at least a small meal before the procedure to minimize vasovagal reactions. The room in which sclerotherapy is performed is kept cool to minimize vasovagal reactions, even though a warm room would cause vasodilatation and permit easier visualization of telangiectases. The first treatment session is usually limited to one or two sites to observe patients for any allergic reactions and the ability to tolerate the burning or cramping of a hypertonic solution, to judge the effectiveness of a particular concentration of sclerosing agent, and to observe for any reactions to the tape used for compression. Patients return in 4 to 6 weeks to compare the test site with pretreatment photographs. At each session, all sites treated are noted in anatomic diagrams (Fig. 69–8).

Cutaneous surgeons frequently see patients with small telangiectases without associated junctional or large perforator incompetence. However, even small telangiectases on the legs have been shown to be enlarged venules on biopsy. Commonly there are scattered groups of telangiectases connected with single or multiple reticular veins (see Fig. 69–4). A reticular vein is a thin-walled blue superficial venulectasia, thought to be a tributary of the main superficial venous system, that appears to drain an area of telangiectasia. These reticular veins are commonly called "feeder" veins, since the assumption is that reflux through them causes the groups of telangiectases. Doppler studies have shown that free reflux with augmentation is usually heard through the reticular veins and sometimes in an upward pattern against the flow of gravity.[109] In approximately 50% of these patients, the reticular veins appear to be tributaries of larger incompetent calf perforators. The reasons for these controversial findings have not yet been explained and may be due to altered hemodynamics during sitting or other activities that are not understood.

It is generally recommended that microsclerotherapy be started with injection of the largest venulectasis and proceeding to the smallest telangiectasis. Occasionally, the sclerosing solution will be observed to enter the telangiectasis directly from the feeder vein, which may eliminate the need to inject the telangiectasia directly. The reverse situation may also be true, so that when injecting groups of telangiectases, the sclerosing solution may enter the feeder vein from the site of injection through a telangiectasis. Practically speaking, the direction of valves in these veins should allow easy flow from smaller to larger veins. However, this method cannot be relied on to treat the reticular vein, as development of extravasation at the site of injection in the telangiectatic vein will often prevent sufficient sclerosant volume or concentration from entering the larger reticular vein.

Treating the source of reflux, the feeder vein, is the most logical initial step. If no clear feeder vessel is seen, then the point at which the telangiectases begin to branch out is the site at which to begin. This saves time, as many telangiectases can be treated with fewer injection sites. A revised, more straightforward classification

of leg varicosities has been developed (Table 69–5), but there is not general agreement with this concept.

The actual injection method[25, 88] uses a sclerotherapy tray prepared by the nurse (Fig. 69–9) with the necessary equipment. The patient is placed in either the prone or supine position on a motorized table with easy height adjustment, thereby allowing easy access to the groups of telangiectases that the patient desires treated. The areas are repeatedly cleansed with cotton balls that are heavily saturated with 70% isopropyl alcohol. This allows better visualization of the vessels by increasing light transmission through otherwise reflective white scale on the epidermal surface. After evaporation of the alcohol, a 30-gauge needle, bent to an angle of 10 to 30 degrees with the bevel up, is placed on the skin so that the needle is parallel to the skin surface. A 3-ml syringe filled with 2 ml of solution is held between the index and middle fingers while the fourth and fifth finger support the syringe against the leg in a fixed position to facilitate accurate penetration of the vessel. The nondominant hand is used to stretch the skin around the needle and may offer additional support for the syringe (see Fig. 69–4). The firmly supported needle is then moved slowly forward 1 to 2 mm, piercing the vein just sufficiently to allow infusion of solution with the most minimal pressure on the plunger. Magnifying lenses (2 to 3×) may help to visualize the cannulation of even the smallest telangiectases.

The technique requires a gentle, precise touch to detect the subtle sensation felt on entering the vessel and to recognize the appearance of the bevel of the needle within the lumen of the telangiectasia. A very sharp needle is critical, and therefore the needle is changed often during the procedure to minimize tearing of the vessel. The use of 32- to 33-gauge needles is not advised, because they are not disposable and dull quickly with sterilization.

Injection of a tiny bolus of less than 0.05 ml of air may help to establish that the needle is within the vein,

TABLE 69–5. **VESSEL CLASSIFICATION**

Type 1. Telangiectasia, or "spider veins"; 0.1–2 mm in diameter; usually red but may rarely be cyanotic.

Type 1A. Telangiectatic matting; <0.2 mm diameter network; bright red.

Type 2. Venulectasis; 1–2 mm diameter; violaceous, cyanotic; usually protrudes; and larger diameter and deeper in color than telangiectases.

Type 3. Reticular veins, also known as "minor" varicose veins or "feeder" veins; 2–4 mm; cyanotic to blue.

Type 4. Nonsaphenous varicose veins (primary varicosity of saphenous tributary, usually related to an incompetent perforator); 2–8 mm; blue to blue-green.

Type 5. Saphenous varicose veins (varicosities associated with reflux at saphenofemoral or saphenopopliteal junction); usually >8 mm in diameter; blue to blue-green.

Modified from Goldman MP: Sclerotherapy treatment for varicose and telangiectatic leg veins. In: Coleman WP, Hanke CW, Alt TH, Asken S (eds): Cosmetic Surgery of the Skin. BC Decker, Philadelphia, 1991, pp 197–211; and Duffy DM: Small vessel sclerotherapy: an overview. In: Callen JP, Dahl MV, Golitz LE, et al (eds): Advances in Dermatology. Vol 3. Year Book, Chicago, 1988, pp 221–242.

SCLEROTHERAPY RECORD

Name_____   Date_____

_____

_____

LEFT LEG

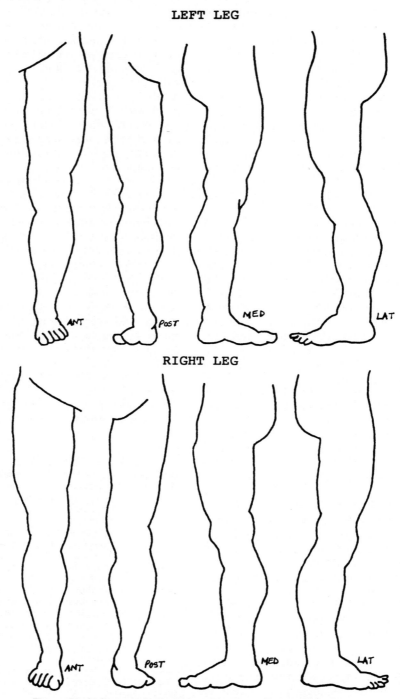

RIGHT LEG

Figure 69–8. Record of sclerotherapy treatment by anatomic sites.

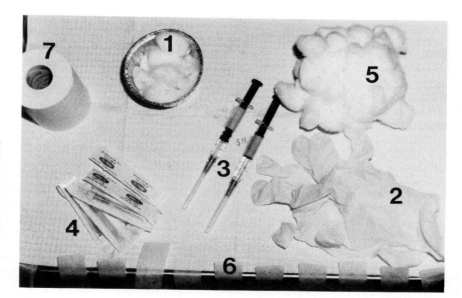

Figure 69–9. Sclerotherapy tray. For treatment of telangiectases and reticular veins, the tray includes the following: 1, cotton balls soaked in 70% isopropyl alcohol; 2, protective gloves to prevent direct contact with blood; 3, sclerosing solutions clearly marked as to type and concentration in 1- to 2-ml aliquots; 4, several 30-gauge needles with transparent hub to allow frequent needle changes; 5, cotton balls or foam pads for larger veins, for compression; 6, multiple strips of paper tape to initially secure the cotton balls rapidly; 7, Microfoam tape to apply sufficient compression over the cotton balls.

as slight clearing 1 to 3 mm ahead of the bevel can be seen. A larger air bolus allows the arborizing vessels to clear instantly, allowing greater spread of the sclerosing solution.[110] Others[3, 25, 88] have found this to occur infrequently and generally find a larger air bolus unnecessary. The sclerosing solution is refrigerated in 2-ml aliquots to enhance vasoconstriction by cold and to sequester the solutions so that the possibility of accidental injection of a sclerosing solution during routine procedures in the office is minimized.

Injection is performed *very slowly* using a small amount (0.1 to 0.5 ml or less) of sclerosant. With minimal or no pressure on a 3-ml syringe, the veins are kept filled with sclerosant for 10 to 15 seconds. Rapid flushing of the vessels with large volumes of sclerosant is not necessary for successful sclerotherapy and is absolutely contraindicated for any varicosity. Particularly when using a hypertonic solution, the injection of sclerosant is stopped when blanching in a radius of 2 cm has occurred or when 15 seconds have passed, which helps to minimize the cramping and burning. When using painless detergent sclerosants, small volumes with small amounts of short-duration blanching will minimize side effects such as telangiectatic matting.[111] Occasionally, no blanching occurs at the site of injection, and the sclerosing solution flows easily through the telangiectasia or can even be seen flowing through adjacent telangiectases or reticular veins several centimeters away from the injection site. In this case the injection is stopped after 0.5 ml of sclerosant has been injected, and immediate manual compression is applied. As a general rule, no more than 0.5 ml is injected into any single site.

By minimizing volume, pressure, and duration of injection, not only pain but also the risks of extravasation are minimized. Multiple areas, up to ten 2- to 4-cm areas of varicosities on one thigh, can be treated with as little as 2 to 3 ml of sclerosant. To minimize skin necrosis, extravasation must be avoided. If resistance to injection of sclerosant or a tiny wheal begins to appear

at the injection site, the injection should be stopped immediately. The injection site should be carefully inspected at all times to detect a wheal at the moment of its occurrence. Some physicians keep a syringe filled with 5 to 10 ml of normal saline nearby to dilute any extravasated sclerosant.

Immediately after injection, the treated area is gently massaged. This may help to reduce pain and hasten the spread of the sclerosant through the vessels. Any vessel larger than 0.5 mm or that protrudes above the surface of the skin will benefit from compression. After massaging for 5 to 10 seconds, cotton balls are secured over the injection sites with paper tape. Compression is maintained by the additional application of Microfoam tape (3M Corp., Medical-Surgical Division, St. Paul, MN) over the cotton balls for 48 to 72 hours. Protuberant telangiectases or telangiectases in association with reticular veins are also treated for 2 weeks with graduated 30- to 40–mm Hg support hose after removal of the tape. Patients are encouraged to walk, with no restriction of activities except for heavy weight lifting with the legs. Treatment intervals may vary, but waiting 4 to 8 weeks between treatments will help minimize the number of treatment sessions.

TREATMENT OF VARICOSE VEINS

The technique for sclerosing varicose veins differs greatly from that used for telangiectasia. There is no universally accepted technique for treating all varicose veins because of the differences in anatomic locations. No method should be accepted as absolute dogma, because techniques are certain to change and improve as knowledge is gained with the application of newer technology such as duplex or intravascular ultrasound.

Doppler ultrasound studies allow evaluation for saphenofemoral, saphenopopliteal, and perforator refluxes. This is absolutely necessary before performing sclerotherapy of varicose veins. When saphenofemoral junction (SFJ) reflux is present, this leak must be blocked initially or recurrences of varicosities treated below that point will result.[112] The French school of sclerotherapy emphasizes the importance of proximal to distal treatment.[113] In the United States, many phlebologists feel uncomfortable with injecting the SFJ without duplex ultrasound guidance, especially because Varigloban, the sclerosant of choice for this site, is unavailable. Surgery with either ligation of the SFJ or ligation with limited stripping is presently the preferred method for treating this area.[33, 42, 112] If the patient refuses surgery or duplex ultrasound is available, sclerotherapy of the SFJ may be attempted with 1 to 3% STS. In the absence of saphenofemoral reflux, varicosities originating from reflux at the saphenopopliteal junction (SPJ) or incompetent perforators may be treated initially by sclerotherapy.

The classic technique,[19] currently employed with minor modifications, begins with the patient sitting at the end of the examining table with the leg to be treated hanging down. The bulging varicosity is cannulated with a needle, being careful to stabilize the 25-, 27-, or 30-gauge needle. The leg is elevated and supported above the level of the patient for about 1 to 2 minutes to allow the drainage of blood. Before injection, blood must be drawn back into the syringe to ensure that the needle remains in the lumen of the vessel. As the injection of approximately 0.5 to 1 ml occurs, finger pressure is applied several centimeters above and below the injection point to confine the action of the sclerosing solution. Finger pressure is maintained for 30 to 60 seconds and followed by immediate compression with a foam pad. The pad is secured by elastic tape or a relatively inelastic wraparound bandage. This method is particularly effective for incompetent perforators. The fascial defects through which perforators course may be palpated and may serve as the site of needle entry. Some believe that injection of multiple puncture sites along the course of a varicosity, independent of the perforators, produces excellent results.[33] When injecting multiple sites along a varicosity, repeat injections are made every 4 to 6 cm until the entire varix has been sclerosed.

One slight variation for large vessel sclerotherapy is the air block technique, in which 0.5 to 1 ml of air is injected initially to clear the varix of blood.[114] Another variation is the foam technique, in which the detergent solution (STS) is shaken for 30 seconds to create a foam.[115] This foam is then injected, thereby allowing less volume of sclerosing solution to be used. Theoretically, these techniques enhance contact with the vessel wall, but whether they actually enhance the efficacy remains to be proved.

One widely used technique consists of marking the varicosities with the patient standing and then inserting the needle with the patient recumbent, which minimizes movement of the leg with the needle in place. The cannulation of a previously marked varicosity is straightforward with the patient supine and helps speed up the technique. Another minor modification is the use of direct finger pressure in a spreading and compressing motion outward from both proximal and distal to the injection site, not only to spread the sclerosing solution

laterally but to promote contact with greater surface area of the varicosity while pushing blood out of the vessel. For compression, bunches of cotton balls may be substituted for foam pads, although the use of foam pads (E pads, S.T.D. Pharmaceuticals, Hereford, United Kingdom) probably allows for the strongest and most complete external compression. Compression hose (30 to 40 mm Hg) may be worn immediately after treatment or after removal of the foam tape, which is left in place for 72 hours. Patients may shower while the waterproof foam tape is in place but not with compression bandages or hose.

Although some authors minimize the importance of compression, several theoretical and practical considerations affirm its necessity. Compression minimizes the flow of blood back into the varicosity, thus minimizing thrombus formation[116] and also the risk for recanalization.[36, 111] Also, compression reduces the risk of thrombophlebitic reaction and postsclerosis pigmentation. For both small and large varicosities, compression has been shown to improve effectiveness with greater resolution per treatment.[117, 118] The use of graduated compression hose also allows the patient complete mobility after treatment and enhances muscle pump function, which can rapidly dilute and remove any sclerosing solution that inadvertently enters the deep system.

The ideal duration of compression is still debated. Although 6 weeks have been recommended,[19] 3 to 5 days of compression have also been suggested as adequate.[112, 119] A trial comparing compression for 1, 3, and 6 weeks concluded that 3 weeks was optimal.[120] Most cutaneous surgeons recommend that patients wear compression hose (30 to 40 mm Hg) for 3 to 6 weeks. However, it is very difficult to obtain patient compliance for more than 2 weeks of compression. One study demonstrated that compression with rubber pads worn under compression hose yielded results equivalent to pads held in place by bandages worn under hose.[118] In this study, compression was carried out for 6 weeks, although 30% of patients removed compression earlier.

TREATMENT OF RETICULAR VEINS

Treatment of reticular veins is very similar to that of large varicose veins, although the concentration, strength, and volume of sclerosing solution are decreased. Reticular veins are treated only after all sources of reflux have been treated by sclerotherapy or surgery. Doppler studies may be used as a guide to demonstrate reflux in the reticular veins and locate those that require treatment.

For this procedure, the patient is recumbent. With the surgeon using a 3-ml syringe with a 27- to 30-gauge needle attached, the superficial and visibly blue reticular vein is cannulated. When the sensation of piercing the vein is felt, the plunger is pulled back gently until blood is seen flowing into the transparent plastic hub, which is possible even with a 30-gauge needle. Usually the volume is no more than 0.5 ml per injection site and often considerably less. With POL solution, a concentration of 0.5 to 1% is most safe in these often fragile, thin-walled vessels. Alternatively, 23.4% HS, hypertonic dextrose–hypertonic saline, or 0.2 to 0.5% STS can also be used. Treatment of reticular veins greatly reduces the recurrence rate of telangiectases associated with them. Studies are currently in progress to further clarify this issue.

Side Effects and Complications

Any therapeutic technique, no matter how effective and safe for most patients, offers some risks. Although an overwhelming number of patients are extremely pleased with the results of sclerotherapy, both the patient and the cutaneous surgeon must be familiar with the type and incidence of expected side effects and unforeseen serious complications. If patients are familiar with and accept the possibility of minor side effects (Fig. 69–10), they are often willing to overlook such effects and continue with treatment.[92] The expected minor and spontaneously resolving side effects include urtication at the needle puncture site and along the treated vessel, a phenomenon that is solution dependent; cutaneous pigmentation along the course of a superficial treated vessel; telangiectatic matting; friction blisters or erosions secondary to compression tape; edema of the ankle; bruising around the injection site; microthrombus or intravascular hematoma; and pain with injection, which is also solution dependent. More serious but rare complications include cutaneous necrosis, superficial thrombophlebitis, arterial injection accompanied by distal necrosis, symptoms of systemic anaphylaxis, and deep vein thrombosis with pulmonary emboli (Table 69–6). Patients should also be reminded that recurrence of a treated area, although not a side effect, is also a possibility.

POSTSCLEROTHERAPY HYPERPIGMENTATION

Postsclerosis pigmentation is defined as the appearance of increased visible pigmentation along the course of a treated vein of any size. This pigmentation may be the result of sclerotherapy but may also be pre-existing. Pretreatment photographs are invaluable in such situations. A histologic study of postsclerosis pigmentation in humans has shown that the pigmentation represents perivascular hemosiderin deposition and not increased melanin production.[121] The incidence of pigmentation is variable and has been reported to be dependent on both the dilution and the type of sclerosing agent, as well as the diameter of the treated vessel;[92] smaller vessels have a decreased frequency. The incidence of postsclerotic hyperpigmentation in the treatment of telangiectases has been reported to be 11 to 30% with HS,[3, 110] 11 to 30% with POL,[25, 88] and 30% with STS.[122] With the use of 1% STS, an incidence of nearly 80% hyperpigmentation has been reported in the treatment of telangiectases.[21] One study using 0.1% STS found a lower incidence of hyperpigmentation (11%) comparable with that of 0.5% POL and HS.[98] One reported risk factor is elevated

TABLE 69–6. SIDE EFFECTS AND COMPLICATIONS OF SCLEROTHERAPY

Side effects
  Frequent and temporary
    Postsclerosis pigmentation (10–30%)
    Telangiectatic matting (10–30%)
    Pain with injection (up to 75% with HS)
    Postinjection urtication (up to 100%)
  Less frequent and temporary
    Blister due to compression tape (<1%)
    Contact dermatitis to tape adhesive (<1%)
    Folliculitis under occlusive tape (<1%)
    Bruising around injection site (<1%)
    Ankle edema (<1%)
Complications
  Less frequent, minor, and temporary
    Microthrombus or intravascular hematoma
  Rare but self-limited
    Cutaneous necrosis
    Superficial thrombophlebitis
  Extremely rare but major
    Arterial injection with distal necrosis
    Systemic allergic reaction
    Deep vein thrombosis
    Pulmonary embolus

serum iron levels with a trend toward higher serum ferritin levels in patients with postsclerotherapy hyperpigmentation.[123]

The type of vessel most susceptible to hyperpigmentation is a thin-walled, blue, venulectasis 1 to 3 mm in diameter that protrudes above the skin surface. Other factors that may influence the incidence of hyperpigmentation are individual patient susceptibility, with more darkly pigmented patients at greater risk[124]; rapidity and extent of compression; predilection for certain body sites, such as the popliteal fossae and ankles; and the existence of reflux proximal to the area of sclerotherapy.

If reflux exists above a sclerotherapy site, higher venous pressure will force more blood to leak into a sclerosed vessel and hence cause more opportunity for hemosiderin accumulation. Because compression influences the occurrence of intravascular thrombi and subsequent organization and intravascular hematoma formation, poor compression would be expected to allow more hemosiderin to be deposited in the sclerosed vessel. However, absolute compression producing complete closure of the lumen is often impossible, leading to trapping or accumulation of blood within the lumen. Therefore, some postsclerosis hyperpigmentation is unavoidable.

MICROTHROMBUS FORMATION AND PIGMENTATION

Coagula trapped in a vein after sclerotherapy should be removed to reduce the amount of hemosiderin and the risk of pigmentation. Palpable lumpy areas may occur after treatment of some veins. Patients may return 2 to 4 weeks after treatment with dark blue sub- or intracutaneous rubbery linear swellings in the outline of

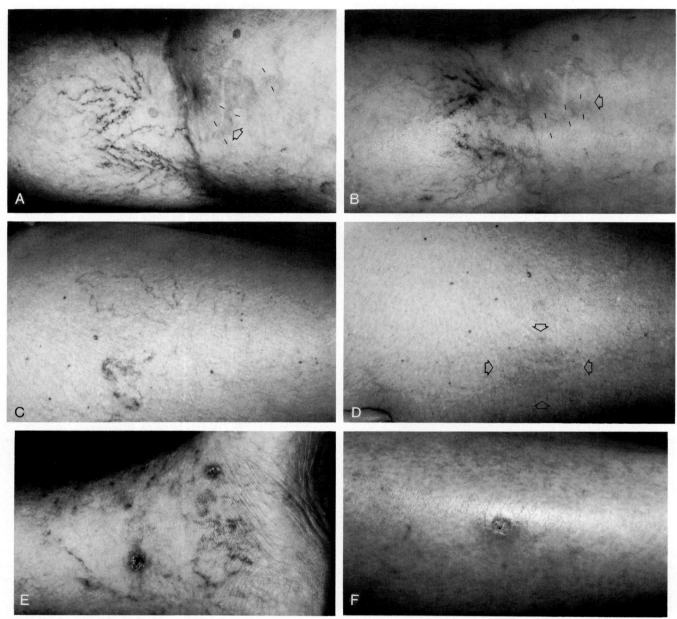

Figure 69–10. Pigmentation, telangiectatic matting, and ulceration. *A,* This patient has multiple groups of telangiectases associated with reticular veins in the popliteal fossa. The reticular vein is indicated by the arrowhead. The long linear scar is from a previous stripping procedure. *B,* One month after treatment with 0.5 ml 1% polidocanol into the telangiectases only, without treatment of the reticular vein, marked hyperpigmentation occurred. The reticular vein *(arrowhead)* is still present, although not easily reproduced in black-and-white photographs. The popliteal fossa is a common location for pigmentation, perhaps because compression is poor during knee flexion. Treatment of the reticular vein initially might have prevented this side effect. The pigmentation resolved spontaneously at 6 months. *C,* A group of telangiectases on the thigh treated with 0.25 ml hypertonic saline. *D,* At 2 months, complete resolution of the treated telangiectases is noted. An area of telangiectatic matting around the treated site *(arrowheads)* has occurred. It consists of a new fine network of bright red vessels with a diameter no greater than 0.2 mm. Spontaneous resolution was noted at 6 months. *E,* Two small healing ulcerations after cutaneous necrosis at the site of injection on the medial ankle. 0.1 ml 0.5% Sotradecol was injected into two small varicosities of the ankle. The ankle is particularly susceptible to ulceration. *F,* A small superficial healing ulcer after cutaneous necrosis at the site of injection of 0.2 ml 1% polidocanol. The site is just above the ankle on the medial aspect of the lower leg. Ulceration after polidocanol use is extremely rare.

the vessel, with very little or no tenderness. No erythema indicative of phlebitis accompanies these. After locating the softest spot and listening for absence of flow by Doppler, an 18- to 22-gauge needle or No. 11 blade puncture will allow the expression of dark, viscous, liquefied clot or intravascular hematoma. Milking the vein by sweeping a cotton-tipped applicator or gloved finger along its length for several centimeters toward the puncture site will help to express the material (Fig. 69–11). Several puncture sites may be necessary to completely expel the liquefied blood. Patients usually report a feeling of relief of pressure after removal, and a palpable decrease in the size of the subcutaneous knob is noted. Compression is applied for an additional 3 days. Several authors have called this technique "microthrombectomy" when used for evacuation of hematomas.[62, 125]

The duration of hyperpigmentation is usually brief, but it may persist for up to 5 years. In one study of 113 patients, 70% of cases of hyperpigmentation resolved within 6 months and only rarely did hyperpigmentation persist for more than 1 year.[92] Attempts to hasten resolution of hyperpigmentation have been mostly unsuccessful, as the pigment is dermal hemosiderin and not epidermal melanin. Bleaching agents, exfoliants such as trichloroacetic acid or phenol, and cryotherapy have been reported as achieving limited success but are not generally useful. The copper vapor laser may be useful in decreasing very superficial postsclerotherapy hyperpigmentation.[123] Informing patients that hyperpigmentation is a positive sign indicating that the varicosities have completely responded to sclerotherapy usually helps to alleviate their concerns.

TELANGIECTATIC MATTING

Telangiectatic matting is defined as the appearance of groups of new, blushlike, fine, telangiectases less than 0.2 mm in diameter surrounding a previously treated area. A reported incidence of 35% was seen initially,[25] but in a more recently published retrospective analysis of more than 2000 patients, an incidence of only 16% was reported in patients treated with HS and POL.[61] Another study of 350 patients indicated an incidence of 11% when using HS only and 16% when using both HS and POL.[92] Resolution usually occurs spontaneously within a 3- to 12-month period,[25] with 70 to 80% spontaneous resolution within the first 6 months.[92] Only 10% of patients with matting require repeat treatment of the area.[25]

Matting may also occur as a result of trauma associated with pregnancy or hormonal therapy or in scars around previous sites of surgical stripping. Sclerotherapy-induced matting has been proposed to be caused by excessive concentrations of sclerosing solution, use of too much sclerosing solution, excessive hydrostatic pressure of injection, too much blanching, or improper compression.[92, 111] Predisposing factors include an individual susceptibility as a result of obesity, previous estrogen therapy, positive family history, and a history of telangiectases.[61] The relative risk factor for development of telangiectatic matting during exogenous hor-

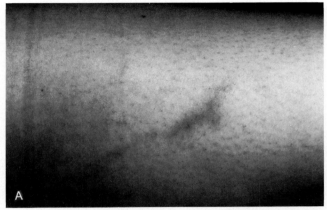

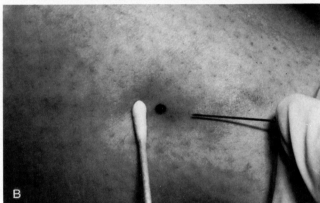

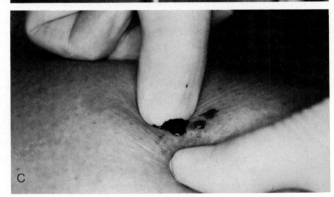

Figure 69–11. Removal of liquefied "microthrombus." *A,* The patient returned several weeks after sclerotherapy of a varicose vein with a slightly tender, raised, dark blue swelling with no surrounding erythema or induration along the course of the treated varicosity. Doppler examination reveals no flow in this vessel, but slight fluctuance is palpable. *B,* To relieve discomfort and reduce the risks of hyperpigmentation, the region is incised with a 22-gauge needle, and dark, viscous blood is expressed. This liquefied intravascular coagulum or hematoma is further expressed by sweeping compression with a cotton-tipped applicator. *C,* Alternatively, finger pressure may be used to expel this coagulum.

monal therapy has been found to be 3.17 times more likely to develop than in women not on hormonal therapy.[92] In many patients on postmenopausal estrogen and progesterone therapy, telangiectatic matting developed in response to sclerotherapy. However, complete clearing can often be accomplished with further sclerotherapy once the exogenous hormones have been discontinued. Because neither estrogen nor progesterone receptors are present in telangiectases, another mechanism may be responsible.[126]

A study of other possible angiogenic factors indicates that inflammation plays an important role,[127] and the goal of sclerotherapy should be to choose the sclerosant concentration that minimizes inflammation. One study[111] indicated that in patients who developed telangiectatic matting with 1% polidocanol, no matting occurred when the concentration was subsequently reduced to 0.5% polidocanol.[92]

The only successful treatment of matting to date has been with the flash lamp–pumped, pulsed-dye laser,[128] although temporary hyperpigmentation usually occurs after laser therapy. In most cases additional treatment is unnecessary, as matting generally resolves spontaneously. However, persistent matting can be treated with a more dilute sclerosing agent. Chromated glycerin, which has rarely been reported to cause matting, may be the ideal agent. Another report recommended the use of 12% salicylate.[107] Stubborn matting can be treated with a reduced concentration of POL (0.25%). At the slightly higher concentration of 0.5%, POL has been proposed as an intradermal sclerosing agent for vessels that cannot be cannulated.[90] When treating the fine vessels of matting, extravasation frequently occurs, which may be therapeutic at low concentrations of POL. Usually patient reassurance and patience are the only therapeutic measures necessary. The initial treatment of a reticular vein in an area of matting has occasionally led to their resolution. The treatment interval of 2 to 3 months is long enough to allow matting to resolve.

PAIN ON INJECTION

Use of the sharpest, most tapered siliconized bevel on a 30-gauge needle, which is changed frequently, minimizes the pain of piercing the skin. Hypertonic solutions produce an intense muscle cramping or burning sensation lasting from 1 to 2 minutes but rarely more than 5 minutes.[3] This can be minimized by slow injection and by injection of volumes of less than 0.1 ml per site. Use of a detergent solution diluted with normal saline to a lower concentration to decrease the concentration of preservative usually allows the injections to be painless.

LOWER EXTREMITY EDEMA

The occurrence of ankle edema is usually related either to the application of nongraduated compression or to constricting pressure at one point by an elasticized bandage without an overlying graduated compression stocking. When no compression hose is worn, the site of sclerotherapy should be compressed only partially with Microfoam tape, being sure to apply the tape noncircumferentially. This avoids the tourniquet effect of complete constriction at any point above the ankle. In addition, the volume of sclerosing solution injected in the ankle should be limited to no more than 1 ml per treatment session.

LOCALIZED URTICATION

Localized urtication is most pronounced with the use of polidocanol, becoming more severe with increasing concentrations. Urtication occurs with other sclerosants as well and is frequently accompanied by pruritus. Swelling, which often appears to be urticarial in nature, occurs commonly with HS, but may be due to edema from the local osmotic gradient, since this is rarely accompanied by itching. The patient must be reassured that the appearance of urtication is not a true allergic reaction but an expected outcome. No treatment is necessary, since spontaneous resolution usually occurs within an hour.

TAPE BLISTER

Blisters or erosions occur unpredictably but are most often seen above the popliteal fossa in response to friction near the knee caused by rubbing against a compression dressing. These do not represent a true allergic response to adhesive; such a response consists of an erythematous patch. Patients who exercise to the point of perspiration or who get the tape wet by showering are more likely to experience a blister. Blisters may occur because of pinching of the skin caused by slippage of the tape at points of overlap, and careful attention must be paid when applying the tape to ensure smoothness. A nonadhesive tape or elastic compression bandage is substituted for tape if the patient repeatedly develops blisters. The blister sites are quite disturbing, because they may remain erythematous or hypopigmented for several months. The initial test visit also serves to gauge tolerance for tape.

CUTANEOUS NECROSIS AND ULCERATION

Avoiding the complication of necrosis is most dependent on the skill of the cutaneous surgeon. Meticulous technique with immediate cessation of injection at the first sign of a wheal, the slightest resistance to injection, or a sudden increase in pain noted by the patient will help to minimize extravasation and resultant ulceration. Use of a solution such as POL at concentrations of less than 0.5% will also help to minimize necrosis.[90] Even when sclerotherapy is performed with the most skilled technique, however, cutaneous ulceration may occur with any sclerosing solution.

Small amounts of extravasation occur even under the best of conditions. Often a tiny amount of sclerosing solution may be left along the needle tract as the needle is withdrawn, or sclerosing solution may leak out into the skin through the small vessel puncture sites. Inadvertent puncture through the entire vessel may result in small perforations in the back wall of the treated vein, through which solution may leak. When the treated vein has a particularly fragile, thin wall, a sclerosant may cause rapid full-thickness injury leading to rupture with perivascular accumulation. In addition, injection may inadvertently occur into a small arteriole associated with a spider telangiectasis, with resultant necrosis and ulceration. Skilled injection technique, although critical, is not a guarantee that extravasation will not occur.

If the cutaneous surgeon recognizes that extravasation has occurred, the risk of necrosis can be minimized by injecting normal saline in a ratio of 10:1 into the site.[25] Also, extensive massage of small subcutaneous blebs to spread the trapped sclerosing agent as quickly as possible will minimize blanching of the area. When erythema replaces the blanch immediately at a site of extravasation, necrosis rarely ensues.

The incidence of necrosis with ulceration is less than 1% for small vessels and possibly even less than this for treatment of large varicosities in deeper locations. Ulcerations are typically smaller than 1 cm and usually heal as small, cosmetically insignificant, hypopigmented patches. However, ulcerations that are extensive and require full-thickness skin grafting have been known to occur. Punctate erosions at the site of needle entry generally heal without scarring. Necrosis with ulceration is most likely to occur with injection of the most superficial vessels, since the more superficial the injection, the more chance that extravasation could cause necrosis. In a review of 13,000 patients, it was found that when small amounts of 0.25 ml of 3% STS are accidently extravasated deeply, the results are not likely to be serious.[19]

SUPERFICIAL THROMBOPHLEBITIS

Superficial thrombophlebitis is most commonly mistaken for the normal nodular fibrosis that occurs with proper sclerotherapy and has also been termed "endosclerosis."[19] After sclerotherapy of large (4- to 8-mm) varicosities, a nontender, nonpigmented, fibrotic cord may be palpable along the course of the vein; this may persist for months. An intravascular coagulum must be excluded by clinical appearance and absence of tenderness. Superficial thrombophlebitis is characterized clinically by a very tender, indurated knot that is surrounded by extensive bright erythema. Its incidence after sclerotherapy is estimated at 0.01 to 1%.[99] A liquefied thrombus usually accompanies superficial thrombophlebitis and should be evacuated using needle puncture under local anesthesia. Treatment also includes leg elevation and compression, as well as regular administration of aspirin or other nonsteroidal anti-inflammatory drugs. Minimization of this complication is best achieved by adequate postsclerotherapy compression.

PULMONARY EMBOLISM

Pulmonary emboli probably occur from extension of a superficial thrombus into the deep venous system. Therefore, superficial thrombus formation or superficial thrombophlebitis should be treated promptly and monitored closely. Fortunately, the incidence of embolism is extremely low, (1 in 40,000 patients) and usually occurs with injection of large quantities of sclerosant at a single site.[129] Exogenous hormonal therapy is known to increase the risk of deep thrombophlebitis and pulmonary embolism, and it has been suggested that oral contraceptive use may increase the risk of emboli for patients undergoing sclerotherapy.[130] Compression followed by immediate ambulation and use of no more than 1 ml of sclerosing solution per site should minimize the risks of emboli.

ARTERIAL INJECTION

Arterial injection is extremely rare but devastating when it occurs. Bright red blood seen on drawing back into the syringe before injection should alert the physician to the possibility of arterial injection. Immediate intense pain far beyond the normal discomfort at the initiation of injection should also be a warning. Immediate, white, cutaneous blanching with progressive cyanosis over a large area is the result of arteriole injection and must be recognized immediately. This complication may be minimized by use of a hand-held Doppler device, which helps identify varicosities close to the arterial signal. Emergency treatment is beyond the scope of this text, but immediate application of ice and injection of 3% procaine to inactivate STS should be considered while the advice of a vascular surgeon is sought. Anticoagulation may need to be employed.

SYSTEMIC ALLERGIC REACTIONS

The incidence of systemic reactions is extremely low and varies with the sclerosing agent. Generalized urticaria may be the only sign and should be treated immediately with antihistamines. Bronchospasm with wheezing, estimated to occur in 0.001% of patients,[25] may be the first sign of impending anaphylaxis and should be treated with injection of 0.2 to 0.5 ml of epinephrine 1:1,000. Patients should be observed carefully for progressive cardiovascular failure so that advanced life support systems can be instituted immediately. Avoiding sclerosing agents with high incidences of allergic reactions (e.g., 3% sodium morrhuate)[131] will help to minimize this complication.

Contraindications to Sclerotherapy

Because ambulation is extremely important after sclerotherapy, a bedridden patient is not a good candidate for sclerotherapy. Patients with severe arterial obstruction in the legs also should not be treated, although patients with mild arterial obstruction have been treated successfully.[19] A history of deep thrombophlebitis should preclude sclerotherapy until the patient has been adequately evaluated by ultrasound or venography, because superficial varicosities may be a mechanism to bypass the internal venous obstruction. Previous urticaria or suspected allergy to a sclerosing agent is a relative contraindication to use of that particular sclerosing agent, although continued use is deemed acceptable by some as long as such use is accompanied by premedication with antihistamines.[96]

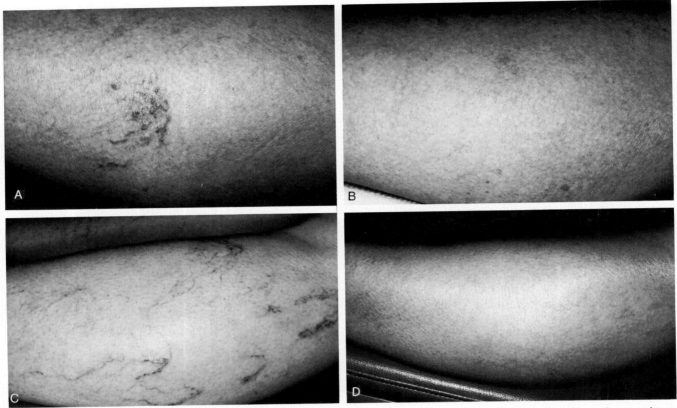

Figure 69–12. Typical results after sclerotherapy. *A,* Grouped telangiectases on the midcalf in a 42-year-old woman, who experienced intermittent focal burning over this area. *B,* After two treatments 2 months apart with 0.5 ml 0.5% polidocanol, the telangiectases completely resolved. Before the complete resolution of the vessels, the patient noted absence of the focal burning. Relief of symptoms often occurs before visual disappearance of the telangiectases. *C,* Multiple telangiectases and reticular veins up to 3 mm in diameter on the calf of a 48-year-old woman. She had experienced focal burning, generalized leg aching, and night cramps for several years. *D,* After three treatment sessions with hypertonic saline 1 month apart, complete resolution was noted, and the patient is now completely symptom free.

Pregnancy is considered a contraindication during the first and second trimester, although extremely painful or bleeding varices may be treated in the last trimester. Fegan does not consider pregnancy to be a contraindication at any time.[19] In our experience, many varicosities and telangiectases resolve spontaneously post partum, so treatment should be postponed until 4 to 6 months after delivery.

Maintaining adequate compression on very obese legs is difficult, and for this reason, gross obesity should be considered a relative contraindication. Sclerotherapy of larger varicosities should be postponed until weight reduction is achieved. During hot summer months, patients may often find thick compression hose intolerable. Patient cooperation is ensured by postponing treatment of larger varicosities until the winter months when the warming effect of compression hose is appreciated.

SUMMARY

Telangiectatic and varicose leg veins often require treatment. Modern sclerotherapy can provide efficacy comparable to or greater than that of surgery with lower cost and lower morbidity, and is preferred by patients.

Symptoms are improved rapidly, with a low risk of side effects and excellent cosmetic results (Fig. 69–12). Sclerotherapy and evaluation of the venous system should become a standard part of the training of American physicians, particularly those with expertise in cutaneous surgery.

REFERENCES

1. Goldman MP: The role of the American dermatologist in phlebology. J Dermatol Surg Oncol 15:135, 1989.
2. Biegeleisen K: Primary lower extremity telangiectasia: relationship of size to color. Angiology 38:760–768, 1987.
3. Weiss RA, Weiss MA: Resolution of pain associated with varicose and telangiectatic leg veins after compression sclerotherapy. J Dermatol Surg Oncol 16:333–336, 1990.
4. Campbell WB: Varicose veins. Br Med J 300:763–764, 1990.
5. Brand FN, Dannenberg AL, Abbott RD, Kannel WB: The epidemiology of varicose veins: the Framingham study. Am J Prevent Med 4:96–101, 1988.
6. Coon WW, Willis PW III: Venous thromboembolism and other venous disease in the Tecumseh Community Health Study. Circulation 48:839–846, 1973.
7. Engel A, Johnson ML, Haynes SG: Health effects of sunlight exposure in the United States: results from the first national health and nutrition examination survey, 1971–1974. Arch Dermatol 124:72–79, 1988.

8. Chant ADB, Magnussen P, Kershaw C: Support hose and varicose veins. Br Med J 290:204, 1985.

9. Orbach EJ: Compression therapy of vein and lymph vessel diseases of the lower extremities. Angiology 30:95–103, 1979.

10. Bloch H: Ambroise Paré (1510–1590): father of surgery as art and science. South Med J 84:763–765, 1991.

11. Browse NL, Burnand KG, Thomas ML: Diseases of the Veins: Pathology, Diagnosis and Treatment. Edward Arnold, London, 1988.

12. Schneider W: Contribution to the history of the sclerosing treatment of varices and to its anatomo-pathologic study. Soc Fran de Phlebol 18:117–130, 1965.

13. Garrison FH: An Introduction to the History of Medicine. WB Saunders, Philadelphia, 1929.

14. Stemmer R: Sclerotherapy of Varicose Veins. AG Ganzoni & Cie, St Gallen, Switzerland, 1990, pp 6–8.

15. Mayo CH: Treatment of varicose veins. Surg Gynecol Obstet 2:385–388, 1906.

16. Cooper WM: Chemical evaluation of sotradecol, a sodium alkyl sulfate solution, in the injection therapy of varicose veins. Surg Gynecol Obstet 83:647–652, 1946.

17. Sigg K: The treatment of varicosities and accompanying complications. Angiology 3:355–379, 1952.

18. Orbach EJ: A new approach to the sclerotherapy of varicose veins. Angiology 1:302–305, 1950.

19. Fegan WG: Continuous compression technique of injecting varicose veins. Lancet 2:109–112, 1963.

20. Biegeleisen HI: Telangiectasia accompanying varicose veins: treatment by a micro-technique. JAMA 102:2092–2094, 1934.

21. Tretbar LL: Spider angiomata: treatment with sclerosant injections. J Kansas Med Soc 79:198–200, 1978.

22. Brauer EW: Cosmetic management of selected skin changes of the legs. South Med J 63:1190–1192, 1970.

23. Foley WT: The eradication of venous blemishes. Cutis 15:665–668, 1975.

24. Alderman DB: Therapy for essential cutaneous telangiectasia. Postgrad Med 61:91–95, 1977.

25. Duffy DM: Small vessel sclerotherapy: an overview. In: Callen JP, Dahl MV, Golitz LE, et al (eds): Advances in Dermatology. Year Book Medical, Chicago, 1988, pp 221–242.

26. Tolins SH: Treatment of varicose veins: an update. Am J Surg 145:248–252, 1983.

27. Dale WA, Cranley JJ, Deweise JA, Meyers TT: Symposium: management of varicose veins. Contemp Surg 6:86–124, 1975.

28. Crane C: The surgery of varicose veins. Surg Clin North Am 59:737–748, 1979.

29. Doran FSA, White M: A clinical trial designed to discover if the primary treatment of varicose veins should be by Fegan's method or by operation. Br J Surg 62:72–76, 1975.

30. Nabatoff RA: Recent trends in the diagnosis and treatment of varicose veins. Surg Gynecol Obstet 90:521–528, 1950.

31. McNamara MF, Takaki HS, Yao JST: Venous diseases. Surg Clin North Am 57:1201–1220, 1977.

32. Hobbs JT: The treatment of varicose veins: a random trial of injection/compression versus surgery. Br J Surg 55:777–780, 1968.

33. Hobbs JT: Surgery and sclerotherapy in the treatment of varicose veins: a random trial. Arch Surg 109:793–796, 1974.

34. Chant ADB, Jones HO, Weddell JM: Varicose veins: a comparison of surgery and injection/compression sclerotherapy. Lancet 2:1188–1191, 1972.

35. Schwartz SI: Year Book of Surgery. Year Book Medical, Chicago, 1979, p 319.

36. Fegan WG, Fitzgerald D, Beasley B: Valvular defect in primary varicose veins. Lancet 2:491–492, 1964.

37. Sigg K, Zelikovski A. "Quick treatment"—a modified method of sclerotherapy of varicose veins. Vasa 4:73–77, 1975.

38. Tretbar LL, Pattison PH: Injection-compression treatment of varicose veins. Am J Surg 120:539–541, 1970.

39. Henry MEF, Fegan WG, Pegum JM: Five year survey of the treatment of varicose ulcers. Br Med J 2:493–494, 1971.

40. Beresford SAA, Chant ADB, Jones HO, et al: Varicose veins: a comparison of surgery and injection/compression sclerotherapy five-year follow-up. Lancet 1:921–924, 1978.

41. Piachaud D, Weddell JM: Cost of treating varicose veins. Lancet 2:1191–1192, 1972.

42. Bergan JJ: Surgical procedures for varicose veins. In: Bergan JJ, Yao JST (eds): Venous Disorders. WB Saunders, Philadelphia, 1991, pp 201–216.

43. Myers TT: Varicose veins. In: Allen EV, Barker NW, Hines EA Jr (eds): Peripheral Vascular Diseases. WB Saunders, Philadelphia, 1962, pp 636–658.

44. Bishara RA, Sigel B, Rocco K, et al: Deterioration of venous function in normal lower extremities during daily activity. J Vasc Surg 3:700–706, 1986.

45. Wells HS, Youmans JB, Miller DG: Tissue pressure, intracutaneous, subcutaneous and intramuscular, as related to venous pressure, capillary filtration and other factors. J Clin Invest 17:489–499, 1938.

46. Reagan B, Folse R: Lower limb venous dynamics in normal persons and children of patients with varicose veins. Surg Gynecol Obstet 132:15–18, 1971.

47. Kerr MG, Scott DB, Samuel E: Studies of the inferior vena cava in late pregnancy. Br Med J 1:532–533, 1964.

48. Barwin BN, Roddie IC: Venous distensibility during pregnancy determined by graded venous congestion. Am J Obstet Gynecol 125:921–923, 1976.

49. McCausland AM, Holmes F, Trotter AD: Venous distensibility during the menstrual cycle. Am J Obstet Gynecol 86:640–645, 1963.

50. Bouissou H, Julian M, Pieraggi M, Louge L: Vein morphology. Phlebology 1:1–8, 1988.

51. Widmer LK: Peripheral venous disorders: prevalence and socio-medical important observations in 4529 apparently healthy persons. Basle Study III. Hans Huber Publishers, Bern, 1978.

52. Galen: Galen on the Affected Parts. Translated by Siegel RE. S Karger, Basel, 1976.

53. Lofgren KA: Varicose veins: their symptoms, complications, and management. Postgrad Med 65:131–139, 1979.

54. Lofgren KA: Stasis ulcer. Mayo Clin Proc 40:564–573, 1965.

55. Burnand KG, Whimster I, Naidoo A, et al: Pericapillary fibrin in the ulcer-bearing skin of the leg: the cause of lipodermatosclerosis and venous ulcerations. Br Med J 285:1071–1072, 1982.

56. Falanga V, Moosa HH, Nemeth AJ, et al: Dermal pericapillary fibrin in venous disease and venous ulceration. Arch Dermatol 123:620–623, 1987.

57. Coleridge Smith PD, Thomas P, Schurr JH, Dormandy JA: Causes of venous ulceration: a new hypothesis. Br Med J 296:1726–1727, 1988.

58. Queral LA, Criado FJ, Lilly MP, Rudolphi D: The role of sclerotherapy as an adjunct to Unna's boot for treating venous ulcers: a prospective study. J Vasc Surg 11:572–575, 1990.

59. Lofgren EP, Lofgren KA: The surgical treatment of superficial thrombophlebitis. Surgery 90:49–54, 1981.

60. Johnson G Jr: Superficial venous thrombosis. In: Rutherford RB (ed): Vascular Surgery. 3rd ed. WB Saunders, Philadelphia, 1989, pp 1518–1520.

61. Davis LT, Duffy DM: Determination of incidence and risk factors for postsclerotherapy telangiectatic matting of the lower extremity: a retrospective analysis. J Dermatol Surg Oncol 16:327–330, 1990.

62. Fronek A: Injection compression sclerotherapy of varicose veins. In: Ernst CB, Stanley JC (eds): Current Therapy in Vascular Surgery. BC Decker, Philadelphia, 1991, pp 961–967.

63. Fronek A: Noninvasive Diagnostics in Vascular Disease. McGraw-Hill, New York, 1989, pp 127–136.

64. Partsch H: Primare Varikose der Vena Saphena Magna und parva. In: Kriessman A, Bollinger A, Keller H (eds): Praxis der Doppler Sonographie. Thieme, Stuttgart, 1982, pp 101–103.

65. Schultz-Ehrenburg U, Hubner H-J: Reflux diagnosis with Doppler ultrasound. Monograph. Schattauer, Stuttgart, 1989, pp 5–10.

66. Evans DS, Cockett FB: Diagnosis of deep-vein thrombosis with an ultrasonic Doppler technique. Br Med J 28:802–804, 1969.

67. Milne RM, Gunn AA, Griffiths MT, Ruckley CV: Postoperative deep venous thrombosis. A comparison of diagnostic techniques. Lancet 2:445–447, 1971.

68. Abramowitz HB, Queral LA, Flinn WR, et al: The use of

photoplethysmography in the assessment of venous insufficiency: a comparison to venous pressure measurements. Surgery 66:434–441, 1979.

69. Orbach EJ: Hazards of sclerotherapy of varicose veins, their prevention and treatment of complications. Vasa 8:170–173, 1979.

70. Szendro G, Nicolaides AN, Zukowski AJ, et al: Duplex scanning in the assessment of deep venous incompetence. J Vasc Surg 4:237–242, 1986.

71. Thibault PK, Bray AE: Cosmetic leg veins: evaluation using duplex venous imaging. J Dermatol Surg Oncol 16:90, 1990.

72. Raymond-Martimbeau P: Duplex ultrasonography, color flow doppler, and magnetic resonance imaging in phlebology. J Dermatol Surg Oncol 16:93, 1990.

73. Shadeck M: Sclerotherapy of great saphenous veins: a 48-month follow-up. J Dermatol Surg Oncol 16:87, 1990.

74. Goldman MP, Kaplan RP, Oki LN, et al: Sclerosing agents in the treatment of telangiectasia: comparison of the clinical and histologic effects of intravascular polidocanol, sodium tetradecyl sulfate, and hypertonic saline in the dorsal rabbit ear vein model. Arch Dermatol 123:1196–1201, 1987.

75. Martin DE, Goldman MP: A comparison of sclerosing agents: clinical and histologic effects of intravascular sodium tetradecyl sulfate and chromated glycerin in the dorsal rabbit ear vein. J Dermatol Surg Oncol 16:18–22, 1990.

76. Goldman MP: Personal communication, 1991.

77. Sarin SK, Kumar A: Sclerosants for variceal sclerotherapy: a critical appraisal. Am J Gastroenterol 85:641–649, 1990.

78. Oscher A, Garside E: Intravenous injection of sclerosing substances: experimental comparative studies of changes in vessels. Ann Surg 96:691–718, 1932.

79. Imhoff E, Stemmer R: Classification and mechanism of action of sclerosing agents. Soc Fran de Phlebol 22:143–148, 1969.

80. Sadick N: Treatment of varicose and telangiectatic leg veins with hypertonic saline: a comparative study of heparin and saline. J Dermatol Surg Oncol 16:24–28, 1990.

81. Goldman MP, Kaplan RP, Oki LN, et al: Extravascular effects of sclerosants in rabbit skin: a clinical and histologic examination. J Dermatol Surg Oncol 12:1085–1088, 1986.

82. Sadick NS: Sclerotherapy of varicose and telangiectatic leg veins: minimal sclerosant concentration of hypertonic saline and its relationship to vessel diameter. J Dermatol Surg Oncol 17:65–70, 1991.

83. Carlin MC, Ratz JL: Treatment of telangiectasia: comparison of sclerosing agents. J Dermatol Surg Oncol 13:1181–1184, 1987.

84. Sclerodex prescribing information. J Dermatol Surg Oncol 17:63–64, 1991.

85. Mantse L: A mild sclerosing agent for telangiectasias. J Dermatol Surg Oncol 11:855, 1985.

86. Mantse L: More on spider veins. J Dermatol Surg Oncol 12:1022, 1986.

87. Eichenberger H: Results of phlebosclerosation with hydroxy-polyethoxydodecane. Zentralbl Phlebol 8:181–183, 1969.

88. Goldman MP: Sclerotherapy of superficial venules and telangiectasias of the lower extremities. Dermatol Clin 5:369–379, 1987.

89. Goldman MP, Bennett RG: Treatment of telangiectasia: a review. J Am Acad Dermatol 17:167–182, 1987.

90. Jaquier JJ, Loretan RM: Clinical trials of a new sclerosing agent, aethoxysklerol. Soc Fran de Phlebol 22:383–385, 1969.

91. Norris MJ, Carlin MC, Ratz JL: Treatment of essential telangiectasia: effects of increasing concentrations of polidocanol. J Am Acad Dermatol 20:643–649, 1989.

92. Weiss RA, Weiss MA: Incidence of side effects in the treatment of telangiectasias by compression sclerotherapy: hypertonic saline vs. polidocanol. J Dermatol Surg Oncol 16:800–804, 1990.

93. Tretbar LL: Injection sclerotherapy for spider telangiectasias: a 20-year experience with sodium tetradecyl sulfate. J Dermatol Surg Oncol 15:223–225, 1989.

94. Passas H: One case of tetradecyl-sodium sulfate allergy with general symptoms. Soc Fran de Phlebol 25:19, 1972.

95. Case report of anaphylaxis and death after injection of 0.5% STS. Proceedings of the 3rd Annual Congress of the North American Society of Phlebology, Phoenix, Arizona, 1990.

96. Fegan WG: Varicose Veins: Compression Sclerotherapy. William Heinemann Medical Books, London, 1967.

97. Fronek H, Fronek A, Saltzbarg G: Allergic reactions to sotradecol. J Dermatol Surg Oncol 15:684, 1989.

98. Weiss MA, Weiss RA: Efficacy and side effects of 0.1% sodium tetradecyl sulfate in compression sclerotherapy of telangiectasias: comparison to 1% polidocanol and hypertonic saline. J Dermatol Surg Oncol 17:90–91, 1991.

99. Goldman MP: Sclerotherapy treatment for varicose and telangiectatic leg veins. In: Coleman WP, Hanke CW, Alt TH, Asken S (eds): Cosmetic Surgery of the Skin. BC Decker, Philadelphia, 1991, pp 197–211.

100. Biegeleisen HI: The evaluation of sodium morrhuate therapy in varicose veins: a critical study. Surg Gynecol Obstet 57:696–700, 1933.

101. Lewis KM: Anaphylaxis due to sodium morrhuate. JAMA 107:1298–1299, 1936.

102. Fearson B, San-Kortsak A: The management of esophageal varices in children by injection therapy of sclerosing agents. Am J Otol Rhinol Laryngol 68:906–915, 1959.

103. Biegeleisen HI: Fatty acid solutions for the injection treatment of varicose veins: evaluation of four new solutions. Ann Surg 105:610–615, 1937.

104. Lindemayr H, Santler R: The fibrinolytic activity of the vein wall. Phlebology 30:151–160, 1977.

105. Raymond-Martimbeau P, Leclerc JR: Activation of blood coagulation after injection sclerotherapy of the lower extremity: a prospective study. J Dermatol Surg Oncol 17:91, 1991.

106. Raymond-Martimbeau P: Two different techniques for sclerosing the incompetent saphenofemoral junction: a comparative study. J Dermatol Surg Oncol 16:626–631, 1990.

107. Ouvry PA: Telangiectasia and sclerotherapy. J Dermatol Surg Oncol 15:177–181, 1989.

108. Nebot F: Quelques points tecniques sur le traitement des varicosities et des telangiectasias. Phlebology 21:133–135, 1968.

109. Tretbar LL: The origin of reflux in incompetent blue reticular/telangiectasia veins. In: Davy A, Stemmer R (eds): Phlebologie '89. John Libbey Eurotext, London, 1989, pp 95–96.

110. Bodian EL: Techniques of sclerotherapy for sunburst venous blemishes. J Dermatol Surg Oncol 11:696–704, 1985.

111. Ouvry PA, Davy A: The sclerotherapy of telangiectasia. Phlebology 35:349–359, 1982.

112. De Groot WP: Treatment of varicose veins: modern concepts and methods. J Dermatol Surg Oncol 15:191–198, 1989.

113. Tournay R, Caille JP, Chatard H, et al: La Sclerose des Varices. 3rd ed. Expansion Scientifique Francaise, Paris, 1980.

114. Orbach EJ: Sclerotherapy of varicose veins: utilization of intravenous air block. Am J Surg 66:362–366, 1944.

115. Orbach EJ, Petretti AK: Thrombogenic property of foam synthetic anionic detergent (sodium tetradecyl sulfate, N.N.R.). Angiology 1:237–243, 1950.

116. Harridge H: The treatment of primary varicose veins. Surg Clin North Am 40:191–202, 1960.

117. Goldman MP, Beaudoing D, Marley W, et al: Compression in the treatment of leg telangiectasia: a preliminary report. J Dermatol Surg Oncol 16:322–325, 1990.

118. Shouler PJ, Runchman PC: Varicose veins: optimum compression after surgery and sclerotherapy. Ann R Coll Surg Engl 71:402–404, 1969.

119. Fraser IA, Perry EP, Hatton M, Watkin DLF: Prolonged bandaging is not required following sclerotherapy of varicose veins. Br J Surg 72:488–490, 1985.

120. Reddy P, Terry T, Lamont P, Dormandy J: What is the correct duration of bandaging following sclerotherapy? In: Negus D, Jantet G (eds): Phlebology '85. John Libbey & Co., London, 1985, pp 141–143.

121. Goldman MP, Kaplan RP, Duffy DM: Postsclerotherapy hyperpigmentation: a histologic evaluation. J Dermatol Surg Oncol 13:547–550, 1987.

122. Tournay PR: Sclerosing treatment of very fine intra or subdermal varicosities. Soc Fran de Phlebol 19:235–241, 1966.

123. Thibault P: Postsclerotherapy pigmentation: the role of serum iron levels and the effectiveness of treatment with the copper vapor laser. J Dermatol Surg Oncol 17:94, 1991.

124. Biegeleisen HI, Biegeleisen RM: The current status of sclerotherapy for varicose veins. Clin Med 83:24–36, 1976.

125. Goldman MP: Polidocanol (aethoxysklerol) for sclerotherapy of

superficial venules and telangiectasias. J Dermatol Surg Oncol 15:204–209, 1989.

126. Sadick NS, Niedt GW: A study of estrogen and progesterone receptors in spider telangiectasias of the lower extremities. J Dermatol Surg Oncol 16:620–623, 1990.

127. Folkman J, Klagsbrun M: Angiogenic factors. Science 235:442–447, 1987.

128. Goldman MP, Fitzpatrick RE: Pulsed-dye laser treatment of leg telangiectasia: with and without simultaneous sclerotherapy. J Dermatol Surg Oncol 16:338–344, 1990.

129. Sigg K: Zur Behandlung der Varizen der Phlebitis und ihrer Komplidationen. Hautarzt 131:443, 1950.

130. Fegan WG: The complications of compression sclerotherapy. Practitioner 207:797–799, 1971.

131. Dick ET: The treatment of varicose veins. NZ Med J 65:310–313, 1966.

CHAPTER 70

Techniques for Tattoo Removal

TIMOTHY J. ROSIO

Historical Aspects of Tattoos

And the Lord set a mark upon Cain . . .
a fugitive and a vagabond in the earth.
BIBLE, OLD TESTAMENT, GENESIS 4:14, 15

Out, damned spot! out, I say!
One; two; why then, 'tis time to do't.
SHAKESPEARE, MACBETH, ACT V

The application method and pigment used for the very first tattoo almost certainly predates recorded history. However, for as long as humans have been acquiring tattoos, removal has also been a concern. The term tattoo comes from the Polynesian word "tatau," which refers to removable body painting, ornamental scars, and dermally implanted pigments, all recognized as forms of tattoos. Beginning with cave dwellers, every major culture has used tattooing for ornamentation, group identity, honors, religious purposes, or political statements.[1] Tattoos have also had less honorable connotations, with slaves, prisoners, criminals, and rebellious and psychologically impaired individuals being identified by or associated with tattoos.[2-7] Traumatic tattoos also result from automobile accidents, explosions, and other penetrating injuries.[8-11]

Prevalence figures for tattoos vary widely, ranging from 65% of individuals in United States federal correctional institutions to 2.5% in the general Swedish population. Even 4% of third grade English schoolchildren have been tattooed.[7] Up to one third of individuals with tattoos report being drunk or in an otherwise compromised state of awareness when receiving their tattoo. Clearly the psychological implications of tattoos must be considered in the societal and cultural context of the patient.[2, 12] Tattoos have been used for quasimedical or therapeutic purposes. They are used for sun protection, as body landmark restoration to re-create eyelashes or eyebrows after trauma or other causes of alopecia, to simulate eyeliner in women who are allergic to mascara, and for areolar reconstruction after mastectomy.[13]

Because of its past, tattooing and tattoo artists have been regulated.[14] Nevertheless, there is little doubt that tattooing will continue into the distant future, given its popularity among music and movie stars, sports figures and their devotees, and military personnel. Correspondingly, as long as tattoos continue to be applied, there will also exist a desire to have them removed. Tattoo removal may also be required for psychiatric reasons, for medical reasons (i.e., inflammatory or allergic reactions or other complications) and for rehabilitative purposes.[4, 6, 7, 15-19] It should be noted that although many people are happy with their tattoos, many people are not. In fact, it has been suggested that for every person thinking of getting a tattoo, there is another person thinking of having a tattoo removed. The majority of physicians are uninterested in tattoos and the techniques used for their removal. Therefore, it is important that cutaneous surgeons be knowledgeable about this problem so that they can provide interested patients with proper assistance.

Approach to the Tattoo Patient

Cutaneous surgeons with experience in tattoo removal realize there is no ideal method for the treatment of all tattoos. Variability in patient selection, tattoo pigments, depth, density, age (Table 70–1), instrumentation, technique, follow-up periods, and wound care requirements all complicate the choice of proper treatment modality (Table 70–2).

PROBLEM AVOIDANCE

Removing a tattoo is an elective decision that is often made after analyzing the cost:benefit:risk ratios. Therefore, the procedure to be utilized for treatment must be fully understood by the patient. The patient must rec-

TABLE 70–1. **VARIABLES THAT AFFECT TATTOO REMOVAL AND HEALING**

Manner of tattooing
Depth
Density
Composition
Color
Age of tattoo
Age of patient
Location
Size
Shape
Direction

ognize that the removal of most tattoos is imperfect, irregular, incomplete, and irreversible. Furthermore, the physician must realize that patients with multiple tattoos often are highly impulsive. If these patients are to be treated successfully, they must fully understand the discomfort, healing time, associated cost, and anticipated final result from treatment; otherwise, a disaster can result. Unfortunately, numerous lawsuits result from removal of tattoos.[20] Therefore, it is important to carefully evaluate each tattoo patient, select only the proper candidates for treatment, know as much as possible about the various forms of treatment available, approach each tattoo and location individually, advise the patient about the best method to use for their particular tattoo and individual goal, and then thoroughly document patient education and informed consent.

PATIENT DESIRES

The cutaneous surgeon should elicit from patients what aspect of the tattoo bothers them most. They should be urged to fully discuss their reasons for seeking removal. These reasons may range from allergic reactions to unpleasant memories engendered by the tattoo or social or professional impairment. Surgeons should

TABLE 70–2. **TECHNIQUES FOR TATTOO REMOVAL**

Full-thickness surgical excision
  Excision and closure
  Serial excision
  Excision and flap or split-thickness skin graft closure
  Punch excision
Split-thickness injury
  Dermabrasion, brushing, curettage
  Tangential excision, overgrafting
  Chemical peeling
    Salabrasion, chemabrasion
  Overtattooing
  Cryosurgery
  Electrofulguration, infrared coagulation
    Electrosurgery
Tattoo supplementation
Laser
  Carbon dioxide laser
  Nd:YAG laser
  Visible light (argon, dye) lasers
  Q-switched ruby laser

avoid projecting their own values and aesthetic judgment onto the patient.

Allergic Reactions or Provocation of Medical Problems

Hypersensitivity to tattoo pigments may cause chronic or recurring dermatitis, adenopathy, or systemic symptoms. Acquired sensitivity to cadium (yellow), chromium (green), cobalt (blue), and mercury (red) has also been noted. Systemic disorders, including erythema multiforme and scleroderma, have been reported in association with tattoos. A wide variety of viral and bacterial infections, including tuberculosis and leprosy, have been seen in association with tattooing. In addition, keloid scars, sarcoidal granulomas, keratoacanthomas, psoriasis, lichen planus, Darier's disease, and chronic discoid lupus erythematosus have localized to tattooed sites.[17, 18] These are striking and exceptional reasons for tattoo removal and are also the most likely situations in which the cost associated with removal may be reimbursed by the insurance carrier.

Professional Impairment

The most commonly cited reason given for tattoo removal is employment. Patients realize that a tattoo often has such a significant negative connotation that it may slow or reduce their chances for occupational advancement. This perception is probably realistic, given the commonly held association of tattoos with violence, drug use, gang membership, and sexual themes.

Cosmesis

Patients who have grown tired of the appearance of a tattoo may want it removed. However, they should be aware that after removal, the tattoo will likely be replaced with some type of visible scar. Some patients may be motivated by the dislike of the tattoo by members of the opposite sex. At least 50% of the men in one study of 50 hospitalized psychiatric patients with tattoos reported having female contacts who admitted to disliking their tattoo. Furthermore, 70% of these patients admitted they would not undergo tattooing again.[2]

Emotional Association

Many tattoos are associated with a particular phase or event in a person's life. People who were members of a gang or counterculture group or who have a tattoo bearing the name of a former loved one often seek removal because of the constant memories the tattoo elicits.

Partial Removal

In a significant number of people, removal of only a portion of a tattoo will provide satisfaction. For large tattoos and those found in anatomic locations prone to abnormal scarring, the option of partially removing or modifying a tattoo should be considered. Examples include the removal of a name or obscene word from a larger tattoo or the conversion of a marijuana leaf into a palm tree using partial excision.

PATIENT CONSULTATION

Nonsurgical Options and Expectations

It is often best to first discuss with the tattoo patient the nonsurgical options that are available, including the use of camouflage makeup. The patient should understand that tattoo removal is performed only for patients who are willing to accept the resultant scar that follows the procedure. Often, more than one office visit is required to ensure that the patient understands the advantages and disadvantages of the various techniques available and the results that are likely to be seen. The obvious reason for lengthy explanations, documentation, and queries about comprehension is that the patient must make an informed decision based on a reasonable understanding of the problem and the available treatment options, including doing nothing, and be totally committed to that decision.

Scarring

The patient's past medical history of wound healing should be fully determined. The cutaneous surgeon should examine any old scars to determine whether the patient is particularly susceptible to atrophy, hypopigmentation, or keloid formation. The patient must recognize the evolution that occurs in scars as wounds mature, including the interim and final appearance, size, texture, color, and sensation. Hypertrophic and keloidal scarring should also be discussed in detail.[20, 21] Often, using a marking pen to illustrate on the patient's skin the range of possible results (e.g., a spread, wide atrophic, or hypertrophic scar) is helpful. Patients must fully understand that individual variations in healing make accurate predictions of the final result impossible, no matter what technique is chosen. Furthermore, they should understand that wounds in some anatomic locations may heal better or worse than wounds in other locations, and the possibility of complications such as wound dehiscence, infection, hematoma formation, or contracture may require intralesional steroid injections or revision of the scar at a later date. Any misconception that the various treatment options are trivial procedures should be fully dismissed.

Incomplete Pigment Removal

Whenever nonexcisional techniques for tattoo removal are considered, the patient must be aware that incomplete pigment removal may occur. The objective for these types of procedures should be defined as making the tattoo less obvious or recognizable than the original tattoo. Patient acceptance is often facilitated by explaining the balance between removal of deep pigment and scar production. Generally, the deeper the pigment that is removed, the greater the risk of adverse scarring.

Cost

The cost of tattoo removal is almost always a personal expense, as it is not likely to be covered by the patient's medical insurance except under very unusual circumstances.[22] The estimated expense should be provided, along with some insight as to the training of the cutaneous surgeon and the cost of the staff, facility, materials, and instrumentation required for performing the proposed procedure. Tattoo patients have a notoriously high rate of failure to keep their appointments. Therefore, it is often advisable to require payment for the procedure before the day of surgery. Many cutaneous surgical practices require 50% payment 4 to 6 weeks before surgery and the remainder 2 weeks preoperatively.

Documentation

Thorough repetition and documentation of patient education is essential, with informed consent preferably signed by both the patient and a witness. Photographs showing ink marks that delineate the possible scar lines and widths may also be helpful.

MANNER OF TATTOOING

The tattoo artist and the equipment used to create the tattoo both strongly influence the depth and quantity of pigment present. The commercial tattoo gun may be adjusted to deliver pigment at a variety of depths. The amateur, using pins, needles, or any other available sharp object freehand, has much less control. Commercial tattoos generally have more pigment that is evenly dispersed in the superficial dermis. Amateur tattoo pigment varies in both quantity and location[23] and may even be found in the deep dermis and fat (Fig. 70–1). Traumatic tattoos vary in depth depending on the type of impact and the composition of the embedded material. Generally, tattoos that follow abrasive injuries deposit pigment superficially, whereas tattoos that follow explosive injuries deposit pigment deeply and have small amounts of pigment that radiate from the entry point.[10]

DEPTH

Commercial tattoos are frequently placed at a depth of 0.5 mm.[24] Outlines and darker colors are usually placed first and may be situated more deeply than brighter colors. Such tattoos vary in depth as a result of factors such as the experience of the tattoo artist and the age of the tattoo. Absolute and relative depths of pigment penetration are also influenced by the thickness, elasticity, and laxity of the skin; the amount of pressure applied on the tattoo gun; and the sharpness and number of needles attached. Usually one to three needle points are used for creating outlines, while 5 to 20 needle points may be used for shading large areas. Varying the amount of electrical current applied to the tattoo motor may also dramatically alter needle excursion and depth of pigment deposition.

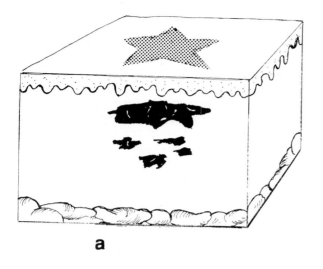 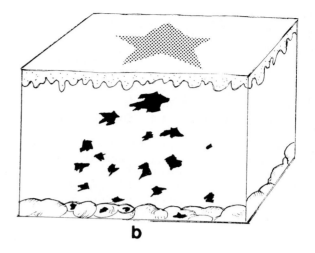

Tattoo Pigment Location: Commercial vs Amateur

Figure 70–1. Commercial tattoos generally have more pigment superficially and evenly dispersed (a), while amateur tattoos have pigment at various depths, including the deep dermis and fat (b).

The depth of amateur tattoos varies greatly, as skill level is lower and less precise instrumentation is utilized. In one study, pigment in amateur tattoos was found at an average depth of 1.04 mm, with a range of 0.48 to 3.2 mm.[25] This range encompasses the upper dermis and the subcutaneous fat. In another study, the mean pigment depth was 1.52 mm.[26] However, in a conflicting study of nine amateur tattoos, pigment was more superficial, occurring at an average depth of 0.88 mm (range, 0.7 to 1.4 mm), whereas in ten professional tattoos, pigment was found at an average depth of 1.17 mm (range, 0.75 to 2.0 mm).[27] The previously mentioned variables help to explain these wide ranges in pigment depths.

Traumatic tattoos are best divided into abrasive and explosive types. Tattoos resulting from abrasions tend to be more superficial, while tattoos from explosions and penetrating trauma place pigment deeply in the skin, with traces left in the entry track.[10]

Depth of pigment, more than any other factor, influences the possibility of tattoo removal with minimal scarring, regardless of the technique used. Gauging the depth of tattoos in advance is difficult. Some cutaneous surgeons advocate performing a punch biopsy on the tattoo before initiating treatment to determine the depth of pigment. However, the sampling error associated with this technique makes the assessment unreliable. If a biopsy is performed and indicates a superficial location for most of the pigment, then thin, split-thickness tangential excision or another superficial technique may be used to minimize scarring. Deep pigmentation favors excision, grafting, or use of one of the newer laser systems.

AGE OF THE TATTOO

Increased age of a tattoo correlates with pigment dispersion horizontally and vertically (Fig. 70–2). The pigment shift occurs gradually over many years. In a commercial tattoo, the majority of pigment initially is quite superficial, usually only 0.05 mm in depth, and densely concentrated. Over time, a significant amount of pigment migrates downward to the mid- and deep dermis. This dispersion accounts for the perceived gradual lightening or black to blue color shift, known as the Tyndall effect, and decreased resolution of tattoo outlines.

Tattoo Pigment Depth Over Time

Figure 70–2. Most pigment is initially superficial and densely concentrated, but with time significant amounts of the pigment migrate downward into the middle and deep dermis, accounting for gradual blurring and lightening.

PIGMENT DENSITY

Local pigment density is also influenced by the original method of administration. Density decreases and dispersion increases with tattoo duration. Pigment localizes near dermal vessels, both in and out of macrophages.[18] Commercial tattoos have a higher pigment density in the outline compared with shaded areas. People with tattoos that have faded after a number of years occasionally have new, dense, superficial pigment added to the less dense areas. Although some amateur tattoos have focal deposits of very high density pigment, they usually contain less pigment that is unevenly distributed. Traumatic tattoos resulting from abrasions vary greatly in pigment density depending on the nature of the original injury and the quantity of pigment that was removed initially as part of the immediate care of the patient. In general, the more localized and superficial the pigment, the easier and more complete will be its removal.

SIZE

The size of a tattoo often dictates the treatment options available. Small tattoos (i.e., less than 2 cm) may be excised with a scalpel or punch and closed with suture or occasionally allowed to heal by second intention. Medium tattoos (2 to 3 cm) may also be excised. However, because large tattoos are commonly found in areas of great tension, excision of them often results in spread, hypertrophic, and atrophic scars. Therefore, split-thickness techniques—including abrasion, caustics, dermal planing, and thermal injury—are frequently chosen for the removal of large tattoos.

SHAPE

Linear tattoos of 5 cm or less in length are often best removed with fusiform excision and primary closure.

Longer tattoos, particularly those not found in close approximation to normal body folds, lines, or creases, are often removed using a broken line or geometric pattern excision. Curvilinear tattoos may be removed with a running W-plasty. In this technique, incisions are made using a more acute angle on the inner aspect of the curved segment than on the corresponding outer aspect to achieve a correct fit. The convex side of the incision line has angles that are more expanded, while angles on the concave side are compressed (Fig. 70–3). A Z-plasty is also beneficial in areas of tension, especially when the direction does not run parallel to an adjacent body line or fold. Many tattoos are round, oval, square, or heart shaped. In these cases, maximal conservation of tissue to achieve closure requires creativity with flap design and tissue movement. An example is an M-plasty or Y-to-V advancement flap, in which two triangles are excised, and the central tissue is advanced with mild or moderate tension. The central tissue is secured with a three-point suture (Fig. 70–4). Other examples of tissue conservation include the O-to-T rotation flap (Fig. 70–5), the A-to-T bilateral advancement flap (Fig. 70–6), and the direct advancement flaps (Figs. 70–6b and 70–7).

LOCATION

Tattoos are rarely found in areas of great skin laxity such as the face or flexural creases. The most common sites are the upper arm, shoulder, and forearm. Excisions in these areas often result in spread scars, and for this reason, some large tattoos found in anatomic locations of high tension are treated with tissue expansion. Although tissue expanders carry a higher risk of complications when used on the extremities than on the head and trunk,[28] their use does permit cautious excision of carefully selected large tattoos in a single-stage pro-

Tattoo Excision: Running W-Plasty

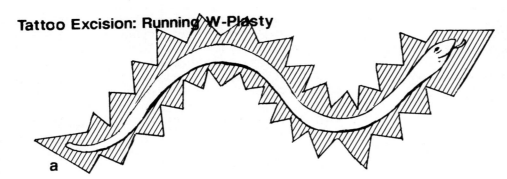

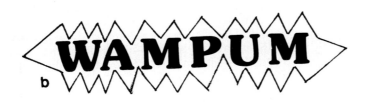

Figure 70–3. *a*, Curvilinear tattoos may be removed with a running W-plasty by making the incisions on the inner aspect more acute or compressed and slightly expanding the corresponding angles of the outer or convex side of the incision line. *b*, Some letters offer an opportunity for tissue conservation and zigzag line excision by placement of peaks and troughs between and within the limbs of each letter.

Heart Tattoo: M-Plasty (Y-V) Advancement

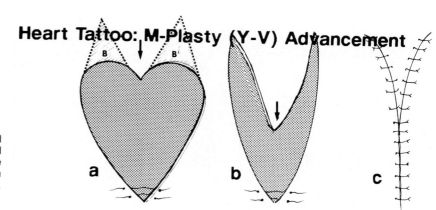

Figure 70–4. The M-plasty makes use of the internal peak of the heart shape so that two triangles, B and B′, are excised to facilitate Y-V advancement of the central tissue, the central tissue being secured with a three-point suture. (From Lindsay DG: Tattoos. Dermatol Clin 7:149–151, 1989.)

cedure. Small superficial tattoos on the digits or digital webs may be treated with excision and primary closure or cryotherapy. Common approaches used to remove tattoos on the extremities when excision is not feasible or desirable include dermabrasion, chemabrasion, dermaplaning or tangential excision, and laser techniques. These approaches all have low rates of surgical complications compared with excisional surgery for large tattoos.

DIRECTION

Determining the best elective incision line is very important in tattoo removal. The likelihood of a thin scar is greatest when the incision line is parallel to relaxed skin tension lines (RSTLs). Relatively linear tattoos that parallel RSTLs or lie close to cosmetic unit boundaries are usually best treated by fusiform excision. More complex excisions should attempt to orient as many lines as possible parallel to RSTLs. Unfavorably directed lines should be made short and oblique to the antitension lines (ATLs). Large tattoos oriented in ATLs are probably best treated by split-thickness injury removal methods, rather than with very large excisions that may produce poor results. Long linear tattoos that run perpendicular to RSTLs may be removed by W-plasty. Tattoos oblique to RSTLs are best revised with a Z-plasty or W-plasty.

COLOR AND COMPOSITION

Composition formulas for commercial tattoos are often secret. However, the main ingredients associated with particular tattoo colors are known. Indian ink or ash is used for black tattoos, cadmium for yellow, chromium for green, cobalt for blue, magnesium and cobalt for violet, mercury for red, and zinc oxide for white; mixtures of these and organic materials are used to make other colors. Ash and Indian ink are carbon-based pigments, whereas the other compounds are metallic or organometallic compounds. Traumatic tattoos are usually composed of tars or petroleum-based products from asphalt. Injuries resulting from close-range gunpowder blasts are generally caused by carbon fragments. Petroleum products vaporize much more easily with the carbon dioxide laser than other substances in the skin. Dark and carbon-based pigments absorb visible and near infrared wavelengths of light much better than do brighter, metallic compounds. Other components of traumatic tattoos include silica, metals, and stones.

AGE OF THE PATIENT

It should be remembered that younger patients are more prone to hypertrophic scarring, especially in areas of high skin tension.

Figure 70–5. For the O-to-T rotation flap, X and Y are advanced and rotated toward the midline, while incisions B and B′ demonstrate two variations of backcuts that allow freer movement of the tissue flaps. (From Lindsay DG: Tattoos. Dermatol Clin 7:149–151, 1989.)

Heart Tattoo: O to T (Rotation)

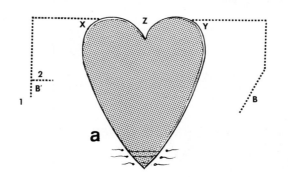
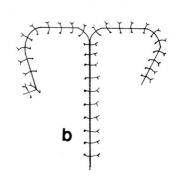

Heart Tattoo: Direct Advancement Flap

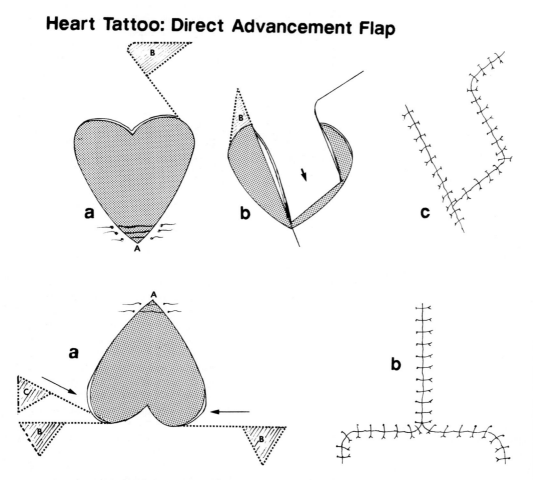

A to T (Bilateral Advancement) Flap

Figure 70–6. *Top*, A standard A-to-T flap is designed with direct advancement of "B" flaps; an alternative method is to make the "C" incision with advancement and rotation. *Bottom*, A direct advancement flap is formed by making two parallel incisions that extend from one outer curve of the heart and from the central peak; the Burow's triangles are made lateral to the advancing flap. (From Lindsay DG: Tattoos. Dermatol Clin 7:149–151, 1989.)

Figure 70–7. *a* to *c*, With a direct advancement flap, the open portions of the "E" define two parallel advancement flaps that are united centrally; laterally based Burow's triangle excisions are performed at B and B'. (From Lindsay DG: Tattoos. Dermatol Clin 7:149–151, 1989.)

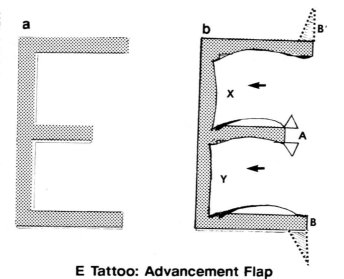

E Tattoo: Advancement Flap

Tattoo Removal and Treatment

Tattoo treatment methods can be grouped into four categories: full-thickness surgical excision, split-thickness injury, tattoo supplementation, and laser surgical techniques.

FULL-THICKNESS SURGICAL EXCISION

Excision With Primary or Flap Closure

The dimension, shape, and location of a tattoo are important considerations in choosing the best form of treatment. Because of varying pigment depth, full-thickness excision offers the only certain method of total pigment removal. Small tattoos (less than 2 cm) usually can be excised and closed in a fusiform shape, with the scar ideally placed in RSTLs. This simple approach is preferable unless tension is excessive or landmark distortion may result. In areas of high tension, such as the ankles or dorsal aspects of the fingers, narrow excision followed by second-intention healing is often better than performing elaborate closures.

This technique is used for simple, small, spread-out groups of letters or figures not amenable to standard excision.[25] A scalpel is used to narrowly trace around the tattoo and excise as superficially as possible above the subcutaneous fat. Second-intention healing occurs in 4 to 8 weeks. The drawback of this technique is the scar, which will be in the shape of the original tattoo. Medium tattoos (2 to 4 cm) may also be excised. However, serial excision, flaps, and zigzag closure techniques may need to be used to distribute tension and improve a lengthy, uninterrupted scar line. Excision and closure of large or medium tattoos in areas where tension is high requires consideration of flaps and zigzag closure. This may include the use of tissue expansion, Z-plasty, W-plasty, and permanent buried suture to provide prolonged wound support.[29–32] For areas of high tension, white, soft, nonabsorbable suture material (e.g., Nurolon) is placed in the deep dermis at least several millimeters from the incision line. This provides prolonged support despite some relaxation from tissue stretch and some gradual cutting of the suture through tissue. For tattoos on the back, smaller scars can be achieved by using narrow excision and second-intention healing, rather than primary closure.[33] It should be remembered that the larger the area excised and the greater the resultant tension, the more likely it is that complications (i.e., dehiscence; hypertrophic, spread, and atrophic scars; and wound contracture) will develop. If excision and closure are not feasible or would result in unacceptable deformity, then split-thickness grafting, laser treatment, or tattoo modifications are the remaining options. These treatments may be safely applied to any size tattoo, but with less chance of complete pigment removal than excision, more discomfort, and slower healing.

Serial Excision

Serial excision typically requires two or more procedures to accomplish complete pigment removal. The surgical risks of a one-stage procedure may be reduced by allowing 8 weeks or more between excisional stages. The drawbacks of a multistage procedure are cost and time. Cumulative temporary disability at work may also be incurred in certain occupations. Several techniques can be used to determine the amount of tissue that can be safely removed at each session. By simply pinching the skin together, a rough but reasonably accurate estimate of the tension present at the anatomic site can be made. Alternatively, after cutting one side of a fusiform incision with the scalpel and undermining, skin hooks or towel clamps are used to pull the tattooed skin across the incision line. The excess tissue is then excised, and the wound is closed primarily.

Full-Thickness Excision and Split-Thickness Skin Graft Closure

Split-thickness skin grafting (STSG) after full-thickness excision is reserved for the removal of large tattoos unsuited to other removal techniques.[24, 34–36] This technique is based on the observation that many tattoos have deep and variably distributed pigment. The tissue is completely removed, and a free skin graft is applied to hasten healing, decrease pain, and reduce wound contraction. Donor tissue may be thin (0.008 inch), intermediate (0.012 inch), or thick (0.024 inch). Thick graft tissue will fill the recipient bed more readily, but the donor site will heal more slowly and result in worse scarring. The technique is rapid, safe, and uses standard skin grafting equipment and techniques. A dermatome may be used to harvest grafts of 3 to 8 cm. Individual grafts may be secured together or meshed in a ratio of up to 3:1 to cover larger areas. Moist healing using occlusive, transparent, nonadherent dressings is fastest and least uncomfortable. This type of dressing is applied a minimum of 2 to 3 cm beyond the donor bed. Excess serous exudate may need to be drained once or twice in the first postoperative week. Healing of the donor site is usually complete in 2 weeks for thin to intermediate grafts, but 3 to 4 weeks may be required for thick donor sites.

The major drawbacks of this technique are the creation of a donor site, which is associated with delayed healing and eventual scar formation; undesirable sunken contour of the recipient site; and poor color and texture of the final scar. Alternative methods such as tangential excision with second-intention healing remove a high percentage of pigment and may provide good cosmetic and functional results.

Punch Excision

Punch excision is a variation of full-thickness excision that uses a biopsy or hair transplant punch to remove small tattoos. Sutured closure, second-intention healing, or punch graft transplantation may be used to repair the defect. This technique is rapid, uses readily available materials, and is easily performed. Most published work on this subject concerns traumatic tattoos,[11] but the technique also has high utility for small facial dot tattoos or small complex figures. Cosmetic results vary from excellent to very good or average, depending on tattoo size, closure technique, and local tension.

SPLIT-THICKNESS INJURY

Chemical Peeling, Salabrasion, Chemabrasion, and Overtattooing

Medical treatment of tattoos first used chemical methods. Ancient Greek and Roman physicians used insect vesicants, garlic, salt, uric acid, citric and acetic acids, lye, sulfuric acid, and other substances to produce an inflammatory reaction.[37] These substances were frequently pricked or scratched into the skin to augment penetration. When applied by tattoo artists, this process is termed overtattooing.

In 1888, a method popularized by Variot and known as the French Method used tannic acid and silver nitrate, which were scratched into the original tattoo. This method was modified by applying tannic acid with superficial dermabrasion and then applying silver nitrate.[38] Dermabrasion was a much quicker way to introduce tannic acid than overtattooing. Results showed that 70 to 80% of patients had complete or nearly complete pigment removal, and 90% had an excellent to very good scar. Another study of overtattooing compared tannic acid with other substances such as oxalic acid. Results with oxalic acid were as good or better than those with tannic acid, which indicated that nonspecific inflammation was the key.[39]

The ancient technique employed by the Greek physician Aetius (543 AD), using table salt, was revived in 1935 and named salabrasion in 1971.[27, 40] Since that time, salabrasion has been advocated as one of several leading methods of tattoo removal.[24, 27, 41–47] Varying the times of salt application and using short application times was reported[27] to cause less scarring but leave far more pigment behind. It is important to recognize the unpredictability of the necrosis depth with prolonged application. Some patients who had undergone 4 hours of salt application had more than double the necrosis depth of patients who had undergone 12 or 24 hours of application. However, the depth of necrosis very clearly correlates with the severity of scarring. In addition, darker tattoos, along with those on the hand, seem to respond poorly.[46]

In this technique, several wet 4 × 4 gauze squares are wrapped tightly around the surgeon's gloved fingers inside a standard surgical glove. Coarse salt is applied to the gauze and vigorously massaged over the tattoo. As the epidermis is removed, the papillary vessels become noticeable, and erythema begins to spread in the adjacent skin. In general, immediate removal of the salt being used for abrasion is advisable. Alternatively, the epidermis can be removed with very superficial dermabrasion using a dermabrader. Salt is then applied under a wet gauze for 3 to 5 minutes to induce a suitable inflammatory response, which is manifested by erythema at the margins and prominent edema of the dermal papillae. Some physicians prefer longer applications for more pigment removal.

The use of trichloroacetic acid or phenol peeling is analagous to the use of other caustics. Familiarity gained with pure agents or mixtures such as Baker's formula in facial peels is helpful. The distal extremities require use of a weaker solution than is used for truncal skin. Standard small, cotton-tipped applicators are used to apply the peeling agent of choice. The depth of the peel injury and the slough are likely defined after 48 hours. The effects of peeling agents[48] are significantly enhanced by tape occlusion. Taping for 24 to 48 hours, followed by painting with 2% gentian violet and daily dry dressing changes, has also been advocated.[49]

Peels are typically helpful only for very superficial tattoos but cause considerable pain and pigmentary abnormalities. Discomfort and healing time are reduced by the use of antibacterial ointment and nonadherent dressings. The advantages of this technique are low cost, ease of application, and simple aftercare. Disadvantages include varying responses, pigmentary changes, and restriction to superficial tattoos.

Urea is a natural product of protein metabolism that produces mild irritation and protein degradation. Uric acid and urea were used in various forms and concentrations in the ancient practice of tattoo removal.

Dermabrasion

Modern mechanical abrasion for tattoos was first reported in 1963.[50] This technique attempted removal of all pigment and, for that reason, often went deeply enough to produce full-thickness injury. Even without penetration to the subcutaneous fat, very deep dermabrasion provokes hypertrophic scar formation frequently. Subsequently, some authors[51, 52] modified the procedure by using only superficial abrasion. Small areas of the tattoo are frozen with spray refrigerant, and the epidermis is removed. The tattoo becomes darker, and the surface tissue glistens. At this point the abrasion is stopped. Various dressings are then applied, but gentian violet painting is no longer a necessary part of the procedure. The inflammatory reaction and exudative process remove a great deal of pigment through the skin surface or into the lymphatic channels. In addition, some is relocated in the deeper dermis. The combined effects of these pathways results in dramatic lightening of the tattoo. Adjunctive procedures can be used to aid pigment removal without increasing the risk of scarring. One of these[53] uses curettage or forceps to remove focal pigment deposits. Studies have shown[24] that dextranomer beads or drying dressings did not lead to appreciably increased pigment removal. This understanding led to refinements in dressing protocols, which resulted in more physiologic wound healing with antibacterial ointments and occlusive synthetic surgical dressings.[54–56]

Dermabrasion for tattoo removal permits graduated margins to feather the treated area into the surrounding normal skin. It also permits the creation of an oval, round, or rectangular shape to help further diguise the original tattoo and make it appear more like a traumatic abrasion injury. Moist healing makes the postoperative period relatively painless, and dressing changes are quick and easy for the patient. The necessary equipment is readily available and relatively inexpensive. The primary disadvantages of dermabrasion include irregular depth; focal scarring; production of potential infectious aerosols from body fluids, which requires the surgeon and all assistants to wear face masks and gowns for protection during the procedure; and meticulous cleaning of the operatory after completion of the procedure.

Electrosurgery and the Infrared Coagulator

Mechanical and thermal techniques are among the oldest and simplest means of tattoo removal. The main instruments used include various types of electrosurgical devices and the infrared coagulator (IRC). Electrofulguration is the most superficial form of electrosurgery. When this technique is used for tattoo removal, the lowest settings are chosen, and continuous movement of the tip provides dispersion of the arc as evenly as possible. The white coagulated tissue is wiped away. Several passes are performed, depending on the tissue thickness and estimated depth of the tattoo. A dressing is then applied. No attempt is made to completely remove the pigment, as significant pigment removal occurs during healing. The risk of scarring with electrosurgery is generally thought to be higher than with most other techniques. The unpredictability of electrical injury and the lack of precision are the primary reasons this technique is rarely used.

The IRC was studied as a comparable but less expensive alternative to the carbon dioxide laser for tattoo treatment. The near-infrared output (900 to 960 nm), timeable pulsed operation, and ability to confine the area of heat damage to the 6-mm sapphire tip[57] all suggested that this might be an effective tool. Preliminary measurements showed that a pulse width of 0.75 seconds produced necrosis to a depth of 0.25 mm, while a pulse of 1.25 seconds produced necrosis to a depth of 1.16 mm. Complete or nearly complete tattoo removal with a single treatment was reported in 66% of treated patients. Retreatment of the remaining patients also had a 66% success rate. Other studies showed that the mechanisms involved direct tissue necrosis, pigment removal by exudate and inflammatory cells, and scar camouflaging of residual pigment as a result of the reduced transparency of scar tissue.[26]

A comparison with the carbon dioxide laser found more complete removal and better visualization with the laser, but with its equivalent scarring, lower cost, and smaller size, the IRC remains a viable treatment modality.[58] Also, because a plume is not created, no smoke evacuator is required. A sterile operative field is also not required, because an open wound is not produced during the procedure. Postoperative dressings are minimal with this technique.

Despite the low cost and ease of use of electrosurgical and IRC devices, dermabrasion, tangential excision, and laser techniques are still preferred. This is primarily a function of the fact that electrosurgery causes worse scarring, and there is better visualization, greater precision and less nonspecific thermal injury with the laser.

Overgrafting and Tangential Excision

The drawbacks of full-thickness excision of tattoos and standard STSG covering of the resultant wound bed prompted the use of a dermatome in a different technique.[34] A thin STSG overlying the tattoo was partially harvested. Then the remaining dermis was excised and the STSG returned back to its original bed. It was hoped that the STSG would not retain tattoo pigment, thereby providing a same-site donor graft for tattoo removals. Instead, this study showed that the pigment was retained throughout the dermis. Just as importantly, the inflammation from wound healing incompletely removed the remaining pigment from the tattooed portion of the STSG.

The next logical step was to perform split-thickness excision and overgraft with a nontattooed STSG. Healing was faster and skin texture improved, with some pigment removed during healing. The white color of the healed graft disguised much, but not all, of the deeper residual pigment, and healing and scarring at the donor site remained problems. It was clear that second-intention healing, as in dermabrasion,[50] allowed more pigment removal. In many cases, better cosmetic and functional results were obtainable from tangential split-thickness excision of the tattoo bed, without incurring a donor site scar.[59] The technique used is that of standard STSG harvesting. Because pigment depth varies greatly, planning is repeated once, after using standard initial dermatome settings, if substantial deeper pigment remains.[54] Recommended settings are 0.008 to 0.014 inches for the forearm and 0.016 to 0.022 inches for the trunk, deltoid, and thigh. Forceps removal of any notable focal pigment deposits is performed at the conclusion of planing, and a polyurethane dressing is placed. Satisfactory scars have been reported, and only occasional minimal pigment has been discernible. Hypertrophic scars requiring steroid treatment have been noted in 10% of patients.

A more recent modification of the tangential excision technique is referred to as epidermal sheet grafting.[60] In this technique, an intermediate to thick (0.2-mm) split-thickness skin graft is removed from the tattoo and meshed. The graft is subjected to dispase enzymatic digestion of hemidesmosomes at the dermal-epidermal junction, resulting in a pure epidermal sheet graft. The epidermal sheet is then applied as a free graft to the wound bed. Healing of the grafted site is complete in 4 days, but the nongrafted portion requires several weeks to heal. The advantages of tangential excision are greater rapidity of healing, lower cost, and reduced surgical risk than with full-thickness excision. Tangential excision with the dermatome appears to have greater precision, control, and predictability as a result of reproducible settings and technique than caustics or dermabrasion. Disadvantages include requirement of a dermatome, familiarity with its use, production of a rectangular scar, and a substantial risk of hypertrophic scarring. In areas of higher scarring risk that require a second pass of the dermatome, overgrafting may remain an option to reduce hypertrophic scar formation and speed healing. In any case, the possible need for intralesional steroid injections should be discussed with the patient before surgery.

Cryosurgery

Cryosurgery using liquid nitrogen[49] for successful tattoo removal has been reported.[61, 62] Liquid nitrogen spray or a cryoprobe chilled to −196°C is applied to the tattooed area. Anesthesia is obtained by the treatment itself, although discomfort is significant during freezing and thawing. In this procedure, a cryoprobe is applied with pressure against the skin for two freeze-thaw cycles of 60 seconds each. In one study,[61] 6 of 11 patients had satisfactory results, but in the remaining patients the tattoo was still obvious. Retreatment later helped only two of these five patients achieve a satisfactory result. The spray technique allows visualization of the area while treating. Movement of the spray may permit a more uniform depth of injury than can be obtained with a probe. When treating areas on the hands, care should be taken to avoid freezing the periosteum and extensor tendons. Multiple dry ice applications have also been tried, with limited success. Atrophy, hypopigmentation, and hyperpigmentation are usual with cryosurgery. Despite the low cost and relative simplicity of cryosurgery, it is generally less effective than other methods and is rarely used except for superficial or digital tattoos.[35]

TATTOO SUPPLEMENTATION

In some tattoos an acceptable result can be obtained by modification with additional tattooing. Variations include changing letters, clothing nude figures, or superimposing pigments to disguise details. Patients may also choose to remove the objectionable parts of a tattoo as much as possible, followed by retattooing to change or further camouflage the offending part. Contact dermatitis to the red dye implanted in a tattoo caused one patient to have only the red pigment removed; and this area was then retattooed using a different color.[63]

LASER SURGICAL TECHNIQUES

Visible Light Lasers

The imperfect results of tattoo removal methods have led to a search for new tools. Since the early 1960s, the laser has been continuously investigated for treating tattoos using a number of different wavelengths, exposure parameters, techniques, and postsurgical care (see Chapters 72 and 73). Trials using the argon laser for tattoo removal soon followed early attempts with the ruby and neodymium:yttrium-aluminum-garnet (Nd:YAG) lasers.[64] The blue-green light from the argon laser, with peak emissions at 488 nm and 514 nm, was demonstrated to be well absorbed by dark pigments, including tattoo dyes.[65] Even in very early studies, argon laser tattoo treatments were noted to cause scarring in virtually all cases.[66] Textural and pigmentary changes may be comparable to those produced by other tech-

niques, but in some cases may be worse.[67] Multiple treatments are typically required, and up to 75% of patients retain a ghost image of the tattoo. The mechanisms proposed for fading of tattoos after argon laser treatment include vaporization of particles in the upper dermis when high-power densities are used,[49, 65] chemical changes of the heated pigment, nonspecific inflammatory removal or relocation of pigment, and optical shielding by scar tissue,[68] which is produced during repair after treatment (Fig. 70–8). An animal study of experimental traumatic tattoos in guinea pigs showed no significant difference between removal by argon or carbon dioxide lasers, overgrafting, and dermabrasion.[69] The argon "chemolaser" technique,[70] which uses topical urea after laser treatment, achieved better results than the argon laser alone. Because of discomfort, lack of pigment removal, the multiple treatments required, the ultimate results achieved, and the price of the equipment, the benefits from using the argon laser for tattoo removal are minimal.

The Carbon Dioxide Laser

The carbon dioxide laser is precisely absorbed by the intracellular and extracellular water of the skin. This precision translates into the removal of a thin layer of tissue (0.1 to 0.2 mm thick) with a surrounding 0.1 to 0.2-mm zone of edema, which signifies reversible cellular injury.[71] These limits of precision theoretically allow removal of a single cell only 30 to 40 microns thick.[72] One method that provides even greater precision is superpulsing, which delivers extremely high-energy pulses as short as 0.0001 second.[73] In one study of 15 tattoo patients, utilization of the carbon dioxide laser resulted in satisfactory to excellent results in 11 of the patients.[72] Despite the precision of this laser technique, scarring does occur and frequently requires intralesional steroid injections and compression to obtain resolution.

Continuous Carbon Dioxide Laser Technique

The first approach to carbon dioxide laser removal of tattoos employed continuous wave delivery of energy.[74–78] Usually, rapid oscillating movements with the handpiece are repeated over the figure until all tattoo pigment is removed (Fig. 70–9). The first layer removed is almost exclusively epidermis, and the underlying tattoo initially appears darker and brighter. The tattoo shape breaks up, and areas become clear as sequential passes remove more pigment.

Pulsed Carbon Dioxide Laser Technique

The pulsed technique offers more safety and precision for thin skin areas, very superficial or small tattoos, and for laser surgeons with less experience in tattoo removal.[72] One drawback of the pulsed technique compared with continuous delivery is the slow rate of tissue removal. Contiguous, slightly overlapping pulses are delivered in repeat pulse mode, moving in a grid follow-

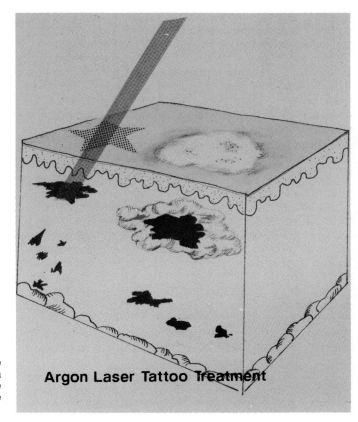

Argon Laser Tattoo Treatment

Figure 70-8. The argon beam causes widespread injury to the epidermis and superficial dermis, so that during tissue repair a superficial band of fibrotic scar forms that optically screens the residual pigment, even though most of it remains unchanged in the dermis.

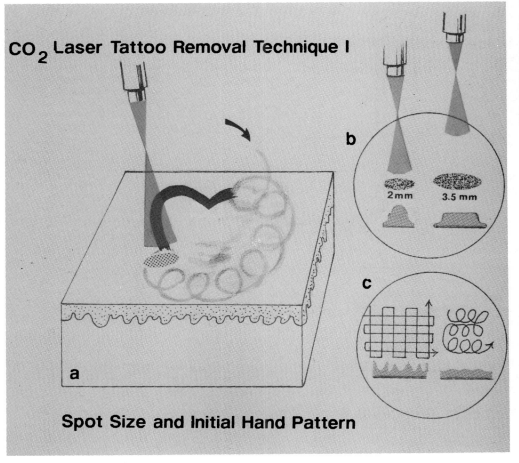

CO_2 Laser Tattoo Removal Technique I

Spot Size and Initial Hand Pattern

Figure 70-9. *a*, The laser handpiece is moved with a rapid, continuous circular motion, using a large beam and adequate power density to achieve instantaneous vaporization. *b*, A larger beam produces a defect with a blunt power profile. *c*, The overlapping circles trace the tattoo shape concentrically or with a grid pattern to yield a more even tissue profile.

ing the outlines of the tattoo. At least three or four passes, covering the entire tattoo, are made. Moist gauze is used to scrub away any adherent char between passes. Subsequent passes become more selective to deeply pigmented areas that remain darker, since more superficial pigment is cleared. Passes continue until all or most pigment is removed. Adjacent tissue is vaporized as necessary to disguise the obvious tattoo design.

Combined Continuous and Pulsed Technique

This technique uses continuous wave delivery of laser energy until approximately 90% of pigment is removed. The beam is then focused to a 0.2-mm spot and a pulse duration of 0.05 second and power settings of 5 to 10 watts are selected. Small amounts of residual pigment are usually shed in the postoperative exudate. By selecting repeat-pulse mode, it is possible to remove specific focal areas of pigment deposition. Magnifying loupes are often beneficial. Spot vaporization of prominent pigment depots is performed thus, but not all pigment is removed (Fig. 70–10). Residual islands of tissue within the original tattoo margins are reduced to intermediate thickness. The outlines of the tattoo are blended into the surrounding skin by graduating the margins. Whenever possible, a simple graphic shape such as an oval, circle, or rectangle is produced, since these shapes appear more natural than a square or triangle and may resemble an accidental traumatic event such as a burn or abrasion.

Combined Carbon Dioxide Laser and Urea Technique

In this technique, the carbon dioxide is used to remove the epidermis, superficial dermis, and only 30 to 50% of the total pigment.[79] The shape of the tattoo margin is then camouflaged, and 50% urea in hydrophilic ointment is applied daily under nonadherent dressings. Ointment application is continued for an average of 10 days or until the pigment is eliminated. The primary mechanism suggested for the action of urea is protein degradation through covalent bond disruption. It has also been suggested that urea acts as a hygroscopic agent that causes the rupture of macrophages and more loss of pigment in the exudate.[80] Advantages of this technique include greater speed and cost effectiveness, as well as improved cosmetic results.

Nd:YAG Laser

The Nd:YAG laser energy is preferentially absorbed by dark pigments, which is the theoretical basis for its use in tattoo removal.[65, 81] However, the non–Q-switched 1064-nm wavelength scatters greatly in cutaneous tissue, causing deep and widespread tissue coagulation and necrosis similar to that caused by the argon laser.[82, 83] The Q-switched Nd:YAG laser can be used to effectively remove black tattoo pigments at its 1064-nm wavelength and red tattoo pigments with its frequency-doubled 532-nm green wavelength without scarring.

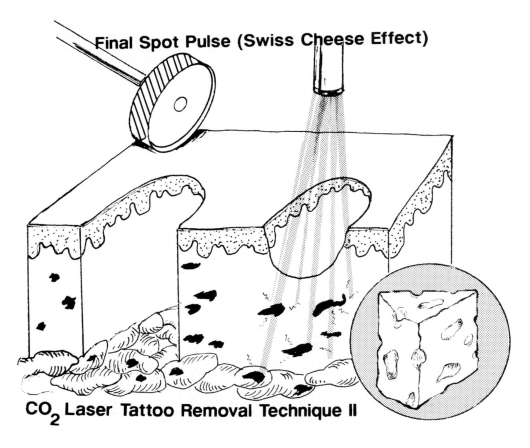

Final Spot Pulse (Swiss Cheese Effect)

CO_2 **Laser Tattoo Removal Technique II**

Figure 70–10. The technique that uses the carbon dioxide laser for tattoo removal employs short pulses with small spot size to vaporize most of the pigment deposits visible in the dermis. The goal is to create a Swiss cheese effect, or an intact dermal framework with only small focal defects.

Ruby and Alexandrite Lasers

The ruby laser was the first laser system to be investigated as a possible useful device for treating tattoos.[64] The 694-nm red light is capable of deep dermal penetration and substantial absorption by melanin and dark pigments. The Q-switched ruby laser allows the delivery of high-energy, short, 20- to 40-nanosecond pulses. Temperature increases measured in peripheral tissue from treatment with the Q-switched ruby laser were limited. Minimal peripheral injury was detected, whereas tattoo pigment fragmentation with rupture of macrophages and subsequent clearance were seen in tattoos.[84-88]

Another solid-state, Q-switched laser system, the alexandrite (755-nm) laser, has properties very similar to those of the ruby laser. It has also been used to effectively remove tattoo pigments without scarring.

The mechanisms offered to explain improvement in tattoos include mechanical or photoacoustic fragmentation and dispersion of pigment, extrusion of pigment fragments through the epidermis or into the fat, removal by the lymphatics, and chemical destruction or transformation to colorless compounds, referred to as photopyrolysis (Fig. 70–11). The mechanisms by which selective damage occurs in tattoo and other pigments have been further verified by looking at lasers other than the Q-switched ruby (e.g., the flashlamp-pumped pulsed dye laser, the picosecond–pulsed mode–locked Nd:YAG laser, and the nanosecond pulsed ultraviolet Excimer laser).[89-91] All of these rapid pulsing lasers can deliver high enough energy in short enough bursts so that selective absorption by the pigment results in mechanical destruction.

Although clinical studies defining optimal protocols are still in progress, energy fluences of from 2 to 8 joules/cm^2 have been found to yield the best results without scarring or permanent pigmentary abnormalities.[92] The threshold dose is indicated by an immediate whitening of the epidermis, and the pulses are administered with a slightly overlapping technique to avoid leaving some pigment untreated. Many patients can tolerate the discomfort readily without a need for local anesthesia. However, it should be available, particularly for large tattoos or those located on sensitive areas. Dressings are usually not necessary. An emollient cream for lubrication decreases post-treatment scaling and possible itching. If any focal erosion develops, antibiotic ointment covered by a nonadherent bandage is sufficient. Residual tattoo pigment can be retreated at 6-week intervals; treatments at 1-week intervals have been documented to cause scarring.[86]

In addition to absorption of ruby laser energy by tattoo pigments, there is also absorption by melanin pigment, which could lead to permanent hypopigmentation. Post-treatment hypopigmentation is more often noticeable in darker patients but usually resolves within 6 months. Postinflammatory hyperpigmentation is more common in patients with darker skin and usually shows gradual improvement. Scarring is a rare event, seen in only one patient who had been retattooed, and even then this only consisted of a very minor textural change.[88]

The number of ruby laser treatments necessary and

Figure 70–11. The Q-switched ruby laser pulses cause photo-acoustic fragmentation and dispersion of pigment from macrophages and fibroblasts, resulting in extrusion of pigment in the crust or into the fat.

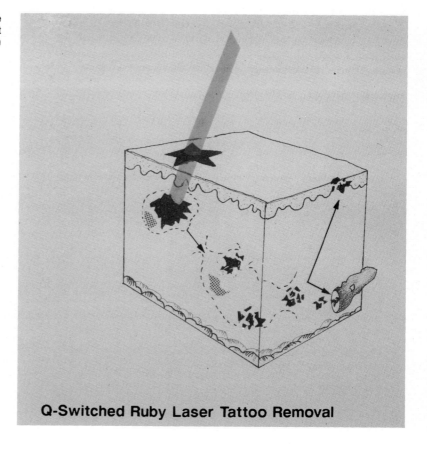

Q-Switched Ruby Laser Tattoo Removal

the degree of success depends on many factors. The most important factor appears to be the tattoo pigment composition. Generally, blue and black carbon-based tattoo pigments will respond best with the fewest treatments. Commercial tattoos with red, yellow, and green colors improve less, even with higher doses of laser energy, perhaps because of poorer absorption or greater stability of these compounds. The end result is variable and cannot be predicted. In addition, older tattoos respond more favorably than new ones.

Advantages of Q-switched ruby, Nd:YAG, and alexandrite laser treatment of tattoos include a more selective, nonscarring approach for large tattoos of any type and for amateur tattoos with deep pigment. The risks of Q-switched ruby laser treatment are minimal in comparison with those posed by other current modalities. Disadvantages include equipment cost and space, multiple retreatments, and incomplete removal in many cases, especially of the organometallic pigments used to produce red, yellow, and bright green colors.

SUMMARY

Selection of the ideal method for tattoo treatment will continue to be a challenging decision for both the cutaneous surgeon and the patient. It requires balancing the degree of pigment removal desired with the scarring risk, cost, number of treatments, availability of modalities, and morbidity. New treatments are being developed, and current therapies are undergoing refinement. At present there is no one right removal technique for all tattoos. The best decision must consider the patient's goals and resource priorities, including cost, time, convenience, and cosmetic appearance of the healed site. This requires a dedicated effort by the cutaneous surgeon to provide detailed information to the patient so that true informed consent can be obtained.

REFERENCES

1. Levy J, Sewell M, Goldstein N: A short history of tattooing. J Dermatol Surg Oncol 5:851–856, 1979.
2. Goldstein N: Psychological implications of tattoos. J Dermatol Surg Oncol 5:883–888, 1979.
3. Bourgeois M, Penaud F: Survey of voluntary tattooing: analytic study of 43 Navy recruits. Ann Med Psychol (Paris) 1:683–705, 1975.
4. Ibrulj PD, Vasiljevic T: Socio-medical aspects of tattooing and motivations for its removal. Med Arh 42:47–49, 1988.
5. Pers M, Herbst TV: The demand for removal of tattoos. A plea for regulations against tattooing of minors. Acta Chir Scand 131:201–204, 1966.
6. Regoje D, Ibrulj PD: Reasons for tattooing, methods of removal and the socio-medical significance of tattooing. Med Arh 36:27–30, 1982.
7. Thomson W, McDonald JC: Self-tattooing by schoolchildren. Lancet 2:1243–1244, 1983.
8. Hanke CW, Conner AC, Probst EL Jr, Fondak AA: Blast tattoos resulting from black powder firearms. J Am Acad Dermatol 17:819–825, 1987.
9. Fuchs T, Zacker KD: Dirt tattooing following an explosion in a chemistry class. Derm Beruf Umwelt 32:138–140, 1984.
10. Agris J: Traumatic tattooing. J Trauma 16:798–802, 1976.
11. Kaufmann R: The mini-punch technic: a method for late removal of traumatic facial tattooing. Hautarzt 41:149–150, 1990.
12. Goldstein N, Sewell M: Tattoos in different cultures. J Dermatol Surg Oncol 5:857–864, 1979.
13. Goldstein N, Muller G, Tuttle L: Modern applications of tattoos. J Dermatol Surg Oncol 5:889–891, 1979.
14. Goldstein N: Laws and regulations relating to tattoos. J Dermatol Surg Oncol 5:913–916, 1979.
15. Blasi B, Caccavari R: Clinico-criminological aspects of tattoo removal. Acta Biomed Ateneo Parmense 52:263–267, 1981.
16. Fisher JC: Development of a plastic surgical teaching service in a women's correctional institution. Am J Surg 129:269–272, 1975.
17. Goldstein N: Complications from tattoos. J Dermatol Surg Oncol 5:869–878, 1979.
18. Goldstein N: Histologic reactions in tattoos. J Dermatol Surg Oncol 5:896–900, 1979.
19. Robinson JK: Tattoo removal. J Dermatol Surg Oncol 11:14–16, 1985.
20. Zimmerman MC: Suits for malpractice based on alleged unsightly scars resulting from removal of tattoos. J Dermatol Surg Oncol 5:911–912, 1979.
21. Brahams D: Affirmation of serious professional misconduct for failure to provide proper care after tattoo removal by laser. Lancet 2:8405, 1984.
22. Meyburg OV: Compensation for removals of tattoos. Lakartidningen 66:970–971, 1969.
23. Grosser A, Konz B, Landthaler M: Possibilities for tattoo removal. Report of experiences. Fortschr Med 100:687–693, 1982.
24. Arellano CR, Leopold DA, Shafiroff BB: Tattoo removal: comparative study of six methods in the pig. Plast Reconstr Surg 70:699–703, 1982.
25. Harrison PV: The surgical removal of amateur tattoos. Clin Exp Dermatol 10:540–544, 1985.
26. Venning VA, Colver GB, Millard PR, Ryan TJ: Tattoo removal using infra-red coagulation: a dose comparison. Br J Dermatol 117:99–105, 1987.
27. Koerber WJ, Price NM: Salabrasion of tattoos. A correlation of the clinical and histological results. Arch Dermatol 114:884–888, 1978.
28. Hallock G: Refinement of the radial forearm flap donor site using skin expansion. Plast Reconstr Surg 81:21–25, 1988.
29. Nordstrom RE, Nordstrom RM: Absorbable versus nonabsorbable sutures to prevent postoperative stretching of wound area. Plast Reconstr Surg 78:186–190, 1986.
30. Nordstrom RE: "Stretch-back" in scalp reductions for male pattern baldness. Plast Reconstr Surg 73:422–426, 1984.
31. Rudolph R: Wide spread scars, hypertrophic scars, and keloids. Clin Plast Surg 14:253–260, 1987.
32. Elliot D: The stretched scar: the benefit of prolonged dermal support. Br J Plast Surg 42:74–78, 1989.
33. Barnett R, Stranc M: A method of producing improved scars following excision of small lesions of the back. Ann Plast Surg 3:391–394, 1979.
34. Gupta SC: An investigation into a method for the removal of dermal tattoos: a report on animal and clinical studies. Plast Reconstr Surg 36:354–361, 1965.
35. Goldstein N, Penoff J, Price N, et al: Techniques of removal of tattoos. J Dermatol Surg Oncol 5:901–910, 1979.
36. Goldstein N: Tattoo removal. Dermatol Clin 5:349–358, 1987.
37. Shie MD: A study of tattooing and methods of removal. JAMA 90:94, 1928.
38. Penoff JH: The office treatment of tattoos: a simple and effective method. Plast Reconstr Surg 79:186–191, 1987.
39. Fogh H, Wulf HC, Poulsen T, Larsen P: Tattoo removal by overtattooing with tannic acid. J Dermatol Surg Oncol 15:1089–1090, 1989.
40. Crittenden FR Jr: Salabrasion: removal of tattoos by superficial abrasion with table salt. Cutis 7:295–300, 1971.
41. Horn W: Effects of tattoo removal and results after salabrasion. Z Hautkr 58:336–342, 1983.
42. Johannesson A: A simplified method of focal salabrasion for removal of linear tattoos. J Dermatol Surg Oncol 11:1004–1005, 1985.
43. Levine H, Bailin P: Carbon dioxide laser treatment of cutaneous hemangiomas and tattoos. Arch Otolaryngol 108:236–238, 1982.
44. Manchester GH: The removal of commercial tattoos by abrasion with table salt. Plast Reconstr Surg 53:517–521, 1974.

45. Shelley WB, Shelley ED: Focal salabrasion for removal of linear tattoos. J Dermatol Surg Oncol 10:216–218, 1984.
46. Strong AM, Jackson IT: The removal of amateur tattoos by salabrasion. Br J Dermatol 101:693–696, 1979.
47. Lindsay DG: Tattoos. Dermatol Clin 7:147–153, 1989.
48. Stegman SJ, Tromovitch TA: Cosmetic dermatologic surgery. Arch Dermatol 118:1013–1016, 1982.
49. Apfelberg DB, Manchester GH: Decorative and traumatic tattoo biophysics and removal. Clin Plast Surg 14:243–251, 1987.
50. Chai KB: The decorative tattoo: its removal by dermabrasion. Plast Reconstr Surg 32:559–563, 1963.
51. Clabaugh W: Removal of tattoos by superficial dermabrasion. Arch Dermatol 98:515–521, 1968.
52. Clabaugh WA: Tattoo removal by superficial dermabrasion. Five-year experience. Plast Reconstr Surg 55:401–405, 1975.
53. Ceilley RI: Curettage after dermabrasion—techniques of removal of tattoos. J Dermatol Surg Oncol 5:905, 1979.
54. Wheeland RG, Norwood OT, Roundtree JM: Tattoo removal using serial tangential excision and polyurethane membrane dressing. J Dermatol Surg Oncol 9:822–826, 1983.
55. Alt TH: Technical aids for dermabrasion. J Dermatol Surg Oncol 13:638–648, 1987.
56. Cramers M: Wound dressing after skin planning. Acta Derm Venereol (Stockh) 69:453–454, 1989.
57. Colver GB, Cherry GW, Dawber RPR, Ryan TJ: Tattoo removal using infra-red coagulation. Br J Dermatol 112:481–485, 1985.
58. Groot DW, Arlette JP, Johnston PA: Comparison of the infrared coagulator and the carbon dioxide laser in the removal of decorative tattoos. J Am Acad Dermatol 15:518–522, 1986.
59. Wheeler ES, Miller TA: Tattoo removal by split thickness tangential excision. West J Med 124:272–275, 1976.
60. Hosokawa K: Treatment of tattoos with pure epidermal sheet grafting. Ann Plast Surg 24:53–60, 1984.
61. Colver GB, Dawber RP: Tattoo removal using a liquid nitrogen cryospray. Clin Exp Dermatol 9:364–366, 1984.
62. Dvir E, Hirshowitz B: Tattoo removal by cryosurgery. Plast Reconstr Surg 66:373–379, 1980.
63. Brodell RT: Retattooing after the treatment of a red tattoo reaction with the CO_2 laser. J Dermatol Surg Oncol 16:771, 1990.
64. Goldman L, Blaney DJ, Kindel DJ, et al: Effect of the laser beam on the skin, preliminary report. J Invest Dermatol 40:121–122, 1963.
65. Goldman L: Laser treatment of tattoos: a preliminary survey of three years' clinical experience. JAMA 201:163–166, 1967.
66. Apfelberg DB, Maser MR, Lash H, et al: Progress report on extended clinical use of the argon laser for cutaneous lesions. Lasers Surg Med 1:71–83, 1980.
67. Landthaler M, Haina D, Waidelich W, et al: A three-year experience with the argon laser in dermatotherapy. J Dermatol Surg Oncol 10:456–461, 1984.
68. Diette KM, Bronstein BR, Parrish JA: Histologic comparison of argon and tunable dye lasers in the treatment of tattoos. J Invest Dermatol 85:368–373, 1985.
69. Sunde D, Apfelberg DB, Sergott T: Traumatic tattoo removal: comparison of four treatment methods in an animal model with correlation to clinical experience. Lasers Surg Med 10:158–164, 1990.
70. Dismukes DE: The "chemo-laser" technique for the treatment of decorative tattoos: a more complete dye-removal procedure. Lasers Surg Med 6:59–61, 1986.
71. Stellar S, Polyani T, Bredemeier H: Lasers in surgery. In: Wolbarsht ML (ed): Laser Applications in Medicine and Biology. Plenum, New York, 1974, p 241.
72. Bailin PL, Ratz JL, Levine HL: Removal of tattoos by CO_2 laser. J Dermatol Surg Oncol 6:997–1001, 1980.
73. Hobbs ER, Bailin PL, Wheeland RG, et al: Superpulsed lasers: minimizing thermal damage with short duration, high irradiance pulses. J Dermatol Surg Oncol 13:955–964, 1987.
74. Reid R, Muller S: Tattoo removal with laser. Med J Aust 1:389, 1978.
75. Reid R, Muller S: Tattoo removal by CO_2 laser dermabrasion. Plast Reconstr Surg 65:717–728, 1980.
76. James SE, Venn GE, Russell RC: Experience using the carbon dioxide laser in the removal of cutaneous tattoos. Br J Surg 72:265–266, 1985.
77. Brady SC, Blokmanis A, Jewett L: Tattoo removal with the carbon dioxide laser. Ann Plast Surg 2:482–490, 1979.
78. Lanigan SW, Sheehan DR, Cotterill JA: The treatment of decorative tattoos with the carbon dioxide laser. Br J Dermatol 120:819–825, 1989.
79. Ruiz-Esparza J, Goldman MP, Fitzpatrick RE: Tattoo removal with minimal scarring: the chemo-laser technique. J Dermatol Surg Oncol 14:1372–1376, 1988.
80. Goldman MP: Discussion of the mode of action of urea ointment. Personal communication, 1991.
81. Kirschner RA: Ablation of tattoos with the Nd:YAG laser. Laser Med Surg News 5:21–25, 1987.
82. Solomon H, Goldman L, Henderson B, et al: Histopathology of the laser treatment of portwine stains. J Invest Dermatol 50:141–146, 1968.
83. Goldman L, Blaney DJ, Kindel DJ, et al: Radiation from a Q-switched ruby laser: effect of repeated impacts of power output of 10 megawatts on a tattoo of man. J Invest Dermatol 40:121–122, 1963.
84. Yules RB, Laub DR, Honey R, et al: The effect of Q-switched ruby laser radiation on dermal tattoo pigment in man. Arch Surg 95:179–180, 1967.
85. Laub DR, Yules RB, Arras M, et al: Preliminary histopathological observations of Q-switched ruby laser radiation on dermal tattoo in man. J Surg Res 8:220–224, 1968.
86. Reid WH, McLeod PJ, Ritchie A, et al: Q-switched ruby laser treatment of black tattoos. Br J Plast Surg 36:455–459, 1983.
87. Dover JS, Margolis RJ, Polla LL, et al: Pigmented guinea pig skin irradiated with Q-switched ruby laser pulses: morphologic and histologic findings. Arch Dermatol 125:43–49, 1989.
88. Taylor CR, Gange RW, Dover JS, et al: Treatment of tattoos by Q-switched ruby laser: a dose-response study. Arch Dermatol 126:893–899, 1990.
89. Goldman AI, Ham WT Jr, Mueller HA: Mechanisms of retinal damage resulting from the exposure of rhesus monkeys to ultra-short laser pulses. Exp Eye Res 21:457–469, 1975.
90. Anderson RR, Parrish JA: Selective photothermolysis: precise microsurgery by selective absorption of pulsed radiation. Science 220:524–527, 1983.
91. Watanabe S, Flotte TJ, McAuliffe DJ, et al: Putative photoacoustic damage in skin induced by pulsed ArF excimer laser. J Invest Dermatol 90:761–766, 1988.
92. Scheibner A, Kenny G, White W, Wheeland RG: A superior method of tattoo removal using the Q-switched ruby laser. J Dermatol Surg Oncol 16:1091–1098, 1990.

CHAPTER 71

Ear Piercing

ALLISON T. VIDIMOS

Earrings have been worn as ornaments, talismans,[1] aids to hearing,[2] and signs of slavery[3] since at least 3500 BC. Silver, gold, nickel, bronze, platinum, gems, plastic, wood, hair, bone, coral, and shell have all been used to make both simple studs and hoop earrings. The predecessor of the pierced earring is the earplug,[1, 4] a type of ear ornament inserted by some primitive tribes into pierced and distended earlobes. These earplugs, made of whale teeth, metal, stone, wood, shells, rags, or bone, may weigh up to three pounds and have a diameter of up to 4½ inches.

In Rosner's English translation of Julius Preuss's historical book, *Biblisch-Talmudische Medizin*,[3] it is noted that a slave would have his ear pierced with an awl in formal court proceedings to profess his dedication to his master. Although current methods of ear piercing have become somewhat more sophisticated, this seemingly simple procedure may be fraught with myriad complications.

Technique

Several different methods for ear piercing have been described. Regardless of the procedure employed, aseptic technique and diligent postoperative care of the pierced earlobes are important in ensuring patient satisfaction and preventing complications. Ear piercing should be restricted to the noncartilaginous portion of the ear (Fig. 71–1), as piercing the cartilaginous portion of the ear may result in chondritis and cartilage necrosis.

Several different options have been described for anesthetizing the earlobe before piercing. The earlobe can be anesthetized with intradermal injection of lidocaine, ethyl chloride spray, firm pressure applied for 30 seconds, or ice cubes applied to the anterior and posterior aspects of the lobes for 1 to 2 minutes. Local anesthetic is not often used with spring-loaded piercing guns because of the relative rapidity and painlessness of the procedure.

One common method of ear piercing uses a simple 21-gauge needle to pierce the earlobe in the anterior-to-posterior direction after first cleansing it with alcohol and marking the desired piercing site on the anterior aspect with ink. Surgical stainless steel or gold-plated post earrings are cold-sterilized in absolute alcohol, benzalkonium chloride, nitromersol, or cetyldimethylethylammonium bromide for 20 to 30 minutes.[5–7] An 18-gauge needle is slipped over the 21-gauge needle, and both are drawn forward through the earlobe. The 21-gauge needle is withdrawn, the earring pin is inserted into the 18-gauge needle lumen, and the pin is drawn posteriorly through the lobe. The 18-gauge needle is then withdrawn, and the earring clasp is fastened.[5]

Many variations on this needle technique have been described. One employs a large 14- or 16-gauge hypodermic needle to pierce the marked lobe in the posterior-to-anterior direction. The cold-sterilized earring pin is then inserted into the lumen of the needle with a sterile pair of forceps; both are then pulled back through the earlobe, the needle is slipped off the post, and the earring clasp is fastened.[8] A similar method substitutes a sterilized, flexible silver or gold wire for the earring pin and clasp.[9] Another technique requires substitution of a 14- or 16-gauge trocar needle antrum for the hypodermic needles.[6]

An ear-piercing instrument can be fashioned from a nonlocking pair of surgical forceps by fitting one jaw with a short segment of a No. 19 needle and forming the second jaw into an anvil with a cut-out area at the tip through which the No. 19 needle can pass.[7] An intravenous cannula and introducer can also be used to pierce the earlobe.[10] The sheathing is trimmed and left in place around the earring pin to act both as a stent to keep the tract open and as possible barrier material to prevent the development of a metal dermatitis.

Various commercial ear-piercing kits are available, two of which are the Steri-Quick ear-piercing instrument (Roman Research, Norwell, MA 02061) and the Debut

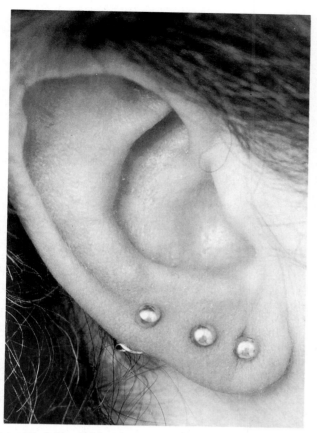

Figure 71–1. Ear piercing should be restricted to the noncartilaginous portion of the ear.

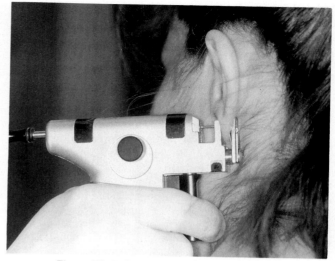

Figure 71–2. Spring-loaded ear-piercing gun.

Prestige ear-piercing kit (H&A Enterprises, Inc., 143–19 Twenty-Fifth Ave., Whitestone, NY 11357). The Steri-Quick kit supplies presterilized, 24-karat, gold-plated studs and clasps that are placed into a spring-loaded piercing gun using sterile forceps. The earlobe is grasped firmly between the anterior portion of the plunger, which contains the piercing pin, and the posterior stop plate, which contains the clasp (Fig. 71–2). Once the surgeon aligns the piercing pin with the inked piercing site, a firing button is depressed, propelling the needle through the lobe and into the posterior clasp. To prevent embedding the earring, care must be taken to ensure that the clasp is fixed securely to the pin but not tightly against the lobe.[11]

After initial placement, the earring stud or wire is left in place at least until the tract has epithelialized, which usually occurs in 10 days to 3 weeks.[7, 9, 12] The patient is instructed to cleanse the earlobes twice daily with 70% isopropyl alcohol to prevent infection. The earrings are rotated 180 degrees twice daily to prevent the formation of adhesions. Potential irritants such as cosmetics, detergents, and hair care products should be kept away from the newly pierced earlobes.[5] Persistent redness or swelling, purulent drainage, or irritation of the earlobe should be reported to the physician. Patients may insert their own earrings after 2 to 6 weeks,[5, 12, 13] preferably using those made with high-grade, low-nickel-content

stainless steel[14] or 14- or 18-karat gold posts to decrease the risk of contact dermatitis.

Complications

Many complications have been reported in association with ear piercing (Table 71–1). Two large groups of patients who underwent ear piercing were found to have complication rates of 52%[12] and 34%.[15] In both series of patients, inflammation, bleeding, drainage and crusting, and infection occurred most frequently. The nature and number of complications were similar regardless of the ear-piercing instrument, the type of initial earring, or the duration that the initial earring was left in the earlobes.[15] However, lack of aseptic piercing technique and improper care of the freshly pierced earlobes contributed significantly to the complication rate, particu-

TABLE 71–1. **COMPLICATIONS OF EAR PIERCING**

Erythema and edema
Bleeding and hematoma formation
Nonpurulent drainage and crusting
Metal allergic dermatitis[12, 13, 16–40]
Infection
    Beta-hemolytic streptococcal infection[43, 44]
    Staphylococcus aureus infection[45–47]
    Pseudomonas chondritis[48]
    Primary tuberculosis of earlobe[49]
    Botryomycosis[50]
    Tetanus[51]
    Hepatitis B[52–57]
Earlobe keloids[58–100, 103]
Embedded earrings[104–110]
Traumatic laceration[71, 107, 111–117, 120]
    Slot earlobe
    Bifid earlobe
Cyst formation
Lipoma formation
Earring ingestion or aspiration[118]
Postauricular pressure sores[119]
"Frostbite" burn secondary to ethyl fluoride spray[121]

larly in cases of metal dermatitis, infection, and embedded earrings.

METAL DERMATITIS

Nickel

Many authors have documented ear piercing as a cause of nickel dermatitis, which can occur in patients of all ages, from infants to adults.[12, 13, 16–34] Ear piercing performed at an early age seems to increase the risk of the development of nickel sensitivity.[19] Approximately 10% of the female population is nickel allergic,[16, 20, 21, 34] and ear piercing is thought to be the most important causative factor.[19, 26] The ability of plasma to leach nickel from earrings,[29] which may be enhanced by bacteria,[23] may explain both the early and late development of nickel sensitivity after ear piercing. This is usually manifested as an eczematous earlobe dermatitis.

Ear piercing does not appear to be a common risk factor for the development of nickel sensitivity in males.[16, 22, 30, 32] Possible explanations for this include the later onset of ear piercing in men and the tendency for men to wear more costly, low-nickel-content jewelry.[30] Another interesting phenomenon noted in two large groups of patients with nickel allergy was that patients with orthodontic devices containing nickel who subsequently underwent ear piercing had a lower frequency of the development of nickel allergy.[17, 18] This supports the premise that oral allergenic exposure to nickel may induce immunologic tolerance.

Approximately 10 to 56% of nickel-allergic patients develop chronic hand eczema, which may be quite debilitating and recalcitrant to treatment.[16, 19, 22, 30, 34] This potential problem underscores the need to take all necessary measures to avoid the development of nickel allergy from ear piercing. Such measures include use of stainless steel needles to pierce the earlobes and insertion of stainless steel earring studs and clasps that have tested negatively with dimethylglyoxime until the newly created tracts have epithelialized.[25]

Various stainless steel and gold- and silver-plated studs and clasps[23] and white gold discs[33] were tested for nickel release after storing them in synthetic sweat. All tested earrings and discs released nickel in varying amounts, the least of which varied from 0.05 to 0.09 μg. When patients with documented nickel allergy were exposed to these particular earrings or discs, they developed earlobe dermatitis and positive patch test reactions. Such reactions are rare in clinical experience,[24] and the dimethylglyoxime test, which will detect nickel release of 10 μg or more, may give false information as to the safety of certain earrings. The nickel content of high-grade stainless steel, such as that used to manufacture surgical instruments, is less than 1%, although other grades may contain up to 36% nickel.[14]

In Denmark, nickel exposure has been regulated by a law that prohibits the manufacture or importation of nickel-containing objects that release more than 0.5 μg/cm^2/week, as indicated by a positive dimethylglyoxime test. Violators of this provision may be charged a fine or imprisoned for up to 1 year.[31]

Gold

The development of gold sensitivity from jewelry is relatively rare,[13, 25, 35–40] probably because of the relative insolubility of gold in tissue fluids.[35–37] The nature of gold sensitivity may be distinctly different from that of nickel dermatitis and persists despite the lack of gold contact.[25, 35, 36, 38, 39] It may present as papules or nodules of the earlobes[35–40] or as an eczematous dermatitis.[35] Histologic examination of these nodules reveals dense lymphohistiocytic infiltrates of the dermal and subcutaneous tissue[35–40] and formation of lymphoid follicles as benign lymphoplasia.[38, 39] The immunomodulatory properties of gold may be responsible for the development of this benign lymphoplasia.[38, 39]

A case of pseudolymphoma of the earlobes after ear piercing has been reported,[41] which emphasizes the need to distinguish these lesions from keloids. A sarcoidal tissue reaction in the earlobes has also been reported[42] after piercing at multiple sites with a gold stud. For this reason, the clinician should also consider sarcoidal granulomas in the differential diagnosis of earlobe nodules. If these are histologically confirmed, the patient should be evaluated for systemic sarcoidosis, although a local sarcoidal tissue reaction is possible.

If metal dermatitis is suspected, patch testing should be performed to elucidate the allergen, which may include nickel, gold, platinum, chromium, or cobalt.[16, 19, 21, 26, 30] Nickel and cobalt allergy may coexist with nickel dermatitis.[12, 27, 28, 30]

INFECTION

Infectious complications are the most common and potentially most serious sequelae of ear piercing. In the two large reported series,[12, 15] infections accounted for 15 to 24% of all reported complications, none of which were serious. However, reported sequelae of beta-hemolytic streptococcal infection after ear piercing include septicemia,[43] acute post-streptococcal glomerulonephritis, and septic arthritis.[44] In addition, liver[45] and chest wall abscesses,[46] septicemia, osteomyelitis,[45] and toxic shock syndrome[47] have also occurred in the wake of *Staphylococcus aureus* earlobe infections. The presence of childhood neutropenia and the accelerated growth of toxin-producing strains secondary to ear piercing were instrumental in the development of toxic shock syndrome reported in a child.[47]

Risk factors for streptococcal and staphylococcal infections include lack of aseptic technique,[2, 43–46] use of nonsterile safety pins or needles, impaired immunologic status,[47] and inadequate postpiercing care. In particular, the relatively underdeveloped immune system in infants may also contribute to the infectious complications reported in this age group.

The onset, within a few days of ear piercing, of dull pain, erythema, tenderness, and warmth and edema of the auricle, with an increased auriculocephalic angle and fever, should alert the cutaneous surgeon to the diagnosis of chondritis. A case of *Pseudomonas* chondritis has been reported[48] in a young woman subsequent to ear piercing. Prompt surgical debridement and antibiotic therapy are necessary in such cases to prevent the development of severe deformity of the ear. *Pseudomonas aeruginosa* is the most frequent offending organism in chondritis, although *S. aureus, Streptococcus,* and *Proteus* may also be causative organisms.[48]

Primary inoculation tuberculosis of the earlobe has been reported in an 18-month-old white infant who had her ears pierced by her mother, who had undiagnosed active pulmonary tuberculosis.[49] Other unusual reported complications include botryomycosis subsequent to intralesional steroid treatments for earlobe keloids[50] and tetanus.[51]

Both individual case reports[52, 53] and large-scale studies[54–57] emphasize the risk of transmission of viral hepatitis when ear piercing is performed under nonsterile conditions. If nondisposable ear-piercing instruments are used, they should be sterilized to destroy any existing hepatitis virus; this is done by boiling them for 20 minutes or autoclaving at 121°C for 15 minutes.[54] Cold sterilization with benzalkonium chloride or 70% alcohol does not kill the hepatitis virus. In addition, although not yet reported, human immunodeficiency virus transmission is another potential hazard of improper ear-piercing methods.

EARLOBE KELOIDS

The earlobe is a common site for keloid formation,[58–60] which usually occurs secondary to the trauma of ear piercing.[60–62] Earlobe keloids do not generally appear until puberty,[63, 64] even though the ear piercing may have been performed in infancy or childhood. Dark-skinned races tend to develop earlobe keloids more frequently than whites; this is also true for keloids elsewhere on the body.[58, 59, 65] However, patients with a history of earlobe keloids only should not be considered

at higher risk for keloid formation elsewhere on the body.[64]

Three varieties of earlobe keloids have been described[63]: the external button variety, which may appear as a nodule on the anterior, posterior, or both aspects of the earlobe, producing a "dumbbell" keloid (Fig. 71–3); the intralobular variety, where the central portion of the earlobe is replaced by the keloidal tissue, thereby obliterating the tract (Fig. 71–4); and the massive nodular keloid, which begins in the center of the earlobe as a slowly enlarging nodule that may grow to partially or totally obscure the auricle (Fig. 71–5). It is unknown why any patient develops one of these types rather than another.

Along with trauma, infection has been implicated as a factor in keloid formation of the earlobe after ear piercing.[60, 66] The preponderance of posterior versus anterior earlobe keloids[61, 63, 67] is probably the result of the direction of piercing trauma, the dissimilarity in biochemical milieu in the two surfaces of the lobe, and possible protective environmental or cosmetic factors. Many different techniques have been employed to treat earlobe keloids, including excision with a scalpel[61, 62, 66, 68–94] or carbon dioxide laser,[95–98] intralesional injection of steroids,[61, 62, 71, 76–82, 87–89, 91, 92, 94, 96, 97, 99] pressure therapy,[83–87] radiation therapy,[60, 61, 66, 68–75, 77] penicillamine,[94] ligation,[61] and cryosurgery either alone[100] or before intralesional steroid injections.[79, 80] As a general rule, combination regimens are often the most efficacious.

Surgical removal of dumbbell earlobe keloids is performed by excising the anterior and posterior nodules along with the keloid core.[90, 91] The anterior and posterior defects are closed with nonabsorbable suture, and intralesional triamcinolone acetonide is injected along the suture line postoperatively. Another method utilizes excision of the loop of skin inferior to the keloid with

Figure 71–3. *A,* Posterior earlobe keloid. *B,* Anterior and posterior earlobe keloids ("dumbbell" keloids).

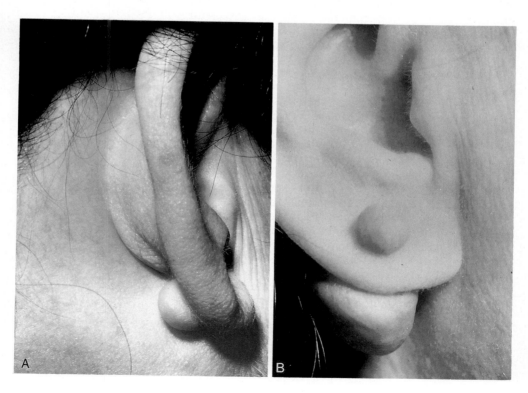

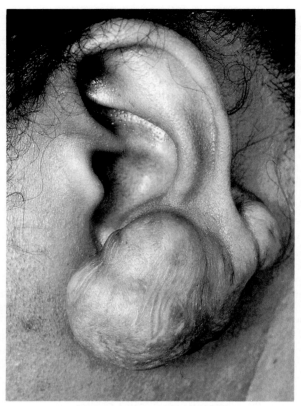

Figure 71–4. Intralobular keloid.

creation of a "V" defect medially and a wedge defect laterally, followed by rotation of the wedge flap into the "V" defect.[90]

Satisfactory results with a maximum of 4 years' follow-up have been reported in 12 patients (19 earlobe keloids) after primary excision and closure followed by intralesional injection of triamcinolone.[81] Another successful method of keloid excision[88] uses a portion of the overlying skin as a flap to cover the defect (Fig. 71–6). Excision of earlobe keloids followed by repair using a full-thickness pedicle flap from the retroauricular skin has also been described.[93]

The carbon dioxide laser, when used as a single modality for treatment of earlobe keloids, has yielded disappointing results in some studies.[95, 97, 98] However, when combined with other adjunctive measures such as intralesional steroid injection, the success rate is improved.[96] Using the carbon dioxide laser in the focused mode with a 0.1- to 0.2-mm spot size permits the incision to be made with minimal thermal damage while sealing small vascular and lymphatic channels.[96, 101] The near-infrared neodymium:yttrium-aluminum-garnet (Nd:YAG) laser has the ability to suppress collagen production by fibroblasts in vitro and in vivo.[102] However, although the carbon dioxide laser is also an infrared laser, its ability to inhibit fibroplasia has not yet been demonstrated. Thus, the role of laser radiation in modulating keloid recurrences remains unclear.

Two large series of surgically excised earlobe keloids noted recurrence rates of approximately 40 to 60%.[68, 70]

The adjunctive use of intralesional steroids has improved the success rate of earlobe keloid treatment remarkably, reducing recurrence rates to 0 to 3%.[76, 81, 82, 89] Steroid-impregnated tape has also been used in conjunction with pressure earrings after excision of recurrent earlobe keloids in 57 patients, resulting in only four recurrences in the 52 patients who were followed for at least 4 years.[83]

Various pressure devices have been applied to the earlobes after keloid excision in an attempt to reduce recurrences. These have included polymethyl methacrylate splints (oyster splints),[85, 87] button compression,[84] and pressure earrings (Fig. 71–7).[83, 86] These pressure devices are worn from 8 to 23½ hours each day, starting 2 weeks postoperatively, for 3 weeks to 24 months.[65, 83–87] The earrings exert approximately 23 to 28 mm Hg of pressure.[83]

In general, concomitant radiation therapy and surgical excision of keloids decrease the recurrence rate by 50%.[74, 75] Recurrence rates between 21 and 36% have been reported in earlobe keloids treated with postoperative radiation therapy.[70, 73] An overall recurrence rate of 8% was achieved in a series of 393 keloids, 79 of which were earlobe keloids.[74] Large keloid size, short duration of growth, and a history of recurrence have been cited as poor prognostic factors.[70, 75]

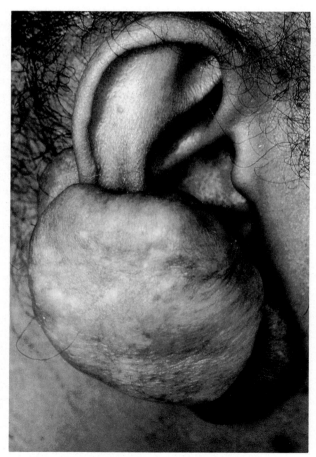

Figure 71–5. Massive nodular keloid of the earlobe.

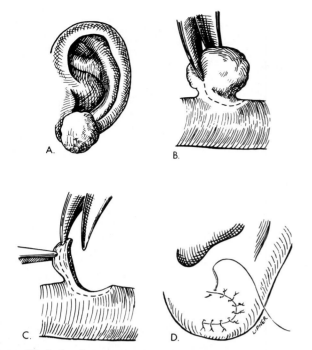

Figure 71–6. A schematic of excision of a keloid on an earlobe. *A,* The keloid before excision. *B,* Excision of the bulk of the keloid with outline of a small portion of skin for a flap with which to cover the defect. *C,* Dissection with iris scissors of residual keloidal tissue from the skin to be used as a flap. *D,* Suture of the flap in place without tension on the suture line. (Reprinted by permission of the publisher from Weimar VM, Ceilley RI: Treatment of keloids on earlobes. J Dermatol Surg Oncol 5:522–523, 1979. Copyright 1979 by Elsevier Science Publishing Co., Inc.)

Bilateral earlobe keloids seen in some patients provide a unique opportunity for controlled investigation of various treatment modalities.[70] As with keloids elsewhere on the body, a minimal follow-up period of at least 2 years is necessary to evaluate accurately the success of any treatment regimen.[75, 87, 91, 103] Surgery, in combination with intralesional steroid injection, pressure therapy, or radiation therapy, tends to be most effective in treating these cosmetically distressing lesions.

EMBEDDED EARRINGS

The problem of embedded earrings has been reported by several authors.[104–110] One 8-year-old girl presented 3 years after ear piercing with hard, tender cysts in both earlobes; on removal these cysts were found to contain the original clasps used for piercing.[104] Although this complication has increased in frequency since the advent of spring-loaded ear-piercing instruments,[105, 109] it has also been reported with manual ear-piercing methods. The risk of embedded earrings can be reduced by confining ear piercing to the earlobe, using larger clasps for the initial ear-piercing studs, employing strict aseptic technique, securing the clasp so that it is loose against the ear, cleaning the earlobes properly after initial insertion, and removing the earrings if purulent drainage and erythema develop.[108, 109] Embedded earrings must always be suspected if small, keloid-like nodules develop on the earlobes.[110] A radiographic examination may be helpful in evaluating such patients.[106, 108]

Figure 71–7. Compression earrings. (*A,* Courtesy of Padgett Instrument Company, Kansas City, MO. *B,* Courtesy of H & A Enterprises, Inc., Whitestone, NY.)

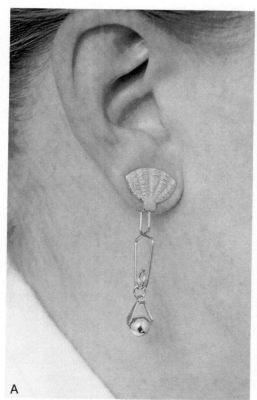

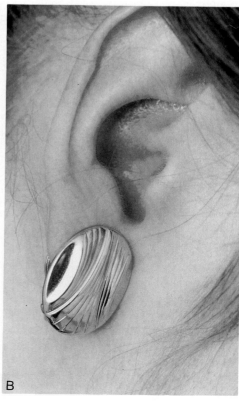

TRAUMATIC LACERATION

Patients may present with elongated earlobe tracts ("slot" lobe) or complete avulsion ("bifid" lobe) secondary to trauma or wearing heavy earrings.[107] The painless pressure necrosis caused by wearing heavy earrings may be exacerbated by exposure to extreme cold.[71] The slot earlobe may be repaired by excising the elongated tract followed by closure with nonabsorbable sutures (Fig. 71–8). The earlobe can be stabilized with a chalazion clamp,[111] while a punch is used to excise the elongated earlobe tracts less than 4 mm in length. The defect is closed with nonabsorbable suture. A wedge excision may also be performed if the intact loop of skin inferiorly is extremely narrow (Fig. 71–9).

The fully avulsed or bifid earlobe may be corrected by a wedge excision made around the cleft in the earlobe, with simple closure of each side of the defect (Fig. 71–10). To prevent an indentation from developing secondary to scar contracture, a Z-plasty may be performed[112–114] at the inferior margin of the lobe (Fig. 71–11). The repaired lobes are allowed to heal for approximately 3 months, at which time the earlobes may be repierced. Alternative methods of repair have been described that enable the original earring canal to be preserved.[115–117]

MISCELLANEOUS COMPLICATIONS

The increasing number of infants and young children who undergo ear piercing has given rise to other complications, including earring ingestion and aspiration[118] and postauricular pressure sores caused by the inability of infants to turn their heads.[119] There is also a documented case of a 1-year-old infant who presented with

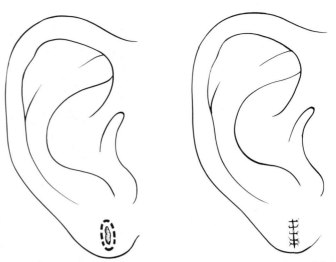

Figure 71–8. Slot earlobe repair with excision of elongated earlobe tract and closure with nonabsorbable sutures.

a torn earlobe secondary to catching her earring on the mesh of her playpen.[120] Temptation on the part of the child or other children to manipulate earrings may also lead to trauma of the earlobe. These potential complications must be seriously considered and discussed with the parents whenever the cutaneous surgeon is asked to pierce the ears of an infant or young child.

Chemical "frostbite" has been reported[121] on the ears of three children who had ear piercing performed by a jeweler who sprayed ethyl chloride for several minutes on each lobe. If this method of topical anesthesia is chosen, the freezing should be limited to approximately 20 seconds.

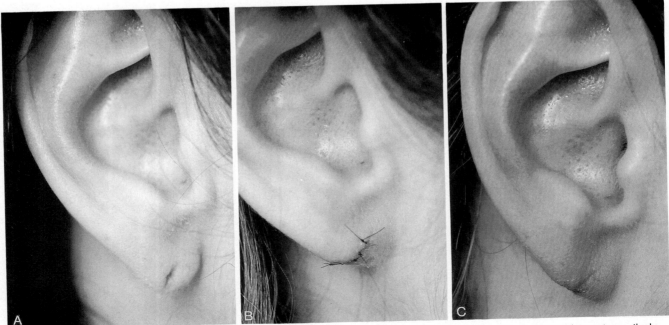

Figure 71–9. Slot earlobe repair with wedge excision. *A,* Preoperative view. *B,* Immediately after repair. *C,* Six weeks postoperatively.

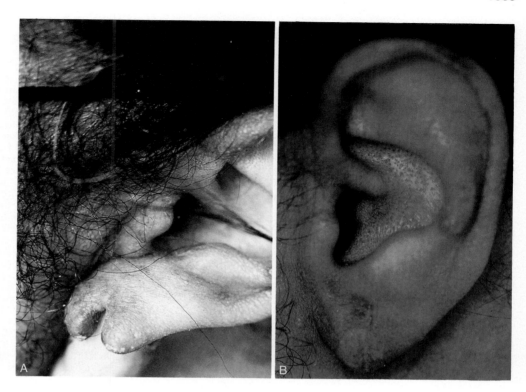

Figure 71–10. Repair of bifid earlobe with wedge excision. *A,* Preoperative view. *B,* Two months postoperatively.

Contraindications

To help minimize the potential complications that can result from this relatively simple procedure, careful screening of patients is required. Patients with local infections, earlobe cysts, deformed earlobes, or a history of keloid formation, metal sensitivity, hemorrhagic diathesis, or immunodeficiency are not candidates for ear piercing.[6, 12, 120] Careful consideration should also be given as to the appropriateness of performing this procedure on patients with a history of rheumatic fever, glomerulonephritis, congenital heart disease, diabetes mellitus, or chronic skin problems such as atopic dermatitis, psoriasis, or lichen planus[12] that may involve the earlobe.

Nose Piercing

Nose piercing is becoming increasingly popular, particularly among Asian women, and may be associated with complications similar to those seen with ear piercing. Four cases of complications from nose piercing have been reported[122]; three consisted of embedded studs or clasps, and one was unilateral nasal obstruction secondary to alar cartilage collapse. The possibility exists of inducing perichondritis and necrosis of the cartilage with piercing through the lateral wall of the nose. Earring clasp aspiration should also be an obvious concern.

Because a significant portion of the population are nasal carriers of *S. aureus,* the likelihood of secondary *S. aureus* infection of a pierced nose is probably greater than on the earlobe. The prospect of developing cavernous sinus thrombosis from a nasal infection after nose piercing is particularly frightening. There is also the possibility of keloid development secondary to nose piercing. This not only is of cosmetic concern, but also can be a significant functional problem because of nasal obstruction.

SUMMARY

Ear piercing is a common procedure performed by medical personnel, jewelers, friends, and family members. This relatively quick and simple procedure may result in both minor and major complications. Suspected metal allergies should be evaluated with patch testing. The dimethylglyoxime test should be used to assess the nickel content of jewelry. Cultures should be obtained

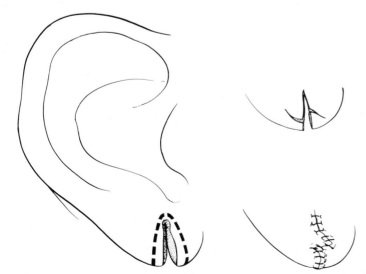

Figure 71–11. Repair of bifid earlobe with wedge excision and Z-plasty at the inferior margin of the lobe.

in suspected cases of infection of the earlobe so that appropriate antibiotic therapy may be prescribed. Nodules at ear-piercing sites should be carefully evaluated, as they may represent the development of keloids, cysts, lipomas, hematomas, embedded studs, benign lymphoplasia, or sarcoidosis.

Careful patient screening, use of sterile ear-piercing technique, thorough education of the patient regarding the nature and potential complications of the procedure, diligent postoperative care of the earlobes, and a method to avoid nickel sensitization are all necessary to ensure patient satisfaction and a complication-free result.

REFERENCES

1. Encyclopedia Americana. Vol 9. Americana Corp, New York, 1989, pp 531–532.
2. Sanders DY: Complications of ear piercing. Woman Physician 26:459, 1971.
3. Rosner F: Otology in the Bible and Talmud. J Laryngol Otol 89:397–404, 1975.
4. The New Encyclopedia Britannica. Vol 4. Encyclopedia Britannica, Chicago, 1986, p 320.
5. Graber RF: Procedures for your practice: ear piercing. Patient Care 24:194–196, 1990.
6. Goff WF: Ear piercing—by whom? Eye Ear Nose Throat Mon 54:319, 1975.
7. Duffy MM: A simple instrument for ear piercing. Plast Reconstr Surg 40:92–93, 1967.
8. Bennett RG: Fundamentals of Cutaneous Surgery. CV Mosby, St Louis, 1988, pp 611–615.
9. Goldman L, Kitzmiller KW: Earlobe piercing with needles and wires. Arch Dermatol 92:305–306, 1965.
10. Zackowski DA: An IV cannula stent for ear piercing. Plast Reconstr Surg 80:751, 1987.
11. Gibson OB: A problem with ear piercing. Br Med J 1:178, 1978.
12. Cortese TA, Dickey RA: Complications of ear piercing. Am Fam Physician 4:66–72, 1971.
13. Fisher AA: Ear piercing and sensitivity to nickel and gold. J Am Acad Dermatol 17:853, 1987.
14. Annual Book of ASTM Standards. American Society for Testing and Materials, Philadelphia, 01.03:43–44, 1988.
15. Biggar RJ, Haughie GE: Medical problems of ear piercing. NY State J Med 75:1460–1462, 1975.
16. Christensen OB: Nickel dermatitis: an update. Dermatol Clin 8:37–40, 1990.
17. van der Burg CK, Bruynzeel DP, Vreeburg KJ, et al: Hand eczema in hairdressers and nurses: a prospective study. Evaluation of atopy and nickel hypersensitivity at the start of apprenticeship. Contact Dermatitis 14:275–279, 1986.
18. Todd DJ, Burrows D: Nickel allergy in relationship to previous oral and cutaneous nickel contact. Ulster Med J 58:168–171, 1989.
19. Rystedt I, Fischer T: Relationship between nickel and cobalt sensitization in hard metal workers. Contact Dermatitis 9:195–200, 1983.
20. Prystowsky SD, Allen AM, Smith RW, et al: Allergic contact hypersensitivity to nickel, neomycin, ethylenediamine, and benzocaine. Relationships between age, sex, history of exposure, and reactivity to standard patch tests and use tests in a general population. Arch Dermatol 115:959–962, 1979.
21. Larsson-Stymne B, Widstrom L: Ear piercing—a cause of nickel allergy in schoolgirls? Contact Dermatitis 13:289–293, 1985.
22. Gawkrodger DJ, Vestey JP, Wong WK, Buxton PK: Contact clinic survey of nickel-sensitive subjects. Contact Dermatitis 14:165–169, 1986.
23. Fischer T, Fregert S, Gruvberger B, Rystedt I: Nickel release from ear piercing kits and earrings. Contact Dermatitis 10:39–41, 1984.
24. Fisher AA: Ear piercing and nickel allergy. Contact Dermatitis 14:328, 1986.
25. Fisher AA: Ear piercing hazard of nickel-gold sensitization. JAMA 228:1226, 1974.
26. Boss A, Menne T: Nickel sensitization from ear piercing. Contact Dermatitis 8:211–213, 1982.
27. Gaul LE: Development of allergic nickel dermatitis from earrings. JAMA 200:186–188, 1967.
28. Gilboa R, Al-Tawil NG, Marcusson JA: Metal allergy in cashiers. An in vitro and in vivo study for the presence of metal allergy. Act Derm Venereol (Stockh) 68:317–324, 1988.
29. Emmett EA, Risby TH, Jiang L, et al: Allergic contact dermatitis to nickel: bioavailability from consumer products and provocation threshold. J Am Acad Dermatol 19:314–322, 1988.
30. Burrows D: Mischievous metals—chromate, cobalt, nickel and mercury. Clin Exp Dermatol 14:266–272, 1989.
31. Menne T, Rasmussen K: Regulation of nickel exposure in Denmark. Contact Dermatitis 23:57–58, 1990.
32. Widstrom L, Erikssohn I: Nickel allergy and ear piercing in young men. First European Symposium on Contact Dermatitis, Heidelberg, May 27–29, 1988.
33. Fischer T, Fregert S, Gruvberger B, Rystedt I: Contact sensitivity to nickel in white gold. Contact Dermatitis 10:23–24, 1984.
34. Peltonen L: Nickel sensitivity in the general population. Contact Dermatitis 5:27–32, 1979.
35. Petros H, Macmillan AL: Allergic contact sensitivity to gold with unusual features. Br J Dermatol 88:505–508, 1973.
36. Fisher AA: Metallic gold: the cause of a persistent allergic "dermal" contact dermatitis. Cutis 14:177–180, 1974.
37. Young E: Contact hypersensitivity to metallic gold. Dermatologica 149:294–298, 1974.
38. Iwatsuki K, Tagami H, Moriguchi T, Yamada M: Lymphadenoid structure induced by gold hypersensitivity. Arch Dermatol 118:608–611, 1982.
39. Iwatsuki K, Yamada M, Takigawa M, et al: Benign lymphoplasia of the earlobes induced by gold earring: immunohistologic study on the cellular infiltrates. J Am Acad Dermatol 16:83–88, 1987.
40. Aoshima T, Oguchi M: Intracytoplasmic crystalline inclusions in dermal infiltrating cells of granulomatous contact dermatitis due to gold earrings. Acta Derm Venereol (Stockh) 68:261–264, 1988.
41. Zilinsky I, Tsur H, Trau H, Orenstein A: Pseudolymphoma of the earlobes due to ear piercing. J Dermatol Surg Oncol 15:666–668, 1989.
42. Mann RJ, Peachey RD: Sarcoidal tissue reaction—another complication of ear piercing. Clin Exp Dermatol 8:199–200, 1983.
43. George J, White M: Infection as a consequence of ear piercing. Practitioner 233:404–406, 1989.
44. Ahmed-Jushuf IH, Selby PL, Brownjohn AM: Acute poststreptococcal glomerulonephritis following ear piercing. Postgrad Med J 60:73–74, 1984.
45. Lovejoy FH Jr, Smith DH: Life-threatening staphylococcal disease following ear piercing. Pediatrics 46:301–303, 1970.
46. Shulman BH: Ear piercing and sepsis. Clin Pediatr 12:27A, 1973.
47. McCarthy VP, Peoples WM: Toxic shock syndrome after ear piercing. Pediatr Infect Dis J 7:741–742, 1988.
48. Turkeltaub SH, Habal MB: Acute Pseudomonas chondritis as a sequel to ear piercing. Ann Plast Surg 24:279–282, 1990.
49. Morgan LG: Primary tuberculous inoculation of an earlobe. J Pediatr 40:482–485, 1952.
50. Olmstead PM, Finn M: Botryomycosis in pierced ears. Arch Dermatol 118:925–927, 1982.
51. Mamtani R, Malhotra P, Gupta PS, Jain BK: A comparative study of urban and rural tetanus in adults. Int J Epidemiol 7:185–188, 1978.
52. Van-Sciver AE: Hepatitis from ear piercing. JAMA 207:2285, 1969.
53. Parry SW: Ear piercing. N Engl J Med 291:1143, 1974.
54. Johnson CJ, Anderson H, Spearman J, Madson J: Ear piercing and hepatitis. Nonsterile instruments for ear piercing and the subsequent onset of viral hepatitis. JAMA 227:1165, 1974.
55. Abdool Karim SS, Coovadia HM, Windsor IM, et al: The prevalence and transmission of hepatitis B virus infection in urban, rural and institutionalized black children of Natal/KwaZulu, South Africa. Int J Epidemiol 17:168–173, 1988.
56. Steigmann F, Dourdourekas D: The asymptomatic HB6-Ag carrier: auto- and heterologous perils. Am J Gastroenterol 65:512–521, 1976.

57. Abdool-Karim SS, Thejpal R, Singh B: High prevalence of hepatitis B virus infection in rural black adults in Mseleni, South Africa. Am J Public Health 79:893–894, 1989.

58. Ketchum LD, Cohen IK, Masters FW: Hypertrophic scars and keloids: a collective review. Plast Reconstr Surg 53:140–154, 1974.

59. Datubo-Brown DD: Keloids: a review of the literature. Br J Plast Surg 43:70–77, 1990.

60. Inalsingh CHA: An experience in treating five hundred and one patients with keloids. Johns Hopkins Med J 134:284–290, 1974.

61. Cheng LH: Keloids of the earlobe. Laryngoscope 82:673–681, 1972.

62. Griffith BH, Monroe CW, McKinney P: A follow-up study in the treatment of keloids with triamcinolone acetonide. Plast Reconstr Surg 46:145–150, 1970.

63. Abdel-Fattah AMA: Three distinct varieties of earlobe keloids in Egypt. Br J Plast Surg 31:261–262, 1978.

64. Kelly AP: Keloids. Dermatol Clin 6:413–424, 1988.

65. Murray JC, Pollack SV, Pinnell SR: Keloids: a review. J Am Acad Dermatol 4:461–470, 1981.

66. Ashbell TS: Prevention and treatment of earlobe keloids. Ann Plast Surg 9:264–265, 1982.

67. Slobodkin D: Why more keloids on back than on front of earlobe. Lancet 335:923–924, 1990.

68. Cosman B, Crikelair GF, Ju DMC, et al: The surgical treatment of keloids. Plast Reconstr Surg 27:335–358, 1961.

69. Cosman B, Wolff M: Correlation of keloid recurrence with completeness of local excision: a negative report. Plast Reconstr Surg 50:163–166, 1972.

70. Cosman B, Wolff M: Bilateral earlobe keloids. Plast Reconstr Surg 53:540–543, 1974.

71. McLaren LR: Surgery of the external ear. J Laryngol Otol 88:23–38, 1974.

72. Ramakrishnan KM, Thomas KP, Sundararajan CR: Study of 1,000 patients with keloids in South India. Plast Reconstr Surg 53:276–280, 1974.

73. Ollstein RN, Siegel HW, Gillooley JF, Barsa JM: Treatment of keloids by combined surgical excision and immediate postoperative x-ray therapy. Ann Plast Surg 7:281–285, 1981.

74. Borok TL, Bray M, Sinclair I, et al: Role of ionizing irradiation for 393 keloids. Int J Radiat Oncol Biol Phys 15:865–870, 1988.

75. Kovalic JJ, Perez CA: Radiation therapy following keloidectomy: a 20-year experience. Int J Radiat Oncol Biol Phys 17:77–80, 1989.

76. Moreno FG, Pennington FR, Bond WR, Morrison WV: Facial keloids and their management. Ear Nose Throat J 60:43–49, 1981.

77. Murray RD: Kenalog and the treatment of hypertrophic scars and keloids in negroes and whites. Plast Reconstr Surg 31:275–280, 1963.

78. Griffith BH: The treatment of keloids with triamcinolone acetonide. Plast Reconstr Surg 38:202–208, 1966.

79. Babin RW, Ceilley RI: The freeze-injection method of hypertrophic scar and keloid reduction. Otolaryngol Head Neck Surg 87:911–914, 1979.

80. Hirshowitz B, Lerner D, Moscona AR: Treatment of keloid scars by combined cryosurgery and intralesional corticosteroids. Aesthetic Plast Surg 6:153–158, 1982.

81. Barton RPE: Auricular keloids: a simple method of management. Ann R Coll Surg Engl 60:324–325, 1978.

82. Shons AR, Press BHJ: The treatment of earlobe keloids by surgical excision and postoperative triamcinolone injection. Ann Plast Surg 10:480–482, 1983.

83. Rauscher GE, Kolmer WL: Treatment of recurrent earlobe keloids. Cutis 37:67–68, 1986.

84. Snyder GB: Button compression for keloids of the lobule. Br J Plast Surg 27:186–187, 1974.

85. Mercer DM, Studd DMM: "Oyster splints": a new compression device for the treatment of keloid scars of the ear. Br J Plast Surg 36:75–78, 1983.

86. Brent B: The role of pressure therapy in management of earlobe keloids: preliminary report of a controlled study. Ann Plast Surg 1:579–581, 1978.

87. Pierce HE: Postsurgical acrylic ear splints for keloids. J Dermatol Surg Oncol 12:583–585, 1986.

88. Weimar VM, Ceilley RI: Treatment of keloids on earlobes. J Dermatol Surg Oncol 5:522–523, 1979.

89. Kelly AP: Surgical treatment of keloids secondary to ear piercing. J Natl Med Assoc 70:349–350, 1978.

90. Howell S, Warpeha R, Brent B: A technique for excising earlobe keloids. Surg Gynecol Obstet 141:438, 1975.

91. Salasche SJ, Grabski WJ: Keloids of the earlobes: a surgical technique. J Dermatol Surg Oncol 9:552–556, 1983.

92. Pollack SV, Goslen JB: The surgical treatment of keloids. J Dermatol Surg Oncol 8:1045–1049, 1982.

93. Bondar VS: Auriculoplasty for keloid scars. Acta Chir Plast 31:101–107, 1989.

94. Mayou BJ: D-Penicillamine in the treatment of keloids. Br J Dermatol 105:87–89, 1981.

95. Apfelberg DB, Maser MR, Lash H, et al: Preliminary results of argon and carbon dioxide laser treatment of keloid scars. Lasers Surg Med 4:283–290, 1984.

96. Kantor GR, Wheeland RG, Bailin PL, et al: Treatment of earlobe keloids with carbon dioxide laser excision: a report of 16 cases. J Dermatol Surg Oncol 11:1063–1067, 1985.

97. Stern JC, Lucente FE: Carbon dioxide laser excision of earlobe keloids. A prospective study and critical analysis of existing data. Arch Otolaryngol Head Neck Surg 115:1107–1111, 1989.

98. Apfelberg DB, Maser MR, White DN, Lash H: Failure of carbon dioxide laser excision of keloids. Lasers Surg Med 9:382–388, 1989.

99. Muir IFK, Wilson HTH: Keloids. Br Med J 4:325, 1968.

100. Shepherd JP, Dawber RPR: The response of keloid scars to cryosurgery. Plast Reconstr Surg 70:677–681, 1982.

101. Kirschner RA: Cutaneous plastic surgery with the CO_2 laser. Surg Clin North Am 64:871–883, 1984.

102. Abergel RP, Meeker CA, Lam TS, et al: Control of connective tissue metabolism by lasers: recent developments and future prospects. J Am Acad Dermatol 11:1142–1150, 1984.

103. Brown LA Jr, Pierce HE: Keloids: scar revision. J Dermatol Surg Oncol 12:51–56, 1986.

104. Smith RB: Earring clasp as a foreign body in the earlobe. Plast Reconstr Surg 62:772, 1978.

105. Cockin J, Finan P, Powell M: A problem with ear piercing. Br Med J 2:1631, 1977.

106. Lazaro CD, Jackson RH: Vanishing earrings. Arch Dis Child 61:606–607, 1986.

107. Jay AL: Ear piercing problems. Br Med J 2:574–575, 1977.

108. Lawrence NW, Skinner JL: Clinical curio: butterfly in the ear. Br Med J 286:1504, 1983.

109. Muntz HR, Pa CDJ, Asher BF: Embedded earrings: a complication of the ear-piercing gun. Int J Pediatr Otorhinolaryngol 19:73–76, 1990.

110. Saleeby ER, Rubin MG, Youshock E, Kleinsmith DM: Embedded foreign bodies presenting as earlobe keloids. J Dermatol Surg Oncol 10:902–904, 1984.

111. Tan EC: Punch technique—an alternative approach to the repair of pierced earlobe deformities. J Dermatol Surg Oncol 15:270–272, 1989.

112. Ellis DA: Complication and correction of the pierced ear. J Otolaryngol 5:247–250, 1976.

113. Casson P: Ask the expert: how do you repair a split earlobe? J Dermatol Surg 2:21, 1976.

114. Harahap M: Repair of split earlobes. A review and new technique. J Dermatol Surg Oncol 8:187–191, 1982.

115. Pardue AM: Repair of torn earlobe with preservation of the perforation for an earring. Plast Reconstr Surg 51:472–475, 1973.

116. Buchan NG: The cleft earlobe: a method of repair with preservation of the earring canal. Br J Plast Surg 28:296–298, 1975.

117. Hamilton R, LaRossa D: Method for repair of cleft earlobes. Plast Reconstr Surg 55:99–101, 1975.

118. Becker PG, Turow J: Earring aspiration and other jewelry hazards. Pediatrics 78:494–496, 1986.

119. Phelan WJ: Complications of earrings in an infant. JAMA 243:2288, 1980.

120. Arevalo R: Ear piercing. N Engl J Med 291:634–635, 1974.

121. Noble DA: Another hazard of pierced ears. Br Med J 1:125, 1979.

122. Watson MG, Campbell JB, Pahor AL: Complications of nose piercing. Br Med J 294:1262, 1987.

CHAPTER 72

Basic Laser Physics and Visible Light Laser Surgery

RONALD G. WHEELAND

Laser surgery represents one of the most important advances that have occurred in cutaneous surgery during the past century. Laser devices provide effective treatment for a number of unrelated skin disorders for which therapy either previously did not exist or was so poor as to be unacceptable. Consequently, laser technology is currently an important, well-established, and respected component of the daily practice of many cutaneous surgeons.

Rapid developments in laser technology have made available increasingly sophisticated instruments offering a wide range of wavelengths capable of providing greater precision and specificity with fewer risks and complications. In addition, better application of basic laser physical principles and concepts to the clinical setting has further improved our understanding of how laser light interacts with living tissue. The number of absolute and relative indications for laser surgery has also been expanded by the many refinements in laser surgical techniques that have been developed during the past several decades. To most appropriately utilize any laser system, it is vital to understand how lasers are constructed and how they generate laser light. A working knowledge of the basic principles of laser-tissue interaction will help the cutaneous surgeon determine the proper clinical indications, associated limitations, potential benefits, and risks that may be encountered when employing each of the various laser systems.

History of Laser Surgery

Laser surgery can be regarded in the simplest of terms as a form of phototherapy. The first laser was not developed until 1960, but the true roots of phototherapy date back to the ancient Egyptians, who worshipped the sun god, Amen-Ra. They developed a therapeutic technique that employed sunlight to activate a naturally occurring photosensitizer found in parsley, psoralen, to stimulate the repigmentation of patches of vitiligo. Since then, many different sources of light have been variously used by physician phototherapists to treat diseases such as cutaneous tuberculosis, psoriasis, eczema, and mycosis fungoides. The first apparent reference to a source of radiant energy that could be interpreted as a laser is found in *War of the Worlds,* written in 1896 by H. G. Wells. In this story, the English countryside is invaded by Martian aliens who use a "heat ray" to destroy the villages. As fanciful as this may seem, Wells may have been ahead of his time by envisioning the subsequent development of the laser.

The theoretic concepts required to understand the principles of both spontaneous and stimulated emission of radiation were developed as part of Albert Einstein's quantum theory, which was published in 1916.[1] However, a long delay occurred before these basic concepts were actually used in the production of light energy. It was not until 1954 that the Microwave Amplification for the Stimulated Emission of Radiation (MASER) was developed by Charles H. Townes and James P. Gordon, using ammonia gas as an optical medium.[2] The first true laser system became operational in 1960 when Theodore Maiman, working for Hughes Corporation, employed microwave energy to stimulate a ruby crystal to generate a red beam of laser light.[3] Many laser systems have since been developed, including both the helium-neon (HeNe) laser by Javan and the neodymium:yttrium-aluminum-garnet (Nd:YAG) by Johnson in 1961, the argon laser in 1962 by Bennet, and the carbon dioxide laser by Patel in 1964.

Characteristics of Laser Energy and Basic Laser Physics

The word laser is an acronym that stands for *l*ight *a*mplification by the *s*timulated *e*mission of *r*adiation. A laser is both a physical process of amplification and an instrument that can be used to perform a variety of surgical procedures. Light, the first word in this acronym, is actually a very complicated system of radiant energy that is composed of both photons, the fundamental units of energy, and waves. It is organized into the electromagnetic spectrum according to the size of waves, usually measured in meters or fractions of a meter, which is the distance between two successive troughs or peaks of the wave form (Fig. 72–1). Each source of electromagnetic energy has a given frequency, which represents the number of waves that pass a fixed point in a second (Fig. 72–2). Because the wavelength and frequency are inversely related to one another, lasers with long wavelengths have low frequency and those with short wavelengths have high frequency. Radiation, the last word in the acronym laser, has been a source of much anxiety for some patients who are being treated with these devices. However, in this context, the word radiation is used to describe how laser energy is propagated in radiant waves and does not imply ionizing radiation. In fact, currently available medical lasers do not generally have sufficient energy to produce ionization. After more than 30 years of clinical experience using a wide variety of different laser systems, no increased risk of malignancy after laser exposure has been demonstrated.

FEATURES OF LASER LIGHT

Laser light has several features that differentiate it from conventional sources of light. One is that the emitted photons are spatially and temporally in phase with one another, a concept known as coherence (Fig. 72–3). A second is that the emitted laser energy is either of only a single wavelength or a very narrow band of wavelengths and conventionally is considered monochromatic. Another unique feature of laser light is collimation, which means the waves travel parallel to one another through space. The properties of coherence and collimation allow laser energy to be transmitted

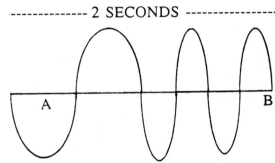

FREQUENCY OF A = WAVES/SECOND = 1
FREQUENCY OF B = WAVES/SECOND = 2

Figure 72–2. The frequency is the number of waves that pass a given point per second; it is inversely proportional to the wavelength.

over long distances without significant divergence of the beam and also permit laser energy to be precisely focused to a very small beam of light. A final property of laser light is its high intensity. The number of photons emitted by a laser per unit area is much greater than that emitted by all other sources of electromagnetic radiation, including sunlight.

COMPONENTS OF A LASER

All lasers have virtually the same four basic components: an optical cavity or resonator, a laser medium, a power source, and a delivery system (Fig. 72–4). The optical cavity surrounds the laser medium and contains the amplification process. The active laser medium usually gives the laser its name and may be composed of a gas, a liquid, or a solid. The gas lasers include the carbon dioxide and argon lasers; the liquid lasers are represented by the dye lasers, as they use liquid rhodamine dye for their active medium; and the solid lasers are represented by the ruby and Nd:YAG and solid-state diode lasers. The power supply, or "pump," excites the electrons found within the active laser medium to initiate the amplification process. This activation can be accomplished by the use of direct electrical current, as in the argon laser; by optical stimulation from another laser or a flashlamp, as in the dye lasers; radiofrequency excitation, as in many carbon dioxide lasers; and by

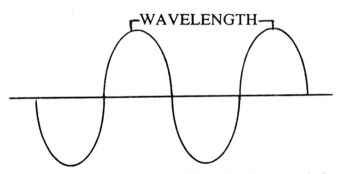

Figure 72–1. The wavelength for all forms of radiant energy is the measured distance between two successive peaks or troughs.

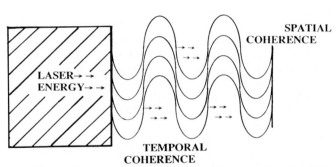

Figure 72–3. One unique feature of laser energy is coherence, both spatial and temporal.

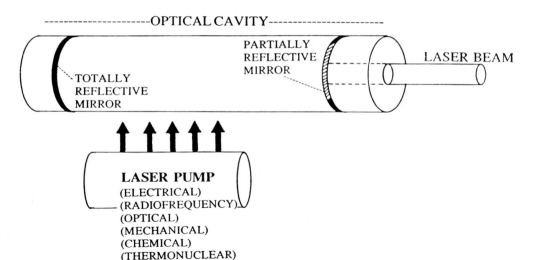

Figure 72–4. An idealized laser system is composed of an optical cavity, the laser medium, and an energizing source or "pump."

chemical reactions in which chemical bonds are made or broken to release energy, as in the hydrogen-fluoride laser. The delivery system may consist of a flexible hollow wave guide, fiberoptics, or an articulating arm with mirrored joints.

PRODUCTION OF LASER ENERGY

In an atom, the electrons occupy specific orbits around the nucleus that correspond to discrete, stable energy levels. When an atom absorbs a photon of energy, one or more electrons will briefly move to a higher energy, outer orbit. Because this excited state configuration is unstable, the atom will rapidly release the absorbed photon of energy, and the energized electron will return to its normal and more stable lower energy configuration, known as the ground energy state. When this decay process occurs under normal circumstances, the photons of energy are released spontaneously in a disorganized and random fashion. In a laser, however, the process of absorption and release of energy by an atom can be stimulated to occur by the delivery of energy from the laser pump.

To generate a laser beam, the molecules or atoms in the active medium must be stimulated by the laser pump in such a way that more molecules exist in their unstable, higher energy configuration than in their resting energy configuration. This phenomenon, known as population inversion, is a necessary requirement for beginning the amplification process. Once population inversion has been achieved, the excited-state electrons can be stimulated by the absorption of a photon of precisely the correct amount of energy to undergo stimulated orbital decay. When this occurs, two photons of identical wavelength and frequency will exit the atom together, traveling in phase and in the same direction as one another. This is the initiating step in the process of amplification and is required for the generation of a laser beam.

The cylindrical shape of the optical cavity or resonator contains the amplification process (Fig. 72–4). Reflective mirrors are placed at both ends of the optical cavity and at right angles to the longitudinal axis of the cylinder.

These mirrors reflect the stimulated photons that are released parallel to the long axis of the optical cavity and perpendicular to the ends back into the active medium. Those photons that are released at an angle to either end of the optical cavity are lost as waste heat. For maximal reflection of photons to occur, parallel transmission must exist; otherwise, amplification will be reduced and more energy will be required to produce a laser beam. Because of this requirement, most laser systems have an efficiency of less than 1%. The carbon dioxide laser, one of the most efficient laser systems, has an efficiency of only 10%. Those photons that are reflected back into the optical cavity will stimulate other excited-state atoms to release two photons of energy. The process of amplification results in a cascade effect; as additional metastable atoms are impacted by ever-increasing numbers of photons, additional coherent photons of energy are released, which further amplifies the process. Once a sufficient intensity has been achieved, complete amplification occurs and a laser beam is generated.

One of the mirrored ends of the optical cavity is only partially reflective, so that between 1% and 3% of the light energy that has been generated by the amplification process is released. Once this beam of energy leaves the resonator tube, it is directed to the target with an appropriate delivery system and focused to the desired beam size using a lens of proper focal length.

LASER-TISSUE INTERACTION

The currently available medical laser systems (Table 72–1) span only a narrow band of the entire electromagnetic spectrum from the ultraviolet to the infrared wavelengths. Despite this fact, it is still possible to produce specific effects in tissue from this relatively limited number of wavelengths. To obtain reproducible results when performing laser surgery, it is important to understand how the treatment parameters—irradiance, energy fluence, spot size, treatment area,[4] pulse duration, and pulse width—and the optical characteristics of the tissue, wavelength, and beam configuration all can influence the results.

TABLE 72–1. **VARIOUS LASER SYSTEMS**

Emission	Laser System	Wavelength (nm)	Mode of Output	Absorption Characteristics
Ultraviolet (100–400 nm)	Argon-fluoride	193	Pulsed	
	Krypton-chloride	222	Pulsed	
	Krypton-fluoride	248	Pulsed	
	Xenon-chloride	308	Pulsed	
	Xenon-fluoride	351	Pulsed	
Visible (400–700 nm)	Argon (blue-green)	488–514	CW	Hemoglobin, melanin
	Dye (pigment)	510	Q-switched	Melanin
	Krypton (green)	521, 530	CW	Hemoglobin, melanin
	Frequency-doubled YAG (green)	532	Q-switched	Melanin, tattoos (red pigments)
	Copper (green)	511	Pulsed	Hemoglobin, melanin
	Krypton (yellow)	568	CW	Hemoglobin
	Copper (yellow)	578	Pulsed	Hemoglobin
	Dye	577, 585	CW, Pulsed	Hemoglobin
	Helium-neon	633	CW	—
	Ruby	694	Q-switched	Melanin, tattoos
	Alexandrite	755	Q-switched	Tattoos, melanin
Infrared (700–100,000 nm)	GaAs	910	CW	—
	Nd:YAG	1,064	CW, Q-switched	Protein, tattoos
	Ho:YAG	2,140	CW, Pulsed	H_2O
	Er:YAG	2,940	CW	H_2O
	CO_2	10,600	CW, SP	H_2O

CW, continuous wave; SP, superpulsed.

Irradiance

Irradiance (IR), also known as the power density (PD), is the power concentration that is incident on tissue.[5, 6] It is calculated by the formula:

$$IR = \frac{\text{laser output (watts)}}{\pi r^2},$$

where r is the radius of the laser beam. The irradiance is inversely proportional to the radius of the beam, so that when the radius of the laser beam is decreased, the IR will be increased (Fig. 72–5). The IR can also be increased by increasing the output of the laser.

Energy Fluence

A second important primary treatment parameter that is used in defining laser beam dosimetry is energy fluence (EF). The EF is the amount of energy delivered to a unit area in a single pulse and is calculated by the formula:

$$EF = \frac{\text{laser output (W)} \times \text{exposure time (sec)}}{\pi r^2} = J/cm^2,$$

where r is the radius of the laser beam. The EF is usually defined for pulsed laser systems.[6] Increasing the laser output, decreasing the beam diameter, or increasing the exposure time will all act to increase the EF. For the continuous-discharge laser systems, EF is not typically used. However, the average amount of the total energy delivered to an entire treatment area, known as the spatial average energy fluence (SAEF), can be calculated for continuous-discharge lasers.

Spot Size and Treatment Area

The diameter of the beam of light influences both the irradiance and the energy fluence. To obtain maximal

Figure 72–5. The irradiance is determined by the incident laser power and the beam diameter.

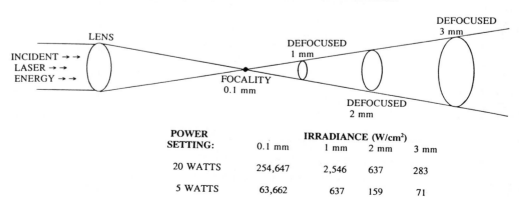

IRRADIANCE AND BEAM DIAMETER

POWER SETTING:	IRRADIANCE (W/cm²)			
	0.1 mm	1 mm	2 mm	3 mm
20 WATTS	254,647	2,546	637	283
5 WATTS	63,662	637	159	71

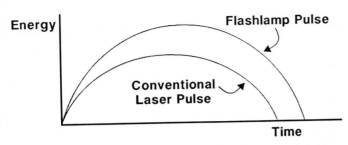

Figure 72–6. The energy-time relationship in a conventional pulsed laser.

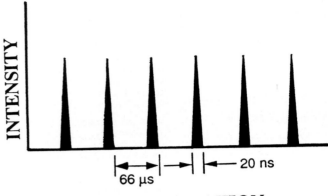

PULSE DURATION

Figure 72–8. The intensity profile of the pulsed metal vapor laser system with short, 20-nsec pulses separated by longer "pauses."

precision when treating small lesions, a beam of light that approximates the size of the lesion is typically utilized. However, when a small laser beam is used, the irradiance will be high unless the power setting of the laser is concomitantly decreased. For the treatment of large lesions, the largest possible beam diameter is used. The size of the beam is typically determined by the output of the laser and the IR required to produce the desired effect. In general, the nature of the condition and the anatomic location being treated, the output and wavelength of the laser being used, the pain tolerance of the patient, and the frequency and number of procedures required to complete the treatment all influence the choice of the beam diameter and the size of the area that is treated in a given session.

Pulse Duration and Pulse Width

The early lasers typically delivered energy in a continuous and sustained fashion, sometimes known as continuous wave (CW) output. The CW laser systems can be electronically or mechanically shuttered to produce interrupted pulses of energy. However, the duration of these pulses is relatively long (e.g., approximately 0.05 to 0.2 second). Newer laser systems have attempted to improve specificity and selectivity by the delivery of much shorter pulses (Figs. 72–6 through 72–9) of laser energy.[7] Two important and highly interrelated factors must be considered when choosing a particular pulsed

laser system for the management of vascular or pigmented lesions. These are the thermal relaxation time (Tr) and selective photothermolysis. The Tr is defined as the time required for an object to cool to 50% of the temperature achieved immediately after laser exposure without conducting heat to the surrounding tissue.[7] To achieve maximum precision, or selective photothermolysis, the exposure time must be shorter than the Tr. If the exposure exceeds or equals the Tr, thermal energy will be transferred by conduction to adjacent tissues, resulting in nonspecific thermal damage. For microvessels, the Tr is on the order of 0.05 to 1.2 milliseconds, and for organelles, it is on the order of nanoseconds.[8, 9]

The newest laser systems have attempted to further improve the precision of the laser-tissue interaction by the delivery of ultrashort, nanosecond pulses of laser energy. These pulses are produced by a process known as Q-switching. In these systems, the light is first polarized to limit propagation in only one direction (Fig. 72–10), and then the amplification process is allowed to

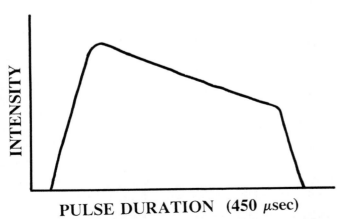

PULSE DURATION (450 μsec)

Figure 72–7. The intensity profile of a conventional pulsed laser system.

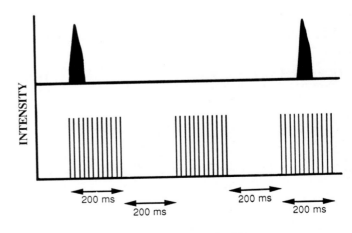

PULSE DURATION

Figure 72–9. Chains of pulses from the metal vapor laser can be delivered to resemble a continuous-discharge laser system.

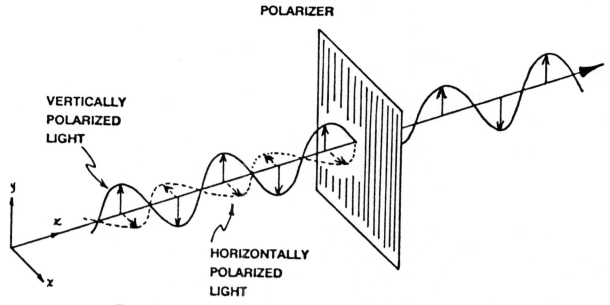

Figure 72–10. The light is polarized to one plane in a Q-switched laser system.

continue within the optical cavity without the release of any energy until a peak power of 10 to 100 megawatts has been reached. The energy is then released by switching the current on a photo-optically activated crystal, known as a Pockels cell (Fig. 72–11), as a single burst having an extremely short pulse width (Fig. 72–12) of 10 to 40 nanoseconds (nsec). The effects of the Q-switched lasers on tissue may be thermal or photoacoustic in nature (Fig. 72–13). These effects will be discussed in more detail under the individual laser systems that employ this technique of pulse production.

Optical Properties of Tissue and the Influence of Wavelength

For laser energy to be useful clinically, it must interact with tissue. However, depending on the optical properties of the target, the incident beam of laser energy can strike tissue (Fig. 72–14) and be reflected, transmitted, scattered, or absorbed.[7] If the light is reflected or transmitted, no interaction will occur with the tissue, and no effect will be produced. Absorption is required for a laser system to produce any photothermal or

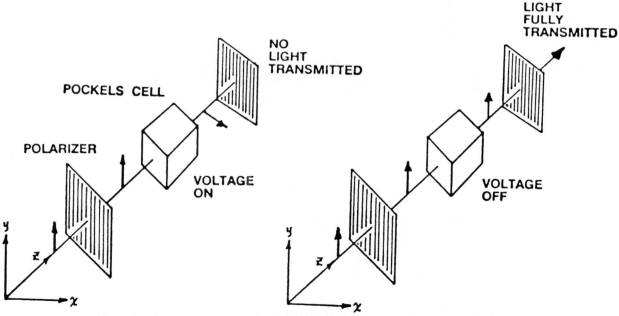

Figure 72–11. The Pockels cell serves as a photo-optical shutter in the Q-switched laser.

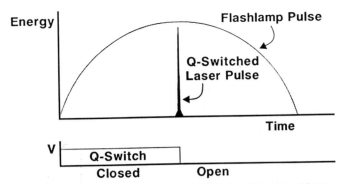

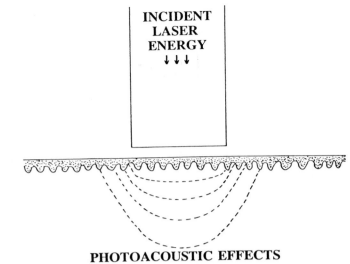

INCIDENT
LASER
ENERGY
↓ ↓ ↓

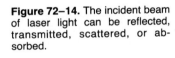

Figure 72–12. The energy-time relationship in a Q-switched laser.

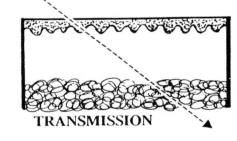

PHOTOACOUSTIC EFFECTS

Figure 72–13. Photoacoustic effects resulting from the impact of a Q-switched laser on tissue.

photochemical effect in tissue. By matching the absorptive characteristics of the targeted tissue with the proper wavelength of laser light, maximal specificity of the laser-tissue interaction will result. If the energy is scattered within the tissue, an imprecise reaction will result in unwanted tissue damage and loss of selectivity.

An understanding of the spectral properties and relative concentration of the various chromophores in the target is also a prerequisite for maximizing the precision of the laser-tissue interaction. For example, it is useful to know, when treating vascular lesions, that the absorption spectrum (Fig. 72–15) for oxygenated hemoglobin ($HgbO_2$) has three main peaks (418, 542, and 577 nm), and thus selection of a laser system that emits one of these wavelengths would likely provide a reasonably precise form of therapy. However, because there is

competitive absorption by melanin in the epidermis and this absorption is greatest at the two shorter absorptive peaks of oxygenated hemoglobin, the best wavelength of light to use in the treatment of vascular lesions is 577 nm. Thus, even though the vascular component of the lesion could be relatively precisely targeted, failure to consider the possible absorption by melanin will result in inadvertent and unwanted epidermal injury, thereby

Figure 72–14. The incident beam of laser light can be reflected, transmitted, scattered, or absorbed.

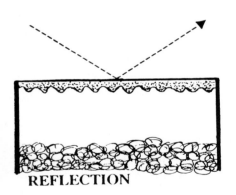

REFLECTION

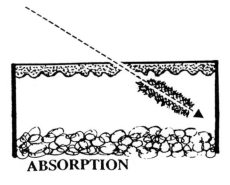

TRANSMISSION

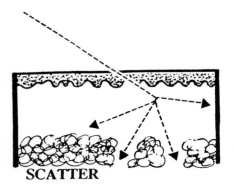

SCATTER

ABSORPTION

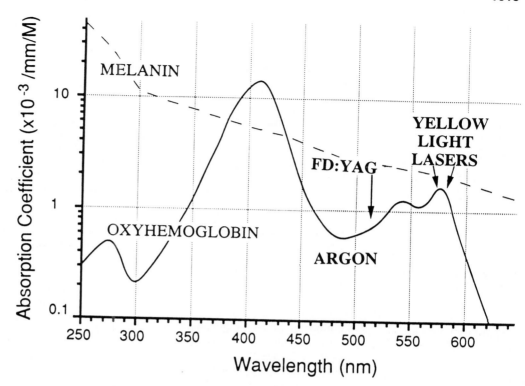

Figure 72–15. The absorption coefficients for the two main chromophores in skin: melanin and oxyhemoglobin.

prolonging healing and possibly causing hypopigmentation, textural changes or scars.

Most of the effects produced by lasers are the result of thermal reactions that are predictably and reproducibly temperature dependent. The only reversible thermal reaction that is produced by laser radiation is protein denaturation, which occurs at tissue temperatures up to 40°C. Irreversible effects are seen at higher temperatures, with coagulation occurring at temperatures up to 68°C (Fig. 72–16), vaporization at 100°C (Fig. 72–17), and carbonization at temperatures of up to 300°C.

Beam Characteristics

The characteristic configuration, or *beam mode,* of the laser determines both the quality of the beam and the spatial distribution of the power within it. The beam mode, also called the transverse electromagnetic mode (TEM), is defined by the profile of the beam and the pattern of the impact it makes on tissue (Fig. 72–18). The most common TEM pattern, known as the TEM_{00} mode, has the greatest concentration of power at the center and lesser amounts at the periphery in a Gaussian distribution. Another type of TEM pattern, the TEM_{01} mode, has a doughnut hole appearance, with greatest power at the periphery and minimal power at the center of the beam impact. Because of this beam mode characteristic, the beam is relatively large and has ill-defined margins.

Visible Light Lasers

Visible light comprises only a relatively small portion of the entire electromagnetic spectrum. However, lasers

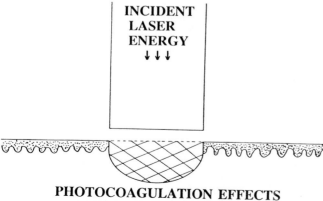

PHOTOCOAGULATION EFFECTS

Figure 72–16. Photocoagulation results from temperatures generated in tissue of up to 68°C by the impact of laser energy.

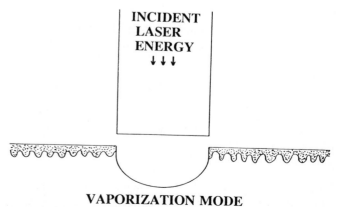

VAPORIZATION MODE

Figure 72–17. Vaporization results from temperatures generated in tissue of 100°C by the impact of laser energy.

IMPACT POWER DISTRIBUTION

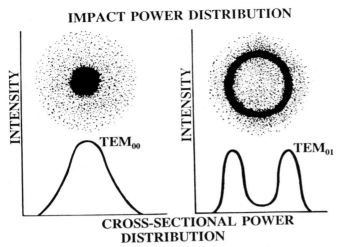

Figure 72–18. Cross-sectional power distribution (transverse electromagnetic mode) for two different beam types.

capable of producing visible light have enabled cutaneous surgeons to manage many conditions for which no effective treatment previously existed.[10] Visible light lasers have been primarily used in the management of vascular (Table 72–2) and inflammatory lesions, pigmented lesions and tattoos, and a host of other uncommon conditions. Each of these conditions will be discussed individually.

VASCULAR LESIONS

There are relatively few absolute indications for performing laser surgery, but one condition that certainly belongs in this category is the port-wine stain. Many of the principles involved in the effective management of port-wine stains can be appropriately applied to the treatment of many other types of vascular lesions. As a consequence, this condition will be used to address the issues involved in the evaluation and selection of the proper laser system and surgical technique to provide the most satisfactory results in treating this common congenital vascular malformation.

Port-Wine Stains

Over the years, a number of ineffective techniques (e.g., excision and grafting, radiation, cryosurgery,[11] and tattooing[12]) have been used to treat port-wine stains (PWS). As a consequence of the inability to provide an acceptable form of treatment for the 0.3% of people born with PWS,[13, 14] many children and adults have suffered significant emotional, psychological, and social difficulties throughout their lives because of this congenital birth defect.[15, 16]

Despite the fact that these lesions are sometimes incorrectly considered to be of only cosmetic importance, a number of predictable changes can be expected to occur within a PWS as the affected individual ages. These changes not only may add to the disfigurement produced by these lesions, but also may cause significant

functional impairment. Many of the changes seen in PWS are the result of progressive dilatation of blood vessels, which develop at an unpredictable rate. One direct effect of this ectasia is a gradual darkening of the color of PWS from faint pink or light red, as seen in infants and children, to a deep red color, as seen in adolescents and young adults, and finally to a blue or even purple color, as seen in older adults. The change in color is frequently seen in association with the development of multiple, elevated, fragile 1- to 3-mm papules,[17] commonly known as blebs. The formation of blebs causes surface irregularities to appear; these are often the source of significant functional impairment,[18] as the lesions may be easily traumatized by minor injuries and bleed or become secondarily infected.[19] The progressive ectasia of the blood vessels may also cause soft tissue hypertrophy, especially of the eyelids and lips, which can also produce additional functional impairment.

Fortunately, the development of laser technology has permitted these progressive changes to be corrected or prevented from occurring, depending on the point at which treatment is initiated. Laser photocoagulation lightens the color of the PWS by reducing the size and number of the ectatic blood vessels. This not only smooths the surface of the PWS, which improves function by reducing the risk of bleeding, but also improves the appearance of the patient.

Argon Laser. As the first laser system used in the management of PWS, the argon laser played an impor-

TABLE 72–2. VASCULAR LESIONS TREATED WITH VISIBLE LIGHT LASERS

Acne rosacea
Adenoma sebaceum
Angiokeratoma
    Fabry's
    Fordyce
Angiolymphoid hyperplasia
Angioma serpiginosa
Angiosarcoma
Blue rubber bleb syndrome
Capillary hemangioma
Carcinoid
Cavernous hemangioma
Cherry angioma
Glomus tumor
Hemangiolymphangioma
Kaposi's sarcoma
Poikiloderma of Civatte
Port-wine stain
Pyogenic granuloma
Rhinophyma
Telangiectasia
    Actinic
    Connective tissue disorders
    Essential
    Nasolabial
    Osler-Weber-Rendu
    Postrhinoplasty red nose
    Postsclerotherapy matting
    Radiation dermatitis
    Rosacea
    Spider
Venous lake

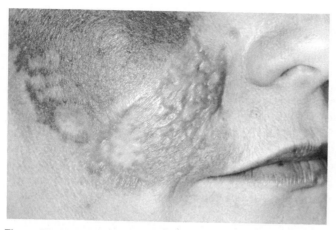

Figure 72–19. Hypertrophic scarring on the cheek that resulted from argon laser photocoagulation.

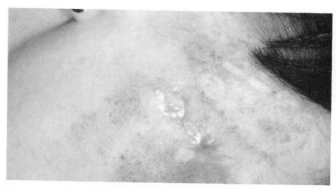

Figure 72–21. Textural changes on the cheek that resulted from argon laser photocoagulation.

tant role in the evolutionary process that has occurred in the treatment of this vascular disorder. Laser surgery for PWS has evolved rapidly, largely as a result of new technology that has provided greater precision in the laser-tissue interaction. However, it was the development of the argon laser that originally sparked the interest of cutaneous surgeons in treating PWS. Initially, when the argon laser became available, there was great anticipation that this blue-green light, with two major emission peaks at 488 and 514 nm, would produce selective damage to blood vessels.[20–23] Because a substantial overlap existed between the emission spectrum for the argon laser and the absorption spectrum for oxyhemoglobin (see Fig. 72–15), it was hoped that the amount of injury to nonvascular tissues would be minimal and the thermal effects would be precisely confined to the vasculature. Unfortunately, these high expectations were not achieved clinically with the argon laser, and a number of significant limitations, side effects, and complications were soon identified.

The most common limitation was the inability to effectively treat children,[24–26] and the most common complications were the development of hypertrophic scars (Figs. 72–19, 72–20) and textural changes (Fig. 72–21) after treatment of certain anatomic locations[27–29] and the creation of permanent hypopigmentation[5] (Figs. 72–22, 72–23). The incidence of scarring from treatment of port-wine stains was found in numerous studies to range from 5 to 20%.[22, 30] It is currently recognized that these effects are largely due to a lack of precision in the laser-tissue interaction, specifically the fact that the energy emission for the argon laser occurs at a trough in the absorption spectrum for oxyhemoglobin (see Fig. 72–15), which causes heat to be distributed more widely throughout the dermis and not strictly confined to the targeted blood vessels. In addition, at these wavelengths considerable absorptive interference by melanin is found

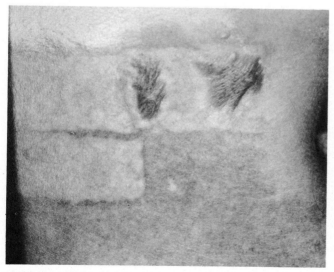

Figure 72–20. Hypertrophic scarring on the neck that resulted from argon laser photocoagulation.

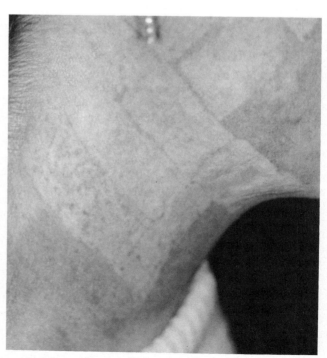

Figure 72–22. Permanent hypopigmentation that followed argon laser photocoagulation.

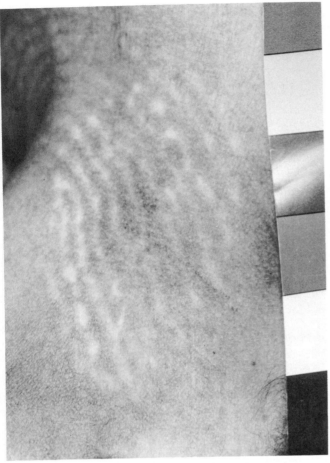

Figure 72–23. Permanent linear hypopigmentation resulted from use of the argon laser and a striping technique.

complications, its role in cutaneous surgery has been at least tentatively defined. Based on considerations such as patient age, anatomic location, and physical appearance of the lesion, several generalizations can be made. In patients more than 37 years of age with deep red or purple lesions, a favorable response can be anticipated with the argon laser.[37] However, patients with lesions located on the upper lip, jawline, nasolabial folds, eyelids, or extremities or those individuals younger than 12 years or with light-colored lesions are more likely to obtain an unfavorable response.[30] Using these suggested guidelines, patients with a potential for poor results can frequently be identified and offered some other form of treatment, resulting in an overall success rate as high as 85%.[30]

Yellow Light Lasers. Because of the many limitations of the argon laser in the treatment of patients with PWS, a concerted attempt was made to identify alternate forms of laser surgery that could reduce the risk of scarring and hypopigmentation while also improving the response, especially in children. Even though the argon laser could effectively treat children when low power and meticulous postoperative wound care were used, the incidence of scarring still remained unacceptably high at 8%.[38]

The net result of this research was the development of a diverse group of lasers capable of producing yellow light with wavelengths varying from 568 to 585 nm, but with marked differences in their active media, mode of delivery, and clinical indications. It has shown that yellow light with an approximate wavelength of 577 nm can provide a more precise form of treatment for vascular lesions, since this energy is maximally absorbed by oxyhemoglobin at its beta-absorption peak.[39, 40] There is also deeper penetration at this longer wavelength, as well as less absorptive interference caused by the main competing chromophore, melanin. The mechanism of

within the overlying epidermis. When selective photocoagulation of dermal blood vessels is attempted,[31] unwanted thermal damage to the epidermis occurs as the light energy is absorbed by it. The effects of this interaction are vesicle formation, crusting, and a reduction in the amount of energy that reaches the dermal blood vessels.

A number of different treatment techniques have been used with the argon laser in an attempt to improve the results and reduce the complication rate. In one of these techniques, several small representative areas are treated as tests using different irradiances to determine the best laser parameters for subsequent treatment of the patient.[32, 33] Other techniques to decrease thermal damage have recommended the delivery of the laser energy with either a slightly overlapping polka-dot pattern[34] (Fig. 72–24) or a spaced striping pattern.[35] Attempts were also made to pre-chill the skin with ice or cool compresses before argon laser exposure.[36] Although the argon laser offered a major advance over older techniques used in the treatment of port-wine stains, its potential usefulness rapidly diminished with the introduction of newer laser systems. Despite the argon laser's significant limitations and well-recognized

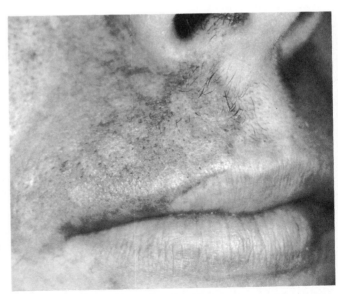

Figure 72–24. Polka-dot pattern used with the argon laser to reduce the risk of hypertrophic scarring during the treatment of port-wine stains.

this laser-tissue interaction is the conversion of light energy to thermal energy after absorption by oxyhemoglobin within the erythrocyte. This energy is then conducted to the endothelial cells within the wall of the blood vessel, causing coagulation and sometimes rupture of the vessel. This selectivity for vascular structures improves precision, reduces epidermal injury, speeds healing, and reduces the risks of nonspecific thermal damage.[41] This minimizes scarring, pigment alteration, and textural changes and maximizes the effectiveness of the treatment of PWS, even in children. Because of these benefits, a number of yellow light lasers have been developed and approved for the treatment of cutaneous vascular lesions, including PWS.

Argon-Pumped Tunable Dye Laser. The argon-dye or tunable dye laser utilizes an argon laser to energize a solution containing one of a number of different organic dyes. This allows the production of an immediately adjustable broad band of light energy with wavelengths varying from 488 nm (blue) to 638 nm (red). This energy is discharged in continuous fashion or is mechanically or electronically shuttered to produce relatively long pulses of light of from 0.05 to 0.3 second. Because of the absorptive characteristics of hemoglobin, this laser is most commonly "tuned" to maximize its output of yellow light at a wavelength of either 577 or 585 nm.[42, 43]

The original technique used to treat PWS with the argon-dye laser was identical to that employing the older argon laser technology. This consisted of the delivery of slightly overlapping pulses in a polka-dot pattern with a 1-mm diameter beam and a pulse duration of 0.05 to 0.2 second. A tracing technique that employs magnified vision to identify and treat individual blood vessels within a PWS has also been described. In this technique, minimal power and a 100-μ beam are used to trace out and photothermally seal individual blood vessels.[42, 43] Perhaps the most innovative technique for treating PWS delivers the laser energy with a robotic optical scanning device. These devices temporally separate individual pulses from one another to minimize thermal damage.

Each of these techniques can utilize the argon-dye laser to effectively treat PWS. The primary advantages of the argon-dye laser over the argon laser are reduced epidermal injury, a lack of permanent postoperative hypopigmentation, and improved responsiveness because of the more precise delivery of laser energy to the vasculature. This precision is sufficient to permit treatment of children, as well as of anatomic locations that are at increased risk for scarring (e.g., the upper lip, jawline, and lateral neck). The primary disadvantage of the tracing technique is the somewhat tedious nature of the procedure, which permits treatment of only small areas per session.

Flashlamp-Pumped Pulsed Dye Laser. This laser system, commonly known as the pulsed dye laser (PDL), also utilizes an organic dye to produce yellow light. This system differs from the argon-dye laser in that the dye is energized by pulses of white light from a flashlamp (see Fig. 72–6). The laser can only be "tuned" to emit different wavelengths of light by changing the organic dye solution within the optical cavity. Used initially at a wavelength of 577 nm,[44] the pulsed dye laser is currently used almost exclusively to produce yellow light with a wavelength of 585 nm. Another unique feature of this laser is that it discharges the energy only in short pulses having a duration of 450 microseconds (see Fig. 72–7). This pulse duration was chosen to provide selective photothermolysis of the small blood vessels in the PWS.[8, 45–47] Selective photocoagulation is possible if the duration of the laser pulse is short enough that thermal diffusion from the blood vessel to the surrounding tissues does not occur.[48] In this way, thermal damage can be very precisely restricted to just the targeted blood vessels.

Treatment of a PWS with the PDL requires determination of the proper energy fluence to be used. Small representative areas are treated as tests with different energy fluences (EF). The minimum EF that will provide clearing of the blood vessels can be determined by evaluating the test sites after 6 to 8 weeks when fading has slowly occurred. Once the proper EF has been established by testing, larger areas can be effectively treated by delivering slightly overlapping pulses. Bruising develops immediately after treatment, and the patient often experiences a sunburn-like sensation that can be reduced by the topical application of aloe vera gel or ice.

The primary benefit of pulsed yellow light in the treatment of PWS is its ability to treat infants, children (Fig. 72–25), and anatomic locations that are normally at high risk for scar formation.[49, 50] It appears, from the collective experience of many cutaneous laser surgeons, that treatment may be initiated early in life with the PDL.[51–54] Treatment of PWS during early infancy may also be associated with such hidden benefits as smaller areas of involvement and fewer treatments required to obtain substantial lightening.[53, 54] Another benefit of the PDL is the ability to rapidly treat large areas because of the 5-mm beam of light that is produced by these systems (Fig. 72–26).

Unfortunately, there are also some disadvantages associated with PDL treatment of PWS. The biggest disadvantage is the immediate ecchymosis that occurs after exposure and persists for 7 to 10 days. In most cases there is also a need for multiple retreatments, performed at 4- to 6-week intervals, to obtain maximal clearing. The number of retreatments required to obtain the desired level of improvement is unpredictable, largely because of the marked variability in blood vessel size, depth within the dermis, and flow rate.[55] The discomfort of the procedure is sufficient that most children will require sedation or general anesthesia for safe and effective treatment. Use of occluded topical anesthetic agents, such as 30 to 40% lidocaine in acid mantle cream and a eutectic mixture of local anesthetics (EMLA), a mixture of prilocaine and lidocaine, has helped reduce the need for sedation and general anesthesia in some individuals.[56–58] A "Swiss cheese" appearance can also result if the pulses are not sufficiently overlapped to provide uniform photocoagulation of the dermal blood vessels (Fig. 72–27). Finally, apparently because of intense competition by melanin for dye laser energy, patients with very dark skin color cannot be effectively treated with the PDL.[59]

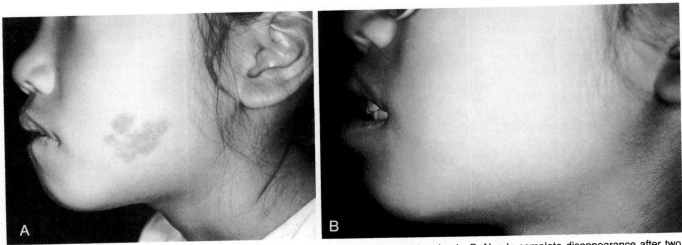

Figure 72–25. *A,* Preoperative appearance of a young girl with a port-wine stain on the cheek. *B,* Nearly complete disappearance after two treatments with the pulsed dye laser.

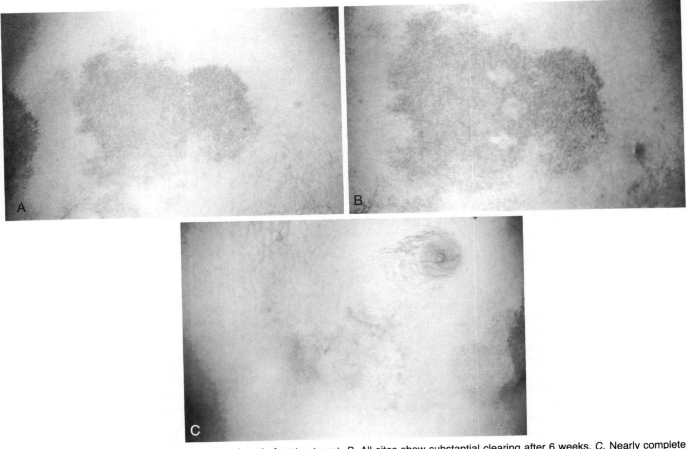

Figure 72–26. *A,* Large port-wine stain on the chest before treatment. *B,* All sites show substantial clearing after 6 weeks. *C,* Nearly complete removal has been accomplished after two treatments with the pulsed dye laser.

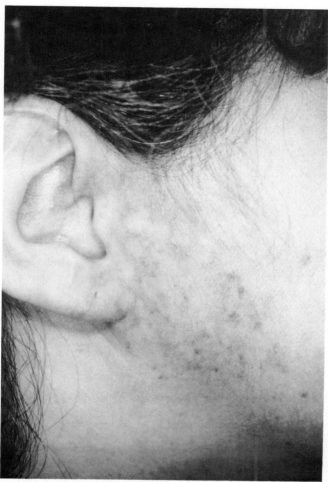

Figure 72–27. An obvious "Swiss-cheese" pattern is produced if the pulses are not slightly overlapped.

Copper Vapor Laser. The copper vapor laser is a heavy metal laser that uses copper as its active medium, instead of the toxic organic dyes and solvents found in some other lasers, to produce yellow light with a wavelength of 578 nm.[60] This laser produces a peak power of 9 kW within the optical cavity and releases this energy in pulses like those produced by the pulsed dye laser (see Fig. 72–8), but only 20 to 40 nanoseconds in duration.[61, 62] Although these lasers are pulsed, the repetition rate of 15 kHz is so fast (see Fig. 72–9) that the light appears to be emitted in continuous fashion, often referred to as "quasicontinuous." Despite marked differences in the time profiles of the copper vapor and pulsed dye lasers,[62] histologic studies have found that exposure to the copper vapor laser produces selective vascular effects with only moderate perivascular changes and preservation of the epidermis.[61, 63, 64]

The chain of copper vapor laser pulses can be electronically "gated" to treat PWS in a polka-dot pattern using a 0.267- to 1.0-mm spot and a short series of 0.075- to 0.3-second pulses. A tracing technique such as that used with the argon-dye laser, with delivery of minimal power and a 0.1-mm spot, can also be used. Finally, this laser can be coupled to a robotic scanner

(Fig. 72–28) so that larger areas can be rapidly and simply treated. This laser has advantages and disadvantages similar to those previously described for the argon-dye laser.

Krypton Laser. The krypton laser has been used clinically in ophthalmology for some time,[65–71] but modifications have been made in this system that allow it to be used in the management of PWS. Because this laser utilizes a gas medium to produce yellow light with a wavelength of 568 nm, the hazards of the toxic solvents and organic substances found in the dye lasers can be avoided. Two bands of green light with wavelengths of 521 and 530 nm are simultaneously produced by this laser, but they are filtered out when only the yellow band of light is desired for treatment. The light from this laser can be delivered using a polka-dot pattern, a tracing technique, or a robotic scanner. Long-term studies of the efficacy of this laser system in the treatment of PWS have not been performed because of the relative newness of this device.

Robotic Optical Scanners and Automated Handpieces. The effectiveness of the polka-dot and the minimal power tracing techniques has been well established in the treatment of PWS, but these methods are somewhat tedious to perform, require maximum attention to detail, and may be difficult to reproduce without a significant amount of experience. For these reasons, techniques using robotic optical scanners and automated handpieces that attach to the laser by fiberoptics have been developed.[72–74] These devices employ microprocessor-controlled automated programs to deliver pulses of light in a predetermined, geometric pattern. This provides a reproducible form of treatment for PWS that reduces the risk of inadvertent thermal injury to nonvascular tissue.

Currently there are three available types of robotic scanners (Scanall, Multiscan, and Autolase) and two types of automated handpieces (Hexascan, CC-Scan).[75] The most widely available of these systems (Hexascan) utilizes a 1-mm beam of light; an adjustable pulse duration of 30 to 990 milliseconds, which varies according to the selected energy fluence; a pause interval of 50 milliseconds; and different sizes of hexagonal grids from 1 to 13 mm in diameter (Fig. 72–29). The time required to deliver the 127 pulses necessary to treat a 13-mm-diameter hexagon is 20 seconds. The latest of the scanning devices, the Autolase, can vary the density of the pulse pattern so that the center of one pulse may be separated from the next pulse by as little as 550 μm for the treatment of pigmented lesions or by as much as 750 μm to 1000 μm for the treatment of vascular lesions (see Fig. 72–28). The majority of these devices can be adapted to connect to a number of different visible light lasers, including the argon, argon-dye, copper vapor, krypton and frequency-doubled Nd:YAG laser.

Telangiectasia

The argon laser remains a very useful instrument for the management of isolated facial telangiectases, especially on the nose,[76, 77] either alone or in association with rhinoplasty.[78] In some patients, the greater thermal

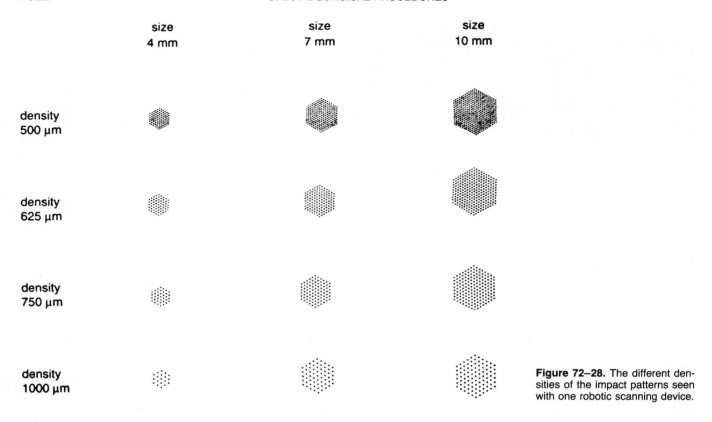

Figure 72–28. The different densities of the impact patterns seen with one robotic scanning device.

injury produced by the reduced specificity of the green light from this laser can seal large blood vessels and vessels with high flow rates (e.g., on the nasal alae) (Fig. 72–30). One effective technique uses a 1-mm beam of light to deliver 0.1- to 0.2-second pulses at spaced intervals along the length of each vessel (Fig. 72–31). This segmental approach often seals the blood vessels without having to treat the entire vessel length. Because only the blood vessels are photocoagulated and the intervening normal skin is spared, the risk of developing permanent hypopigmentation or scarring is substantially reduced compared with that seen with the treatment of PWS. Crusting of the skin surface typically develops postoperatively but is usually of only short duration. Gradual disappearance of the treated vessels can be expected to occur over a period of 4 to 6 weeks, but persistent lesions commonly require retreatment.

Using a similar treatment technique, the argon-dye, copper vapor,[79] and krypton lasers can also be used to treat facial telangiectasia (Fig. 72–32). For laser systems

Figure 72–29. The various densities of the impact patterns seen with a different robotic scanning device.

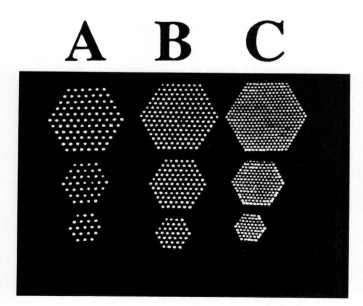

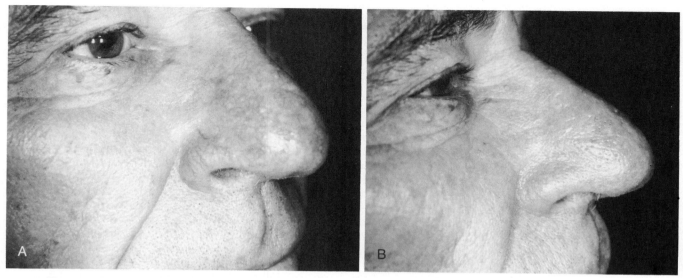

Figure 72–30. *A,* Multiple telangiectases on the nose seen preoperatively. *B,* Nearly complete clearing after one treatment.

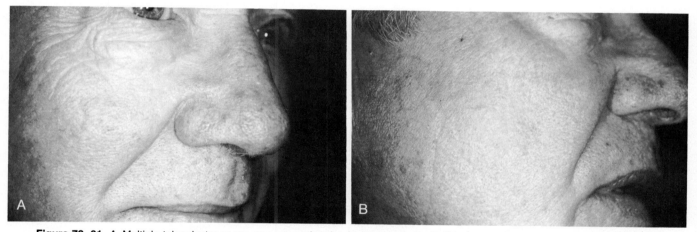

Figure 72–31. *A,* Multiple telangiectases are present on the cheek preoperatively. *B,* Nearly complete clearing after one treatment.

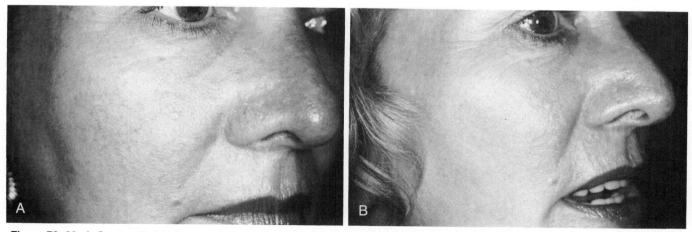

Figure 72–32. *A,* Scattered telangiectases are present on the cheek preoperatively. *B,* Nearly complete clearing is seen after one treatment.

that are capable of producing yellow as well as green light, an attempt is often made to first treat the fine blood vessels with yellow light. If resolution does not occur, green light is subsequently used to improve the results.

For telangiectases that involve large areas, such as poikiloderma of Civatte,[80] severe facial solar telangiectasia (Fig. 72–33), and extensive acne rosacea[81] (Fig. 72–34), a different technique is often required to be successful. In these patients, the confluence of blood vessels makes the risk of scarring or hypopigmentation substantial unless maximum precision of the laser-tissue interaction is accomplished. For this reason, yellow light is most often utilized in the management of these patients and is delivered with one of the robotic scanning devices or with a pulsed dye laser.[76] Poor responsiveness has been seen using a variety of lasers to treat red telangiectases 0.2 mm or larger on the legs. However, the PDL does seem to be beneficial in the management of the small matlike telangiectases that form in some individuals after traditional sclerotherapy.[82]

Tattoos

Over the years, cutaneous surgeons have used a multitude of different techniques for removing decorative tattoos. These have included salabrasion,[83] derma-brasion,[84] split-thickness tangential excision,[85] chemical scarification,[86] cryosurgery,[87] excisional surgery,[88] infrared coagulation,[89] and ablation using the argon[22] and carbon dioxide lasers.[90–92] However, none of these techniques could ensure complete tattoo pigment removal in a single procedure without also producing irregularities in the texture or color of the skin or scarring. In addition, 18 to 24 months were typically required before the final cosmetic result was achieved.

Q-Switched Ruby Laser. As a consequence of the poor results provided by the existing forms of treatment for decorative tattoos, new techniques were constantly being sought.[93, 94] A successful technique was described in 1983 using the Q-switched ruby laser[95] to remove blue and black tattoos without causing scarring or producing permanent textural changes. These obvious advantages helped re-establish the ruby laser as a valuable clinical tool for cutaneous surgeons.[96–98]

Characteristics. The ruby laser produces high-intensity red light with a wavelength of 694 nm. Within the flashlamp-pumped optical cavity (Fig. 72–35), the peak energy often reaches 100,000,000 W. Because the laser is Q-switched (see Fig. 72–12), the energy is emitted in extremely short pulses of only 20 to 40 nanoseconds.

Mechanism of Action. The ruby laser energy is well absorbed by carbon particles, moderately absorbed by melanin, and minimally, if at all, absorbed by oxyhemoglobin.[99, 100] Very selective injury to only the tattoo

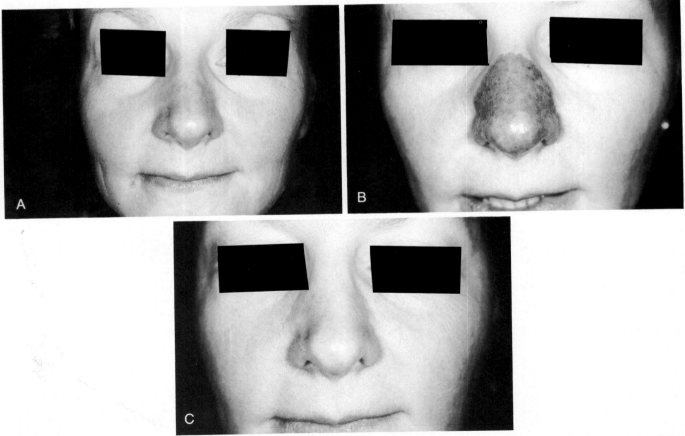

Figure 72–33. *A,* Diffuse telangiectases on the nose before treatment. *B,* Immediate ecchymosis occurs after treatment with the pulsed dye laser. *C,* Substantial lightening is present 6 weeks after treatment.

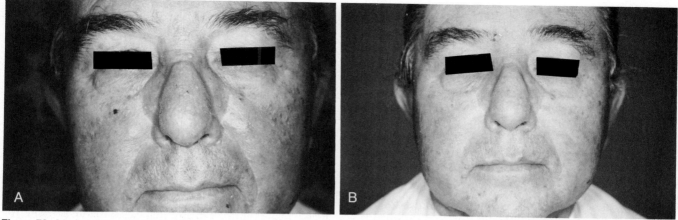

Figure 72–34. *A*, Diffuse "blushed" appearance owing to severe and uncontrolled acne rosacea. *B*, Substantial lightening has been accomplished after treatment with the pulsed dye laser.

pigments is produced by the ruby laser, probably as a result of selective photothermolysis.[8] Transepidermal elimination of tattoo pigment does occur and is often evident in the healing crust, but this probably plays only a minor role in the resolution of the tattoo. Biopsies of successfully treated tattoos have shown a large amount of residual pigment,[100] but the treated tattoo pigment granules are altered in both size and shape and are also often found in macrophages located beneath areas of mild fibrosis. This fibrosis may sufficiently alter the optical properties of the skin to improve the clinical appearance of the tattoo.

The alteration in the size, shape, and appearance of the tattoo pigments after treatment with the ruby laser has been partially attributed to the thermoacoustic properties of this system.[101–103] The high-energy pulses produced by the ruby laser generate photoacoustic waves in soft tissue that fragment the pigment granules[104–106]

by a process known as cavitation (see Fig. 72–13). The average size of the tattoo pigment clusters before ruby laser treatment typically varies from 147 to 180 μm in diameter. However, immediately after treatment, these clusters become superheated to 300°C, which causes them to fragment into much smaller particles. Macrophages can engulf these smaller pigment clusters and remove them through the lymphatics. In addition, some of the pigment is lost through the epidermis by transepidermal elimination, and some of the pigment is redistributed within the dermis, where it is no longer clinically visible.

Treatment Technique. Small test sites that are representative of the tattoo are often treated first using different EFs to determine the ideal laser parameters for subsequent treatment. Most commonly, the tests are performed at EFs of 2 to 3 J/cm² and increased by 0.5 J/cm² until a uniform whitening of the skin surface is

Figure 72–35. Schematic of the optical cavity for the ruby laser.

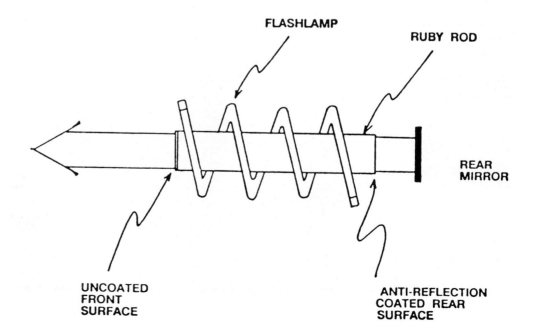

FLASHLAMP

RUBY ROD

REAR MIRROR

UNCOATED FRONT SURFACE

ANTI-REFLECTION COATED REAR SURFACE

produced.[98] The test procedure is usually well tolerated, with no local anesthesia needed. However, anesthesia may be required when treatment is actually begun, especially for large tattoos and those located on sensitive anatomic sites such as the fingers or breast. The evanescent white discoloration, which is the result of steam generated within the dermis by the photoacoustic wave, is always greatest overlying the tattooed areas. It typically lasts only 20 minutes and is replaced by a wheal-and-flare reaction. At higher EFs, petechiae are commonly seen after treatment. The typical EF for tattoo treatment using the ruby laser ranges from 2 to 10 J/cm^2, with the most common being between 4 and 8 J/cm^2.[97]

Because several weeks are commonly required for the tattoo to fade, retreatment should not begin until sufficient lightening has occurred to justify the procedure and to ensure that scarring and textural or pigmentary changes have not resulted. Treatment is commonly performed on an ambulatory basis and requires local anesthesia in approximately 20 to 50% of patients. Pulses are delivered so that they overlap by approximately 10 to 20% and produce uniform whitening of the entire surface of the tattoo. Any hair within the treatment area should be shaved before treatment to avoid the strong malodor that will otherwise result.

After completion of treatment, there may be significant redness and swelling that may feel like a mild sunburn for 30 to 60 minutes. This mild postoperative pain can be lessened by immediate topical application of 100% aloe vera gel and ice. Although bleeding and exudation are not common, petechiae occur at higher EFs. Superficial crusting typically replaces the minor vesiculation that is occasionally seen. Only minimal postoperative wound care is normally required, since the treated areas heal completely in 10 to 14 days. While fading of the tattoo pigment in most cases occurs gradually over a period of 4 to 6 weeks after each treatment,[98] residual erythema and transient hypopigmentation may persist for 2 to 6 months.

Results. Even though an accurate estimation of the likely response of a tattoo to ruby laser treatment is impossible, several generalizations can be made. The best results are obtained in amateur and blue-black tattoos. Although amateur tattoos require lower EFs and fewer retreatments to obtain maximal improvement, an average of four retreatments may still be required (Fig. 72–36). In contrast, professional multicolored tattoos, especially those with red, green, and yellow pigments, fade more slowly and may require an average of six retreatments (Fig. 72–37) to obtain satisfactory lightening.[96, 98, 107] This poorer response may be due to the higher pigment density, larger particle size, and greater stability or variable energy absorption by the many metals and organic compounds that are used to produce the different colors found in some tattoos. Despite these facts, professional tattoos that have been present for more than 10 years can be expected to respond more favorably than tattoos that have only recently been applied. One very important consideration should be kept in mind when evaluating patients who desire removal of cosmetic tattoos of the eyebrows, lips, and eyelids with the ruby laser. The tattoo pigments used in these patients to camouflage areas of alopecia or scars are typically composed of titanium or ferrous salts. Exposure of these tattoo pigments to the Q-switched ruby laser light commonly results in oxidation of these metals, which causes them to immediately turn black. This black discoloration may be very resistant to subsequent treatment and can be permanent. As a consequence of this finding, small test sites should be performed on these types of tattoos before initiating complete treatment. Regardless of the nature of the tattoo, the incidence of scarring is very low, approximately 2%,[99] and appears to be least common when treatment is performed at lower EFs.

The natural color of the patient's skin can also influence the outcome of treatment. Individuals with dark complexions develop immediate whitening at lower EFs and obtain less fading of the tattoo. Despite some limitations, the benefits resulting from ruby laser treatment of tattoos are substantial and certainly make it a

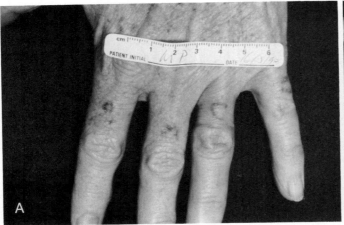
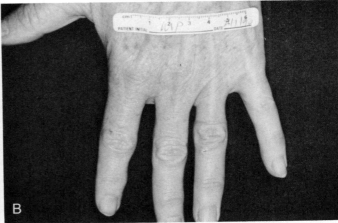

Figure 72–36. *A,* Preoperative appearance of an amateur tattoo. *B,* Clearing without textural changes or scarring has been accomplished by multiple treatments with the ruby laser.

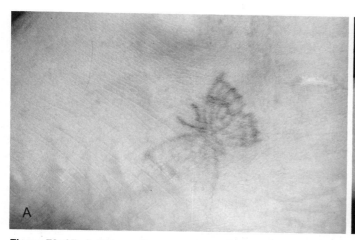 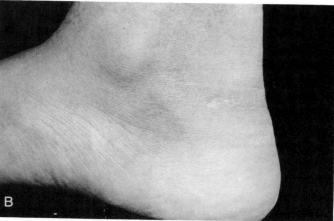

Figure 72–37. *A,* Preoperative appearance of a professional tattoo. *B,* Clearing without textural changes or scarring has been accomplished by multiple treatments with the ruby laser.

viable consideration for many patients with large tattoos or tattoos located in anatomic locations susceptible to adverse scarring and for those who seek tattoo removal without scarring as the ultimate cosmetic goal.

Nd:YAG Laser

Characteristics. The Nd:YAG laser produces invisible, near-infrared light with a wavelength of 1064 nm. Because it is poorly absorbed by any particular chromophore,[108] energy from this laser penetrates to a depth of 5 to 8 mm and results in the production of a diffuse zone of thermal injury and substantial scarring. For this reason, it has been used primarily in the treatment of thicker vascular lesions such as cavernous hemangiomas, finding only limited use in cutaneous surgery before the development of the contact scalpel.[109] In the treatment of PWS, Nd:YAG systems have been used to reduce the soft tissue hypertrophy that develops as blood vessels slowly dilate.[110, 111]

The conventional Nd:YAG laser has been modified by a Q-switching technique to produce high peak energies and short pulse durations (10 nanoseconds) similar to those of the ruby laser. In a modification of the Nd:YAG laser, the near-infrared light passes through an optical crystal composed of potassium titanyl phosphate (KTP), doubling the frequency and halving the wavelength. This converts the invisible infrared energy to green light with a wavelength of 532 nm.[112, 113] Both the regular and the modified technique have been used to successfully treat amateur and professional tattoos.

Mechanism of Action. The mechanisms that have been proposed to explain the usefulness of the ruby laser in the treatment of tattoos are probably also responsible for the results seen with the Q-switched Nd:YAG laser. However, there are two inherent benefits provided by the Nd:YAG laser. First, because the 1064-nm light is poorly absorbed by melanin, there is less absorptive interference within the epidermis compared with that seen with the red light produced by the ruby laser. Also, because of the longer wavelength, this light can penetrate deeper into tissue, which may increase its effectiveness in the treatment of some tattoos.

Treatment Techniques. It appears from the limited amount of published information on the use of this laser[114, 115] that EFs of 6 to 12 J/cm^2 at a wavelength of 1064 nm are very effective in fading blue, black, and green tattoos. This is especially impressive, because many of the original tattoos that were treated with this laser system had failed to clear with previous ruby laser treatments.[115] Orange and red tattoos will respond favorably to the frequency-doubled Nd:YAG laser with a wavelength of 532 nm, often requiring only one to two treatments. Slightly overlapping pulses are generally performed without anesthesia in an ambulatory setting. Retreatments are done at 4- to 6-week intervals until satisfactory fading or clearing has been achieved.

Results. Lightening of more than 50% has been observed after only one treatment, and the best results are generally obtained at higher EFs. Unlike treatment with the ruby laser, capillary bleeding usually develops within a few minutes after treatment. However, there is considerably less vesiculation and pain postoperatively with the Nd:YAG laser than with the ruby laser. No significant side effects of scarring or textural and pigmentary changes have occurred, and the incidence of hypopigmentation is less than that seen with the ruby laser.

Alexandrite Laser. Another laser used in the treatment of amateur and professional tattoos is the solid-state alexandrite laser. This Q-switched laser uses flash-lamp excitation of an alexandrite rod to produce a peak pulse power of 5.65 gigawatts at a wavelength of 755 nm and a pulse duration of 100 nanoseconds.[116, 117] As in treatment with other Q-switched lasers, the treated area becomes white immediately after exposure but returns to normal color in 10 to 20 minutes. The treated site first becomes erythematous and edematous, then pinpoint areas of bleeding develop, and crusting forms. Transient hypopigmentation has been reported after treatment, but spontaneous recovery can be expected over time.

The initial reports of the efficacy of this laser system in the treatment of tattoos suggest that the high-energy laser pulse fragments the tattoo pigment on impact, which stimulates tissue macrophages to engulf the pigment particles and remove them from the dermis. Sequential treatments performed at 4- to 6-week intervals using increased EFs provides the greatest degree of improvement without scarring or changes in texture.[116] Amateur tattoos can be expected to respond more rapidly than professional tattoos, but the number of treatments required to obtain the desired response remains unpredictable. This is probably related to the density and color of the pigment present. Between three and ten treatments may be necessary to completely clear some tattoos.

BENIGN PIGMENTED LESIONS

A number of different benign pigmented lesions[118] have been successfully treated (Table 72–3) using a variety of different laser systems.

Q-Switched Ruby Laser. The ruby laser has also been used to effectively treat a variety of pigmented lesions,[93, 94, 118, 119] presumably because the 30- to 40-nanosecond pulse duration is within the range of the thermal relaxation time for both melanocytes (1 microsecond) and melanosomes (50 nanoseconds).[120–122]

Mechanism of Action. The endogenous chromophore, melanin, has a broad absorption spectrum that ranges from the ultraviolet through the visible wavelengths to the near-infrared regions of the electromagnetic spectrum (EMS); this range overlaps the emission of the ruby laser.[120] In addition, there is minimal absorption by oxyhemoglobin, so the effects can be precisely confined to melanin-containing cells of the epidermis or upper dermis.[120] The melanosomes can be targeted for selective photothermolysis[121–124] by the 20- to 40-nanosecond pulses of the ruby laser because they approximate the thermal relaxation time for melanosomes (50 to 100 nanoseconds) and are shorter than the Tr for melanocytes (1000 nanoseconds). Microscopic photodisruption occurs in both pigmented lesions[125] and normal skin[122] when densely melanized melanosomes are exposed to the short pulses from the ruby laser.

TABLE 72–3. PIGMENTED LESIONS TREATED WITH VISIBLE LIGHT LASERS

Café au lait macule
Ephelides
Epidermal nevus
Lentigo benigna
Lentigo maligna
Melasma
Nevocellular nevus
Nevus of Ito
Nevus of Ota
Peutz-Jeghers spot
Pigmented basal cell carcinoma
Postinflammatory hyperpigmentation
Seborrheic keratosis
Tattoo
    Traumatic
    Decorative
    Medical
    Cosmetic

Treatment Techniques. The ruby laser has been used to treat lentigines, ephelides, café au lait spots, Becker's nevus, melasma, nevus of Ota,[126] postinflammatory hyperpigmentation, and Peutz-Jeghers spots.[125] The treatment technique is very similar to that used for the treatment of tattoos, except a wider range of EFs (2 to 10 J/cm²) may be necessary. The number of retreatments required for maximal improvement is extremely variable, except for lentigines, in which one to four treatments can generally be expected to provide excellent results.[126, 127] Except when treating larger pigmented lesions such as café au lait spots, delivery of overlapping pulses is not required.

Results. Many pigmented lesions can be effectively managed with the ruby laser to provide excellent lightening without scarring or textural or permanent pigmentary changes. However, the best results can be expected in nevus of Ota,[126] Becker's nevus, lentigines, and café au lait spots. Unfortunately, melasma and postinflammatory hyperpigmentation often prove to be resistant to treatment or show rapid recurrence after initial clearing.[128] Additional controlled clinical investigations are currently under way and will help define the proper indications for this laser system.

Frequency-Doubled, Q-Switched Nd:YAG Laser. The Q-switched Nd:YAG laser has also been effectively used to treat pigmented lesions by employing the same concept of selective photothermolysis. However, a modification of the normal Nd:YAG laser, known as frequency doubling, has been shown to further improve the specificity of this laser for treating pigmented lesions. In this laser system, the invisible, near-infrared Nd:YAG laser light of 1064 nm is passed through an optical crystal, doubling the frequency and halving the wavelength to yield green light with a wavelength of 532 nm.

Because the frequency-doubled green light overlaps the absorption spectrum for melanin, this laser system can be appropriately used to treat benign pigmented lesions. Furthermore, the 10-nanosecond pulse duration is shorter than the established thermal relaxation times for both melanosomes and melanocytes, which permits selective photothermolysis.[113]

Treatment Technique. To determine the ideal treatment parameters, small tests are performed on inconspicuous but representative pigmented lesions at EFs ranging from 2 to 5 J/cm². Uniform whitening of the skin surface develops immediately after exposure but disappears spontaneously in 15 to 20 minutes and is replaced by painless petechial or purpuric lesions, which typically fade after 3 to 4 days.

Results. The treated lesions often become much darker in color until the skin surface desquamates after about 5 to 7 days (Figs. 72–38 through 72–40). Slight erythema commonly remains for about 4 to 6 weeks but then gradually fades. Persistent hypopigmentation, scarring, and textural changes have not been reported.

Copper Vapor Laser. Superficial benign pigmented lesions such as lentigines and ephelides can be treated using the 511-nm green band from the copper vapor laser.[129, 130] A slightly overlapping, polka-dot delivery in short pulses of 0.1 to 0.2 seconds is most commonly

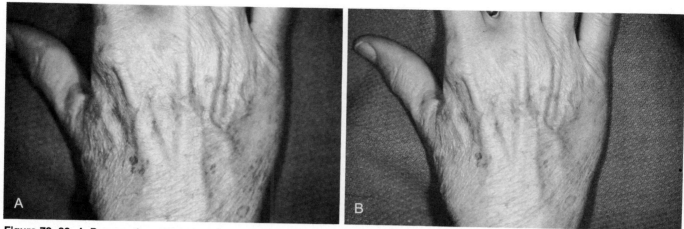

Figure 72-38. *A,* Preoperative appearance of multiple lentigines on the dorsal aspect of a man's hand. *B,* Substantial clearing without scarring or textural changes is seen after one treatment with the frequency-doubled, Q-switched Nd:YAG laser.

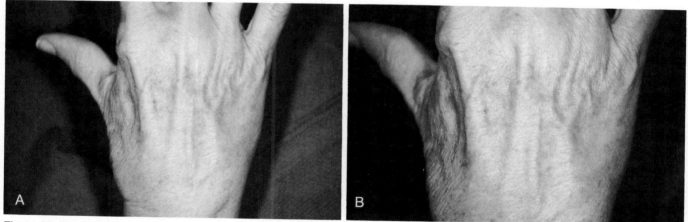

Figure 72-39. *A,* Preoperative appearance of multiple lentigines on the dorsal aspect of a woman's hand. *B,* Substantial clearing without scarring or textural changes is seen after one treatment with the frequency-doubled, Q-switched Nd:YAG laser.

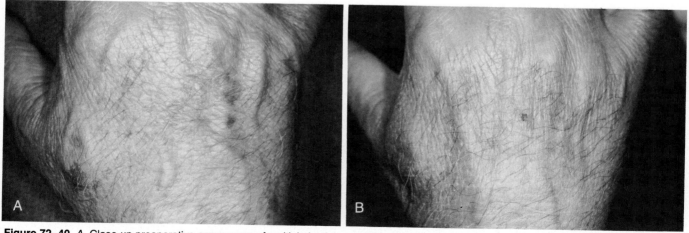

Figure 72-40. *A,* Close-up preoperative appearance of multiple lentigines on the dorsal aspect of a man's hand. *B,* Substantial clearing without scarring or textural changes has been accomplished after one treatment with the frequency-doubled, Q-switched Nd:YAG laser.

utilized. However, these types of lesions can also be treated with the Autolase robotic scanning device set to deliver closely spaced pulses with a density of 500 μm. The hyperpigmentation that develops on the legs from the deposition of hemosiderin in the superficial dermis after traditional injection sclerotherapy for telangiectasia can be substantially lightened in 69% of patients with the copper vapor laser.[131]

Pulsed Dye Laser for Pigmented Lesions. A different type of flashlamp-pumped pulsed dye laser has been developed for the treatment of pigmented lesions.[132] This system delivers green light with a peak pulse power of 2.25 MW at a wavelength of 510 nm in short pulses of 300 nanoseconds. In general, EFs of 2 to 3 J/cm² are used. Again, because the green color is selectively absorbed by melanized tissues and the short pulses limit nonspecific thermal damage by selective photothermolysis, this system can provide a very selective and precise form of treatment for lentigines, ephelides, melasma, nevus spilus, nevus of Ota, postinflammatory hyperpigmentation, seborrheic keratoses, and café au lait spots.[133] Vesiculation and crusting may appear postoperatively[134]; purpura can be expected to occur in about 60% of patients and result in transient pigmentation from hemosiderin, but no scarring has been reported. One treatment will clear approximately 50% of epidermal pigmented lesions, and three treatments will clear approximately 90% of these lesions.[133]

In approximately 10 to 30% of patients who undergo injection sclerotherapy, temporary hyperpigmentation will develop at the treatment site from the deposition of hemosiderin, which occurs as a result of the extravasation of red blood cells. Topical medications used to fade this pigment have yielded poor results. However, the delivery of overlapping pulses of green light from the pulsed dye laser at EFs of 2 to 3 J/cm² can provide substantial lightening in some patients.[135]

Krypton Laser. Even though the gas-medium krypton laser has been primarily used as a source of yellow light to treat vascular lesions, it also simultaneously produces two bands of green light with wavelengths of 521 and 530 nm.[65] These bands of light can be used to treat pigmented lesions, but because this system is only capable of producing "long" pulses of light, there is a significant risk of producing unwanted thermal damage and scarring. As a consequence, treatment of pigmented lesions with the krypton laser is typically limited to smaller lesions such as lentigines. However, similar to the way the green band of light from the copper vapor laser is used, this system could be coupled to a robotic scanning device to improve the specificity of the laser-tissue interaction and reduce the risk of complications.

Alexandrite Laser. Preliminary results of treatment of benign pigmented lesions with the alexandrite laser appear promising, with the best response seen in lentigines and café au lait macules. Deeper penetration into the dermis can be expected with this laser because of its slightly longer wavelength compared with that of other lasers used to treat pigmented lesions. This may serve to improve the results in the treatment of dermal pigmented lesions such as nevus of Ota.[136]

MISCELLANEOUS VASCULAR LESIONS

Many vascular lesions less common than the port-wine stain have also been effectively treated with visible light lasers. Of these treatments, pulsed dye laser treatment of capillary and mixed hemangiomas, which are present in 1 to 2.6% of newborns and 10 to 12% of infants,[137, 138] remains the most controversial. Much of the debate in this regard is a result of the unpredictable course these lesions tend to follow, with spontaneous involution occurring in 50 to 65% of patients by 5 years of age, in 70% by 7 years of age, and in 90% by 9 years of age.[139, 140] However, when complications such as ulceration,[141] bleeding, infection, visual impairment, and other functional problems develop, medical or surgical intervention is indicated. High-dose systemic steroids, cryosurgery (see Chap. 61), radiotherapy, and excision are also associated with numerous complications that may make these forms of treatment contraindicated. Based on the established safety and efficacy of the pulsed dye laser in the treatment of port-wine stains, this laser system has been used to treat a large number of patients. From this work it appears that the pulsed dye laser treatment is capable of providing an effective form of treatment for a highly selected group of patients. The best response can be anticipated in patients with thin lesions (less than 3 mm thick), especially during the early proliferative period. Treatment should also be considered when the hemangioma interferes with normal function (e.g., with involvement of the hands or feet or around the eyes and mouth). Furthermore, when large areas are affected and may cause disfigurement or be subject to secondary infection, bleeding, or trauma, the pulsed dye laser may be useful in promoting involution or even complete elimination.[142, 143] It also appears to be effective in controlling active capillary proliferations and preventing rapid enlargement in expanding lesions.[144]

Another relatively common vascular condition that has been successfully managed with various laser systems is the pyogenic granuloma.[145] These idiopathic, rapidly growing, benign vascular lesions often develop at sites of trauma, especially in children, and commonly recur after treatment with curettage and electrosurgery, excision, and cryosurgery. However, the pulsed dye laser has been shown to provide excellent therapeutic and cosmetic results with only one treatment.[145]

Another uncommon vascular condition that frequently resists conventional surgical treatment with excision, dermabrasion, and skin grafting is lupus pernio.[146] This rare form of cutaneous sarcoidosis usually affects the nose, cheeks, ears, and eyelids and may cause significant disfigurement as well as septal perforation as a result of granulomatous inflammation. Treatment with the pulsed dye laser eliminates the erythematous component of this condition as well as the telangiectasia.[146]

A final vascular lesion that has been treated with various lasers is Kaposi's sarcoma (KS). Unfortunately, KS lesions seen in association with the acquired immunodeficiency syndrome (AIDS) failed to show long-term clearing after treatment with the pulsed dye laser.[147] However, the argon laser has been used to successfully treat the nonepidemic lesions of KS that are typically found on the legs of elderly men.[148] Whether the same technique using the argon laser would provide similar beneficial results in treating the epidemic forms of KS awaits further clinical trials.

MISCELLANEOUS LESIONS

There are a number of relative indications for laser surgery; these include some rare cutaneous conditions that have been successfully treated with one or more of the visible light lasers (Table 72–4). The success of treating one of these, lymphangioma circumscriptum,[149] is primarily dependent on the presence of a sufficient amount of hemoglobin to provide the degree of specificity of the laser-tissue interaction necessary to limit

thermal injury to the abnormal tissue while simultaneously minimizing injury to the surrounding normal skin. In several of the inflammatory conditions treated with the visible light lasers (e.g., lymphocytoma cutis and granuloma faciale), the vasodilation that occurs as a secondary event provides the necessary target for the blue, green, or yellow light lasers to produce the desired thermal effects.

Low-Energy Lasers

A low-energy laser (LEL), also called "cold," "soft," low-level, low-power, and low-output laser, is one that produces a temperature elevation of less than 0.1° to

TABLE 72–4. INDICATIONS FOR LASER SURGERY

	Condition	Lasers Utilized
Absolute indications	Port-wine stain (photocoagulation)	Argon Argon-dye Flashlamp pulsed dye Copper vapor Krypton

	Tattoos
	  Decorative
	    Amateur
	    Professional
	  Traumatic
	  Medical
	  Cosmetic
		Ruby
		Q-switched Nd:YAG
		Frequency-doubled (FD):YAG
		Alexandrite

Relative indications	Vascular lesions (photocoagulation) Kaposi's sarcoma	 Argon, argon-dye, copper vapor, flashlamp pulsed dye, krypton
	Angiokeratoma	As above
	Adenoma sebaceum	As above
	Venous lakes	As above
	Pyogenic granuloma	As above
	Angiolymphoid hyperplasia	As above
	Cavernous hemangioma	As above, plus Nd:YAG
	Glomus tumors	As above

	Telangiectases
	    Osler-Weber-Rendu
	    Solar
	    Rosacea
	    Essential
	    Collagen-vascular
	    Postrhinoplasty
	    Nevus araneus
		As above

	Pigmented lesions (photocoagulation)	
	Adenoma sebaceum	Argon, argon-dye, copper vapor, carbon dioxide, flashlamp pulsed dye
	Nevus of Ota	Ruby, FD:YAG, alexandrite
	Café au lait	Ruby, FD:YAG, alexandrite
	Becker's nevus	Ruby, FD:YAG, alexandrite
	Ephelides	Ruby, dye, FD:YAG, alexandrite
	Lentigo senilis	Argon, ruby, dye, FD:YAG, pulsed dye, krypton, copper vapor, alexandrite
	Granuloma faciale	Argon, argon-dye, copper vapor, pulsed dye

	Miscellaneous conditions
	  Actinic cheilitis (vaporization)
	  Warts
	    Recurrent
	    Paronychial
	    Plantar (vaporization)
		
		Carbon dioxide
		Carbon dioxide

	Anticoagulated patients (excision)	Carbon dioxide

Table continued on following page

TABLE 72–4. **INDICATIONS FOR LASER SURGERY** *Continued*

	Condition	Lasers Utilized
Advantageous indications	Appendigeal tumors	Carbon dioxide
	Vaporization mode	
	Vellus hair cysts	
	Steatocystoma	
	Digital myxoid cysts	
	Trichoepitheliomas	
	Tricholemmomas	
	Adenoma sebaceum	
	Sebaceous hyperplasia	
	Syringoma	
	Vascular leions or locations	
	Lymphangioma	Carbon dioxide (vaporization)
	Nail surgery	Carbon dioxide (excision)
	Cavernous hemangiomas	Carbon dioxide, Nd:YAG (contact)
	Miscellaneous conditions	
	Xanthelasma	Carbon dioxide (vaporization)
	Granuloma faciale	Carbon dioxide (vaporization)
	Rhinophyma (excision)	Carbon dioxide
	Keloids	Carbon dioxide (excision)
	Stromal-independent tumors	
	Squamous cell carcinoma	Carbon dioxide, Nd:YAG (contact)
	Melanoma	
	Basal cell nevus syndrome	Carbon dioxide (vaporization)
Experimental indications	Basal cell nevus syndrome (photodynamic therapy)	Argon-dye, gold vapor
	Tissue welding	Carbon dioxide, dye, Nd:YAG
	Biostimulation	Low-energy lasers

0.5°C in tissue with exposure to the laser.[150] This temperature increase is so neglible that any effects are not the result of a photothermal reaction but are the direct result of the radiation itself. The most common LEL systems (Table 72–5) are the helium-neon (HeNe) and the diode lasers (gallium-arsenide [GaAs] and the gallium-aluminum-arsenide [GaAlAs] lasers). The most controversial area of LEL research in cutaneous surgery has been the reported ability of these lasers to modulate various aspects of wound healing.[151–161]

The use of cell cultures has helped to identify the mechanisms by which LELs exert their effects on wound healing. In these models, LEL irradiation has been shown to increase the rate of DNA and RNA synthesis,[162–164] which increases fibroblast proliferation and collagen synthesis.[165, 166] The proposed mechanism for these effects is activation of a porphyrin-containing enzyme,[167] which stimulates the mitochondrial synthesis of adenosine triphosphate (ATP). However, fibroblast DNA replication and procollagen synthesis can also be inhibited by LEL irradiation from the Nd:YAG laser, prob-

ably as a result of selective suppression of fibroblast procollagen production.[168, 169] This may prove to be useful in the management of some patients with hypertrophic scars and keloids.[156]

Stimulation of keratinocyte motility can also result from exposure to LEL.[170, 171] In addition, the stimulatory effects of LEL on wound healing have been documented both in wounds allowed to heal by second intention[153, 154] and in sutured wounds.[159, 160] These effects are mediated by increases in the levels of procollagen messenger RNA (mRNA) and may also cause systemic effects.[161] Using different techniques, the LELs have also been used to close skin incisions[172] by using protein coagulation as the sealing material (see Chap. 78). Finally, by stimulating a photosensitizing drug that attaches preferentially to malignant cells with red light from various types of LEL, a revolutionary form of cancer therapy has evolved. This technique, known as photodynamic therapy (PDT),[173, 174] can be used for the palliation of certain types of respiratory and urinary tract malignancies (see Chap. 79). It is currently being studied in the management of some refractory forms of cutaneous malignancies as well.

TABLE 72–5. **COMMON LOW-ENERGY LASERS**

Laser System	Wavelength (nm)	Color of Emission
Helium-neon (HeNe)	632	Red
Gallium-arsenide (GaAs)	904	Near-infrared
Gallium-aluminum-arsenide (GaAlAs)	830	Near-infrared
Neodymium:yttrium-aluminum-garnet (Nd:YAG)	1064	Near-infrared

SUMMARY

During its relatively short history, the laser has become widely accepted as a valuable addition to the arsenal of tools available to the cutaneous surgeon. Visible light lasers currently provide successful treatment for some disorders for which no form of therapy previously existed. In some cases, they have been incorporated into existing conventional surgical techniques to provide revolutionary solutions to problems that previously carried significant complications for the patient. However, to most successfully utilize lasers in cutaneous surgery, a complete understanding of basic laser characteristics and principles is required. As more sophisticated and refined devices become available in the future, surgeons who have learned how to determine the proper indications and contraindications for laser surgery will be able to provide their patients with the optimal care possible.

REFERENCES

1. Einstein A: Zur quantentheorie der strahlung. Physiol Z 18:121–128, 1917.
2. Bromberg JL: The Laser in America, 1950–1970. The MIT Press, Cambridge, 1991, pp 19–23.
3. Maiman TH: Stimulated optical radiation in ruby. Nature 187:493–494, 1960.
4. Adams S, Swain C, Mills T, et al: The effect of wavelength, power and treatment pattern on the outcome of laser treatment of portwine stains. Br J Dermatol 117:487–494, 1987.
5. Arndt K, Noe J, Northam D, et al: Laser therapy: basic concepts and nomenclature. J Am Acad Dermatol 5:649–654, 1981.
6. Sliney D: Laser-tissue interactions. Clin Chest Med 6:203–208, 1985.
7. Anderson R, Parrish J: The optics of human skin. J Invest Dermatol 77:13–19, 1981.
8. Anderson R, Parrish J: Selective photothermolysis: precise microsurgery by selective absorption of pulsed radiation. Science 220:524–527, 1983.
9. Parrish J, Anderson R, Harris T, et al: Selective thermal effects with pulsed irradiation from organ to organelle. J Invest Dermatol 80:75–80, 1983.
10. Wheeland RG, Walker NPJ: Lasers—25 years later. Int J Dermatol 25:209–216, 1986.
11. Hidano A, Ogihara Y: Cryotherapy with solid carbon dioxide in the treatment of nevus flammeus. J Dermatol Surg Oncol 3:213–216, 1977.
12. Conway H, Montry RE: Permanent camouflage of capillary hemangioma of the face by intradermal injection of insoluble pigments (tattooing): indications for surgery. NY St J Med 65:876–885, 1965.
13. Pratt AG: Birthmarks in infants. Arch Dermatol 67:302–305, 1953.
14. Jacobs AH, Walton RG: The incidence of birthmarks in the neonate. Pediatrics 58:218–222, 1976.
15. Malm M, Calberg M: Port-wine stain—a surgical and psychological problem. Ann Plast Surg 20:512–516, 1988.
16. Lanigan SW, Cotterill JA: Psychological disabilities amongst patients with port wine stains. Br J Dermatol 121:209–215, 1989.
17. Barsky SH, Rosen S, Geer D, Noe JM: The nature and evaluation of port wine stains: a computer-assisted study. J Invest Dermatol 74:154–157, 1980.
18. Wagner K, Wagner R: The necessity for treatment of childhood portwine stains. Cutis 5:317–318, 1990.
19. Geronemus RG, Ashinoff R: The medical necessity of evaluation and treatment of port-wine stains. J Dermatol Surg Oncol 17:76–79, 1991.
20. Goldman L: The argon laser and the port wine stain. Plast Reconstr Surg 65:137–139, 1980.
21. Cosman B: Experience in the argon laser therapy of port wine stains. Plast Reconstr Surg 65:119–129, 1980.
22. Apfelberg DB, Maser MR, Lash H, et al: The argon laser for cutaneous lesions. JAMA 245:2073–2075, 1981.
23. Arndt KA: Argon laser therapy of small cutaneous vascular lesions. Arch Dermatol 118:220–224, 1982.
24. Noe JM, Barsky SH, Geer DE, et al: Port-wine stains and the response to argon laser therapy: successful treatment and the predictive role of color, age, and biopsy. Plast Reconstr Surg 65:130–136, 1980.
25. Brauner GJ, Schliftman A: Laser surgery for children. J Dermatol Surg Oncol 13:178–186, 1987.
26. Dixon JA, Rotering RH, Huether SE: Patients' evaluation of argon laser therapy of port-wine stain, decorative tattoo, and essential telangiectasia. Lasers Surg Med 4:181–190, 1984.
27. Cotterill JA: Laser treatment of portwine stains. Br Med J 284:766–767, 1982.
28. Dixon JA, Huether S, Rotering R: Hypertrophic scarring in argon laser treatment of port wine stains. Plast Reconstr Surg 73:771–777, 1984.
29. Landthaler M, Haina D, Waidelich W, Braun-Falco O: A three-year experience with the argon laser in dermato-therapy. J Dermatol Surg Oncol 10:456–461, 1984.
30. Dixon J, Huether S, Rotering R: Hypertrophic scarring in argon laser treatment of portwine stains. Plast Reconstr Surg 73:771–777, 1984.
31. Keller GS, Doiron D, Weingarten C: Advances in laser skin surgery for vascular lesions. Arch Otolaryngol 111:437–440, 1985.
32. Touquet VLR, Carruth JAS: Review of the treatment of port wine stains with the argon laser. Lasers Surg Med 4:191–199, 1984.
33. Yanai A, Fukuda O, Soyano S, et al: Argon laser therapy of portwine stains: effects and limitations. Plast Reconstr Surg 75:520–525, 1985.
34. Apfelberg DB, Smith T, Maser MR, et al: Dot or pointillistic method for improvement in results of hypertrophic scarring in the argon laser treatment of portwine hemangiomas. Lasers Surg Med 6:552–558, 1987.
35. Apfelberg DB, Flores JT, Maser MR, et al: Analysis of complications of argon laser treatment of port wine hemangiomas with reference to the striped technique. Lasers Surg Med 2:357–371, 1983.
36. Gilchrest BA, Rosen S, Noe JM: Chilling port wine stains improves the response to argon laser therapy. Plast Reconstr Surg 69:278–283, 1982.
37. Noe J, Barsky S, Geer D, et al: Port wine stains and the response to argon laser therapy: successful treatment and the predictive role of color, age, and biopsy. Plast Reconstr Surg 65:130–136, 1980.
38. Brauner G, Schliftman A, Cosman B: Evaluation of argon laser surgery in children under 13 years of age. Plast Reconstr Surg 87:37–43, 1991.
39. Greenwald J, Rosen S, Anderson RR, et al: Comparative histological studies of the tunable dye (at 577 nm) laser and argon laser: the specific vascular effects of the dye laser. J Invest Dermatol 77:305–310, 1981.
40. Landthaler M, Haina D, Brunner R, et al: Effects of argon, dye, and Nd:YAG lasers on epidermis, dermis, and venous vessels. Lasers Surg Med 6:87–93, 1986.
41. Malm M, Rigler R, Jurell G: Continuous wave (CW) dye laser vs CW argon laser treatment of portwine stains (PWS). Scan Plast Reconstr Surg Hand Surg 22:241–244, 1988.
42. Scheibner A, Wheeland RG: Argon-pumped tunable dye laser therapy for facial port-wine stain hemangiomas in adults—new technique using small spot size and minimal power. J Dermatol Surg Oncol 15:277–282, 1989.
43. Scheibner A, Wheeland RG: Use of the argon-pumped tunable dye laser for port-wine stains in children. J Dermatol Surg Oncol 17:735–739, 1991.
44. Garden J, Tan O, Parrish J: The pulsed dye laser: its use at 577 nm wavelength. J Dermatol Surg Oncol 13:134–139, 1987.
45. Anderson RR, Parrish JA: Microvasculature can be selectively damaged using dye lasers: a basic theory and experimental evidence in human skin. Lasers Surg Med 1:263–276, 1981.
46. Anderson RR, Jaenicke KF, Parrish JA: Mechanism of selective vascular changes caused by dye lasers. Lasers Surg Med 3:211–215, 1983.
47. Van Gemert MJC, Welch AJ, Amin AP: Is there an optimal laser treatment for port wine stains? Lasers Surg Med 6:76–83, 1986.
48. Garden JM, Tan OT, Kerschmann R, et al: Effect of dye laser pulse duration on selective cutaneous vascular injury. J Invest Dermatol 87:653–657, 1986.
49. Garden JM, Polla LL, Tan OT: The treatment of port-wine stains by the pulsed dye laser. Arch Dermatol 124:889–896, 1988.

50. Tan OT, Sherwood K, Gilchrest BA: Treatment of children with port-wine stains using the flashlamp-pulsed tunable dye laser. N Engl J Med 320:416–421, 1989.

51. Tan OT, Gilchrest BA: Laser therapy for selected cutaneous vascular lesions in the pediatric population: a review. Pediatrics 82:652–662, 1988.

52. Nelson J, Applebaum J: Clinical management of portwine stain in infants and young children using the flashlamp-pulsed dye laser. Clin Pediatr 29:503–508, 1990.

53. Reyes BA, Geronemus R: Treatment of port-wine stains during childhood with the flashlamp-pumped pulsed dye laser. J Am Acad Dermatol 23:1142–1148, 1990.

54. Ashinoff R, Geronemus RG: Flashlamp-pumped pulsed dye laser for port-wine stains in infancy: earlier versus later treatment. J Am Acad Dermatol 24:467–472, 1991.

55. Polla L, Tan O, Garden J, et al: Tunable pulsed dye laser for the treatment of benign cutaneous vascular ectasia. Dermatologica 174:11–17, 1987.

56. Lanigan SW, Cotterill JA: Use of a lidocaine-prilocaine cream as an analgesic in dye laser treatment of portwine stains. Lasers Med Sci 2:87–89, 1987.

57. Ashinoff R, Geronemus RG: Effect of the topical anesthetic EMLA on the efficacy of pulsed dye laser treatment of port-wine stains. J Dermatol Surg Oncol 16:1008–1011, 1990.

58. Tan OT, Stafford TJ: EMLA for laser treatment of portwine stains in children. Lasers Surg Med 12:543–548, 1992.

59. Ashinoff R, Geronemus RG: Treatment of a port-wine stain in a black patient with the pulsed dye laser. J Dermatol Surg Oncol 18:147–148, 1992.

60. Lancer HA: Clinical summary of copper vapor laser treatment of dermatologic disease: a private practice viewpoint. Am J Cosmet Surg 8:1–4, 1991.

61. Walker E, Butler P, Pickering J, et al: Histology of portwine stains after copper vapor laser treatment. Br J Dermatol 121:217–223, 1989.

62. Pickering J, Walker E, Butler P, et al: Copper vapor laser treatment of portwine stains and other vascular malformations. Br J Plast Surg 43:272–282, 1990.

63. Tan OT, Stafford TJ, Murray S, Kurban AK: Histologic comparison of the pulsed dye laser and copper vapor laser effects on pig skin. Lasers Surg Med 10:551–558, 1990.

64. Neumann RA, Knobler RM, Leonshartsberger H, Gebhart W: Comparative histochemistry of port-wine stains after copper vapor laser (578 nm) and argon laser treatment. J Invest Dermatol 99:160–167, 1992.

65. Loh RCK: Uses of krypton laser. Singapore Med J 29:66–67, 1988.

66. Grossniklaus HE, Frank KE, Green WR: Subretinal neovascularization in a pseudophakic eye treated with krypton laser photocoagulation. A clinicopathologic case report. Arch Ophthalmol 106:78–81, 1988.

67. Kremer I, Gilad E, Ben-Sira I: Juxtapapillary exophytic retinal capillary hemangioma treated by yellow krypton (568 nm) laser photocoagulation. Ophthalmic Surg 19:743–747, 1988.

68. Singerman LJ, Ferris FL III, Mowery RP, et al: Krypton laser for proliferative diabetic retinopathy: the krypton-argon regression of neovascularization study. J Diabet Complicat 2:189–196, 1988.

69. Menchini U, Scialdone A, Pietroni C, et al: Argon versus krypton panretinal photocoagulation side effects on the anterior segment. Ophthalmologica 201:66–70, 1990.

70. Olk RJ: Argon green (514 nm) versus krypton red (647 nm) modified grid laser photocoagulation for diffuse diabetic macular edema. Ophthalmology 97:1101–1112, 1990.

71. Fine SL, Hawkins BS, Maguire MG: Krypton laser photocoagulation for neovascular lesions of age-related macular degeneration. Arch Ophthalmol 109:614–615, 1991.

72. Rotteleur G, Mordon S, Buys B, et al: Robotized scanning laser handpiece for the treatment of port wine stains and other angiodysplasias. Lasers Surg Med 8:283–287, 1988.

73. Mordon SR, Rotteleur G, Buys B, Brunetaud JM: Comparative study of the "point-by-point technique" and the "scanning technique" for laser treatment of port-wine stain. Lasers Surg Med 9:398–404, 1989.

74. McDaniel DH, Mordon S: Hexascan: a new robotized scanning laser handpiece. Cutis 45:300–305, 1990.

75. Chambers IR, Clark D, Bainbridge C: Automation of laser treatment of port-wine stains. Phys Med Biol 7:1025–1028, 1990.

76. Dicken CH: Treatment of the red nose with the argon laser. Mayo Clin Proc 61:893–895, 1986.

77. Dicken CH: Argon laser treatment of the red nose. J Dermatol Surg Oncol 16:33–36, 1990.

78. Noe JM, Finly J, Rosen S, Arndt K: Post-rhinoplasty "red nose": differential diagnosis and treatment by laser. Plast Reconstr Surg 67:661–664, 1981.

79. Key JM, Waner M: Selective destruction of facial telangiectasia using a copper vapor laser. Arch Otolaryngol Head Neck Surg 118:509–513, 1992.

80. Wheeland RG, Applebaum J: Flashlamp-pumped pulsed dye laser therapy for poikiloderma of Civatte. J Dermatol Surg Oncol 16:12–16, 1990.

81. Lowe NJ, Behr KL, Fitzpatrick R, et al: Flash lamp pumped dye laser for rosacea-associated telangiectasia and erythema. J Dermatol Surg Oncol 17:522–525, 1991.

82. Goldman MP, Fitzpatrick RE: Pulsed-dye laser treatment of leg telangiectasia: with and without simultaneous sclerotherapy. J Dermatol Surg Oncol 16:338–344, 1990.

83. Koerber WA Jr, Price NM: Salabrasion of tattoos. A correlation of the clinical and histological results. Arch Dermatol 114:884–888, 1978.

84. Clabaugh W: Removal of tattoos by superficial dermabrasion. Arch Dermatol 98:515–521, 1968.

85. Wheeland RG, Norwood OT, Roundtree JM: Tattoo removal using serial tangential excision and polyurethane membrane dressing. J Dermatol Surg Oncol 9:822–826, 1983.

86. Scutt RWB: The chemical removal of tattoos. Br J Plast Surg 25:189–194, 1972.

87. Dvir E, Hirshowitz B: Tattoo removal by cryosurgery. Plast Reconstr Surg 66:373–378, 1980.

88. Bailey BN: Treatment of tattoos. Plast Reconstr Surg 40:361–371, 1967.

89. Groot DW, Arlette JP, Johnston PA: Comparison of the infrared coagulator and the carbon dioxide laser in the removal of decorative tattoos. J Am Acad Dermatol 15:518–522, 1986.

90. Bailin PL, Ratz JL, Levine HL: Removal of tattoos by CO_2 laser. J Dermatol Surg Oncol 6:997–1001, 1980.

91. Apfelberg DB, Maser MR, Lash H, et al: Comparison of argon and carbon dioxide laser treatment of decorative tattoos: a preliminary report. Ann Plast Surg 14:6–15, 1985.

92. Reid R, Muller S: Tattoo removal by CO_2 laser dermabrasion. Plast Reconstr Surg 65:717–728, 1980.

93. Goldman L, Blaney DJ, Kindel DJ, et al: Effect of the laser beam on the skin: preliminary report. J Invest Dermatol 40:121–122, 1963.

94. Goldman L, Wilson RG, Hornby P, et al: Radiation from a Q-switched ruby laser. Effect of repeated impacts of power output of 10 megawatts on a tattoo of man. J Invest Dermatol 44:69–71, 1965.

95. Reid WH, McLeod PJ, Ritchie A, et al: Q-switched ruby laser treatment of black tattoos. Br J Plast Surg 36:455–459, 1983.

96. Vance CA, McLeod PJ, Reid WH, et al: Q-switched ruby laser treatment of tattoos: a further study. Lasers Surg Med 5:179, 1985.

97. Taylor CR, Gange RW, Dover JS, et al: Treatment of tattoos by Q-switched ruby laser. Arch Dermatol 126:893–899, 1990.

98. Scheibner A, Kenny G, White W, Wheeland RG: A superior method of tattoo removal using the Q-switched ruby laser. J Dermatol Surg Oncol 16:1091–1098, 1990.

99. Taylor C, Gange W, Dover J, et al: Treatment of tattoos by Q-switched ruby laser: a dose response study. Arch Dermatol 126:893–899, 1990.

100. Taylor C, Anderson R, Gange R, et al: Light and electron microscopic analysis of tattoos treated by Q-switched ruby laser. J Invest Dermatol 97:131–136, 1991.

101. Carome SF, Hamrick PE: Laser-induced acoustic transients in the mammalian eye. J Acoust Soc Am 46:1037–1044, 1969.

102. Sigrist MW, Kneubuhl FK: Laser generated stress waves in liquids. J Acoust Soc Am 64:1652–1663, 1978.

103. Mainster MA, Sliney DH, Belcher D, et al: Laser photodisruptors. Damage mechanism, instrument design, and safety. Ophthalmology 99:973–991, 1983.

104. Goldman AI, Ham WT Jr, Mueller HA: Mechanisms of retinal

damage resulting from the exposure of rhesus monkeys to ultra-short laser pulses. Exp Eye Res 21:457–469, 1975.

105. Boulnois JL: Photophysical processes in recent medical laser developments: a review. Lasers Med Sci 1:47–66, 1986.

106. Watenebe S, Flotte TJ, McAuliffe DJ, et al: Putative photoacoustic damage in skin induced by pulsed ArF excimer laser. J Invest Dermatol 90:761–766, 1988.

107. Reid W, Miller I, Murphy M, et al: Q-switched ruby laser treatment of tattoos: a 9 year experience. Br J Plast Surg 43:663–669, 1990.

108. Landthaler M, Haina D, Brunner R, et al: Neodymium-YAG laser therapy for vascular lesions. J Am Acad Dermatol 14:107–117, 1986.

109. Hukki J, Krogerus L, Castren M, Schroder T: Effects of different contact laser scalpels on skin and subcutaneous fat. Lasers Surg Med 8:276–282, 1988.

110. Dixon JA, Gilbertson JJ: Argon and neodymium YAG laser therapy of dark nodular port-wine stains in older patients. Lasers Surg Med 6:5–11, 1986.

111. Apfelberg DB, Smith T, Lash H, et al: Preliminary report on use of the neodymium-YAG laser in plastic surgery. Lasers Surg Med 7:189–198, 1987.

112. Apfelberg DB, Bailin P, Rosenberg H: Preliminary investigation of KTP/532 laser light in the treatment of hemangiomas and tattoos. Lasers Surg Med 6:38–42, 1986.

113. Kilmer SL, Anderson RR: Clinical use of the Q-switched ruby and the Q-switched Nd:YAG (1064 nm and 532 nm) lasers for treatment of tattoos. J Dermatol Surg Oncol 19:330–338, 1993.

114. Anderson RR, Margolis RJ, Watenabe S, et al: Selective photothermolysis of cutaneous pigmentation by Q-switched Nd:YAG laser pulses at 1064, 532, and 355 nm. J Invest Dermatol 93:38–42, 1989.

115. Kilmer SL, Lee M, Farinelli W, et al: Q-switched Nd:YAG laser (1064 nm) effectively treats Q-switched ruby laser resistant tattoos. Lasers Surg Med 4S:72, 1992.

116. Fitzpatrick RE, Ruiz-Esparza J, Goldman MP: The alexandrite laser for tattoos: a preliminary report. Lasers Surg Med 4S:72, 1992.

117. Tan OT, Lizek R: Alexandrite (760 nm) laser treatment of tattoos. Lasers Surg Med 4S:72–73, 1992.

118. Ohshiro T, Maruyama Y: The ruby and argon lasers in the treatment of naevi. Ann Acad Med Singapore 12:388–395, 1983.

119. Scheibner A: Removal of tattoos and benign pigmented lesions using the ruby laser. Lasers Surg Med 2S:51, 1990.

120. Dover JS, Margolis RJ, Polla LL, et al: Pigmented guinea pig skin irradiated with Q-switched ruby laser pulses. Arch Dermatol 125:43–49, 1989.

121. Polla LL, Margolis RJ, Dover JS, et al: Melanosomes are the primary target of Q-switched ruby laser irradiation in guinea pig skin. J Invest Dermatol 89:281–286, 1986.

122. Hruza GJ, Dover JS, Flotte TJ, et al: Q-switched ruby laser irradiation of normal human skin. Arch Dermatol 127:1799–1805, 1991.

123. Murphy GF, Shepard RS, Paul BS, et al: Organelle-specific injury to melanin-containing cells in human skin by pulsed laser irradiation. Lab Invest 49:680–685, 1983.

124. Goldman L, Igelman JM, Richfield DF: Impact of the laser on nevi and melanomas. Arch Dermatol 90:71–75, 1964.

125. Ohshiro T, Maruyama Y, Makajima H, Mimi M: Treatment of pigmentation of the lips and oral mucosa in Peutz-Jeghers syndrome using ruby and argon lasers. Br J Plast Surg 33:346–349, 1980.

126. Goldberg DJ, Nychay SG: Q-switched ruby laser treatment of nevus of Ota. J Dermatol Surg Oncol 18:817–821, 1992.

127. Goldberg DJ: Benign pigmented lesions of the skin: treatment with the Q-switched ruby laser. J Dermatol Surg Oncol 19:376–379, 1993.

128. Ashinoff R, Geronemus RG: Q-switched ruby laser treatment of benign epidermal pigmented lesions. Lasers Surg Med 4S:73, 1992.

129. McMeekin TO, Goodwin D: Comparison of Q-switched ruby, pigmented lesion dye laser and copper vapor laser treatment of benign pigmented lesions of the skin. Lasers Surg Med 4S:74, 1992.

130. Goldberg DJ: Benign pigmented lesions of the skin: treatment with Q-switched ruby, copper vapor, and pigmented lesion lasers. Lasers Surg Med 4S:74, 1992.

131. Thibault P, Wlodarczyk J: Postsclerotherapy hyperpigmentation: the role of serum ferritin levels and the effectiveness of treatment with the copper vapor laser. J Dermatol Surg Oncol 18:47–52, 1992.

132. Tan OT, Morelli JG, Kurban AK: Pulsed dye laser treatment of benign cutaneous pigmented lesions. Lasers Surg Med 12:538–542, 1992.

133. Fitzpatrick RE, Goldman MP, Ruiz-Esparza J: Laser treatment of benign pigmented epidermal lesions using a 300 nsecond pulse and 510 nm wavelength. J Dermatol Surg Oncol 19:341–347, 1993.

134. Grekin RC, Shelton RM, Geisse JK, Frieden I: 510 nm pigmented lesion dye laser: its characteristics and clinical uses. J Dermatol Surg Oncol 19:380–387, 1993.

135. Goldman MP: Postsclerotherapy hyperpigmentation: treatment with a flashlamp-excited pulsed dye laser. J Dermatol Surg Oncol 18:417–422, 1992.

136. Brauner GJ: Treatment of pigmented lesions of the skin with alexandrite laser. Lasers Surg Med 4S:72, 1992.

137. Holmdahl K: Cutaneous hemangiomas in premature and mature infants. Acta Paediatr 44:370–379, 1955.

138. Easterly NB: Cutaneous hemangiomas, vascular stains and associated syndromes. Curr Probl Pediatr 17:1–69, 1987.

139. Bowers RE, Graham EA, Tomlinson KM: The natural history of the strawberry nevus. Arch Dermatol 83:667–680, 1960.

140. Margileth AM, Mussles M: Current concepts in diagnosis and management of congenital cutaneous hemangiomas. Pediatrics 36:410–416, 1965.

141. Morelli J, Tan O, Weston W: Treatment of ulcerated hemangiomas with the pulsed tunable dye laser. Am J Dis Child 145:1062–1064, 1991.

142. Sherwood KA, Tan OT: The treatment of a capillary hemangioma with the flashlamp pumped-dye laser. J Am Acad Dermatology 22:136–137, 1991.

143. Ashinoff R, Geronemus RG: Capillary hemangiomas and treatment with the flash lamp-pulsed dye laser. Arch Dermatol 127:202–205, 1991.

144. Garden JM, Bakus AD, Paller AS: Treatment of cutaneous hemangiomas by the flashlamp-pumped pulsed dye laser: prospective analysis. J Pediatr 120:555–560, 1992.

145. Goldberg DJ, Sciales CW: Pyogenic granuloma in children. J Dermatol Surg Oncol 17:960–962, 1991.

146. Goodman MM, Alpern K: Treatment of lupus pernio with the flashlamp pulsed dye laser. Lasers Surg Med 12:549–551, 1992.

147. Tappero JW, Grekin RC, Zanelli GA, Berger TG: Pulsed-dye laser therapy for cutaneous Kaposi's sarcoma associated with acquired immunodeficiency syndrome. J Am Acad Dermatol 27:526–530, 1992.

148. Wheeland RG, Bailin PL, Norris MJ: Argon laser photocoagulative therapy of Kaposi's sarcoma: a clinical and histologic evaluation. J Dermatol Surg Oncol 11:1180–1185, 1985.

149. Weingold D, White P, Burton C: Treatment of lymphangioma circumscriptum with tunable dye laser. Cutis 45:356–366, 1990.

150. Basford JR: Low-energy laser therapy: controversies and new research findings. Lasers Surg Med 9:1–5, 1989.

151. Mester E, Spiry T, Szende B, Tota JG: Effect of laser rays on wound healing. Am J Surg 122:532–535, 1971.

152. Mester E, Korenyi-Both A, Spiry T, et al: Stimulation of wound healing by means of laser rays. Acta Chir Acad Sci Hung 14:347–356, 1973.

153. Kana JS, Hutschenreiter G, Haina D, Waidelich W: Effect of low-power density laser radiation on healing of open skin wounds in rats. Arch Surg 116:293–296, 1981.

154. Surinchak JS, Alago ML, Bellamy RF, et al: Effects of low-level energy lasers on the healing of full-thickness skin defects. Lasers Surg Med 2:267–274, 1983.

155. Hunter J, Leonard L, Wilson R, et al: Effects of low energy laser on wound healing in a porcine model. Lasers Surg Med 3:285–290, 1984.

156. Abergel RP, Meeker CA, Lam TS, et al: Control of connective tissue metabolism by lasers: recent developments and future prospects. J Am Acad Dermatol 11:1142–1150, 1984.

157. Mester E, Ludani G, Selyei M, et al: The stimulating effect of low power laser rays on biological systems. Laser Rev 1:3–8, 1968.

158. Longo L, Evangelista S, Tinacci G, Sesti AG: Effect of diodes-laser silver arsenide-aluminium (Ga-Al-As) 904 nm on healing of experimental wounds. Lasers Surg Med 7:444–447, 1987.

159. Lyons RF, Abergel RP, White RA, et al: Biostimulation of wound healing in vivo by a helium-neon laser. Ann Plast Surg 18:47–50, 1987.

160. Abergel RP, Lyons RF, Castel JC, et al: Biostimulation of wound healing by lasers: experimental approaches in animal models and in fibroblast cultures. J Dermatol Surg Oncol 13:127–133, 1987.

161. Braverman B, McCarthy RJ, Ivankovich AD, et al: Effect of helium-neon and infrared laser irradiation on wound healing in rabbits. Lasers Surg Med 9:50–58, 1989.

162. Fava G, Marchesini R, Melloni E, et al: Effect of low energy irradiation by He-Ne laser on mitosis rate of HT-29 tumor cells in culture. Lasers Life Sci 1:135–141, 1986.

163. Karu TI, Kalendo GS, Letokhov VS, Lobko JJ: Biostimulation of HeLa cells by low-intensity visible light: stimulation of DNA and RNA synthesis in a wide spectral range. Il Nuovo Cimento 3:309–318, 1984.

164. Karu TI, Kalendo GS, Letokhov VS, Lobko JJ: Biostimulation of HeLa cells by low-intensity visible light: stimulation of nucleic-acid synthesis in plateau phase cells. Il Nuovo Cimento 3:319–325, 1984.

165. Lam TS, Abergel RP, Meeker CA, et al: Laser stimulation of collagen synthesis in human skin fibroblast cultures. Lasers Life Sci 1:61–77, 1986.

166. Boulton M, Marshall J: He-Ne laser stimulation of human fibroblast proliferation and attachment in vitro. Lasers Life Sci 1:125–134, 1986.

167. Pasarella S, Dechecchi MS, Quagliariello E, et al: Optical and biochemical properties of NADH irradiated by high peak power Q-switched ruby laser or by low power CW He-Ne laser. Bioelectrochem Bioenerg 8:315–319, 1981.

168. Castro DJ, Abergel RP, Meeker CA, et al: Effects of the Nd:YAG laser on DNA synthesis and collagen production in human skin fibroblast cultures. Ann Plast Surg 11:214–222, 1983.

169. Abergel RP, Meeker CA, Dwyer RM, et al: Nonthermal effects of Nd:YAG laser on biological functions of human skin fibroblasts in culture. Lasers Surg Med 3:279–284, 1984.

170. Haas AF, Isseroff RR, Wheeland RG, et al: Low-energy helium-neon laser irradiation increases the motility of cultured human keratinocytes. J Invest Dermatol 94:822–826, 1990.

171. Rood PA, Haas AF, Graves PJ, et al: Low-energy helium neon laser irradiation does not alter human keratinocyte differentiation. J Invest Dermatol 99:445–448, 1992.

172. Robinson JK, Garden JM, Taute PM, et al: Wound healing in porcine skin following low-output carbon dioxide laser irradiation of the incision. Ann Plast Surg 18:499–505, 1987.

173. Pennington DG, Waner M, Knox A: Photodynamic therapy for multiple skin cancers. Plast Reconstr Surg 82:1067–1071, 1988.

174. Bernstein EF, Friauf WS, Smith PD, et al: Transcutaneous determination of tissue dihematoporphyrin ether content—a device to optimize photodynamic therapy. Arch Dermatol 127:1794–1798, 1991.

Infrared, Ultraviolet, and Experimental Laser Surgery

RONALD G. WHEELAND

Of the multitude of medical lasers that are currently available, the infrared lasers have found the widest clinical application in cutaneous surgery. The proven utility of the infrared lasers is largely a result of the precision with which the energy can be controlled and delivered and the reproducible results that can be achieved in the treatment of a variety of cutaneous disorders. One of the infrared lasers, the carbon dioxide laser, has long been considered the workhorse of all the cutaneous surgical lasers. It has become the treatment of choice for many lesions, and in select cases it may represent the only available form of treatment.[1, 2] One of the consequences of the widespread use of these lasers has been the development of many modifications in surgical technique to reduce inadvertent and unwanted thermal injury. In addition, new advances and refinements in the infrared laser equipment have made these systems more compact, lighter, less expensive, and more user friendly.

Carbon Dioxide Laser

ABSORPTION CHARACTERISTICS

The carbon dioxide laser emits an invisible beam of light in the mid-infrared region of the electromagnetic spectrum (wavelength, 10,600 nm).[3] This energy is precisely absorbed by the intracellular and extracellular water found in all living soft tissues and shows no color specificity. Absorption of this laser energy by water results in instantaneous conversion from a liquid state to a gaseous state, which creates a plume of smoke and steam.[4] This process occurs so rapidly that minimal thermal diffusion occurs, and adjacent cells remain viable. The zone of thermal injury created by the carbon dioxide laser in soft tissue is only 0.1 mm thick, which allows very precise and delicate surgery to be performed without unacceptable injury to surrounding vital structures.

DELIVERY SYSTEMS

Unlike many laser systems in which fiberoptics can be employed to deliver the light, current technology does not yet permit effective use of fiberoptics[5] for delivery of light from the carbon dioxide laser. Consequently, the energy is delivered through a system of sealed hollow tubes with mirrored articulating joints (Fig. 73–1) that reflect the light so that it can be used with a sterilizable handpiece that has a built-in focusing lens and an attached stylus to ensure that the beam of light is used at focality (Fig. 73–2). Most of these systems may initially be somewhat awkward to use. Because the carbon dioxide laser energy is invisible to the human eye, a low-energy, red aiming beam is emitted in coaxial fashion from a helium-neon (HeNe) laser to precisely direct the carbon dioxide laser beam to the target. Despite the cumbersome nature of the delivery system, many carbon dioxide laser systems have undergone remarkable miniaturization so that some current models weigh as little as 45 pounds. A major reduction in the size of the carbon dioxide laser equipment resulted from the development of sealed tube technology, which eliminated the need for flow-through gases of the laser medium and improved its portability. Better efficiency also has occurred with the substitution of radiofrequency for electrical excitation.[6]

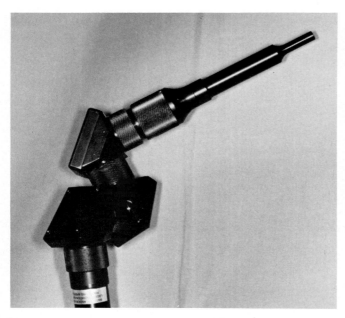

Figure 73–1. Articulating mirrored joints deliver the carbon dioxide laser to the handpiece.

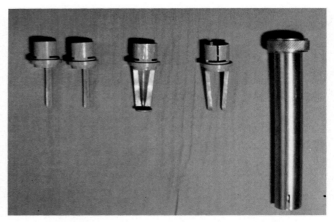

Figure 73–2. A stylus attaches to the end of the handpiece to ensure that the laser energy is being precisely delivered at its focal point.

MODES OF OPERATION

The versatility of the carbon dioxide laser is largely due to the two entirely different operational modes (Fig. 73–3) that permit this system to be used as a cutting instrument or to precisely and superficially ablate tissue.[7] The first mode of operation is the focused mode, which utilizes a lens to focus to a spot size of 0.1 to 0.2 mm (Fig. 73–4), resulting in the creation of a powerful beam of light with a very high irradiance.[8] This is sufficient to cut soft tissues precisely and bloodlessly in most cases. The second technique utilizes the beam of light from the same lens system used for the focused beam but after it has passed its focal point and become divergent. This results in the creation of a larger, 1- to 3-mm beam of light with a concomitant reduction in the irradiance to 500 to 1000 W/cm², which is sufficient to superficially ablate soft tissue.

Carbon Dioxide Laser Excision

The carbon dioxide laser can be used in place of a standard scalpel to make precise incisions when it is operated in its focused mode using a small beam and high laser output. In this mode of operation, the com-bination of small beam diameter (0.1 to 0.2 mm) and high power setting (20 to 35 W) results in the creation of an extremely high irradiance, varying from 50,000 to 100,000 W/cm². This irradiance is sufficient to incise most soft tissues without difficulty. The main advantage of using the carbon dioxide laser to incise the skin is the quality of hemostasis that is provided.[9] Blood vessels up to 0.5 mm in diameter are routinely sealed by the carbon dioxide laser, minimizing blood loss and improving visibility.[10] In addition, lymphatic channels are closed in similar fashion, which has proven beneficial in limiting the spread of tumor cells during certain oncologic surgical procedures.[11] Because this laser also seals cutaneous sensory nerve endings, there frequently is a marked reduction in postoperative pain when the laser is used to perform the excision.[12–14]

In this mode of operation, the depth of the incision made with the carbon dioxide laser is a function of both the irradiance being used and the rate at which the laser is moved along the incision line. Generally, a carbon dioxide laser incision will proceed more slowly than a conventional scalpel incision. However, the additional time is usually compensated for by the improved hemostasis provided by the laser. However, even though the hemostasis provided by the carbon dioxide laser is excellent in most cases, it is always prudent to have an electrosurgical device available to control bleeding that may occur from larger vessels not sealed by the carbon dioxide laser because of a high internal pressure or rapid flow rates. The quality of hemostasis is typically so good that immediate primary closure of a laser-incised wound

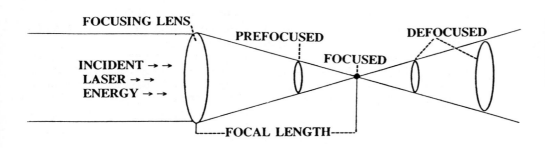

Figure 73–3. After the incident laser energy passes through its focusing lens, it can be used at its focal point to incise tissue or allowed to defocus to vaporize tissue.

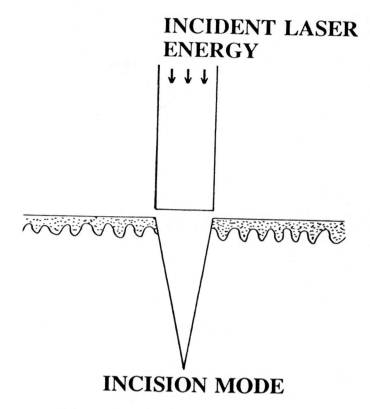

INCIDENT LASER ENERGY

INCISION MODE

Figure 73–4. The incident laser energy is delivered at its focal point to incise tissue.

can be performed with confidence that postoperative bleeding will be unlikely to occur. Similarly, repair of a wound created by carbon dioxide laser excision using a local flap can typically be performed without compromising the result.[15] However, skin graft survival may be somewhat impaired because of the high quality of hemostasis provided by the laser,[16] which may impede formation of a fibrin clot.

Very little modification of the standard scalpel surgical technique is required to perform carbon dioxide laser excisions. The most significant changes that are required are the direct result of important safety measures that must be observed to reduce the risk of injury to the patient, the cutaneous surgeon, and the operating room personnel. First, appropriate eyewear must be worn by

all individuals in the operating room. Second, a specially designed laser smoke evacuator must be employed to eliminate the noxious smell and smoke generated during the procedure. Third, flammable surgical preparations, sterile drapes, and anesthetic gases must be prohibited from the laser operating room to reduce the risk of ignition and fires. When these simple precautions are followed, the risk of complications during laser surgery is minimal.[17]

The final appearance of the carbon dioxide laser–incised wound is typically indistinguishable from that of a wound made using the traditional scalpel technique (Fig. 73–5). There is some controversy regarding the use of the carbon dioxide laser for excisional procedures because of the potentially negative effects it appears to

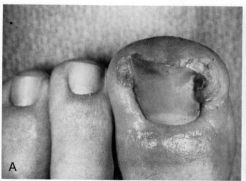
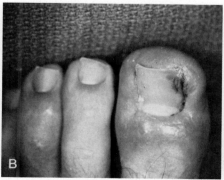
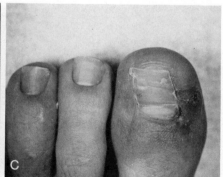

Figure 73–5. *A,* Preoperative appearance of a bilateral ingrown toenail. *B,* Clinical appearance 6 weeks after the lateral nail fold has been excised to produce partial matricectomy using the focused carbon dioxide laser. *C,* The final clinical appearance 3 months after partial matricectomy.

have on some wounds. A demonstrable decrease in tensile strength develops in laser-incised wounds, and delayed contraction and epithelialization of carbon dioxide laser wounds, when compared with scalpel wounds, have been shown.[18, 19] However, the opposite effect has also been described.[20] Despite this apparent conflict, the clinical management of patients treated with laser excision remains identical to that for those treated with the standard scalpel technique. However, it is important to recognize these potential side effects so that necessary steps can be taken to support the wound postoperatively and reduce the risk of complications.

Largely because of its hemostatic ability, the carbon dioxide laser is used in the excision mode of operation to remove highly vascular tumors or lesions found in vascular anatomic locations such as the scalp (Table 73–1).[21] In addition, the carbon dioxide laser can be effectively used in the treatment of anticoagulated patients. Patients with pacemakers that might be adversely affected by electrosurgical cutting devices or those who require cardiac monitoring during surgery can undergo carbon dioxide laser surgery performed without increased risk of complications. The precision with which excisional carbon dioxide laser surgery is performed can be shown by its use in Mohs micrographic surgery.[22] In this procedure, skin cancers that are found in anatomic locations at high risk for recurrence are removed in thin horizontal layers by delivering the focused carbon dioxide laser energy parallel to the skin surface. The excised disk of tissue is immediately processed in the laboratory using frozen sections and examined histologically so that any areas of residual tumor can be treated using a similar technique.

In some studies, the carbon dioxide laser has also been successfully used in its excisional mode to perform numerous cosmetic procedures, including blepharoplasty,[23, 26] rhinophyma,[27, 28] scalp reductions,[21] and removal of keloids from the earlobes[29] (Fig. 73–6) and scalp.[30, 31] The precise role of the carbon dioxide laser in the treatment of refractory keloids remains somewhat unclear. Some reports show a lower recurrence rate of keloid formation after laser excision compared with scalpel excision,[29, 31, 32] while other reports show either

no benefit or no difference between the two surgical techniques.[33–35] A lower recurrence rate of keloids has been shown when laser excision is coupled with intermittent intralesional steroid or hyaluronidase injections.[36] The mechanism by which the carbon dioxide could theoretically reduce the risk of recurrent keloid formation relates to the proven inhibitory effect that near-infrared laser energy exerts on fibroblasts grown in culture.[37]

Carbon Dioxide Laser Vaporization

In cutaneous surgery, the carbon dioxide laser is most frequently used in its vaporizational mode of operation, as superficial ablation of soft tissues such as the skin can be performed very precisely when the carbon dioxide laser is operated at relatively low irradiances.[8] It is a simple procedure to obtain the required low irradiances in most common carbon dioxide laser systems. In these systems, the beam can be made larger by pulling the handpiece away from the target, making it defocus to a much larger beam size (1 to 3 mm in diameter) without requiring a change of lenses (see Fig. 73–3). While it is possible to perform vaporization by using the large prefocused beam of light before its focal point, control is suboptimal, as deeper penetration will occur after the superficial tissue has been ablated.

TABLE 73–1. INDICATIONS FOR EXCISIONAL SURGERY WITH THE CARBON DIOXIDE LASER

Anticoagulation
Vascular tumor
Vascular anatomic location
Keloids
Rhinophyma
Malignant melanoma
Squamous cell carcinoma
Cardiac pacemaker
Cardiac monitoring
Perforation of cranial bone
Blepharoplasty
Nail surgery

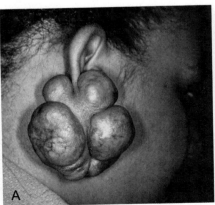
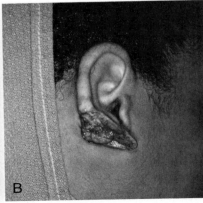
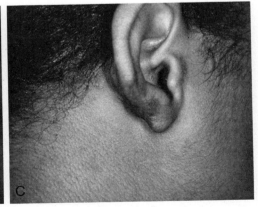

Figure 73–6. *A,* Preoperative appearance of a large, recurrent multilobular keloid on the right ear. *B,* Bloodless defect seen immediately after completion of carbon dioxide laser excision. *C,* Appearance 3 months after the defect was allowed to heal by second intention with nearly constant external pressure.

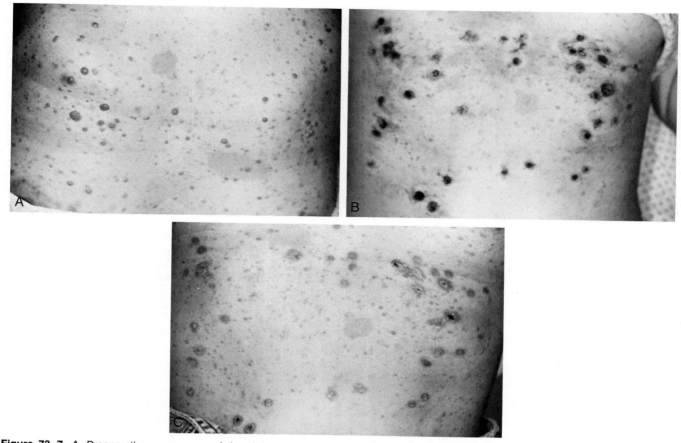

Figure 73–7. *A*, Preoperative appearance of the abdomen of a patient with neurofibromatosis. *B*, Multiple large lesions were excised in bloodless fashion using the focused carbon dioxide laser. *C*, Nearly all treated sites healed by second intention in 3 weeks.

A large number of inflammatory lesions,[38–41] infiltrative conditions,[42] cysts,[43–45] and benign tumors[46–48] (Fig. 73–7) have been successfully treated using the defocused carbon dioxide laser in its vaporizational mode of operation (Table 73–2).

Appendigeal Tumors. This technique is extremely beneficial in the treatment of multiple small, benign appendigeal tumors such as trichoepitheliomas,[49] syringomas,[50–52] and porokeratoses.[53] Local anesthesia must be used with this technique so that the short pulses (0.1 to 0.2 second) and low irradiance (400 to 600 W/cm²) can be delivered to the surface of each individual lesion without discomfort (Fig. 73–8). The precision of this technique stems from the fact that each pulse has the same irradiance and duration, which provides a constant depth of tissue ablation. For treating larger areas of involvement, such as adenoma sebaceum,[54, 55] the laser may be used in its continuous discharge mode, in a

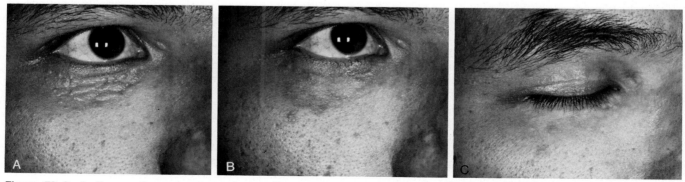

Figure 73–8. *A*, Preoperative appearance of a patient with multiple syringomas of the infraorbital area. *B*, Slight postinflammatory hyperpigmentation is present 6 weeks after carbon dioxide laser vaporization. *C*, Treated area 6 months later showing normal color without textural changes or scarring.

TABLE 73–2. CUTANEOUS CONDITIONS TREATED WITH VAPORIZATIONAL SURGERY USING THE CARBON DIOXIDE LASER

Acne scars (pitted)
Actinic cheilitis
Adenoma sebaceum
Balanitis xerotica obliterans
Basal cell carcinoma (superficial variant)
Chondrodermatitis nodularis helicis
Digital mucous cyst
Epidermal nevus
Erythroplasia of Queyrat
Granuloma faciale
Infectious lesions
   Cutaneous deep fungal infections
   Verrucae
      Condyloma
      Immunosuppressed individuals
      Periungual
      Plantar warts
Lentigines
Lichen sclerosus et atrophicus
Lymphangioma circumscriptum
Nail matricectomy
Neurofibroma
Nodular amyloidosis
Ochronosis
Porokeratosis
Rhinophyma
Steatocystoma
Syringoma
Tattoo
Trichoepithelioma
Tricholemmoma
Vascular lesions
   Angiokeratoma
   Cherry angioma
   Lymphangioma circumscriptum
   Port-wine stain (adults only)
   Pyogenic granuloma
   Telangiectasia (hereditary hemorrhagic)
   Venous lake
Vellus hair cyst
Xanthelasma
Zoon's balanitis

fashion analogous to conventional dermabrasion, so that the procedure may be performed more quickly. This technique has been erroneously called laser abrasion, an obvious misnomer, as the tissue is vaporized and not abraded. When treating acne scars[56] and other superficial processes, this technique employs a 1- to 3-mm, low-irradiance beam with continuous discharge to ablate thin layers of the lesion with each pass.

The surface char that is produced by vaporization is always removed by lightly scrubbing the surface with a clean wet gauze or a cotton-tipped applicator soaked in normal saline or 3% hydrogen peroxide to provide better visibility. This treatment process is repeated in a stepwise layer-by-layer process using similar laser parameters and interval cleansing until all remaining abnormal tissue has been removed. Because there is typically no bleeding during this procedure, the residual tumor islands can be identified by their differences in texture or color compared with the surrounding normal tissue. Wound healing occurs by second intention over a period of 7 to 10 days with good wound care.

Decorative Tattoos. The carbon dioxide laser is also commonly used in its vaporizational mode to remove decorative tattoos.[57–60] Again, local anesthesia must be employed, as the discomfort from the laser exposure would otherwise be intolerable. Although it is possible to precisely remove a tattoo with the carbon dioxide laser, this is frequently not desirable, as the resulting scar would duplicate the original appearance of the tattoo. Consequently, tattoos that consist of distinctive patterns or letters are removed by creating a different geometric shape or design during the vaporization process to make the appearance of the scar unidentifiable (Fig. 73–9). By vaporizing successive layers with interval cleansing using 3% hydrogen peroxide, areas of persistent tattoo pigment can be readily identified and treated until all pigment has been completely removed. The wound is allowed to heal by second intention, which takes 4 to 12 weeks depending on the size of the tattoo, its anatomic location, the depth of the wound, and the degree of patient compliance (Fig. 73–10). Amateur tattoos are generally more difficult to remove with the carbon dioxide laser, because the pigment is deposited at different depths within the dermis and may even extend into the subcutaneous fat. Professional tattoos typically have pigment deposited at a uniform depth, even though the different colors may be injected at different levels.

This technique offers a major advantage over most other forms of tattoo treatment, such as dermabrasion or salabrasion, in that only a single procedure is required to effect complete removal of the tattoo pigment (Fig. 73–11). Unlike the Q-switched lasers, the carbon dioxide laser can remove all tattoo pigments with equal effectiveness and can also be used to remove tattoo pigments that have resulted in allergic reactions from the injection of mercury. The main disadvantages of this technique are the resultant permanent scar and the relatively long time required for complete healing. All patients must be told in advance that the final cosmetic result will likely not be obtained for 12 to 18 months after carbon dioxide laser treatment.

Premalignant and Malignant Lesions

Actinic Cheilitis. Actinic cheilitis can be very successfully treated using the carbon dioxide laser.[61–63] In the past, this disorder was poorly treated using conventional surgical excision and oral mucosal advancement. With local anesthesia, the carbon dioxide laser can be used in its vaporizational mode to precisely remove the abnormal mucosal epithelium. After vaporization, the surface char is removed by cleansing with hydrogen peroxide. Any areas of abnormal epithelial cells will appear slightly yellow or white when compared with normal tissue, which is red or pink. Additional thin layers of tissue are then immediately vaporized until all the gross abnormal epithelium has been totally removed.

Minimal wound care is required during the postoperative period, and patients can be expected to have nearly normal function when eating, drinking, or talking. Healing by second intention occurs over a period of several weeks, and the cosmetic result obtained in most cases is excellent, with a return of normal color, texture, and sensation.

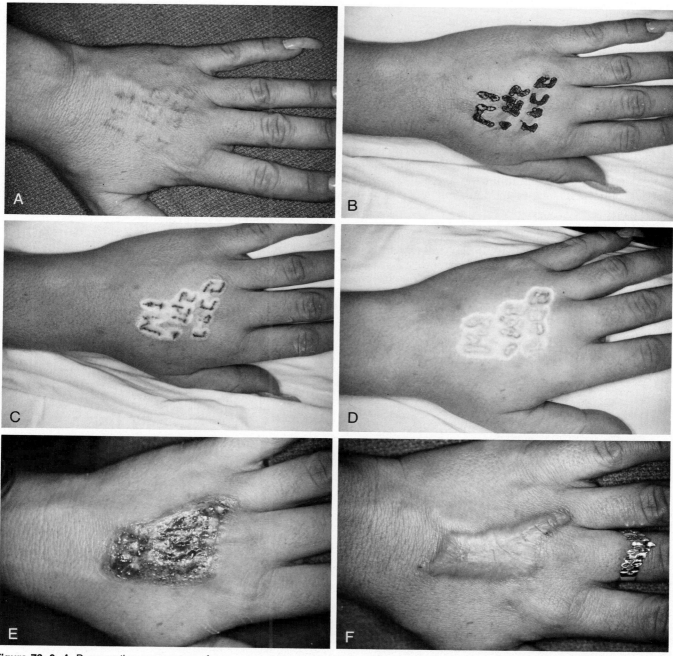

Figure 73–9. *A,* Preoperative appearance of an amateur tattoo on the back of the hand. *B,* Surface char forms where the tattoo pigment has been precisely vaporized. *C,* One superficial pass is made over the nontattooed skin so that the resultant scar will not duplicate the original appearance of the tattoo. *D,* At the completion of the procedure, all tattoo pigment has been removed. *E,* Granulation tissue has formed by 10 days as the wound heals by second intention. *F,* A slightly hypertrophic scar is present 4 months after carbon dioxide laser vaporization.

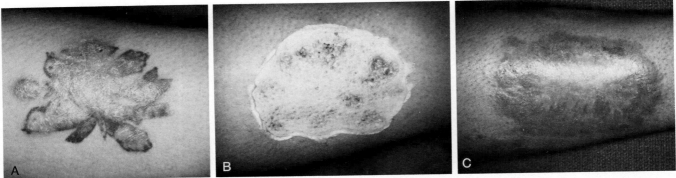

Figure 73–10. *A,* Preoperative appearance of a large, multicolored, professional tattoo on the leg. *B,* Oval defect produced by carbon dioxide laser vaporization. *C,* A flat, soft, slightly erythematous scar had formed 3 months after healing by second intention.

Erythroplasia of Queyrat. The vaporization mode of operation has also been used to treat erythroplasia of Queyrat.[64] Careful medical follow-up and self-examination are important factors in detecting any areas of recurrence.

Basal Cell Carcinoma (Superficial Type). A number of different surgical techniques have been used to successfully manage patients with basal cell carcinomas (BCC). However, patients with the superficial variant of BCC are often afflicted with multiple lesions in low-risk areas for recurrence (e.g., the trunk and extremities). In these situations, the carbon dioxide laser can be used in its vaporizational mode combined with standard curettage to rapidly treat large numbers of lesions without bleeding, significant postoperative pain, or excessive wound care.[65] In carefully selected patients, the risk of recurrence is low and the cosmetic results are comparable to those obtained using older, more established techniques.

Verrucae. Another commonly refractory disorder that

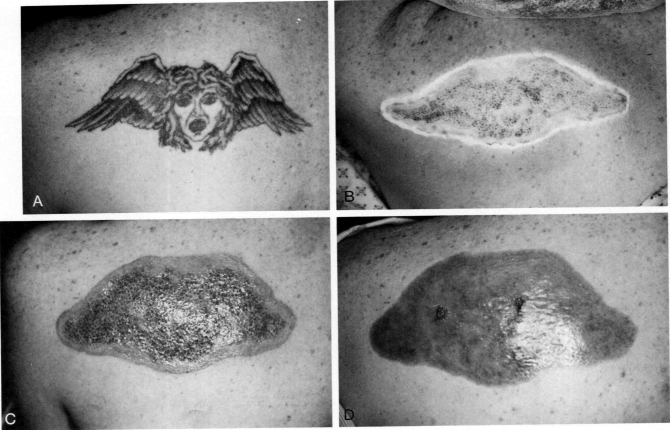

Figure 73–11. *A,* Preoperative appearance of a large, black, professional tattoo on the back. *B,* Irregularly shaped defect produced by carbon dioxide laser vaporization. *C,* Granulation tissue had formed by 12 days. *D,* Nearly complete reepithelialization had occurred by 8 weeks.

has been successfully treated using the carbon dioxide laser is papilloma virus infections or verrucae.[66, 67] The technique for the removal of warts is very similar to that described for the removal of tattoos and is also performed under local anesthesia. The wart is vaporized using either short pulses of 0.1 to 0.2 second for smaller lesions or continuous discharge for larger warts. Typically, the power setting is between 4 and 10 W, the beam diameter is 1 to 3 mm, and the irradiance is 360 to 1250 W/cm². After a single pass has been made, the surface char is removed using a cotton-tipped applicator soaked in 3% hydrogen peroxide. After two to three repetitions, the wart typically separates from the normal underlying skin during cleansing. With careful visual assessment, areas of persistent infection can be grossly identified by disturbance in the normal dermatoglyphic pattern. Because the hemostasis provided by this technique is virtually complete, residual areas of infection can be better visualized and precisely treated so that inadvertent injury to normal skin is minimized. Postoperatively, there is usually only minimal discomfort, and depending on the size, depth, and location of the verrucae, healing is usually complete in 2 to 5 weeks. Permanent changes in the texture of the skin can be anticipated after carbon dioxide laser vaporization.

The biggest difficulty associated with any existing treatment for verrucae is the inability to accurately determine the true extent of the infection. Residual viral particles can exist in normal-appearing skin and lead to apparent recurrent infection if they are not eliminated.[68] Unfortunately, the carbon dioxide laser vaporization technique used in the treatment of verrucae limits the injury to the adjacent tissue—unlike the more diffuse effects produced by cryosurgery or chemical destruction—which may allow these focal areas of infection to persist and result in recurrence (Fig. 73–12).

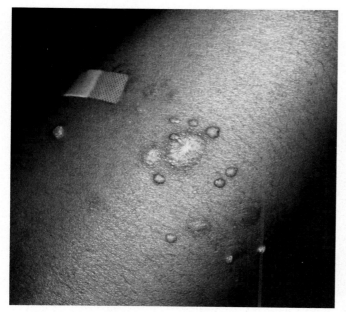

Figure 73–12. Multiple new verrucae that appeared around the residual scars from previous carbon dioxide laser vaporization.

Vascular Lesions

Lymphangioma Circumscriptum. The traditional surgical management of lymphangiomas is often followed by either superficial or deep recurrence because of the inability to accurately determine the true extent of this vascular disorder. In its vaporizational mode of operation, the carbon dioxide laser can be used to successfully ablate the superficial lymphangiomatous components.[69, 70] Although this technique is not particularly useful in eliminating the deeper lymphatic cisterns, marked functional improvement can often be obtained by removing those lesions that rupture with minor external trauma. Furthermore, superficial ablation of fragile superficial lymphangiomas also often reduces the recurrence rate of the soft tissue infections commonly seen in this condition.

Port-wine Stains. Because of its precise absorption by intracellular and extracellular water and limited depth of penetration,[71] the carbon dioxide laser has also been used in its vaporizational mode to treat some port-wine stains.[72–74] This technique should not be used to treat macular port-wine stains or port-wine stains in children.[75, 76] However, the CO_2 laser can be a useful tool in the removal of surface irregularities, known as blebs, that result from progressive dilatation of blood vessels as the patient ages. In most cases, it is desirable to perform a series of test treatments using both visible and infrared laser light (Fig. 73–13). After 6 to 8 weeks, the results can be evaluated, and the laser system that provided the greatest degree of improvement can be used to initiate treatment. If the surface of the lesion largely consists of ectatic blood vessels or blebs, resulting in an irregular surface, these areas of hypertrophic soft tissue can often be eliminated by carbon dioxide laser vaporization. Additional lightening of the port-wine stain, if desired, can often be accomplished by selectively photocoagulating the residual small blood vessel component with one of the visible light laser systems (see Chap. 72).

Hereditary Hemorrhagic Telangiectasia. Telangiectases are typically treated using one of the visible light lasers because of the precise absorption of light energy by oxyhemoglobin, which results in rapid clearing and an associated low risk of scarring. However, the carbon dioxide laser has also been used to ablate the telangiectatic blood vessels found on the mucosal surfaces in patients with hereditary hemorrhagic telangiectasia or Osler-Weber-Rendu syndrome.[77]

Miscellaneous Lesions. A number of unrelated conditions have also been treated with the carbon dioxide laser in its vaporizational mode. One of the more intriguing applications has been in the removal of benign lentigines using either very low energy fluences[78] or conventional vaporizational parameters.[79] Laser surgery of the nail unit has also proved to be very beneficial,[80] especially in matricectomies,[81] in which improved visibility and precise delivery of the laser energy yield excellent results. The limited thermal injury produced by the precise absorption of the carbon dioxide laser energy has been successfully exploited to manage patients with the painful condition of the ear known as

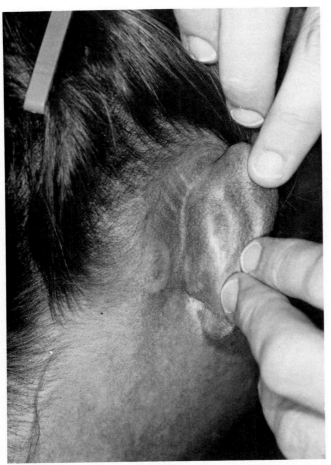

Figure 73–13. Lightening of the color of a port-wine stain can be seen at multiple test sites in the retroauricular area after treatment using a visible light laser (superior sites) and the carbon dioxide laser (inferior sites) in its vaporizational mode of operation.

chondrodermatitis.[82] Finally, carbon dioxide laser vaporization has also been used to effectively treat hypertrophic forms of epidermal nevi (Fig. 73–14), with good cosmetic and functional results.[83]

Combined Excisional and Vaporizational Modes

In some cases, both modes of operation for the carbon dioxide laser may be used in the treatment of the same lesion. For example, in the treatment of patients with massive lesions such as large trichoepitheliomas[49] or rhinophymas,[27, 28] excess tissue is first excised in relatively bloodless fashion using the focused laser. Once the gross architectural shape and contours have been created, the final shape is achieved by precisely vaporizing thin layers of tissue.

Superpulsed Mode

The carbon dioxide laser can also be used in a third mode of operation, the superpulsed mode (Fig. 73–15). In these systems, the high-intensity laser energy (150 to 500 W) is delivered in short pulses of 0.2 to 0.3 millisecond at a frequency of 250 to 5000 Hz. The pulses are separated from one another by brief pauses so that the duty cycle, or "on" time, is only 10%, and the average power delivered is only 30% of that delivered by a continuous discharge system (Fig. 73–16A). These pulsed systems take advantage of heat conduction to minimize thermal injury and reduce nonspecific thermal damage by allowing the targeted tissue to cool (Fig. 73–16B) between successive pulses.[84] When superpulsed lasers are used in the vaporization mode to precisely ablate tissue, the incidence of adverse scarring is reduced[48, 51] and the cosmetic results are often better than those obtained using the carbon dioxide laser in continuous discharge.[48] In the excisional mode of operation, the superpulsed carbon dioxide laser delivers less total energy per unit of time than the continuous discharge carbon dioxide laser, thereby reducing the thermal injury. However, this also reduces the rate at which tissue can be excised[84] and provides less coagulation. For these reasons, the exact role for the superpulsed carbon dioxide laser systems still remains to be defined,[71] despite the apparent advantages that would seem to result from their use.

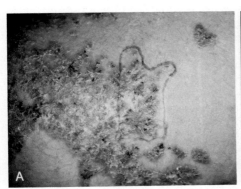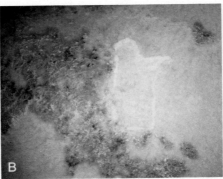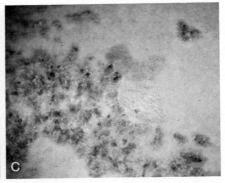

Figure 73–14. *A,* Preoperative appearance of a keratotic, verrucous epidermal nevus. *B,* Clinical appearance immediately after carbon dioxide laser vaporization of a small test site. *C,* A flat, soft, textural scar had formed 6 weeks after healing by second intention without evidence of recurrent growth.

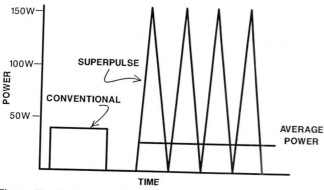

Figure 73–15. A comparison of the average power delivered using conventional and superpulsed carbon dioxide lasers.

Neodymium:Yttrium-Aluminum-Garnet (Nd:YAG) Laser

A second type of infrared laser is the neodymium:yttrium-aluminum-garnet (Nd:YAG) laser, a near-infrared light source with a wavelength of 1064 nm. As is clear from its name, the optical medium for the Nd:YAG laser is a crystal composed of neodymium, yttrium, aluminum, and garnet. This system can emit energy in continuous fashion or in pulses. Because its emission is in the near-infrared portion of the electromagnetic spectrum, it is invisible to the human eye. Developed in 1964, this laser has been primarily used in the photocoagulation of large vascular lesions of the skin and internal organs, as it can be delivered by fiberoptics through endoscopes. Energy from this laser system is not well absorbed by any particular chromophore in the skin, but rather is volume absorbed by protein.[85] This characteristic results in the Nd:YAG laser causing a relatively wide zonal type of destruction as a result of diffuse thermal damage. The 5- to 8-mm depth of penetration by the Nd:YAG laser has resulted in its use being largely restricted to the treatment of large, deep vascular lesions with significant volume.[86–89]

SAPPHIRE TIPS FOR Nd:YAG INCISIONS

Synthetic sapphire tips that focus the Nd:YAG laser energy to a precise point[90, 91] can be coupled to the optical fiber. By using different sizes and shapes of sapphire tips, both diffuse photocoagulation[87–89] and precise and bloodless incisions can be performed with this laser (Fig. 73–17).

FREQUENCY DOUBLING

The near-infrared energy from the Nd:YAG laser can be passed through an optical crystal that doubles the frequency and halves the wavelength. This results in the production of green visible light with a wavelength of 532 nm. Because this wavelength of light matches the absorption spectrum for melanin, the frequency-doubled Nd:YAG laser can be used to treat benign pigmented lesions when delivered in short Q-switched pulses (see Chap. 72). This output also overlaps the absorption spectrum for oxyhemoglobin, and so this laser system has also been used in the treatment of vascular lesions.[92]

BIOINHIBITION

Convincing laboratory research has demonstrated that low energy from the Nd:YAG laser can inhibit human fibroblasts grown in tissue culture without producing thermal injury.[93] It appears that this wavelength of light inhibits the production of collagen and elastin by fibroblasts and also inhibits fibroblast proliferation.[94–97] The clinical usefulness of this effect on tissue has yet to be fully substantiated, but it could provide an effective form of treatment for a variety of fibrotic conditions, including keloids,[98, 99] hypertrophic scars, and scleroderma.

LASER WELDING

Low-energy output from several different laser systems, including the Nd:YAG laser, has been used to thermally weld tissues together by the creation of a

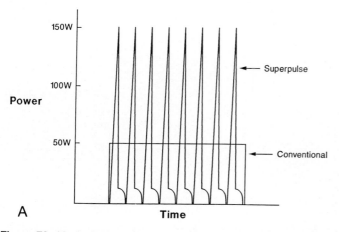

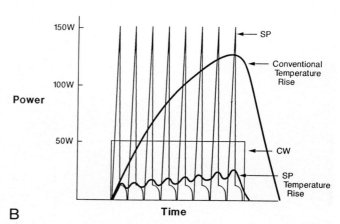

Figure 73–16. *A,* A comparison of the peak power delivered using conventional and superpulsed carbon dioxide lasers. *B,* A comparison of the temperature increase seen during delivery of conventional and superpulsed carbon dioxide laser energy.

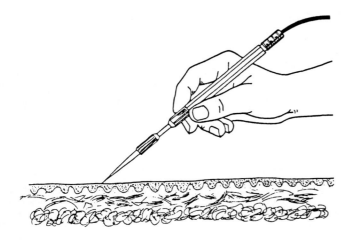

Figure 73–17. Schematic showing the contact mode Nd:YAG laser.

protein coagulum.[100–102] However, a number of obstacles, such as difficulty of delivery, dosimetric factors, and the expense of the equipment, must be overcome before this technique achieves wide clinical usefulness (see Chap. 78).

Laser Safety

Although lasers have proved to be extremely beneficial in various conditions, there are also some potential problems associated with their use. To reduce the risk of inadvertent complications during laser surgery and permit procedures to be performed with greatest safety, several precautions must be closely observed.

OCULAR INJURY

Probably the greatest safety issue related to laser surgery concerns the potential risk of ocular injury to the physician, operating room personnel, and the patient. Many common laser systems can cause permanent loss of visual acuity or blindness. For this reason, special protective eyewear must be worn by all members of the operating room team and by the patient. In addition, appropriate signs should be placed outside the operating room door describing the wavelength(s) of the laser in operation and the type of exposure. Each pair of laser glasses or goggles should be stamped on the arm (Fig. 73–18A) or face plate (Fig. 73–18B) with the optical density (OD) provided by the eyewear. This information should also indicate the particular wavelengths of laser light for which this protection is provided.[91] With the large number of currently available laser systems that can simultaneously produce multiple bands of visible laser light, it is a potentially hazardous practice to select a pair of laser glasses based merely on the color of the lenses. Before initiating each procedure, the laser surgeon should always first determine the optical density that will be provided by the eyewear, since many of the current products provide adequate protection for only a relatively narrow band of wavelengths.

Because carbon dioxide laser energy cannot pass through plastic, glass, or polycarbonate, simple prescription glasses, nonprescription lenses with protective side shields, or goggles all provide adequate protection (Fig. 73–19). However, special eye protection is required for the invisible light from the Nd:YAG laser. While these glasses may appear colorless (Fig. 73–20A), they have special optical coatings that provide adequate eye protection (Fig. 73–20B) while permitting maximal visibility. For patients undergoing laser surgery on the eyelids or inner canthus, sterile stainless steel eyeshields (Fig. 73–21) can be placed directly on the cornea after ob-

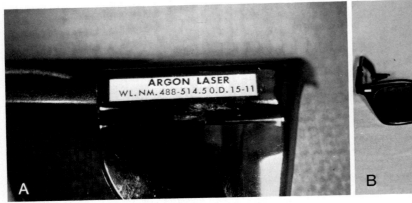

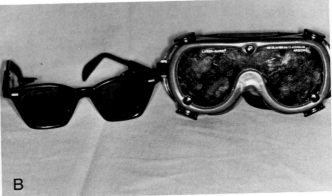

Figure 73–18. A, Optical density (O.D.) is indicated on the arm of the glasses used for performing argon laser surgery. B, "O.D." is also stamped on the face plate of the goggles used for performing argon laser surgery *(right)*.

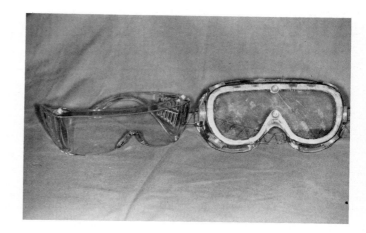

Figure 73–19. Simple polycarbonate glasses with side shields *(left)* or plastic goggles provide appropriate protection during carbon dioxide laser surgery.

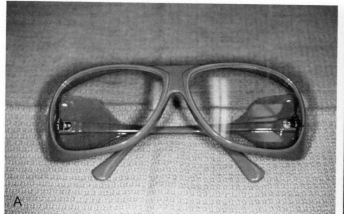

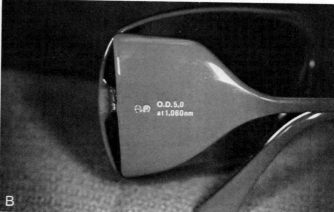

Figure 73–20. *A,* The glass used in the Nd:YAG glasses is treated with special optical coatings so that they remain clear. *B,* Optical density ("O.D.") indicated on the arm of the glasses used for performing Nd:YAG laser surgery.

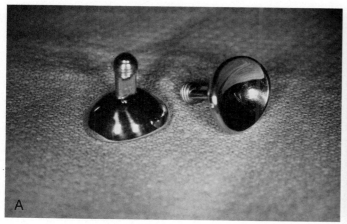

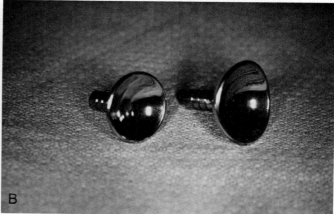

Figure 73–21. *A,* Stainless steel scleral eye shields permit safe performance of laser surgery on the eyelids. *B,* Scleral eye shields are available in pediatric *(left)* and adult *(right)* sizes.

taining topical anesthesia with proparacaine eye drops to protect the eye from inadvertent exposure to laser energy.[103] Alternatively, single (Fig. 73–22*A*) or double stainless steel eye cups (Fig. 73–22*B, C*) can be placed on the external surface of the eyelid to provide eye protection when laser surgery is being performed in the immediate vicinity of the eye but not directly on the eyelids themselves.

FLAMMABILITY

There is a risk of igniting dry surgical drapes, flammable surgical skin preparation agents, bowel gas, and certain anesthetic gases during carbon dioxide laser surgery. For this reason, flammable materials should be excluded from the laser operating room at all times to reduce the risk of an accidental fire. When a sterile surgical field is required for performing laser excisions, the standard cloth surgical drapes must be kept moist by the application of sterile saline or sterile water (Fig. 73–23). Nonflammable, disposable laser surgical drapes are also available.

REFLECTION

Reflection of laser light during a cutaneous surgical procedure by shiny, flat surgical instruments represents a potential risk to the patient, the surgeon, and the operating room personnel. Depending on the anatomic site and the irradiance being used, reflection of this light could result in inadvertent injury to the normal surrounding tissue, ignition of surgical drapes or cloth garments, or ocular injury. For this reason, laser surgical tools that have been specially burnished or anodized to decrease the amount of light reflected from the surface are available. For the carbon dioxide laser, the intensity of the reflected light is relatively limited, since the beam rapidly diverges after leaving its focal point and travels through space.

LASER PLUME

Laser systems that are capable of vaporizing or incising soft tissues all have the ability to generate a plume of smoke and steam. Studies have shown that papilloma viral DNA fragments can be recovered from the carbon dioxide laser plume during the treatment of warts.[104] This is also true for the plume generated during electrosurgical procedures.[105] While the infectiousness of these viral particles has not been established, this finding must be considered seriously, since other studies have shown that certain bacterial spores can survive carbon dioxide laser vaporization.[106, 107] Current technology has produced a laser smoke evacuation system that can filter particles as small as 0.01 μ with very high efficiency (Fig. 73–24). However, the sterile nozzle (Fig. 73–25)

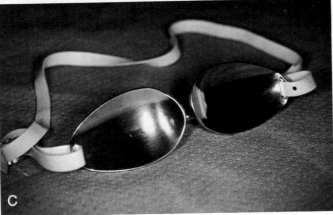

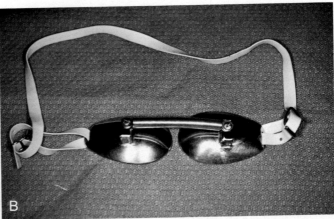

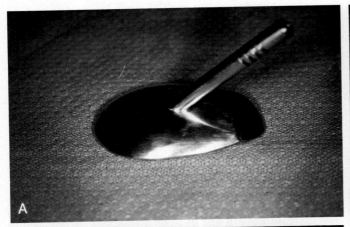

Figure 73–22. *A,* A single stainless steel eye cup can be placed on the external surface of the eyelid to provide protection during periorbital laser surgery. *B,* A pair of stainless steel eye cups with an elasticized head band can be worn over the external surfaces of the eyelids to provide protection during periorbital laser surgery. *C,* The concave surface of the stainless steel eye cups fits comfortably against the external surface of the eyelid.

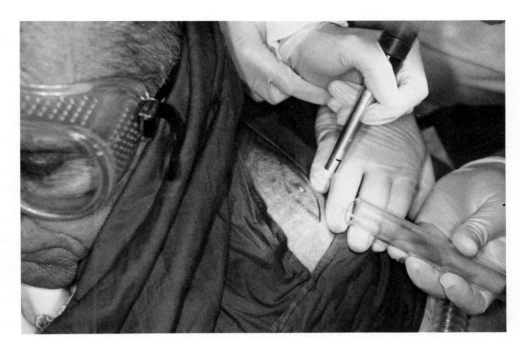

Figure 73–23. During carbon dioxide laser excisional surgery, wet sterile surgical drapes are placed around the excision site to prevent ignition during inadvertent exposure to the laser beam. (*Note:* The sterile laser smoke evacuator nozzle is held close to the surgical field.)

must be kept close to the treatment site or a significant amount of the plume will escape. In addition, special surgical masks have been developed that can further reduce the potential risk of transmission of infectious agents during laser surgery by filtering particles as small as 0.3 μ. The potential risk of exposure to the human immunodeficiency virus (HIV) during laser surgical procedures has not been determined. However, one study using the simian immunodeficiency virus (SIV) was unable to demonstrate any persistent viral particles in the laser plume collected during carbon dioxide laser vaporization performed at several different irradiances.[108] For these reasons, appropriate safety precautions should always be observed, including the use of surgical masks or other safe-breathing devices, proper eye protection, and surgical gowns and gloves.[109]

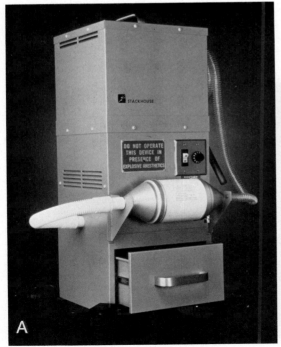

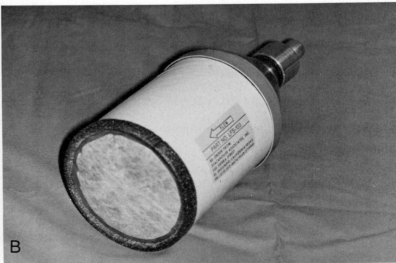

Figure 73–24. *A,* High-efficiency laser smoke evacuation system. *B,* The special filter within the smoke evacuator.

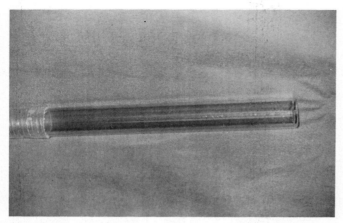

Figure 73–25. The plastic smoke evacuator nozzle can be sterilized so that it can be held close to the operative site.

CARCINOGENICITY

Despite long-term use of many different medical lasers in a wide variety of different organ systems, there has been no evidence that exposure to laser light results in neoplastic changes.[110] Among the currently available experimental laser systems, the excimer lasers could conceivably increase the risk of malignant degeneration, because they emit various wavelengths of ultraviolet light. However, this potential risk has been recognized, and the use of these systems is being closely monitored to determine the true extent of this possibility.

Experimental Laser Systems and Techniques

EXCIMER LASERS

A group of ultraviolet lasers known as the excimer lasers get their name from *excited dimer,*[111] which signifies the nature of their rare gas and halogen composition. This group of five laser systems emits light ranging from 193 to 351 nm, with very high energy and extremely short pulse duration. Standard pulse widths range from 1 to 10 nanoseconds with peak powers from 1 to 50 MW. These pulsed laser systems can incise tissue very cleanly, because they have very little thermal effect on the tissues.[112, 113] In addition, because the pulse duration is so short, the xenon-fluoride laser with its wavelength of 351 nm has been used for selective photothermolysis of the subcellular melanosomes within a melanocyte without causing injury to other cellular subcomponents.[114] The current application of these systems in medicine is very limited at present, but additional research using these lasers will likely define new possibilities in the near future.

LASER DOPPLER

Low-energy light from the helium-neon laser in the form of a laser Doppler device has been used to non-invasively measure the contours of skin,[115] as well as blood flow.[116–118] Laser Dopplers have been used to determine the amount of blood flow in an extremity or digit with compromised vascularity and also the viability of a surgical flap being used to reconstruct a cutaneous defect. They have also been used to study the amount of blood flow in a port-wine stain before laser surgery in an attempt to determine the most ideal treatment parameters.

LOW-ENERGY LASERS AND PHOTODYNAMIC THERAPY

Photodynamic therapy (PDT) is a form of cancer treatment that utilizes low levels of laser energy to activate various photosensitizers that have accumulated in neoplastic cells from intravenous or topical application.[119–122] One of these photosensitizers, hematoporphyrin derivative (HpD), is activated by red laser light with a wavelength of 630 nm that has been generated by an tunable argon-dye or gold vapor laser.[123] The laser exposure results in a photochemical reaction that causes release of singlet oxygen and superoxide radicals.[124, 125] These products are injurious to both the cell membrane and subcellular organelles, as well as to the endothelium of blood vessels that supply tumors.[126] The initial studies on PDT for cutaneous malignancies have shown many beneficial effects (see Chap. 79) but the proper clinical indications and ideal laser parameters must still be determined.[127, 128] New agents,[129] especially those that can be applied topically,[134] await further development.

GOLD VAPOR LASER

This laser system is very similar to the copper vapor laser. The use of high temperatures in the optical cavity to vaporize elemental gold results in the production of red light with a wavelength of 632 nm.[131] Although it is still experimental, this laser will likely be another source of red light for use in performing photodynamic therapy.

HOLMIUM:YAG LASER

The holmium:YAG laser, like the carbon dioxide laser, is a mid-infrared laser system with a wavelength of 2140 nm. The energy from this laser, which is precisely absorbed by intracellular and extracellular water, can be delivered by fiberoptics in a continuous fashion or in short pulses. This system has been approved for arthroscopic and laparoscopic surgical procedures in which ablation of tissue by vaporization or coagulation is required. Because of the precise absorption of this energy by soft tissues, its depth of penetration is 0.4 to 0.5 mm. Additional studies are currently under way to determine whether this system might also be beneficial in performing cutaneous surgical procedures.

ERBIUM:YAG LASER

The erbium:YAG laser, which has a wavelength of 2940 nm, is a third type of mid-infrared laser. The energy from this laser is emitted at the exact maximum absorption peak for water, which makes it an appropriate device for limiting nonspecific thermal injury during the treatment of soft tissues. This laser can be operated in continuous fashion or used to deliver short pulses. Further work is required to establish the potential usefulness of this system in cutaneous surgery.

TITANIUM:SAPPHIRE LASER

The laser medium in the experimental titanium:sapphire laser consists of a solid-state rod that is composed of titanium-doped sapphire $Ti:Al_2O_3$.[132, 133] This pulsed laser system is tunable over a relatively narrow spectrum of wavelengths but is commonly operated at 800 nm. This system is exceedingly powerful, with peak intensities of 10 terrawatts (10^{12}), and also has very short pulse durations of less than 120 femtoseconds (10^{-15}). These short pulses are generated by a mechanism known as "chirped" pulse amplification, which requires two passes through a diffraction-grating pulse stretcher that acts to disperse the 100-femtosecond pulses to 450 picoseconds. A pulse slicer then extracts 1-nJ pulses from the 82-MHz train before it enters a regenerative amplifier, which amplifies the pulse to 10 mJ. This action is "pumped" by a 70-mJ, Q-switched, frequency-doubled Nd:YAG laser. Another pass through a pulse slicer removes any pulses that leak from the regenerative amplifier. The beam is then amplified to 80 mJ in a $Ti:Al_2O_3$ amplifier pumped by a Q-switched, frequency-doubled Nd:YAG laser. A parallel grating pulse compressor acts to compress 10-Hz pulses temporally and changes the pulse duration to 120 femtoseconds. The pulse energy increases to 50 mJ before passing through a saturable absorber of IRI-40 dye in methanol, which absorbs 25% of incident energy to generate pulses with clean leading edges that are less than 120 femtoseconds in duration.

One of the most interesting features of this laser system is its ability to precisely ablate tissue without causing any thermal injury. This ablative process results in the formation of a "plasma,"[134] which forms as high-energy photons from the laser break molecular bonds through the production of photoacoustic shock waves[135] and cavitation bubbles. This process results in ablative photodecomposition[136] and causes the ejection of fragments from the impact site.

In this technique, an atmosphere of helium is required to prevent distortion of the temporal fidelity of the pulse caused by the nonlinear breakdown of air. The production of the laser-induced plasma results in the generation of a white spark and an ablation crater with sharply defined smooth walls. The optimal pulse threshold has been determined to be 2 mJ, or an intensity of 2.5 terrawatts/cm². Subthreshold pulses produce no tissue ablation, and suprathreshold pulses result in creation of plasma without tissue ablation. The ablation depths vary with the pulse energy, but at threshold, 0.1 μm of tissue is ablated. It is possible to produce precise ablation only of the epidermis by controlling the number and energy of pulses delivered. Nonthermal, collateral damage is minimal and ranges from 0 to 30 μm.[132, 137, 138] The potential clinical uses of tissue ablation by laser-induced plasma formation remain to be defined. However, the possibility of making precise incisions without causing thermal injury in certain cosmetic surgical procedures should serve the dual purpose of allowing rapid healing while also minimizing scarring.

DIODE LASERS

High-powered semiconductor diode lasers, made from small chips of gallium-aluminum-arsenide (GaAlAs), have been developed that emit energy at a wavelength of 805 nm in continuous or pulsed fashion.[139] Light from this laser can be transmitted by fiberoptics and delivered using synthetic sapphire tips in a contact mode to incise or vaporize soft tissue. In this way, this laser can provide clinical results that are similar to those obtained with the Nd:YAG laser. Additional basic clinical research is necessary to determine the usefulness of these relatively small devices in cutaneous surgery.

FREE ELECTRON LASERS

The free electron laser is an expensive experimental device with an average power level of 1×10^{15} W. A linear accelerator is used in a vacuum to generate free electrons of 3.5 to 100 MeV. Because the free electrons are not bound to atoms or molecules, they can be forced to vibrate at different frequencies by being passed through an alternating series of magnetic fields. This device is the focus of much current laser research activity because of its short pulse duration, high power, and ability to be adjusted over a relatively wide range of wavelengths (200 to 20,000 nm).[140]

The potential medical uses of the free electron laser have yet to be fully explored. However, the unique features of this laser system could be exploited in cutaneous surgery by performing precise tissue welds, ablating minute volumes of tissue through photovaporization, and destroying pigment-containing cells or removing tattoos through its photoacoustic effects.

SUMMARY

Although absolute indications for lasers have been clearly established only in very limited circumstances, the infrared and ultraviolet lasers will play an increasingly important future role in the surgical management of many cutaneous disorders. Furthermore, laser systems offering greater specificity in interacting with living tissue will also likely be developed. Determination of standard laser treatment parameters will provide the ideal wavelength and type of exposure for the management of many cutaneous disorders. Current technology is certain to be replaced with more efficient and precise instrumentation in the future, but this evolutionary process will occur more rapidly as more physicians become knowledgeable and skilled in the uses of currently available laser surgical instruments.

REFERENCES

1. Wheeland RG, Walker NPJ: Lasers—twenty-five years later. Int J Dermatol 25:209–216, 1986.
2. Garden JM, Geronemus RG: Dermatologic laser surgery. J Dermatol Surg Oncol 16:156–168, 1990.
3. Polanyi TG: Laser physics: medical applications. Otolaryngol Clin North Am 16:753–774, 1983.
4. Sliney DH: Laser-tissue interactions. Clin Chest Med 6:203–208, 1985.
5. Fuller TA: Mid-infrared fiber optics. Lasers Surg Med 6:399–403, 1986.
6. Goldman L, Perry E, Stefanovsky D: A flexible sealed tube transverse radiofrequency excited carbon dioxide laser for dermatologic surgery. Lasers Surg Med 2:317–322, 1983.
7. Polanyi TG: Physics of surgery with lasers. Clin Chest Med 6:179–202, 1985.
8. Arndt KA, Noe JM, Northam DBC, Itzkan I: Laser therapy basic concepts and nomenclature. J Am Acad Dermatol 5:649–654, 1981.
9. Slutzki S, Shafir R, Bornstein LA: Use of the carbon dioxide laser for large excisions with minimal blood loss. Plast Reconstr Surg 60:250–255, 1977.
10. Guerry TL, Silverman S Jr, Dedo HH: Carbon dioxide laser resection of superficial oral carcinoma: indications, technique, and results. Ann Otol Rhinol Laryngol 95:547–555, 1986.
11. Lanzafame RJ, Rogers DW, Naim JO, et al: Reduction of local tumor recurrence by excision with the CO_2 laser. Lasers Surg Med 6:439–441, 1986.
12. Ascher PW, Ingolitsch E, Walter G, et al: Ultrastructural findings in CNS tissue with CO_2 laser. In: Kaplan I (ed): Laser Surgery II. Jerusalem Academic Press, Jerusalem, 1978, pp 81–90.
13. Kamat BR, Carney JM, Arndt KA, et al: Cutaneous tissue repair following CO_2 laser irradiation. J Invest Dermatol 87:268–271, 1986.
14. Koranda FC, Grande DJ, Whitaker DC, et al: Laser surgery in the medically compromised patient. J Dermatol Surg Oncol 8:471–474, 1982.
15. Sacchini V, Lovo GF, Arioli N, et al: Carbon dioxide laser in scalp tumor surgery. Lasers Surg Med 4:261–269, 1984.
16. Lejeune F, Van Hoof G, Gerard A: Impairment of skin graft after CO_2 laser surgery in melanoma patients. Br J Surg 67:318, 1980.
17. Olbricht SM, Stern RS, Tang SV, et al: Complications of cutaneous laser surgery: a survey. Arch Dermatol 123:345–349, 1987.
18. Buell BR, Schuller DE: Comparison of tensile strength in CO_2 laser and scalpel skin incisions. Arch Otolaryngol 109:465–467, 1983.
19. Jarmuske M, Stranc M, Stranc L: The effect of carbon dioxide laser on wound contraction epithelia regeneration in rabbits. Br J Plast Surg 43:40–46, 1990.
20. Finsterbush A, Rousso M, Ashur H: Healing and tensile strength of CO_2 laser incisions and scalpel wounds in rabbits. Plast Reconstr Surg 70:360–362, 1982.
21. Wheeland RG, Bailin PL: Scalp reduction surgery with the carbon dioxide CO_2 laser. J Dermatol Surg Oncol 10:565–569, 1984.
22. Bailin PL, Ratz JL, Lutz-Nagey L: CO_2 laser modification of Mohs' surgery. J Dermatol Surg Oncol 7:621–623, 1981.
23. Bakers SS, Muenzler WS, Small RG, Leonard JE: Carbon dioxide laser blepharoplasty. Ophthalmology 91:238–244, 1984.
24. Davis L, Sanders G: CO_2 laser blepharoplasty: a comparison to cold steel and electrocautery. J Dermatol Surg Oncol 13:110–114, 1987.
25. Korn E: Use of a carbon dioxide laser for lesions extending into the lashes. Ophthalmic Surg 21:581–584, 1990.
26. Morrow DM, Morrow LB: CO_2 laser blepharoplasty: a comparison with cold-steel surgery. J Dermatol Surg Oncol 18:307–313, 1992.
27. Wheeland RG, Bailin PL, Ratz JL: Combined carbon dioxide laser excision and vaporization in the treatment of rhinophyma. J Dermatol Surg Oncol 13:172–177, 1987.
28. Haas A, Wheeland R: Treatment of massive rhinophyma with the carbon dioxide laser. J Dermatol Surg Oncol 16:645–649, 1990.
29. Kantor GR, Wheeland RG, Bailin PL, et al: Treatment of earlobe keloids with carbon dioxide laser excision. J Dermatol Surg Oncol 11:1063–1067, 1985.
30. Glass F, Berman B, Laub D: Treatment of perifolliculitis capitis abscedens et suffodiens with the carbon dioxide laser. J Dermatol Surg Oncol 15:673–676, 1989.
31. Kantor GR, Ratz JL, Wheeland RG: Treatment of acne keloidalis nuchae with carbon dioxide laser. J Am Acad Dermatol 14:263–267, 1986.
32. Henderson DL, Cromwell TA, Mes LG: Argon and carbon dioxide laser treatment of hypertrophic and keloid scars. Lasers Surg Med 3:271–277, 1984.
33. Stern J, Lucente F: Carbon dioxide laser excision of earlobe keloids: a prospective study and critical analysis of existing data. Arch Otolaryngol Head Neck Surg 115:1107–1111, 1989.
34. Norris J: The effect of carbon dioxide laser surgery on the recurrence of keloids. Plast Reconstr Surg 87:44–49, 1991.
35. Apfelberg DB, Maser M, White D, Lash H: Failure of carbon dioxide laser excision of keloids. Lasers Surg Med 9:382–389, 1989.
36. Stucker FJ, Shaw GY: An approach to management of keloids. Arch Otolaryngol Head Neck Surg 118:63–67, 1992.
37. Abergel RP, Dwyer RM, Meeker CA, et al: Laser treatment of keloids: a clinical trial and an in vitro study with Nd:YAG laser. Lasers Surg Med 4:291–295, 1984.
38. Wheeland RG, Ashley JA, Smith DA, et al: Carbon dioxide CO_2 laser treatment of granuloma faciale. J Dermatol Surg Oncol 10:730–733, 1984.
39. Dinehart S, Gross D, Davis C: Granuloma faciale: comparison of different treatment modalities. Arch Otolaryngol 116:849–851, 1990.
40. Don P, Carney P, Lynch W, et al: Carbon dioxide laserabrasion: a new approach to management of familial benign chronic pemphigus (Hailey-Hailey disease). J Dermatol Surg Oncol 13:1187–1194, 1987.
41. Baldwin H, Geronemus R: Carbon dioxide laser vaporization of Zoon's balanitis: a case report. J Dermatol Surg Oncol 15:491–494, 1989.
42. Apfelberg D, Maser M, Lash H, et al: Treatment of xanthelasma palpebrarum with the carbon dioxide laser. J Dermatol Surg Oncol 13:149–151, 1987.
43. Huerter C, Wheeland R: Multiple eruptive vellus hair cysts treated with carbon dioxide laser vaporization. J Dermatol Surg Oncol 13:260–263, 1986.
44. Huerter CJ, Wheeland RG, Bailin PL, et al: Treatment of digital myxoid cysts with carbon dioxide laser vaporization. J Dermatol Surg Oncol 13:723–727, 1987.
45. Bickley L, Goldberg D, Imaeda S, et al: Treatment of multiple apocrine hidrocystomas with the carbon dioxide laser. J Dermatol Surg Oncol 15:599–602, 1989.
46. Roenigk RK, Ratz JL: CO_2 laser treatment of cutaneous neurofibromas. J Dermatol Surg Oncol 13:187–190, 1987.
47. Becker D: Use of the carbon dioxide laser in treating multiple cutaneous neurofibromas. Ann Plast Surg 26:582–588, 1991.
48. Wheeland RG, McGillis ST: Cowden's disease—treatment of cutaneous lesions using carbon dioxide laser vaporization: a comparison of conventional and superpulsed techniques. J Dermatol Surg Oncol 15:1055–1059, 1989.
49. Wheeland RG, Bailin PL, Kronberg E: Carbon dioxide (CO_2) laser vaporization for the treatment of trichoepitheliomata. J Dermatol Surg Oncol 10:470–475, 1984.
50. Wheeland RG, Bailin PL, Reynolds OD, Ratz JL: Carbon dioxide (CO_2) laser vaporization of multiple facial syringomas. J Dermatol Surg Oncol 12:225–228, 1986.
51. Apfelberg DB, Maser MR, Lash H, et al: Superpulse CO_2 laser treatment of facial syringomata. Lasers Surg Med 7:533–537, 1987.
52. Fleming MG, Brody N: A new technique for laser treatment of cutaneous tumors. J Dermatol Surg Oncol 12:1170–1175, 1986.
53. Hunziker T, Bayard W: Carbon dioxide laser in the treatment of porokeratosis. J Am Acad Dermatol 16:625, 1987.
54. Wheeland RG, Bailin PL, Kantor GR, et al: Treatment of

adenoma sebaceum with carbon dioxide laser vaporization. J Dermatol Surg Oncol 11:861–864, 1985.

55. Janniger C, Goldberg D: Angiofibromas in tuberous sclerosis: comparison of treatment by carbon dioxide and argon laser. J Dermatol Surg Oncol 16:317–320, 1990.

56. Garrett A, Dufresne R, Ratz J, et al: Carbon dioxide laser treatment of pitted acne scarring. J Dermatol Surg Oncol 16:737–740, 1990.

57. Reid R, Muller S: Tattoo removal by CO_2 laser dermabrasion. Plast Reconstr Surg 65:717–728, 1980.

58. Levine H, Bailin P: Carbon dioxide laser treatment of cutaneous hemangiomas and tattoos. Arch Otolaryngol 108:236–238, 1982.

59. Apfelberg DB, Maser MR, Lash H, et al: Comparison of argon and carbon dioxide laser treatment of decorative tatoos: a preliminary report. Ann Plast Surg 14:6–15, 1985.

60. Ruiz-Esparza J, Goldman M, Fitzpatrick R: Tattoo removal with minimal scarring. The chemo-laser technique. J Dermatol Surg Oncol 14:1372–1376, 1988.

61. David LM: Laser vermilion ablation for actinic cheilitis. J Dermatol Surg Oncol 11:209–212, 1985.

62. Whitaker DC: Microscopically proven cure of actinic cheilitis by CO_2 laser. Lasers Surg Med 7:520–523, 1987.

63. Stanley RJ, Roenigk RK: Actinic cheilitis: treatment with the carbon dioxide laser. Mayo Clin Proc 63:230–235, 1988.

64. Greenbaum S, Glogau R, Stegman S, Tromovitch T: Carbon dioxide laser treatment of erythroplasia of Queyrat. J Dermatol Surg Oncol 15:747–754, 1989.

65. Wheeland RG, Bailin PL, Ratz JL, et al: Carbon dioxide laser vaporization and curettage in the treatment of large or multiple superficial basal cell carcinomas. J Dermatol Surg Oncol 13:119–225, 1987.

66. Mueller TJ, Carlson BA, Lindy MP: The use of the carbon dioxide surgical laser for the treatment of verrucae. J Am Podiatr Assoc 70:136–141, 1980.

67. McBurney EI, Rosen DA: Carbon dioxide laser treatment of verrucae vulgares. J Dermatol Surg Oncol 10:45–48, 1984.

68. Ferenczy A, Mitas M, Nigai N, et al: Latent papilloma virus and recurring genital warts. N Engl J Med 313:784–788, 1985.

69. Bailin PL, Kantor GR, Wheeland RG: Carbon dioxide laser vaporization of lymphangioma circumscriptum. J Am Acad Dermatol 14:257–262, 1986.

70. Eliezri Y, Sklar J: Lymphangioma circumscriptum: review and evaluation of carbon dioxide vaporization. J Dermatol Surg Oncol 14:357–364, 1988.

71. Fitzpatrick RE, Ruiz-Esparza J, Goldman MP: The depth of thermal necrosis using the CO_2 laser: a comparison of the super-pulsed mode and conventional mode. J Dermatol Surg Oncol 17:340–344, 1991.

72. Ratz JL, Bailin PL, Levine HL: CO_2 laser treatment of port-wine stains: a preliminary report. J Dermatol Surg Oncol 8:1039–1044, 1982.

73. Buecker JW, Ratz JL, Richfield DF: Histology of port wine stain treated with carbon dioxide laser: a preliminary report. J Am Acad Dermatol 10:1014–1019, 1984.

74. Ratz JL, Bailin PL: The case for use of the carbon dioxide laser in the treatment of port-wine stains. Arch Dermatol 123:74–75, 1987.

75. Tan OT, Carney JM, Margolis R, et al: Histologic responses of port-wine stains treated by argon, carbon dioxide, and tunable dye lasers: a preliminary report. Arch Dermatol 122:1016–1022, 1986.

76. van Gemert MJC, Welch AJ, Tan OT, Parrish JA: Limitations of carbon dioxide lasers for treatment of port-wine stains. Arch Dermatol 123:71–73, 1987.

77. Ben-Bassat M, Kaplan I, Levy R: Treatment of hereditary haemorrhagic telangiectasia of the nasal mucosa with the carbon dioxide laser. Br J Plast Surg 31:157–158, 1978.

78. Dover J, Smoller B, Stern R, et al: Low-fluence carbon dioxide laser irradiation of lentigines. Arch Dermatol 124:1219–1224, 1988.

79. Benedict LM, Cohen B: Treatment of Peutz-Jeghers lentigines with the carbon dioxide laser. J Dermatol Surg Oncol 17:954–955, 1991.

80. Geronemus RG: Laser surgery of the nail unit. J Dermatol Surg Oncol 18:735–743, 1992.

81. Leshin B, Whitaker DL: Carbon dioxide laser matriectomy. J Dermatol Surg Oncol 14:608–611, 1988.

82. Taylor MB: Chondrodermatitis nodularis chronica helicis: successful treatment with the carbon dioxide laser. J Dermatol Surg Oncol 17:862–864, 1991.

83. Ratz JL, Bailin PL, Wheeland RG: CO_2 laser treatment of epidermal nevi. J Dermatol Surg Oncol 12:567–570, 1986.

84. Hobbs ER, Bailin PL, Wheeland RG, et al: Superpulsed lasers: minimizing thermal damage with short duration, high irradiance pulses. J Dermatol Surg Oncol 13:955–964, 1987.

85. Landthaler M, Haina D, Brunner R, et al: Neodymium-YAG laser therapy for vascular lesions. J Am Acad Dermatol 14:107–117, 1986.

86. Dixon JA, Gilbertson JJ: Argon and neodymium YAG laser therapy of dark nodular port wine stains in older patients. Lasers Surg Med 6:5–11, 1986.

87. Apfelberg DB, Smith T, Lash H, et al: Preliminary report on use of the neodymium-YAG laser in plastic surgery. Lasers Surg Med 7:189–198, 1987.

88. Rosenfeld H, Wellisz T, Teinisch JF, et al: The treatment of cutaneous vascular lesions with the Nd:YAG laser. Ann Plast Surg 21:223–230, 1988.

89. Parkin JL, Dixon JA: Laser photocoagulation in hereditary hemorrhagic telangiectasia. Otolaryngol Head Neck Surg 89:204–208, 1981.

90. Hukki J, Krogerus L, Castren M, et al: Effects of different contact laser scalpels on skin and subcutaneous fat. Lasers Surg Med 8:276–282, 1988.

91. Goldman L, Stefanovsky D, Gregory RO, et al: Research and development of additional aids for dermatologic and plastic surgery. Lasers Surg Med 2:323–330, 1983.

92. Apfelberg DB, Bailin PL, Rosenberg H: Preliminary investigation of KTP/532 laser light in the treatment of hemangiomas and tattoos. Lasers Surg Med 6:38–42, 1986.

93. Castro DJ, Abergel RP, Meeker C, et al: Effects of the Nd:YAG laser on DNA synthesis and collagen production in human skin fibroblast cultures. Ann Plast Surg 11:214–222, 1983.

94. Castro DJ, Abergel RP, Johnston KJ, et al: Wound healing: biological effects of Nd:YAG laser on collagen metabolism in pig skin in comparison to thermal burn. Ann Plast Surg 11:131–140, 1983.

95. Abergel RP, Meeker CA, Lam TS, et al: Control of connective tissue metabolism by lasers: recent developments and future prospects. J Am Acad Dermatol 11:1142–1150, 1984.

96. Abergel RP, Meeker CA, Dwyer RM, et al: Nonthermal effects of Nd:YAG laser on biological functions of human skin fibroblasts in culture. Lasers Surg Med 3:279–284, 1984.

97. Abergel RP, Zaragoza EJ, Dwyer RM, et al: Differential effects of Nd:YAG laser on collagen and elastin production by chick embryo aortae in vitro. Biochem Biophys Res Comm 131:462–468, 1985.

98. Abergel RP, Dwyer RM, Meeker CA, et al: Laser treatment of keloids: a clinical trial and an in vitro study with Nd:YAG laser. Lasers Surg Med 4:291–295, 1984.

99. Sherman R, Rosenfeld H: Experience with the Nd:YAG laser in the treatment of keloid scars. Ann Plast Surg 21:231–235, 1988.

100. Garden JM, Robinson JK, Taute PM, et al: The low-output carbon dioxide laser for cutaneous wound closure of scalpel incisions: comparative tensile strength studies of the laser to the suture and staple for wound closure. Lasers Surg Med 6:67–71, 1986.

101. Abergel RP, Lyons R, Dwyer R, et al: Use of lasers for closure of cutaneous wounds: experience with Nd:YAG, argon and CO_2 lasers. J Dermatol Surg Oncol 12:1181–1185, 1986.

102. Abergel RP, Lyons RF, White RA, et al: Skin closure by Nd:YAG laser welding. J Am Acad Dermatol 14:810–814, 1986.

103. Wheeland RG, Bailin PL, Ratz JL, et al: Use of scleral eye shields for periorbital laser surgery. J Dermatol Surg Oncol 13:156–158, 1987.

104. Garden JM, O'Banion MK, Schelnitz LS, et al: Papillomavirus in the vapor of carbon dioxide laser-treated verrucae. JAMA 259:1199–1202, 1988.

105. Sawchuk WS, Weber PJ, Lowy DR, et al: Infectious papillomavirus in the vapor of warts treated with carbon dioxide laser

or electrocoagulation: detection and protection. J Am Acad Dermatol 21:41–49, 1989.

106. Mullarky MB, Norris CW, Goldberg ID: The efficacy of the CO_2 laser in the sterilization of skin seeded with bacteria: survival at the skin surface and in the plume emissions. Laryngoscope 95:186–187, 1985.

107. Walker NPJ, Matthews J, Newsom SWB: Possible hazards from irradiation with the carbon dioxide laser. Lasers Surg Med 6:84–86, 1986.

108. Starr JC, Kilmer SL, Wheeland RG: Analysis of the carbon dioxide laser plume for simian immunodeficiency virus. J Dermatol Surg Oncol 18:297–300, 1992.

109. Sawchuk WS, Felten RP: Infectious potential of aerosolized particles. Arch Dermatol 125:1689–1692, 1989.

110. Apfelberg DB, Mittelman H, Chadi B, et al: Investigation of carcinogenic effects of in vitro argon and CO_2 laser exposure of fibroblasts. Lasers Surg Med 4:173–179, 1984.

111. Parrish JA: Ultraviolet-laser ablation. Arch Dermatol 121:599–600, 1985.

112. Lane RJ, Linsker R, Wynne JJ, et al: Ultraviolet-laser ablation of skin. Arch Dermatol 121:609–617, 1985.

113. Lane RJ, Wynne JJ, Geronemus RG: Ultraviolet laser ablation of skin: healing studies and a thermal model. Lasers Surg Med 6:504–513, 1987.

114. Parrish JA, Anderson RR, Harrist T, et al: Selective thermal effects with pulsed irradiation from lasers: from organ to organelle. J Invest Derm 80(6 suppl):755–805, 1983.

115. Braverman IM, Schechner JS: Contour mapping of the cutaneous microvasculature by computerized laser doppler velocimetry. J Invest Dermatol 97:1013–1018, 1991.

116. Sundberg S: Acute effects and long-term variations in skin blood flow measured with laser doppler flowmetry. Scand J Clin Lab Invest 44:341–345, 1984.

117. Bisgaard H: Laser doppler flowmeter. Int J Dermatol 26:511–512, 1987.

118. Braverman IM, Keh A, Goldminz D: Correlation of laser doppler wave patterns with underlying microvascular anatomy. J Invest Dermatol 95:283–286, 1990.

119. Dougherty TJ, Kaufman JE, Goldfarb A, et al: Photoradiation therapy for the treatment of malignant tumors. Cancer Res 38:2628–2633, 1978.

120. McCaughan JS, Guy JT, Hawley P, et al: Hematoporphyrin-derivative and photoradiation therapy of malignant tumors. Lasers Surg Med 3:199–209, 1983.

121. Evensen J, Sommer S, Moan J, et al: Tumor localizing and photosensitizing properties of main components of hematoporphyrin derivative. Cancer Res 44:482–486, 1984.

122. Berns MW, McCullough JL: Porphyrin sensitized phototherapy. Arch Dermatol 122:871–874, 1986.

123. Carruth JAS: Photodynamic therapy: the state of the art. Lasers Surg Med 6:404–407, 1986.

124. Grossweiner LI: Optical dosimetry in photodynamic therapy. Lasers Surg Med 6:462–466, 1986.

125. Henderson BW, Dougherty TJ, Malone PB: Studies on the mechanism of tumor destruction by photoradiation therapy. Prog Clin Biol Res 170:601–612, 1984.

126. Gluckman JL, Waner M, Shumrick K, et al: Photodynamic therapy. Arch Otolaryngol Head Neck Surg 112:949–952, 1986.

127. Gregory RO, Goldman L: Applications of photodynamic therapy in plastic surgery. Lasers Surg Med 6:62–66, 1986.

128. Keller GS, Doiron DR, Fisher GU: Photodynamic therapy in otolaryngology—head and neck surgery. Arch Otolaryngol 111:758–761, 1985.

129. Bown SG, Tralau CJ, Coleridge Smith PD, et al: Photodynamic therapy with porphyrin and phthalocyanine sensitisation: quantitative studies in normal rat liver. Br J Cancer 54:43–52, 1986.

130. McCullough JL, Weinstein GD, Lemus L, et al: Development of a topical hematoporphyrin derivative formulation: characterization of photosensitization effects in vivo. J Invest Dermatol 81:528–532, 1983.

131. Goldman L, Taylor A, Putnam T: New developments with the heavy metal vapor lasers for the dermatologist. J Dermatol Surg Oncol 13:163–165, 1987.

132. White WE, Hunter JR, Van Woerkom L, et al: 120-fs terrawatt $Ti:Al_2O_3/Cr:LiSrAlF_6$ laser system. Opt Lett 17:219–221, 1992.

133. Goodberlet J, Wang J, Fujimoto JG: Femtosecond passively mode-locked $Ti:Al_2O_3$ laser with a nonlinear external cavity. Opt Lett 14:1125–1127, 1989.

134. Steinert RF, Puliafito CA, Trokel S: Plasma formation and shielding by three ophthalmic neodymium-YAG lasers. Am J Ophthalmol 96:427–434, 1983.

135. Yashima Y, McAuliffe DJ, Jacques SL, Flotte TJ: Laser-induced photoacoustic injury of skin: effect of inertial confinement. Lasers Surg Med 11:62–68, 1991.

136. Srinivasan R, Leigh WJ: Ablative photodecomposition: action of far-ultraviolet (193 nm) laser radiation on poly (ethylene terephthalate) films. J Am Chem Soc 104:6784–6785, 1982.

137. Fujimoto JG, Lin WZ, Puliafito CA, Steinert RF: Time-resolved studies of Nd:YAG laser-induced breakdown. Invest Ophthalmol Vis Sci 26:1771–1777, 1985.

138. Stern D, Schoenlein RW, Puliafito CA, et al: Corneal ablation by nanosecond, picosecond, and femtosecond lasers at 532 and 625 nm. Arch Ophthalmol 107:587–592, 1989.

139. Wyman A, Duffy S, Sweetland HM, et al: Preliminary evaluation of a new high power diode laser. Lasers Surg Med 12:506–509, 1992.

140. Brau CA: Free-electron lasers. Science 236:1115–1121, 1988.

CHAPTER 74

Podiatric Soft Tissue Surgical Procedures

JOHN C. STEPHENS and RODNEY L. TOMCZAK

The foot and lower extremity are common sites for a number of primary skin conditions that frequently require surgical intervention. Unfortunately, cutaneous surgery training in treatment of conditions at these anatomic locations is often neglected in favor of acquiring greater knowledge and experience in properly dealing with the more cosmetically important facial lesions. However, because a significant degree of dysfunction and even incapacitation can result from soft tissue disorders found on the feet and toes, the cutaneous surgeon should be knowledgeable in the proper management of such skin diseases.

Anesthesia for Surgery on the Toes and Foot

LOCAL ANESTHESIA FOR MATRICECTOMIES

Local anesthesia for performing matricectomies is generally obtained by infiltrating 1% or 2% plain lidocaine[1] just distal to the metatarsal head of the affected toe. In the presence of marked digital inflammation, the metabolism and pH of the soft tissues will often be sufficiently altered that the injection of more anesthetic agent than normal,[2] often 6 to 7 ml, may be required. However, care must always be taken not to inject such a large volume into the affected digit that vascular compromise results from compartment syndrome.

DIGITAL NERVE BLOCK

The technique used for performing digital nerve blocks on the toes is identical to that previously described for the fingers (see Chap. 9).[3]

ANKLE OR FOOT BLOCK

When treating large lesions such as plantar warts[4–7] that involve extensive areas on the sole,[8] local infiltration may be associated with significant discomfort. An alternative method to obtain effective anesthesia of the foot in these situations is an ankle or foot block.[9] In this technique, a total of five nerves must be blocked at the level of the ankle to provide total anesthesia of the foot. These five nerves are the superficial peroneal nerve, the saphenous nerve, the deep peroneal nerve, the posterior tibial nerve, and the sural nerve. The superficial peroneal nerve, a branch of the common peroneal nerve, supplies all five toes and the dorsal aspect of the foot. This nerve is blocked with superficial injection of a local anesthetic on the dorsal aspect of the foot, just lateral to the flexor hallucis longus (Fig. 74–1A). The saphenous nerve, a terminal branch of the femoral nerve, provides superficial sensation to the anteromedial foot, is the only one of the sensory nerves supplying the foot that is not a part of the sciatic system, and travels with the greater saphenous vein. It crosses the ankle lateral to the medial malleolus and medial to the anterior tibial tendon. It is blocked with a superficial injection of local anesthetic just lateral to the saphenous vein and just anterior to the medial malleolus (Fig. 74–1B). The deep peroneal nerve, a continuation of the common peroneal nerve, supplies the sensation for the medial half of the dorsal foot. It travels with the dorsalis pedis artery distal to the ankle and can often be palpated along with it. The deep peroneal nerve is blocked by injecting deep through the anesthetic area provided by the saphenous nerve block, lateral to the pulsation of the dorsalis pedis artery and the tendon of the extensor hallucis longus muscle (Fig. 74–1C). The injection is continued slowly until the periosteum has been reached. The posterior

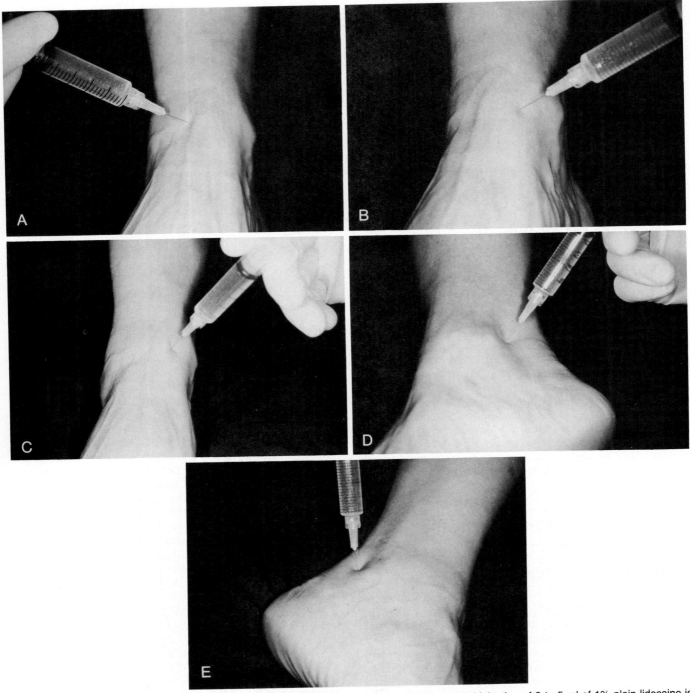

Figure 74–1. Technique for performing ankle blocks. *A,* Superficial peroneal nerve: A superficial injection of 3 to 5 ml of 1% plain lidocaine is performed just lateral to the flexor hallucis longus. *B,* Saphenous nerve: A superficial injection of 3 to 5 ml of 1% plain lidocaine is performed just anterior to the medial malleolus. *C,* Deep peroneal nerve: A deep injection of 4 to 8 ml of 1% plain lidocaine is made to the periosteum through the anesthetic area from the injection of the saphenous nerve, just lateral to the tendon of the extensor hallucis longus muscle and lateral to the anterior tibial artery. *D,* Posterior tibial nerve: A deep injection of 4 to 6 ml of 1% plain lidocaine is made down to the level of the periosteum just posterior to the medial malleolus and the posterior tibial artery. *E,* Sural nerve: A deep fanlike injection of 3 to 6 ml of 1% plain lidocaine is performed between the Achilles tendon and the lateral malleolus.

tibial nerve, providing sensation for the medial sole and heel as well as part of the lateral sole, is located posterior to the medial malleolus and travels with the posterior tibial artery and vein. The nerve can be found by palpating the posterior tibial artery, as it travels just posterior to it. To block this nerve, anesthetic agent is injected deeply in an inferior direction, just posterior to the posterior tibial artery (Fig. 74–1*D*). The sural nerve courses with the lesser saphenous vein just posterior to the lateral malleolus. Although it normally lies rather deeply, this nerve can frequently be isolated by palpating just posterior to the lateral malleolus. It is blocked by injecting deeply, in a fanlike pattern, between the lateral malleolus and the Achilles tendon (Fig. 74–1*E*).

When performing the ankle block, a 27- or 30-gauge needle is used to inject a solution of 1% plain lidocaine. In patients without evidence of vascular compromise, 1% lidocaine with epinephrine can be used to prolong the duration of anesthesia. Its rapid onset of action makes lidocaine the preferred agent for performing cutaneous surgery on the foot. However, for very painful procedures in which longer periods of anesthesia may be advantageous, compounds such as etidocaine mixed with epinephrine can provide total anesthesia for up to 24 hours.

Toenail Trauma

Trauma to the great toenail is one of the most common foot injuries and is usually the result of a blunt injury to the nail or nailbed. The injury may result in mild inflammation, moderate ecchymosis, or even an open compound fracture of the distal phalanx. In severe nail injury, radiologic studies of the affected digit should be obtained to exclude a possible phalangeal fracture (Fig. 74–2) that might delay healing if left undiagnosed.

Blunt soft tissue injuries to the nailbed commonly result either from the toe striking an object or from an object falling on the end of the toe. A relatively minor

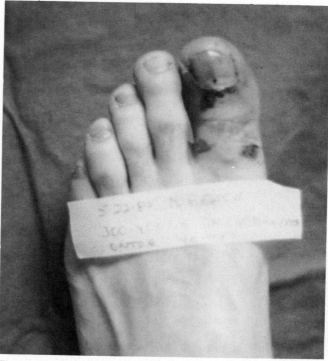

Figure 74–3. Subungual hematoma that developed after blunt trauma.

injury may result in mild inflammation and subungual hematoma (Fig. 74–3) without nail plate detachment, while more serious injuries can result in partial or complete nail plate detachment (Fig. 74–4). The initial treatment for minor injuries resulting in subungual hematoma formation typically consists of drilling a hole or perforating the nail with a hot lancet to release the pressure caused by the accumulation of blood and serous fluid beneath the plate. This is a virtually painless procedure that provides almost immediate relief.

Surgical management of extensive blunt injuries to the great toe that result in avulsion of 25% or more of the nail plate from the nailbed consists of completely removing the toenail using digital nerve block anesthe-

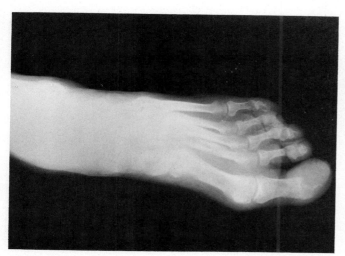

Figure 74–2. Radiograph of a fracture of the distal phalanx after blunt trauma to the great toe.

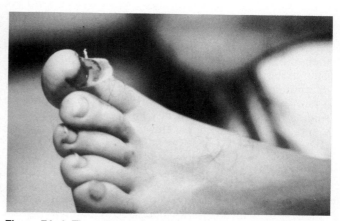

Figure 74–4. The nail plate has been completely avulsed after blunt trauma.

sia. If an organized hematoma has formed in the nailbed, it can easily be removed by performing gentle lavage with normal saline. In very extensive blunt injuries, it is common to find small fragments of the nail plate remaining in the eponychial area after surgical nail avulsion has been performed. It is important to carefully examine this area and remove these nail fragments, because if they are allowed to remain in place, they cause a foreign body reaction that delays wound healing.

The nailbed should also be examined for the presence of lacerations, deep gouges, or tissue defects. Larger fragments are simply placed back in their normal anatomic position and immobilized using a compressive bandage. The digit is kept immobile while the wound is allowed to heal by second intention. For large tissue defects, it may be exceedingly difficult at times to free sufficient amounts of soft tissue to allow primary wound closure, as the nailbed is very thin and is firmly attached to the dorsal aspect of the distal phalanx. However, mobilization, if required, should be undertaken by undermining down to the dorsal aspect of the proximal phalanx in the most atraumatic fashion possible to avoid scar formation and flap necrosis. If meticulous technique is not utilized, the resulting scar may prevent reattachment of the nail plate to the nailbed.

Healing of minor and moderate blunt injuries to the great toe usually requires 14 to 21 days. However, it may take 6 to 9 months for the nail plate to completely regrow and become reattached to the nailbed. Periodic examination should be performed during healing to check for ingrowth of the lateral nail margins. Two full nail growth cycles may be required to properly determine the extent of viable nail tissue. After trauma, the nail often becomes slightly dystrophic or markedly thicker than normal. If the injury is so severe that the damaged nail plate does not regrow properly or does not reattach to the nailbed, permanent matricectomy may be required to return the patient to maximal function as rapidly as possible.

Congenital Defects

A number of congenital soft tissue defects of the foot (e.g., accessory digits, skin tags, and accessory toes) are commonly found on the great toe. Patients with these congenital defects may present with an irritation of the second toe caused by the protrusion of soft tissue or a toenail from the medial aspect of the adjacent great toe. This irritation is typically associated with a history not of trauma, but of slowly progressive growth noted over a period of several months. On physical examination, a spicule of toenail can typically be seen protruding from a small, fibrotic lesion on the lateral aspect of the toe (Fig. 74–5).

SURGICAL TECHNIQUE

Surgical treatment consists of simple fusiform excision (Fig. 74–6), which is performed using digital nerve block anesthesia with 1% lidocaine. The procedure should be done as atraumatically as possible to minimize injury to

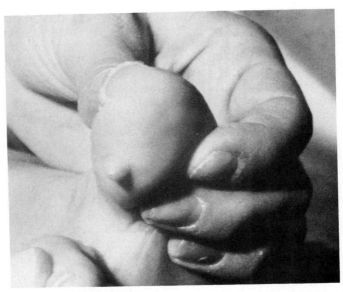

Figure 74–5. A small, fibrotic accessory toe is located on the lateral aspect of the great toe.

the surrounding tissues. After the excision has been completed, the deeper tissues should be carefully inspected for the presence of residual abnormal structures (Figs. 74–7, 74–8). The excised tissue should routinely be sent for histologic processing and evaluation. Hemostasis should be obtained by suture ligation of all blood vessels greater than 1 mm in diameter and by electrocoagulation of any smaller bleeding vessels. Any dead space created by the procedure should be precisely closed to avoid hematoma or seroma formation postoperatively. Dogears should be repaired using a V-Y incision. Standard primary closure using low reactive sutures such as nylon, polypropylene, or stainless steel wire can usually be accomplished without difficulty. The

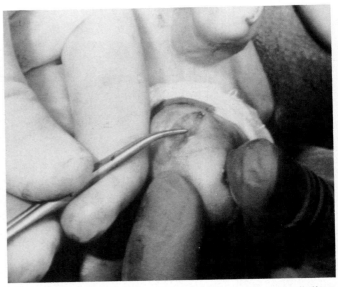

Figure 74–6. The accessory toe has been removed by simple fusiform excision.

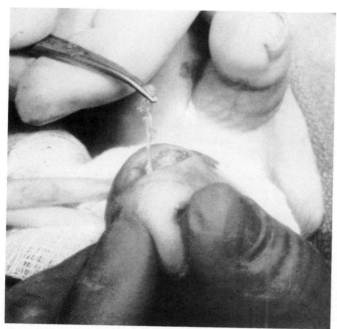

Figure 74–7. After performing excision, a small connecting strand extends into the deep soft tissues.

sutures should be placed so that they do not strangulate tissue and yet provide tensionless wound closure.

POSTOPERATIVE WOUND CARE

The rate of wound healing after any surgical procedure on the foot is determined by multiple factors. The time required for a patient to recover full ambulation after surgery is influenced by the torsional, rotational, longitudinal, and perpendicular forces that may disrupt the surgical wound margins. To facilitate wound healing, it is best to minimize these external forces by immobilizing the foot and limiting postoperative ambulation. Healing will occur most rapidly when the foot is kept in a fixed position. It is especially important to minimize weight bearing after treatment of plantar lesions to avoid keloid formation, wound dehiscence, and hypertrophic scar formation.

The first postoperative dressing change should be performed within 24 to 48 hours after the completion of surgery. This is especially important on the foot because of the potential contamination that can occur during bathing or from maceration caused by perspiration. The initial dressing change involves cleansing the treatment site lightly with 3% hydrogen peroxide, followed by application of a topical antibiotic ointment. Thereafter, the patient is instructed to change the dressing twice daily until the sutures are removed approximately 14 days later. After suture removal, the incision should be supported for an additional 7 to 14 days using externally applied adhesive sterile tape strips.

Subungual Exostosis

Another relatively common growth that may occur on or around the toenail is subungual exostosis. This

growth, which may occur spontaneously or follow a traumatic injury, is often misdiagnosed as an ingrown toenail that does not respond to conventional conservative medical treatment (Fig. 74–9). With continued growth, subungual exostoses may result in nail dystrophy and pain. Treatment, which consists of removing the bony growth, allows the nail to return to a normal configuration over time.

Gouty Tophi

Tophaceous gout deposits of the toes may mimic soft tissue masses and be confused with a host of other cutaneous conditions (Fig. 74–10). Accurate diagnosis is usually suggested by a history of arthritis and can be easily confirmed by obtaining a blood uric acid level or by performing needle aspiration of the deposit. On microscopic examination, typical birefringent crystals can be identified. After obtaining appropriate medical consultation, the painful tophus can be simply excised under local anesthesia without difficulty.

Cutaneous Malignancies

Cutaneous malignancies[10] on the lower extremity or foot or around or under the nail plate should be suspected when a minor injury fails to heal in a normal period of time, when an ulceration appears without predisposing cause, when a pigmented[11-13] or nonpig-

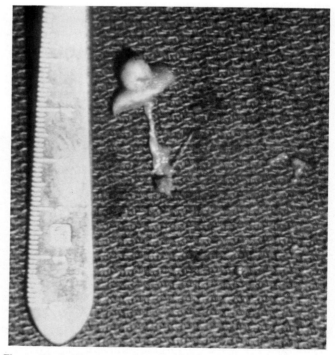

Figure 74–8. The gross specimen with the accessory toe and the deep connecting strand of ductal tissue.

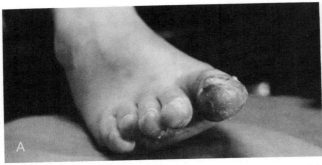
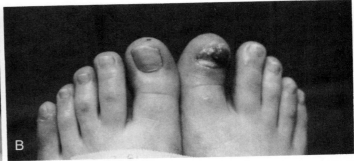

Figure 74–9. *A,* Chronic inflammation of the great toe caused by a subungual exostosis that was misdiagnosed as an ingrown nail. *B,* Comparison of the normal great toe *(left)* and the chronic inflammation produced by the subungual exostosis *(right).*

mented lesion causes pain or discoloration beneath the nail plate or adjacent to it (Fig. 74–11), or if changes occur in a pre-existing pigmented lesion. Differential diagnoses that must be considered include Bowen's disease, squamous cell[14, 15] and basal cell carcinomas, malignant melanoma, and metastatic cancers from distant sources. Performing a punch or excisional biopsy will typically provide sufficient tissue to establish a definitive pathologic diagnosis.[16, 17] Once the diagnosis of malignancy has been confirmed histologically, appropriate treatment may consist of simple surgical excision, Mohs micrographic surgery,[18] radiotherapy, or even amputation, depending on the nature of the cancer and its long-term prognosis.

Skin Lesions Associated With Structural Deformities

HELOMA

Hyperkeratotic lesions that arise in the skin on the toes have a variety of different names. When present over the proximal or distal interphalangeal joints or the distal tips of the toes, they are commonly referred to as heloma durum, or hard corns.[19] When found between the toes, they are commonly referred to as heloma

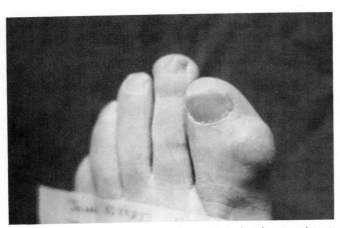

Figure 74–10. A painful, slow-growing gouty tophus is present as a soft tissue mass on the great toe.

molle, or soft corns. When associated with neural or vascular components, they are known as heloma neurofibrosim or heloma vascularis, respectively, and may be extremely painful. The amount of hyperkeratosis present may vary from only a mild, diffuse thickening to a very focal, keratotic lesion with a hard central nucleated core. The cause of these lesions is generally an underlying structural deformity related to a weakness in the intrinsic musculature of the foot and lower extremity. This weakness results in fatigue and musculoskeletal imbalance that leads to contracture of the metatarsophalangeal, proximal, and distal interphalangeal joints, which is associated with the formation of a hammer toe deformity and heloma. Conservative palliative treatment, consisting of local debridement of the hyperkeratotic tissue and application of a protective pad, will provide effective short-term pain relief. An underlying periostitis or bursitis, often seen in association with the hyperkeratosis, is diagnosed through clinical examination of the proximal or distal interphalangeal joints and the palpation of a small painful bursal sac. Effective treatment of the bursitis or periostitis is accomplished by intralesional injection of a local anesthetic agent in combination with corticosteroids. This mixture is infiltrated in a fanlike pattern into the lesion and periarticular areas. Surgical correction of the hammer toe may be required if conservative measures do not alleviate the pain. The treatment is virtually certain to fail if only the reactive hyperkeratosis is excised and the underlying bony deformity is not corrected.

TYLOMA

The terms used to describe a painful keratotic lesion found on the sole of the foot in association with an abnormality of the underlying metatarsal head include tyloma,[20] plantar callus, or intractable plantar keratosis (IPK). Tylomas are a common cause of pain and typically progress in both size and symptomatology over time; they commonly result from a combination of abnormal bone structure and intrinsic muscle weakness in the foot. This abnormality allows the metatarsal head to become plantarflexed below the level of the adjacent metatarsal heads, resulting in disproportionate weight bearing. Identification of the exact location of the lesion is extremely important in making an accurate clinical

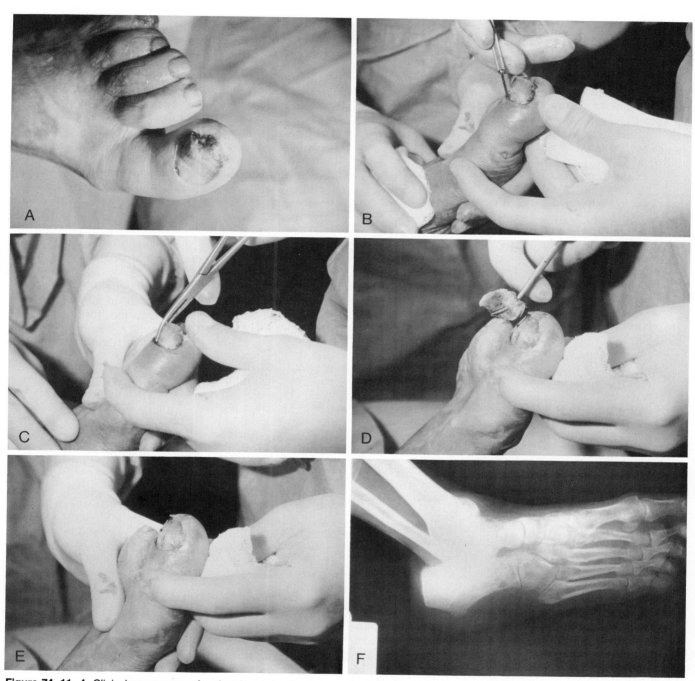

Figure 74–11. *A,* Clinical appearance of a chronic, nonhealing ingrown toenail that was subsequently diagnosed as a primary squamous cell carcinoma. *B,* The nail plate is freed from the proximal nail fold for nail avulsion. *C,* The nail plate is grasped with blunt hemostats. *D,* The nail plate is atraumatically avulsed. *E,* A friable tumor is identifiable after nail plate avulsion. *F,* Radiologic examination shows metastatic lesions to the heel with erosion of several digits.

diagnosis. Although the hyperkeratotic lesion may be proximal, distal, medial, or lateral to the metatarsal head, there must be some direct pressure or contact with it to establish the diagnosis. When the lesion does not contact the metatarsal head, the differential diagnostic possibilities include verruca, porokeratosis, granuloma, encapsulated cyst, foreign body reaction, keloid, and hypertrophic scar.

Depending on the amount of plantarflexion or declination of the metatarsal head, the reactive hyperkeratosis can be mild and diffuse in nature or may appear as a nucleated, deeply keratinizing lesion that causes significant pain on ambulation. When the lesion is located adjacent to a metatarsal head, there is often an associated underlying bursitis, capsulitis, tendinitis, or neuroma.

The initial treatment for managing tylomas includes topical use of keratolytic agents applied under occlusive dressings, conservative surgical debridement, and enucleation. Custom-designed orthotic devices also sometimes help control the associated discomfort and permit nearly normal physical activities. To prevent recurrence when excision of the lesion is considered as a primary form of treatment, the underlying bony abnormality must also be corrected by means of a plantar metatarsal head condylectomy or elevational metatarsal osteotomy. Simple surgical excision of the reactive hyperkeratosis is rarely effective and usually results in recurrence of the lesion. In addition, there is the added risk that this technique will produce a painful scar on the weight-bearing aspect of the foot that may be more uncomfortable than the original lesion.

GLOMUS TUMORS

Glomus tumors of the foot are benign lesions that arise from dermal arteriovenous shunts and may occur under the nail plate or on any skin surface of the foot.[21] These tumors are frequently painful because of their involvement with smooth muscles and free nerve endings. This neuromuscular structure is commonly accepted as being important for temperature regulation in the dermis. Additional studies are currently under way to determine whether there are any other functional activities associated with this structure.

Clinical Presentation

The usual clinical presentation of a glomus tumor is the acute onset of a red, blue, or violaceous lesion beneath the nail plate or on the sole of the foot. This is usually associated with pain that is disproportionate to the size of the lesion and may radiate to the leg, knee, hip, and even the arm on occasion. These friable tumors may be papular, nodular, or pedunculated but typically do not rapidly increase in size.

Treatment

Effective treatments for glomus tumors range from topical application of silver nitrate to stop the bleeding

to simple surgical excision. Laser photocoagulation surgery has also been recommended as a form of treatment for this tumor.[22]

Surgical Treatment of Ingrown Hallus Nails

GENERAL TYPES OF INGROWN NAILS

Three different types of ingrown nails have been described: the simple ingrown nail, the incurvated nail, and the hypertrophic ungualabia. The simple ingrown nail results from improper trimming of the nail plate that produces a small fragment of nail resembling a fish hook. This spicule of nail grows into the lateral nail fold, where it irritates the tissue and may result in foreign body reaction and secondary infection. Trauma to the distal hallux is also thought to result in the development of a subungual exostosis that increases the curvature of the nail, producing the second type of ingrown nails, the incurvated nail. The third type, hypertrophic ungualabia, is usually a result of chronic irritation and inflammation caused by either the incurvated nail or the ingrown nail itself. If the ingrown nail is removed, some cases of hypertrophic ungualabia will resolve spontaneously.

SURGICAL MATRICECTOMY

A number of different techniques (see Chap. 31) have been utilized for the management of chronic ingrowing nails,[23-28] including electrocautery[29-31] and laser ablation.[32] However, in a standard partial surgical matricectomy, only that portion of the matrix involved with the incurvated portion of the nail is dissected and removed along with a portion of the affected nailbed. The hypertrophic tissue that develops in response to the ingrown nail often resolves spontaneously when the offending nail spicule is removed, and thus it is not always necessary to include these tissues in the surgical excision. The offending portion of the nail is removed using an English anvil nail cutter. The nailbed is then incised to approximately 0.5 cm proximal to the eponychium, where a perpendicular incision is made to expose the matrix. The matrix is then dissected free, and the affected portion is removed. The wound is either closed primarily with sutures or reapproximated with adhesive sterile tape strips.

CHEMICAL MATRICECTOMY

Many cutaneous surgeons prefer chemical matricectomy using phenol.[33-38] In this technique, a tourniquet is wrapped around the base of the toe to provide hemostasis. The offending portion of the nail plate is first removed by performing partial nail avulsion. Then a cotton-tipped applicator, with most of the cotton removed, is dipped into a solution of 89% liquid phenol. The applicator is then inserted under the posterior nail fold in meticulous fashion to the appropriate part of the nail matrix. The applicator is rotated in place for approximately 15 seconds and then removed. This same procedure is repeated twice before the treated area is irrigated with a copious amount of 70% isopropyl alcohol. The alcohol does not neutralize the phenol solution, but rather dilutes it or removes it by irrigation. After alcohol irrigation has been completed, the tourniquet is released, and hemostasis is achieved. A small dressing is applied, and the patient is allowed to ambulate on a limited basis immediately.

The patient is instructed to soak the toe in a warm solution of salt water or magnesium sulfate (Epsom salt) for 15 minutes twice daily, followed by application of an antibacterial ointment and a small bandage. The patient should be seen 3 days after surgery to evaluate wound healing and ensure that secondary infection has not occurred. Because phenol acts as a disinfectant, the risk of infection is generally minimal. Some cutaneous surgeons also have the patient apply a fluorinated topical steroid to the treatment site to reduce the inflammation caused by the phenol.

An alternate technique that replaces phenol with a 10% solution of sodium hydroxide has also been described.[39] In this procedure, sodium hydroxide is applied in the same manner used to apply phenol, but once the nailbed capillaries have been coagulated, the solution is neutralized by applying a solution of 5% acetic acid. Because the sodium hydroxide can be immediately neutralized, there is often much less local tissue reaction than with phenol. However, no controlled studies have been performed comparing the relative inflammatory responses with each of these two techniques.

Miscellaneous Conditions

DIABETIC ULCERS

A special area of concern for cutaneous surgeons is the treatment of patients with diabetic ulcers on the sole of the foot. Because diabetics frequently suffer from sensory nerve loss, they may be unaware of the rate of evolution of a foot ulcer. In addition, because of the extensive small blood vessel disease seen in diabetics, obtaining an adequate tissue level of antibiotics to eliminate infectious processes is often very difficult. Finally, the nearly constant trauma and shearing forces that occur during normal ambulation make the treatment of plantar ulcers even more difficult in diabetics.

The natural progression of lower extremity ulcerations[40] follows a rather predictable clinical course (Table 74–1). The basic cornerstone of treatment is proper assessment of ischemia, which is measured by Doppler ultrasound. This index is presented as the ratio of the systolic brachial pressure to the systolic pressures at various levels in the leg and foot. A high degree of success can generally be anticipated in healing ulcers if this index is 0.45 or greater at the level of the ulceration. However, if the ischemic index is below 0.45, further vascular evaluation is generally necessary.

The management of patients with ulcers having an ischemic index of 0.45 or greater generally consists of surgical debridement, resection of any underlying bony prominences, application of skin grafts, and use of

TABLE 74–1. CLASSIFICATION OF DIABETIC ULCERS

Grade 0: Skin intact
Grade 1: Localized superficial ulcer
Grade 2: Deep ulcer to tendon, bone, ligament, or joint
Grade 3: Deep abscesses or osteomyelitis
Grade 4: Gangrene of toes or forefoot
Grade 5: Gangrene of whole foot

immobilizing walking casts. Debridement can be most effectively accomplished with a carbon dioxide laser. The laser is used to precisely excise the necrotic tissue under local anesthesia. Once a clean, well-vascularized base has been reached, the laser is used in a defocused mode to coagulate any small persistent bleeding points. The fresh clean base will accept a skin graft as long as an immobilizing, weight-bearing cast is applied.

OVERLAPPING FIFTH TOE

A relatively common congenital deformity of the foot is a varus deformity of the fifth toe that causes it to overlap the fourth toe. This deformity can be corrected by placing the toe in an abducted and plantarflexed position while a V-shaped incision is made. The extensor tendon is tenotomized, and the joint capsule is released. As the toe is further plantarflexed, the skin will slide, allowing a V-Y closure to be performed.[41] Occasionally, it is necessary to remove two semielliptical wedge-shaped pieces of tissue on the plantar aspect of the toe and tenotomize the flexor tendon if the correction is not satisfactory.

MORTON'S NEUROMA

A Morton's neuroma is a degenerative intraneural fibrosis that most commonly involves the third interdigital nerve, which is a branch of the medial plantar nerve.[42, 43] This condition occurs more often in individuals whose second digit is longer than the hallux. Although this neuroma is most common in the third interspace, it can occur in the second interspace as well. Conservative treatment has not been able to provide a satisfactory level of success, and as a result, surgical removal of the neuroma through a dorsal incision is the most common treatment. However, the dorsal incision requires transection of the intermetatarsal ligament and may possibly result in damage to the lumbricales and interossei muscles, which can result in formation of an iatrogenic hammer toe deformity. For this reason, these neuromas are also sometimes removed through a plantar incision, which respects the anatomy of the plantar aspect of the foot and avoids making transverse incisions on major weight-bearing portions of the sole. Incisions that parallel Langer's lines do not generally exhibit much tension and heal without excessive scarring.[44]

The main advantages to the plantar approach are minimal tissue disruption, excellent exposure, decreased pain and edema, decreased risk of adhesions, preservation of the deep transverse metatarsal ligament, and a reduced chance of hammer toe formation. The plantar incision is placed between the metatarsal heads and courses from just proximal to the toes to just proximal to the metatarsal heads. The adipose tissue is bluntly dissected so that the nerve can be identified and transected proximal to the metatarsal heads. The wound is closed in normal fashion, and the patient is allowed to ambulate with special shoes that help to distribute the weight more evenly over the heel and hindfoot without placing any weight on the surgical incision.

SUMMARY

A number of different cutaneous lesions and conditions not found in other anatomic sites commonly occur on the feet and toes. However, many of the surgical procedures performed elsewhere on the body can be easily modified for the effective management of many individuals with disorders that involve the soles, toes, or nail units. Mastery of some basic concepts and principles is required for the cutaneous surgeon to perform proper soft tissue surgery on the lower extremity and foot.

REFERENCES

1. Grekin RC, Auletta MJ: Local anesthesia in dermatologic surgery. J Am Acad Dermatol 19:599–614, 1988.
2. Cohen EN, Levine DA, Colliss JE, Gunther RE: The role of pH in the development of tachyphylaxis to local anaesthetic agents. Anesthesiology 29:994–1001, 1968.
3. Albom MJ: Digital block anesthesia. J Dermatol Surg 2:366–367, 1976.
4. Mueller MJ, Carlson BA, Lindy MP: The use of the carbon dioxide surgical laser for the treatment of verrucae. J Am Podiatr Assoc 70:136–141, 1980.
5. Borovoy M, Klein JT, Fuller TA: Carbon dioxide laser methodology for ablation of plantar verrucae. J Foot Surg 24:431–437, 1985.
6. Cacciaglia GB, Regellhaupt RW: Effectiveness of lasers on plantar papillomas: a preliminary study. J Foot Surg 24:71–75, 1985.
7. Lavery LA, Cutler JM, Galinski AW, Gastwirth BW: The efficacy of laser surgery for verruca plantaris: report of a study. Clin Podiatr Med Surg 5:377–383, 1988.
8. Lewis G, Gatti A, Barry LD, et al: The plantar approach to heel surgery: a retrospective study. J Foot Surg 30:542–546, 1991.
9. Schurman DJ: Ankle block anesthesia for foot surgery. Anesthesiology 44:342–348, 1976.
10. Salasche SJ, Garland LD: Tumors of the nail. Dermatol Clin 3:501–519, 1985.
11. Kopf A, Waldo E: Melanonychia striata. Aust J Dermatol 21:59–70, 1980.
12. Baran R, Haneke E: Diagnosis and therapy of streaked nail pigmentation. Hautarzt 35:359–365, 1984.
13. Tom DWK, Scher RK: Melanonychia striata in longitudinem. Am J Dermatopathol 7:161–163, 1985.
14. Mauro JA, Maslyn R, Stein AA: Squamous cell carcinoma of the nail bed in hereditary ectodermal dysplasia. NY St J Med 72:1065–1066, 1972.
15. Attiyeh FF, Shah J, Booher RJ, et al: Subungual squamous cell carcinoma. JAMA 241:262–263, 1979.
16. Scher RK: Punch biopsies of nails: a simple, valuable procedure. J Dermatol Surg Oncol 4:528–530, 1978.
17. Kechijian P: Nail biopsy vignettes. Cutis 40:331–335, 1987.
18. Zitelli JA: Mohs micrographic surgery for skin cancer. Prin Pract Oncol 8:1–10, 1992.
19. Laine W: Benign neoplasia of the foot. In: McCarthy DJ, Montgomery R (eds): Podiatric Dermatology. Williams & Wilkins, Baltimore, 1986, pp 53–73.
20. Jimenez A, McGlamry E, Green D: Lesser ray deformities. In: McGlamry E, Dalton E (eds): Comprehensive Textbook of Foot Surgery. Williams & Wilkins, Baltimore, 1987, pp 57–113.
21. Shelley ED, Shelley WB: Exploratory nail plate removal as a diagnostic aid in painful subungual tumors: glomus tumor, neurofibroma, and squamous cell carcinoma. Cutis 39:310–312, 1986.
22. Barnes L, Estes S: Laser treatment of hereditary multiple glomus tumors. J Dermatol Surg Oncol 12:912–915, 1986.
23. Winograd AM: A modification in the technic of operation for ingrown toenail. JAMA 92:229, 1929.
24. Boll OF: Surgical correction of ingrowing nails. J Am Podiatr Assoc 35:8–9, 1945.
25. Subotnick SI: How I manage ingrown toenails. Physician Sportsmed 11:65–68, 1983.
26. Murray WR, Bedi BS: The surgical management of ingrowing toenails. Br J Surg 62:409–412, 1975.
27. McGlamry ED: Management of painful toes from distorted toenails. J Dermatol Surg Oncol 5:554–556, 1979.
28. Haneke E: Surgical treatment of ingrowing toenails. Cutis 39:251–256, 1986.
29. Andrew T, Wallace WA: Nail bed ablation: excise or cauterize? A controlled study. Br Med J 1:1539, 1979.
30. Polokoff M: Ingrown toenail and hypertrophied nail lip surgery by electrolysis. J Am Podiatr Assoc 51:805–806, 1961.
31. Abbott WW, Geho EH: Partial matricectomy via galvanic current. J Am Podiatr Assoc 70:239–243, 1980.
32. Leshin B, Whitaker DC: Carbon dioxide laser matricectomy. J Dermatol Surg Oncol 14:608–611, 1988.
33. Nyman SP: The phenol-alcohol technique for toenail excision. J NJ Chiropract Soc 5:4–6, 1956.
34. Suppan RJ, Ritchlin JD: A non-debilitating surgical procedure for ingrown toenail. J Am Podiatr Assoc 52:900–902, 1962.
35. Greene AA: A modification of the phenol-alcohol technique for toenail correction. Curr Podiatr 13:20–23, 1964.
36. Wee GC, Tucker GL: Phenolic cauterization of the matrix in the surgical care of ingrown toenails. Mo Med 66:802–803, 1969.
37. Yale JF: Phenol-alcohol technique for correction of infected ingrown toenail. J Am Podiatr Assoc 64:46–53, 1974.
38. Brown FC: Chemocautery for ingrown toenails. J Dermatol Surg Oncol 7:331–333, 1981.
39. Travers GR, Ammon RG: The sodium hydroxide chemical matricectomy procedure. J Am Podiatr Assoc 70:476–478, 1980.
40. Mooney V, Wagner FW: Neurocirculatory disorders of the foot. Clin Orthop 122:53–59, 1977.
41. Wilson JN: V-Y correction for varus deformity of the fifth toe. Br J Surg 41:133–135, 1953.
42. Morton TG: A peculiar and painful affection of the fourth metatarsophalangeal articulation. Am J Med Sci 71:35–36, 1876.
43. Gaynor R, Hake D, Spinner SM, Tomczak RL: A comparative analysis of conservative versus surgical treatment of Morton's neuroma. J Am Podiatr Assoc 79:27–30, 1989.
44. Lewis G, Gatti A, Barry LD, et al: The plantar approach to heel surgery: a retrospective study. J Foot Surg 30:542–546, 1991.

CHAPTER 75

The Art of Cutaneous Scalpel Surgery

LAWRENCE M. FIELD

It has often been said that "there are many roads to Rome." However, the roads are often uneven, and progress is sometimes made with uncertain difficulty. In cutaneous surgery, that progress is often measured by both the patient's functional performance and the final cosmetic appearance. For cutaneous surgeons to continue to improve their technique, it is important to learn not only from one's own errors, but also from others. Awareness of the tremendous knowledge that has been gained by other cutaneous surgeons through many years of experience can be effectively and advantageously used to help avoid some of the common errors or difficulties encountered when performing surgery on the skin. It is important to stress that the "art" of cutaneous surgery is an intrinsic component of performing aesthetically pleasing cutaneous scalpel surgery.

Preplanning and Marking

The most magnificent surgical technique is doomed to fail unless considerable thought is given to the preliminary design of the procedure being performed.[1] Only in this way will the most appropriate procedure be chosen to meet the needs of the individual patient. Thus, a great deal of thought should be given to the procedure before initiating even the simplest of skin incisions.[1] Recognition and consideration of a variety of important factors that can influence the surgical decisions are absolutely mandatory before an incision is ever made. In this regard, one of the simplest but most important aspects of skin surgery that is frequently overlooked is preliminary marking of the incision. Of course, this also requires that the anticipated closure be simultaneously planned.[2] The planned incision should be marked on the patient with a surgical marking solution or pen, taking special care to also mark the adjacent wrinkle lines, folds, scars, regional junction lines, current or anticipated future gravitational lines, and any asymmetries that could influence the final closure. If possible, preoperative surgical marking should be performed with the patient positioned so that maximal gravitational pull can be fully appreciated.

The overriding principle guiding this preliminary marking and planning approach is to place the resultant final scar in as unobtrusive a location as possible and then to undermine an adequate amount of tissue to accomplish closure without tension. Only the tissue that is to be moved is undermined to help preserve and maintain the vascular supply in its normal and intact position; this, in turn, aids flap movement. Regardless of whether buried, horizontal[3] or vertical "dermal tuck,"[4] half-buried or full horizontal mattress, or vertical mattress sutures are used, the flap can be precisely attached to the underlying tissue bed to limit the amount of movement. Conversely, by invoking movement of the deeper superficial musculoaponeurotic system (SMAS), easier surface approximation can be obtained. In either situation, the principal tissue movement and attachment of the flap can be accomplished. When adequate tissue is available and tension on the anastomotic line is avoided by appropriate closure techniques, fine surgical scars in the preplanned configuration result. This preliminary planning and marking approach, with preplanned tissue movement and fixation, allows an aesthetically superior result when compared with the random final scar line position that results from relative forces of tension exerted on the scar after total peripheral undermining.

After the tissue to be removed has been delineated,

blunt undermining is performed beneath the entire amount of tissue to be excised. The undermining is also continued at the same level into the adjacent perilesional skin.[5] When undermining is performed in this manner, the tissue used to close the excision is the same thickness as the tissue that was removed. To further facilitate this, especially in elliptical or fusiform excisions, a small attached segment is allowed to remain at each tip (Fig. 75-1) to anchor the excisional specimen until all the undermining can be done beneath it and at the periphery.[6] When the flap is undermined to close a particular defect, the blunt dissection should extend to the delineated excisional site. The final dissection to free the flap is performed using scissors.

Injection of Local Anesthetic Agents

Administration of any anesthetic solution should be delayed until appropriate landmarks have been identified and considered in the planning process. Once the anesthetic solution has been instilled and the epinephrine effect achieved, potentially critical observations regarding wound closure can no longer be accurately made. This concept is especially important when performing Mohs micrographic surgery, since wound closure cannot, in most cases, be adequately preplanned. The end result is that many of the anatomic features important to evaluate to obtain the best aesthetic and functional reconstruction possible are obscured. A tu-

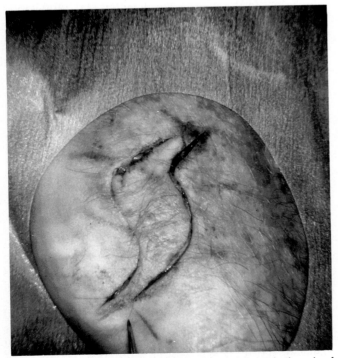

Figure 75–1. A small isthmus of intact skin remains at both ends of this "S"-shaped ellipse to stabilize the wound during undermining and permit precise incision of the wound tips.

mescent technique for obtaining anesthesia, described primarily for liposuction procedures,[7, 8] can also be beneficially used in excisional and flap surgery, where the "ballooning" effect serves to protect the underlying blood vessels and nerves from injury.

Hemostatic Techniques

Because postoperative bleeding is the major cause of a variety of postoperative complications, it is extremely important to pay strict attention to hemostasis. The least traumatic method of accomplishing hemostasis is by applying external pressure against some subjacent firm tissue. Manual pressure with moistened gauze produces excellent results, although it should be remembered that a warm compress evokes more vascular dilatation and bleeding than does a cold compress. Cotton-tipped applicator sticks may be used both to remove blood and to apply gentle external pressure for hemostasis. If cotton-tipped applicators are used, it should be recognized that they may be a source of contamination of the wound and may result in foreign body granuloma formation.

SUTURES

A great variety of suture ligatures and ties have been described over the years. Clear nylon is sometimes preferred for buried sutures or for tying off larger blood vessels.[9] Silk sutures have been promoted for epidermal wound closures, if they are removed within 7 days, because of their handling qualities, knot security, and aesthetic accuracy. Nevertheless, all surgeons eventually develop their own favorite suture material and techniques for ligating large and deep vessels.

ELECTROSURGERY

Cautery insults to tissues are frequently misapplied, with resultant desiccation of large areas by the direct introduction of cautery tips into bleeding wounds. It must be stressed that only the most distal aspect of a severed vessel needs coagulation, and bipolar cautery forceps are the most meticulous method presently available to control small vessel bleeding. Larger vessels may require the use of jeweler's forceps or even a small mosquito clamp applied to the vessel tip. A monopolar current may then be applied to the shaft of the occluding forceps close to the occlusion point, with passage of the current interrupted at the instant visible coagulation begins. Although the cautery tip may be applied directly to vessels, more peripheral tissue destruction occurs with this technique than is necessary. Direct cautery application is even more hazardous in thin-skinned areas, where perforation and necrosis may occur, or in proximity to critical nerves and vessels.

Wound Closure Techniques

Just as all surgeons develop their own individual suturing techniques, so, too, does a particular type of

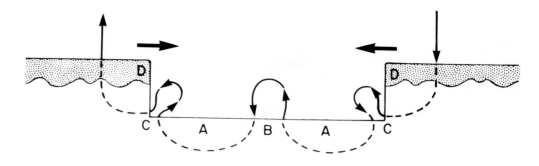

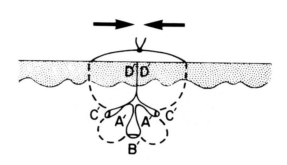

Figure 75–2. A double-lobed "basting" stitch employs two equidistant tacking maneuvers to invert soft tissue to fill deep defects and simultaneously close the skin surface. (Note: The corresponding points A, C, and D are closely approximated with this suturing technique.)

suturing material become a personal favorite. However, no one suture material or suturing technique can be used to solve all problems for all surgeons in all tissues (Fig. 75–2). Each surgeon must seek his or her own level of security and comfort, which includes an acceptance or rejection of the principles of multilayered closures, tensionless closures, and closures under tension. Each approach has its place, but many surgeons prefer to either make additional incisions or lengthen the excision as necessary to provide adequate tissue movement for tensionless wound closure. This is known as the "draping effect."[10] While each approach has its proponents, many surgeons feel that, unless the wound or tissue defect is very deep and will require movement of the SMAS for wound closure, use of buried sutures is rarely indicated. This is particularly true when performing reconstructive surgery on thin skin (e.g., the face).

The combination of alternating horizontal dermal tuck sutures,[3, 4] which attach the moving flap edge to the dermis on the nonundermined, fixed side,[4] and several vertical mattress sutures is the mainstay of wound closure. After the dermis has been incorporated[4] and the anastomotic line everted, a continuous 5-0 or 6-0 nylon suture running at 2-mm intervals in the high dermis gives excellent results (Fig. 75–3). Some surgeons prefer continuous fast-absorbing 6-0 chromic suture.[11] Continuous sutures require constant variation of the depth of needle passage so that the surface approximation is precise. As the continuous suture traverses the surface, occasional deep bites are taken to fix the tissues to the defect bed. Dermal approximation is critical, for precise epidermal approximation is its natural consequence. Contrary to frequent practice, "subcuticular" sutures should never be placed in a superficial dermis.[12] To do

so invites suture extrusion, infection, or lumpy or irregular healing and thus dissatisfied patients. Subcuticular sutures are most valuable in closing skin on parts of the body with thick dermal layers (Fig. 75–4) or when the skin is firmly attached to strong subdermal fascia that will hold sutures well. Whenever the dermis is thin,

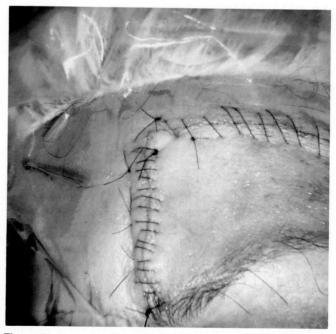

Figure 75–3. A variety of suture materials and suturing techniques, including half-buried mattresses, horizontal "dermal tuck" sutures, and continuous running sutures, can be used for wound closures in complicated repairs.

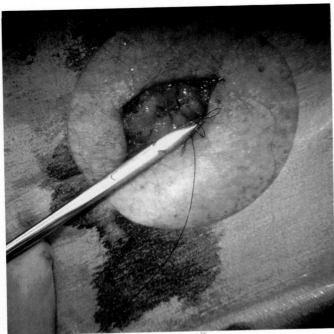

Figure 75–4. Deep "tacking" sutures may be employed to eliminate "dead space" or establish the final point of flap movement before fixation.

superficial subcuticular sutures should be avoided.[12] Whenever possible, the knot should be placed on or moved to the nonundermined side, as pressure necrosis is less likely to occur where the blood supply has not been interrupted or disturbed.

In cervical facial rhytidectomy, both plication and imbrication techniques may be employed to reposition the SMAS for lessened tension on the final anastomotic line. Scalp reductions also may benefit from the use of galeal sutures,[13] although even when these are used in combination with stainless steel staples, the depressed trough defect that so frequently follows is not always prevented.

Equipment and Instrumentation

To obtain the best results, all surgeons must use the very finest instrumentation possible, and no expense should be spared in achieving that goal. Lower quality equipment will eventually result in a lower level of surgical execution. However, it must be remembered that no instrument can replace the experience and good judgment of a skilled surgeon, the visual impact of the intended surgical site and its environment, the tactile ability of the surgeon's fingers in assessing the skin and its potential for movement, and an understanding of wound healing abilities. Gentle handling of tissue during wound closure or to assess the movement of a local flap is always an appropriate concern in performing cutaneous surgery.

Platform forceps are an infrequently used but excellent tool to help grasp the suture needle as it exits the skin after having traversed the wound. When held across the palm in the nondominant hand, the flat platform grasps the needle at a right angle to its curvature and a supination-pronation movement of the wrist then delivers the needle. This instrument helps to preserve both the sharpness and normal shape of the needle, whereas grasping the needle with a pair of needle holders or regular forceps can blunt the tip or bend it. Furthermore, use of the platform forceps also reduces the potential risk of inadvertent needle sticks or glove perforations, which is extremely important to surgeons.

Proper Scalpel Technique

The most common errors made by many beginning cutaneous surgeons relate to improperly holding the scalpel handle, maintaining its position, and providing stable peripheral support while the incisions are made. These principles hold true whether using a rectangular handle (e.g., Bard-Parker); the smaller, rounded Beaver handle; or the larger, similarly rounded (Fig. 75–5) Field handle (Padgett Instruments, Kansas City, MO).[14] Scalpel handles must be firmly grasped and held in position without any wavering, change in angulation, or variation in depth of penetration unless specifically desired otherwise. A rounded pencil-like handle works better for some surgeons, undoubtedly as a consequence of the decades of using pens and pencils on a daily basis. Most cutaneous surgeons use a No. 10 or 15 blade for larger procedures and a No. 67 blade or razor blade fragment on a smaller handle for finer work.

Unlike an abdominal surgeon, who grasps the scalpel handle so as to use the horizontal rounded surface of larger blades, cutaneous surgeons initially pierce the epidermis to the level of the dermis or fat by using the pointed tip of the chosen blade. After entrance at a 75- to 90-degree angle, the angle of the handle is then

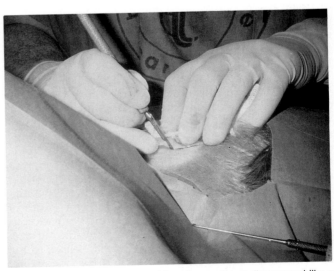

Figure 75–5. A rounded scalpel handle can be easily grasped like a pen or pencil while the nondominant hand provides pressure and stabilizes the skin in the immediate area.

changed so that the distal end is lowered, enabling the most inferior, curved aspect to be incised at a 30- to 45-degree handle angle. The surgeon must learn to *feel* the exact level of blade penetration and maintain the proper angulation and depth throughout the procedure, unless there is a specific indication for depth variation. This control is best accomplished by precise placement of the middle, fourth, and fifth fingers on the patient directly beneath the handle. As the incision continues, this fulcrum of support must be repositioned smoothly. If this is not accomplished, an irregular incision line will result. Timid superficial strokes, clinically manifested as unaesthetic multiple slashes, are frequently made by neophyte cutaneous surgeons.

Simultaneously, the most rigorous attention must be paid to stabilization of the incisional platform. While the scalpel-holding hand presses downward, the surgeon's other hand is employed to press and position the skin immediately adjacent to the blade. The thumb and index finger separate the incision line by exerting force in both directions away from the incision line. Visual and tactile control are both employed, maintaining precise separation at varying levels of dermis, subdermis, upper fat, and fascia.[1] As the finger fulcrum is changed beneath the scalpel handle, the peripheral support and stabilization by the opposite hand must follow. On a moist or bleeding surface, increased traction may be obtained by placing gauze beneath the gloved hand. For free-edged surfaces such as the lip or earlobe, better fixation can be obtained by firmly grasping the tissue with gauze that has been rolled between the surgeon's thumb and index finger, while the area from the cutting edge of the scalpel blade to the opposite surface is constantly palpated. Integration of these interdependent movements will help guarantee the finest results from incisional movements.

Scissors, Incisions, and Dissection

Additional skills are frequently acquired with a variety of scissors that are available. Very thin skin (e.g., the eyelid) is preferentially incised with scissors after an undermining plane has been established. Scissors that are blunt on the end and on both external blade margins, such as Stevens tenotomy scissors, may be utilized for safer establishment of a skin-muscle flap in the eyelid and frequently for flaps involving the lip vermillion. Thicker areas of skin may require an initial shallow incision into the epidermis followed by appropriate undermining. The final step in the development of the flap margin is to join the bluntly undermined plane with the surface scalpel incision by using scissors.[15] Because scissors exert focal pressure on tissue as the incision is made, very small vessels may stop bleeding. This is in contrast to an incision made with a scalpel, which may allow bleeding to continue.

It is important to remember that each type of tissue has its own specific requirements and levels for undermining, and the most appropriate technique will vary

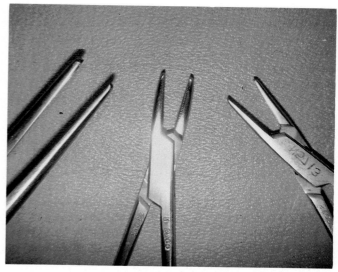

Figure 75–6. The blunt tips of some common instruments (*left*, Iconoclast; *center*, small needle holders; *right*, large needle holders) used for performing fast, effective, and safe undermining.

according to the tissue type and location. Because random-pattern flaps rely on the diffuse dermal and subdermal plexuses for their blood supply, care must be taken when these types of flaps are undermined. Rather than randomly selecting the level at which to begin undermining, use of the blunt ends of the needle holder (Fig. 75–6)[15] or, in special circumstances, the Iconoclast,[16] a superb instrument for undermining,[10] is often appropriate for finding the most natural and relatively avascular plane of separation. The use of a needle holder (Fig. 75–7) is excellent for accomplishing undermining, as a blunt instrument serves to identify the most avascular level of cleavage for the dissection.[5] An appropriate protective pad of subcutaneous fat is left on the undersurface of the flap; this helps prevent necrosis. Also, the bluntness of the needle holder offers reliably safe dissection.[5] Furthermore, both straight and curved

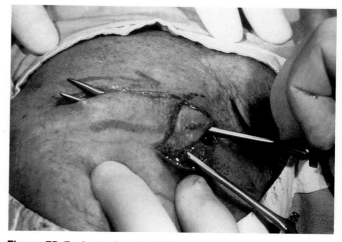

Figure 75–7. A small pair of blunt needle holders are used to simultaneously undermine both the tissue to be excised and the flap that has been designed to close the defect.

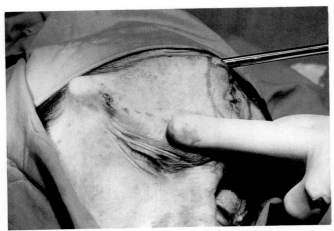

Figure 75–8. The blunt, spatula-type liposuction cannula can be used as a superb dissecting and undermining instrument.

liposuction cannulas with flattened, blunt, or rounded tips (Fig. 75–8) have been increasingly used for undermining after the proper entrance plane has been found with the tips of the needle holder.[17] These flat cannulas are ideal instruments with which to accomplish a remarkable degree of undermining and flap mobilization while leaving neurovascular septa between the subjacent bed and the suprajacent flap intact.

On many occasions, the beginning cutaneous surgeon will attempt to dissect a flap free from its underlying attachments by using curved iris scissors. If the concave surface positions the tips of the scissors upward, the cutting action of the instrument will be directed into the dermal plexus of blood vessels. For this reason, the convex surface of the curved scissors should be positioned parallel to the surface beneath the flap so as to minimize the risk of vascular injury.[5] If the anatomic contours at the site of the procedure are variable, the surgeon must pay constant attention to redirect the cutting action of the scissors throughout the undermining or dissection procedure.

Finally, it should be remembered that the finger has excellent undermining and dissecting ability and carries with it the tactile sensibility necessary to detect tissues such as larger blood vessels and nerves that should be avoided.

Skin-Handling and Stabilization Techniques

It is extremely important that tissue be handled gently. Every additional injury to a cell increases the risk to that cell and may compromise the final aesthetic results. Flaps or grafts may fail partially or even completely because the underlying tissues have been unnecessarily traumatized by pressure, electrosurgery, or improper handling. Excess tension on wound closures results in tissue necrosis and often produces a widened scar. Nothing can replace the surgeon's hands and fingers as the primary tools of surgery. Thin, fine-quality surgical

gloves increase the ability to perceive a variety of tactile stimuli while preserving a sterile surgical environment.

It is extremely important for the cutaneous surgeon to learn early how to work with skin hooks. This involves learning to place the fingers or forceps on either side of the hook, rather than directly over it. Most cutaneous surgeons try to avoid the use of forceps whenever possible. When traction on tissue is necessary, it is generally best to grasp the subepidermal tissue with a weighted skin hook or forceps in such a way that permanent surface marks are not left by the teeth. In some cases, a single tooth of a two- or three-toothed forceps can be used to hook a flap from below and atraumatically lift it upward. Some surgeons prefer to use double hooks, blunted hooks, or hooks with a springlike action, but a small, single-toothed hook remains the most common choice for most. Use of the weighted skin hook (Fig. 75–9) allows an undermined flap to be pulled open, toward the surgeon, by placing it on the inside margin of the wound. This assists the surgeon in visually inspecting a wound and simultaneously provides a degree of hemostasis. The weighted skin hook may also be used at the inferior margin of a fusiform excision to put some tension at the apex of a wound, permitting more precise wound edge approximation and placement of sutures. Finally, the weighted skin hook can be used like an extra pair of hands to help drape loose tissue into a defect as a flap is being created.[18]

SUMMARY

The high-technology world of modern medicine has often shown a tendency to solve problems through the use of a series of dogmatic and often idealized equations

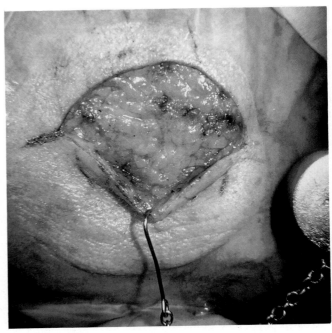

Figure 75–9. The weighted skin hook improves visibility while stabilizing the wound margin with simple traction.

that frequently fail to take into account the individual variations that are inherent to each patient. This stylized, formulaic approach to surgical care can also be found in cutaneous surgery, where premeasured,[19] rigidly constructed flaps[20] and preplanned geometric surgical excisions[21] are often employed haphazardly, without any thought for the likely final functional or cosmetic result. Fortunately, even though the "artful" aspects of cutaneous surgery are frequently overlooked in the education of physicians, these skills can be learned and put to appropriate use. It is possible to improve these skills by carefully reviewing and learning from each procedure performed, by talking with more experienced surgeons about problems encountered, and by extensively reviewing old techniques and reading about new techniques as they become available. Only with this type of dedicated effort will the "art" of cutaneous surgery become a standard part of the surgical armamentarium, allowing true progress to be made.

REFERENCES

1. Field LM: The power of surgical thinking. J Dermatol Surg Oncol 12:1021–1022, 1986.
2. Field LM: Make your incision where you want your final scar line to be: a surgical philosophy. J Dermatol Surg Oncol 16:1062–1063, 1990.
3. Field LM: The "dermal tuck." J Dermatol Surg Oncol 11:671–673, 1985.
4. Field LM: The "dermal tuck" revisited. J Dermatol Surg Oncol 12:392, 1986.
5. Field LM: Finding, developing, and maintaining a proper undermining plane. In: Robins P (ed): Surgical Gems in Dermatology. Journal Publishing Group, New York, 1988, pp 103–109.
6. Field LM: A helpful support system for precise tip dissections. J Dermatol Surg Oncol 8:1010–1011, 1982.
7. Klein JA: Tumescent technique for regional anesthesia permits lidocaine doses of 35 mg/kg for liposuction: peak plasma lidocaine levels are diminished and delayed 12 hours. J Dermatol Surg Oncol 16:248–263, 1990.
8. Lillis PJ: The tumescent technique for liposuction surgery. Dermatol Clin 8:439–450, 1990.
9. Edgerton M: Modern methods of arresting bleeding. In: Edgerton M: The Art of Surgical Technique. Williams & Wilkins, Baltimore, 1988, pp 76–100.
10. Field LM: The "draping effect" movement for aesthetic flap reconstruction. Presented at the American Academy of Dermatology meeting, December, 1979.
11. Grekin R: Verbal communication. San Francisco, August, 1990.
12. Edgerton M: Subcuticular sutures. In: Edgerton M: The Art of Surgical Technique. Williams & Wilkins, Baltimore, 1988, pp 122, 124.
13. Alt T: Verbal communication. Minneapolis, February, 1990.
14. Field LM: A new, rounded scalpel handle. J Dermatol Surg Oncol 8:918, 1982.
15. Costenares S: Modifications of the face lift procedure. In: Masters F, Lewis J (eds): Symposium on Aesthetic Surgery of the Face, Eyelid and Breast. Educational Foundation of the American Society of Plastic and Elective Surgery. CV Mosby, St Louis, 1972, pp 48–49.
16. Luikart R: The "Iconoclast," a superb instrument for undermining. J Dermatol Surg Oncol 6:274–277, 1980.
17. Field LM, Skouge J, Anhalt TS, et al: Blunt liposuction cannulae dissection with and without suction-assisted lipectomy in reconstructive surgery. J Dermatol Surg Oncol 14:1116–1122, 1988.
18. Field L: A weighted retraction hook. J Dermatol Surg Oncol 8:531, 1982.
19. Field L: A criticism of premeasured excision and surgical mathematics. Ann Plast Surg 7:257, 1981.
20. Field L: A further criticism of geometric surgery. Ann Plast Surg 10:340, 1983.
21. Field L: Inappropriate geometric surgical applications. Plast Reconstr Surg 76:157, 1985.

PART FIVE

Future Advances in Cutaneous Surgery

CHAPTER 76

Autologous Skin Grafting

R. RIVKAH ISSEROFF and ANNE E. MISSAVAGE

The ready availability of unlimited amounts of a permanent synthetic skin to facilitate wound repair has always been a surgeon's dream. In recent years that dream has nearly become reality. The currently accepted "gold standard" for material to resurface wounds is the split-thickness skin graft (STSG).[1] However, for patients with little normal skin available to harvest for STSG (e.g., those with extensive burns), obtaining enough tissue becomes problematic. When more than 60 to 70% of the total body surface area (TBSA) is lost, even repeated harvesting of available donor sites for STSG will not provide resurfacing rapidly enough to prevent significant mortality.[1] Although materials such as pig skin and cryopreserved human cadaveric skin have been used for early wound coverage in these situations, these materials must be primarily considered biologic dressings, as they are invariably rejected. The patient must then undergo subsequent regrafting with autologous material. Additionally, human allografts carry the unfortunate associated risk of disease transmission, most significantly hepatitis and human immunodeficiency virus (HIV).[2, 3] Attempts to create a totally synthetic, "nonliving" skin graft devoid of cellular elements led to the recognition that all such grafts must ultimately be resurfaced with the patient's own epidermal cells. Until relatively recently, these cells were ordinarily derived from the patient's normal skin and applied in either a thin or meshed STSG, leaving unanswered the clinical problem of the patient with few available donor sites.

History

In the early 1970s, as techniques for the in vitro cultivation of human keratinocytes were being described,[4–7] the possibility of using cultured keratinocytes to form the epidermal component of a skin graft was considered.[4, 8, 9] These early keratinocyte culture systems were hampered, however, by their inability to produce long-term proliferation of the cultured cells, which prevented large-scale propagation. In the late 1970s, with innovative culture techniques, epithelial keratinocytes were finally able to be cultured in large numbers. A 1975 landmark paper[10] described a method for human keratinocyte cultivation that circumvented the difficulties in the continued multiplication of these cells. Some of the innovations in this technique included the plating of keratinocytes on a feeder layer of irradiated 3T3 murine fibroblasts and the use of a medium supplemented with growth promoters such as epidermal growth factor, hydrocortisone, and cholera toxin. Subsequently, other techniques for large-scale cultivation of keratinocytes have evolved, including propagation in an acidic medium[11] and the development of a "serum-free" culture system.[12]

The increase in the accessibility of large quantities of cultured epithelial cells has consequently spawned multiple methods for creating an epithelium-containing synthetic skin substitute. Investigators have endeavored to create in the laboratory a physiologically functional skin, ideally possessing properties such as easy drapablity and conformability to the wound bed, resiliency to stress, elasticity, the ability for self-renewal, and the water-permeable characteristics of the normal epidermis. Clearly, the availability of cultured, viable epithelial cells is a key element for achieving at least the last two of these properties.

Types of Cultured Skin Grafts

AUTOLOGOUS EPITHELIAL GRAFTS

In 1975, Rheinwald and Green proposed that large expanses of skin could be resurfaced with cultured keratinocytes.[10] Small (2 cm²) biopsies of normal skin were harvested from patients soon after admission, and over the course of 3 to 4 weeks, the epidermal cells from the biopsy specimens were cultivated in the laboratory and expanded 10,000-fold. Shortly thereafter, the use of cultured epithelial autografts (CEAs) in two patients with 40% and 80% TBSA burns was reported.[13] Others[14] subsequently reported successful, lifesaving engraftment with CEAs of two pediatric patients who had suffered extensive burns (more than 90% TBSA).

Numerous additional reports[15-19] have confirmed the utility of this procedure. In fact, this CEA technique has been the most extensively used grafting procedure, with at least 200 documented cases.[20] However, the procedure is not without significant shortcomings. The absence of any dermal elements in the initial cultured graft makes the final resulting skin appear somewhat atrophic and will accentuate contour defects. The best "takes" are often achieved when the graft is applied to freshly excised muscle fascia or fresh granulation tissue.[17] More seriously, unlike the STSG, in which the bond between graft and patient occurs at the level of the dermis, in CEAs, the bond forms at the level of the epidermal-dermal interface. Although all the parameters

necessary for the formation of this bond are not yet clear, studies have demonstrated delayed reformation of at least one parameter: the anchoring fibrils.[21, 22] These fibrils are not seen before 12 to 14 weeks after engraftment (Table 76–1), which may account in part for CEAs' increased susceptibility to shearing and their propensity to form spontaneous blisters at the level of the dermal-epidermal junction.[23] Nevertheless, this laboratory technique, with its ability to manufacture the extensive amounts of epidermis ultimately necessary for wound coverage, has proved to be a major contribution to the surgical sciences.

A variation of the pure CEA system has also been described.[24] While the original methods used bovine serum and murine fibroblast feeder cells, the newer system uses no feeder cells and is based on a "serum-free" keratinocyte medium.[12] Harvested keratinocytes are first cultivated in a low-calcium medium (MCDB 153, 0.3 mM Ca^{2+}, containing epidermal growth factor, insulin, ethanolamine, phosphoethanolamine, hydrocortisone, bovine pituitary extract, and other supplements),[24] in which they grow as a nonstratifying monolayer composed of proliferative basaloid cells. To induce

TABLE 76–1. CHARACTERISTICS OF ENGRAFTED CULTURED EPITHELIAL AUTOGRAFTS (CEAS)*

	In Vitro CEA	Engrafted CEA (E-CEA)	Meshed STSG Interstices
Epidermis	1–12 cell layers thick; disorganized	9–15 cell layers Normal strata	9–15 cell layers Normal strata
Keratohyalin	Absent	At 1 week: normal granular layer with keratohyalin granules	At 1 week: no granules granular layer
Lamellar bodies	Absent	At 1 week: present	Not reported
Stratum corneum	Absent	At 1 week: present; normal basketweave pattern	At 1 week: present; parakeratotic
Melanocytes	Present at a relative density as initial cell suspension	Repigmentation variable (26 days to 7 mo)	Repigmentation variable: weeks to 2–3 yr
Langerhans cells	Rare in primary culture, none in secondary culture	At 1 wk to 1 yr: normal numbers At >1 yr: 2–3 times increased over normal	At <1 yr: same as CEA At >1 yr: 3–5 times increased over normal
Merkel cells†	Absent	At 21 days: present in CEA originating from sole skin only At 21 days–5 yr: density decreased over normal	Absent
Cytokeratins	Keratin 19 (characteristic of hyperproliferative epidermis)	Keratins 1, 10 (characteristic of normal differentiated epidermis)	Not reported
Rete ridges	Absent	At 1 week: absent At 21 wk–1 yr: present	Up to 5 yr: absent
Appendages	Absent	Absent	Absent
Hemidesmosomes	Immature	At 1 wk: forming At 2 wk: present but smaller than normal	At 1 wk: forming At 2 wk: present but smaller than normal
Basal lamina	Absent	At 2 wk: 50% complete At 3–4 wk: complete	At 2 wk: 50% complete At 3–4 wk: complete
Anchoring fibrils	Absent	At 3 wk: sparser and thinner than normal At 1–2 yr: resemble normal	At 3 wk: sparser and thinner than normal At 1–2 yr: resemble normal
Wound bed		At 2 wk: granulation tissue At 3 mo: collagen oriented parallel to epidermis At 6–18 mo: pattern of collagen At 2–3 yr: bilayered dermis with subepithelial fine collagen fibers and thicker woven fibers below development of a superficial plexus At 3 yr: elastic fibers develop At 4–5 yr: fine elastic fibers in papillary dermis	Up to 5 yr: collagen remains dense, uniformly distributed, typical of scar; no elastin seen

*From ref. 22.
†From ref. 70.

stratification and differentiation of the cultures, bovine serum–containing medium is added in the final phase of cultivation. The keratinocyte sheets are then enzymatically removed from the culture dish and transferred to the patient.

The major innovation with this newer method lies in the first culture phase, in which serum-free medium that promotes a highly proliferative cell type is utilized. However, because the time from harvesting the initial biopsy until final engraftment to the patient is similar in both techniques (3 to 4 weeks), it is unclear what advantage this new technique offers. The addition of bovine serum to the culture medium in this and the previously described technique also raises the question of possible allergic reactions to foreign proteins in recipient patients. Although no clinical reactions have yet been reported, an increase in titres of anti–bovine serum protein antibodies in recipient patients has been discovered.[25] Rabbits immunized with bovine serum albumin who develop anti–bovine albumin antibodies have demonstrated alterations in the synthesis of components of their dermal matrix.[26] The relationship of this finding to the human clinical situation, however, is not clear. Long-term follow-up of patients who develop the anti–bovine albumin antibodies is clearly required to determine their ultimate clinical significance.

ALLOGENEIC EPITHELIAL GRAFTS

One of the drawbacks of the CEA technique is the 3- to 4-week delay from the time of biopsy until the graft is ready for placement on the patient. Indeed, as the age of the patient increases, so does the time necessary for cultivation and expansion of the donor site keratinocytes,[17] making autologous epithelial grafting a lengthy procedure for elderly patients. This, coupled with the ready availability of neonatal foreskins from which epithelial cultures can be initiated, cryopreserved, and banked, has resulted in study of the use of unrelated allogenic epithelial grafts. Early studies reported enhanced healing of wounds grafted with the epithelial allografts,[27–30] and investigators postulated that the allogeneic keratinocytes persisted in the healed wound because the major histocompatibility complex (MHC) class II HLA-DR–bearing Langerhans cells were lost during the cultivation process.[31] Subsequent studies, however, using Y-chromosome analysis in sex-mismatched grafts[32, 33] and DNA fingerprinting[17] have provided strong evidence that allografted keratinocytes do not survive and are ultimately replaced with those of the recipient.[34]

However, despite that fact, more rapid healing has been demonstrated in second-degree burns[17, 27, 30, 35] and chronic ulcers[29, 36, 37] treated with allogeneic epithelial grafts, without signs of clinical rejection. In a review of 99 skin ulcers grafted with allogeneic keratinocytes,[37] a mean healing time of 4.5 weeks was noted along with a remarkable diminution in pain within 24 hours of application of the graft. These authors and others[38] have postulated that the allografted keratinocytes stimulate wound healing by promoting reepithelialization from the dermal appendageal remnants. One study[39] has demonstrated that factors secreted by cultured keratinocytes into the culture medium can enhance wound healing by stimulating keratinocyte proliferation in the wound bed dermal appendages. This study also reported that the cultured epidermal cell–derived factors strongly diminish the capability of fibroblasts to contract a collagen sponge in vitro, implying an additional role for the cultured epithelial grafts in the reduction of wound contraction. Potential paracrine factors known to be secreted by cultured keratinocytes may include, but are certainly not limited to, interleukins,[40, 41] transforming growth factor α,[42] and fibronectin.[43, 44] Although it remains to be determined which, if any, of these factors are important in the enhancement of wound healing noted with cultured allografted keratinocytes, this procedure appears to hold promise in the management of wound healing.

A caveat for the use of allogeneic autografts is the possibility of disease transmission. Rigorous screening[36, 37] has included testing of the mothers of foreskin donors both at the time of birth and 6 months later for HIV antibodies by enzyme-linked immunosorbent assay (ELISA), as well as testing the cultured cells for cytomegalovirus (CMV), herpes simplex virus type I, hepatitis B surface antigen, and bacterial contaminants. With the advent of polymerase chain reaction (PCR) technology and the development of probes for many of these transmissible diseases, this may become the most sensitive method with which to screen potential allogeneic cultured grafts. One report indicates that HIV could be detected using PCR in the skin of at least 45% of patients with known HIV positivity.[45]

HUMAN ALLODERMIS-CEA COMPOSITE GRAFTS

Early literature suggested that engrafted cryopreserved dermis is not rejected by the recipient,[46–48] and as a result, allogeneic dermis has been used as a substrate for cultured autologous epithelial cells.[49, 50] Allogeneic, cryopreserved skin was engrafted after excision of burn eschar. The grafts remained viable, and before signs of epidermal rejection appeared at day 27 to 32, the alloepidermis was removed by dermabrasion and replaced with CEA sheets. The dermal allograft appeared to remain, although it was extensively remodeled by ingrowth of host fibrovascular elements. Electron micrographic analysis revealed the synthesis of a basement membrane and anchoring fibrils 4 months after placement of the epithelial grafts. As in the epidermal allografts, DNA analysis of the dermal cells 5 weeks after engraftment revealed that the allogeneic cells were ultimately replaced by those of the recipient.[51] A similar composite grafting technique has been used successfully.[52]

This graft system confers the advantage of inclusion of a dermal bed, which may diminish contracture formation and enhance graft take. Disadvantages include the requirement of two separate patient procedures and possible disease transmission through the dermal autograft. The ultimate utility of the allodermis-CEA procedure will become increasingly evident as more patients receive these grafts and can be extensively evaluated.

SYNTHETIC DERMIS–AUTOLOGOUS CULTURED KERATINOCYTES COMPOSITE GRAFTS

To circumvent the problems surrounding cadaveric dermal allografts, a number of systems for the creation of a totally synthetic skin have been proposed. In one system,[53, 54] autologous cultured keratinocytes, instead of being cultivated as isolated epidermal sheets, are seeded as a single-cell suspension on a dermal substitute; this system is already in wide clinical use.[55] Although the original method[53, 54] utilized a model of an acellular, synthetic, porous membrane of cross-linked collagen and glycosaminoglycans as the dermal equivalent,[56] the procedure was subsequently modified to incorporate autologous cultured fibroblasts into the artificial dermis.[57] Hansbrough and coworkers reported a total of seven burn patients successfully engrafted with this material[57, 58] and noted remodeling of the synthetic dermis by ingrowth of native fibrovascular tissue.

Other composite graft systems employ a dermal component consisting of a contracted collagen gel of either bovine[59] or rat[60, 61] origin, seeded with either autologous[60] or allogeneic[61] cultured fibroblasts. The prototype for this approach is known as the "living skin equivalent."[62, 63] The fate of the allogeneic dermal fibroblasts incorporated into the grafts is unclear, but some work[51] suggests that the fibroblasts probably do not survive. Although these composite graft systems show great promise, the limited numbers of patients who have received these grafts so far (see Table 76–1) makes judgment of the ultimate potential of the method premature.

Thus far, the described composite grafts all use non-human collagen in the dermal component, which carries the risk of patient reaction to the foreign proteins. Presumably, antibodies directed against the foreign collagen may develop in these patients, as they do in patients who receive intradermal injections of bovine-derived collagen (Zyderm) for cosmetic correction of scars and rhytides.[64, 65] The prognostic or clinical significance of these antibodies has not yet been fully ascertained.

Laboratory Technique of CEA

Successful development of any of these cultured grafts requires a fully equipped tissue culture facility and well-trained laboratory personnel. For the cultivation of epithelial autografts, the method developed by Rheinwald and Green[10] has received the widest use thus far and is the one used, with some modifications, in our facility (Fig. 76–1). A small sample (2 to 4 cm^2) of the patient's skin, harvested as either full-thickness excisional biopsy specimen or as a split-thickness keratome sample, is transported to the laboratory in sterile Dulbecco's modification of Eagle's medium (DMEM) containing antibiotics and amphotericin B (Fungizone). All dermis, if present, is trimmed from the biopsy specimen, and the trimmed skin is floated overnight at 4°C on a calcium-free buffer containing 0.25% trypsin. The following day the epidermis easily separates from the dermis and is minced and further disaggregated to a single-cell suspension by agitation in a calcium-free buffer. Released keratinocytes are collected by centrifugation and plated in DMEM supplemented with 10% fetal bovine serum, cholera toxin 10^{-10}, and hydrocortisone (0.4 µg/ml) in a culture dish containing 3T3 murine fibroblasts (American Type Culture Collection, Rockville, MD) that were previously treated with mitomycin C[66] to prevent their multiplication. Keratinocytes attach and begin to replicate, forming small colonies on the plate that push the 3T3 feeder cells into a rim at their periphery. After the third day of culture, epidermal growth factor (10 ng/ml) is added to the culture; earlier addition reduces the frequency of colony formation.[66] When the culture dish reaches 50% confluence, the remaining 3T3 cells are removed from the culture dish by spraying the surface of the dish with a buffered 2-mM ethylenediaminetetra-acetic acid (EDTA) solution that selectively releases fibroblasts but not the more adherent keratinocytes.[10] Before the cultures are totally confluent, usually 10 days after initial plating, the plates are treated with trypsin to release the keratinocytes, which are either cryopreserved for future use or put into secondary culture, again using mitomycin-treated 3T3 cells as a feeder layer. When these plates are 50% confluent, the process is repeated and tertiary cultures initiated. Alternatively, the secondary cultures can be maintained until they reach confluence, at which time they can be used for grafting.

Secondary or tertiary cultures, which will be ultimately used as grafts, are most conveniently plated into rectangular flasks because of the ease with which rectangular grafts can be placed on the wound bed. Once these cultures reach a confluent, multilayered stage, usually 20 to 25 days after initial biopsy, they are washed in a buffered saline solution to remove most of the bovine serum present in the culture medium and treated with the neutral protease Dispase (Boehringer Mannheim Biochemicals, Indianapolis, IN) at 2.5 mg/ml to release the cultured cells from the flask as a single sheet (Fig. 76–2). To facilitate removal of the sheet of cultured cells from the flask, the top of the flask is removed either by cutting with a hot soldering iron or by using convenient special "tear top" flasks (Accell Flasks, Costar, Van Nuys, CA) (Fig. 76–3). Because the released keratinocyte sheet is only two to eight cells thick[14] and thus quite fragile, it is clipped to a sheet of petrolatum (Vaseline) gauze (Chesebrough-Ponds, Inc, Greenwich, CT) using hemoclips (Weck Surgical, Research Triangle Park, NC) to facilitate manipulation. The epidermal sheet is then inverted, basal cell side up, in a culture dish with fresh serum-free medium (Fig. 76–4). To maintain appropriate pH of the culture medium, the epidermal sheets are transported to the operating room in small portable incubators (Billup-Rothenberg, Del Mar, CA) equilibrated with 5% CO_2 (Fig. 76–5).

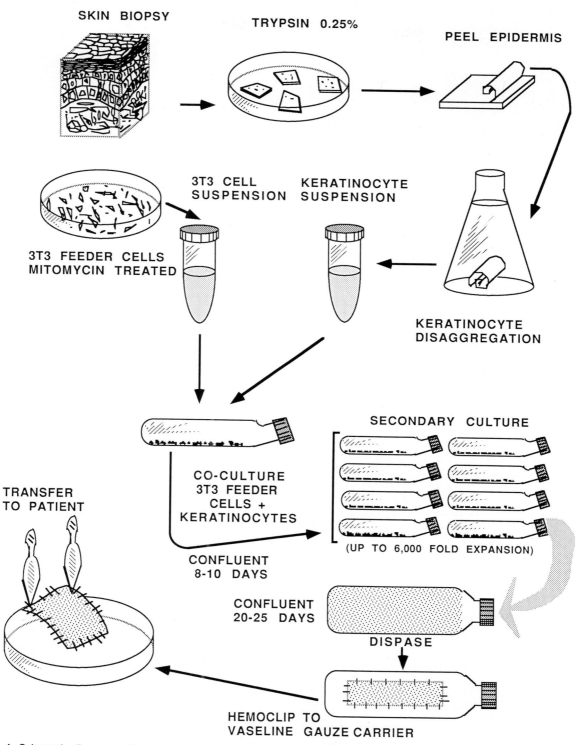

Figure 76–1. Schematic diagram of the steps from the isolation of human keratinocytes from a skin biopsy through the harvesting of intact epithelial sheets for grafting.

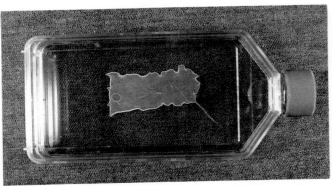

Figure 76–2. Cultured epidermal sheet after enzymatic detachment from the culture flask. The resultant membrane is thin, virtually transparent, and fragile.

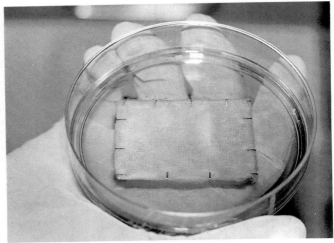

Figure 76–4. Cultured epidermal sheet hemoclipped to a Vaseline gauze carrier (basal cells facing upward, carrier gauze below).

Physiology of Cultured Grafts

Extensive studies have followed the evolution of engrafted cultured epithelium[22] by analyzing more than 400 skin biopsies in 19 graft recipients for a period of 5 years. This work (Table 76–2) compares cultured epithelial autografts with split-thickness grafts in the rate of acquisition of characteristics of epidermal differentiation, formation of the dermal-epidermal junction, cellular population of the grafts, and the formation of connective tissue beneath the graft.

Other investigators[22, 24, 28] have found that the epidermis develops normal strata and organization rapidly, typically by 1 week after grafting, but that rete ridges remain absent even 6 months[18] to 1 year[22] after engraftment. The majority of the components of the dermal-epidermal junction were present by 3 weeks, with type IV collagen, laminin, and bullous pemphigoid antigen immunolocalized in a linear pattern to the area as early as 5 days after graft placement.[28] Although hemidesmosomes and anchoring fibrils are present as early as 2 weeks,[22] more than 1 year may be necessary for these structures to resemble a normal epidermis. One study[21] suggests that until at least 5 months after engraftment, the anchoring fibrils are structurally abnormal, which

may account for the greater susceptibility to shear stress and spontaneous blister formation observed in some patients. It is interesting to note, however, that an almost identical temporal evolution of the dermal-epidermal junction has been noted in the interstices of STSGs[22] and that spontaneous blister formation has also been noted to occur in these graft sites as well.[67, 68]

Nonkeratinoycte epithelial cells found in the normal epidermis eventually repopulate the cultured autograft. Melanocytes are transferred in the culturing methodology and are present in the initial autograft, although in diminished numbers, and repigmentation eventually proceeds in a variable course.[22] Langerhans cells, which are lost during the process of keratinocyte cultivation, repopulate the engrafted epidermis, presumably from bone marrow–derived precursors, and occur in increased numbers relative to normal epidermis.[22, 28, 69] Merkel cells appear to repopulate those cultured epithelial grafts originally derived from sole skin, a location ordinarily rich in these cells.[70]

Perhaps the most interesting finding[22, 69] is that a connective tissue structure, very like normal dermis,

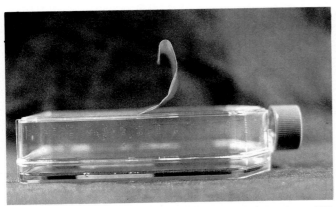

Figure 76–3. "Tear top" flasks (Accell, Costar, Van Nuys, CA) facilitate the removal of the epidermal sheet from the culture vessel.

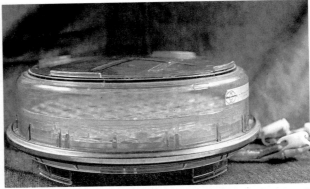

Figure 76–5. A portable incubator (Billup-Rothenberg, Del Mar, CA) to maintain proper pH and humidity during transport of cultured grafts to the operating room.

TABLE 76–2. **ULCERS TREATED WITH
ALLOGENEIC CULTURED EPITHELIAL GRAFTS**

Diagnosis	Number of Ulcers	Healed Completely (%)	Mean Time to Healing (Wk)
Venous ulcer	24	67	4.4
Rheumatoid ulcer	17	71	2.9
Sarcoidosis	25	88	6.0
Surgical wounds	8	100	2.8
Donor sites	7	100	1.8
Scleroderma	6	17	6.0
Decubitus ulcer	4	100	4.5
Amputation stump ulcer	3	67	6.0
Buerger's disease	2	100	7.0
Pyoderma gangrenosum	1	100	8.0
Trauma	2	100	4.5
Total	99	78	4.5

Modified by permission of the publisher from Phillips TJ, Gilchrest BA: Cultured allogenic keratinocyte graft in the management of wound healing: prognostic factors. J Dermatol Surg Oncol 15:1169–1176, 1989. Copyright 1989 by Elsevier Science Publishing Co., Inc.

forms gradually over 4 to 5 years beneath the grafted epithelium. This "neodermis" has a bilayered architecture with a collagen and elastin network and vasculature characteristic of nonscarred, normal dermis. Histologic analysis does not allow precise discrimination between the possibility that this dermis reforms from the remnants of the allografted dermis originally placed as a temporary dressing on the wound and the possibility that the dermis forms newly. The long induction time would seem to suggest that the latter possibility is the correct one.

Clinical Uses

BURN PATIENTS

Although cultured grafts have been used in a number of clinical situations, they offer by far the most potential for saving lives in patients with extensive thermal burns. These patients present significant problems for the surgeon. When patients have limited donor sites for autologous skin grafting, the surgeon must choose between artificial or temporary skin substitutes to close the wound and then must replace the temporary cover with autologous skin grafts when donor sites heal sufficiently for reharvesting. Some patients may have insufficient donor sites available, either because the burn wounds involve most of the appropriate areas for autograft harvest or because it may not be possible to recrop the donor sites enough times to provide sufficient autograft skin. Large meshed expansion has frequently been required for these patients to extend the available donor sites most effectively. However, the results are often cosmetically poor, and hypertrophic scarring and graft contraction can be significant. In these patients, CEA may be the best alternative. Advantages of CEA include the ready expansion of donor skin to cover even large wounds and the rapid availability of the CEA material, despite insufficient availability of normal split-thickness autologous grafts. The wound can be covered with intact epidermis relatively quickly, and the chance of burn wound infection is decreased. Because meshed expansion of the CEA is not required, the increased risk of hypertrophic scarring of the large, meshed autologous skin graft is avoided, and the cosmetic appearance of the wound is improved.

Two considerations involved in patient selection include the percentage of TBSA lost and the location of the burns. Available donor sites are assessed, and the area of uninjured donor skin is compared with that of the full-thickness wound that will require grafting. For example, burns to both arms and hands, both feet, legs, thighs, and face may constitute almost 60% of the TBSA. However, the anterior and posterior torso donor areas will provide enough split-thickness skin grafts to cover most of the wound without large meshed expansion. The wounds can be excised, autologous grafts placed, and the wounds closed in the first 3 weeks after injury. In comparison, another patient with burns to the torso, face, scalp, thighs, and arms may also have burns to about 60% of the TBSA, but with significantly less autologous skin graft donor area, and thus may be considered a good candidate for CEA.

Another point that should be considered is the general physical status of the burn patient. Patients with severe inhalation injuries may succumb to pulmonary failure before the grafts are applied, and patients with significant pre-existing internal disease may not survive until the CEAs are ready. A secondary consideration for the use of CEA is the location of the wound. In some anatomic locations the grafts may be difficult to secure or to nurse because of the possibility of shear. The grafts are best applied to large surfaces, where they are easily secured, and to anterior surfaces so that the patient can be cared for in the supine position after surgery. If the wounds include the posterior surface, the patient may require special positioning and nursing care to prevent shear and graft loss. The perineal area may be too heavily contaminated to allow take of CEA and is probably best repaired with split-thickness autograft skin.

In general, suitable candidates for CEA are patients in whom the large burn size is a significant threat to survival, donor sites are limited, and associated injuries or pre-existing medical problems are not expected to cause death or to prevent CEA application. In addition, patients should be cooperative and should fully understand the need for postoperative immobilization or be capable of being sedated sufficiently to prevent motion of the grafts. A burn center, with resources available to provide the extra hours of medical and nursing supervision of the CEA dressing changes, is generally the ideal environment for rendering this type of care.

Preparation of the Burn Patient

Initial care of the burn patient proceeds in the usual fashion depending on the extent of the injury. Fluid resuscitation and respiratory support are initiated and modified according to the patient response. The decision to use CEA can be made during the first 24 hours of care and biopsy specimens of unburned skin obtained for delivery to the laboratory.

While awaiting graft cultivation, the burn surgeon proceeds with the usual care of the patient, including early excision or debridement of the eschar, preliminary grafting from available donor sites to close a portion of the wounds, and use of temporary synthetic dressings or biologic dressings such as cadaveric allograft or porcine xenograft to reduce infection and desiccation. For larger burns, cadaveric allografts offer the best results for coverage. They frequently adhere to the wound and usually persists at least 7 days before being rejected. In patients with large burns that cause significant immunosuppression, the allograft may persist and protect the wound for several weeks. However, there is a potential for transmission of viral infection, including HIV and hepatitis. Porcine xenografts are cheaper and more readily available than cadaveric allografts but will invariably begin to be rejected within 5 to 7 days after application, requiring replacement. Synthetic dressings may be applied to protect the wound from desiccation, but these do not function as well as allografts or xenografts in preventing infection.

Attention must also be paid to provision of sufficient nutritional support, which is judged by estimates from the burn wound and modified with indirect calorimetry. In most patients, the enteral feeding route is preferred to prevent bacterial translocation and ameliorate multisystem organ failure. Tube feeding into the intestine is tolerated in most burn patients but presents the problem of defecation and the potential risk of contamination of wounds of the posterior surfaces of the buttocks and thighs. Cleansing these areas may dislodge grafts or dressings, which may promote infection in the adjacent wounds.

Infection is monitored using routine culture techniques in all burn patients. Cultures are obtained from the sputum and urine at least weekly and from the wounds twice weekly. Cultures can be obtained with culture swabs, but contact culture plates or quantitative culture biopsies will give a more consistent picture of the bacterial balance in the wound. The dressings should protect the excised wound from bacterial overgrowth, which could impair the adherence of the CEA. Before placement of the CEA, multiple quantitative cultures are recommended to confirm that bacterial counts remain below 100,000 organisms per gram of tissue. It is unclear how many bacteria in a wound a CEA will tolerate, but the number is almost certainly less than that tolerated by a split-thickness skin graft.

Before CEA placement, in the fourth week after burn injury, the wound should be clean, with well-vascularized granulation tissue and minimal evidence of infection. Any areas of eschar adjacent to the proposed area for CEA placement should be removed, because the wound care for the eschar will promote shear and may allow leaching of topical antibiotics onto the CEA, causing cell death. Sufficient staff must be available to provide the intensive postoperative care required with this grafting procedure.

Surgical Technique for CEA Graft Application

Preoperative planning for surgery includes appropriate surgical consent, with risks of surgery and anesthesia adequately documented. Blood may be ordered if the preoperative hematocrit is depressed, but platelets and plasma are infrequently required for these patients, who generally have elevated platelet counts and increased clotting factors. Rarely will large excisions or significant blood loss be expected at the time of CEA application, because the wound will have been previously excised while awaiting CEA production. Because the wound will undergo some manipulation during this procedure, perioperative antibiotics should be ordered based on the most recent cultures obtained from the wound. Most often, antistaphylococcal and gram-positive coverage is combined with coverage against gram-negative bacilli. These antibiotics are continued for at least 24 hours after surgery.

The surgical technique may require modifications in anesthesia, monitoring devices, and vascular access. Paralysis and deep anesthesia are not usually required for CEA placement, since little of the manipulation is expected to be painful. After appropriate anesthesia is obtained, the wound is prepared with povidone-iodine solution, carefully rinsing with sterile saline, since povidone-iodine has been shown to be toxic to CEA. Sterile drapes are arranged in the usual fashion.

Surgery begins by removing any adherent dressings, allograft, or xenograft, along with debridement of poorly vascularized or necrotic tissue and exuberant granulation tissue. Bleeding should be minimal if excision is not required and is controlled with topical thrombin spray and topical epinephrine (1:10,000 dilution). The wound is meticulously reinspected immediately before CEA placement.

The CEA is delivered to the operating room in tissue culture dishes with only a sterile interior. This precludes transfer to the sterile field or instrument tray. Each individual culture dish is opened by the circulating nurse or a surgical assistant, and the surgeon removes the graft for placement with two forceps. By grasping the graft carefully at the edges of the petrolatum gauze carrier, the graft can be inspected to ensure that the cells are on top of the carrier gauze and that they are not folded. The CEA is properly oriented and placed exactly in the desired position on the wound bed. The CEA and carrier must not be moved or slid after positioning, because any movement will shear the keratinocytes and may destroy them. Small gaps of less than 2 to 3 mm between carriers will epithelialize, and overlapping grafts will also survive and adhere without problems. Circumferential placement of CEA on an extremity is facilitated by suspension by hooks to allow access to the posterior dependent portion. After the graft is dropped into place, the carrier is stapled into position to adjacent carriers or intact adjacent skin (Figs. 76–6, 76–7).

After all the grafts have been applied, a bulky dressing is placed on the surface. The innermost layer should be

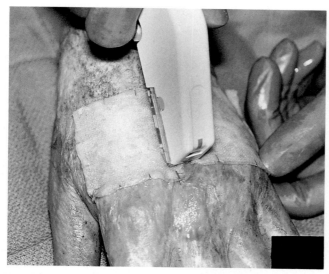

Figure 76–6. A cultured epidermal graft is placed on the wound bed (basal cells side applied to the wound, carrier gauze above). The graft and carrier gauze are stapled into place.

a nonabsorbent, nonadherent permeable gauze, such as sterilized dressmaker's nylon netting, bridal veil, or a synthetic surgical dressing made as a permeable monofilament nylon mesh (N-terface, Winfield Laboratories, Inc, Richardson, TX). This is stretched over the CEA carriers and secured snugly into place. This layer of dressing protects the CEA from dislodgement when dressings are changed.

Next, bulky, loose, mesh gauze absorbent layers are applied to a thickness of about 2 to 3 cm and secured in place with gauze rolls on extremities or burn dressings for larger surfaces. A stretchable net can be used as the outer layer to maintain the integrity of the dressing. The patient is transferred from the operating room table to an appropriate therapeutic bed to reduce any motion of the grafts or dressings and to decrease pressure on the graft or the dependent posterior surface. The anesthetic termination should allow good pain control so that patients do not move as they emerge from the effects of anesthesia.

Postoperative Care

If there is no evidence of excessive drainage, it is desirable to leave the dressing undisturbed for 24 to 48 hours after CEA application. Dressings with evidence of exudation must be changed earlier. All layers of the dressing, except the inner nylon mesh, are removed at 48 hours and the CEA inspected. The carrier petrolatum gauze should look dry, with minimal drainage, and should have developed a crusted, golden appearance similar to that of a potato chip. If the carrier gauze is still moist, the bulky gauze dressing will require changing every 12 hours, but if the grafts are dry, the time interval for dressing changes can be extended. Purulent drainage is never expected.

Nursing care can become very important after placement of the CEA.[71] The grafted areas must be kept immobilized. Inadvertent patient motion may dislodge grafts, and any movement associated with pruritus may rapidly destroy the immature keratinocytes. Sedation and analgesics should be administered as necessary to maximize patient comfort, and antihistamines should be used for pruritus. Daily nursing care for patient comfort and hygiene is limited by the requirement that any shifting of the graft and dressing must be prevented. Turning or lifting of the patient will require additional nursing personnel to prevent shearing and dislodgement of the CEA. Nutritional support is reinstituted to help heal the wound but may promote stool production and make cleansing of the patient difficult. Sufficient personnel must be allocated to meet the needs of skin care and hygiene.

Before formation of an intact stratum corneum in the CEA, at about 7 to 8 days after engraftment,[16] the grafts are very susceptible to desiccation and must be protected by occlusive petrolatum gauze dressings. These dressings are usually removed between the tenth and fourteenth days after graft application. The confluent keratinocytes will appear as a dull, pale pink film, in contrast to areas where the keratinocytes are not adherent, which are shiny and dark pink (Fig. 76–8). The epidermal sheet will still be very friable, and a nonadherent petrolatum gauze dressing should be reapplied for wound protection and changed daily for about 1 month after graft application. Eventually, when the grafts are stable, a pressure garment should be applied.

Complications of CEA

Infection. Because CEAs take several days to adhere and are very fragile, any infection may destroy the keratinocytes. Infection is cited as the major cause for graft failure,[13, 72] and prevention of this problem is facilitated by controlling infection before graft placement. However, infection may develop after placement of the CEA, and if it is not rapidly treated, the graft

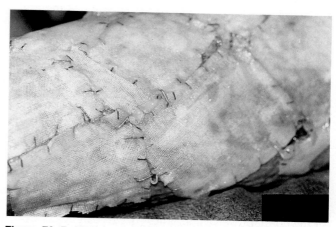

Figure 76–7. Multiple grafts are applied to the wound bed. Small gaps of less than 2 to 3 mm between adjacent grafts are tolerated and will epithelialize from the edges of the grafts.

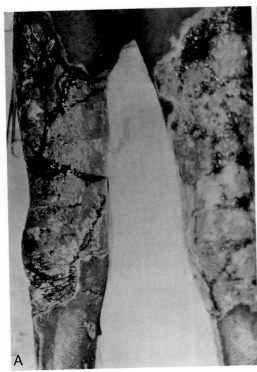
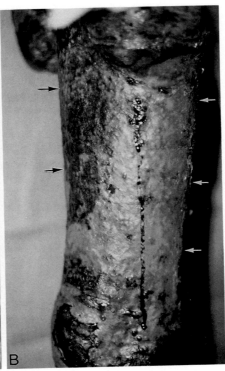

Figure 76–8. Appearance of cultured epithelial autografts placed on a burn wound. *A,* 14 days after graft placement. Areas of "take" appear as a dull pink film. *B,* 2½ months after graft placement. The areas engrafted by cultured epithelium have a light pink appearance *(white arrows).* Areas grafted with conventional split-thickness skin grafts *(dark arrows)* have a darker, mottled appearance.

will be lost. Many of the more commonly used topical antimicrobials are toxic to the cultured keratinocytes, including povidone-iodine, silver nitrate, and silver sulfadiazine,[18] mafenide (Sulfamylon),[73–75] bacitracin-polymyxin B (Polysporin), gentamicin sulfate, modified Dakin's solution (25%), and acetic acid (0.25%).[73, 75] Agents proved to be nontoxic to the keratinocytes (Neosporin G. U. Irrigant, aqueous solutions of penicillin, aminoglycosides, and vancomycin) should be used to control wound infection. The solution is applied to the bulky gauze dressing and changed at least twice daily. A week or more of therapy may be required until the keratinocytes are either lost or grow to confluence.

Graft Shear. Another mechanism for CEA loss is mechanical shear. Because of the fragility of the grafts, no motion between the grafts and the wound bed can be tolerated. To prevent shear, it must be understood that any patient care activity or patient motion may destroy the CEA. The patient is supported in a therapeutic bed to prevent pressure sore development. If graft loss occurs because of shear, either additional CEA will have to be applied or skin grafting with autologous split-thickness skin must be performed.

Bullae. The spontaneous occurrence of bullae in CEAs has been noted and is possibly due to the delayed and abnormal formation of anchoring fibrils.[21, 22] These bullae can be prevented by protecting the patient from shear and by use of a pressure garment as soon as the skin is sufficiently stable for placement. Scratching, one of the common ways that bullae occur, can be controlled with antihistamine administration. It is of interest to note that spontaneous bullae formation has also been observed in STSG.[67, 68]

GIANT CONGENITAL NEVI

Because of the possible development of melanoma, giant congenital nevi are generally excised as soon as feasible. As in patients with extensive burns, the areas of normal skin available as donor sites may be limited. Other considerations in pediatric patients are the risks of anesthesia and loss of blood volume that are engendered by repeated reharvesting of donor sites for conventional STSG. CEA has been used in eight pediatric patients for engraftment of excised giant congenital nevi.[15] The technique used was similar to that described for burn wound patients, except that all wounds were freshly excised down to muscle fascia at the time of graft application. The blood loss was considerably diminished (fourfold) when compared with estimated blood loss for grafting of an equivalent percentage of TBSA using STSG. The mean reported rate of take was 68%, and contraction was noted to be similar to that seen in equivalent anatomic sites grafted with STSG.

CHRONIC SKIN ULCERS

CEAs, both autologous[76, 77] and allogeneic,[23, 28, 29, 35, 36] have been applied in the treatment of skin ulcers. The most extensive series reported treatment of 99 ulcers in 41 patients with allogenic CEA.[36] The patients in this series all had ulcers of diverse etiologies and of least 2 months' duration that had not responded to conventional therapy (see Table 76–2). Allogeneic CEAs were established from neonatal foreskin keratinocytes and were applied to the patient using standard methods, except that grafts, instead of being stapled to the wound bed, were secured with a zinc oxide–impregnated bandage (Dome-Paste Unna's Boot (Miles Inc., West Haven, CT) or restrictive bandage. The procedures were performed primarily on an outpatient basis, although results may be improved by a 24- to 48-hour hospitalization period immediately after graft placement. In this report, a mean healing time of 4.5 weeks and total healing in 77% of treated patients were observed.

Prognostic factors included ulcer depth (i.e., the deeper the ulcer, the poorer the result) and etiology, with clean surgical wounds healing best and ulcers secondary to connective tissue disorders faring worst. Of note, there was no correlation between the age of the patient and time to healing.[36]

MISCELLANEOUS CONDITIONS

The ready availability of neonatal foreskin-derived allogeneic CEA has led to its use in other clinical situations (Table 76–3). These include the closure of STSG donor sites,[28, 30, 78] sites of excision[33] or CO_2 laser removal of tattoos,[23] Mohs micrographic surgical wounds, and desiccation and curettage sites.[36] As techniques for ensuring the absence of transmitted disease in the autografts improve, this procedure is certain to have more applications in the future.

HYPERTROPHIC SCARS AND KELOIDS

A decrease in hypertrophic scarring and contracture of CEA-grafted wounds, when compared with wounds grafted with traditional large, meshed autograft techniques, has been described.[79] Because this technique has been available for only a short time, a sufficient number of patients has not yet been accumulated to evaluate the potential decrease in scarring. If this phenomenon is substantiated, prevention of hypertrophic scarring may make this the preferred technique for coverage of most full-thickness wounds.

In addition, in eight patients with existing keloids and established hypertrophic scars, excision of the hypertrophic scar or keloid and resurfacing of the wound with autologous CEA resulted in resolution of the hypertrophic scar or keloid, with no recurrence up to 40 months after grafting. The experience in our institution with the resurfacing of keloids with CEA has demonstrated equally impressive results.[80]

A novel variation of the CEA technique has been reported[81] in two patients who had autologous CEA derived from a 2-mm² biopsy specimen of urethral

TABLE 76–3. CLINICAL APPLICATIONS FOR CULTURED SKIN GRAFTS

Thermal burn injury
Skin ulcers
Surgical wound repair
Large congenital nevus excision/repair
Scar/keloid reduction
Hypospadias repair
Gene therapy

mucosa used as a graft to repair posterior hypospadias. The cultures were initiated and maintained in standard fashion, with the graft placed as a lining on a newly constructed dermal bed on the ventral aspect of the penis to form a new urethra.

GENE THERAPY

Another exciting innovative use for CEA is gene therapy. Two groups of investigators have suggested that CEAs could be genetically engineered in vitro and transplanted into a recipient, where they would then deliver secreted gene products into the systemic circulation.[82–84] In an experimental model of human cultured keratinocytes grafted onto athymic mice, research[84] has demonstrated that a graft of 10⁶ keratinocytes transfected with the human growth factor gene can secrete about one seventh of the total daily average production of the hormone by the human pituitary gland. Keratinocytes may be ideal for gene introduction because of the ease of harvest, cultivation, and grafting into the recipient. Although this procedure has not yet been used in humans, use of a grafted patch of genetically engineered autologous keratinocytes could become a relatively noninvasive method to correct certain genetic deficits.

New Developments

CEA technology is currently available commercially through BioSurface Technology, Inc. (Cambridge, MA). This company, initiated by some of the originators of the CEA technique,[14] provides biopsy kits for the harvesting of patient skin from which the CEA is subsequently derived. The biopsy specimen is transported to the company's laboratories and expanded to provide the amount of CEA needed for the individual patient. These grafts are then transported to the operating room for patient application. In this way institutions without available tissue culture facilities can also utilize CEA.

Other biotechnical advances are on the horizon. Integra (Marion Merrell Dow, Inc., Kansas City, MO), a wholly synthetic skin substitute[56] that has had extensive, multisite clinical trials, is in premarket approval stage. This skin substitute has a dermal component composed of cross-linked collagen and chondroitin sulfate and may prove to be a good substrate on which to cultivate epithelial cells.[53] A cellular, wholly allogeneic synthetic skin is also currently in clinical trials. The product, Graftskin (Organogenesis, Inc., Cambridge, MA), is based on a "living skin equivalent."[62, 63] Allogeneic keratinocytes are seeded on a contracted collagen gel containing allogeneic dermal cells. Finally, an absorbable dermal substitute, composed of a polyglycolic mesh that is populated with allogeneic dermal fibroblasts actively secreting dermal structural components (DermaGraft, Marrow-Tech, Inc., La Jolla, CA) is currently in clinical trials and may be available for clinical use by 1993. This dermal substitute may also prove to be a good substrate for cultured autologous or allogeneic epithelial grafts.

SUMMARY

The availability of novel technologies since the 1980s has allowed for the generation of a number of types of cultured skin substitutes. Thus far, cultured epithelial autografts have been the most widely used, primarily for patients with extensive burn wounds. Despite some significant drawbacks, these skin substitutes have offered the surgeon access to virtually unlimited amounts of epithelium for wound repair. New technologies are rapidly evolving that may address some of the deficits associated with the epithelial autografts. Unlimited availability of a physiologically functional synthetic skin may soon become a reality.

REFERENCES

1. Gallico GG III: Biologic skin substitutes. Clin Plast Surg 17:519–526, 1990.
2. Clarke JA: HIV transmission and skin grafts. Lancet 1:983, 1987.
3. Hammond J, Buck BE, Malinin T: Human immunodeficiency virus and cadaver skin allografts: reducing the risk. Proc Am Burn Assoc 21:162, 1989.
4. Yuspa SH, Morgan DL, Walker RJ, Bates RR: The growth of fetal mouse skin in cell culture and transplantation to F1 mice. J Invest Dermatol 55:379–389, 1970.
5. Fusenig NE, Worst PKM: Mouse epidermal cell cultures. II. Isolation, characterization, and cultivation of epidermal cells from perinatal mouse skin. Exp Cell Res 93:443–457, 1975.
6. Karasek MA, Charlton ME: Growth of postembryonic skin epithelial cells on collagen gels. J Invest Dermatol 56:205–210, 1971.
7. Mareclo CL, Kim YG, Kaine JL, Voorhees JJ: Stratification, specialization and proliferation of primary keratinocyte cultures. J Cell Biol 79:356–370, 1978.
8. Karasek MA: Growth and differentiation of transplanted epithelial cell cultures. J Invest Dermatol 51:247–252, 1968.
9. Igel HJ, Freeman AE, Boeckman CR, Kleinfeld KL: A new method for covering large surface area wounds with autografts. II. Surgical application of tissue culture and expanded rabbit skin autografts. Arch Surg 108:724–729, 1974.
10. Rheinwald J, Green H: Serial cultivation of strains of human keratinocytes. Cell 6:331–344, 1975.
11. Eisinger M, Lee JS, Hefton JM, et al: Human epidermal cell cultures: growth and differentiation in the absences of dermal components or medium supplements. Proc Natl Acad Sci USA 76:5340–5344, 1979.
12. Boyce ST, Ham RG: Calcium-regulated differentiation of normal human epidermal keratinocytes in chemically defined clonal culture and serum-free serial culture. J Invest Dermatol 81:33s–40s, 1983.
13. O'Connor NE, Mulliken JB, Banks-Schlegel S, et al: Grafting of burns with cultured epithelium prepared from autologous epidermal cells. Lancet 1:75–78, 1981.
14. Gallico GG III, O'Connor NE, Compton CC, et al: Permanent coverage of large burn wounds with autologous cultured human epithelium. N Engl J Med 311:448–451, 1984.
15. Gallico GG III, O'Connor NE, Compton CC, et al: Cultured epithelial autografts for giant congenital nevi. Plast Reconstr Surg 84:1–9, 1989.
16. O'Connor NE, Gallico G, Compton C, et al: Grafting of burns with cultured epithelium prepared from autologous epidermal cells. II: intermediate term results on three pediatric patients. In: TK Hunt, RB Heppenstall, E Pines, D Rovee (eds): Soft and Hard Tissue Repair. Praeger Scientific, New York, 1984, pp 283–292.
17. De Luca M, Albanese E, Bondanza S, et al: Multicentre experience in the treatment of burns with autologous and allogenic cultured epithelium, fresh or preserved in a frozen state. Burns 15:303–309, 1989.
18. Eldad A, Burt A, Clarke JA, Gusterson B: Cultured epithelium as a skin substitute. Burns 13:173–180, 1987.
19. Bettex-Galland M, Slongo T, Hunziker T, et al: Use of cultured keratinocytes in the treatment of severe burns. Z Kinderchir 43:224–228, 1988.
20. BioSurface Technology, personal communication, Mark Smith, September 1991.
21. Woodley DT, Peterson HD, Herzog SR, et al: Burn wounds resurfaced by cultured epidermal autografts show abnormal reconstitution of anchoring fibrils. JAMA 259:2566, 1988.
22. Compton CC, Gill JM, Bradford DA, et al: Skin regenerated from cultured epithelial autografts on full-thickness burn wounds from 6 days to 5 years after grafting. Lab Invest 60:600–612, 1989.
23. Phillips TJ: Cultured skin grafts. Arch Dermatol 124:1035–1038, 1988.
24. Pittelkow MR, Scott RE: New techniques for the in vitro culture of human skin keratinocytes and perspectives on their use for grafting of patients with extensive burns. Mayo Clin Proc 61:771–777, 1986.
25. Meyer AA, Manktelow A, Johnson M, et al: Antibody response to xenogeneic proteins in burned patients receiving cultured keratinocyte grafts. J Trauma 28:1054–1059, 1988.
26. Jensen BA, Lorenzen I: Immune-induced dermal connective tissue alterations in rabbits chronically immunized with bovine serum albumin: biochemical studies on collagen, glycosamino-glycans, RNA and DNA. Clin Immunol Immunopathol 41:66–74, 1986.
27. Hefton JM, Finkelstein JL: Grafting of burn patients with allografts of cultured epidermal cells. Lancet 2:428–430, 1983.
28. Faure M, Mauduit G, Schmitt D, et al: Growth and differentiation of human epidermal cultures used as auto- and allografts in humans. Br J Dermatol 116:161–170, 1987.
29. Leigh IM, Purkis PE, Navsaria HA, Phillips TJ: Treatment of chronic venous ulcers with sheets of cultured allogenic keratinocytes. Br J Dermatol 117:591–597, 1987.
30. Madden M, Finkelstein JL, Staiano-Coico L, et al: Grafting of cultured allogeneic epidermis on second- and third-degree burn wounds on 26 patients. J Trauma 26:955–962, 1986.
31. Morhenn VB, Benike CJ, Cox AJ, et al: Cultured human epidermal cells do not systhesize HLA-DR. J Invest Dermatol 78:32–37, 1982.
32. Burt AM, Pallett CD, Sloane JP, et al: Survival of cultured allografts in patients with burns assessed with probe specific for Y chromosome. Br Med J 298:915–917, 1989.
33. Brain A, Purkis P, Coates P, et al: Survival of cultured allogeneic keratinocytes transplanted to deep dermal bed assessed with probe specific for Y chromosome. Br Med J 298:917–919, 1989.
34. Gielen V, Faure M, Mauduit G, et al: Progressive replacement of human cultured epithelial allografts by recipient cells as evidenced by HLA class I antigens expression. Dermatologica 175:166–170, 1987.
35. Thivolet J, Faure M, Demidem A, et al: Cultured human epidermal allografts are not rejected for a long period. Arch Dermatol Res 278:252–254, 1986.
36. Phillips TJ, Gilchrest BA: Cultured allogenic keratinocyte graft in the management of wound healing: prognostic factors. J Dermatol Surg Oncol 15:1169–1176, 1989.
37. Phillips TJ, Kehinde O, Green H, Gilchrest BA: Treatment of skin ulcers with cultured epidermal allografts. J Am Acad Dermatol 21:191–199, 1989.
38. Regauer S, Compton CC: Cultured keratinocyte sheets enhance spontaneous re-epithelialization in a dermal explant model of partial-thickness wound healing. J Invest Dermatol 95:341–346, 1990.
39. Eisinger M, Sadan S, Silver IA, Flick RB: Growth regulation of skin cells by epidermal cell-derived factors: implications for wound healing. Proc Natl Acad Sci USA 85:1937–1941, 1988.
40. Luger TA, Wirth U, Kock A: Epidermal cells synthesize a cytokine with interleukin 3 like properties. J Immunol 134:915–919, 1985.
41. Kupper TS, Ballard DW, Chua AO, et al: Human keratinocytes contain mRNA indistinguishable from interleukin 1 alpha and beta mRNA. J Exp Med 164:2095–2100, 1986.

42. Coffey RJ, Derynck R, Wilcox JN, et al: Production and auto-induction of transforming growth factor alpha in human keratinocytes. Nature 328:817–820, 1987.

43. Kubo M, Norris DA, Howell SE, et al: Human keratinocytes synthesize, secrete, and deposit fibronectin in the pericellular matrix. J Invest Dermatol 82:580–586, 1984.

44. O'Keefe EJ, Woodley DT, Castillo G, et al: Production of soluble and cell-associated fibronectin by cultured keratinocytes. J Invest Dermatol 82:150–155, 1984.

45. Wainwright DJ, Luetchke D, Jordan R, Parks DH: The use of polymerase chain reaction to detect human immunodeficiency virus in human skin. Proc Am Burn Assoc 22:79, 1990.

46. Medawar PB: A second study of the behavior and fate of skin homografts in rabbits. J Anat 79:157, 1945.

47. Abbott WM, Hembree JS: Absence of antigenicity in freeze-dried skin allografts. Cryobiology 6:416, 1969.

48. Heck EL, Bergstresser PR, Baxter CR: Composite skin graft: frozen dermal allografts support the engraftment and expansion of autologous epidermis. J Trauma 25:105–112, 1985.

49. Cuono C, Langdon R, McGuire J: Use of cultured epidermal autografts and dermal allografts as skin replacement after burn injury. Lancet 1:1123–1124, 1986.

50. Cuono CB, Langdon R, Birchall N, et al: Composite autologous allogeneic skin replacement: development and clinical application. Plast Reconstr Surg 80:628–635, 1987.

51. Young D, Langdon R, Kahn R, et al: Analysis of the fate of allografted dermis using a DNA fingerprinting technique. Proc Am Burn Assoc 21:71, 1989.

52. Pittelkow MR: Cultured epidermal cells for skin replacement. Perspect Plast Surg 3:101–122, 1989.

53. Boyce ST, Hansbrough JF: Biologic attachment, growth, and differentiation of cultured human epidermal keratinocytes on a graftable collagen and chondroitin-6-sulfate substrate. Surgery 103:421–431, 1987.

54. Boyce ST, Christianson DJ, Hansbrough JF: Structure of a collagen-GAG dermal skin substitute optimized for cultured human epidermal keratinocytes. J Biomed Mater Res 22:939–957, 1988.

55. Heimbach D, Luterman A, Burke J, et al: Artificial dermis for major burns. A multi-center randomized clinical trial. Ann Surg 208:313–320, 1988.

56. Burke JF, Yannas IV, Quinby WC, et al: Successful use of a physiologically acceptable artificial skin in the treatment of extensive burn injury. Ann Surg 194:413–428, 1984.

57. Hansbrough JF, Boyce ST, Cooper ML, Foreman TJ: Burn wound closure with cultured autologous keratinocytes and fibroblasts attached to a collagen-glycosaminoglycan substrate. JAMA 262:2125–2130, 1989.

58. Cooper M, Hansbrough J, Foreman T, et al: Early formation of basement membrane with an autologous dermal-epidermal composite cultured skin substitute: a clinical series. Proc Am Burn Assoc 22:1, 1990.

59. Wasserman D, Schlotterer M, Toulon A, et al: Preliminary clinical studies of a biological skin equivalent in burned patients. Burns 14:326–330, 1988.

60. Nanchahal J, Otto WR, Dover R, Dhital SK: Cultured composite skin grafts: biological skin equivalents permitting massive expansion. Lancet 22:191–193, 1988.

61. Hull BE, Finley RK, Miller SF: Coverage of full-thickness burns with bilayered skin equivalents: a preliminary clinical trial. Surgery 107:496–502, 1989.

62. Bell E, Erlich HP, Sher S, et al: Development and use of a living skin equivalent. Plast Reconstr Surg 67:386–392, 1981.

63. Bell E, Sher S, Hull B, et al: The reconstruction of living skin. J Invest Dermatol 81:2s–10s, 1983.

64. Delustro F, Smith ST, Sundsmo J, et al: Reaction to injectable collagen: results in animal models and clinical use. Plast Reconstr Surg 79:581–594, 1987.

65. McCoy JP Jr., Schade W, Siegle RJ, et al: Immune responses to bovine collagen implants. J Am Acad Dermatol 16:955–960, 1987.

66. Rheinwald JG: Serial cultivation of normal human epidermal keratinocytes. In: Prescott DM (ed): Methods in Cell Biology. Academic Press, New York, 1980, pp 229–254.

67. Baran R, Juhlin L, Brun P: Bullae in skin grafts. J Dermatol 3:221–225, 1984.

68. Epstein A, Hendrick S, Sanchez R, et al: Persistent dermal blistering in split thickness skin graft sites. Arch Dermatol 124:244–248, 1988.

69. Petersen MJ, Lessane B, Woodley DT: Characterization of cellular elements in healed cultured keratinocyte autografts used to cover burn wounds. Arch Dermatol 126:175–180, 1990.

70. Compton CC, Regauer S, Seiler GR, Landry DB: Human merkel cell regeneration in skin derived from cultured keratinocyte grafts. Lab Invest 62:233–241, 1990.

71. Bayley EW: Wound healing in the patient with burns. Nurs Clin North Am 25:205–222, 1990.

72. Hancock K, Leigh IM: Cultured keratinocytes and keratinocyte grafts. BMJ 299:1179–1180, 1989.

73. Cooper M, Laxer J, Foreman T, Hasbrough J: Assessing cytotoxicity of topical antimicrobial agents used in burn care to human keratinocytes with a direct bioassay. Proc Am Burn Assoc 22:8, 1990.

74. McCauley RL, Poole B, Heggers JP, et al: Differential in vitro toxicity of topical antimicrobial agents to human keratinocytes. Proc Am Burn Assoc 22:2, 1990.

75. Cooper ML, Hansbrough JF, Foreman TJ: In vitro effects of matrix peptides on a cultured dermal-epidermal skin substitute. J Surg Res 48:528–533, 1990.

76. Hefton JM, Caldwell D, Biozes DG, et al: Grafting of skin ulcers with cultured autologous epidermal cells. J Am Acad Dermatol 14:399–405, 1986.

77. Leigh IM, Purkis PE: Culture grafted leg ulcers. Clin Exp Dermatol 11:650–652, 1986.

78. Nakano M: Clinical application of cultured autologous epithelium to donor sites for split-thickness skin graft. Hokkaido J Med Sci 65:56–66, 1990.

79. O'Connor NE, Gallico GG, Compton CC: Modification of hypertrophic scars and keloids with cultured epithelial autografts. Proc Am Burn Assoc 22:7, 1990.

80. Thaller S, personal communication, September 1991.

81. Romagnoli G, De Luca M, Bandelloni R, et al: Treatment of posterior hypospadias by the autologous graft of cultured urethral epithelium. N Engl J Med 323:527–530, 1990.

82. Fenjves ES, Gordon DA, Pershing LK, et al: Systemic distribution of apolipoprotein E secreted by grafts of epidermal keratinocytes: implications for epidermal function and gene therapy. Proc Natl Acad Sci 86:8803–8807, 1989.

83. Morgan JR, Barrandon Y, Green H, Mulligan RC: Expression of exogenous growth hormone gene by transplantable human epidermal cells. Science 237:1476–1479, 1987.

84. Teumer J, Lindahl A, Green H: Human growth hormone in the blood of athymic mice grafted with cultures of hormone-secreting human keratinocytes. FASEB J 4:3245–3250, 1990.

CHAPTER 77

Surgical Repigmentation of Leukoderma

RAFAEL FALABELLA

S table leukoderma is a nonprogressive pigmentary disorder occurring as a result of ill-defined endogenous factors that cause a local destruction of melanocytes. The final expression of this condition is total or partial absence of melanocytes and pigmentation, manifested clinically as macules of different sizes and skin tones in many different anatomic locations.[1] Skin depigmentation is an aesthetic problem that commonly provokes major emotional disturbances.[2, 3] It is particularly important in dark-skinned individuals, because the lesions are more noticeable. Because of the prevalence of leukoderma,[4] surgical alternatives to restore the normal pigmentation have become well established.

Causes and Treatments of Leukoderma

When dealing with skin depigmentation, it is important to determine the nature of the condition. If the ailment arises spontaneously (e.g., vitiligo), medical therapies to induce repigmentation should be used first. Photochemotherapy using psoralens and ultraviolet light (PUVA),[5–11] topical[12, 13] or intralesional steroids,[14] topical 5-fluorouracil,[15, 16] or phenylalanine plus ultraviolet light[17, 18] should be tried initially. Surgical transplantation of melanocytes should be attempted only after medical therapies have failed. However, when leukoderma occurs as a consequence of chemical, thermal, or physical trauma and destruction of the melanocytes has occurred, failure of medical therapies can be anticipated, and the surgical technique of melanocyte transplantation becomes the only way to restore normal pigmentation.

Physiology of Repigmentation

Under normal conditions, melanocytes play an important role in aesthetic appearance in addition to serving as a protective barrier against ultraviolet light radiation. Melanin, produced by melanocytes, absorbs much of the solar energy reaching the skin and prevents significant photodamage from occurring.[19] When superficial melanocytes are destroyed through trauma, the deeper melanocytes recolonize the epidermis by migrating from the hair bulb to the basal cell layer of the epidermis.[20–23] If the hair follicles have been destroyed as a result of disease or trauma, the repigmentation process will not take place even after adequate stimulation with nonsurgical therapies, and melanocyte transplantation then becomes the only method capable of replacing the lost pigment cells. In vitiligo, repigmentation is possible only after the disorder becomes stable and the pathogenic mechanisms that caused the melanocyte damage are no longer active.

Patient Selection

Not every patient with a depigmented lesion is a good candidate for surgical melanocyte transplantation. A number of considerations must be taken into account before deciding to proceed with surgical intervention (Table 77–1).

Failure of Medical Therapy. Because every invasive surgical procedure is associated with potential complications, risks, and side effects, every effort should first be made to repigment leukoderma using established medical techniques. Once nonsurgical therapies have

TABLE 77–1. **PATIENT SELECTION CRITERIA FOR SURGICAL REPIGMENTATION**

Failure with medical therapies
Visible anatomic location
Small area of involvement
Skin types III or IV
Lesions with distinct, well-defined margins
Presence of complete achromia
Reasonable patient expectations
Psychological stability
Emotional maturity
Negative history of keloid formation
Negative history of prolonged postinflammatory
    hyperpigmentation
Stable disease activity

failed, the patient should be considered for possible surgery.

Anatomic Location. Although any anatomic area may be surgically treated using melanocyte transplantation, the visible areas of the face, neck, hands, arms, and feet should be given highest priority for treatment.

Lesion Size. Small areas of involvement are relatively easy to repigment surgically. However, very extensive defects are often impractical to effectively treat with currently available procedures. The severely affected patient should be made aware of this fact before a long or comprehensive treatment plan is initiated.

Race and Skin Type. Dark-skinned individuals with skin types III and IV are generally good candidates for surgical melanocyte transplantation. These patients show more vigorous repigmentation and obtain a better degree of improvement.

Color Tone of Leukodermic Lesions. Results are usually better when complete achromia is present rather than only hypopigmentation. Monochromic defects show better degrees of improvement than leukodermic macules of different skin tones. Well-defined lesions are also more effectively treated than those that are poorly circumscribed.

Patient Expectations. Anxious patients or those who are excessively preoccupied with only small areas of involvement or minimal amounts of pigment loss may have unrealistic expectations about what can be accomplished with surgical repigmentation techniques. Despite obtaining substantial improvement, these patients may be dissatisfied with the final result. For these reasons, a thorough psychological evaluation of each patient should be part of the initial consultation before beginning surgical repigmentation.

Past History of Keloids or Hyperpigmentation. It is important to establish whether the patient has a tendency to develop keloidal scars or long-lasting postinflammatory hyperpigmentation. If so, surgical repigmentation should be avoided because of an increased risk of these complications occurring with this technique.

Activity of Disease. Patients with progressive leukoderma are not suitable candidates for surgical repigmentation. However, a long-standing stable achromic lesion that has shown no progression over time is usually associated with a high probability of success. This can

be verified by performing a small test by implanting four to five autologous grafts 1 to 1.2 mm in diameter into the achromic test area. If pigmentation occurs around these test grafts in three to four months, the stable nature of the leukoderma is confirmed, and surgical melanocyte transplantation can then be performed.[24]

Surgical Techniques

Four different surgical techniques for performing melanocyte transplantation have been effectively used to repigment areas of leukoderma. These include thin Thiersch grafts, epidermal grafts, minigrafts, and in vitro culture of epidermis-bearing melanocytes.

THIN THIERSCH GRAFTS

This technique was first described in 1964[25] in the treatment of patients with long-standing, quiescent vitiligo, as well as other leukodermas. More than 85% of affected individuals were found to be satisfied with the level of repigmentation achieved, even though hypertrophic scars occurred in some cases.[26, 27] The procedure has also been employed to treat patients with leukoderma after burn injuries.[28] In this group, 95 to 100% repigmentation was attained, but hyperpigmentation and hypertrophic scars occurred in 13% of patients.

Technique

Under local anesthesia, the small achromic areas are denuded to a thickness of 0.2 to 1.0 mm using a hand dermatome to produce a uniformly bleeding surface. The depigmented skin is discarded, and the area is covered with compresses wet with normal saline solution until the grafts have been placed. This controls bleeding and keeps the recipient site both moist and free from possible contamination.

Pigmented skin is harvested at a thickness of 0.1 to 0.2 mm (Fig. 77–1A) using the hand dermatome. Each graft is cut to an approximate size of 3–4 × 5–6 cm and placed in chilled physiologic saline until all the grafts are ready to be placed. The grafts are applied as close to one another as possible, sometimes so that the adjacent edges even overlap slightly, to help prevent the formation of achromic fissures (Fig. 77–1B). The grafted surface is then covered with petrolatum-impregnated gauze, followed by dry gauze and an external elastic compression wrap, for 5 to 6 days. The donor sites are treated in a similar fashion. The dressings are removed after first soaking them in normal saline. This process is continued until complete reepithelialization occurs.

Results

Repigmentation begins soon after grafting, but the associated swelling and erythema may persist for several weeks.

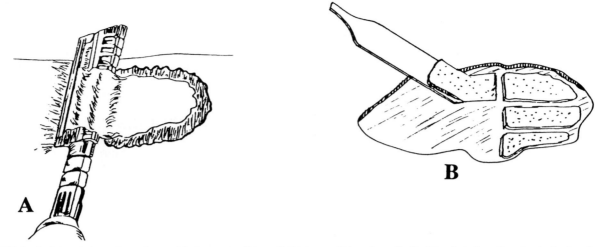

Figure 77–1. *A,* A hand dermatome is used to harvest a thin split-thickness Thiersch graft. *B,* After first denuding the leukodermic area, the grafts are applied using a grafting spatula.

EPIDERMAL GRAFTING

First described in 1971,[29] this technique obtains normal pigmented epidermis by the application of prolonged suction at a negative pressure of 200 to 300 mm Hg for 2 to 4 hours. Epidermal blisters are produced by continuous suction[30] because of complete dermoepidermal separation.[31] The epidermal sheet contains melanocytes and is used as a pigment cell graft to replace the achromic epithelium of the leukodermic areas.[29] Epidermal grafting has been used to treat leukodermas resulting from burns,[32] vitiligo and other types of stable leukoderma,[33, 34] piebaldism,[35] and segmental vitiligo.[36]

Technique

Epidermal grafting requires two stages to prepare both the recipient and the donor sites. Two days before grafting is performed, the achromic area is frozen with liquid nitrogen for 4 to 5 seconds (Fig. 77–2A). Although a bulla develops in a few hours, grafting is delayed for 48 hours until the inflammation and edema subside (Fig. 77–2B). The bulla should be left intact until the day of melanocyte grafting, when the surface is removed (Fig. 77–2C).

On the day of grafting, a multiple-cup suction device is placed on the donor site, typically the upper and medial aspect of the thigh. If suction is continuously applied at 200 to 300 mm Hg, donor bullae usually form within 2 to 4 hours. The size of each graft is about 2 cm, and the total number of grafts required is determined by the size of the lesion to be treated.

Grafting Maneuvers

Once the donor bullae have been produced by the suction device, they are ready for harvesting (Fig. 77–2D). The pigmented epidermal grafts are harvested using iris scissors and fine forceps (Fig. 77–2E). One technique that can be used to facilitate placement of the

grafts is to stretch them on a glass slide using jeweler's forceps. The epithelial graft is then positioned on the recipient bed with the two dermal surfaces placed in direct contact with one another (Fig. 77–2F). After all grafts have been placed, a nonadherent dressing is applied to cover the wound surface. This is followed by application of a dry gauze and an elastic bandage to ensure complete apposition of the grafts to the wound bed for a period of 5 to 6 days. After that interval, the dressings are removed to permit inspection of the grafts. Normal saline compresses are applied for 2 to 3 additional days until healing is complete. The grafts gradually repigment the treated area over 3 to 4 months. During this period, narrow achromic fissures may be present between the grafts, but these disappear with extension of pigment over time. Further improvement in color will continue for several months.

The donor site is covered with a similar dressing until healing is complete, approximately 7 to 8 days. The same donor site can be reused for additional grafts once reepithelialization is complete. Scarring does not occur at either the donor or recipient sites, as the dermis is not injured by this surgical procedure. Slight hyperpigmentation sometimes occurs at the recipient site, as with other types of skin grafts.[37, 38] Good results can be obtained using this technique in appropriately selected patients (Figs. 77–3, 77–4).

MINIGRAFTING

The technique of minigrafting using punch grafts to treat a small area of leukoderma was first reported in 1972.[39] The successful repigmentation of leukodermic skin by stimulating punch grafts with PUVA in patients with residual achromia and vitiligo has also been described.[40, 41] The technique of minigrafting, developed in 1978,[42] has been shown to be a very effective and simple office procedure capable of providing excellent cosmetic results. It has been used in the treatment of leukoderma resulting from burns, exposure to mono-

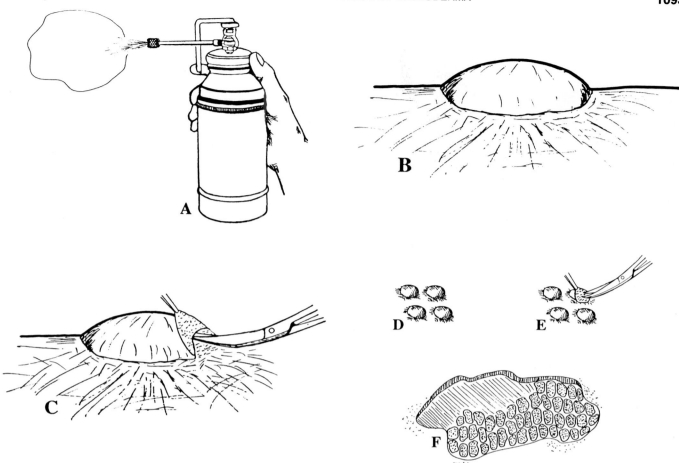

Figure 77–2. *A,* The recipient leukodermic defect is frozen using a liquid nitrogen spray technique or a cotton-tipped applicator. *B,* Bulla formation occurs after 48 hours and separates the achromic epidermis from the dermis. *C,* Immediately before epidermal grafting, the depigmented bullous epidermis is unroofed using iris scissors. *D,* Suction bullae are produced at the donor site to create the grafts. *E,* The pigmented epidermal grafts are harvested using iris scissors and fine forceps. *F,* The epidermal grafts are placed on the recipient site with their dermal sides down.

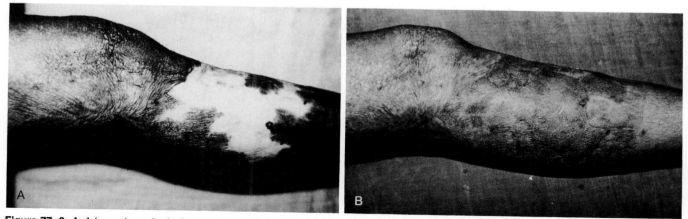

Figure 77–3. *A,* A large, irregular leukodermic area that resulted from a previous burn injury. *B,* Satisfactory repigmentation has been achieved after autologous epidermal grafting. (Reprinted by permission of the publisher from Repigmentation of leukoderma by autologous epidermal grafting, by R. Falabella, Journal of Dermatologic Surgery and Oncology, vol. 10, pp. 136–144. Copyright 1984 by Elsevier Science Publishing Co., Inc.)

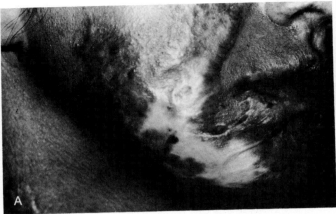
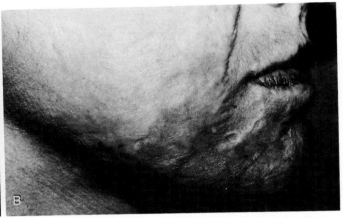

Figure 77–4. *A,* An area of leukoderma developed after dermabrasion of hypertrophic burn scars. *B,* Complete repigmentation is seen 5 years after epidermal grafting. (Reprinted by permission of the publisher from Postdermabrasion leukoderma, by R. Falabella, Journal of Dermatologic Surgery and Oncology, vol. 13, pp. 44–48. Copyright 1987 by Elsevier Science Publishing Co., Inc.)

benzyl ether of hydroquinone, piebaldism,[1] segmental vitiligo,[1, 24] dermabrasion[43] and discoid lupus erythematosus.[1] The repigmentation induced by minigrafting develops as melanocytes migrate from the epidermis of the minigrafts into the adjacent achromic epidermis, with subsequent coalescence of the pigmented islands.[1, 42] In general, a 1-mm minigraft repigments an area of about 5 mm, or an area approximately 25 times larger than the original implant. This figure is determined by calculating the relationship between the area of the graft and the area of the repigmented spot, using the formula

$$a = \pi r^2,$$

where a = area and r = radius of the graft for determining the area of a circle.[1]

Technique

The procedure is performed on an ambulatory basis under local anesthesia. Epinephrine should not be used when treating lesions resulting from traumatic injuries such as burns, as residual fibrosis may impair the microcirculation, making it susceptible to excess vasoconstrictive effects that can result in necrosis.

The recipient site is prepared in routine fashion, and local anesthesia is obtained. Wounds 1 to 1.2 mm in diameter and separated from one another by 3 to 4 mm are made using a punch. The number of recipient sites is counted to ensure that the proper number of minigrafts are taken from the donor site. The achromic skin plugs are removed using fine-tipped jeweler's forceps and iris scissors. The recipient site is kept covered with wet compresses moistened with normal saline until grafting is completed to keep the wounds clean and free of plasma and blood clots.

Although many different areas are suitable as donor sites, the gluteal region is often preferred because it can normally be hidden. However, other sites may also be used, since the minute scars that result from this procedure become less noticeable with time.

After infiltration with local anesthesia, punch incisions of the same size as the recipient site are made. They are positioned very close to each other (Fig. 77–5A) in rows of eight to ten grafts each so that they can be easily counted. The donor minigrafts are harvested using fine forceps and iris scissors and then transferred to a Telfa gauze pad moistened with normal saline solution. Once all grafts have been harvested, the donor site is covered with a sterile dressing.

The recipient site is cleansed using normal saline to

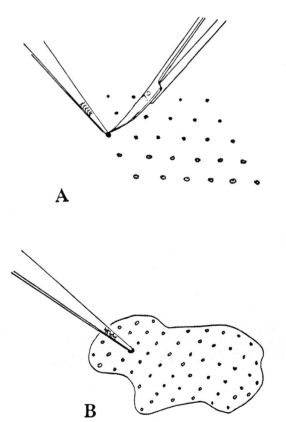

Figure 77–5. *A,* Small donor minigrafts are cut at close intervals using a 1- or 1.2-mm punch and harvested with fine forceps and iris scissors. *B,* The minigrafts are then placed in the recipient sites at greater intervals.

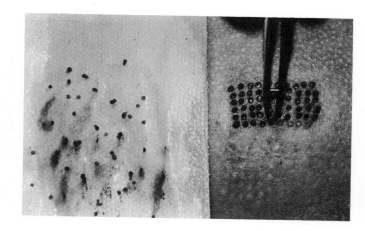

Figure 77-6. Multiple minigrafts being harvested and transferred to gauze moistened with normal saline solution.

eliminate all blood from the surface. The minigrafts are placed in the recipient holes, ensuring that the dermal side of the graft is in direct contact with the recipient dermis (Fig. 77-5B). When all grafts have been transferred, a compression bandage is applied on top of a dry gauze dressing to secure the minigrafts in place. Monsel's solution is then applied to the surface of each minigraft at the periphery to prevent leakage of serum during the postoperative period. The ferric salts do not cause pigmentation in this procedure as sometimes occurs in open wounds.[44] After drying the surgical area, Micropore adhesive tape is placed directly on the grafted surface to secure the minigrafts. Normally, immobilization provides a high degree of graft survival, and the resulting repigmentation is very satisfactory. Sessions in which about 100 to 150 minigrafts are transferred are generally recommended. Magnifying loupes are of great value in the proper performance of this procedure.

The tape is gently removed after 15 days, and the patient then exposes the treated zone to natural sunlight for a few minutes each day to stimulate melanogenesis. Pigment spread results in the coalescence of all minigrafts gradually over a period of 3 to 6 months. The graft procedure can be repeated until complete repigmentation is achieved (Figs. 77-6 through 77-9).

Side Effects and Complications

A "cobblestone" appearance of the minigrafts is one of the major side effects of this procedure and is mainly seen in young patients. This complication can be minimized by using a 1-mm punch rather than the normal 1.2-mm punch and by placing the implants at the same level as the adjacent skin.

IN VITRO CULTURED EPIDERMAL AUTOGRAFTS BEARING MELANOCYTES

Successful transplantation of cultured autografts and allografts for the treatment of thermal burns,[45-48] leg ulcers,[49-52] and dystrophic epidermolysis bullosa[53, 54] is possible. This same technique has also been applied in the treatment of vitiligo.[55-58] With a variety of different surgical techniques, melanocytes found within autologous cultured epithelium can be successfully transplanted to treat patients with stable vitiligo.[59] Long-term

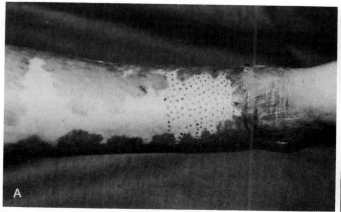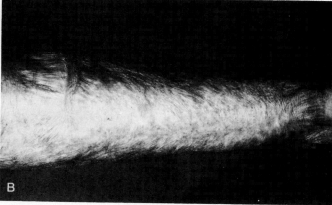

Figure 77-7. A, Clinical appearance of leukoderma after a thermal burn during the process of minigrafting with pigmented autologous skin. B, Complete repigmentation has been achieved after minigrafting. (Reprinted by permission of the publisher from Repigmentation of leukoderma by minigrafts of normally pigmented, autologous skin, by R. Falabella, Journal of Dermatologic Surgery and Oncology, vol. 4, pp. 916-919. Copyright 1978 by Elsevier Science Publishing Co., Inc.)

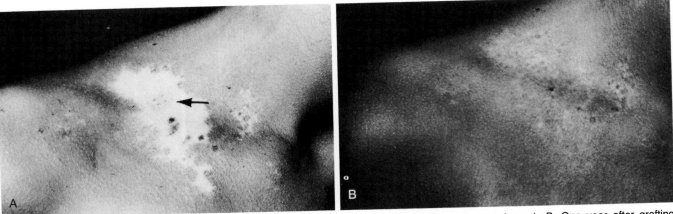

Figure 77–8. *A,* Clinical appearance of segmental vitiligo showing autologous minigrafting test area *(arrow). B,* One year after grafting, repigmentation remains complete. (From Falabella R: Repigmentation of segmental vitiligo by autologous minigrafting. J Am Acad Dermatol 9:514–521, 1983.)

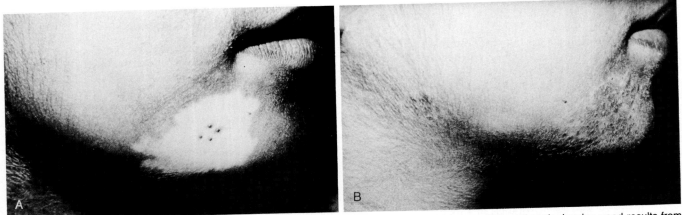

Figure 77–9. *A,* A 16-year-old girl with three achromic spots from segmental vitiligo on the right mandible and neck showing good results from 4 minigrafts placed within the largest leukodermic lesion. *B,* Clinical appearance after two minigrafting procedures showing complete repigmentation. (From Falabella R: Treatment of localized vitiligo by autologous minigrafting. Arch Dermatol 124:1649–1655, 1988. Copyright 1988, American Medical Association.)

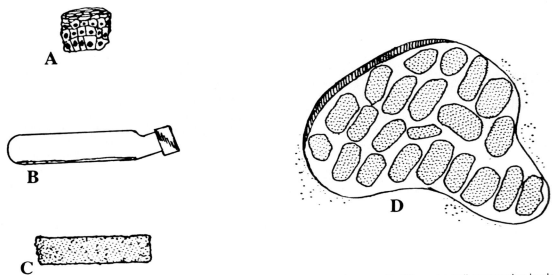

Figure 77–10. A small piece of donor skin is obtained for growing cultured epidermal autografts *(A),* and a cell suspension is plated in culture flasks *(B).* By 21 days, the cultured epidermal sheet *(C)* is ready for placement on the denuded recipient site *(D).*

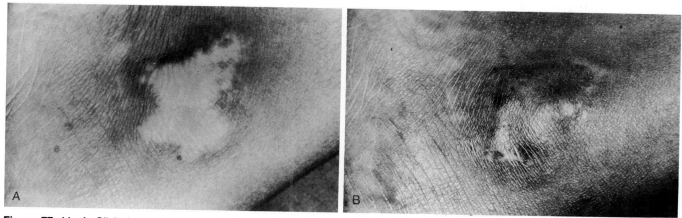

Figure 77–11. *A,* Clinical appearance of refractory focal vitiligo of the left ankle. *B,* Nearly complete repigmentation was achieved after transplantation of epidermis-bearing melanocytes grown in vitro. (*Note:* Two small areas show slight hyperpigmentation.) (From Falabella R, Escobar C, Borrero I: Transplantation of in vitro cultured epidermis bearing melanocytes for repigmenting vitiligo. J Am Acad Dermatol 21:257–264, 1989.)

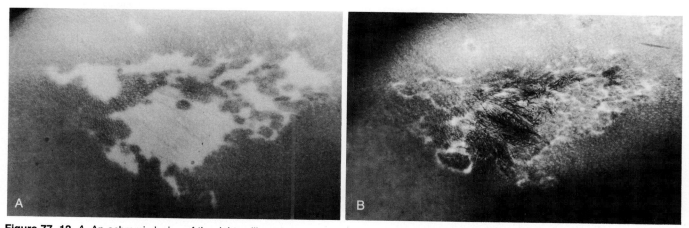

Figure 77–12. *A,* An achromic lesion of the right axilla approximately 10 × 7 cm in size. *B,* Clinical appearance 8 months after transplantation with in vitro cultured epidermis-bearing melanocytes showing more than 95% repigmentation. (From Falabella R, Borrero I, Escobar C: Cultivo in vitro de epidermis portadora de melanocitos y su aplicación en el tratamiento del vitiligo y las leucodermias estables. Med Cutan Ibero Lat Am 17:193–198, 1989.)

TABLE 77–2. CONSIDERATIONS BEFORE PERFORMING SURGICAL REPIGMENTATION OF LEUKODERMA

1. Do not consider surgical repigmentation as a first therapeutic option, as some types of leukoderma may respond to medical treatment.
2. Do not treat hypopigmented lesions, since they may become more noticeable as hyperpigmented macules.
3. Do not try to solve psychological problems caused by leukoderma.
4. Do not begin any repigmenting procedure without first performing a small minigraft test and evaluating the results 3 to 4 months later.
5. Do not underestimate the patient's expectations of the results of repigmentation surgery. Always warn the patient of possible side effects and unexpected risks or complications.
6. Do not use minigrafts larger than 1.2 mm, as "cobblestoning" may result.
7. Do not use local anesthetics containing epinephrine in areas of leukoderma with residual dermal fibrosis, as skin necrosis can occur.
8. Do not use Thiersch grafts thicker than 0.2 mm, as they may result in unaesthetic hypertrophic grafts.
9. Do not use exposed anatomic areas as donor sites.
10. Do not offer the patient better results than can be anticipated in most cases. A "variegated" and slightly hyperpigmented appearance is not uncommon, and peripheral hypopigmentation may also occur around the grafts.

production of pigment and remarkable improvement of the achromic lesions typically occurs with this technique.

The cultured epithelium (Fig. 77–10) is transplanted onto areas of leukoderma that may have been superficially dermabraded or frozen with liquid nitrogen in a manner similar to that used for epidermal grafting (Figs. 77–11, 77–12). One of the most important advantages of this method is that the epithelium can be expanded many times during the culture process, making the treatment of even large defects possible, with only a small amount of donor tissue required.

SUMMARY

Repigmentation of leukoderma is possible with a variety of different surgical techniques. A number of important considerations must be kept in mind when deciding on using this procedure (Table 77–2). The method selected for each patient is largely a function of the expertise of the cutaneous surgeon. Although minigrafting and epidermal grafting are often attractive alternatives, they also have striking limitations when large areas of leukoderma are being treated. In these cases, although thin Thiersch grafts may provide a faster solution, they always produce unwanted scars, which must be taken into consideration. In vitro cultured grafts remain experimental at present. Future use of these grafts will be dependent on the development of a simplified technique[60] that will allow the procedure to be performed in a cost-effective fashion.

REFERENCES

1. Falabella R: Repigmentation of stable leukoderma by autologous minigrafting. J Dermatol Surg Oncol 12:172–179, 1986.
2. Porter J, Beuf AH, Nordlund JJ, et al: Psychological reaction to chronic skin disorders: a study of patients with vitiligo. Gen Hosp Psychiatry 1:73–77, 1979.
3. Porter JR, Beuf AH, Lerner AB, et al: Psychosocial effect of vitiligo: a comparison of vitiligo patients with "normal" control subjects, with psoriasis patients, and with patients with other pigmentary disorders. J Am Acad Dermatol 15:220–224, 1986.
4. Lerner AO, Nordlund JJ: Vitiligo. What is it? Is it important? JAMA 239:1183–1187, 1978.
5. Fulton JE Jr, Leyden J, Papa C: Treatment of vitiligo with topical methoxalen and blacklight. Arch Dermatol 100:224–229, 1969.
6. Bleehen SS: Treatment of vitiligo with 4,5,8-trimethylpsoralen (Trisoralen). Br J Dermatol 86:54–60, 1972.
7. Parrish JA, Fitzpatrick TB, Shea C, et al: Photochemotherapy of vitiligo: use of orally administered psoralen and a high-intensity long-wave ultraviolet light system. Arch Dermatol 112:1531–1534, 1976.
8. Lassus A, Kalme K, Eskelinen A, et al: Treatment of vitiligo with oral methoxalen and UVA. Photodermatology 1:170–173, 1984.
9. Ortel B, Tanew A, Honingsmann H: Treatment of vitiligo with khellin and ultraviolet A. J Am Acad Dermatol 18:693–701, 1988.
10. Pathak MA, Mosher DB, Fitzpatrick TB, et al: Relative effectiveness of three psoralens and sunlight in repigmentation of 365 vitiligo patients. J Invest Dermatol 74:252, 1980.
11. Africk J, Fulton J: Treatment of vitiligo with topical trimethylpsoralen and sunlight. Br J Dermatol 84:151–156, 1971.
12. Van Dorp BK, van Bigk BG, Neerung H, et al: Treatment of vitiligo by local application of betamethasone 17-valerate in a dimethyl sulfoxide cream base. Dermatologica 146:310–314, 1973.
13. Kumari J: Vitiligo treated with topical clobetasol propionate. Arch Dermatol 120:631–635, 1984.
14. Kandil E: Treatment of localized vitiligo with intradermal injections of triamcinolone acetonide. Dermatologica 140:195–206, 1970.
15. Tsuji T, Hamada T: Topically administered fluorouracil in vitiligo. Arch Dermatol 119:722–727, 1983.
16. Szekeres E, Morvay M: Repigmentation of vitiligo macules treated topically with Efudex cream. Dermatologica 171:55–59, 1985.
17. Cormane RH, Siddiqui AH, Westerhof W, et al: Phenylalanine and UVA light for the treatment of vitiligo. Arch Dermatol Res 277:126–130, 1985.
18. Kuiters GRR, Middelkamp HJ, Siddiqui AH, et al: Oral phenylalanine loading and sunlight as source of UVA irradiation in vitiligo on the Caribbean Island of Curaçao SA. J Trop Med Hyg 89:149–155, 1986.
19. Fenske NA, Lober CW: Structural and functional changes of normal aging skin. J Am Acad Dermatol 15:571–585, 1986.
20. Staricco RG: Mechanisms of migration of the melanocytes from the hair follicle into the epidermis following dermabrasion. J Invest Dermatol 36:99–104, 1961.
21. Staricco RG: Amelanotic melanocytes in the outer sheath of the human hair follicle and their role in the repigmentation of regenerated epidermis. Ann NY Acad Sci 100:239–255, 1963.
22. Ortonne JP, MacDonald DM, Micoud A, et al: PUVA-induced repigmentation of vitiligo: a histochemical (split-dopa) and ultrastructural study. Br J Dermatol 101:1–12, 1979.
23. Ortonne JP, Schmitt D, Thivolet J: PUVA-induced repigmentation of vitiligo: scanning electron microscopy of hair follicles. J Invest Dermatol 74:40–42, 1980.
24. Falabella R: Repigmentation of segmental vitiligo by autologous minigrafting. J Am Acad Dermatol 9:514–521, 1983.
25. Behl PN: Treatment of vitiligo with homologous thin Thiersch skin grafts. Curr Med Pract 8:218–221, 1964.
26. Behl PN: Repigmentation of leukoderma. J Dermatol Surg Oncol 10:669–670, 1984.
27. Behl PN: Repigmentation of segmental vitiligo by autologous minigrafting. J Am Acad Dermatol 12:118–119, 1985.
28. Taki T, Kosuka S, Izawa Y, et al: Surgical treatment of skin depigmentation caused by burn injuries. J Dermatol Surg Oncol 11:1218–1221, 1985.
29. Falabella R: Epidermal grafting: an original technique and its application in achromic and granulating areas. Arch Dermatol 104:592–600, 1971.
30. Kiistala U, Mustakallio KK: In vivo separation of epidermis by production of suction blisters. Lancet 1:1444, 1964.

31. Kiistala U: Suction blister device for separation of viable epidermis from dermis. J Invest Dermatol 50:129–137, 1968.
32. Falabella R: Repigmentation of leukoderma by autologous epidermal grafting. J Dermatol Surg Oncol 10:136–144, 1984.
33. Hatchome N, Kato T, Tagami H: Therapeutic success of epidermal grafting in generalized vitiligo is limited by the Koebner phenomenon. J Am Acad Dermatol 22:87–91, 1990.
34. Suvanprakorn P, Dee-Ananlap S, Pongsomboon CH, et al: Melanocyte autologous grafting for treatment of leukoderma. J Am Acad Dermatol 13:968–974, 1985.
35. Selmanowitz VJ, Rabinowitz AD, Orentreich N, et al: Pigmentary correction of piebaldism by autografts: procedures and clinical findings. J Dermatol Surg Oncol 3:615–622, 1977.
36. Koga M: Epidermal grafting using the tops of suction blisters in the treatment of vitiligo. Arch Dermatol 124:1656–1658, 1988.
37. Mir y Mir: The problem of pigmentation in the cutaneous graft. Br J Plast Surg 14:303–307, 1961.
38. Tsukada S: The melanocytes and melanin in human skin autografts. Plast Reconstr Surg 53:200–207, 1974.
39. Orentreich N, Selmanowitz VJ: Autograft repigmentation of leukoderma. Arch Dermatol 105:736–784, 1972.
40. Lobuono P, Shatin H: Transplantation of hair bulbs and melanocytes into leukodermic scars. J Dermatol Surg Oncol 2:53–55, 1976.
41. Bonafé JL, Lassere J, Chavoin JP, et al: Pigmentation induced in vitiligo by normal skin grafts and PUVA stimulation: a preliminary study. Dermatologica 166:113–116, 1983.
42. Falabella R: Repigmentation of leukoderma by minigrafts of normally pigmented, autologous skin. J Dermatol Surg Oncol 4:916–919, 1978.
43. Falabella R: Postdermabrasion leukoderma. J Dermatol Surg Oncol 13:44–48, 1987.
44. Olmstead M, Lund H, Leonard D: Monsel's solution: a histologic nuisance. J Am Acad Dermatol 3:492–498, 1980.
45. O'Connor NE, Mulliken JB, Banks-Schlegel S, et al: Grafting of burns with cultured epithelium prepared from autologous epidermal cells. Lancet 1:75–78, 1981.
46. Gallico GG, O'Connor NE, Compton CC, et al: Permanent coverage of large burn wounds with autologous cultured human epithelium. N Engl J Med 311:448–451, 1984.
47. Cuono C, Langdon R, McGuire J: Use of cultured epidermal autografts and dermal allografts as skin replacement after burn injury. Lancet 1:1123–1124, 1986.
48. Eldad A, Burt A, Clarke JA: Cultured epithelium as a skin substitute. Burn 13:173–180, 1987.
49. Hefton JM, Caldwell D, Biozes DG, et al: Grafting of skin ulcers with cultured autologous epidermal cells. J Am Acad Dermatol 14:399–405, 1986.
50. Leigh IM, Purkis PE, Navsaria HA, et al: Treatment of chronic venous ulcers with sheets of cultured allogenic keratinocytes. Br J Dermatol 117:591–597, 1987.
51. Phillips TJ, Kehinde O, Green H, et al: Treatment of skin ulcers with cultured epidermal allografts. J Am Acad Dermatol 21:191–199, 1989.
52. Mol MA, Nanninga PB, van Eendenburg JP, et al: Grafting of venous ulcers. J Am Acad Dermatol 24:77–82, 1991.
53. Carter DM, Lin AN, Varghese MC, et al: Treatment of junctional epidermolysis bullosa with epidermal autografts. J Am Acad Dermatol 17:246–250, 1987.
54. McGuire J, Birchal N, Cuono C, et al: Successful engraftment of allogeneic keratinocytes in recessive dystrophic epidermolysis bullosa. Clin Res 35:702A, 1987.
55. Falabella R, Escobar C, Borrero I: Transplantation of in vitro-cultured epidermis bearing melanocytes for repigmenting vitiligo. J Am Acad Dermatol 21:257–264, 1989.
56. Falabella R, Borrero I, Escobar C: Cultivo in vitro de epidermis portadora de melanocitos y su aplicación en el tratamiento del vitiligo y las leucodermias estables. Med Cutan Ibero Lat Am 17:193–198, 1989.
57. Brysk MM, Newton RM, Rajaraman S, et al: Repigmentation of vitiliginous skin by cultured cells. Pigment Cell Res 2:202–207, 1989.
58. Plott RT, Brysk MM, Newton R, et al: A surgical treatment for vitiligo: transplantation of autologous cultured epithelial grafts. J Dermatol Surg Oncol 15:1161–1166, 1989.
59. Falabella R, Escobar C, Borrero I: Treatment of refractory and stable vitiligo by in-vitro cultured epidermal autografts bearing melanocytes. J Am Acad Dermatol 26:230–236, 1992.
60. Falabella R: Grafting and transplantation of melanocytes for repigmenting vitiligo and other types of stable leukoderma. Int J Dermatol 28:363–369, 1989.

CHAPTER 78

Low-Energy Lasers for Wound Healing and Tissue Welding

JUNE K. ROBINSON

S urgeons have found many applications for laser systems, which generate heat to destroy tissues, in the treatment of tumors, tattoos, and vascular lesions. New areas of laser research suggest the possible value of using low-energy lasers in accelerating wound healing, speeding neural regeneration, and relieving pain. The mechanism of biostimulation, or biomodulation, remains unclear[1] at the present time, and a much greater understanding of the photobiology and photochemistry of irradiated cells is required before laser light can be routinely used to fuse wounds and speed healing.

Laser-Tissue Interactions

One of the most important goals of laser therapy is the precise control of thermal damage by the accurate delivery of energy to the tissue. It is necessary to understand what effect a rise in temperature has on the tissue being irradiated. For temperature rises between 37° and 60°C, the tissue retracts, and conformational changes are seen. Above 60°C, protein denaturation and coagulation occurs, which is followed by carbonization and burning of tissue. Above 100°C, the tissue is vaporized and ablated (Table 78–1).[2]

TABLE 78–1. **CLINICAL AND BIOLOGIC EFFECTS OF TISSUE HEATING**

Temp (°C)	Visual Change	Biologic Change
100+	Smoke plume	Vaporization
	Blackening	Carbonization
90–100	Puckering	Drying
60–65	Blanching	Denaturation of protein
37–60	None	Heating, welding

THERMAL EFFECT

Tissue changes can usually be visually discerned by the effects of thermal energy from a number of physical sources, including electrocautery and a variety of lasers. The therapeutic process can be stopped at the desired point, thereby limiting the destruction of tissue. In general, the primary use of thermal energy has been to destroy diseased tissue; only recently has it been used to promote wound healing.

In delivering this energy, heat radiates in all directions from the point of impact, which produces circumambient zones of carbonization, vacuolization, and edema as the heat dissipates. The zones of vacuolization and edema may be reversibly or irreversibly affected and eventually become necrotic and slough off or are repaired. Thus, when the carbon dioxide laser is used as a cutting tool, it can never produce a perfectly clean cut, because there is some unavoidable and inadvertent minimal damage to the adjacent tissues. The actual width of this zone of damage depends on the tissue being treated, the irradiance of the beam, and the rate of movement along the incision line.

THERMAL RELAXATION TIME

One way to minimize thermal injury is to use a pulsed laser that has a pulse width on the order of the thermal relaxation time (Tr) of the tissue. The Tr is defined as the time it takes for the target to cool to one half of its initial temperature without heating the surrounding or adjacent tissues. Shorter pulse durations confine the laser energy to progressively smaller targets, while longer pulses cause more generalized heating and less spatial selectivity.[3]

Interactions of laser radiation with living tissue are complex phenomena influenced not only by laser parameters (e.g., energy fluence, exposure times, spot size, and wavelength), but also by tissue properties. In the case of the carbon dioxide (CO_2) laser, for which water is the absorbing molecule, the state of hydration of the tissue is a significant variable. In well-hydrated tissue, the superficial ablation possible with the CO_2 laser can be compared with that produced by dermabrasion, which is capable of removing a thin layer of tissue at a time. The CO_2 laser does this by the volatilization of water present in the tissue. However, other lasers, such as the neodymium:yttrium-aluminum-garnet (Nd:YAG) laser, do not have this selectivity in skin, since these photons are poorly absorbed by hemoglobin, water, and body pigments. Thus, the Nd:YAG laser energy penetrates more deeply into tissue and affects a greater volume of tissue than the CO_2 laser.

Lasers and Wound Healing

Although lasers have been reported clinically to stimulate wound healing and cell growth, there are conflicting reports about the ability of low-energy lasers to heal wounds and ulcers, to stimulate wound healing in vitro, and to modulate other biologic processes. Part of the confusion that exists in comparing the results of these studies relates to the use of different laser systems with different exposures, different fluences, and different animal models, cell systems, and culture media that may each change the nature of the laser-tissue interaction.

LOW-ENERGY LASERS

Low-energy laser therapy occurs at irradiation intensities so low that any biologic effects occur because of the direct effect of the irradiation and not as the result of heating.[1, 4] This means that irradiation-induced temperature elevations should be less than 0.1° to 0.5°C. For practical purposes, this limits treatment energies to a few joules per square centimeter and laser powers to less than 50 mW. Clear guidelines for the use of low-energy laser irradiation are lacking, and difficulty in measuring the end result makes it hard to isolate the true laser effect.[5]

Most of the claims for laser stimulation of wound healing state that such stimulation occurs during the proliferative phase. During the initial phase of wound healing (i.e., the first 3 to 4 days), inflammatory and vascular cells appear. The wound is stabilized by a fibrin clot, and the process of cellular debridement, neovascularization, and epithelialization begins. During the next 10 to 14 days, the proliferative phase begins in which the predominant factor is the entrance of fibroblasts into the wound, which begins the synthesis of collagen. In the final, or remodeling, phase, the original deposited collagen is replaced with a more stable form, and wound contraction occurs.

IN VITRO VERSUS IN VIVO EFFECTS

Several reports show in vitro effects of low-energy lasers on various aspects of wound healing, including fibroblast proliferation, increased synthesis of collagen, acceleration of production of extracellular matrix proteins, and stimulation of macrophages.[6–10] However, other authors have not been able to reproduce these findings,[11, 12] and these cellular effects do not necessarily translate to documentable clinical responses in animals or humans.[13, 14] Acceleration of wound healing in the early stages is most prominent in small, loose-skinned animals.[15] Enhanced healing is less apparent in animals such as pigs,[16] which have skin similar to that of humans. Thus, even if accelerated healing does occur in rodents, it is unclear how well this response is reproduced in humans.

Irradiation with monochromatic light in the blue, red, and infrared regions of the electromagnetic spectrum can enhance metabolic processes in the cell. The photobiologic effects of stimulation depend on the wavelength, dose, and intensity of the light. In theory, photoreception occurs at the level of the mitochondria by intensifying the respiratory metabolism of the excited cell.

There are isolated case reports of low-energy laser irradiation modifying a disease process both in vitro and in vivo. Cell growth as measured by tritiated thymidine incorporation is decreased in cultured scleroderma fibroblasts when compared with normal skin fibroblasts after irradiation. Cell proliferation of scleroderma fibroblasts is also decreased, but normal fibroblasts show no change in thymidine incorporation or cell proliferation. Low-energy, defocused, pulsed CO_2 laser irradiation treatments of the fingertips at 20 to 35 J/cm^2 three times a week improved Raynaud's phenomenon of the fingertips of scleroderma patients.[17]

RESULTS OF EARLY RESEARCH

Eastern European,[18–21] Italian,[22] and Chinese[23, 24] investigators have all sought clinically beneficial effects of low-level laser irradiation. The first studies were largely uncontrolled, and the reports appeared in journals that were not available for review in the United States. The methodology problems in the early experiments were corrected as the field matured, but many other investigators have failed to confirm earlier findings of stimulation of wound healing.[11] Research in humans has emphasized soft tissue wound healing, as well as healing in other conditions such as osteoarthritis, trigeminal neuralgia, radiculopathy, vascular headaches, rheumatoid arthritis, tendinitis, dental disease, Peyronie's disease, Sjögren's syndrome, and diabetic neuropathy. While some of these wound healing studies have involved hundreds of patients in open trials, the initial positive reports[25] have not been confirmed in smaller restricted studies.[14, 26] At present, the most convincing evidence of low-energy laser biostimulation of wound healing is found at the cellular level.[9] Results in animals and humans have been too disparate to predict the expected outcome, but there is enough tantalizing information about low-intensity laser stimulation at the cellular level to justify continued investigation.

Tissue Welding

CHEMICAL WELDING

For many years surgeons have searched for an adhesive to close surgical wounds without sutures or staples. Cyanoacrylate derivates with shorter methyl- and ethyl chains are more histotoxic than longer derivatives such as butyl- and isobutyl-cyanoacrylate. Ethyl-2-cyanoacrylate (Krazy Glue) has been shown to be more toxic than butyl-2-cyanoacrylate (Histoacryl) in bone graft–cartilage binding in the rabbit ear. The Krazy Glue–treated ears developed seromas with histologic evidence of acute inflammation, tissue necrosis, and chronic foreign body reaction. The Histoacryl-treated ears showed mild acute inflammation and foreign body reaction.[27]

LASER WELDING

General Principles

Because all tissue "glues" can be expected to induce an inflammatory reaction, it was concluded that welding tissue with low-energy laser irradiation might provide a useful alternative. A specially designed CO_2 laser that produces low energy has been used to "weld" vascular anastomoses[28] by causing heating without vaporization. Laser welding is thought to occur from denaturation of protein and fusion of collagen fibers. Typically, adequate tissue seals occur only when the tissues are directly opposed by buried stay sutures. One problem is that blood in the wound selectively absorbs the energy and rapidly forms a fibrin bridge that is too weak to withstand the removal of the stay sutures. Additional problems include the considerable expense of the laser equipment and the difficulties associated with learning a new technique. For laser welding to have wide clinical application, it must have healing characteristics superior to those of conventional suture.

Use in the Lung and Blood Vessels

The low-power CO_2 laser guided by an operating microscope has been used in different animal models to study wound healing. In the lung and vascular systems, the potential benefits of a "no-touch" technique to provide sealing deep within body cavities are very attractive, the goal being to decrease the operative time by speeding closure. Unfortunately, the technique did not live up to its promise in any of the model systems. Clinically, the laser did not appear to completely seal leaks in diseased human lung.[29, 30] Also, in vascular anastomosis there was an unacceptably higher rate of arterial aneurysm after laser fusion than with conventional suturing methods.[31, 32] The laser-assisted vascular anastomosis involves full-thickness injury of the vessel wall. An anastomosis cannot be performed with less power output than 40 to 50 mW (less than 50 W/cm^2 total energy in the rabbit femoral artery). Whether the energy was delivered in a continuous fashion or in 0.5-second pulses, the results were not discernibly different. It is unlikely that any change in method designed to produce less heat (e.g., prechilling the site or shortening the pulse duration) will be effective, because to produce the seal, a certain heating intensity must be achieved to denature the protein. Such heat damages the muscular arterial wall and produces extensive scarring and a wider area of elastic tissue loss than seen with other methods.[33]

Use in the Skin

Wound healing in the skin of minipigs has been studied by comparing sutured wounds, low-energy CO_2 laser–sealed wounds, and skin staples.[34] It was anticipated that low-energy CO_2 laser wound closure might stimulate fibrin clot formation and result in an accelerated repair process, with more rapid activation of fibroblasts, earlier formation of fibronectin, and more rapid epithelialization, but this did not prove to be the case. In a comparison of all wound closure modalities, there was no difference in the onset of deposition or in the initial and final distribution patterns of fibronectin or any of the basement membrane components studied.

Laser wound closure and healing were found to be clinically and histopathologically similar to conventional wound closure and healing in the minipig model in this study.[34] The surface crusting that was produced by laser wound closure adhered to the incision line longer than that produced by other methods. This eschar is a dehydrated, fully contracted blood clot that prevents physical trauma, drying, hemorrhage, and external contamination and is the standard against which moist wound healing under occlusive dressings is measured. The benefits of occlusive wound healing in reducing the time to reepithelialization have been recognized since 1962.[35] Thus, it is unlikely that low-energy CO_2 wound closure will offer any benefit over occlusive wound healing. Although laser wound closure of skin incisions produces results equivalent to those produced by standard surgical methods, there is no practical reason for the surgeon to abandon current methods of skin closure and adopt this technique.

SUMMARY

Much basic research remains to be done in the areas of laser biostimulation, wound healing, and bioinhibition. A new international medical journal concerned with these topics has been established, and several books have been published,[36] which should help to facilitate the dissemination of new techniques and improve the collaborative efforts by the many scientists who are working in these areas. This should ultimately help to determine the mechanisms by which the proven in vitro responses occur so that they can be applied to many human clinical situations in the very near future.

REFERENCES

1. Basford JR: Low energy laser therapy: controversies and new research findings. Lasers Surg Med 9:1–5, 1989.
2. Nelson JS, Berns MW: Basic laser physics and tissue interactions. Contemp Dermatol 2:12–32, 1988.
3. Anderson RR, Parrish JA: Selective photothermolysis: precise microsurgery by selective absorption of pulsed radiation. Science 220:524–527, 1983.
4. Abergel RP, Meeker CA, Dwyer RM, et al: Non-thermal effects of Nd YAG laser on biological functions of human skin. Lasers Surg Med 3:279–284, 1984.
5. Karu T: Photobiology of low power laser effects. Health Phys 56:591–704, 1989.
6. Lyons RF, Abergel RP, White RA, et al: Biostimulation of wound healing in vivo by a helium neon laser. Ann Plast Surg 18:47–50, 1987.
7. Young S, Bolton P, Dyson M, et al: Macrophage responsiveness to light therapy. Lasers Surg Med 9:497–505, 1989.
8. Bosatre M, Jucci A, Olliari P, et al: In vitro fibroblast and dermis fibroblast activation by laser irradiation at low energy. Dermatologica 168:157–162, 1984.
9. Haas AF, Isseroff RR, Wheeland RG, et al: Low energy helium-neon laser iradiation increases the motility of cultured keratinocytes. J Invest Dermatol 94:822–826, 1990.
10. Lamm TS, Abergel RP, Meeker CA, et al: Laser stimulation of collagen synthesis in human skin fibroblast cultures. Lasers Life Sci 1:61–77, 1986.
11. Surinchak JS, Alago ML, Bellamy RF, et al: Effects of low level energy lasers on the healing of full thickness skin defects. Lasers Surg Med 2:267–274, 1983.
12. Hollman HO, Basford JR, O'Brien JF, Cummins LA: Does low energy helium neon laser irradiation alter "in vitro" replication of human fibroblast? Lasers Surg Med 8:125–129, 1988.
13. Jongsma FHM, Bogaard AEJM, van Genert MJC, Huhlsbergen-Henning JP: Is closure of open skin wounds in rats accelerated by argon laser exposure? Lasers Surg Med 3:75–80, 1983.
14. Santorianni P, Monfrecola G, Martellota D, Ayala F: Inadequate effects of helium neon laser on venous leg ulcers. Photodermatology 1:245–249, 1984.
15. Anneroth G, Hall G, Ryden H, Zetterquist L: The effect of low energy infrared laser radiation on wound healing in rats. Br J Oral Maxillofac Surg 26:12–17, 1988.
16. Hunter J, Leonard L, Wilson R, et al: Effects of low energy laser on wound healing in a porcine model. Lasers Surg Med 3:285, 1984.
17. Campolmi P, Loni T, Bonan P, et al: In vivo (scleroderma) and in vitro (cultured fibroblasts) effects of defocused CO_2 laser. Presented at American Academy of Dermatology Annual Meeting, December, 1990.
18. Auerbakh MM, Sorkin MZ, Dobkin VG, et al: The effect of helium-neon laser on the healing of asceptic experimental wounds. Eksp Khir Anesteziol 3:56, 1976.
19. Kovacs IB, Mester E, Gorog P: Stimulation of wound healing with laser beam in the rat. Experientia 30:1275, 1974.
20. Mester E, Jaszsagi-Nagy E: The effect of laser radiation on wound healing and collagen synthesis. Stud Biophys 35:227, 1973.
21. Mester E, Korenyi-Both A, Kovacs I, et al: Laser in the locoregional treatment of tumors. Panminerva Med 17:229, 1975.
22. Marschesini R, Dasdia T, Melloni E, Pocco A: Effect of low-energy laser irradiation on colony formation capability in different human tumor cells in vitro. Lasers Surg Med 9:59, 1989.
23. He F, Oupingan KH: Irradiation effect of low power laser on the healing of experimental animal wounds. Laser J 7:53, 1980.
24. Hu R: Argon laser in the treatment of 45 cases of traumatic paraplegia. Laser J 7:37, 1980.
25. Mester E, Mester AF, Mester A: The biomedical effects of laser application. Lasers Surg Med 5:31–35, 1985.
26. Brunner R, Haina D, Landthaler M, et al: Applications of laser light of low power density: experimental and clinical investigations. Curr Probl Dermatol 15:111, 1986.
27. Toriumi DM: Histotoxicity of cyanoacrylate tissue adhesives: a comparative study. Arch Otolaryngol Head Neck Surg 116:546–550, 1990.
28. Serure A, Withers EH, Thomsen S, Morris J: Comparison of carbon dioxide laser-assisted microvascular anastomosis and conventional microvascular sutured anastomosis. Surg Forum 34:634–636, 1983.
29. LoCicero J, Hartz RS, Frederiksen JW, Michaelis LL: New applications of the laser in pulmonary surgery: hemostasis and sealing of air leaks. Ann Thorac Surg 40:546–550, 1985.
30. LoCicero J, Frederiksen JW, Hartz RS, et al: Experimental air leaks in lung sealed by low-energy carbon dioxide laser irradiation. Chest 87:820–822, 1985.
31. McCarthy WJ, Hartz RS, Yao JST, et al: Vascular anastomoses with laser energy. J Vasc Surg 3:32–41, 1986.
32. Hartz RS, McCarthy WJ, LoCicero J, Shih SR: Arterial aneurysm model using laser energy. J Surg Res 43:109–113, 1987.
33. Gandy KL, Hartz RS, Shih SR, Roth SI: CO_2 laser radiation damage of the arterial wall. Virchows Arch (Cell Pathol) 58:411–416, 1990.
34. Robinson JK, Garden JM, Taute PM, et al: Wound healing in porcine skin following low-output carbon dioxide laser irradiation of the incision. Ann Plast Surg 18:499–505, 1987.
35. Winter GD: Formation of scab and rate of epithelialization of superficial wounds in the skin of the domestic pig. Nature 193:293, 1962.
36. Oshiro T: Low Reactive-Level Laser Therapy: Practical Application. John Wiley & Sons, Chichester, 1991.

CHAPTER 79

Photodynamic Therapy for Cutaneous Malignancies

B. DALE WILSON

Photodynamic therapy (PDT) is an experimental treatment modality that combines a photosensitizing drug, light, and oxygen to destroy cancer cells. The relatively selective retention of the photosensitizing drug by tumor cells compared with normal tissues, as well as their favorable photobleaching kinetics yields a high therapeutic ratio for most patients. In PDT, light stimulates the electronic excitation of the photosensitizer, resulting in subsequent energy transfer to endogenous molecular oxygen,[1] producing the highly reactive singlet oxygen (Table 79–1). While the exact mode of action of PDT has yet to be determined, the formation of singlet oxygen has been shown to cause irreversible oxidation of critical cellular components, primarily the membranous structures of the cell,[2–4] as a result of the localization of the drug within the cell membranes. Further studies in animal models have demonstrated secondary damage to tumor microvasculature that is rapid in onset and results in ischemic necrosis of the tumor.[4]

Characteristics of the Photosensitizers

Although a number of potential photosensitizers are available (Table 79–2) that could be used in PDT, hematoporphyrin derivative (Photofrin) is presently the only drug approved by the U.S. Food and Drug Administration (FDA) for investigational trials. Hematoporphyrin derivative (HpD) is an oligomeric mixture of porphyrins linked by ether bonds. The precise mechanism for the uptake and retention of HpD by living tissue has not been completely discerned, although phagocytosis by reticuloendothelial cells and a concom-

itant slow clearance from tumor interstitial fluid have been demonstrated. Subsequent uptake in the lipophilic or membranous structures of the tumor suggests that another mechanism is likely to be responsible for increased retention.[5, 6] PDT has been applied to the treatment of tumors of the bladder, bronchus, esophagus, and the skin,[5] and studies have demonstrated its efficacy and safety in the eradication of early cancers and as curative and palliative treatment for advanced cancers.[7, 8]

Side Effects

Photosensitivity is the major side effect of PDT. Patients may have prolonged photosensitivity to any bright visible light source, including sunlight and operating room lights. For that reason, patients should avoid or minimize light exposure for 4 to 6 weeks after PDT, as even normal skin has the potential to be reversibly damaged. A mild phototoxic or sunburn-like reaction, with erythema, edema, blistering, and scarring in the

TABLE 79–1. **MECHANISM OF PHOTODYNAMIC REACTIONS**

Absorption	$D + hv = D^* (S)$
Intersystem crossing	$D^* (S) = D^* (T)$
Energy transfer	$D^* (T) + O_2 (T) = D + O_2^* (S)$
Deactivation	$O_2^* (S) = O_2 (T)$
	or
Reaction	$O_2^* (S) + X = X'$

D, Dye; $D^* (S)$, dye in excited singlet state; $D^* (T)$, dye in excited triplet state; hv, light energy at 630 nm; $O_2^* (S)$, oxygen in excited singlet; $O_2 (T)$, oxygen in ground (triplet) state; X, biologic substrate; X', oxidized biologic substrate.

TABLE 79-2. TARGETS OF DIFFERENT PHOTOCHEMOTHERAPEUTIC AGENTS

Photosensitizer	Site of Damage
HpD and anionic dyes	Tumor cells
	Possibly vasculature
Cationic dyes	Mitochondria
Monoclonal antibody-photosensitizer conjugates	Cell surfaces
Merocyanine 540	Leukemic cell surfaces
Psoralens	DNA

extreme case, can occur, particularly when tolerable light doses are exceeded.

Treatment Parameters

The amount of light delivered to a tumor is largely dependent on the drug dosage given to the patient. The upper light dose is approximately 36 J/cm^2 after administration of 2 mg/kg of HpD.[9] Studies have demonstrated in vivo photodestruction of HpD by photobleaching during illumination.[9–11] Thus the differential concentration of porphyrins in tumor cells compared with the surrounding normal tissue offers a potential advantage. Destruction or consumption by the photobleaching process of the small amount of drug that is deposited in normal tissue occurs before irreparable photodynamic damage, which allows continued delivery of light to produce the desired therapeutic effect in tumor cells without producing significant injury to the adjacent normal tissue. As a theoretical consequence of the photobleaching process, an unlimited amount of light could be delivered to the surface of a tumor to cause necrosis at a greater depth within it.

A potential disadvantage of the photobleaching consumption of porphyrins within the tumor is that tissue concentrations of the drug may be inadequate to induce a complete response to PDT. The optimal drug dose of porphyrins for skin that should allow maximal normal tissue sparing, or reversible photodynamic damage, has been estimated to be between 0.5 and 1 mg/kg.[10] To test this hypothesis, a phase II pilot study has been performed in patients with nonmelanoma skin tumors using an injected dose of HpD of 1 mg/kg with increasing light doses. This combination resulted in higher tissue doses and deeper tumor necrosis.[6]

Therapeutic Technique

To participate in PDT clinical trials, all patients must be informed of the investigative nature of the studies and sign a consent form in accordance with FDA guidelines. Current studies have been limited to nonmelanoma skin tumors, including squamous cell and basal cell carcinomas, either primary or recurrent after previous therapy with simple excision, cryosurgery, ionizing radiation, or desiccation and curettage. To initiate

treatment, the photosensitizer, dihematoporphyrin ether (DHE), is administered in sterile saline by intravenous bolus injection at a dose of 1 mg/kg body weight. Patients are irradiated approximately 48 hours after injection using red laser light with a wavelength of 630 nm. This is delivered from an argon-pumped tunable dye laser through a 400-micron quartz fiber. A diverging lens at the distal end of the fiberoptic provides uniform light illumination at the skin surface. The size of the treatment field is approximately twice that of the clinically measured lesion. Patients with extensive or multiple tumors over large portions of the body may require multiple treatment sessions.

A complete response is defined as complete clinical absence of tumor as confirmed by post-treatment biopsies whenever appropriate. A partial response is defined as a tumor that shows at least a 50% reduction in size on biopsy 4 to 6 weeks after therapy. In one study, after a 24-month follow-up period of 151 treated tumors, a complete response rate of 92% was achieved, including initial partial responders who required subsequent retreatment. A disproportionate number of recurrences were found on the nose, which had an overall recurrence rate of 32%, compared with only 4% for all other sites. Most recurrences were found to be morpheaform basal cell carcinomas (BCCs), while only 11% of all the treated tumors were of this histologic subtype.

Adverse Reactions

Approximately 20% of patients experience a mild sunburn-like reaction which consists of erythema, 3 to 12 weeks after injection. This may occur despite the fact that patients are advised to avoid exposure to sunlight and other sources of visible light for 4 to 6 weeks, which is generally sufficient to avoid this type of reaction.

Facial edema occurs (Fig. 79–1) when extensive or multiple facial tumors are treated. These reactions can be greatly minimized by the administration of systemic corticosteroids immediately after PDT. However, preoperative use of systemic corticosteroids or nonsteroidal anti-inflammatory agents such as indomethacin or aspirin could diminish or block the photodynamic effect and consequently should be avoided.

All patients develop an eschar at the treatment site (Figs. 79–2 to 79–5). However, the cosmetic results are generally excellent after sloughing of the eschar and reepithelialization of the treated surfaces. Postinflammatory hyperpigmentation is usually transient and occurs predominantly on the trunk. Hypertrophic scarring on the nose has also been reported.

Lesions on the nose have been shown to respond less well to PDT than do lesions at other sites on the face or trunk.[12] This lower response rate may be a result of the thicker skin of the nose compared with that at other facial locations or possibly a result of light scattering by the sebaceous glands. The multiple angles required to treat the varied contours of the nose may result in uneven illumination, which may be partially responsible for some treatment failures. Irradiation with implanted

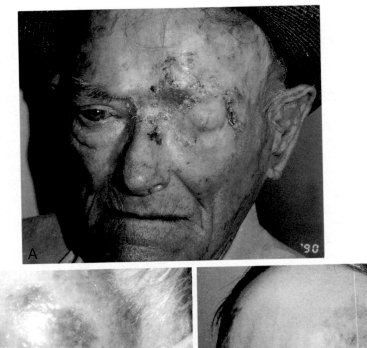

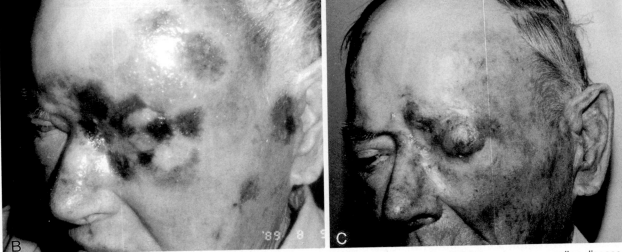

Figure 79–1. *A,* Pretreatment appearance of an elderly man with multiple basal cell carcinomas (BCCs) and severe cardiac disease, which makes him an unsuitable surgical candidate. Previous treatment with ionizing radiation also eliminates that treatment option. *B,* Severe facial edema has developed 48 hours after photodynamic therapy (PDT). *C,* Final clinical appearance after three PDT sessions.

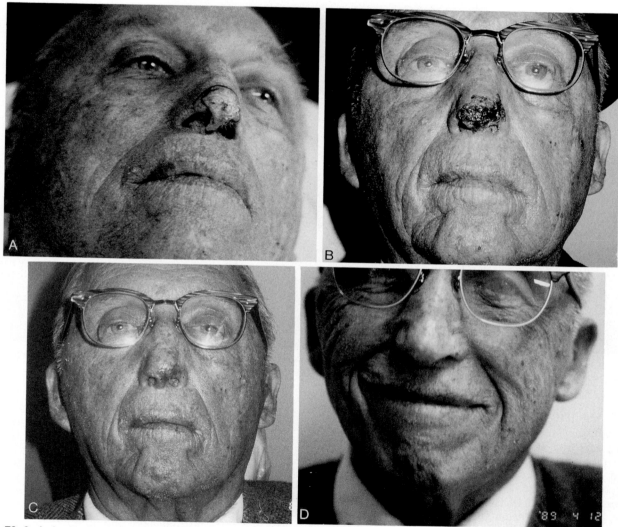

Figure 79–2. *A,* An 87-year-old man with a BCC involving the entire distal nasal tip and left septum. *B,* An eschar has formed 2 weeks after PDT. *C,* Granulation tissue has developed 5 weeks after treatment. *D,* Final clinical appearance without evidence of recurrence 3 years after treatment.

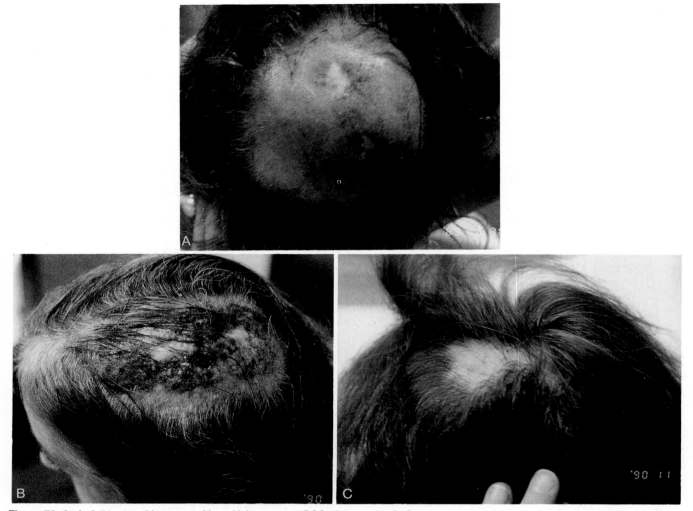

Figure 79–3. *A,* A 51-year-old woman with multiply recurrent BCC of the scalp. *B,* Crusting is seen at the overlapping treatment fields 2 days after PDT. *C,* Long-term follow-up 3 years after treatment showing no sign of recurrence.

interstitial fibers before surface illumination is currently being evaluated to improve light delivery.

Morpheaform BCCs are more difficult to control[13, 14] than other tumor subtypes, since these tumors may extend into the tissue and be two to three times their apparent clinical size. For this reason, the size of the treatment field with PDT may be inadequate for this tumor. The fibrous stroma and the location of the tumor may also result in treatment failure.

Recurrent tumors or BCCs found in high-risk locations for recurrence[15, 16] may require interstitial fiber implantation in addition to surface illumination to achieve an adequate treatment response with PDT. The tissue planes near bone, muscle, and cartilage can allow wide transit of tumor cells that may be clinically inapparent before deep invasion,[17] and inadvertent inadequate treatment with PDT can result.

Topical PDT Agents

Topical porphyrins have been found to be of little use in treating cutaneous malignancies. However, PDT with endogenous protoporphyrin has been reported in preliminary studies using a precursor of photoporphyrin in the biosynthetic pathway for hemoglobin, δ-aminolevulinic acid (ALA).[18] The long-term efficacy of this form of treatment has not been demonstrated, but the initial response rates in the treatment of BCCs, Bowen's disease, and superficially invasive squamous cell carcinomas (SCCs) are encouraging.

By contrast, normal skin and nonmalignant lesions such as warts and seborrheic keratoses do not appear to take up ALA. These early studies also demonstrate ALA to be ineffective for thick, hyperkeratotic, and ulcerated BCCs; invasive SCCs; and cutaneous metastases from breast carcinomas.

Other Tumors Treated With PDT

Kaposi's sarcoma (KS) was previously a rare disease that occurred primarily in elderly people of Italian or Jewish ancestry,[19] with a 3:1 to 15:1 male-to-female ratio.[20] However, with the acquired immunodeficiency syndrome (AIDS) epidemic, a new virulent form of this

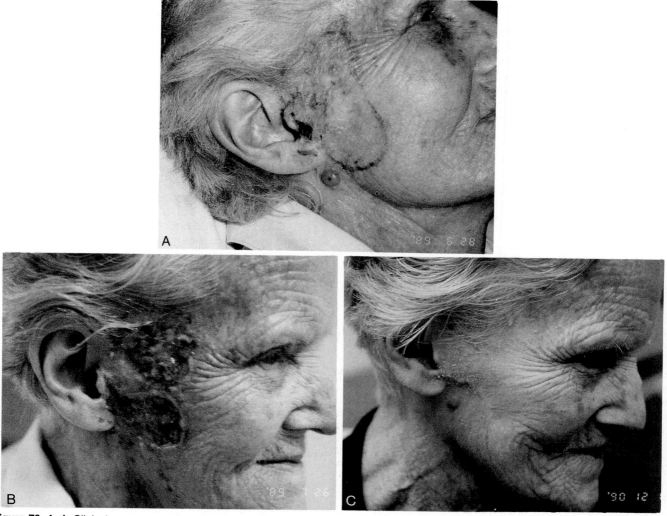

Figure 79–4. *A,* Clinical appearance of a 74-year-old woman who refused radiation and surgical treatment of a large nodular BCC in the right preauricular area. *B,* Extensive necrosis and granulation tissue formation is evident 4 weeks after PDT. *C,* Clinical appearance. The patient remains tumor free 3 years after treatment.

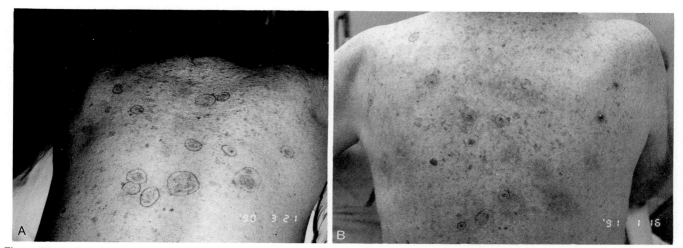

Figure 79–5. *A,* This patient has numerous superficial and nodular BCCs on the trunk that can be treated without anesthesia or pain in a single PDT session. *B,* Postinflammatory hyperpigmentation and multiple new lesions that will require treatment can be seen after PDT.

tumor has been identified. AIDS-associated KS with disseminated visceral lesions, including involvement of the skin and oral cavity, has been reported since 1981.[21, 22] Approximately 25 to 35% of AIDS patients develop KS, and most cases in homosexual males occur as the initial clinical manifestation of the disease.[23] In these patients, standard treatment with ionizing radiation, chemotherapy, or surgery may not be appropriate because of their immunocompromised status.[24, 25]

PDT has been effectively applied as palliative treatment in some cases of oral KS.[26] In addition, treatment of a small number of patients with tumors on the extremities has shown objective responses after several years of follow-up. PDT appears to be a potentially nontoxic treatment modality for these patients. However, the treatment parameters used for cutaneous malignancies may not be ideal for patients with KS, so additional studies are required before valid recommendations can be made.

Other vascular tumors (e.g., angiosarcomas) also appear to respond to PDT in a fashion similar to that shown by KS. However, the long-term cure and survival rates cannot be accurately determined at present because of the small number of patients treated thus far. For the treatment of vascular tumors, patients currently receive HpD in a dose of 2 mg/kg with light doses based on the thickness of the plaques or tumors. Lesions less than 5 mm thick are treated with surface illumination using a power density of 50 to 200 mW/cm² and an energy fluence of 25 to 50 J/cm². Thicker lesions are treated with both surface and interstitial irradiation using a power density of 200 to 400 mW/cm² and an energy fluence of 100 to 400 J/cm². Again, further studies must be performed to determine the true efficacy of this treatment protocol.

SUMMARY

PDT appears to be efficacious in the treatment of nonmelanoma cutaneous malignancies either as adjuvant therapy or when other forms of treatment are contraindicated. Prolonged photosensitivity with an average duration of 4 to 6 weeks remains the most important side effect of this treatment. A moderate photosensitivity reaction typically includes erythema and superficial blistering (Fig. 79–6) and may begin immediately after injection of HpD, which makes the patient at high risk for severe sunburns, edema, and blistering, even with only short exposures to sunlight. Unfortunately, standard sunscreen agents are of little value in preventing this reaction.

PDT also appears to be effective in the treatment of some internal malignancies of the lung, bladder, and esophagus. It may also be useful in certain types of brain tumor (e.g., glioblastomas), certain types of metastatic breast cancer, laryngeal papillomatosis, some head and neck tumors, melanomas, and gynecologic tumors. The main advantages of PDT are that it is safe, has no significant adverse side effects (other than photosensitivity), and, unlike ionizing radiotherapy, can be repeated on multiple occasions. In addition, it can be used concomitantly with or after chemotherapy. When used in combination with radiotherapy, it is desirable to wait approximately 90 days before use of PDT, since radiation therapy can augment the phototoxic effect.

Currently, the main disadvantages of PDT include photosensitization, the expense of the equipment required to deliver the laser energy, and the need for specially trained personnel to perform the treatments. Although much remains to be learned about PDT, early clinical studies suggest that this new form of therapy will become a useful diagnostic and therapeutic tool in the effective management of certain cutaneous malignancies.

REFERENCES

1. Weishaupt KR, Gomer CJ, Dougherty TJ: Identification of singlet oxygen as the cytotoxic agent in photodynamic inactivation of a murine tumor. Cancer Res 36:2326–2329, 1976.
2. Henderson BW, Waldow SM, Mang TS, et al: Tumor destruction and kinetics of tumor cell death in two experimental mouse tumors following photodynamic therapy. Cancer Res 45:572–576, 1985.
3. Selman SH, Kreimer-Birnbaum M, Klaunig JE, et al: Blood flow in transplantable bladder tumors treated with hematoporphyrin derivative and light. Cancer Res 44:1924–1927, 1984.
4. Star WM, Marijnissen HPA, Hans AE, et al: Destruction of rat mammary tumor and normal tissue microcirculation by hematoporphyrin derivative photoradiation observed *in vivo* in sandwich observation chambers. Cancer Res 46:2532–2540, 1986.
5. Dougherty TJ: Photosensitization of malignant tumors. Semin Surg Oncol 2:2427–2437, 1986.
6. Wilson BD, Mang TS, Cooper M, Stoll H: Use of photodynamic therapy for the treatment of extensive basal cell carcinomas. Facial Plast Surg 6:185–189, 1990.
7. Dubbelman TMAR, Degoeij AFPM, vanStevenick J: Protoporphyrin-induced photodynamic effects on transport processes across the membrane of human erythrocytes. Biochem Biophys Acta 595:133, 1980.
8. Hilf R, Murant RS, Narayanan U, Gibson SL: Relationship of mitochondrial function and cellular adenosine triphosphate levels to hematoporphyrin derivative-induced photosensitization in R3230AC mammary tumor. Cancer Res 46:211–217, 1986.
9. Mang TS, Dougherty TJ, Potter WR, et al: Photobleaching of porphyrins used in photodynamic therapy and implications for therapy. Photochem Photobiol 45:501–506, 1987.
10. Potter WR: The theory of PDT dosimetry: consequences of photodestruction of sensitizer. Photochem Photobiol 46:97–101, 1987.

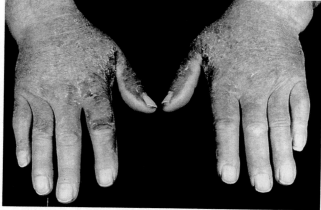

Figure 79–6. Moderate photosensitivity reaction after PDT consists of erythema, blistering, and crusting of the dorsum of the hands.

11. McCaughan JR Jr: Overview of experience with photodynamic therapy for malignancy in 192 patients. Photochem Photobiol 46:903–909, 1987.
12. Pennington DG, Waner M, Knox A: Photodynamic therapy for multiple skin cancers. Plast Reconstr Surg 82:1067–1071, 1988.
13. Lang PG Jr: Indications and limitations of Mohs micrographic surgery. Dermatol Clin 7:627–644, 1989.
14. Mohs FE: Chemosurgery—Microscopically Controlled Surgery for Skin Cancer. Charles C Thomas, Springfield, IL, 1978, pp 30–105.
15. Panje WR, Ceilley RI: The influence of embryology of the midface on the spread of epithelial malignancies. Laryngoscope 89:1914–1920, 1979.
16. Bailin PL, Levine HL, Wood BJ, et al: Cutaneous carcinoma of the auricular and periauricular region. Arch Otolaryngol 106:692–696, 1980.
17. Swanson NA: Mohs surgery. Arch Dermatol 119:761–773, 1983.
18. Kennedy JC, Pottier RH, Pross DC: Photodynamic therapy with endogenous protoporphyrin. J Photochem Photobiol 6:143–148, 1990.
19. Kaposi M: Idiopathisches multiples pigmensarkim der haut. Arch Dermatol Syphilol 4:265–273, 1872.
20. Cox FH, Helwig EB: Kaposi's sarcoma. Cancer 12:289–298, 1959.
21. Centers for Disease Control: Kaposi's sarcoma and *Pneumocystis* pneumonia among homosexual men—New York City and California. MMWR 30:305–308, 1981.
22. Friedman-Kien AE, Laubenstein LJ, Rubenstein P, et al: Disseminated Kaposi's sarcoma in homosexual men. Ann Intern Med 96:693–700, 1983.
23. Blattner WA, Hoover RN: Cancer in the immunosuppressed host. In: Devita V, Hellman S, Rosenberg S (eds): Principles and Practice of Oncology. JB Lippincott, Philadelphia, 1985, pp 2002–2005.
24. Mitsuyasu RT, Groopman JE: Biology and therapy of Kaposi's sarcoma. Semin Oncol 11:53–59, 1984.
25. Nisce L, Safai B: Radiation therapy of Kaposi's sarcoma in AIDS. Front Radiat Ther Oncol 19:133–137, 1985.
26. Schweitzer VI, Visscher D: Photodynamic therapy for treatment of AIDS-related oral Kaposi's sarcoma. Otolaryngol Head Neck Surg 102:639–649, 1990.

APPENDIX

Surgical Suppliers

Accurate Surgical and Scientific Instruments Corporation
300 Shames Drive
Westbury, New York 11590
516-333-2570
Electrosurgical equipment

Acme United Corporation
Medical Products Division
Fairfield, Connecticut 06430
800-835-2263
Op-Site and LYOfoam synthetic surgical dressings

Acuderm, Inc.
5370 NW 35th Terrace
Fort Lauderdale, Florida 33309
800-327-0015
Disposable punches and curets; blades, needles, and cautery devices

Aesculap Instruments Corporation
875 Stanton Road
Burlingame, California 94010
415-692-6022
Surgical instruments

Allerderm Laboratories
P.O. Box 931
Mill Valley, California 94942
800-365-6868
Flesh-tone paper tape and vinyl gloves

Alpha Pro Tech, Inc.
903 W. Center Street
Building E
North Salt Lake, Utah 84054
801-298-3240
Surgical masks and facial shields

American Optical, Inc.
P.O. Box 537
Sturbridge, Massachusetts 01566
617-765-9711
Surgical eyewear

American Sterilizer Company
2424 W. 23rd Street
Erie, Pennsylvania 16514
814-452-3100
Instrument washers, surgical tables, and autoclaves

American Surgical Laser, Inc.
600 W. Cummings Park
Suite #3050
Woburn, Massachusetts 01801
617-933-8116
Carbon dioxide laser

Ansell Medical
446 State Highway 35
Eatontown, New Jersey 07724
908-542-9500
Hypoallergenic surgical gloves

Anthony Products, Inc.
7711 Records Street
Indianapolis, Indiana 46226
317-545-6196
Surgical eyeware, microsurgical loupes, and surgical headlamps

Arista Surgical Supply Company, Inc.
67 Lexington Avenue
New York, New York 10010-1898
800-223-1984
Surgical instruments

Arjo Hospital Equipment Company
6380 W. Oakton Street
Morton Grove, Illinois 60053
708-967-0360
Ultrasonic cleansers

Aseptico, Inc.
P.O. Box 3209
Kirkland, Washington 98083-3209
206-487-3157
Halogen headlamps and surgical lights

Astra Pharmaceutical Products, Inc.
50 Otis Street
Westborough, Massachusetts 01581-4500
508-366-1100
Topical and local anesthetic agents, absorbable hemostatic collagen material

Aurora Medical
2211 Post Street
Suite #404
San Francisco, California 94115
800-547-1133
Suction lipectomy dressings

Baker-Cummins Dermatologicals, Inc.
8800 N.W. 36th Street
Miami, Florida 33178-2404
800-735-2315
Disposable biopsy punches

Banyan International Corporation
2118 E. Interstate 20
Abilene, Texas 79604-1779
800-351-4530
Emergency life support equipment

Barriers for Diseases
2724 7th Avenue South
Birmingham, Alabama 35233
205-252-0075
Disposable eye and face shields

Baxter Healthcare Corporation
O.R. Division
1500 Waukegan Rd.
McGraw Park, Illinois 60085
312-473-1500
Laser peripherals: masks, goggles, filters, and anodized instruments

Becton Dickinson AcuteCare
One Becton Drive
Franklin Lakes, New Jersey 07147
201-848-6800
Gloves, scalpel blades, Beaver blade system, and scrub brushes

Beiersdorf, Inc.
360 Dr. Martin Luther King Drive
Norwalk, Connecticut 06856-5529
203-853-8008
Coverlet elasticized tape and dressings, wound closure strips, and Aquaphor gauze

Belair Instrument Company
88 South Avenue
Fanwood, New Jersey 07023
908-322-4800
Cryostats, microscopes, and histology products

Bernsco Surgical Supply, Inc.
6653 N.E. Windermere Road
Seattle, Washington 98115
800-231-8409
Complete line of cutaneous surgical supplies

Biomed Supply
18530 Mack Avenue
Grosse Pointe Farms, Michigan 48236
800-526-1309
Surgical gloves

Bio-Medical Service Associates
825 East Acosta Avenue
Glendora, California 91740
818-914-5011
Monitoring and anesthesia equipment

Bio-Rad Micromeasurements, Inc.
19 Blackstone Street
Cambridge, Massachusetts 02139
617-864-5820
Dermascope video microscope

Birtcher Corporation
4501 North Arden Drive
P.O. Box 4399
El Monte, California 91734
800-423-4889
Electrosurgery equipment

Boundary Healthcare Products Corporation
549 Yorkville Park Square
Columbus, Mississippi 39702
601-327-8011
Disposable operating room linens and gowns

Boyd Industries, Inc.
12275 75th Street North
Largo, Florida 34643-3031
800-255-2693
Surgical tables and stools

Britt Corporation
2231 S. Barrington Avenue
Los Angeles, California 90064
800-344-9751
Carbon dioxide and Nd:YAG lasers

Brymill Corporation
P.O. Box 2392
Vernon, Connecticut 06066
203-875-2460
CRY-AC cryosurgical spray devices

Burton Medical Products
7922 Haskell Avenue
Van Nuys, California 91406
800-444-9909
Electrosurgical device, surgical lights

Byron Medical
3280 E. Hemisphere Loop
Suite 100
Tucson, Arizona 85706
800-777-3434
Surgical clogs, dermabrasion equipment, and local anesthesia injection system

Calgon Vestal Laboratories
Merck and Company, Inc.
Box 147
St. Louis, Missouri 63166
800-325-8005
Mitraflex wound dressing

Cameron-Miller, Inc.
3949 S. Racine
Chicago, Illinois 60609
312-523-6360
Electrosurgical devices

Camp International, Inc.
P.O. Box 89
Jackson, Michigan 49204
517-789-3280
Lymphatic compression gradient system

Candela Laser Corporation
530 Boston Post Road
Wayland, Massachusetts 01778
508-358-7637
Pulsed dye lasers

Caromed International, Inc.
308-D West Millbrook Rd.
Raleigh, North Carolina 27609
800-833-2237
Postsurgical garments, compression stockings

CNH Pillow, Inc.
P.O. Box 1247
Abilene, Texas 79604
Pillow for chondrodermatitis patients

Coherent, Inc.
3270 West Bayshore Road
Palo Alto, California 94303
800-227-1914
Carbon dioxide and argon-dye lasers; laser scanner

Colin Medical Instruments Corporation
University Technology Park
5850 Farinon Drive
San Antonio, Texas 78249-9969
800-829-6427
Blood pressure/pulse monitor

Collagen Biomedical
1850 Embarcader Road
Palo Alto, California 94303
415-856-0200
Zyderm injectable collagen

Concept, Inc.
11311 Concept Blvd.
Largo, Florida 34543
813-392-6464
Electrosurgical devices

Continuum Biomedical, Inc.
547 Rhea Way
Livermore, California 94550
800-532-1064
Q-switched Nd:YAG laser

ConvaTec
E.R. Squibb and Sons, Inc.
Princeton, New Jersey 08540
800-422-8811
DuoDerm surgical dressing

Criticare Systems, Inc.
P.O. Box 26556
Milwaukee, Wisconsin 53226
414-797-0356
Pulse oximeter and patient monitoring devices

CUI Corporation
1160 Mark Avenue
Carpinteria, California 93013
805-684-7617
Tissue expanders; silicone implants and drainage catheters; liposuction equipment

DMI—Division of the Health Chair Corporation
2601 South Constitution Blvd.
West Valley City, Utah 84119-1988
801-972-3165
Surgical tables, stools, chairs, and lights

D.R. Labs
P.O. Box 419
Millbrae, California 94030-9902
800-533-7522
Omiderm surgical dressing, patient wound care kits

Davis and Geck
1 Casper Street
Danbury, Connecticut 06810
203-796-9580
Suture materials, surgical scrubs and instruments

Davol, Inc.
P.O. Box 8500
Cranston, Rhode Island 02920
401-463-7000
Davol-Simon dermatome

Dermacare Products, Inc.
7651 National Turnpike
Louisville, Kentucky 40214
502-368-1654
Disposable operating room products, electrosurgical devices, laser safety equipment

Derma-Lase, Inc.
3 Main Street
Hopkinton, Massachusetts 01748
508-435-0277
Q-switched ruby laser

Dermatologic Lab & Supply Company
608 13th Avenue
Council Bluffs, Iowa 51501
712-323-3269
Complete line of cutaneous surgical supplies

Detrex Corporation
P.O. Box 5111
Southfield, Michigan 48086
313-358-5800
Ultrasonic cleaners

Devon Industries, Inc.
9530 DeSoto Avenue
Chatsworth, California 91311
818-709-6880
Surgical marking and sharps disposal systems

Lester A. Dine, Inc.
PGA Commerce Park
351 Hiatt Drive
Palm Beach Gardens, Florida 33418
407-624-9103
Medical photographic equipment

Diomed Limited
King's Court
Kirkwood Road
Cambridge, Great Britain
CB4 2PF
44-223-425006
Surgical diode laser

Directed Energy, Inc.
2 Goodyear
Irvine, California 92718
714-707-2800
Carbon dioxide lasers

Dow Corning Wright
5677 Airline Road
Arlington, Tennessee 38002
901-867-4546
Tissue expanders; Silastic gel sheets for topical dressings

Du Pont Company
P.O. Box 80-705
Wilmington, Delaware 19880-0705
302-744-1000
Disposable operating room gowns and surgical drapes

Ellman International Mfg., Inc.
1135 Railroad Avenue
Hewlett, New York 11557
800-569-5355
Surgical eye shields, Surgitron electrosurgical instrument

Envision Imaging Technologies
8910 Purdue Road, Suite 690
Indianapolis, Indiana 46268
317-879-8700
Computer imaging system

Esma Chemicals, Inc.
P.O. Box 162
Highland Park, Illinois 60035
708-433-6116
Ultrasonic cleaning devices

Ethicon, Inc.
P.O. Box 151
Route 22
Somerville, New York 08876
908-218-2465
Suture and staplers; wound closure tapes

Euro-Med, Inc.
Cooper Surgical
8561 154th Avenue NE
Redmond, Washington 98052-3557
206-861-9008
Disposable biopsy punches

Fashion Seal Uniforms
10099 Seminole Blvd.
Seminole, Florida 34642
813-397-9611
Operating room apparel

Felco Products, Inc.
1928 Mears Parkway
Margate, Florida 33063
305-973-6599
Prone pillow head support for scalp surgery

Ferndale Laboratories, Inc.
780 West Eight Mile Road
Ferndale, Michigan 48220
313-548-0900
Mastisol liquid adhesive; Detachol adhesive remover

Freeman Health Care Products
900 W. Chicago Road
Sturgis, Michigan 49091
800-253-2091
Compression stockings

Frigitronics
Box 855
770 River Road
Shelton, Connecticut 06484
800-243-2974
Cryosurgical instruments

Gebauer Company
9410 Saint Catherine Avenue
Cleveland, Ohio 44104
800-321-9348
Fluro-ethyl spray

GEM Nonwovens, Inc.
2800-E Bob Wallace Ave.
Huntsville, Alabama 35805
205-539-9559
Disposable operating room clothing

Glendale Protective Technologies
130 Crossways Park Drive
Woodbury, New York 11797
516-921-5800
Laser eyewear

Glenwood, Inc.
83 N. Summit Street
Tenafly, New Jersey 07670
201-569-0050
Bichloracetic acid kit

H&A Enterprises, Inc.
143-19 25th Avenue
P.O. Box 489
Whitestone, New York 11357-0489
718-767-7770
Pressure earrings

HGM Medical Laser Systems, Inc.
3959 West 1820 South
Salt Lake City, Utah 84104-4996
801-972-0500
Argon and krypton lasers

Hammill Medical International
2328 N. Batavia
Suite 105
Orange, California 92665
714-637-0344
Operating room shoes

Havel's Incorporated
3726 Lonsdale Avenue
Cincinnati, Ohio 45227
800-638-4770
Scalpel blades and handles

Health Communications Productions
255 E. Brown
Suite 400
Birmingham, Michigan 48009
313-540-6006
Patient information videos

Healthfirst Corporation
Box 279
Edmonds, Washington 98020
800-331-1984
Cardiopulmonary resuscitation emergency kit

Heine Optotechnik USA
3500 Regency Parkway
Suite C
Cary, North Carolina 27511-8569
913-380-8090
Magnifying loupes, magnifying dermatoscope

Heraeus LaserSonics, Inc.
3420 Central Expressway
P.O. Box 58005
Santa Clara, California 95052
800-227-8372
Carbon dioxide, argon, argon-dye, and Nd:YAG lasers

Hermal Pharmaceutical Labs, Inc.
Route 145
Oak Hill, New York 12460
518-475-0175
Scanpor tape, Vigilon surgical dressing, Elastyren hypoallergenic gloves

Dow B. Hickam, Inc.
P.O. Box 2006
Sugar Land, Texas 77487
713-240-1000
Sorbsan wound dressing

Hinkel Company
11760 Roscoe Blvd.
Building E
Sun Valley, California 91352
800-982-1600
Electrology equipment

Hi-Tech Medical Lasers, Inc.
1105 Chestnut Street
Burbank, California 91506
213-849-1554
Carbon dioxide laser

International Equipment Company
300 Second Avenue
Needham Heights, Massachusetts 02194
617-455-9728
Microtome-cryostat

Iomed, Inc.
1290 W. 2320 South
Salt Lake City, Utah 84119
801-975-1191
Iontophoretic delivery device for local anesthesia

Jarit Instruments
9 Skyline Drive
Hawthorne, New York 10532
914-592-9050
Surgical instruments

Jamar Medical Systems
3956 Sorrento Valley Blvd.
San Diego, California 92121
619-597-8860
Portable carbon dioxide laser

Jobst Institute, Inc.
P.O. Box 653
Toledo, Ohio 43694
800-537-1063
Postsurgical garments

Johnson and Johnson
Patient Care Division
New Brunswick, New Jersey 08903-2400
908-524-0400
Bioclusive surgical dressing

Johnson and Johnson Medical, Inc.
2500 Arbrook Blvd.
Arlington, Texas 76014
817-465-3141
Surgical gloves, Cidex sterilization solution, wound care products

Keeler Instruments, Inc.
456 Parkway
Broomall, Pennsylvania 19008
800-523-5620
Magnifying loupes, surgical headlamps, and video headlamps

Kells Medical, Inc.
136 Shore Drive
Burr Ridge, Illinois 60521
312-789-3790
Evertor-Strip adhesive wound closure device

Kendall Healthcare Products Company
15 Hampshire Street
Mansfield, Massachusetts 02048
800-346-7197
Pneumatic compression devices

Kentek Laser Components
4 Depot Street
Pittsfield, New Hampshire 03263
603-435-7201
Laser eyewear

Kimberly-Clark Corporation
1400 Holcomb Bridge Rd.
Roswell, Georgia 30076
404-587-8000
Surgical gowns

L&R Manufacturing Company
577 Elm Street
Kearny, New Jersey 07032
201-991-5330
Ultrasonic cleansing system

Lase, Inc.
7209 E. Kemper Road
Cincinnati, Ohio 45249
800-543-2070
Smoke evacuation systems, laser safety devices

Lasercomp
16630 Aston
Irvine, California 92714
800-777-1421
Carbon dioxide laser

Lasermatic
10575 Newkirk Street
Suite 740
Dallas, Texas 75220
800-992-5504
Carbon dioxide and Nd:YAG lasers

LaserMed International
810 Office Park Circle
Suite 102
Lewisville, Texas 75057
214-420-8611
Diode laser pointer

Laser Peripherals, Inc.
10395 West 70th Street
Eden Prairie, Minnesota 55344
612-944-1159
Laser eyewear and safety signs

Laserscope, Inc.
3052 Orchard Dr.
San Jose, California 95134
408-943-0636
Frequency-doubled:YAG laser

Lihtan Technologies, Inc.
901 E Street, Suite 210
San Rafael, California 94901
415-459-1085
Argon-dye laser and Hexascan laser dosing device

Look, Inc.
80 Washington Street
Norwell, Massachusetts 02061
617-878-8220
Suture and needles

Luxar Corporation
11816 North Creek Parkway North
Suite 102
Bothell, Washington 98011-8205
206-483-4142
Carbon dioxide laser

3M Health Care
Medical-Surgical Division
3M Center Building 225-5S-01
St. Paul, Minnesota 55144-1000
800-228-3957
Laser surgical mask

Mada Equipment Company, Inc.
60 Commerce Road
Carlstadt, New Jersey 07072
201-460-0454
MadaJet air injection system

Marion Merrell Dow Labs, Inc.
Wound Care Division
Kansas City, Missouri 64137
816-966-4000
Envisan wound cleaning pads

M.D., Inc.
6008 Fort Henry Drive
Kingsport, Tennessee 37663
615-239-3410
Neutra-caine—local anesthetic neutralizer

Medasonics
P.O. Box 4903
Fremont, California 94539-4903
415-623-0626
Doppler ultrasound

Medi USA, L.P.
76 W. Seegers Road
Arlington Heights, Illinois 60005
708-640-8400
Compression stockings

Medical Art Resources, Inc.
2021 Pleasant Street
Wauwatosa, Wisconsin 53213
414-453-6929
Mohs surgery instructional model

Medical Choice, Inc.
P.O. Box 354
Etobicoke Station "D"
Etobicoke, Ontario
Canada M9A 4X4
416-762-2021
Reusable electrosurgical electrodes

Mentor Corporation
5425 Hollister
Santa Barbara, California 93111
805-681-6000
Fibrel collagen implant

Meshtel
957 15th Street
Santa Monica, California 90403
800-729-3094
Diode laser pointers

Metalaser Technologies, Inc.
1244 Quarry Lane
Pleasanton, California 94566
415-846-3030
Vasculase copper vapor laser

Micropigmentation Devices, Inc.
Permark Division
450 Raritan Center Parkway
Edison, New Jersey 08837
908-225-3700
Cosmetic tattooing device

Midmark Corporation
Medical Products
Versailles, Ohio 45380
800-643-6275
Surgical tables

Miltex Instrument Company, Inc.
6 Ohio Drive
Lake Success, New York 11042
800-645-8000
Surgical instruments

Navitar AV Division
D.O. Industries, Inc.
200 Commerce Drive
Rochester, New York 14623
716-359-4999
Diode laser pointers

Nellcor Inc.
25495 Whitesell Street
Hayward, California 94545
415-887-5858
Pulse oximeters

NiiC USA, Inc.
460 Seaport Court
Redwood City, California 94063
800-992-6442
Carbon dioxide laser

Ohmeda
1315 W. Century Drive
Louisville, Colorado 80027
800-652-2469
Pulse oximeter and patient monitoring devices

On-Gard Systems, Inc.
1900 Grant Street
Suite 710
Denver, Colorado 80203
303-825-5210
Needle handling systems

Orascoptic Magnification Systems
7 North Pinckney Street
Suite 305
Madison, Wisconsin 53703
608-256-0344
Surgical magnifiers

Ormed Corporation
70 Santa Felicia Dr.
Santa Barbara, California 93117
805-968-1921
Epigard temporary wound coverage material

Ortho Pharmaceutical Corporation
P.O. Box 300
Route 202
Raritan, New Jersey 08869-0602
908-218-6571
Topical retinoic acid

Osada Electric Company, Inc.
8242 W. Third Street
Suite 150
Los Angeles, California 90048
800-426-7232
Dermabrasion and hair transplantation electric motor unit

Owen/Galderma Laboratories, Inc.
6201 South Freeway
P.O. Box 6600
Fort Worth, Texas 76115
817-293-0450
CRY-AC cryosurgical spray devices

Padgett Dermatome Division
2838 Warwick Trafficway
Kansas City, Missouri 64108
Dermatomes

PBI Medical
35 McArthur Lane
Smithtown, New York 11787
516-543-6780
Copper vapor laser

Perimed
200 Centennial Avenue
Piscataway, New Jersey 08854-9960
201-457-9111
Laser Doppler flowmeter

Personna Medical
American Safety Razor Company
Medical Products Division
P.O. Box 500
Staunton, Virginia 24401
703-248-8000
Surgical scalpel blades, disposable scalpels, prep razors

Pilling Company
420 Delaware Drive
Ft. Washington, Pennsylvania 19034
215-643-2600
Surgical lights

Polaroid Corporation
2625 S. Roosevelt Street
Tempe, Arizona 85282-9701
800-428-0238
Instant color photography

Porex Medical
500 Bohannon Road
Fairburn, Georgia 30213
800-241-0195
Surgical drainage systems, silicone implants, surgical markers

Premier Laser Systems
3 Morgan
Irvine, California 92718
800-844-8044
Carbon dioxide laser

Preven-A-Stik, Inc.
P.O. Box 272664
Houston, Texas 77277-2664
800-648-4588
Surgical instrument tray

Propper Manufacturing Company, Inc.
36-04 Skillman Ave.
Long Island City, New York 11101
718-392-6650
Surgical blades

Quick Notes/HSP Associates, Inc.
2470 Windy Hill Road
Suite 161
Marietta, Georgia 30067
404-984-1447
Medical record barcode scanning system

Redfield Corporation
210 Summit Avenue
Montvale, New Jersey 07645
201-391-0494
Infrared coagulator

Robbins Instruments, Inc.
P.O. Box 441
2 North Passaic Avenue
Chatham, New Jersey 07928
201-635-8972
Surgical instruments

Rockwell Associates, Inc.
P.O. Box 43010
Cincinnati, Ohio 45243
513-271-1568
Laser signs

Scientech, Inc.
5649 Arapahoe Ave.
Boulder, Colorado 80303
303-444-1361
Laser power meters

Sharplan Lasers
Advanced Surgical Technologies
1 Pearl Court
Allendale, New Jersey 07401
201-327-1666
Carbon dioxide and Nd:YAG lasers

Sherwood Medical
P.O. Box 14738
St. Louis, Missouri 63178
800-325-7472
Synthetic surgical dressings: Viabsorb Ultec, and BlisterFilm

Siamed STAR Foundation
8441 SE 68th Street
Suite 343
Mercer Island, Washington 98040
800-888-8417
Latex examination gloves

Siemens Medical Systems
186 Wood Avenue South
Iselin, New Jersey 08830
908-321-3400
Surgical lights

Sigvaris, Inc.
P.O. Box 570
Branford, Connecticut 06405
203-481-5588
Compression stockings

SmartPractice
3400 E. McDowell Road
Phoenix, Arizona 85008-7889
800-822-8956
Nonlatex surgical gloves

Smith and Nephew, Inc.
1920 S. Jefferson Avenue
St. Louis, Missouri 63104-2621
800-325-8860
Surgical lights

Solar Protective Factory, Inc.
2524 North Lincoln Avenue, Suite 197
Chicago, Illinois 60614-2389
800-786-2562
Ultraviolet light protective clothing

Sorenson Laboratories, Inc.
2495 South West Temple
Salt Lake City, Utah 84115
800-851-5227
Laser smoke filtration system

Southeastern Medical Associates
4927 Mystere Circle
Lilburn, Georgia 30247
404-413-7372
Derma-Shield hand barrier for latex-sensitive individuals

Spectrum Medical Technologies, Inc.
15 Meadowbrook Road
Sherborn, Massachusetts 01770
508-650-4640
Q-switched ruby laser

Sporicidin International
5901 Montrose Road
Rockville, Maryland 20852
301-231-7700
Disinfectant solution

Stackhouse, Inc.
150 Sierra Street
El Segundo, California 90245
213-322-6676
Smoke filtration system, surgical helmet, and glove liners

Stefanovsky and Associates
30150 Royalview
Willowick, Ohio 44094
215-944-4482
Laser surgical eye shields

Storz Instrument Company
3365 Tree Court Industrial Blvd.
St. Louis, Missouri 63122
800-325-9500
Surgical instruments

Surgical Laser Technologies
1 Great Valley Parkway
Malvern, Pennsylvania 19355
800-772-5273
Nd:YAG laser system, sapphire laser tips, optical fibers

Surgilase
1 Richmond Square
Providence, Rhode Island 02906
401-272-4950
Carbon dioxide laser, Nd:YAG laser fibers

Surgimedics
2828 N. Crescent Ridge Dr.
The Woodlands, Texas 77381
800-669-9001
Smoke evacuators

George Tiemann and Company
84 Newtown Plaza
Plainview, New York 11803-4506
516-694-6283
Surgical instruments

Triangle Biomedical Sciences
2604-G Carver Street
Durham, North Carolina 27705
919-477-9283
Tissue marking dyes

Ultracision, Inc.
25 Thurber Blvd.
Unit #3
Smithfield, Rhode Island 02917
401-232-7660
Ultrasonic scalpel device

UniPlast Imaging
United Digital Systems, Inc.
4305 Enterprise Drive
Suite G
Winston-Salem, North Carolina 27106
800-336-5484
Computer software imaging systems for cosmetic surgical procedures

United States Surgical Corporation
150 Glover Ave.
Norwalk, Connecticut 06856
203-845-1000
Sutures and staples

Uvex Safety, Inc.
10 Thurber Blvd.
Smithfield, Rhode Island 02917
401-232-1200
Laser eyewear

Valleylab
5920 Longbow Drive
Boulder, Colorado 80301
303-449-2340
Electrosurgical instruments, ultrasonic systems

Vasamedics Inc.
2963 Yorkton Blvd.
St. Paul, Minnesota 55117-1064
612-490-0999
Laserflow Doppler flowmeter

Viaderm Pharmaceuticals, Inc.
2195 Faraday Avenue
Suite B
Carlsbad, California 92008
619-431-9904
Alginate surgical dressing material

Edward Weck, Inc.
85 Orchard Road
Princeton, New Jersey 08543-5251
908-359-9700
Surgical instruments, skin staplers, and electrosurgical devices

Welch Allyn Medical Division
4341 State Street Road
P.O. Box 220
Skaneateles Falls, New York 13153-0220
315-685-4560
Skin surface microscope

Wells Company
8075 E. Research Ct.
Suite 101
Tucson, Arizona 85710
602-298-6069
Liposuction equipment

Wimex, Inc.
P.O. Box 3481
New York City, New York 10008
800-368-6650
Surgical masks, caps, gowns

Winfield Laboratories, Inc.
1303 Columbia Drive
Suite 207
Richardson, Texas 75081
214-783-6493
N-terface surgical dressing

World Medical Supply Inc.
4340 Stevens Creek Blvd.
Suite 110
San Jose, California 95129
800-545-5475
Pristine powder-free surgical gloves

Xomed
6743 S. Point Drive North
P.O. Box 1900F
Jacksonville, Florida 32216
904-737-7900
Surgical drapes

Carl Zeiss, Inc.
One Zeiss Drive
Thornwood, New York 10594
914-747-1800
Surgical microscopes, optical loupes

Zimmer
1800 W. Center St.
P.O. Box 708
Warsaw, Indiana 46581-0708
219-267-6131
Brown electrodermatome

Julius Zorn, Inc.
80 Chart Road
P.O. Box 1088
Cuyahoga Falls, Ohio 44223
800-222-4999
Compression stockings

Index

Note: Pages in *italics* indicate illustrations; those followed by t refer to tables.